July 1998
Volume 208 • Number 1
RADLAX 208 (1) 1–280

1923-1998 75th ANNIVERSARY

Radiology

From the Editor	1
Subspecialty Society Messages	3
Annual Oration	9
Editorial	17
Health Policy and Practice	19
Review	25
Pediatric Imaging	35
Musculoskeletal Imaging	43
Diagnosis Please: Case 4	63
Experimental Studies	65
Genitourinary Imaging	87
Ultrasound	111
Emergency Radiology	125
Neuroradiology	129
Signs in Imaging	143
Vascular and Interventional Radiology	145
Cardiac Imaging	167
Radiation Oncology	173
Thoracic Imaging	187
Gastrointestinal Imaging	217
Breast Imaging	245
Technical Developments	261
Letters to the Editor	266
In Memoriam	273

THE RADIOLOGICAL SOCIETY OF NORTH AMERICA

RSNA **84th Scientific Assembly and Annual Meeting**
Chicago, November 29–December 4, 1998

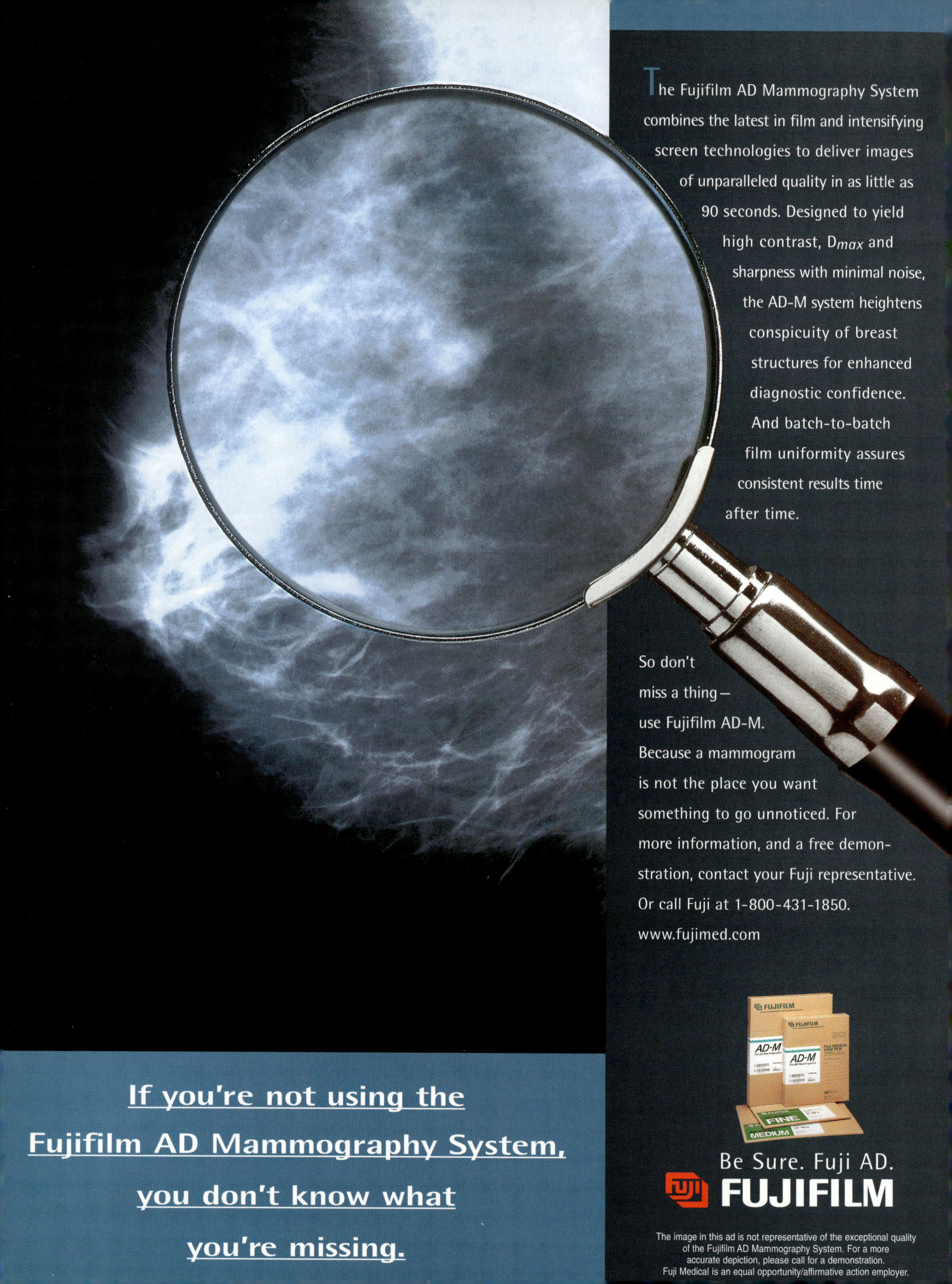
The Fujifilm AD Mammography System combines the latest in film and intensifying screen technologies to deliver images of unparalleled quality in as little as 90 seconds. Designed to yield high contrast, Dmax and sharpness with minimal noise, the AD-M system heightens conspicuity of breast structures for enhanced diagnostic confidence. And batch-to-batch film uniformity assures consistent results time after time.
So don't miss a thing—use Fujifilm AD-M. Because a mammogram is not the place you want something to go unnoticed. For more information, and a free demonstration, contact your Fuji representative. Or call Fuji at 1-800-431-1850.
www.fujimed.com
FUJIFILM
AD-M
FINE
MEDIUM
If you're not using the Fujifilm AD Mammography System, you don't know what you're missing.
Be Sure. Fuji AD.
FUJIFILM
The image in this ad is not representative of the exceptional quality of the Fujifilm AD Mammography System. For a more accurate depiction, please call for a demonstration.
Fuji Medical is an equal opportunity/affirmative action employer.

Radiology

July 1998
Volume 208
Number 1

RSNA
A monthly journal devoted to clinical radiology and allied sciences, owned and published by THE RADIOLOGICAL SOCIETY OF NORTH AMERICA, INC.

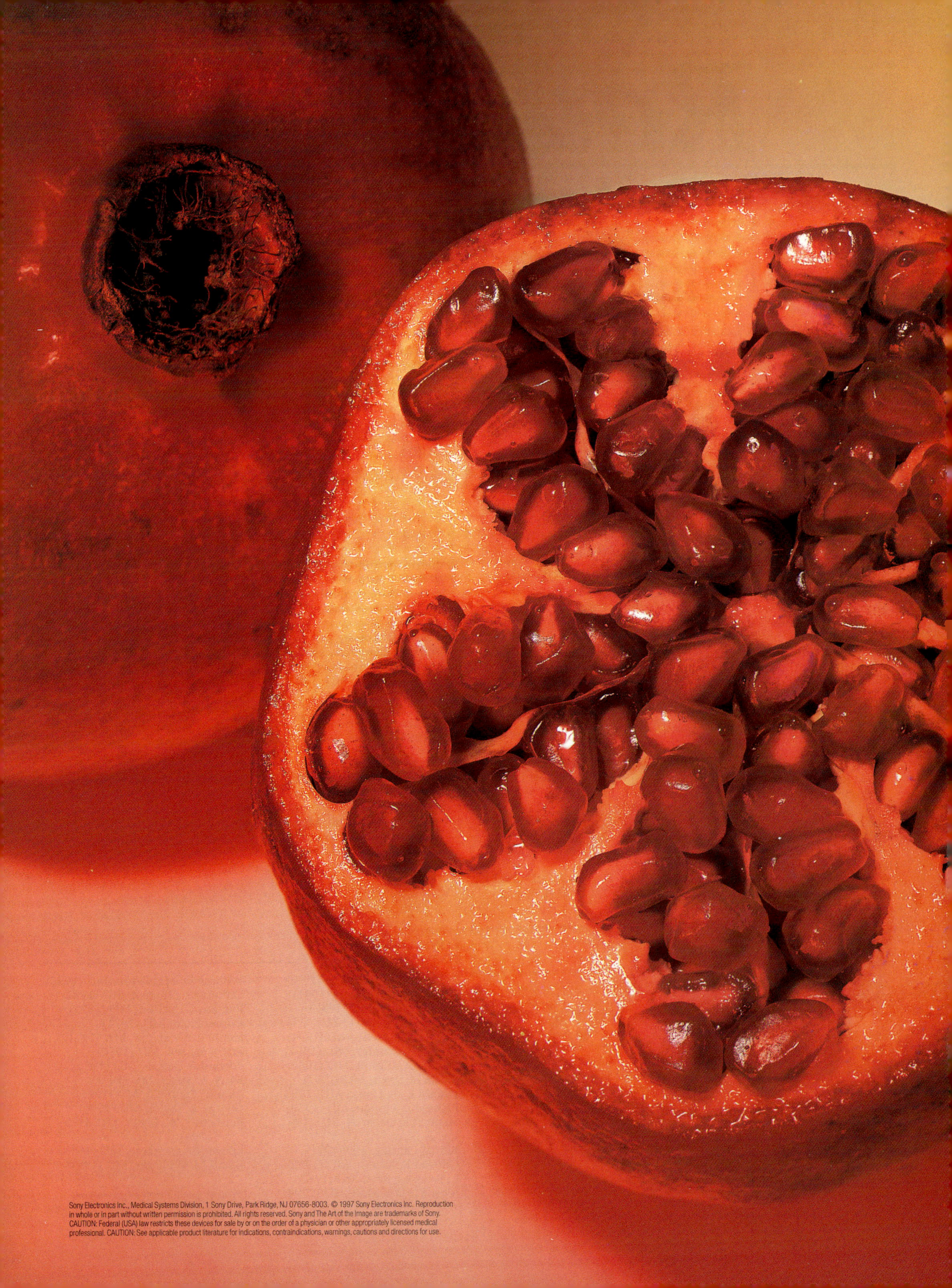

July 1998
Volume 208 • Number 1

Radiology

A monthly journal devoted to clinical radiology and allied sciences, owned and published by the Radiological Society of North America, Inc.

RSNA

From the Editor

1 *Radiology* 1998—Change in Deputy Editor
Anthony V. Proto

Future Directions of Imaging Research: Subspecialty Society Messages

3 *The Society of Nuclear Medicine*—
Predictions for Nuclear Medicine in the Next Decade
Michael L. Goris and H. William Strauss

The practice of nuclear medicine in 2008 is likely to use gamma cameras that employ lenses in place of collimators, scintillators that will allow novel modular detector shapes, and computers capable of real-time iterative reconstruction to characterize lesions in anticipation of using the most effective therapy.

6 **Commentary**
Predictions for Nuclear Medicine in the Next Decade: Commentary
R. Edward Coleman

We will see more emphasis placed on registering the biochemical information from nuclear medicine with the anatomic information from CT and MR imaging.

1997 RSNA Annual Oration in Diagnostic Radiology

9 **The Genesis of Modern Science: Contributions of Scientific Societies and Scientific Journals**
Stanley S. Siegelman

Scholarly journals made many important contributions to the genesis of modern science.

Editorial

17 **Imaging-guided Gene Therapy in the Central Nervous System**
David J. Seidenwurm and Howard A. Rowley

Radiologic monitoring of the site of delivery of a potentially effective vector for gene therapy has been accomplished in vivo.

Health Policy and Practice

19 **U.S. Radiologists' Workload in 1995–1996 and Trends Since 1991–1992**
Jonathan H. Sunshine, Gerald R. Busheé, and Rajiv Mallick

Our best point estimate is that, on average, diagnostic radiologists were performing approximately 5% more procedures per full-time equivalent in 1995–1996 than in 1991–1992 and that the average relative value unit per procedure increased from 0.693 to 0.748, so that the total workload increase was approximately 13% ($1.05 \times 1.08 = 1.34$), as measured in terms of relative value units.

Continued—

Review

25 **Kawasaki Disease: A Review**
Charles J. Chung and Leonard Stein
This article reviews the pathologic, epidemiologic, clinical, and radiologic findings of Kawasaki disease and discusses the possible etiology and therapeutic management options.

Pediatric Imaging

35 **US of the Painful Hip in Childhood: Diagnostic Value of Cartilage Thickening and Muscle Atrophy in the Detection of Perthes Disease**
Simon G. F. Robben, Morteza Meradji, Ad F. M. Diepstraten, and Wim C. J. Hop
Patients with a painful hip who have cartilage thickening, muscle atrophy, or both at US are highly suspected of having Perthes disease, regardless of the duration of the symptoms.

Musculoskeletal Imaging

43 **Hip Joint Fluid: Detection and Distribution at MR Imaging and US with Cadaveric Correlation**
Steven G. Moss, Mark E. Schweitzer, Jon A. Jacobson, Joachim Brossmann, Joseph V. Lombardi, Steven M. Dellose, Jeffrey R. Coralnick, Kathleen N. Standiford, and Donald Resnick
Fluid adjacent to the entire length of the femoral neck, measuring at least 5 mm in width, is compatible with a joint effusion.

49 **Quantitative MR Imaging Evaluation of Chondropathy in Osteoarthritic Knees**
Jean-Luc Drapé, Eric Pessis, Guy-Robert Auleley, Alain Chevrot, Maxime Dougados, and Xavier Ayral
The quantification of chondropathy of the knee with MR imaging is feasible by using the French Society of Arthroscopy arthroscopic scoring and grading systems.

57 **Evaluation of Patellar Cartilage with a Low-Field-Strength Extremity-only Magnet: Comparison of MR Imaging Sequences, with Marcoscopic Findings as the Standard**
Joong Mo Ahn, Sandy M. Kwak, Heung Sik Kang, Claus Muhle, Robert A. Pedowitz, Lawrence R. Frank, Debra Trudell, Parviz Haghighi, and Donald Resnick
High-grade cartilaginous lesions can be evaluated reliably with low-field-strength MR imaging by using a combination of imaging sequences.

Diagnosis Please

63 **Case 4**
David Karasick and Mark E. Schweitzer

Experimental Studies

65 **MR Imaging of Gene Delivery to the Central Nervous System with an Artificial Vector**
Giovanni de Marco, Alexei Bogdanov, Edgardo Marecos, Anna Moore, Maria Simonova, and Ralph Weissleder
A model DNA vector has been attached to dextran particles and expression both in cell culture and in vivo, neuronal and glial accumulation, and MR detection have been demonstrated.

73 **Excitotoxin-induced Cerebral Hyperemia in Newborn Piglets: Regional Cerebral Blood Flow Mapping with Contrast-enhanced Power Doppler US**
George A. Taylor, Carol E. Barnewolt, and Patricia S. Dunning
Contrast-enhanced power Doppler US can be used to create accurate regional blood flow maps in the newborn brain.

81 **Intraoperative Assessment of Microsurgery with Three-dimensional Optical Coherence Tomography**
Stephen A. Boppart, Brett E. Bouma, Costas Pitris, Gary J. Tearney, James F. Southern, Mark E. Brezinski, and James G. Fujimoto
Optical coherence tomography should improve intraoperative diagnostics by providing high-resolution, subsurface, cross-sectional imaging of vessels and nerves in real time.

Continued—

Radiology is published monthly by the Radiological Society of North America, Inc, 2021 Spring Rd, Suite 600, Oak Brook, IL 60523 (ISSN 0033-8419). Printed in USA. Periodical class postage paid at Oak Brook, Ill, and additional mailing offices. The nonmember subscription rate for the USA is $215.00 per year; for all other countries, $260.00 (includes postage). Information about subscription rates for residents is available on request. (Air freight is available; rates are furnished on request.) Single copies are $25.00 ($36.00 to a non-U.S. address). Notice of missing issues or change of address (include old mailing label and new address) should be sent to RSNA Subscriptions Department, 2021 Spring Rd, Suite 600, Oak Brook, IL 60523. Inquiries via e-mail should be directed to *subscrib@rsna.org.* POSTMASTER: Send address correction “changes” to: *Radiology,* RSNA, 2021 Spring Rd, Suite 600, Oak Brook, IL 60523.

Claims for copies lost in the mail are allowed within 90 days of the date of issue. Claims are not allowed for issues lost as a result of insufficient notice of change of address.

Membership in the Radiological Society of North America is by formal application. Membership information should be secured from the Executive Director, the Radiological Society of North America, Inc, 2021 Spring Rd, Suite 600, Oak Brook, IL 60523. Dues are payable annually in January. In accordance with U.S. postal regulations, $107.50 of active membership dues is allocated to a subscription to *Radiology.*

"KODAK MIN-R 2000 Film and the 2190 Screen set a standard."

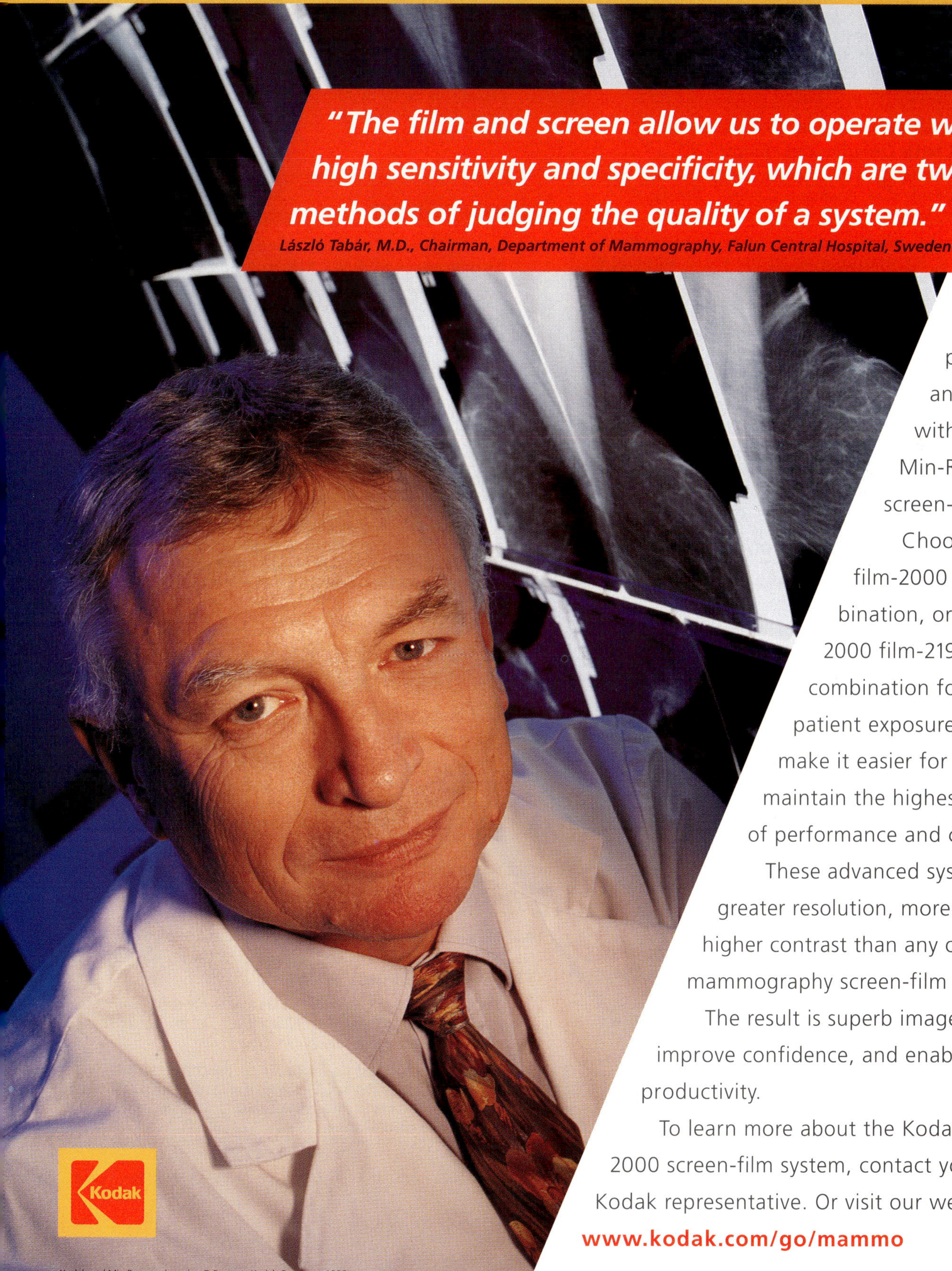

"The film and screen allow us to operate with high sensitivity and specificity, which are two methods of judging the quality of a system."

László Tabár, M.D., Chairman, Department of Mammography, Falun Central Hospital, Sweden

Maximize performance and productivity with the Kodak Min-R 2000 screen-film system. Choose the 2000 film-2000 screen combination, or the faster 2000 film-2190 screen combination for reduced patient exposure. Each can make it easier for you to maintain the highest standards of performance and care.

These advanced systems yield greater resolution, more detail, and higher contrast than any other Kodak mammography screen-film system. The result is superb images to improve confidence, and enable increased productivity.

To learn more about the Kodak Min-R 2000 screen-film system, contact your Kodak representative. Or visit our web site:

www.kodak.com/go/mammo

Kodak

Genitourinary Imaging

87 **Myelolipoma: CT and Pathologic Features**
Philip J. Kenney, Brent J. Wagner, Padma Rao, and Clara S. Heffess
Myelolipoma most often occurs in the adrenal glands, but myelolipomatous foci can be found within other adrenal pathologic conditions or in extra-adrenal locations.

97 **Ureterolithiasis: Can Clinical Outcome Be Predicted with Unenhanced Helical CT?**
Naoki Takahashi, Akira Kawashima, Randy D. Ernst, Illya C. Boridy, Stanford M. Goldman, George S. Benson, and Carl M. Sandler
CT findings of a smaller stone size and a higher degree of perinephric fat stranding or an increased amount of perinephric fluid are associated with a higher likelihood of spontaneous passage.

103 **Benign and Malignant Ovarian Masses: Selection of the Most Discriminating Gray-Scale and Doppler Sonographic Features**
Douglas L. Brown, Peter M. Doubilet, Frank H. Miller, Mary C. Frates, Faye C. Laing, Donald N. DiSalvo, Carol B. Benson, and Mark H. Lerner
The four sonographic features that, as a group, are statistically significant contributors to the distinction between benign and malignant adnexal masses are (*a*) presence and nature of any solid component, (*b*) presence and location of flow at conventional color Doppler imaging, (*c*) presence and amount of free intraperitoneal fluid, and (*d*) presence and thickness of septations.

Ultrasound

111 **Deep Pelvic Abscesses: Transperineal US-guided Drainage**
David C. Sperling, Laurence Needleman, David J. Eschelman, David M. Hovsepian, and Anna S. Lev-Toaff
US-guided transperineal abscess drainage may be successfully performed in patients who cannot undergo traditional transabdominal, transvaginal, or transrectal catheter drainage.

117 **Lymphadenopathy: Differentiation of Benign from Malignant Disease—Color Doppler US Assessment of Intranodal Angioarchitecture**
Alexander Tschammler, German Ott, Thomas Schang, Birgit Seelbach-Goebel, Konrad Schwager, and Dietbert Hahn
The assessment of intranodal angioarchitecture with color Doppler US is a reliable and reproducible method to help differentiate between reactive and malignant lymphadenopathy in superficial lymph nodes.

Emergency Radiology

125 **Head Trauma: CT Scan Interpretation by Radiology Residents versus Staff Radiologists**
Michael G. Wysoki, Carlos J. Nassar, Robert A. Koenigsberg, Robert A. Novelline, Scott H. Faro, and Eric N. Faerber
We found a low discrepancy rate of 5.3% between interpretations made by radiology residents and those by staff neuroradiologists of CT scans of the head in trauma patients.

Neuroradiology

129 **Small, Patent Cerebral Aneurysms: Atypical Appearances at 1.5-T MR Imaging**
Paul B. Rolen and Gordon Sze
In most instances, small patent aneurysms are characterized by a signal void on MR images obtained with typical pulse sequences, as seen in 53% of the cases in our series; however, in 47% of the cases in our series, variable signal intensities were seen.

137 **Guillain-Barré Syndrome: MR Imaging Findings of the Spine in Eight Patients**
Woo Mok Byun, Won Kyu Park, Bok Hwan Park, Sang Ho Ahn, Mi Soo Hwang, and Jay Chun Chang
Although contrast material enhancement of the spinal nerve roots is a nonspecific finding that can be seen in neoplastic or other inflammatory processes, enhancement of only the anterior nerve roots is suggestive of Guillain-Barré syndrome.

Signs in Imaging

143 **The Sugarcoating Sign**
Alan J. Holz
It is the striking contrast between nonenhancing neural tissue, sheetlike enhancing tumor implants, and dark cerebrospinal fluid that produces the sugarcoating sign seen in patients with leptomeningeal carcinomatosis.

Vascular and Interventional Radiology

145 **Hypocalcemic Stimulation and Nonselective Venous Sampling for Localizing Parathyroid Adenomas: Work In Progress**
John L. Doppman, Monica C. Skarulis, Richard Chang, H. Richard Alexander, David Bartlett, Steven K. Libutti, Stephen J. Marx, and Allen M. Spiegel
Nonionic contrast material is an effective stimulus for releasing parathyroid hormone and simplified the procedure by confining the imaging and sampling study to a single injection.

Continued—

153 **Dual-Helical CT for Detecting Aortic Atheromas as a Source of Stroke: Comparison with Transesophageal Echocardiography**
Alexander Tenenbaum, Alexander Garniek, Joseph Shemesh, Enrique Z. Fisman, Chaim I. Stroh, Yacov Itzchak, Zvi Vered, and Michael Motro
Unenhanced dual-helical CT may become complementary, and occasionally even superior, to transesophageal echocardiography in the rapid, noninvasive detection of protruding aortic plaques in areas not well visualized with the latter technique.

159 **Percutaneous Drainage of Fluid Collections in the Extremities**
Herman P. Wu and Thomas M. Vesely
The results of this study of patients with fluid collections of varying size, depth, and complexity at presentation suggest that percutaneous drainage of fluid collections in the extremities is as effective as percutaneous drainage of abdominal or pelvic fluid.

Cardiac Imaging

167 **Coronary Artery Stenoses: Assessment with Contrast-enhanced Electron-Beam CT and Axial Reconstructions**
Gautham P. Reddy, Daniel M. Chernoff, James R. Adams, and Charles B. Higgins
This study and prior reports demonstrate that electron-beam CT angiography can readily image the coronary arteries and can depict coronary artery stenoses.

Radiation Oncology

173 **Brachytherapy for Prophylaxis of Restenosis after Long-Segment Femoropopliteal Angioplasty: Pilot Study**
Erich Minar, Boris Pokrajac, Ramazanali Ahmadi, Thomas Maca, Wolfgang Seitz, Andreas Stümpflen, Richard Pötter, and Herbert Ehringer
Considering the negative selection of patients with a high risk of restenosis, the results of this pilot study are promising concerning the possibility of reduction of restenosis by means of endovascular brachytherapy after long-segment femoropopliteal percutaneous transluminal angioplasty without stent implantation.

181 **Bronchial Carcinoid Tumors: Importance of Prognostic Factors That Influence Patterns of Recurrence and Overall Survival**
Perry M. Gould, James A. Bonner, Timothy E. Sawyer, Claude Deschamps, Carla M. Lange, and Hongzhe Li
Atypical histologic findings were associated with higher rates of local recurrence and of regional recurrence than were typical histologic findings in this group of patients with bronchial carcinoid tumors.

Thoracic Imaging

187 **Hypertrophied Bronchial Artery at Thin-Section CT in Patients with Bronchiectasis: Correlation with CT Angiographic Findings**
Jae-Woo Song, Jung-Gi Im, Young-Soo Shim, Jae Hyung Park, Kyung Mo Yeon, and Man Chung Han
Within the mediastinum and around the central airway, nodular and tubular structures with an appearance unlike that of lymph nodes or normal vessels on thin-section CT scans in patients with bronchiectasis can be suggestive of hypertrophied bronchial arteries.

193 **Ventilator-associated Pneumonia in Patients with Adult Respiratory Distress Syndrome: CT Evaluation**
Helen T. Winer-Muram, Robert M. Steiner, Jud W. Gurney, Rosita Shah, S. Gregory Jennings, Kristopher L. Arheart, Mahmoud A. Eltorky, and G. Umberto Meduri
In patients who are not deteriorating clinically, CT findings suggesting the absence of infection may delay or preclude invasive procedures, so bronchoscopy may be reserved for patients who are more likely to have pneumonia.

201 **Pulmonary Embolism: Diagnosis with Spiral CT and Ventilation-Perfusion Scanning—Correlation with Pulmonary Angiographic Results or Clinical Outcome**
Kavita Garg, Carol H. Welsh, Angela J. Feyerabend, Stephen W. Subber, Paul D. Russ, Robert J. Johnston, Janette D. Durham, and David A. Lynch
Our results confirm the usefulness of spiral CT as a noninvasive screening examination for the diagnosis of pulmonary embolism.

209 **Unsuspected Pulmonary Embolism: Prospective Detection on Routine Helical CT Scans**
Mark V. Gosselin, Geoffrey D. Rubin, Ann N. Leung, Judy Huang, and Norman W. Rizk
The prevalence of incidental pulmonary embolism was six times higher in inpatients with underlying malignancy (9%).

Gastrointestinal Imaging

217 **Initially Unresectable Hilar Cholangiocarcinoma: Hepatic Regeneration after Transarterial Embolization**
Thomas J. Vogl, Jörn O. Balzer, Kai Dette, Rainer Hintze, Wassilios Pegios, Jürgen Mäurer, Heinrich Keck, Peter Neuhaus, and Roland Felix
Preoperative embolization of affected hepatic lobes results in a marked increase in the volume of noninvolved liver parenchyma.

Continued—

223 **Hepatic Infarction Secondary to Arterial Insufficiency in Native Livers: CT Findings in 10 Patients**
Gail S. Smith, Bernard A. Birnbaum, and Jill E. Jacobs
Hepatic infarction may occur in native livers despite the liver's dual blood supply and propensity to develop collateral blood flow.

231 **Mucin-producing Pancreatic Tumors: Comparison of MR Cholangiopancreatography with Endoscopic Retrograde Cholangiopancreatography**
Kazumitsu Koito, Tsutomu Namieno, Takeshi Ichimura, Naoya Yama, Masato Hareyama, Kazuo Morita, and Motoi Nishi
MR cholangiopancreatography is more effective and less invasive than endoscopic retrograde cholangiopancreatography in the evaluation of the changes in size and extent of mucin-producing pancreatic tumors and the determination of whether new lesions will appear, and the former may replace the latter in the evaluation of these tumors, for which follow-up is necessary.

239 **Gastric Mucosa-associated Lymphoid Tissue Lymphoma: Radiographic Findings in Six Patients**
Charles C. Yoo, Marc S. Levine, Emma E. Furth, Kevin E. Salhany, Stephen E. Rubesin, Igor Laufer, and Hans Herlinger
When low-grade mucosa-associated lymphoid tissue lymphoma is suspected on the basis of barium study findings, endoscopic biopsy specimens should be obtained for a definitive diagnosis so these patients can be treated before the development of high-grade gastric lymphoma.

Breast Imaging

245 **Screening Behavior of Women after a False-Positive Mammogram**
Etta D. Pisano, JoAnne Earp, Michael Schell, Kathryn Vokaty, and Amy Denham
A false-positive mammogram that leads to open surgical biopsy does not inhibit most women from undergoing subsequent screening mammography, nor does it increase their fear of mammography or their worry about their future risk of breast cancer.

251 **Calcification Retrieval at Stereotactic, 11-gauge, Directional, Vacuum-assisted Breast Biopsy**
Laura Liberman, Jennifer H. Smolkin, D. David Dershaw, Elizabeth A. Morris, Andrea F. Abramson, and Paul Peter Rosen
Stereotactic, 11-gauge, directional, vacuum-assisted breast biopsy resulted in successful calcification retrieval in 95% of cases.

Technical Developments

261 **Vogele-Bale-Hohner Mouthpiece: Registration Device for Frameless Stereotactic Surgery**
Arno Martin, Reto J. Bale, Michael Vogele, Andreas R. Gunkel, Walter F. Thumfart, and Wolfgang Freysinger
The Vogele-Bale-Hohner mouthpiece is a device that offers precisely defined external correlation points for patient-image registration in computer-assisted frameless stereotactic surgeries with any three-dimensional navigation system.

Letters to the Editor

266 **Pneumothorax after Fine-Needle Aspiration Biopsy**
Piergiorgio Solli, Leonardo Cattelani, Michele Rusca, and Alessandra Ganzetti

266 **Reply**
Karen T. Brown, Lynn A. Brody, and George I. Getrajdman

267 **Liver Hemangioma: US-guided Core-Needle Biopsy**
Robert D. Harris

267 **Reply**
Arne Heilo

268 **A Reviewer Responds**

268 **A Reviewer Responds**

269 **Editor's Response**

269 **Specimen Weights Obtained with 14- and 11-gauge Breast Biopsy Probes**
Fred Burbank

270 **Reply**
Wendie A. Berg and Thorsten L. Krebs

270 **Hard- versus Soft-Copy Readings of Computed Radiographs**
Paula W. Brill and Patricia Winchester

270 **Reply**
Harold L. Kundel, Wallace T. Miller, Sr, Wallace T. Miller, Jr, Judith Aronchick, and Warren B. Gefter

271 **Human Chorionic Gonadotropin Levels in the Evaluation of Ectopic Pregnancy**
Faye C. Laing and Douglas L. Brown

272 **Reply**
Deborah Levine and Teas S. Mehta

Continued—

In Memoriam

273 B. Leonard Holman, MD
Steven E. Seltzer, MD

273 Lucy Frank Squire, MD
Joshua A. Becker, MD

274 Cyrus Paul Klein, MD
W. Richard Seibold, Jr, MD

Book Reviews

34 Naked to the Bone: Medical Imaging in the Twentieth Century

96 Atlas of Infertility: Diagnostic and Therapeutic Radiology

124 Duke Radiology Case Review: Imaging, Differential Diagnosis, and Discussion

142 Nuclear Medicine Physics: The Basics. 5th ed.

180 Radiotherapy of Ocular Disease

Interludes

8 A True Dinner-Fork Deformity of the Wrist?

56 Radiography of the Queen Elizabeth Rose

80 Digital Photographs

Departments

275 Abstracts of Current Literature

16A Advertisers' Index

15A RSNA Quick Reference

48A *Radiology* Business Information

23A Announcements and Books, Audiovisual Materials, and Software Received

28A Continuing Medical Education

53A Publication Information for Authors

57A *Radiology* Manuscript Categorization Terms

52A Copyright and Certifications Agreement

59A Classified Services

73A RSNA Bulletin Board

50A Associated Sciences Workshop 1998

RSNA | Radiological Society of North America Founded in 1915 | 2021 Spring Road, Suite 600 Oak Brook, Illinois 60523 630/571-2670 FAX: 630/571-7837

Quick Reference

RSNA PURPOSE

The purpose of the Radiological Society of North America is to promote and develop the highest standards of radiology and related sciences through education and research. The Society seeks to provide radiologists and allied health scientists with educational programs and materials of the highest quality, and to constantly improve the content and value of these educational activities. The Society seeks to foster closer fellowship among all radiologists and greater cooperation among radiologists and members of other branches of medicine and allied health care professionals.

RSNA OFFICERS FOR 1998

President, **David B. Fraser, MD,** Halifax, NS

President-Elect, **Seymour H. Levitt, MD,** Minneapolis, MN

First Vice-President, **Carol B. Stelling, MD,** Houston, TX

Second Vice-President, **Miguel E. Stoopen, MD,** Mexico City, Mexico

Third Vice-President, **Guy H. Simmons, Jr, PhD,** Lexington, KY

Historian, **William R. Eyler, MD,** Beverly Hills, MI

RSNA BOARD OF DIRECTORS FOR 1998

C. Douglas Maynard, MD, Chairman of the Board, Winston-Salem, NC

Jerry P. Petasnick, MD, Liaison for Education, Northbrook, IL

R. Nick Bryan, MD, PhD, Liaison for Publications, Baltimore, MD

Peggy J. Fritzsche, MD, Liaison for Annual Meeting Arrangements, Riverside, CA

Brian C. Lentle, MD, Liaison Designate for Education, Vancouver, BC

David B. Fraser, MD, President, Halifax, NS

Seymour H. Levitt, MD, President-Elect, Minneapolis, MN

Delmar J. Stauffer, Executive Director

RSNA IMPORTANT TELEPHONE NUMBERS

MAIN TELEPHONE	(630) 571-2670	MEMBERSHIP	(630) 571-7873
FAX	(630) 571-7837	RESEARCH DEVELOPMENT	(630) 368-3756
ACCOUNTING	(630) 571-7812	PROGRAM SERVICES	(630) 571-7874
EXECUTIVE	(630) 571-7866	RESEARCH & EDUCATION FUND	(630) 571-7816
LEARNING CENTER	(630) 368-3753	ADVERTISING	(630) 571-7817
MARKETING COMMUNICATIONS	(630) 571-7830	CLASSIFIED ADVERTISING	(630) 571-7817
MEETINGS	(630) 571-7850	RSNA LINK	http://www.rsna.org
PERMISSIONS	(630) 571-7829	SUBSCRIPTIONS	(630) 571-7873 e-mail: subscrib@rsna.org

RSNA MEETING DATES AND LOCATIONS

1998 November 29 to December 4
McCormick Place, Chicago

1999 November 28 to December 3
McCormick Place, Chicago

2000 November 26 to December 1
McCormick Place, Chicago

RSNA YEAR-AT-A-GLANCE

July 1, 1998
Deadline for receipt of Education Editor Applications

September 1–2, 1998
R&E Fund Trustee Meeting

September 9–10, 1998
RSNA Board of Directors Meeting

September 15, 1998
Third Seed Grant Deadline

October 30, 1998
Deadline for Advance Registration Forms for RSNA Scientific Assembly

November 29 to December 4, 1998
RSNA 84th Scientific Assembly and Annual Meeting

January 1, 1999
Call for Scientific Papers, Scientific Exhibits, and *info*RAD Exhibits

January 9, 1999
Deadline for receipt of all RSNA R&E Fund Grant Materials

January 15, 1999
First Seed Grant Deadline

February 19–21, 1999
RSNA Board of Directors Meeting

March 1, 1999
Roentgen Centennial Fellow "Preliminary Letter of Interest" Deadline

March 23-24, 1999
R&E Fund Trustee Meeting

April 15, 1999
Deadline for Submission of Scientific Paper, Scientific Exhibit, and *info*RAD Applications

May 15, 1999
Second Seed Grant Deadline

June 16–20, 1999
RSNA Board of Directors Meeting

Advertisers' Index

RSNA Advertising Policy

According to the advertising policy of the Radiological Society of North America, the information describing radiological equipment, products, and services offered by vendors in their advertisements should be ethical, educational, professional, of value in furthering the radiologic evaluation and treatment of patients and furthering the education of the radiologists and allied scientists. The guidelines below should be followed for advertising in RSNA journals.

- All advertising must be directed to radiologic diagnosis, therapy, research, communication and/or to the professional and managerial roles of radiologists and allied scientists. Advertising material should be consistent with the highest standards of professionalism.

- RSNA reserves the right to reject copy which, in its opinion, is not in good taste, is unprofessional, or is inappropriate for a radiology publication, or offers products or services not in the best interest of the patient or the Society. Advertisements that are constructed to resemble the journal's editorial pages will not be accepted in that form.

- Acceptance of advertising does not mean endorsement by RSNA of the products or services advertised, the advertisers, or the claims made.

For media kits and questions about advertising ONLY, contact:

Jim Drew, *Director of Advertising*
RSNA Publications
2021 Spring Road, Suite 600
Oak Brook, IL 60523
(630) 571-2670
FAX (630) 571-7837

For all other RSNA department telephone numbers, see "RSNA Quick Reference"; consult "Departments" in the Table of Contents for page.

Aloka 9A

Bioscan 33A

CompHealth 67A

Daniel & Yeager 61A
Diversified Diagnostic Products, Inc 11A, 38A, 44A

Eastman Kodak Company 7A

Fuji Medical Systems IFC

GE Medical Systems 39A–42A, OBC
Gundersen Lutheran 64A, 71A

Harvard Medical School 33A
Hitachi Medical Systems America, Inc 34A–35A

Imation 37A
InterAmerican Congress of Radiology 45A

Jackson & Coker 69A

Maimonides Medical Center 71A
Marshfield Clinic 71A
Mayo Clinic Scottsdale 65A
MetroHealth Medical Center 69A
Mount Sinai Medical Center 67A

Nationwide Medical Services, Inc 66A
NDC Health Information Services 25A
Northwest Mississippi Regional Medical Center 64A

Ochsner Clinic 63A
Osler Institute 33A

Picker 13A, 19A–22A

RadioGraphics 216
Radiology 200
Radiology Resources 63A
RADX 43A
RSNA Associated Sciences 50A
RSNA Committee on International Radiology Education 250
RSNA *EJ* 166, IBC
RSNA Learning Center 24A, 75A–78A, 152, 186, 192
RSNA *Link* 46A
RSNA Membership 51A
RSNA Online Journals 72
RSNA ORD 116
RSNA Research & Education Fund 26A–27A, 238
RSNA Resident Membership 17A–18A

S&S X-Ray Products Inc 47A
W.B. Saunders Company 31A
Society of Nuclear Medicine 29A
Sony Medical Systems 2A–3A
SUNY Health Science Center at Syracuse 65A, 66A

Team Health 66A
Toshiba 4A
Trex Medical 244

U.S. Army Reserve 31A

VA Chicago Health Care System 67A
Vista Staffing Solutions 61A

PICKER

Announcements and Books, Audiovisual Materials, and Software Received

Announcements

Associated Sciences to Present Program at RSNA '98

The RSNA Associated Sciences Consortium is sponsoring a workshop on Saturday, November 28, from 10:15 AM to 3:00 PM during the RSNA Scientific Assembly and Annual Meeting in Chicago. The theme of the workshop is "Integrating Science into Practice." Four speakers will discuss a variety of issues currently affecting radiology departments. The keynote presentation, "Impact of Telematic Technologies on Image-guided Medicine," will be given by Heinz U. Lemke, PhD, of Berlin, Germany. Dr Lemke will discuss issues such as digital imaging, multimedia, virtual reality, and computational intelligence in medicine.

Bruce Johnson, BSEE, of Plano, Tex, will present a special luncheon program entitled "Networking for the New Millennium: Important Factors to Consider." Mr Johnson will review the basics of networking and identify some of the key criteria to consider when planning a networking purchase. New advances in storage technology and the associated trade-offs will also be presented.

The workshop will conclude with a panel presentation on "The Reality of Computerization." The panel will be composed of Heinz Lemke, PhD; Robert Seely, MBA, RT(R), director of diagnostic imaging at Western Baptist Hospital in Paducah, Ky; and Richard Carlton, MS, RT(R), assistant professor of radiologic science, Arkansas State University, State University, Ark. The panel will discuss a variety of issue related to computerization in the radiology department, including the future direction of information systems and computerization, the financial needs that will accompany the transition to computerization, and the educational needs and skill sets that will be needed by radiographers of the future.

The Associated Sciences program also includes a series of eight refresher courses of interest to managers and supervisors of radiology departments and radiologists. Four new courses will be introduced this year: "Specialized Accreditations: A Cost of Doing Business," "Managing a Multisite Radiology Network," "Multidisciplinary Standards for the New Millennium," and "Marketing Radiology: Getting the Message Out."

The Consortium is composed of the American Health Care Radiology Administrators, American Institute of Architects Committee on Architecture for Health, American Radiological Nurses Association, American Society of Radiologic Technologists, Association of Educators of Radiologic Sciences, Radiology Business Management Association, Society for Diagnostic Medical Sonography, Society of Nuclear Medicine—Technologists' Section, Society for Radiation Oncology Administrators, Association of Vascular and Interventional Radiographers, and Society of Magnetic Resonance Technologists.

Members of the participating organizations, physicians, physicists, and exhibitors are encouraged to attend the Associated Sciences program. Registration for the RSNA Scientific Assembly and Annual Meeting (November 29–December 4) is required for admission. Registration may be made in advance by mail before October 24 or on site at the assembly. Advance registration brochures will be available through the office of each association beginning the 1st week of July. Free bus transportation is provided by the RSNA all hotels participating in the official RSNA Hotel Block to McCormick Place beginning Saturday morning.

Detailed information on the Associated Sciences program appears in this issue of *Radiology* and in the RSNA *Scientific Program,* a supplement to the November issue of *Radiology.*

South African Society of Nuclear Medicine

The Eighth Biennial Congress of the South African Society of Nuclear Medicine will be held on October 7–9, 1998, at the Civic Centre, Cape Town, South Africa. Topics include general nuclear medicine, medical physics, radiopharmacy, and radiochemistry. In addition, a pre-congress workshop on orthopedic nuclear medicine will be held on October 6. Congress chairperson: Ellmann. Workshop organizer: Klopper. Fee: $180. For further information, contact Dr Sietske Rubow, congress secretariat, Department of Nuclear Medicine (C10A), Tygerberg Hospital, Tygerberg 7505, South Africa; telephone 27 21 938 4265 or 27 21 938 4350; fax 27 21 938 4694; e-mail *SMR@maties.sun.ac.za; http://www.nac.ac.za/congress.html.*

Royal Australasian College of Radiologists

The Royal Australasian College of Radiologists (RACR) will hold its 49th Annual General and Scientific Meeting on October 16–20, 1998, at the Brisbane Convention Centre, Brisbane, Australia. The meeting will serve as a forum for the presentation and discussion of new developments in the fields of radiology and radiation oncology. Convenor: Lisle. Guest faculty: Brada, Charboneau, Kricun, Mendenhall, Mould, Naidich, Reznek, Smirniotopoulos, Stevenson, Weir. For further information, contact Michelle Fok, RACR 1998 conference secretariat, C/-Convention Network, 224 Rouse St, Port Melbourne, Victoria 3207, Australia; telephone 613 9646 4122; fax 613 9646 7737; e-mail *convnet@peg.apc.org.*

6th International Magnetic Resonance Imaging Course

The 6th International Magnetic Resonance Imaging Course will be held on October 26–28, 1998, at the Armed Forces Hospital, Riyadh, Saudi Arabia. The course will provide an overview of magnetic resonance (MR) technology and basic principles, as well as current and future applications of MR in the whole body. Topics include MR physics, neurology, and musculoskeletal radiology. Chairman: Al Thagafi. Faculty: Ball, McNamara, Mafee, Modic, Osborn, Recht, Schild. Fee: SR 1,500 (SR 750 for physicians in training; SR 450 for radiographers and technologists). For further information, contact the Department of Postgraduate and Academic Affairs, Armed Forces Hospital, PO Box 7897, Riyadh 11159, Saudi Arabia; telephone 966 1 477 7714 or 966 1 479 1000, ext 4933 or 4937; fax 966 1 476 0853.

2nd Heidelberg Conference on Dynamic and Functional Radiological Imaging of the Brain

The Department of Radiology, University of Heidelberg Medical School, is sponsoring the 2nd Heidelberg Conference on Dynamic and Functional Radiological Imaging of the Brain on October 29–31, 1998, in Heidelberg, Germany. The conference will focus on radiologic techniques with regard to normal and abnormal cerebral physiology. Topics include dynamic and functional magnetic resonance imaging, dynamic spiral computed tomography, single photon emission computed tomography, positron-emission tomography, and magnetic source imaging. Fee: DM 350. For further information, contact Diana Brinkmann, Department of Neuroradiology, University of Heidelberg Medical School, Im Neuenheimer Feld 400, D-69120 Heidelberg, Germany; telephone 49 6221 567566; fax 49 6221 564673; e-mail *Diana_Brinkmann@ukl.uni-heidelberg.de.*

Books, Audiovisual Materials, and Software Received

Radiology carries a complete listing of all books, CD-ROMs, and other material received by the Radiological Society of North America. If the material is later reviewed, the reviews of books will be printed in *Radiology* and the reviews of CD-ROMs and electronic material will appear in *RadioGraphics.*

Send publications for review to Richard A. Szucs, MD, Book Review Editor, *Radiology* Editorial Office, 1001 E Broad St, Suite 310, Richmond, VA 23219.

AIDS Imaging: A Practical Clinical Approach. Edited by Jacques W. A. J. Reeders, MD, PhD, John R. Mathieson, MD, FRCPC. Hardcover, $140.00; 342 pp, 244 illustrations. ISBN: 0-7020-1904-6. Philadelphia, Pa: Saunders, 1998.

Basic Clinical Radiobiology. 2nd ed. Edited by G. Gordon Steel. Hardcover, $45.00; 262 pp, 181 illustrations. ISBN: 0-340-70020-3. New York, NY: Oxford University Press, 1997.

Announcements and Books, Audiovisual Materials, and Software Received

Color and Power Doppler Sonography: A Teaching File. R. Brooke Jeffrey, Jr, Philip W. Ralls. Hardcover, $135.00; 314 pp, 153 illustrations. ISBN: 0-397-51779-3. Philadelphia, Pa: Lippincott-Raven, 1998.

Computed Body Tomography with MRI Correlation. Vol 2. 3rd ed. Edited by Joseph K. T. Lee, MD, Stuart S. Sagel, MD, Robert J. Stanley, MD, Jay P. Heiken, MD. Hardcover, $245.00; 1,610 pp, 2,110 illustrations. ISBN: 0-7817-0291-7. Philadelphia, Pa: Lippincott-Raven, 1998.

Current and Future Applications of Magnetic Resonance in Cardiovascular Disease. Edited by Charles B. Higgins, MD, Joanne S. Ingwall, PhD, Gerald M. Pohost, MD. From the American Heart Association Monograph Series. Hardcover, $130.00; 576 pp, 188 illustrations. ISBN: 0-87993-681-9. Armonk, NY: Futura, 1998.

Diagnostic Ultrasound: Principles and Instruments. 5th ed. Frederick W. Kremkau, PhD. Hardcover, $49.95; 602 pp, 358 illustrations. ISBN: 0-7216-7148-8. Philadelphia, Pa: Saunders, 1998.

Essentials of Nuclear Medicine Imaging. 4th ed. Fred A. Mettler, Jr, MD, MPH, Milton J. Guiberteau, MD. Hardcover, $69.00; 484 pp, 301 illustrations. ISBN: 0-7216-5121-6. Philadelphia, Pa: Saunders, 1998.

Imaging of Anorectal Diseases. Shahid M. Hussain, MD. Hardcover, £69.50; 164 pp, 95 illustrations. ISBN: 1-900151-36-7. Oxford, England: Oxford Medical Publications, 1998.

Neuroimaging and the Psychiatry of Late Life. Edited by David Ames, Edmond Chiu. Hardcover, $95.00; 251 pp, 67 illustrations. ISBN: 0-521-49505-9. New York, NY: Cambridge University Press, 1997.

Osteonecrosis: Etiology, Diagnosis, and Treatment. Edited by James R. Urbaniak, MD, John Paul Jones, Jr, MD. Hardcover, price not available; 472 pp, 194 illustrations. ISBN: 0-89203-174-3. Rosemont, Ill: American Academy of Orthopaedic Surgeons, 1997.

Radiology. Bradford J. Wood, MD, Sangeeta Desai Wood, MD. Hardcover, $24.95; 245 pp, 138 illustrations. ISBN: 0-683-30363-5. Baltimore, Md: Williams & Wilkins, 1998.

X-ray Repair: A Comprehensive Guide to the Installation and Servicing of Radiographic Equipment. Joseph J. Panichello, CBET. Hardcover, $59.95; 276 pp, 45 illustrations. ISBN: 0-398-06815-1. Springfield, Ill: Charles C. Thomas, 1998.

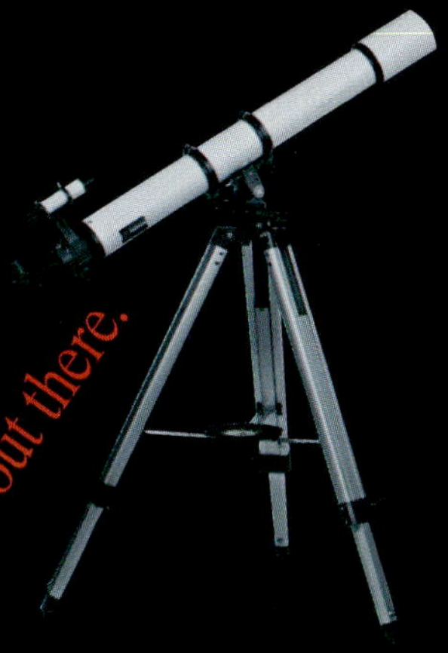

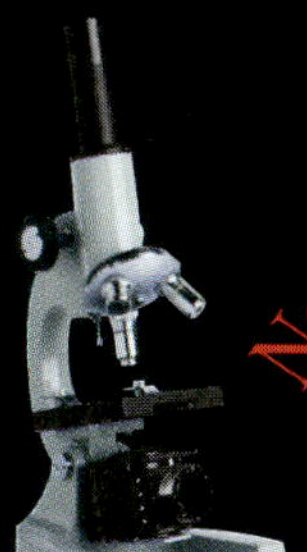

RSNA®

Research & Education Fund

Now Available

Application/Nomination Information

The deadline for most 1999 Grant Programs is January 8, 1999. Most grants begin on July 1, 1999.

Seed Grant Program and Roentgen Centennial Fellow Program have additional deadlines and start dates. See the respective sections for details.

For additional information and application/ nomination materials, please contact the RSNA Research and Education Fund office at 630-368-7885.

Scholar

Purpose –To support young faculty members by freeing at least one–half of their time to gain experience in research early in their academic careers.

Amount –$60,000 annually for two years, payable to the institution, to be used exclusively as stipend.

Requirements –Nominee should:
- have advanced training completed, including residency, fellowship, doctorate, etc.;
- be Board Certified or eligible to sit for certifying exams;
- be a faculty member of a North American educational institution at time of award commencement;
- be within five years of initial faculty appointment;
- and have not served as principal investigator on a major ($50,000 or more) grant.

Only one nominee per department.

Medical Student/Scholar Assistant

Purpose –To provide promising medical students an opportunity to experience radiology research while assisting second year RSNA Scholars.

Amount –$5,000 per year payable to the institution.

Requirements –Candidates must be nominated by a current RSNA Scholar grant recipient and must be medical students at the time of nomination. Medical students who receive this award will devote 100% of their time to the research activity during an initial period of vacation or elective time, and will continue on a part–time basis throughout the academic year.

Notes: Parties from institutions that are hosts to current RSNA Research and Education Fund Scholars and Fellows interested in applying for these awards, should be aware that the Trustees have developed policies regarding the equitable distribution of awards. Please contact the Society office for details on these policies.

Awards, with the exception of the Seed grant award, are restricted to citizens of North American countries and to individuals in the process of becoming citizens of the same.

Medical Student Department Program

Purpose –To enable departments of diagnostic radiology/radiation oncology/nuclear medicine allied with medical schools to provide research opportunities to medical students.

Amount –$1,000 per month to be matched by department for a period of 3 or more months.

Requirements –Awards restricted to departments of diagnostic radiology/radiation oncology/nuclear medicine allied with fully accredited North American medical schools. Departments must describe the following: commitment to research, student project that will require 100% of student's time, and proposed benefit for both medical student and the designated scientific advisor/project manager. The method by which student will be selected must also be identified.

Note: Name of student must be advised prior to grant disbursement.

Research Fellow

Purpose –To provide educational opportunities for young investigators not yet professionally established in radiologic sciences to gain further insight into scientific investigation, or to develop competence in research and educational techniques and methods.

Amount –$35,000 Fellow stipend for one year, with opportunity to renew for a second year at $40,000. Upon request, $5,000 is given to the institution to be applied directly to expenses.

Requirements –Nominee should:
- hold a degree of MD, DO, DVM, DDS, DMD, or the equivalent as recognized by the American Medical Association, and
- be nearing the end of prescribed training and/or have completed the prerequisite training to sit for certifying exams.

It is expected that Fellows will devote, essentially, their full time to research under the guidance of a scientific advisor of their choice.

Research Resident

Purpose –To provide educational opportunities for radiology residents to gain further insight into scientific investigation, or to develop competence in research and educational techniques and methods.

Amount –$30,000 grant for one year, payable to the department, to be used as stipend.

Requirements –Nominee should:
- possess an academic degree acceptable for the radiology residency, and
- at time of nomination, be in a residency program.

It is expected that the Research Resident will devote 90% of his or her time to the program outlined.

Seed Grant

Purpose –To assist young investigators in testing hypotheses and defining objectives before they apply for major grants from corporations, foundations, or government agencies.

Amount –One-year grant of $25,000 or less, payable to the department in equal installments.

Requirements –Applicant should hold full–time faculty position,
- have completed all advanced training, and
- have not served as principal investigator in a major ($50,000 or more) grant.

Any area of radiology–related research is eligible, including basic, clinical, developmental, health care planning and delivery, efficacy studies, and education.

Note: Applicant need not be citizen/resident of a North American country.

The Seed Grant Program will be offered three times each year. Deadlines are:
January 15 for July 1 start date
May 15 for November 1 start date
September 15 for March 1 start date

Roentgen Centennial Fellow Program

Purpose –To permit experienced practitioners the opportunity to explore and apply innovative solutions to key issues facing the radiology community. Such activity may include, but is not limited to: research studies, or program delivery focusing on topics such as health care policy/economics; educational methodology; evaluation methodology/outcomes research; basic or clinical research; rural health care delivery; or technology assessment.

Amount –This $100,000 award is designed to support a one–year program of study and/or research.

Requirements –Nominee should be beyond initial radiologic training and have several years of experience.

The individual who receives this award will devote a majority of his or her time to the proposed activity for a period of one year.

Application details differ for this program. Detailed letter of interest outlining applicant's innovative idea should be received at the Fund's office by March 1 each year.

Outstanding Researcher Award

Purpose –To honor one senior physician or radiology researcher who has made a career of significant contributions to the field of radiology or radiologic sciences through research.

Amount –$25,000 award payable to the recipient.

Requirements –Nominee must demonstrate a long–term commitment to radiology research.

Nomination packets must include:
- letter of nomination that addresses individual's appropriateness for award;
- corroborating letter of support; and
- nominee's CV, which includes a summary of candidate's grant support and research activities.

Nominations must be made by June 15. Nominee need not be a member of the RSNA.

Roentgen Resident/Fellow Research Award

Purpose –To recognize and encourage outstanding residents and fellows in radiologic research.

Recognition Award –Each participating residency program will receive an award plaque. Plaque includes place for additional names. Each year the Fund will provide a memento for the department to present to the selected resident or fellow.

Requirements –The director of the residency program or the department chair will identify an individual based on the following criteria:
- presentations or scientific papers at regional or national meetings,
- publication of scientific papers in peer-reviewed journals,
- receipt of a research grant, or
- other research activities.

The R&E Fund does not make the selections. Each department simply submits the name and address of the resident/fellow selected with a description of the individual's research activities. Nomination is to be submitted no later than April 1.

Continuing Medical Education

NOTE: Notices of continuing medical education programs will be considered for publication in *Radiology* if the program is directly relevant to medical imaging and if the following information is included: (*a*) dates and location, (*b*) a brief description of the course, (*c*) a listing of local and visiting faculty, (*d*) fees, and (*e*) number of category 1 credits that are available. Such notices should be submitted *at least* 5 months before the meeting date. Announcements of CME programs we consider not pertinent will not be published. We assume no responsibility for the content of CME programs appearing here. **Address announcements to** Julie Pietryla, RSNA Publications, 2021 Spring Rd, Suite 600, Oak Brook, IL 60523.

Continuing medical education programs are listed according to diagnostic discipline; interdisciplinary programs are grouped under the predominant or first-listed specialty.

Diagnostic Imaging

International Skeletal Society 25th Annual Refresher Course

The International Skeletal Society and the University of California–San Diego are co-sponsoring the society's 25th Annual Refresher Course, to take place on September 9–12, 1998, at the Jury's Hotel, Dublin, Ireland. The program will present current knowledge and future trends in the diagnosis and management of a wide range of musculoskeletal disorders to practicing physicians and trainees interested in this area of medicine. A systemic approach correlating etiologies and regional anatomy will be enhanced by focus sessions on emerging techniques and modalities, works in progress, and newer interventional procedures in both radiology and orthopedic surgery. At the conclusion of the course, participants will have received a balance of critical reviews of current standards and introductions to the newer methods for diagnosis and treatment of musculoskeletal disease. Fee: $650 ($425 for residents, fellows, and technologists); 25 hours of category 1 credit will be available. For further information, contact Ryals & Associates, Inc, PO Box 1925, Roswell, GA 30077-1925; telephone (770) 641-9773; fax (770) 552-9859; e-mail *webmaster@ryalsmeet.com; http://www.ryalsmeet.com.*

Radiology in Spain

The Cleveland Clinic Foundation, Radiology International, Inc, and the Sociedad Española de Radiología Médica are co-sponsoring "Radiology in Spain," a course to take place on October 4–11, 1998, in Santiago de Compostela and Madrid, Spain. The purpose of this congress is to bring together radiologists from around the world to discuss the latest advances in diagnostic radiology and allied subjects, discuss the place of these advances in the everyday practice of radiology, give radiologists from different countries the opportunity to compare and contrast their practice of radiology, and encourage mutual cooperation among radiologists of various nationalities. Topics include magnetic resonance imaging of bone, joints, abdomen, chest, and central nervous system; helical computed tomography; mammography; Doppler ultrasound; and neuroradiology. Program chairmen: Crawford, Jiménez. Assistant chairman: Birchenough. Faculty: Cardenosa, Cáceres, Cosgrove, Crues, Drayer, Ferreiros, McGuinness, L. Ros, P. Ros, Ross, Spackman, Vilar. Fee: $895; 32 hours of category 1 credit will be available. For further information, contact Betsy Birchenough, director, Radiology International, Inc, 340 Cleverdale Rd, PO Box 95, Cleverdale, NY 12820; telephone (888) 656-3104 or (518) 656-3104; fax (518) 656-9815; e-mail *betsy@radiologyintl.com; http://www.radiologyintl.com.*

12th Annual Imaging Seminar during Vermont Fall Foliage

The "12th Annual Imaging Seminar during Vermont Fall Foliage," co-sponsored by the Department of Radiology, University of Vermont, and Fletcher Allen Health Care, will be held on October 9–11, 1998, at the Sheraton Burlington Hotel & Conference Center, Burlington, Vt. This program has been specifically designed with the practicing radiologist in mind in hopes of combining an intensive course with the convenience of a weekend timetable. A nationally recognized faculty with supplementary talks from the University of Vermont radiology faculty will review current topics in body imaging, including ultrasound and computed tomography. Each session will be organized so that there is a brief question-and-answer period to permit interaction of participants and faculty. Guest faculty: Dershaw, Goldstein, Pugatch. Local faculty: Klein, Mindell, Oppenheimer, Pappas, Zeman. Fee: $350 until August 1, $395 thereafter ($200 for residents and technologists); 11 hours of category 1 credit will be available. For further information, contact Linda Saia, Continuing Medical Education, University of Vermont College of Medicine, 75 University Heights, PO Box 52025, Burlington, VT 05405-2025; telephone (802) 656-2292; fax (802) 656-1925.

Mt Sinai 1998 Body Imaging Update

The "Mt Sinai 1998 Body Imaging Update," sponsored by the International Institute for Continuing Medical Education, will be held on October 10–13, 1998, at the Plaza Hotel, New York, NY. This is a comprehensive course that covers current imaging concepts of the most important subspecialty areas in the field of body imaging. Basic anatomy and recent advances in the various subspecialty areas will be reviewed. Emphasis is placed on the practical relationship between imaging and the clinical problems presented by the patients. Program directors: Drayer, Som. Faculty: Dalinka, Mendelson, Naidich, Schnall, Shapiro. Fee: $695 ($450 for residents, fellows, and technologists); 22.5 hours of category 1 credit will be available. For further information, contact Ryals & Associates, Inc, PO Box 1925, Roswell, GA 30077-1925; telephone (770) 641-9773; fax (770) 552-9859; e-mail *webmaster@ryalsmeet.com; http://www.ryalsmeet.com.*

Mt Sinai 1998 Brain, Spine, Neurovascular and ENT Imaging Update

The International Institute for Continuing Medical Education is sponsoring the "Mt Sinai 1998 Brain, Spine, Neurovascular and ENT Imaging Update" on October 14–18, 1998, at the Plaza Hotel, New York, NY. This course is designed for neuroradiologists, general radiologists, and clinicians with an interest in imaging of the brain, spine, and head and neck. The case material shown will include examples of both common and uncommon diseases that affect these areas. Program directors: Drayer, Som. Faculty: Curtin, Naidich, Sze, Zimmerman. Fee: $675 ($375 for residents, fellows, and technologists); 25.5 hours of category 1 credit will be available. For further information, contact Ryals & Associates, Inc, PO Box 1925, Roswell, GA 30077-1925; telephone (770) 641-9773; fax (770) 552-9859; e-mail *webmaster@ryalsmeet.com; http://www.ryalsmeet.com.*

6th Multidisciplinary Conference: Osteoporosis

The Division of Radiologic Sciences, Wake Forest University School of Medicine, is sponsoring a course entitled "6th Multidisciplinary Conference: Osteoporosis" on October 22–25, 1998, at the Greenbrier, White Sulphur Springs, WVa. This conference has been designed for all physicians with an interest in the diagnosis and treatment of osteoporosis. Family medicine physicians, gynecologists, endocrinologists, orthopedic surgeons, radiologists, and rheumatologists will benefit from this multidisciplinary approach to osteoporosis. Problems in patient management will be discussed; emphasis will be placed on the integration of key considerations from each contributing discipline. Program director: Lenchik. Faculty: Jayo, Linville, Monteleone, Sollenberger, Snyder, Sutej. Fee: $425; 15 hours of category 1 credit will be available. For further information, contact Pat Rice, Department of Radiology, Wake Forest University School of Medicine, Medical Center Boulevard, Winston-Salem, NC 27157-1088; telephone (800) 277-7654 or (336) 716-2470; fax (336) 716-2029; e-mail *ricep@rad.wfubmc.edu.*

13th Annual Economics of Diagnostic Imaging

Educational Symposia, Inc, is sponsoring the "13th Annual Economics of Diagnostic Imaging 1998: National Symposium" on October 22–25, 1998, at the Hyatt Regency Washington Hotel, Washington, DC. A faculty of internationally known authorities will discuss how to react to current economic pressures and how to develop strategies to meet the challenges of successfully practicing medicine in the 21st century. Topics include mergers, networks, and group aggregation; health reform and managed care; the new economics; and PACS, RIS, and teleradiology. Fee: $695; 27 hours of category 1 credit will be available. For further information, contact Lawrence R. Muroff, MD, FACR, Educational Symposia, Inc, 1527 S Dale Mabry Hwy, Tampa, FL 33629-5808; telephone (800) 338-5901 or (813) 254-4608; fax (800) 344-0668 or (813) 254-9773; e-mail *information@edusymp.com; http://www.edusymp.com.*

Breast Imaging

Breast Intervention and Diagnosis

"Breast Intervention and Diagnosis: Stereotaxis and Ultrasound in the Mammography Lab," a course sponsored by the Institute for Advanced Medical Education, will take place on October 2–4, 1998, at the Renaissance Chicago Hotel, Chicago, Ill. This program provides an update on the use of stereotaxis and ultrasound in mammography. Every attendee will attend hands-on workshops on stereotactic and ultrasound-guided biopsy techniques, as well as on ultrasound imaging of the breast. Fee: $515; 18 hours of category 1 credit will be available. For further information, contact Penney Margeotes, Institute for Advanced Medical Education, 14 Elm Pl, Rye, NY 10580; telephone (914) 921-5700; fax (914) 921-6048; e-mail *info@iame.com.*

Advanced Breast Imaging at Tysons Corner

The Department of Radiology, Stanford University School of Medicine, is sponsoring "Advanced Breast Imaging at Tysons Corner," to be held on October 16–18, 1998, at the Ritz-Carlton Hotel, Tysons Corner, Va. This course, intended for practicing radiologists, will review the current state of the art in mammography. Topics include mammographic analysis of breast calcifications, differential diagnosis of breast masses, and physiologic changes in the breast. Course director: Ikeda. Guest faculty: Bassett, Mendelson, Rubin. Local faculty: Birdwell, Jeffrey. Fee: $550 until September 14, $605 thereafter ($455 [$510] for Stanford alumni and military personnel; $355 [$410] for residents and fellows); 17.5 hours of category 1 credit will be available. For further information, contact Sharon Pollio or Mary Anne Pleskach, Department of Radiology, Postgraduate Education Program, Stanford University Medical Center, 300 Pasteur Dr, Rm S-058A, Stanford, CA 94305-5105; telephone (888) 556-2230; fax (650) 498-4335; *http://www-radiology.stanford.edu/education/CME.html.*

Master Class in Histologic-Mammographic Correlation

Mammography Education, Inc, will sponsor a course entitled "Master Class: Histologic-Mammographic Correlation with Therapeutic Implications" on October 20–23, 1998, at the Ritz-Carlton Buckhead Hotel, Atlanta, Ga. Designed for radiologists, surgeons, and pathologists, this course will emphasize the proper mammographic-pathologic mapping of breast diseases in order to arrive at a correct therapeutic decision. Upon completion of the course, participants should be able to (*a*) understand the complex relationship between the histopathologic and mammographic representations of breast diseases, (*b*) refine their understanding of the capabilities and limitations of mammography, (*c*) analyze the mammographic image properly and determine which adjunctive methods will be most appropriate for each of the subgroups of breast diseases, (*d*) appreciate the importance of weekly tumor board meetings and cooperation with the pathologist, and (*e*) understand the value and interrelationship of the main prognostic factors in order to predict the outcome of the disease. Faculty: Lagios, Tabár, Tot. Fee: $695 for physicians and administrators ($545 for residents, fellows, and military personnel; $395 for technologists); 20 hours of category 1 credit will be available. For further information, contact Mammography Education, Inc, 15436 N 50th St, Scottsdale, AZ 85254; telephone (602) 788-6836 or (602) 788-0064; fax (602) 482-4955.

Breast Imaging and Interventions Update

A "Breast Imaging and Interventions Update," sponsored by the University of California–San Diego, will take place on October 30 to November 1, 1998, at the Hotel del Coronado, San Diego, Calif. This course will provide a practical overview of breast imaging and interventions by leaders in the field. Topics include diagnosis of breast disease using mammography, ultrasound, and magnetic resonance imaging; evaluation of the male breast; and interventions including fine needle and core biopsies. Program director: Bergin. Fee: $450 ($275 for residents, fellows, and technologists); 15 hours of category 1 credit will be available. For further information, contact Ryals & Associates, Inc, PO Box 1925, Roswell, GA 30077-1925; telephone (770) 641-9773; fax (770) 552-9859; e-mail *webmaster@ryalsmeet.com; http://www.ryalsmeet.com.*

Computed Tomography

Clinical Essentials of Spiral CT

The Institute for Advanced Medical Education is sponsoring the "Clinical Essentials of Spiral CT" course on October 2–4, 1998, at the Renaissance Chicago Hotel, Chicago, Ill. This course is designed for practicing radiologists and technologists who want to enhance their knowledge of spiral and helical computed tomography. It provides a comprehensive review of the principles, applications, and chief topics needed to maximize the benefit of this modality in today's practice. Fee: $425; 18 hours of category 1 credit will be available. For further information, contact Cheryl Ann DeLena, Institute for Advanced Medical Education, 14 Elm Pl, Rye, NY 10580; telephone (914) 921-5700; fax (914) 921-6048; e-mail *info@iame.com.*

Health Policy and Practice

Society of Health Services Research in Radiology

The Department of Radiology, University of Pennsylvania Medical Center, is sponsoring a "Health Services Research Meeting" on October 23–24, 1998, at the Providence Biltmore Hotel, Providence, RI. This meeting, which will coincide with the annual meeting of the Society of Health Services Research in Radiology (SHSRR), is designed for physicians, scientists, and administrators interested in health services as they relate to radiology. The program covers a broad spectrum of topics ranging from radiology research methods to management and policy issues. Course director: Langlotz. Fee: $425 ($275 for SHSRR members; $150 for residents and fellows); 16 hours of category 1 credit will be available. For further information, contact Janice Ford Benner, Department of Radiology, University of Pennsylvania Medical Center, 3400 Spruce St, 1 Founders Bldg, Philadelphia, PA 19104; telephone (215) 662-7825; fax (215) 349-5925.

Interventional Radiology

Practical Training in Interventional Radiology

A 5-day course entitled "Practical Training in Interventional Radiology" will be held on October 5–9, 1998, at the M. D. Anderson Cancer Center, Houston, Tex. The emphasis of this course will be on interventional procedures using the pig as a model. Guest faculty: Cho, Lunderquist. Local faculty: Wallace, Wright. Fee: $2,000; 40 hours of category 1 credit will be available. For further information, contact Anders Lunderquist, MD, Svenska vägen 48, S-226 39 Lund, Sweden; telephone and fax 46 46 211 56 56.

Review of Vascular and Interventional Radiology

The School of Medicine, University of California–San Diego, is sponsoring the "18th Annual Comprehensive Review of Vascular and Interventional Radiology" on October 23–25, 1998, at the Hotel del Coronado, San Diego, Calif. This course will provide a comprehensive review of vascular and interventional radiology. It is intended for interventionists and interventional fellows, general radiologists who perform invasive procedures, and radiology residents. Program directors: D'Agostino, Oglevie. Fee: $500 ($300 for residents, fellows, and technologists); 18.75 hours of category 1 credit will be available. For further information, contact Ryals & Associates, Inc, PO Box 1925, Roswell, GA 30077-1925; telephone (770) 641-9773; fax (770) 552-9859; e-mail *webmaster@ryalsmeet.com; http://www.ryalsmeet.com.*

Magnetic Resonance

Internal Derangements of Joints: Advanced and Intensive MR Imaging

"Internal Derangements of Joints: Advanced and Intensive MR Imaging," a course sponsored by the International Institute for Continuing Medical Education, will be held on October 9–11, 1998, at the Westin River North Hotel, Chicago, Ill. This course will provide a comprehensive review of current knowledge with regard to magnetic resonance imaging in the assessment of musculoskeletal disorders. Program director: Resnick. Faculty: Resnick, Sundaram. Fee: $695 ($495 for residents, fellows, and technologists); 19 hours of category 1 credit will be available. For further information, contact Ryals & Associates, Inc, PO Box 1925, Roswell, GA 30077-1925; telephone (770) 641-9773; fax (770) 552-9859; e-mail *webmaster@ryalsmeet.com; http://www.ryalsmeet.com.*

10th Annual Advances in Mid & Low Field Magnetic Resonance Imaging

Educational Symposia, Inc, is sponsoring the "10th Annual Advances in Mid & Low Field Magnetic Resonance Imaging" course on October 15–18, 1998, at the Buena Vista Palace Resort and Spa at Walt Disney World Village, Orlando, Fla. This symposium is designed for physicians, technologists, and administrators currently using or contemplating the purchase of mid- or low-field magnetic resonance imaging equipment. Fee: $625 ($445 for residents, fellows, technologists, nurses, and military personnel); 25 hours of category 1 credit will be available. For further information, contact the program committee, Educational Symposia, Inc, 1527 S Dale Mabry Hwy, Tampa, FL 33629-5808; telephone (800) 338-5901 or (813) 254-4608; fax (800) 344-0668 or (813) 254-9773; e-mail *information@edusymp.com;http://www.edusymp.com.*

Musculoskeletal MR

"Musculoskeletal MR," a course sponsored by the School of Medicine, University of California–San Diego, will be held on October 22–25, 1998, at the Westin Resort Hotel, Hilton Head, SC. This course is designed for radiologists and allied health personnel involved in the diagnosis of musculoskeletal disorders. Emphasis is placed on the clinical application of magnetic resonance imaging, with particular regard to the internal derangement of joints. Program directors: Pathria, Resnick. Faculty: Boutin, Deutsch, Pathria, Resnick. Fee: $650 ($450 for residents, fellows, and technologists); 18 hours of category 1 credit will be available. For further information, contact Ryals & Associates, Inc, PO Box 1925, Roswell, GA 30077-1925; telephone (770) 641-9773; fax (770) 552-9859; e-mail *webmaster@ryalsmeet.com; http://www.ryalsmeet.com.*

Neuroradiology

Neuroradiology for the Practicing Radiologist

The International Institute for Continuing Medical Education is sponsoring a course entitled "Neuroradiology for the Practicing Radiologist" on October 12–15, 1998, at the Hotel Loretto, Santa Fe, NM. This course, designed for the practicing radiologist, will be a practical review of various aspects of neuroradiology. Program directors: Brant-Zawadzki, Hesselink. Fee: $695 ($495 for residents, fellows, and technologists); 20 hours of category 1 credit will be available. For further information, contact Ryals & Associates, Inc, PO Box 1925, Roswell, GA 30077-1925; telephone (770) 641-9773; fax (770) 552-9859; e-mail *webmaster@ryalsmeet.com; http://www.ryalsmeet.com.*

2nd Annual Intensive Review of Neuro, Head, and Neck Radiology

The "2nd Annual Intensive Review of Neuro, Head, and Neck Radiology," sponsored by the University of California–Irvine, will be held on October 29 to November 1, 1998, at the Four Seasons Resort Hotel, Newport Beach, Calif. This update course is designed to expand the appropriateness criteria of the American College of Radiology. Most of the lecture topics are structured with subtopics that define the appropriate imaging procedures for a variety of common patient complaints. Program director: Hasso. Fee: $725 ($450 for residents, fellows, and technologists); 28 hours of category 1 credit will be available. For further information, contact Ryals & Associates, Inc, PO Box 1925, Roswell, GA 30077-1925; telephone (770) 641-9773; fax (770) 552-9859; e-mail *webmaster@ryalsmeet.com; http://www.ryalsmeet.com.*

Ultrasound

Principles and Instruments

"Principles and Instruments," a course sponsored by and being held at the Center for Medical Ultrasound, Wake Forest University School of Medicine, will take place on September 9–11, 1998. The course, intended for physicians in training and allied health students, will allow participants to gain an understanding of the physical principles and instruments of ultrasound and how these principles apply to clinical practice. Topics include transducers, sonographic instruments, spectral and color-flow Doppler instruments, artifacts, performance, and safety. Fee: $495; 16 hours of category 1 credit will be available. For further information, contact the Center for Medical Ultrasound, Wake Forest University School of Medicine, Medical Center Boulevard, Winston-Salem, NC 27157-1039; telephone (800) 277-7654 or (336) 716-4505; fax (336) 716-4204; *http://www.wfubmc.edu/bgsm/ultrasound.*

Peripheral Vascular Ultrasound

"Peripheral Vascular Ultrasound," a course sponsored by and being held at the Center for Medical Ultrasound, Wake Forest University School of Medicine, will take place on September 14–17, 1998. Participants will learn how ultrasound is used to detect and evaluate disorders of the blood vessels of the extremities and abdomen. Topics include interpretation of test results, clinical manifestations of peripheral arterial and venous diseases, and vascular anatomy and physiology. Fee: $795; 27 hours of category 1 credit will be available. For further information, contact the Center for Medical Ultrasound, Wake Forest University School of Medicine, Medical Center Boulevard, Winston-Salem, NC 27157-1039; telephone (800) 277-7654 or (336) 716-4505; fax (336) 716-4204; *http://www.wfubmc.edu/bgsm/ultrasound.*

Obstetrical Ultrasound

"Obstetrical Ultrasound," a course sponsored by and being held at the Center for Medical Ultrasound, Wake Forest University School of Medicine, will take place on September 21–25, 1998. About 15 hours are dedicated to lectures by experienced sonologists, with the remaining time spent in scanning laboratories with obstetric and gynecologic patients. Fee: $945; 30 hours of category 1 credit will be available. For further information, contact the Center for Medical Ultrasound, Wake Forest University School of Medicine, Medical Center Boulevard, Winston-Salem, NC 27157-1039; telephone (800) 277-7654 or (336) 716-4505; fax (336) 716-4204; *http://www.wfubmc.edu/bgsm/ultrasound.*

Abdominal Ultrasound

"Radiological Ultrasound (Abdominal)," a course sponsored by and being held at the Center for Medical Ultrasound, Wake Forest

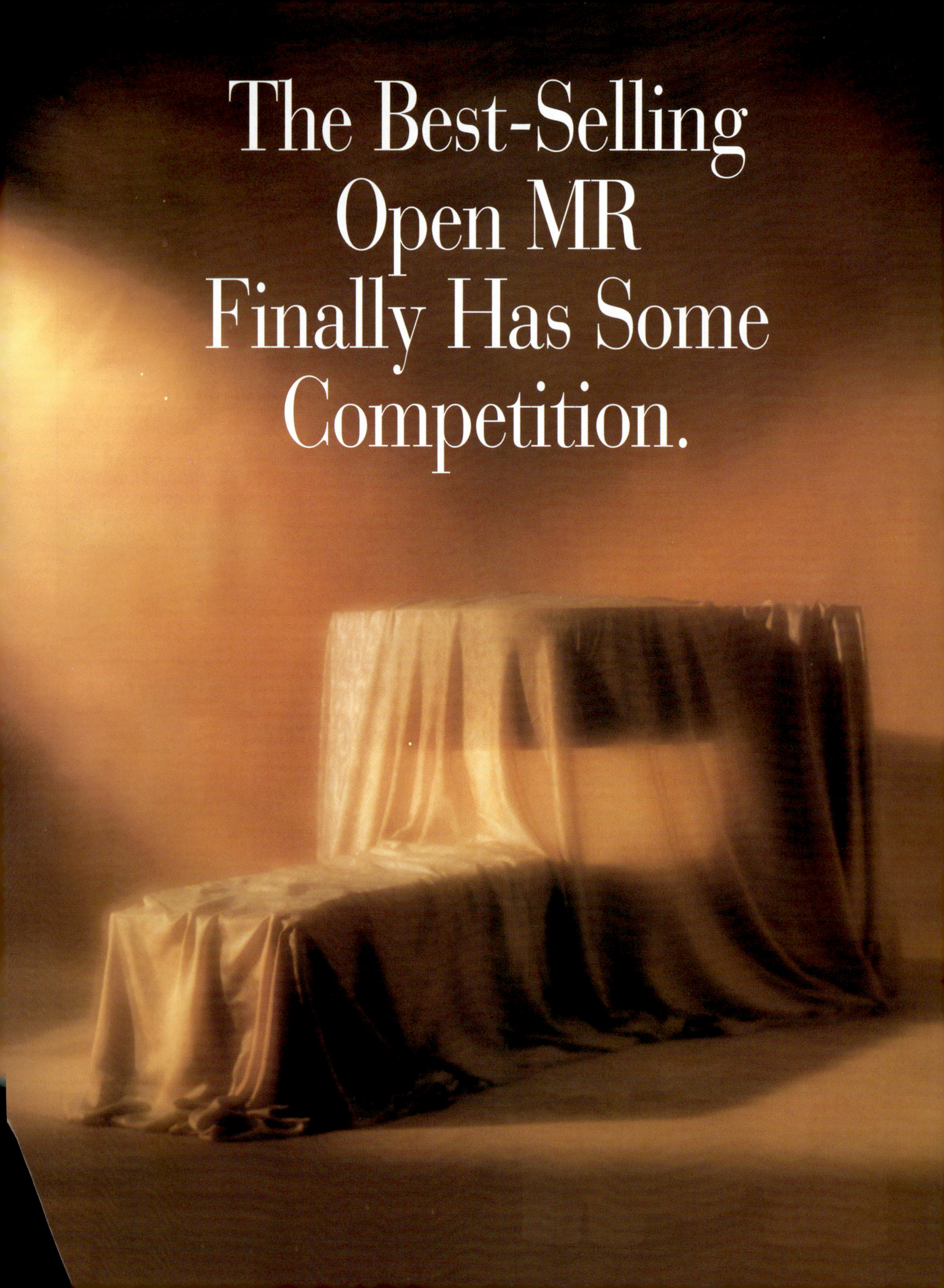
The Best-Selling Open MR Finally Has Some Competition.

University School of Medicine, will take place on September 28 to October 2, 1998. Topics include ultrasound physics and artifacts, sonographic anatomy and pathology of the abdomen, male and female pelvis, and the breast. Hands-on scanning laboratory sessions, conducted with various clinical instruments, will be featured. Fee: $895; 28 hours of category 1 credit will be available. For further information, contact Center for Medical Ultrasound, Wake Forest University School of Medicine, Medical Center Boulevard, Winston-Salem, NC 27157-1039; telephone (800) 277-7654 or (336) 716-4505; fax (336) 716-4204; *http://www.wfubmc.edu/bgsm/ultrasound.*

Neurovascular Ultrasound

"Neurovascular Ultrasound (Carotid and TCD)," a course sponsored by and being held at the Center for Medical Ultrasound, Wake Forest University School of Medicine, will take place on October 5–9, 1998. This course will examine basic principles of ultrasound physics and technology, as well as anatomy, pathophysiology, and hemodynamics with regard to extra- and intracranial cerebral circulation. Duplex sonography, color Doppler flow imaging, transcranial Doppler imaging, and new developments in ultrasonographic methods will be presented during lecture and hands-on scanning laboratory sessions. Fee: $895; 32 hours of category 1 credit will be available. For further information, contact Center for Medical Ultrasound, Wake Forest University School of Medicine, Medical Center Boulevard, Winston-Salem, NC 27157-1039; telephone (800) 277-7654 or (336) 716-4505; fax (336) 716-4204; *http://www.wfubmc.edu/bgsm/ultrasound.*

Adult Echocardiography

"Adult Echocardiography," a course sponsored by and being held at the Center for Medical Ultrasound, Wake Forest University School of Medicine, will take place on October 12–16, 1998. The course will provide an introduction to basic cardiac ultrasound techniques, including two-dimensional and m-mode echocardiography and spectral and color Doppler flow imaging. While brief overviews of advanced techniques such as transesophageal and stress echocardiography are provided, emphasis will be placed on fundamental and practical aspects of adult echocardiography. Several small scanning laboratory sessions will be conducted, featuring up-to-date equipment from many major manufacturers, to provide practical hands-on experience. Fee: $895; 32 hours of category 1 credit will be available. For further information, contact Center for Medical Ultrasound, Wake Forest University School of Medicine, Medical Center Boulevard, Winston-Salem, NC 27157-1039; telephone (800) 277-7654 or (336) 716-4505; fax (336) 716-4204; *http://www.wfubmc.edu/bgsm/ultrasound.*

Clinical Innovations in OB-GYN Ultrasound

The Institute for Advanced Medical Education is sponsoring the "Clinical Innovations in OB-GYN Ultrasound" course on October 16–18, 1998, at the Aldolphus Hotel, Dallas, Tex. This program brings together leading speakers in ultrasound and obstetrics and gynecology. In addition to talks on the various clinical aspects of ultrasound, there will be presentations on newer imaging technologies and lab accreditation. Fee: $575; 15 hours of category 1 credit will be available. For further information, contact Penney Margeotes, Institute for Advanced Medical Education, 14 Elm Pl, Rye, NY 10580; telephone (914) 921-5700; fax (914) 921-6048; e-mail *info@iame.com.*

Current Practice of Vascular Ultrasound

"Current Practice of Vascular Ultrasound," a course sponsored by the Institute for Advanced Medical Education, will take place on October 23–25, 1998, at the Grand Hyatt Buckhead, Atlanta, Ga. This program will emphasize carotid, peripheral, and abdominal applications, and will include individual hands-on instruction along with live demonstrations using the latest in ultrasound equipment. Physician interpretation sessions include panel discussion and practice cases. Live scanning of patients with known disease is also featured. Fee: $525; 21 hours of category 1 credit will be available. For further information, contact Penney Margeotes, Institute for Advanced Medical Education, 14 Elm Pl, Rye, NY 10580; telephone (914) 921-5700; fax (914) 921-6048; e-mail *info@iame.com.*

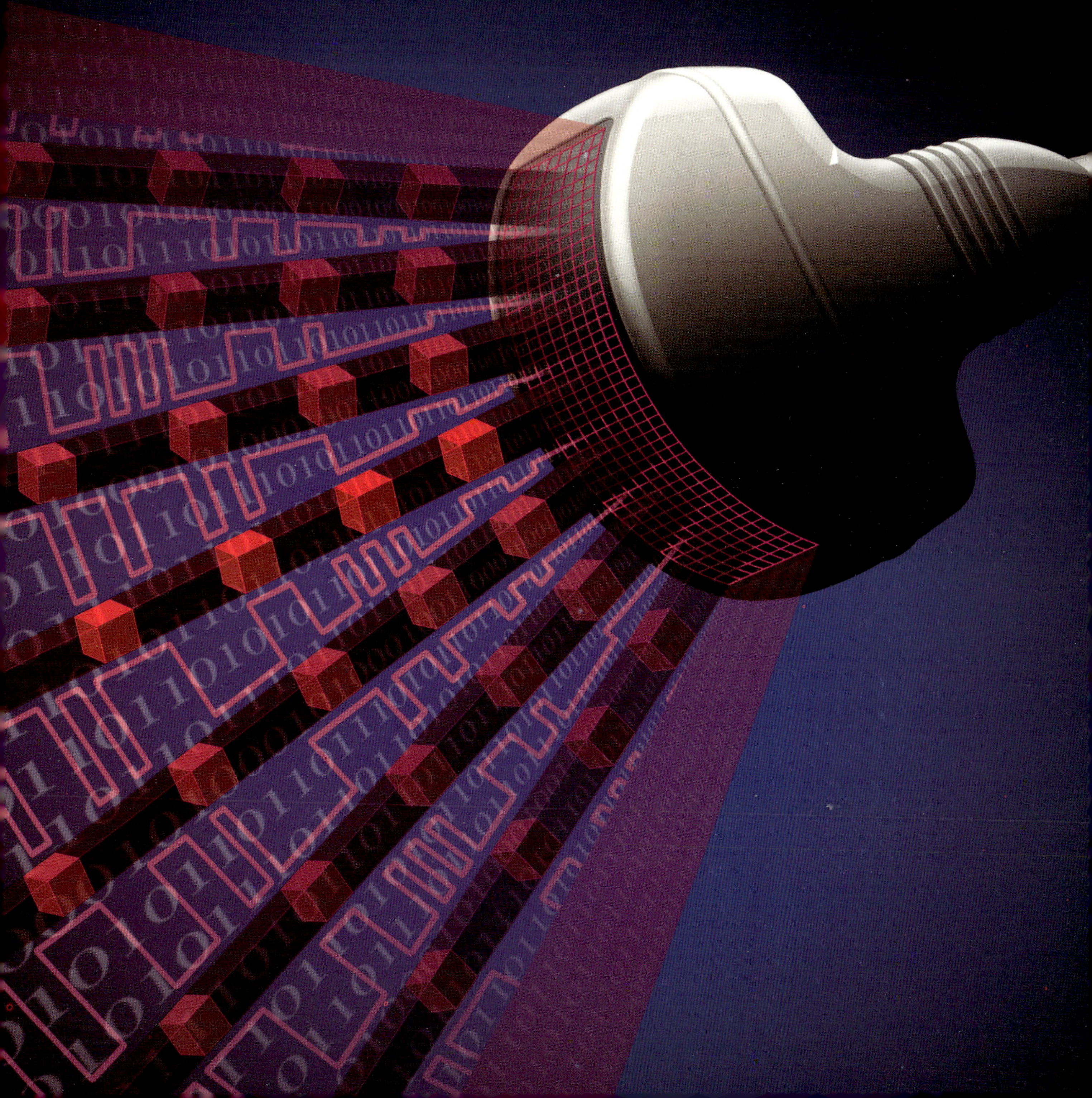

Radiology Business Information

Radiology, a monthly journal devoted to clinical radiology and allied sciences, is owned and published by

The Radiological Society of North America, Inc (RSNA)
2021 Spring Road, Suite 600
Oak Brook, IL 60523 USA
(630) 571-2670 • FAX (630) 571-7837
RSNA Link *http://www.rsna.org*

Delmar J. Stauffer, *Executive Director and Business Manager for Publications*

■ JOURNAL BUSINESS

Send new manuscripts to the address given in the Publication Information for Authors.

Correspondence concerning accepted or published material should be addressed to

Anthony V. Proto, MD–Editor, *Radiology*
Radiology Editorial Office • 1001 East Broad Street
Suite 310 • Richmond, VA 23219
(804) 644-5667 FAX (804) 644-5672
e-mail: *proto@rsna.org*

■ COPYRIGHT AND PERMISSIONS

■ PHOTOCOPYING

Authorization to photocopy items for internal or personal use, or the internal or personal use of specific clients and educators, is granted by RSNA, provided that the appropriate fee is paid directly to Copyright Clearance Center, Inc (CCC), 222 Rosewood Dr, Danvers, MA 01923 (phone 978-750-8400; FAX 978-750-4744).

Consent for photocopying does not extend to copying for general distribution, resale, or advertising and promotional purposes, or for creating new collective works. Permission for the latter categories may be sought by writing to the Permissions Coordinator, RSNA Publications, Oak Brook, IL (address above).

■ SUBSCRIPTION INFORMATION

The nonmember subscription rate for the USA is $215.00 per year; for outside USA, $260.00 (includes postage). (Air freight is available; rates are furnished on request.) Residents who are members of the RSNA may subscribe to **both** *Radiology* and *RadioGraphics* for a special rate of $80.00 (for North American addresses; residents from outside North America, add $60.00 for postage). Single copies are $25.00 (air freight, $11.00). Orders for subscriptions, remittances, and questions about subscriptions should be sent to

RSNA Subscriptions Department
2021 Spring Road, Suite 600
Oak Brook, IL 60523 USA
(630) 571-7873
FAX (630) 571-7837
e-mail: *subscrib@rsna.org*

■ CHANGE OF ADDRESS

The Post Office will not forward your journal to a new address. To avoid missing any issues, you must notify us of a change in address. At least 5 weeks before you move, please send (*a*) your **new address**, with zip code, and (*b*) your **current mailing label** with your old address to the address above.

■ MISSING ISSUES AND BACK COPIES

Claims for copies lost in the mail are allowed within 90 days of issue. Claims are not allowed for issues lost as a result of insufficient notice of change of address. To replace a missing issue or order a back copy contact RSNA Subscriptions Department at the address above. Back copies cost $25.00 (air freight, $11.00).

■ REPRINTS

The first footnote on the first page of each *Radiology* article contains the name and address of the author who answers requests for reprints. For reprint orders of 100 or more, contact

(continued)

The page containing advertising information (Advertisers' Index) may be located by consulting the Departments section in the Table of Contents.

RSNA DEPARTMENT TELEPHONE NUMBERS

Accounting	(630) 571-7812
Advertising	(630) 571-7817
Copyrights and Permissions	(630) 571-7829
Executive	(630) 571-7866
Learning Center	(630) 368-3753
Meetings	(630) 571-7850
Membership	(630) 571-7873
Office of Research	(630) 368-3756
Permissions	(630) 571-7829
Program	(630) 571-7874
Research and Education Fund	(630) 571-7816
Reprints	(610) 250-7244
Subscriptions	(630) 571-7873
Syllabus sales	(800) 272-2920
Main telephone	(630) 571-2670
FAX	(630) 571-7837

Radiology Business Information

Radiology Reprints
1991 Northampton St
Easton, PA 18042-3189 USA
(610) 250-7244

For reprints of advertisements, contact the Advertising Production Manager (address under Advertising).

■ MICROFORM

Radiology is available in microfilm and microfiche from

University Microforms International
300 N Zeeb Road
Ann Arbor, MI 48106 USA
(800) 521-3044

■ INDEXES

Radiology is included in the *RSNA Index to Imaging Literature,* a 3-year cumulative subject and author index of *Radiology* and 41 radiologic journals, available for $35.00 per copy (air freight, $11.00). Subscribers to the Journal receive the index free of charge. *Radiology* is indexed in *Current Contents/Clinical Medicine,* available from the Institute for Scientific Information, and *Index Medicus,* available from the National Library of Medicine.

■ BOOK REVIEWERS AND BOOKS FOR REVIEW

Any person who would like to help in reviewing books for *Radiology* should contact

Richard A. Szucs, MD, Book Review Editor
Radiology Editorial Office
1001 E Broad St
Suite 310
Richmond, VA 23219

Publishers wishing to have books reviewed should send them to the same address.

■ PUBLISHERS' ROW

As a service to readers and colleagues in medical publishing, *Radiology* publishes a list of current imaging publications of interest to radiologists and allied scientists. Complete addresses and phone numbers of participating publishers are included. Publishers' Row is featured quarterly, in the March, June, September, and December issues. For information on publishing a list, contact Mary Ann Morrissey at RSNA Publications (address under Journal Business).

■ ADVERTISING

The advertising policy appears on the Advertisers' Index of each issue. Questions about advertising and billing, advertising contracts, and insertion orders and requests for media kits should be addressed to

James F. Drew, *Director of Advertising*
RSNA Publications
2021 Spring Road, Suite 600
Oak Brook, IL 60523 USA
(630) 571-7819
FAX (630) 571-7837

Questions about advertising production should be addressed to:

Pat Hollingsworth, *Advertising Production Manager*
RSNA Advertising Department
2021 Spring Rd, Suite 600
Oak Brook, IL 60523 USA
(630) 571-7818
FAX (630) 571-7837

■ CLASSIFIED ADVERTISING

As a service to readers, *Radiology* accepts classified advertising, and every effort is made to ensure that the ads are relevant to the practice of radiology. For more details on the classified advertising policy and procedures, see the Classified Advertising section in each issue (consult the Departments section in the Table of Contents for page number) or contact the Advertising Production Manager (address under Advertising).

CHANGE OF ADDRESS FORM

Please allow 90 days for change to take effect

Name: ______________________________

Previous Address

Address: ______________________________

____

____

City/State/Zip: ______________________________

New Address

Address: ______________________________

____

____

City/State/Zip: ______________________________

Mail to:
RSNA Subscriptions Department • 2021 Spring Road • Suite 600 • Oak Brook, IL 60523 USA **FAX:** (630) 571-7837

Science to Practice RSNA '98

Integrating Science Into Practice

Associated Sciences Program at RSNA 1998

Workshop: Saturday, Nov. 28, 1998, 10:15 am - 4:30 pm, McCormick Place Sout

Refresher Courses: Sunday, Nov. 29, 1998 through Friday, Dec. 4, 1998

Credits: 4¼ hours and an additional 1½ hours credit for attendance at the Basic Physics Lecture

Welcome and Introduction
10:15 am
Samuel L. Hissong, MD, Chair, Associated Sciences Consortium and Committee
Eugene D. Frank, MA, RT(R), Coordinator, Associated Sciences Consortium

Keynote Presentation
10:30 - 11:50 am
Impact of Telematic Technologies on Image-Guided Medicine (AIA-AAH)
Heinz U. Lemke, PhD

Break
11:50 am - 12:10 pm

Special Luncheon Program
12:10 - 1:20 pm
Networking for the New Millennium - Important Factors to Consider (SMRT)
Bruce Johnson, BSEE

Break
1:20 - 1:30 pm

Panel Presentation
1:30 - 2:50 pm
The Reality of Computerization (AERS, AHRA, SROA)
Richard Carlton, MS, RT(R)
Robert Seely, MBA, RT(R)
Heinz U. Lemke, PhD

AAPM/RSNA Basic Physics Lecture for the Radiologic Technologist: Vascular Imaging Physics
Organized by Gerald A. White, Jr., MS
3:00 - 4:30 pm
1½ hours credit

Refresher Courses

(Each Refresher Course is approved for 1½ hours credit)

Sunday RC 124
Organizational Culture and Health System Change
Cornelius J. Rater, MD (AERS)
Harry J. Granito, MS (RBMA)
Douglas R. Hanson (ASRT)

Monday RC 224
Liability Issues Arising from the Changing Health Care Environment
Ann Obergfell, JD, RT(R) (ASRT)
Perry Smith, JD, RDMS (SDMS)

Monday RC 324
Organizational Change In Radiology: Preparing Radiology for the Next Millennium
Monte G. Clinton (AHRA)
Donna L. Wright, EdD, RT(R) (AERS)
Loretta L. Hanwell, MPA (AHRA)

Tuesday RC 424
Competency, Continuity, and Compliance
Susan S. Weiss, CNMT (SNM-TS)
Kate Little, RN (ARNA)

Wednesday RC 524
Managing a Multisite Radiology Network
Larry Ranahan, MBA (RBMA) Moderator
Sherry Rader (RBMA)
Charles Deschamps, RT(R)(MR) (SMRT)
Rebecca Shanahan, JD (RBMA)

Thursday RC 624
Specialized Accreditations: A Cost of Doing Business
Luann J. Culbreth, MEd, RT(R)(MR) (SMRT) Moderator
John Kovelski, RT(R)(MR) (SMRT)
Karol Handrahan, RT(R) (SMRT)
Linda Zanin, MS, PhD (SDMS)
Ronald F. Bernardi, BA, RT(R)(N) (AHRA)

Thursday RC 724
Multidisciplinary Standards for the New Millennium
Susan S. Weiss, CNMT (SNM-TS), Moderator
William R. Poller, MD (SNM-TS)
Michael R. Bloyd, RT(R), BSN (ASRT)
Liz Anderson, MBA (AVIR)

Friday RC 824
Marketing Radiology: Getting the Message Out
Ronald F. Bernardi, BA, RT(R)(N), Moderator
Cherrill Farnsworth (AHRA)
Michael R. Favreau, FAHRA (AHRA)

Registration Information

Advance registration for the RSNA Scientific Assembly ends October 30. Onsite registration begins at 12:00 noon on Saturday, November 28, at McCormick Place. RSNA shuttle bus service to McCormick Place will be available beginning at 10:00 am on Saturday. Advance registration is not required for the Saturday workshop; however, to receive continuing education credit, you must register.

Advance registration information appears in the July issue of *Radiology.* Brochures are also available from your association or from the RSNA, 2021 Spring Road, Suite 600, Oak Brook, IL 60523-1860. Phone: 630/571-7862.

Registration for the RSNA Scientific Assembly includes registration for the Associated Sciences Workshop. A box lunch will be available for purchase to facilitate your attendance at the workshop. These lunches must be purchased with your advance registration for the RSNA Meeting. **If you wish to purchase a box lunch, please check the appropriate box on the RSNA Advance Registration form and enclose your $11.50 payment.**

If you would like a copy of the published Associated Sciences Proceedings, please call 630/571-7877.

Sponsoring Organizations

- American Healthcare Radiology Administrators (AHRA)
- American Institute of Architects — Academy on Architecture for Health (AIA-AAH)
- American Radiological Nurses Association (ARNA)
- American Society of Radiologic Technologists (ASRT)
- Association of Educators in Radiological Sciences (AERS)
- Association of Vascular and Interventional Radiographers (AVIR)
- Radiological Business Management Association (RBMA)
- Society for Radiation Oncology Administrators (SROA)
- Society of Diagnostic Medical Sonographers (SDMS)
- Society of Magnetic Resonance Technologists (SMRT)
- Society of Nuclear Medicine — Technologists Section (SNM-TS)

RSNA® Radiological Society of North America Founded in 1915

2021 Spring Road, Suite 600
Oak Brook, Illinois 60523-1860
630/571-2670 FAX: 630/571-7837
www.rsna.org

Associated Sciences

Transfer of Copyright and Certifications Agreement

Manuscript No. (for Editorial Office use only)____________________

Complete copyright to the article entitled:

____

____

is hereby transferred to the Radiological Society of North America (for **U.S. government employees:** to the extent transferable), effective if and when the article is accepted for publication in ***Radiology,*** printed or electronic format. In the case of authors who are officers or employees of the U.S. government, the Radiological Society of North America recognizes that works prepared by them as part of their official government duties are in the public domain.

Authors reserve the following rights:

A. Other than copyright, all proprietary rights including patent rights relating to the subject matter of the article.
B. The license for personal use in lectures, lecture notes, and exhibits.

Please return this form as soon as possible. The signed statement **must** be received by the Editor **before** the manuscript can be processed for publication.

A. All authors certify that this material or similar material has not been and will not be submitted by them or by colleagues in their institution to any other publication prior to its appearance in ***Radiology.***

B. All authors certify that they have read the Publication Information for Authors found in the most recently published issue of ***Radiology*** at the time the manuscript is submitted. They further certify their compliance with the various requirements found therein.

C. All authors certify that they have submitted all required permissions and that all required statements have been inserted in the text where appropriate.

D. All authors certify that all individuals who have participated sufficiently in the conception and design of this work, in the analysis of the data, and in the writing of the manuscript have been listed as authors. All authors further certify that they have read the final version of the manuscript and approve it for submission for publication.

E. All authors certify that the Editor may correspond with the designated *corresponding author* regarding acceptance, rejection, revision of the manuscript and that the corresponding author is responsible for informing all other authors of the same.

F. All authors certify that responses, revisions received by the Editor from the designated *corresponding author* will be treated as if from all authors and that the corresponding author is responsible for informing all other authors of the same.

G. All authors certify that: **(must check one)**

- ❐ they have no direct or indirect financial interest in the products under investigation or subject matter discussed in this manuscript, or
- ❐ one or more (please name) authors do have a direct or indirect financial interest in the products under investigation or subject matter discussed in this manuscript. A separate statement is attached that details this proprietary interest, and the authors hereby grant permission to publish this information or an appropriate summary thereof with the manuscript if the manuscript is published.

TO BE SIGNED BY ALL AUTHORS:

Name (print) (First) ____________________ Signature ____________________

Name (print) ____________________ Signature ____________________

Name (print) ____________________ Signature ____________________

Name (print) ____________________ Signature ____________________

Name (print) ____________________ Signature ____________________

Name (print) ____________________ Signature ____________________

Use additional page if necessary.

This signed form (a photocopy is acceptable) must be submitted with all proffered works.

Radiology Publication Information for Authors

Radiology is published under the supervision of the Board of Directors of the Radiological Society of North America, Inc, which appoints the Editor who selects all material submitted for publication, including advertisements. No responsibility is accepted by the Board of Directors or the appointed Editor for the opinions expressed by the contributors. Please note that the instructions below are in accord with the *Uniform Requirements for Manuscripts Submitted to Biomedical Journals* (*Annals of Internal Medicine* 1997; 126:36-47). Although *Radiology* will receive material prepared and submitted according to these instructions, the right is reserved to introduce any changes necessary to make the contributions conform to the individual editorial standards of this Journal.

Full manuscripts should be addressed to:
Anthony V. Proto, MD—Editor, *Radiology*
Radiology Manuscripts • RSNA Publications
2021 Spring Road, Suite 600 • Oak Brook, IL 60523 USA
FAX (630) 571-7837

All other submissions and correspondence concerning accepted or published material should be addressed to:
Anthony V. Proto, MD—Editor, *Radiology*
Radiology Editorial Office • 1001 East Broad Street
Suite 310 • Richmond, VA 23219
(804) 644-5667 FAX (804) 644-5672
e-mail: *proto@rsna.org*

Assistant to the Editor: Deborah L. Hogan
Office Coordinator: Donna L. Schulze, Beth A. Stephenson

Inquiries about manuscript status and preparation, as well as letters to the editor, can be directed to *radiolog@ rsna.org*

The page containing advertising information (Advertisers' Index) may be located by consulting the Departments section in the Table of Contents.

■ TRANSFER OF COPYRIGHT AND CERTIFICATIONS AGREEMENT

Please send the copyright and certifications agreement with the initial submission of all proffered works. This may be accomplished by using a copy of the form that appears in this issue. **All** authors of any single composition must sign this agreement. In the case of officers or employees of the U.S. government, the Society recognizes that works prepared as part of their official government duties are in the public domain, but they must still sign the copyright and certifications agreement.

■ FINANCIAL INTEREST

Authors must describe any direct or indirect financial interest they may have in the subject matter of a submitted manuscript, and they must authorize the Society to publish this financial disclosure with the article if deemed appropriate. The Society's Financial Disclosure policy is as follows:

"Each author shall describe (*a*) any direct financial interest that author has in the subject matter discussed in the submitted manuscript, and (*b*) any affiliation or financial involvement that author has with or in any organization having a direct financial interest in the subject matter discussed in the submitted manuscript. Such information will be held in the confidence of the journal Editor during the review process. If necessary, in the Editor's view, this information may be shared with reviewers after discussion between the Editor and author. The submission of a manuscript to *Radiology* grants permission for RSNA to publish the financial information described above, or an appropriate summary thereof, with the manuscript if the manuscript is accepted for publication."

■ MANUSCRIPT PREPARATION

Original writings will be accepted only with the understanding that they are contributed solely to *Radiology*. Manuscripts should be typewritten and **double-spaced (all pages)** on only one side of the paper with at least 3-cm margins. Each manuscript component should begin on a **new page** in this order: title pages, abstract, text, acknowledgments, references, tables (each on a separate page), and captions for illustrations. The title pages and abstract page should not be numbered. Sequential numbering should begin with the text. To ensure anonymity in the review process, authors' names should appear on only the full title page; names of authors or the institution should **not** be given in the text or on the illustrations. **Three copies** of the manuscript and three complete sets of mounted illustrations should be submitted. The author should retain a complete copy of the manuscript, since accepted manuscripts will not be returned and only the illustrations of rejected manuscripts will be returned. All manuscripts are acknowledged; please allow 2-3 weeks from the time you mailed the manuscript for receipt of an acknowledgment.

■ TITLE PAGES, AUTHOR CONTRIBUTIONS

Full Title Page: This page should include the title of the manuscript, the first and last names, middle initials, and degrees of all authors, the name and street address (not a postal box) of the institution from which the work originated, the telephone number, the FAX or Telex number, and the e-mail address (if available) of the **corresponding author**, and information concerning grants. The address for reprint requests should include

(continued)

the **complete** name, street address (not a postal box), and zip code. It is important to indicate on this title page whether your paper has been presented at an RSNA meeting (please give year) or has been accepted for presentation at a future meeting.

Abbreviated Title Page: This page should include only the title of the manuscript so as to allow for anonymity during the review process.

Author Contributions: Authors are required to identify their manuscript contributions, for which they are responsible. The author(s) responsible for the integrity of the entire study should also be identified. Please list the following phrases on a separate page, to follow the "*Abbreviated Title Page,*" and beside each indicate the name(s) of the author(s) to whom these phrases apply:

- guarantor of integrity of entire study
- study concepts
- study design
- definition of intellectual content
- literature research
- clinical studies
- experimental studies
- data acquisition
- data analysis
- statistical analysis
- manuscript preparation
- manuscript editing
- manuscript review

For those phrases that do not apply, please list them and so indicate.

■ ABSTRACT, KEY WORDS, CATEGORIZATION TERMS, AND SUMMARY STATEMENT

An abstract of 200 words or less must be submitted with each manuscript of a major paper. The abstract must be divided into four paragraphs with the following headings.

Purpose: State the hypothesis being tested or the procedure being evaluated.

Materials and Methods: Briefly state what was done and what materials were used, including number of subjects. Also include the methods used to assess the data and to control bias.

RESULTS: Provide the findings of the study, including indicators of statistical significance. Include actual numbers, as well as percentages.

CONCLUSION: Summarize in one or two sentences the conclusion made on the basis of the findings.

Below the abstract, please list three to six key words as derived from the terms used in the most recent 3-year *RSNA Index to Imaging Literature.* Also, on the Manuscript Categorization Terms form provided at the end of these instructions, please select as many terms as are appropriate for your manuscript. It is important that you comply with this request, since the terms you select are utilized to match your manuscript with the appropriate reviewers.

On the reverse side of the Manuscript Categorization Terms form, the *author should reproduce from the text the one statement that best conveys or summarizes the message of the study.*

An abstract of 60 words or less must be submitted for each case report or Technical Developments paper. The abstract must state (*a*) what was done, (*b*) what was found, and (*c*) what was concluded.

■ TEXT

The text of observational and experimental studies is arranged in sections with the headings Introduction, Materials and Methods, Results, and Discussion. Lengthy papers may need subheadings within some sections to clarify their content, especially within the Results and Discussion sections.

Introduction: Clearly state the hypothesis or purpose of the study. Give only strictly pertinent references, and do not review the literature extensively.

Materials and Methods: Describe clearly the number and selection of the subjects studied (patients or experimental animals, including controls). Identify the methods, instrumentation (manufacturer's name and address in parentheses), and procedures in sufficient detail to allow other workers to reproduce the results. To ensure anonymity in the review process, do **not** include the name of the institution where the work was performed, either within the text or at the top of each manuscript page. Give references to established methods, including statistical methods that have been published but are not well known; describe new or substantially modified methods and give reasons for using these techniques. Include numbers of observations and the statistical significance of the findings when appropriate. Detailed statistical analyses, mathematical derivations, and the like should be presented in one or more appendixes.

Results: Present the results in logical sequence in the text, along with tables, and illustrations. Do not repeat in the text all the data in the tables and/or illustrations; summarize only important observations.

Discussion: Emphasize the new and important aspects of the study and conclusions that follow from them. Do not repeat in detail the data given in the Results section. Include in the Discussion the implications of the findings and their limitations, in particular with reference to the use of modified methods, statistical or otherwise. Relate the observations to other relevant studies. Link the conclusions with the goals of the study, but avoid unqualified statements and conclusions not supported completely by the data. Avoid claiming priority and alluding to work that has not been completed. State new hypotheses when warranted, but clearly label them as such. Recommendations, when appropriate, may be included.

For experimental studies, please describe the potential importance of your conclusions as they relate to future practical applications. Please identify this paragraph with the title "Practical Application(s)."

■ ACKNOWLEDGMENTS

List here those who have contributed substantially to the work reported in the manuscript, such as editorial and writing assistance, but who are not authors of the study. Authors are expected to obtain written permission of those acknowledged, and to submit the same, as readers might interpret that those acknowledged agree with the data and conclusions of the study.

■ REFERENCES

Number references consecutively in the order in which they are first mentioned. The abbreviations used for periodicals cited in the references should follow the style of *Index Medicus.* For journal articles, list surnames and initials of all authors when six or less, such as:

1. Stuart MJ, Elrad H, Graeber JE, Hakanson DO, Sunderji SG, Barvinchak MK. Increased synthesis of prostaglandin endoperoxides and platelet hyperfunction in infants of mothers with diabetes mellitus. J Lab Clin Med 1979; 94:12–26.

When seven or more authors are listed, only the first three names need to be identified, followed by "et al," such as:

1. Hibbard CT, Campbell S, Sabbagha RE, et al. Demonstration of tissue interfaces within the body by ultrasonic echo sounding. Br J Radiol 1961; 34:539–549.

Abstracts, editorials, and letters to the Editor should be noted as such. In the case of books, the authors of a chapter, title of the chapter, editor(s), title of the book, edition, city, publisher, year, and specific pages must be provided.

1. Brown M, Gray L. Indications for hematology. In: Wintrobe MM, ed. Clinical hematology. 3rd ed. Philadelphia, Pa: Lea & Febiger, 1975; 1146–1167.

It is the responsibility of the author(s) to ensure that all references are listed accurately.

■ TABLES

Tables should be numbered in Arabic numerals and should have a title. All abbreviations used in the table should be explained in a footnote.

Tables should be presented in the style used in recent issues of the Journal. No vertical lines or shading should be included. Avoid excessive use of horizontal lines within the table.

■ CAPTIONS FOR ILLUSTRATIONS

A caption must be supplied for each illustration, including drawings and graphs. It should not duplicate text material and should follow the style used in recent issues of the Journal. All captions should appear collectively on one or more pages separate from the text, and each caption should also appear below the corresponding illustration. It is essential that the caption describes all labels placed on the print of an illustration.

■ ILLUSTRATIONS

Illustrations should be limited to those required to show the essential features described in the manuscript. Space constraints prevent us from publishing redundant or excessive illustrations. Unretouched glossy prints no larger than 12.7 × 17.8 cm (5 × 7 inches) are desirable. Prints to be combined into one array, such as posteroanterior and lateral views, should be the same height or the same width to facilitate reproduction. They should correspond in appearance to the tonal relations of the original radiograph (ie, showing the bones white on a dark background, with the patient's right to the observer's left; computed tomograms and MR images should employ the "view from below"). If an image has been enhanced electronically, explain the alterations that have been made and send an original image along with the enhanced one. Drawings and charts should be rendered professionally in India ink on white paper. In computer-generated artwork, shading should be done in continuous tones (ie, solid black, solid gray, solid white): **Do not use dotted shadings.**

Since the size of the illustration printed in the Journal is typically smaller than that submitted by the author(s), it is essential that each submitted illustration show only the area(s) of interest with enough surrounding area for orientation puposes (e.g., to illustrate a cavity at the right lung apex, show only that area with enough surrounding area for orientation, rather than the entire chest).

All illustrations must be numbered and the top indicated on the back. For protection against loss or damage, each illustration should then be neatly attached to paper (one illustration per page), and the number and top should be reindicated on this page. For attachment, **avoid using glue, staples, or corner mounts.** Because it holds the illustration securely to the page without damage, we recommend Scotch Removable Magic Tape (3M, St Paul, Minn). **Please** do not add letters or numbers to the **face** of the illustration to identify the figure (such as 1A or 1B).

Arrows and other labels should be placed only on the final print, should be of professional quality, and should be **removable.** Professional artist service for such items is available to authors without charge. The desired additions may simply be indicated on tissue or a transparent overlay attached securely to the print.

Illustrations of accepted manuscripts become the property of the RSNA and will be stored for 2 years after publication. Illustrations will be returned only upon receipt of a written request from the corresponding author. We suggest that authors make and keep a set of illustrations in addition to the three sets submitted to the Journal.

■ UNITS AND ABBREVIATIONS

Radiation measurements and laboratory values should be given in the *International System of Units (SI)* (resources: SI Units in Radiation Protection and Measurements, NCRP Report no. 82 [August 1985]; "Now Read This: The SI Units Are Here," *JAMA* 1986; 255:2329–2339). Abbreviations should be spelled out when first used in the text, such as "cerebrospinal fluid (CSF)." Laboratory slang, clinical jargon, and uncommon abbreviations should be avoided.

■ INFORMED CONSENT

Manuscripts reporting the results of experimental studies on human subjects must include a statement in Materials and Methods to the effect that informed consent was obtained after the nature of the procedure(s) had been fully explained. In addition, a statement affirming approval of the appropriate institutional review board is required. If a review board does not exist, then the Declaration of Helsinki principles should be followed and a statement affirming the same should be made (41st World Medical Assembly. Declaration of Helsinki: recommendations guiding physicians in biomedical research involving human subjects. Bull Pan Am Health Organ 1990; 24: 606-609).

The maintenance and care of experimental animals to provide humane treatment and to ensure reliable results are described in the National Institutes of Health guidelines for use of laboratory animals. Authors must affirm compliance with these guidelines or approval of the appropriate institutional review board in the Materials and Methods section.

■ RIGHTS AND PERMISSIONS

Written permission (we require a copy) must be granted by the publisher and author to reproduce any previously published figures, including permission to reproduce in both print and electronic formats; any such material must be clearly noted and its source given in the manuscript. A signed letter of permission must be included with your manuscript for any individual who might be identified due to written descriptions, photographs (masking the eyes in photographs is not sufficient protection of anonymity), or otherwise. Informed consent, which requires that the individual be shown the manuscript, should be affirmed in the Materials and Methods section.

If reference is made in the text to personal communication (oral or written) as a source of information, a signed statement of permission is required from each such source.

■ AUTHOR RESPONSIBILITY

Authors must be certain that no manuscript on the same or similar material has been or will be submitted to another journal by themselves or others at their institution before their work appears in *Radiology*. The submission by authors of similar material to advertising media must be indicated at the time *Radiology* receives the manuscript.

■ ELECTRONIC SUBMISSION OF ACCEPTED MANUSCRIPTS

Manuscripts that have been **accepted** for publication must be submitted on computer disk (required for text, desirable for illustrations). A hard copy should accompany the disk and should match the disk file exactly. The disk should be labeled with its assigned manuscript number, the first author's last name, the word processing program used, and the file name.

Text File: Submit text on high-density 3½-inch disk prepared with an IBM- or Macintosh-compatible computer. Manuscripts should be prepared in WordPerfect 6.1 or Microsoft Word for PC (7.0) or Mac (5.0 or higher). Files prepared in any other word-processing program should be saved in an unformatted, text-only ASCII file and the program used should be indicated.

The entire article should be submitted as a single text file, with the elements in the standard order: title pages, abstract, text, acknowledgments, references, tables, captions. Only the final version of the article should be on the submitted disk. Keep the text file as free from formatting codes as possible: Do not use boldface, italic, underlining, strange fonts, codes for centering, unnecessary line spacing, etc. Use the default settings of the word-processing program; especially do not use right-justified margins. Use tabs to indent at the beginnings of paragraphs, and insert only one space after end punctuation marks. Use hard returns only at the ends of paragraphs or between sections of the manuscript; do not insert them mid-paragraph. Do not insert tabs in references; use only one hard return at the end of each reference.

Illustrations File: Although not required, submission of illustrations on 3½" disk, ZIP disk, or Syquest cartridge will improve image quality. For black and white images, we require that they be submitted in PC Tiff or PC eps format with a dot range of 5%–95% and resolution of 500 dpi. Four-color images should also be PC Tiff or PC eps format with a maximum of 280% total tonal density and resolution of 300 dpi. Each image file should be named, and with the disk or cartridge the following should be provided: a hard-copy inventory with specific information on the image, two sets of proofs obtained at 800–1,800 dpi, and one set of proofs obtained with a laser printer to be used as a reference set.

■ BOOK REVIEWERS

Any person who would like to help in reviewing books for *Radiology* should contact

Richard A. Szucs, MD, Book Review Editor
Radiology Editorial Office
1001 E Broad St
Suite 310
Richmond, VA 23219

■ BOOKS FOR REVIEW

Publishers wishing to have books reviewed should send them to the address above.

✔ Checklist of Requirements:

❐ 1. Send 3 copies of manuscript and 3 copies of illustrations.
❐ 2. Mount each illustration on a separate page, 8½ × 11 inches. Indicate figure number and top.
❐ 3. Double space all parts of manuscript.
❐ 4. Send copyright and certifications agreement with signatures of all authors.
❐ 5. Send institutional affiliation for each author and corresponding author's name, address, phone number, FAX or Telex number, and e-mail address.
❐ 6. Send a **brief** abstract: 200 words or less for regular articles, 60 words or less for case reports and Technical Developments papers.
❐ 7. Give SI units for radiation measurements and laboratory values.
❐ 8. Send copy of letter of permission to reprint any figure that was published previously or for any other reasons as noted in the instructions found above.
❐ 9. Send a completed copy of the Manuscript Categorization Terms form. Please remember to reproduce from the text the one statement that best conveys or summarizes the message of your study.

Radiology Manuscript Categorization Terms

Please PRINT your name: ____________________

Please print the title of your manuscript ____________________

____

For each section, please categorize your manuscript by checking off **as many terms as are appropriate.**

Modalities/Techniques

- ___ Absorptiometry/ Bone Densitometry
- ___ Angiography
- ___ Arthrography
- ___ Conventional Radiography
- ___ CT
- ___ CT-Angiography
- ___ CT-Electron Beam
- ___ CT-High Resolution
- ___ CT-Spiral
- ___ Dacryocystography
- ___ Defecography
- ___ Digital Radiography
- ___ Echocardiography
- ___ Fluoroscopy
- ___ Hysterosalpingography
- ___ Image Manipulation/ Reconstruction
- ___ Lymphography
- ___ MR-Angiography
- ___ MR-Diffusion/Perfusion
- ___ MR-Functional Imaging
- ___ MR-Imaging
- ___ MR-Spectroscopy
- ___ Neural Networks
- ___ PACS
- ___ PET
- ___ Radionuclide Studies
- ___ Sialography
- ___ SPECT
- ___ Ultrasound
- ___ Ultrasound-Color Doppler
- ___ Ultrasound-Doppler
- ___ Ultrasound-Power Doppler
- ___ Ultrasound-Spectral Doppler

Procedures

- ___ Angioplasty
- ___ Angioscopy
- ___ Balloon Insertions
- ___ Biopsy/Drainage
- ___ Dilation
- ___ Embolization
- ___ Endoscopy
- ___ Filter Insertions
- ___ Interventional Other ____________
- ___ Intraoperative
- ___ Laser
- ___ Lithotripsy
- ___ Localization
- ___ Myelography
- ___ Percutaneous
- ___ Radiation Therapy/Oncology
- ___ Radionuclide Therapy
- ___ Shunts
- ___ Stents
- ___ Thrombolysis

Areas/Systems

- ___ Abdomen
- ___ Biliary
- ___ Breast
- ___ Cardiac
- ___ CNS
- ___ Ear/Nose/Throat
- ___ Genital/Reproductive
- ___ GI
- ___ Head/Neck
- ___ Hematologic
- ___ Lymphatic
- ___ Muscular
- ___ Nervous-Peripheral
- ___ Skeletal-Appendicular
- ___ Skeletal-Axial
- ___ Soft Tissues/Skin
- ___ Thorax
- ___ Urinary
- ___ Vascular

Structures

- ___ Adrenal
- ___ Ankle
- ___ Anus
- ___ Aorta
- ___ Appendix
- ___ Arteries
- ___ Bile Ducts
- ___ Bladder
- ___ Brain/Brain Stem
- ___ Breast
- ___ Cervix
- ___ Diaphragm
- ___ Duodenum
- ___ Ear
- ___ Elbow
- ___ Esophagus
- ___ Extremities
- ___ Eye
- ___ Face
- ___ Fallopian Tubes
- ___ Foot
- ___ Gallbladder
- ___ Hand
- ___ Heart
- ___ Hip
- ___ Jaw
- ___ Joints
- ___ Kidney
- ___ Knee
- ___ Lacrimal Glands
- ___ Large Bowel
- ___ Larynx
- ___ Ligaments
- ___ Liver
- ___ Long Bones
- ___ Lung
- ___ Marrow
- ___ Mediastinum
- ___ Meninges
- ___ Mesentery
- ___ Omentum
- ___ Orbit
- ___ Ovaries
- ___ Pancreas
- ___ Paranasal Sinuses
- ___ Parathyroid
- ___ Pelvis
- ___ Pelvocalyceal
- ___ Penis
- ___ Pericardium
- ___ Peritoneum
- ___ Pharynx
- ___ Pineal
- ___ Pituitary
- ___ Pleura
- ___ Prostate
- ___ Pylorus
- ___ Rectum
- ___ Retina
- ___ Retroperitoneum
- ___ Ribs
- ___ Salivary Glands
- ___ Scrotum
- ___ Shoulder
- ___ Skull
- ___ Small Bowel
- ___ Spinal Cord
- ___ Spine-Cervical
- ___ Spine-Lumbar

Continued

Structures, continued

- ___ Spine-Sacrum/Coccyx
- ___ Spine-Thoracic
- ___ Spleen
- ___ Stomach
- ___ Tendons
- ___ Testes
- ___ Thymus
- ___ Thyroid
- ___ Tongue
- ___ Tracheobronchial Tree
- ___ Ureters
- ___ Urethra
- ___ Uterus
- ___ Vagina
- ___ Valves
- ___ Veins
- ___ Vena Cava
- ___ Wrist

Topics

- ___ Abscess
- ___ Acceptance Testing
- ___ Acute
- ___ Adults
- ___ AIDS
- ___ Anatomy
- ___ Aneurysms
- ___ Animal Investigations
- ___ Arteriosclerosis
- ___ Arthritides
- ___ Artifacts
- ___ Atelectasis
- ___ Athletic Injuries
- ___ AVM
- ___ Axilla
- ___ Biological Effects
- ___ Biostatistics
- ___ Blood
- ___ Calcifications/Calculi
- ___ Cardiac Assist Devices
- ___ Catheters
- ___ Cavitation
- ___ Cerebral Palsy
- ___ Chemistry
- ___ Chronic Obstructive Airways Disease
- ___ Cirrhosis
- ___ Comparative Studies
- ___ Complications
- ___ Computer Applications-3D
- ___ Computer Applications-Teleradiology
- ___ Computer Applications-Virtual Imaging
- ___ Computer Applications-Other____________________
- ___ Congenital
- ___ Connective Tissue Disorders
- ___ Contrast Agents-Intravenous
- ___ Contrast Agents-Oral
- ___ Cost-effectiveness
- ___ CSF
- ___ Cysts
- ___ Dementia
- ___ Demineralization-Bone
- ___ Dilatation
- ___ Dissection
- ___ Diverticula
- ___ Dosimetry
- ___ Drugs/Reactions
- ___ Dysplasias
- ___ Eating Disorders
- ___ ECMO
- ___ Edema
- ___ Education
- ___ Efficacy Studies
- ___ Embolism
- ___ Endocrine Disorders
- ___ Equipment
- ___ Ethics
- ___ Experimental Investigations
- ___ Fetus
- ___ Fistula
- ___ Foreign Bodies
- ___ Forensics
- ___ Genetic Defects
- ___ Grafts
- ___ Health Policy and Practice
- ___ Hemangioma
- ___ Hematologic Diseases
- ___ Hemodynamics/Flow Dynamics
- ___ Hemorrhage
- ___ Hernia
- ___ History
- ___ Hyperplasia/Hypertrophy
- ___ Hypertension
- ___ Imaging Sequences
- ___ Infection
- ___ Inflammation
- ___ Instrumentation
- ___ Ischemia/Infarction
- ___ Laboratory Tests
- ___ Leukemia
- ___ Lymphoma
- ___ Medicolegal Issues
- ___ Metabolic Disorders
- ___ Metastases
- ___ Monoclonal Antibodies
- ___ Motility
- ___ Neoplasms-Primary
- ___ Normal Variants
- ___ Observer Performance
- ___ Obstetrics
- ___ Obstruction/Occlusion
- ___ Occupational/Environmental Hazards
- ___ Outcomes Analysis
- ___ Parasites
- ___ Pathology
- ___ Pediatric Population-Adolescents
- ___ Pediatric Population-Children
- ___ Pediatric Population-Infants
- ___ Pediatric Population-Neonates
- ___ Physics
- ___ Physiological Studies
- ___ Pregnancy
- ___ Prostheses
- ___ QA/QC
- ___ Radiation Effects
- ___ Radiation Safety
- ___ Radiobiology
- ___ Safety
- ___ Screening
- ___ Sedation
- ___ Seizure Disorders
- ___ Socioeconomic Issues
- ___ Speech Disorders
- ___ Staging
- ___ Statistics
- ___ Surgery
- ___ Technical Aspects
- ___ Technology Assessments
- ___ Tissue Characterization
- ___ Transplantation
- ___ Trauma
- ___ Treatment Effects
- ___ Tropical Diseases
- ___ Varices
- ___ Volvulus

Please reproduce here the **one sentence** from the text that best conveys or summarizes the message of your study.

____

____

Please provide author initials by appropriate author contribution category.

- ________ Guarantor of integrity of entire study
- ________ Study concepts
- ________ Study design
- ________ Definition of intellectual content
- ________ Literature research
- ________ Clinical studies
- ________ Experimental studies
- ________ Data acquisition
- ________ Data analysis
- ________ Statistical analysis
- ________ Manuscript preparation
- ________ Manuscript editing
- ________ Manuscript review

This form *must be* included with your manuscript submission.

Anthony V. Proto, MD

Radiology 1998—Change in Deputy Editor

In the January 1998 issue of *Radiology* (1), I introduced our new Deputy Editors, whose names appear on our masthead. It has been my good fortune to work with these four talented individuals, Panos P. Fatouros, PhD, Ann S. Fulcher, MD, Curtis W. Hayes, MD, and Wendy R. K. Smoker, MD, over the past several months. They have provided me with invaluable input and assistance regarding manuscript decision category (accept, under consideration, reject), required manuscript revisions, and manuscript processing activities before final manuscript acceptance and subsequent preparation for publication. Unfortunately, one of them, Dr Curtis Hayes, will no longer serve as Deputy Editor as of July 1, 1998. Dr Hayes is joining the Department of Radiology at the University of Michigan, Ann Arbor, as Director of the Division of Musculoskeletal Radiology. No doubt that department will soon recognize its good fortune in having Dr Hayes as a faculty member.

Index terms:
Editorials
Radiology (journal)

Radiology 1998; 208:1

Dr Hayes's insights into musculoskeletal and trauma radiology have proved highly valued assets to me as Editor. I will miss the meticulous approach he exercised during each of the many phases of manuscript review we have implemented in the Richmond, Va, office. As he leaves our *Radiology* Editorial Office and the masthead as a Deputy Editor, we wish him every success during the continuation of his career and the practice of his specialty. We are fortunate that Dr Hayes will remain one of our reviewers.

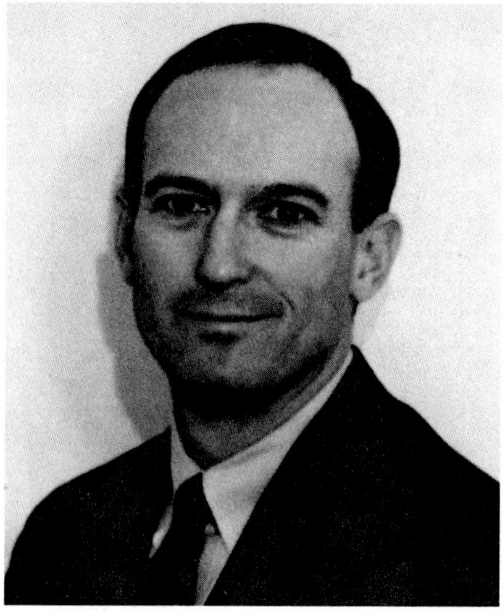

Curtis W. Hayes, MD

Reference

1. Proto AV. New deputy editors. Radiology 1998; 206:3–4.

Michael L. Goris, MD, PhD ▮ H. William Strauss, MD

The Society of Nuclear Medicine

Predictions for Nuclear Medicine in the Next Decade[1]

The difficulty lies not in the new ideas, but in escaping from the old ones, which ramify, for those brought up as most of us have been, into every corner of our minds.

John Maynard Keynes

Where We Come From

Nuclear medicine was born out of the fertile marriage of the tracer principle to the study of pathophysiology. The offspring of this marriage, radionuclide imaging, used advances in physics and electronics to record images of the distribution of physiologic activities such as renal cortical function, integrity of the blood-brain barrier, and the rate and distribution of iron in the bone marrow. Seminal determinations of the body's compartments, pools, and spaces led to evaluation of the distribution of the reticuloendothelial system and its function, evaluation of the distribution of perfusion and air in the lungs, and detection of increased cerebral perfusion associated with brain activation, to name a few of the early measurements that were made with radiopharmaceuticals. Rapid growth in biochemistry and cell physiology provided an impetus to develop commercial radiopharmaceuticals to make clinically important measurements of function. Similar strides were made in instrumentation, with the development of the multihole collimator (1), the application of filtered back projection to depict transverse section tomographic techniques in the early 1960s (2), the application of computers to record and display the distribution of radiopharmaceuticals in 1962 (3), and the genesis of functional imaging (4,5) to depict the change in tracer distribution as a single image.

Now the revolutions in physics, computer sciences, medicinal chemistry, molecular biology, and clinical care have positioned nuclear medicine for the development of new procedures that will enhance its role in patient care. The paradigm of care today is treating the sick. The paradigm of health care of tomorrow is maintaining health. Since health maintenance and early intervention is less expensive in the long run and results in more productive individuals, it is the model to address. The health maintenance approach is not popular in the current environment because people change health care payers frequently enough that the up-front investment does not pay off before the patient leaves the system. In the presence of a single-payer system, or if patients had an inducement to remain with one payer for more than a few years, the paradigm shift would be worthwhile. Coronary revascularization, for example, in a patient who has coronary disease, is, at best, a temporary solution to an inexorable problem. Coronary bypass surgery has a warranty of about 10 years, whereas angioplasty has a warranty of about 5 years (5,7,8). When the warranty expires and the patient manifests recurrent disease, the therapeutic options are limited, often associated with increasing risk, complexity, and cost. It is more logical to address the problem when atheromatous plaque is in its early stages, before the onset of angina or infarction. To this end, imaging needs to evolve procedures that address the status of tissue.

Where We Are Going

Contemplating the scintillating crystal ball of the next decade from the perspective of the twilight of a century of major technologic and biologic revolution, with the assistance of Nostradamus, the future we "see" has the following characteristics.

Instrumentation

First, there will be a major change in collimation. The collimator, a necessary evil for single photon imaging, robs our images of more than 1,000 photons for each photon it allows to reach the detector. Since photons with energies between 50 and 500 keV cannot be focused, photons traveling in inappropriate directions are eliminated by the collimator to create an image. High-energy physicists have known for many years that photons with energies less than 5 keV can be focused with fiberoptic principles. Despite major efforts, the fiberoptic principle has not worked effectively for higher energy photons. In a recent report, Golovchenko and Liu (9) suggest that the problem may be addressable. These investigators used a "grazing principle" with highly polished silicon to focus gamma rays of up to 200 keV. If this principle can be adapted to produce a useful lens, images of current

Index terms:
Radiology and radiologists, research
Radionuclide imaging
Subspecialty society messages

Radiology 1998; 208:3–5

[1] From the Division of Nuclear Medicine, University of California, San Francisco—Stanford Healthcare, 300 Pasteur Dr, Stanford, CA 94062. Received December 8, 1997; accepted February 11, 1998. **Address reprint requests to** M.L.G.

See also the article by Coleman (pp 6–7) in this issue.

quality could be obtained in seconds instead of minutes, or the image count density could be increased by a factor of 1,000 with an accompanying increase of resolution to the range of cycles per millimeter to permit detection of subtle changes in tracer distribution, highlighting changes in pathophysiology at an earlier stage.

Comparable changes are occurring in the area of detector material. For the past 50 years, radionuclide imaging has used sodium iodide as the major scintillator. Sodium iodide is hydroscopic, and although it meets the criteria for high density and good light output, it cannot be readily fabricated to shapes that conform to the contours of the body. An agent with greater density and light output that is not hydroscopic and that is fabricated with solid-state light-detecting material (to replace the current phototubes) will allow the fabrication of thin flexible detectors. Lutetium silicon oxide and yttrium silicon oxide meet these criteria as scintillators (10). These agents have high density, high light output, and fast scintillation times. This combination makes the agents valuable for imaging both 511- and 140-keV photons. Mating these scintillators with folded, square, position-sensitive phototubes permits the design of small, flat detector modules. A modular design will allow multiple parts to be fit together to make nearly any field size desired. Individual parts will be lightweight, minimizing the constraints on the design of detector mounts that plague current instrument designers. An additional bonus is that this detector-collimator design could be built to follow the contours of the body, permitting contact imaging with its enhanced resolution. Contact imaging with a detector that is W-shaped could be particularly useful in the breast, for example, where compression views from medial and lateral perspectives of both breasts could be recorded simultaneously. The thin, large-field-of-view detectors will have only millimeters of dead space around the perimeter, instead of the 2–3 cm typically encountered in today's devices.

Enhancements in computer capability will allow the routine application of iterative reconstruction algorithms. These algorithms will provide higher fidelity data, even in the presence of existing count densities. When this approach is married to a lens-based imaging device with its enhanced count rate, the quality and fidelity of in vivo radionuclide images will approach that of autoradiography.

Radiopharmaceuticals

It has been said that the cell requires about 15–20 minutes to respond to a stimulus with the activation of a genomic switch to code a new protein (11). As molecular biology identifies the key interactions, it is likely that molecular stress tests will be designed to determine if a tissue responds normally to a given stimulus. At our current level of understanding, it is now appreciated that vast changes in the cell, such as neoplasia, require thousands of changes in the genome. Many of these changes are common to multiple types of neoplasms, some of which will be amenable to imaging. One area where this appears to be the case is apoptosis. Programmed cell death is a mechanism employed by cells under a number of circumstances. A few conditions associated with apoptosis are (*a*) cells that are about to undergo division but recognize that they have an incomplete or abnormal compliment of DNA, (*b*) cells under attack by the immune system, (*c*) cells that are exposed to a hypoxic environment on the periphery of an ischemic zone with borderline oxygen concentration to maintain a hostile environment, and (*d*) cells that are infected with certain viral particles. Cancer cells typically downregulate apoptosis, whereas connective tissue disorders upregulate apoptosis. An imaging approach to detect and quantify this condition would offer substantial insights into the cellular status of these diseases and allow a prompt determination of the effectiveness of therapy. Among other changes, cells undergoing apoptosis express phosphatidylserine on their surface, probably as a signaling mechanism. An endogenous human protein, annexin V, binds with high affinity to phosphatidylserine expressed on the outer leaflet of the cell membrane of cells undergoing apoptosis. Blankenberg and colleagues (12) demonstrated the utility of radiolabeled annexin V as a radiopharmaceutical to localize in tissues undergoing apoptosis in vivo.

Two agents are currently in the process of human trials for the localization of venous and arterial clots. These agents both localize at sites of increased expression of the arginine-glycine-aspartate sequence (called the RGD sequence, based on the shorthand for the amino acids recognized by the agents). This sequence is expressed by activated platelets and by tissue undergoing a severe inflammatory response. The agents, DMP 444 (13) from Dupont Merck (Billerica, Mass) and P280 (14) from Diatide (Londonderry, NH) both appear to localize at sites of thrombus in preliminary clinical trials. Comparable advances are being made with the clinical testing of small radiolabeled molecules to detect receptor sites for hormones and neurotransmitters and to localize specific pump mechanisms in tissues.

One of the original dreams of radionuclide imaging was to use the imaging technique in anticipation of therapy. This is now being realized with the use of bone-localizing agents such as strontium-89 for the palliation of intractable bone pain (15). A more elusive goal has been the effective use of radiolabeled antibodies for therapy of tumors. Recent publications from investigators such as Kaminski et al (16), Knox et al (17), and Corcoran et al (18) suggest this approach will work in patients with leukemia and lymphoma. Some patients, even in these preliminary drug trials, have achieved long-term remission of their disease.

Imaging of inflammation will evolve with the development of techniques to specifically label activated populations of white cells in vivo. Laboratory studies have defined the rapid localization of chemotactic peptides at sites of active granulocyte chemotaxis (19). Although it is unclear whether these agents will come to clinical trials because intravenous injection is associated with a mild, transient leukopenia, other peptides have been identified for monocytes (such as monocyte chemotactic peptide 1) and for lymphocytes. As a result, it will be possible to identify specific cell migration in vivo. Other nonspecific approaches to characterizing the degree of inflammation in human tissues including radiolabeled liposomes (20) or radiolabeled immunoglobulin G (21) have also proved effective.

In this article, we have connected current trends in technology with clinical and basic research in biology to define how radionuclide methodology will bring these opportunities to the bedside. In summary, the practice of nuclear medicine in 2008 is likely to use gamma cameras that employ lenses in place of collimators, scintillators that will allow novel modular detector shapes, and computers capable of real-time iterative reconstruction to characterize lesions in anticipation of using the most effective therapy. When possible, imaging procedures will be ordered after genetic testing demonstrates a propensity for an illness.

References

1. Richards P, Atkins HL. A collimator system for scanning at low energies. J Nucl Med 1967; 8:143–153.
2. Kuhl DE. Brain scanning of children using body section techniques and pertechnetate 99m-Tc. Acta Radiol 1966; 5:843–854.
3. Brown DW. The role of the computer in nuclear medicine (abstr). J Nucl Med 1967; 8:376.
4. Kaihara S, Natarajan TK, Maynard CD, Wagner HN Jr. Construction of a functional image from spatially localized rate constants obtained from serial camera and rectilinear scanner data. Radiology 1969; 93:1345–1348.
5. DeRoo MJK, Goris M, Cosemans J, et al. Computerized dynamic scintigraphy of the lungs. J Belge Radiol 1968; 51:339–348.
6. Weintraub WS, Stein B, Kosinski A, et al. Outcome of coronary bypass surgery versus coronary angioplasty in diabetic patients with multivessel coronary artery disease. J Am Coll Cardiol 1998; 31:10–19.
7. Hasdai D, Bell MR, Grill DE, et al. Outcome 10 years after successful percutaneous transluminal coronary angioplasty. Am J Cardiol 1997; 79:1005–1011.
8. Bourassa MG, Wilson JW, Detre KM, Kelsey SF, Robertson T, Passamani ER. Long-term follow-up of coronary angioplasty: the 1977–1981 National Heart, Lung, and Blood Institute registry. Eur Heart J 1989; 10(suppl G):36–41.
9. Golovchenko J, Liu C. Surface trapped x-ray whispering gallery modes at wavelengths of 0.7 A. Phys Rev Lett 1997; 79:788–791.
10. Shao Y, Cherry SR, Farahani K, et al. Simultaneous PET and MR imaging. Phys Med Biol 1997; 42:1965–1970.
11. Lyall F, Deehan MR, Greer IA, Boswell F, Brown WC, McInnes GT. Mechanical stretch increases proto oncogene expression and phosphoinositol turnover in vascular smooth muscle cells. J Hypertens 1994; 12:1139–1145.
12. Blankenberg FG, Katsikis PD, Tait JF, et al. Increased localization of 99m-Tc hydrazino nicatinamide (HYNIC) labeled annexin V lipocortin in lymphatic tissue of animals treated with dexamethasone (abstr). J Nucl Med 1997; 38:268P–289P.
13. Barrett JA, Crocker A, Hemingway S, et al. DMP-444: a technetium-labeled platelet GPIIb-IIIa antagonist for the detection of arterial thrombi. J Nucl Med 1997; 38(suppl 5):18P–19P.
14. Lister-James J, Moyer BR, Dean T. Small peptides radiolabeled with 99mTc. Q J Nucl Med 1996; 40:221–233.
15. Porter AT, McEwan AJB, Powe JE, et al. Results of a randomized phase III trial to evaluate the efficacy of strontium-89 adjuvant to local field external beam irradiation in the management of endocrine resistant metastatic prostate cancer. Int J Radiat Oncol Biol Phys 1993; 25:805–813.
16. Kaminski MS, Zasadny KR, Francis IR, et al. Radioimmunotherapy of B-cell lymphoma with I-131 anti B1 (anti CD20) antibody. N Engl J Med 1993; 329:459–465.
17. Knox SJ, Goris ML, Trisler K. Ninety-Y labeled anti-CD20 monoclonal antibody therapy of recurrent B cell lymphoma. Clin Cancer Res 1996; 2:457–470.
18. Corcoran MC, Fary J, Bernstain I, Press OW. Radioimmunotherapy strategies for non-Hodgkins lymphomas. Ann Oncol 1997; (suppl 1):133–138.
19. Fischman AJ, Babich JW, Barrow SA, et al. Detection of acute bacterial infection within soft tissue injuries using a 99mTc-labeled chemotactic peptide. J Trauma 1995; 38:223–227.
20. Boerman OC, Oyen WJ, van Bloois L, et al. Optimization of technetium-9mm labeled PEG liposomes to image focal infection: effects of particle size and circulation time. J Nucl Med 1997; 38:489–493.
21. Rubin RH, Fischman AJ, Callahan RJ, et al. Indium-111–labeled nonspecific immunoglobulin scanning in the detection of focal infection. N Engl J Med 1989; 321:935–940.

R. Edward Coleman, MD

Commentary

Predictions for Nuclear Medicine in the Next Decade: Commentary[1]

Drs Goris and Strauss have predicted the future of nuclear medicine in the next decade (1). I am in the much more desirable position of being asked to comment on their predictions rather than being asked to do the predicting, although I am permitted to provide predictions of my own. The use of the quote from John Maynard Keynes is particularly appropriate for some of their predictions because they did not let old ideas keep them from making some fantastic predictions for nuclear medicine in the next decade.

In the same format used by Goris and Strauss (1), I will comment on the topics Where We Come From and Where We Are Going from my perspective along with my impression of their perspectives.

Where We Come From

Nuclear medicine is the specialty that uses radionuclides and the tracer technique to diagnose and treat disorders of physiology and/or biochemistry in the human body. The ability to help accurately characterize and quantify normal and abnormal physiologic and biochemical processes is the strength of nuclear medicine. Nuclear medicine has made major advances since the use of iodine-131 sodium iodide for determining thyroid function to the use of receptor and metabolic imaging for characterizing masses and staging malignancy, techniques that are available to every nuclear medicine practitioner today. The tracer technique permits detection of administered radiolabeled agents at the picomolar level, whereas computed tomography (CT) and magnetic resonance (MR) imaging are able to depict changes in attenuation or signal intensity, respectively, from administered agents at the micromolar and millimolar levels (2). Thus, the radionuclide techniques provide opportunities to probe disorders of biochemistry that are not available to CT or MR imaging. MR spectroscopy provides biochemical information on steady-state processes, and the information from MR spectroscopy has not replaced the kinetic and metabolic information from nuclear medicine techniques.

The combination of anatomic information from high-resolution CT or MR imaging and the metabolic information from nuclear medicine provides unique information that is important from both a diagnostic and a therapeutic standpoint. Imaging of glucose metabolism by using 2-[fluorine-18]fluoro-2-deoxy-D-glucose (FDG) and positron emission tomography (PET) has become a routine procedure in institutions with PET scanners for several indications, including the characterization of brain tumors and lung nodules and the staging of lung cancer. Image registration permits the accurate characterization of the metabolic status of an anatomic lesion. The metabolic information permits the determination of whether tumor is present in the anatomic lesion, and the metabolic extent of tumor can be used by the radiotherapist in treatment planning.

The devices used for imaging the distribution of single photon–emitting and positron-emitting radiopharmaceuticals provide important diagnostic information. Gamma cameras with 3/8-inch-thick sodium iodide crystals are used to perform planar and single photon emission CT (SPECT) imaging. Dedicated PET scanners typically used bismuth germinate block detectors. An alternative to the bismuth germinate block detection design is the use of large-area, 1-inch-thick sodium iodide crystals in a hexagonal array. More recently, every manufacturer of gamma cameras is offering coincidence detection for their two-head or three-head systems for imaging with FDG (3). These systems are able to produce diagnostic quality images of FDG uptake, and the quality of images is improving rapidly because of changes in both hardware and software (2). The use of the new iterative reconstruction algorithms is particularly promising for making major improvements in image quality. The availability of FDG commercially and the use of camera-based PET make these studies of glucose metabolism available to most departments performing nuclear medicine imaging.

Where We Are Going

Imaging instrumentation will improve. I like the concept of the use of a lens for focusing gamma rays instead of the use of collimators (1), but I doubt this technique will be available in the next decade. We are seeing the development of solid-state detectors and proposals for dedicated systems to image specific regions, such as the breast, and these systems will be evaluated for use during the next decade. I am also optimistic about the use of the new rare-earth oxyorthosilicates, lutetium oxyorthosilicate and yttrium oxyorthosilicate, for imaging both positron- and single photon–emitting radionuclides. Furthermore, instruments that

Index terms:
Radiology and radiologists, research
Radionuclide imaging
Subspecialty society messages

Radiology 1998; 208:6–7

[1] From the Department of Radiology, Duke University Medical Center, Box 3949, Durham, NC 27710. Received January 9, 1998; accepted February 11. **Address reprint requests to** the author.

Research grant and consulting, Elgems and Elscint; Stockholder, PETNet Pharmaceuticals.

See also the article by Goris and Strauss (pp 3–5) in this issue.

combine SPECT and/or PET with CT will become available. This new and improved instrumentation will be used to image the biochemical reactions that occur normally and abnormally in our bodies. Molecular biology is providing the framework on which tracers can be developed to probe abnormalities in the genome that result in disease. Much of the initial research will be in oncology (4), but the techniques will be applicable to other disorders resulting from the genetic structure. Studies have demonstrated the ability to quantify different levels of marker gene expression in tumor-bearing animals with use of PET imaging (5). The results of these studies suggest that the technique could be used to monitor the delivery and expression of therapeutic genes in target tissues.

As discussed by Goris and Strauss (1), peptides will play an important role in imaging various disease states. I am less optimistic about the use of systemically administered radiolabeled antibodies for diagnostic and therapeutic purposes. Perhaps the use of fragments or the use of the avidin-biotin system will make their use feasible. For a therapeutic purpose, the direct administration of radionuclide therapy into the tumor will be used for localized malignancy. Preliminary results with use of I-131–labeled monoclonal antibodies administered into postoperative cystic cavities of patients with malignant primary brain tumors have been encouraging (6).

During the next decade, we will see an increase in the use of PET imaging combined with molecular biologic techniques to characterize disease processes. The techniques will permit the early evaluation of therapy for these disorders. We will see more emphasis placed on registering the biochemical information from nuclear medicine with the anatomic information from CT and MR imaging.

References

1. Goris M, Strauss HW. Predictions for nuclear medicine in the next decade. Radiology 1998; 208:3–5.
2. Eckelman WC. The development of 99mTc radiopharmaceuticals for perfusion and biochemistry. In: Nicolini M, Bandoli G, Mazzi V, eds. Technetium and rhenium in chemistry and nuclear medicine. 3rd ed. Verona, Italy: Cortina International, 1990; 571–580.
3. Coleman RE. Camera-based PET: the best is yet to come. J Nucl Med 1997; 38:1796–1797.
4. Britton KE. Towards the goal of cancer-specific imaging and therapy. Nucl Med Comm 1997; 18:992–1007.
5 Tjuvajev J, Avril N, Safer M, et al. Quantitative PET imaging of HSV1-tk gene expression with [I-124]-FIAU (abstr). J Nucl Med 1997; 5:239.
6. Bigner DD, Brown MT, Friedman AH, et al. Iodine-131 labeled antitenascin monoclonal antibody 81C6 treatment of patients with recurrent brain tumors: phase I trials. J Clin Oncol (in press).

A True Dinner-Fork Deformity of the Wrist?

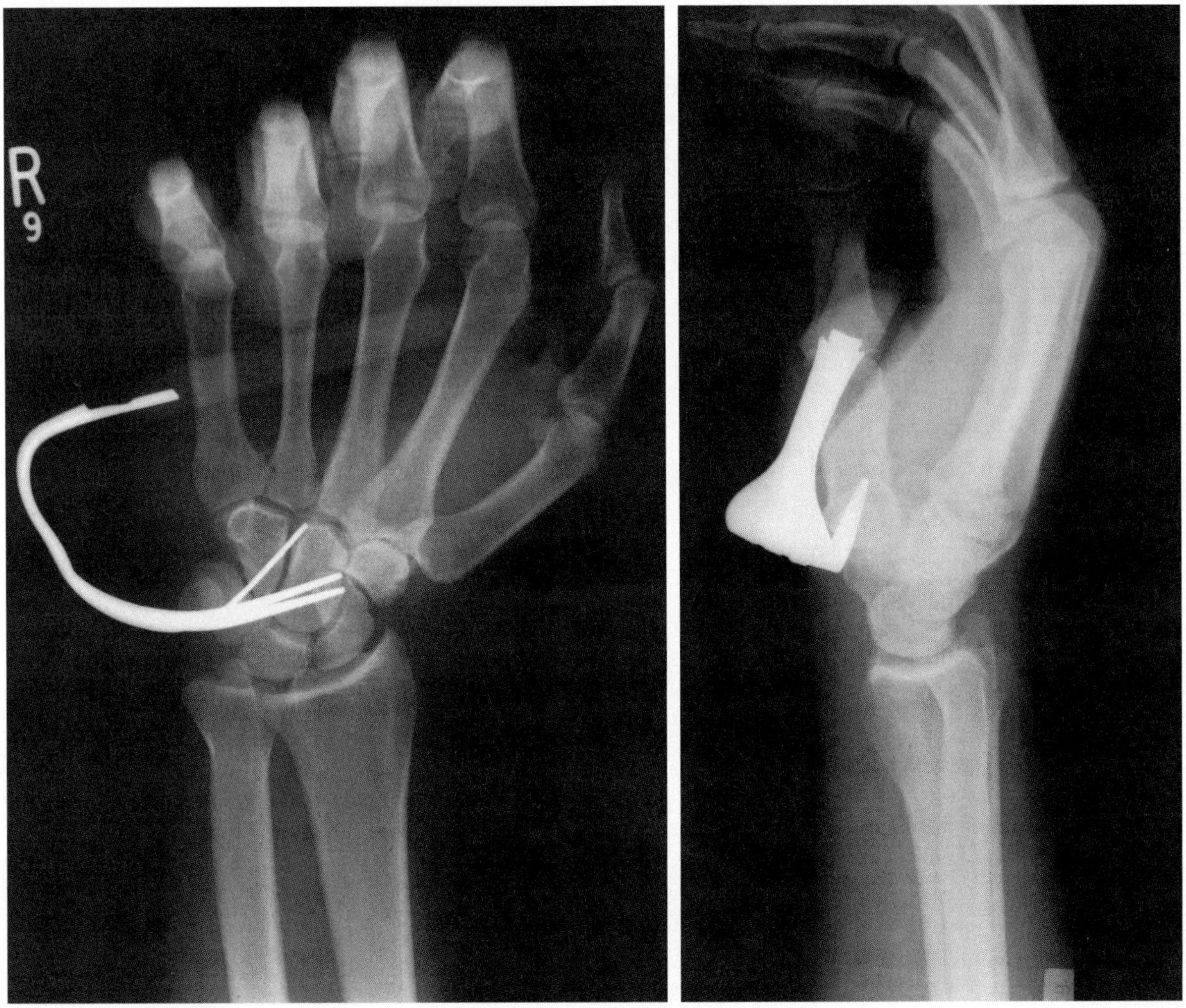

A somewhat unusual way of obtaining a dinner-fork deformity of the wrist, although not by means of a Colles fracture. So, don't persist with heated dinner table conversation!

Courtesy of Ioannis G. Kolovos, MB, ChB, MMed, Southall, England

Stanley S. Siegelman, MD

Index term:
Radiology and radiologists, history

Radiology 1998; 208:9–16

[1] From the Russell H. Morgan Department of Radiology and Radiological Science, the Johns Hopkins Medical Institutions, 600 N Wolfe St, Baltimore, MD 21287. Received December 30, 1997; revision requested February 4, 1998; revision received February 27; accepted March 2. **Address reprint requests to** the author.

The Genesis of Modern Science: Contributions of Scientific Societies and Scientific Journals[1]

Let us go then, you and I,
When the evening is spread out against the sky
Like a patient etherized upon a table
—T. S. Eliot, *The Love Song of Alfred Prufrock*

ARISTOTLE, THE MIDDLE AGES

The opening lines of T.S. Eliot's poem, with a striking image of a flattened sky, evoke the cosmology of Aristotle. Aristotle (384–322 BC), whose nickname was "The Genius," dealt with every aspect of human experience in his lectures and writings on logic, rhetoric, music, poetry, ethics, economics, politics, physics, metaphysics, anatomy, natural history, physiology, and astronomy (1). Aristotle saw the universe as a series of concentric transparent spheres that revolved about the earth. The stars were presumed to be situated on a single sphere that circled the earth every 24 hours. The system implied only modest astronomic distances. Observatories were placed in tall towers in an attempt to get considerably closer to the objects regularly viewed in the night sky (1). In the 13th century, Thomas Aquinas incorporated Aristotle's cosmology into the teachings of the Catholic Church. Throughout the Middle Ages, scholars were quite comfortable with the legacy of the Greek philosophers; indeed, ancient conclusions were accepted with reverence. Even though vigorous discussions and debates abounded, all probing thinking presumed that the Church, and what it had embraced from the ancient Greeks, was a final, definitive authority.

THE RENAISSANCE, ANTI-ARISTOTELIAN THINKING, GALILEO

During the Renaissance, Aristotle's theories were challenged. Galileo (1564–1642), a key figure in the emergence of modern science, was born to a distinguished but impoverished Italian family (2,3). His father, Vicenzio, a mathematician and musician, was outraged by the rigidity of the rules for musical composition drawn from the teachings of Aristotle. Vicenzio had discovered, by using instruments with greater range, that he could fashion more esthetically pleasing works by avoiding arbitrary classical restrictions. Again and again he cautioned his son to think for himself, to avoid blind acceptance of authority, and to make judgments only after tests and observations. Deeply affected by his father's admonitions, Galileo devoted his life to observation and experimentation. He did not hesitate to question and to doubt traditional conclusions supported by the weight of ancient authority but not verifiable by experimentation. His schoolmates called him "The Wrangler" (2,3).

Galileo was interested in motion and in the force of attraction between objects. In his early years, he conducted experiments that showed Aristotle had been wrong when he held that different objects composed of the same material would fall at different rates in direct proportion to their weight. Galileo established himself as a scientific genius when he correctly inferred that the motion of weights swinging on a string and of balls descending an inclined plane were completely analogous to objects falling in space (4). Galileo showed that the rate of fall was independent of weight. In 1632, he formulated a mathematic formula to describe the acceleration and the rate of descent of falling bodies (5). Aristotle had maintained that rest was the natural state and that moving objects tended to come to rest. Galileo disagreed. By reducing friction, he demonstrated that objects in motion tended to remain in motion unless an external force was applied. (This concept was later developed as Newton's first law.)

Galileo was particularly adept at designing scientific devices and fashioning equipment for experiments. He invented the thermometer. At age 45 years (1609), Galileo learned that the telescope had been developed by lens makers in Holland. He immediately grasped the concept of its operation and constructed an increasingly sophisticated series of such instruments. Galileo began to view the night sky, and his observations led to an explosion of astronomic knowledge (1). Galileo is widely viewed as the most seminal figure of his time. Indeed, Einstein has said, "Pure logical thinking cannot yield us any knowledge of the empirical world; all knowledge of reality starts from experience and ends in it....Because Galileo saw this, and particularly because he drummed it into the scientific world, he is the father of modern physics—indeed, of modern science altogether" (1).

FRANCIS BACON

Francis Bacon (1561–1626), born 3 years earlier than Galileo, was also a seminal figure in the genesis of modern science. He was the son of Sir Nicholas Bacon, lord keeper of the great seal, and a popular and influential insider in the court of Queen Elizabeth (6). Intellectually precocious, he attended Cambridge and graduated at age 15 years. After training as a barrister, he spent his life in the practice of law, heavily involved with duties on behalf of the monarchy (7). He was knighted (1603), appointed Lord Chancellor (1618), Baron Verulam (1618), and Viscount St Albans (1621). Bacon had a talent for writing with style and grace. His books on history, law, morals, and philosophy were widely circulated and extremely influential. It has even been suggested that Bacon was the actual author of Shakespeare's plays.

Although he was not a scientist, Bacon's writings had a profound influence throughout Europe during the Renaissance. Bacon's philosophy consisted of a number of recurring themes (6,7).

Emphasis on the Practical

Bacon, dating from his studies at Cambridge, was disappointed in the paucity of practical applications of the philosophy of Aristotle. Societies that espoused Aristotle, hobbled by a suffusion of speculative information, did nothing to exploit the potentially rich resources of nature. Bacon was excited by items such as printing, gunpowder, and the compass, which offered a means for mastering nature to improve the quality of human life. In Bacon's view, society was misguided in consuming too much of its intellectual vigor with theology and philosophy. He urged a turning toward more practical matters. The effecting of this important change in focus has led many to consider Bacon as the spiritual father of the Industrial Revolution (7).

Inductive Rather than Deductive Reasoning

Aristotle's analytic approach began with a series of postulates: presumptions assumed to be valid based on faith but not verified by observation or investigation. He then built an orderly system based on deductions from the postulates. Bacon advised a fresh start to build a new system of knowledge without assumptions. Groups of men, called natural philosophers, would make original observations of natural phenomena. Where reproducible findings were obtained, theories would be developed (hypotheses) to explain the observations. Finally, the hypotheses would be tested by further experimentation to obtain final verification. A book outlining the new logic (*Novum Organum*) appeared in 1620 (8). Thus, Bacon preferred an inductive as opposed to a deductive approach. "If a man will begin with certainties, he shall end in doubts; but if he will consent to begin with doubts, he shall end in certainties" (8).

"Communism"

The discovery of scientific truth was to be a dynamic process requiring the efforts and combined skills of many investigators. Bacon wrote that progress could best be achieved by the cooperative efforts of groups who communicated freely with one another. Mastery over nature would come only by this sharing of experiences, a phenomenon that he called "communism."

Bacon described an ideal research institution that he called Solomon's House (9,10). It would consist of a team of natural philosophers with varying expertise and assignments. (*a*) Merchants of Light would determine the focus of investigation in academies and research institutions around the world. (*b*) Mystery Men would be responsible for reviewing the literature to summarize the previously published information. (*c*) Dowry Men or Benefactors would be charged with obtaining the funds needed to support ongoing research and development. (*d*) Inoculators were the laboratory technicians who specialized in the actual performance of experiments. (*e*) Compilers would study the data to see if one could draw inferences from the results. (*f*) Lamps would plan additional experiments of a more penetrating nature (of a higher light) to gain additional insights. (*g*) Interpreters of nature were the theorists who would analyze the data and develop axioms or mathematic formulas to characterize the basic principles uncovered.

The regular personnel of the institution would be augmented by novices, apprentices, and advanced students who would obtain additional training while assisting with the ongoing programs.

It is amazing that this analysis by Bacon, the nonscientist, which resonates with the actual operation of a modern laboratory, was written 375 years ago! (*Solomon's House*, a section in the *New Atlantis*, was published in 1626 after Bacon's demise; the material was actually written several years earlier.)

SCIENTIFIC SOCIETIES

Scientific societies flourished in a golden period during the 17th century. Educated men, anxious to participate in the awakening of interest in natural phenomena, willingly devoted their time and energy to the enterprise. The movement began in Italy, which had 171 academies, and spread to England, France, and Germany (4,11). Although the societies varied widely in conception and function, it is possible to characterize them with some general principles. (*a*) Societies were extremely popular because they were fashionable. Attendance often bestowed a social éclat. They offered an opportunity to regularly gather with the intellectually and socially elite, and even to rub elbows with nobility. Chique names such as "the Pensive," "the Intrepid," and "the Fiery" were chosen (4). Attendance was frequently limited to those with documented intellectual achievement, a factor that augmented desire for membership. (*b*) The scope and the mission of groups varied greatly; many were simply weekly discussion clubs that carried out no original investigation. The most ambitious enterprises were located in the largest cities. (*c*) To be productive, a society needed a patron, generally a wealthy nobleman who sponsored the operation and provided space for the meetings and funds for acquiring scientific instruments and conducting experiments. Such patrons were proud to be considered "natural philosophers," and often they actively participated in the proceedings. Even with large, ambitious, successful societies, death or departure of the sponsor invariably resulted in cessation of activities. (*d*) Organizers of scientific assemblies were invariably au courant with the writings of Francis Bacon and completely in concert with his grand philosophy. Thus, secretaries were appointed to record the results of experiments and the substance of discussions. Such information was shared through regular correspondence with other societies. Although many of the most active participants in the society held university appointments, the universities as institutions did nothing to support the new science. However, the Pan-European network of communicating scholars and investigators constituted what was frequently referred to as "an invisible college" (12). (*e*) Societies were in peril unless they managed to deal with the powerful, omnipresent officials of the church. This was especially true in Italy. Giambattista della Porta (1538–1615) presided over an academy that met at his home in Naples. The Academia Secretorum Naturae experimented with magnetism and a primitive steam engine. The academy was shut down by ecclesiastical authorities because members were accused of delving into the occult (5). Most societies excluded the clergy from membership. The Italian academies were barely tolerated. Their minutes were diligently monitored for activities or speculations that might be considered heresy. Accordingly, Italian investigators focused on scientific instrumentation and objective reporting of observations. They had to be extremely circumspect and thus were restrained from analyzing the implications of their work. (*f*) The goals of the 17th century societies were to examine and to discuss the phenomena of nature. The most popular topics were heat, light, weight, motion, magnetism, the behavior of gases, tides, metallurgy, optics, astronomy, and physiology.

INITIAL SCIENTIFIC SOCIETIES: ITALY

The initial serious, successful scientific societies were in Italy. The Academia del Lincei (Academy of the Lynx) was organized in Rome by Duke Federigo Cesi in 1601 (4). In an abortive start, the society was censured for heretic practices and disbanded. After reorganization on a grander scale, activities resumed in 1609 and continued until the death of the duke in 1620. The membership focused on studies of plants and animals. Galileo, a corresponding member, crafted a microscope for the society. The proceedings of the society were recorded as *Gesta Lynceorum*, which in 1609 constituted the initial formal recordings of a Renaissance society. The academy published two of Galileo's early astronomic works.

The Academia del Cimento (Academy of Experimentation) in Florence from 1657 to 1667 was a first-rate scientific academy with nine scientists. The patron was Prince Leopold Medici, brother of Grand Duke Ferdinand II. Leopold financed the operation and actively participated in the biologic and chemical investigations. Galileo was the spiritual inspiration since the principal investigators were his disciples Viviani and Torricelli. The group possessed mathematic knowledge and technical experimental skills. Areas of investigation included the effects of heat and cold, the effects of a vacuum, and the development of thermometers, hygrometers, and other scientific instruments. The published proceedings of the academy, containing descriptions of laboratory procedures and experimental techniques, were translated from Italian into English, French, and German and became the standard laboratory manual for subsequent groups of investigators (4). Leopold became a cardinal in 1667, and the academy was disbanded.

THE ROYAL SOCIETY OF LONDON

The most successful of the 17th century societies was the Royal Society of London. Every conceivable aspect of its antecedents, organization, and operation has been documented and preserved (4,5,11–14). Like many of the current radiologic societies (eg, the Society of Cardiovascular and Interventional Radiology, the International Skeletal Society), before its official establishment the Royal Society began as a small club of individuals with shared interests. It met weekly in London beginning in 1645 (13). The group included John Wallis, a mathematician (widely regarded as the greatest English mathematician before Newton); John Wilkins, a mathematician and astronomer; and several physicians with special interests in chemistry, pharmacology, physiology, and botany (4,13). In 1648, the weekly meetings of the club were moved to Oxford where John Wallis had become Savilian professor of mathematics and Wilkins had received an appointment as warden of Wadham College.

The newly constituted Philosophical Society of Oxford quickly attracted additional active members including Robert Boyle, son of one the wealthiest men in Ireland, the Earl of Cork. Boyle, a prototypic gentleman–amateur scientist could live quite comfortably without concern for employment. His scientific talent and financial resources were an important asset. Boyle set up an experimental laboratory, and numerous investigations were conducted by the members of the society.

In 1658, London again became the central focus of activity. In his will, Sir Thomas Gresham established a college in his spacious mansion. The faculty consisted of seven professors who lectured daily to the public on astronomy, geometry, physics, law, divinity, music, and rhetoric. Christopher Wren, professor of astronomy, and Lawrence Rooke, professor of geometry, had been active members of the Oxford Society before moving to London. The reconstituted group began meeting regularly at Gresham College, and in 1660 the Royal Society was organized. From 1649 to 1660, the monarchy had been dissolved, but in 1660 the restoration brought Charles II back to the throne. In 1662, the society was granted an official king's charter.

The Royal Society was an immediate success. Initially the society had two salaried employees: The first was Robert Hooke (1635–1702) who was appointed curator of experiments. Hooke had special mechanical skills. After training at Oxford in mathematics, astronomy, and chemistry, he had been engaged by Boyle to prepare equipment and carry out studies for the Oxford Society. Hooke's assignment was to prepare three or four experiments and demonstrations for the weekly meetings. He obtained various available scientific instruments; many he modified, others he designed and built on his own. His armamentarium included a mechanical pump for compressing and rarifying air used to produce a vacuum, an effective compound microscope that was employed in weekly demonstrations on plants and animals, instruments for keeping time, several telescopes, and a variety of meteorologic instruments (4,11). Henry Oldenberg, a scholar and diplomat, fluent in Latin, English, French, Italian, and German, was hired as secretary. Oldenberg, a native of Bremen, with a classical education, had been dispatched as an emissary to negotiate with the English government on ongoing maritime conflicts. He had then remained as a tutor at Oxford where he met and was befriended by Boyle. Oldenberg prepared the minutes of the weekly meeting and corresponded with scientific groups throughout Europe.

Success was definitely multifactorial, but three items appear to have had the most critical impact: (*a*) Educated English gentlemen were eager to follow Francis Bacon's admonition to pursue natural philosophy. (*b*) Wisely, religion and politics were excluded from all discussions. (*c*) There was a liberal membership policy.

MEMBERSHIP POLICY

Fortuitously, the Royal Society initiated a membership policy that differed from the prototypic approach of other institutions: Anyone was eligible for membership. The approach was not based on egalitarian principles but rather on financial necessity since no rich patron was available. The king was extremely enthusiastic, but the Royal coffers were bare, drained by the expenses of fighting a long civil war. An important paradigm for future societies was established: The dues and initiation fees of a large membership could serve as a substitute for the largesse of a noble patron. The fees for new members were 20 shillings for commoners and five pounds for peers (one pound was 24 shillings). Thereafter, the dues were one shilling per week (14). There were 96 founding fellows. Hunter has analyzed the composition of the 479 British members from 1660 through 1699. Physicians were the largest group (16%). Other fellows included courtiers and politicians (16%), gentlemen of independent means (15%), aristocrats (14%), scholars and writers (12%), divines (8%), merchants and tradesmen (7%), lawyers (4%), civil servants (4%), and all other unclassified individuals (1%). In addition, 72 foreign fellows were elected (14).

The Royal Society was spared difficulties with ecclesiastical authorities, which plagued so many of its European counterparts. After all, the bishops of the most important dioceses in the country were active members, as was the Archbishop of Canterbury. Church authorities relaxed with the knowledge that prudent eyes and ears were monitoring the weekly activities. Educated clergymen were proud to be enlisted as natural philosophers. Included in the philosophy of Francis Bacon, spiritual father of this society, was the concept that an understanding of nature would reveal "the footprints of the Creator imprinted on its creatures" (6). Thus, he contended that the pursuit of natural philosophy was a religious duty.

The Royal Society from its inception served a social function. Merchants, physicians, aristocrats, and landed gentlemen would dine together before the meetings or gather over coffee after the sessions to network and to socialize with the scientists. In this sense, the society was criticized by some as a mere gentlemen's club. However, there was always a corps of dedicated investigators led by Boyle, Hooke, Wren, and Wallis who carried out serious science each week. The informal fraternizing by the serious members yielded many benefits. The coffeehouse discussions often included an issuance of friendly challenges. Isaac Newton was encouraged, and even prodded, to attend regularly after he devised and demonstrated a reflecting telescope to the group. Newton was stimulated and encouraged by members Wren, Halley, and Hooke. For some, the opportunities for social interaction were the most valuable aspect of society activities.

The French Academie des Sciences in Paris was a 17th century society that could claim parity with the Royal Society of London. Again, the genesis of the society began with more than a decade of clublike weekly informal gatherings at the homes of leading scientists (4,15). France had a number of talented mathematicians, including Paul Fermat, Blaise Pascal, and Pierre Gassendi. Christian Huygens (1629–1695) was Dutch, but he lived in France for many years. Huygens, a mathematician, astronomer, and designer of scientific instruments, provided an opportunity to conduct studies with his air pump and telescope. The Academie des Sciences was formally organized in 1666 under the sponsorship of King Louis XIV. Unlike the English monarch, Louis XIV was at his prime and was able to provide sumptuous laboratory space and equipment and stipends for full-time scientific investigators. (The inaugural meeting was held in his private library.) The society also financed astronomic observatories, data-gathering expeditions, and translators. The early activities of the Paris Academy included perfection of the telescope, dissections of human cadavers, blood transfusions between dogs, calculations on the velocity of light, and studies of the properties of phosphorous (5).

SCIENTIFIC JOURNALS, 333rd ANNIVERSARY

The first two scientific journals originated 333 years ago in 1665.

Journal des Scavans

The *Journal des Scavans* appeared in Paris in January 1665. The impetus for the innovative, learned periodical was the first editor, Denis de Sallo, a counselor of the French court of parliament. de Sallo, an energetic, scholarly gentleman, with diverse interests, wanted a regular compendium of contemporary intellectual activity (16,17). The journal was like a *Reader's Digest* for cultured men with interests in natural science, affairs of state, trade, law, and theology. The first 20-page issue contained 10 articles plus several letters and notes. It dealt with reviews of books published in Europe, current events, decisions of civil and religious courts, plus results of experiments in physics, chemistry, and anatomy from the group of Parisian scientists about to formally initiate the French Academie des Sciences (16,17). The journal was published weekly. Officials of the court of King Louis XIV were displeased with several political and theologic items in the early issues, and after 4 months, permission for publication was withdrawn. The journal reappeared, however, in 1666 with a new editor. It contained frequent contributions from the French Academie. Publication with scholarly book reviews and literary materials admixed with scientific reports continued until 1816 when it became the *Journal des Savants*, a purely literary periodical.

Philosophical Transactions of the Royal Society

In March 1665, the second scientific journal, the *Philosophical Transactions of the Royal Society*, was published in London. Legal and theologic matters were excluded. The project was spurred by the first editor, Henry Oldenburg, secretary of the Royal Society (5,16,17). In his role as secretary, Oldenburg communicated extensively with a host of scientists who were keenly interested in learning of the activities of the Royal Society. He regularly corresponded with over 30 individuals in England and Europe. An official collection of Oldenburg's correspondence fills 28 volumes. In 1664, a committee was appointed to assist with the arduous task of selecting, preparing, and distributing the materials and responding to the correspondence. Eventually Oldenburg decided that Bacon's admonition for sharing of knowledge by various groups of natural philosophers would be greatly facilitated by regular issuance of a scientific journal.

Although the Royal Society officially approved of the publication of the *Transactions*, it was unwilling to serve as formal sponsor or to bear any financial responsibility for the venture. Oldenburg was forced reluctantly into an entrepreneurial role; receipts from subscriptions would likely exceed expenses, but no income was guaranteed. As financier of the operation, Oldenburg had almost no success. The inaugural year of publication, 1665, was notably inauspicious because London was beset with an epidemic of plague. Members of the society dispersed to the countryside, and so meetings were curtailed. Initial subscriptions were disappointing, but Oldenburg hoped to recoup with sales of back issues (for which there was eventually some demand). Unfortunately, all reserve copies were destroyed by the great fire of London in 1666. As a final blow to Oldenburg, he was suspected of being a spy because of his extensive multilingual correspondence. (England had been at war with Holland.) He was imprisoned in the Tower of London for 3 months in 1667 until his influential friends secured his release. One of Oldenburg's successors as editor, Robert Peele, agreed to assume the position only after the society agreed to purchase 60 subscriptions. *Transactions* eventually became an official society-sponsored publication in 1753.

The first issue, which appeared in March 1665, consisted of 16 pages containing nine articles and extracts of Oldenburg's foreign correspondence. The contents included a manuscript from Rome dealing with improvement in opera glasses, observations on details of the planet Jupiter from Britain, descriptions of lead ore from Germany, and a paper from America dealing with the motion of whales. (Oldenburg corresponded regularly with Governor Winthrop of Connecticut [17].)

OVERVIEW OF SCIENTIFIC JOURNALS

The scholarly journals made many contributions to the genesis of modern science.

Fostering of Communication

A strong desire to communicate with fellow scientists has been and continues to be a considerable force in the scientific world. Researchers want to monitor the landscape in their areas of interest to ensure that their investigations are properly focused in the issues of greatest moment. Knowledge that their competitors are pursuing a pressing question imparts a sense of urgency. They also derive a deep sense of fulfillment when they can convey word of their successful efforts to respected colleagues.

In Europe, an extensive system of communication was already in place. Guttenburg's invention of movable type in the middle of the 15th century had been a key factor in producing greater enlightenment. By the end of the 16th century, there were over 10 million copies of 50,000 books in print (18). Booklets, pamphlets, and broadsides abounded. Natural philosophers communicated by means of scientific letters, generally written in Latin (19,20). In Oldenburg's view, the new scientific journals were simply a practical means of distributing multiple detailed "erudite letters."

The items published in the new journals were much shorter than the communications offered in a book. Harvey's book on the circulation of blood, which appeared in 1628, had 72 pages. As previously noted, individual issues of journals usually consisted of fewer than 20 pages. Thus, it became possible to communicate bits of information. Brief snippets, inadequate for a book, often proved valuable particularly when combined with complementary matter from other sources (20). A seminal fragment, by serving as a small piece in a jigsaw puzzle, could help to achieve a corporate collective power (21).

Replacing Secrecy with Public Disclosure

Before the emergence of scientific journals, a rather standard practice in the 17th century had been to announce a scientific discovery with a cryptogram or cipher: an encoded message. The purpose was to establish priority but to maintain an advantage by withholding useful information from competitors (17,18). Acceptance by scientific journals required public disclosure.

SECRETS IN THE SKY

The annoying practice of announcing important discoveries without disclosing useful information was especially prevalent among astronomers. Galileo, Tycho Brahe (1546–1601), and Johannes Kepler (1571–1630) corresponded by letter. Galileo had written initially to discuss his sympathy with the work of Copernicus. When Kepler determined that the orbits of each of the planets passed through the sun, he reported the information with an unintelligible Latin cryptogram. Galileo was no less forthcoming when he discovered the phases of Venus (powerful evidence that Venus rotated around the sun). Similarly other observations by Galileo, including the rings of Saturn and the moons of Jupiter, were initially presented in code. Public disclosure came months to years later with the publication of their books. Tycho Brahe, the greatest observational astronomer of the 16th century, was convinced by his colleagues that the planets revolved about the sun. However, he conceived a system in which the sun with the orbiting planets all rotated around the earth. Tycho Brahe reasoned correctly that if the earth were circling the sun the stars should appear to be moving in the opposite direction (1). The stars did not appear to move. Hence, either the earth was not orbiting the sun or the stars were so far away that their minute shifts could not be detected. Of course, the latter was true, but stellar parallax could not be accurately measured until the 19th century (22).

Tycho Brahe could not fathom a system in which the stars were thousands of times more distant than the outer planet Jupiter. Such a void, he reasoned, "would be a tremendous sign of wastefulness on the part of the Creator" (23).

The emergence of scientific journals led to an eventual discarding of coded communications. To gain the advantage conferred by publication, authors had to clearly disclose the nature of their observations.

Transforming "Printing" into "Publication": Peer Review

Inclusion of one's work in a scientific journal offered an advantage over having the material appear as a monograph.

"Printing was transformed into publication" (24). Editors were quite aware that the act of publication legitimized a selection by conferring the imprimatur of the sponsoring society (24,25). They also realized that official approval of a dubious paper could compromise the reputation of the society. Thus, the Royal Society had a system whereby submissions of papers presented at sessions of the society were referred by the editor for review and criticism by qualified referees. Material was published only if it was judged to be worthy and, hence, endorsed by the editor and referees. The French Academie had similar policies. Academy members acquired the habit of placing "academician" after their name in published papers and books. A rule was instituted to prevent use of the term unless the material had been reviewed and approved by an official committee. Despite assurances that all papers had passed muster, readers were quick to write critical letters to protest publication of questionable material (24). Seventeenth century peer review was a general success; scientists welcomed competent assessment of their efforts. Referees, on occasion, would advise that a manuscript appeared logical and reasonable, but they were unable to actually verify the work. In these instances, the editor published the paper with the inscription "Sit penes authorum fides" (let the author take responsibility for it) (24).

Establishing Priority

Articles in current scientific journals list the date of submission of the manuscript and the date of acceptance. This practice, initiated in the 17th century, established priority. Before the emergence of journals, quarrels over the issue of priority were a growing impediment to communication among investigators. Codiscovery of new information is an extremely common phenomenon. Independent investigators pursuing similar lines of inquiry observed the same phenomena, or designed similar experiments, or reached the same conclusions. This led to anger, to shouts of philosophical robbery, and often to a cessation of communication between scientists in the same field. Hooke in London and Huygens in Paris each developed a balancing spring for watches, and there were multiple conflicting claims for priority in the matter of blood transfusions in animals.

Merton studied the issue and documented an unusually high prevalence of codiscovery (10). An analogy has been made to apples growing on a tree. They do not drop to the ground randomly. Rather, ripening after a period of growth, two or three apples falling within a very short period is the rule rather than the exception (18). Original scientific insight that produces a major advance is always based on the foundation of prior knowledge and observation. The principle that all advances, including apparent revolutionary disclosures, are invariably based on a foundation of earlier publications is often called "the Ortega Hypothesis" (20,26). Many contend that with very rare exceptions, pivotal scientific evidences would have come to light eventually even without the contribution of the famous lead scientists responsible for their discovery. A sense of urgency with a need to report results rapidly propels those who recognize the steady progression of science. Happily, the need to claim priority usually results in prompt publication of seminal work.

Credit for a scientific advance is accorded to a single individual or a small group of individuals. This was not always the case. Bacon had stressed that progress would come from efforts of a network of communicating teams of scientists. This proved to be true to a large extent, but Bacon underestimated the importance of the creative act of discovery, which was often the product of a single mind (15). In the *Proceedings of the Academy de Cimento*, collective findings were presented without the listing of individual contributors. Initially, the French Academie under Baconian influence favored anonymous publication. Most of the reports from Paris from 1667 to 1692 excluded or minimized credit for individual scientists. Before the 17th century ended, however, it became apparent that the most important ingredient of discovery is personal and that proud men responsible for creative acts require specific recognition (15).

Journals were perceived as having real value and as fulfilling important needs; thus, they received strong support from the scientific community. Scientific investigators need intellectual property. To be successful, they must obtain financial support to provide sufficient leisure for sustained work. In the 17th century, sponsorships came to those who had received official recognition of their work and particularly to those with certification of priority. This phenomenon remains true today. The supporting agencies are universities, national institutes, and industry rather than kings and princes, but funding is most readily available to those with documented priority for original work. Journals can function efficiently because of an effective system of quid pro quo. Investigators are willing to devote many hours to provide constructive criticism in reviews of their colleagues' manuscripts because they know that they will receive similar assistance with their own submissions (27).

ISAAC NEWTON

Isaac Newton (1642–1727) was a key figure in 17th century science. During his lengthy career, he had several notable and illuminating interactions with scientific societies and scientific journals. Newton, a brilliant student, trained in mathematics at Cambridge. The outbreak of the plague in London in 1665 sent him home to the countryside for an 18-month period in which he discovered important properties of light, developed calculus, and formed his earliest thoughts about the nature of gravity (1,6,28).

On returning to Cambridge, he was given the tenured, supported position of Lucasian Professor of Mathematics when Isaac Barrow (the initial Lucasian professor) resigned in his favor. Accounts of the transfer are vague. If Barrow relinquished the position because he had recognized Newton's talents and wished to advance the career of his former pupil, his resignation would stand as a great act of mentorship (28). His motives are uncertain, however, because he assumed a more lucrative position as royal chaplain. Newton occupied the chair in mathematics for 33 years. Stephen Hawking is the current Lucasian professor.

Bolstered by financial security at an early age, Newton felt no pressure to publish. He formulated a description of his system of calculus, which he termed "fluxions," but issued only a cryptogram to document his discovery. Gottried Wilhelm Leibniz (1646–1716), a German diplomat, lawyer, historian, mathematician, and philosopher, also developed a system of calculus. The material was published in *Acta Eruditorum*, an early German scientific journal that first appeared in 1682 (4). Because his work was published, Leibniz received primary recognition for the discovery of calculus even though Newton's work clearly had occurred at an earlier date. This was an important lesson for future mathematicians.

Newton's friends in the Royal Society urged him to prepare a manuscript detailing his work on the nature of light. He had determined correctly that light could be separated by a prism into a spectrum (Newton's word) of red, orange, yellow, green, blue, indigo, and violet. Looking at the spectrum, one wonders why Newton made a special designation for indigo; the other six colors easily would have sufficed. Newton chose seven colors because there are seven notes in the musical scale. Like Plato, he believed in the harmony of the universe and anticipated that studies of nature would reveal elegant symmetries. Kepler had pursued and successfully found harmonious order in the location and motion of the planets. Milton and Shakespeare, Newton's contemporaries, also espoused the concept of a harmonious universe in their writings (1,28). Newton's paper on light was reviewed by Hooke, who recommended that it be rejected (29). Newton contended that light behaved as if it were composed of tiny particles. Hooke and Huygens held that light consisted of waves. Oldenburg decided to publish Newton's paper along with Hooke's dissenting comments. The paper aroused great interest. Newton was required to respond to 12 letters to the editor, a task that vexed him to declare that he would be loathe to submit another manuscript. "It had sacrificed my peace, a matter of real substance" (1,28).

With the security of his tenured position, there was no pressure to produce, and for a number of years he published nothing. Celestial mechanics, the nature of the motion of the heavenly bodies, was a key question for 17th century natural philosophers. Thomas Aquinas had written that the angels directed the motion of the planets around the earth. Copernicus held that rotation was an innate feature of perfect spheres, that rotation in a circular orbit was an inherent property of the planets (30). Tycho Brahe had great difficulty in explaining irregularities in his observations of the orbit of Mars. When Kepler joined him in Prague, he was given the task of resolving the nature of Mars' orbit. Tremendously pleased with the assignment, Kepler promised an answer within 8 days. It took him 8 years. Kepler determined that the paths of the planets traced an ellipse with the sun situated at one of the foci.

Kepler's revelation of the elliptic orbits of the planets was discussed by the members of the Royal Society in London. Hooke had intuited that the force of attraction between heavenly bodies behaved as if it were inversely related to the square of the distance between objects. In informal discussions, members pondered whether this could be proved mathematically for planets in an elliptic orbit. A challenge to produce the proof was issued by Christopher Wren who offered a reward (28). Hooke was unable to solve the problem. Newton, however, came upon the solution. Stimulated and pressed by his colleagues, Newton worked on the principles of celestial mechanics for 18 months. Completely possessed by the subject, he worked ceaselessly on the matter, often going for several days without sleeping or eating. Newton's efforts reflect Edison's maxim that genius is 1% inspiration and 99% perspiration.

Newton's *Principia, Mathematical Principles of Natural Philosophy,* was published in 1682. Newton is widely quoted as having written, "If I have seen further than others, it is because I was standing on the shoulders of giants" (28). It is often presumed that this remark referred to Galileo and Kepler, whose work was a vital contribution to *Principia*. Actually, the statement came from Newton's letter to Hooke, discussing their mutual interest in the study of light (29). Hooke was the Rodney Dangerfield of 17th century scientists. Working at the cutting edge of scientific endeavor, Hooke was extremely versatile, constantly filled with original ideas and germinal concepts. Unfortunately, despite his extraordinary ingenuity, he was overwhelmed by the scope of his extremely diverse interests and never focused sufficiently on projects to bring them to fruition (29). Thus, credit went to others for advances for which Hooke supplied the initial stimulus.

During his productive years, Newton was considered by many to be an unsympathetic and difficult individual. "Standing on the shoulders of giants" was an expression that dates from the 11th century (31). Newton's use of the phrase in a letter to Hooke was possibly a cruel, calculated gesture since Hooke was quite short because of severe kyphoscoliosis.

Newton was also a devoted chemist and alchemist. Six years after completing his masterpiece, he suffered through an illness that some have attributed to mercury intoxication. Unfortunately, Newton never regained his intellectual vigor. He moved to London, resigned his Lucasian professorship, and enjoyed a successful second career as master of the mint. In the last 25 years of his life, he served as president of the Royal Society. This was an ironic turn for the great scientist. The presidency of the society had not been a role filled by elite scientists. Almost all of his predecessors had been gentlemen politicians. In his early years, Newton had expressed a disdain for the political aspects of society activities. His position is similar to that of Einstein who once remarked, "To punish me for my contempt for authority, fate made me an authority myself" (1). Nevertheless, Newton's stature strengthened the reputation of the Royal Society, and he was a very successful president.

The natural philosophers of the 17th century made an incalculable contribution to the genesis of modern science. One would anticipate that they would have earned the deep respect of their contemporaries and, in their final years, would have been treated with reverence and honor. This, however, was generally not the case. Galileo's plight is well known. He was forced to recant his heretical heliocentric speculations and was sentenced to house arrest for life. He was finally forgiven by the Catholic Church in 1982 (3). Kepler's mother was imprisoned for over a year after being accused of being a witch. Kepler's defense of her honor exhausted his savings. Later, Kepler was pressured by the Counter-Reformation to renounce his religion and adopt Catholicism. He died penniless and forlorn. Bacon was accused of accepting bribes. The standard practice of the times had been for both parties in a litigation to make a gift to the presiding judge. This system was in place because judges otherwise received little compensation. Naturally, the judges claimed that they were above being influenced and were capable of delivering proper verdicts. Initially, Bacon responded that, "There are vita temporis and vita hominis" (there are evils of the time and evils of the man). That is, if there was a problem, the system was at fault, not the judges (7). He later reconsidered, confessed his guilt, and suffered dismissal and brief imprisonment in the Tower of London.

We have briefly revisited the spirits of the early natural philosophers. The principles that they espoused resonate with present late–20th century concerns. Communication among scientists through professional societies and scientific journals remains an essential element in scientific progress. We salute the natural philosophers who established such an effective system for scientific communication. It is our hope that should some future scholars reflect on current scientific societies such as the Radiological Society of North America and scientific journals such as *Radiology*, they will conclude that we have made a contribution by honoring and refining the standards set in the 17th century.

Acknowledgments: I am grateful to Christine A. Ruggere, curator, Institute of the History of Medicine, Johns Hopkins University, for important suggestions and criticism and to Ian Isherwood, Professor of Diagnostic Radiology, University of Manchester, for additional review.

References

1. Ferris T. Coming of age in the Milky Way. New York, NY: Morrow, 1988.
2. Fahie JJ. Galileo: his life and work. London, England: Murray, 1903.
3. Hitzeroth D, Heerboth S. The importance of Galileo Galilii. San Diego, Calif: Lucent, 1992.
4. Ornstein M. The role of scientific societies in the seventeenth century. (Reprinted, 1st edition 1913) Hamden, London: Archon, 1963.
5. Purver M. The royal society: concept and creation. London: Routledge & Kegan, 1967.
6. Gillespie CC. Dictionary of scientific biography. New York, NY: Scribner's Sons, 1970.
7. Farrington B. Francis Bacon: philosopher of industrial science. New York, NY: Schuman, 1949.
8. Bacon F. Novum Organum with other parts of the great instauration. Urbach P, Gibson J, trans and eds. Chicago, Ill: Open Court, 1994.
9. Bacon F. The advancement of learning and New Atlantis. 1974 printing. London, England: Oxford Press, 1906.
10. Merton R. Singletons and multiples in scientific discovery: chapter in the sociology of science. Proc Am Philos Soc 1961; 105:470–486.
11. Weld CR. A history of the Royal Society. London, England: Parker, 1848.
12. Anderson FH. Francis Bacon: his career and his thought. Westport, Conn: Greenwood, 1957.
13. Andrade EN da C. A brief history of the Royal Society. London, England: Royal Society, 1960.
14. Hunter M. The Royal Society and its fellows, 1660–1700: the morphology of an early scientific institution—British Society for the History of Science. Great Britain: Chalfont St Giles, 1982.
15. Hahn R. The anatomy of a scientific institution: the Paris Academy of Sciences, 1666–1803. Berkeley, Calif: University of California Press, 1971.
16. Houghton B. Scientific periodicals: their historical development, characteristics, and control. Hamden, Conn: Linnet Books & Clive Bingley, 1975.
17. Porter JR. The scientific journal: 300th anniversary. Bacteriol Rev 1964; 28:211–230.
18. De Solla P, Derek J. Little science, big science. New York, NY: Columbia University Press, 1963.
19. Booth CC. The development of medical journals in Britain. Br Med J 1982; 285:105–108.
20. Kronick DA. The literature of the life sciences. Philadelphia, Pa: ISI, 1985.
21. Ziman JM. Information, communication, and knowledge. Nature 1969; 224:318–324.
22. Ferris T. The whole shebang: a state of the universe report. New York, NY: Simon & Shuster, 1997.
23. Gade JA. The life and times of Tycho Brahe. Princeton, NJ: Princeton University Press, 1947.
24. Zuckerman H, Merton RK. Patterns of evaluation in science: institutionalization, structure and functions of the referee system. Minerva 1971; 9:66–100.
25. Ziman JM. Public knowledge: the social dimension of science. Cambridge, England: Cambridge University Press, 1966.
26. Ortega Y, Gasset J. Revolt of the masses. New York, NY: Norton, 1932.
27. Siegelman SS. Valediction: secret sorrow. Radiology 1997; 205:647–648.
28. Ipsen DC. Isaac Newton: reluctant genius. Hillside, NJ: Enslow, 1985.
29. Espinasse M. Robert Hooke. Berkeley, Calif: University of California Press, 1956.
30. DeSantillana G. Dialogue on the great world systems. Chicago, Ill: University of Chicago Press, 1953.
31. Merton RK. On the shoulders of giants. New York, NY: Free Press, 1965.

Editorial

David J. Seidenwurm, MD ■ Howard A. Rowley, MD

Imaging-guided Gene Therapy in the Central Nervous System[1]

Gene therapy, broadly defined, consists of any deliberate alteration of somatic or germ line genetic material, with the goal of alleviating the symptoms of disease or curing disease. Introduced with great fanfare in the previous decade, human gene therapy is evolving into a realistic approach to difficult medical problems previously thought hopeless. The therapeutic potential is enormous: Inherited diseases caused by defective genes are now prime targets for cure by means of gene replacement, whereas acquired infections or cancers can be selectively marked for destruction with genetic methods (1–3).

Difficulties in delivering genes, sustaining beneficial effects, and, of course, isolating and correcting the specific genetic defects responsible for previously incurable diseases remain challenges. The collective efforts of many investigators have led to the discovery and cloning of genes that may be manipulated for therapeutic purposes. Once isolated, the selected gene can be inserted into a target cell by means of a variety of techniques (eg, with a modified viral vector that will carry the gene into cells but will not replicate itself). Such genetic engineering may have any of several purposes: alteration of the native immune response, up- or down-regulation of cell surface receptors, direct replacement of faulty genes, or insertion of "suicide genes" into unwanted cell types. Selectable markers can be co-transferred into cells along with the genes of interest, to allow efficient monitoring of the process, and may permit selective eradication of transfected cells if untoward effects develop. Ethical concerns have limited enthusiasm for germ line therapies, but they are largely irrelevant to somatic treatments (4–6).

In this edition of *Radiology*, de Marco and colleagues (7) provide us with a tantalizing glimpse into the future of gene therapy and the potential for radiologic techniques and radiologists to play a crucial role. Although the topic may seem arcane and distant from clinical relevance at present, it ought to be viewed as a harbinger. The authors describe their model for documentation of the site of a DNA delivery system with poly-L-lysine–conjugated dextran chains anchored with a magnetic resonance (MR) imaging–detectable superparamagnetic substance. They demonstrate that radiologic monitoring of the site of delivery of a potentially effective vector for gene therapy has been accomplished in vivo. Needless to say, this is a bit removed from everyday clinical experience, but the demonstration of feasibility is a critical step in the development of gene therapy for somatic gene alteration in localized tissues with low turnover rates.

This is important because the central nervous system is an organ system in which the cell turnover is low or absent, especially among the neuron populations. Gene therapy replacement strategies often exploit fast cell turnover rates to remove, alter, and then reintroduce genetically re-engineered cells to cure disease (eg, use of bone marrow stem cells for severe combined immunodeficiency). The structural integrity of the brain and the fact that mature neurons do not divide has made neurogenetic therapy especially challenging. However, among the 100–150 reasonably common disorders targeted for the development of new therapies are a number of common, disabling, expensive, currently incurable disorders that are diseases of the brain and spinal cord (1,2,8).

Huntington disease, Tay-Sachs disease, adrenoleukodystrophy, the neurofibromatoses, and some of the inborn errors of metabolism are already considered to be targets for gene therapy because the genes responsible have been located and, in some cases, even cloned. This not only permits identification of presymptomatic carriers but also holds promise for functional correction of the disease discovered. Genetic targets could be the defective gene itself or the genes that regulate or code the production of downstream products or provide for their metabolism (6,9). For example, in Parkinson disease, one might imagine a therapeutic approach based on alteration of the genetic regulation of L-dopa in the nigrostriatal system. In Alzheimer disease, alteration of the expression of activity in cholinergic cell populations or alteration of genes involved in regulation of cholinergic pathways might be considered. Hereditary disorders such as Tay-Sachs disease might be dealt with by means of somatic cell approaches in which the defective gene is replaced in the entire neuron population.

Malignant and infectious diseases targeted for genetic treatment also present unique circumstances in the central nervous system. Ingenious strategies have been developed to circumvent the obstacles to successful treatment (6,10–12). Gene therapy for malignancy may involve the addition of genes to lympho-

Index terms:
Editorials
Genes and genetics
Magnetic resonance (MR), utilization

Radiology 1998; 208:17–18

[1] From the Radiological Associates of Sacramento, 1800 I St, Sacramento, CA 95814 (D.J.S.), and the Departments of Radiology and Neurology, University of California, San Francisco (H.A.R.). Received March 17, 1998; accepted March 26. **Address reprint requests to** D.J.S.

See also the article by de Marco et al (pp 65–71) in this issue.

cytes to produce or augment the host immune response to the tumor, down-regulate gene expression at various points in the genetic pathway of the tumor cell, or replace the oncogene or mutant tumor suppressor genes themselves. Another approach involves introduction of genes into the dividing tumor cells, thus conferring vulnerability to chemotherapeutic agents ordinarily ineffective against brain tumors and harmless to normal cells. Interestingly, transfection need occur in only a small percentage of cells to result in therapeutic effect, perhaps as a result of a bystander effect from toxic metabolites transferred among nearby tumor cells.

The central nervous system provides challenges and opportunities for genetic therapy. Owing to the precise anatomic localization of many disorders, specific delivery of the gene vector may be required (13,14). To the extent that this may be accomplished with minimal disruption of normally functioning surrounding tissues, radiologic guidance will be essential. Because of the risks involved in delivery, be it via direct stereotactically guided injection, intrathecal administration, or intravascular administration of the vector, confirmation of the effect at the genome or phenotypic level would be desirable.

The need for precision in introduction of gene therapy vectors in the nervous system is magnified by the anatomic and functional complexity of the brain (6). A degenerative disease might be manifest as loss of function in a discrete cell population. Targeted vector delivery would prevent unintended alteration in the function of healthy neurons or damage to eloquent areas along the delivery pathway. The approach of de Marco et al (7) provides an example that may be used to target a specific anatomically defined cell population.

Structural and functional radiologic techniques will each play a role in gene therapy. Ideally, the presence or expression of the gene itself would be directly imaged. Owing to small quantities and intracellular location, this is not feasible at present. Structural findings may help select candidates for treatment and assess response to therapy on the basis of the anatomic patterns, receptor status, size of lesion, or stage of disease. Because gene transfer can be performed with a variety of markers independent of the active gene, MR imaging, functional MR imaging, MR spectroscopy, single photon emission computed tomography, and positron emission tomography are candidates for noninvasive confirmation of transfection and gene expression. Assessments may be based on serial volume measurements, magnetic susceptibility changes, metabolic consequences of therapy, permeability factors, blood volumes, receptor activity, or specific ligands (15–17). Increasingly, such noninvasive radiologic techniques are being employed to provide surrogate end points in clinical trials.

As new therapeutic modalities are developed, it is tempting to be both unrealistically optimistic or overly skeptical and fearful. Findings in the study of de Marco et al (7) suggest that the role of radiologists in gene therapies will be similar to our role in conventional therapies. We will diagnose the diseases, monitor and quantify the effectiveness of initial treatments, and monitor for recurrence or cure. The potential for gene therapy in neurologic disorders will be realized only through a concentrated cooperative effort involving all the disciplines of the basic and clinical sciences. de Marco and colleagues demonstrate persuasively that imaging techniques will provide a vehicle for clinical implementation of gene therapy in the central nervous system.

Acknowledgments: We thank Denette Cook and Casey Robbins for their assistance in preparing the manuscript for this editorial, and Carol Diamond, MD, for her thoughtful comments.

References

1. Goldspiel BR, Green L, Calis KA. Clinical frontiers: human gene therapy. Clin Pharm 1993; 12:488–505.
2. McCade ER. Clinical application of gene therapy: emerging opportunities and current limitations. Biochem Med Metab Biol 1993; 50:241–253.
3. Wolff JA, Lederberg J. An early history of gene transfer and therapy. Hum Gene Ther 1994; 5:469–480.
4. Ledley FD. Are contemporary methods for somatic gene therapy suitable for clinical applications? Clin Invest Med 1993; 16:78–88.
5. Crystal RG. Transfer of genes to humans: early lessons and obstacles to success. Science 1995; 270:404–410.
6. Fick J, Israel MA. Gene therapy for diseases of the nervous system. West J Med 1994; 161:260–263.
7. de Marco G, Bogdanov A, Marecos E, Moore A, Simonova M, Weissleder R. MR imaging of gene delivery to the central nervous system with an artificial vector. Radiology 1998; 208:65–71.
8. Drews J. Genomic sciences and the medicine of tomorrow. Nat Biotechnol 1996; 14:1516–1518.
9. Rosenberg RN. Molecular neurogenetics: the genome is settling the issue. JAMA 1997; 278:1282–1283.
10. Izquierdo M, Cortes ML, Martin V, et al. Gene therapy in brain tumours: implications of the size of glioblastoma on its curability. Acta Neurochir Suppl (Wien) 1997; 68:111–117.
11. Tjuvajev JG, Finn R, Watanabe K, et al. Noninvasive imaging of herpes virus thymidine kinase gene transfer and expression: a potential method for monitoring clinical gene therapy. Cancer Res 1996; 56:4087–4095.
12. Gorlich M, Jandrig B. Steroid hormone receptors and antineoplastic chemotherapy in human breast cancer. J Exp Clin Cancer Res 1997; 16:95–103.
13. Marshall E. Gene therapy's growing pains. Science 1995; 269:1050–1055.
14. Kelly PJ. Stereotactic procedures for molecular neurosurgery. Exp Neurol 1997; 144:157–159.
15. Moretti JL, Caglar M, Duran-Cordobes M, Morere JF. Can nuclear medicine predict response to chemotherapy? (editorial). Eur J Nucl Med 1995; 22:97–100.
16. Fabry ME, Kennan RP, Paszty C, et al. Magnetic resonance evidence of hypoxia in a homozygous alpha-knockout of a transgenic mouse model for sickle cell disease. J Clin Invest 1996; 98:2450–2455.
17. Oshiro EM, Viola JJ, Oldfield EH, et al. Toxicity studies and distribution dynamics of retroviral vectors following intrathecal administration of retroviral vector-producer cells. Cancer Gene Ther 1995; 2:87–95.

Jonathan H. Sunshine, PhD
Gerald R. Busheé, PhD
Rajiv Mallick, PhD

Index terms:
Radiology and radiologists
Radiology and radiologists, socioeconomic issues

Radiology 1998; 208:19–24

Abbreviations:
ACR = American College of Radiology
BMAD = Part B Medicare Annual Data
CPT = *Physicians' Current Procedural Terminology*
FTE = full-time equivalent
RVS = relative value scale
RVU = relative value unit

[1] From the Research Department, American College of Radiology, 1891 Preston White Dr, Reston, VA 20191 (J.H.S., G.R.B.), and PraCon, a Division of Excerpta Medica, Reston, Va (R.M.). Received November 10, 1997; revision requested January 29, 1998; revision received February 27; accepted March 10. **Address reprint requests to** J.H.S.

Author contributions:
Guarantor of integrity of entire study, J.H.S.; study concepts and design, J.H.S.; definition of intellectual content, J.H.S., G.R.B.; literature research, G.R.B.; data acquisition, G.R.B., R.M.; data analysis, J.H.S., G.R.B., R.M.; statistical analysis, G.R.B., R.M.; manuscript preparation and editing, J.H.S., G.R.B.; manuscript review, J.H.S.

U.S. Radiologists' Workload in 1995–1996 and Trends since 1991–1992[1]

PURPOSE: To measure U.S. radiologists' workload and the variation and trends in workload.

MATERIALS AND METHODS: A stratified, random sample of 794 radiology practice groups were surveyed about hiring and workload in 1996; 78% responded. Responses were weighted to represent all U.S. radiologists. Types of procedures performed in Medicare patients in 1991 and 1995 were analyzed.

RESULTS: In 1995–1996, the average workload per full-time equivalent diagnostic radiologist was 11,600 procedures ± 200 (standard error) annually, an apparent (but not statistically significant) 5% increase from 4 years earlier. Average relative value units per Medicare procedure increased by 8%, due to the increasing role of magnetic resonance imaging, computed tomography, and interventional radiology. The annual average number of procedures varied substantially by group type (eg, 13,200 procedures ± 500 in groups of two to four radiologists vs 10,300 ± 300 in groups of 11 or more radiologists). Within any group type, radiologists at the 75th percentile in terms of workload typically performed at least 50% more procedures than did radiologists at the 25th percentile.

CONCLUSION: Given the large variability in the annual number of procedures within and across group types, averages should not be taken as norms. Contrary to concerns about a possible surplus of radiologists, the workload per radiologist has increased substantially in the past few years.

The operational and organizational characteristics of radiologists' practices can play an important role in ensuring both high-quality patient care and financial soundness in a practice. One important operational characteristic is workload. Indeed, the single most frequently asked question of the research department of the American College of Radiology (ACR) is, "What is a typical radiologist's workload?" The answer is important for individual practices, the members of which want to know how they compare with others.

Workload analysis is also important for the profession as a whole. The rate of growth of the number of radiologists in practice (approximately 2.5% annually) exceeds the growth rate of the U.S. population (approximately 1% annually) (1), and a declining workload may signal that this difference in growth rates is creating a surplus of radiologists. There has been much concern among radiologists about a weak employment market, and the trend in workload is one core indication of whether a surplus is developing.

To provide the most up-to-date information about radiologists' workload and other aspects of the profession, the ACR conducts periodic surveys of both radiology groups and individual radiologists (2–12). This article continues the long-standing practice of the ACR of providing regular updates on critical issues. Our purpose was to measure the workload of diagnostic radiologists and radiation oncologists in various regions of the country, practice types, practice locations, and group sizes. By means of comparisons with previous data (6,8), we also sought to identify trends.

MATERIALS AND METHODS

Data

The 1995–1996 workload data are drawn from the ACR's 1996 Survey of Hiring by Groups, which has been described in detail elsewhere (13). In brief, questionnaires for this survey were mailed in August 1996 to a stratified, random sample of 794 radiology groups, approximately one-fourth of the estimated 3,286 radiology groups in the United States. Between August and October 1996, up to three follow-up mailings, with the last sent by means of Priority Mail, were sent to those who had not responded. The survey encompassed all types of radiology groups, including academic departments, radiology units in multispecialty groups, private groups, and the staff of government facilities. Telephone calls were made to clarify ambiguous responses to the most important questions.

The sample was drawn from the ACR's master list of radiology practices and was stratified to mirror the known distribution of groups in five size categories (two, three to four, five to seven, eight to 10, and 11 or more radiologists) and four census regions (Northeast, Midwest, South, and West). We received 617 responses, for an overall response rate of 78%; seven groups that were no longer in existence were excluded (ie, 617/[794 − 7] = 0.78, or 78%). Nine respondents who reported that they were solo practices were excluded from the analyses. The remaining 608 responses were weighted to represent what the responses would be had all radiology groups in the United States been surveyed and responded to the survey. To ensure that the data on workload were representative of radiologists, not groups, we multiplied these weights by the number of radiologists in each group. This special weighting method has been described elsewhere (8).

Because of the nature of the survey questions about workloads, it was possible to analyze workload data solely on the basis of diagnostic radiology–only and radiation oncology–only groups (hereafter, diagnostic-only and oncology-only, respectively). The 59 groups that reported that they provided both types of services were omitted from our study of workload. We also omitted groups that failed to indicate what types of services they provided or omitted other data needed for the analysis. Our analysis of the survey is based on the remaining 457 diagnostic-only groups and 52 radiation oncology-only groups.

To study trends over time, we compared the 1995–1996 data with previously published (8) data for 1991–1992 obtained from an earlier survey, the ACR's 1992 Group Practice Survey.

Some procedures involve more work than others. Therefore, a count of procedures does not provide a full analysis of workload. To address this issue, we carried out analyses of the 1991 and 1995 Part B Medicare Annual Data (BMAD) procedure files. These files contain reasonably complete and consistent data on all physician services rendered to Medicare patients. Medicare patients constitute approximately one-third of the total workload of U.S. physicians (14).

From the BMAD procedure files for 1991 and 1995, we first selected, for each year, all procedures related to diagnostic radiology. These are *Physicians' Current Procedural Terminology* (CPT) (15) codes 70000–79999, except for radiation oncology, which is composed of CPT codes 77000–77999, as well as ultrasound (US) and interventional imaging procedures, which are found among CPT codes 93307–93981. All procedures not performed by diagnostic radiologists, nuclear medicine specialists, or interventional radiologists were then deleted.

Some of the BMAD analyses involved relative value units (RVUs). For all observations from both the 1991 data and the 1995 data, other than the interventional supervision and interpretation codes, RVUs were measured with the 1995 Medicare resource-based relative value scale (RVS) professional-component relative value. For the approximately 85 supervision and interpretation codes, we developed resource-based RVS professional values that represented a "complete procedure." For interventional procedures that had existed earlier than 1992, the relative value assigned to the supervision and interpretation code was set to equal that of the corresponding "complete procedure" code by using Medicare's 1989–1991 radiology RVS multiplied by 0.285, the factor needed to convert from Medicare's 1989–1991 radiology scale to the 1995 Medicare resource-based RVS. For procedures first listed in the CPT in 1992 or later, the RVU used for the supervision and interpretation code was the sum of the resource-based RVS relative value for that code plus the relative value (or values) for the other code (or codes) judged most frequently to be part of the complete procedure by the ACR's in-house coding and nomenclature expert (Mabry M, written communication, 1997).

Analysis Methods

Survey findings for 1995–1996 and 1991–1992 are presented as averages ± the standard error of the annual workload of a full-time equivalent (FTE) radiologist (Table 1). Standard errors were calculated to measure the uncertainty (sampling variability) in these means due to the use of data from a sample of groups rather than from all groups in the United States. Although all data collected by means of the sampling procedures are subject to sampling variability, the relatively large sample size used in the 1996 Survey of Hiring by Groups minimized this effect. Table 1 also reports the 25th, 50th, and 75th percentiles, to indicate the variability among groups within each response category.

To assess whether average workloads varied according to practice type, practice size, how urban the practice was, geographic region, and year, we used Student *t* tests, analysis of variance, and correlation coefficients. Student *t* tests were used to compare workload statistics whenever a comparison involved only two categories, for example, hospital-only versus office-only practices in 1995–1996, or hospital-only practices in 1995–1996 versus the same type of practice in 1991–1992. Analysis of variance was used to compare three or more categories, for example, to determine whether there were statistically significant differences among workloads in the four regions of the United States. Because the original data on group size were the actual number of radiologists in each group, rather than the categories of group size mentioned earlier, we used a correlation analysis to examine the relationship between group size and workload. For all analyses, a two-tailed P value of .05 or less served as the level of significance needed to conclude that an observed difference reflected a real difference in workload rather than a difference due to sampling variability.

The BMAD data were used to conduct separate analyses by (*a*) year; (*b*) place of service, namely hospitals (inpatient, outpatient, and emergency room) versus offices and imaging centers; and (*c*) modality, namely, angiography and interventional radiology, computed tomography (CT) and magnetic resonance (MR) imaging combined, nuclear medicine, US, and general radiology (all other procedures).

RESULTS

1995–1996 Findings

In diagnostic-only practices, the annual average number of procedures performed in 1995–1996 by an FTE radiologist was 11,600 ± 200 (Table 1). However, there was much variation from one prac-

TABLE 1
Annual Workload per FTE Radiologist: 1995–1996 and 1991–1992

Group Characteristic	1995–1996 Mean*	1995–1996 Percentile 25th	50th	75th	1991–1992 Mean*	Difference between 1995–1996 and 1991–1992 Means
Diagnostic-only Groups (n = 457)†						
All groups	11.6 (0.2)	9.2	11.6	14.7	11.1 (0.2)	0.5
No. of radiologists in group						
Two to four	13.2 (0.5)	9.6	12.9	16.0	11.2 (0.5)	2.0‡
Five to seven	12.6 (0.4)	9.4	11.5	14.4	12.0 (0.4)	0.6
Eight to 10	11.7 (0.5)	9.4	11.5	14.4	11.8 (0.7)	−0.1
11 or more	10.3 (0.3)	8.5	10.8	13.3	10.0 (0.4)	0.3
Practice type						
Primarily academic	8.0 (0.8)	6.2	7.8	9.7	7.8 (0.6)	0.2
Nonacademic multispecialty	10.6 (0.8)	8.6	11.0	13.8	11.8 (0.7)	−1.2
Nonacademic private, radiology only	12.3 (0.2)	9.9	12.0	15.0	11.5 (0.3)	0.8§
Practice location						
Hospital	12.9 (0.4)	10.0	12.5	15.0	11.1 (0.3)	1.8‡
Office or imaging center	9.6 (0.9)	7.8	10.0	11.2	7.4 (0.9)	2.2
Region‖						
Midwest	13.5 (0.5)	11.7	13.3	15.9	13.4 (1.1)	0.1
Northeast	10.9 (0.5)	8.9	11.0	13.1	11.6 (0.4)	−0.7
South	13.4 (0.5)	10.3	13.2	16.0	12.8 (0.7)	0.7
West	10.8 (0.5)	8.3	10.5	14.4	10.9 (0.5)	−0.1
Oncology-only Groups (n = 52)						
No. of new patients	209 (9)	183	211	250	188 (11)	21

* Number in parentheses is the standard error.
† Data are thousands of procedures.
‡ Difference between 1995–1996 data and 1991–1992 data was significant (P < .01).
§ Difference between 1995–1996 data and 1991–1992 data was significant (P < .05).
‖ Data are for private, nonacademic, non-multispecialty groups with both hospital and office or imaging center activity.

tice to another, as the percentile values indicate. For example, one-fourth of all diagnostic radiologists were in groups that performed 9,200 or fewer procedures annually per FTE radiologist (25th percentile), whereas another one-fourth were in groups that performed at least 14,700 procedures per year per FTE radiologist (75th percentile). Thus, those at the 75th percentile or higher performed at least 60% more procedures annually than did those at the 25th percentile.

Per FTE radiologist per year, groups of two to four FTE radiologists performed an average of 13,200 procedures ± 500, groups of five to seven performed an average of 12,600 procedures ± 400, groups of eight to 10 performed an average of 11,700 procedures ± 500, and groups of 11 or more performed an average of 10,300 procedures ± 300. The median (50th percentile) number of procedures also decreased with increasing group size. The correlation between actual (uncategorized) group size and the annual number of procedures per FTE radiologist in a group was r = −.21, which indicates only a modest relationship between group size and the average number of procedures performed annually; nonetheless, the correlation was highly significant (P < .001).

In private, nonacademic, non-multispecialty practices, diagnostic radiologists performed an average of 12,300 procedures ± 200 per year per FTE radiologist. Those working in nonacademic multispecialty groups and in primarily academic settings performed fewer procedures per year per FTE radiologist (10,600 ± 800 and 8,000 ± 800, respectively). The difference between any two of these three practice types was significant (P < .05).

Because academic groups typically are large, the preceding finding means that the overall association of large group size with fewer procedures per year may be a reflection of academic status, not group size. To investigate this possibility, we analyzed data for nonacademic groups. Among nonacademic groups, we found the average annual number of procedures per FTE radiologist in groups of 11 or more radiologists was 1,500 fewer than that in groups of two to four radiologists, or approximately half the difference found when academic groups were included in the analysis. The correlation between group size and annual number of procedures was r −.09 for nonacademic groups, again approximately half that found when academic groups were included. This correlation was at the margin of statistical significance (two-tailed P = .06).

Diagnostic radiologists in hospital-only practices performed an average of 12,900 procedures ± 400 per year, compared with 9,600 procedures ± 900 for those in practices that had no hospital activity. (These are referred to as "office or imaging center" practices in Table 1.) The difference of 3,300 procedures per year was significant (P < .001).

In 1995, the overall average professional-component RVU per radiology procedure (measured by using the Medicare 1995 resource-based RVS) for procedures performed in Medicare patients by diagnostic radiologists was 0.75 (Table 2). The average was 0.75 for procedures performed at hospitals and 0.74 for procedures performed at offices or imaging centers. Forty-three percent of all hospital procedures were one- or two-view chest radiography examinations, compared with 23% of such procedures in offices or imaging centers.

There was considerable geographic variation with regard to workload, even after we controlled for group characteristics. Diagnostic radiologists in private, nonacademic, non-multispecialty groups that had both hospital and office or imaging center activity performed an average of 13,500 procedures ± 500 annually in the Midwest and 13,400 procedures ± 500 in the South, compared with 10,900 procedures ± 500 in the Northeast and 10,800 procedures ± 500 in the West (Table 1). These regional differences of approximately 2,500 procedures performed annually were significant (P < .001).

Within practice types, practice sizes, and geographic locales, there were wide variations in workload from one diagnostic-only practice to another. In general, the workload of diagnostic radiologists at the 75th percentile was more than 50% greater than the workload of those at the 25th percentile. For example, the 75th percentile workload in practices with two to four radiologists was 16,000 procedures per year per FTE radiologist compared with the 25th percentile workload of 9,600 procedures per FTE radiologist per year.

Radiation oncologists in oncology-only practices averaged 209 new patients ± 9 per FTE radiologist per year. Radiation oncologists at the 25th percentile averaged 183 new patients per FTE radiologist per year, and those at the 75th percentile averaged 250 new patients, a difference of more than one-third. As will be noted in the Discussion, because of the omission of groups in which both diagnostic radiology and radiation oncology procedures are performed, these findings may not be representative of most radiation oncologists.

Comparisons between 1995–1996 and 1991–1992 Data

The average annual number of procedures performed per FTE diagnostic radiologist apparently increased from 11,100 in 1992 to 11,600 in 1995–1996 (Table 1). However, this difference of 500 procedures was not large in percentage terms (4.5%), nor was it statistically significant. For most (but not all) group size categories, practice types, and geographic areas, the pattern was similar. Workload in 1995–1996 was slightly higher than that in 1991–1992, but the difference generally was not statistically significant.

Most of the variations among categories found in the 1995–1996 data were also found in the 1991–1992 data. For example, in both periods, the average number of procedures per FTE diagnostic radiologist was lower for academic groups than for other types of groups and higher for hospital-only practices than for office or imaging center–only practices. However, differences within categories in 1995–1996 were often greater than those reported for 1991–1992.

The overall average professional-component RVU per radiology procedure (for procedures performed in Medicare patients by diagnostic radiologists) increased from 0.693 to 0.748 RVU, or 8%, between 1991 and 1995 (Table 2). (Note that we used the 1995 resource-based RVS for the analysis of both the 1991 and the 1995 data.) During the same period, the percentage of these procedures that were interventional increased from 1.5% to 2.2%, the percentage that were CT and MR imaging increased from 11% to 13%, and the percentage that were general radiology decreased from 77% to 74%. More detailed analysis showed that at least nine-tenths of the increase in the overall average RVU per procedure resulted from a change in the share of each modality in the total, rather than from a change in the average RVU per procedure within modalities.

TABLE 2
Selected Medicare Data

Description	1995	1991
All sites		
Average RVUs per procedure	0.75	0.69
Procedures by modality (%)		
Interventional	2.2	1.5
CT and MR imaging	12.9	10.5
Nuclear medicine	4.1	4.6
US	6.9	5.8
General radiology	74.0	77.0
Hospitals*		
Average RVUs per procedure	0.75	0.69
One- and two-view chest radiographs (%)†	43	44
Procedures by modality (%)		
Interventional	2.4	2.0
CT and MR imaging	12.6	10.5
Nuclear medicine	4.3	4.8
US	6.5	5.5
General radiology	74.0	77.0
Offices and imaging centers		
Average RVUs per procedure	0.74	0.72
One- and two-view chest radiographs (%)†	23	23
Procedures by modality		
Interventional	0.4	0.3
CT and MR imaging	15.0	12.5
Nuclear medicine	2.8	3.4
US	9.5	8.0
General radiology	72.0	75.0

Note.—Data are for approximately 71 million procedures in 1995 and 65 million procedures in 1991.
* Includes inpatient, outpatient, and emergency services.
† As a percentage of all procedures.

In 1991, the average RVU per procedure was 0.69 in hospitals and 0.72 in offices. Forty-four percent of hospital procedures were chest radiography examinations, compared with 23% of the procedures in offices or imaging centers.

DISCUSSION

Strengths and Weaknesses of the Data

As is true of all survey data, the data from the 1996 Survey of Hiring by Groups have strengths and weaknesses. The strengths derive from the large, carefully drawn sample (n = 794), high response rate (78%), and accurate weighting of responses to reflect the total population of radiologists. Our effort to clarify ambiguous answers by means of follow-up telephone calls also minimized potential errors.

Despite these factors, some weaknesses remain. First, by excluding groups that provide both diagnostic radiology and radiation oncology services from the analyses, we omitted more than half of the responding groups that perform radiation oncology procedures. Thus, our radiation oncology data may be atypical. Workload data from the ACR's Patterns of Care Study facilities surveys (16,17) include all radiation oncology facilities and are therefore more representative and reliable than ours.

Second, despite the large size of the survey, the standard errors—which measure how much uncertainty there is in our estimates due to the use of a sample—are nontrivial, and this limits our ability to detect relatively small differences. For example, the estimated average number of procedures per FTE diagnostic radiologist increased by slightly less than 5% from 1991–1992 to 1995–1996. Given the standard errors of the estimates, we cannot be 95% confident that this difference of less than 5% is real rather than due merely to sampling variability.

Third, the BMAD data provide accurate, detailed, and complete information about Medicare services but may not be representative of the services to non-Medicare patients, which constitute about two-thirds of radiologists' workload. However, trends over time, such as the 8% increase in average RVU per procedure, should at least be broadly generalizable to the non-Medicare population. Data from radiology groups that measured radiologists' workload in terms of RVUs, not in terms of the number of procedures, would

TABLE 3
Changes in Workload between 1991–1992 and 1995–1996

Parameter	Change (%)
Change in no. of diagnostic radiologists*	$(1 + 0.025)^4$
Change in average no. of procedures per diagnostic radiologist	× 1.05
Change in average RVUs per procedure	× 1.08
Equals total 1995–1996 workload measured in RVUs	1.25
Change due to growth and aging of U.S. population†	$\div (1 + 0.015)^4$
Total 1995–1996 radiologic work of diagnostic radiologists per typical U.S. patient relative to 1991–1992‡	1.18

* Change is approximately + 2.5% annually.
† Change is approximately + 1.5% annually.
‡ Data are adjusted for aging.

presumably be more informative and accurate than the data we obtained; however, we found that only a small percentage of groups can provide the necessary data to measure RVUs.

Interpretation of Findings

Norms.—Our data show that in every practice group category (large and small, academic and nonacademic, in the East and in the West, etc) there is substantial variation in workload, with radiologists at the 75th percentile of workload typically performing approximately one and one-half times as many procedures as those at the 25th percentile (Table 1). Hence, there should be no presumption that the average or median represents a workload that is somehow normatively "right." Not only are there major variations in workload, but there are also multiple reasons for such variations.

Increasing workload and technologic change.—The number of diagnostic radiologists in practice in the United States increases by approximately 2.5% annually while the growth and aging of the U.S. population generate an increase in "requirements" for health care services of only approximately 1.5% annually (1). In light of the rapid growth of managed health care and some evidence of a relatively weak job market for radiologists that has been seen in recent years, this disparity has generated concerns that there will not be enough work for the increasing number of diagnostic radiologists.

Our findings should somewhat allay this concern, for they present clear evidence that, on average, diagnostic radiologists' workload is not declining and, most likely, is increasing. Specifically, our best point estimate is that, on average, diagnostic radiologists were performing approximately 5% more procedures per FTE radiologist in 1995–1996 than in 1991–1992 (Table 1), and that the average RVU per procedure increased from 0.693 to 0.748 (Table 2), so that the total workload increase was approximately 13% (1.05 × 1.08 = 1.34), as measured in terms of RVUs.

The conclusion that the number of procedures per diagnostic radiologist is not declining can probably be extended backward to a somewhat longer time horizon. The results from a 1989 ACR survey (6), although methodologically weak (the response rate was only 37%), showed an average annual number of procedures that was, for each group size category (two to four radiologists, five to seven, etc), no higher than that found in the 1996 survey.

As Table 3 shows, our data indicate that, on average, a patient in the United States was receiving approximately 18% more radiologic services from diagnostic radiologists in 1995–1996 than in 1991–1992. (For this result, again measured as RVUs per year, increases due to the increase in the average age of U.S. patients were subtracted.) This increase, which amounts to approximately 4% annually, is the increase usually attributed to "technology" or "technologic progress" when the growth of spending on health care is tabulated in the United States. It represents a substantial growth rate. (In principle, the 4% annual increase could be due to a shift of radiologic work from nonradiologists to radiologists; however, we have other, unpublished data that show that such a shift has not occurred.)

The observed increase in radiologists' workload and in the quantity of radiologic services per patient are probably somewhat conditional on the current character of managed health care. At present, most Americans have health care coverage through some form of a managed health care organization. Thus far, however, managed care has done little that would affect radiologists' workload. Managed care organizations have achieved cost containment mostly (*a*) by heavily discounting fee-for-service payments and (*b*) by discouraging the use of the inpatient hospital setting. Other forms of utilization management have been uncommon, as has been capitation payment. For example, the latest available data (18) show that in 1996 only 5% of radiologists' revenue was from capitation payments.

The strategies used in managed care to control costs may or may not change. In 1996 and 1997, many managed care firms incurred losses, probably because they were keeping prices low to try to increase market share. To return to profitability, these firms may expand the use of capitation payment, which creates incentives to reduce workload, and they may try to apply additional utilization-management controls directly to radiologic services, which would also put downward pressure on workload. However, the more intensive use of current cost-control mechanisms—that is, by cutting prices further and reducing inpatient care more—represents another strategy for a return to profitability. This strategy has the advantage of familiarity to managed care organizations, whereas greater use of capitation payment and broader application of utilization management would be something of a venture into the unknown. Another possible strategy is to raise the prices charged to employers and others who purchase coverage. This would not greatly affect radiologists' workload. In short, the future effect of managed care on radiologists' workload is quite uncertain, because the strategies managed care organizations will use to regain profitability may or may not heavily affect radiologists' workload.

Our data on the percentage of total procedures in each imaging modality (Table 2) generally show an increase in the share for high-technology modalities, particularly interventional radiology and CT and MR imaging, and a decline in the percentage share for general radiology. This trend is not unexpected, but we do not believe it has previously been reported for so broad a database. (Recall that the BMAD data cover approximately one-third of the work of all radiologists in the United States.) It is interesting that a change in the share for modalities in total procedures, rather than a change in the mix of procedures *within* modalities, almost completely accounts for the increase in the average complexity of procedures. Also interesting is the declining percentage of total procedures that are nuclear medicine studies; this result is counter to the general pattern of high-technology procedures becoming an increasing percentage of the total.

Differences among types of groups.—It is not surprising that diagnostic radiologists in academic groups perform, on average, fewer procedures annually per FTE radiologist than do other diagnostic radiologists (Table 1). Presumably, (*a*) procedures performed in an academic setting tend to be more complex, and (*b*) academic radiologists spend more of their time in activities other than clinical work, particularly research and teaching. We have no direct information on the first of these two points and, indeed, would hesitate to assert that it is certain, given the findings to be discussed later in this article. As regards the second point, the results of another ACR survey (12) show that, on average, academic radiologists report more time spent on teaching and research (26%) and administration and management (7%) than do nonacademic radiologists (2% and 3%, respectively).

Approximately half the decrease in the average number of procedures per diagnostic radiologist found with increasing group size (Table 1) reflects the relatively large size of academic groups. They form a greater portion of larger-sized groups, and radiologists in such groups perform relatively few procedures annually. The other half of the decrease in annual procedures with group size must have other causes.

It is puzzling that diagnostic radiologists in office or imaging center–only practices perform about one-fourth to one-third fewer procedures annually than do those in hospital-only practices (Table 1). We sought a possible explanation in terms of the differences in procedure complexity between the two settings, but this difference was very small in 1995 (Table 2).

Readers may be surprised to learn that the average hospital procedure is no more complex (as measured in terms of professional-component RVUs) than the average procedure in an office or imaging center (Table 2). Certainly, many high-complexity procedures—most notably interventional and nuclear medicine procedures—are typically associated with the hospital setting. Our data show, however, that a much larger percentage of hospital procedures than office or imaging center procedures are one- or two-view chest radiography examinations. Consequently, general radiology procedures, which average the lowest RVU per procedure of any modality, form a slightly larger percentage of hospital procedures than of procedures at offices or imaging centers, as Table 2 shows. Also, Table 2 shows (*a*) that nuclear medicine procedures are only slightly concentrated in the hospital setting and (*b*) that CT and MR imaging, which average a relatively high RVU per procedure, constitute a larger percentage of procedures at offices or imaging centers than at hospitals. These factors explain why the complexity of a typical hospital procedure is only about the same as that of a typical office or imaging center procedure.

We earlier reported (8) the same unexpected finding—that hospital procedures were not more complex, on average, than office or imaging center procedures—for 1992. Indeed, at that time, the average office or imaging center procedure was somewhat more complex than the average hospital procedure.

Acknowledgments: We thank George Kamp, MD, chair of the ACR's Commission on General and Pediatric Radiology, for oversight and helpful comments. We thank the groups that responded to our survey; their response makes information available to the entire profession.

References

1. Janower ML, Sunshine JH. Too many radiologists? update. Radiology 1996; 200: 545–549.
2. Bansal S, Sunshine JH. Basic characteristics of radiology groups in the United States: results of a 1991–1992 census. AJR 1994; 162:263–270.
3. Bansal S, Sunshine JH. Hospital activities of radiology groups in the United States: results of a 1992 ACR survey. AJR 1995; 165:453–465.
4. Deitch CH, Sunshine JH, Bansal S. Diagnostic radiologists' non-hospital practice: high technology and other characteristics of radiology offices. AJR 1996; 167:591–595.
5. Deitch CH, Sunshine JH, Chan WC, Shaffer KA. Women in the radiology profession: data from a 1995 national survey. AJR 1998; 170:263–270.
6. Sunshine JH, Bansal S. Operational, professional, and business characteristics of radiology groups in the United States. Radiology 1992; 183:535–540.
7. Bansal S, Sunshine JH. Hospital and office practices of radiology groups. Radiology 1992; 183:729–736.
8. Sunshine JH, Bansal S. Operational characteristics of radiology groups in the United States in 1992. Radiology 1994; 193:613–618.
9. Sunshine JH, Bansal S. Professional and business characteristics of radiology groups in the United States: 1992. Radiology 1995; 194:365–371.
10. Chan WC, Sunshine JH, Owen JB, Shaffer KA. Radiologists' satisfaction in their profession. Radiology 1995; 194:649–656.
11. Deitch CH, Chan WC, Sunshine JH, Shaffer KA. Profile of U.S. radiologists at mid-decade: overview of findings from the 1995 survey of radiologists. Radiology 1997; 202:69–77.
12. Chan WC, Sunshine JH, Kunkle LM, Shaffer KA. Characteristics of radiology groups and of diagnostic radiologists and radiation oncologists in different types of practices. Radiology 1998; 207:443–453.
13. Mallick R, Leader SG, Sunshine JH, Shaffer KA. Hiring by radiology groups in 1996. Radiology 1997; 205:479–486.
14. Sunshine JH, Swartzman J. Medicare's share in U.S. physicians' revenues: background paper 89-4. Washington, DC: Physician Payment Review Commission, 1989.
15. Kirschner CG, Burkett RC, Kotowicz GM, et al. Physicians' current procedural terminology: CPT '95. Chicago, Ill: American Medical Association, 1994.
16. Owen JB, Coia LR, Hanks GE. Recent patterns of growth in radiation therapy facilities in the United States: a patterns of care study report. Int J Radiat Oncol Biol Phys 1992; 24:983–986.
17. Owen JB, Coia LR, Hanks GE. The structure of radiation oncology in the United States in 1994. Int J Radiat Oncol Biol Phys 1997; 39:179–185.
18. Gonzalez ML, ed. Physician marketplace statistics 1996. Chicago, Ill: American Medical Association, 1997.

Kawasaki Disease: A Review[1]

Charles J. Chung, MD
Leonard Stein, MD

Index terms:
Coronary vessels, diseases, 54.629
Heart, diseases, 51.629
Kawasaki disease, **.629[2], 51.629, 99.629
State-of-art reviews

Radiology 1998; 208:25–33

Abbreviation:
MHC = major histocompatibility complex

[1] From the Departments of Radiology (C.J.C.) and Pediatrics (L.S.), University of North Carolina School of Medicine, CB 7510, Chapel Hill, NC 27599-7510. Received October 29, 1997; revision requested November 18; final revision received February 23, 1998; accepted March 3. **Address reprint requests to** C.J.C.

[2] **. Multiple body systems

Kawasaki disease, or acute infantile febrile mucocutaneous lymph node syndrome, was originally described as a distinct clinical entity in Japanese children by Dr Tomisaku Kawasaki in 1967 (1), then in the English literature in 1974 (2). The disease is now recognized as an acute febrile illness of unknown etiology that predominantly affects young children of all races and produces histologic changes of a systemic vasculitis (2–6). Although the disease is generally a self-limited endemic illness, epidemics may occur. The illness may be associated with considerable morbidity and mortality, mostly due to coronary artery and myocardial involvement (7–12). In this article, we review the pathologic, epidemiologic, clinical, and radiologic findings of Kawasaki disease and discusses the possible etiology and therapeutic management options.

PATHOLOGIC FINDINGS

The histologic changes of Kawasaki disease are consistent with a systemic vasculitis affecting medium and small arteries, and veins to a lesser extent, with inflammatory lesions in virtually all organs. There is a severe exudative change with infiltration of lymphocytes and large mononuclear cells into the media and adventitia of the vessels with endothelial necrosis (Fig 1). With the exception of arterial lesions, inflammatory lesions heal without residual structural changes. In arteries, reactive proliferation of medial smooth-muscle cells, medial disruption, intraluminal thrombosis, and aneurysmal dilatation of vessels may be seen, with the most severe and consistent changes seen in the coronary arteries (13–15).

In the heart, perivasculitis and endarteritis are seen during the first 10 days of clinical illness and progress during the subsequent 2 weeks to panvasculitis. Development of aneurysms and intraluminal thrombi, as well as phlebitis, myocarditis, coagulation necrosis, pericarditis, endocarditis, and valvulitis, is also seen during days 12 through 25 of clinical illness. Subsequently, vasculitic changes subside, and granulation can be seen followed by scarring, stenosis, fibrosis, coagulation necrosis, and endocardial fibroelastosis (15,16).

In an autopsy series (14), the inflammatory changes of the lungs, spleen, lymph nodes, and salivary glands remained more than 61 days after onset of the clinical illness in the majority of cases, whereas elsewhere in the body, the inflammatory changes persisted for less than 60 days. Also, there is a predilection for involvement of duct systems, such as the prostate (75%), pancreas (53%), bile ducts (49%), and salivary glands (81%) (14). In the central nervous system, aseptic leptomeningitic and choriomeningitic findings are similar to those seen in acute viral meningitis (14,17). Essentially, these histologic changes are similar to those of infantile periarteritis nodosa; the two diseases cannot be differentiated by means of pathologic findings alone (14).

EPIDEMIOLOGY AND ETIOLOGY

Kawasaki disease predominantly affects children younger than 5 years and has a slight increased prevalence in the late winter and spring (2,4,5,12,18,19). Nationwide surveys of Kawasaki disease carried out every 2 years by the Japan Kawasaki Disease Research Committee have documented over 116,848 cases of Kawasaki disease in Japan as of 1992, with a male-to-female ratio of 1.3–1.5:1. During the survey period of 1970 to 1992, the incidence of Kawasaki disease in children younger than 5 years increased from approximately four per 100,000 in 1970 to approximately 76 per 100,000 in 1992. Additionally, epidemics were also observed in 1979, 1982, and 1986, with peak incidence of 196.1 per 100,000 children noted in 1982 (19).

Since the first report of Kawasaki disease outside Japan in 1976 (3), studies have demonstrated similar epidemiologic findings whether inside or outside Japan. Outside Japan, however, the overall incidence of Kawasaki disease is less than that observed in Japan, varying from three per 100,000 to seven per 100,000 in children younger than 5 years. In the United States, 80% of Kawasaki disease cases manifest by 5 years of age. The peak incidence is in children 1–2 years of age, as compared to 6–12 months of age in Japan (6,12,18–27). The ages of reported cases range from a 20-day-old girl (28) to adults (29,30). It is thought, however, that many of the reported cases in adults are actually toxic shock syndrome, a disease with clinical signs and symptoms, as well as a possible cause, very similar to those of Kawasaki disease (6,12).

The mortality rate associated with Kawasaki disease was reported to be greater than 1% in the 1970s in Japan; however, this rate has declined steadily since the 1970s to approximately 0.04% in the 1990s (19). The standardized mortality ratio of boys with Kawasaki disease is 1.78, whereas that of the girls is 1.16 compared with an age-matched general population during the same time period. The increased mortality rate in boys is seen only during the acute phase and returns to baseline thereafter (31,32). These findings likely reflect the fact that cardiac and coronary artery abnormalities occur more frequently in boys than in girls, and that most deaths from Kawasaki disease are due to acute-phase coronary disease or cardiac complications (32). However, sequelae of Kawasaki disease do account for many of the acquired cardiovascular diseases (33). In Japan as well as in the United States, Kawasaki disease is a leading cause of acquired heart disease in children (5,12,34,35).

Several studies have demonstrated other epidemiologic risk factors: (*a*) Kawasaki disease appears to occur more frequently in children of middle and upper-middle socioeconomic status. (*b*) Children with Kawasaki disease have increased prevalence of recent exposure to freshly shampooed carpets and rugs and antecedent respiratory illness. (*c*) Children with Kawasaki disease live closer to bodies of water than do children in the control group (36–39). Of interest, the children of Asian ancestry living outside Japan have a higher prevalence of the disease compared with that in black children, with the lowest prevalence seen among white children (6,12,18,19). Also, person-to-person transmission has not been clearly documented. In one study, however, the prevalence of Kawasaki disease was 2.1% among siblings of patients with Kawasaki disease, compared with the overall prevalence of 0.19% in the general study population (3,19,40). These results suggest the role of a common infectious agent and/or genetic predisposition in the development of Kawasaki disease.

There has been no single organism demonstrated or a unique toxin repeatedly found in children with Kawasaki disease. Although group A β-hemolytic streptococci, staphylococci, and leptospirae are known to cause illnesses with similar clinical signs and symptoms in the acute phase, early studies have not revealed an association with these common organisms. Although there have been numerous reports suggesting infectious agents such as retroviruses, other viruses, *Propionibacterium acnes*, rickettsiae, and dust mites, none of these infectious agents have been seen consistently in children with Kawasaki disease (6,41).

IMMUNE SYSTEM INVOLVEMENT

Activation of the immune system has been well documented in the acute phase of disease. White blood cell count is increased, with a lymphocytosis, and the percentage of activated $CD4^+$ helper T cells is increased. The percentage of $CD8^+$ suppressor cytotoxic T cells is relatively decreased. There is macrophage activation. The levels of macrophage- and T cell–derived cytokines are increased. For example, serum levels of interleukin-1β, tissue necrosis factor-α, and interleukin-2 are increased. There is also evidence of B-cell activation with an increased number of DR-positive B cells and an increased number of spontaneously secreting B cells. There are reports of the presence of antibodies against vascular endothelial cell antigens and neutrophil cytoplasmic antigens (12,42–45).

The results of recent immunologic, microbiologic, and molecular studies have suggested that superantigen-producing agents (certain staphylococci or streptococci) may be the cause for Kawasaki disease. Superantigens are chemicals such as staphylococcal enterotoxins, which cause food poisoning and toxic shock syndrome. They circumvent the usual recognition-activation system of T cells, either causing them to replicate excessively or to be destroyed (12,34, 43,46).

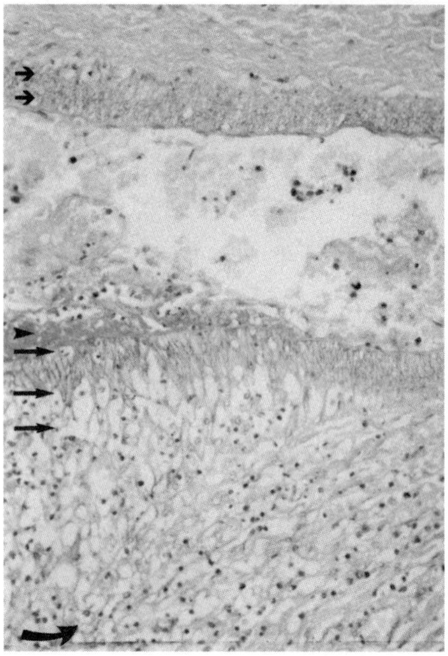

Figure 1. Histologic characteristics of Kawasaki vasculitis in a coronary artery. Photomicrograph of a longitudinal section of a small coronary artery demonstrates the edematous and necrotic muscularis (long arrows) with leukocyte infiltration. Normal muscularis for comparison is visible at the top of the vessel (short arrows). Small thrombus is seen in the lumen (arrowhead), and perivascular inflammation is also visible (curved arrow). (Hematoxylin-eosin stain; original magnification, ×300.) (Case courtesy of Charles Jennette, MD, University of North Carolina School of Medicine, Department of Pathology.)

Ordinarily, when a conventional protein antigen is introduced into body tissues, it is consumed by a macrophage and processed into peptides. The macrophage then presents the peptide pieces (antigens) by holding them within major histocompatibility complex (MHC) molecules on the cell membrane. A T cell can then bind to the peptide but only if the T-cell receptor site is appropriate for that antigen. The T-cell receptor protein-binding site is formed from a combination of elements of the two chains (αβ chains or γδ chains). Differences in the amino acid sequences of areas of these chains and their combining abilities bestow the diversity and specificity of the T-cell receptor antigen recognition. Thus, when MHC-presented antigens bind to selective T-cell receptors via the protein-binding site, only a very small number of T cells recognize a particular antigen, participate in this specific interaction, and become activated. It has been estimated that this occurs in only 0.01% of an individual's T cells with typical antigens (47).

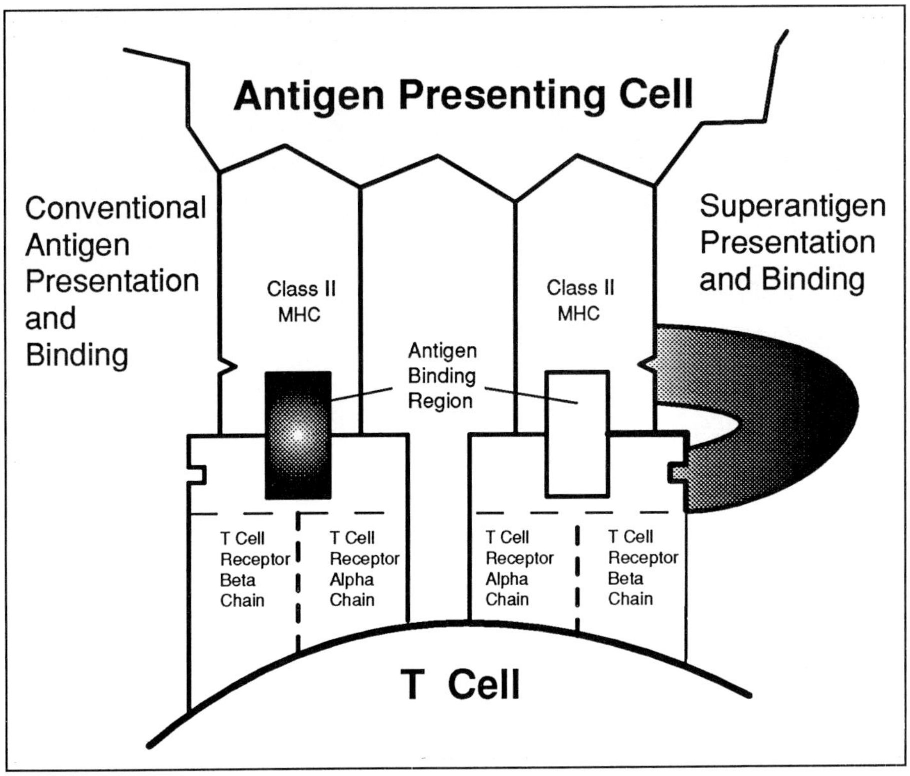

Figure 2. Conventional antigen versus superantigen presentation by class II MHC receptors and binding to T-cell receptor. Conventionally processed peptide antigen is bound to the T-cell receptor in the antigen-binding region of the T-cell receptor. Alternatively, superantigen does not require intracellular procession and binds to areas of T-cell receptor outside the conventional antigen-binding receptor. (Artwork courtesy of D. D. Gellatly.)

A. Fever lasting for at least 5 days*
B. Presence of four of the following five conditions
   1. Bilateral conjunctival injection
   2. Changes of mucosa of the oropharynx, including injected pharynx, injected and/or dry fissured lips, strawberry tongue
   3. Changes of the peripheral extremities, such as edema and/or erythema of hands and/or feet, desquamation usually beginning periungually
   4. Rash, primarily truncal; polymorphous but nonvesicular
   5. Cervical lymphadenopathy
C. Illness not explained by other known disease process

Figure 3. Diagnostic criteria for Kawasaki Disease (4). *Many experts believe that, in the presence of classic features, the diagnosis of Kawasaki disease can be made (and treatment instituted) by experienced individuals before the 5th day of fever.

Measles
Group A streptococcal infection
Other viral infections, drug reactions
Juvenile rheumatoid arthritis
Scarlet fever
Staphylococcal scalded skin syndrome
Toxic shock syndrome
Rocky Mountain spotted fever
Leptospirosis
Stevens-Johnson syndrome

Figure 4. Differential diagnoses of Kawasaki disease (6,53).

A superantigen is also bound to an MHC molecule on the antigen-presenting cell but does not require internal processing by the presenting cell. In addition, rather than the conventional antigen-binding groove of the T cell, a superantigen binds to the outer hypervariable 4 region (V_β) of the β chain (Fig 2), an area with a relatively small number of variability. Thus, superantigens may stimulate a much larger number of T cells expressing particular β chain gene sequences (estimated at 10%–40%). In this manner, superantigens activate large numbers of T cells instead of the very small number that conventional antigen presentation activate through the T-cell protein-binding groove (47,48). These activated T cells produce cytokines, such as interleukin-2, which are thought to be mediators of the systemic signs and symptoms of disease, such as fever, malaise, nausea, and shock (47,49).

Supporting this theory has been the discovery that the levels of T cells that bear $V_\beta 2$ and $V_\beta 8$ (sites associated with binding of superantigens) are increased in the first 2 weeks of disease and are subsequently reduced to normal at later stages (43). V_β^+ T cells were found in the myocardium and coronary tissue of an infant who died of acute Kawasaki disease (50). Additionally, studies of the small-bowel mucosa demonstrated selective increase in the population of $V_\beta 2^+$ T cells, especially within the lamina propria (51). These findings suggest the possible role of the small intestine as the portal of entry site for presentation of the superantigen and further implicate superantigen-producing gram-positive cocci as an infectious agent of Kawasaki disease. Some investigators (48) have found superantigen-secreting staphylococcal or streptococcal strains in the pharynx, small bowel, or rectum of a high percentage of patients with Kawasaki disease (13 of 16 patients) but not in those of control subjects (one of 15 subjects) (34,52). Thus, there are immunologic and microbiologic data supporting the theory that the clinical findings of Kawasaki disease may be caused by a superantigen.

CLINICAL MANIFESTATION AND DIAGNOSIS

Kawasaki disease manifests as an acute febrile illness that can be delineated into acute, subacute, and convalescent phases. The acute phase lasts 7–14 days, the subacute phase extends from days 10 to 24 of illness, and the convalescent stage typically lasts 6–8 weeks. During the acute phase, the diagnosis can be established when a fever of 5 days duration is accompanied by four of five clinical findings of the major criteria (Fig 3) and when other causes for the fever (Fig 4) have been excluded (6,53). The North American criteria differ only slightly from the Japanese diagnostic criteria (4,5). The other five clinical diagnostic criteria are peripheral extremity skin changes, conjunctivitis, mucosal changes, rash, and cervical lymphadenopathy.

Fever, usually the earliest sign, is remittent, spiking to 104°F (40°C) or higher and returning to lower but still elevated levels. It lasts 1–2 weeks without therapy or 2–3 days with aspirin or intravenous gamma globulin therapy. Conjunctival injection primarily involves the bulbar conjunctivae, is rarely exudative, and

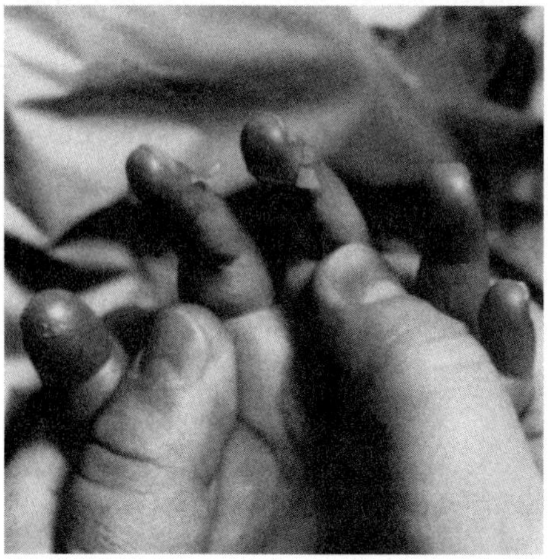

Figure 5. Photograph shows skin changes of Kawasaki disease in a 6-month-old child. Desquamation of the fingertips is visible involving the thumb and the index and middle fingers; this is one of the diagnostic criteria for Kawasaki disease.

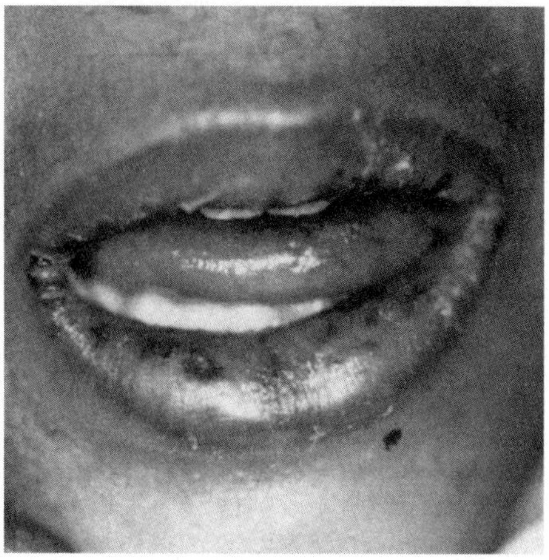

Figure 6. Photograph shows fissuring and bleeding of the lips in a child with Kawasaki disease. These changes are seen more often than other clinical diagnostic criteria.

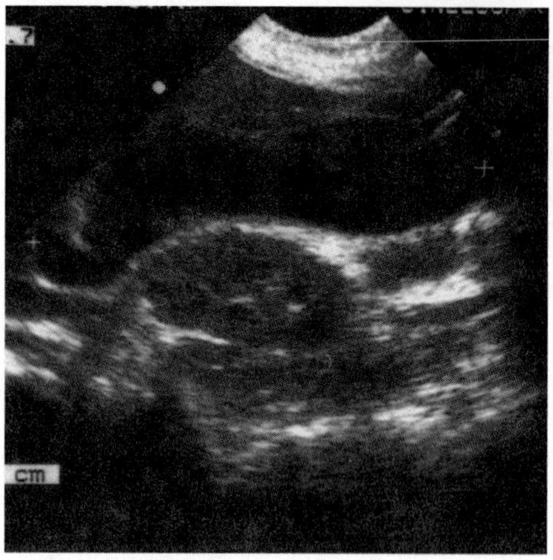

Figure 7. Gallbladder hydrops in a child with Kawasaki disease. Sagittal US image shows an 11-cm gallbladder (between cursors), without evidence of wall thickening or pericholecystic fluid collection. Gallbladder hydrops is the second most commonly described imaging finding other than vascular aneurysm and occurs in approximately 5% of children with Kawasaki disease. (Case courtesy of Lakshmana Das Narla, MD, Medical College of Virgina of Virginia Commonwealth University; reprinted with permission from Advance Newsmagazines [70].)

usually follows the onset of fever. Oral changes involve erythema of the lips, mucosa, and tongue without ulceration. Peeling, fissuring, and bleeding of the lips and a strawberry tongue are common. The hands and feet typically become swollen and erythematous, with desquamation beginning approximately 10–20 days after the onset of illness in the periungual region and extending to the palms and soles (Figs 5, 6). Transverse grooves across the nails (Beau lines) develop approximately 1–2 months later. The rash of Kawasaki disease is nonspecific and generally develops within 5 days of the onset of fever. It may be urticarial exanthem or a maculopapular rash, may have target lesions, or may be micropustular. The rash typically involves the trunk and the extremities with prominence of the perineum. The least common of the major clinical criteria is cervical lymphadenopathy, which is seen 50%–75% of the time, as compared with 90% for the other major criteria. The adenopathy is usually unilateral, may be firm and tender, or have overlying erythema, but in general it is not suppurative, although peritonsillar abscess, acute mastoiditis, neck abscess, parapharyngeal abscess, and retropharyngeal mass have been reported (4,54,55).

Although the diagnostic criteria require fever of 5 days duration, many experts prefer to treat otherwise classic Kawasaki disease before the 5th day. In addition, some children have disease that does not meet the diagnostic criteria but have a similar clinical course with development of coronary artery aneurysms. It is likely that many of these children, especially the infants, have incomplete or atypical Kawasaki disease (4). Some experts in North America will consider a child with fever, two of five diagnostic criteria, and coronary arteritis to have atypical disease, whereas in Japan a child with any three of five diagnostic criteria (with or without coronary arteritis) would be considered to have atypical Kawasaki disease (5). Thus, Kawasaki disease may be considered as a diagnosis in a child with unexplained fever and no other definable cause so the child may be treated appropriately to reduce the frequency of and screen for possible cardiac complications (4,56–58).

Recurrent episodes, defined as a new onset of illness after 3 months, can occur in 1% of the children. If fever returns accompanied by at least one other acute diagnostic feature, the child is considered to have clinical rebound, which most often occurs within a few weeks of initial onset (4–6).

CLINICAL AND IMAGING FEATURES

The underlying systemic vasculitis of Kawasaki disease may present as a wide spectrum of clinical and radiologic findings.

General and Head and Neck Features

During the acute phase of Kawasaki disease, children are extremely irritable and also may develop aseptic meningitis (10%–25%), hyperemic tympanic membrane (27%), or uveitis (17%) (59). During the subacute phase, the fever, rash, and lymphadenopathy generally resolve, while conjunctival injection, irritability, and anorexia persist. Neurologic complications, which may be seen in 1% of the children with Kawasaki disease, include facial nerve palsy, seizures, ataxia, encephalopathy, hemiplegia, and cerebral infarction (3,6,21–24,27,46,53,60–63). Less common findings include erythema and induration at a recent bacille Calmette-Guérin, or BCG, vaccination site (6), thrombocytosis, and histiocytic hemophagocytosis (53,54).

Abdominal features

Renal involvement includes urethritis, priapism (65), epididymo-orchitis (66), cystitis, prostatitis (14), acute renal failure, interstitial nephritis, and nephrotic syndrome (67,68). Isolated azotemia may be seen in up to 3% of children (69). At ultrasound (US) examination, enlarged kidneys with increased renal echoes and enhanced corticomedullary differentiation may be seen in children who have associated elevation of creatinine, blood urea nitrogen, and proteinuria (68).

Acute gastrointestinal findings include diarrhea (15%), hepatic dysfunction with elevated liver function test results (5%), and gallbladder hydrops (5%) (Fig 7).

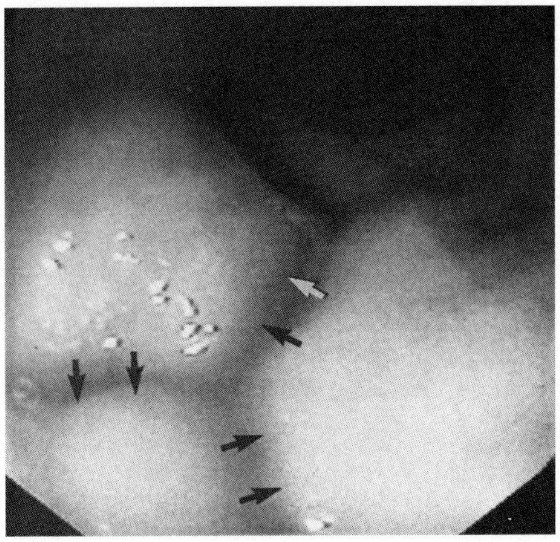

a.

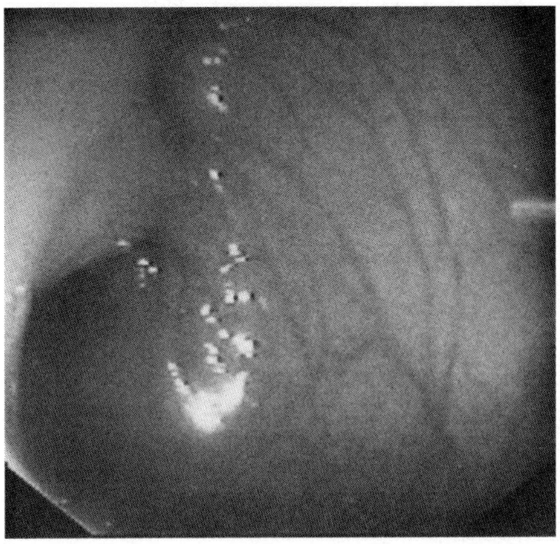

b.

Figure 8. Colonic edema visible at colonoscopy in a 4-year-old child with Kawasaki disease. **(a)** Image from colonoscopy demonstrates multiple nodular areas (arrows) in the colon that are consistent with mucosal and submucosal edema of the colon. **(b)** Another image from the same colonoscopic examination shows a normal area of the colon.

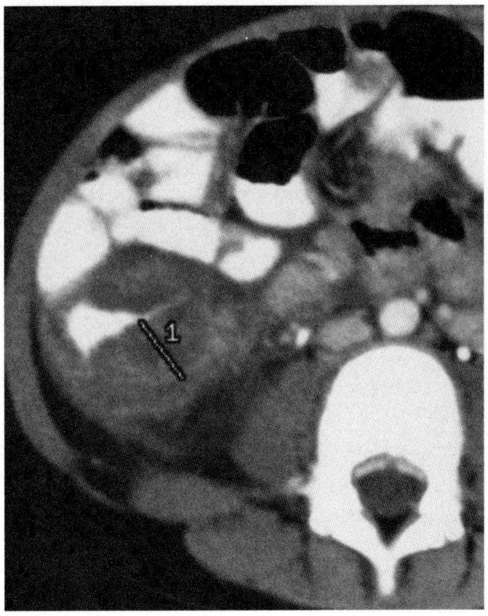

Figure 9. Computed tomography (CT) of colonic edema in a 4-year-old child with Kawasaki disease. Axial CT scan of the lower abdomen demonstrates considerable colonic wall thickening (*1 line*) in the right colon. Stranding of the pericolonic fat is most consistent with edema. Although patients with Kawasaki disease often may present with abdominal pain or diarrhea, abscess formation or superinfection is rare and surgery may be contraindicated.

Whereas gallbladder hydrops is thought to occur due to extension of periportal inflammation to the cystic duct and is generally self-limited, cholecystectomy may be required in very rare cases (71). Surgery, however, is discouraged, and serial US to evaluate for hydrops is recommended because the surgical mortality rate is reported to be as high as 25%, presumably secondary to the superimposed cardiovascular abnormalities of Kawasaki disease (72–74). Other gastrointestinal findings that may be seen include splenic infarct (75), pancreatitis (76), jejunal stricture and adhesion (77), colonic obstruction (78), intussusception (69), intestinal pseudo-obstruction (Fig 8) (79), bowel edema (Fig 9) (80), ascites, adenopathy, and cholangitis (81,82). The specific frequencies of these findings are not certain, but in one autopsy series (14), vasculitis of the renal artery was seen in 50% of cases, intestinal and hepatic vessels in over 75%, and splenic artery in 50%.

Chest Features

Although clinical pulmonary symptoms generally do not occur or may simulate influenza (14), radiographic changes are common (Fig 10). In one review (83), 14.7% of children with Kawasaki disease had abnormal findings on chest radiographs, including reticulogranular pattern in 89.5%, peribronchial cuffing in 21.1%, pleural effusion in 15.8%, atelectasis in 10.5%, and air trapping in 5.3%. Radiographic abnormalities were present within 10 days after initial onset and resolved 10–50 days after onset.

Musculoskeletal and Extremity Features

Arthritis and arthralgia have been commonly noted (30%) in the acute phase, although less commonly seen since the introduction of intravenous gamma globulin therapy. Other musculoskeletal findings include sacroiliitis (84), myositis (85), and avascular necrosis of the femoral head (86). Periungual desquamation and peripheral gangrene may also develop during the subacute phase (3,6,21–24,27,46,61,63,87,88).

CARDIOVASCULAR INVOLVEMENT

Kawasaki disease is known to be a major cause of acquired heart disease in children and will likely be an important cause of acquired heart disease of adults in whom the occurrence of Kawasaki disease is common. A study of 598 children with Kawasaki disease demonstrated that 4.7% developed ischemic heart disease, 1.9% developed myocardial infarction, and 0.8% died of cardiac complications (8). Kawasaki disease also likely accounts for a large percentage of coronary disease in young adults (33). In one study of 130 adults with coronary aneurysms, 21 had definite or suspected history of Kawasaki disease during childhood, and 82% of these patients presented with myocardial infarction during strenuous exercise (7,89). Because cardiac lesions account for most of the mortality and morbidity, much of the treatment, imaging, and follow-up of children with Kawasaki disease is focused on reducing the prevalence of cardiac complications (19).

Coronary aneurysm is said to occur in 20%–25% of children with Kawasaki disease not treated with intravenous gamma globulin therapy and aspirin (Fig 11a) (8,9). In one review (63), the frequency of coronary artery aneurysms was 79% in infants with Kawasaki disease who were younger than 6 months compared with 44% in infants 6–12 months of age. Most of the aneurysms occurred within 3–6 months of acute illness. Involvement was in the left coronary artery in 12% of cases, right coronary artery in 3%, and both arteries in 8% (8). Coronary artery aneurysms are classified as small if less than 5 mm in internal diameter, medium if 5–8 mm, or giant if larger than 8 mm (35). These aneurysms can be seen on echocardiograms, magnetic resonance (MR) images, or coronary angiograms, although the external diameter of the aneurysm may be underestimated on the angiogram due to intraluminal clot or intimal hyperplasia (90). Small coronary aneurysms regress, but medium and giant aneurysms may remain unchanged or even progress to stenosis (9). In addition, ring calcification of coronary artery aneurysms (Fig 12) is seen on the chest radiograph in 36.4% of adults with history of Kawasaki disease (89).

Although coronary artery aneurysm is the best known cardiovascular lesion as-

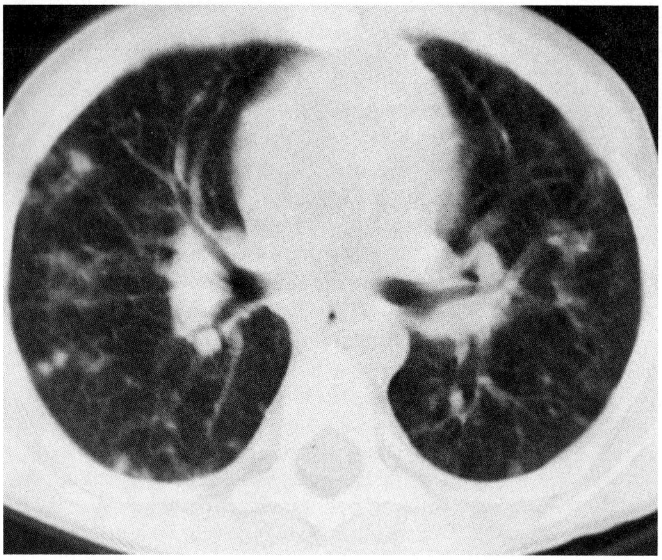

Figure 10. Pulmonary nodules at CT in a 4-year-old child with Kawasaki disease. Helical, 5-mm (pitch 1) CT scan of the thorax demonstrates multiple, ill-defined, mostly peripheral small nodules in the lungs. These lesions did not enhance visibly with contrast material so as to exclude aneurysms. Also, diffuse increased interstitial markings are seen bilaterally, a common finding in patients with Kawasaki disease. The prominent soft-tissue areas in the hila correspond to enlarged pulmonary arteries.

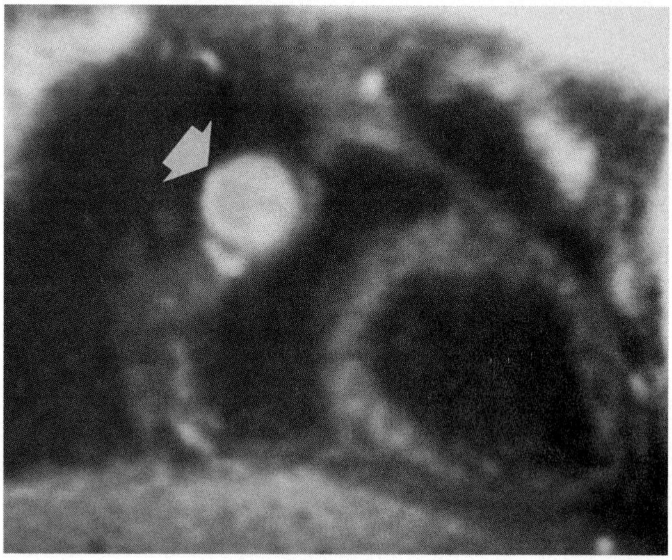

a.

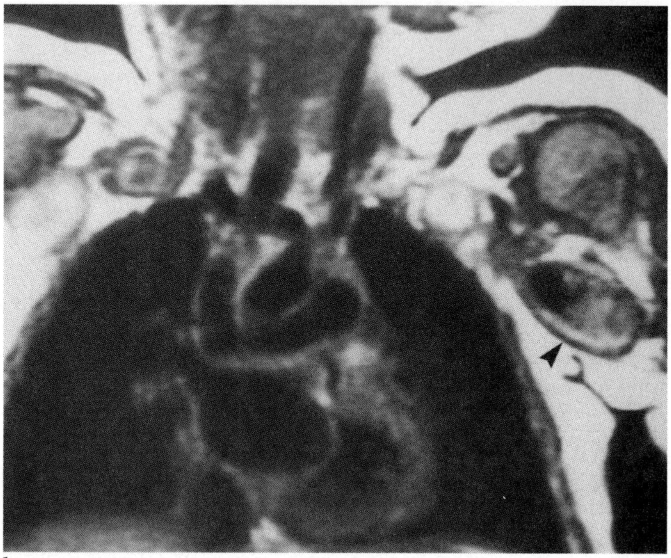

b.

Figure 11. Aneurysms at MR imaging in a 7-month-old child with Kawasaki disease. **(a)** Gated coronal spin-echo MR image (cardiac gated; repetition time, 500 msec; echo time, 20 msec) of the chest demonstrates a focal hyperintense area (arrow) within the coronary artery consistent with a coronary artery aneurysm. **(b)** Coronal MR image of the thorax shows fusiform dilatation (arrowhead) of the axillary artery consistent with peripheral aneurysm. (Case courtesy of George Bisset III, MD, Duke University, Durham, NC.)

sociated with Kawasaki disease, myocarditis and development of coronary artery stenosis are likely more clinically important. Stress myocardial perfusion studies have demonstrated that perfusion defects are not strongly associated with aneurysms but are probably associated with stenosis (91). A study of segmental wall motion abnormalities in 53 children with Kawasaki disease failed to demonstrate a statistically significant correlation of coronary abnormalities and wall motion abnormalities, suggesting that wall motion abnormalities may be due to myocarditis, which may be seen on radiolabeled leukocyte scans (11,92). Other cardiac manifestations of Kawasaki disease include pericarditis with pericardial effusions, wall motion abnormality, valvulitis or papillary muscle dysfunction, and acute mitral regurgitation secondary to rupture of chordae tendineae (6,11,35, 93). Findings seen in the noncoronary vascular system are similar to those seen with coronary arteries, including stenosis, thrombosis, and aneurysm formation (Fig 11b), particularly in the axillary artery (87,88).

TREATMENT AND PROGNOSIS

Treatment of Kawasaki disease should be viewed as a therapeutic and management plan for the acute, subacute, and convalescent phases of disease. The plan in each phase differs depending on which pathologic processes are present, the severity of disease, systems involved, and outcome expected. In the acute phase of the disease, the primary objectives are to make a definitive diagnosis, to provide supportive care as needed (eg, fluid and electrolytes), and to decrease the inflammatory process. Evaluation of the cardiovascular system is obtained by means of an initial echocardiogram, which is particularly sensitive in depicting the presence of aneurysms in the coronary arteries (35). Electrocardiogram and chest radiographs are also usually obtained in the acute phase.

Early treatment of Kawasaki disease with aspirin and high-dose intravenous gamma globulin has been proved to be effective in reducing the clinical symptoms, as well as the prevalence of coronary aneurysms to approximately 5% (94–96). Since intravenous gamma globulin prescribed as 2 g per kilogram of body

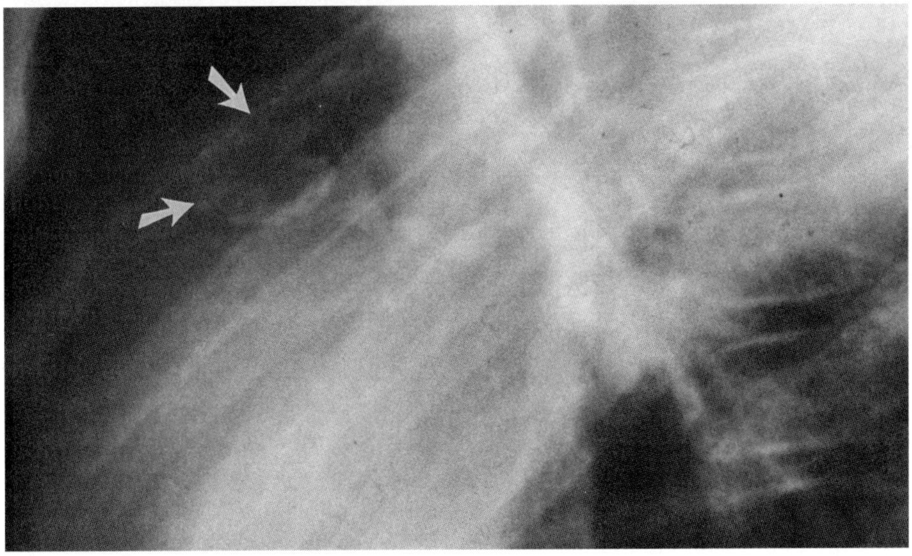

Figure 12. Coronary aneurysm ring calcification in a young adult with history of Kawasaki disease as a child. Lateral chest radiograph shows a ring-shaped opacity (arrows) consistent with a coronary artery aneurysm calcification. This finding may be seen in up to 36.4% of adults with a history of Kawasaki disease.

weight per day given as a single long infusion has been shown to be more effective than multiple doses, this regimen is now the standard recommended initial therapy (93). Treatment with aspirin in the acute phase is generally begun at antiinflammatory doses (100 mg/kg per day in divided doses) and continued until 48–72 hours after resolution of fever or until approximately day 14 of illness. Most patients who receive the intravenous gamma globulin and aspirin treatment regimen experience defervescence within 24 hours, and by 48 hours almost 90% are afebrile (94).

If therapy is successful in the acute phase, the management goals in the subacute phase are to decrease platelet adhesiveness (usually with low-dose aspirin at 3–5 mg/kg per day), to provide supportive care if still needed, and to monitor in case of cardiovascular involvement. In both the subacute and convalescent phases, management plans including activity and follow-up diagnostic testing are based on the presence or absence of coronary artery involvement and risk level present, individualized for each patient (35). Patients with mild arterial abnormalities (ectasias) may be followed up at widely spaced intervals, whereas those with aneurysms are currently followed up at more frequent intervals and by a cardiologist for an indefinite period. Coronary angiography is recommended in a patient who has or has had multiple aneurysms or a giant aneurysm, if stenosis is suggested at echocardiography or stress testing (35). At times, coronary artery bypass grafting may be necessary. The results of at least one multicenter study suggest that the patency rate for internal thoracic or gastroepiploic artery graft is higher (77%) than that for saphenous vein grafts (46%) at 85 months after the operation (97). Obviously, supportive care, emotional support, and a liberal amount of patience are required to help the child and family through the acute phase. As with any chronic rheumatologic disease, education of the family is necessary for optimal success of any management plan.

Approximately 10% of patients do not respond fully or have fever recrudescence after initial treatment with intravenous gamma globulin. To our knowledge, no study has formally examined the comparative efficacies of therapeutic options for these patients. Repeat treatment with intravenous gamma globulin (1–2 g/kg) has been reported successful in approximately 69% (nine of 13 patients) after the second treatment and 85% (11 of 13 patients) after the third treatment (98). The reason for pharmacologic effectiveness of higher doses of intravenous gamma globulin is not yet clear, but the clinical response to the higher single dose may be related to competitive binding of intravenous gamma globulin. The repeat dose is thus usually given with a different manufacturer's brand of intravenous gamma globulin to maximize competitive binding (50,99).

The treatment of patients who are refractory after repeat treatment with intravenous gamma globulin continues to be controversial. An early study (100) found a greater frequency of coronary disease in subjects receiving steroids alone; however, in one small recent report (101), methylprednisolone was used successfully to treat four patients with illness resistant to intravenous gamma globulin. The role of steroids in the treatment of Kawasaki disease is currently being reevaluated.

CONCLUSION

Kawasaki disease is a pediatric febrile vasculitis that may be caused by superantigens. The illness may manifest in any body organ, with clinical and imaging findings of inflammation and edema of the involved organs. There is a predilection for coronary vessels, however, with cardiovascular inflammatory changes such as aneurysms, stenosis, and secondary ischemia responsible for the majority of the morbidity and mortality of the illness. Treatment with aspirin and intravenous gamma globulin has improved the overall outcome; however, Kawasaki disease remains a major cause of acquired heart disease in children and may become a substantial problem for adults who had Kawasaki disease during their childhood.

References

1. Kawasaki T. Acute febrile mucocutaneous syndrome with lymphoid involvement with specific desquamation of the fingers and toes in children: clinical observation of 50 cases. Jpn J Allerg 1967; 16:178–222.
2. Kawasaki T, Kosaki F, Okawa S, Shigematsu I, Yanagawa H. A new infantile acute febrile mucocutaneous lymph node syndrome prevailing in Japan. Pediatrics 1974; 54:271–276.
3. Melish CE, Hicks RM, Larson EJ. Mucocutaneous lymph node syndrome in the United States. Am J Dis Child 1976, 130:599–607.
4. Shulman ST, Bass JL, Bierman F, et al. Management of Kawasaki syndrome: a consensus statement prepared by North American participants of the third international Kawasaki disease symposium, Tokyo, Japan, December, 1988. Pediatr Infect Dis J 1989; 8:663–665.
5. Kawasaki T. Kawasaki disease. Acta Paediatr 1995, 84:713–715.
6. Shulman ST, De Inocencio J, Hirsh R. Kawasaki disease. Pediatr Clin North Am 1995; 42:1205–1222.
7. Kato H, Inoue O, Kawasaki T, Fujiwara H, Watanabe T, Toshima H. Adult coronary artery disease probably due to childhood Kawasaki disease. Lancet 1992; 340:1127–1129.
8. Kato H, Sugimura T, Akagi T, et al. Long-term consequences of Kawasaki disease: a 10 to 21 year follow-up study of 594 patients. Circulation 1996; 94:1379–1385.
9. Fukushige J, Takahashi N, Ueda K, Hijii T,

Ohshima A. Long-term outcome of coronary abnormalities in patients after Kawasaki disease. Pediatr Cardiol 1996; 17:71–76.
10. Takahashi N, Fukushige J, Htii T, Igarashi H, Ooshima A, Ueda K. Occlusion of the right coronary artery as sequelae of Kawasaki disease: the clinical features of nine cases. Cardiology 1995; 86:207–210.
11. Vogel M, Smallhorn JF, Freedon RM. Serial analysis of regional left ventricular wall motion by two-dimensional echocardiography in patients with coronary artery enlargement after Kawasaki disease. J Am Coll Cardiol 1992; 20:915–919.
12. Leung DYM. Kawasaki disease. Curr Opin Rheumatol 1993; 7:455–458.
13. Masuda H, Shozawa T, Naoe S, Tanaka N. The intercostal artery in Kawasaki disease. Arch Pathol Lab Med 1986; 110:1136–1142.
14. Amano S, Hazama F, Kubagawa H, Tasaka K, Haebara H, Hamashima Y. General pathology of Kawasaki disease: on the morphological alterations corresponding to the clinical manifestations. Acta Pathol Jpn 1980; 30:681–694.
15. Fujiwara H, Hamashima Y. Pathology of the heart in Kawasaki disease. Pediatrics 1978; 61:100–107.
16. Masuda H, Naoe S, Tanaka N. A pathological study of coronary artery in Kawasaki disease (MCLS) with special reference to morphogenesis of aneurysm. J Jpn Coll Angiol 1981; 21:899–912.
17. Amano S, Hazama F. Neural involvement in Kawasaki disease. Acta Pathol Jpn 1980; 30:365–373.
18. Rauch AM. Kawasaki syndrome: critical review of US epidemiology. Prog Clin Biol Res 1987; 250:33–44.
19. Yanagawa H, Yashiro M, Nakamura Y, Kawasaki T, Dato H. Results of 12 nationwide epidemiological incidence surveys of Kawasaki disease in Japan. Arch Pediatr Adolesc Med 1995; 149:779–783.
20. Smith PK, Goldwater PN. Kawasaki disease in Adelaide: a review. J Paediatr Child Health 1993; 29:126–131.
21. Salo E. Kawasaki disease in Finland in 1982–1992. Scand J Infect Dis 1993; 25:497–502.
22. Windsor AMB, Schell WL, Davis JP. Kawasaki syndrome in Wisconsin. Wis Med J 1991; 90:227–231.
23. Casey F, Craig B, Shanks D, Jackson P, Mulholland HC. Kawasaki disease: the Northern Ireland experience. Ir J Med Sci 1993; 162:397–400.
24. St John MA, Ishmael RG. Outcome of Kawasaki disease in Barbados. West Indian Med J 1992; 41:68–71.
25. Meade RH, Brandt L. Manifestations of Kawasaki dsease in New England outbreak of 1980. J Pediatr 1982; 100:558–562.
26. Tizard EJ, Suzuki A, Levin M, Dillon MJ. Clinical aspects of 100 patients with Kawasaki disease. Arch Dis Child 1991; 66:185–188.
27. Schiller B, Fasth A, Bjorkhem G, Elinder G. Kawasaki disease in Sweden: incidence and clinical fetures. Acta Paediatr 1995; 84:769–774.
28. Tsuchida S, Yamanaka T, Tsuchida R, Nakamura Y, Yashiro M, Yanagawa H. Epidemiology of infant Kawasaki disease with a report of the youngest neonatal case ever reported in Japan. Acta Paediatr 1996; 85:995–997.
29. Paira SO, Roverano S. Kawasaki syndrome in a young adult. J Rheumatol 1992; 19:488–490.
30. Jackson JL, Kunkel MR, Libow L, Gates RH. Adult Kawasaki disease. Arch Intern Med 1994; 154:1398–1404.
31. Nakamura T, Yanagawa H, Kawasaki T. Mortality among children with Kawasaki disease in Japan. N Engl J Med 1992; 326:1246–1249.
32. Nakamura Y, Yanagawa H, Kato H, Kawasaki T. Mortality rates for patients with a history of Kawasaki disease in Japan. J Pediatr 1996; 128:75–81.
33. Taubert KA, Rowley AH, Shulman ST. Nationwide survey of Kawasaki disease and acute rheumatic fever. J Pediatr 1991; 119: 279–282.
34. Leung DYM, Meissner HC, Fulton DR, Murray DL, Kotzin BL, Schlievert PM. Toxic shock syndrome toxin-secreting *Staphylococcus aureus* in Kawasaki syndrome. Lancet 1993; 342:1385–1388.
35. Dajani AS, Taubert KA, Takahashi M, et al. Guidelines for long-term management of patients with Kawasaki disease: report from the Committee on Rheumatic Fever, Endocartitis, and Kawasaki Disease, Council on Cardiovascular Disease in the Young, American Heart Association. Circulation 1994; 89:916–922.
36. Patriarca PA, Rogers M, Morens D, et al. Kawasaki syndrome: association with the application of rug shampoo. Lancet 1982; ii:578–580.
37. Rauch AM. Kawasaki syndrome: review of new epidemiologic and laboratory developments. Pediatr Infect Dis J 1987; 6:1016–1021.
38. Rauch AM, Kaplan SL, Nihill MR, Pappas PG, Hurwitz ES, Schonberger LB. Kawasaki syndrome clusters in Harris County, Texas and Eastern North Carolina: a high endemic rate and a new environmental risk factor. Am J Dis Child 1988; 142:441–444.
39. Rauch AM, Glode MP, Wiggins JW, et al. Outbreak of Kawasaki syndrome in Denver, Colorado: association with rug and carpet cleaning. Pediatrics 1991; 87:663–669.
40. Fujita Y, Nakamura T, Sakata K, et al. Kawaski disease in families. Pediatrics 1989; 84:666–669.
41. Nigro G, Pisano P, Krzysztofiak A. Recurrent Kawasaki disease associated with co-infection with parvovirus B19 and HIV-1. AIDS 1993; 7:288–290.
42. Leung DYM. Immunologic aspects of Kawasaki disease: implications for pathogenesis and therapy. Clin Cardiol 1991; 14(suppl 2):11–15.
43. Abe J, Kotzin Bl, Jujo K, et al. Selective expansion of T cells expressing T-cell receptor variable regions $V_\beta 2$ and $V_\beta 8$ in Kawasaki disease. Proc Natl Acad Sci USA 1992; 89: 4066–4070.
44. Lang BA, Silverman ED, Laxer RM, Rose V, Nelson DL, Rubin LA. Serum-soluble interleukin-2 receptor levels in Kawasaki disease. J Pediatr 1990; 116:592–596.
45. Furukawa S, Matsubara T, Tsuji K, Motohashi T, Okumura K, Yabuta K. Serum soluble CD4 and CD8 levels in Kawasaki disease. Clin Exp Immunol 1991; 86:134–139.
46. Meissner HC, Leung DYM. Kawasaki syndrome. Curr Opin Rheumatol 1995; 7:455–458.
47. Drake CG, Kotzin BL. Superantigens: biology, immunology, and potential role in disease. J Clin Immunol 1992; 12:149–162.
48. Leung DYM. Superantigens related to Kawasaki syndrome. Springer Semin Immunopathol 1996; 17:385–396.
49. Resnick SD. Toxic shock syndrome: recent developments in pathogenesis. J Pediatr 1990; 116:321–328.
50. Leung DYM. Kawasaki syndrome: immunomodulatory benefit and potential toxin neutralization by intravenous immune globulin. Clin Exp Immunol 1996; 104(suppl 1):49–54.
51. Yamashiro Y, Nagata S, Oguchi S, Shimizu T. Selective increase of $V_\beta 2^+$ T cells in the small intestinal mucosa in Kawasaki disease. Pediatr Res 1996; 39:264–266.
52. Yamashiro Y, Nagata S, Ohtsuka Y, Ogushi S, Shimizu T. Microbiologic studies on the small intestine in Kawasaki disease. Pediatr Res 1996; 39:622–624.
53. Burns JC, Mason WH, Glode MPS, et al. Clinical and epidemiologic characeristics of patients referred for evaluation of possible Kawasaki disease. J Pediatr 1991; 118:680–686.
54. Hester TO, Harris JP, Kenny JF, Albernaz MS. Retropharyngeal cellulitis: a manifestation of Kawasaki disease in children. Otolaryngol Head Neck Surg 1993; 109:1030–1033.
55. Pontell J, Rosenfeld RM, Kohn B. Kawasaki disease mimicking retropharyngeal abscess. Otolaryngol Head Neck Surg 1994; 110:428–430.
56. Fukushige J, Takahashi N, Ueda Y, Ueda K. Incidence and clinical features of incomplete Kawasaki disease. Acta Paediatr 1994; 83:1057–1060.
57. Joffe A, Kabani A, Jadavji T. Atypical and complicated Kawasaki disease in infants: do we need criteria? West J Med 1995; 162:322–327.
58. Boven K, DeGraeff-Meeder ER, Spliet W, Kuis W. Atypical kawasaki disease: an often missed diagnosis. Eur J Pediatr 1992; 151:577–580.
59. Lacroix J, Lapointe N, Weber M, et al. Prospective study of 64 cases of Kawasaki's disease. Arch Fran Pediatr 1985; 42:771–776.
60. Terasawa K, Ichinose E, Matsuishi T, Kato H. Neurological complications in Kawasaki disease. Brain Dev 1993; 5:371–374.
61. Gallagher PG. Facial nerve paralysis and Kawasaki disease. Rev Infect Dis 1990; 12:403–405.
62. Kryzer T, Derkay DS. Kawasaki disease: five-year experience at Children's National Medical Center. Int J Pediatr Otorhinolaryngol 1992; 23:211–220.
63. Rosenfeld EA, Corydon KE, Shulman ST. Kawasaki disease in infants less than one year of age. J Pediatr 1995; 126:524–529.
64. Ohga S, Ooshima A, Fukushige J, Ueda K. Histiocytic haemophagocytosis in a patient with Kawasaki disease: changes in the hypercytokinaemic state. Eur J Pediatr 1995; 154:539–541.
65. Waring NP, Ortenberg J, Galen WK, Robinson C, Baker A. Priapism in Kawasaki disease. JAMA 1989; 261:1730–1731.
66. Sacco M, Meleleo D, Castriota Scanderbeg A. Hydrocele in Kawasaki disease. Pediatr Med Chir 1995; 17:279–280.
67. Lee B, Yap H, Yip W, Giam Y, Tay J. Nephrotic syndrome in Kawasaki disease. Aust Pediatr J 1989; 25:241–242.
68. Nardi P, Haller J, Friedman A, Slovis T, Schaffer R. Renal manifestations of Kawasaki's disease. Pediatr Radiol 1985; 15:116–118.
69. Huang Y, Lin T, Su W. Unusual manifestations in children with Kawasaki disease. J Formos Med Assoc 1997; 96:451–456.
70. Dunn MM, Das Narla L, Spiegle JB, Spottswood SE, Hingsbergen EA. Under-

standing and imaging pediatric patients with Kawasaki syndrome. Adv Administrators Radiol Radiat Oncol 1996; May:21–24.
71. Falcini F, Trpani S, Pampaloni A, Ienuso R, Pollini I, Bartolozzi G. Hydrops of gallbladder requiring cholecystectomy in Kawasaki syndrome. Clin Exp Rheumatol 1990; 11:99–100.
72. Mercer S, Carpenter B. Surgical complications of Kawasaki disease. J Pediatr Surg 1981; 16:444–448.
73. Wheeler R, Najmaldin A, Soubra M, Griffiths D, Burge D, Atwell J. Surgical presentation of Kawasaki disease (mucocutaneous lymph node syndrome). Br J Surg 1990; 77:1273–1274.
74. Waldron RJ. Kawasaki disease and anaesthesia. Anaesth Intensive Care 1993; 21:213–217.
75. Huong D, Gatfosse M, Papo T, Barjonet G, Lacombe P, Godeau P. Symptomatic splenic infarction complicating adult Kawasaki disease. Br J Rheumatol 1995; 34:579–580.
76. Lanting W, Muinos W, Kamani N. Pancreatitis heralding Kawasaki disease. J Pediatr 1992; 21:743–744.
77. Murphy DJ, Morrow WR, Harberg FJ, Hawkins EP. Small bowel obstruction as a complication of Kawasaki disease. Clin Pediatr 1987; 26:193–196.
78. Fan S, Lau W, Wong K. Ischemic colitis in Kawasaki disease. J Pediatr Surg 1986; 21:964–965.
79. Franken E, Kleiman M, Norins A, Smith J, Smith W. Intestinal pseudo-obstuction in mucocutaneous lymph-node syndrome. Radiology 1979; 130:649–651.
80. Chung CJ, Rayder S, Meyers W, Long J. Kawasaki disease presenting as focal colitis. Pediatr Radiol 1996; 26:455–457.
81. Gear J, Meyers K, Steele M. Kawasaki disease manifesting with acute cholangitis. S Afr Med J 1991; 81:31–33.
82. Bader-Meunier B, Hadchouel M, Fabre M, Arnoud MD, Dommergues JP. Intrahepatic bile duct damage in children with Kawasaki disease. J Pediatr 1992; 120:750–752.
83. Umezawa T, Saji T, Matsuo N, Odagiri K. Chest x-ray findings in the acute phase of Kawasaki disease. Pediatr Radiol 1989; 20:48–51.
84. Herrero J, Ornia N, Serrano O, et al. Kawasaki's syndrome in the adult and bilateral sacroiliitis. Ann Med Interne 1995; 12:549–545.
85. Koutras A. Myositis with Kawasaki's disease. Am J Dis Child 1982; 136:78–79.
86. Yanagitani Y, Fujita M. Avascular necrosis of the femoral head associated with mucocutaneous lymph node syndrome. J Pediatr Orthop 1986; 6:107–109.
87. von Planta M, Fasnacht M, Holm C, Fanconi S, Seger R. Atypical Kawasaki disease with peripheral gangrene and myocardial infarction: therapeutic implications. Eur J Pediatr 1995; 154:830–834.
88. Tomita S, Chung K, Mas M, Gidding S, Shulman ST. Peripheral gangrene associated with Kawasaki disease. Clin Infect Dis 1992; 14:121–126.
89. Burns JC, Shike H, Gordon JB, Malhotra A, Schoenwetter M, Kawasaki T. Sequelae of Kawasaki disease in adolescents and young adults. J Am Coll Cardiol 1996; 28:253–257.
90. Bisset GS, Strife JL, McCloskey J. MR imaging of coronary artery aneurysms in a child with Kawasaki disease. AJR 1989; 152:805–807.
91. Hijazi ZM, Udelson JE, Snapper H, et al. Physiologic significance of chronic coronary aneurysms in patients with Kawasaki disease. J Am Coll Cardiol 1994; 24:1633–1638.
92. Kao CH, Hsieh KS, Chen YC, Wang YL, Wang SJ, Yeh SH. Labeled WBC cardiac imaging and two-dimensional echocardiography to evaluate high-dose gamma globulin treatment in Kawasaki disease. Clin Nucl Med 1995; 20:813–816.
93. Mishima A, Asano M, Saito T, et al. Mitral regurgitation caused by ruptured chordae tendineae in Kawasaki disease. J Thorac Cardiovasc Surg 1996; 111:895–896.
94. Newburger JW, Takahashi M, Beiser AS, et al. A single intravenous infusion of gamma globulin as compared with four infusions in the treatment of acute Kawasaki syndrome. N Engl J Med 1991; 324:1633–1639.
95. Hsu CH, Chen MR, Hwang FY, Kao HA, Hung HY, Hsu CS. Efficacy of plasmin-treated intravenous gamma-globulin for therapy of Kawasaki syndrome. Pediatr Infect Dis J 1993; 12:509–511.
96. Durongpistkul D, Gururaj V, Park JM, Martin CF. The prevention of coronary artery aneurysm in Kawasaki disease: a meta-analysis on the efficacy of aspirin and immunoglobulin treatment. Pediatrics 1995; 96:1057–1061.
97. Kitamura S, Yoichi K, Seki T, et al. Long-term outcome of myocardial revascularization in patients with Kawasaki coronary artery disease. J Thorac Cardiovasc Surg 1994; 107:663–674.
98. Sundel RP, Burns JC, Baker A, Beiser AS, Newburger JW. Gamma globulin re-treatment in Kawasaki disease. J Pediatr 1993; 123:657–659.
99. Wolf HM, Eibl MM. Immunomodulatory effect of immunoglobulins. Clin Exp Rheumatol 1996; 14(suppl 15):17–25.
100. Kato H, Koike S, Yokomaya T. Kawasaki disease: effect of treatment on coronary involvement. Pediatrics 1976; 63:175–179.
101. Wright DA, Newburger JW, Baker A, Sundel RP. Treatment of immune globulin resistant Kawasaki disease with pulsed doses of corticosteroids. J Pediatr 1996; 128:146–149.

Book Review

Naked to the Bone: Medical Imaging in the Twentieth Century

Bettyann Holtzmann Kevles
New Brunswick, NJ: Rutgers University Press, 1997. ISBN 0-8135-2358-3.
Hardcover, $35.95; pp 392; 74 figures.

The recent centennial of the discovery of x rays has prompted a spate of interest in radiation history. Books on the subject have ranged from fact-laden chronicles to more interpretive works that explore the cultural effect of radiation. *Naked to the Bone* incorporates both approaches in dealing with the history of medical imaging.

The first half of the book deals with radiography. Wilhelm C. Roentgen's discovery and the resultant furor in the scientific community and lay press are discussed in a standard chronologic format. There are some interesting sidelights, however. Philipp Lenard's acrimonious tiff with Roentgen over primacy in the discovery of x rays provides a personal, if unseemly, glimpse of the conflict between these two men that belies the calm, scientific façade of their investigational treatises. So, too, Alexander Graham Bell's attempt to localize the bullet within assassinated President James A. Garfield's body is a fascinating bit of imaging history. In addition, the story of early forensic radiology is spiced with tales of infidelity, murder, and medical misdeed.

Because this book does not aim to be an exhaustive historical treatise, some topics are discussed in less depth. The events leading to recognition of the dangers of radiation, the story of early radiation safety standards, and the steady stream of radiographic innovations (eg, Coolidge tube, Bucky-Potter grid, contrast materials) are among these topics.

The second half of the book details the origins of imaging modalities beyond basic radiography, such as computed tomography, magnetic resonance imaging, mammography, and positron emission tomography. The contest between Paul C. Lauterbur and Raymond V. Damadian for "father of MRI" honors makes for some colorful reading. Otherwise, these chapters essentially are a chronologic overview of the people and places important in the early years of these fledgling modalities. Since the author is a science journalist and not a radiation sciences worker, the few errors in this more technical portion of the book are forgivable: "Spiral CT ... is usually used without any contrast media."

The lengthy section on the revolutionary effect of medical imaging on art offers a lively and eclectic assortment of works inspired by the new "transparency" that radiation provides. The tone of the text becomes a bit more pointed in the chapter on radiation and popular culture: "The X-rays ... penetrated the flesh of human women, unveiling their age-old secrets.... Since much of the unveiling was done by men, it can be construed as a kind of visual deflowering." And similarly, "male doctors experimented by 'poking X-ray projectors and radioactive substances into every part of their patient's bodies ... with a special interest in irradiating the vagina and the uterus.'" By highlighting this perceived misogyny in the history of our specialty, the author clearly has not sought to sidestep controversy.

For the reader seeking a thumbnail sketch of how medical imaging came to be (in particular, one who loves contemporary art and feminism), this book is a good choice. From a purely historical standpoint, it cannot compete with the more encyclopedic and lavishly illustrated tomes—nor is it meant to. Its strength is that it emphasizes just how deeply medical imaging has been incorporated into the fabric of our culture.

Reviewed by David J. DiSantis, MD

US of the Painful Hip in Childhood: Diagnostic Value of Cartilage Thickening and Muscle Atrophy in the Detection of Perthes Disease[1]

Simon G. F. Robben, MD
Morteza Meradji, MD
Ad F. M. Diepstraten, MD
Wim C. J. Hop, PhD

Index terms:
Bones, necrosis, 442.443
Cartilage, 442.1298, 442.443
Cartilage, US, 442.1298
Hip, diseases, 44.443
Hip, US, 44.1298
Joints, fluid, 44.254
Muscles, US, 44.1298

Radiology 1998; 208:35–42

Abbreviation:
SCFE = slipped capital femoral epiphysis

[1] From the Departments of Pediatric Radiology (S.G.F.R., M.M.) and Pediatric Orthopedic Surgery (A.F.M.D.), Sophia Children's Hospital, University Hospital Rotterdam, Dr Molewaterplein 60, 3015 GJ Rotterdam, The Netherlands, and the Department of Epidemiology and Biostatistics, Erasmus University, Rotterdam, The Netherlands (W.C.J.H.). Received April 14, 1997; revision requested June 3; final revision received February 2, 1998; accepted March 5. **Address reprint requests to** S.G.F.R.

PURPOSE: To evaluate the combined use of several ultrasonographic (US) criteria in the detection of Perthes disease.

MATERIALS AND METHODS: In a prospective study, 144 consecutive children with a painful hip underwent US. The thicknesses of the (*a*) anterior recess of the joint capsule, (*b*) cartilage of the femoral head, and (*c*) quadriceps muscle were assessed. Sixty-eight children with no symptoms, the control group, were also examined.

RESULTS: The final diagnosis was transient synovitis (n = 58), Perthes disease (n = 21), slipped capital femoral epiphysis (SCFE; n = 5), or miscellaneous (n = 6). Fifty-four patients had no US or radiographic abnormalities, and symptoms disappeared during follow-up. The anterior recess in patients with transient synovitis was significantly wider than that in the other patients and control subjects ($P < .001$). Patients with Perthes disease showed significant cartilage thickening in the symptomatic hip compared with the other patients and control subjects ($P < .001$). Patients with Perthes disease and patients with SCFE showed significant atrophy of the ipsilateral quadriceps muscle compared with all other groups ($P < .001$). The combined use of these US criteria for the diagnosis of Perthes disease resulted in a positive predictive value of 95%, a negative predictive value of 95%, a sensitivity of 71%, and a specificity of 99%.

CONCLUSION: The combination of several US criteria increases the diagnostic value of US of the painful hip in patients with Perthes disease.

The pediatric hip is susceptible to a large variety of diseases that may manifest as localized or referred pain, limping, refusal to bear weight, and limitation of movement of the hip. These symptoms, however, are nonspecific, and many diseases produce the same clinical picture (eg, Perthes disease, septic arthritis, slipped capital femoral epiphysis [SCFE], osteomyelitis, juvenile chronic arthritis, neoplasm, trauma, and nonaccidental injury).

Some authors recommend ultrasonography (US) as the examination of choice for painful hips, omitting radiography in uncomplicated cases (1–6). Unfortunately, the role of US has been limited to the detection of effusion; moreover, because several diseases are accompanied by effusion, the discriminatory value of US is limited. Other US criteria, however, such as cartilage thickening and muscle atrophy, have the potential to be useful. Thickening of articular cartilage is recognized as an early US sign of Perthes disease (5,7). Muscle atrophy is important because muscular components respond rapidly to changes in activity patterns (8), and clinical studies have reported considerable muscle atrophy in patients with Perthes disease (9,10).

In this prospective study, the thicknesses of the musculature, joint cartilage, and anterior joint capsule were assessed in all patients presenting with a painful hip. We performed this study to determine whether the use of a combination of these criteria increased the US capacity to help

Author contributions:
Guarantor of integrity of entire study, S.G.F.R.; study concepts and design, S.G.F.R., M.M.; definition of intellectual content, S.G.F.R., M.M.; literature research, S.G.F.R.; clinical studies, A.F.M.D., S.G.F.R.; data acquisition, S.G.F.R.; data analysis, S.G.F.R., W.C.J.H.; statistical analysis, W.C.J.H.; manuscript preparation and editing, S.G.F.R.; manuscript review, M.M., A.F.M.D.

differentiate between various diseases and to help detect Perthes disease in a population of children with painful hips.

MATERIALS AND METHODS

Between January 1994 and August 1995, 144 consecutive children with clinical symptoms of hip disease were examined in a prospective study. There were 88 boys and 56 girls aged 1.1–15.6 years (mean, 6.4 years). Patients with bilateral symptoms were excluded. We also examined 68 children without symptoms or previous orthopedic disease. This control group comprised 45 boys and 23 girls aged 1.6–14.3 years (mean, 6.7 years).

The study was approved by the institutional medical ethical review board. Informed consent was obtained from parents and children before the examination.

All patients and control subjects were examined with US by the same investigator (S.G.F.R.); 7–10-MHz (Ultramark 9 HDI; Advanced Technology Laboratories, Bothell, Wash) and 7-MHz (model 128 XP10; Acuson, Mountain View, Calif) linear-array transducers were used. Patients were examined in the supine position with hips in a neutral position. Both hips were examined; the contralateral, asymptomatic hip was used as a normal reference. The thicknesses of the (*a*) anterior recess of the joint capsule, (*b*) articular cartilage of the femoral head, and (*c*) quadriceps muscle were assessed.

To evaluate the anterior recess of the joint capsule, an anterior approach along the long axis of the femoral neck was used to depict the anterior recess of the synovial membrane. The anterior recess of the hip joint is seen as a hyperechoic stripe of tissue between the anterior femoral neck and the fascia of the iliopsoas muscle. It consists of two layers of synovial membrane that in the case of an effusion are separated by an anechoic space (Fig 1). The maximal width of the recess perpendicular to the femoral neck was measured (11).

To evaluate the articular cartilage of the femoral head, the transducer was placed on the anterior femoral head and aligned parallel to the femoral neck. Subsequently, it was moved laterally and simultaneously angulated slightly in the anterior oblique plane to depict the cartilage of the femoral head at the level of the labrum to the best extent possible (Fig 2). The cartilage was seen as a hypoechoic rim around the femoral head, and the thickness of it was measured perpendicularly to the femoral head at the level of the labrum.

To evaluate the quadriceps muscle, the transducer was placed on the anterior thigh in the transverse plane, at the midpoint between the superior border of the patella and the anterior superior iliac spine. Any pressure of the transducer on the skin was eliminated by using an excess amount of

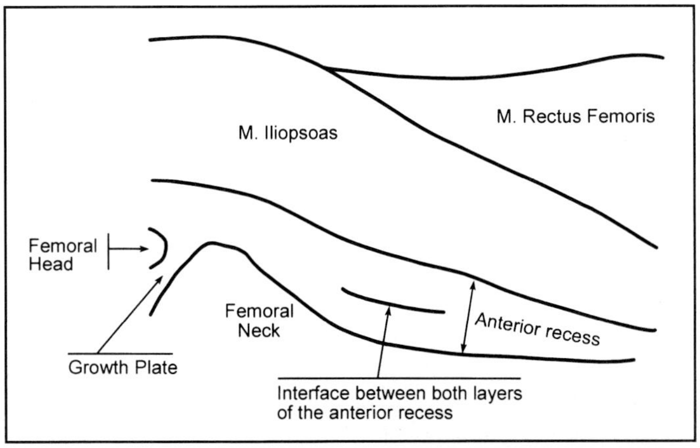

a.

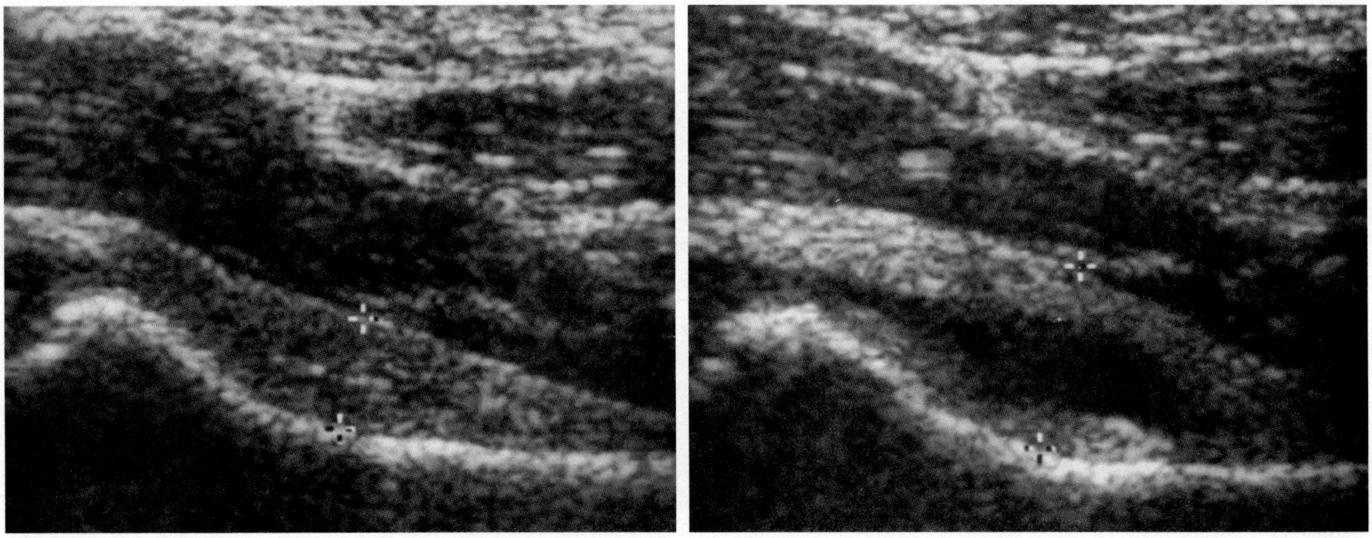

b. c.

Figure 1. (**a**) Schematic shows the anterior recess of a normal right hip. *M.* = musculus. (**b, c**) Parasagittal US scans of (**b**) the normal right hip and (**c**) the left hip with effusion (anechoic space) that caused widening of the anterior recess of the joint capsule in a 4-year-old boy with transient synovitis. The width of the anterior recess was measured with the calipers.

ultrasound gel to prevent compression of the muscle. Moreover, the patient's attention was diverted to optimize muscle relaxation. The distance from the femoral cortex to the anterior fascia of the rectus femoris muscle was measured (Fig 3).

All measurements were performed in both hips, and the differences between the asymptomatic and the symptomatic hips were calculated.

Additional Imaging Studies

Additional radiographs of both hips (frontal and lateral frog-leg views [Lauenstein views; anteroposterior radiographs with the thighs in abduction and external rotation, projecting the hips in a lateral fashion]) were obtained in all patients immediately after US examination. In selected cases, radiographs of the upper and lower parts of the leg were also obtained.

If no abnormalities were found and the symptoms persisted after a period of rest, additional imaging studies were performed (eg, control radiography, bone scintigraphy, magnetic resonance [MR] imaging, computed tomography [CT]); the choice of imaging study depended on the individual symptoms.

In patients with classic signs of transient synovitis (eg, acute onset of symptoms, irritable hip, effusion at US, absence of fever, age of 4–10 years) (12), however, radiography was not performed at the initial examination. Radiographs were obtained only if the symptoms persisted for more than 4 weeks.

Diagnostic Criteria

Patients with an irritable hip were considered to have had transient synovitis if US depicted effusion of any size (or a difference in the thickness of the anterior recess between both hips of more than 2 mm), the symptoms subsided completely within 4 weeks without specific therapy, and the patient remained symptom-free for at least 6 months thereafter. If the symptoms persisted, radiographs of the hips (frontal and lateral views) were obtained.

Perthes disease was diagnosed with radiography. A patient was considered to have Perthes disease if the typical changes of avascular necrosis appeared on serial radiographs (ie, condensation, subchondral fracture, collapse, and, eventually, fragmentation) (Table 1). SCFE was diagnosed if the epiphysis slipped at radiography of the hip. In patients with fever, septic arthritis was diagnosed with bacteriologic analysis of aspirated fluid. Neoplasm (eg, osteoid osteoma) was diagnosed with histologic analysis. The final clinical diagnosis was established 6 months after presentation by reviewing the medical and radiologic records.

Six patients with the tentative diagnosis of transient synovitis did not show up for regular checkups. To confirm the assumption that the symptoms had disappeared, the parents were interviewed by telephone. All patients appeared to have had a fast and complete recovery and stayed symptom-free thereafter.

Statistical Analysis

For statistical evaluation of measurements among different patient groups, the Kruskal-Wallis one-way analysis of variance and the Mann-Whitney rank sum test were used. The correlation between measure-

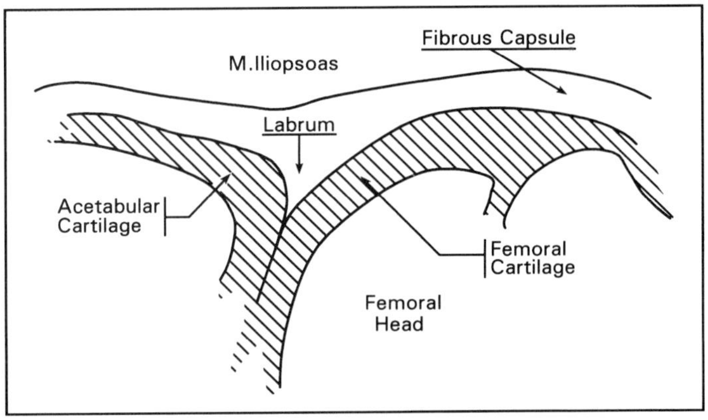

a.

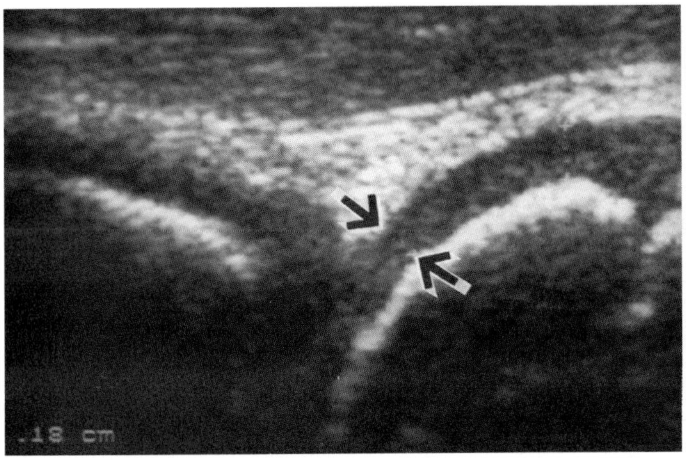

b.

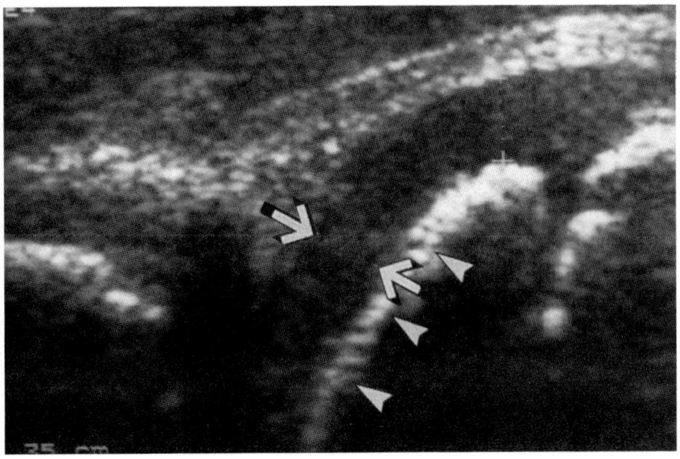

c.

Figure 2. (a) Schematic shows a normal right hip. *M.* = musculus. (b, c) Parasagittal US scans of (b) the normal right hip and (c) the affected left hip in a 5-year-old boy with Perthes disease. The cartilage thickness (arrows) was 1.8 mm in **b** and 3.5 mm in **c**. Note the mild flattening of the osseous nucleus (arrowheads) in **c**.

ments and age was analyzed by using Pearson correlation coefficients. A *P* value of less than .05 was considered statistically significant. Multivariate analysis (logistic regression) was used to differentiate between groups. This analysis proceeded in two stages. At the first stage, patients with Perthes disease were differentiated from both those with no visible abnormality and those with transient synovitis. At the second stage, the latter two groups were differentiated from each other.

RESULTS

The final clinical diagnoses are given in Table 2. Fifty-four patients had no joint effusion at US, normal radiographs, and spontaneous resolution of symptoms without specific therapy.

Five patients with Perthes disease showed no osseous abnormalities on initial radiographs (Table 1). These patients had symptoms that persisted and changes typical of avascular necrosis on serial radiographs.

Two patients had an occult fracture: One patient, a 15-year-old boy, had an avulsion fracture of the minor trochanter, and the other, a 2-year-old boy, had a fissure of the fibula. These fractures were diagnosed with radiography.

One patient with hemophilia had a large hyperechoic effusion after a minor trauma. The tentative diagnosis of articular hemorrhage was made, and the patient recovered completely after intravenous administration of coagulation factor VIII.

The numbers of patients with occult fracture, articular hemorrhage, septic arthritis, or osteoid osteoma were too small for statistical analysis.

Difference between Hips in Anterior Recess Thickness

Patients with transient synovitis and patients with Perthes disease showed statistically significant thickening of the anterior recess as compared with the control subjects and the patients with no visible abnormality ($P < .001$) (Table 3). Moreover, the difference between the symptomatic and asymptomatic hips in the mean thickness of the anterior recess in patients with transient synovitis was significantly different from that in patients with Perthes disease ($P < .001$). No significant difference was present among other groups.

Difference between Hips in Femoral Articular Cartilage Thickness

The femoral articular cartilage of the symptomatic hip was significantly thicker in patients with Perthes disease than it was in the other patient groups and control subjects ($P < .001$) (Fig 4, Table 4). The other patient groups did not show statistically significant cartilage thickening. Figure 4 shows that all but one patient

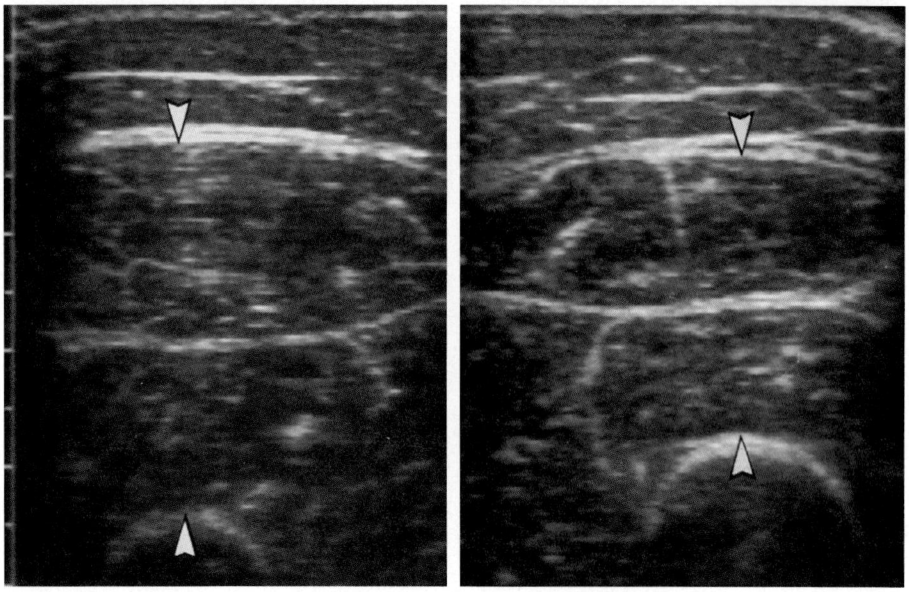

a. b.

Figure 3. Transverse US scans of the quadriceps muscles (arrowheads) in a 9-year-old boy with a left hip affected by Perthes disease. **(a)** US scan of the normal right quadriceps muscle (muscle thickness, 31.9 mm). **(b)** US scan of the left quadriceps muscle demonstrates muscle atrophy (muscle thickness, 23.7 mm).

TABLE 1
Summary of Data for 21 Patients with Perthes Disease

Patient No./Sex/ Age (y)	Duration of Complaints (d)	Stage*	Remarks	Difference in Cartilage Thickness (mm)†	Difference in Quadriceps Muscle Thickness (mm)†
1/M/7.0	10	Initial	Small subchondral fissure	0.4	0.0
2/M/6.6	14	Initial	No osseous abnormalities	0.2	−0.9
3/M/4.4	14	Initial	No osseous abnormalities	0.9	1.0
4/M/3.9	14	Initial	No osseous abnormalities	0.7	4.3
5/M/6.6	36	Initial	Small subchondral fissure	0.3	2.6
6/M/7.1	51	Initial	Small subchondral fissure	0.4	3.7
7/M/4.9	60	Initial	No osseous abnormalities	0.0	1.5
8/F/6.4	70	Initial	Height loss	0.6	4.5
9/F/5.1	90	Initial	Subchondral fissure	0.6	5.1
10/M/5.9	90	Initial	Subchondral fissure	1.7	4.3
11/F/11.7	90	Initial	Height loss	1.5	−2.0
12/M/4.7	90	Initial	Height loss, sclerosis	−0.1	3.4
13/M/3.2	120	Initial	Height loss, sclerosis	0.8	1.2
14/F/5.7	150	Initial	Subchondral fissure	1.5	3.5
15/F/5.2	150	Initial	Incipient sclerosis, height loss	0.4	5.0
16/M/4.9	150	Initial	Sclerosis, height loss	1.8	0.7
17/F/3.9	180	Initial	Incipient sclerosis, anterior collapse	1.1	4.4
18/M/9.3	180	Initial	Incipient sclerosis, height loss	0.1	6.8
19/M/4.7	180	Initial	Height loss, sclerosis	0.6	3.1
20/M/8.0	180	Fragmentation	Fragmentation, sclerosis, collapse	0.3	1.9
21/M/6.5	360	Initial	No osseous abnormalities	1.4	3.4

* According to Edgren (13).
† Difference between the two hips.

TABLE 2
Final Diagnoses and Descriptive Data

Final Diagnosis	Mean Age (y)	Duration of Symptoms before US (d)	
		Mean	Range
Transient synovitis (n = 58)	6.1	7.2	1–69
No visible abnormality (n = 54)	6.6	67.4	0–720
Perthes disease (n = 21)	5.9	108.5	10–360
SCFE (n = 5)	12.6	49.2	21–100
Occult fracture (n = 2)	8.5	2.5	. . .
Septic arthritis (n = 2)	3.7	3.7	. . .
Articular hemorrhage (n = 1)	11.5	1.0	. . .
Osteoid osteoma (n = 1)	3.2	90.0	. . .

TABLE 3
Mean Thickness of the Anterior Recess according to Diagnosis

Diagnosis	Mean Thickness of the Anterior Recess (mm)		Difference between Hips (mm)*
	Painful Hip	Normal Hip	
Transient synovitis (n = 58)	8.8	4.8	4.0 (1.9)
No visible abnormality (n = 54)	4.5	4.5	0.0 (0.6)
Perthes disease (n = 21)	6.8	4.9	1.9 (1.5)
SCFE (n = 5)	5.7	4.5	1.3 (0.6)
Occult fracture (n = 2)	4.0	4.0	0.0 (0.3)
Septic arthritis (n = 2)	8.0	4.9	3.1 (.05)
Articular hemorrhage (n = 1)	15.7	9.3	6.4
Osteoid osteoma (n = 1)	3.5	2.8	0.7

Note.—In the 68 control subjects, the mean thickness of the anterior recess was 4.6 mm for the left hip and 4.7 mm for the right hip (difference, −0.1 mm ± 0.4 [standard deviation]).
* Number in parentheses is the standard deviation.

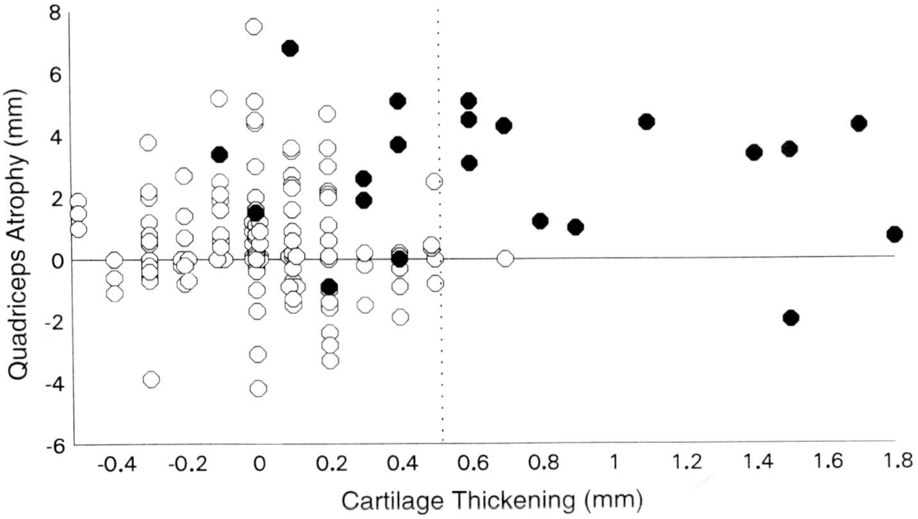

Figure 4. Graph shows the difference in quadriceps muscle thickness versus the difference in articular cartilage thickness between the painful hip and the normal hip for all patients (n = 144). ● = patients with Perthes disease, ○ = other patients. The dotted line indicates the threshold of a 0.5-mm difference in articular cartilage thickness.

with cartilage thickening greater than 0.5 mm had Perthes disease. The patient with thickening and no Perthes disease was a 1.7-year-old boy who had unexplained cartilage thickening and an uneventful recovery.

Use of the threshold of 0.5-mm cartilage thickening to diagnose Perthes disease resulted in a specificity of 99% (122 of 123). The sensitivity was 57% (12 of 21), the negative predictive value was 93% (122 of 131), and the positive predictive value was 92% (12 of 13). No statistically significant correlation was found between the difference in cartilage thickness between hips and age for all groups, including control subjects.

Difference between Hips in Quadriceps Muscle Thickness

Statistically significant ipsilateral muscle wasting was present in the patients with Perthes disease and in the patients with SCFE as compared with muscle wasting in the other patients and the control subjects (P < .001) (Fig 5, Table 5). The difference in muscle wasting between patients with Perthes disease and those with SCFE showed a trend but was not statistically significant (P = .079). The patients with no visible abnormality did not differ significantly from those with transient synovitis (P = .93) or control subjects (P = .33) in terms of muscle wasting. The difference between the transient synovitis group and the control group, however, was statistically significant (P = .02). No statistically significant correlation was found between the change in quadriceps muscle thickness and age for all groups, including control subjects.

When we compared the patients with Perthes disease with the patients with no visible abnormality and the patients with transient synovitis combined, we found that the optimal combination of the difference between hips in cartilage thickness and the difference between hips in quadriceps muscle thickness that enabled differentiation of both groups could be written as follows: $6 \times (\Delta\text{cartilage}) + 0.75 \times (\Delta\text{quadriceps})$, where Δcartilage is the difference between hips in the cartilage thickness (symptomatic hip minus asymptomatic hip) and Δquadriceps is the difference between hips in the quadriceps muscle thickness (asymptomatic side minus symptomatic side).

When we compared patients with transient synovitis with those with no visible abnormalities, we found that only the difference in anterior recess thickness had a discriminatory value. Figure 6 shows the total (in millimeters) derived with the formula (vertical axis) versus the difference between hips in the anterior recess thickness (horizontal axis) for all patient groups.

As shown in Figure 6, all but one patient with a total of at least 5 mm had Perthes disease. One patient with SCFE had considerable muscle atrophy. Therefore, the positive predictive value for Perthes disease was 94% when the total of 6 × (△cartilage) + 0.75 × (△quadriceps) was at least 5 mm. The sensitivity was 71%, the specificity was 99%, and the negative predictive value was 95% (Table 6).

DISCUSSION

US of the joint was first described by Kramps and Lenschow in 1979 (12). One year later, Seltzer et al (14) showed that fluid collections as small as 10 mL could be demonstrated in the hip with US. Subsequently, the results of several studies confirmed that US is more sensitive for detecting hip effusion than is plain radiography (6,15–20). Although there is excellent correlation between US and CT for the detection of intraarticular effusion (21,22), US is preferable because it is less expensive, requires no sedation, and is not associated with ionizing radiation. Although US is operator-dependent, the anatomic landmarks in the present study are easy to depict.

The present study depends heavily on comparison of the abnormal hip joint with the contralateral normal hip joint; therefore, patients with bilateral disease were excluded. This is a limitation of the study; however, the number of patients with bilateral hip pain was negligible. Moreover, bilateral synchronous involvement is very rare in Perthes disease and transient synovitis, with reported frequencies of 0.4% and 1%, respectively (23,24).

Hip Joint Effusion

Until recently, the role of US in patients with a painful hip has been limited to the detection of joint capsule thickening as evidence of joint effusion. Unfortunately, many diseases cause an increase in the capsular joint space (eg, transient synovitis, Perthes disease, SCFE, rheumatoid or septic arthritis) (3,5,18,25–31). Although the mean capsular joint widths in Perthes disease, transient synovitis, and septic arthritis differ significantly, there is considerable overlap in individual patients (5,28,32). In the present study, all patients with Perthes disease had capsular joint widths within the range seen in patients with transient synovitis.

The duration of the effusion can be of help in differentiating transient synovitis from other diseases. An effusion lasting 3–6 weeks is suggestive of Perthes disease

TABLE 4
Mean Articular Cartilage Thickness according to Diagnosis

Diagnosis	Mean Articular Cartilage Thickness (mm): Painful Hip	Normal Hip	Difference between Hips (mm)*
Transient synovitis (*n* = 58)	2.4	2.4	0.0 (0.2)
No visible abnormality (*n* = 54)	2.3	2.3	0.0 (0.2)
Perthes disease (*n* = 21)	3.2	2.5	0.7 (0.6)
SCFE (*n* = 5)	1.5	1.4	0.1 (0.1)
Occult fracture (*n* = 2)	2.0	2.0	0.0 (0)
Septic arthritis (*n* = 2)	3.0	3.0	0.0 (0)
Articular hemorrhage (*n* = 1)	1.5	1.5	0.0
Osteoid osteoma (*n* = 1)	2.4	2.5	−0.1

Note.—In the 68 control subjects, the mean articular cartilage thickness was 2.3 mm for both the left and right hips (standard deviation, 0.2 mm).
* Number in parentheses is the standard deviation.

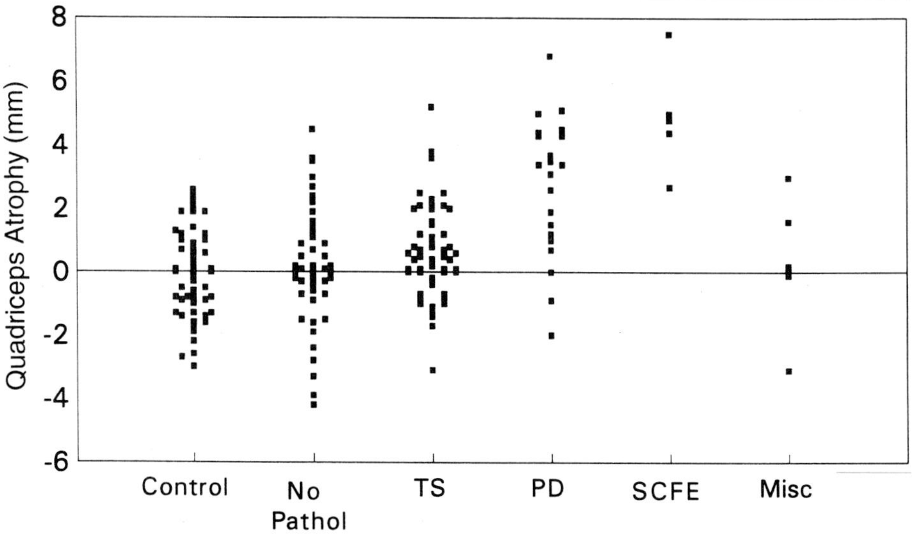

Figure 5. Graph shows the difference in quadriceps muscle thickness between the painful hip and the normal hip in all groups. *Control* = control subjects, *No Pathol* = patients with no visible abnormality, *TS* = patients with transient synovitis, *PD* = patients with Perthes disease, *SCFE* = patients with SCFE, *Misc* = patients with miscellaneous abnormalities.

TABLE 5
Mean Quadriceps Muscle Thickness according to Diagnosis

Diagnosis	Mean Quadriceps Muscle Thickness (mm): Painful Hip	Normal Hip	Difference between Hips (mm)*
Transient synovitis (*n* = 58)	23.8	24.4	0.6 (1.4)
No visible abnormality (*n* = 54)	24.0	24.2	0.2 (1.7)
Perthes disease (*n* = 21)	22.4	25.1	2.7 (2.1)
SCFE (*n* = 5)	28.4	33.3	4.9 (1.5)
Occult fracture (*n* = 2)	30.6	32.6	2.0 (1.0)
Septic arthritis (*n* = 2)	23.1	22.5	−0.6 (2.5)
Articular hemorrhage (*n* = 1)	30.5	31.0	0.5
Osteoid osteoma (*n* = 1)	20.0	21.6	1.6

Note.—In the 68 control subjects, the mean quadriceps muscle thickness was 28.1 mm for the left hip and 28.2 mm for the right hip (difference, −0.1 mm ± 1.4 [standard deviation]).
* Number in parentheses is the standard deviation.

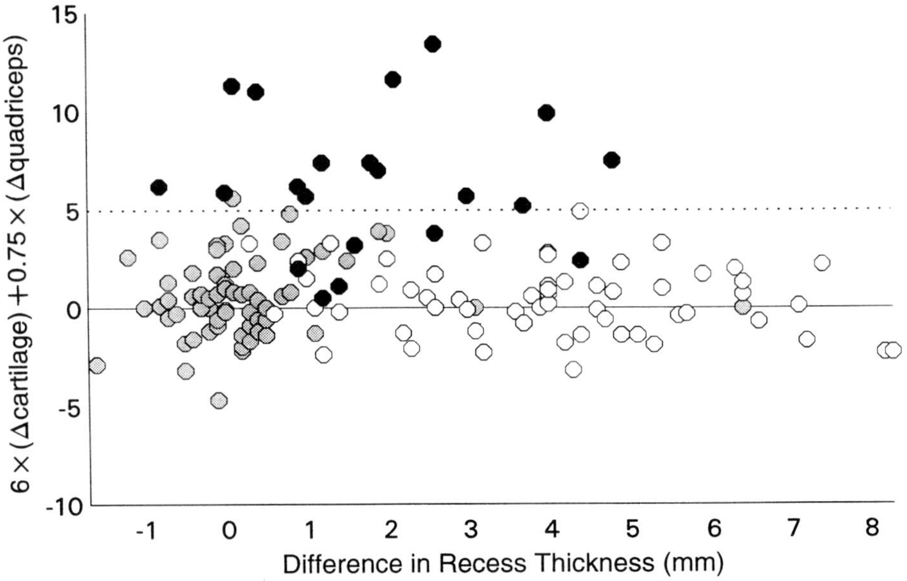

Figure 6. Graph shows the total of 6 × (△cartilage) + 0.75 × (△quadriceps), where △cartilage is the difference in cartilage thickness (symptomatic hip minus asymptomatic hip) and △quadriceps is the difference in quadriceps thickness (asymptomatic hip minus symptomatic hip) between the painful hip and the normal hip, versus the difference in the anterior recess thickness between the painful hip and the normal hip. All but one patient with a total of at least 5 mm had Perthes disease. Black circles = patients with Perthes disease, white circles = patients with transient synovitis, gray circles = other patients.

TABLE 6
Value of the Formula 6× (Δ Cartilage) + 0.75 × (Δ Quadriceps) in the Diagnosis of Perthes Disease, with a Total of 5 mm as a Threshold

Total (mm)	No. of Patients with Perthes Disease	No. of Patients without Perthes Disease	Total
≥5	15	1	16
<5	6	122	128
Total	21	123	144

(2–4,33–35); however, this observation cannot be applied at presentation. Moreover, other diseases, such as rheumatoid arthritis, show effusions that persist.

Therefore, the US detection of effusion is useful for identifying the hip joint as the source of the symptoms, but the discriminatory role of US is limited when only the presence of effusion, the amount of effusion, or both are evaluated.

Cartilage Thickness

The cartilage of the femoral head also can be depicted with US. There is a good correlation between bone age and cartilage thickness (36). Thickening of the articular cartilage in Perthes disease is a well-known phenomenon in both experimental and clinical studies (37–40). This cartilage thickening is attributed to swelling (41,42), hyperplasia (39,43,44), or ceased endochondral ossification in combination with continued cartilaginous growth (40,45,46).

To our knowledge, few reports have emphasized the importance of cartilage thickening in the differential diagnosis of the painful hip (5,7). Unfortunately, in all of those studies, Perthes disease was compared with transient synovitis. Other entities that cause a hip to be painful were not included.

To overcome that drawback, we included all patients with a painful hip in our study and correlated the US criteria with the final diagnosis. Patients with Perthes disease showed a statistically significant increase in the cartilage thickness of the symptomatic hip compared with the other patient groups; cartilage thickening in other patients was virtually absent. Among the patients with cartilage thickening of more than 0.5 mm, all but one—a 1.7-year-old boy with cartilage thickening of 0.7 mm—had Perthes disease (Fig 4). At this age, cartilage thickening can be caused by irregular mineralization of the osseous nucleus of the femoral head.

A threshold of more than 0.5 mm seems, therefore, to be a reliable discriminator for Perthes disease (positive predictive value, 92%; negative predictive value, 93%; specificity, 99%). Unfortunately, some patients with Perthes disease had no evident cartilage thickening, resulting in a sensitivity of 57% (Table 1).

Muscle Atrophy

US of normal skeletal muscle has been described in healthy children and adults (47,48). US assessment of muscle wasting has been performed in children with neuromuscular disease (49–52) and in children with acute leukemia (53). To our knowledge, however, there are no reports in the US literature about muscle atrophy in patients with a painful hip. Muscle atrophy in patients with a painful hip probably results from decreased ipsilateral postural and locomotor activity.

In our study, the maximal difference between the left and right quadriceps muscles in the control group was 3 mm (Fig 5). Therefore, a decrease of more than 3 mm on the side with the symptomatic hip can be considered atrophy.

Patients with Perthes disease and patients with SCFE showed a statistically significant decrease in ipsilateral quadriceps muscle thickness compared with patients with transient synovitis, patients with no visible abnormality, and control subjects. In addition, patients with transient synovitis showed slight, although statistically significant, muscle wasting compared with the control subjects. According to Wills et al (54), several factors can influence the degree of muscle atrophy, including the duration and degree of inactivity. These factors probably contribute to the differences in muscle atrophy among patients with transient synovitis, Perthes disease, and SCFE. Apparently, muscle atrophy can be a potential US criterion for detecting abnormalities. There was considerable overlap, however, among the groups (Fig 5), so it is hazardous to extrapolate these findings to individual patients.

Twenty-four patients had muscle atrophy (quadriceps muscle wasting at the ipsilateral side of ≥3 mm), 17 of whom had a severe abnormality (12 had Perthes disease, four had SCFE, and one had an occult fracture) and seven of whom had self-limiting diseases (three had transient synovitis and four had no visible abnormality). Therefore, a threshold of at least 3 mm for muscle wasting results in a positive predictive value of 50% (12 of 24) for Perthes disease, a negative predictive value of 92% (111 of 120), and a specificity of 90% (111 of 123). The relatively low sensitivity of 57% (12 of 21), however, indicates that many cases of Perthes disease will go undetected.

The results of the present study show that each US criterion (thickness of the anterior recess, thickness of the cartilage, and muscle atrophy) can be useful for differentiating among various diseases. Combining these criteria and applying thresholds for muscle atrophy ($\geq$3 mm) and cartilage thickening (>0.5 mm) can improve the diagnostic performance of US.

Multivariate analysis optimizes this multiparameter approach with use of the formula $6 \times (\triangle\text{cartilage}) + 0.75 \times (\triangle\text{quadriceps})$. All patients with a total of at least 5 mm had a severe hip abnormality (15 had Perthes disease, and one had SCFE). This results in a positive predictive value for Perthes disease of 94%, a negative predictive value of 95%, a sensitivity of 71%, and a specificity of 99% (Table 6).

US of the hip joint is very sensitive in the detection of even small amounts of synovial effusion. Several frequently encountered diseases (eg, transient synovitis, Perthes disease and SCFE), however, can manifest as hip joint effusion. The results of this study show that the role of US should not be limited to the detection of effusion.

Patients with a painful hip who have ipsilateral cartilage thickening, muscle atrophy, or both at US are highly suspected of having Perthes disease, regardless of the duration of symptoms. Plain radiography should be performed in these patients to confirm Perthes disease. If the plain radiographs are negative, additional investigations, such as radionuclide studies or MR imaging, are justified to confirm or rule out early Perthes disease.

Acknowledgments: The authors thank Teun Rijsdijk and Andries Zwamborn for preparing the illustrations and photographs.

References

1. Castriota-Scanderbeg A, Orsi E, de Micheli V, Pedrazzi G, Letico M, Coppi M. Ultrasound in the diagnosis and follow-up of hip disorders in children. Radiol Med 1993; 86:808–814.
2. Bickerstaff DR, Neal LM, Booth AJ, Brennan PD, Bell MJ. Ultrasound examination of the irritable hip. J Bone Joint Surg [Br] 1990; 72:549–553.
3. Dörr U, Zieger M, Hauke H. The painful hip: diagnostic possibilities of sonography. ROFO 1988; 148:487–491.
4. Terjesen T, Osthus P. Ultrasound in the diagnosis and follow-up of transient synovitis of the hip. J Pediatr Orthop 1991; 11:608–613.
5. Futami T, Kasahara Y, Suzuki S, Ushikubo S, Tsuchiya T. Ultrasonography in transient synovitis and early Perthes' disease. J Bone Joint Surg [Br] 1991; 73:635–639.
6. Meradji M, Diepstraten AFM. Coxitis fugax, sonografisches und radiologisches bild in 65 fallen. Radiologe 1988; 28:473–478.
7. Wirth T, LeQuesne GW, Paterson DC. Ultrasonography in Legg-Calve-Perthes' disease. Pediatr Radiol 1992; 22:498–504.
8. Booth FW, Gollnick PD. Effects of disuse on the structure and function of skeletal muscle. Med Sci Sports Exerc 1983; 15:415–420.
9. Ferguson AB Jr. Synovitis of the hip and Legg-Perthes' disease. Clin Orthop 1954; 4:180–188.
10. Schiller MG, Axer A. Legg-Calve-Perthes' syndrome (L.C.P.S.): a critical analysis of roentgenographic measurements. Clin Orthop 1972; 86:34–42.
11. Rohrschneider WK, Fuchs G, Tröger J. Ultrasonographic evaluation of the anterior recess in the normal hip: a prospective study on 166 asymptomatic children. Pediatr Radiol 1996; 26:629–634.
12. Kramps HA, Lenschow E. Einsatzmoglichkeiten der ultraschalldiagnostik am bewegungsapparat. Zeitschrift Orthopedie Grenzgebiete 1979; 118:355–364.
13. Edgren W. Coxa plana. Acta Orthop Scand 1965; 84(suppl):1–129.
14. Seltzer S, Finberg H, Weissma BA. Arthrosonography: technique, sonographic anatomy and pathology. Invest Radiol 1980; 15:19–28.
15. Wilson DJ, Green DJ, MacLarnon JC. Arthrosonography of the painful hip. Clin Radiol 1984; 35:17–19.
16. Adam R, Hendry GM, Moss J, Wild SR, Gillespie I. Arthrosonography of the irritable hip in childhood: a review of 1 year's experience. Br J Radiol 1986; 59:205–208.
17. Marchal GJ, Holsbeeck MT, Raes M, et al. Transient synovitis of the hip in children: role of US. Radiology 1987; 162:825–828.
18. Miralles M, Gonzales G, Pulpeiro JR, et al. Sonography of the painful hip in children: 500 consecutive cases. AJR 1989; 152:579–582.
19. Peck RJ. Ultrasound of the painful hip in children. Br J Radiol 1986; 59:293–294.
20. Rosenborg M, Mortensson W. The validity of radiographic assessment of childhood transient synovitis of the hip. Acta Radiol Diagn 1986; 27:85–89.
21. Wingstrand H, Egund N. Ultrasonography in hip joint effusion. Acta Orthop Scand 1984; 55:469–471.
22. Egund N, Wingstrand H, Forsberg L, Petterson H, Sunden G. Computed tomography for the diagnosis of hip joint effusion in children. Acta Orthop Scand 1986; 57:211–215.
23. Nevelös AB. Bilateral Perthes' disease. Acta Orthop Scand 1980; 51:649–654.
24. Haueisen DC, Weiner DS, Weiner SD. The characterization of "transient synovitis of the hip" in children. J Pediatr Orthop 1986; 6:11–17.
25. Shiv VK, Jain AK, Taneja K, Bhargava SK. Sonography of hip joint in infective arthritis. J Can Assoc Radiol 1990; 41:76–78.
26. Sell S, Zacher J, Konig J, Goethe S. Ultrasound in inflammatory rheumatic joint disease. Ultraschall Med 1993; 14:63–67.
27. Koski JM, Antilla P, Hamalainen M, Isomaki H. Hip joint ultrasonography: correlation with intraarticular effusion and synovitis. Br J Rheumatol 1990; 29:189–192.
28. Kallio P, Ryoppy S, Jappinen S, Siponmaa AK, Jaaskelainen J, Kunnamo I. Ultrasonography in hip disease in children. Acta Orthop Scand 1985; 56:367–371.
29. Konermann W, de Pelligrin M. The differential diagnosis of juvenile hip pain in the ultrasonographic picture: transient synovitis, Legg-Calve-Perthes' disease, epiphysiolysis capitis femoris. Orthopade 1993; 22:280–287.
30. Castriota-Scanderbeg A, Orsi E. Slipped capital femoral epiphysis: ultrasonographic findings. Skeletal Radiol 1993; 22:191–193.
31. Kallio PE, LeQuesne GW, Paterson DC, Foster BK, Jones JR. Ultrasonography in slipped capital femoral epiphysis. J Bone Joint Surg [Br] 1991; 73:884–889.
32. Alexander JE, Seibert JJ, Glasier CM, et al. High-resolution hip ultrasound in the limping child. JCU 1989; 17:19–24.
33. Terjesen T. Ultrasonography in the primary evaluation of patients with Perthes' disease. J Pediatr Orthop 1993; 13:437–443.
34. Kallio P, Ryoppy S. Hyperpressure in juvenile hip disease. Acta Orthop Scand 1985; 56:211–214.
35. Linnenbaum FJ, Woltering H, Karbowski A, Harle A. Ultrasonography of the hip for Perthes's disease. Arch Orthop Trauma Surg 1989; 108:166–172.
36. Castriota-Scanderbeg A, de Micheli V. Ultrasound of femoral head cartilage: a new method of assessing bone age. Skeletal Radiol 1995; 24:197–200.
37. Rush BH, Bramson RT, Ogden JA. Legg-Calve-Perthes' disease: detection of cartilaginous and synovial changes with MR imaging. Radiology 1988; 167:473–476.
38. Katz JF. Arthrography in Legg-Calve-Perthes' disease. J Bone Joint Surg [Am] 1968; 60:467–472.
39. Gershuni DH, Axer A, Hendel D. Arthrographic findings in Legg-Calve-Perthes' disease and transient synovitis of the hip. J Bone Joint Surg [Am] 1978; 60:457–464.
40. Zahir A, Freeman MAR. Cartilage changes following a single episode of infarction of the capital femoral epiphysis in the dog. J Bone Joint Surg [Am] 1972; 54:125–136.
41. Gershuni DH, Amiel D, Gonsalves M. The biochemical response of rabbit articular cartilage to an induced talcum synovitis. Acta Orthop Scand 1981; 52:599–603.
42. Ueo T, Tsutsumi S, Yamamuro T, Okumura H. Biomechanical analysis of Perthes' disease using the finite element method: the role of swelling of articular cartilage. Arch Orthop Trauma Surg 1987; 106:202–208.
43. Axer A, Schiller MG. The pathogenesis of the early deformity of the capital femoral epiphysis in Legg-Calve-Perthes' syndrome (L.C.P.S.): an arthrographic study. Clin Orthop 1972; 84:106–115.
44. Larsen E, Reimann J. Calve Perthes' disease with special reference to histological observations. Acta Orthop Scand 1973; 44:426–438.
45. Singleton WB, Jones EL. The experimental induction of subclinical Perthes' disease in the puppy following arthrotomy and intracapsular tamponade. J Comp Pathol 1979; 89:57–71.
46. Kemp HBS, Bolero JL. Radiological changes in Perthes' disease. Br J Radiol 1966; 39:744–760.
47. Heckmatt JZ, Pier N, Dubowitz V. Measurement of quadriceps muscle thickness and subcutaneous tissue thickness in normal children by realtime ultrasound imaging. JCU 1988; 16:171–176.
48. Weiss LW, Clark FC. Ultrasonic protocols for separately measuring subcutaneous fat and skeletal muscle thickness in the calf area. Phys Ther 1985; 65:477–481.
49. Heckmatt JZ, Pier N, Dubowitz V. Real-time ultrasound imaging of muscle. Muscle Nerve 1988; 11:56–65.
50. Dock W, Happak W, Grabenwöger F, Toilf K, Bittner R, Gruber H. Neuromuscular diseases: evaluation with high-frequency sonography. Radiology 1990; 177:825–828.
51. Kamala D, Suresh S, Githa K. Real-time ultrasonography in neuromuscular problems of children. JCU 1985; 13:465–468.
52. Heckmatt JZ, Pier N, Dubowitz V. Assessment of quadriceps femoris muscle atrophy and hypertrophy in neuromuscular disease in children. JCU 1988; 16:177–181.
53. Koskelo EK, Saarinen UM, Siimes MA. Skeletal muscle wasting and protein energy malnutrition in children with newly diagnosed acute leukemia. Cancer 1990; 66:373–376.
54. Wills CA, Caiozzo VJ, Yasakuwa DI, Prietto CA, McMaster WC. Effect of immobilisation of human skeletal muscle. Orthop Rev 1982; 11:57–64.

Hip Joint Fluid: Detection and Distribution at MR Imaging and US with Cadaveric Correlation[1]

Steven G. Moss, MD
Mark E. Schweitzer, MD
Jon A. Jacobson, MD
Joachim Brossmann, MD
Joseph V. Lombardi, MD
Steven M. Dellose, MD
Jeffrey R. Coralnick, MD
Kathleen N. Standiford, MD
Donald Resnick, MD

Index terms:
Hip, arthritis, 442.254, 442.70
Hip, fractures, 442.41
Hip, MR, 442.121411, 442.121415
Hip, US, 442.1298
Joints, fluid, 442.254

Radiology 1998; 208:43–48

[1] From the Department of Radiology, Thomas Jefferson University Hospital, 132 S 10th St, 1096 Main Bldg, Philadelphia, PA 19107 (S.G.M., M.E.S., J.V.L., S.M.D., J.R.C., K.N.S.), and the Department of Radiology, San Diego Veterans Administration Medical Center, San Diego, Calif (J.A.J., J.B., D.R.).
Received August 13, 1997; revision requested October 23; revision received January 27, 1998; accepted February 11. **Address reprint requests to** M.E.S.

Author contributions:
Guarantors of integrity of entire study, S.G.M., M.E.S.; study concepts and design, S.G.M., M.E.S.; definition of intellectual content, S.G.M., M.E.S.; literature research, S.G.M.; clinical studies, S.G.M., M.E.S.; data acquisition, S.G.M., M.E.S., J.A.J., J.B., J.V.L., S.M.D., J.R.C., K.N.S., D.R.; data and statistical analyses, S.G.M., M.E.S.; manuscript preparation, editing, and review, S.G.M., M.E.S.

PURPOSE: To define the magnetic resonance (MR) imaging appearance of a hip effusion.

MATERIALS AND METHODS: Fifty-two asymptomatic hips in 26 volunteers aged 20–37 years and five fractured hips were imaged at 1.5 T with T2-weighting in three planes. Images were computer digitized and analyzed for hip fluid volume and visually assessed for the presence and width of fluid pockets (in millimeters) seen in the acetabular notch; recesses anterior, posterior, and lateral to the femoral head; and recesses anterior, posterior, and medial to the femoral neck. Cadaveric hips were also injected with graduated amounts of saline (1–20 mL), and sequential MR and ultrasound images were obtained.

RESULTS: Computer analysis yielded an average fluid volume of 2.7 mL (range, 0.7–5.6 mL) in asymptomatic and 6.1 mL (range, 1.7–11.6 mL) in symptomatic hips. The mean difference between the right and left hips was 0.8 mL (range, 0.0–2.9 mL). Discrete fluid pockets, sometimes measuring greater than 5 mm in width, were commonly seen in asymptomatic hips. Distention of the capsule by at least 5 mm along the length of the femoral neck was almost always seen after injection of 5 mL of saline and was consistently seen after injection of 10 mL of saline into cadaveric hips.

CONCLUSION: Fluid adjacent to the entire length of the femoral neck, measuring at least 5 mm in width, is compatible with a joint effusion.

The magnetic resonance (MR) imaging appearance of normal joint fluid and MR definitions of effusions, although initially anecdotally described, have been scientifically evaluated more recently in several articulations including the glenohumeral (1), acromioclavicular (2), knee (3), and ankle joints (4,5). Despite the hip being a common joint affected by arthritis, avascular necrosis, and trauma, the normal volume, distribution, and clinical relevance of hip joint fluid have been investigated, to our knowledge, only preliminarily with MR imaging (6,7). Because disorders of the hip are common and the diagnosis of an effusion is an important ancillary finding, the distribution and appearance of hip joint fluid in normal, asymptomatic hips must be understood to avoid mistaking normal fluid for a pathologic effusion. Consequently, the purpose of our study was to define the normal appearance of hip joint fluid and to evaluate the MR and ultrasonographic (US) appearance of increasing amounts of fluid injected into cadaveric hips to aid in the development of criteria for detection of hip effusions.

MATERIALS AND METHODS

Asymptomatic Volunteers

From August 1994 through December 1994, 26 volunteers were recruited to undergo MR imaging of their hips. Each volunteer was told the purpose of the study and then questioned about medical history as it related to the hips. Volunteers were excluded if they had any previous medical condition or current symptoms involving either hip, including

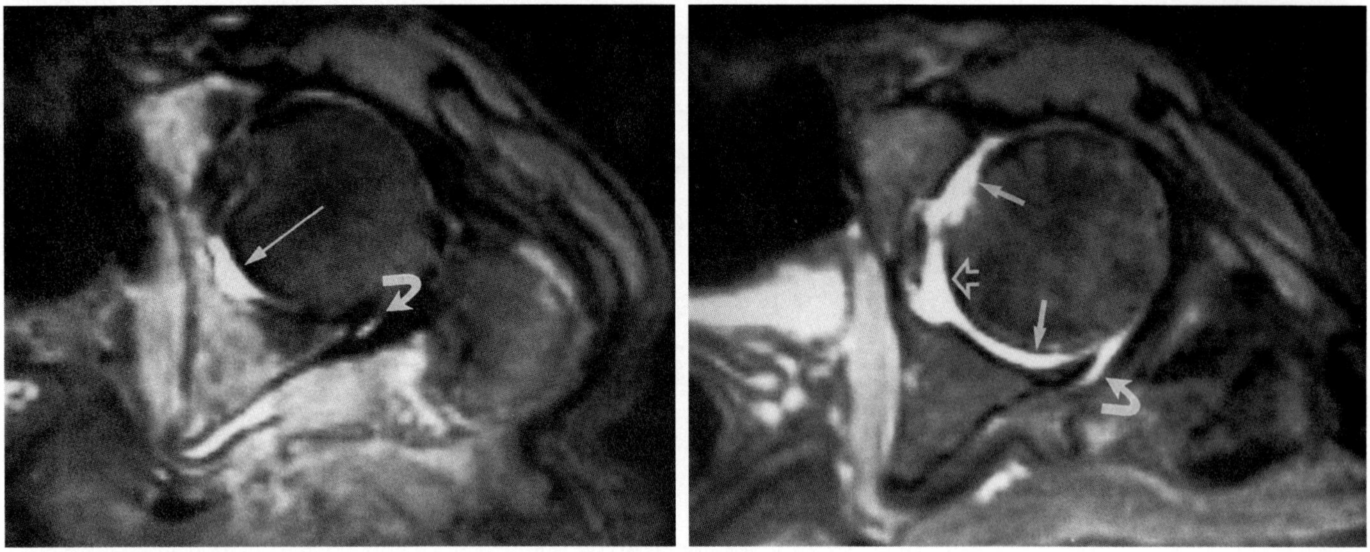

a. b.

Figure 1. Axial fast spin-echo, fat-saturated images (3,500/85) of cadaveric hips at the level of the femoral head were obtained after the injection of **(a)** 5 mL and **(b)** 10 mL of saline. **(a)** Only a small amount of fluid is seen between the femoral head and the acetabulum (straight arrow) and adjacent to the posterior labrum (curved arrow). **(b)** Compared with **a**, more fluid is seen between the femoral head and the acetabulum (solid straight arrows) and posterior to the labrum (curved arrow). Fluid also almost completely fills the acetabular notch (open arrow).

any past or present hip pain. The study was performed under approval from the institutional review board, and written informed consent was obtained from each of the volunteers. A total of 52 hips in 26 asymptomatic volunteers (13 men, 13 women) aged 20–37 years (mean age, 25.5 years) were studied with MR imaging. The imaging was performed with a 1.5-T unit (Signa; GE Medical Systems, Milwaukee, Wis) and either a body coil or a phased-array coil. All imaging was performed in the axial, coronal, and sagittal planes with a T2-weighted, fast spin-echo, fat-saturated sequence (5,500/85 [repetition time msec/echo time msec], 32-cm field of view, and 256 × 256 matrix).

Symptomatic Patients

Because acute fractures are known to be associated with effusions, five patients (one man, four women) aged 70–82 years (mean age, 76 years) who had acutely fractured hips underwent imaging between January 1, 1988, and March 15, 1995. The imaging findings in these five patients were retrospectively analyzed. All of these hips were imaged in the axial plane. Three of the five were also imaged in the coronal plane, whereas the other two were imaged in the sagittal plane.

Image Analysis

Computer analysis.—With the T2-weighted images in all three planes, one observer (S.G.M.) identified all of the visible fluid on each image in each patient and volunteer. Each image was then digitized by three computer operators (S.G.M., J.V.L., S.M.D.) who used the CUE-2 image analysis software package (Galai Production, Migdal Haemek, Israel). Each operator analyzed the images of approximately one-third of the 57 hips (26 volunteers and five patients). Once the image was digitized, the computer operator selected the previously identified visible fluid on that section for the computer to analyze. The area of the fluid on each section was then determined by the image analysis software, and the total sum of the area of all fluid on each section in the given plane was calculated. The total area was converted to a total volume of joint fluid by multiplying by the total section thickness, which was defined as the image section thickness plus the gap thickness. This procedure was performed separately for each of the three imaging planes.

Visual analysis.—In addition, axial images in the volunteers were visually assessed by two independent observers (J.R.C., K.N.S.) for the amount of fluid (measured in millimeters) seen in specific locations of the hip joint. Each observer was blinded to the computer analysis of fluid volume for each volunteer. We visually quantified fluid in the following locations within the hip joint: the acetabular notch, adjacent to the acetabular fat pad; recesses anterior, posterior, and lateral to the femoral head; and recesses anterior, posterior, and medial to the femoral neck. Fluid in each location was graded as 0 = no fluid, 1 = 0–5 mm of fluid, and 2 = greater than 5 mm of fluid. We chose to apply our grading scheme to the axial images because the fluid was most easily located in the axial plane and because clinically MR imaging is almost universally performed in the axial plane.

TABLE 1
Average Fluid Volume (milliliters) in the Hips of Asymptomatic Volunteers (52 Hips)

View	Hip: Right	Hip: Left	Range
Axial	3.2	2.4	0.4–6.2
Coronal	2.6	1.9	0.0–6.9
Sagittal	2.8	2.9	0.6–7.1
Total average volume in each hip	2.9	2.4	0.7–5.6

Note.—Mean absolute difference between right and left hips = 0.8 mL (range, 0.0–2.9 mL).

Appearance of Progressive Distention of Normal Volumes

One hip of an additional asymptomatic volunteer, who was 32 years of age, was imaged in the axial plane with a

TABLE 2
Location of Fluid in Asymptomatic Hips by Grade (percentage of total)

	Femoral Head Recesses				Femoral Neck Recesses		
Grade*	Ant	Post	Notch	Lat	Ant	Post	Med
0	79	32	4	7	13	29	8
1	20	66	54	78	60	50	34
2	1	2	42	15	27	21	58

Note.—Ant = anterior, post = posterior, notch = acetabular notch, lat = lateral.
* 0 = no fluid, 1 = 0–5-mm width of fluid, 2 = greater than 5-mm width of fluid.

TABLE 3
Interobserver Variation of Grade at Each Location

Location	Percentage with Exact Agreement	Percentage Differing by One Grade
Femoral head		
Anterior	79	21
Posterior	60	40
Lateral	86	14
Acetabular	76	24
Femoral neck		
Anterior	73	27
Posterior	60	38
Medial	77	21

TABLE 4
Average Fluid Volume (milliliters) in Patients with Occult Hip Fractures (Five Hips)

View	Volume	Range
Axial	7.7	4.0–11.6
Coronal	3.9	2.0–6.1
Sagittal	5.7	4.4–6.9
Total average volume in each hip	6.1	2.0–11.6

TABLE 5
Distention (millimeters) of the Anterior Hip Joint Capsule Seen with US

Volume Injected (mL)	Right Hip	Left Hip
First cadaveric pelvis		
0	2.5	2.1
2	2.7	2.5
5	4.8	5.1
10	5.2	6.6
20	5.8	10.0
Second cadaveric pelvis		
0	1.0*	1.0*
1	2.1*	2.0*
3	2.5*	2.3*
5	3.2*	2.9
10	3.6	4.1
20	4.2	4.0

* Estimated.

T2-weighted, fast spin-echo, fat-suppressed sequence. An MR imaging–compatible 20-gauge titanium needle was then inserted into the hip with fluoroscopic guidance. The needle was confirmed to be within the hip joint by injecting 0.3 mL of iohexol (Omnipaque; Nycomed, Princeton, NJ) during fluoroscopic observation. Once the intra-articular position of the needle was confirmed, an additional 0.7 mL of sterile saline was injected to equal 1 mL of fluid injected into the hip joint. Axial MR images with the same sequence described earlier were then obtained with the needle remaining in the hip joint. After the first set of images was obtained, an additional 2 mL of saline was injected through the needle into the hip joint and, again, axial MR images were obtained with the same pulse sequence. This procedure was repeated one more time after injecting an additional 5 mL of fluid. A direct comparison of the pre- and postinjection images was performed.

Cadaveric Hips

Two freshly thawed cadaveric pelves (four hips) were initially imaged with a Signa 1.5-T magnet (GE Medical Systems) and a shoulder coil. A fast spin-echo, fat-saturated sequence (3,500/85) was used with the following parameters: 16×16-cm field of view, echo train length of eight, 256×256 matrix, two signals acquired, and a 16-kHz bandwidth. Each hip was imaged individually in the axial, coronal, and sagittal planes.

US of each hip joint was also performed in the oblique sagittal plane from an anterior approach with 5.0-MHz curvilinear and 7.5-MHz linear transducers (Acoustic Imaging Technologies, Phoenix, Ariz). A 20-gauge spinal needle was then inserted into each hip joint with the anteroinferior approach and US guidance. Once the needle came into contact with the femoral neck, the needle was retracted 1 mm. One milliliter of saline was injected into each hip joint. Verification of intra-articular placement was based on low resistance to injection. The needle was then removed, and repeat MR imaging and US of each hip joint were performed as described earlier. This process was repeated after the injection of an additional 2 mL, 2 mL more, then 5 mL more, and then 10 mL more. Therefore, imaging was performed at baseline and sequentially after instillation of a total of 1, 3, 5, 10, and 20 mL of saline. A similar procedure was performed on the second pelvis, with imaging performed at baseline and after the injection of 2, 5, 10, and 20 mL of saline. The MR images were then visually inspected by two observers (S.G.M., M.E.S.). Consensus was attained with respect to the presence and distribution of fluid in each hip in each imaging plane, and the results were recorded. Correlation of MR imaging and US findings was also performed. For each volume of fluid injected, the width of fluid distending the capsule was measured anterior to the femoral neck on the axial and sagittal images and inferior to the femoral neck on the coronal images. Measurements were made perpendicular to the femoral neck on the images on which the femoral neck was seen in the long axis.

RESULTS

Fluid was seen in 50 of 52 asymptomatic hips (24 of 26 volunteers) in each of the three imaging planes (two of these hips were imaged in only the axial and the sagittal planes). In the two remaining hips (two volunteers), fluid was visible in the axial and sagittal planes but not the coronal plane. Computer digital analysis yielded an average volume of fluid present in all three imaging planes, which combined to be 2.9 mL in the right hip and 2.4 mL in the left hip with a range of 0.7–5.6 mL (Table 1). Although up to 7.1 mL was seen in the sagittal plane in one hip, the largest volume of fluid observed in any hip when averaging all three planes was 5.6 mL. In asymptomatic hips, discrete intra-articular fluid pockets, sometimes measuring greater than 5 mm in width, were commonly seen. These results are summarized in Table 2. Table 3 demonstrates interobserver variation with respect to grading the presence of fluid in the various locations.

The average volume of fluid seen in the fractured hips was 6.1 mL (range, 2.0–11.6 mL). Fluid was seen in every hip in all planes imaged (Table 4). Figures 1–3

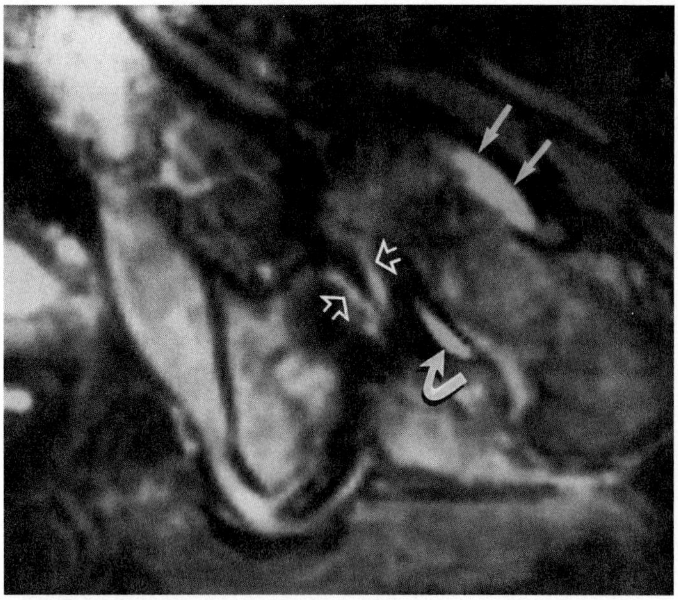

a.

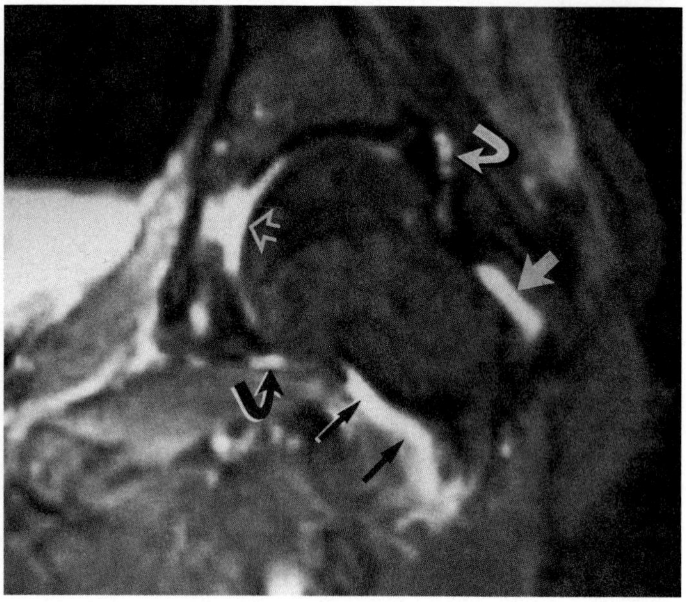

c.

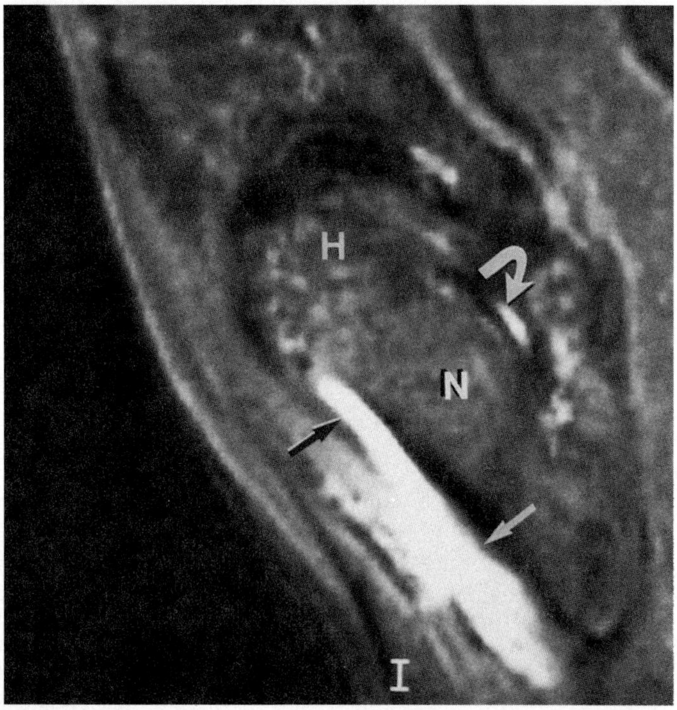

b.

Figure 2. Fast spin-echo, fat-saturated images (3,500/85) obtained at the level of the femoral neck after injection of 5 mL of saline into cadaveric hips show findings compatible with a joint effusion. **(a)** Axial image shows fluid measuring 5 mm in width anterior to the femoral neck (solid straight arrows) and a smaller amount of fluid posterior to the femoral neck (curved arrow). Open arrows = volume averaging with intracapsular fluid posterior to the femoral head better seen on an adjacent image (not shown). **(b)** Sagittal image shows fluid anterior to the femoral neck measuring 7 mm in width (straight arrows). A small amount of fluid is also seen posterior to the femoral neck (curved arrow). *H* = lateral femoral head, *I* = inferior, *N* = femoral neck, anterior is to the left. **(c)** Coronal image shows fluid measuring 5 mm in width inferior to the femoral neck (straight black arrows). Fluid is also seen in the region of the acetabular notch (open arrow) and superior to the femoral neck (straight white arrow). A tiny amount of fluid is also seen adjacent superiorly (curved white arrow) and inferiorly (curved black arrow) to the labrum.

illustrate the MR appearance of various volumes of fluid within cadaveric hip joints in the axial, sagittal, and coronal planes. After the injection of 5 mL of saline, fluid pooled adjacent to the femoral neck, measuring 5 mm in width anterior to the femoral neck on the axial and sagittal images and inferior to the femoral neck on the coronal images in all but one of the cadaveric hips, in which it measured 4 mm in these locations. Fluid measured 5 mm or more in width in these locations in all cadaveric hips after the injection of 10 and 20 mL of saline. US demonstrated progressive distention of the hip joint capsule anterior to the femoral neck (Fig 4). US measurements are shown in Table 5.

DISCUSSION

The appearance of fluid in the hip joint on MR images was initially described by Beltran et al (6) in healthy volunteers and patients with clinical hip effusions and by Mitchell et al (8) in patients with avascular necrosis. More recently, Bogost et al (9) concluded that a hip joint effusion was found in 13 of 26 patients with hip fracture and four of 44 without hip fracture. Their definition of an effusion was "greater than physiologic amounts of joint fluid." To our knowledge, our study is the first to quantify and describe the MR appearance of physiologic fluid in the normal, asymptomatic hip joint and to establish MR criteria for hip effusions.

Anatomic correlation reveals that normally only a thin film of fluid separates the articular surfaces in synovial joints (10). Our findings of average volumes of 2.5–3.0 mL of fluid in asymptomatic hips correlate well with estimates of the volume in large joints, primarily the knee, which range from less than 1 mL to less than 4 mL (11–13). Various systemic and articular disorders, as well as trauma and

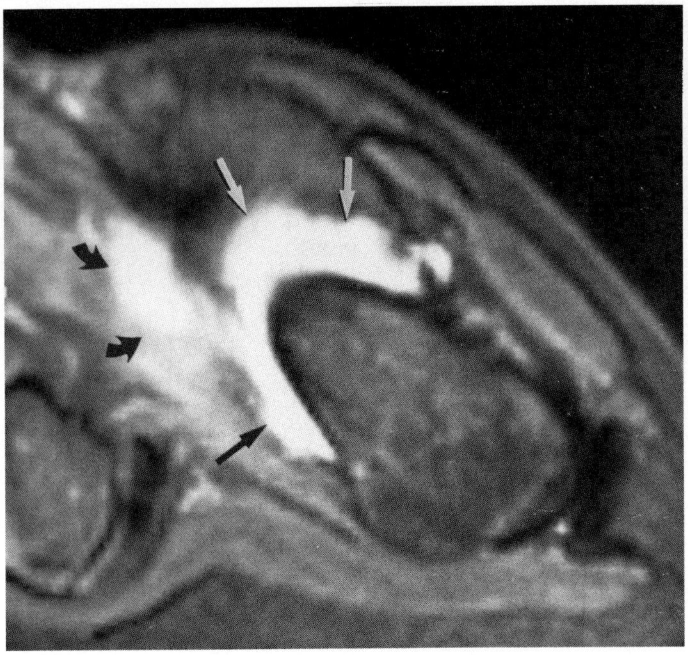

a.

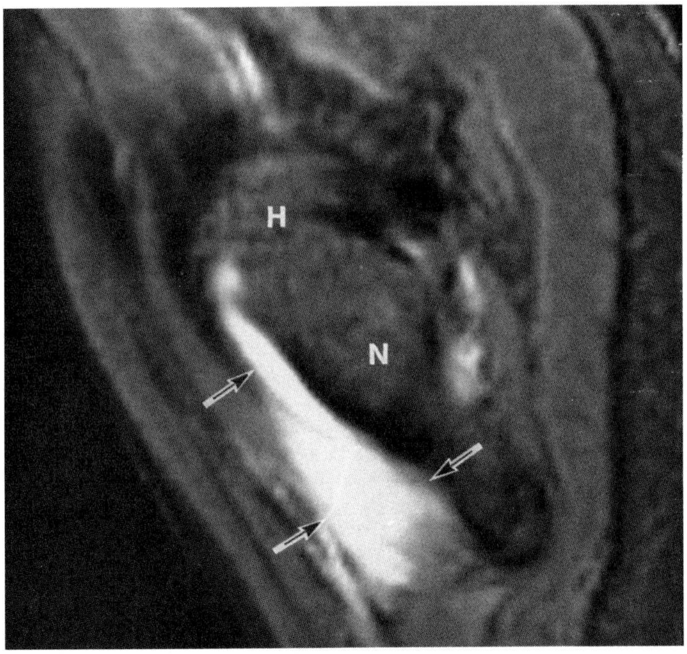

b.

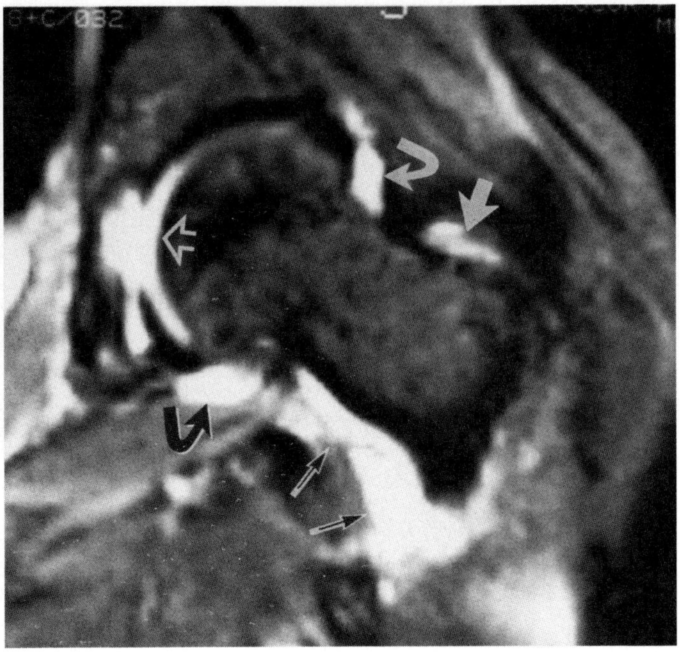

c.

Figure 3. Fast spin-echo, fat-saturated images (3,500/85) of cadaveric hips were obtained after injection of 20 mL of saline. **(a)** Axial image at the inferior femoral neck shows pooling of fluid in the inferior portion of the joint capsule (straight arrows) measuring 10 mm in width. Curved arrows = volume averaging of intracapsular fluid better seen on an adjacent image (not shown). **(b)** Sagittal image shows pooling of fluid anterior to the femoral neck (arrows) measuring 15 mm in maximum width at the base of the femoral neck. *H* = lateral femoral head, *N* = femoral neck, anterior is to the left. **(c)** Coronal image shows fluid pooling around the inferior femoral neck (small straight arrows) measuring 10 mm in width. Fluid adjacent superiorly (curved white arrow) and inferiorly (curved black arrow) to the labrum measure 5 mm. Fluid is completely filling the acetabular notch (open arrow), and a small amount of fluid is seen superior to the femoral neck (large straight arrow).

avascular necrosis, cause an increase in joint fluid. Effusions of sufficient volume can alter the biomechanics of the joint, causing decreased stability (10) and pain in both children (14) and adults (6,15). US has a high sensitivity for detection of hip effusions but is operator dependent; therefore, the volume of synovial fluid may be underestimated if excessive compression is applied on the joint capsule by the transducer (16) or if the fluid is within recesses that are obscured by adjacent bone. Our US images of the cadaveric hips showed progressive distention of the hip joint capsule as more fluid was injected into the joint. However, there was wide variation in the measurement from the anterior capsule to the anterior femoral neck. Although it was tempting to explain this by postulating that more fluid pooled posterior to the femoral neck secondary to gravity (the cadavers were in the supine position during saline injection and imaging), slightly more fluid was usually seen anterior to the femoral neck, possibly related to the saline injection.

Most of the fluid in the asymptomatic hips was seen as small, discrete pockets adjacent to the femoral neck on MR images. Furthermore, as progressive amounts of fluid were injected into the cadaveric hip joints, most of the fluid was noted to pool around the femoral neck. These findings correlate well with what has been observed at arthrography. It is unclear why there was a difference in the volume of fluid measured in the right and left hips, but this may be secondary to leg dominance or error in measurement. Because only five of our asymptomatic hips had more than 5 mL of fluid according to our computer analysis and because estimates of normal volumes in large joints are less than 4 mL, we based our criteria for hip effusions on findings in the cadaveric hips in which 5 mL of saline was injected. Since all but one cadaveric hip had fluid measuring 5 mm in width anterior to the femoral neck on the axial and sagittal images and inferior to the femoral neck on the coronal images, fluid pooling around the femoral neck measuring 5 mm in width in these locations is compatible with an effusion. Although fluid in one hip measured only 4 mm in width in these locations after the injection of 5 mL of fluid, we chose a measurement of 5 mm instead of 4 mm to decrease the frequency of considering maximal normal volumes of fluid an effusion. Furthermore, after the injection of 10 mL of fluid, the width of fluid pooling around the femoral neck in these locations was always at least 5 mm and often greater (Fig 2).

Our study has several limitations. We had a relatively small number of hips in our study and very few patients with fractured hips. It is possible that the volume of fluid would be different or have a more uniform distribution among the three imaging planes if a larger number of patients were studied. Furthermore, imaging of the fractured hips was not performed in all three imaging planes. In addition, all of the volunteers were young, healthy, and asymptomatic. These findings may have been different in a population with a wider age range, with clinical symptoms referable to the hip, or in aggressive athletes; however, previous studies have shown either no detectable change (17) or only a mild increase in joint fluid (18) in runners. The quantitative analysis of the fluid volume also has some inherent, albeit small, approximations. Even though all MR images were obtained with a 1-mm gap between sections, we incorporated the gap into the total thickness for each section and therefore assumed that the fluid seen within each section was also representative of the fluid in the 1-mm gap. Also, some variation may have been introduced by the three separate operators of the image analyzer. Finally, distribution of fluid in cadaveric hips may not simulate distribution of fluid in living patients.

In conclusion, asymptomatic hip joints average 2.5–3.0 mL of fluid within the hip joint itself, occasionally exceeding 5 mL, and may contain small, discrete pockets of fluid within the hip joint capsule. By comparing the appearance of fluid in the cadaveric hips after injection of 5 and 10 mL of saline with the appearance of fluid in our asymptomatic hips, we developed criteria for effusions. Our findings suggest that pooling of fluid adjacent to the entire length of the femoral neck, measuring at least 5 mm in width, is compatible with a joint effusion.

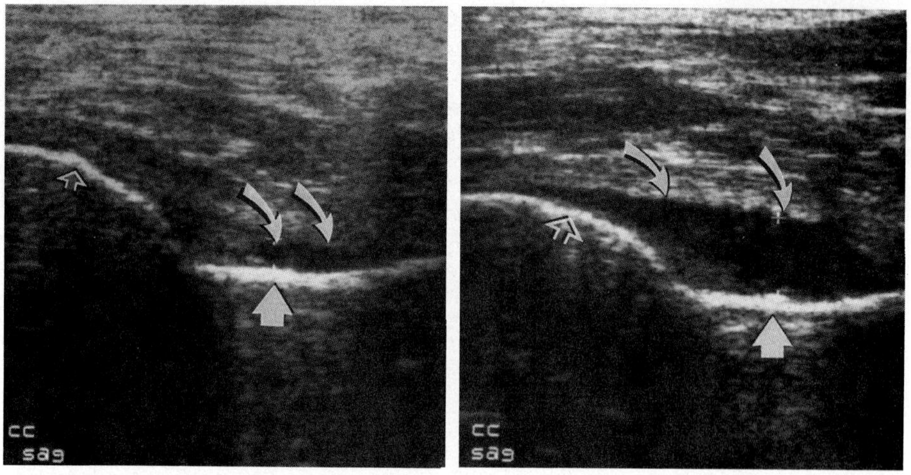

a. b.

Figure 4. Sagittal oblique US images of cadaveric hips obtained with an anterior approach after injection of **(a)** 2 mL and **(b)** 10 mL of saline. **(a)** Anechoic fluid (curved arrows) measuring 2.7 mm in width is seen anterior to the femoral neck (straight solid arrow). Open arrow = femoral head. **(b)** Anechoic fluid (curved arrows) measures 6.6 mm in width anterior to the femoral neck (straight solid arrow). A small amount of anechoic fluid extends anterior to the femoral head (open arrow).

References

1. Schweitzer ME, Magbalon MJ, Fenlin JM, Frieman BG, Ehrlich S, Epstein RE. Effusion criteria and clinical importance of glenohumeral joint fluid: MR imaging evaluation. Radiology 1995; 194:821–824.
2. Schweitzer ME, Magbalon MJ, Frieman BG, Ehrlich S, Epstein R. Acromioclavicular joint fluid: determination of clinical significance with MR imaging. Radiology 1994; 192:205–207.
3. Schweitzer ME, Falk A, Berthoty D, Mitchell M, Resnick D. Knee effusion: normal distribution of fluid. AJR 1992; 159:361–363.
4. Schweitzer ME, van Leersum M, Ehrlich SS, Wapner K. Fluid in normal and abnormal ankle joints: amount and distribution as seen on MR images. AJR 1994; 162:111–114.
5. Nazarian LN, Rawool NM, Martin CE, Schweitzer ME. Synovial fluid in the hindfoot and ankle: detection of amount and distribution with US. Radiology 1995; 197: 275–278.
6. Beltran J, Noto AM, Herma LJ, et al. Joint effusions: MR imaging. Radiology 1986; 158:133–137.
7. Mitchell DG. MR of the normal and ischemic hip. In: Kressell HY, ed. Magnetic resonance annual. New York, NY: Raven, 1988; 37–69.
8. Mitchell DG, Rao V, Dalinka M, et al. MRI of joint fluid in the normal and ischemic hip. AJR 1986; 146:1215–1218.
9. Bogost GA, Lizerbram EK, Crues JV III. MR imaging in evaluation of suspected hip fracture: frequency of unsuspected bone and soft-tissue injury. Radiology 1995; 197:263–267.
10. Simkin PA. Synovial physiology. In: McCarty DJ, ed. Arthritis and allied conditions. 12th ed. Philadelphia, Pa: Lea & Febiger, 1989; 209–211.
11. Schumacher HR Jr. Synovial fluid analysis and synovial biopsy. In: Kelly WN, Harris ED Jr, Ruddy S, Sledge CB, eds. Textbook of rheumatology. 4th ed. Vol 1. Philadelphia, Pa: Saunders, 1993; 562–578.
12. McCarty DJ. Synovial fluid. In: McCarty DJ, ed. Arthritis and allied conditions. 12th ed. Philadelphia, Pa: Lea & Febiger, 1993; 64–65.
13. Gatter RA. A practical handbook of joint fluid analysis. Philadelphia, Pa: Lea & Febiger, 1984.
14. Miralles M, Gonzalez G, Pulpeiro JR, et al. Sonography of the painful hip in children: 500 consecutive cases. AJR 1989; 152:579–582.
15. Foldes K, Balint P, Gaal M, Buchanan WW, Balint GP. Nocturnal pain correlates with effusions in diseased hips. J Rheumatol 1992; 19:1756–1758.
16. Chhem RK, Kaplan PA, Dussault RC. Ultrasonography of the musculoskeletal system. Radiol Clin North Am 1994; 32:275–289.
17. Shellock FG, Mink JH. Knees of trained long-distance runners: MR imaging before and after competition. Radiology 1991; 179:635–637.
18. Kursunoglu-Brahme S, Schwaighofer B, Gundry C, Ho C, Resnick D. Jogging causes acute changes in the knee joint: an MR study in normal volunteers. AJR 1990; 154:1233–1235.

Quantitative MR Imaging Evaluation of Chondropathy in Osteoarthritic Knees[1]

Jean-Luc Drapé, MD, PhD
Eric Pessis, MD
Guy-Robert Auleley, MD
Alain Chevrot, MD
Maxime Dougados, MD
Xavier Ayral, MD

Index terms:
Arthroscopy, 4521.1269
Cartilage, 4521.4851
Cartilage, MR, 4521.12146, 4521.12117, 4521.121412
Knee, arthritis, 452.77
Magnetic resonance (MR), comparative studies
Magnetic resonance (MR), volume measurement, 4521.12146

Radiology 1998; 208:49–55

Abbreviation:
SFA = French Society of Arthroscopy

[1] From the Departments of Radiology (J.L.D., E.P., A.C.) and Rheumatology (G.R.A., M.D., X.A.), Hôpital Cochin, 27 rue du Fg Saint-Jacques 75679, Paris 14, France. Received October 6, 1997; revision requested November 26; revision received February 11, 1998; accepted March 10. **Address reprint requests to** J.L.D.

PURPOSE: To determine the validity and the reliability of T1-weighted three-dimensional gradient-echo magnetic resonance (MR) imaging for quantification of articular cartilage abnormalities of osteoarthritic knees.

MATERIALS AND METHODS: Forty-three patients (mean age, 63 years) with knee osteoarthritis (American College of Rheumatology criteria) of the medial tibiofemoral compartment underwent a prospective, cross-sectional study. Knees were examined with a T1-weighted three-dimensional gradient-echo sequence (1.4-mm contiguous sections), with use of a 0.2-T dedicated MR unit, before arthroscopic exploration. The tibiofemoral articular cartilage abnormalities were quantified blindly on both the MR and arthroscopic images with the French Society of Arthroscopy (SFA) score (0–100) and grading scheme (five grades).

RESULTS: There was a statistically significant correlation between the SFA-arthroscopic score and the SFA-MR score ($r = .83$) and between the SFA-arthroscopic grade and the SFA-MR grade (weighted $\kappa = 0.84$). The deepest cartilage lesions graded with arthroscopy and MR imaging showed correlation in the medial femoral condyle (weighted $\kappa = 0.83$) and in the medial tibial plateau (weighted $\kappa = 0.84$). The intraobserver reliability of the SFA-MR score was higher ($r = .94$) than the interobserver reliability ($r = .80$).

CONCLUSION: Quantification of chondropathy with MR imaging is feasible and well correlated with anatomic cartilage breakdown.

Osteoarthritis frequently affects the knee and is characterized by cartilage fissuring and erosions, osteophytes, subchondral sclerosis, and cysts, often in combination with synovial changes and meniscal degeneration. Magnetic resonance (MR) imaging is capable of providing evaluation of the entire joint. In addition to depiction of surface abnormalities and the thickness and signal intensity of the cartilage, MR imaging depicts the synovial membrane and signal intensity of subchondral bone.

From numerous articles (1–15), we found a wide range of MR imaging accuracies (50%–97%) for detection of chondral lesions of the knee. Various study designs have been used, from in vitro models with human cadaveric joints (4,11,15) to in vivo correlations with arthroscopy or arthrotomy (1–3,5–8,10,12–14). The tibiofemoral compartments were much less often investigated than was the femoropatellar joint (2,5,6,9,12,14). The authors of several recent studies propose three-dimensional gradient-echo MR imaging with fat suppression as one of the most accurate sequences for imaging cartilage (9,12,13,15).

In time, progression of cartilage ulcerations, in both depth and extent, causes a decrease in the amount of articular cartilage. This parameter probably is the most clinically pertinent and useful for assessment of the natural history of osteoarthritis and for evaluation of potential structure-modifying drugs. In this field, the medial tibiofemoral compartment is most often evaluated.

Several methods have been proposed to evaluate the amount of articular cartilage. Measurement of joint space narrowing on weight-bearing plain radiographs represents a simple technique to assess the severity of chondropathy (16–19). However, radiographic assessment of an affected knee remains an indirect approach and is still tainted by false-positive and false-negative findings (20). Hyaline cartilage appears anechoic at ultrasonography, and its thickness may be measured. The entire articular cartilage of the

Author contributions:
Guarantors of integrity of entire study, J.L.D., A.C., M.D.; study concepts, J.L.D., M.D.; study design, J.L.D., X.A., M.D.; definition of intellectual content, J.L.D., X.A.; literature research, J.L.D.; clinical and experimental studies, J.L.D., E.P., X.A.; data acquisition and analysis, J.L.D., E.P., X.A.; statistical analysis, G.R.A.; manuscript preparation, J.L.D., X.A.; manuscript editing, J.L.D.; manuscript review, J.L.D., X.A., G.R.A.

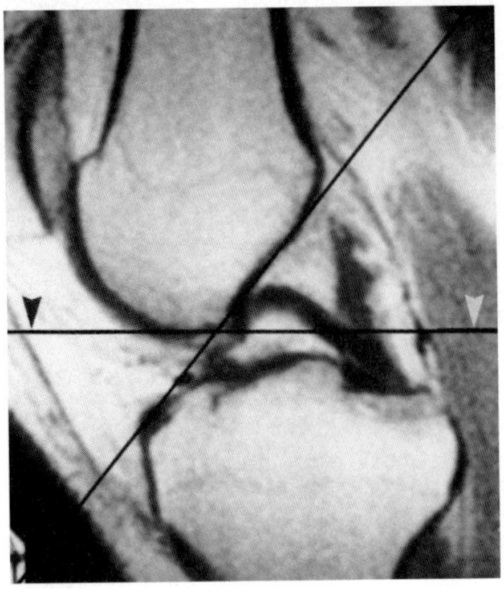

Figure 1. Anterior limit of the femoral condyles. Sagittal T1-weighted MR image of the knee shows the anterior limit defined by the intersection of the horizontal line (arrowheads) and the foot of the intercondylar notch. The oblique line corresponds to the Blumensaat line.

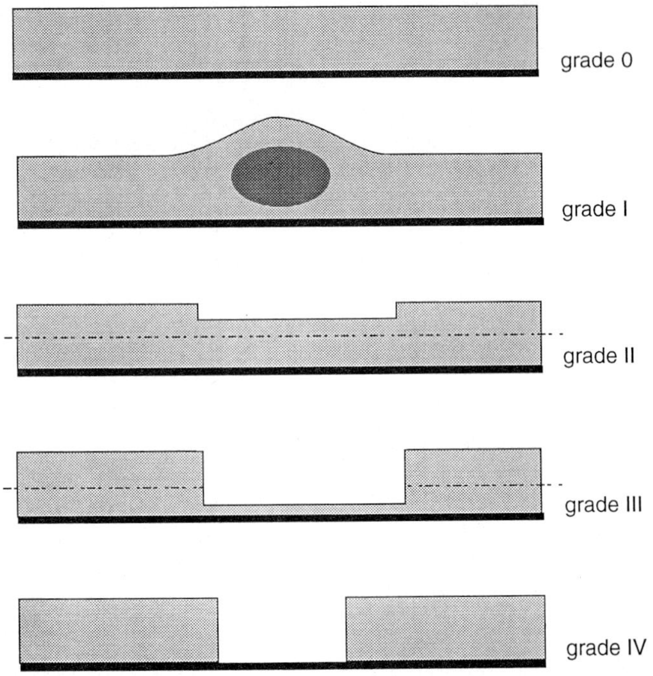

Figure 2. MR grading system of chondral lesions: *grade 0*, normal cartilage; *grade I*, focal blistering and intracartilaginous low-signal-intensity area; *grade II*, superficial irregularities and loss of thickness of less than 50%; *grade III*, deep ulceration with loss of thickness of more than 50%; *grade IV*, exposure of subchondral bone.

knee is not attainable with the probe, however, and the cartilage interfaces become less distinct with wear and degenerative changes. Arthroscopy provides a direct magnified view of the cartilage surface and is still considered as the standard of reference for assessing cartilage lesions (20–22). Even with a detailed analysis of the cartilage, a composite index that takes into account the three baseline characteristics of location, depth, and size of the chondral lesions was required. Such an index of severity of chondropathy was established by the French Society of Arthroscopy (SFA) and is known as the SFA scoring and grading systems (18,23). The SFA systems have been validated (24–26). However, the arthroscopic procedure remains invasive and time-consuming, even with use of local anesthesia and a small arthroscope (24).

A few previous MR imaging studies took a quantitative approach to the articular cartilage by focusing on measurements of the thickness or the volume of cartilage (27–35). MR imaging appeared as a reproducible method of measurement of the cartilage of the knee in human specimens (27,31,34,35) or animal models (32,35). In several study designs, however, a complex three-dimensional imaging postprocessing technique on a dedicated workstation was necessary (27,28,30,32,34,35), and only one in vivo study concerned a small series of osteoarthritic knees (27).

The aim of our study was to evaluate the validity of this MR imaging method of grading articular cartilage abnormalities by comparing arthroscopic and MR imaging findings in a population with medial tibiofemoral osteoarthritis, and to evaluate the intra- and interobserver reliability of manual MR scoring and grading systems derived from the SFA systems.

MATERIALS AND METHODS

Patients

Forty-three patients (30 women, 13 men; age range, 53–78 years; mean age, 63 years) were included in the study. All patients were examined by the same rheumatologist (X.A.) and had active medial tibiofemoral osteoarthritis with indication for a joint lavage by means of arthroscopy. They were enrolled in the study after providing informed consent. They fulfilled the American College of Rheumatology clinical and radiographic criteria for knee osteoarthritis (36). Other inclusion criteria were (*a*) clinical involvement (pain) of the medial tibiofemoral compartment, (*b*) active disease (inadequate pain control certified by prior failure of intraarticular glucocorticoid injection, physical exercises, analgesics, and nonsteroidal anti-inflammatory drugs), (*c*) mild radiologic osteoarthritis of the medial compartment (medial tibiofemoral joint space ≥ 2 mm on a weight-bearing extended anteroposterior view), and (*d*) lack of contraindication for MR imaging and arthroscopic procedures.

Study Design

This single-center prospective cross-sectional study was approved by the ethics committee of our hospital. MR imaging and arthroscopy were successively performed the same day.

MR Data Collection

Patients underwent MR imaging with a 0.2-T musculoskeletal dedicated MR unit (Artoscan; Esaote Biomedica, Genoa, Italy). Knees were placed in a receive-only, cylindric solenoid coil. Two successive three-dimensional gradient-echo sequences (repetition time msec/echo time msec, 60/24; 45° flip angle) were acquired in the sagittal and coronal planes with, respectively, 40 and 32 contiguous 1.4-mm-thick sections. The field of view was 150 mm, the matrix was 192 × 160, and voxels were anisotopic with a size of

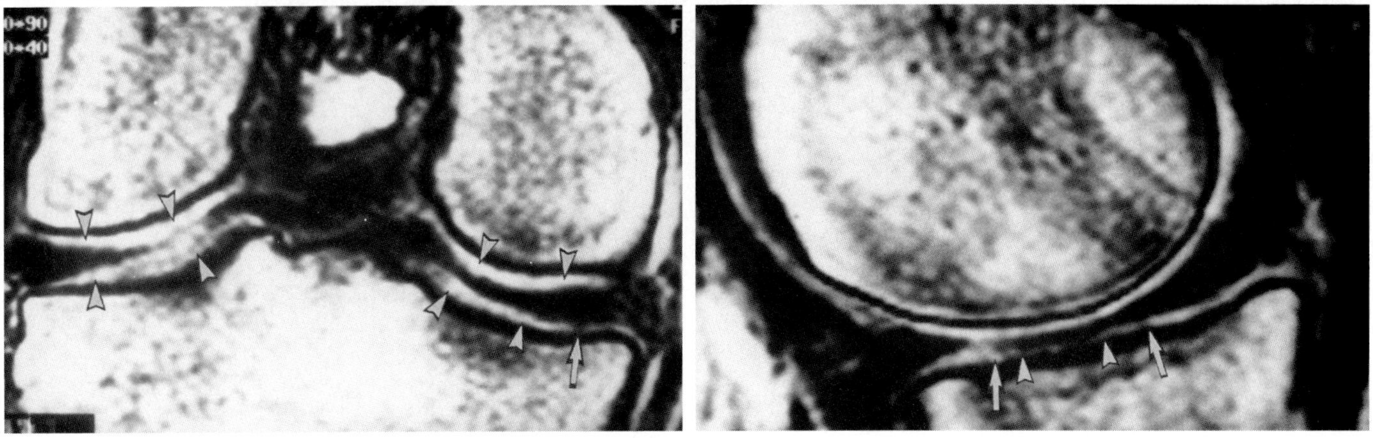

a. b.

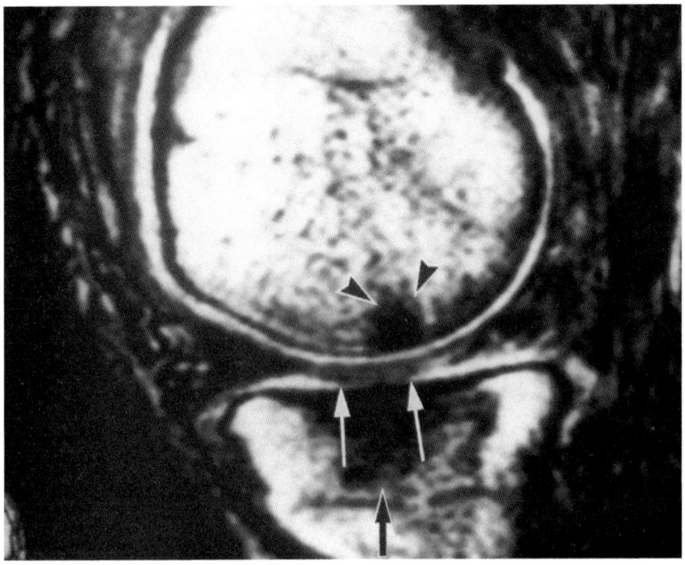

c.

Figure 3. Three-dimensional gradient-echo 1.4-mm-thick MR images (60/24, 45° flip angle) of the tibiofemoral compartments in three different patients. **(a)** Coronal view shows cartilage that was normal at arthroscopy. Articular cartilage shows high signal intensity (arrowheads). The thin, low-signal-intensity intracartilaginous line of the lateral tibial plateau is not relevant and may be due to truncation artifacts. Note the tiny focal chondral area of low signal intensity (arrow) below the medial meniscus. **(b)** Sagittal view of the medial tibiofemoral compartment shows a deep ulceration (grade III)(arrowheads) surrounded by a rim of grade II abnormalities (arrows). **(c)** Sagittal view of the medial tibiofemoral compartment shows a grade IV ulceration of the tibial plateau (white arrows) with a large low-signal-intensity area in the underlying subchondral bone (black arrow). Note the focal low-signal-intensity area (arrowheads) on the subchondral bone of the femoral condyle, with only grade II lesions of the overlying cartilage.

0.78 × 0.94 × 1.4 mm. The acquisition time of each sequence ranged from 6 minutes 26 seconds to 5 minutes 9 seconds, with one signal acquired.

Arthroscopic Data Collection

The arthroscopic exploration was performed immediately after MR imaging and focused on the medial tibiofemoral compartment. Arthroscopy was performed by a trained arthroscopist (X.A.), with use of local anesthesia, without tourniquet hemostasis. A 2.7-mm Storz arthroscope (Storz, Paris, France) with a 30° angled view was used with an inferolateral approach. The medial femoral condyle was explored from 0° to 90° of knee flexion. Each arthroscopic examination was recorded on videotape in a standardized manner.

Arthroscopic Data Evaluation

Qualitative study.—The severity of cartilage breakdown was studied for the medial femoral condyle and medial tibial plateau. The depth of cartilage abnormalities was graded 0–IV according to the classification proposed by Beguin and Locker (37): grade 0, normal cartilage; grade I, swelling and/or softening; grade II, superficial fibrillations; grade III, deep fibrillations down to bone; grade IV, exposure of subchondral bone.

Quantitative study.—The first step consisted in recording on an articular diagram of the knee the observed chondropathy with three main baseline variables: (*a*) location: medial femur and medial tibia; (*b*) depth based on the classification of chondropathy proposed by Beguin and Locker; and (*c*) size from 0% to 100% of the involved articular surface. The size of the lesions was estimated by the arthroscopist as a percentage of the entire articular surface and was recorded on a special form (18,24).

The composite index of severity of chondropathy taking into account location, depth, and size of cartilage lesions consisted of two variables: (*a*) SFA score. This is a continuous variable between 0 and 100 obtained for the medial tibiofemoral compartment as follows (23): SFA score = $S_{I} \times 0.14 + S_{II} \times 0.34 + S_{III} \times 0.65 + S_{IV} \times 1.00$, where S_I through S_{IV} are the sizes (expressed as percentages) of grades I–IV lesions. The size (as a percentage) of grade x (where x is 0 to IV) corresponded to the mean value of the size of grade x of the medial femoral condyle and the medial tibial plateau. (*b*) SFA grade (or category of chondropathy severity of the compartment). This is a semiquantitative variable that includes five grades (18). SFA grade 0 indicates the lack of chondropathy, and SFA grade 4 indicates a severe chondropathy. The above numbers (size as a percentage) for grades 0 to IV, according to Beguin and Locker, were placed in a formula to provide SFA grades. For the medial tibiofemoral compartment, the SFA grades were calculated as follows: SFA grade 0 if grade 0 = 100%; SFA grade 1 if grade IV = 0% and grade 0 ≥ 80% but < 100%; SFA grade 2 if grade IV = 0%, grade 0 < 80%, and grade III < 15%; SFA grade 3 if grade IV = 0%, grade 0 < 80%, and grade III ≥ 15% or if

TABLE 1
Case Record Form Used to Record Lesion Size

MR Grade*	Lesion Size in Femur (%)	Lesion Size in Tibia (%)	Mean Value† (%)
0	67	87.5	77.25
I	0	0	0
II	21	0	10.50
III	0	12.5	6.25
IV	12	0	6.00

Note.—The numbers represent the size of the corresponding MR grade expressed as a percentage of the corresponding entire articular surface. The percentage is established by recording the involved surface on the entire surface on the knee diagram (Fig 4). Each column totals 100%.

* MR grades are defined in Figure 2.

† Medial SFA-MR score = 10.5 × 0.34 + 6.25 × 0.65 + 6 × 1.00 = 13.63. Medial SFA-MR grade = 3 (MR grade IV ≥ 1% and MR grade 0 ≥ 65%). (See text for explanations of SFA score and grade.)

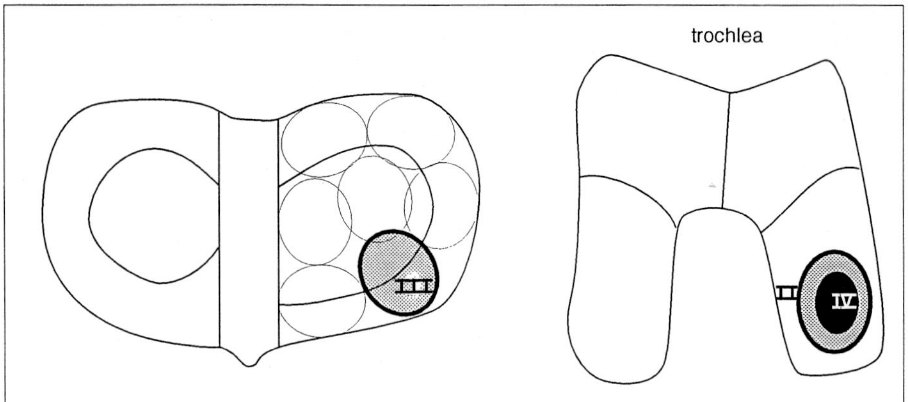

Figure 4. Example of articular cartilage lesions of the medial tibiofemoral compartment visualized with MR imaging and recorded on this knee diagram (right knee). *II*, *III*, and *IV* are the MR grades of chondral lesions described in Figure 2. (See Table 1 for calculation of SFA-MR score and SFA-MR grade.)

grade IV ≥ 1% and grade 0 ≥ 65%; and SFA grade 4 if grade IV ≥ 1% and grade 0 < 65%.

In this study, the SFA score and grade obtained arthroscopically are called SFA-arthroscopic score and SFA-arthroscopic grade. The calculation of these scores and grades was performed by a trained arthroscopist (X.A.) blinded from the patient identity and MR findings.

MR Imaging Data Evaluation

Qualitative study.—The severity of cartilage lesions was also noted for each articular surface of the medial tibiofemoral compartment. The limits of the condyles were defined to match with the arthroscopic field of investigation: The anterior limit was defined by the foot of the intercondylar notch (Fig 1) and the posterior limit was the posterior end of the condylar cartilage. The depth of cartilage abnormalities were graded 0–IV (MR grade), derived from the arthroscopic classification of Beguin and Locker (37)(Figs 2, 3).

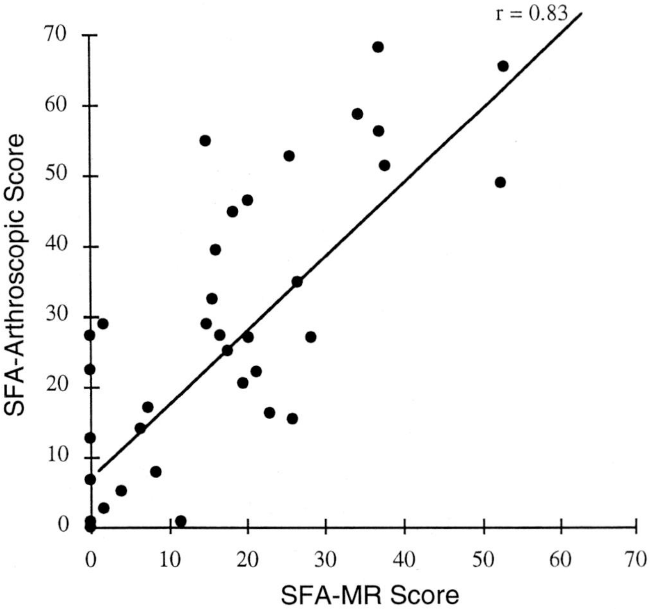

Figure 5. Validity of MR imaging quantification of chondropathy. Correlation between SFA-MR and SFA-arthroscopic scoring systems in 43 patients with osteoarthritis of the medial tibiofemoral compartment.

Quantitative study.—Two scoring methods were used: the SFA-MR scoring system and the SFA-MR grading system derived from the SFA scoring and grading systems. As with arthroscopy, the observed chondropathy was recorded on the same articular diagram of the knee (Fig 4). The SFA-MR score and the SFA-MR grade were calculated by using the mathematic formula described for arthroscopy and taking into account the depth of chondral lesions, seen on MR images, and their size (Table 1). The calculation of these scores and grades was performed by two musculoskeletal radiologists (E.P., J.L.D.) blinded from the arthroscopic scores and grades and blinded from the patient identity.

Statistical Analysis

Statistical analyses were performed to evaluate the validity of this method of MR quantification of the cartilage, and the intra- and interobserver reliability.

Validity of MR imaging.—The extrinsic validity of MR quantification of chondral lesions was evaluated by calculating the correlation between SFA-arthroscopic score and SFA-MR score on the one hand and between SFA-arthroscopic grade and SFA-MR grade on the other (coefficient of correlation [*r*] and weighted κ statistic, respectively). Equal weighting was given for each grade of disagreement. Moreover, qualitative comparison between the two techniques was assessed by comparing the deepest chondral lesions seen at MR images and at arthroscopy (weighted κ statistic).

Test-retest reliability.—For this purpose, MR examinations were read twice by a

TABLE 2
MR Validity: Correlation between SFA-MR and SFA-Arthroscopic Grades in 43 Patients with Osteoarthritis of the Medial Compartment

SFA-Arthroscopic Grade	SFA-MR Grade 0	1	2	3	4
0	1	4	2	0	0
1	0	4	3	0	0
2	1	2	4	1	0
3	0	2	2	1	0
4	0	0	0	6	10

Note.—Weighted κ = 0.84.

TABLE 3
MR Validity: Correlations between MR and Arthroscopy for Depiction of the Deepest Cartilage Lesion of the Medial Femoral Condyle and the Medial Tibial Plateau in 43 Patients

Arthroscopic Maximum Grade	MR Maximum Grade 0	II	III	IV
	Medial Femoral Condyle*			
0	8	0	0	0
II	5	3	5	0
III	1	1	4	2
IV	1	0	3	10
	Medial Tibial Plateau†			
0	11	0	1	0
II	5	2	1	2
III	2	0	2	3
IV	0	0	1	13

Note.—Maximum grade is according to the classification of Beguin and Locker (37).
* Weighted κ = 0.83.
† Weighted κ = 0.84.

single musculoskeletal radiologist (E.P.) after an interval of 2 months (for intraobserver reliability) and independently by two trained musculoskeletal radiologists (E.P., J.L.D.) in the same period (for interobserver reliability).

Reliability of the SFA-MR scores was evaluated by calculating the intraclass correlation coefficient (38). This coefficient was calculated from a one-way analysis of variance table and could theoretically range from 0 to 1, with higher values indicating stronger agreement. The distribution of differences in scores was based on the technique proposed by Bland and Altman (39). This technique consisted of calculation of the differences in the result of a variable (SFA-MR score) obtained in a single patient by two different observers and/or at two different times by a single observer. Since several MR studies were analyzed, it was possible to calculate the mean ± standard deviation of these differences. The distribution of differences (ie, mean ± 2 standard deviations) indicated the range of the changes related to the variability of the technique. In other words, it permits evaluation of the cutoff above which the changes observed in a single subsequent patient could be reasonably attributed to disease progression.

Reliability of the SFA-MR grades was evaluated by calculating the weighted κ value.

RESULTS

MR Validity

The mean SFA-arthroscopic score was 23.5 ± 21.0 (standard deviation). The mean SFA-MR score was 15.39 ± 11.27 and 14.69 ± 15.32 for the two observers (E.P. and J.L.D., respectively). There was a statistically significant correlation between the SFA-arthroscopic score and the SFA-MR score of the medial tibiofemoral compartment (r = .83)(Fig 5). There was also a highly statistically significant correlation between the SFA-arthroscopic grade and the SFA-MR grade of the medial tibiofemoral compartment (weighted κ = 0.84)(Table 2). However, there was complete agreement between the two methods for only 20 of the 43 patients. In five patients, there was a disagreement of two categories, with SFA-arthroscopic grades 0, 2, or 3, and with either under- or overestimation of the lesions with MR imaging compared with arthroscopic findings. In the same way, there was a statistically significant correlation between the deepest cartilage lesion of the medial femoral condyle or tibial plateau seen at arthroscopy and at MR imaging (weighted κ = 0.83 and 0.84, respectively)(Table 3). However, there was complete agreement between the two methods in 25 patients for the femoral condyle and in 28 patients for the tibial plateau. There was a disagreement of two grades in two patients, with condylar arthroscopic grades III and IV (according to the classification proposed by Beguin and Locker) not detected with MR imaging, and in five patients with tibial arthroscopic grade 0, II, or III, with either underestimation (two patients) or overestimation (three patients) at MR imaging.

MR Reliability

Figure 6 and Tables 4 and 5 summarize the results of intra- and interobserver reliability. Detailed analysis of the standard deviation of the changes clearly shows that intraobserver reliability was better than interobserver reliability. The minimum interval changes of SFA-scores that could be measured were about 12% for the same observer and 19% for two different observers.

DISCUSSION

In this study, MR imaging appeared as an effective noninvasive method of quantification of chondral lesions of the knee in a large series of patients. An outcome measure is usually considered relevant when such measure fulfills the following characteristics: simplicity, validity, reliability, and responsiveness (38). The results of this study suggest that MR imaging could fulfill simplicity, validity, and reliability. Evaluation of responsiveness requires a longitudinal study with MR imaging and arthroscopic follow-up. The MR examination took less than ½ hour and did not require injection of a contrast medium. Low-cost MR examinations were available with a low-field-strength, dedicated MR unit. A three-dimensional gradient-echo sequence was performed in this study because it offered thin (1.4-mm) sections. Thin sections were essential to decrease partial volume averaging artifacts and to limit the errors of assessment of the cartilage thickness, which can be as high as 40% (28,29,32). Fat suppression has been used by most authors to quantify cartilage (11,27,30,32,33,35), but it is not available at low field strength, the fat and water peaks being too close. Cartilage appeared spontaneously with a high signal intensity at 0.2 T, and there was high contrast between the cartilage and the subchondral bone and the surrounding soft tissues. With high field strength, fat suppression is useful to eliminate chemical shift artifacts at the interface between the cartilage and the subchondral bone. These artifacts are minimized with low-field-strength MR units.

Our results confirm the validity of the SFA-MR scoring and grading systems, with a statistically significant correlation with the arthroscopic quantification. The SFA-MR score takes into account only articular cartilage lesions and is not influenced by osteophytes, subchondral signal intensity abnormalities, degenerative meniscal lesions, or synovial or ligamentous abnormalities. The SFA-MR scores were very close between the two observers but lower than the SFA-arthroscopic scores. This shift may be due to the

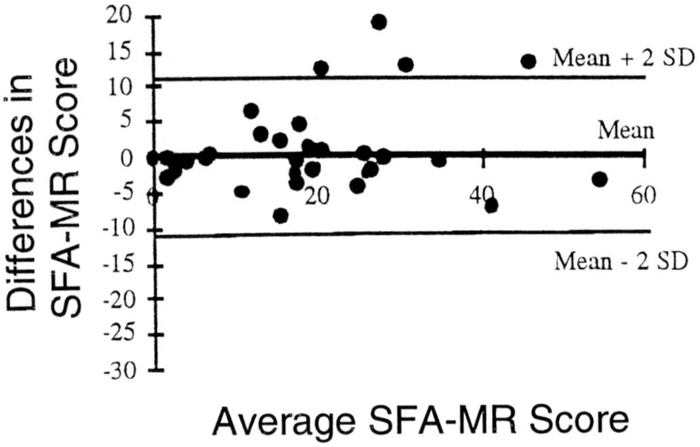

a.

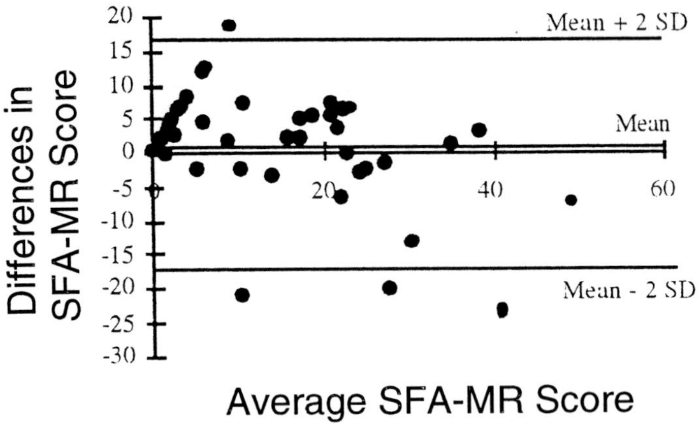

b.

Figure 6. Test-retest reliability evaluated for the MR examinations of 43 patients with osteoarthritic knees (medial tibiofemoral compartment). **(a)** Intraobserver reliability. The y axis is the differences in SFA-MR score between two readings for the same observer. **(b)** Interobserver reliability. The y axis is the differences in SFA-MR score between two readings for the two observers.

TABLE 4
MR Reliability: Differences in SFA-MR Grades in 43 Patients

A: Intraobserver Reliability*

SFA-MR Grade at Second Evaluation	SFA-MR Grade at First Evaluation				
	0	1	2	3	4
0	13	0	0	0	0
1	1	4	1	0	0
2	0	1	0	1	0
3	0	1	0	7	7
4	0	0	0	3	4

B: Interobserver Reliability†

SFA-MR Grade per Investigator B	SFA-MR Grade per Investigator A				
	0	1	2	3	4
0	1	9	4	0	0
1	0	3	3	0	0
2	0	0	1	0	0
3	1	0	3	5	2
4	0	0	0	3	8

* Weighted κ = 0.91.
† Weighted κ = 0.82.

TABLE 5
MR Reliability: Differences in SFA-MR Scores in 43 Patients

A: Intraobserver Reliability

Outcome Measure	First Evaluation	Second Evaluation	Differences	Reliability Coefficient
SFA-MR score (0–100)	14.69 ± 15.32	13.57 ± 13.69	1.12 ± 5.47	.94

B: Interobserver Reliability

Outcome Measure	Investigator A	Investigator B	Differences	Reliability Coefficient
SFA-MR score (0–100)	15.39 ± 11.27	14.69 ± 15.32	0.70 ± 8.98	.80

difference of the areas explored with the two methods. We tried to match the anterior limit, but the posterior edge of the condyles and the peripheral area of the tibial plateau below the meniscus were not always attainable by the arthroscopist. The area investigated with MR imaging was larger than that visible at arthroscopy, which decreased systematically the SFA-MR scores. Moreover, the surface of the cartilage was only visible with arthroscopy, and chondral lesions could have been overgraded in comparison with MR imaging.

Our results confirm also that intraobserver reliability of the SFA-MR quantification of cartilage lesions is satisfactory and better than interobserver reliability, regardless of the method used. The minimum interval change in SFA-MR score for the same observer that could be measured was about 12%, and the same accuracy was noted in volumetric assessment of the cartilage (27). Reviewing MR images is time-consuming (about 20 minutes per patient), but even in a multicenter study dealing with a large population of patients, the interpretation of MR images should be centralized and reviewed by a single, trained radiologist.

The comparison between the deepest cartilage lesions seen with arthroscopy and MR imaging showed discrepancies of more than one grade in seven of 86 examinations (43 condyles, 43 plateaus). These misinterpretations concerned superficial but also deep arthroscopic lesions, which were under- or overestimated with MR imaging. Earlier stages of cartilage thinning with tiny focal defects are often occult and responsible of overestimation of the thickness of the cartilage with MR imaging (31). MR grade I lesions were not found in this study. Artifacts, such as magic angle phenomenon or truncation artifact, may interfere (40,41). The accuracy of MR depiction of natural or artificial lesions in cadaveric models (28,29,31–33,35) may be higher but is not representative of clinical actuality. Isotonic saline solution is often injected and mimics synovial fluid and may improve the detectability of surface abnormalities. High-resolution imaging with long acquisition times is often performed, but this quality of imaging is not representative of what is generally available clinically.

Our global quantitative and semiquantitative assessment of the articular cartilage presents some advantages over MR measurements of the thickness or the volume of the cartilage. Results of thickness measurements are not reproducible without a position marker to identify the same location on the cartilage every time. Measurements of the volume may be more reproducible but need a dedicated three-dimensional workstation or custom software (27,30,32,34,35), which is not necessary with the SFA-MR method. However, volumetric quantification with three-dimensional reconstructions may be less sensitive than single-section data or the SFA-MR method in identifying tiny focal defects in the cartilage. Semiquantitative scoring methods, in which the experienced observer can compensate for slight variations in section location and orientation, may be more reliable for longitudinal evaluation of focal chondral defects than are volume measurements.

In conclusion, our results suggest that the quantification of chondropathy of the knee with MR imaging is feasible by using the SFA-arthroscopic scoring and grading systems. Further longitudinal studies to evaluate the responsiveness of this method (ie, the capacity of MR imaging to depict statistically significant deterioration of cartilage breakdown over time) are required. If MR scoring is then validated, this noninvasive method could be used as an outcome measure of cartilage lesions in clinical trials to evaluate potential structure-modifying drugs in patients with osteoarthritis.

References

1. McCauley TR, Kier R, Lynch KJ, Jokl P. Chondromalacia patellae: diagnosis with MR imaging. AJR 1992; 158:101–105.
2. Heron CW, Calvert PT. Three-dimensional gradient-echo MR imaging of the knee: comparison with arthroscopy in 100 patients. Radiology 1992; 183:839–844.
3. Brown TR, Quinn SF. Evaluation of chondromalacia of the patellofemoral compartment with axial magnetic resonance imaging. Skeletal Radiol 1993; 22:325–328.
4. Recht MP, Kramer J, Marcelis S, et al. Abnormalities of articular cartilage in the knee: analysis of available MR techniques. Radiology 1993; 187:473–478.
5. Kramer J, Recht MP, Imhof H, Stiglbauer R, Engel A. Postcontrast MR arthrography in assessment of cartilage lesions. J Comput Assist Tomogr 1994; 18:218–224.
6. Broderick LS, Turner DA, Renfrew DL, Schnitzer TJ, Huff JP, Harris C. Severity of articular cartilage abnormality in patients with osteoarthritis: evaluation with fast spin-echo MR vs arthroscopy. AJR 1994; 162:99–103.
7. Rose PM, Demlow A, Szumowki J, Quinn SF. Chondromalacia patellae: fat-suppressed MR imaging. Radiology 1994; 193:437–440.
8. Gagliardi JA, Chung EM, Chandnani VP, et al. Detection and staging of chondromalacia patellae: relative efficacies on conventional MR imaging, MR arthrography, and CT arthrography. AJR 1994; 163:629–636.
9. Disler DG, McCauley TR, Wirth CR, Fuchs MD. Detection of knee hyaline cartilage defects using fat-suppressed three-dimensional spoiled gradient-echo MR imaging: comparison with standard MR imaging and correlation with arthroscopy. AJR 1995; 165:377–382.
10. Vallotton JA, Meuli RA, Leyvraz PF, Landry M. Comparison between magnetic resonance imaging and arthroscopy in the diagnosis of patellar cartilage lesions. Knee Surg Sports Traumatol Arthrosc 1995; 3:157–162.
11. Van Leersum M, Schweitzer ME, Gannon F, Vinitski S, Finkel G, Mitchell DG. Thickness of patellofemoral articular cartilage as measured on MR imaging: sequence comparison of accuracy, reproducibility, and interobserver variation. Skeletal Radiol 1995; 24:431–435.
12. Disler DG, McCauley TR, Kelman CG, et al. Fat-suppressed three-dimensional spoiled gradient-echo MR imaging of hyaline cartilage defects in the knee: comparison with standard MR imaging and arthroscopy. AJR 1996; 167:127–132.
13. Recht MP, Piraino DW, Paletta GA, Schils JP, Belhobek GH. Accuracy of fat-suppressed three-dimensional spoiled gradient-echo FLASH MR imaging in the detection of patellofemoral articular cartilage abnormalities. Radiology 1996; 198:209–212.
14. Shahabpour M, Tebache C, Casteleyn PP, et al. IRM du cartilage: comparaison IRM arthroscopie a propos de 320 cas. In: Bard H, Drapé JL, Goutallier D, Laredo JD, eds. Le genou traumatique et degeneratif. Paris, France: Sauramps Médical, 1997; 161–176.
15. Brossmann J, Frank LR, Pauly JM, et al. Short echo time projection reconstruction MR imaging of cartilage: comparison with fat-suppressed spoiled GRASS and magnetization transfer contrast MR imaging. Radiology 1997; 203:501–507.
16. Ravaud P, Giraudeau B, Auleley GR, et al. Radiographic assessment of knee osteoarthritis: reproducibility and sensitivity to change. J Rheumatol 1996; 23:1756–1764.
17. Dougados M, Gueguen A, Nguyen M, et al. Longitudinal radiologic evaluation of osteoarthritis of the knee. J Rheumatol 1992; 19:378–384.
18. Dougados M, Ayral X, Listrat V, et al. The SFA system for assessing articular cartilage lesions at arthroscopy of the knee. Arthroscopy 1994; 10:69–77.
19. Conrozier T, Tron AM, Balbanc JC, et al. Measurement of the hip joint space using computerized image analysis. Rev Rhum Mal Osteoartic (Engl ed) 1995; 60:105–111.
20. Fife RS, Brandt KD, Braunstein EM, et al. Relationship between arthroscopic evidence of cartilage damage and radiographic evidence of joint space narrowing in early osteoarthritis of the knee. Arthritis Rheum 1991; 34:377–382.
21. Chan WP, Lang P, Stevens MP, et al. Osteoarthritis of the knee: comparison of radiography, CT, and MR imaging to assess extent and severity. Am J Rheumatol 1991; 157:799–806.
22. Blackburn WD Jr, Bernreuter WK, Rominger M, Loose LL. Arthroscopic evaluation of knee articular cartilage: a comparison with plain radiographs and magnetic resonance imaging. J Rheumatol 1994; 21:675–679.
23. Ayral X, Gueguen A, Listrat V, et al. Simplified arthroscopy scoring system for chondropathy of the knee (revised SFA score). Rev Rhum Mal Osteoartic (Engl Ed) 1994; 61:97–99.
24. Ayral X, Dougados M, Listrat V, et al. Chondroscopy: a new method for scoring chondropathy. Semin Arthritis Rheum 1993; 22:289–297.
25. Ayral X, Dougados M, Listrat V, Bonvarlet JP, Simonnet J, Amor B. Arthroscopic evaluation of chondropathy in osteoarthritis of the knee. J Rheumatol 1996; 23:698–706.
26. Listrat V, Ayral X, Patarnello F, et al. Arthroscopic evaluation of potential structure modifying activity of hyaluronan (Hyalgan) in osteoarthritis of the knee. Osteoarthritis Cartilage 1997; 5:153–160.
27. Peterfy CG, Dijke van CF, Janzen DL, et al. Quantification of articular cartilage in the knee with pulsed saturation transfer subtraction and fat-suppressed MR imaging: optimization and validation. Radiology 1994; 192:485–491.
28. Pilch L, Stewart C, Gordon D, et al. Assessment of cartilage volume in the femorotibial joint with magnetic resonance imaging and 3D computer reconstruction. J Rheumatol 1994; 21:2307–2319.
29. Hodler J, Loredo RA, Longo C, Trudell D, Yu JS, Resnick D. Assessment of articular cartilage thickness of the humeral head: MR-anatomic correlation in cadavers. AJR 1995; 165:615–620.
30. Peterfy CG, Dijke van CF, Lu Y, et al. Quantification of the volume of articular cartilage in the metacarpophalangeal joints of the hand: accuracy and precision of three-dimensional MR imaging. AJR 1995; 165:371–375.
31. Van Leersum M, Schweitzer ME, Gannon F, Finkel G, Vinitski S, Mitchell DG. Chondromalacia patellae: an in vitro study—comparison of MR criteria with histologic and macroscopic findings. Skeletal Radiol 1996; 25:727–732.
32. Lavid NE, DePaolis DC, Pope TW, et al. Analysis of three-dimensional computerized representations of articular cartilage lesions. Invest Radiol 1996; 31:577–585.
33. Tan TCF, Wilcox DM, Frank L, et al. MR imaging of articular cartilage in the ankle: comparison of available imaging sequences and methods of measurement in cadavers. Skeletal Radiol 1996; 25:749–755.
34. Sittek H, Eckstein F, Gavazzeni A, et al. Assessment of normal patellar cartilage volume and thickness using MRI: an analysis of currently available pulse sequences. Skeletal Radiol 1996; 25:55–62.
35. Piplani MA, Disler DG, McCauley TR, Holmes TJ, Cousins JP. Articular cartilage volume in the knee: semiautomated determination from three-dimensional reformations of MR images. Radiology 1996; 198:855–859.
36. Altman R, Asch E, Bloch D, et al. Development of criteria for the classification and reporting of osteoarthritis: classification of osteoarthritis of the knee. Arthritis Rheum 1986; 29:1039–1049.
37. Ayral X. Quantitative arthroscopy. Baillieres Clin Rheumatol 1996; 10:477–494.
38. Bartko JJ. Measure of agreement: a single procedure. Stat Med 1994; 13:737–745.
39. Bland JM, Altman DG. Statistical methods for assessing agreement between two methods of clinical measurement. Lancet 1986; 1:307–310.
40. Rubenstein J, Recht M, Disler DG, Kim J, Henkelman R. Laminar structures on MR images of articular cartilage. Radiology 1997; 204:15–16.
41. Erickson SJ, Prost RW. Laminar structures on MR images of articular cartilage (reply). Radiology 1997; 204:16–18.

Radiography of the Queen Elizabeth Rose

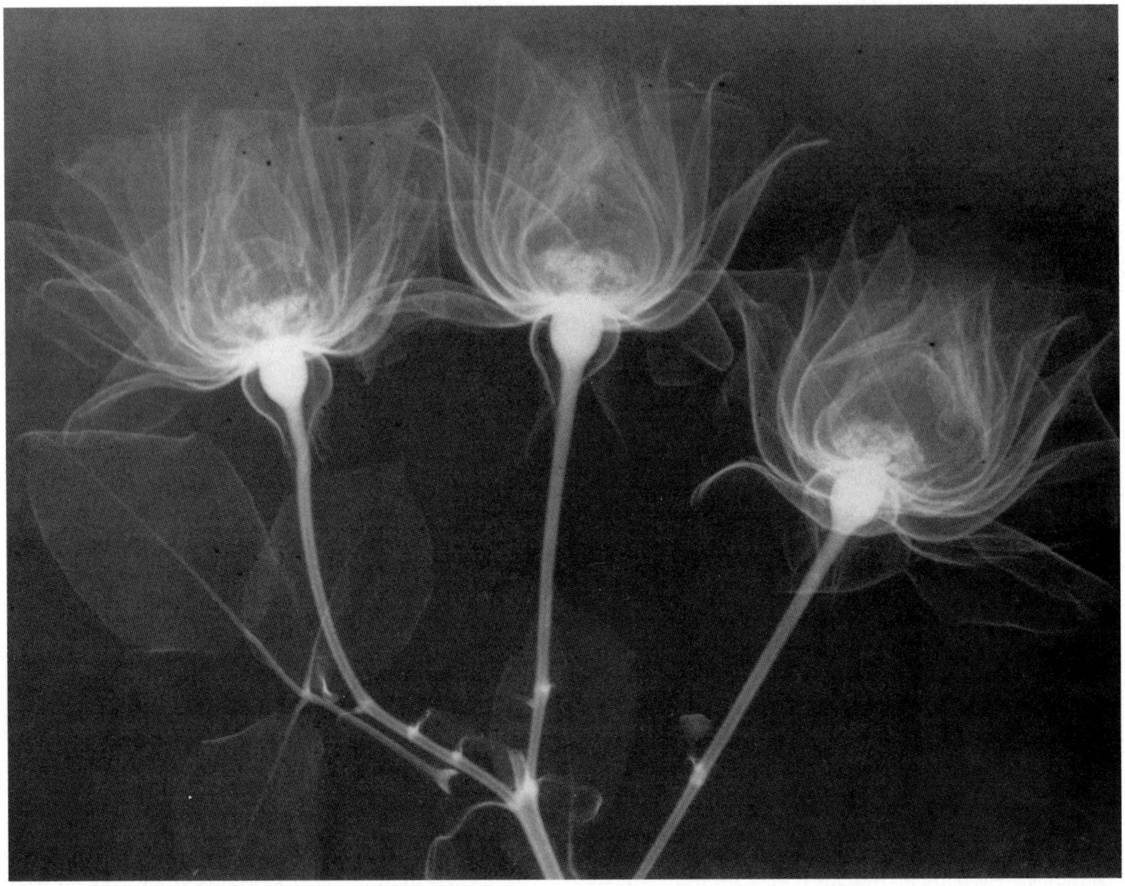

This radiograph, taken with mammographic equipment (22 kV, 8 mAs), illustrates the intricate internal structure of three Queen Elizabeth (QE) roses. The radiograph reveals the stalks bearing the sepals, the petals, and the separate male and female parts.

The QE rose was developed in 1954 by horticulturist Walter E. Lammerts in Los Angeles from the hybrid tea "Charlotte Armstrong" and the floribunda "Floradora," and it was named in honor of Queen Elizabeth II (1926–). It is in a class of its own and has been designated a grandiflora. The QE rose was voted "the best rose in the world" in 1980 by the World Federation of Rose Societies. The carmine-pink blooms are 8¾–10 cm wide, and the petals vary from high-centered to cupped. The growth is vigorous, tall, and upright, with large, abundant foliage; it is capable of making a hedge 6 feet (1.8 m) tall. The QE rose is very resistant to changes in weather, but, unfortunately, the scent is only slight.

Queen Elizabeth I (1533–1603) was a great admirer of roses, and almost all her portraits feature her posed wearing or holding a rose. It is remarkable that the stalk of the QE rose has almost no thorns and that the motto of Queen Elizabeth I was "rosa sine spina" (rose without thorns). At the time of her reign, the medicinal and pharmaceutical value of roses was greatly appreciated: "The infusion or decoction of them is of the kinde of soft and gentle medicines, which loose and open the belly and may be taken without danger. It purgeth downward cholerique humours and openeth the stoppings of the liver, strengthening and clensing the same; also is good against hoate fevers and against the Jaunders" (attributed to Rembert Dodoens [1517–1585], a notable Belgian botanist and writer of the Elizabethan era). Spiritual cures were available to those parts of the human body accorded mythical functions, such as the heart, breasts, and genitals. Dried rose petals when "boyled in wine were said to be good against ... the Mother of Women's secretes, eyther poured in or annoyted with a feather" (Dodoens).

Is it possible in our sophisticated medical world today that some of these ancient remedies could be rediscovered? If not, they still make suitable subjects for the eye of the "Roentgen ray."

Courtesy of Fred van Gelderen, MD, New Plymouth, New Zealand

Joong Mo Ahn, MD[2]
Sandy M. Kwak, MD
Heung Sik Kang, MD
Claus Muhle, MD
Robert A. Pedowitz, MD, PhD
Lawrence R. Frank, PhD
Debra Trudell, RA
Parviz Haghighi, MD
Donald Resnick, MD

Index terms:
Cartilage, 4521.92
Knee, MR, 4521.1214
Magnetic resonance (MR), comparative studies, 4521.121412, 4521.121413, 4521.121416, 4521.121417, 4521.12149
Patella, 453.92

Radiology 1998; 208:57–62

Abbreviations:
GRE = gradient echo
MTC = magnetization transfer contrast
SE = spin echo
STIR = short inversion time inversion recovery
TSE = turbo spin echo
2D = two-dimensional
3D = three-dimensional

[1] From the Departments of Radiology (J.M.A., S.M.K., C.M., L.R.F., D.T., D.R.), Orthopedic Surgery (R.A.P.), and Pathology (P.H.), Veterans Affairs Medical Center, 3350 La Jolla Village Dr, San Diego, CA 92161, and the Department of Radiology, Seoul National University Hospital, Korea (H.S.K.). Received Sep 2, 1997; revision requested Nov 13; revision received Jan 6, 1998; accepted Mar 3. Supported in part by VA grant SA-360. **Address reprint requests to** D.R.

[2] Current address: Department of Radiology, Samsung Medical Center, Sung Kyun Kwan University, Seoul, Korea.

Author contributions:
Guarantors of integrity of entire study, J.M.A., D.R.; study concepts, D.R.; study design, J.M.A., S.M.K., D.R.; definition of intellectual content, D.R.; literature research, L.R.F.; experimental studies, J.M.A., D.T., P.H., R.A.P.; data acquisition, H.S.K.; data analysis, S.M.K.; statistical analysis, C.M.; manuscript preparation, J.M.A.; manuscript editing and review, D.R.

Evaluation of Patellar Cartilage in Cadavers with a Low-Field-Strength Extremity-Only Magnet: Comparison of MR Imaging Sequences, with Macroscopic Findings as the Standard[1]

PURPOSE: To assess a low-field-strength extremity-only magnet in the evaluation of patellar cartilage abnormalities.

MATERIALS AND METHODS: Four regions in each of 10 patellae from cadavers were examined in the transaxial plane with a 0.2-T extremity-only magnet and the following sequences: T1-weighted spin echo, proton density– and T2-weighted turbo spin echo, short inversion time inversion recovery, and two- and three-dimensional gradient echo with and without magnetization transfer contrast subtraction. Lesions depicted with MR imaging and seen in anatomic sections of the patellae were classified according to a modified standardized arthroscopic grading system. MR imaging and pathologic correlation was then analyzed.

RESULTS: On the basis of macroscopic findings, 14 of 40 cartilage regions were found to be intact, grade 2A lesions were present in eight regions, grade 2B lesions in eight, and grade 3 lesions in 10. For the various MR imaging techniques, sensitivity was 25%–62% for grade 2A lesions, 50%–75% for grade 2B lesions, and 60%–90% for grade 3 lesions. Specificity was 81%–97% for grades 2A and 2B lesions, and 80%–97% for grade 3 lesions. Accuracy was 75%–82% for grade 2A lesions, 75%–92% for grade 2B lesions, and 80%–92% for grade 3 lesions.

CONCLUSION: High-grade cartilaginous lesions can be evaluated reliably with low-field-strength MR imaging by using a combination of imaging sequences.

Articular cartilage abnormality is an important component of many common conditions including osteoarthritis, rheumatoid arthritis, and osteochondritis dissecans. Advances in surgical and pharmacologic techniques for treating and preventing cartilage abnormalities are creating a demand for an accurate and noninvasive imaging method for evaluating articular cartilage (1). The most promising method in this regard is magnetic resonance (MR) imaging, which has been used widely in the evaluation of cartilage lesions (1–16). A multitude of pulse sequences have been advocated as optimal methods for the analysis of cartilage abnormalities: T1-weighted (2–5), proton density–weighted, and T2-weighted (5–7) spin-echo (SE) sequences; two-dimensional (2D) and three-dimensional (3D) gradient-echo (GRE) sequences (8–10); inversion-recovery sequences (11); fat-suppressed sequences (7,12–14); and the magnetization transfer contrast (MTC) sequence (15,16). Few communications, however, have specifically addressed the capabilities of low-field-strength MR imaging in the evaluation of patellar cartilage. Low-field-strength extremity-only magnets make claustrophobic patients more comfortable and cost less than high-field-strength magnets (17).

The objectives of the present study were to assess the capabilities of a low-field-strength extremity-only magnet in evaluating patellar cartilage abnormalities and to compare available MR imaging sequences in the assessment of chondral abnormalities.

MATERIALS AND METHODS

Ten knees, sectioned across the distal third of the femur and the proximal third of the tibia, were derived from nonembalmed cadavers (four male, six female; age range at time of death, 78–97 years; mean, 85 years). The specimens were immediately deep-frozen at −40°C (Forma Bio-Freezer; Forma Scientific, Marietta, Ohio). All specimens were examined with routine radiography to exclude those with obvious arthritic deformity. The specimens were allowed to thaw for 24 hours at room temperature prior to MR imaging.

MR images were obtained with a 0.2-T extremity-only magnet (Artoscan; Esaote, Genoa, Italy) with use of a standard knee coil supplied by the manufacturer. T1-weighted SE, proton density– and T2-weighted turbo SE (TSE), short inversion time inversion recovery (STIR), 2D GRE, 3D GRE, 2D GRE with MTC subtraction (2D MTC), and 3D MTC images were acquired. Only transaxial images were obtained because of previous reports that transaxial images are most useful in the assessment of patellar cartilage (4,5,9). MTC was achieved by application of a train of five radio-frequency pulses. To produce MTC subtraction images, the 2D and 3D GRE images with and without the magnetization transfer pulse were subtracted online. The MR imaging protocols are summarized in Table 1.

TABLE 1
MR Imaging Protocols

Sequence	TR (msec)	TE (msec)	T/G (mm)	NSA	FOV (cm)	Matrix	TI (msec)	FA
SE T1	500	20	4/1	4	16	192 × 160	NA	NA
TSE PD	4,000	34	4/1	2	16	192 × 160	NA	NA
TSE T2	4,000	90	4/1	2	16	192 × 160	NA	NA
STIR	2,000	20	4/1	2	16	192 × 160	65	NA
2D GRE	500	16	4/1	4	16	192 × 160	NA	75°
3D GRE	60	16	4/0	1	16 × 16 × 13	192 × 160 × 48	NA	45°
2D GRE MTC	500	16	4/1	4	16	192 × 160	NA	75°
3D GRE MTC	60	16	4/0	1	16 × 16 × 13	192 × 160 × 48	NA	45°

Note.—FA = flip angle, G = intersection gap, NA = not applicable, NSA = number of signals acquired, PD = proton density–weighted, T = section thickness, TE = echo time, TI = inversion time, TR = repetition time, T1 = T1-weighted, T2 = T2-weighted.

TABLE 2
Grading Systems for Macroscopic Inspection of Articular Cartilage Lesions and MR Image Interpretation

Grade	Macroscopic Findings	MR Imaging Findings
0	Intact cartilage	Homogeneous, without surface irregularity
1	Cartilage softening with intact surface	Focal signal intensity changes without surface irregularity
2A	Damage involves less than half of cartilage thickness	Thinning involves less than half of cartilage thickness
2B	Damage involves more than half but less than full thickness of cartilage	Thinning involves more than half but less than full thickness of cartilage
3	Exposed bone with or without cavitation	Exposed bone with or without bone surface irregularity

Source—Reference 18.

After MR imaging, the specimens were again frozen and sectioned, with a band saw, parallel to the imaging plane into 4-mm-thick sections. Each patella was subdivided into four regions: proximal medial, proximal lateral, distal medial, and distal lateral. In each region, the anatomic section that best demonstrated cartilage abnormalities was chosen. Representative MR images, obtained with each of the imaging sequences, that corresponded to this section location were then evaluated.

A total of 320 MR images were graded by two experienced observers (J.M.A., S.M.K.), who were blinded to the results of macroscopic inspection, findings obtained with other imaging sequences, and relative frequency of normal or pathologic cases in randomized images (ie, images from all specimens were viewed in random order). Differences of opinion were resolved by consensus. For MR image interpretation, a modified Noyes classification system (18), proposed by Recht et al (19), was adopted, as it more closely corresponded to the arthroscopic grading system used by the referring arthroscopist (Table 2).

The patellar sections were graded after macroscopic inspection by an experienced arthroscopist (R.A.P.) who had no knowledge of the imaging findings. The system used to grade the patellar cartilage at macroscopic inspection was again the modification of the Noyes classification scheme (18) (Table 2). The most severe grade for the patellar cartilage as recorded by the arthroscopist was matched with the MR imaging interpretations. The macroscopic findings from inspection of the anatomic sections were used as a reference standard.

Histologic examinations were performed in 10 random regions to evaluate the correlation of the inspection grades of the gross sections with the histopathologic findings. Small rectangular blocks of patellar cartilage containing adjacent subchondral bone were obtained from the defined regions for histologic evaluation. All histologic slides were examined by an experienced pathologist (P.H.) blinded to the MR imaging findings and the results of inspection of the gross sections. For quantitative grading of the histopathologic findings, a previously described point system (20,21) was adopted (Table 3). By adding the point scores of the various histopathologic changes (Table 3), a point score for each region was obtained. Also, a point scale was used for the inspection grading of the gross specimens; each grade was given a value that ranged from 0 to 4 (grade 0: 0, grade 1: 1, grade 2A: 2, grade 2B: 3, and grade 3: 4).

The sensitivity, specificity, and accuracy of each MR imaging sequence for determining the grade of cartilage abnormality were calculated. The sensitivity for a particular grade of cartilage abnormality was calculated by using the number of regions with a specific imaging grade that correlated with that of macroscopic inspection as the true-positive value. The number of regions with a particular grade at macroscopic inspection that did not

TABLE 3
Point System for Evaluation of Histopathologic Changes in Cartilage

Histopathologic Change	Grade	Points
Surface irregularities	None	0
	Mild	1
	Advanced	2
Vertical clefts extending into transitional zone	None	0
	Mild	1
	Advanced	2
Vertical clefts extending into radial zone	None	0
	Mild	1
	Advanced	2
Transverse clefts	None	0
	Mild	1
	Advanced	2
Transverse clefts with tissue loss	None	0
	Mild	1
	Advanced	2
Cloning	None	0
	Mild	1
	Moderate	2
	Advanced	3
Hypocellularity	None	0
	Mild	1
	Moderate	2
	Advanced	3

Source—Reference 21.

TABLE 4
Calculation of Specificity

	Macroscopic Inspection	
MR Imaging	*X*	Non-*X*
X	*a*	*b*
Non-*X*	*c*	*d*

Note.—*a* = no. of true-positive regions, *b* = no. of false-positive regions, *c* = no. of false-negative regions, *d* = no. of true-negative regions. Specificity = *d*/(*b* + *d*). For a particular grade *X*, the number of regions with non-*X* at macroscopic inspection that were graded *X* at imaging was used as the false-positive value (*b*). The number of regions with non-*X* at macroscopic inspection that were graded non-*X* at imaging was used as the true-negative value (*d*).

TABLE 5
Most Useful MR Sequences for Each Grade of Cartilage Lesion with Extremity-Only Magnet

Cartilage Grade	Best MR Sequences
0	2D GRE, 3D GRE
2A	2D GRE, 2D MTC
2B	2D GRE
3	2D GRE

correlate with the imaging grade was used as the false-negative value. The specificity for a particular grade was calculated by using the number of regions with other than the particular grade noted at macroscopic inspection that were graded a particular grade at imaging as the false-positive value. The number of regions with other than the particular grade at macroscopic inspection that were graded differently than the particular grade derived from imaging was used as the true-negative value (Table 4). Differences between the imaging techniques were tested for statistical significance by using the McNemar test for matched data if the total number of differences exceeded 10; if the number of differences was less than 10, the binomial test was used (22). Correlation of the gross specimen inspection grades and histopathologic findings was per the Spearman rank correlation coefficient (23). The results were considered statistically significant at $P < .05$.

RESULTS

On the basis of macroscopic findings at gross specimen inspection, 14 of 40 cartilage regions were found to be intact; grade 2A lesions were present in eight regions, grade 2B lesions in eight regions, and grade 3 lesions in 10 regions. None of the lesions was considered grade 1.

Of the 14 regions considered intact at macroscopic inspection, 11 (79%) appeared normal with 2D and 3D GRE sequences, 10 (71%) appeared normal with the T1-weighted SE sequence, seven (50%) appeared normal with STIR and 2D and 3D MTC sequences, six (43%) appeared normal with proton density–weighted TSE sequences, and five (36%) appeared normal with T2-weighted TSE sequences (Table 5) (Fig 1). In assessment of cartilage considered normal at macroscopic inspection, the accuracy of 2D and 3D GRE sequences was significantly better than that of proton density– and T2-weighted TSE sequences ($P < .05$). The MR imaging grade of the intact regions graded abnormal ranged from grade 1 to grade 3. Twelve (86%) of 14 intact regions were graded normal with at least one imaging sequence.

The sensitivity of MR imaging was 25%–62% for grade 2A lesions, 50%–75% for grade 2B lesions, and 60%–90% for grade 3 lesions. The specificity was 82%–97% for grade 2A and 2B lesions and 80%–97% for grade 3 lesions. The accuracy was 75%–82% for grade 2A lesions, 75%–92% for grade 2B lesions, and 80%–92% for grade 3 lesions.

The most sensitive MR techniques were the 2D MTC sequence (62%) for the detection of grade 2A lesions (Table 5) (Fig 2); the T1-weighted SE, 2D GRE, and 3D MTC sequences (75%) for the detection of grade 2B lesions; and the proton density– and T2-weighted TSE, STIR, and 2D GRE sequences (90%) for the detection of grade 3 lesions (Fig 2). No significant differences in sensitivity for the detection of grade 2A, 2B, or 3 lesions between the MR imaging techniques were found.

The most specific MR imaging techniques were the 2D GRE sequence (97%) for grades 2A and 2B lesions and the T1-weighted SE, 3D GRE, and 3D MTC sequences (97%) for grade 3 lesions. No significant differences in specificity for the detection of grade 2A, 2B, or 3 lesions between the MR imaging techniques were found.

The most accurate MR imaging technique was the 2D GRE sequence for grade 2A lesions (82%), grade 2B lesions (92%), and grade 3 lesions (92%) (Fig 2). No significant differences in accuracy for the diagnosis of grade 2A, 2B, or 3 lesions between the MR imaging techniques were found. Six (75%) of eight grade 2A lesions and all of the grade 2B and grade 3 lesions were identified with at least one type of sequence. There was a significant association between the macroscopic inspection grades and histopathologic findings ($r = .006$, $P < .05$).

DISCUSSION

Our results show that 2D and 3D GRE sequences are better (78.6% sensitivity) than other sequences (35.7%–71.5% sensitivity) for depiction of normal patellar cartilage with a low-field-strength extremity-only magnet (Table 5). The better correlation between GRE sequences and macroscopic inspection in assessment of normal cartilage is believed to be related principally to the ease with which visualization of patellar cartilage can be accomplished with GRE sequences.

For the detection of grade 2A lesions, the most sensitive technique was the 2D MTC sequence (62.5%), followed by the 3D MTC sequence (50%). However, the specificity of these two techniques (81.3%) was poorer than that of other imaging sequences (93.8%– 96.9%).

For the detection of grade 2B lesions,

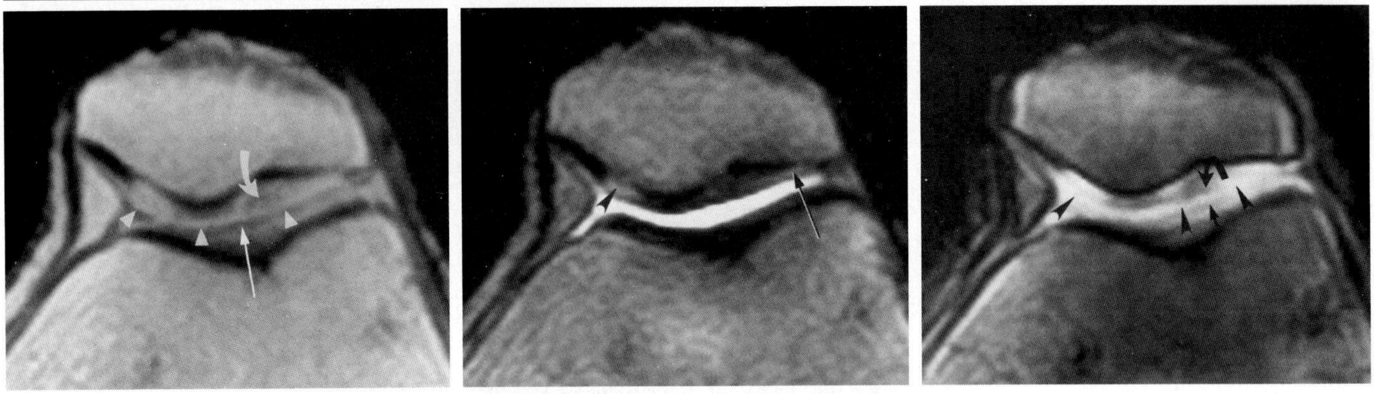

a. b. c.

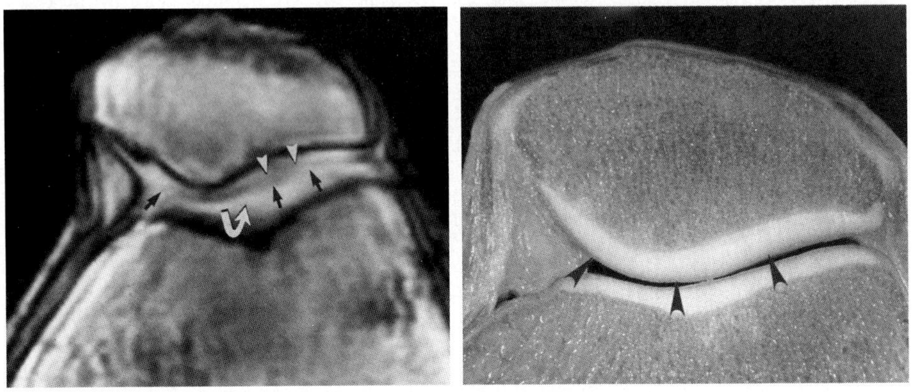

d. e.

Figure 1. Normal patellar cartilage, as determined at macroscopic inspection. **(a)** T1-weighted SE transaxial image (repetition time msec/echo time msec = 500/20) shows the patellar cartilage with a subtle bilaminar appearance (curved arrow) and smooth cartilage surface (arrowheads) in the medial and lateral regions. Note the small amount of joint fluid of low signal intensity (straight arrow). The medial and lateral regions were considered normal at MR image interpretation. **(b)** T2-weighted TSE transaxial image (4,000/90) obtained at the same level as in **a** shows focal areas with increased signal intensity in medial (arrowhead) and lateral (arrow) regions. Both areas were considered grade 1. **(c)** Two-dimensional GRE image (500/16, 75° flip angle) at the same level as in **a** shows patellar cartilage with subtle bilaminar appearance (curved arrow) and smooth cartilage surface (arrowheads) in the medial and lateral regions. Note the small amount of joint fluid of low signal intensity (straight arrow) due to the use of the long repetition time (500 msec) and large flip angle. The medial and lateral regions were considered normal at MR image interpretation. **(d)** Three-dimensional GRE image (60/16, 45° flip angle) at the same level as in **a** shows a subtle bilaminar appearance (arrowheads) and smooth cartilage surface (straight arrows). There is associated joint effusion of high signal intensity (curved arrow). The medial and lateral regions were considered normal at MR image interpretation. **(e)** Corresponding anatomic section from the same cadaveric specimen reveals normal, smooth articular cartilage of the patella (arrowheads) in the medial and lateral regions.

the 2D GRE sequence was the most useful technique (Table 5), because it was the most specific (96.9%) and the most sensitive (75%). Gagliardi et al (24) found that the sensitivity and specificity of spoiled 2D GRE acquisition in the steady state with fat saturation were 20% and 98%, respectively, for intermediate stage cartilage lesions, consisting of stage II (bulge or blister lesions) and stage III (ulceration and fragmentation of larger area of cartilage) lesions according to Shahriaree's classification (25). Although a different grading system was used in our study, we believe that the sensitivity and specificity of the 2D GRE sequence for the detection of grade 2B lesions in our study are comparable with those in the report of Gagliardi et al.

For the detection of grade 3 lesions, proton density– and T2-weighted TSE, STIR, and 2D GRE sequences were the most sensitive (90%); however, with regard to specificity, T1-weighted SE, 3D GRE, and 3D MTC sequences (96.7%) were better than the other techniques (80%–93.3%). In previous studies (6,7), sensitivity and specificity of proton density–weighted images for depicting cartilage abnormalities have been poor: Sensitivity has ranged from 26% to 62%, and specificity has varied from 78% to 80% in these studies. Sensitivities and specificities of T2-weighted sequences for detecting cartilage abnormalities have been reported as 48%–72% and 58%–87%, respectively (6,7). In our study, however, proton density– and T2-weighted TSE sequences showed promise for the detection of grade 3 lesions. Unlike the experience of McCauley et al (6), who used a 1.5-T magnet, we found that proton density–weighted images were equivalent to T2-weighted images for evaluation of patellar cartilage with regard to sensitivity, specificity, and accuracy.

In previously reported studies (2,5,8–10,26), although the investigators used different grading systems, MR imaging and arthroscopy showed excellent correlation in the assessment of patellar cartilage in cases of advanced degeneration causing cartilage thinning. Our observations are similar. Grade 2B and grade 3 lesions were identified with higher sensitivity (50%–90%) than grade 2A lesions (25%–62%). Accurate identification of grades 2 and 3 lesions is important clinically. Orthopedic surgeons may consider subchondral perforation or abrasion arthroplasty for these more severe grades of patellar cartilage abnormality. In comparison, no surgical treatment may be necessary for grade 1 lesions (8,12,25). In the present study, we were unable to analyze the results of MR imaging for grade 1 lesions, because no grade 1 lesions were found at macroscopic inspection of the cartilage.

The present study has several potential limitations. First, the study was performed in cadavers rather than in living subjects derived from a clinical popula-

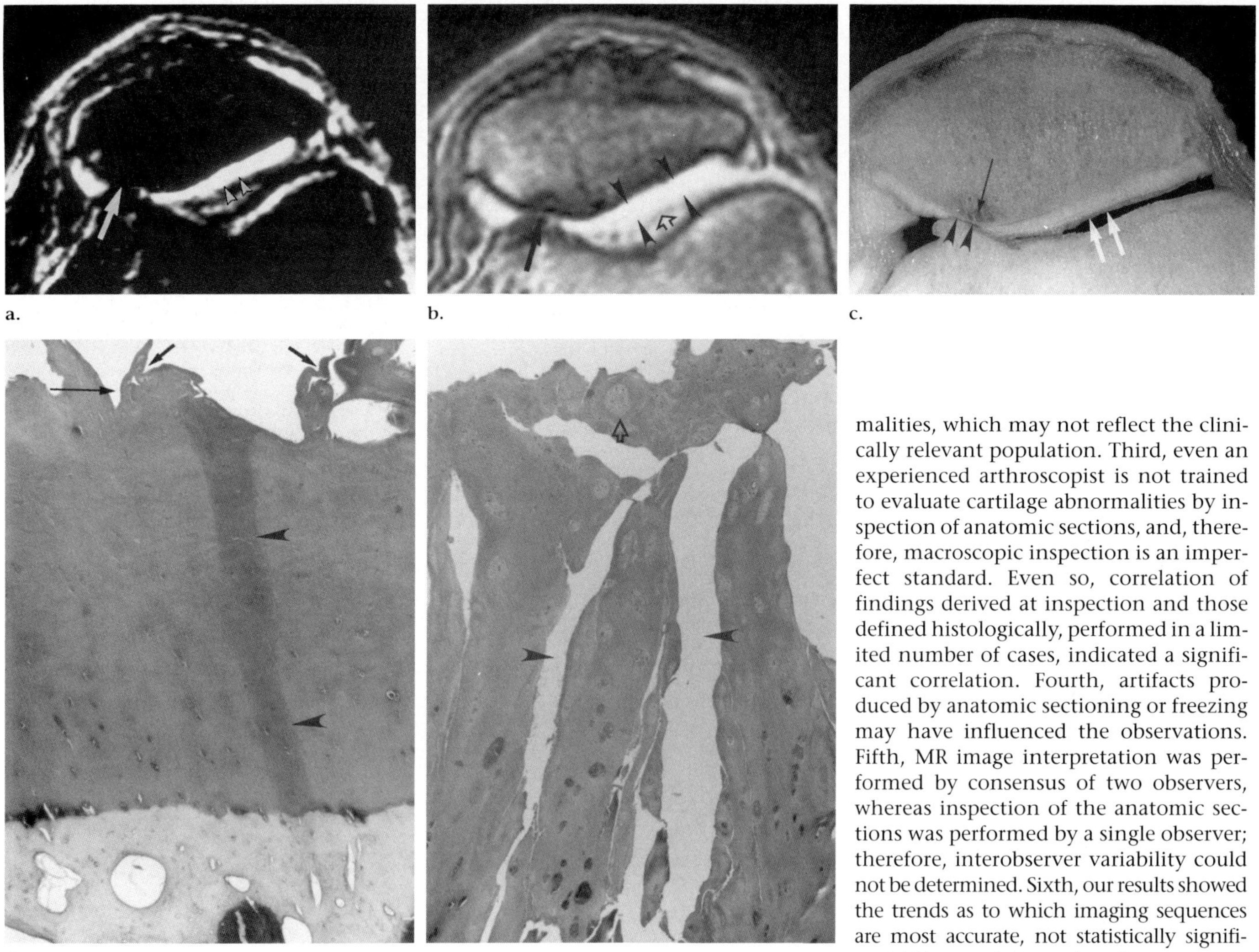

a. b. c. d. e.

Figure 2. Patellar cartilage with grade 2A and grade 3 lesions, as determined at macroscopic inspection. **(a)** Two-dimensional GRE image with MTC (500/16, 75° flip angle) shows minimal thinning of patellar cartilage (arrowheads) in the lateral region, involving less than half of the thickness of the cartilage and, therefore, considered a grade 2A lesion. Note a focal cartilage defect (arrow) extending from the articular surface to the bone in the medial region; it was judged to be a grade 3 lesion. **(b)** Two-dimensional GRE image (500/16, 75° flip angle) at the same level as in **a** shows patellar cartilage with homogeneous appearance and high signal intensity (arrowheads) in the lateral regions, which was considered normal. The cartilage defect (solid arrow) involving the full thickness of the patellar cartilage in the medial region was considered a grade 3 lesion. Note the joint fluid of low signal intensity (open arrow). **(c)** Corresponding anatomic section from the same cadaveric specimen reveals cartilage thinning (white arrows) involving less than half of the entire thickness of the cartilage in the lateral region, and a focal cartilage defect (arrowheads) extending from the articular surface to the bone, with subchondral cysts (black arrow), in the medial region. The lesions were considered to be grade 2A and grade 3, respectively, at macroscopic inspection. **(d)** Photomicrograph of specimen obtained from the lateral region of the patella depicted in **c** shows surface irregularity (short arrows) with superficial vertical clefts (long arrow). The dark transchondral bandlike appearance (arrowheads) is caused by cutting artifact. (Hematoxylin-eosin stain; original magnification, ×16.) **(e)** Photomicrograph of specimen obtained from the medial region of the patella depicted in **c** shows severe cartilage abnormalities including deep transchondral clefts (arrowheads) with chondrocyte cloning (arrow). (Hematoxylin-eosin stain; original magnification, ×16.)

tion. However, each lesion studied was a naturally occurring lesion and was not produced artificially. Second, because of the limited availability of cadavers of young persons, all specimens were obtained from cadavers of patients older than 78 years, a population expected to have a high prevalence of cartilage abnormalities, which may not reflect the clinically relevant population. Third, even an experienced arthroscopist is not trained to evaluate cartilage abnormalities by inspection of anatomic sections, and, therefore, macroscopic inspection is an imperfect standard. Even so, correlation of findings derived at inspection and those defined histologically, performed in a limited number of cases, indicated a significant correlation. Fourth, artifacts produced by anatomic sectioning or freezing may have influenced the observations. Fifth, MR image interpretation was performed by consensus of two observers, whereas inspection of the anatomic sections was performed by a single observer; therefore, interobserver variability could not be determined. Sixth, our results showed the trends as to which imaging sequences are most accurate, not statistically significant differences between imaging sequences. Finally, observer awareness of cartilage lesions probably was higher in the present study than it would be in clinical practice, which may have led to improved sensitivity for detecting lesions.

In summary, various imaging techniques obtainable with a low-field-strength extremity-only magnet seem to be sensitive and specific for the evaluation of patellar cartilage, although the results depend on the grade of cartilage abnormality. Our observations suggest that high-grade patellar cartilage lesions can be evaluated reliably with low-field-strength MR imaging by using a combination of imaging sequences. The 2D GRE sequence can be generally recommended for the evaluation of patellar cartilage, and the 2D MTC sequence might be useful for the detection of grade 2A lesions.

References

1. Recht MP, Resnick D. MR imaging of articular cartilage: current status and future directions. AJR 1994; 163:283–290.

2. Hayes CW, Sawyer RW, Conway WF. Patellar cartilage lesions: in vitro detection and staging with MR imaging and pathologic correlation. Radiology 1990; 176:479–483.
3. Karvonen RL, Negendank WG, Fraser SM, Mayes MD, An T, Fernandez-Madrid F. Articular cartilage defects of the knee: correlation between magnetic resonance imaging and gross pathology. Ann Rheum Dis 1990; 49:672–675.
4. Conway WF, Hayes CW, Loughran T, et al. Cross-sectional imaging of the patellofemoral joint and surrounding structures. RadioGraphics 1991; 11:195–217.
5. Yulish BS, Montanez J, Goodfellow DB, Bryan PJ, Mulopulos GP, Modic MT. Chondromalacia patellae: assessment with MR imaging. Radiology 1987; 164:763–766.
6. McCauley MR, Kier R, Lynch KJ, Jokl P. Chondromalacia patellae: diagnosis with MR imaging. AJR 1992; 158:101–105.
7. Recht MP, Kramer J, Marcelis S, et al. Abnormalities of articular cartilage in the knee: analysis of available MR techniques. Radiology 1993; 187:473–478.
8. Tyrrell RL, Gluckert K, Pathria M, Modic MT. Fast three-dimensional MR imaging of the knee: comparison with arthroscopy. Radiology 1988; 166:865–872.
9. Reiser MF, Bongartz G, Erlemann R, et al. Magnetic resonance in cartilaginous lesions of the knee joint with three-dimensional gradient-echo imaging. Skeletal Radiol 1988; 17:465–471.
10. Heron CW, Calvert PT. Three-dimensional gradient-echo MR imaging of the knee: comparison with arthroscopy in 100 patients. Radiology 1992; 183:839–844.
11. Lehner KB, Rechl HP, Gmeinwieser JK, Heuck AF, Lukas HP, Kohn HP. Structure, function, and degeneration of bovine hyaline cartilage: assessment with MR imaging in vitro. Radiology 1989; 170:495–499.
12. Chandnani VP, Ho C, Chu P, Trudell D, Resnick D. Knee hyaline cartilage evaluated with MR imaging: a cadaveric study involving multiple imaging sequences and intraarticular injection of gadolinium and saline solution. Radiology 1991; 178:557–561.
13. Leersum M, Schweitzer ME, Gannon F, Finkel G, Vinitski S, Mitchell DG. Chondromalacia patellae: an in vitro study comparison of MR criteria with histologic and macroscopic findings. Skeletal Radiol 1996; 25:727–732.
14. Disler DG, McCauley TR, Kelman CG, et al. Fat-suppressed three-dimensional spoiled gradient-echo MR imaging of hyaline cartilage defects in the knee: comparison with standard MR imaging and arthroscopy. AJR 1996; 167:127–132.
15. Wolff SD, Chesnick S, Frank JA, Lim KO, Balaban R. Magnetization transfer contrast: MR imaging of the knee. Radiology 1991; 179:623–628.
16. Brossmann J, Frank LR, Pauly JM, et al. Short echo time projection reconstruction MR imaging of cartilage: comparison with fat-suppressed spoiled GRASS and magnetization transfer contrast MR imaging. Radiology 1997; 203:501–507.
17. Peterfy CG, Roberts T, Genant HK. Dedicated extremity MR imaging: an emerging technology. Radiol Clin North Am 1997; 35:1–20.
18. Noyes FR, Stabler CL. A system for grading articular cartilage lesions at arthroscopy. Am J Sports Med 1989; 17:505–513.
19. Recht MP, Piraino DW, Paletta GA, Schils JP, Belhobek GH. Accuracy of fat-suppressed three-dimensional spoiled gradient-echo FLASH MR imaging in the detection of patellofemoral articular cartilage abnormalities. Radiology 1996; 198:209–212.
20. Mankin HJ. Biochemical and metabolic aspects of osteoarthritis. Orthop Clin North Am 1971; 2:19–31.
21. Shapiro F, Glimcher MJ. Induction of osteoarthrosis in the rabbit knee joint: histologic changes following meniscectomy and meniscal lesions. Clin Orthop 1979; 147:287–295.
22. Siegel S, Castellan NJ. The case of one sample, two measures or paired replicates. In: Siegel S, Castellan NJ, eds. Nonparametric statistics for the behavioral sciences. 2nd ed. New York, NY: McGraw-Hill, 1988; 73–87.
23. Conover WJ. Contingency tables. In: Conover WJ, ed. Practical nonparametric statistics. 2nd ed. New York, NY: Wiley, 1980; 143–170.
24. Gagliardi JA, Chung EM, Chandnani VP, et al. Detection and staging of chondromalacia patellae: relative efficacies of conventional MR imaging, MR arthrography, and CT arthrography. AJR 1994; 163:629–636.
25. Shahriaree H. Chondromalacia. Contemp Orthop 1985; 11:27–39.
26. Brown TR, Quinn SF. Evaluation of chondromalacia of the patellofemoral compartment with axial magnetic resonance imaging. Skeletal Radiol 1993; 22:325–328.

Diagnosis Please

David Karasick, MD
Mark E. Schweitzer, MD

Case 4[1]

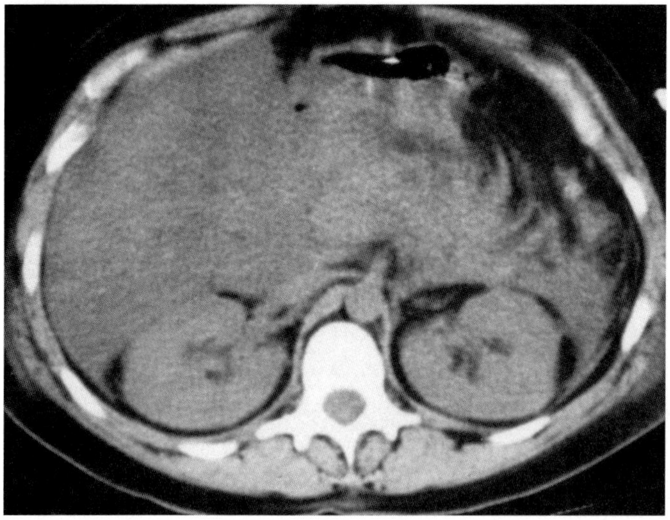

Figure 1. Unenhanced CT scan of the abdomen.

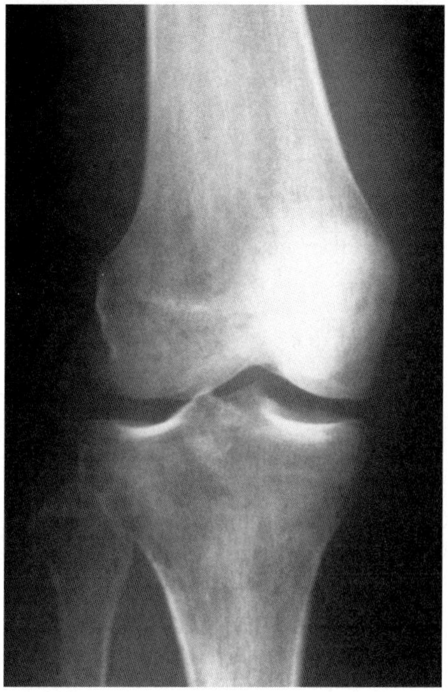

Figure 2. Anteroposterior radiograph of the left knee.

HISTORY

A 33-year-old woman presented with severe abdominal pain and vomiting. The results of physical examination revealed increased abdominal girth and severe abdominal tenderness. Abdominal computed tomography (CT) was performed without contrast material enhancement (Fig 1).

Four months later, the patient noted the development of multiple subcutaneous nodules on her extremities and multiple swollen and painful joints. A diagnostic left knee aspiration was performed. Imaging studies performed at this time included radiography of the shoulders, elbows, wrists, knees (Fig 2), and ankles (Figs 3, 4). Magnetic resonance (MR) imaging of the left knee (Fig 5) was performed 2 weeks later. Follow-up ankle radiography (Fig 6) was performed 2 years later. The patient experienced recurrent joint symptoms, and consequently 10 years after initial presentation, MR imaging of the left elbow was performed (Fig 7).

(continued)

Index term:
Diagnosis please

Radiology 1998; 208:63–64

[1]From the Department of Radiology, Thomas Jefferson University Hospital, 111 S 11th St, Philadelphia, PA 19107. Received November 21, 1997; revision requested December 30; revision received January 14, 1998; accepted January 23. **Address reprint requests to** D.K.

Submit the most likely diagnosis to *dxplease@rsna.org* (use **only** for submission of diagnosis). Include case number, your name (as you would want it to appear in the journal), address, phone and fax numbers. Multiple diagnoses, multiple submissions, submissions without a case number will not be considered. **Deadline**: September 18, 1998. Answer will appear in the November issue. See also the editorial by Proto (p 1) in the April 1998 issue.

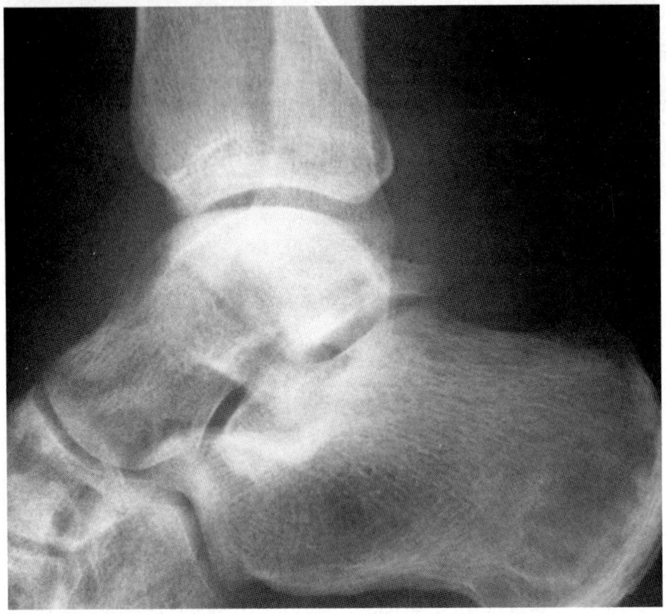

Figure 3. Lateral radiograph of the left ankle.

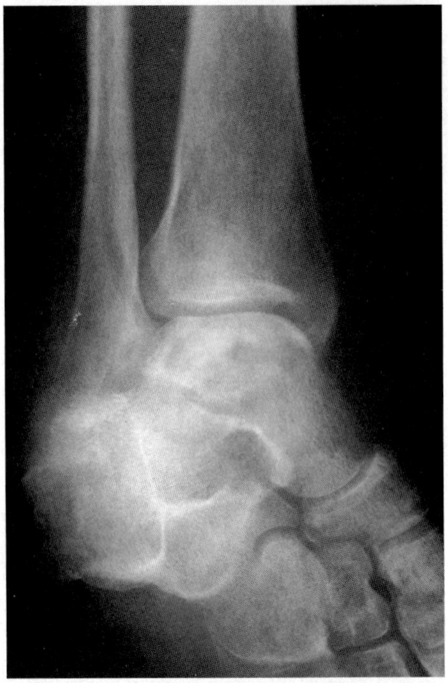

Figure 4. Mortise view radiograph of the right ankle.

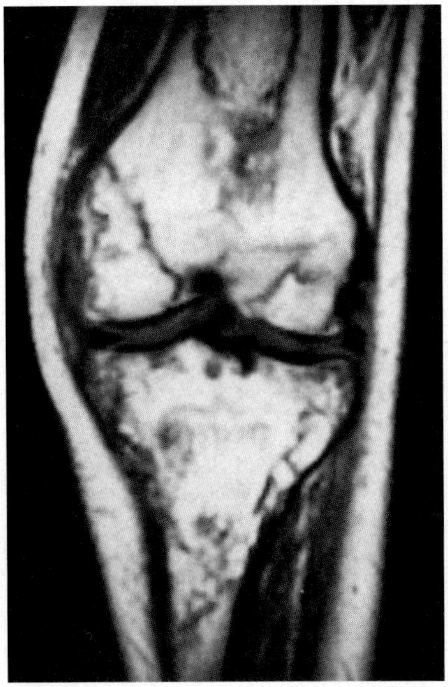

Figure 5. Coronal T1-weighted MR image (600/20 [repetition time msec/echo time msec]) of the left knee.

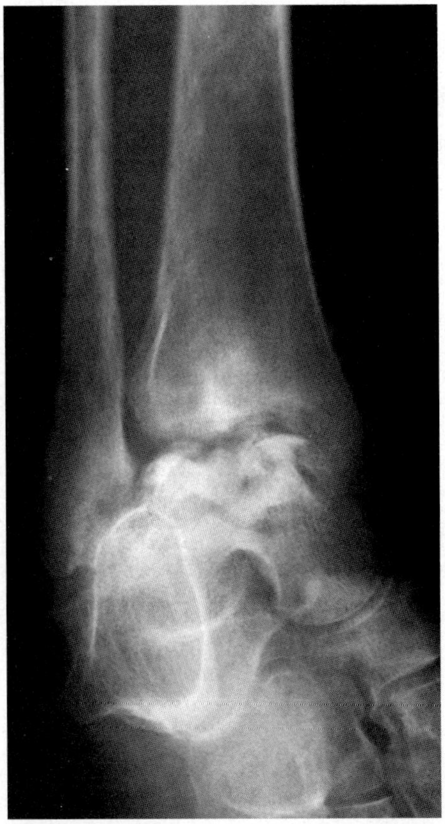

Figure 6. Mortise view radiograph of right ankle.

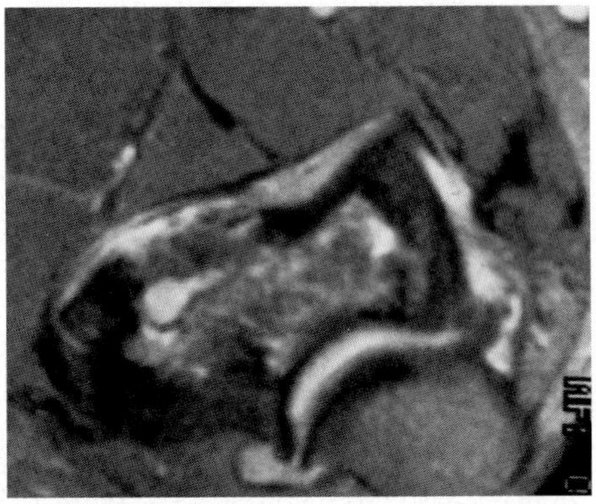

Figure 7. Axial fat-suppressed intermediate-weighted MR image (2,216/40 effective) of the left elbow.

Giovanni de Marco, PhD
Alexei Bogdanov, PhD
Edgardo Marecos, MD
Anna Moore, PhD
Maria Simonova, PhD
Ralph Weissleder, MD, PhD

Index terms:
Genes and genetics
Magnetic resonance (MR), utilization

Radiology 1998; 208:65–71

Abbreviations:
cDNA = complementary DNA
dCTP-33 = 2′-deoxycytidine 5′-triphosphate
DEAE = diethylaminoethyl
GFP = green fluorescent protein

[1] From the Department of Radiology, Center for Molecular Imaging Research, Massachusetts General Hospital, 149 13th St, Rm 5403, Charlestown, MA 02129. Received October 21, 1997; revision requested December 31; revision received January 22, 1998; accepted February 12. Supported in part by National Institutes of Health grant 5RO1-NS35258-02. G.d.M. supported by the Association pour la Récherche sur le Cancer (Paris, France) and Ligue Nationale contre le Cancer (Angers, France). **Address reprint requests to** R.W.
See also the editorial by Seidenwurm and Rowley (pp 17–18) in this issue.

Author contributions:
Guarantor of integrity of entire study, R.W.; study concepts, A.B., M.S., R.W.; study design, A.B., A.M., R.W.; definition of intellectual content, R.W.; literature research, G.d.M., E.M., R.W.; experimental studies, G.d.M., E.M., A.M., M.S., R.W.; data acquisition, G.d.M., E.M., A.M., R.W.; data analysis, G.d.M., E.M., A.M., R.W.; statistical analysis, R.W.; manuscript preparation, G.d.M., A.B., A.M., M.S., R.W.; manuscript editing, R.W.; manuscript review, R.W.

MR Imaging of Gene Delivery to the Central Nervous System with an Artificial Vector[1]

PURPOSE: To determine whether gene delivery by means of a synthetic nonviral DNA delivery system that is capable of gene transfer can be mapped with magnetic resonance (MR) imaging.

MATERIALS AND METHODS: The DNA delivery system consisted of aminated (poly-L-lysine–conjugated) dextran chains anchored together with a central superparamagnetic core. Three different types of constructs were synthesized that differed in their amino content and, thus, DNA-loading capacity. The model plasmid consisted of complementary DNA encoding for humanized green fluorescent protein. Constructs were tested in cell culture and in vivo in a rat model.

RESULTS: All three constructs were capable of transfecting human cells in culture with transfection efficiencies ranging from 0.3% to 4.1%, which is similar to that of diethylaminoethyl-dextran. MR imaging experiments showed that DNA constructs induced signal intensity changes that co-localized with phosphorus-33–labeled plasmid distribution at autoradiography. After injection of the constructs into the corpus callosum of rats, weak green fluorescent protein expression of neuronal and glial cells could be detected at immunohistologic examination.

CONCLUSION: Dextran-based nonviral DNA delivery systems are capable of transfecting cells and can be visualized with MR imaging.

Gene delivery to the central nervous system would have a major medical effect in the treatment of late-onset neurodegenerative diseases (eg, Parkinson and Huntington diseases) (1), inherited enzymatic deficiency diseases (eg, Tay-Sachs disease) (2), or brain tumors (3). The basic paradigm for gene therapy of these diseases is that it can correct a genetic defect or introduce a new function to cells. Currently, more than 4,000 human diseases have been classified as genetic in origin (4). Therapeutic genes are typically delivered into mammalian cells by means of one of three methods: (*a*) by packaging of DNA cloned into viral expression cassettes ("viral vectors"), (*b*) by attaching DNA to a synthetic delivery system ("artificial vectors"), or (*c*) by means of electric pulse discharge into a cell-containing solution ("electroporation"). Despite the ability to efficiently transfect cells (ie, gene transfer into mammalian cells), viral methods for human gene therapy may have certain limitations (5,6): (*a*) Viral particles are often unstable; (*b*) viruses are frequently immunogenic, making repeated administrations problematic; and (*c*) viral genomic elements can incorporate into the human genome with the potential for oncogene activation (7). Thus, gene delivery approaches with nonviral artificial carriers are being actively investigated (8). The pros and cons of novel vector systems are described in more detail elsewhere (6,8).

The arsenal of nonviral synthetic gene therapy vectors (delivery systems) has included a variety of carriers: cationic liposomes, poly-L-lysine–DNA complexes, DNA-coated microprojectiles (gold particles), and dendrimers (5,6,9–14). There is also evidence that free expression vectors ("naked DNA") can transfect some mammalian cells, although not very efficiently. On the other hand, diethylaminoethyl (DEAE)-dextran–mediated transfection is very efficient but not applicable for in vivo use because of rapid elimination and toxicity (15). We have previously described and characterized the cellular delivery and pharmacokinetics of modified dextran nanoparticles that have magnetic properties. Such particles can potentially be used for different applications such as in vivo magnetic resonance (MR) imaging of drug delivery (16), magnetic DNA targeting, or DNA isolation (17,18). The nanoparticles are readily taken up by neuronal and glial cells after injection into the central nervous system (18,19), and they may undergo axonal transport (20).

In the current study, we built on prior observations and designed different dextran-DNA constructs to determine if (*a*) gene transfer occurs in vivo and (*b*) distribution of such a gene delivery system can be mapped with MR imaging. Experiments were designed to characterize these constructs, investigate their ability to transfect cells, correlate their central nervous system distribution by means of MR imaging in vivo and autoradiography, and determine whether DNA results in gene expression in vivo.

TABLE 1
Characterization of Constructs

Constructs	NH_2/ Dextran Molar Ratio*	DNA Content (DNA/dextran [wt/wt])	Size† (nm) of Unloaded Construct	Size (nm) of DNA-loaded Construct	No. of DNA Molecules per Particle
Dextran-coated particle	NA	NA	20.0 ± 2.0	NA	NA
Construct 1	4.2 ± 1.2	0.03 ± 0.01	22.5 ± 1.2	70.0 ± 16.9	1.2
Construct 2	8.3 ± 2.8	0.04 ± 0.02	26.0 ± 1.3	139.0 ± 61.2	1.7
Construct 3	10.0 ± 4.0	0.05 ± 0.01	33.5 ± 1.3	171.0 ± 67.7	2.8

Note.—Data are the mean ± standard deviation. NA = not applicable.
* Value reflects the positive charge of the carrier and, thus, DNA-binding capacity.
† Volume-weighted mean particle diameter determined by means of laser light scattering.

MATERIALS AND METHODS

Plasmid

The model plasmid used in this study contained a humanized green fluorescent protein (GFP) coding complementary DNA (cDNA) sequence obtained as a gift (Seed B, Massachusetts General Hospital, Boston, Mass). The cDNA was subcloned into the pcDNA3 vector (Invitrogen, Carlsbad, Calif) at the *HindIII-NotI* sites and was positioned under control of the cytomegalovirus promoter. To produce the amount of plasmid necessary for transfection experiments, competent bacteria (*Eschericia coli*, strain DH5-α) were transformed by means of an established heat-shock procedure (21). The plasmid was purified by using a commercially available kit (Qiagen, Chatsworth, Calif). The purity of the plasmid was verified by means of DNA electrophoresis in 0.8% agarose. To label the DNA vector with 2′-deoxycytidine 5′-triphosphate (dCTP-33), a commercially available nick translation kit was used (Gibco Life Technologies, Gaithersburg, Md). Labeled DNA was purified on spin columns (Sephadex G50; Pharmacia Biotech, Gaithersburg, Md) equilibrated with 10 mmol/L tris HCl (pH, 8), 50 mmol/L NaCl, and 0.1 mmol/L Na_2 ethylenediaminetetraacetic acid, or EDTA. The specific activity of the nick translated pcDNA3 GFP was 4.8 μCi/μg (177.6 μBq).

Synthesis of Constructs

The dextran carriers were synthesized similarly as previously described (22) but with additional purification to remove all free dextran and other by-products or stabilizers. Briefly, dextran particles were prepared by means of NH_4OH co-precipitation of triple crystallized divalent and trivalent iron chloride (Sigma, St Louis, Mo) in the presence of high concentrations of pharmaceutical-grade dextran (dextran/Fe^{2+}/Fe^{3+} = 39.6/1.0/2.7, wt/wt [B-512 dextran; molecular mass, 11 kd]; Pharmacia, Piscateway, NJ). The product was fractionated (YM-300 membrane; Amicon, Danvers, Mass) and concentrated by means of ultrafiltration. The dextran particles (each particle contained an average of 25 dextran chains) were then modified with poly-L-lysine (molecular mass, 35 kd; Sigma, St Louis, Mo). For this purpose, 4-mg dextran particles were partially oxidized with 0.1 mg (construct 1), 0.4 mg (construct 2), or 0.6 mg (construct 3) of sodium periodate (Sigma) at pH 6 for 40 minutes in the dark to yield different amounts of aldehyde groups. The oxidation was terminated by adding 10 μL of ethylene glycol (Aldrich Chemical, Milwaukee, Wis). After additional purification by means of dialysis in NaCl (0.15 mol/L) at pH 6.5, the aldehyde groups were reacted with amino groups of poly-L-lysine (0.1 mol/L $NaHCO_3$, pH 8.5) at a ratio of 5 mg of poly-L-lysine per 4 mg of dextran particles. After 1 hour of incubation, Schiff bonds were reduced with 1 mg/mL sodium cyanoborohydride (Sigma) at pH 8.5. Finally, particles were purified in sodium citrate buffer (10 mmol/L citrate, 0.15 mol/L NaCl, pH 7) by using concentrators (Centricon 100; Amicon, Beverly, Mass). The pcDNA3 GFP dissolved in 1 mol/L NaCl was then added to the poly-L-lysine–modified dextran constructs (construct 1, 14.3 ng of DNA per microgram of dextran particle; construct 2, 20.0 ng/μg DNA; construct 3, 33.3 ng/μg DNA).

Characterization of Constructs

The DNA-loading capacity of dextran–poly-L-lysine particles was determined by means of fluorescence spectrophotometry (model F-4500; Hitachi, Danbury, Conn). Ten-microliter aliquots (2 mg/mL poly-L-lysine dextran particles) were added to propidium iodide (1 μg) and pcDNA3 GFP plasmid (4 μg); the loading capacity was then determined by measuring changes in emission as cDNA bound to dextran particles. Dextran concentrations were established by means of a colorimetric technique, as previously described (23), measuring the optical density at 490 nm. The iron content of the different samples was determined by UV absorption at 410 nm (Spectronic, Rochester, NY) (22).

The hydrodynamic diameter of particles was measured by means of laser light scattering (N4MD Nanosizer; Coultronics, Hialeah, Fla) and expressed as unimodal size distribution. Magnetic properties of the constructs were measured by determining T1 and T2 by using a MR spectrometer (NMS-120 Minispec; Bruker Instruments, Toronto, Ontario, Canada) operating at 0.47 T (20 MHz) and 37°C. T1 was measured with an inversion-recovery pulse sequence, yielding 20 data points that were then fit to a monoexponential regression curve. T2 was measured from 75 data points generated with a Carr-Purcell-Meiboom-Gill pulse sequence with a 90°–180° pulse separation of 250 μsec. Then 1/T1 and 1/T2 were expressed per 1 second to determine relaxivities (R1 and R2).

To determine the effect of the different constructs on MR signal intensity, a phantom experiment was performed. Construct 1 was dissolved in water at DNA concentrations ranging from 0 to 25 μg/mL DNA, and phantoms were imaged with a 1.5-T superconducting magnet system (System 5X; GE Medical Systems, Milwaukee, Wis). Coronal images were acquired with an extremity coil (repetition time msec/echo time msec = 300/10, 20 and 2,000/20; four signals acquired;

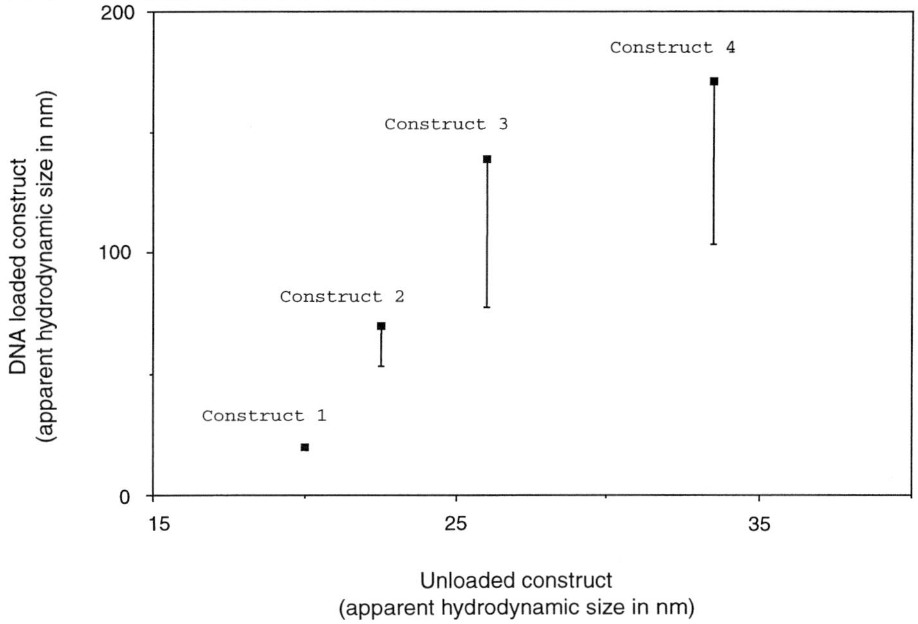

Figure 1. Size distribution of carrier and constructs. The size of DNA-loaded construct is plotted against the size of DNA-free (*unloaded*) construct. Data are presented as mean apparent hydrodynamic diameter and −1 standard deviation. The smaller a given construct, the more likely it is to be useful for systemic use.

TABLE 2
Relaxivity Values of Constructs

Constructs	Before DNA Attachment		After DNA Attachment	
	R1	R2	R1	R2
Dextran-coated particle	20.0 ± 2.1	41.4 ± 1.8	NA	NA
Construct 1	18.9 ± 1.0	40.4 ± 1.2	17.9 ± 1.6	38.9 ± 2.1
Construct 2	19.1 ± 0.9	39.3 ± 1.4	15.1 ± 2.4	38.2 ± 6.4
Construct 3	18.2 ± 1.8	38.1 ± 1.1	15.6 ± 1.7	40.1 ± 4.9

Note.—Data are the mean ± standard deviation ($mmol^{-1} \cdot L \cdot sec^{-1}$) at 0.47 T and 37°C. R2 values are not significantly different ($P > .1$) among constructs before or after DNA attachment.

256 × 192 matrix; 12-cm field of view; and 3-mm section thickness.

Transfection

Transfection experiments were performed in human 293 embryonal kidney cells (CRL-1573; American Tissue Culture Collection, Rockville, Md). Cells were plated at 10^5 per well in 24 well plates (Falcon; Becton Dickinson, Lincoln Park, NJ) in Dulbecco modified Eagle medium (DMEM Cellgro; Mediatech, Washington, DC) supplemented with 10% fetal bovine serum (FBS Cellgro; Mediatech) 24 hours before transfection. Transfection was carried out by incubating cells with the constructs or DNA alone for 24 hours. Cells were then propagated for another 48 hours with change of medium every 24 hours. Transfection efficiency was determined by acquiring fluorescence images on an inverted fluorescence microscope (Axiovert 100 TV; Zeiss, Wetzlar, Germany) equipped with a filter set (XF 22; Omega Optical, Brattleboro, Vt) and a charge coupled device (Photometrics, Tuscon, Ariz) connected to a computer (Power Macintosh 7600/120; Apple Computers, Cupertino, Calif). For each experiment, five high-power fields (magnification, ×630) were selected, and the ratio of fluorescent to nonfluorescent cells was determined in bright field (total cells) and fluorescent (transfected cells) channels. Automated quantitative image segmentation analysis (mean, standard deviation, and range of fluorescence) was performed with commercially available software (IP LAB SPECTRUM; Signal Analytics, Vienna, Va) on 12-bit data. Each experiment was performed in triplicate. Standard DEAE-dextran– and $CaPO_4$-mediated transfections (15) served as a positive control and mock-transfected cells served as a negative control.

Animal Imaging Experiments

To directly compare the distribution of the constructs with MR imaging and autoradiography, animals received corpus callosum injections of dCTP-33–labeled construct 1. All injections were made stereotactically into the corpus callosum of 10 anesthetized (intraperitoneal ketamine, 50 mg per kilogram of body weight, Park-Davis, Morris Plains, NJ; xylazine, 2 mg/kg, Miles, Shawnee Mission, Kan) adult Sprague Dawley rats. The head was shaved, and the rat was placed in a stereotactic frame (David Kopf Instruments, Jujunga, Calif). A midline incision was then made to expose the frontal bone, and a 1-mm-diameter burr hole was drilled. The tip of a 27-gauge needle attached to a 10-μL syringe (Hamilton; Reno, Nevada) was then lowered into the right corpus callosum with use of stereotactic coordinates (bregma, −0.6 mm; vertical, −2.0 mm; right lateral, −2.0 mm). A maximum 10 μL ($n = 3$ [2 μL, $n = 2$; 1 μL, $n = 3$; 0.5 μL, $n = 2$]) of the test compounds was administered over 10–20 minutes. The needle was withdrawn over 10 minutes, the burr hole was closed with bone wax, and the skin was closed in a single layer.

All animals underwent MR imaging 12–96 hours after inoculation with use of the same pulse sequences that were used for the phantom experiment. The animal imaging experiments were adapted to ensure the best spatial resolution and signal-to-noise ratio (3-inch surface coil; 8-cm field of view; spatial resolution, 312 × 312 × 3,000 μm). Spin-echo images (1,500/40) were acquired. After MR imaging, the animals were sacrificed with an overdose of phenobarbital and frozen in liquid nitrogen. Brains were later removed for histologic and autoradiographic examinations. All animal experiments were conducted in accordance with institutional and national guidelines.

Histologic and Autoradiographic Examinations

Twenty-four hours after intracerebral injection of construct 1, three rats were sacrificed with an overdose of pentobarbital and quickly immersed in liquid nitrogen and stored at −86°C. Prior to sectioning, brains were removed and cryocut into 8-μm-thick sections (2800 Frifocut-E; Leica Instruments, Nussloch, Germany).

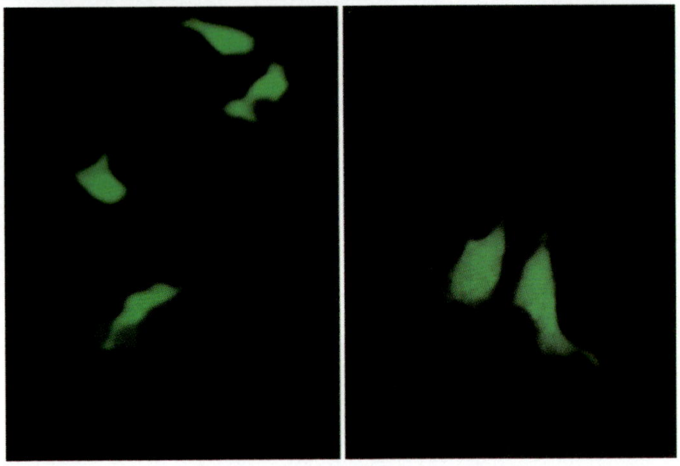

2.

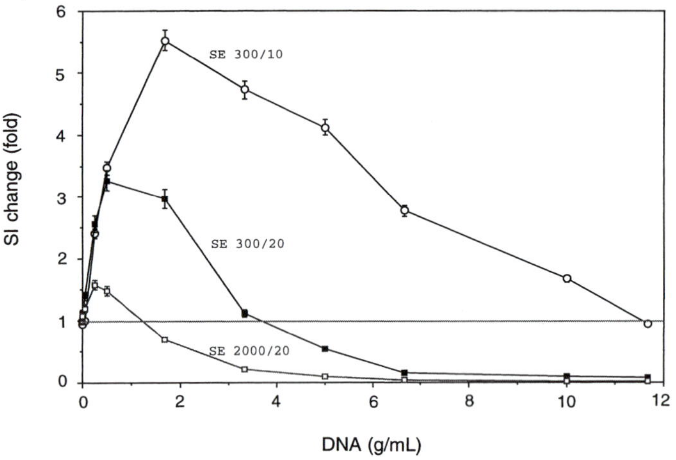

3.

Figures 2, 3. (2) Transfection in cell culture. Transfection of human 293 cells with construct 1 (left, 2 μg of DNA per 10^5 cells) or the $CaPo_4$ method (right). Transfected cells express GFP with little morphologic difference. **(3)** Signal intensity (*SI*) changes as a function of DNA concentration in human 293 cells and as a function of construct concentration in phantoms. At lower DNA concentrations, signal intensity increases (T1 effect) whereas at higher concentrations it decreases (T2 effect).

Unstained slices were exposed to phosphor screens that were then read with a digital phosphor image analyzer (Molecular Dynamics, Sunnyvale, Calif). Digital images of corresponding MR sections were then juxtaposed for analysis.

Histologic slices were also stained for iron (to visualize the magnetic carrier) with a Perls stain. Slides were incubated for 30 minutes in equal parts of 2% HCl and 2% potassium ferrocyanide, followed by rinsing for 30 minutes in double distilled water. Slides were counterstained with weak eosin (Fisher Scientific, Fair Lawn, NJ).

Slices were also stained for GFP by using a commercially available anti-GFP polyclonal antibody (Clontech, Palo Alto, Calif). Slides were incubated with the primary antibody for 30 minutes and then with an avidin-biotin complex (Vectastain ABC kit; Vector Laboratories, Burlingame, Calif) as described by the manufacturer. Sections were dehydrated and lightly counterstained with hematoxylin.

Statistical Analysis

Differences in relaxation times or fluorescence between experimental groups was tested with a Student *t* test, and *P* less than .1 was considered to indicate a statistically significant difference.

RESULTS

Physicochemical Properties of Different Conjugates

Three different constructs were synthesized that had variable amounts of DNA attached with poly-L-lysine (Table 1). The moles per liter ratio of amino groups per dextran chain ranged from 4.2 (construct 1) to 10 (construct 3). As expected, the hydrodynamic diameter of the carrier increased with increasing poly-L-lysine attachment from 20.0 to 33.5 nm (Table 1). DNA attachment further increased the mean diameter of constructs from 70.0 to 171.2 nm (Table 1, Fig 1). Determination of DNA-to-dextran ratios indicate that there were between 1.2 and 2.8 DNA molecules associated with each dextran nanoparticle (Table 1).

The relaxation properties of the constructs are listed in Table 2. Neither poly-L-lysine modification nor DNA attachment to the magnetic carrier significantly altered R2 relaxation rates ($P > .1$). This observation is consistent with the fact that the relaxation properties are mainly determined by the sterically shielded central iron oxide crystal whose size or structure is little affected by surface modification.

Transfection

To prove that the modified dextran particles are capable of transfection, cell culture experiments were performed. Constructs 1–3 resulted in measurable levels of GFP gene expression in human 293 cells (Fig 2) whereas DNA alone or dextran particle (no DNA attached) did not. Among the three constructs, there were differences in transfection efficiency (Table 3). Construct 1 had the highest transfection efficiency (4.1% of cells transfected), which was slightly higher than that of construct 2 (2.9%), and construct 3 had the lowest transfection efficiency (0.3%). Interestingly, the transfection efficiency of construct 1 was similar to that of DEAE-dextran (4.1% vs 6.0%, respectively). Transfection efficiency with $CaPO_4$ (positive control) was highest (52.1% of cells transfected). Differences were not statistically significant ($P > .1$) in the mean fluorescence of transfected cells (Table 3). The range of cellular fluorescence was slightly higher for constructs 1 and 2 than for other experimental constructs owing to the presence of a few intensely bright cells.

Imaging Findings

Figure 3 shows MR signal intensity as a function of DNA concentration and pulse sequences used for measurement. As expected on the basis of findings in prior calibration and phantom studies (24), observed signal intensity depended on concentration of constructs, with high signal intensity at low concentrations and low signal intensity at high concentrations, as predicted by theory (25). Signal intensity changes occurred in the range of approximately 0.005–10.000 μg/mL DNA with the spin echo pulse sequences. At DNA concentrations of more than 15 μg/mL, quantitation (but not detection) appears unreliable because of the predominating T2* effect and susceptibility artifacts.

In vivo imaging showed the distribution of local vector concentrations after callosal injection (Fig 4). As expected, local concentrations of the construct were highest at the center of the injection site

TABLE 3
Transfection Efficiency

Constructs	Quantity of DNA (μg/10^5 cells)	Transfection Efficiency (% of cells transfected)	Fluorescence (signal intensity value)*		
			Mean	Standard Deviation	Range
Dextran-coated particle	None	0.0	NA	NA	NA
Construct 1	2	4.1	503	311	210–1,426
Construct 2	2	2.9	539	301	208–1,698
Construct 3	2	0.3	316	51	209–500
DEAE-dextran	2	6.0	394	220	213–1,195
$CaPO_4$	2	52.1	385	220	211–1,115
DNA alone	2	0.0	NA	NA	NA

Note.—NA = not applicable.
* Measure of expression of GFP transfected into human 293 cells.

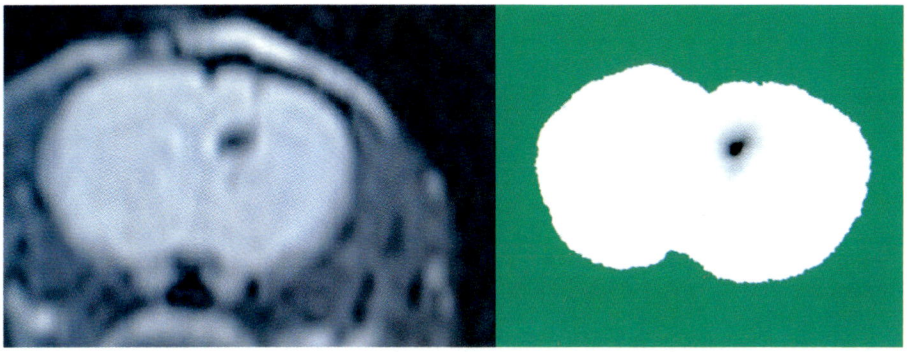

Figure 4. Cerebral DNA distribution in vivo. Correlation of spin-echo (1,500/40) MR image (left) and autoradiograph (P-33–labeled construct) superimposed on histologic outline of corresponding brain section (right). There is good correlation between the in vivo imaging appearance of the construct and the autoradiographic distribution of the construct (section thickness for MR image, 300 μm; autoradiograph, 30 μm).

and decreased toward the periphery. In some animals, axonal transport, diffusion, or both across the corpus callosum could also be seen as dark bands crossing to the contralateral hemisphere. Autoradiographs showed distribution volumes and local concentrations of construct nearly identical to those depicted on MR images (Fig 4).

Histologic Findings

Histologic evaluation of brain specimens showed the administered constructs to be located adjacent to the injection site both within the interstitium and in neuronal and glial cells. Constructs were also detectable in cells as far as 2 mm from the injection site. Fluorescence microscopy and immunohistochemistry with anti-GFP antibody showed scant GFP staining in neuronal and glial cells (Fig 5).

DISCUSSION

The development of injectable, stable, and efficient constructs for gene delivery to the central nervous system has been challenging. Viral vectors are often efficient in gene transfer, but toxicity and immunogenicity can be substantial obstacles to their use (8). Nonviral gene delivery systems (eg, particulates, conglomerates, or lipophilic compounds) on the other hand are often not efficient (8) or face major barriers to delivery in vivo. Certain dextran carriers have been found to be an alternative to viruses for shuttling plasmid DNA into neuronal and glial cells (18,19), as well as other cells in vivo (24). In this study, a model DNA vector has been attached to dextran particles and expression both in cell culture and in vivo, neuronal and glial accumulation, and MR detection have been demonstrated. These constructs can thus theoretically be used to image gene delivery (distribution maps, local concentration) to the central nervous system in vivo.

Properties of the Construct

B-512 dextran produced from sucrose by *Leuconostoc mesenteroides* has been characterized previously (26). The polyglucosan molecule utilized in this study has an average molecular mass of 11 kd. It consists of 21 1,6–linked linear glucose units, one nonreducing end group, and only one 1,3,6–linked residue (branch point) and is thus 95% linear. Each assembled 20-nm-diameter dextran particle contains an average of 25 dextran molecules held together by a central, sterically shielded iron oxide core. To attach and condense DNA, the particle surface was modified with poly-L-lysine at different stochiometric amounts. Prior research had shown that dextran particle modification with poly-L-lysine, wheat germ agglutinin, or rhodamine (27) still results in neuronal uptake (20,28–31).

Some of the physical properties of the different constructs are listed in Tables 2 and 3. The size of the poly-L-lysine–modified dextran particles ranged between 22.5 and 33.5 nm with small standard deviations indicative of tight size distribution similar to the parent monodispersed dextran particle. After incubation of the poly-L-lysine–modified dextran particles with DNA, the size of resultant constructs ranged from 70.0 to 171.2 nm in mean diameters small enough for local and systemic use. The standard deviation of size distribution of the constructs was considerably wider than that of dextran particles, indicating heterogeneous particle populations. Calculations based on DNA-loading capacity and particle size indicate that on average there are one to three plasmids associated with each dextran particle, depending on construct (Table 2).

Cellular Uptake

After stereotactic injection into the brain, dextran particles were taken up by neurons in sufficiently high quantities to be detectable at histologic examination, similar to that described after intravenous administration and blood-brain-barrier disruption (19). Neuronal and glial cells were labeled predominantly adjacent to the injection site after stereotactic injection, but axonal transport was also observed as in prior studies (20).

With use of cell culture techniques, it has previously been shown that dextran constructs accumulate in tubular lysosomes and endosomes in a variety of cells as corroborated by means of double staining with an antibody against LGP-A, a lysosomal glycoprotein (32,33). The cellular capacity of dextran particle uptake is relatively high in cell culture (10^4–10^5 particles per cell), and no adverse effects on cellular morphology or replication could previously be demonstrated (24). Nuclear uptake from the endosomal, lysosomal, or cytoplasmic compartment has not been observed directly, but findings in our study clearly show marker gene expression indicative of such transport.

The current results show that the dextran-based DNA carrier could be used to transfect human 293 cells in culture with an efficiency similar to that with DEAE-dextran, a commonly used transfection technique in cell culture (Table 3). Histologic evaluation of the injected brains also confirmed that transfection occurs in vivo (Fig 5), although scant and faint. The difference in transfection efficiency in cell culture and in vivo is most likely related to the fact that most cells in vivo are differentiated and nondividing, whereas those in cell culture are dividing. Immunohistochemistry with anti-GFP antibody showed GFP staining to be most marked adjacent to the injection site in glial and neuronal cells. Cells as far as 1–2 mm from the injection site were also occasionally faintly positive for GFP.

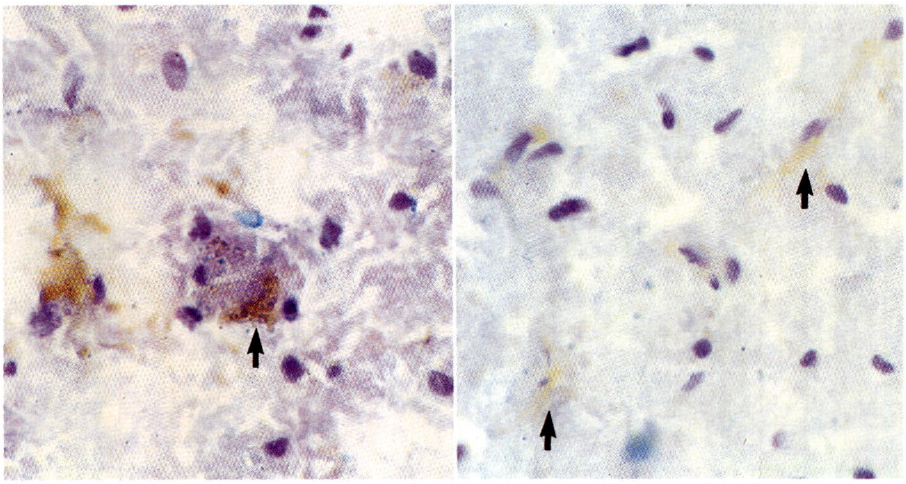

Figure 5. Histologic findings. Photomicrographs depict anti-GFP immunohistologic specimens counterstained with hematoxylin (original magnification, ×1,000). Left: slice adjacent to injection site shows brown GFP staining product in the cytoplasm of cells (arrow). Right: slice approximately 1 mm away from the injection site shows weak brown GFP staining in several cells (arrows). GFP expression was also demonstrated at fluorescence microscopy (not shown).

Imaging of Gene Delivery

Gene delivery vehicles that can be identified with in vivo imaging techniques may be useful to objectively assess delivery to in vivo macro- and microenvironments. These environments can represent major barriers to efficient gene delivery. Barriers are cellular (transport across plasma membrane) and subcellular (transport across nuclear membrane) or posed by in vivo macroenvironments (organ barriers, flow) and microenvironments (tissue inhomogeneities, pressure differences, convection heterogeneities, inactivation of constructs by the body's immunonologic machinery, metabolism) (34). Transport across a cell membrane barrier is best tested in cell culture, but evaluation of other barriers requires testing in an intact organism with carriers detectable by means of imaging techniques. The choice of imaging techniques is currently limited to MR imaging (35), scintigraphy, or optical imaging (36).

The amount of dextran-coated iron oxide particles in brain tissue necessary for detection has previously been determined by means of in vivo MR imaging (18). At 1.5 T, the detection threshold is roughly 86 ng of iron per cubic millimeter with a gradient-echo pulse sequence (50/6, 60° flip angle) corresponding to approximately 4.5×10^4 particles per gram of tissue (18). Extrapolated to the current study, the detection threshold of locally injected DNA would thus be 4.1 ng of DNA, well below amounts used for gene therapy (milligram range). Indeed, these imaging studies show a remarkable concordance between in vivo DNA distribution determined at MR imaging and autoradiography.

The artificial gene delivery constructs developed in this study can be used in applications other than the imaging of gene delivery or the noninvasive estimation of gene concentrations. For example, the magnetic DNA carriers may also be useful for site-specific DNA delivery by means of application of external magnets (37).

Practical Application: The current research is proof that gene delivery can be imaged with MR imaging. The developed constructs may be useful for in vivo gene transfer in central nervous system disease.

References

1. Horellou P, Bilang-Bleuel A, Mallet J. In vivo adenovirus-mediated gene transfer for Parkinson's disease. Neurobiol Dis 1997; 4:280–287.
2. Lacorazza H, Flax J, Snyder E, Jendoubi M. Expression of human beta-hexosaminidase alpha-subunit gene. Nat Med 1996; 2:424–429.
3. Breakefield X. Gene delivery into the brain using virus vectors. Nat Genet 1993; 3:187–189.
4. McKusick V. Mendelian inheritance of man: catalogs of autosomal dominant, autosomal recessive, and x-linked phenotypes. Baltimore, Md: Johns Hopkins University Press, 1988.
5. Curiel D. High-efficiency gene transfer mediated by adenovirus-polylysine-DNA complexes. Ann NY Acad Sci 1994; 176:36–58.
6. Mulligan R. The basic science of gene therapy. Science 1993; 260:926–932.
7. Boris-Lawrie K, Temin H. The retroviral vector: replication cycle and safety considerations for retroviral mediated gene therapy. Ann NY Acad Sci 1994; 176:59–71.
8. Hodgson C. The vector void in gene therapy: can viral vectors and transfection be combined to permit safe, efficacious, and targeted gene therapy? Biotechnology 1995; 13:222–226.
9. Wu G, Wilson J, Shalaby F, Grossman M, Shafritz D, Wu C. Receptor-mediated gene delivery in vivo: partial correction of genetic analbumenia in nagase rats. J Biol Chem 1991; 266:14338–14342.
10. Goldspiel B, Green L, Calis K. Clinical frontiers: human gene therapy. Clin Pharm 1993; 12:488–505.
11. Ledley F. Review: are contemporary methods for somatic gene therapy suitable for clinical applications? Clin Invest Med 1993; 16:78–88.
12. McCabe E. Minireview: clinical application of gene therapy—emerging opportunities and current limitations. Biochem Med Metab Biol 1993; 50:241–253.
13. Schreier H. The new frontier: gene and oligonucleotide therapy. Pharm Acta Helv 1994; 68:145–159.
14. Haensler J, Szoka F. Polyamidoamine cascade polymers mediate efficient transfection in cells in culture. Bioconjug Chem 1993; 4:372–379.
15. Sambrook J, Fritsch E, Maniatis T, eds. Transfection of coprecipitates of calcium phosphate and DNA. In: Molecular cloning: a laboratory manual. New York, NY: Cold Spring Harbor Laboratory Press, 1989; 16.32–16.41.
16. Shen T, Bogdanov A Jr, Bogdanova A, Poss K, Brady T, Weissleder R. Magnetically labeled secretin retains receptor affinity to pancreas acinar cells. Bioconjug Chem 1996; 7:311–316.
17. Bosnes M, Deggerdal A, Rian A, Korsnes L, Larsen F. Magnetic separation in molecu-

lar biology. In: Häefeli U, Schütt W, Teller J, Zborowski M, eds. Scientific and clinical applications of magnetic carriers. New York, NY: Plenum, 1997; 269–285.
18. Zimmer C, Weissleder R, O'Connor D, LaPointe L, Brady T, Enochs W. Cerebral iron xoide distribution: in vivo mapping with MR imaging. Radiology 1995; 196: 521–527.
19. Kneeled E, Weissleder R, Nilaver G, et al. Delivery of virus-sized iron oxide particles to rodent CNS neurons. Neurosurgery 1994; 34:777–784.
20. van Everdingen K, Enochs W, Bhide P, et al. Determinants of in vivo MR imaging of slow axonal transport. Radiology 1994; 193:485–491.
21. Sambrook J, Fritsch E, Maniatis T, eds. Plasmid vectors. In: Molecular cloning: a laboratory manual. New York, NY: Cold Spring Harbor Laboratory, 1989; 1.7–1.22.
22. Shen T, Weissleder R, Papisov M, Bogdanov A, Brady T. Monocrystalline iron oxide nanocompounds (MION): physicochemical properties. Magn Reson Med 1993; 29:599–604.
23. Dubois M, Gilles K, Hamilton J, Rebers P, Smith F. Colorimetric method for determination of sugars and related substances. Anal Chem 1956; 28:350–356.
24. Weissleder R, Cheng H, Bogdanova A, Bogdanov A. Magnetically labeled cells can be detected by MR imaging. JMRI 1997; 7:258–263.
25. Bulte J, Brooks R. Magnetic nanoparticles as contrast agents for MR imaging. In: Häfeli U, Schütt W, Teller J, Zborowski M, eds. Scientific and clinical applications of magnetic carriers. New York, NY: Plenum, 1997; 527–543.
26. Van Cleve J, Schaefer W, Rist C. The structure of NRRL B-512 dextran: methylation studies. J Am Chem Soc 1956; 78: 4435–4438.
27. Keifer J, Vyas D, Houk J. Sulforhodamine labeling of neural circuits engaged in motor pattern generation in the in vitro turtle brainstem-cerebellum. J Neurosci 1992; 12:3187–3199.
28. Fritzsch B, Niemann U, Bleckmann H. A discrete projection of the sacculus and legens to a distinct brainstem nucleus in a catfish. Neurosci Lett 1990; 111:7–11.
29. Nance D, Burns J. Fluorescent dextrans as sensitive anterograde neuroanatomical tracers: applications and pitfalls. Brain Res Bull 1990; 25:139–145.
30. Schmued L. In vivo anterograde and retrograde axonal transport of the fluorescent rhodamine-dextran-amine, fluoro-ruby, within the CNS. Brain Res 1990; 526:127–134.
31. Olsson T, Kristensson K. A simple histochemical method for double labeling of neurons by retrograde axonal transport. Neurosci Lett 1978; 8:265–268.
32. Rabinowitz S, Horstmann H, Gordon S, Griffiths G. Immunocytochemical characterization of the endocytic and phagolysosomal compartments in peritoneal macrophages. J Cell Biol 1992; 116:95–112.
33. Schulze E, Ferrucci J, Poss K, LaPointe L, Bogdanova A, Weissleder R. Cellular uptake and trafficking of a prototypical magnetic iron oxide label in vitro. Invest Radiol 1995; 30:604–610.
34. Jain R. Vascular and interstitial barriers to delivery of therapeutic agents in tumors. Cancer Metastasis Rev 1990; 9:253–266.
35. Jacobs R, Fraser S. Magnetic resonance microscopy of embryonic cell lineages and movements. Science 1994; 263:681–684.
36. Tearney G, Brezinski M, Bouma B, et al. In vivo endoscopic optical biopsy with optical coherence tomography. Science 1997; 276:2037–2039.
37. Häfeli U, Pauer G, Roberts W, Humm J, Macklis R. Magnetically targeted microspheres for intracavitary and intraspinal Y-90 radiotherapy. In: Häfeli U, Schütt W, Teller J, Zborowski M, eds. Scientific and clinical applications of magnetic carriers. New York, NY: Plenum, 1997; 501–516.

George A. Taylor, MD
Carol E. Barnewolt, MD
Patricia S. Dunning, RT

Index terms:
Cerebral blood vessels, flow dynamics, 17.919
Cerebral blood vessels, US, 17.12988
Ultrasound (US), contrast media, 17.12988
Ultrasound (US), power Doppler studies, 17.12984, 17.12988

Radiology 1998; 208:73–79

Abbreviations:
ANOVA = analysis of variance
NMDA = *N*-methyl-D-aspartic acid

[1] From the Department of Radiology, Children's Hospital and Harvard Medical School, 300 Longwood Ave, Boston, MA 02115. Supported in part by Alliance Pharmaceutical, San Diego, Calif, and Acuson, Mountain View, Calif. Received November 6, 1997; revision requested January 22, 1998; revision received February 4; accepted February 11. **Address reprint requests to** G.A.T.

Excitotoxin-induced Cerebral Hyperemia in Newborn Piglets: Regional Cerebral Blood Flow Mapping with Contrast-enhanced Power Doppler US[1]

PURPOSE: To create regional cerebral blood flow maps with contrast material–enhanced power Doppler ultrasound (US).

MATERIALS AND METHODS: In six anesthetized newborn piglets, cerebral hyperemia was induced after intrastriatal injection of 5 μmol of *N*-methyl-D-aspartic acid. Coronal power Doppler US was performed with a microbubble-based contrast agent, and cerebral blood flow was determined before and at 15, 30, and 60 minutes after injection. Images were digitized and analyzed for changes in mean pixel intensity. A bolus injection curve was constructed by plotting mean pixel intensity versus time, and the area under this normalized curve was compared with cerebral blood flow.

RESULTS: Hemispheric cerebral blood flow increased from 40 mL/min/100 g ± 1 (mean ± standard error) to 90 ± 12, 86 ± 8, and 85 ± 12 at 15, 30, and 60 minutes after injection, respectively ($P < .0001$ [analysis of variance]). Hemispheric mean pixel intensity at peak contrast also increased from 69 units ± 5 to 120 ± 4, 112 ± 6, and 98 ± 13 at 15, 30, and 60 minutes after injection, respectively ($P < .003$). The area under the normalized curve correlated well with changes in hemispheric and striatal cerebral blood flow ($r = .73$, $P = .0001$; $r = .62$, $P = .0001$, respectively).

CONCLUSION: In the newborn brain, regional blood flow maps can be created accurately with contrast-enhanced power Doppler US.

Birth asphyxia is one of the most common causes of severe brain injury in full-term infants worldwide. The incidence of birth asphyxia in the United States has been reported to be between 2.9 and nine cases per 1,000 deliveries (1). Abnormalities in cerebral blood flow have been implicated as a key factor in the development of hypoxic ischemic brain injury in the newborn (2).

Techniques for determining regional blood flow in infants that can be performed at the bedside and are safe, reliable, and reproducible are currently lacking. Although color Doppler ultrasound (US) has been useful at the crib side in showing some qualitative changes in neonatal brain blood flow, quantification of blood flow has been difficult due to aliasing and the angle dependence of frequency shift information (3–5). Power Doppler US has been recently developed in an attempt to overcome some of these limitations (6,7). This technique, based on the Doppler US autocorrelation function, encodes the integral of the Doppler US signal amplitude as a color map, in which pixel brightness is proportional to the number of moving reflectors in the field, and velocity and directional information are not depicted. The main advantage of power Doppler US is that electronic noise can be reduced without loss of sensitivity to low-flow states (7). Findings in studies with power Doppler US have shown an improved ability to detect brain hyperemia after injection of an excitotoxic amino acid into the basal ganglia of newborn lambs (8). Unfortunately, power Doppler US is highly susceptible to flash artifact from tissue motion, and detection of blood flow is often impossible in subjects receiving high-frequency ventilation or otherwise

Author contributions:
Guarantor of integrity of entire study, G.A.T.; study concepts, G.A.T.; study design, G.A.T., C.E.B., P.S.D.; definition of intellectual content, G.A.T.; literature research, G.A.T.; experimental studies, G.A.T., C.E.B., P.S.D.; data acquisition, G.A.T., C.E.B., P.S.D.; data analysis, G.A.T., C.E.B.; statistical analysis, G.A.T.; manuscript preparation, G.A.T., C.E.B.; manuscript editing and review, G.A.T., C.E.B., P.S.D.

unable to remain motionless during the examination. In addition, power Doppler US does not measure tissue perfusion but rather depicts an estimate of fractional moving blood volume. True perfusion measurements require estimates of how rapidly a volume of blood moves through tissue (9,10).

Findings in preliminary studies have shown that the combination of power Doppler US and microbubble-based contrast agents can further improve the ability to detect signal from flowing blood and distinguish it from background clutter and may be used to create regional blood flow maps of the brain (11,12). In addition, contrast agent transit time through tissue can be observed and quantified. In the current study, we used contrast material–enhanced power Doppler US to study changes in regional cerebral perfusion induced by injecting *N*-methyl-D-aspartic acid (NMDA) into the basal ganglia of newborn piglets. NMDA is a synthetic analogue of glutamate that has been used as a chemical model that replicates important factors of perinatal hypoxic-ischemic injury (13). Local intracerebral injection of NMDA acts as a potent cerebral vasodilator in experimental animals (4,14). Our goals were to further explore the feasibility of this technique for creating regional cerebral blood flow maps and for quantifying physiologic conditions of regional blood flow that mimic clinically relevant situations in the newborn.

MATERIALS AND METHODS

This study was approved by our institutional animal care and use committee, and it complied with the guidelines of the National Institutes of Health for care and handling of animals.

Six newborn Yorkshire piglets were anesthetized with 20 mg of ketamine hydrochloride per kilogram of body weight and 5 mg/kg of xylazine by means of intramuscular injection followed by inhalation anesthesia with halothane until venous access could be secured. Thereafter, a continuous intravenous infusion of diprivan 1% (Propofol; Stuart Pharmaceuticals, Wilmington, Del) diluted in 5% dextrose at a dose of 0.002 mg/kg/min was used for the remainder of the experiment. Controlled ventilation was maintained via an oral endotracheal tube, and supplemental oxygen was administered to maintain Pa_{O_2} at 80–200 mm Hg and Pa_{CO_2} at 30–45 mm Hg. Polyvinyl chloride catheters were placed in the left ventricle via the right femoral artery for administration of radiolabeled microspheres; in the left femoral artery for continuous blood pressure monitoring and microsphere reference sample withdrawal; and in both femoral veins for administration of intravenous fluids, medications, and US contrast material. A 1 × 2-cm craniotomy was performed across the midline, at the level of the coronal suture, leaving the dura intact for US access.

Arterial blood pressure, heart rate, and core (rectal) temperature were monitored continuously (model 76 physiologic monitoring system; Hewlett Packard, Andover, Mass). Arterial P_{O_2}, P_{CO_2}, pH, and hematocrit were intermittently measured throughout the experiment.

A 27-gauge needle was placed into the left striatum under direct US visualization, and 5 μmol of NMDA in 0.2 mL of buffered saline were injected into the striatum over a 2-minute period. The needle was left in place for an additional minute before removal. This dose was determined on the basis of previous experience with this model (4).

US guidance for needle placement and brain imaging were performed with a 7.0-MHz vector transducer (model 128 XP; Acuson, Mountain View, Calif) held in place by an articulated mechanical holder during the entire experiment. Serial coronal power Doppler US images of the brain were obtained before, during, and after injection of contrast material. Imaging parameters were set to standardize the dynamic range of the image by using the lowest temporal averaging settings. The lowest Doppler US power settings were used (estimated in situ spatial peak temporal average, <50 mW). Nonlinear image pre- and postprocessing (input-output conversion) curves were not used. In previous experiments, we had used the method of Rubin et al (6) to set the color gain so that vascular signal was maximized and spurious tissue motion artifacts were reduced. With use of this technique, we found that the color gain setting was always between 48%–52% of maximum. In the current study, color gain was set at 50% of maximum and left unchanged throughout the experiment.

The contrast agent (Imagent US, formulation AF0150; Alliance Pharmaceutical, San Diego, Calif) was reconstituted according to the manufacturer's directions. A dispersion of surfactant-coated perfluorohexane and nitrogen-containing microbubbles with a median diameter of approximately 5 μm is formed after reconstitution. Elimination from the blood is accomplished by means of evaporation through the lungs (15). The contrast material was administered at a dose of 0.2 mL/kg. Each dose was injected intravenously over a 1–2-second interval. This dose range was determined on the basis of previous brain blood flow experiments with this agent (16). At least 15 minutes elapsed between injections, and the catheter and stopcock were flushed with enough saline solution to fill the catheter dead space three times after each dose to clear any residual contrast material from the delivery system.

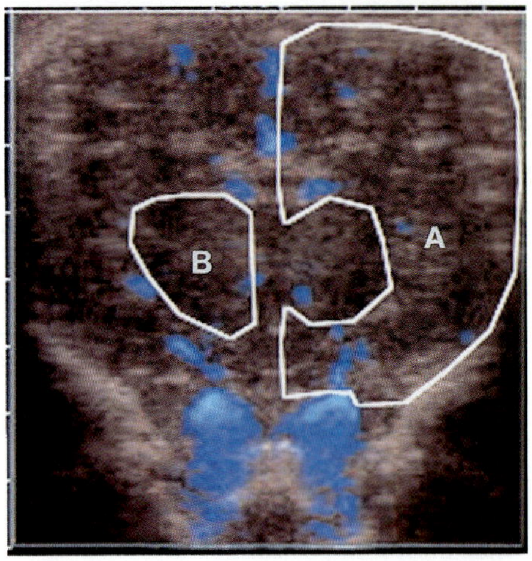

Figure 1. Coronal power Doppler US image obtained at the level of the basal ganglia shows regions of interest for mean pixel intensity analysis for cerebral hemisphere (*A*) and basal ganglia (*B*).

Acquisition of images of the brain was timed to coincide with the onset of intravenous injection of contrast material, and images were electronically captured every 0.4 second for the first 10 seconds of injection. The images were recorded by using a digital image processing unit (Aegis QV200; Acuson) and saved in an 8-bit tagged image file format, or TIFF. Images were then transferred onto a computer (Power MacIntosh; Apple Computers, Cupertino, Calif) and analyzed (PHOTOSHOP 4.0; Adobe Systems, Mountain View, Calif). Serial images were saved as separate layers within each file. Regions of interest were drawn over each cerebral hemisphere and basal ganglia (Fig 1). Each region of interest was identified on images obtained before the administration of contrast material and electronically superimposed on subsequent anatomically registered images obtained after the administration. Thus, region of interest of the same size was used to determine mean pixel intensity in each part of a given experiment so differences in inten-

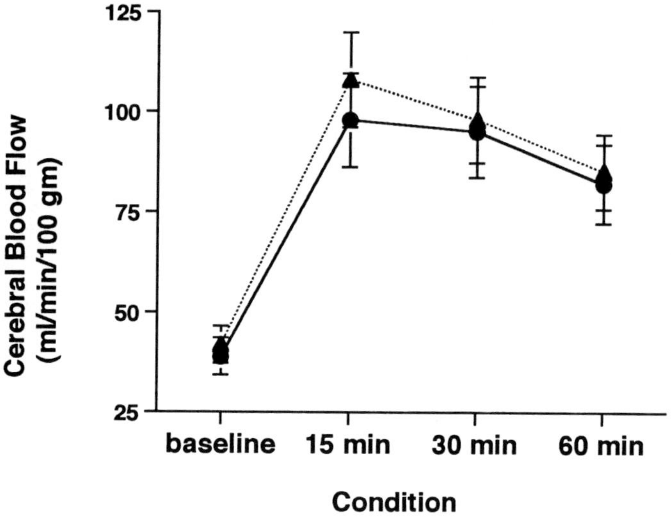

2.

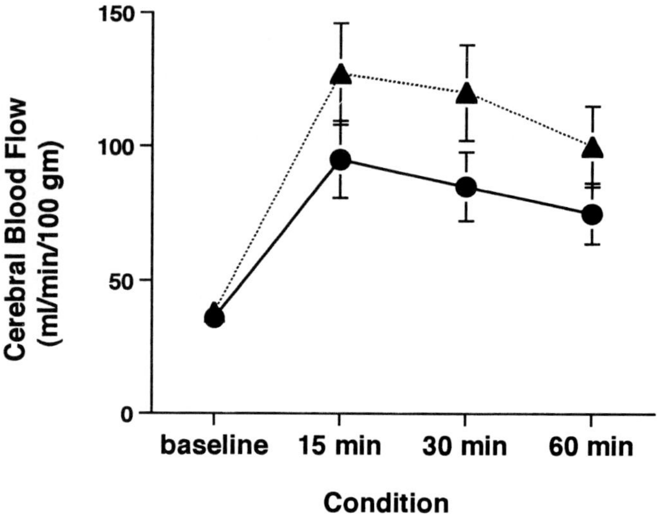

3.

Figures 2, 3. (2) Line graph shows regional cerebral blood flow for each hemisphere (● = right, ▲ = left) before (*baseline*) and at 15, 30, and 60 minutes after injection of NMDA into the left basal ganglion. Flow increases markedly to both hemispheres ($P < .0001$ compared with baseline, ANOVA). **(3)** Line graph shows regional cerebral blood flow for each basal ganglion (● = right, ▲ = left) before (*baseline*) and at 15, 30, and 60 minutes after injection of NMDA into the left basal ganglion. Flow increases markedly to both basal ganglia ($P < .0001$ compared with baseline, ANOVA). Flow to the left basal ganglion was higher than to the right basal ganglion after NMDA injection ($P < .004$)

TABLE 1
Changes in P_{CO_2} and Mean Arterial Blood Pressure

Condition	Arterial P_{CO_2} (mm Hg)	Mean Arterial Blood Pressure (mm Hg)
Baseline	39 ± 4	72 ± 11
Time (min) after NMDA injection		
15	48 ± 1*	110 ± 25*
30	45 ± 3	100 ± 13*
60	34 ± 9	92 ± 11*

Note.—Data are the mean ± standard error.
* Differences from baseline were significant at $P < .05$, ANOVA.

sity were related to changes in mean pixel value and not to variations in the size of the area measured. The number of pixels and mean pixel value for each region of interest were calculated by means of the program's histographic function. Time-intensity curves were generated, and the area under the initial wash-in phase of the curve (area under the normalized curve [in pixels]) was calculated and compared with flow in milliliters per minute per 1 g of tissue for each cerebral hemisphere and basal ganglia by means of linear regression. The area under this normalized curve and the mean pixel intensity at peak enhancement for each area of brain were recorded at each interval.

Regional cerebral blood flow was determined by using a radiolabeled microsphere technique in every animal (17). We used 16-mm ± 0.5 microspheres labeled with four separate isotopes: cerium-141, tin-113, ruthenium-103, and scandium-46 (Dupont–New England Nuclear Products, Boston, Mass). Each isotope has a different photon energy that allows it to be measured independently of other isotopes. For each blood flow determination, a volume containing 1.5×10^6 microspheres labeled with one of the isotopes was injected into the left ventricle and flushed with 5 mL of saline solution over a period of 20 seconds. This allows distribution of spheres throughout the body according to regional blood flow. A reference blood sample was withdrawn from a femoral catheter at a rate of 2 mL/min beginning 30 seconds before microsphere injection and continuing for 90 seconds after the infusion of flush solution was complete. Microsphere injection did not alter mean arterial blood pressure. At the end of each experiment, the animals were euthanized with an intravenous injection (2 mL/kg) of pentobarbital (euthanasia solution), and the brain was harvested. The brain was immediately sectioned in coronal orientation along a plane correlating to the region identified on the US image. After sectioning, tissue samples from basal ganglia and cerebral hemispheres were dissected, weighed, and placed in 15-mL vials for analysis in an autogamma scintillation spectrometer (Cobra II Gamma Counter; Packard Instruments, Meriden, Conn). Blood flow is determined by comparing counts for each radiolabel in each tissue sample and comparing the counts with those in the reference blood samples. Cerebral blood flow is expressed in milliliters per minute per 100 g of tissue by normalizing for tissue weight.

Cerebral blood flow determinations, contrast-enhanced power Doppler US images, and blood pressure and arterial blood gas levels were obtained at baseline, after a 30-minute equilibration period after surgery, and at 15, 30, and 60 minutes after intracerebral injection of NMDA.

Statistical significance of differences was determined by means of analysis of variance (ANOVA) or paired *t* test.

RESULTS

Cerebral Blood Flow Studies

Injection of NMDA into the left basal ganglion resulted in marked global cerebral hyperemia for at least 1 hour after injection as measured on the basis of radiolabeled microspheres. Supratentorial blood flow increased from 40 mL/min/100 g ± 2 (baseline) to 103 mL/min/100 g ± 7, 97 mL/min/100 g ± 8, and 84 mL/min/100 g ± 8 at 15, 30, and 60

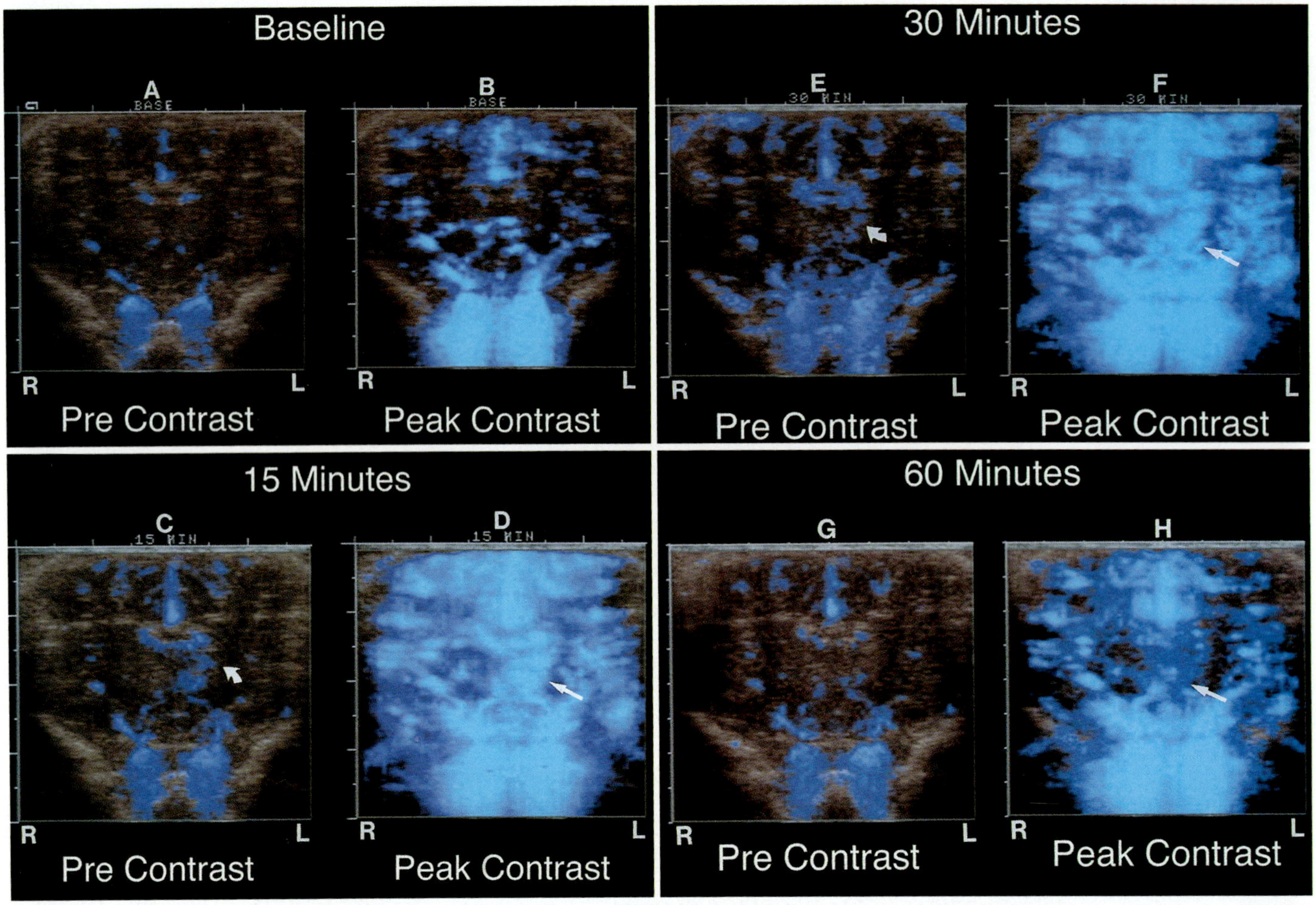

Figure 4. In one piglet, serial coronal power Doppler US images (*A–H*) were obtained at the level of the basal ganglia before administration of NMDA (*Pre Contrast*) and at peak contrast effect after injection (*15, 30, 60 Minutes*) into the left basal ganglion. Note increased symmetric enhancement to both hemispheres and greater focal enhancement of the left basal ganglion (straight arrow in *D, F,* and *H*) compared with that on the right. Only minimally increased power Doppler US signals (curved arrow in *C* and *E*) are identified in the left basal ganglion 15 and 30 minutes after NMDA injection on precontrast images. *L* = left, *R* = right.

minutes after NMDA injection, respectively ($P < .0001$ compared with baseline). Cerebral blood flow was symmetrically increased to both hemispheres, with no statistically significant differences in flow between right and left cerebral hemispheres at any time interval (Fig 2) ($P = .35$). Blood flow to the basal ganglia was also markedly elevated after injection of NMDA, but the hyperemia was asymmetric, with more marked increases in blood flow to the left compared with the right basal ganglion after NMDA injection (Fig 3) ($P < .001$). In addition, NMDA injection was associated with significant elevations in Pa_{CO_2} and mean arterial blood pressure (Table 1) ($P < .01$).

Power Doppler US

On contrast-enhanced power Doppler US images, cerebral hyperemia was characterized by an increase in number and brightness of pixels containing color information (mean pixel intensity), as well as increases in the area under the curve during the initial injection of the bolus of contrast material. The degree of enhancement in power Doppler US intensity varied with increasing cerebral blood flow after NMDA injection. Figure 4 shows a series of power Doppler US images obtained before contrast material administration and at peak contrast effect for one animal. NMDA injection resulted in increased symmetric enhancement to both hemispheres and asymmetric enhancement of the basal ganglia, with greater focal enhancement of the left basal ganglion compared with that on the right.

Figure 5 shows changes in the area under the curve and mean pixel intensity in the cerebral hemispheres of six animals. Both measures increased significantly after NMDA injection ($P < .0009$) with no left-right differences in enhancement ($P > .5$). Enhancement was elevated for at least 30 minutes and approached baseline levels at 60 minutes after NMDA injection. Similarly, the area under the curve and mean pixel intensity were increased in both basal ganglia after NMDA injection ($P < .001$). Although both measures were higher for the left basal ganglion at every interval after NMDA injection, these differences did not reach statistical significance ($P < .09$) (Fig 6). Basal ganglia values for area under the curve and mean pixel intensity during maximal NMDA hyperemia (15 and 30 minutes after injection) were combined and analyzed for right-left differences. Power Doppler US enhancement after NMDA injection was significantly higher for left basal ganglion compared with that on the right. These results are shown in Table 2.

Images obtained without contrast en-

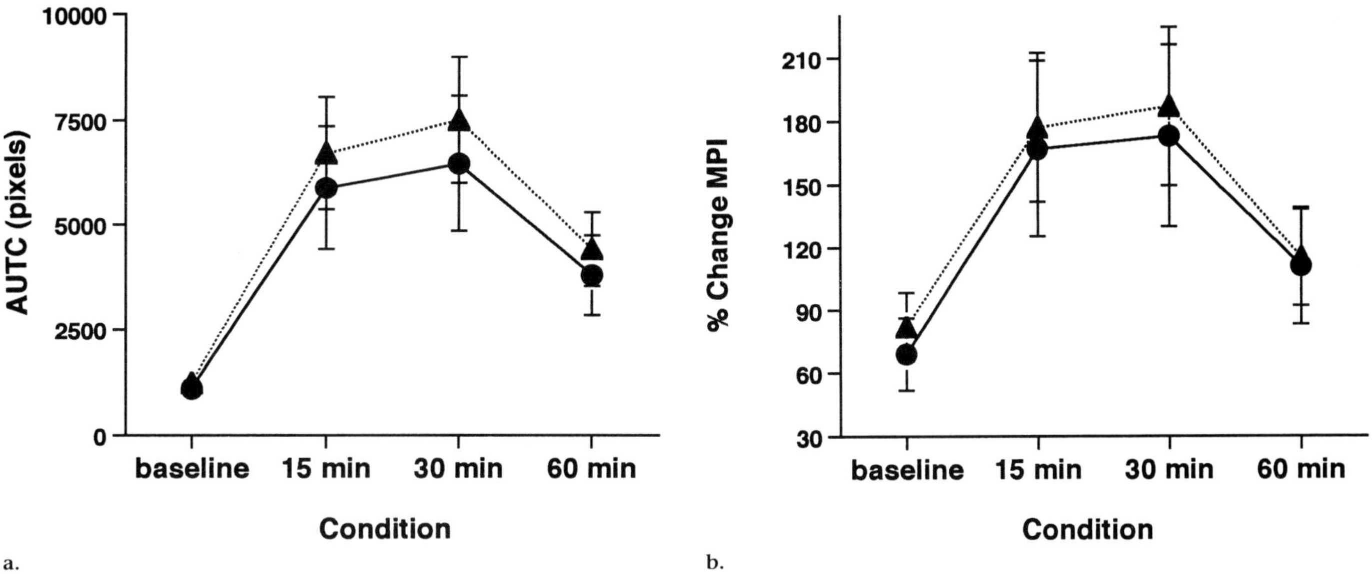

Figure 5. Line graphs show changes in **(a)** area under the curve (*AUTC*) and **(b)** mean pixel intensity (*MPI*) for cerebral hemispheres before (*baseline*) and at 15, 30, and 60 minutes after injection of NMDA into the left basal ganglion. Both measures increased significantly after NMDA injection ($P <$ .0009) with no left-right differences in enhancement ($P >$ .5, two-factor ANOVA). ● = right, ▲ = left.

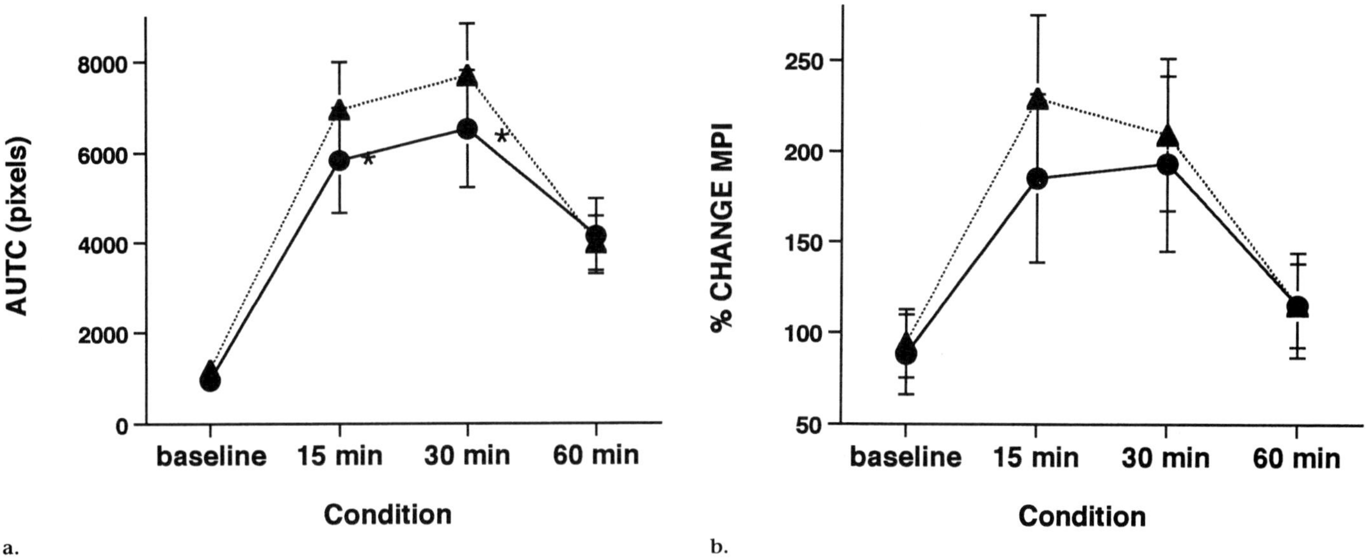

Figure 6. Line graphs show changes in **(a)** area under the curve (*AUTC*) and **(b)** mean pixel intensity (*MPI*) for the basal ganglia before (*baseline*) and at 15, 30, and 60 minutes after injection of NMDA into the left basal ganglion. The area under the curve increased significantly at 15 and 30 minutes after NMDA injection ($P <$ .0001 [* in **a**]). Left-right differences in mean pixel intensity did not reach statistical significance ($P <$ .09, two-factor ANOVA). ● = right, ▲ = left.

hancement showed little if any changes in apparent flow after NMDA injection as determined on the basis of differences in mean pixel intensity ($P >$ .1).

Quantification of Flow

Figure 7 compares area under the curve to regional blood flow determined on the basis of radiolabeled microspheres for cerebral hemispheres and basal ganglia in six animals. The area under the curve values correlated well with changes in hemispheric and striatal blood flow (r = .73, P = .0001; r = .62, P = .0001, respectively).

DISCUSSION

During an hypoxic ischemic insult, some neurons die immediately or during the reperfusion-reoxygenation period. In animal models, resuscitation after mild to moderate ischemia is accompanied by an initial period of hyperemia during which a number of processes occur that eventually lead to neuronal injury (18). These include the production of reactive oxygen metabolites and the excessive release or diminished reuptake of endogenous excitatory amino acids, such as glutamate and aspartate (19,20). A latent period begins between 2 and 12 hours after the insult and may persist for several days. This is followed by a second period of metabolic failure and neuronal death (21).

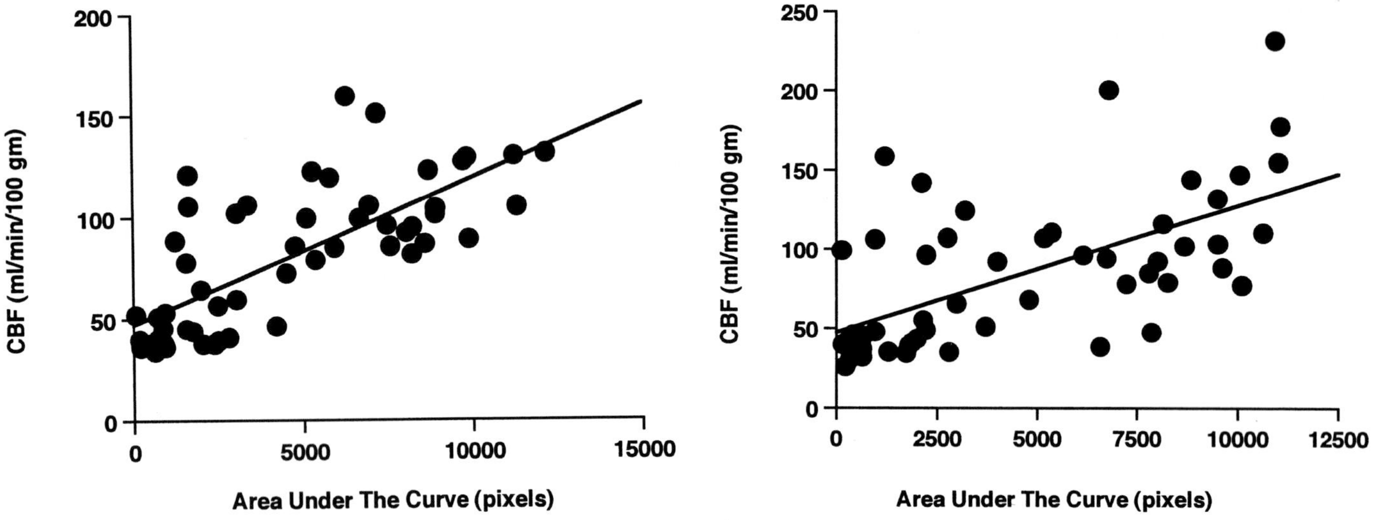

a. b.

Figure 7. Scatterplots show correlation between area under the curve and regional cerebral blood flow (*CBF*) on the basis of radiolabeled microspheres for **(a)** cerebral hemispheres and **(b)** basal ganglia. The area under the curve correlated well with changes in hemispheric and striatal blood flow ($r = .73$, $P = .0001$; $r = .62$, $P = .0001$, respectively).

Global cerebral blood flow is increased during this secondary phase and is associated with a rise in extracellular glutamate levels. This pattern of hyperemia has also been demonstrated in asphyxiated newborns by means of a variety of techniques including duplex Doppler US (22), near infrared spectroscopy (23), and xenon-133 extraction techniques (24). Although the mechanism by which glutamate (or its analogue, NMDA) exerts its vasodilatory effect is not well understood, it is thought to be mediated in part by increased production of nitric oxide and in part by prostaglandins, and it may be associated with loss of autoregulation and acidosis (14,21,25).

TABLE 2
Findings in Basal Ganglia after NMDA Injection

Finding	Basal Ganglia Right	Basal Ganglia Left	P*
Area under the curve (pixels)	6,194 ± 848	7,347 ± 782	<.03
Pixel intensity (units)	103 ± 8	121 ± 7	<.0001

Note.—Data are the mean ± standard error.
* Paired *t* test.

Findings in this study confirm the marked hyperemia associated with intrastriatal injection of NMDA and show that contrast-enhanced power Doppler US can be used as a noninvasive method for depicting regional changes in cerebral blood flow.

In prior experimental studies with intrastriatal NMDA injections, cerebral hyperemia could be detected as areas of increased color-containing pixels and higher mean pixel intensity on unenhanced power Doppler US scans. Mean pixel intensities correlated well with changes in cerebral blood flow measured by means of the radiolabeled microsphere technique. However, increased power Doppler US signal could be detected only in regions of brain in which blood flow was markedly elevated, such as the area immediately surrounding the NMDA injection site (8). In the current study, similar focal areas of increased signal could be detected after NMDA injection near the injection site on the unenhanced power Doppler US images (Fig 4). However, the presence of cerebral hyperemia elsewhere in the brain was apparent on only contrast-enhanced images. In addition, contrast-enhanced images depicted a diminution of contrast enhancement as the degree of cerebral hyperemia decreased over time. These changes were not visible on unenhanced images.

Although depiction of regional changes in cerebral blood flow is markedly improved by enhancement with intravenous contrast material, quantification of blood flow remains an elusive goal with current signal processing techniques. Video signal compression is used in the creation of the final display of all US images, including power Doppler US scans. This results in a nonlinear relationship between Doppler US signal intensity and pixel brightness. The use of different color maps may also have a marked effect on the linearity of response (26). Additional limiting factors include variable rates of bubble destruction by the Doppler US pulse, differences in backscatter attenuation at different tissue depths, and the lack of calibration of ultrasound measurements with true flow. These factors are likely to have contributed to the wide variability in values for area under the curve for any given level of cerebral blood flow to either hemisphere or basal ganglion. Absolute quantification would require a variety of features not yet developed, including an input function, depth-dependent calibration of contrast material–related backscattered signal, and noncompressed Doppler US signal.

Nonetheless, findings in our study show that despite the presence of systematic errors related to nonlinear video signal compression, differences in regional cerebral blood flow can be effectively demonstrated with contrast-enhanced power Doppler US. Furthermore, contrast material administration allowed perfusion maps to be created while using the lowest Doppler US intensity settings (spatial peak temporal average, <50 mW/cm²), low frame rates, and approximately 50% gain settings with no noticeable interference by flash or blooming artifacts. We are currently exploring the possibility of image capture before final video compression, as well as the use of harmonic imaging for further refinement of this technique.

Practical Application: Contrast-enhanced power Doppler US can be used to create accurate regional blood flow maps in the newborn brain. Potential clinical applications of this new technique include the early noninvasive identification of focal areas of brain ischemia, the depiction of altered cerebral perfusion in infants with hypoxic ischemic injury, and the monitoring of effectiveness of therapies designed to preserve or improve cerebral perfusion in the critically ill infant.

Acknowledgments: The authors thank Kimberly Eaton, BA, and Christopher Contois, BS, for their help in preparing the manuscript for this article.

References

1. Levene MI. The asphyxiated newborn infant. In: Levene MI, Bennett MJ, Punt J, eds. Fetal and neonatal neurology and neurosurgery. New York, NY: Livingstone, 1988; 357–369.
2. Volpe JJ, Herscovitch P, Perlman JM, Raichle ME. Positron emission tomography in the newborn: extensive impairment of regional cerebral blood flow with intraventricular hemorrhage and hemorrhagic intracerebral involvement. Pediatrics 1983; 72:589–601.
3. Taylor GA. Alterations in regional cerebral blood flow in neonatal stroke: imaging with color Doppler. Pediatr Radiol 1994; 24:111–115.
4. Taylor GA, Trescher WH, Traystman RJ, Johnston MV. Acute experimental neuronal injury in the newborn lamb: US characterization and demonstration of hemodynamic effects. Pediatr Radiol 1993; 23: 268–275.
5. Taylor GA, Short BL, Walker LK, Traystman RJ. Quantification of intracranial blood flow with duplex Doppler and color flow imaging. Radiology 1990; 176:231–236.
6. Rubin JM, Bude RO, Carson PL, Bree RL, Adler RS. Power Doppler: a potentially useful alternative to mean-frequency–based color Doppler sonography. Radiology 1994; 190:853–856.
7. Newman JS, Adler RS, Bude RO, Rubin JM. Detection of soft-tissue hyperemia: value of power Doppler sonography. AJR 1994; 163:335–339.
8. Taylor GA. Regional cerebral blood flow estimates in newborn lamb using amplitude mode color Doppler ultrasound. Pediatr Radiol 1996; 26:282–286.
9. Rubin JM, Adler RS, Fowlkes JB, et al. Fractional moving blood volume: estimation with power Doppler US. Radiology 1995; 197:183–190.
10. Dymling SO, Persson HW, Hertz CH. Measurement of blood perfusion in tissue using Doppler ultrasound. Ultrasound Med Biol 1991; 17:433–444.
11. Schrope B, Newhouse VL, Uhlendorf V. Simulated capillary blood flow measurement using a nonlinear ultrasonic contrast agent. Ultrason Imaging 1992; 14: 134–158.
12. Greenberg RS, Taylor GA, Stapleton JC, Hillsley CA, Spinak D. Analysis of regional cerebral blood flow in dogs, with an experimental microbubble-based US contrast agent. Radiology 1996; 201:119–123.
13. McDonald JW, Johnston MV. Physiological and pathophysiological roles of excitatory amino acids during central nervous system development. Brain Res Rev 1990; 15:41–70.
14. Taylor GA, Trescher WH, Johnston MV, Traystman RJ. Experimental neuronal injury in the newborn lamb: a comparison of *N*-methyl-D-aspartic acid receptor blockade and nitric oxide synthesis inhibition on lesion size and cerebral hyperemia. Pediatr Res 1995; 38:644–651.
15. Goldberg BB, Liu JB, Forsberg F. Ultrasound contrast agents: a review. Ultrasound Med Biol 1994; 20:319–333.
16. Taylor GA, Ecklund K, Dunning P. Renal cortical perfusion in rabbits: visualization with color amplitude imaging and an experimental microbubble-based US contrast agent. Radiology 1996; 201:125–129.
17. Heymann MA, Payne BD, Hoffman JIE, Rudolph AM. Blood flow measurements with radionuclide-labeled particles. Prog Cardiovasc Dis 1977; 20:55–77.
18. Fellman V, Raivio KO. Reperfusion injury as the mechanism of brain damage after perinatal asphyxia. Pediatr Res 1997; 41: 599–606.
19. Dugan LL, Choi DW. Excitotoxicity, free radicals, and cell membrane changes. Ann Neurol 1995; 35(suppl):S17–S21.
20. Lipton SA, Rosenberg PA. Mechanisms of disease: excitatory amino acids as a final common pathway for neurological disorders. N Engl J Med 1994; 330:613–622.
21. Gluckman PD, Gunn AJ. Neuroprotection in hypoxic-ischemic encephalopathy. In: Bar PR, Beal SE, eds. Neuroprotection in CNS diseases. New York, NY: Dekker, 1977; 409–424.
22. Archer LNJ, Levene MI, Evans DH. Cerebral artery Doppler ultrasonography for prediction of outcome after perinatal asphyxia. Lancet 1986; 2:1116–1118.
23. Wyatt JS. Near-infrared spectroscopy in asphyxial brain injury. Clin Perinatol 1993; 20:369–378.
24. Frewen TC, Kissoon N, Kronick J, et al. Cerebral blood flow, cross-brain oxygen extraction, and fontanelle pressure after hypoxic-ischemic injury in newborn infants. J Pediatr 1991; 118:265–271.
25. Northington FJ, Tobin JR, Koehler RC, Traystman RJ. In vivo production of nitric oxide correlates with NMDA-induced cerebral hyperemia in newborn sheep. Am J Physiol 1995; 269(suppl):H215–H221.
26. Taylor GA, Greenberg RS. Can relative contrast agent concentration be measured in vivo with color Doppler US?: reply (letter). Radiology 1997; 204:280–281.

Interlude

Digital Photographs

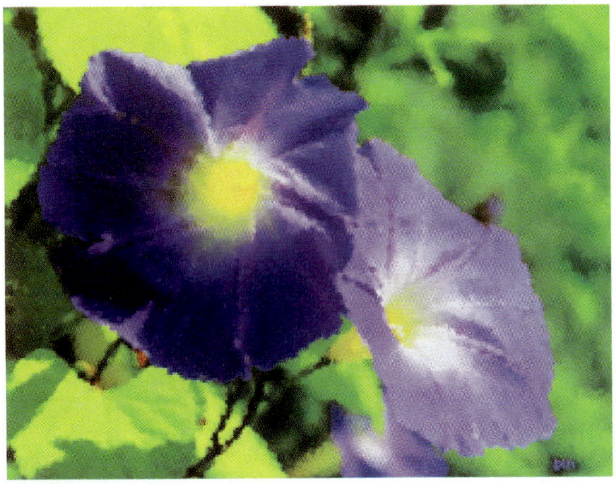

Flowers
Giverny, France

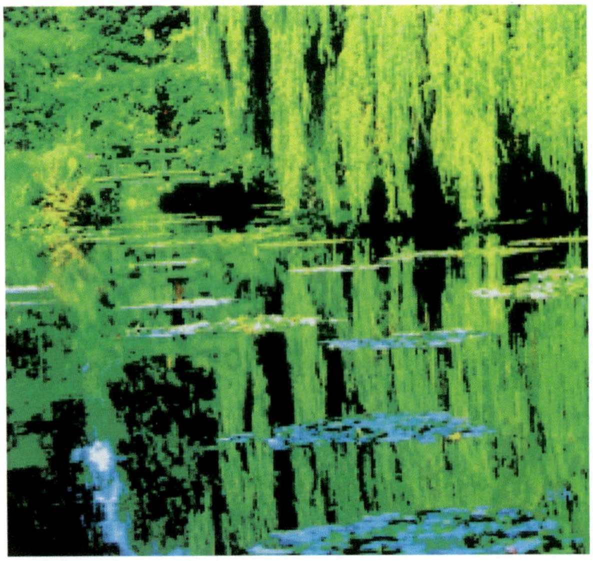

Lily Pond
Giverny, France

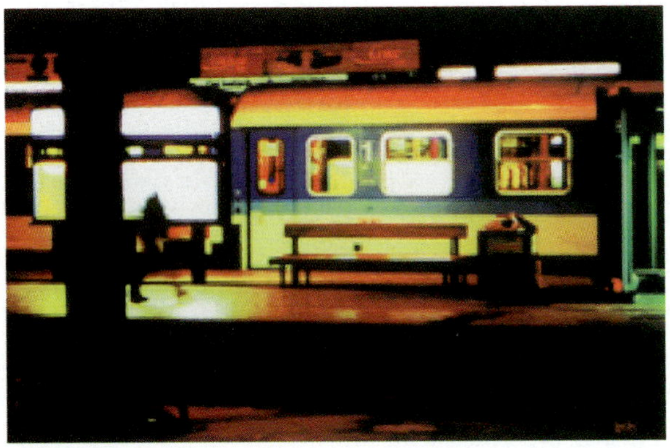

Train Station
Karlsruhe, Germany

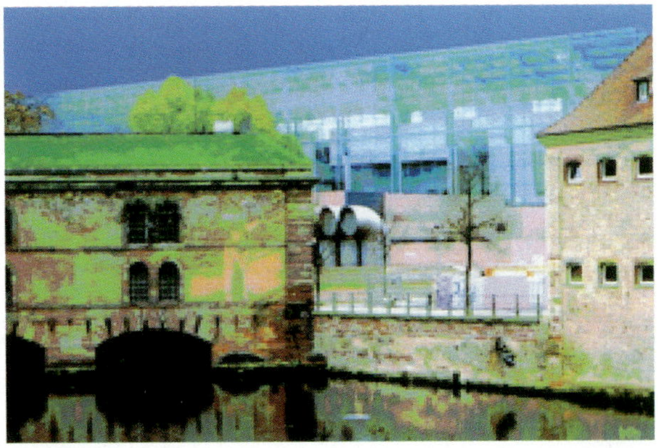

Progress
Strasbourg, France

Photographs by B. Leonard Holman, MD, Boston, Mass

Stephen A. Boppart, MSEE
Brett E. Bouma, PhD
Costas Pitris, MSEE
Gary J. Tearney, PhD
James F. Southern, MD, PhD
Mark E. Brezinski, MD, PhD
James G. Fujimoto, PhD

Index terms:
Blood vessels, stenosis or obstruction, 92.92, 9*.721[2], 9*.92[2]
Lasers
Nerves, injuries, 40.40, 40.92
Optical coherence tomography, 9*.1299[2]
Surgery

Radiology 1998; 208:81–86

Abbreviations:
OCT = optical coherence tomography
2D = two-dimensional
3D = three-dimensional

[1] From the Dept of Electrical Engineering and Computer Science, Research Laboratory of Electronics, Massachusetts Institute of Technology, 77 Massachusetts Ave, Rm 36-345, Cambridge, MA 02139 (S.A.B., B.E.B., C.P., G.J.T., J.G.F.); Div of Health Sciences and Technology, Harvard–Massachusetts Institute of Technology (S.A.B., C.P.); Dept of Pathology, Children's Hospital, Boston (J.F.S.); and Cardiac Unit, Massachusetts General Hospital and Harvard Medical School (M.E.B.). Received Oct 1, 1997; revision requested Dec 24; revision received Jan 20, 1998; accepted Mar 3. Supported in part by grants from Office of Naval Research Medical Free Electron Laser Program grant (N00014-94-1-0717), U.S. Air Force Office of Scientific Research grant (F49620-95-1-0221), and U.S. Air Force Palace Knight Program; National Institutes of Health contracts NIH-9-RO1-EY11289-11 (J.G.F), NIH-1-R01-CA75289-01 (J.G.F., M.E.B.), and NIH-1-R29-HL55686-01A1 and NIH-RO1-AR44812-01 (M.E.B.); and Whittaker Foundation contract 96-0205 (M.E.B.). **Address reprint requests to** S.A.B.

[2] 9*. Vascular system, location unspecified

Author contributions:
Guarantors of integrity of entire study, S.A.B., J.G.F., M.E.B.; study concepts, S.A.B., M.E.B.; study design, S.A.B., J.G.F.; definition of intellectual content, S.A.B., M.E.B.; literature research, M.E.B.; experimental studies, S.A.B., B.E.B., G.J.T.; data acquisition, S.A.B., C.P., J.F.S.; data analysis, S.A.B.; manuscript preparation, S.A.B.; manuscript editing, S.A.B., M.E.B., J.G.F.; manuscript review, M.E.B., J.G.F.

Intraoperative Assessment of Microsurgery with Three-dimensional Optical Coherence Tomography[1]

PURPOSE: To evaluate three-dimensional optical coherence tomography (OCT) for use in the assessment of the microsurgical anastomoses of vessels and nerves.

MATERIALS AND METHODS: OCT is an optical analogue of ultrasonography and is capable of imaging nontransparent biologic tissue by detecting backscattered infrared light. Cross-sectional in vitro images of rabbit and human vessels and nerves were obtained in as little as 125 msec at 10-μm resolution by using a solid-state laser as a light source. A surgical microscope was integrated with OCT to perform simultaneous imaging with en face visualization. Cross-sectional images were assembled to produce three-dimensional reconstructions of microsurgical specimens.

RESULTS: Three-dimensional OCT reconstructions depicted the structure within an arterial anastomosis and helped identify sites of luminal obstruction. The longitudinal spatial orientation of individual nerve fascicles was tracked in three dimensions to identify changes in position. In vitro human arteries and nerves embedded in highly scattering tissue and not visible at microscopy were located and imaged with OCT at eight frames per second.

CONCLUSION: The three-dimensional, micrometer-scale, diagnostic imaging capabilities of OCT permit rapid feedback for assessment of microsurgical procedures. OCT technology can be readily integrated with surgical microscopes and has potential for intraoperative monitoring to improve patient outcome.

Optical instruments have become well integrated into the surgical setting to visualize tissue and improve patient outcome. Surgical microscopes and loupes magnify tissue to help prevent iatrogenic injury and guide delicate surgical techniques. The repair of injured vessels and nerves is necessary to restore sensory and motor function after traumatic injury (1). Although the repair of sensitive structures is performed with the aid of surgical microscopes and loupes to magnify the surgical field (2), surgeons are limited to the en face view that these devices provide. A technique capable of subsurface, three-dimensional (3D), micrometer-scale imaging in real-time would permit the intraoperative monitoring of microsurgical procedures, offering immediate feedback to the surgeon and likely improvement in patient outcome.

Optical coherence tomography (OCT) is an optical imaging technology (3) ideally suited for the rapid acquisition of micrometer-scale–resolution two-dimensional (2D) and 3D images of biologic tissues such as small vessels and nerves. OCT was first used to image the transparent structures of the human eye (4,5) and has been used to help diagnose and track various macular diseases in a clinical setting (5,6). More recently, the use of longer wavelengths, which are absorbed and scattered less in biologic tissue, has permitted imaging in nontransparent tissues (7–9), for example, in the preliminary assessment of vessels and nerves (10). OCT is well suited for integration with medical and surgical optical instruments, and imaging has been performed with a radial-imaging, flexible catheter-endoscope (11), as well as a handheld surgical probe and laparoscope (12). Recently, catheter-endoscope–based OCT imaging of the gastrointestinal and respiratory tracts has been demonstrated in vivo in an animal model (13). OCT can function as a type of "optical biopsy" by permitting the in vivo imaging of biologic morphology with micrometer-scale resolution without the need to excise and process a tissue specimen as in conventional biopsy.

The purpose of this study was to determine the capabilities of OCT for the intraoperative assessment of microsurgical procedures. We integrated the high-speed OCT technology with a surgical microscope and performed micrometer-scale 3D imaging of microsurgical specimens.

MATERIALS AND METHODS

OCT is a noninvasive imaging technology that does not necessitate contact with tissue; it works on the principle of the detection of optical backscatter of near-infrared light from biologic tissue (3,6). The technique is somewhat analogous to ultrasound (US) B-mode imaging, except reflections of light are detected rather than those of sound. Whereas ultrasound pulse propagation and detection can be described in terms of time delays, the echo delay time of light returning to the OCT instrument from the specimen cannot be measured directly with electronic methods due to the high speeds associated with the propagation of light. Therefore, a technique known as interferometry is used, in which a reference and a sample arm are used. A schematic of the instrument is shown in Figure 1. A chromium (Cr^{4+}):forsterite laser is used as a low-coherence light source for OCT imaging (14). Because the infrared imaging beam (wavelength, 1,280 nm) cannot be seen, a visible aiming beam (wavelength, 632 nm) is combined for guidance and tissue registration. The imaging beam is split in equal parts by means of a fiberoptic coupler, with half the beam sent to the reference arm and half sent to the sample arm of the fiberoptic Michelson interferometer.

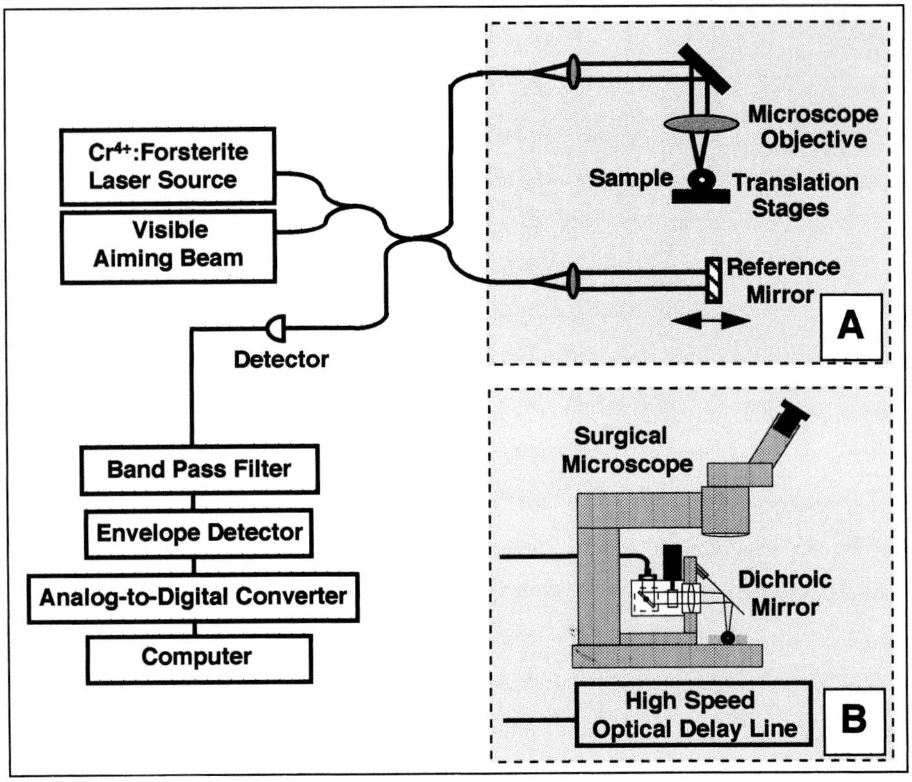

Figure 1. Schematic of the OCT instrument and surgical microscope shows two imaging configurations that use a Cr^{4+}:forsterite laser source. *A,* Configuration used to acquire cross-sectional and 3D images of microsurgical specimens: Sample arm includes a fixed microscope objective and micrometer-precision, computer-controlled stages to translate specimens. Reference arm mirror scanning is performed with a mechanical galvanometer. *B,* Configuration used for high-speed data acquisition: Specimens are imaged and visualized simultaneously with an integrated surgical microscope.

Two configurations are shown in Figure 1. The first configuration (Fig 1, *A*) was used for in vitro imaging of rabbit arteries and nerves. The reference arm contained a mirror on a mechanical translating galvanometer to perform axial scanning. The position of the reference arm mirror was used to set the depths at which backscatter would be measured, because interference between the two arms only occurs when their path lengths are matched to within the coherence length of the laser source. The imaging beam in the sample arm was focused by means of a lens to a 30-μm-diameter spot, which corresponds to a 1.1-mm depth of field. The spot size determined the transverse resolution of the image, and the axial resolution was determined by means of the coherence length of the laser source. The laser source has a center wavelength of approximately 1,280 nm and provides an axial resolution of 10 μm.

The specimens to be imaged were placed on a 2D micrometer-precision translational stage used to position and translate the specimen under a stationary imaging beam. Reflections from each arm were combined and detected with a photodiode. The reference arm mirror was translated at a known linear velocity. This translation imparts a Doppler shift to the reflected light. The electronic detection filter, with a center frequency at this known Doppler shift frequency, permits a high sensitivity and dynamic range (110 dB).

The second configuration (Fig 1, *B*) was used for in vitro imaging of human arteries and nerves at high speeds through a surgical microscope. The reference arm contained a high-speed optical delay line to permit more rapid axial imaging (13). The fiber of the sample arm was connected to a surgical microscope that had been modified for the simultaneous performance of OCT imaging and en face visualization. The infrared imaging beam and the visible aiming beam were directed by means of a pair of orthogonal galvanometer scanners to a focusing lens. A dichroic mirror coated to reflect the imaging and aiming beams was used to align the beams with the viewing axis of the microscope and to direct the beams onto the specimen. The OCT imaging beam was focused to a 30-μm-diameter spot, which corresponds to a 1.1-mm depth of field. The working distance of 60 mm beneath the dichroic mirror provided ample room for manual manipulation of microsurgical specimens. The specimen and image location were viewed through the microscope with the eye or were digitally imaged with a charge-coupled–device camera.

To demonstrate the use of OCT imaging for help in the diagnostic assessment of microsurgical procedures, in vitro microsurgical specimens were first acquired

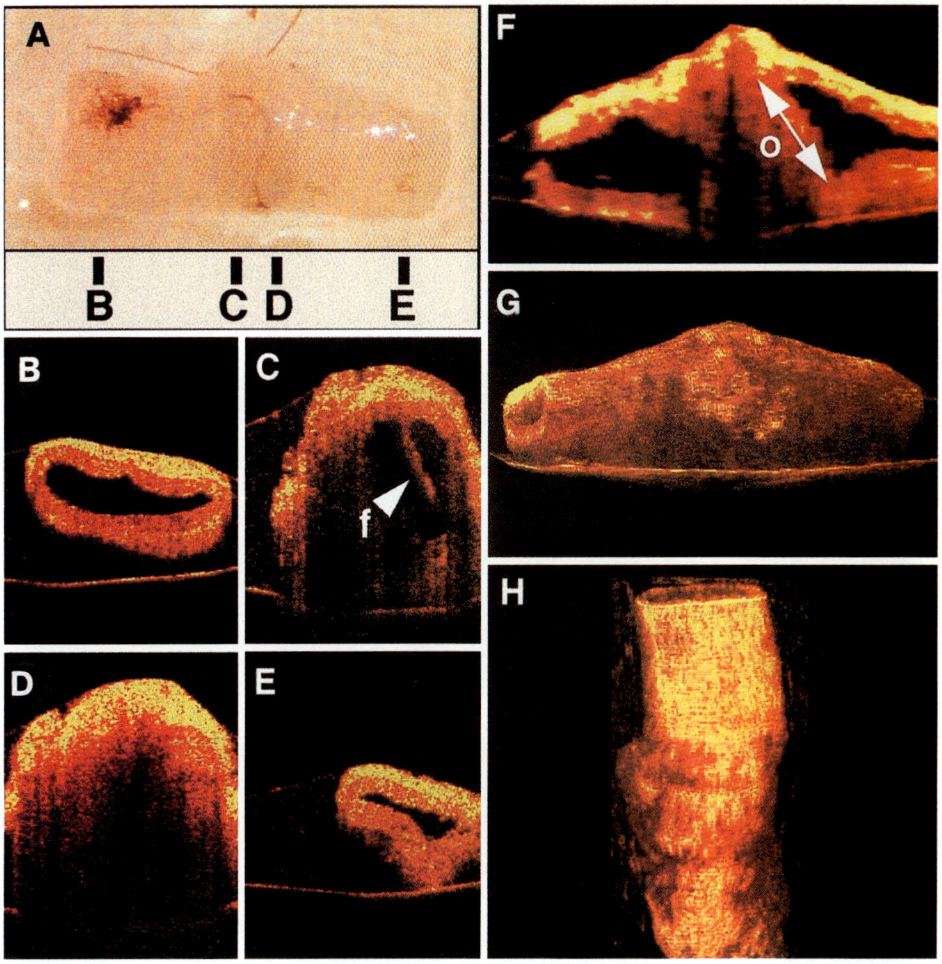

Figure 2. Three-dimensional OCT imaging of an anastomosis in a rabbit artery. *A,* Digital image obtained with a charge-coupled–device camera shows the 1-mm-diameter artery, which was anastomosed with a continuous suture. Lines labeled *B, C, D,* and *E* indicate planes from which corresponding cross-sectional OCT images were obtained. *B* and *E,* At the opposite ends of the anastomosis, the multilayered structure of the artery is visible, and the lumen is patent. *C,* Lumen is partially obstructed and a thrombogenic flap (arrowhead, *f*) is present. *D,* Fully obstructed portion of the anastomotic site is seen. Intraluminal features such as those in *C* and *D* are not observable on the en face view in *A. F,* Longitudinal section of the artery shows the obstruction (double-headed arrow, *o*). *G* and *H,* 3D projections can be arbitrarily constructed in any orientation, such as the horizontal (*G*) and vertical (*H*) orientations.

from animal and human tissue. Segments of inguinal-area arteries and nerves were resected from a 3.5-kg New Zealand White rabbit immediately after the rabbit was euthanized with a 5-mL injection of pentobarbital sodium (65 mg/mL). The specimens were immediately placed in 0.9% normal saline and were stored at 0°C. An artery segment was bisected cross-sectionally with a scalpel and was then re-anastomosed. A 10-0 nylon suture with a 50-μm-diameter needle was used to place a continuous suture and to perform an end-to-end anastomosis.

For the precise registration of 3D images, the anastomosed segment was positioned on a micrometer-stepping, computer-controlled, motorized translational stage in the sample arm of the OCT instrument (Fig 1, *A*). The OCT imaging beam was held fixed as motorized stages translated the specimen. A series of 40 cross-sectional images were acquired perpendicular to the long axis at 100-μm intervals. Imaging was performed through the anastomotic site and several millimeters on either side of the anastomosis. After OCT imaging, the en face image of the specimen was digitally recorded with a charge-coupled–device camera. Three-dimensional imaging of the peripheral nerve was performed by using the same parameters as described for the artery. The animal used in this study was cared for and maintained under the established protocols of the Massachusetts Institute of Technology committee on animal care.

To demonstrate the ability of OCT to depict vessels and nerves embedded in highly scattering tissue in real time, a 1-cm^3 block of human tissue was removed from the left lateral ankle of an amputated foot, immediately placed in 0.9% normal saline, and stored at 0°C. The ankle had been amputated as a result of complications associated with vascular insufficiency secondary to diabetes mellitus. The block of tissue was manually manipulated under the surgical microscope (Fig 1, *B*) while OCT imaging was performed at eight frames per second in a single cross-sectional plane. Images were acquired and stored directly to S-VHS videotape while they were viewed on a monitor. The magnified imaging location was directly viewed through the surgical microscope as various locations were imaged in search of subsurface morphology. Specimens to be processed for histologic comparison were placed in 5% buffered formaldehyde immediately after imaging and were later embedded in paraffin, sectioned, and stained with hematoxylin-eosin. The protocol to use discarded tissue was approved by the committee on the use of human subjects at Massachusetts General Hospital.

Cross-sectional OCT images and 3D data-set projections were processed and displayed by using rendering software (NIH Image version 1.60; National Institutes of Health, Bethesda, Md). A false-color scale was assigned to the logarithm of the data in each image in a manner analogous to that used in US. For the 40 images obtained in the peripheral nerve, a single fascicle was manually segmented and colored white on the images to enable tracking through the multiple sections and 3D volume. The multiple sections for each specimen were assembled into a stack and used to generate projections from the 3D data set. The projections were rotated in the x, y, and z planes to view particular features and to determine planes at which arbitrary sections could be displayed.

RESULTS

The ability to assess the internal structure and the luminal patency within an arterial anastomosis by using OCT was demonstrated by acquiring cross-sectional OCT images (2.2 × 2.2 mm, 250 × 600 pixels) and 3D projections of a 1-mm-diameter rabbit inguinal artery. A digitized image of the arterial anastomotic segment is shown in *A* in Figure 2. Cross-sectional 2D images in *B–E* in Figure 2 were acquired from the locations labeled in *A* in Figure 2. *B* and *E* in Figure 2 were acquired from each end of the anastomosis. These images clearly show the arterial morphology that corresponds to the intimal, medial, and adventitial layers of the elastic artery. The muscular media exhibits less backscatter than the adventitia, which merges with the surrounding collagenous tissue. The patent lumen is readily apparent. This is in contrast to *C* in Figure 2, where a tissue flap is seen in cross section at the site of anastomosis. *D* in Figure 2 reveals an obstruction within the arterial lumen. Note that the presence of additional tissue has attenuated the signal from the lower wall and, hence, reduces the ability to resolve individual layers.

By assembling a series of cross-sectional 2D images, a 3D data set was produced. From this data set, arbitrary planes could be selected, and corresponding sections could be displayed. For an arterial anastomosis, it is often more informative to image longitudinally along the axis of the artery and through the site of the anastomosis. *F* in Figure 2 is a longitudinal section from the 3D data set, which confirms the occlusion within the anastomotic site.

G and *H* in Figure 2 show 3D projections of the arterial anastomosis. These horizontally and vertically rotated projections comprised 80 sections at 50-μm intervals. At this high section density, the internal structure shown in *B–F* in Figure 2 is difficult to visualize. However, high section densities are necessary if the 3D data set is to be sectioned at arbitrary planes, as shown in *F* in Figure 2. In addition, micrometer-scale surface features that were not readily apparent on the 2D sections are more prominent.

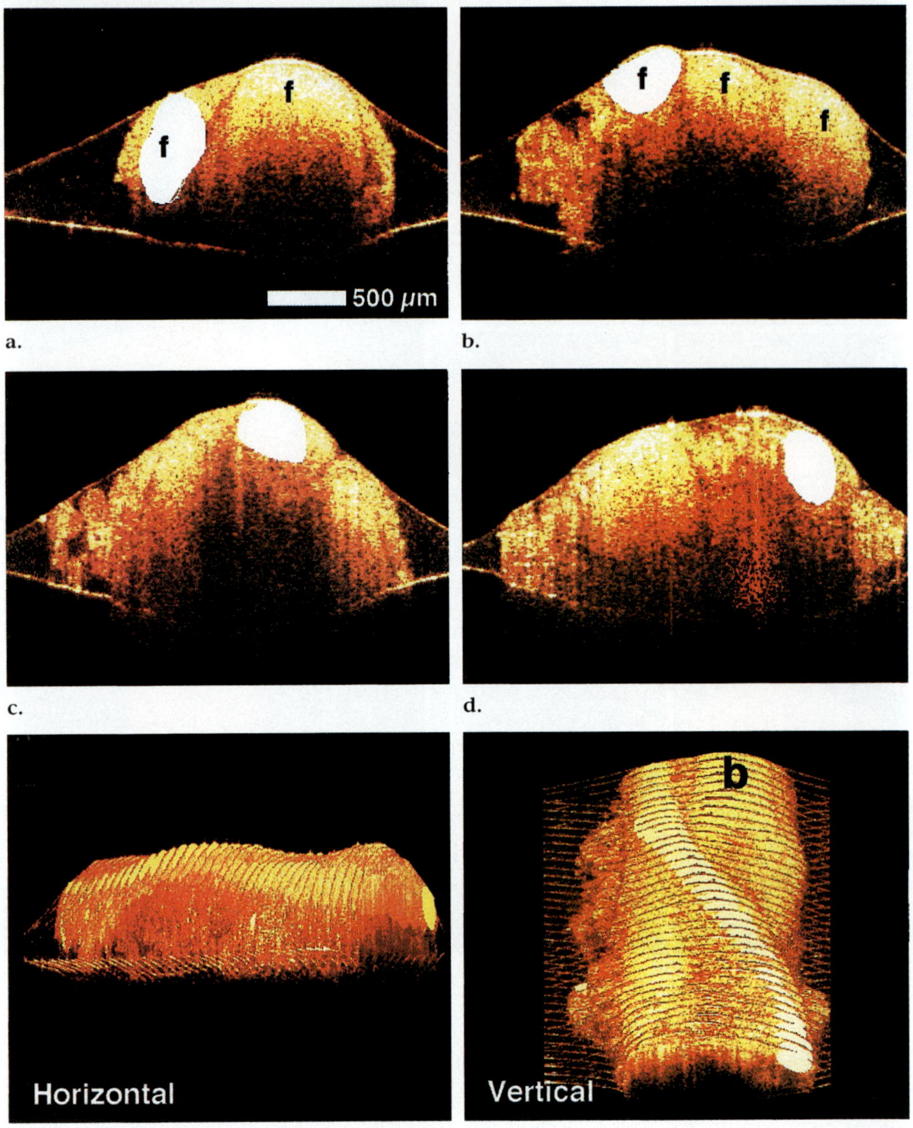

a. b. c. d. e. f.

Figure 3. Three-dimensional OCT imaging of a peripheral nerve. Multiple fascicles (*f* in **a** and **b**) are evident within the peripheral nerve. **(a–d)** A single fascicle was followed longitudinally along the axis of the nerve, manually segmented, and colored white. **(e)** Horizontally and **(f)** vertically oriented 3D projections illustrate the spatial arrangement of individual fascicles and a bifurcation (*b* in **f**) not previously appreciated on 2D cross sections.

Longitudinal tracking of the spatial orientation of peripheral nerve fascicles is demonstrated in Figure 3. Representative cross-sectional images (3.0 × 2.2 mm, 300 × 600 pixels) of the peripheral nerve are shown in Figure 3a–3d. For each section, one fascicle was manually segmented, colored white, and tracked through the acquired volume of data. Forty images at 100-μm intervals were assembled for the 3D projections shown in Figure 3e and 3f. The horizontally and vertically rotated projections of the peripheral nerve dramatically reveal the twisted path of the segmented fascicle along the longitudinal axis of the nerve. In addition, a branch in another, unsegmented fascicle can be seen in Figure 3f. This feature was not recognized at the examination of the 2D images.

OCT image data was correlated with corresponding histology. Figure 4 shows cross-sectional images acquired from a rabbit arterial bifurcation and from a human retroperitoneal nerve. The arterial segment was imaged with OCT distal to the bifurcation, and two independent lumina are shown (Fig 4a). The OCT images clearly resolve individual layers within the arterial wall and demonstrate

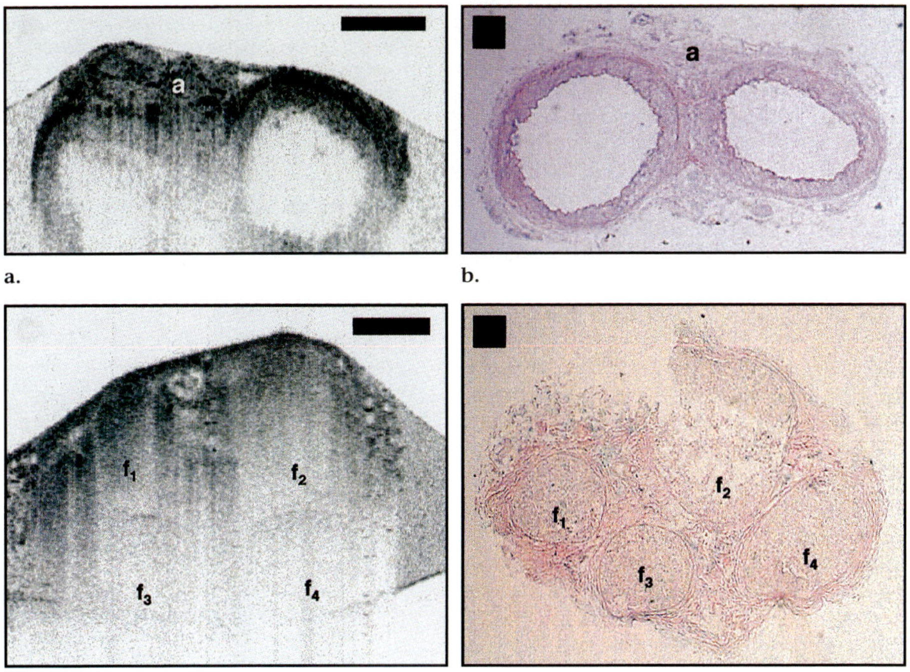

a. b. c. d.

Figure 4. OCT images and corresponding histology of microsurgical specimens for correlation of image features with architectural morphology. The black bar in **a** and **c** represents 500 μm. (Disregard the black squares in **b** and **d.**) **(a)** OCT image and **(b)** photomicrograph show a bifurcation of a rabbit femoral artery, with adjacent adipose tissue (*a* in **b**). (Hematoxylin-eosin stain; original magnification, ×20.) **(c)** OCT image and **(d)** photomicrograph show multiple fascicles (f_1, f_2, f_3, f_4) in a human retroperitoneal nerve. (Hematoxylin-eosin stain; original magnification, ×20.)

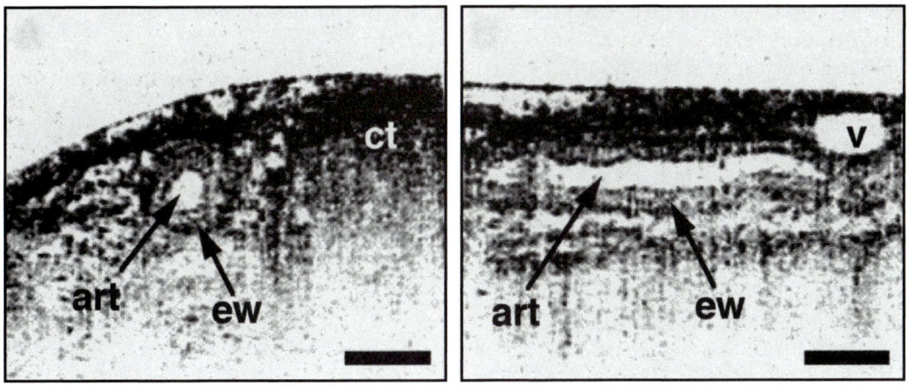

a. b.

Figure 5. OCT images of a subsurface, in vitro human artery were acquired with an integrated surgical microscope at high speed (eight frames per second). The black bar in **a** and **b** represents 500 μm. **(a)** Cross-sectional image of the artery (*art*) illustrates the thick elastic wall (*ew*) and patent lumen. The artery is surrounded by adipose tissue and is adjacent to dense connective tissue (*ct*). **(b)** Longitudinal cross section of the same artery (*art*) with the thick elastic wall (*ew*) shows a thin-walled vein (*v*) in oblique cross section.

patent lumina. Above the arteries is a region of adipose tissue, which appears to have less backscatter in the OCT image, except for the nuclei and cell walls. The images of the human retroperitoneal nerve illustrate OCT imaging of individual fascicles, which correlates well with the histology (Fig 4c, 4d). Because of the larger diameter of this nerve, the OCT optical beam is attenuated, and deeper fascicles (f_3 and f_4 in Fig 4) are difficult to resolve, except for the sheath surrounding each fascicle.

The OCT instrument was integrated with a surgical microscope (Fig 1, *B*) to obtain the images shown in Figure 5. Because the OCT imaging beam and visible aiming beam were co-aligned with the optical axis of the microscope, the image location on the specimen could be directly viewed through the microscope. A block of tissue was manually manipulated under the microscope while images (3.00 × 2.75 mm, 256 × 256 pixels) were acquired at eight frames per second. Subsurface microsurgical structures were immediately identified, including numerous small arteries, veins, and nerves and even a vascular clip from previous surgical repair. All structures were embedded in adipose and connective tissues. Figure 5a illustrates a cross section of an artery located 500 μm below the surface and surrounded by adipose tissue. This artery could not be visualized with the microscope alone. The image clearly shows the characteristic thick wall and multiple layers of the artery. To the right of the artery is a portion of dense connective tissue that does not have the clear, low-backscatter regions present in adipose tissue. Figure 5b shows a longitudinal section of the same artery after the tissue block was rotated 90°. The thick arterial wall is readily identified. The right edge of Figure 5b shows an oblique cross section of a vein with its characteristic thin wall.

DISCUSSION

During microsurgical procedures, patient outcome can be substantially influenced by the ability of the surgeon to assess tissue microstructure (15). The in vitro arterial anastomosis shown in Figure 2 demonstrates the ability of OCT to help assess internal structure within an anastomotic site and evaluate patency. Precision realignment of individual nerve fascicles increases the likelihood that end-organ function will be restored after peripheral nerve reconstruction (16). With Figures 3 and 4, we showed that OCT can image peripheral nerves in cross section and that individual fascicles can be identified and segmented. The use of OCT to acquire multiple cross-sectional images and perform 3D reconstructions of the peripheral nerve offers the opportunity to determine the relative diameters of individual fascicles, as well as track their spatial orientation. The 3D projection of the segmented peripheral nerve in Figure 3f not only revealed the twisted course of one fascicle but also revealed a bifurcation of a second fascicle, a feature not previously appreciated on the 2D images.

Future work will focus on methods to increase the rate of data acquisition, to increase the resolution, and to combine structural imaging with OCT Doppler techniques. The rapid acquisition rate of eight frames per second enabled immediate feedback for repositioning of the specimen and tracking of the vessels and nerves. The current limitation to acquisition speed is the axial scanning mechanism. Use of the high-speed optical delay line has decreased image acquisition times from 30 seconds to 125 msec compared with the acquisition time achievable with a mechanical scanning galvanometer. Acquisition time can also be improved by decreasing the number of pixels in an image. We chose to acquire images with a higher resolution (256 × 256 pixels) at the expense of speed. Further improvements in axial imaging technology will enable video-rate (30 frames per second) and high-speed volume acquisition.

The image resolutions achieved in this study are as high as 10 μm and exceed the performance of clinical US, computed tomography, and magnetic resonance imaging. By using broader-bandwidth laser sources such as a titanium:sapphire Kerr-lens modelocked laser (17,18) or a Cr^{4+}: forsterite laser (14), resolutions as high as 2–5 μm may be achieved. Higher resolutions would further improve the identification of morphologic features within the anastomotic site. The maintenance of these high resolutions during performance of high-speed imaging is a current technical pursuit.

In a manner analogous to Doppler US, OCT may be configured to perform laser-Doppler velocimetry. This technique has been used for the in vivo measurement of blood flow velocities in animal models (19,20) and may be useful for the assessment of perfusion after vascular anastomosis.

Potential limitations of OCT imaging are the maximal penetration and the effect of blood on imaging. When longer wavelengths (in the near infrared range) have been used, imaging depths have increased from 1 mm up to 2–3 mm due to decreased optical absorption and scattering in tissue. These depths may appear limiting. However, the majority of microsurgical complications occur in vessels and nerves less than 2 mm in diameter and are suitable for OCT imaging. The presence of blood in the surgical field may influence the quality of OCT images. Future studies will assess the influence of blood on OCT imaging.

Practical applications: The use of a surgical microscope serves to magnify the tissue but provides only a surface, or en face, view. OCT should improve intraoperative diagnostics by providing high-resolution, subsurface, cross-sectional imaging of vessels and nerves in real time. The extension of imaging to three dimensions permits the assessment of the longitudinal spatial orientation of morphologic features such as individual peripheral nerve fascicles. Intraoperative assessment of luminal obstructions is crucial to the successful performance of a procedure. OCT can be used to identify the location and longitudinal extent of the obstruction. This would include the presence of a thrombogenic adventitial flap or intimal inversion, which predisposes the site to postoperative subacute occlusion.

We have demonstrated the capabilities of an integrated surgical microscope by acquiring in vitro images of subsurface human vessels and nerves at eight frames per second. The integration of high-speed OCT imaging components with a surgical microscope was a challenge. An aberration-free beam had to be tightly focused at a long working distance and maintained throughout the entire imaging range. Integration with the surgical microscope permitted not only en face visualization but also simultaneous cross-sectional OCT imaging. The microscope-based OCT system is a practical application of OCT technology and was used to demonstrate the potential for prevention of iatrogenic injuries during surgical procedures. Vessels and nerves, which could not be identified on en face images, were clearly identified on OCT images. Performance of many fine surgical procedures in vulnerable tissues would likely benefit from high-resolution subsurface imaging findings.

In this article, we have shown the 3D imaging capabilities of OCT and how acquired images can provide diagnostic feedback for the assessment of microsurgical anastomoses. This previously unavailable diagnostic ability offers the potential to directly affect and improve patient outcome by incorporating high-speed, high-resolution, intraoperative imaging of microsurgical procedures.

Acknowledgments: The authors thank Eric A. Swanson, MS, of Massachusetts Institute of Technology Lincoln Laboratories for helpful technical discussions and contributions and Cindy Kopf of the Massachusetts Institute of Technology for helping to assemble this manuscript.

References

1. Zhong-wei C, Dong-yue Y, Di-Sheng C, eds. Microsurgery. New York, NY: Springer-Verlag, 1982; 68–92.
2. Rooks MD, Slappey J, Zusmanis K. Precision of suture placement with microscope and loupe assisted anastomoses. Microsurgery 1993; 14:547–550.
3. Huang D, Swanson EA, Lin CP, et al. Optical coherence tomography. Science 1991; 254:1178–1181.
4. Hee MR, Izatt JA, Swanson EA, et al. Optical coherence tomography of the human retina. Arch Ophthalmol 1995; 113: 326–332.
5. Puliafito CA, Hee MR, Lin CP, et al. Imaging of macular diseases with optical coherence tomography. Ophthalmology 1995; 120:217–229.
6. Puliatifo CA, Hee MR, Schumann JS, Fujimoto JG. Optical coherence tomography of ocular diseases. Thorofare, NJ: SLACK, 1995.
7. Fujimoto JG, Brezinski ME, Tearney GJ, et al. Optical biopsy and imaging using optical coherence tomography. Nat Med 1995; 1:970–972.
8. Schmitt JM, Yadlowsky M, Bonner RF. Subsurface imaging of living skin with optical coherence microscopy. Dermatology 1995; 191:93–98.
9. Brezinski ME, Tearney GJ, Bouma BE, et al. Optical coherence tomography for optical biopsy: properties and demonstration of vascular pathology. Circulation 1996; 93: 1206–1213.
10. Brezinski ME, Tearney GJ, Boppart SA, Swanson EA, Southern JF, Fujimoto JG. Optical biopsy with optical coherence tomography: feasibility for surgical diagnostics. J Surg Res 1997; 71:32–40.
11. Tearney GJ, Boppart SA, Bouma BE, et al. Scanning single-mode fiber optic catheter-endoscope for optical coherence tomography. Opt Lett 1996; 21:543–545.
12. Boppart SA, Bouma BE, Pitris C, Tearney GJ, Fujimoto JG, Brezinski ME. Forward-imaging instruments for optical coherence tomography. Opt Lett 1997; 22:1618–1620.
13. Tearney GJ, Brezinski ME, Bouma BE. In vivo endoscopic optical biopsy with optical coherence tomography. Science 1997; 276:2037–2039.
14. Bouma BE, Tearney GJ, Bilinsky IP, Golubovic B, Fujimoto JG. Self-phase modulated Kerr-lens modelocked Cr^{4+}: forsterite laser source for optical coherence tomography. Opt Lett 1996; 21:1839–1841.
15. Culbertson JH, Rand RP, Jurkiewicz MJ. Advances in microsurgery. Adv Surg 1990; 23:57–88.
16. Wyrick JD, Stern PJ. Secondary nerve reconstruction. Microsurgery 1992; 8:587–598.
17. Bouma BE, Tearney GJ, Boppart SA, Hee MR, Brezinski ME, Fujimoto JG. High resolution optical coherence tomographic imaging using a modelocked $Ti{:}Al_2O_3$ laser source. Opt Lett 1995; 20:1486–1488.
18. Clivaz X, Marquis-Weible F, Salathe RP. Optical low coherence reflectometry with 1.9 μm spatial resolution. Electronics Lett 1992; 28:1553–1555.
19. Chen Z, Milner TE, Srinivas S, Wang X. Noninvasive imaging of in vivo blood flow velocity using optical Doppler tomography. Opt Lett 1997; 22:1119–1121.
20. Izatt JA, Kulkami MD, Yazdanfar S, Barton JK, Welch AJ. In vivo bidirectional color Doppler flow imaging of picoliter blood volumes using optical coherence tomography. Opt Lett 1997; 22:1439–1441.

Myelolipoma: CT and Pathologic Features[1]

Philip J. Kenney, MD
Brent J. Wagner, MD
Padma Rao, MD
Clara S. Heffess, MD

Index terms:
Adrenal gland, CT, 86.1211
Adrenal gland, neoplasms, 86.3141
Myelolipoma, 86.3141, 87.3141
Retroperitoneal space, neoplasms, 87.3141

Radiology 1998; 208:87–95

[1] From the Department of Radiologic Pathology (P.J.K., B.J.W., P.R.) and the Division of Endocrine Pathology (C.S.H.), Armed Forces Institute of Pathology, Washington, DC. From the 1996 RSNA scientific assembly. Received August 19, 1997; revision requested November 13; revision received January 21, 1998; accepted March 3. Supported in part by the American Registry of Pathology, Washington, DC. **Address reprint requests to** P.J.K., Department of Radiology, University of Alabama at Birmingham, 619 S 19th St, Birmingham, AL 35233-6830.

The opinions are those of the authors and do not necessarily reflect the views of the Department of the Air Force or the Department of Defense.

PURPOSE: To correlate clinical and pathologic patterns of myelolipoma with the computed tomographic (CT) appearance.

MATERIALS AND METHODS: All cases of myelolipoma accessioned by the Armed Forces Institute of Pathology from 1981 through 1997 were reviewed. CT images were scored for the location and size of each myelolipoma and the presence of calcification, hemorrhage, fat, and pseudocapsule. Pathologic findings for the pattern of fat and bone marrow elements were correlated with CT findings.

RESULTS: In 74 patients, 86 myelolipomas were found, of which 72 were in an adrenal gland (eight were bilateral), and 14 extra-adrenal masses were found in 10 patients. Four clinicopathologic patterns emerged: (*a*) isolated adrenal myelolipoma in 37 patients (fat evident at CT, no other disorders present); (*b*) myelolipoma with hemorrhage in nine patients (imaging features similar to those of isolated adrenal myelolipomas but larger [mean diameter, 14.2 vs 9.9 cm; $P = .01$]; (*c*) extra-adrenal myelolipoma in 10 patients (imaging findings similar to those of adrenal myelolipomas, found most often in the retroperitoneum); and (*d*) myelolipomatous foci within other adrenal pathologic conditions in 18 patients (smaller, lower fat content, more heavily calcified).

CONCLUSION: Myelolipomas are adrenal or extra-adrenal masses, with hemorrhage more common in larger lesions (diameter, >10 cm). The CT appearance of myelolipomatous foci, which can be found within other pathologic adrenal conditions, is different from that of isolated adrenal myelolipomas.

Myelolipoma is an uncommon tumorlike lesion composed of a variable mixture of mature fat and hematopoietic elements that resembles bone marrow (1). The lesion was described by Gierke in 1905 (2). The term "myelolipoma" was used by Oberling in 1929 (3). Numerous reports of this entity have since been published. Although several theories have been proposed, the origin remains uncertain (1,4).

Myelolipoma has been most often found in the adrenal gland, but there have been reports of extra-adrenal locations (5–7). The lesion itself does not cause an endocrine disorder, but there have been a few reports of the presence of myelolipomatous tissue in patients with a variety of adrenal functional disorders, such as Cushing syndrome, congenital adrenal hyperplasia, and Conn syndrome (8,9). No malignant potential has been demonstrated. The frequency has been determined at autopsy as between 0.08% and 0.2% (10). With the widespread use of noninvasive imaging, particularly ultrasonography (US), computed tomography (CT), and magnetic resonance imaging, incidental detection of a myelolipoma is becoming more commonplace. In one study of 210 incidental adrenal tumors, 7% were myelolipomas (11). The majority of such incidental adrenal myelolipomas are small and asymptomatic and usually do not undergo pathologic examination.

There have been several descriptions of this entity in the literature, including several regarding the imaging appearance, but most publications are case reports or involve a small study from a single institution (12–17). A few larger reviews have been published, but these are primarily a compilation of prior reports with a few new cases added (4,6,8,10). In such studies, the full spectrum of pathologic and imaging data was not available. The purpose of this study was to correlate the clinicopathologic patterns and imaging findings of myelolipoma on the basis of the large collection of pathologically proved cases in the archives of the Armed Forces Institute of Pathology.

Author contributions:
Guarantor of integrity of entire study, P.J.K.; study concepts, P.J.K.; study design, P.J.K.; literature research, P.J.K.; data acquisition, P.J.K., B.J.W., C.S.H.; data analysis, P.J.K.; statistical analysis, P.J.K.; manuscript preparation, P.J.K., P.R.; manuscript editing, B.J.W.; manuscript review, C.S.H., B.J.W.

MATERIALS AND METHODS

This study was based on an analysis of all cases of myelolipoma accessioned into the archives of the Armed Forces Institute of Pathology from 1981 through 1997 in which CT was among the diagnostic procedures. The imaging data for each case were correlated with the gross and microscopic findings.

Clinical data regarding age, sex, symptoms, and evidence of an endocrine disorder or acute hemorrhage were tabulated for each case. The CT images were independently reviewed and scored by two experienced abdominal radiologists (P.J.K., B.J.W.); disagreements were resolved in consensus conference (P.J.K., B.J.W., P.R.). Imaging features recorded included location and size of the myelolipoma, presence or absence of calcification, imaging evidence of hemorrhage, and the relation of the tumor margin to the surrounding tissue. A thin soft-tissue margin around the mass was recorded as a partial or complete pseudocapsule (this term was selected because the pathology literature is inconsistent about whether myelolipoma typically has a capsule). CT attenuation values were recorded when they were available (24 cases). Each reader independently scored the lesions for the relative proportion of fat to soft tissue within the mass on the basis of visual assessment of the CT scan (no visible fat; <10%, <50%, 50%–90%, or >90% fat). In the absence of attenuation values, fat was identified as an area that was visually similar to subcutaneous or retroperitoneal fat or had clearly lower attenuation than water. Disagreements about the initial score were resolved by consensus in conference (P.J.K., B.J.W., P.R.).

Pathologic findings were compared with CT appearance to assess the pattern of fat and bone marrow elements, the relation of the myelolipoma cells to the residual adrenal cortex, and evidence of hemorrhage and other disease in the adrenal gland.

Characteristics of Patients and Myelolipomas

Characteristic	Isolated Adrenal Myelolipoma (*n* = 37)	Adrenal Myelolipoma with Hemorrhage (*n* = 9)	Extra-adrenal Myelolipoma (*n* = 10)	Myelolipoma in Other Pathologic Condition (*n* = 18)
Patients (*n* = 74)				
Mean age (y)	55	48	64*	55
Sex				
Male	19 (51)	8 (89)	4 (40)	5 (27)*
Female	18 (49)	1 (11)	6 (60)	13 (81)*
Myelolipomas (*n* = 86)				
Location				
Right adrenal gland	30 (73)	9 (90)	. . .	14 (67)
Left adrenal gland	11 (27)	1 (10)	. . .	7 (33)
Bilateral	4	1	. . .	3
Presacral	. . .	. . .	4	. . .
Retroperitoneal	. . .	. . .	4	. . .
Other	. . .	. . .	6	. . .
Mean diameter (cm)	9.9	14.2*	8.2	7.1*
Calcification	10 (24)	1 (10)	0 (0)	11 (52)*
Median fat content	50%–90%	50%–90%	<50%	<10%*
Pseudocapsule	31 (75)	10 (100)	9 (90)	7 (33)*

Note.—Data are number of patients or myelolipomas. Numbers in parentheses are percentages.
*Differences are statistically significant compared with isolated adrenal myelolipoma.

RESULTS

Eighty-six lesions identified as myelolipomas were found in 74 patients (35 men, 39 women; age range, 28–77 years), and these lesions formed the basis of this study (Table).

The CT scans available in these 74 cases were obtained on a variety of scanners: Only contrast material–enhanced images were available in 51 cases, only unenhanced images in six, and both unenhanced and contrast-enhanced images in 17. As required by the entry criteria, pathologic specimens were available in all 74 cases. A resected surgical specimen was available in 70 of the cases, including 61 specimens obtained at adrenalectomy and nine obtained at resection of an extra-adrenal mass. In the remaining four cases, only specimens obtained at fine needle aspiration were available (from three adrenal masses and one extra-adrenal mass). In one case, a patient with bilateral adrenal tumors had undergone surgical resection of the lesion on the left and fine needle aspiration of that on the right. In two cases, the patients had adrenal masses and initially underwent fine needle aspiration with nondiagnostic findings; definitive diagnosis was then made at surgical resection. Seventy-two of the myelolipomas occurred in an adrenal gland (right, 53; left, 19). In eight cases, bilateral adrenal myelolipomas were found. In 10 cases, myelolipoma was found outside the adrenal glands with multiple extra-adrenal myelolipomas in one case. In nine cases, acute hemorrhage from an adrenal myelolipoma was present. In 18 cases, myelolipomatous tissue was found in other pathologic adrenal conditions, including an endocrine disorder. Four distinct clinicopathologic patterns emerged.

Isolated Adrenal Myelolipoma

In the majority of the cases, myelolipomas were found in an adrenal gland that was otherwise normal (in 37 patients [19 men and 18 women; mean age, 55 years; age range, 28–79 years]). In none of these cases were symptoms directly attributable to the myelolipoma, and none of the patients had an endocrine disorder. The myelolipoma occurred in only the right adrenal gland in 26 patients, in only the left adrenal gland in seven, and bilaterally in four, for a total of 30 right (30 of 41 [73%]) and 11 left (11 of 41 [27%]) masses. The mean diameter of these tumors was 9.9 cm (range, 2.5–20.0 cm).

Individual image appearance and proportions varied, but all CT scans in this group demonstrated an area of clearly recognizable fat attenuation (Figs 1, 2). In some cases, rather sharply marginated areas of fat and soft-tissue attenuation were seen. In most cases, however, margins were not clearly defined and ill-defined areas of fat attenuation shaded gradually into areas of higher attenuation (Figs 2, 3). Frequently, the areas of higher attenuation were not of true soft-tissue attenuation and had a wispy appearance or an appearance reminiscent of partial volume averaging (Fig 2). Attenuation measurements were available in 24 cases. Measurements in areas that visually appeared to be fat ranged from −130 to −23 HU (mean, −74 HU). Measurements in areas that visually appeared to be soft tissue ranged from −33 to +53 HU (mean, 18 HU). Average increased attenuation of 26 HU was found when pre- and postcontrast measurements were compared.

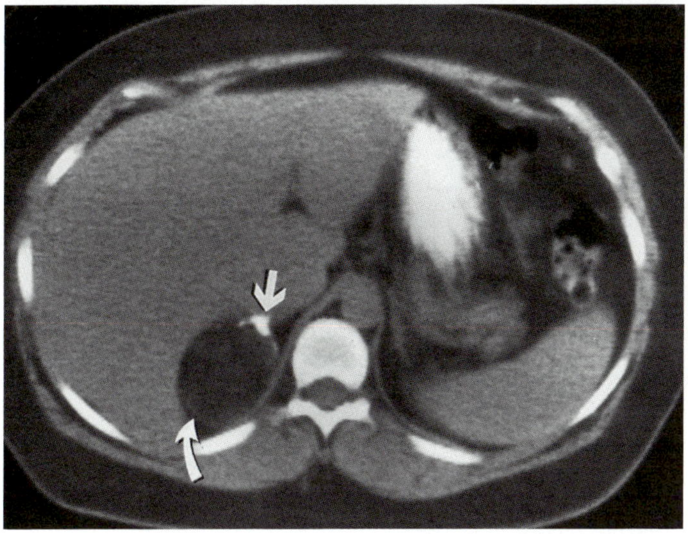

a.

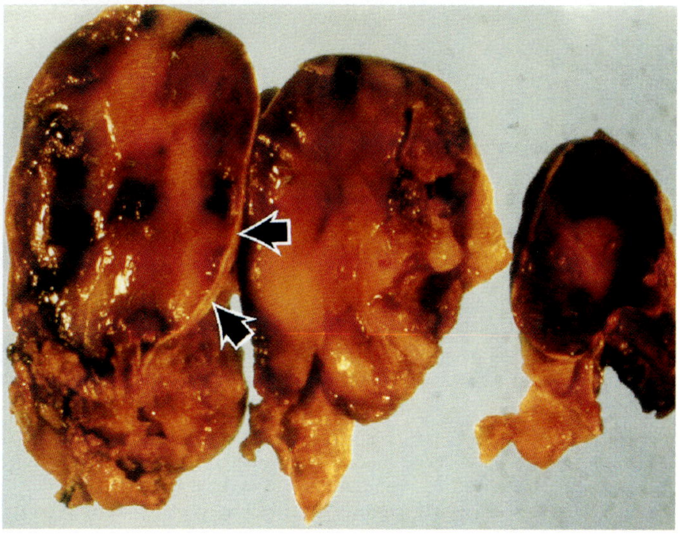

b.

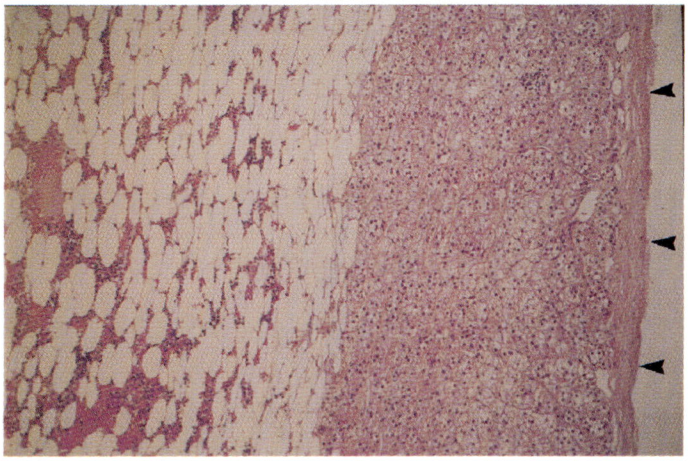

c.

Figure 1. Right adrenal mass in a 40-year-old woman evaluated for hypertension. Findings at biochemical testing were negative. **(a)** CT scan depicts 6-cm-diameter mass with peripheral calcification (straight arrow) and partial apparent capsule (curved arrow) that was scored as having 50%–90% fat. **(b)** Photograph of specimen of the mass in **a** shows an isolated adrenal myelolipoma with typical variegated appearance. Yellowish areas contain predominantly fat, and dark red areas contain predominantly marrow. Residual adrenal cortex is seen at the periphery (arrows). **(c)** Photomicrograph depicts the myelolipoma (left) with residual adrenal cortex bounded by the adrenal capsule (arrowheads). (Hematoxylin-eosin stain; original magnification, ×40.)

Thirty-three of the 41 isolated adrenal myelolipomas were scored as having at least 50% fat, with 13 having more than 90% fat. In the initial reading, five cases were scored as having less than 10% fat. Review of these five cases showed that although only a small proportion of the mass demonstrated true fat attenuation, most of the lesion was of intermediate attenuation (from −20 to +20 HU), presumably as a result of a diffuse admixture of fat and soft-tissue elements. Ten (24%) of the isolated adrenal myelolipomas demonstrated some calcification at CT, usually in small amounts (Fig 1). In 31 (75%), either a partial or complete pseudocapsule could be identified between the mass itself and surrounding retroperitoneal fat (Fig 1). Examination of the pathologic specimens showed a consistent pattern except for variation in the proportion of fat and bone marrow elements. In each adrenal gland, a single central focal mass was surrounded by a rim of residual adrenal cortical cells (sometimes only a few layers thick), which in turn was surrounded by the capsule of the adrenal gland (Figs 1, 3). The myelolipoma was in direct contact with the residual adrenal cortex at the periphery. Within the myelolipoma, only fat cells, myeloid elements, and sometimes lymphocytes and calcification were seen. Although there was considerable variation, some fat was usually seen microscopically even in areas that contained predominantly myeloid tissue. There was a gradual transition to areas with a greater proportion of fat (Fig 3), which accounts for the poor demarcation between fat and higher attenuation areas at CT. The apparent pseudocapsule seen at CT correlated with the thin rim of residual cortex with attached adrenal capsule rather than to a true capsule of the myelolipoma itself.

Myelolipoma with Acute Hemorrhage

Nine patients (eight men and one woman; mean age, 48 years; age range, 33–66 years) presented with clinical evidence of an acute hemorrhage, usually with sudden onset of pain, nausea and vomiting, hypotension, or laboratory documentation of a low hematocrit level. In two of these cases, an adrenal myelolipoma had been incidentally discovered earlier and the hemorrhage occurred subsequently (Fig 4). Mean tumor diameter was 14.2 cm (range, 8.5–18.0 cm). In all cases, an adrenal mass containing fat was clearly evident, as was acute hemorrhage. (The diameter of the mass measured without the hemorrhage correlated well with findings in the specimen.) The fat content was scored as more than 50% in all but one case and as more than 90% in three cases. Only one of the lesions was calcified.

Extra-adrenal Myelolipoma

Ten patients (four men and six women; mean age, 64 years; age range, 44–76 years) had an extra-adrenal myelolipoma. Findings on all CT scans that included the adrenal glands showed they were

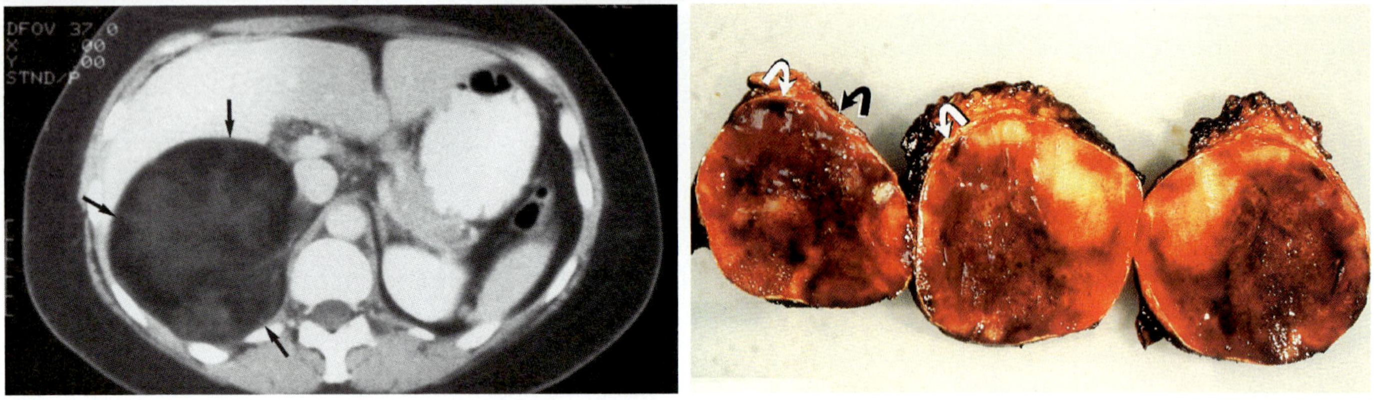

a. b.

Figure 2. Lucent right upper quadrant mass was noted incidentally on a scout radiograph (not shown) obtained before upper gastrointestinal examination in a 45-year-old man. (a) Contrast-enhanced CT scan depicts a 10 × 14-cm mass (arrows) that is largely fatty (50%–90%) with areas of higher attenuation within. Attenuation in the mass ranged from −105 HU peripherally to −37 HU centrally. Findings at biochemical testing were negative. (b) Photograph of specimen of the mass in **a** shows typical variegated appearance with peripheral residual adrenal cortex (arrows). Note lack of sharp margination between regions of predominantly marrow (red areas) and predominantly fat (yellow areas).

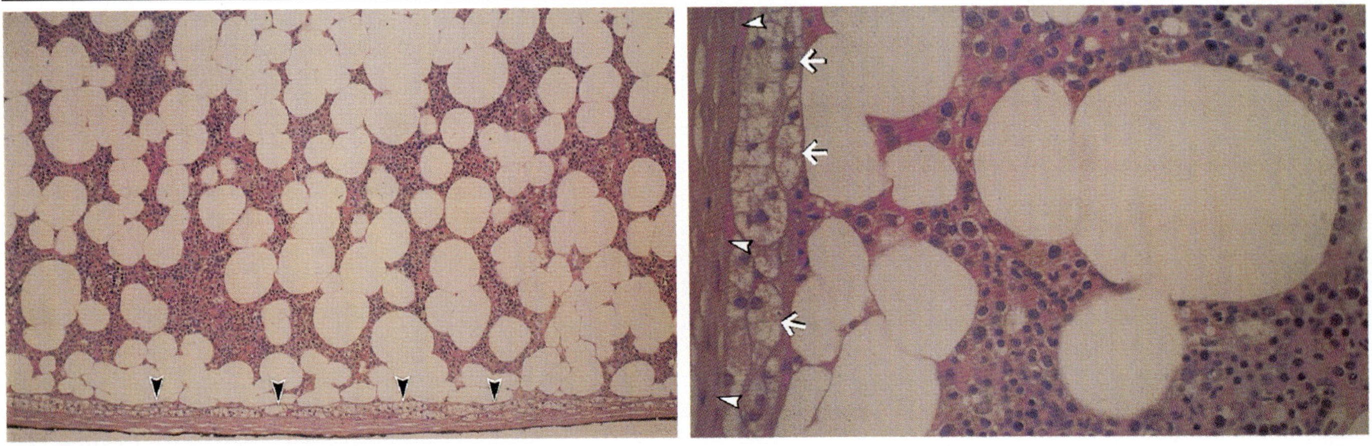

a. b.

Figure 3. (a) Photomicrograph from a typical isolated adrenal myelolipoma demonstrates elements of fat (round clear spaces) and marrow (cellular regions interspersed between fat) that abut a thin rim of residual adrenal cortex (arrowheads), which forms an apparent capsule. Cellularity in the myelolipoma varies gradually with no sharp margins. (Hematoxylin-eosin stain; original magnification, ×40.) (b) Higher power photomicrograph shows myelolipoma abutting a very thin rim of adrenal cortical cells (arrows) bounded by the adrenal capsule (arrowheads). (Hematoxylin-eosin stain; original magnification, ×200.)

normal. None of these patients had an endocrine disorder or a clinically evident acute hemorrhage (although some areas of hemorrhage and necrosis were seen in the specimens). The myelolipoma was in the presacral retroperitoneal space in four cases, in the peri- or infrarenal retroperitoneal space in four cases, and in the low pelvis in one case. In one case, a retroperitoneal myelolipoma was discovered synchronously with four intrathoracic myelolipomas. In another case, a solitary thoracic myelolipoma was present. Mean diameter of the extra-adrenal myelolipomas was 8.2 cm (range, 4–15 cm). None of the myelolipomas demonstrated calcification at CT. The imaging features at CT were otherwise similar to those of isolated adrenal myelolipomas (Fig 5). Median fat content was less than 50%, although the content was less than 10% in only two cases and was more than 90% in only one case. Nine of the lesions were well circumscribed with a partial or complete apparent pseudocapsule seen at CT. A true capsule was not seen at pathologic examination, but many of the lesions were well circumscribed with a condensation of connective tissue surrounding them that apparently accounted for the appearance of a pseudocapsule (Fig 5c). The appearance of a pseudocapsule is not caused by the presence of residual adrenal tissue in these cases, because in only one presacral myelolipoma was adrenal cortical tissue present. (This case may represent an ectopic adrenal gland with myelolipoma; the contributor did not include a CT scan of the adrenal bed and the status of the ipsilateral adrenal gland is unknown.) In the nine other patients, the adrenal glands were normal at CT and no ectopic adrenal tissue was found at histologic examination of the resected extra-adrenal mass.

Myelolipomatous Foci with Other Pathologic Conditions

In 18 patients (five men and 13 women; mean age, 55 years; age range, 28–83

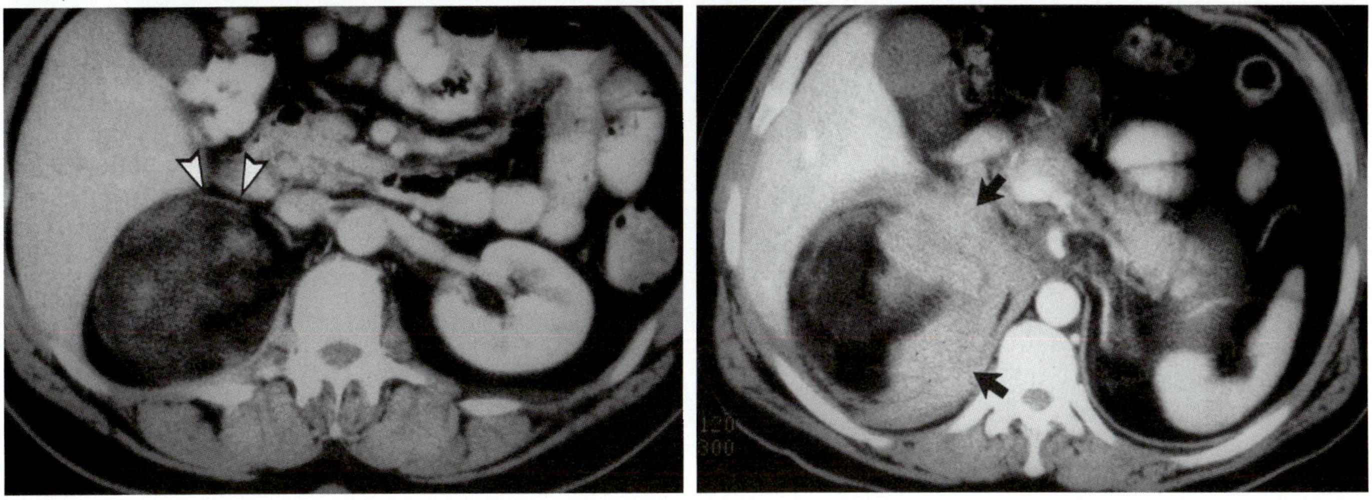

a. b.

Figure 4. US (not shown) performed in a 42-year-old man to evaluate vague right upper quadrant pain revealed a hyperechoic right suprarenal mass. **(a)** Contrast-enhanced CT scan obtained to follow up for presumed myelolipoma demonstrates a 8 × 10-cm mass with partial capsule (arrowheads) that was scored as having 50%–90% fat. **(b)** CT scan obtained after **a** (when the patient developed acute pain with weakness, dizziness, and hypotension) shows an acute hemorrhage (arrows).

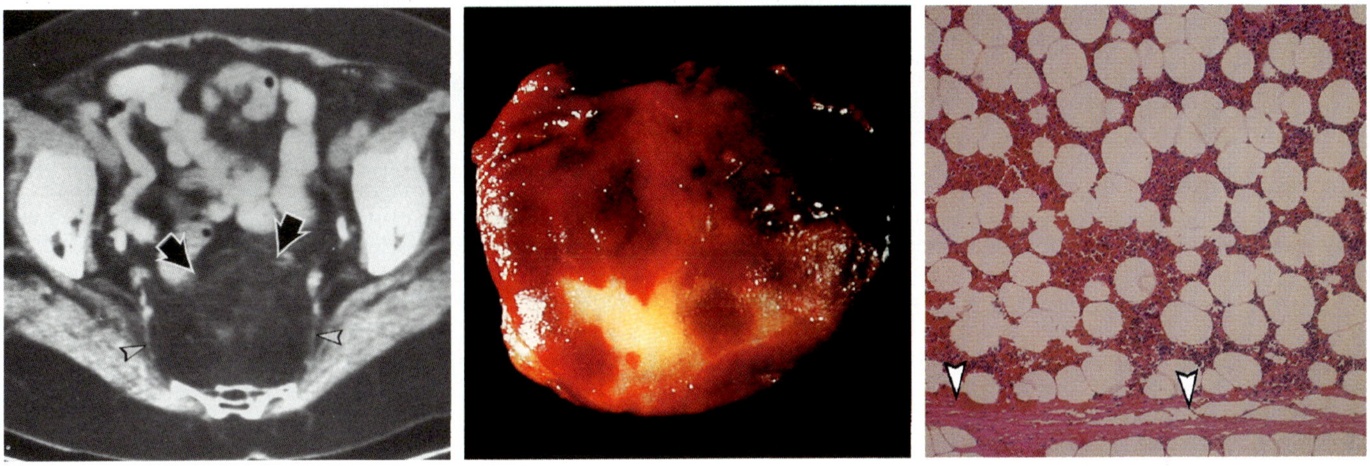

a. b. c.

Figure 5. Evaluation for fecal incontinence in a 76-year-old woman with history of lower back pain for 16 years. **(a)** Contrast-enhanced CT scan depicts a 7 × 8-cm presacral mass (arrows) scored as having 50%–90% fat with a partial apparent capsule (arrowheads). **(b)** Photograph of the specimen of the mass in **a**, which appears to be an adrenal myelolipoma (cf Fig 2b) except for the absence of adrenal cortex at the periphery. **(c)** Photomicrograph from a different case reveals the cells of fat (round, clear spaces) and marrow (red-blue regions interspersed between fat) of a typical extra-adrenal myelolipoma, which is identical to an adrenal myelolipoma but does not have any adrenal cortex. The connective tissue condenses at the periphery (arrowheads) to form an apparent capsule. (Hematoxylin-eosin stain; original magnification, ×40.)

years), lesions that had been archived as "myelolipoma" at review were found to contain myelolipomatous foci within other pathologic conditions in the adrenal gland. In three cases, bilateral disease was present (including congenital adrenal hyperplasia due to 21-hydroxylase deficiency in two cases) (Fig 6). In six cases, the patient had an endocrine disorder (hypercortisolism due to hyperfunctioning adenomas in two patients and due to hyperplasia in one patient, and 21-hydroxylase deficiency in three patients). In the remaining 12 cases of myelolipomatous foci in nonhyperfunctioning adenomas (with one case of bilateral adenomas), pathologic examination revealed an adenoma but there was no clinical or biochemical evidence of an endocrine disorder.

Mean diameter of the lesions was 7.1 cm (range, 2–15 cm). In cases of myelolipomatous foci within an adenoma, the diameter of the overall adrenal mass was measured and not just of the myelolipomatous foci (Fig 7). The diameter ranged from 2.0 to 13.0 cm, and all masses were readily seen at CT. The mass was in the right adrenal gland in 14 cases. Calcification was found in 11 cases and was often very extensive (Fig 7). Fat content was relatively scant. In four cases, no fat was recognizable at CT. The median fat content was less than 10%; in only two cases was the score more than 50%. As a rule, a pseudocapsule was not evident.

In these cases, pathologic examination showed a very different pattern from that seen in isolated adrenal myelolipomas.

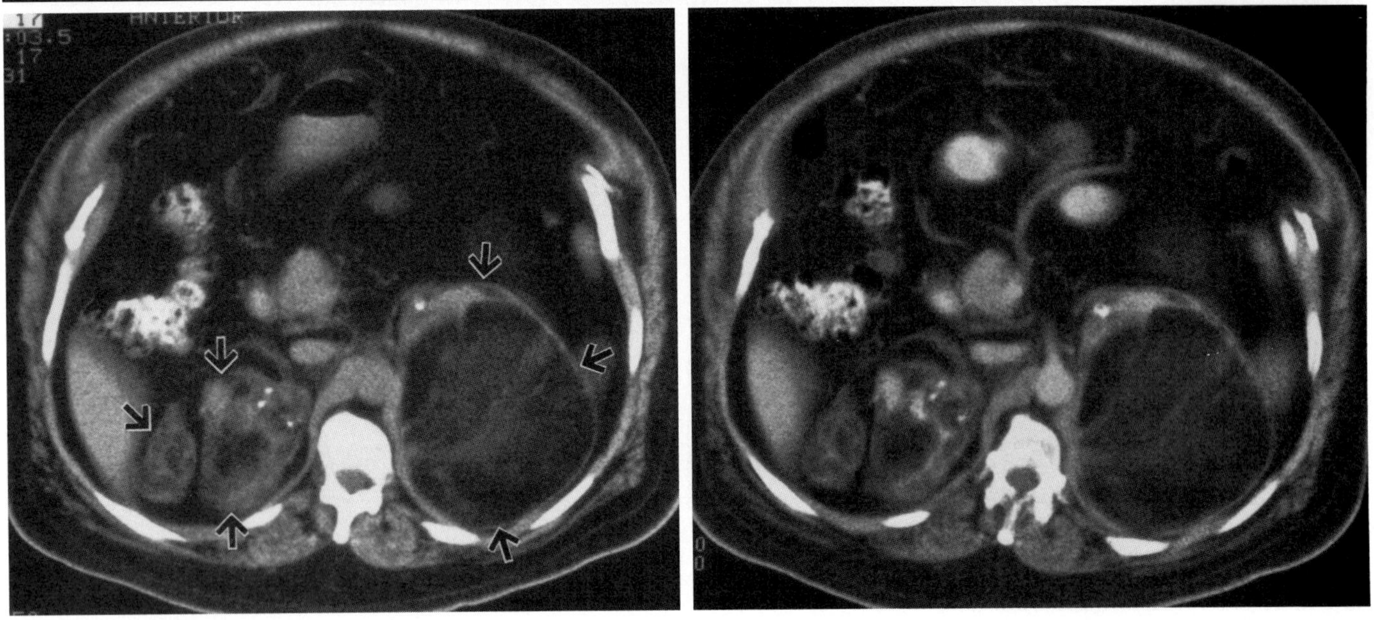

a. b.

Figure 6. Evaluation of a 39-year-old woman with known congenital adrenal hyperplasia (21-hydroxylase deficiency) and increasing abdominal girth. **(a)** Precontrast CT scan reveals bilateral adrenal masses (arrows) with fat and stippled calcification. **(b)** Postcontrast CT scan obtained at approximately the same level shows little enhancement in the wispy central soft tissue. Attenuation ranged from −61 to −7 HU.

Interspersed within the abnormal cortical tissue were small foci of myelolipomatous tissue composed of adenomatous or hyperplastic cells (Fig 7b). The intermixed myelolipomatous foci and abnormal cortical cells were surrounded by the residual normal adrenal tissue, which in turn was surrounded by the adrenal capsule. In many cases, the myelolipomatous foci composed only a small proportion of the abnormal tissue and did not directly contact the peripheral residual normal adrenal glands. Although findings were variable at microscopic examination, calcification was often found to occur in areas of old hemorrhage or degeneration within an adenoma rather than within the myelolipomatous foci.

Statistical Analysis

Statistical analysis was performed to identify significant differences between subgroups of the full study: adrenal myelolipoma alone (group 1), myelolipomas that hemorrhaged (group 2), extra-adrenal myelolipomas (group 3), and adrenal myelolipomatous foci in other pathologic adrenal conditions (group 4). The characteristics of groups 2, 3, and 4 were compared with those of group 1. The Wilcoxon rank sum test was used to compare groups with respect to age and size. The Fisher exact test and the χ^2 test were used to compare groups with respect to categorical data. The following statistically significant differences were found: age, group 3 vs group 1 (P = .007); sex, group 2 vs group 1 (P = .013) and group 4 vs group 1 (P = .003); diameter, group 2 vs group 1 (P = .010) and group 4 vs group 1 (P = .003); calcification, group 4 vs group 1 (P = .017); fat content, group 3 vs group 1 (P = .016) and group 4 vs group 1 ($P \leq$ .001); pseudocapsule, group 4 vs group 1 (P = .001).

The Mantel-Haenszel relative risk and its 95% confidence interval were used to compare the risk of a hemorrhage in larger and smaller lesions. A cutoff diameter of 10 cm was arbitrarily selected to assess relative risk of hemorrhage versus size in group 1. Of the 20 isolated myelolipomas with diameter less than 10 cm, one (5%) experienced hemorrhage. Of the 33 isolated myelolipomas with diameter of 10 cm or more, eight (24%) experienced hemorrhage. The relative risk in larger compared with smaller isolated myelolipomas was 4.848. The 95% confidence interval was from 0.86 to 27.27 (and included unity); therefore, the relative risk was not significantly different from unity.

DISCUSSION

Myelolipomas have been somewhat of a medical curiosity for many years, as they are uncommon, benign, and usually asymptomatic. They are discovered incidentally rather frequently, however, as a result of widespread noninvasive adrenal imaging (11). Many of the clinical and pathologic characteristics have been well described, but mostly in nonradiology literature. Myelolipomas consist of mature fat and hematopoietic elements (usually including erythroid, myeloid, megakaryocyte types and, often, lymphocytes) (1). Myelolipoma is distinct from true bone marrow because no reticular sinusoids or bone spicules are present. Myelolipoma is also distinct from extramedullary hematopoietic tissue, which (unlike myelolipoma) occurs in concert with hematologic disease and splenomegaly, does not contain fat, and usually is multifocal with a propensity to occur in the mediastinum (6,7). The origin of myelolipoma remains obscure although various theories have been proposed including development from embryonic mesenchymal rests in the adrenal glands, development from hematogenously seeded bone marrow emboli, and metaplasia of reticuloendothelial cells as a result of chronic stress (1,4,10,18).

The most common pattern of myelolipoma is the isolated adrenal lesion, which probably occurs more often in the general population than the 62% of patients seen in this study. In all such cases in this study, some fat was recognizable at CT although the amount was quite variable.

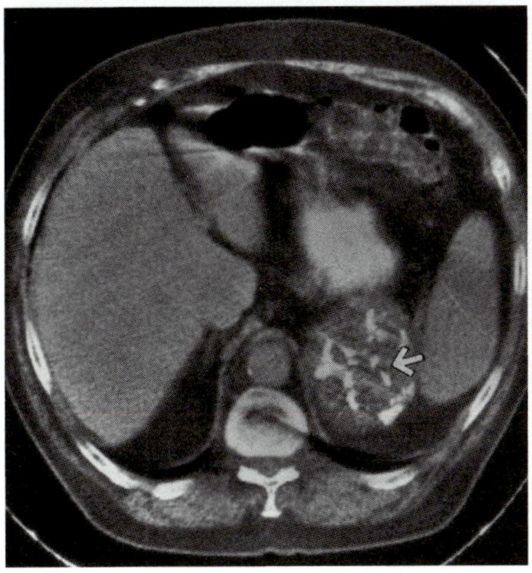

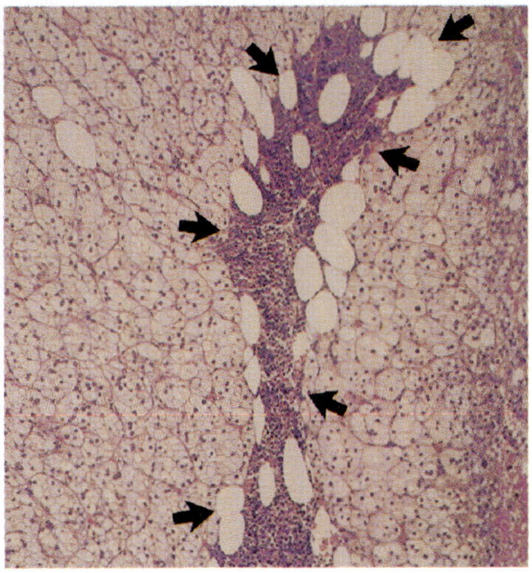

a. b.

Figure 7. Calcified left upper quadrant mass was identified on an upper gastrointestinal series (not shown) obtained to evaluate epigastric pain in a 73-year-old man with negative findings at endocrine testing. **(a)** Contrast-enhanced CT scan reveals a heavily calcified 9 × 10-cm left adrenal mass scored as having less than 10% fat. A few tiny possible foci of fat (arrow) are seen, but no capsule is evident. **(b)** Photomicrograph demonstrates a small focus of myelolipomatous cells (arrows) within an adenoma. (Hematoxylin-eosin stain; original magnification, ×100.)

Some higher attenuation areas were typically seen, often with attenuation readings less than that of true soft tissue, as well as indistinct margins because of the irregular intermixture of fat and myeloid elements seen microscopically (Figs 2, 3). Myelolipomas commonly demonstrate an apparent pseudocapsule, which histologically correlates with a rim of residual adrenal cortex and the adrenal capsule. The pathologic pattern was that of a benign tumorlike mass within or replacing an otherwise normal adrenal gland.

A rather striking right-sided predominance (53 of 72 adrenal myelolipomas [74%]) was noted in this study. Although speculative, a possible explanation is that asymptomatic right-sided adrenal masses are more likely to be detected incidentally, particularly at US, because the right adrenal region is seen clearly during US examination of the gallbladder. A right-sided predominance (63%) was noted in a study of incidental adrenal masses detected at US (11). In another study (13), all the myelolipomas detected at US were in the right adrenal gland. In a large surgical study (8), however, only 47% of 59 myelolipomas were on the right side.

The most dramatic clinical presentation of myelolipomas is that of an acute hemorrhage. Patients present with typical clinical signs and symptoms of an abdominal hemorrhage, usually with pain localizing to the flank or back. In all nine such cases in our study, CT readily demonstrated acute hemorrhage as well as a fat-containing adrenal mass. These cases in fact represent a subset of the usual isolated adrenal myelolipomas, except that they hemorrhaged. It is thus not surprising that the imaging features of the myelolipomas that bled were similar in most ways to isolated adrenal myelolipomas that had not bled. The most important difference in the myelolipomas that bled was size—lesions that bled were statistically significantly larger than those that had not bled. The smallest lesion that bled had a diameter of 8.5 cm; all the others had a diameter greater than 10 cm. One unexplained demographic feature is the male preponderance among those with a hemorrhage (89% [eight of nine men]) versus 47% overall [35 of 74 patients]). The specific cause of the bleeding in these cases is unclear. On the basis of information reported with the contributed specimens, none of the patients had a history of trauma. It is possible that a history of trauma could have been omitted, but this is not likely in all cases; in five of the nine cases, the clinical history clearly stated that the episode was spontaneous without antecedent trauma.

Most adrenal myelolipomas are asymptomatic, especially when small. Nonspecific pain is often reported with large lesions. Acute hemorrhage has been reported only sporadically (8,12,19). In the report of 59 surgical cases by Dieckmann et al (8), only three myelolipomas had acute retroperitoneal hemorrhage. These lesions were 12, 18, and 30 cm in greatest dimension. Numerous "giant" myelolipomas, however, have been reported that have not bled. In this study, the diameter of 22 adrenal myelolipomas was more than 10 cm at the time they were removed, but they had no sign of acute hemorrhage. Risk of hemorrhage in our study was calculated as more than four times greater with lesions more than versus less than 10 cm in diameter (24% vs 5%), but this did not exceed 95% confidence intervals. Because myelolipoma can be presumptively diagnosed at CT on the basis of fat demonstrated in an adrenal mass, patients with large lesions are often followed up instead of undergoing resection. In one case report, an increase in size of an adrenal myelolipoma was seen over a 4-year follow-up period (from 6 × 10 to 8 × 14 cm) (15). In our study, two myelolipomas (10.5 and 12 cm in diameter) that were being followed up conservatively after incidental discovery developed a clinically evident hemorrhage (Fig 4). Because of the risk of hemorrhage and the potential for further growth, elective removal of large myelolipomas (>10 cm) might still be considered.

Although myelolipomas have been reported to occur outside the adrenal glands (5–7), this is unusual and the possibility may not be well known. Ten patients with extra-adrenal myelolipomas were included in this study, including one with multiple extra-adrenal lesions. The patients tended to be slightly older (mean age, 64 years), with mild female predominance (six of 10 patients [60%]). The imaging features were the same as those for adrenal myelolipoma, with a mixture of fat and soft tissue, often with a capsule. Similar findings were noted in a prior review of 25 published cases of extra-adrenal myelolipomas (7): Twenty-three were solitary; female-to-male ratio was 2:1; 50% were presacral, and retroperitoneal, thoracic, and pelvic locations were observed less commonly. Clinically evident hemorrhage was not noted. The differential diagnosis of a fat-containing extra-adrenal mass must include liposarcoma, teratoma, and an exophytic angiomyolipoma of the kidney. Because the pathologic characteristics of myelolipoma are so distinctive, needle biopsy might be considered in patients with such masses if they are poor surgical candidates (20). However, none of the patients with an extra-adrenal myelolipoma in this study underwent percutaneous biopsy. In this study, six patients underwent percutaneous fine needle aspiration biopsy of adrenal myelolipomas; results were diagnostic in four but yielded only fat in one and only adrenal cortical cells in the other.

An intriguing subset of patients in this study is the 18 patients with foci of myelolipomatous tissue in association with adrenal adenomas and hyperplasia. Previous articles reported the occasional discovery of "myelolipoma" in conjunction with functional disorders, including cortical adenomas and cortical hyperplasia resulting in congenital adrenal hyperplasia (due to 21- and 17-hydroxylase deficiency), hypercortisolism, or hyperaldosteronism or Addison disease (9,17,21–23). A case of myelolipoma and pheochromocytoma has been reported, but this appears to be a coincidence of two separate masses in the same adrenal gland (24). Nevertheless, only 5% of the 59 patients with myelolipomas in the study by Dieckmann et al (8) had associated pathologic adrenal conditions. Our study also included 11 patients with myelolipomatous foci within a nonhyperfunctioning adrenal adenoma.

In the cases of myelolipomatous foci associated with other pathologic adrenal conditions, careful examination of the specimens showed a consistent pattern that was distinctly different from that seen in the myelolipomas in otherwise normal adrenal glands. One or more small clusters of myelolipomatous foci were embedded within large regions of hyperplastic or adenomatous cells (Fig 7b), with residual normal adrenal cortex surrounding the entire intermixed abnormal tissue. This has been commented on but not emphasized in previous pathologic reports (9,17,21,22). The appearance is not that of a tumor but that of foci of degeneration within another pathologic condition.

Perhaps more important for radiologists is the fact that the imaging features of myelolipomatous foci within hyperplastic or adenomatous lesions are different from those of typical isolated myelolipomas. The former were significantly smaller than the latter (mean diameter, 7.1 vs 10.9 cm, respectively). Frequency of calcification was greater with the latter (53% vs 26%), and the calcification was often more extensive (Fig 7). In the former, calcification is frequently within the adenomatous component. Although benign adenomas are not commonly calcified, the presence of hemorrhage or degeneration within adenomas is accompanied by a greater likelihood of calcification, and many of the benign adenomas associated with myelolipomatous foci in this study were degenerated. The amount of fat evident at CT was significantly less than in the group of isolated adrenal myelolipomas. In four myelolipomas associated with nonhyperfunctioning adenomas, no definite fat was seen at CT. Prior reports of myelolipomatous foci associated with other pathologic adrenal conditions have not emphasized imaging features, although review of those images shows that calcification and scant amounts of fat were present (9,21,25). A prior report of five cases of "myelolipoma" emphasized the appearance of tiny amounts of fat and extensive calcification (26). Findings on those CT scans were identical to those in our cases of mixed myelolipomatous foci and nonhyperfunctioning adenomas, but full pathologic correlation was not available in that study. The explanation for the difference in the imaging features is that the myelolipomatous foci compose only a portion of the abnormality, in addition to abnormal tissue (adenoma or hyperplasia) with the attenuation of soft tissue and, frequently, calcifications. In any case, the presence of myelolipomatous foci in these associated adrenal lesions is not particularly important: The treatment of the patient should be determined on the basis of the other adrenal pathologic condition and not on the basis of the myelolipomatous foci. Myelolipomatous foci may coexist with these other lesions, however, and a knowledge of the imaging appearance is helpful.

This study has several possible limitations that are largely a result of the selection process of the case material available in the archives of the Armed Forces Institute of Pathology. All cases are pathologically proved; thus, cases are accrued only after surgical removal or percutaneous biopsy. Large masses (with which concern for malignancy is greater), symptomatic lesions, and lesions with hemorrhage are probably overrepresented. Cases voluntarily submitted to the Armed Forces Institute of Pathology are often unusual or diagnostically difficult. A greater proportion of extra-adrenal lesions and lesions associated with endocrine disorders are included in this study than would be seen generally. This study does not include the typical small, asymptomatic adrenal myelolipoma commonly seen in busy CT practices because such lesions rarely have pathologic proof. Also, a study such as this cannot validate a prospective radiologic diagnosis of myelolipoma, including the accuracy of distinction of a myelolipoma from other fat-containing lesions such as angiomyolipoma or liposarcoma. Last, the CT scans in this study were obtained on a variety of CT scanners with variable technique dependent on the protocol used by the contributor at the time of the examination. Nevertheless, the ability to review a large collection of cases including unusual types and to directly correlate the clinical and imaging findings with the pathologic findings helps understanding of the disease process and development of a diagnostic approach for patients with masses that may be myelolipomas.

This review of a large number of pathologically proved myelolipomas reveals several characteristics of this lesion. Myelolipoma most often occurs in the adrenal glands, but myelolipomatous foci can be found within other adrenal pathologic conditions or in extra-adrenal locations. Most myelolipomas occur in an otherwise normal adrenal gland. These are not associated with endocrine disorders or other pathologic adrenal conditions and have a histologic pattern of a benign tumor. Fat is nearly always clearly evident at CT. Acute hemorrhage can result from an adrenal myelolipoma. This is more common in men and in larger lesions. Statistical analysis did not, however, definitively prove a significantly greater risk with myelolipomas more than 10 cm in diameter. Myelolipomas occur in extra-adrenal locations, most commonly the presacral and other retroperitoneal areas. The clinical and imaging characteristics are similar to those of adrenal myelolipomas but are not clearly distinct from those of other fat-containing retroperitoneal masses. Myelolipomatous foci can be found within other pathologic conditions (including hyperplasia and adenomas) in the adrenal glands, whether they are functioning or nonfunctioning. Such cases occur more frequently in women, and the lesions have a tendency to be smaller, are more frequently calcified, and have a lower proportion of fat (occasionally demonstrating no recognizable fat at CT). Histologically, the pattern is that of degeneration within the other pathologic condition.

Acknowledgments: Statistical analysis was performed by Jeannette Y. Lee, PhD, of the University of Alabama at Birmingham. Advice and critique were provided by Alan J. Davidson, MD.

References

1. Plaut A. Myelolipoma in the adrenal cortex. Am J Pathol 1958; 34:487–515.
2. Gierke E. Uber knochenmarksgewebe in der nebenniere. Beitr Path Anat 1905; 7:311–325.
3. Oberling C. Les formations myelolipomatouses. Bull Cancer 1929; 18:234–246.
4. Rubin HB, Hirose F, Benfield JR. Myelolipoma of the adrenal gland: angiographic

findings and review of the literature. Am J Surg 1975; 130:354–358.

5. Chen KTK, Felix EL, Flam MS. Extra-adrenal myelolipoma. Am J Clin Pathol 1982; 78:386–389.
6. Fowler MR, Alba JM, Williams RR, Byrd CR. Extra-adrenal myelolipomas compared with extra medullary hematopoietic tumors. Am J Surg Pathol 1982; 6:363–374.
7. Brietta LK, Watkins D. Giant extra-adrenal myelolipoma. Arch Pathol Lab Med 1994; 118:188–190.
8. Dieckmann KP, Hamm B, Pickartz H, Jonas D, Bauer HW. Adrenal myelolipoma: clinical, radiologic, and histologic features. Urology 1987; 29:1–8.
9. Oliva A, Duarte B, Hammadeh R, Ghosh L, Baker RJ. Myelolipoma and endocrine dysfunction. Surgery 1988; 103:711–715.
10. Olsson CA, Krane RJ, Klugo RC, Selikowitz SM. Adrenal myelolipoma. Surgery 1973; 73:665–670.
11. Aso Y, Homma Y. A survey on incidental adrenal tumors in Japan. J Urol 1992; 147:1478–1481.
12. Vick CW, Zeman RK, Mannes E, Cronan JJ, Walsh JW. Adrenal myelolipoma: CT and ultrasound findings. Urol Radiol 1984; 6:7–13.
13. Musante F, Derchi LE, Zappasodi F, et al. Myelolipoma of the adrenal gland: sonographic and CT features. AJR 1988; 151: 961–964.
14. Musante F, Derchi LE, Bazzocchi M, Avataneo T, Gandini G, Mucelli RSP. MR imaging of adrenal myelolipomas. J Comput Assist Tomogr 1991; 15:111–114.
15. Meaglia JP, Schmidt JD. Natural history of an adrenal myelolipoma. J Urol 1992; 147:1089–1090.
16. Casey LR, Cohen AJ, Wile AG, Dietrich RB. Giant adrenal myelolipomas: CT and MRI findings. Abdom Imaging 1994; 19: 165–167.
17. Goetz SP, Niemann TH, Robinson RA, Cohen MB. Hematopoietic elements associated with adrenal glands. Arch Pathol Lab Med 1994; 118:895–896.
18. Wooley PA. Heteroplastic bone and bone marrow formation associated with tuberculosis in the adrenal. J Lab Clin Med 1915; 1:502–508.
19. Goldman HB, Howard RC, Patterson AL. Spontaneous retroperitoneal hemorrhage from a giant adrenal myelolipoma. J Urol 1996; 155:639.
20. Dunphy CH. Computed tomography: guided fine needle aspiration biopsy of adrenal myelolipoma—case report and review of the literature. Acta Cytol 1991; 35:353–356.
21. Kanj HA, Noronha J, D'Aguillo AF, Amorosa JK, Amorosa LF. Bilateral adrenal myelolipomas with Cushing's syndrome. JAMA 1988; 259:3034–3036.
22. Vyberg M, Sestoft L. Combined adrenal myelolipoma and adenoma associated with Cushing's syndrome. Am J Clin Pathol 1986; 86:541–545.
23. Escuin F, Gomez P, Martinez I, Perez-Fontan M, Selgas R, Sanchez-Sicillia L. Angiomyelolipoma associated with bilateral adrenocortical hyperplasia and hypertension. J Urol 1985; 133:655–657.
24. Ukimura O, Inui E, Ochiai A, Kojima M, Watanabe H. Combined adrenal myelolipoma and pheochromocytoma. J Urol 1995; 154:1470.
25. Whaley D, Becker S, Presbrey T, Shaff M. Adrenal myelolipoma associated with Conn syndrome: CT evaluation. J Comput Assist Tomogr 1985; 9:959–960.
26. Rofsky NM, Bosniak MA, Megibow AJ, Schlossberg P. Adrenal myelolipomas: CT appearance with tiny amounts of fat and punctate calcification. Urol Radiol 1989; 11:148–152.

Book Review

Atlas of Infertility: Diagnostic and Therapeutic Radiology

Amy S. Thurmond, MD
Malden, Mass: Blackwell Science, 1998. ISBN 0-63204-305-9.
Hardcover, $75.00; pp 110; 160 figures; one table.

This book presents a multimodality approach for diagnosing infertility in women, which includes hysterosalpingography, sonography, and magnetic resonance (MR) imaging. It discusses some of the interventional options available for treatment, particularly from a radiologic standpoint. It is intended for radiologists, gynecologists, nurses, and technologists who work in this rapidly changing field.

The book is divided into five basic chapters, the first three of which cover the anatomy, pathologic conditions, and congenital variations of the cervix and uterus, the fallopian tube, and the ovary and adnexa. The fourth chapter concerns imaging for assisted reproductive technologies, and the last chapter deals with procedures for diagnosis and treatment of infertility.

The first three chapters are the strength of the book and contain many examples of uterine anomalies and abnormalities. The fallopian tubes, ovaries, and adnexal regions are also discussed well. The section on assisted reproductive technologies is quite short and provides only cursory information on this topic. The last chapter is somewhat repetitive, as the technique of hysterosalpingography and examples of disease are discussed; this constitutes a partial review of what was covered in the first three chapters. It then concludes with interventional procedures involving fallopian tube recanalization, which may have warranted a separate chapter.

In general, the figures are of good quality. There are many examples of most of the pathologic characteristics usually identified in hysterosalpingography. It would have been beneficial if there had been more examples of abnormalities demonstrated with sonography, especially sonohysterography, and MR imaging. Perhaps more space can be devoted to these modalities in the next edition. There are no major errors, although the words "therapeutic radiology" are usually reserved for radiation therapy, and the "therapy" that is being described in the book is normally termed "interventional radiology."

This book is useful to anyone imaging women with infertility. Unlike many textbooks in the field, this one introduces sonography and MR imaging. The cost is modest and well within reach. Expansion of the chapter on assisted reproductive technologies, as well as further development of sonography and MR imaging, will enhance this already excellent book.

Reviewed by Joseph H. Tashjian, MD

Naoki Takahashi, MD
Akira Kawashima, MD
Randy D. Ernst, MD
Illya C. Boridy, MD
Stanford M. Goldman, MD
George S. Benson, MD
Carl M. Sandler, MD

Index terms:
Kidney, stenosis or obstruction, 81.899
Ureter, calculi, 82.811
Ureter, CT, 82.12111, 82.12115

Radiology 1998; 208:97–102

Abbreviation:
ROC = receiver operating characteristic

[1] From the Department of Radiology, Lyndon B. Johnson General Hospital, 5656 Kelley St, Houston, TX 77026 (N.T., A.K., R.D.E., I.C.B., C.M.S.), and the Departments of Radiology (N.T., A.K., R.D.E., I.C.B., S.M.G., C.M.S.) and Urology (S.M.G., G.S.B., C.M.S.), University of Texas Houston Medical School. From the 1997 RSNA scientific assembly. Received August 15, 1997; revision requested October 27; revision received December 29; accepted March 3, 1998. **Address reprint requests to** A.K.

Author contributions:
Guarantor of integrity of entire study, N.T.; study concepts and design, N.T.; definition of intellectual content, N.T., A.K.; literature research, N.T.; clinical studies, N.T., A.K., R.D.E., I.C.B.; data analysis, N.T., A.K.; statistical analysis, N.T., A.K.; manuscript preparation, N.T., A.K., C.M.S.; manuscript editing, C.M.S.; manuscript review, C.M.S., S.M.G., G.S.B.

Ureterolithiasis: Can Clinical Outcome Be Predicted with Unenhanced Helical CT?[1]

PURPOSE: To evaluate the use of helical computed tomography (CT) without contrast material enhancement for prediction of a favorable outcome in ureterolithiasis.

MATERIALS AND METHODS: CT studies were reviewed in 69 patients with a single ureteral stone not located at the ureteropelvic junction. CT findings (tissue rim sign, hydronephrosis, perinephric fat stranding, perinephric fluid collections, and thickening of renal fascia) were graded on a scale of 0–3. Stone diameter and renal parenchymal enlargement were also measured.

RESULTS: Twenty-two patients had spontaneous passage, 12 did not respond to conservative treatment, and 35 were lost to follow-up. When the latter 35 patients were excluded, perinephric fat stranding ($P = .044$) and perinephric fluid collections ($P = .021$) were graded significantly higher in patients with spontaneous stone passage. Mean stone diameter was significantly larger ($P < .001$) in patients in whom conservative treatment failed (mean, 7.8 mm) than in patients with spontaneous stone passage (mean, 2.9 mm). The presence of a tissue rim sign and the grade of hydronephrosis, renal fascial thickening, and renal parenchymal enlargement were not significantly different between the two groups.

CONCLUSION: In addition to stone size, the degree of perinephric fat stranding and the presence of perinephric fluid collections are useful ancillary signs for help in predicting the likelihood of stone passage.

Since Smith et al (1) first reported the use of helical computed tomography (CT) without contrast material enhancement in patients with acute flank pain, the value of this modality in the demonstration of ureteral stones has been well established (2–7). Unenhanced helical CT has been reported (1,3) to be more sensitive than excretory urography for the demonstration of ureteral stones. The role of secondary CT findings such as stranding of perinephric fat, hydronephrosis, the tissue rim sign, and nephromegaly in the diagnosis of ureterolithiasis has been documented (1,4–7). The advantages of unenhanced helical CT over excretory urography include speed, no need for intravenously administered contrast material, and the potential ability to reveal extraurinary causes of acute flank pain (1–3).

Smaller stone size (8–10), location of the stone in the distal part of the ureter (8,10), shorter duration of flank pain (8,10), and the presence of pyelosinus extravasation at excretory urography (11) have been reported to correlate with spontaneous stone passage. To our knowledge, little work has been done in the evaluation of CT for help in predicting a favorable clinical outcome in patients with ureteral stones. The purpose of our study was to evaluate the use of unenhanced helical CT in patients with ureterolithiasis for prediction of a favorable clinical outcome.

MATERIALS AND METHODS

The study group comprised 174 patients who underwent unenhanced helical CT because of possible ureterolithiasis between August 1995 and December 1996. Unenhanced helical CT was performed with a HiSpeed Advantage CT scanner (GE Medical Systems, Milwaukee, Wis), with a collimation of 5 mm and a pitch of 1.5 or 1.6. Scans were obtained during two to three breath holds. Images were reconstructed at 3-, 5-, or 8-mm intervals and were reproduced on hard copy with a soft-tissue window setting (window width, 450 HU; window level, 50 HU).

Among the 174 patients, CT scans depicted 79 ureteral stones in 79 patients. The stones were in the ureteropelvic junction in 10 patients and in non–ureteropelvic junction locations in 69. Ninety-five patients had no ureteral stones. The 10 patients with ureteropelvic junction stones were excluded from the analysis because such stones rarely pass spontaneously (8), and, in our series, the stones in three patients were associated with pyonephrosis and needed emergent intervention.

Sixty-nine patients (48 men and 21 women), aged 17–63 years (mean, 36.4 years), with non–ureteropelvic junction stones formed the study population. None of the study patients had clinical evidence of pyonephrosis at the time of CT.

The CT scans obtained in these 69 patients were retrospectively reviewed by two radiologists (A.K., R.D.E.) without knowledge of the clinical outcome. The location (proximal part of the ureter, distal part of the ureter, or ureterovesical junction) and maximal diameter of the stones in the axial plane were recorded from the hard copy, as was the presence of the following secondary CT findings: the presence of the tissue rim sign; the degree of hydronephrosis, perinephric fat stranding, renal parenchymal enlargement, and thickening of the renal fascia; and the amount of perinephric fluid.

The tissue rim sign was graded as follows: 0 = definitely absent, 1 = probably absent, 2 = probably present, and 3 = definitely present. Hydronephrosis was graded as follows: 0 = absent, 1 = mild (prominence of the intrarenal pelvis or mild dilatation of the ureter), 2 = moderate (dilatation of the renal calices or moderate dilatation of the ureter), and 3 = severe (marked dilatation of the collecting system). Perinephric fat stranding was defined as linear areas of soft-tissue attenuation in the perinephric space and was graded as follows: 0 = absent, 1 = mild (a few thin strands), 2 = moderate (between stranding grades 1 and 3), and 3 = severe (many thick strands). Renal parenchymal enlargement was recorded as the ratio of the short axis diameter (in the axial plane) of the affected kidney to that of the contralateral kidney. Thickening of the renal fascia was graded as follows: 0 = absent, 1 = mild (thin), 2 = moderate (thick but not circumferential), and 3 = severe (thick and circumferential). Perinephric fluid collections were defined as discrete, rounded areas of fluid attenuation in the perinephric space and were graded as follows: 0 = absent, 1 = mild (one or two small [<1-cm-diameter] fluid collections), 2 = moderate (between fluid collection grades 1 and 3), and 3 = severe (more than two large [≥1-cm-diameter] fluid collections).

When a disagreement between the two observers occurred with regard to location, agreement was reached by consensus. For other parameters, the mean of the two grading scores was used as the representative value.

Medical records and follow-up imaging studies were reviewed for clinical outcome. The patients with non–ureteropelvic junction stones were subdivided into three categories: (*a*) patients with documented spontaneous stone passage, (*b*) patients in whom conservative treatment failed (with resultant intervention or presence of a stone after 4 weeks), and (*c*) patients who were lost to follow-up.

The size of the ureteral stone and the associated secondary CT findings were correlated with the clinical outcome (patients with documented passage of stones vs patients in whom conservative treatment failed) by using the nonpaired Student *t* test and the Mann-Whitney *U* test, respectively. The patients who were lost to follow-up were excluded from the statistical analysis.

The sensitivity, specificity, and positive predictive value were calculated for parameters identified as statistically significant (ie, with a P value of less than .05) to assess the value of each parameter in the prediction of passage of the ureteral stone. Receiver operating characteristic (ROC) curves were constructed for the same parameters. The programs LABROC and ROCFIT, developed by Rockette et al (12), were used for the quantitative and the qualitative parameters, respectively.

Spearman correlation coefficients were calculated to test the relationships among stone diameter and the other parameters identified as statistically significant.

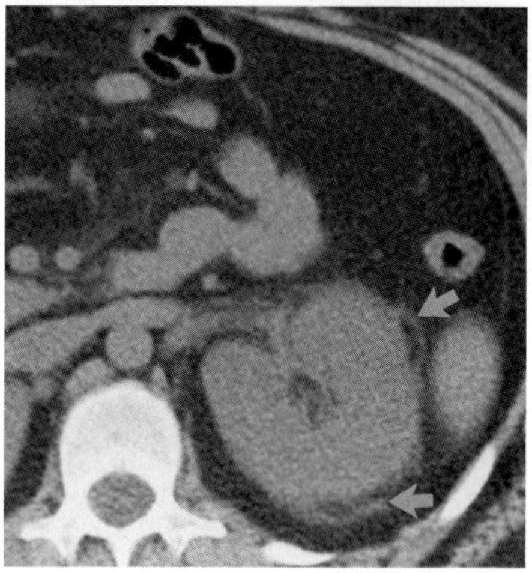

Figure 1. Unenhanced helical CT scan in a 40-year-old woman with a 1-mm-diameter ureteral stone located at the ureterovesical junction on the left reveals a severe degree of perinephric fat stranding (arrows) on the left. The stone passed spontaneously.

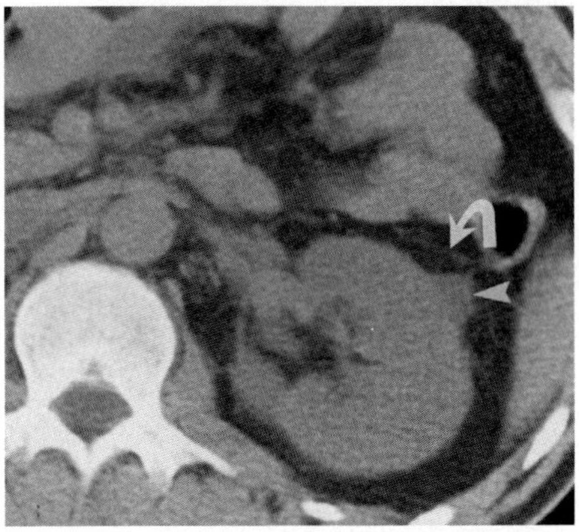

Figure 2. Unenhanced helical CT scan in a 32-year-old man with a 2-mm-diameter ureteral stone at the ureterovesical junction on the left reveals a large perinephric fluid collection (arrowhead) on the left. Mild thickening of the renal fascia (arrow) is also seen. The stone passed spontaneously.

RESULTS

Of the 69 stones in 69 patients, 22 (32%) passed spontaneously, 12 (17%) did not respond to conservative management, and 35 (51%) were lost to follow-up. Passage of the 22 stones was confirmed by means of passage through the urethra in two patients, with follow-up abdominal plain radiography or excretory urography in 19 patients, and with clinical examination results in one patient. Of the 12 stones in which conservative management failed, nine needed surgical intervention, and three were still present after 4 weeks.

Of 14 stones in the proximal ureter, two (14%) passed spontaneously, six (43%) did not respond to conservative management, and six (43%) were lost to follow-up. Of 17 stones in the distal ureter, four (24%) passed spontaneously, three (18%) did not respond to conservative management, and 10 (59%) were lost to follow up (the percentages do not total 100% due to rounding). Of 38 stones at

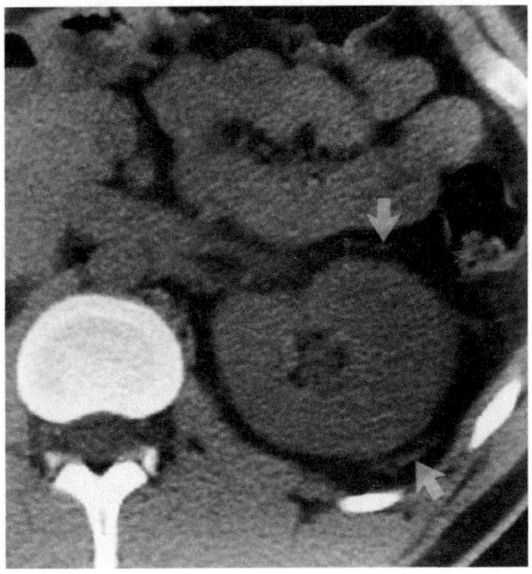

Figure 3. Unenhanced helical CT scan in a 22-year-old man with a 6-mm-diameter ureteral stone in the left distal part of the ureter shows a few thick strands (arrows), graded as moderate, in the left perinephric space. Mild renal enlargement and mild hydronephrosis (intrarenal pelviectasis) are also present. The stone passed spontaneously.

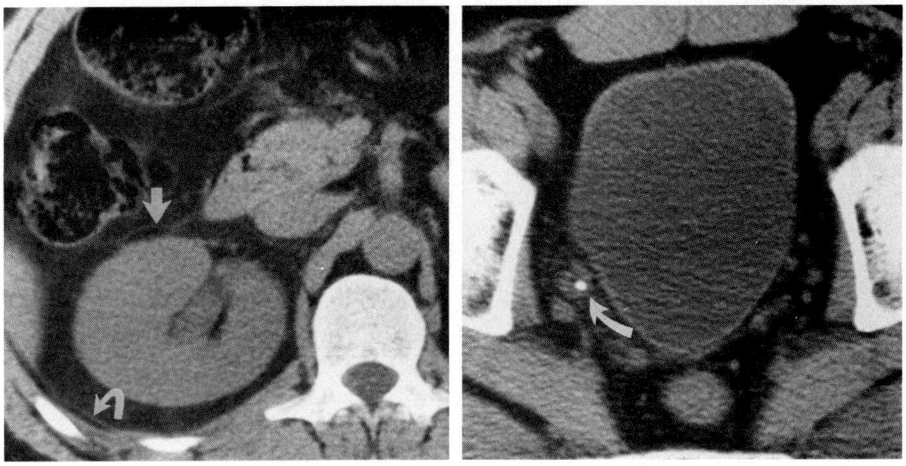

a. b.

Figure 5. Unenhanced helical CT scans in a 42-year-old man with a 4-mm-diameter ureteral stone at the right ureterovesical junction that failed to pass spontaneously. **(a)** CT scan through the level of the kidneys demonstrates mild perinephric fat stranding (straight arrow) and mild thickening of the renal fascia (curved arrow) on the right. Mild renal enlargement and mild hydronephrosis (intrarenal pelviectasis) are also present. **(b)** CT scan obtained through the lower pelvis reveals a stone (arrow) in the right ureterovesical junction surrounded by a halo of soft-tissue attenuation (tissue rim sign).

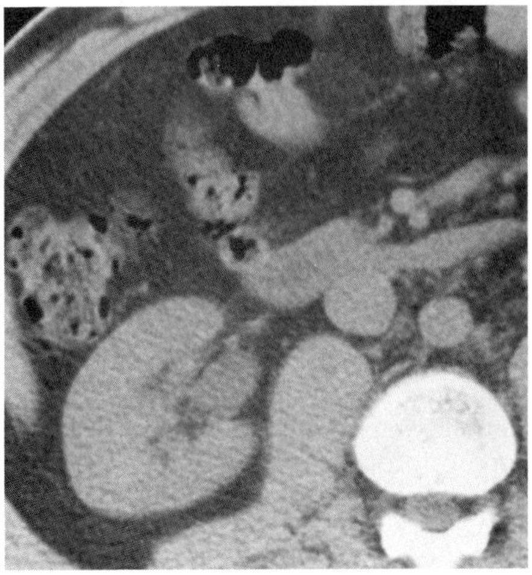

Figure 4. Unenhanced helical CT scan in a 25-year-old man with a 3.5-mm-diameter ureteral stone in the right proximal part of the ureter reveals no perinephric fat stranding or perinephric fluid collections. The stone failed to pass spontaneously.

the ureterovesical junction, 16 (42%) passed spontaneously, three (8%) did not respond to conservative management, and 19 (50%) were lost to follow-up.

The degree of perinephric fat stranding (grade: 2.0 ± 0.7 [mean ± 1 standard deviation] vs 1.4 ± 0.7; $P = .044$) and the amount of perinephric fluid (grade: 1.6 ± 0.9 vs 0.9 ± 0.7; $P = .021$) were significantly more severe in cases of stones that passed spontaneously than in cases of stones that did not respond to conservative management (Figs 1–5). Spontaneous stone passage also correlated with a significantly smaller stone diameter (mean: 2.9 mm ± 2.0 [range, 1.0–8.5 mm] vs 7.8 mm ± 3.3 [range: 3.0–11.5 mm]; $P < .001$). Presence of the tissue rim sign (grade: 1.2 ± 0.6 vs 1.3 ± 0.8; $P = .79$), hydronephrosis (grade: 1.2 ± 0.3 vs 1.6 ± 0.8; $P = .18$), thickening of the renal fascia (grade: 1.1 ± 0.5 vs 1.0 ± 0.8; $P = .31$), or renal parenchymal enlargement (ratio: 1.2 ± 0.1 vs 1.3 ± 0.3; $P = .72$) were not significantly different between the two groups. No strong correlation was found between the diameter of the stone and the degree of perinephric fat stranding or the amount of perinephric fluid ($\rho = -0.37$ and -0.40, respectively).

Patient outcome (stone passage vs nonpassage) with respect to stone diameter, perinephric fat stranding, and perinephric fluid collection is presented in Tables 1–3. When a stone diameter of 3 mm or smaller was used as a predictor of stone passage, the sensitivity, specificity, and positive predictive value were 77%, 92%, and 94%, respectively. When grade 3 perinephric stranding was used as a predictor of stone passage, the sensitivity, specificity, and positive predictive value were 18%, 100%, and 100%, respectively. When a grade 2 or higher perinephric fluid collection was used as a predictor of stone passage, the sensitivity, specificity, and positive predictive value were 45%, 92%, and 91%, respectively. When a stone diameter of larger than 7 mm was used as a predictor of unsuccessful medical management, the sensitivity, specificity, and positive predictive value were 58%, 95%, and 88%, respectively.

ROC curves were constructed for stone diameter, the degree of perinephric fat stranding, and the amount of perinephric fluid in the prediction of stone passage (Fig 6). The areas under the ROC curves (± 1 standard deviation) for stone diameter, degree of perinephric fat stranding, and amount of perinephric fluid were 0.93 ± 0.04, 0.73 ± 0.09, and 0.76 ± 0.08, respectively.

DISCUSSION

Our results show that, in addition to a small stone diameter, secondary CT findings of an increased degree of perinephric fat stranding and the presence of perinephric fluid collections are useful in the prediction of spontaneous stone passage. The finding of a stone diameter of 3 mm or smaller was both sensitive and specific for the prediction of stone passage (77% and 94%, respectively). In the absence of clinical evidence of infection, a moderate to severe perinephric fluid collection (grade 2 or higher) and a severe degree of perinephric fat stranding (grade 3) were specific (92% and 100%, respectively) but not sensitive (45% and 18%, respectively) for the prediction of stone passage. A stone diameter of larger than 7 mm was specific (95%) for the prediction of unsuccessful medical management.

The degree of perinephric fat stranding and the presence of perinephric fluid collections were not useful in the prediction of unsuccessful medical management because of substantial overlap of the grading score between the two groups. The degree of hydronephrosis, although not statistically significant, tended to be less severe in cases of passed stones than in cases of stones that did not respond to conservative management. The presence of a tissue rim sign, thickening of the renal fascia, and enlargement of the renal parenchyma were not useful for prediction of the clinical outcome.

The CT findings of perinephric stranding were first described by Winfield et al (13) as filiform, curvilinear areas of soft-tissue attenuation in the perinephric space in patients with renal venous thrombosis. These areas of soft-tissue attenuation were attributed to venous collateral vessels in the perinephric space. Later, perinephric stranding was reported (14) in patients with an inflammatory or a neoplastic condition. Kunin (15) reported that the perinephric space is divided into multiple compartments by means of fibrous lamellae, or "bridging septa," which become thickened in the presence of disease and become readily visible in that state. These bridging septa may serve as a conduit for the spread of fluid, inflammation, or neoplasm from the kidney to outside the perinephric space (16). In addition to the bridging septa, a rich network of lymphatic channels is present in the perinephric space (17). These lymphatic channels provide potential pathways for the spread of disease or fluid to or from the perinephric space (16,18).

Perinephric stranding has been reported (1,4,5) as an important secondary sign for the unenhanced helical CT diagnosis of ureterolithiasis (1,4,5). Although perinephric stranding is a nonspecific finding, in the clinical setting of acute flank pain it proved to have relatively high sensitivity (82%) and specificity (94%) for the presence of a ureteral calculus (5).

Immediately after acute ureteral obstruction, the intraluminal pressure of the collecting system is increased. One hour after obstruction, the pressure becomes three to five times greater than the pressure before the obstruction (19–21). At this point, coaptation of the ureteral walls does not occur. Smooth muscle fibers in the urinary tract respond to the increase in pressure by contracting, which increases the tension. The frequency and amplitude of peristalsis also increase. With persistent obstruction, the smooth muscles of the urinary tract contract less forcefully, the tension of the walls of the obstructed tract decreases, and dilation of the collecting system ensues. The intraluminal pressure normalizes and peristalsis decreases, after prolonged obstruction (22).

Decompression of the obstructed urinary tract, however, cannot be entirely accounted for by dilatation and decreased smooth muscle tone in the walls of the urinary tract. The glomerular filtration pressure and renal blood flow are also reduced. The escape of urine into the renal interstitium (pyelotubular backflow), across the renal pelvis into the renal sinus (pyelosinus backflow), or into the lymphatic system (pyelolymphatic backflow) or the renal venous system (pyelovenous backflow) plays a role in decompression of the intraluminal pressure (20,21). An increase in the lymphatic flow in the perinephric space also results from the elevated intrarenal venous pressure and venous stasis (23).

Perinephric stranding seen at CT is probably a manifestation of the increased pressure in the collecting system during the acute phase of ureteral obstruction, which in turn causes increased lymphatic flow in the perinephric space secondary to pyelolymphatic backflow and elevation of the intrarenal venous pressure. Pyelosinus and pyelovenous backflow of urine may also contribute to perinephric stranding. A perinephric fluid collection probably represents a similar pathophysiologic process, with confluent fluid trapped most noticeably along the renal surface.

Increased pressure in the collecting system is considered to be the most important propelling force that causes a stone to move down the ureter, at least during the acute phase of obstruction (24,25). This is probably why an increased degree of perinephric fat stranding and the presence of perinephric fluid collections were associated with an increased rate of spontaneous stone passage. Chapman et al (11) reported an association between pyelosinus extravasation at excretory urography and a higher rate of spontaneous stone passage. Perinephric fat stranding and perinephric fluid collections seen at CT occur as a result of a pathophysiologic condition similar to that seen at urography in cases of pyelosinus extravasation. Indeed, our data support the findings of Chapman et al that increased pressure in

TABLE 1
Patient Outcome with Respect to Stone Size

Outcome	Stone Diameter (mm)							
	≤1	>1 to 2	>2 to 3	>3 to 4	>4 to 5	>5 to 6	>6 to 7	>7
Passage (n = 22)	2	8	7	1	1	1	1	1
Nonpassage (n = 12)	0	0	1	2	1	1	0	7

TABLE 2
Patient Outcome with Respect to Perinephric Fat Stranding

Outcome	Grade						
	0	0.5	1.0	1.5	2.0	2.5	3.0
Passage (n = 22)	0	1	2	7	3	5	4
Nonpassage (n = 12)	0	2	4	2	2	2	0

TABLE 3
Patient Outcome with Respect to Perinephric Fluid Collection

Outcome	Grade						
	0	0.5	1.0	1.5	2.0	2.5	3.0
Passage (n = 22)	1	4	2	5	4	4	2
Nonpassage (n = 12)	3	2	3	3	1	0	0

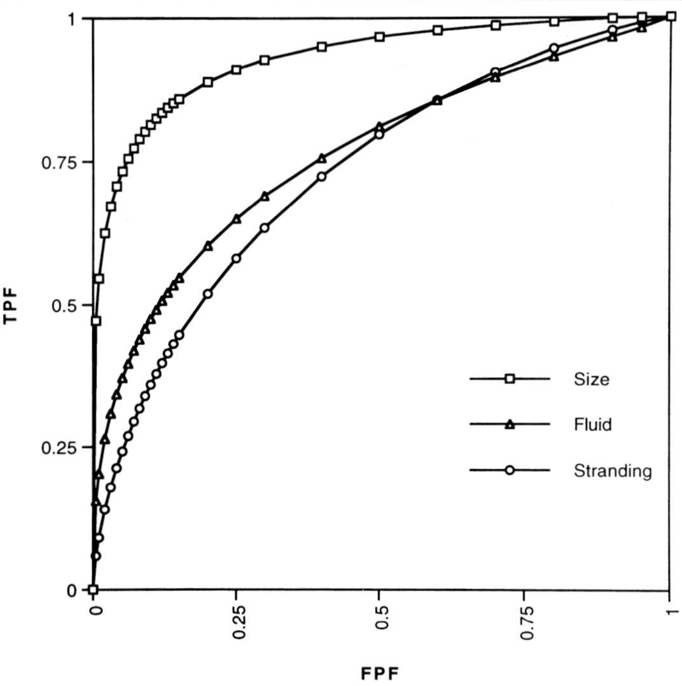

Figure 6. ROC curves for stone diameter, degree of perinephric fat stranding, and degree of perinephric fluid collection in the prediction of passage of ureteral stones. The areas under the ROC curves for stone size (ie, diameter), degree of perinephric fat stranding, and amount of perinephric fluid were 0.93, 0.73, and 0.76, respectively. *FPF* = false-positive fraction, *TPF* = true-positive fraction.

the collecting system as manifested by pyelosinus extravasation is associated with a high likelihood of spontaneous stone passage. Our data contradict the popular notion that a high degree of obstruction suggests the need for urgent intervention.

Hydronephrosis probably reflects a subacute to chronic phase of obstruction, when the intraluminal pressure has normalized and the peristalsis has decreased (22). Patients who present with a longer duration of pain are known to have a lower rate of stone passage (8,10). Our results showed that hydronephrosis tended to be less severe in cases of passed stones than in cases of stones that did not respond to conservative management, although this result was not statistically significant. Difficulty in the accurate evaluation of the degree of hydronephrosis at CT may account for the lack of statistical significance.

Thickening of the renal fascia (26) and enlargement of the renal parenchyma (5), although pathophysiologically similar to perinephric fat stranding and the presence of perinephric fluid, were not useful in the prediction of the clinical outcome in cases of ureteral stones. These changes may be less sensitive to increased pressure in the collecting system. In addition, renal parenchymal enlargement, measured as the short axis diameter of the kidney, may not truly represent thickening of the renal parenchyma because the measurement includes the collecting system, which may be dilated.

The tissue rim sign was originally described by Smith et al (1) as a circumferential rim of soft-tissue attenuation around the ureteral stone; this sign probably represents local inflammation and edema of the ureteral wall. Although not sensitive (50%–77%), the rim sign is highly specific (92%–100%) for the presence of a ureteral stone and for differentiation from a phlebolith (6,7). The rim sign can be thought of as analogous to excretory urographic findings of edema in the bladder wall at the ureterovesical junction around an impacted stone. Clinical and experimental evidence suggest that local inflammation and edema of the ureteral wall are important for arresting the passage of ureteral stones (27,28). Anti-inflammatory agents have been shown to facilitate stone passage by means of reduction of ureteral edema (28–30). Our results failed to demonstrate this correlation, probably because the prevalence of the tissue rim sign seen at CT is not high. Also, the tissue rim sign is more frequently observed at CT in cases of smaller stones (6,7).

The importance of the size of the stone to the prediction of clinical outcome has been well documented with excretory urography (8–10). The larger the stone, the less likely it is to pass and the more likely it is to necessitate intervention. We obtained similar results with CT by using the stone diameter measured in the axial plane.

Prediction of the outcome in a case of a ureteral stone becomes important in the decision about when to intervene. The clinical decision is dependent not only on the likelihood of passage but also on the degree of pain, impairment of renal function, the presence of a superimposed infection, and the presence of coexistent morbidity (31). The degrees of perinephric stranding and perinephric fluid collection were considered to be independent of stone diameter in the prediction of outcome because a strong correlation was not found in our study. We believe, therefore, that additional predictive information can be gained with the use of these parameters. The areas under the ROC curves for the degree of perinephric fat stranding and the amount of perinephric fluid, however, were relatively low (0.73 and 0.76, respectively). Therefore, the actual effect of these parameters in clinical decision making is not certain. The area under the ROC curve for stone diameter was 0.93, and stone diameter remains the most important factor in the prediction of clinical outcome.

One limitation of our study was that a relatively large number of patients (35 [51%] of 69) were excluded from the statistical analysis because they were lost to follow-up. One could argue that the reason for this large number was that stone passage occurred in the majority of the patients, and the patients therefore did not return for follow-up. If we assume that all stones 2 mm or smaller in diameter in the distal ureter passed spontaneously, an additional 11 patients from the group lost to follow-up would be included in the passed stone group. When we recalculated our data with this assumption, the perinephric fluid collections remained significantly more severe in cases of stones that passed spontaneously than in cases of stones that did not respond to conservative management (P = .043). The degree of perinephric fat stranding tended to be more severe and hydronephrosis tended to be less severe in cases of stones that passed spontaneously (P = .054 and .086, respectively).

Although the assessment of the degree of perinephric changes (fat stranding and fluid collections) is somewhat subjective, we attempted a semiquantitative assessment by means of a grading system. In addition, caution should be used in the interpretation of the secondary CT findings of increased perinephric fat stranding and perinephric fluid collections as indicators of a favorable outcome in cases of a ureteral stone when the patient has signs of a superimposed infection. Patients with pyonephrosis may have similar perinephric changes. Clinical correlation is essential to avoid this misinterpretation.

Fielding et al (32) found that the presence of perinephric changes seen at CT was not useful for the prediction of stone passage. We semiquantitatively assessed the perinephric changes by using a four-point grading system; we also excluded cases of ureteropelvic stones and of pyonephrosis, which may account for the difference between our results and those of Fielding et al.

In summary, CT findings of a smaller stone size and a higher degree of perinephric fat stranding or an increased amount of perinephric fluid are associated with a higher likelihood of spontaneous passage. A higher degree of perinephric fat stranding or an increased amount of perinephric fluid are believed to reflect increased intraluminal pressure of the collecting system. This additional information may aid in the prediction of clinical outcome in cases of a ureteral stone, although the actual clinical effect of this information has yet to be determined in a large, prospective series.

References

1. Smith RC, Rosenfield AT, Choe KA, et al. Acute flank pain: comparison of non-contrast-enhanced CT and intravenous urography. Radiology 1995; 194:789–794.
2. Sommer FG, Jeffrey RB Jr, Rubin GD, et al. Detection of ureteral calculi in patients with suspected renal colic: value of reformatted noncontrast helical CT. AJR 1995; 165:509–513.
3. Smith RC, Verga M, McCarthy S, Rosenfield AT. Diagnosis of acute flank pain: value of unenhanced helical CT. AJR 1996; 166:97–101.
4. Katz DS, Lane MJ, Sommer FG. Unenhanced helical CT of ureteral stones: incidence of associated urinary tract findings. AJR 1996; 166:1319–1322.
5. Smith RC, Verga M, Dalrymple N, McCarthy S, Rosenfield AT. Acute ureteral obstruction: value of secondary signs on helical unenhanced CT. AJR 1996; 167:1109–1113.
6. Kawashima A, Sandler CM, Boridy IC, Takahashi N, Benson GS, Goldman SM. Unenhanced helical CT of ureterolithiasis: value of the tissue rim sign. AJR 1997; 168:997–1000.
7. Heneghan JP, Dalrymple NC, Verga M, Rosenfield AT, Smith RC. Soft-tissue "rim" sign in the diagnosis of ureteral calculi with use of unenhanced helical CT. Radiology 1997; 202:709–711.
8. Sandegard E. Prognosis of stone in the ureter. Acta Chir Scand 1956; 219(suppl):1–67.
9. Ueno A, Kawamura T, Ogawa A, Takayasu H. Relation of spontaneous passage of ureteral calculi to size. Urology 1977; 10:544–546.
10. Morse RM, Resnick MI. Ureteral calculi: natural history and treatment in an era of advanced technology. J Urol 1991; 145:263–265.
11. Chapman JP, Gonzalez J, Diokno AC. Significance of urinary extravasation during renal colic. Urology 1987; 30:541–545.
12. Rockette HE, Gur D, Metz CE. The use of continuous and discrete confidence judgements in receiver operator characteristic studies of diagnostic imaging techniques. Invest Radiol 1992; 27:169–172.
13. Winfield AC, Gerlock AJ Jr, Shaff MI. Perirenal cobwebs: a CT sign of renal vein thrombosis. J Comput Assist Tomogr 1981; 5:705–708.
14. Feuerstein IM, Zeman RK, Jaffe MH, Clark LR, David CL. Perirenal cobwebs: the expanding CT differential diagnosis. J Comput Assist Tomogr 1984; 8:1128–1130.
15. Kunin M. Bridging septa of the perinephric space: anatomic, pathologic, and diagnostic considerations. Radiology 1986; 158:361–365.
16. Aizenstein RI, Wilbur AC, O'Neil HK. Interfascial and perinephric pathways in the spread of retroperitoneal disease: refined concepts based on CT observations. AJR 1997; 168:639–643.
17. Meyers MA. The extraperitoneal spaces: normal and pathological anatomy. In: Dynamic radiology of the abdomen. 4th ed. New York, NY: Springer-Verlag, 1994; 220–342.
18. Wilbur AC, Turk JN, Capek V. Perirenal metastases from lung cancer: CT diagnosis. J Comput Assist Tomogr 1992; 16:589–591.
19. Rose JG, Gillenwater JY. Pathophysiology of ureteral obstruction. Am J Physiol 1973; 225:830–837.
20. Gillenwater JY. The pathophysiology of urinary tract obstruction. In: Walsh PC, Retik AB, Stamey TA, Vaughan ED Jr, eds. Campbell's urology. 6th ed. Philadelphia, Pa: Saunders, 1992; 499–532.
21. Klahr S. Urinary tract obstruction. In: Schrier RW, Gottschalk CW, eds. Diseases of the kidney. 6th ed. Boston, Mass: Little, Brown, 1997; 709–738.
22. Holden D, George NJ, Rickards D, Barnard RJ, O'Reilly PH. Renal pelvic pressures in human chronic obstructive uropathy. Br J Urol 1984; 56:565–570.
23. Holmes MJ, O'Morchoe PJ, O'Morchoe CCC. The role of renal lymph in hydronephrosis. Invest Urol 1977; 15:215–219.
24. Sivula A, Lehtonen T. Spontaneous passage of artificial concretions applied in the rabbit ureter. Scand J Urol Nephrol 1967; 1:259–263.
25. Algood CB, Sood N, Fairchild T, Mayo ME. Experimental study of ureteral calculus disease: effects of calculus size, obstruction, and hydration. J Urol 1983; 130:999–1004.
26. Parienty RA, Pradel J, Picard JD, Ducellier R, Lubrano JM, Smolarski N. Visibility and thickening of the renal fascia on computed tomograms. Radiology 1981; 139:119–124.
27. Holmlund D, Hassler O. A method of studying the ureteral reaction to artificial concrements. Acta Chir Scand 1965; 130:335–343.
28. Borghi L, Meschi T, Amato F, et al. Nifedipine and methylprednisolone in facilitating ureteral stone passage: a randomized, double-blinded, placebo-controlled study. J Urol 1994; 152:1095–1098.
29. Holmlund D. Oxyphenbutazone in the treatment of acute ureteral stone disease. Scand J Urol Nephrol 1968; 1(suppl 1):63–66.
30. Nygard A, Bjorneby S. Oxyphenbutazone in the treatment of acute ureteral stone disease. Scand J Urol Nephrol 1975; 9:36–38.
31. Drach GW. Urinary lithiasis: etiology, diagnosis, and medical management. In: Walsh PC, Retik AB, Stamey TA, Vaughan ED Jr, eds. Campbell's urology. 6th ed. Philadelphia, Pa: Saunders, 1992; 2085–2156.
32. Fielding JR, Silverman SG, Samuel S. Spiral CT of ureteral stones: predicting the need for intervention (abstr). Radiology 1997; 205(P):508.

Benign and Malignant Ovarian Masses: Selection of the Most Discriminating Gray-Scale and Doppler Sonographic Features[1]

Douglas L. Brown, MD
Peter M. Doubilet, MD, PhD
Frank H. Miller, MD[2]
Mary C. Frates, MD
Faye C. Laing, MD
Donald N. DiSalvo, MD
Carol B. Benson, MD
Mark H. Lerner, MD

Index terms:
Ovary, neoplasms, 852.30
Receiver operating characteristic curve (ROC)
Ultrasound (US), Doppler studies, 852.12984

Radiology 1998; 208:103–110

Abbreviations:
PI = pulsatility index
RI = resistance index
ROC = receiver operating characteristic

[1] From the Department of Radiology, Brigham and Women's Hospital, Harvard Medical School, 75 Francis St, Boston, MA 02115. From the 1995 RSNA scientific assembly. Received October 15, 1997; revision requested December 30; revision received January 26, 1998; accepted February 6. **Address reprint requests to** D.L.B.

[2] Current address: Department of Diagnostic Radiology, Northwestern Memorial Hospital and Northwestern University Medical School, Chicago, Ill.

PURPOSE: To determine the gray-scale and Doppler sonographic features that best enable discrimination between malignant and benign ovarian masses and develop a scoring system for accurate diagnosis with these features.

MATERIALS AND METHODS: Gray-scale and Doppler sonographic features of 211 adnexal masses were correlated with the final diagnosis; the most discriminating features for malignancy were selected with stepwise logistic regression.

RESULTS: Twenty-eight masses were malignant and 183 benign. All masses with a markedly hyperechoic solid component or no solid component were benign. For masses with a nonhyperechoic solid component, additional features that allowed statistically significant discrimination of benignity from malignancy were, in decreasing order of importance, (*a*) location of flow at conventional color Doppler imaging, (*b*) amount of free intraperitoneal fluid, and (*c*) presence and thickness of septations. A scoring formula that made use of values based on the logistic regression equation had an area under the receiver operating characteristic curve of 0.98 ± 0.01. The cutoff score with the highest accuracy had a sensitivity of 93% and specificity of 93%.

CONCLUSION: A solid component is the most statistically significant predictor of a malignant ovarian mass. A multiparameter scoring system that uses three gray-scale and one Doppler feature, developed by means of stepwise logistic regression, has high sensitivity and specificity for predicting malignancy.

A number of gray-scale and Doppler sonographic features have been studied for the ability to allow distinction between benign and malignant ovarian masses. Initial reports suggested a high degree of accuracy for some of these features, such as the pulsatility index (PI) or resistance index (RI) (1–4). Further experience revealed, however, that no single parameter has sufficiently high sensitivity, specificity, or predictive values to allow confident diagnosis or exclusion of malignancy (5–20). Subsequently, most investigators have found gray-scale sonography to be as good as or better than Doppler sonography in allowing distinction between benign and malignant ovarian masses (6,11,15–17, 20–27).

Some investigators, in an effort to improve the accuracy of sonography in discriminating benign from malignant ovarian masses, have proposed scoring systems based on several gray-scale and/or Doppler sonographic features (8,23,26,28–34). A scoring system works by assigning a numeric value to each of several features that may be present. For any adnexal mass visualized at ultrasound, one determines which features are present, adds the corresponding numeric values to yield a score for that mass, and diagnoses malignancy or benignity according to whether the score is greater or less than a cutoff score.

Most of the scoring systems that have appeared in the literature, however, have important shortcomings. Although the optimal way to develop a scoring system from a set of data is to use statistical regression analysis to determine which features to include and what numeric values to assign them, we are aware of only one published study in which this was done (32), and that study did not include Doppler sonography. Furthermore,

Author contributions:
Guarantor of integrity of entire study, D.L.B.; study concepts and design, D.L.B., P.M.D.; definition of intellectual content, D.L.B., P.M.D.; literature research, D.L.B.; clinical studies, D.L.B., P.M.D., M.C.F., F.C.L., D.N.D., C.B.B., M.H.L.; data acquisition, D.L.B., P.M.D., F.H.M., M.C.F., F.C.L., D.N.D., C.B.B., M.H.L.; data analysis, D.L.B., P.M.D., F.H.M.; statistical analysis, D.L.B., P.M.D.; manuscript preparation, D.L.B.; manuscript editing and review, D.L.B., P.M.D., F.H.M., M.C.F., F.C.L., D.N.D., C.B.B.

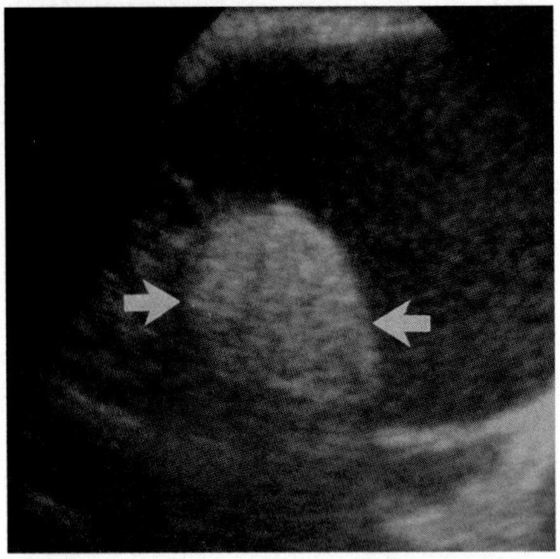

Figure 1. Ovarian mass with a hyperechoic solid component. Sagittal gray-scale sonogram shows a highly echogenic nodule (arrows) within a mature cystic teratoma.

most scoring systems fail to account for the echogenicity of the solid portion of a mass, despite the fact that a highly echogenic solid component is strong evidence of a teratoma (32,35–44).

The purpose of our study was to determine which gray-scale and/or Doppler sonographic features best enable discrimination of benign from malignant ovarian masses and to develop a scoring system based on these features by using stepwise logistic regression analysis.

TABLE 1
Gray-Scale Sonographic Features of 211 Ovarian Masses

Gray-Scale Feature	Benign Masses	Malignant Masses	P Value
Solid component*			<.001
None	98	0	
Hyperechoic	27	0	
Nonhyperechoic	58	28	
Fluid component			<.001
Anechoic	67	13	
Echogenic†	107	6	
None	9	9	
Septations			.02
Thin (<3 mm)	47	1	
Thick (≥3 mm)	32	4	
None	104	23	
Wall			<.001
Thin (<3 mm)	91	8	
Thick (≥3 mm)	78	9	
None discernible	14	11	
Free fluid‡			<.001
Normal	179	19	
Abnormal	4	9	
Unilateral or bilateral§			.23
Unilateral	157	20	
Bilateral	13	4	
Size, average‖ (cm)#	5.1 ± 2.7	5.9 ± 3.2	.17
Size, maximum (cm)#	6.0 ± 3.3	6.9 ± 3.8	.24

*The term *solid component* refers to any focal solid area, regardless of its shape, or to an entire mass if it is uniformly solid; this term does not refer to septations or diffuse wall thickening. The term *hyperechoic solid component* refers to a highly echogenic nodule or a mass that is composed entirely of highly echogenic material, both of which are characteristic of teratomas (35,37–46). Any other solid component was considered nonhyperechoic. Care was taken not to designate a nodule as highly echogenic solely because of enhanced sound transmission due to fluid between the nodule and the transducer (16). Calcifications alone were not considered highly echogenic nodules.

†Fluid was considered echogenic if, while we attempted to keep gain settings at a subjectively appropriate level, there were echoes within the fluid, including diffuse low-level echoes typical of an endometrioma (36,47–50) or a reticular or "fishnet" pattern typical of fibrin strands in a hemorrhagic cyst (16,21,36,51). Such fibrin strands were not considered septations.

‡In a premenopausal patient, no free intraperitoneal fluid or a small amount in the cul-de-sac was considered normal; free intraperitoneal fluid that filled the cul-de-sac or extended around the ovaries, above the uterus, into the paracolic gutters, or into the upper abdomen was considered abnormal. In a postmenopausal patient, any amount of free intraperitoneal fluid was considered abnormal.

§Values are number of patients.

‖Average of maximum diameter and the two orthogonal diameters.

#Values are mean ± standard deviation.

MATERIALS AND METHODS

Our study set consisted of all adnexal masses scanned at our institution between July 1991 and July 1996 in which (*a*) both gray-scale and Doppler sonography had been performed and (*b*) a histopathologic diagnosis had been made or a follow-up sonogram had demonstrated resolution of the mass. We excluded masses in pregnant women, masses in premenopausal patients who were scanned more than 10 days after a known last menstrual period, simple cysts less than 2 cm in greatest diameter in premenopausal women, and masses that were clearly extraovarian at sonography (eg, pedunculated leiomyoma, hydrosalpinx). We excluded women beyond the 10th day of the menstrual cycle in an attempt to avoid low-resistance flow associated with the corpus luteum; such flow may be similar to the low-resistance flow associated with malignant neoplasms.

The study population included 194 patients with 211 masses (17 patients had bilateral masses). The mean patient age was 39.9 years ± 12.7 (standard deviation) (range, 16–78 years). The Doppler features in 44 of the masses were reported previously (5); the remaining 167 masses were evaluated since that study.

Transvaginal sonography with a 5-MHz transducer was performed unless the mass was judged to be adequately imaged with transabdominal sonography performed with a 3.5-MHz transducer (generally when the mass was relatively large or superiorly located) or the patient declined transvaginal sonography. A model 128 or XP unit (Acuson, Mountain View, Calif) was used. Of the 211 masses, 83 (39%) were evaluated with both transvaginal and transabdominal sonography, 75 (36%) with transvaginal sonography alone, and 53 (25%) with transabdominal sonography alone.

Several gray-scale, Doppler, and clinical features were analyzed for each mass. Gray-scale features (Table 1) included the presence and nature of the solid component (Figs 1–3), fluid component, septations (Fig 2), and wall, as well as the presence of free fluid and the size of the mass. Doppler features (Table 2) included the presence and location of flow detected with conventional color Doppler sonography (Fig 3), as well as the lowest and average values of RI and PI, the highest peak systolic velocity, and the presence of a diastolic notch. The sonograms were obtained prospectively to evaluate all of the preceding gray-scale and Doppler features of each mass. Recording of each feature for statistical analysis was performed later by one investigator (D.L.B.), who

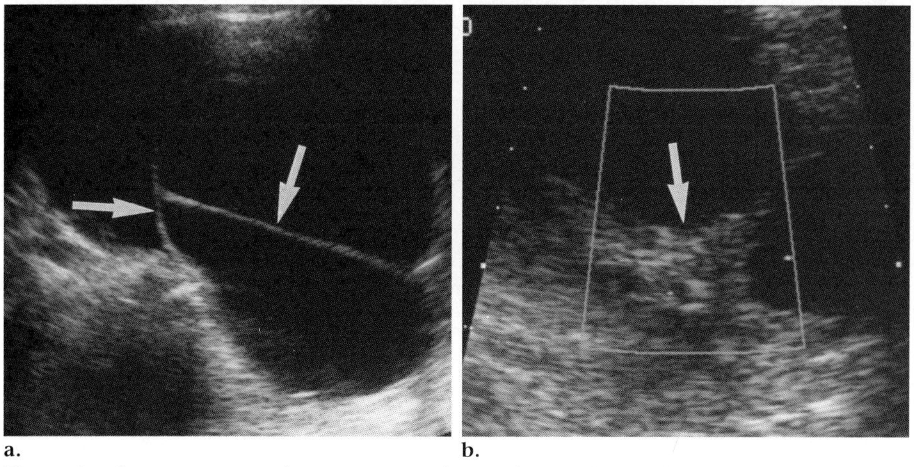

Figure 2. Ovarian mass with septations and a nonhyperechoic solid component. **(a)** Grayscale sonogram shows two thin septations (arrows) within a cystic mass. **(b)** Black-and-white representation of a color Doppler sonogram shows no flow in a small, nonhyperechoic solid component (arrow). There was also no detectable flow in the septations (shown in **a**), and there was a trace (normal) amount of free intraperitoneal fluid. From Table 4, the malignancy score was 394, correctly predictive of benignity; from Table 5, there was a less than 1% probability of malignancy. The mass was a mucinous cystadenoma.

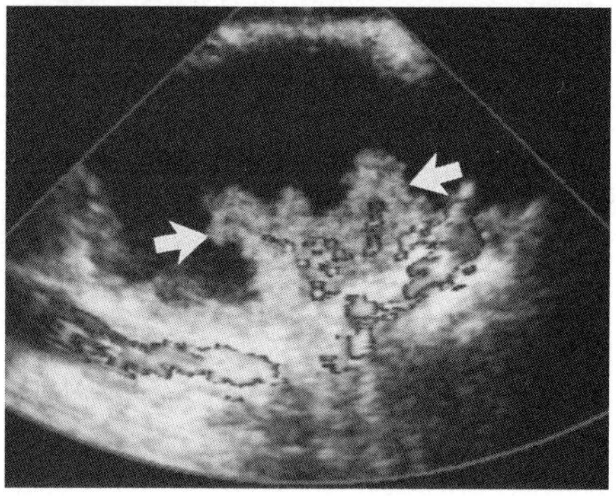

Figure 3. Ovarian mass with a nonhyperechoic solid component. Black-and-white representation of a color Doppler sonogram shows central flow within a nonhyperechoic solid component (between arrows). There was no associated free intraperitoneal fluid and no septations in this serous cystadenoma of borderline malignancy. The malignancy score was 469 (Table 4), above the cutoff of 453 and correctly predictive of malignancy, and there was a 75% probability of malignancy (Table 5).

TABLE 2
Doppler Sonographic and Clinical Features in 211 Ovarian Masses

Doppler or Clinical Feature	Benign Masses	Malignant Masses	*P* Value
Doppler features			
Location of flow at color imaging*			<.001
Central (and peripheral in some cases)	31	24	
Peripheral only	90	2	
None detected	62	2	
Pulsed Doppler features			
RI, lowest†	0.59 ± 0.17	0.45 ± 0.14	<.001
RI, average†	0.63 ± 0.15	0.51 ± 0.12	<.001
PI, lowest†	1.16 ± 0.76	0.67 ± 0.40	<.001
PI, average†	1.34 ± 0.84	0.79 ± 0.38	<.001
Peak systolic velocity (m/sec)‡	0.20 ± 0.16	0.20 ± 0.15	.70
Diastolic notch§			.12
Present	21	1	
Absent	95	24	
Clinical features			
Age (y)‖	38.8 ± 12.0	48.0 ± 15.4	.01
Menopausal status#			.06
Premenopausal	122	13	
Peri- or postmenopausal	29	9	
Had undergone hysterectomy	19	2	

*Flow was considered central if it was within any solid component, as described in Table 1, or within a septation. Flow was considered peripheral if it was within or immediately adjacent to the wall of the mass. Flow in both locations was recorded as central. Although arterial flow was always sought, in six masses all pulsed Doppler waveforms were venous; five of these masses were benign and one was malignant. In these six masses, flow was considered to be present. Before a mass was recorded as having no flow, Doppler settings were optimized to detect slow flow.

†Values in masses in which arterial flow was detected. Values are mean ± standard deviation.

‡The highest peak systolic velocity obtained for each mass was analyzed, but this value was not a true velocity because no angle correction for direction of flow could be performed due to the small size and short length of vessels seen. Values are mean ± standard deviation.

§If a diastolic notch (18,52) was present in any of the waveforms from a mass, a diastolic notch was considered present for that mass. Torsion was present in the single malignant mass with a diastolic notch.

‖Values are mean ± standard deviation.

#Values are number of patients.

had 10 years experience in gynecologic sonography and who was unaware of the final results.

Each patient's age and menopausal status were also recorded (Table 2). The serum level of CA-125 was not included in the analysis because it had been obtained in only 73 patients.

For each mass, we recorded the final diagnosis, which was categorized as benign or malignant. This diagnosis was based on histopathologic evaluation of a surgical specimen whenever one was available. Borderline tumors (53) were considered malignant. In cases in which surgery was not performed and a follow-up sonogram demonstrated resolution of the mass, the lesion was considered benign.

Each gray-scale, Doppler, and clinical feature was assessed individually with regard to its relationship with the final diagnosis (benign vs malignant) by using the Mann-Whitney *U* test for continuous variables, the Fisher exact test for categorical variables with two values, and the χ^2 test (with the Yates correction, as appropriate) for categorical variables with more than two values (StatView; Abacus Concepts, Berkeley, Calif). A *P* value of less than .05 was considered to indicate a statistically significant difference.

To assess the variables jointly, stepwise logistic regression analysis was used to identify the group of features that allowed the best prediction of benignity versus malignancy. Each variable that was individually significant was included in the regression analysis. Logistic regression analysis was used because it deals with prediction of a binary outcome variable (benign vs malignant) from a collection of continuous and categorical variables. The stepwise analysis was performed as an upward stepping procedure, with a P value of less than .05 required for inclusion, by using the SYSTAT Logit statistical software package (SYSTAT, Evanston, Ill). The stepwise regression process identifies the group of variables that is the best predictor of outcome. This process also yields a regression formula with a coefficient for each variable that can be used as the basis for a scoring system. Analysis of receiver operating characteristic (ROC) curves for the scoring system and for the pulsed Doppler indexes was performed (54,55). If a particular variable is not selected for inclusion with the stepwise regression procedure, this result does not mean that the feature by itself is not a statistically significant discriminator between malignancy and benignity. This result does mean, however, that the feature fails to add any statistically significant additional information over and above that provided by previously selected features.

TABLE 3
Final Diagnoses in 211 Ovarian Masses

Final Diagnosis	No. of Masses
Malignant masses (n = 28)	
Cystadenocarcinoma of ovary	
Serous	9
Endometrioid	2
Clear cell (arose within an endometrioma)	1
Mixed	3
Borderline cystadenoma of ovary	
Serous	6
Mucinous	1
Mixed	1
Metastatic carcinoma (gastric)	1
Granulosa cell tumor	2
Sertoli-Leydig cell tumor	1
Malignant mixed müllerian tumor	1
Benign masses (n = 183)	
Masses that resolved at follow-up sonography (no surgery)	43
Masses histopathologically diagnosed from surgical specimen	
Endometrioma	31
Mature cystic teratoma (one with coexisting mucinous cystadenoma)	27
Hemorrhagic ovarian cyst	20
Cystadenofibroma, serous	11
Simple ovarian cyst (undetermined type)	9
Tubo-ovarian abscess	8
Cystadenoma	
Mucinous	6
Serous	2
Follicular ovarian cyst	5
Hydrosalpinx (one with coexisting hemorrhagic cyst)	5
Paratubal cyst	3
Fibroma	3
Peritoneal inclusion cyst	2
Cystadenofibroma and endometrioma	1
Brenner tumor and hemorrhagic cyst	1
Epidermoid cyst	1
Fibroma and Brenner tumor	1
Leiomyoma of fallopian tube	1
Paraovarian neoplasms	
Paraovarian cyst with papillary adenofibroma	1
Paraovarian cystadenofibroma	1
Paraovarian cystadenoma	1

RESULTS

Twenty-eight (13%) of the 211 masses were malignant, and 183 were benign (Table 3). Of the 17 patients with bilateral masses (13 premenopasual, three postmenopausal, and one who had undergone hysterectomy), four had bilateral malignancies (three premenopausal, one postmenopausal) and 13 had bilateral benign masses. The most common malignancy was primary cystadenocarcinoma; endometrioma, teratoma, and hemorrhagic cyst were the most common histopathologically proved benign lesions.

Evaluation of individual features revealed that most of the gray-scale, Doppler, and clinical features were significantly associated with malignancy versus benignity (Tables 1, 2). Mass size (both mean and maximum) and unilaterality versus bilaterality were the only gray-scale features not significantly associated with malignancy (Table 1).

The only Doppler features not significantly associated with malignancy were peak systolic velocity and diastolic notch (Table 2). The average and lowest values of both RI and PI were significantly associated with malignancy. To assess and compare the performance of lowest RI, average RI, lowest PI, and average PI, ROC curves were generated (Fig 4). There was no significant difference between the areas (54,55) under these four curves (P > .29 for all comparisons), suggesting that these four Doppler indexes do not differ significantly in performance. As for the two clinical features, age was significantly associated with malignancy, but the association of menopausal status did not quite reach statistical significance (Table 2).

Stepwise logistic regression was used to determine which subset of sonographic and clinical features allows the best discrimination between malignancy and benignity. Because this form of statistical analysis requires that each variable have a value in every case, two modifications of the pulsed Doppler indexes were necessary. First, masses with no detectable arterial flow were assigned a lowest and average RI of 1.0. This value was chosen because it is the maximum possible value of RI (unless there is reversed diastolic flow) and both absence of detectable flow and a high RI generally correlate with benignity. Second, PI was not included in the regression analysis because there was no obvious value to assign to PI when there was no flow; furthermore, there was no statistically significant difference in performance for PI versus RI.

The stepwise logistic regression revealed that four features, as a group, were significantly associated with malignancy (Table 4). In decreasing order of importance, these features were as follows: (*a*) solid component (a nonhyperechoic solid component is associated with malignancy); (*b*) location of flow at color Doppler imaging (central flow has a stronger association with malignancy than does solely peripheral flow, which has a stronger association than no flow);

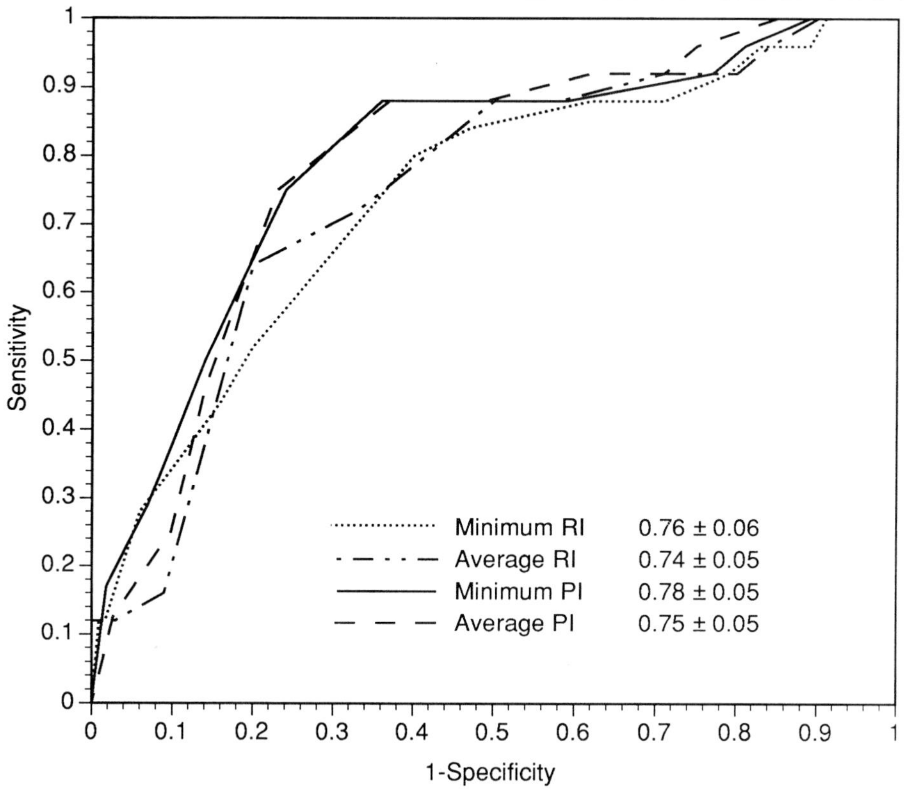

Figure 4. ROC curves for PI and RI. Diagram shows the ROC curves for the minimum and average values of both PI and RI; the curves are based on masses in which arterial flow was detected. The area under each curve (mean ± standard deviation) is also given.

TABLE 4
Results of Stepwise Logistic Regression and Malignancy Scoring System

Sonographic Feature	Regression Coefficient*	Subscore Value†
Solid component		
Any nonhyperechoic solid component	0	394
No solid component	−38.1	13
Markedly hyperechoic solid component	−39.4	0
Flow location		
Central	3.7	37
Peripheral only	0.1	1
None detected	0	0
Free intraperitoneal fluid		
Abnormal amount	3.8	38
Normal amount	0	0
Septation		
None	3.8	38
Thick	2.2	22
Thin	0	0

*This column represents the coefficient of each feature from the logistic regression analysis. The constant term of the regression equation was −6.4.

†Although the coefficients themselves could have been used for the scoring system, we converted all the coefficients to positive integers by multiplying each coefficient by 10 and adding 394 to each of the coefficients for the solid component. The malignancy score of a mass is obtained by assigning the appropriate subscore value for each of the four individual sonographic features and then summing those four values. The constant term of the regression equation was not used in the scoring system. The *P* values for inclusion in the stepwise logistic regression were as follows: (*a*) solid component ($P < 10^{-8}$), (*b*) flow location ($P < 10^{-6}$), (*c*) free intraperitoneal fluid ($P = .0002$), and (*d*) septation ($P = .004$).

(*c*) free intraperitoneal fluid (an abnormal amount is associated with malignancy); and (*d*) septations (absence of septations has a stronger association with malignancy than do thick septations, which have a stronger association than thin septations). None of the remaining gray-scale or Doppler features added any additional statistically significant information about malignancy versus benignity over and above that provided by these four features.

The presence and nature of a solid component demonstrated the most statistically significant association. In particular, all masses without a solid component or with a markedly hyperechoic solid component were benign. Among the 27 masses with a markedly hyperechoic solid component, there were 24 teratomas, two endometriomas, and one combined Brenner tumor and fibroma.

For masses with a nonhyperechoic solid component ($n = 86$), the presence and location of flow was the next most helpful feature. Twenty-four of 40 masses (60%) with a nonhyperechoic solid component and central flow were malignant, but only four of 46 masses (9%) with a nonhyperechoic solid component and peripheral or no flow were malignant.

The regression equation was used as the basis for a malignancy score (Table 4). This score was calculated by omitting the constant term of the regression equation and by converting the regression coefficients to positive integers. The malignancy score ranged from 0 to 507, with higher scores favoring malignancy and lower scores favoring benignity. The ROC curve for the scoring system (Fig 5) was well above the main diagonal, with an area under the curve of 0.98 ± 0.01 (mean ± standard deviation) (55). This result indicates excellent performance of the malignancy score in distinguishing malignant from benign lesions. The highest accuracy (93%) was achieved with a cutoff score of 453 (a cutoff of 469 has essentially equivalent accuracy but a lower sensitivity). A malignancy score of 453 or higher had a sensitivity of 93%, specificity of 93%, positive predictive value of 67%, and negative predictive value of 99% for malignancy. To achieve a sensitivity (and negative predictive value) of 100%, a malignancy score of 433 or higher was required; the specificity then dropped to 86% and the positive predictive value to 52%.

The regression equation can also be used to calculate the probability of malignancy for a given mass (Table 5). This table indicates, for example, that an adnexal mass with a nonhyperechoic solid component, peripheral flow only, no free fluid, and no septations has an 8% probability of being malignant.

DISCUSSION

An adnexal mass is a fairly common finding on a pelvic sonogram. Although there are several reasons to consider surgical removal of an adnexal mass, concern about malignancy is probably the major reason. Most adnexal masses are benign (48), however, and numerous studies have examined whether gray-scale or Doppler sonographic criteria can allow distinction between benign and malignant ovarian masses. As a whole, the literature indicates that no single gray-scale or Doppler sonographic feature allows reliable distinction between benignity and malignancy. Despite the now-extensive literature on the subject, the choice of which sonographic feature(s) to use, and in particular the role of Doppler sonography, in predicting malignancy remains controversial. Although most comparison studies have found gray-scale sonography to be superior to Doppler sonography (11,16,17, 21,22) or that Doppler sonography offers no significant improvement over gray-scale sonography (6,15,20,23–25), a minority of studies report Doppler features to be superior (26,27).

Our study, which made use of logistic regression analysis, provides answers to these controversial issues. The four sonographic features that, as a group, are statistically significant contributors to the distinction between benign and malignant adnexal masses are (*a*) presence and nature of any solid component, (*b*) presence and location of flow at conventional color Doppler imaging, (*c*) presence and amount of free intraperitoneal fluid, and (*d*) presence and thickness of septations. The first of these four features was by far the most significant. Masses without a solid component or with a markedly hyperechoic solid component were always benign, regardless of any other gray-scale or Doppler feature. When a nonhyperechoic solid component was present, the three other features (two gray-scale and one Doppler) aided in the distinction of benignity from malignancy.

The location of any flow detected in the mass was the only statistically significant Doppler feature in our logistic regression analysis. This result suggests that color Doppler sonography should be used to evaluate the presence and location of flow in masses with a solid component. The pulsed Doppler indexes add no further predictive information.

The results of our analysis can be used clinically in several ways. First, the regression equation can be used to calculate a malignancy score to discriminate between malignant and benign masses (Table 4). Second, the regression equation can also be used to calculate the probability that a mass is malignant on the basis of its sonographic features (Table 5). Third, and perhaps most simply, one can qualitatively assess the likelihood of malignancy using only the four selected features. For example, consider the mass shown in Figure 3. The malignancy score

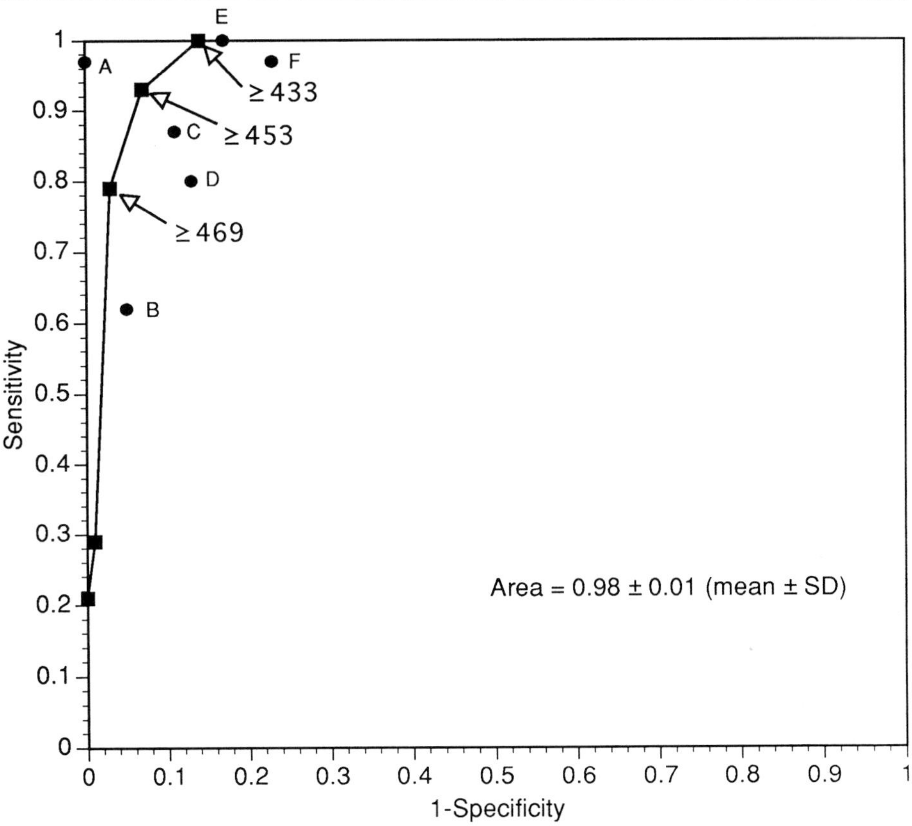

Figure 5. ROC curve for the malignancy scoring system. Diagram shows malignancy score cutoff values used to determine performance (solid squares labeled with numbers). The solid circles represent the reported performance of other scoring systems that evaluated both pre- and postmenopausal patients. *A* represents a combined Doppler and gray-scale sonographic scoring system (26); *B* (29), *D* (30), *E* (28), and *F* (32) represent gray-scale sonographic scoring systems; and *C* represents a combined gray-scale sonographic and clinical scoring system (34).

TABLE 5
Probability of Malignancy for Masses with a Nonhyperechoic Solid Component

Gray-Scale Sonographic Findings	Central Flow	Peripheral Flow Only	No Flow
Abnormal amount of free fluid			
No septation	0.99	0.79	0.77
Thick septation	0.96	0.43	0.40
Thin septation	0.75	0.08	0.07
Normal amount of free fluid			
No septation	0.75	0.08	0.07
Thick septation	0.38	0.02	0.01
Thin septation	0.06	<0.01	<0.01

Note.—The probability p of malignancy is calculated with the following formula (56): $p = e^{VRE}/(1 + e^{VRE})$, where e is the base of natural logarithms and VRE is the value of the regression equation. The value of the regression equation was obtained by summing the appropriate regression coefficient for each of the sonographic features (Table 4) and subtracting the constant term of 6.4. This table does not include masses with no solid component or with a hyperechoic solid component because all such masses in our series were benign.

(Table 4) is 469, the sum of 394 (for a nonhyperechoic solid component), 37 (for central flow), 0 (for normal free fluid), and 38 (for no septation). This score is above the cutoff of 453, suggesting that the mass is malignant. Alternatively, Table 5 indicates that there is a 75% probability that the lesion is malignant. Qualitatively, the mass would be highly suspicious for malignancy, primarily on the basis of the nonhyperechoic solid component with central flow.

Unlike in most earlier scoring systems, which usually selected features and scores on the basis of educated assumptions, the group of features in our system and the values assigned to each were selected on the basis of stepwise logistic regression analysis. The features included in our scoring system are not surprising, as each has previously been used to distinguish benign from malignant masses. In particular, the most statistically significant feature, a solid component, has long been recognized as strongly associated with malignancy in both gross pathologic and sonographic studies (17,31,57–59). Although a solid component is highly sensitive for malignancy, this feature does not have high specificity, being present in 20%–58% of benign masses (57–59). A nonhyperechoic solid component was present in 32% of the benign masses in our series (58 of 183). Color Doppler sonography may help distinguish solid tumor tissue from clot by demonstrating flow in a solid component, but use of this technique still does not allow perfect distinction between malignancy and benignity.

Our scoring system performed better than most other scoring systems (Fig 5) that evaluated both premenopausal and postmenopausal women. One scoring system was reported to have better performance than ours (26), although to our knowledge these results have not been confirmed by others and the RI cutoff of 0.4 used in that study has not been found reliable by other investigators (5,10–13,15,16,18,21). Furthermore, because our methods allowed us to identify the features that, as a group, enabled statistically significant distinction between malignancy and benignity, our system requires one to assess only four features rather than the numerous features used in that system (26).

Our study had a few limitations. Interobserver variability, although unlikely to be significant for the four sonographic features in our scoring system, was not assessed. The relatively small number of malignancies is also a limitation but is likely a reflection of the low prevalence of ovarian malignancy in the general population. In addition, to avoid low-resistance corpus luteal flow, we excluded premenopausal patients when it was known that they were past day 10 of the menstrual cycle; therefore, our results may not be applicable to patients scanned after cycle day 10. Also, some other potentially useful features such as CA-125 level were not assessed.

In summary, our statistical methods yielded a scoring system for adnexal masses that has high sensitivity and specificity for malignancy. Malignancy can be virtually excluded in masses that have no solid component or a markedly hyperechoic solid component typical of a teratoma. For other masses, information concerning flow location, free intraperitoneal fluid, and septations can be used to help in the diagnosis of ovarian malignancy.

Acknowledgments: CLABROC and LABROC5 software for ROC curve analysis was provided by Charles E. Metz, MD.

References

1. Bourne T, Campbell S, Steer C, Whitehead MI, Collins WP. Transvaginal colour flow imaging: a possible new screening technique for ovarian cancer. Br Med J 1989; 299:1367–1370.
2. Fleischer AC, Rodgers WH, Rao BK, et al. Assessment of ovarian tumor vascularity with transvaginal color Doppler sonography. J Ultrasound Med 1991; 10:563–568.
3. Kurjak A, Zalud I, Alfirevic Z. Evaluation of adnexal masses with transvaginal color ultrasound. J Ultrasound Med 1991; 10:295–297.
4. Weiner Z, Thaler I, Beck D, Rottem S, Deutsch M, Brandes JM. Differentiating malignant from benign ovarian tumors with transvaginal color flow imaging. Obstet Gynecol 1992; 79:159–162.
5. Brown DL, Frates MC, Laing FC, et al. Ovarian masses: can benign and malignant lesions be differentiated with color and pulsed Doppler US? Radiology 1994; 190:333–336.
6. Hata K, Hata T, Manabe A, Sugimura K, Kitao M. A critical evaluation of transvaginal Doppler studies, transvaginal sonography, magnetic resonance imaging, and CA 125 in detecting ovarian cancer. Obstet Gynecol 1992; 80:922–926.
7. Kawai M, Kano T, Kikkawa F, Maeda O, Oguchi H, Tomoda Y. Transvaginal Doppler ultrasound with color flow imaging in the diagnosis of ovarian cancer. Obstet Gynecol 1992; 79:163–167.
8. Timor-Tritsch IE, Lerner JP, Monteagudo A, Santos R. Transvaginal ultrasonographic characterization of ovarian masses by means of color flow–directed Doppler measurements and a morphologic scoring system. Am J Obstet Gynecol 1993; 168:909–913.
9. Tekay A, Jouppila P. Validity of pulsatility and resistance indices in classification of adnexal tumors with transvaginal color Doppler ultrasound. Ultrasound Obstet Gynecol 1992; 2:338–344.
10. Hamper UM, Sheth S, Abbas FM, Rosenshein NB, Aronson D, Kurman RJ. Transvaginal color Doppler sonography of adnexal masses: differences in blood flow impedance in benign and malignant lesions. AJR 1993; 160: 1225–1228.
11. Levine D, Feldstein VA, Babcook CJ, Filly RA. Sonography of ovarian masses: poor sensitivity of resistive index for identifying malignant lesions. AJR 1994; 162:1355–1359.
12. Prompeler HJ, Madjar H, Sauerbrei W, Lattermann U, Pfleiderer A. Quantitative flow measurements for classification of ovarian tumors by transvaginal color Doppler sonography in postmenopausal patients. Ultrasound Obstet Gynecol 1994; 4:406–413.
13. Lin PY, Lai JI, Wu CC, et al. Color Doppler ultrasound in the assessment of ovarian neoplasms. J Med Ultrasound 1993; 1:172–176.
14. Salem S, White LM, Lai J. Doppler sonography of adnexal masses: the predictive value of the pulsatility index in benign and malignant disease. AJR 1994; 163:1147–1150.
15. Buy J, Ghossain MA, Hugol D, et al. Characterization of adnexal masses: combination of color Doppler and conventional sonography compared with spectral Doppler analysis alone and conventional sonography alone. AJR 1996; 166:385–393.
16. Stein SM, Laifer-Narin S, Johnson MB, et al. Differentiation of benign and malignant adnexal masses: relative value of gray-scale, color Doppler, and spectral Doppler sonography. AJR 1995; 164:381–386.
17. Valentin L, Sladkevicius P, Marsal K. Limited contribution of Doppler velocimetry to the differential diagnosis of extrauterine pelvic tumors. Obstet Gynecol 1994; 83:425–433.
18. Maly Z, Riss P, Deutinger J. Localization of blood vessels and qualitative assessment of blood flow in ovarian tumors. Obstet Gynecol 1995; 85:33–36.
19. Sladkevicius P, Valentin L, Marsal K. Transvaginal Doppler examination for the differential diagnosis of solid pelvic tumors. J Ultrasound Med 1995; 14:377–380.
20. Sengoku K, Satoh T, Saitoh S, Abe M, Ishikawa M. Evaluation of transvaginal color Doppler sonography, transvaginal sonography, and CA 125 for prediction of ovarian malignancy. Int J Gynaecol Obstet 1994; 46:39–43.
21. Jain KA. Prospective evaluation of adnexal masses with endovaginal gray-scale and duplex and color Doppler US: correlation with pathologic findings. Radiology 1994; 191:63–67.
22. Alcazar JL, Ruiz-Perez ML, Errasti T. Transvaginal color Doppler sonography of adnexal masses: which parameter performs best? Ultrasound Obstet Gynecol 1996; 8:114–119.
23. Bromley B, Goodman H, Benacerraf BR. Comparison between sonographic morphology and Doppler waveform for the diagnosis of ovarian malignancy. Obstet Gynecol 1994; 83:434–437.
24. Schneider VL, Schneider A, Reed KL, Hatch KD. Comparison of Doppler with two-dimensional sonography and CA 125 for prediction of malignancy of pelvic masses. Obstet Gynecol 1993; 81:983–988.
25. Anandakumar C, Chew S, Wong YC, Chia D, Ratnam SS. Role of transvaginal ultrasound color flow imaging and Doppler waveform analysis in differentiating between benign and malignant ovarian tumors. Ultrasound Obstet Gynecol 1996; 7:280–284.
26. Kurjak A, Predanic M. New scoring system for prediction of ovarian malignancy based on transvaginal color Doppler sonography. J

Ultrasound Med 1992; 11:631–638.
27. Zanetta G, Vergani P, Lissoni A. Color Doppler ultrasound in the preoperative assessment of adnexal masses. Acta Obstet Gynecol Scand 1994; 73:637–641.
28. Sassone AM, Timor-Tritsch IE, Artner A, Westhoff C, Warren WB. Transvaginal sonographic characterization of ovarian disease: evaluation of a new scoring system to predict malignancy. Obstet Gynecol 1991; 78:70–76.
29. Finkler NJ, Benacerraf B, Lavin PT, Wojciechowski C, Knapp RC. Comparison of serum CA 125, clinical impression, and ultrasound in the preoperative evaluation of ovarian masses. Obstet Gynecol 1988; 72:659–664.
30. Benacerraf BR, Finkler NJ, Wojciechowski C, Knapp RC. Sonographic accuracy in the diagnosis of ovarian masses. J Reprod Med 1990; 35:491–495.
31. DePriest PD, Shenson BS, Fried A, et al. A morphology index based on sonographic findings in ovarian cancer. Gynecol Oncol 1993; 51:7–11.
32. Lerner J, Timor-Tritsch I, Federman A, Abramovich G. Transvaginal ultrasonographic characterization of ovarian masses with an improved, weighted scoring system. Am J Obstet Gynecol 1994; 170:81–85.
33. Kurjak A, Schulman H, Sosic A, Zalud I, Shalan H. Transvaginal ultrasound, color flow, and Doppler waveform of the postmenopausal adnexal mass. Obstet Gynecol 1992; 80:917–921.
34. Davies AP, Jacobs I, Woolas R, Fish A, Oram D. The adnexal mass: benign or malignant? evaluation of a risk of malignancy index. Br J Obstet Gynaecol 1993; 100:927–931.
35. Mais V, Guerriero S, Ajossa S, Angiolucci M, Paoletti AM, Melis GB. Transvaginal ultrasonography in the diagnosis of cystic teratoma. Obstet Gynecol 1995; 85:48–52.
36. Filly RA. Ovarian masses . . . what to look for . . . what to do. In: Callen PW, ed. Ultrasonography in obstetrics and gynecology. Philadelphia, Pa: Saunders, 1994; 625–640.
37. Bronshtein M, Yoffe N, Brandes JM, Blumenfeld Z. Hair as a sonographic marker of ovarian teratomas: improved identification using transvaginal sonography and simulation model. JCU 1991; 19:351–355.
38. Cohen L, Sabbagha R. Echo patterns of benign cystic teratomas by transvaginal ultrasound. Ultrasound Obstet Gynecol 1993; 3:120–123.
39. Laing FC, Van Dalsem VF, Marks WM, Barton JL, Martinez DA. Dermoid cysts of the ovary: their ultrasonographic appearances. Obstet Gynecol 1981; 57:99–104.
40. Quinn SF, Erickson S, Black WC. Cystic ovarian teratomas: the sonographic appearance of the dermoid plug. Radiology 1985; 155: 477–478.
41. Sheth S, Fishman EK, Buck JL, Hamper UM, Sanders RC. The variable sonographic appearances of ovarian teratomas: correlation with CT. AJR 1988; 151:331–334.
42. Atri M, Reinhold C, Bret PM. Ovarian dermoid: correlation of endovaginal sonographic and MR imaging findings (abstr). Radiology 1994; 193(P):309.
43. Atri M, Kintzen GM, Ye S, Reinhold C, Aldis AE, Bret PM. How accurate is endovaginal US in the diagnosis of ovarian dermoid? (abstr). Radiology 1994; 193(P):145.
44. Caspi B, Appelman Z, Rabinerson D, Elchalal U, Zalel Y, Katz Z. Pathognomonic echo patterns of benign cystic teratomas of the ovary: classification, incidence, and accuracy rate of sonographic diagnosis. Ultrasound Obstet Gynecol 1996; 7:275–279.
45. Owre A, Pedersen JF. Characteristic fat-fluid level at ultrasonography of ovarian dermoid cyst. Acta Radiol 1991; 32:317–319.
46. Malde HM, Kedar RP, Chadha D, Nayak S. Dermoid mesh: a sonographic sign of ovarian teratoma (letter). AJR 1992; 159:1349–1350.
47. Fried AM, Kenney CM, Stigers KB, Kacki MH, Buckley SL. Benign pelvic masses: sonographic spectrum. RadioGraphics 1996; 16: 321–334.
48. Mais V, Guerriero S, Ajossa S, Angiolucci M, Paoletti AM, Melis GB. The efficiency of transvaginal ultrasonography in the diagnosis of endometrioma. Fertil Steril 1993; 60:776–780.
49. Kupfer MC, Schwimer SR, Lebovic J. Transvaginal sonographic appearance of endometriomata: spectrum and findings. J Ultrasound Med 1992; 11:129–133.
50. Athey PA, Diment DD. The spectrum of sonographic findings in endometriomas. J Ultrasound Med 1989; 8:487–491.
51. Okai T, Kobayashi K, Ryo E, Kagawa H, Kozuma S, Taketani Y. Transvaginal sonographic appearance of hemorrhagic functional ovarian cysts and their spontaneous regression. Int J Gynaecol Obstet 1994; 44:47–52.
52. Fleischer AC, Rodgers WH, Kepple DM, Williams LL, Jones HW III. Color Doppler sonography of ovarian masses: a multiparameter analysis. J Ultrasound Med 1993; 12:41–48.
53. Chambers JT, Merino MJ, Kohorn EI, Schwartz PE. Borderline ovarian tumors. Am J Obstet Gynecol 1988; 159:1088–1094.
54. Metz CE, Wang PL, Kronman HB. A new approach for testing the significance of differences between ROC curves measured from correlated data. In: Deconinck F, ed. Information processing in medical imaging. The Hague, The Netherlands: Nijhoff, 1984; 432–445.
55. Metz CE, Shen JH, Herman BA. New methods for estimating a binormal ROC curve from continuously-distribued test results. Presented at the Joint Statistical Meetings of the American Statistical Society and the Biometric Society, Anaheim, Calif, 1990.
56. Rosner B. Fundamentals of biostatistics. 2nd ed. Boston, Mass: Duxbury, 1986; 404–408.
57. Granberg S, Wikland M, Jansson I. Macroscopic characterization of ovarian tumors and the relation to the histological diagnosis: criteria to be used for ultrasound evaluation. Gynecol Oncol 1989; 35:139–144.
58. Granberg S, Norstrom A, Wikland M. Tumors in the lower pelvis as imaged by vaginal sonography. Gynecol Oncol 1990; 37:224–229.
59. Herrmann UJ Jr, Locher GW, Goldhirsch A. Sonographic patterns of ovarian tumors: prediction of malignancy. Obstet Gynecol 1987; 69:777–781.

David C. Sperling, MD
Laurence Needleman, MD
David J. Eschelman, MD
David M. Hovsepian, MD[2]
Anna S. Lev-Toaff, MD

Deep Pelvic Abscesses: Transperineal US-guided Drainage[1]

Index terms:
Abscess, percutaneous drainage, 875.1263
Pelvic organs, abscess, 875.211
Pelvic organs, interventional procedure, 875.1262, 875.1263
Pelvic organs, US, 875.12985, 875.12986, 875.12989
Surgery, complications, 875.458
Ultrasound (US), guidance, 875.12985

Radiology 1998; 208:111–115

Abbreviation:
APR = abdominoperineal resection

[1] From the Department of Radiology, Thomas Jefferson University Hospital, Jefferson Medical College, 132 S 10th St, Philadelphia, PA 19107. Received August 19, 1997; revision requested November 13; revision received February 10, 1998; accepted March 9. **Address reprint requests to** L.N.

[2] Current address: Division of Vascular and Interventional Radiology, Mallinckrodt Institute of Radiology, St Louis, Mo.

Author contributions:
Guarantor of integrity of entire study, L.N.; study concepts and design, L.N., D.M.H., D.C.S.; definition of intellectual content, L.N.; literature research, D.C.S., L.N., D.J.E.; clinical studies, L.N., D.J.E., D.M.H., A.S.L., D.C.S.; data acquisition, L.N., D.C.S., D.M.H.; data analysis, L.N., D.C.S., D.J.E.; manuscript preparation, D.C.S.; manuscript editing and review, L.N., D.J.E., D.M.H., D.C.S., A.S.L.

PURPOSE: To examine the efficacy of transperineal sonographically guided drainage of deep pelvic abscesses.

MATERIALS AND METHODS: Twelve drainage procedures were performed in 11 adults with symptoms of infection and cross-sectional images demonstrating a deep pelvic abscess. Eight patients had recently undergone abdominoperineal resection, seven of whom underwent preoperative radiation therapy. Two had chronic osteomyelitis with adjacent fluid collections, and one developed an infected hematoma after trauma. With ultrasound (US) guidance for initial access, catheters were placed for drainage in 11 procedures. One patient was treated with aspiration alone. Patients underwent clinical follow-up and subsequent imaging as necessary.

RESULTS: Transperineal needle placement was successful in 12 of 12 patients (100%). In procedures that required catheter placement, 10 of 11 placements (91%) were achieved with the transperineal approach. One patient required fluoroscopic transvaginal catheter placement after opacification of the collection transperineally. Catheter drainage was maintained for 2–146 days (mean, 40 days; median, 21 days). Clinical success was achieved in nine of 10 patients (90%) by means of transperineal drainage. There were no complications, although premature catheter removal occurred in two patients.

CONCLUSION: US-guided transperineal abscess drainage may be successfully performed in patients who cannot undergo conventional transabdominal, transvaginal, or transrectal catheter drainage.

Drainage of deep pelvic abscesses guided by ultrasound (US), computed tomography (CT), or fluoroscopy may be accomplished by using a variety of approaches, most commonly transabdominal, transvaginal, transrectal, and transgluteal. The transperineal route has been described for biopsy of the prostate gland with US guidance (1,2). As an adaptation of this technique, we report our experience with US-guided transperineal drainage of deep pelvic abscesses, typically in patients for whom conventional routes cannot be used.

MATERIALS AND METHODS

Eleven patients (eight men and three women), aged 21–78 years (mean age, 59 years), were referred between December 1989 and August 1996 for transperineal percutaneous aspiration and drainage of pelvic fluid collections. Written informed consent was obtained from all patients. Patients had clinical symptoms consistent with infection, including elevated white blood cell counts (range, 5,100–23,500/mm^3 [5.1–23.5 $\times$ 10^9/L]; mean, 15,100/mm^3 [15.1 $\times$ 10^9/L]), fevers, and/or symptoms such as erythema or tenderness in the perineal or sacral regions. Eight patients (six men and two women) had recently undergone an abdominoperineal resection (APR) for rectal carcinoma, and seven of these eight patients had previously received local radiation therapy. Two patients had chronic osteomyelitis complicated by adjacent fluid collections, and one man had a posttraumatic infected hematoma.

All patients had CT scans or sonograms showing fluid collections in the pelvis that were inaccessible with the transabdominal approach because of an overlying bowel or bladder

(Figs 1a, 2a). A transperineal approach was selected for the following reasons. The transvaginal and transrectal approaches were precluded in six patients because they were men and had undergone APR. In one man who had not undergone colorectal surgery, the transperineal approach was chosen because visualization of the collection was better than with transrectal US. The other man who had not undergone colorectal surgery preferred this transperineal approach rather than a transrectal drainage catheter. He was our initial patient, and transrectal US guidance was used only in this patient. In the two women who had undergone APR, the transperineal approach was chosen over the transvaginal route because of the patient's preference in one case and the physician's preference in the other case, on the basis of accessibility of the collection. A transvaginal approach was planned for one elderly woman, but her vaginal canal could not accommodate the US transducer. The collection was initially accessed and opacified with contrast material by means of a US-guided transperineal approach.

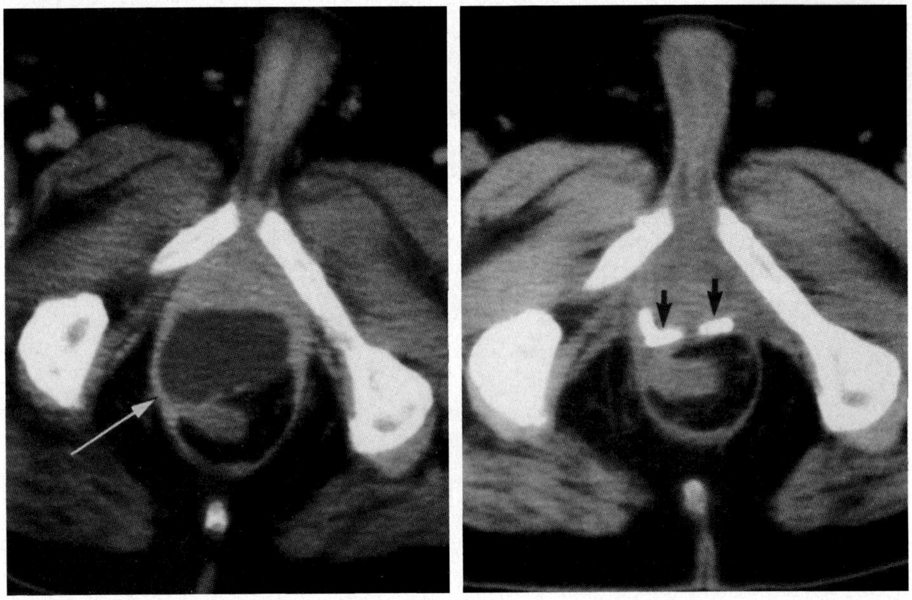

a. b.

Figure 1. **(a)** CT scan in a 52-year-old man shows a deep pelvic abscess (arrow) after APR and radiation therapy. **(b)** After US-guided transperineal aspiration and 8 days of catheter drainage, CT scan shows the collection is completely resolved. Only the indwelling catheter (arrows) remains.

All patients received intravenous antibiotics before the procedure. The patients were placed in the lithotomy position. US guidance was provided by means of various 3.0–7.5-MHz end-firing sector probes (Acuson, Mountain View, Calif; Acoustic Imaging, Tempe, Ariz; and Advanced Technology Laboratories, Bothell, Wash) applied to the perineum (Figs 2b, 3a), except for the first patient, who underwent transrectal US with a 7-MHz side-firing linear probe (Acuson), which was used to guide transperineal needle placement.

After the fluid collection was localized, the perineum was prepared with povidone-iodine solution and sterile drapes were applied. Midazolam and fentanyl citrate were administered intravenously for conscious sedation. Lidocaine 2% (Abbott Laboratories, North Chicago, Ill) was administered for local anesthesia with a 25-gauge needle. Needle guidance was usually performed through a biopsy guide (Fig 2c), although a freehand approach was occasionally used according to physician preference. An 18-gauge trocar needle or 20-gauge spinal needle was directed into the fluid collection under continuous US observation (Fig 3b). Because the window for perineal visualization was usually small, the distance of the needle from the transducer was minimized. This was accomplished by keeping the angle of the needle as low as possible relative to the transducer. Needle placement was as close to the midline as possible, thus avoiding the pudendal nerves located laterally in the ischiorectal fossa. Needle placement was confirmed by means of sonographic observation and aspiration of fluid, which was sent to the pathology department for culture. In the 11 procedures that progressed to catheter drainage, a stiff guide wire (Cook, Bloomington, Ind) was placed under US or fluoroscopic guidance or both.

Twelve procedures were performed. In nine procedures (eight patients), locking drainage catheters were placed with fluoroscopic guidance after fascial dilation (Fig 2d). On the basis of the character of the aspirate, the following catheters were placed: six 8-F locking all-purpose drainage catheters (Medi-tech/Boston Scientific, Watertown, Mass), two 10-F locking all-purpose drainage catheters (Medi-tech), and one 12-F locking vanSonnenberg sump catheter (Medi-tech). One patient required catheter replacement after the original catheter was unintentionally removed by a nurse before resolution of the collection. Passing fascial dilators through the scarred perineum of the elderly woman who could not accommodate a transvaginal probe was quite difficult and created much discomfort for the patient. Because the fluid collection was opacified with contrast material after the initial transperineal needle was placed, an 18-gauge trocar needle was advanced with fluoroscopic guidance from a transvaginal approach into the abscess directly posterior to the vaginal fornix. A 10-F locking all-purpose drainage catheter was then easily placed. In one patient, an 8.3-F Sacks locking drainage catheter (Medi-tech) was placed with sonographic guidance. In another patient, the small collection was completely aspirated during US examination, so a drainage catheter was not placed.

All catheters were attached to a 30-cm-long tube (Cook) and a leg bag (Professional Medical Products, Greenwood, SC) for gravity drainage. All catheters were initially flushed daily with 10 mL of normal saline solution to maintain catheter patency. For very thick collections, two to three daily flushes of normal saline were recommended. Daily bedside evaluation of catheter function was performed, with additional catheter checks and changes as clinically indicated. The decision to remove the drainage catheter was based on the patient's clinical status, and abscess resolution was confirmed by means of injection of contrast material through the catheter under fluoroscopic or cross-sectional imaging guidance (Fig 1b). In patients discharged with an indwelling catheter, follow-up was performed on an outpatient basis until catheter removal.

Review of the medical records was performed as follow-up to assess for

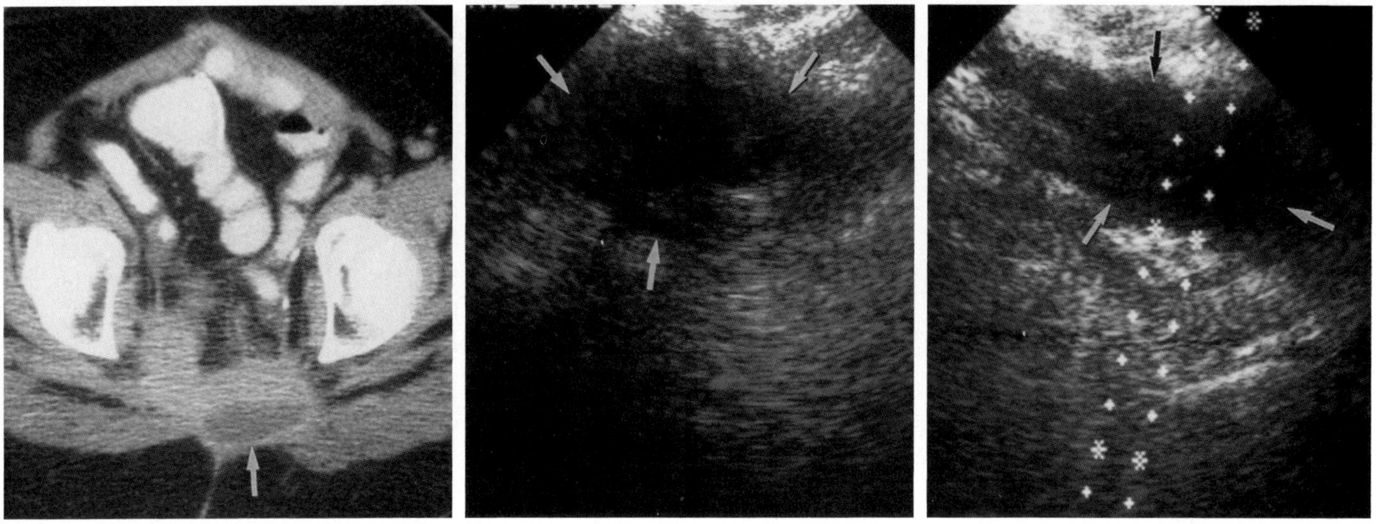

a. b. c.

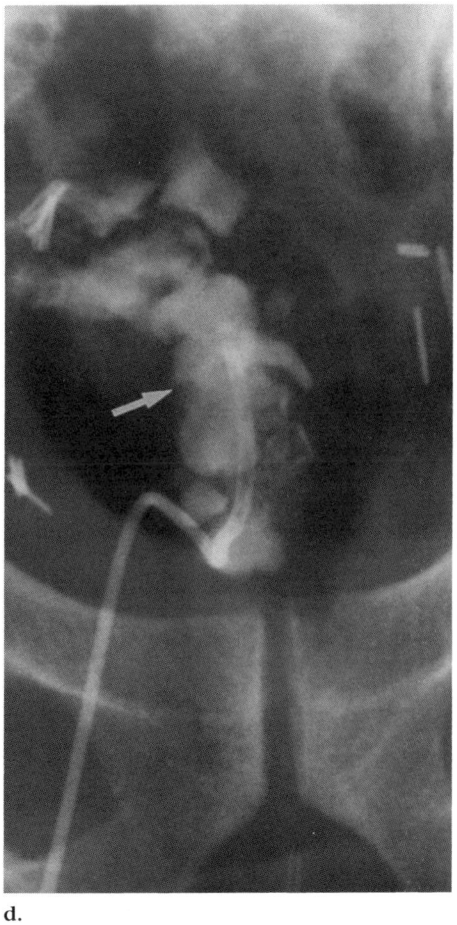

d.

Figure 2. (a) CT scan in a 45-year-old man shows a deep pelvic collection (arrow) after APR and radiation therapy. (b) Transperineal coronal US image of the presacral area shows the complex fluid collection (arrows). (c) Transperineal sagittal US image of the complex fluid collection (arrows) shows the biopsy guide (+ and ∗). (d) Radiograph obtained immediately after injection of contrast material shows placement of a drainage catheter into the abscess cavity (arrow). The locking loop was formed later (not shown).

delayed recurrences of abscess or surgical intervention for treatment failures. Statistical analysis with the paired Student t test was performed by using StatView (Abacus Concepts, Berkeley, Calif) to evaluate the association between radiation therapy and drainage catheter duration.

RESULTS

The fluid collections were successfully accessed with the US-directed transperineal approach in 100% of patients (11 of 11) and procedures (12 of 12). Purulent fluid was aspirated from eight patients, and cultures confirmed that these collections were abscesses. Infected serosanguinous fluid was aspirated on two separate occasions from a patient with chronic osteomyelitis. Dark hemorrhagic fluid was obtained in two patients, but results of culture were negative for infection. Treatment with multiple antibiotics before the procedure may have prevented bacterial growth in the cultures from these two collections. Because of the high clinical suspicion for infection, a drainage catheter was placed in each of these patients even though purulent aspirates were not present.

Catheter placement was accomplished with the transperineal approach in nine of 10 patients (90%) and 10 of 11 procedures (91%). A catheter was placed with the transvaginal approach in one patient. In another patient, a small collection was completely aspirated with sonographic observation, and catheter placement was not necessary. Transperineal catheter drainage was maintained for 2–146 days (mean, 40 days; median, 21 days). On average, transperineal catheters were removed after 59 days in those patients who previously underwent pelvic radiation therapy and after 12 days in those who did not receive radiation ($P = .16$).

Premature drainage catheter removal occurred in two patients, at 2 and 3 days after placement. In one patient, the tube was mistakenly removed by a caregiver, and a new drainage catheter was placed by using a similar approach 8 days later because of a persistent collection and symptoms of infection. The abscess subsequently resolved. The catheter spontaneously fell out of the other patient, and she underwent surgical incision and drainage. In the other eight patients, transperineal abscess drainage or aspiration was complete without recurrence. Clinical success, defined as abscess resolution, was achieved in nine of 10 patients (90%) and nine of 11 procedures (82%) with the transperineal approach. Successful treatment was also achieved in the patient whose abscess was drained with a transvaginal approach. There were no complications or deaths resulting from transperineal aspiration or drainage catheter placement. The catheters were well tolerated without local pain or perineal neuralgia.

One patient did not return to the interventional radiology department or to the surgeon for follow-up as scheduled after hospital discharge. When he returned 146 days after catheter placement, the drain was removed. There had been no output from the catheter for a long time, and he experienced no complications from this prolonged catheter placement.

Specimens from two patients produced no microbial growth. On the basis of clinical presentation, one patient was treated as if the collection were infected despite the negative results of cultures, and the drain remained in place for 23 days until the cavity resolved. The second patient developed a ureteral leak and a perforated gallbladder unrelated to the drainage procedure. Despite appropriate placement of percutaneous nephrostomy and cholecystostomy catheters, there was persistent drainage of urine and bile through the dependent perineal drain, so it was left in place for 115 days until resolution of these other complications occurred.

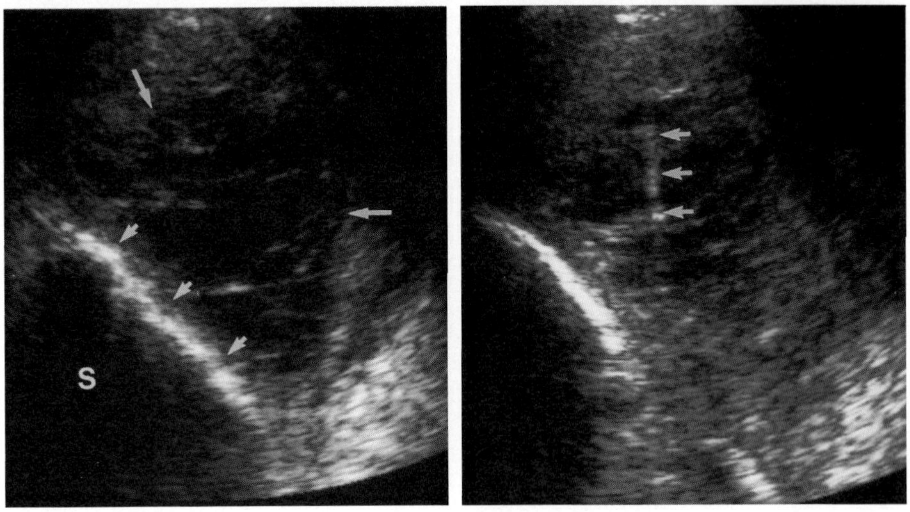

a. b.

Figure 3. **(a)** Transperineal sagittal oblique US image in a 46-year-old man with chronic osteomyelitis of the left hip shows a multiseptated collection (large arrows) abutting the adjacent inferior pubic ramus (small arrows). S = shadow from the pubic bone. **(b)** US image in the same patient depicts a needle (arrows) placed into the fluid collection. Note the low angle of the needle with respect to the ultrasound beam, which allows the distance between the needle and the transducer to be minimized.

DISCUSSION

Deep pelvic abscesses may occur as a complication of surgery, trauma, or infectious processes in the abdomen and pelvis (3). Rates of occurrence of pelvic abscess after APR of 0.6% (4) and 1.8% (5) have been reported, although Stevens et al (6) noted that 3.5% of patients developed a perineal abscess after rectosigmoid resection and radiation therapy. Traditional surgical drainage has been largely superseded by image-directed percutaneous procedures (3). Fluoroscopy, CT, and US can be used to guide abscess drainage (3,7–13). The percutaneous transabdominal approach is usually preferred because of the high success rate, ease of catheter care, and high level of patient acceptance and comfort. However, many pelvic abscesses are inaccessible by this approach because of overlying bowel, bladder, reproductive organs, or vascular and osseous structures.

The transvaginal route offers a useful alternative in many women (12). However, presacral collections may be inaccessible because of interposed rectum, and the approach is often inappropriate in young girls. Also, as demonstrated by one patient in our series, the vagina in an elderly woman may be unable to accommodate the transvaginal US probe. Transrectal drainage is an alternative route that is especially useful in men and for drainage of presacral collections in women (11). The transgluteal approach (10), commonly achieved with CT guidance, risks injury to neurovascular structures in the greater sciatic foramen and elsewhere in the pelvis (14). Catheters in this location cause discomfort and are prone to kinking, especially when patients lie supine. As an alternative to transgluteal drainage in patients who have undergone colorectal surgery, paracoccygeal drainage with CT guidance has been successfully employed in six patients (15).

The transperineal approach had been used routinely for biopsy of the prostate gland with use of transrectal US guidance (1) before the development of transrectal biopsy techniques. Transperineal US-guided biopsy of the prostate may be used in men who have undergone APR (2). The physicians in our group also had experience with using transrectal US-guided transperineal aspiration for other pelvic collections such as postprostatectomy cysts, seminal vesicle cysts, and rectal dermoid cysts. Abscess drainage was a natural extension of these techniques. Although a transrectal probe was used to guide drainage in our first patient, the availability of end-firing sector probes provided a more direct approach from the perineum in the remaining patients. Other small series of transperineal abscess drainage guided by fluoroscopy (16), CT (17), and transrectal US (18) have been reported to have had good success. To our knowledge, only a single case of transperineal US-guided catheter drainage of a pelvic abscess has been reported in the English literature (19).

Transperineal abscess drainage was achieved safely with US guidance. The procedures were performed with the patients under conscious sedation, and the catheters were well tolerated. The catheter was taped to the patient's inner thigh and posed no marked impediment to walking or sitting. There were no instances of perineal neuralgia that could be caused by impingement of the pudendal nerve (the Alcock canal syndrome) (20). Some patients preferred this approach as opposed to having a catheter in their vagina or rectum.

Our technical and clinical success rates compare favorably with those in other series describing abscess drainage (3,7, 11,12). As with transvaginal and transrectal drainage catheters, the transperineal approach often offers a short, direct access route to deep pelvic fluid collections and excellent needle visualization (13). This catheter position is dependent, allowing complete drainage by means of gravity. This site also offers an extraperitoneal approach. Unlike transvaginal or transrectal drains, the transperineal catheter can generally be secured to the skin in the perineum near the entry site. Despite this and the use of self-retaining catheters, an occasional catheter may be expelled before abscess resolution.

Catheter drainage was performed in most of our patients, but aspiration of purulent material without catheter drainage produced symptom resolution in one patient. The utility of aspiration without catheter placement has been demonstrated (12,21).

The duration of catheter drainage in our study was substantially longer than the mean of 13 days reported for transvaginal drainage procedures (12) or 7 days reported for transrectal drainage procedures (11). There was a trend toward longer times for the catheter to remain in place in the group of patients who had undergone APR and who had received preoperative radiation therapy. However, this trend was not statistically significant, probably because of the small patient population. Delayed healing after radiation therapy has been noted (22,23), and this corresponds to our overall experience with abscess drainage in irradiated fields. Despite these prolonged catheter placements, we still consider catheter drainage preferable to a complicated surgical procedure for abscess drainage. Outpatient catheter management may allow patients to leave the hospital earlier because they do not need to recover from a surgical procedure.

In conclusion, US-guided transperineal abscess drainage may be successfully performed in patients who cannot undergo traditional transabdominal, transvaginal, or transrectal catheter drainage. The US-guided approach is useful for percutaneous catheter treatment of deep pelvic abscesses not accessible with other approaches, especially in men who have undergone APR.

Acknowledgment: We thank Kevin L. Sullivan, MD, for statistical analysis.

References

1. Rifkin MD, Kurtz AB, Goldberg BB. Sonographically guided transperineal prostatic biopsy: preliminary experience with a longitudinal linear-array transducer. AJR 1983; 140:745–747.
2. Fornage BD, Dinney CP, Troncoso P. Ultrasound-guided transperineal needle biopsy of the prostate after abdominoperineal resection. JCU 1995; 23:263–265.
3. vanSonnenberg E, D'Agostino HB, Casola G, Halasz NA, Sanchez RB, Goodacre BW. Percutaneous abscess drainage: current concepts. Radiology 1991; 181:617–626.
4. Rothenberger DA, Wong WD. Abdominoperineal resection for adenocarcinoma of the low rectum. World J Surg 1992; 16: 478–485.
5. Danzi M, Ferulano GP, Abate S, Dilillo S, Califano G. Survival and locations of recurrence following abdomino-perineal resection for rectal cancer. J Surg Oncol 1986; 31:235–239.
6. Stevens KR Jr, Allen CV, Fletcher WS. Preoperative radiotherapy for adenocarcinoma of the rectosigmoid. Cancer 1976; 37:2866–2874.
7. vanSonnenberg E, D'Agostino HB, Casola G, Goodacre BW, Sanchez RB, Taylor B. US-guided transvaginal drainage of pelvic abscesses and fluid collections. Radiology 1991; 181:53–56.
8. Nosher JL, Winchman HK, Needell GS. Transvaginal pelvic abscess drainage with US guidance. Radiology 1987; 165:872–873.
9. Nosher JL, Needell GS, Amorosa JK, Krasna IH. Transrectal pelvic abscess drainage with sonographic guidance. AJR 1986; 146:1047–1048.
10. Butch RJ, Mueller PR, Ferrucci JT Jr, et al. Drainage of pelvic abscesses through the greater sciatic foramen. Radiology 1986; 158:487–491.
11. Alexander AA, Eschelman DJ, Nazarian LN, Bonn J. Transrectal sonographically guided drainage of deep pelvic abscesses. AJR 1994; 162:1227–1230.
12. Feld R, Eschelman DJ, Sagerman JE, Segal S, Hovsepian DM, Sullivan KL. Treatment of pelvic abscesses and other fluid collections: efficacy of transvaginal sonographically guided aspiration and drainage. AJR 1994; 163:1141–1145.
13. Hovsepian DM. Transrectal and transvaginal abscess drainage. JVIR 1997; 8:501–515.
14. Malden ES, Picus D. Hemorrhagic complication of transgluteal pelvic abscess drainage: successful percutaneous treatment. JVIR 1992; 3:323–328.
15. Longo JM, Bilbao JI, deVilla VH, et al. CT-guided paracoccygeal drainage of pelvic abscesses. J Comput Assist Tomogr 1993; 17:909–914.
16. Michalson AE, Brown BP, Warnock NG, Simonson TM. Presacral abscesses: percutaneous transperineal drainage with use of bone landmarks and fluoroscopic guidance. Radiology 1994; 190:574–575.
17. Karnel FJ, Schurawitzki H, Teleky B, Walter R, Gebauer A. Transperineal pelvic abscess drainage after rectal amputation: a new access. JVIR 1992; 3:22–23.
18. Bachor R, Gottfried HW, Hautmann R. Minimal invasive therapy of prostatic abscess by transrectal ultrasound-guided perineal drainage. Eur Urol 1995; 28:320–324.
19. Place C, Nolan RL, Nickel JC. Alternate approaches to pelvic abscess drainage after cystectomy. Urol Radiol 1989; 11:161–164.
20. Oberpenning F, Roth S, Leusmann DB, van Ahlen H, Hertle L. The Alcock syndrome: temporary penile insensitivity due to compression of the pudendal nerve within the Alcock canal. J Urol 1994; 151:423–425.
21. Kuligowska E, Keller E, Ferrucci JT. Treatment of pelvic abscesses: value of one-step sonographically guided transrectal needle aspiration and lavage. AJR 1995; 164:201–206.
22. Kraybill WG, Reinsch J, Puckett CL, Bricker EM. Pelvic abscess following preoperative radiation and abdominoperineal resection: management with a free flap. J Surg Oncol 1984; 25:18–20.
23. Fortier GA, Krochak RJ, Kim JA, Constable WC. Dose response to preoperative irradiation in rectal cancer: implications for local control and complications associated with sphincter sparing surgery and abdominoperineal resection. Int J Radiat Oncol Biol Phys 1986; 12:1559–1563.

Lymphadenopathy: Differentiation of Benign from Malignant Disease—Color Doppler US Assessment of Intranodal Angioarchitecture[1]

Alexander Tschammler, MD
German Ott, MD
Thomas Schang, MD
Birgit Seelbach-Goebel, MD
Konrad Schwager, MD
Dietbert Hahn, MD

Index terms:
Lymphatic system, flow dynamics
Lymphatic system, neoplasms, 99.23, 99.833, 99.834
Lymphatic system, US, 99.12981, 99.12983

Radiology 1998; 208:117–123

[1] From the Departments of Radiology (A.T., D.H.); Pathology (G.O.); Surgery (T.S.); Gynecology and Obstetrics (B.S.G.); and Ear, Nose, and Throat Medicine (K.S.), University of Würzburg, Josef-Schneider-Strasse 2, D-97080 Würzburg, Germany. Received October 23, 1997; revision requested January 5, 1998; revision received February 12; accepted March 9. **Address reprint requests to** A.T.

Author contributions:
Guarantors of integrity of entire study, D.H., A.T.; study concepts and design, A.T.; definition of intellectual content, D.H., A.T.; literature research, A.T.; clinical studies, A.T., G.O., T.S., B.S.G., K.S.; data acquisition, A.T., G.O.; data analysis, A.T.; statistical analysis, A.T.; manuscript preparation and editing, A.T.; manuscript review, D.H., A.T.

PURPOSE: To differentiate reactive from malignant lymphadenopathy by using color Doppler ultrasonographic (US) findings of intranodal blood vessels.

MATERIALS AND METHODS: Color Doppler US was performed in 117 lymph nodes in 100 consecutive patients before performance of surgical biopsy (47 nodes), neck dissection (62 nodes), or high-speed core biopsy (eight nodes). The presence of malignant changes in intranodal angioarchitecture (focal perfusion defects, aberrant course of central vessels, displacement of intranodal vessels, subcapsular vessels) was evaluated in each node. Inter- and intraobserver variability were evaluated.

RESULTS: Histopathologic examination demonstrated 48 reactive lymph nodes (longest diameter ± standard deviation, 13.5 mm ± 6.0), 56 nodal metastases (longest diameter, 19.2 mm ± 8.8), 12 malignant lymphomas (longest diameter, 23.2 mm ± 10.5), and one node infiltrated by Langerhans cell histiocytosis. At color Doppler US, 103 (88%) nodes were classified correctly, with a specificity of 77% and a sensitivity of 96%. Reproducibility was 90%–96% (κ = 0.79–0.91, $P < .001$).

CONCLUSION: Color Doppler US is a reliable and reproducible method for help in the differentiation between reactive and malignant alterations of superficial lymph nodes by using findings of intranodal angioarchitecture.

In a previous article (1), we described the typical angioarchitecture of the blood vessels in 130 reactive or malignant lymph nodes as demonstrated with color Doppler ultrasonography (US). In the meantime, the results of this retrospective study were confirmed with results reported in two other publications (2,3) in which similar criteria were used for the classification of the intranodal angioarchitecture. The purpose of the present prospective study was to test the value of our published criteria for the differential diagnosis of reactive versus malignant lymphadenopathy of superficial lymph nodes, with histopathologic correlation.

MATERIALS AND METHODS

Patients

One hundred consecutive patients (35 female and 65 male patients; average age, 53.2 years; age range, 13–80 years) were included in the study after oral informed consent had been obtained. The study complied with the principles of the Declaration of Helsinki. Clinical diagnoses served as the indication for 47 surgical lymph node biopsies, 45 neck dissections (62 lymph nodes), and eight US-guided high-speed core biopsies (Magnum Biopsy Instrument with 16-gauge needle; Bard, Covington, Ga). The diagnoses are summarized in Table 1. Usually, one lymph node in each patient was included in the study. A second lymph node was included only if there were lymph nodes with different sonomorphologies in the region of the planned surgical intervention (17 lymph nodes). Two patients who underwent two interventions at different dates are included twice in the study. Most lymph nodes were located in the cervical, submandibular, and supraclavicular regions (n = 67). Altered lymph nodes included 33 axillary nodes and 17 inguinal nodes.

The size and exact location of each assessed lymph node were reported to the surgeon. In addition, skin marks were applied if necessary. After excision, we compared the size and shape of the excised nodes with the US results to ensure that exactly the same lymph nodes were assessed both histopathologically and with US. Discrepancies between the gross morphology of the specimen and US results were found for seven lymph nodes, which were excluded from the study. In 12 additional patients, no lymph nodes were seen at US; histopathologic examination results revealed two abscesses and one granuloma in three lesions seen at US and confirmed nine cases of normal US findings in the axilla of patients with breast cancer. All eight histopathologic results from core biopsy specimens revealed malignant lymphadenopathy.

TABLE 1
Clinical Diagnoses and Histopathologic Results in 117 Lymph Nodes in 100 Patients

Pathologic Condition	Clinical Diagnosis	Histopathologic Result
Reactive lymph node	2	48
Nonspecific	0	45
Tuberculosis	0	3
Lymph node metastases	96	56
Squamous cell carcinoma	39	20
Malignant melanoma	33	22
Breast cancer	16	10
Other	8	4
Malignant lymphoma	15	12
High-grade non-Hodgkin lymphoma	0	2
Low-grade non-Hodgkin lymphoma	0	6
Hodgkin lymphoma	0	4
Langerhans cell histiocytosis	0	1*
Lymph node enlargement of unknown cause	4	0

* For purposes of statistical evaluation, this node was included in the group of malignant lymphomas because a disseminated and very aggressive form of Langerhans cell histiocytosis was seen at histopathologic examination.

US Methods

Color Doppler US (model QAD1, Quantum Medical Systems, Issaquah, Wash, distributed by Philips Medical Systems, Eindhoven, The Netherlands; or model Q2000, Versa, or Elegra, Siemens, Erlangen, Germany) was performed with a 7.5-MHz linear-array transducer and standardized parameter settings that were optimized for the detection of slow flow velocities in small vessels (1). Criteria for optimized adjustment of the power, threshold, persistence, and wall filter were the detection of small vessels in the perinodal tissues, the appearance of the first color artifacts located at the same depth as the lymph node, or both. Focus position was optimal when the depth was the same as the lower boundary of the lymph node.

Each lymph node was assessed completely by means of transverse movement of the transducer in both planes to obtain a virtually three-dimensional depiction of the intranodal angioarchitecture. Color Doppler signals were regarded as intranodal flow signals only if they could be located intranodally in both planes. All color Doppler studies were performed by the same examiner (A.T.) and were documented either digitally or on video tape.

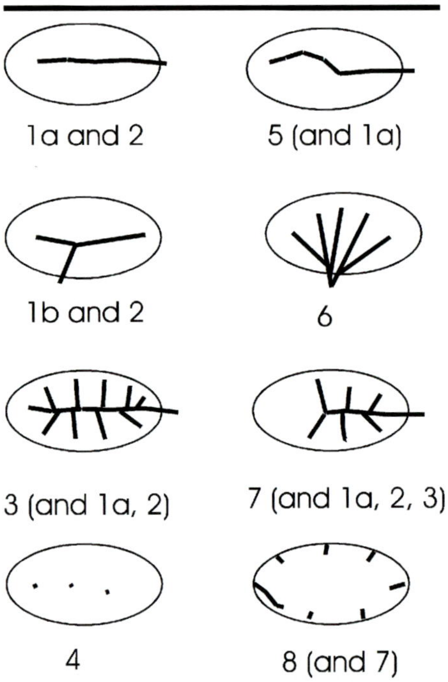

Figure 1. Schematic of the angioarchitecture in reactive (left) and malignant (right) lymph nodes. The description of the perfusion patterns is detailed in the text.

The angioarchitecture in reactive lymph nodes (Fig 1, left) was classified in hilar vessels (*1a* and *1b* in Fig 1), longitudinal vessels (*2* in Fig 1), and peripheral branches that originated from the longitudinal vessels (*3* in Fig 1; Fig 2). Some hypovascularized lymph nodes showed only small intranodal color dots, which represented short vessel segments (*4* in Fig 1).

Malignant lymph node alterations (Fig 1, right) showed typical distortions

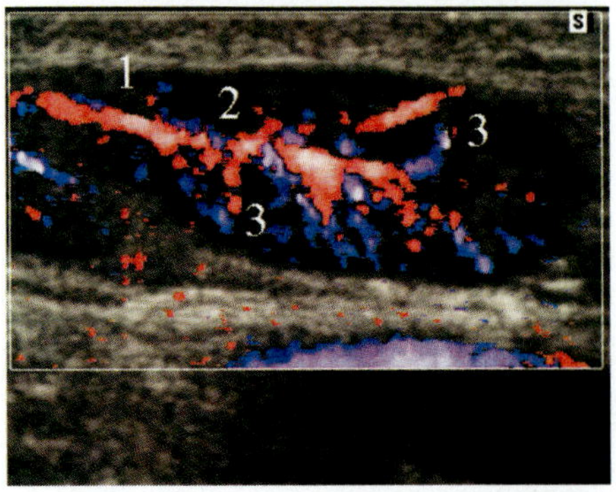

Figure 2. Color Doppler US scan shows the angioarchitecture in a hypervascularized reactive lymph node. *1* = hilar vessel, *2* = longitudinal vessel, *3* = peripheral branches.

of this angioarchitecture, which were classified by using the following four criteria: (i) displacement (*5* in Fig 1), characterized by the curved course of intranodal vessels (Fig 3a); (ii) aberrant vessels (*6* in Fig 1), characterized by one or more central vessels (no branches of a longitudinal vessel) that formed an angle of more than 30° with the skin surface or with the longitudinal axis of the lymph node (Fig 3b); (iii) focal absence of perfusion (*7* in Fig 1), characterized by intranodal regions with missing flow signals in lymph nodes that demonstrated high vascularization of the remaining intranodal tissue (Fig 3c). (iv) Subcapsular vessels (*8* in Fig 1), characterized by mostly short vessel segments in the periphery of the lymph node that do not originate from hilar or longitudinal vessels (see the Discussion) (Fig 3d).

The presence of one of these four criteria of malignancy led to the classifica-

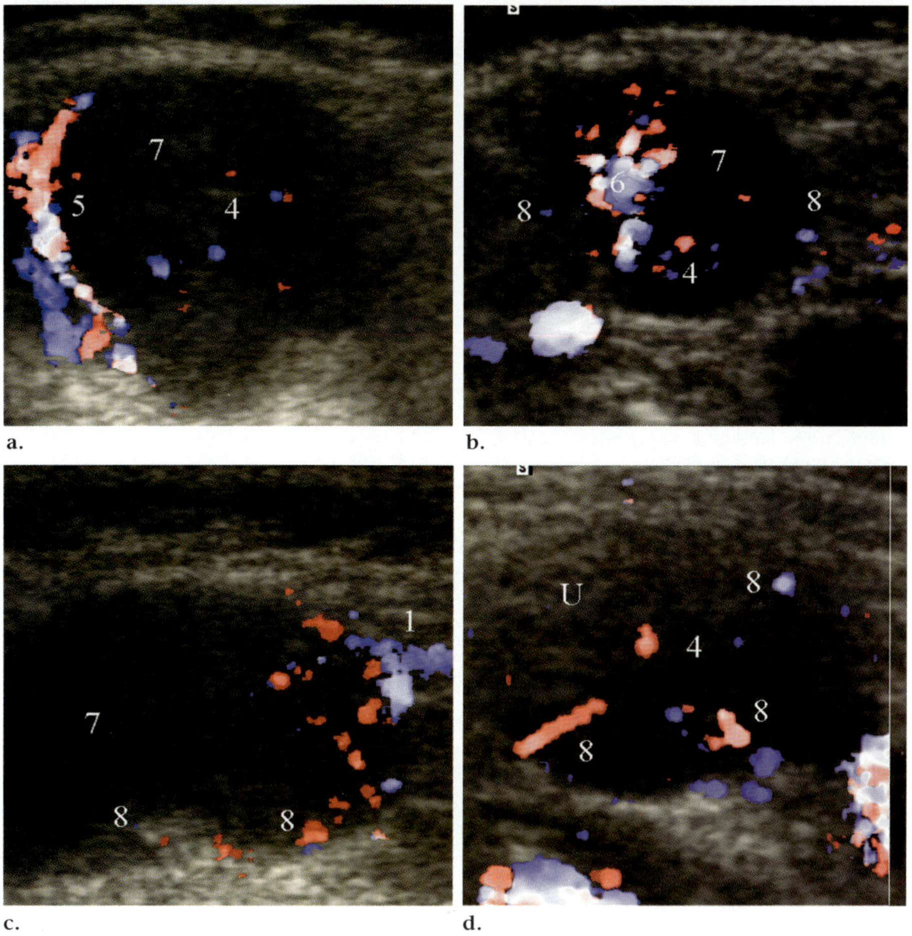

Figure 3. Color Doppler US scans show the angioarchitecture in malignant lymph nodes. **(a)** Displacement of intranodal vessels (*5*), which have an aberrant course. There is a small area with no perfusion (*7*). In the center of the lymph node, disseminated short vessel segments (*4*) can be seen. **(b)** Aberrant course of intranodal vessels (*6*) is visible; these vessels form an angle of about 90° with the skin surface. Additional findings include subcapsular vessels (*8*), a focal area of perfusion (*7*), and some short vessel segments (*4*). **(c)** A focal area of no perfusion (*7*) is shown in 80% of the lymph node tissue, and strong flow signals are present in the remaining tissue. A hilar vessel (*1*) enters the lymph node at one pole. Multiple subcapsular vessels (*8*) are present. **(d)** Subcapsular vessels (*8*) are visible. In addition, there are some short vessel segments (*4*) in the center of the lymph node. The indistinct contour (*U*) of the lymph node is a sign of perinodal tumor infiltration.

tion "malignant lymph node." Avascular lymph nodes were defined as having a benign, reactive, or regressive lymph node alteration. Documentation was standardized and included location, size, shape, echostructure, vascularization, and angioarchitecture of the lymph nodes.

In addition to the assessment of the intranodal angioarchitecture, we tested the correlation between the defined criteria of malignancy and the sonomorphology by using a multivariate regression analysis and dichotomous variables (except diameters) to search for a possible bias of the sonomorphology in the assessment of nodal angioarchitecture.

To assess the intra- and interobserver variability, a high-quality, real-time documentation of the complete lymph node study is necessary. Recording of the US studies on VHS or S-VHS video tape, which was possible with three US units, is insufficient for a detailed analysis of the intranodal angioarchitecture. Real-time storage of the digital data was possible with only one US unit (model QAD1). For this reason, reproducibility was tested with a different group of 134 lymph nodes, which were assessed consecutively and documented digitally by one observer (A.T.), who used this equipment. The final histologic or clinical diagnosis was not known for all of these 134 lymph nodes. The interobserver variability was calculated on the basis of the results of two observers (including A.T.) by using the digitally archived lymph node studies. For intraobserver variability, we compared the results of one examiner, which were documented immediately after the real-time examination and after the review of the digitally archived study performed at least 3 months later.

TABLE 2
Sonomorphology of Reactive and Malignant Lymph Nodes

Criterion	Reactive Nodes (n = 48)	Metastases (n = 56)	Malignant Lymphoma (n = 13)
Length (mm)*	13.5 ± 6.0 (6–34)	19.2 ± 8.8 (6–43)	23.2 ± 10.5 (12–50)
Thickness (mm)*	6.0 ± 2.9 (3–17)	11.6 ± 5.4 (4–29)	16.2 ± 9.9 (9–45)
Width (mm)*	9.1 ± 3.8 (4–24)	15.6 ± 7.4 (4–42)	19.4 ± 8.9 (10–45)
Shape			
Oval†	34 (71)	8 (14)	3 (23)
Round†	14 (29)	48 (86)	10 (77)
Echoic center			
Present†	26 (54)	6 (11)	4 (31)
Absent†	22 (46)	50 (89)	9 (69)

Note.—Differences among criteria between reactive nodes, metastases, and malignant lymphoma were significant ($P < .001$).
* Data are the mean ± 1 standard deviation. Numbers in parentheses are the range.
† Data are the number of lymph nodes. Number in parentheses is the percentage.

RESULTS

Sonomorphology and Angioarchitecture

Histopathologic examination yielded 48 reactive lymph nodes, 56 lymph node metastases, and 13 malignant lymphomas (Table 1). Malignant lymph nodes had larger diameters in all three axes than did reactive lymph nodes (Table 2). A missing echogenic center and a round shape were further signs of malignancy.

Thirteen lymph nodes showed no intranodal perfusion, 45 lymph nodes showed low vascularization, and 59 lymph nodes were hypervascularized compared with the vascularization of the adjacent fat and soft tissues. Twelve of 13 lymph nodes without intranodal flow signals were reactive. There was no significant difference between vascularized reactive and malignant lymph nodes in the subjective, semiquantitative assessment of lymph node perfusion.

Of the 69 malignant lymph nodes, 66 (96%) showed at least one criterion of malignancy in the assessment of the intranodal angioarchitecture (Table 3). In the 48 reactive lymph nodes, 12 (25%) showed no perfusion, 25 (52%) had a normal angioarchitectural features, and 11 (23%) were classified as false-positive, three of which were affected by tuberculosis. If perfusion defects were present, the average size of the region with missing perfusion in relation to the total volume of the lymph node was 54% in reactive lymph nodes ($n = 5$), 59% in lymph node metastases ($n = 50$), and 58% in malignant lymphomas ($n = 10$) ($P > .05$ for all three).

In those lymph nodes that were classified as malignant at color Doppler US, there were an average of 2.6 criteria of malignancy (mean ± standard deviation: reactive nodes, 2.3 criteria ± 1.0 [ie, false-positive]; metastases, 2.7 criteria ± 0.9; malignant lymphoma, 2.8 criteria ± 1.1). The negative predictive value was 93%. The positive predictive value was 86% when at least one criterion of malignancy was found. If exactly one criterion of malignancy ($n = 9$) was found, the positive predictive value was only 67%. If all four criteria of malignancy were present in a node, the positive predictive value increased to 94% (Table 4).

There was no statistically significant correlation between the criteria used to classify the intranodal angioarchitecture and the size and shape of the lymph nodes. The echogenicity of the center of the lymph nodes, which represents multiple interfaces between medullary tissue and central vessels (4), was the only sonomorphologic criterion that was correlated with the angioarchitecture (Table 5).

TABLE 3
Vascularization and Angioarchitechture in 117 Reactive and Malignant Lymph Nodes

Criterion	Reactive Lymph Nodes ($n = 48$)	Metastases ($n = 56$)	Malignant Lymphoma ($n = 13$)
Longitudinal vessel with peripheral branches	12 (25)	25 (45)	9 (69)
Longitudinal vessel without branches	28 (58)	33 (59)	11 (85)
Hilar vessels	31 (65)	30 (54)	11 (85)
Short vessel segments*	4 (8)	14 (25)	2 (15)
Focal absence of perfusion†	5 (10)	50 (89)	10 (77)
Subcapsular vessels†	10 (21)	43 (77)	7 (54)
Displacement†	4 (8)	25 (47)	6 (46)
Aberrant course†	6 (13)	28 (50)	10 (77)
No perfusion†	12 (25)	1 (2)	0 (0)
Only benign criteria†	25 (52)	1 (2)	1 (8)
One or more criteria of malignancy†	11 (23)	54 (96)	12 (92)
One criterion of malignancy	3 (6)	4 (7)	2 (15)
Two criteria of malignancy	3 (6)	20 (36)	2 (15)
Three criteria of malignancy	4 (8)	18 (32)	5 (38)
Four criteria of malignancy	1 (2)	12 (21)	3 (23)

Note.—Data are number of nodes. Numbers in parentheses are percentages.
* Difference between reactive and malignant nodes was significant ($P < .05$).
† Difference between reactive and malignant was significant ($P < .001$).

TABLE 4
Positive and Negative Predictive Values according to Number of Criteria of Malignancy in 48 Reactive and 69 Malignant Lymph Nodes

No. of Criteria	No. of Lymph Nodes	Negative Predictive Value (%)	Positive Predictive Value (%)
None	40	93	...
One or more	77	...	86
One	9	...	67
Two	25	...	88
Three	27	...	86
Four	16	...	94

Reproducibility

The reproducibility of the assessment of the intranodal angioarchitecture was tested with a different group of 134 lymph nodes. Results were documented by observer A immediately after the real-time US examination. Results obtained at independent review of the digitally stored images by observers A and B were also documented (Table 6). The rate of lymph nodes classified as malignant was equal to that found in the study of 117 nodes with histopathologic correlation, but the number of pathologic criteria found was lower.

The reproducibility of the four single criteria was 85%–90% for the evaluation of the intraobserver variability. Of the 134 lymph nodes, 129 (96%) were classified identically by observer A immediately after US and 3 months later. The κ value of 0.91 indicates nearly perfect agreement between the two observations (Table 7).

The interobserver variability (Table 8) was slightly higher than the intraobserver variability; 121 (90%) of the 134 lymph nodes were classified identically by both observers. The κ value of 0.79 indicates very good agreement between the two observers. The reproducibility with regard to a single criterion (84%–87%) was in the same range as that for the assessment of intraobserver variability.

TABLE 5
Correlation between Malignant Angioarchitecture and Echogenicity of the Center in 117 Lymph Nodes

Angioarchitecture	Echogenicity: Normal	Narrow	Absent
Focal absence of perfusion*			
No	13	17	22
Yes	3	3	59
Aberrant course†			
No	10	8	15
Yes	3	4	37
Displacement‡			
No	12	10	28
Yes	0	2	33
Subcapsular vessels§			
No	13	17	24
Yes	3	2	55

* Difference between the presence of normal or narrow echogenicity and the absence of echogenicity was significant ($P < .001$).
† Difference between the presence of normal or narrow echogenicity and the absence of echogenicity was significant ($P < .01$). There were no data for 40 nodes.
‡ Difference between the presence of normal or narrow echogenicity and the absence of echogenicity was significant ($P < .001$). There were no data for 32 nodes.
§ Difference between the presence of normal or narrow echogenicity and the absence of echogenicity was significant ($P < .001$). There were no data for three nodes.

DISCUSSION

Color Doppler US is the only method that can display the angioarchitecture of

TABLE 6
Frequency of Malignancy Criteria in 134 Lymph Nodes Assessed by Two Observers

	Initial Reading	Review	
Criterion	Observer A	Observer A	Observer B
Focal absence of perfusion	64 (48)	57 (43)	58 (43)
Subcapsular vessels	56 (42)	55 (41)	47 (35)
Displacement	34 (25)	34 (25)	47 (35)
Aberrant course	49 (37)	47 (35)	55 (41)
One or more criteria	75 (56)	73 (54)	74 (55)

Note.—Results of the initial reading were documented immediately after US. Results of the review of digitally stored images took place at least 3 months after US. Numbers in parentheses are percentages.

TABLE 7
Intraobserver Variability in Assessment of 134 Lymph Nodes

Criterion	Identical Assessment	Contradictory Assessment	κ Value*
Focal absence of perfusion	119 (89)	15 (11)	0.77
Subcapsular vessels	119 (89)	15 (11)	0.77
Displacement	120 (90)	14 (10)	0.72
Aberrant course	114 (85)	20 (15)	0.68
One or more criteria of malignancy	129 (96)	6 (4)	0.91

Note.—Numbers in parentheses are percentages.
* Difference from chance agreement was significant ($P < .001$).

TABLE 8
Interobserver Variability in Assessment of 134 Lymph Nodes

Criterion	Identical Assessment	Contradictory Assessment	κ Value*
Focal absence of perfusion	116 (87)	18 (13)	0.73
Subcapsular vessels	113 (84)	21 (16)	0.67
Displacement	114 (85)	20 (15)	0.65
Aberrant course	113 (84)	21 (16)	0.67
One or more criteria of malignancy	121 (90)	14 (10)	0.79

Note.—Numbers in parentheses are percentages.
* Difference from chance agreement was significant ($P < .001$).

lymph nodes in daily practice (5–10). There are only a few case reports about intranodal vessels depicted at angiography (11) or computed tomography (CT) (12). Color Doppler US will not show all intranodal blood vessels. The relatively low number of backscattering erythrocytes in the tiny peripheral vessels decreases the signal intensity (13), which may not surpass the noise level. Low flow velocities or high Doppler angles result in a low Doppler frequency shift, which may be suppressed by the high-pass or wall filter. Postprocessing functions that suppress flow signals in echogenic tissues to reduce motion artifacts may also suppress flow signals in the echogenic center of the lymph node. Consequently, absent flow signals do not mean perfusion is absent. Lymphatic vessels are not displayed at color Doppler sonography due to the low flow velocity and the lack of backscattering erythrocytes.

To our knowledge, in 1988 Morton et al (14) were the first to describe flow signals in the hilum of lymph nodes by using color Doppler US. Further studies (6,7,15–18) described flow signals in the hilum or center of reactive lymph nodes. If the intranodal vessels are assessed meticulously, reactive lymph nodes display the angioarchitecture known from histopathologic (19–24) and microangiographic (23) studies (*1–4* in Fig 1). The main arteries and veins enter the lymph node at the hilum and spread in bundles of arterioles and venules that course in alignment with the long axis of the lymph node (23,25). The cortex of the lymph node is fed by capillaries originating from these hilar and medullary vessels.

First described in 1991 (5), focal absence of perfusion was the first criterion of a distorted angioarchitecture in malignant lymph nodes. Later, the value of this criterion for the differential diagnosis of lymph node alterations was confirmed with the results of two other studies (6,7). Perfusion deficits and the displacement of vessels (26–28) are well known angiographic criteria for pathologic perfusion in tumors and metastases. Further angiographic criteria for pathologic perfusion patterns, such as irregular vessel diameters, stenoses, occlusions, arteriovenous shunts, or dilated veins (26, 27,29–32), were not depicted at color Doppler US, probably because of the low spatial resolution of color Doppler US in relation to the diameter of the intranodal vessels. Lacunar vessels that are striking at angiography cannot be displayed at color Doppler US due to their slow flow velocity.

Aberrant central vessels do not correlate with the angiographic findings of pathologic vessels, which have been described as starlike, tortuous, or chaotic (26–30). With color Doppler US, this criterion describes only an increased angle (>30°, usually near 90°) between large central vessels and the skin surface. If the lymph node has an obvious longitudinal axis, this axis should be chosen as the anatomic reference instead of the skin surface. In reactive lymph nodes, the angle between longitudinal vessels and the skin surface or longitudinal axis is near 0°. The limit of 30° was determined on the basis of clinical experience, to reduce errors caused by inaccurate measurements of the angle.

Subcapsular vessels are the only criterion of malignancy that can be applied to hypovascularized lymph nodes with only short intranodal vessel segments. Subcapsular vessels were originally called accessory vessels because it was thought they would correlate with neovascularization (1). Preliminary results of a study of the US-histopathologic correlation (33) show that these vessels are located in residual subcapsular lymphatic tissue after central malignant lymph node infiltration.

There were a higher number of false-positive classifications in the present prospective study than in our previous retrospective study (1), which decreased the specificity and the positive predictive value. The sensitivity and the negative predictive value were greater than 95%. The increase in false-positive results may have been caused by overinterpretation of peripheral flow signals that were better depicted with the newer US equipment, which provides better image resolution. (Morphologic causes for false-positive results are discussed in the next paragraph.) We could not assess whether the results of our color Doppler studies could have had any effect on further diagnostic or therapeutic procedures because the clinical indication to perform a lymph node biopsy was the main inclusion criterion for our study.

The presence of subcapsular vessels was the criterion that led to the highest number of false-positive results. This criterion was positive in two lymph nodes that were suspected of being a conglomerate of two reactive nodes, but there was no clear boundary between the nodes. In both lymph nodes, there were major and minor vessels with regular branches to the periphery that had to be classified as subcapsular vessels, according our definition. These false-positive results could have been avoided if the definition of subcapsular vessels were changed to "the presence of at least two vessels in the periphery of the lymph node that do not originate from hilar or central vessels." Tuberculous infiltration of lymph nodes leads to destruction of the lymph node architecture in a manner similar to tumor infiltration. In consequence, these lymph nodes show a sonomorphology (34) and angioarchitecture similar to that found in malignant lymph nodes.

One of the three false-negative results was a lymph node infiltrated by low-grade non-Hodgkin lymphoma. This type of lymphoma less frequently shows distortions of the angioarchitecture (1). The two remaining false-negative results occurred in metastases of squamous cell carcinoma. One of these two lymph nodes displayed a normal intranodal angioarchitecture; the other showed no perfusion. Avascularity was defined as a sign of benignancy, although it is known that acute reactive alterations of lymph nodes lead to hypervascularity (35,36). However, no flow signals were found in 17%–100% of benign lymph node alterations described by several authors (6–9,18,37,38). This was probably caused by regressive tissue alterations, which have low perfusion.

In lesions that show no or only tiny flow signals, power Doppler US may detect more flow signals than color Doppler US (39). Power Doppler US was not used in the present study because only one of the four US units was equipped with this technology. Our preliminary experience with the assessment of lymph node alterations shows no advantages for power Doppler US if color Doppler US clearly depicts intranodal flow signals. The results of one study (40) in which power Doppler US was used for the differential diagnosis of lymph node alterations showed insufficient diagnostic accuracy. It is possible that the use of US contrast media may increase the sensitivity of flow detection in lymph nodes (41), but at the present we are aware of no information on the effect of such contrast media on diagnostic accuracy.

In a study with color Doppler US, a bias caused by the sonomorphology of the lesions can never be excluded. Sonomorphologic changes are known to be nonspecific, however, and proved to result in lower accuracy than changes in the angioarchitecture of lymph nodes (1). In the present study, we evaluated the correlation between angioarchitecture and sonomorphology but found no statistically significant evidence for a bias as a result of the sonomorphology. The echogenicity of the center of the lymph nodes was the only sonomorphologic criterion that correlated with the angioarchitecture. That result was to be expected, because the echogenic center is known to represent multiple interfaces between central blood vessels, the lymphatic sinus, and medullary tissues (4).

In numerous publications on the imaging of superficial lymph nodes with the use of US, CT, or magnetic resonance imaging, there are no reports on inter- or intraobserver variability, to our knowledge. In our study, intraobserver variability was lower than interobserver variability, as expected. The κ value of 0.91 indicates nearly perfect agreement between a single observer's two observations separated by an interval of at least 3 months. Agreement was a very good (κ = 0.79) between the two observers, which indicates high reproducibility of the criteria for the assessment of the intranodal angioarchitecture.

The criteria for malignancy are valid only for the assessment of superficial lymph node alterations. The angioarchitecture cannot be assessed reliably in lymph nodes located in the mediastinum or abdomen because of the increased attenuation of the ultrasound beam with increased depth. The assessment of mediastinal lymph nodes is additionally impaired by means of pulsations originating from the heart and great vessels. Mesenteric lymph nodes have a specific angioarchitecture, with a vascular supply from vessels that penetrate the capsule at multiple extrahilar sites (21,23).

In conclusion, the assessment of intranodal angioarchitecture with color Doppler US is a reliable and reproducible method to help differentiate between reactive and malignant lymphadenopathy in superficial lymph nodes.

Acknowledgment: We thank Stefan Schmitt, MD, for interpreting US studies for the assessment of interobserver agreement.

References

1. Tschammler A, Wirkner H, Ott G, Hahn D. Vascular patterns in reactive and malignant lymphadenopathy. Eur Radiol 1996; 6:473–480.
2. Omlor G, Dill-Mueller D, Gross G, et al. Elektive lymphknotendissektion (ELND) beim malignen melanom: stellenwert des farbdopplerbefundes. Zentralbl Chir 1996; 121: 469–473.
3. Na DG, Lim HK, Byun HS, Kim HD, Ko YH, Haek JH. Differential diagnosis of cervical lymphadenopathy: usefulness of color Doppler sonography. AJR 1997; 168:1311–1316.
4. Rubaltelli L, Proto E, Salmaso R, Bortoletto P, Candiani F, Cagol P. Sonography of abnormal lymph nodes in vitro: correlation of sonographic and histologic findings. AJR 1990; 155:1241–1244.
5. Tschammler A, Gunzer U, Reinhart E, et al. Dignitaetsbeurteilung vergroesserter lymphknoten durch qualitative und semiquantitative auswertung der lymphknotenperfusion mit der farbkodierten duplexsonographie. ROFO 1991; 154:414–418.
6. Schreiber J, Mann W, Lieb W. Farbduplexsonographische messung der lymphknotenperfusion: ein beitrag zur diagnostik der zervikalen metastasierung. Laryngorhinootologie 1993; 72:187–192.
7. Steinkamp HJ, Rausch M, Maeurer J, et al. Farbkodierte duplexsonographie in der differentialdiagnostik zervikaler lymphknotenvergroesserungen. ROFO 1994; 161: 226–232.
8. Steinkamp HJ, Maeurer J, Cornehl M, Knoebber D, Hettwer H, Felix R. Recurrent cervical lymphadenopathy: differential diagnosis with color-duplex sonography. Eur Arch Otorhinolaryngol 1994; 251:404–409.
9. Chang DB, Yuan A, Yu CJ, Luh KT, Kuo HS, Yang PC. Differentiation of benign and malignant cervical lymph nodes with color Doppler sonography. AJR 1994; 162:965–968.
10. Choi MY, Lee YW, Kyung JJ. Distinction between benign and malignant causes of cervical, axillary and inguinal lymphadenopathy: value of Doppler spectral waveform analysis. AJR 1995; 165:981–984.
11. Bjoerk L, Leven H. Intra-arterial DSA and duplex-sonography in detection of vascularized inguinal lymph node. Acta Radiol 1990; 31:106–107.
12. Sakai F, Sone S, Kiyono K, et al. Computed tomography of neck lymph nodes involved

with malignant lymphoma: comparison with ultrasound. Radiat Med 1991; 9:203–208.
13. Nakayama K, Furuhata H. Necessary requirements for blood flow-metering by ultrasonic Doppler method. Electronics Commun Jpn 1974; 57:82–92.
14. Morton MJ, Charboneau JW, Banks PM. Inguinal lymphadenopathy simulating a false aneurysm in color flow Doppler sonography. AJR 1988; 151:115–116.
15. Turlington BS, Reading CC, Charboneau JW. Color Doppler US in the neck: differentiating neoplastic from nonneoplastic lymphadenopathy (abstr). Radiology 1991; 181(P):177.
16. Ohnesorge I, Koenig H, Schill S, Wolf KJ. Color-coded duplex sonography of pathologically enlarged lymph nodes (abstr). Radiology 1991; 181(P):177.
17. Swischuk LE, Desai PB, John SD. Exuberant blood flow in enlarged lymph nodes: findings on color flow Doppler. Pediatr Radiol 1992; 22:419–421.
18. Raffaelli C, Bruneton JN, Padovani B, Belaidi M, Chanalet S. Normal cervical and inguinal lymph nodes: color Doppler evaluation (abstr). J Ultrasound Med 1996; 15(suppl):83.
19. His. Beitraege zur kenntnis der zum lymphsystem gehoerigen druesen. Z Wissensch Zool 1860; 10:333–357.
20. Calvert WJ. The blood vessels of the lymphatic gland. Anat Anz 1897; 13:174–180.
21. Darbelow A. Die blutgefaessversorgung der lymphatischen organe. Verh Anat Gesellsch 1939; 46:179–224.
22. Herman PG, Ohba S, Mellins HZ. Blood microcirculation in the lymph node. Radiology 1969; 92:1073–1080.
23. Semeraro D, Davies JD. The arterial blood supply of human inguinal and mesenteric lymph nodes. J Anat 1986; 144:221–233.
24. Bélisle C, Saint-Marie G. Blood vascular network of the rat lymph node: tridimensional studies by light and scanning electron microscopy. Am J Anat 1990; 189:111–126.
25. Gadre A, Briner W, O'Leary M. A scanning electron microscope study of the human cervical lymph node. Acta Otolaryngol 1994; 114:87–90.
26. Baum S, Roy R, Finkelstein AK, Blakemore WS. Clinical application of selective celiac and superior mesenteric arteriography. Radiology 1965; 84:279–294.
27. Sammons BP, Neal MP, Armstrong RH, Hager HG. Ten years experience with celiac and upper abdominal superior mesenteric arteriography. AJR 1967; 101:345–360.
28. Nebesar RA, Pollard JJ, Stone DL. Angiographic diagnosis of malignant disease of the liver. Radiology 1966; 56:284–291.
29. Anacker H, Gaul A, Bernett P. Die arteriographie des mammakarzinoms. ROFO 1970; 113:448–456.
30. Feldmann F, Habif DV, Fleming RJ, Kanter IE, Seaman WB. Arteriography of the breast. Radiology 1967; 89:1053–1061.
31. Ney FG, Feist JH, Altemus LR, Ordinario VR. The characteristic angiographic criteria of malignancy. Radiology 1972; 104:567–570.
32. Viamonte M, Roen S, LePage J. Nonspecificity of abnormal vascularity in the angiographic diagnosis of malignant neoplasms. Radiology 1973; 106:59–63.
33. Tschammler A, Haeuser B, Ott G, Hahn D. Colour Doppler sonography of superficial lymph nodes: histopathological correlation (abstr). Eur Radiol 1997; 7(suppl):155.
34. Evans RM, Ahuja A, Metreweli C. The linear echogenic hilus in cervical lymphadenopathy: a sign of benignity or malignancy? Clin Radiol 1993; 47:262–264.
35. Hay JB, Hobbs BB. The flow of blood to lymph nodes and its relation to lymphocyte traffic and the immune response. J Exp Med 1977; 145:31–44.
36. Herman PG, Lyonnet D, Fingerhut R, Tuttle RN. Regional blood flow to the lymph node during the immune response. Lymphology 1976; 9:101–104.
37. Giovagnorio F, Rusticali A, Araneo AL. Color and pulsed Doppler evaluation of benign and malignant adenopathy. Clin Imaging 1997; 21:163–169.
38. Bruneton JN, Balu-Maestro C, Marcy PY, Melia P, Mourou MY. Very high frequency (13 MHz) ultrasonographic examination of the normal neck. J Ultrasound Med 1994; 13:87–90.
39. Hosoki T, Mitomo M, Chor S, Miyahara N, Ohtani M, Morimoto K. Visualization of tumor vessels in hepatocellular carcinoma: power Doppler compared with color Doppler and angiography. Acta Radiol 1997; 38:422–427.
40. Giovagnorio F, Caiazzo R, Avitto A. Evaluation of vascular patterns of cervical lymph nodes with power Doppler sonography. J Clin Ultrasound 1997; 25:71–76.
41. Tschammler A, Krahe T, Wittenberg G, Jenett M. Contrast enhanced color Doppler flow imaging of superficial lymph nodes and correlation with dynamic MRI (abstr). Echocardiography 1993; 10:682.

Book Review

Duke Radiology Case Review: Imaging, Differential Diagnosis, and Discussion

Edited by James M. Provenzale, MD, and Rendon C. Nelson, MD
Philadelphia, Pa: Lippincott-Raven, 1997. ISBN 0-397-51613-4.
Softcover, $75.00; pp 596; 275 figures.

Duke Radiology Case Review: Imaging, Differential Diagnosis, and Discussion was prepared by the Duke University Department of Radiology as a resource for radiology residents to use in preparation for the American Board of Radiology (ABR) oral examination. This book is specifically designed to simulate the way radiology residents are typically taught, with information organized in a case-presentation format.

This book is divided into the 10 major subsections of the ABR oral examination: chest, breast, gastrointestinal, genitourinary, musculoskeletal, neuroradiology, vascular, pediatric, ultrasound, and nuclear medicine. Nearly 30 cases are presented in each chapter. Each case presentation includes a one- or two-sentence clinical history, followed by several images of the entity that were obtained by using different modalities. The radiographic findings for each image are briefly described. Discussion for each case includes a differential diagnosis, final diagnosis, and key clinical and radiologic facts. The discussion is not meant to be exhaustive but serves more as a framework on which the resident can build. Included is a brief suggested reading list that directs the reader to more extensive reference material.

The editors have created a visually appealing textbook. The selected images are, for the most part, of high quality. However, the more subtle findings, especially in the chest and musculoskeletal sections, are often difficult to appreciate. The important radiographic features of each image are discussed without the benefit of arrows on the figures to guide the reader.

The book is clearly written for all resident levels. The case-presentation format allows the reader to approach each case as an unknown diagnosis. The strengths of this book, which set it apart from other review resources, are the extensive list of differential diagnoses for each case and the reasonable arguments for exclusion of incorrect diagnoses. This is especially important for the resident preparing for the ABR oral examination.

This review textbook efficiently covers a large number of important entities in a well-organized manner. Reasonably priced at $75.00, this review will greatly benefit radiology residents preparing for the ABR oral examination, as well as residents who simply want a quick review prior to starting a new rotation.

Reviewed by Karen L. Killeen, MD

Head Trauma: CT Scan Interpretation by Radiology Residents versus Staff Radiologists[1]

Michael G. Wysoki, MD
Carlos J. Nassar, MD
Robert A. Koenigsberg, DO
Robert A. Novelline, MD
Scott H. Faro, MD
Eric N. Faerber, MD

Index terms:
Brain, injuries, 13.1211, 13.433
Diagnostic radiology, observer performance, 13.1211
Education
Head, injuries, 10.1211, 10.41, 10.433
Images, interpretation, 13.1211

Radiology 1998; 208:125–128

[1] From the Department of Radiology, Allegheny University Hospital, 3300 Henry Ave, Philadelphia, PA 19129 (M.G.W., C.J.N., R.A.K., S.H.F.); the Department of Radiology, Massachusetts General Hospital, Boston (R.A.N.); and the Department of Radiology, St Christopher's Hospital for Children, Philadelphia, PA (E.N.F.). Received October 23, 1997; revision requested December 23; final revision received February 25, 1998; accepted March 4. **Address reprint requests to** M.G.W.

PURPOSE: To determine the rate and clinical outcome of discrepancies in interpretation by radiology residents and staff neuroradiologists of posttraumatic cranial computed tomographic (CT) scans.

MATERIALS AND METHODS: Prospective evaluation was performed for 419 consecutive emergency posttraumatic cranial CT studies that had been interpreted by radiology residents on call over a 16-month period. Discrepancies between the interpretations made by residents and those made by staff radiologists were divided into two groups: failure to recognize an abnormality (false-negative finding) and interpretation of normal as abnormal (false-positive finding). Discrepancies were considered major if they could affect patient care in the emergency setting and minor if they could not.

RESULTS: Major and minor discrepancies were 1.7% and 2.6%, respectively, among interpretations made by residents and those by staff radiologists. Major discrepancies were four subdural hematomas, one pneumocephalus, one hemorrhagic contusion, and one subarachnoid hemorrhage. Minor discrepancies included six skull and five facial fractures. The discrepancy rate was statistically significantly higher (12.2%) when CT findings were abnormal than when they were normal (1.5%). No change in treatment was attributed to the delay in diagnosis.

CONCLUSION: A low discrepancy rate was found between interpretations made by radiology residents and those made by staff neuroradiologists of posttraumatic cranial CT scans. There were no adverse clinical outcomes.

Trauma is the leading cause of death in children and young adults, with head trauma contributing to the cause of death in more than 50% of trauma patients (1). Although some hospitals may have immediate interpretation by trained radiologists or neuroradiologists available at all hours every day, many centers do not always have this capability. In many institutions, radiology residents interpret all radiologic studies after working hours; these studies include the emergency trauma computed tomographic (CT) scans of the head.

Cranial CT is currently the modality of choice in the initial work-up of head trauma (2). Therefore, misinterpretation of posttraumatic cranial CT scans has potential for substantial morbidity and mortality. Among trauma patients who undergo neurosurgery, those who have fewer symptoms ultimately have the best prognosis (3–5). Therefore, accurate CT scan interpretation is particularly important, since it allows identification of traumatic lesions at an early stage, when patients have fewer symptoms and clinical suspicion is low (6,7).

Test misinterpretation rates have been suggested as a quality assurance indicator (8,9). Our study was designed to assess the discrepancy rate between interpretations made by radiology residents on call and those made by attending neuroradiologists. In addition, the clinical relevance of the discrepancies was determined.

Author contributions:
Guarantors of integrity of entire study, M.G.W., C.J.N.; study concepts, M.G.W., C.J.N., R.A.K., S.H.F.; study design, M.G.W., C.J.N.; literature research, M.G.W.; clinical studies, M.G.W., C.J.N., R.A.K., S.H.F.; data acquisition, M.G.W., C.J.N., R.A.K., S.H.F.; data analysis, M.G.W., C.J.N.; statistical analysis, M.G.W.; manuscript preparation, M.G.W., C.J.N.; manuscript editing, R.A.N., E.N.F.; manuscript review, R.A.K., S.H.F., R.A.N., E.N.F.

MATERIALS AND METHODS

Four hundred nineteen consecutive emergency posttraumatic CT studies of the head were performed after working hours (Saturday and Sunday and 5 PM to 8 AM Monday through Friday) at a level one trauma center over a 16-month period (October 1995 through February 1997). Each scan was interpreted by the radiology resident on call. All studies were performed with a single CT scanner (PQ 2000; Picker International, Cleveland, Ohio) and a protocol of contiguous axial 5-mm sections through the posterior fossa and contiguous axial 10-mm sections to the vertex. Brain (window width, 80 HU; level, 40 HU), subdural (width, 350 HU; level, 40 HU), and bone (width, 3,500 HU; level, 500 HU) windows were scanned in each patient. No contrast material was administered.

Sixteen radiology residents who were on call during that time participated in the study. Before being on call, all residents had at least 1 month of neuroradiology training, 3 additional months of general radiology training, and 3 h/wk of dedicated neuroradiologic conferences. In Allegheny University Hospital, residents are on call during their 1st, 2nd, and 3rd years of radiology training.

For each patient who underwent trauma-related cranial CT, the resident recorded the patient information, the date, a short history, and the findings. This information was written and presented to the attending neuroradiologist the next morning. The staff neuroradiologist reviewed the scans and documented any discrepancies between interpretations made by the radiology resident and those made by the neuroradiologist.

Discrepancies were divided into two groups: failure to recognize an abnormality (false-negative finding) and interpretation of scans that were negative for traumatic injury as positive (false-positive finding). The false-negative findings were further divided into two groups: major discrepancies if they could affect emergency patient care or minor discrepancies if immediate care could not be affected.

Findings considered major discrepancies included an intracranial hemorrhage and pneumocephalus. Findings considered minor discrepancies were nondisplaced skull fracture, facial fracture, sinus and/or mastoid fluid, and soft-tissue hematoma or laceration. The clinical follow-up was based on communication with the clinical staff and imaging findings.

TABLE 1
Discrepancies among Residents by Type of Discrepancy and Year of Training

Year of Training	Total No. of Cases	Correct Diagnosis	False-Negative Finding: Minor Discrepancy	False-Negative Finding: Major Discrepancy	False-Positive Finding	Total No. of Discrepancies
1st	164	150 (91.5)	8 (4.9)	4 (2.4)	2 (1.2)	14 (8.5)
2nd	176	174 (98.9)	1 (0.6)	0	1 (0.6)	2 (1.1)
3rd	79	73 (92)	2 (2)	3 (4)	1 (1)	6 (8)
Total	419	379 (90.4)	11 (2.6)	7 (1.7)	4 (1.0)	22 (5.2)

Note.—Numbers in parentheses are percentages.

RESULTS

Discrepancies

The overall discrepancy rate for false-positive and false-negative findings was 22 in 419 studies (5.2%). Among the false-negative findings, major discrepancies were identified in seven of 419 patients (1.7%). These discrepancies included four subdural hematomas, one hemorrhagic contusion, one pneumocephalus, and one subarachnoid hemorrhage. Minor discrepancies were identified in 11 of 419 patients (2.6%). These included six skull fractures and five facial bone fractures. The discrepancies among the false-positive findings included three normal scans that were interpreted as subdural hemorrhages and one arteriovenous malformation that was misinterpreted as an intracranial hemorrhage (four of 419 [1%]). Table 1 presents the number and type of discrepancies for each training level. The total discrepancy rate was highest for 1st-year residents (8.5%), followed by the 3rd-year residents (8%). The 2nd-year residents had the lowest rate (1.1%). The difference between the discrepancies among the 3rd- and 1st-year residents was not statistically significant ($P > .05$, Fisher exact test). The discrepancy rate for the 2nd-year residents was significantly lower when compared with that for the other residents ($P < .05$, Fisher exact test).

Table 2 contains the discrepancy rates among scans positive and negative for traumatic injury: Discrepancy was found in 12.2% of the positive scans (false-negative findings). This number was statistically significantly higher ($P < .0001$, Fisher exact test) than the discrepancy rate of 1.5% for the negative scans (false-positive findings).

A total of 69 intracranial hemorrhages were found in 57 patients. Six intracranial hemorrhages were not identified by the resident (9%). A total of 63 facial and cranial fractures were found in 57 patients. Eleven fractures were not identified by the resident (17%). No statistically significant difference between discrepancy rates for identification of fractures or hemorrhages was found ($P > .05$, Fisher exact test).

TABLE 2
Discrepancy Rates among Scans Positive and Negative for Traumatic Injury

Finding	Discrepancy	No Discrepancy	Total
Positive	18 (12.2)	129 (87.8)	147 (35.1)
Negative	4 (1.5)	268 (98.5)	272 (64.9)
Total	22 (5.2)	397 (94.7)	419 (100)

Note.—Data are the number of scans. Numbers in parentheses are percentages.

All unidentified fractures were clearly seen with bone window settings. The unidentified subdural hemorrhages were seen clearly with the subdural window settings. The pneumocephalus was clearly seen with both subdural and bone window settings. Sixteen of 18 discrepancies (89%) were clearly discernible with subdural or bone settings.

Clinical Outcome

None of the patients in whom diagnosis was delayed required surgery; the intracranial hemorrhages missed by the resident were too small to necessitate any surgical intervention. Two patients with false-positive findings were transferred to a pediatric hospital for further observation. The other two patients with false-positive findings were admitted for observation for a few hours, pending scan interpretation by a staff neuroradiologist.

DISCUSSION

To our knowledge, no studies examining discrepancy rates in the evaluation of CT

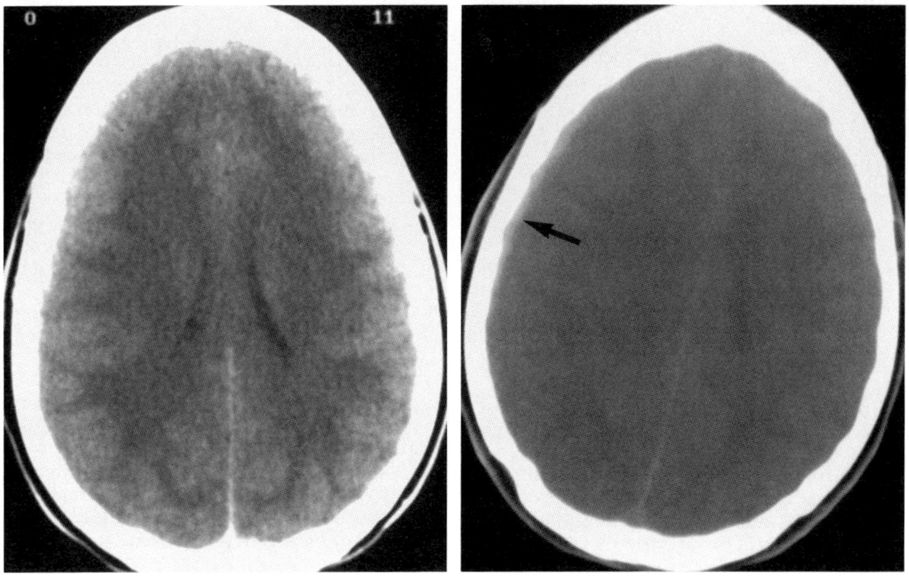

a. b.

Figure 1. False-negative finding in an 18-year-old man injured in a motor vehicle accident. **(a)** Axial unenhanced cranial CT scan obtained at the level of the roof of the lateral ventricles with a brain window setting (width, 80 HU; level, 40 HU) shows no abnormalities. **(b)** Axial unenhanced cranial CT scan obtained with a subdural window setting (width, 350 HU; level, 40 HU) in the same patient shows a right convex subdural hematoma (arrow) that was not identified by the resident on call.

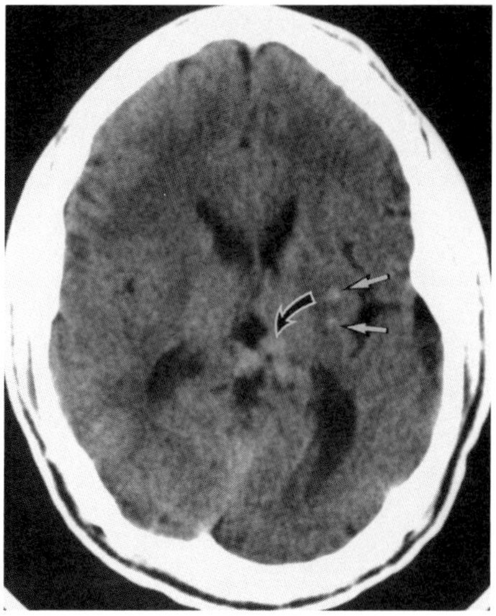

Figure 2. False-positive finding in a 66-year-old woman with trauma to the head. Axial unenhanced cranial CT scan obtained at the level of the roof the foramen of Monro with a brain window setting (width, 80 HU; level, 40 HU) shows two small, focal hyperattenuating areas (straight arrows) in the left subinsular white matter that were initially interpreted as intracranial hemorrhage by the resident on call. The staff neuroradiologist interpreted the areas as an arteriovenous malformation. Note the enlarged draining vein in the region of the vein of Galen (curved arrow).

scans obtained in patients with head trauma have been reported. We found a low discrepancy rate (5.3%) between the interpretation of posttraumatic cranial CT scans by radiology residents and that by staff neuroradiologists, with no adverse clinical outcome. Discrepancies in interpretation have been reported for a variety of radiologic examinations (8,10). For instance, the disagreement rate for interpretation by two different staff radiologists has been reported to be 10%–23% with mammography and 13%–19% with barium enema studies (11,12). Discrepancy rates for interpretation by residents and by staff were 26% for chest radiography and 13.7% for body CT (13,14). These discrepancy rates are higher than the discrepancy rate in our study. However, Alfaro et al (15) found a discrepancy rate of 38.7% between staff emergency medicine physicians and staff radiologists in the interpretation of emergency CT scans of the head. Potentially clinically relevant discrepancies were found in 24.1%. This rate is much higher than the discrepancy rate among radiology residents and staff neuroradiologists in our study.

A significant difference was found in discrepancy rates among various levels of training. The discrepancy rate among 1st-year residents was the highest (8.5%). The discrepancy rate among 3rd-year resident was almost as high (8%). The lowest rate of discrepancies was among 2nd-year residents (1.1%). The higher discrepancy rate for 1st-year residents could be explained on the basis of inexperience. Overconfidence and lack of thorough examination of the CT scan are possible explanations for the relatively high discrepancy rate found among 3rd-year residents. These results are in concordance with those of Herman and Hessel (9), who state that beyond a basic level of training, experience is overshadowed by the individual reading characteristics.

Sixteen of the 18 false-negative discrepancies were clearly discernible with subdural or bone windows. For example, all the intracranial hemorrhages, including subdural hematomas, were clearly seen with the subdural window settings (Fig 1). No statistically significant difference was found between the discrepancy rate in identification of bone fractures and that of intracranial hemorrhages. It has been reported that the likelihood of missing a finding in a radiologic study increases if another finding is identified first (13). Therefore, a possible explanation for these false-negative discrepancies is that the residents first looked carefully at scans obtained with brain window settings; after finding those scans negative, examination of scans obtained with bone and subdural window settings was performed less thoroughly.

Four false-positive discrepancies were found: three subdural hematomas and one arteriovenous malformation. All of the suspected subdural hematomas were misinterpretations of beam-hardening artifacts that caused increased attenuation adjacent to the inner calvaria, thus mimicking a subdural hematoma. The arteriovenous malformation was misinterpreted as an intracranial hemorrhage. Review of this case by a neuroradiologist revealed a negative mass effect and a large draining vessel (Fig 2), consistent with an arteriovenous malformation.

Table 2 shows a higher discrepancy rate in positive studies compared with that in negative ones. This has been reported previously by authors who investigated various imaging modalities (9,10,14).

No change in treatment or prognosis was attributed to the delay in diagnosis. Most major discrepancies involved subdural hematomas. Acute subdural hematomas have an overall mortality rate of 60%–90% (16). Mortality and morbidity in acute subdural hematoma is not attributed to the presence of blood or its mass effect alone but also to co-existing axonal injury (16). The effect of a missed small subdural hematoma is difficult to assess, because of the lack of follow-up and its potential for uneventful resolution. However, patients in our study with major as well as minor discrepancies had no adverse clinical outcome. In our series, all acute traumatic injuries that necessitated immediate neurosurgical intervention were identified by the resident on call and were clearly seen with all window settings.

The clinical relevance of unidentified nondisplaced cranial fractures is questionable. Only 20% of linear skull fractures are known to be demonstrated at CT (17). Isolated nondisplaced skull fractures require no treatment (7).

In this study, we measured discrepancies between interpretations made by residents and those made by staff neuroradiologists. We did not measure the rate of true diagnosis. The hemorrhages that were identified by staff neuroradiologists and missed by radiology residents did not require surgical intervention and resolved uneventfully. The total discrepancy rate of 5.3% for interpretations made by residents and staff is lowest among all discrepancy rates for radiologists at any level of training, including staff radiologists, with any imaging modality (12,13,18,19).

In conclusion, we found an overall discrepancy rate of 5.3% between interpretations made by radiology residents and those by staff neuroradiologists of CT scans of the head in trauma patients. This rate is much lower than the one between staff emergency medicine physicians and staff radiologists (38.7%). A possible cause of discrepancies in our series was the lack of thorough examination scans obtained with "nonbrain" settings. Therefore, examination of images obtained with all settings should be emphasized during residency training. No adverse clinical outcome was found in cases in which a discrepancy occurred, possibly indicating that a delay of up to 15 hours in interpretation by staff neuroradiologists does not compromise patient care.

References

1. Castillo M, Harris JH. Skull and brain. In: Harris JH, Harris WH, Novelline AR, eds. The radiology of emergency medicine. 3rd ed. Baltimore, Md: Williams & Wilkins, 1993.
2. Stein SC, Ross SE. Mild head injury: a plea for routine early CT scanning. J Trauma 1992; 33:11–13.
3. Shackford SR, Wald SL, Ross SE, et al. The clinical utility of computed tomographic scanning and neurologic examination in the management of patients with minor head trauma. J Trauma 1992; 33:385–394.
4. Jeret JS, Mandell M, Anziska B, et al. Clinical predictors of abnormality disclosed by computed tomography after mild head trauma. Neurosurgery 1993; 32:9–15.
5. Miller EC, Derlet RW, Kinser D. Minor head trauma: is computed tomography always necessary? Ann Emerg Med 1996; 27:290–294.
6. Dacey RG, Alves WM, Rimel RW, et al. Neurosurgical complications after apparently minor head injury. J Neurosurg 1986; 65:203–210.
7. Klauber MR, Marshal LF, Luerssen T, Frankowski R, Tabaddor K, Eisenberg HM. Determinants of head injury mortality: importance of the low risk patient. Neurosurgery 1989; 24:31–36.
8. Rhea JT, Potsaid MS, DeLuca AS. Errors of interpretation as elicited by a quality audit of an emergency radiology facility. Radiology 1979; 132:277–280.
9. Herman PG, Hessel SJ. Accuracy and its relationship to experience in interpretation of chest radiographs. Invest Radiol 1975; 10:62–67.
10. Berlin L. Reporting the "missed" radiologic diagnosis: medicolegal and ethical considerations. Radiology 1994; 192:183–187.
11. Randall T. Varied mammogram reading worries researchers. JAMA 1993; 269: 2616–2617.
12. Markus JB, Somers S, O'Malley BP, Stevenson GW. Double-contrast barium enema: effect of multiple readings on perception error. Radiology 1990; 175:155–156.
13. Seltzer SE, Hessel SJ, Herman PG, Swenson RG, Sherrif CR. Resident film interpretation and staff review. AJR 1981; 137:129–133.
14. Wechsler RJ, Spettell CM, Kurtz AB, et al. Effects of training and experience in interpretation of emergency body CT scans. Radiology 1996; 199:717–720.
15. Alfaro D, Levitt MA, English DK, Williams V, Eisenberg R. Accuracy of interpretation of cranial computed tomography scans in an emergency medicine residency program. Ann Emerg Med 1995; 25: 169–174.
16. Wilberger JE, Harris M, Diamond DL. Acute subdural hematoma: morbidity, mortality and operative timing. J Neurosurg 1991; 74:212–218.
17. Orrison WW. Introduction to neuroimaging. Boston, Mass: Little, Brown, 1989; 61.
18. Hessel SJ, Herman PE, Swensson RG. Improving performance by multiple interpretations of chest radiographs. Radiology 1978; 127:589–594.
19. Renfrew DL, Franken EA, Berbaum KS, Weigelt FH, Abu-Yousef MM. Error in radiology: classification and lesions in 182 cases presented at a problem case conference. Radiology 1992; 183:145–150.

Paul B. Rolen, MS, MD
Gordon Sze, MD

Small, Patent Cerebral Aneurysms: Atypical Appearances at 1.5-T MR Imaging[1]

Index terms:
Aneurysm, cerebral, 17.73
Angiography, comparative studies, 10.124
Aneurysm, MR, 17.121411, 17.12142, 17.12143
Brain, MR, 13.121411, 13.12142, 13.12143

Radiology 1998; 208:129–136

Abbreviation:
TR = repetition time

[1] From the Department of Diagnostic Radiology, Section of Neuroradiology, Yale University School of Medicine, PO Box 208042, New Haven, CT 06520-8042. From the 1996 RSNA scientific assembly. Received August 20, 1997; revision requested October 28; revision received February 26, 1998; accepted March 10. **Address reprint requests to** G.S.

PURPOSE: To determine the frequency and characteristics of small cerebral aneurysms with atypical appearances on magnetic resonance (MR) images.

MATERIALS AND METHODS: MR imaging studies (n = 117) obtained at 1.5 T of small aneurysms (<1 cm diameter) were prospectively and retrospectively analyzed. Signal intensity characteristics and gadolinium-enhancement patterns in 84 aneurysms (62 patients) were evaluated. The patency of all aneurysms was confirmed at angiography or at the time of surgery.

RESULTS: A characteristic signal void was seen on 62 (53%) of 117 studies. On the remaining 55 (47%) studies, aneurysms had atypical signal intensity that was isointense, heterogeneous, or hyperintense. Contrast-enhanced aneurysms were seen on 27 (53%) of 51 gadolinium-enhanced studies.

CONCLUSION: Atypical MR imaging characteristics were seen in roughly half of cases. These atypical-appearing aneurysms may erroneously be considered to be thrombosed or be mistaken for other common lesions such as small tumors and be dismissed as nonvascular.

The reported prevalence of aneurysms in the general population is approximately 5% (prevalence range, 0.8%–9.0%) (1–3), with a prevalence of familial aneurysms occurring in the second generation as high as 30% (4,5). Also, up to 30% of patients have multiple aneurysms (1,6,7).

According to reports (8–12) of accumulated data, the annual risk of aneurysm rupture is 1%–2% per year—6.25% if the aneurysms produce symptoms (13). Even with improved surgical procedures and management, there is a 60%–75% mortality rate and an 18%–25% severe neurologic morbidity rate for ruptured aneurysms (14–18). Because of these dismal statistics and because the morbidity rate in cases of surgical repair of non–symptom-producing aneurysms is relatively low (6.5%) (19), many aneurysms are now aggressively pursued by surgeons and interventional neuroradiologists rather than being followed until symptoms develop (10,20). Hence, the exclusion and characterization of aneurysms remain a mainstay of neurovascular imaging.

A single, cost-effective, noninvasive modality to exclude and follow cerebral aneurysms is still being pursued (21,22). Magnetic resonance (MR) imaging and MR angiography are considered by many to be screening examinations for the identification of aneurysms in high-risk patients, such as those with familial aneurysms, as well as for serial follow-up studies, although not in the acute setting of subarachnoid hemorrhage (23,24). The reported sensitivity of MR imaging and MR angiography in the evaluation of aneurysms is approximately 67%–93% but varies depending on the technique, software, and imaging parameters, with aneurysms smaller than 5 mm in diameter most often among those that are overlooked (24–26).

The failure to document small aneurysms aggressively is no longer permissible in light of recent data on rupture and aneurysm growth. Size was once considered to be the most important risk factor for aneurysm rupture: In several large early series (11,27), no rupture

Author contributions:
Guarantor of integrity of entire study, P.B.R.; study concepts and design, G.S.; definition of intellectual content, G.S.; literature research, P.B.R.; clinical studies, P.B.R.; data acquisition and analysis, P.B.R.; statistical analysis, P.B.R.; manuscript preparation, P.B.R.; manuscript editing and review, G.S.

was reported for aneurysms smaller than 10 mm in diameter, although in several large autopsy series (28,29) the average diameter of a ruptured aneurysm was reported to be smaller than 10 mm. In more recent studies (12,30), however, no differences in rupture rates have been reported on the basis of aneurysmal size. In fact, in the Cooperative Aneurysm Study (31), 71% of ruptured aneurysms were smaller than 10 mm in diameter, and Inagawa and Hirano (1) reported that 63% of ruptured aneurysms were smaller than 9 mm in diameter. Reports (5,32,33) of ruptured aneurysms as small as 3 mm in diameter are becoming more frequent. Furthermore, familial aneurysms may rupture at a smaller size, especially in female patients (34) and in patients with multiple aneurysms (35,36).

The issue of the "critical size" for rupture may be moot, because most aneurysms followed to rupture increase in size (10), although growth rates are not stable (37). Giant aneurysms may develop from small, saccular aneurysms (38), and the probability of the de novo development of aneurysms after a screening study is 2.2% per year as a patient ages (10). Therefore, an analysis of the typical appearance on MR images of small aneurysms deserves consideration. Moreover, the characterization of which of the 20% of non–symptom-producing aneurysms are likely to rupture is an important corollary to screening (27).

Although giant aneurysms often display characteristic laminated or heterogeneous features on traditional spin-echo MR images (39), small, patent aneurysms are thought to produce a signal void on typical images obtained with a long or a short repetition time (TR). This study was performed to determine the frequency of unusual imaging characteristics of small, patent aneurysms.

TABLE 1
Distribution of Aneurysms and Frequency of Typical and Atypical Appearances

Location of Aneurysm	No. of MR Studies	Typical Appearance*	Atypical Appearance
Cavernous segment of internal carotid artery	21	16 (76)	5 (24)
Ophthalmic segment of internal carotid artery	6	2 (33)	4 (66)
Supraclinoid segment of internal carotid artery	3	2 (66)	1 (33)
Superior hypophyseal segment of internal carotid artery	4	3 (75)	1 (25)
Middle cerebral artery bifurcation or trifurcation	24	7 (29)	17 (71)
M1 segment of middle cerebral artery	2	1 (50)	1 (50)
Distal branch of middle cerebral artery	1	0 (0)	1 (100)
Anterior communicating artery	14	8 (57)	6 (43)
Anterior cerebral artery	7	5 (71)	2 (29)
Posterior communicating artery	17	10 (59)	7 (41)
Basilar summit	7	7 (100)	0 (0)
Vertebral basilar junction	1	0 (0)	1 (100)
Posterior cerebral artery	6	0 (0)	6 (100)
Superior cerebellar artery	2	2 (100)	0 (0)
Anterior inferior cerebellar artery	1	0 (0)	1 (100)
Posterior inferior cerebellar artery	1	0 (0)	1 (100)
Total	117	54 (46)	63 (54)

Note.—Numbers in parentheses are percentages.
* Typical appearance was a signal void on spin-echo MR images acquired with short or long TR and no contrast enhancement.

TABLE 2
MR Imaging Characteristics of Aneurysms

MR Imaging Characteristic	Long TR MR Studies	Gadolinium-enhanced MR Studies
Signal void on short TR studies (*n* = 81)		
Signal void	62	2 of 21
Isointense	0	0
Heterogeneous	17	7 of 8
Hyperintense	2	2 of 2
Isointense on short TR studies (*n* = 17)		
Signal void	5	1 of 3
Isointense	1	1 of 1
Heterogeneous	5	2 of 2
Hyperintense	6	4 of 4
Heterogeneous on short TR studies (*n* = 10)		
Signal void	3	0 of 2
Isointense	0	0
Heterogeneous	6	1 of 1
Hyperintense	1	1 of 1
Hyperintense on short TR studies (*n* = 9)		
Signal void	0	0
Isointense	0	0
Heterogeneous	2	2 of 2
Hyperintense	7	4 of 4
Total	117	27 of 51

MATERIALS AND METHODS

The radiology records of patients who underwent both angiography and MR imaging between 1987 and 1997 were reviewed at our teaching hospital. Only patients with small (diameter < 1 cm), angiographically confirmed aneurysms were evaluated. In all, 84 aneurysms in 62 patients (18 male patients, 44 female patients), aged 17–89 years, were evaluated. Because 15 patients had multiple aneurysms and several patients were examined two to four times, a total of 117 MR imaging appearances of aneurysms were evaluated. Aneurysm locations as seen on MR imaging studies are shown in Table 1.

MR imaging was performed with 1.5-T units (Horizon EchoSpeed; GE Medical Systems, Milwaukee, Wis) equipped with version 4.5 and version 5.5 software. Cerebral angiograms were obtained on film or digitally by using Advantx equipment (GE Medical Systems). MR images were obtained with short (400–500/11–20 [TR msec/echo time msec]) and long (2,000–2,400/80–90) TRs in all patients. Sagittal short TR and axial long TR images were routinely obtained in all patients, and coronal images were also obtained in 16 patients. Images were obtained in at least two orthogonal planes with a 256 × 192 matrix, one or two signals acquired, and a section thickness of 3–5 mm. Flow compensation was used in all long TR sequences.

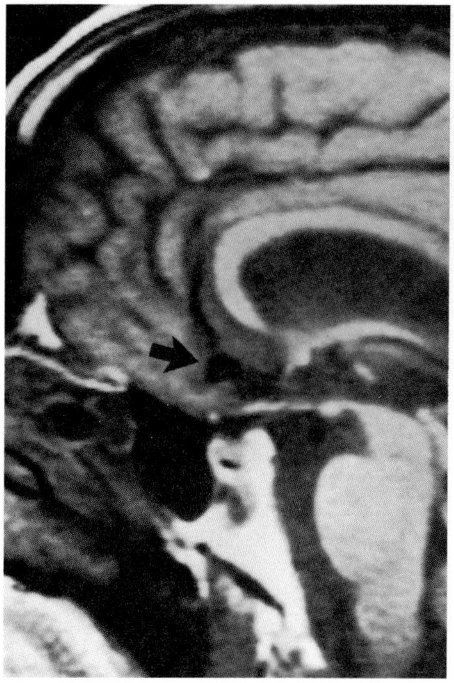

a.

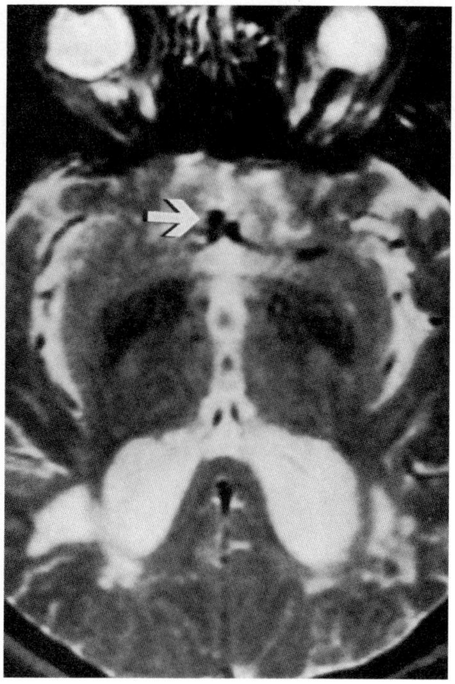

b.

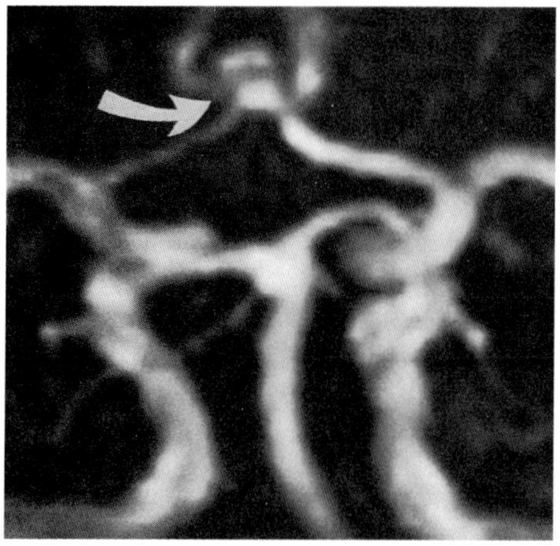

c.

Figure 1. Incidentally discovered aneurysm of the anterior communicating artery in a 73-year-old man. The characteristic signal void (arrow in **a–c**) was seen on **(a)** the sagittal T1-weighted, or short TR, MR image (500/12) and **(b)** the axial T2-weighted, or long TR, MR image (2,000/80) and was confirmed on **(c)** the three-dimensional time-of-flight MR angiogram (47/6.9, 20° flip angle) and subsequent conventional angiogram (not shown).

Short TR sequences were performed in the axial and coronal planes in 30 patients and in 36 of 70 studies both before and after the administration of contrast material. Therefore, 51 of 117 total images of aneurysms were evaluated with contrast material enhancement. Patients received a standard dose (0.1 mmol/kg) of gadopentetate dimeglumine (Magnevist; Berlex Laboratories, Wayne, NJ). In 53 patients, MR imaging findings were also correlated with axial three-dimensional time-of-flight MR angiographic (47/6.9, 20° flip angle) findings.

MR images were reviewed by the authors, who are both neuroradiologists, after aneurysm patency and position had been determined by using concurrent angiograms, MR angiographic data, and surgical reports. Lesions not seen on angiograms and presumed to be thrombosed were excluded. The size of the lesion, the feeding vessel, the shape, and the appearance were documented. Aneurysm appearances were categorized according to the following MR imaging characteristics: (*a*) presence of a signal void, (*b*) signal intensity that was isointense or hyperintense to gray matter, or (*c*) heterogeneous appearance in comparison with adjacent parenchyma. Heterogeneous-appearing aneurysms displayed a hyperintense or isointense center, with a signal void of the peripheral rim (Table 1).

RESULTS

Among the 117 studies of aneurysms that we evaluated, short TR studies revealed the characteristic signal void in 81 cases. However, 17 short TR studies depicted isointense aneurysms; 10 depicted aneurysms with heterogeneous, mixed signal intensity; and nine depicted hyperintense aneurysms (Table 2). The signal intensity of the aneurysms on short TR images was used as a framework for the classification of aneurysms on the long TR images.

Signal Void on Short TR Studies

Of the 81 short TR studies of aneurysms with a signal void, 62 corresponding long-TR studies also showed a signal void, which is the classic appearance of a patent aneurysm on spin-echo images (Fig 1). With regard to the 19 remaining short-TR studies of aneurysms with a signal void, 17 corresponding long TR studies depicted heterogeneous signal intensity, and two depicted hyperintense aneurysms.

With regard to the 81 short TR studies of aneurysms with a signal void, 31 corresponding gadolinium-enhanced studies were obtained. Two of 21 gadolinium-enhanced studies of aneurysms with a signal void on the corresponding long TR studies showed contrast-enhanced aneurysms, whereas seven of the eight gadolinium-enhanced studies of aneurysms with a heterogeneous appearance on long TR images showed enhancement, and two of two gadolinium-enhanced studies with hyperintense aneurysms on long TR images showed enhancement. An example of an aneurysm with a signal void on short TR images, heterogeneous signal intensity on long TR images, and contrast enhancement on gadolinium-enhanced images is shown in Figure 2.

Isointensity on Short TR Studies

With regard to the 17 short TR studies of aneurysms that were isointense, five had a signal void on the corresponding long TR study, one was isointense, five had heterogeneous signal intensity, and six were hyperintense.

With regard to the 17 images of aneurysms in this category, 10 corresponding gadolinium-enhanced studies were obtained. One of three gadolinium-enhanced studies of aneurysms with a signal void on long TR images showed a contrast-enhanced aneurysm. The remaining seven gadolinium-enhanced studies showed enhanced aneurysms regardless of their appearance on corresponding long TR images. An example of an aneurysm that was atypically isointense on short TR images, hyperintense on long TR images, and enhanced on gadolinium-enhanced images is shown in Figure 3.

Heterogeneous Signal Intensity on Short TR Studies

With regard to the 10 short TR images of aneurysms with a heterogeneous appearance, three corresponding long TR images depicted a signal void, six depicted heterogeneous signal intensity, and one depicted a hyperintense aneurysm.

With regard to the 10 studies of aneurysms in this category, four corresponding gadolinium-enhanced studies were obtained. Neither of the two gadolinium-enhanced studies of aneurysms with a signal void on long-TR images depicted an enhanced aneurysm. One of one gadolinium-enhanced study of an aneurysm that was heterogeneous on long TR images depicted an enhanced aneurysm. One of one gadolinium-enhanced study of an aneurysm that was hyperintense on long TR images depicted an enhanced aneurysm.

Hyperintensity on Short TR Studies

With regard to the nine short TR studies of aneurysms that were hyperintense, two corresponding long TR studies depicted aneurysms with heterogeneous signal intensity, and seven depicted hyperintense aneurysms. Contrast enhancement was seen in all six of the cases in this category that were imaged with gadolinium enhancement. An example of an aneurysm that was hyperintense on both short and long TR images and was enhanced on gadolinium-enhanced images is shown in Figure 4.

Aneurysm Distribution and Appearance

As demonstrated in Table 1, an atypical appearance of an aneurysm often, but not invariably, correlated with an atypical location of the aneurysm that involved smaller vessels or was outside the circle of Willis proper. For example, aneurysms that arose from the internal carotid artery and basilar summit usually displayed the classic signal void and did not enhance. Most aneurysms in the common locations—the anterior communicating and posterior communicating arteries—also had a typical appearance. Aneurysms of smaller vessels or at more peripheral locations, such as the posterior cerebral artery, however, were frequently associated with an atypical appearance.

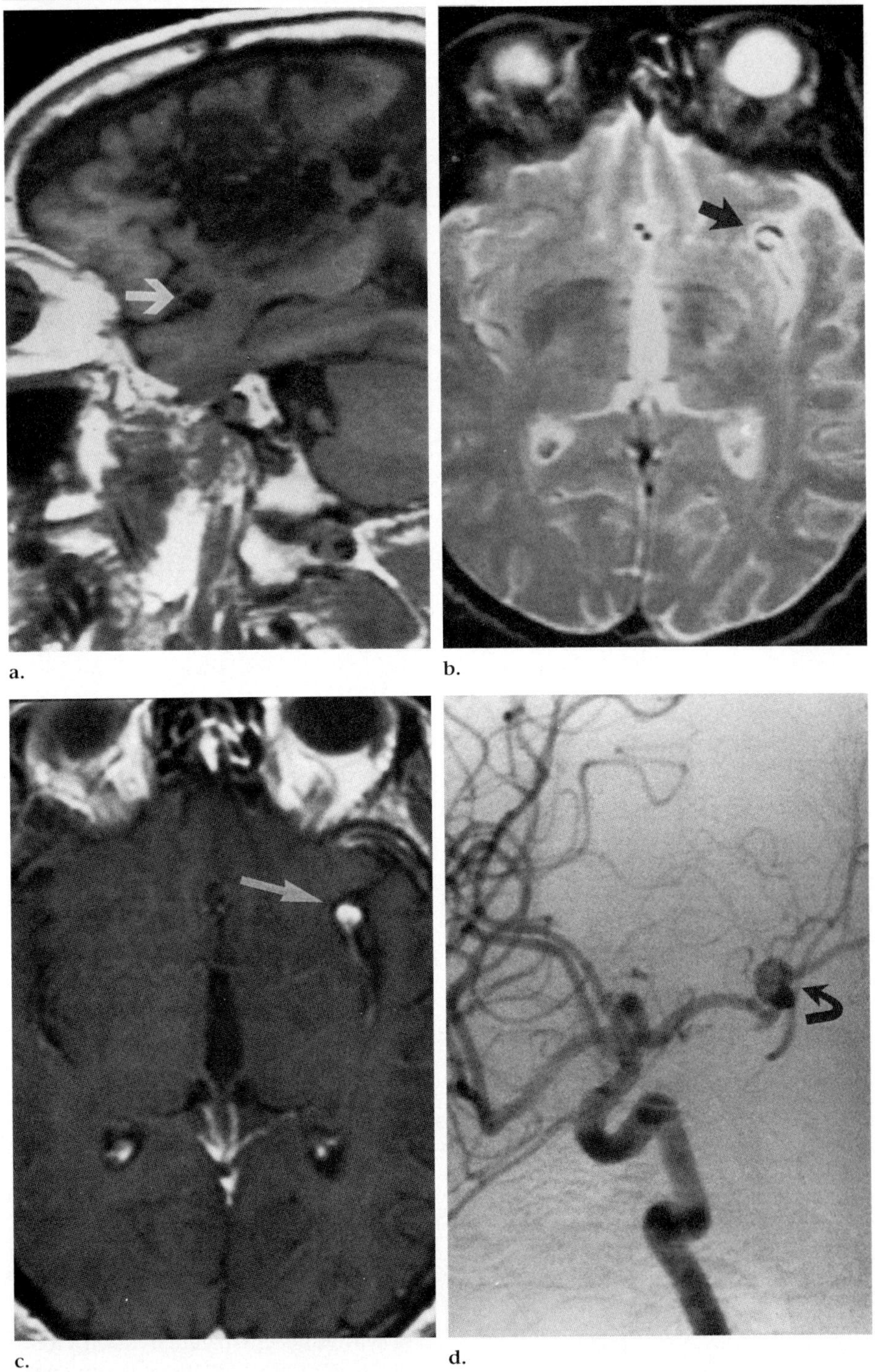

Figure 2. Aneurysm of the left middle cerebral artery bifurcation in a 53-year-old man. **(a)** A 5-mm-diameter lesion (arrow) appears as a signal void on the sagittal unenhanced T1-weighted, or short TR, MR image (500/11). **(b)** The same lesion (arrow) has heterogeneous signal intensity, with a hyperintense center and a peripheral rim of signal void, on the axial T2-weighted, or long TR, image (2,000/80). **(c)** On the axial gadolinium-enhanced T1-weighted image (516/26), the aneurysm (arrow) is enhanced. **(d)** Subsequent conventional angiogram (right internal carotid injection, right anterior oblique projection) confirmed a left middle cerebral artery bifurcation aneurysm (arrow).

DISCUSSION

In general, the lumina of patent arteries display a signal void on both short- and long TR spin-echo images. Flow within patent aneurysms can be visualized due to signal void, as well (23,40). Indeed, signal void has been cited as a criterion of patency at the performance of serial follow-up studies for the evaluation for thrombosis. This signal void has been attributed to various mechanisms, includ-

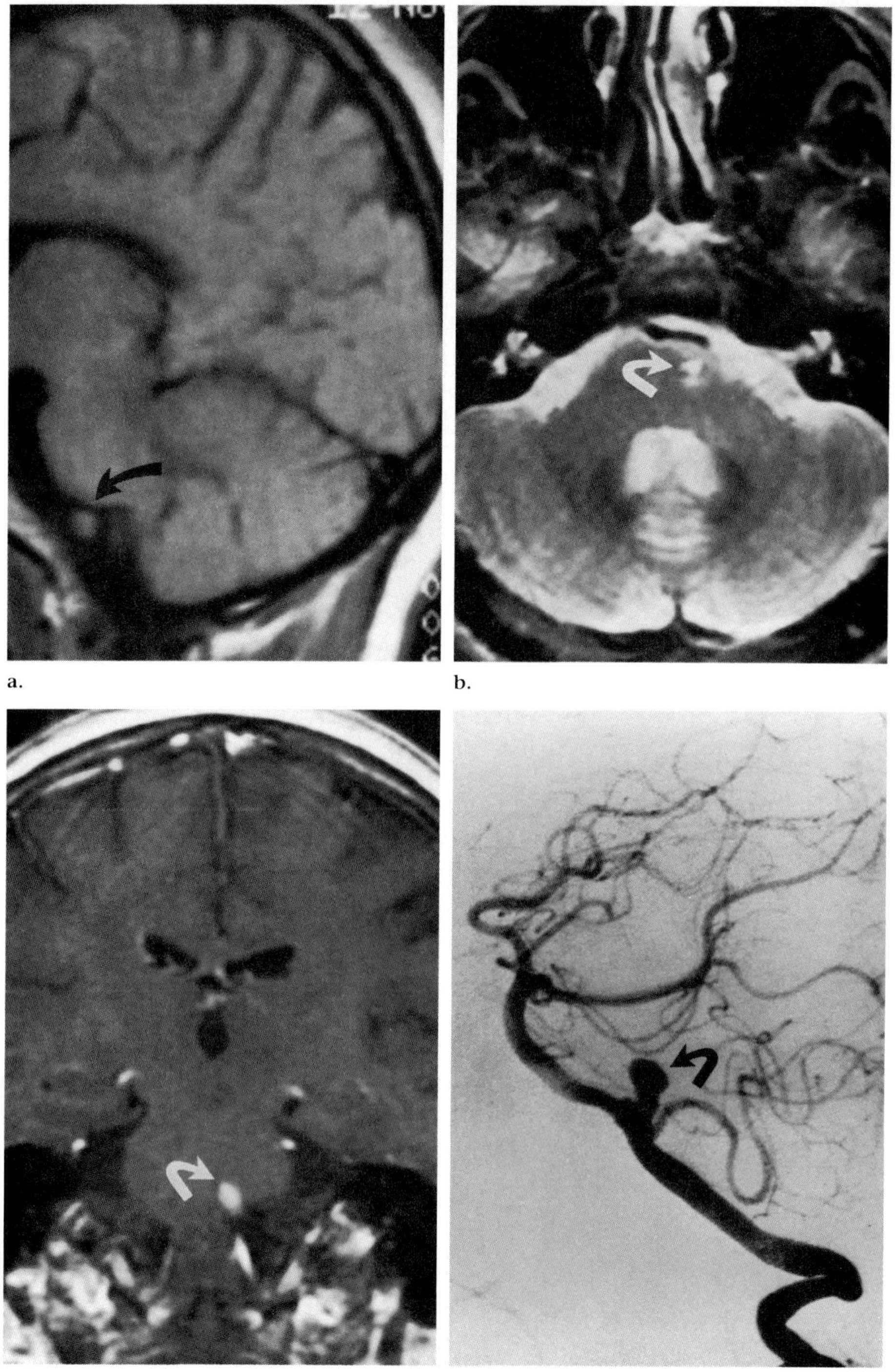

Figure 3. Aneurysm of the left posterior inferior cerebellar artery in a 48-year-old woman with a lesion scalloping the left brachium pontis. **(a)** The aneurysm (arrow) is isointense on the unenhanced T1-weighted, or short TR, sagittal MR image (500/12). **(b)** On the T2-weighted, or long TR, MR image (2,000/80), the aneurysm (arrow) is hyperintense. **(c)** The aneurysm (arrow) is enhanced on the gadolinium-enhanced coronal T1-weighted MR image (416/20). **(d)** Subsequent conventional angiogram (left vertebral injection, lateral view) revealed a 6-mm-diameter left posterior inferior cerebellar artery aneurysm (arrow).

ing time-of-flight effects of rapidly flowing blood, turbulence related to randomly fluctuating flow velocities, vessel wall irregularities, or branching and, in earlier studies, possible signal loss during odd-numbered echoes due to dephasing phenomena (41,42). In our study, 62 (53%) of 117 cases had this classic appearance of a signal void on both short and long TR images (Fig 1).

Some early investigators (41,42), however, have noted that not all arterial vessels display a signal void. The results of both flow phantom and clinical studies (41,42) have shown that intravascular flow may result in high or heterogeneous signal intensity. The factors responsible for this increased signal intensity may include flow-related enhancement, gradient moment nulling, or even, as noted in earlier work, echo-rephasing effects, diastolic pseudogating, or stagnation effects of decelerating or nonmoving blood (43,44).

Similar factors may be at play in producing a variable signal intensity in some patent aneurysms. Relatively little work has addressed the variable signal intensity in small aneurysms, despite their relatively common frequency. With regard to smaller aneurysms, Biondi et al (45) noted "one medium" patent aneurysm with inhomogeneous signal intensity and recognized that the thrombosis and flow effects may be responsible for the variable signal intensity. Schwaighofer et al (46) noted heterogeneous or high signal intensity in two aneurysms 1 cm or smaller in diameter, but these aneurysms were seen on subsequent angiograms to be completely or partially thrombosed.

Several factors may be responsible for the atypical signal intensity in small patent aneurysms, including artifact due to flow effects or misregistration and slowed or aberrant flow patterns within the aneurysm lumen due to the origin of the aneurysm or to the position and size of the ostium versus the volume of the aneurysm lumen. Although blood degradation products in thrombosed aneurysms may produce mixed signal intensities, in our cases, the patency of the aneurysm lumen was documented within an interval close to the time of MR imaging. Although a partially thrombosed aneurysm may have recanalized by the time angiography was performed, this is an unusual scenario and would not account for the large number of atypical aneurysms we observed.

To our knowledge, no MR imaging studies have been performed to demonstrate intact flow models of small aneurysms. However, aberrant flow patterns at the neck of the aneurysm or within the aneurysm lumen may result in atypical signal intensity patterns. Aberrant flow at the neck may result from nonlaminar flow patterns when the aneurysm origi-

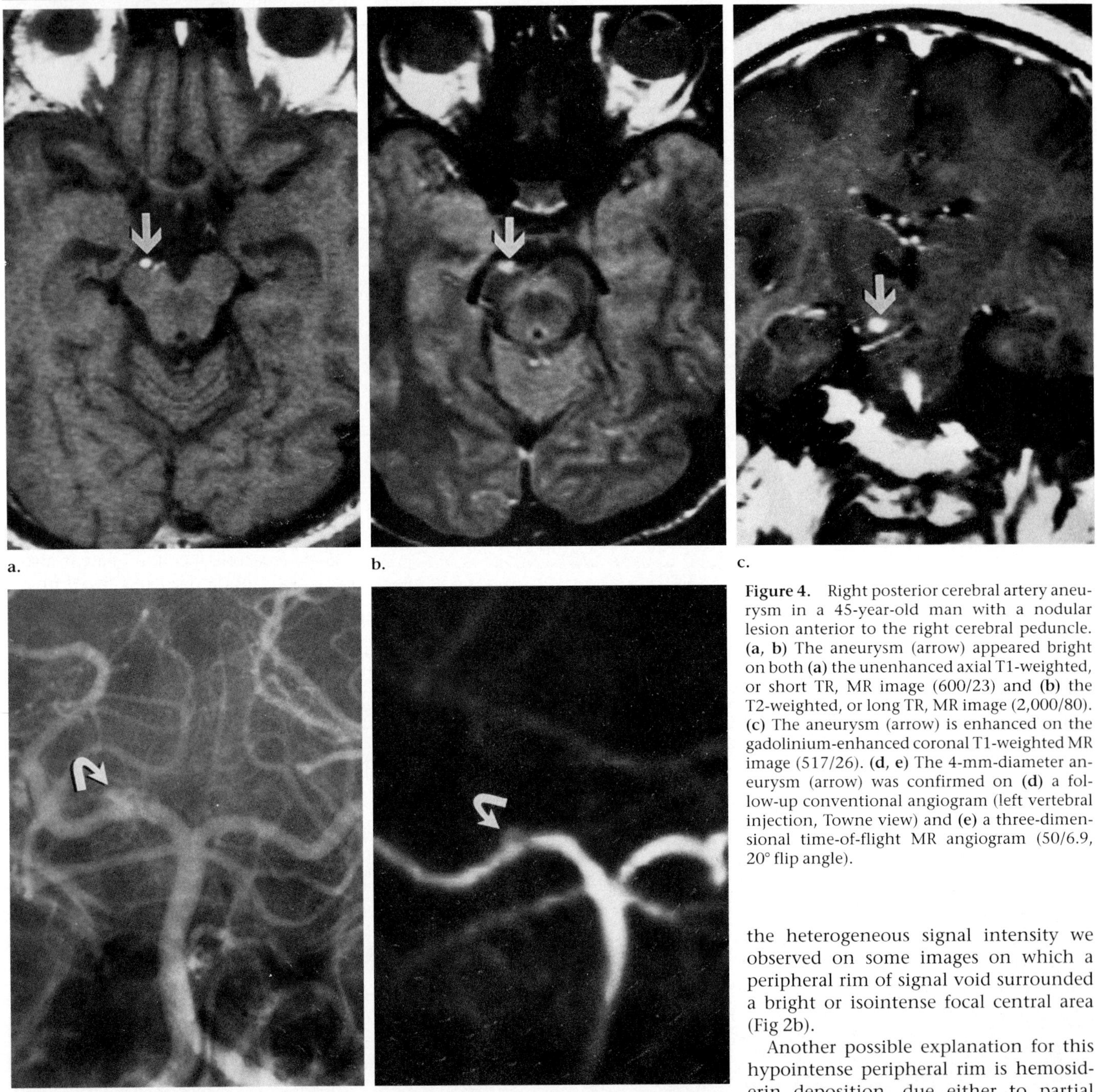

Figure 4. Right posterior cerebral artery aneurysm in a 45-year-old man with a nodular lesion anterior to the right cerebral peduncle. **(a, b)** The aneurysm (arrow) appeared bright on both **(a)** the unenhanced axial T1-weighted, or short TR, MR image (600/23) and **(b)** the T2-weighted, or long TR, MR image (2,000/80). **(c)** The aneurysm (arrow) is enhanced on the gadolinium-enhanced coronal T1-weighted MR image (517/26). **(d, e)** The 4-mm-diameter aneurysm (arrow) was confirmed on **(d)** a follow-up conventional angiogram (left vertebral injection, Towne view) and **(e)** a three-dimensional time-of-flight MR angiogram (50/6.9, 20° flip angle).

nates at a loop, bend, or branch point of a vessel. An aneurysm with a narrow neck may also distort laminar flow patterns. In addition, flow patterns within the aneurysm itself may result in atypical signal intensity. In distinction to the parabolic distribution of laminar flow within arteries, which is faster centrally than at the luminal wall, flow in aneurysms is thought to be slower centrally and faster at the luminal margins (21,47). As seen in simulation studies, the inflow and the volume of this low-flow central recirculation zone depends on many factors, including the volume of the aneurysm versus the size of the ostium and the flow rate in the parent artery. Likewise, the residence time of blood in the aneurysm lumen is highly variable (48,49). Therefore, a centripetal flow pattern and a variable residence time may explain the loss of the typical signal void or explain the heterogeneous signal intensity we observed on some images on which a peripheral rim of signal void surrounded a bright or isointense focal central area (Fig 2b).

Another possible explanation for this hypointense peripheral rim is hemosiderin deposition, due either to partial thrombosis or to previous rupture or leakage. Hemosiderin, however, tends to have a "smudged" appearance, unlike the sharp outlines seen in the aneurysms in our series, and seems less likely.

Visualization on MR images of variable flow patterns in aneurysms or in their parent arteries may indicate hemodynamic flow patterns that predispose to growth or future formation of additional aneurysms or that even presage rupture. The results of pathologic studies (50,51) have shown that not only does shear stress directly damage the vascular endothelium, but zones of both high shear stress and recirculation promote damaging platelet activation and impair metabolic activity. The clinical association of vascular hemodynamic alterations and aneurysm formation and rupture has also been studied previously. For example, aneurysms have been seen to arise from a previously normal carotid artery after ligation of the contralateral carotid artery (52), as well as in cases of aplasia of the anterior cerebral or internal carotid artery (53,54). Likewise, a strong association has been described (55–57) between hemodynamic alterations and aneurysms proximal to or in the feeding vessel to an arteriovenous malformation.

Hemodynamic stresses may be inferred from MR imaging findings. The results of studies (43) have shown that acceleration or deceleration and variable velocity of blood may result in varying signal intensity within an aneurysm, as is the case within major vessels. Turbulence, due either to nonlinear flow or to vessel irregularity, results in variations in the net longitudinal velocity and a random distribution of phase shifts. The irregular distribution of phase and signal intensity is especially prominent during late systole, as has been shown with flow phantom models (43,44). Nussel et al (21) attributed to turbulence the bandlike appearance of heterogeneous signal intensity in the center of larger aneurysms.

Slowed or nonmoving blood, as found in aneurysms with a high residence time, may also render variable appearances on MR images. Nonthrombosed stationary blood has been shown (58) to be of intermediate signal intensity on short-TR images and bright on long-TR images. Indeed, this isointense-hyperintense pattern was seen in several instances in our study (Fig 3). Such a pattern may presage complete thrombosis, or because of decreased wall stress, a lower frequency of rupture. Further longitudinal studies would be helpful for confirmation of this more fortunate possibility in this class of patients.

Flow-related enhancement is also a particular issue in larger aneurysms, where flow velocities are slower and a large portion of the protons remain within the imaging plane for both the excitation and the signal-generation phases and where there is partial replacement with a variable volume of unsaturated blood. As noted earlier in this article, nonlaminar flow patterns at the neck or branching point of a vessel also may slow blood flow. Such a microclimate may also exist in smaller aneurysms, where turbulent flow slows incoming nonmagnetized or partially magnetized protons, resulting in heterogeneous, concentric-ring signal intensity patterns or relatively homogeneous high signal intensity on both short and long TR images, as seen in Figure 4. Concentric-ring patterns in laminar flow models, which represent parabolic phase distributions, are a frequently seen phenomenon in carotid arteries and have been well described in earlier studies (42,43,59,60). Such a phenomenon also may explain a similar pattern observed in our study, namely, the heterogeneous-appearing aneurysms.

Recognition of the variable signal intensity possibilities of intraluminal blood flow, especially in aneurysms, is important and may be of consequence to the patient. Intraluminal high signal intensity may represent thrombus or variable blood flow, and vessel or aneurysm patency should be verified by using other techniques such as phase-contrast MR angiography or conventional angiography. Although some authorities (23) regard a flow void on spin-echo images as pathognomonic for the patency of aneurysms, the finding of variable signal intensity within an aneurysm may invite a specious conclusion of complete thrombosis. High or intermediate signal intensity within a small aneurysm may represent either true flow or blood degradation products in cases of partial thrombosis and needs correlation.

In a worse scenario, a focal area of aberrant signal intensity may preclude consideration of a vascular cause altogether. Although mixed and high signal intensity within the patent aneurysm lumen, as well as contrast enhancement, may be attributed to the flow-related factors mentioned above, confusion with other pathologic entities that produce variable signal intensity (eg, schwannoma, meningioma, tuberculous or sarcoid granuloma) is also possible. On a screening study, atypical signal intensity patterns and contrast enhancement may mimic the appearance of other types of small lesions.

In conclusion, in most instances, small patent aneurysms are characterized by a signal void on MR images obtained with typical pulse sequences, as was seen in 53% of the cases in our series; however, in 47% of the cases in our series, variable signal intensities were seen. Patent aneurysms appeared isointense, heterogeneous, or hyperintense on short and long TR images, and enhanced with contrast material. Such atypical MR imaging appearances may be falsely presumed to represent aneurysm thrombosis or mimic the appearance of other common lesions, such as small tumors, granulomas, or even metastases. Further longitudinal studies may aid in the evaluation of the hemodynamic stresses that are important in the formation of aneurysms or in the prediction of those patent aneurysms that are more likely to rupture.

References

1. Inagawa T, Hirano A. Ruptured intracranial aneurysms: an autopsy study of 133 patients. Surg Neurol 1990; 33:117–123.
2. Winn HR, Almaani WS, Berga SL, Jane JA, Richardson AK. The long-term outcome in patients with multiple aneurysms: incidence of late hemorrhage and implications for treatment of incidental aneurysms. J Neurosurg 1983; 59:642–651.
3. McCormick WE, Acosta-Rua GJ. The size of intracranial saccular aneurysms: an autopsy study. J Neurosurg 1970; 33:422–427.
4. Obuchowski NA, Modic MT, Magdinec M. Current implications for the efficacy of noninvasive screening for occult intracranial aneurysms in patients with a family history of aneurysms. J Neurosurg 1995; 83:42–49.
5. Schievink WI, Piepgras DO, Wirth FP. Rupture of previously documented small asymptomatic saccular intracranial aneurysms: report of three cases. J Neurosurg 1992; 76:1019–1024.
6. Sekhar LN, Heros RC. Origin, growth, and rupture of saccular aneurysms: a review. Neurosurgery 1981; 8:248–260.
7. Teresi LM. Cerebrovascular malformations. In: Stark BW, ed. Magnetic resonance imaging. 2nd ed. St Louis, Mo: Mosby–Year Book, 1992; 963–987.
8. Heiskanen O, Vilkki J. Intracranial arterial aneurysms in children and adolescents. Acta Neurochir 1981; 59:55–63.
9. Jane JA, Kassell NF, Torner JC, Winn HR. The natural history of aneurysms and arteriovenous malformations. J Neurosurg 1985; 62:321–323.
10. Juvela S, Porras M, Heiskanen O. Natural history of unruptured intracranial aneurysms: a long-term follow-up study. J Neurosurg 1993; 79:174–182.
11. Wiebers DO, Whisnant JP, O'Fallon WM. The natural history of unruptured intracranial aneurysms. N Engl J Med 1981; 304:696–698.
12. Winn HR, Richardson AK, Jane JA. The long-term prognosis in untreated cerebral aneurysms. I. The incidence of late hemorrhage in cerebral aneurysm: a 10-year evaluation of 364 patients. Ann Neurol 1977; 1:358–370.
13. Kassell NF, Torner JC. The International Cooperative Study on Timing of Aneurysm Surgery: an update. Stroke 1984; 15:566–570.
14. Pakarinen S. Incidence, aetiology, and prognosis of primary subarachnoid haemorrhage: a study based on 589 cases diagnosed in a defined urban population during a defined period. Acta Neurol Scand 1967; 43:(suppl 29):1–28.
15. Phillips LHD, Whisnant JP, O'Fallon WM, Sundt TM Jr. The unchanging pattern of subarachnoid hemorrhage in a community. Neurology 1980; 30:1034–1040.

16. Drake CG. Progress in cerebrovascular disease: management of cerebral aneurysm. Stroke 1981; 12:273–283.
17. Kassell NF, Drake CG. Timing of aneurysm surgery. Neurosurgery 1982; 10:514–519.
18. Kassell NF, Drake CG. Review of the management of saccular aneurysms. Neurol Clin 1983; 1:73–86.
19. Wirth FP, Laws ER Jr, Piepgras D, Scott RM. Surgical treatment of incidental intracranial aneurysms. Neurosurgery 1983; 12: 507–511.
20. Deruty R, Pelissou-Guyotat I, Mottolese C, Bognar L, Oubouklik A. Surgical management of unruptured intracranial aneurysms: personal experience with 37 cases and discussion of the indications. Acta Neurochir 1992; 119:35–41.
21. Nussel F, Wegmuller H, Huber P. Morphological and haemodynamic aspects of cerebral aneurysms. Acta Neurochir 1993; 120:1–6.
22. Schmid UD, Steiger HJ, Huber P. Accuracy of high resolution computed tomography in direct diagnosis of cerebral aneurysms. Neuroradiology 1987; 29:152–159.
23. Atlas SW. Intracranial vascular malformations and aneurysms. In: Atlas SW, ed. Magnetic resonance imaging of the brain and spine. 2nd ed. Philadelphia, Pa: Lippincott-Raven, 1996; 489–556.
24. Ross JS, Masaryk TJ, Modic MT, Ruggieri PM, Haacke EM, Selman WR. Intracranial aneurysms: evaluation by MR angiography. AJNR 1990; 11:449–455.
25. Schuierer G, Huk WJ, Laub G. Magnetic resonance angiography of intracranial aneurysms: comparison with intra-arterial digital subtraction angiography. Neuroradiology 1992; 35:50–54.
26. Ikawa F, Sumida M, Uozumi T, et al. Comparison of three-dimensional phase-contrast magnetic resonance angiography with three-dimensional time-of-flight magnetic resonance angiography in cerebral aneurysms. Surg Neurol 1994; 42:287–292.
27. Wiebers DO, Whisnant JP, Sundt TM Jr, O'Fallon WM. The significance of unruptured intracranial saccular aneurysms. J Neurosurg 1987; 66:23–29.
28. McCormick W, Nofzinger J. Saccular intracranial aneurysms: an autopsy study. J Neurosurg 1964; 22:155–159.
29. Chason J, Hindman W. Berry aneurysms of the circle of Willis: results of a planned autopsy study. Neurology 1958; 8:41–44.
30. Juvela S. Prevalence of risk factors in spontaneous intracerebral hemorrhage and aneurysmal subarachnoid hemorrhage. Arch Neurol 1996; 53:734–740.
31. Kassell NF, Torner JC. Size of intracranial aneurysms. Neurosurgery 1983; 12:291–297.
32. Asari S, Ohmoto T. Natural history and risk factors of unruptured cerebral aneurysms. Clin Neurol Neurosurg 1993; 95: 205–214.
33. Solomon RA, Correll JW. Rupture of a previously documented asymptomatic aneurysm enhances the argument for prophylactic surgical intervention. Surg Neurol 1988; 30:321–323.
34. Lozano AM, Leblanc R. Familial intracranial aneurysms. J Neurosurg 1987; 66:522–528.
35. Mount L, Brisman R. Treatment of multiple asymptomatic aneurysms. In: Schmidek H, Sweet W, eds. Operative neurosurgical techniques: indications, methods, and results. Vol 2. New York, NY: Grune & Stratton, 1983; 765–769.
36. Heiskanen O. Risk of bleeding from unruptured aneurysm in cases with multiple intracranial aneurysms. J Neurosurg 1981; 55:524–526.
37. Allcock JM, Canham PB. Angiographic study of the growth of intracranial aneurysms. J Neurosurg 1976; 45:617–621.
38. Barrow DL, Alleyne C. Natural history of giant intracranial aneurysms and indications for intervention. Clin Neurosurg 1995; 42:214–244.
39. Atlas SW, Grossman RI, Goldberg HI, Hackney DB, Bilaniuk LT, Zimmerman RA. Partially thrombosed giant intracranial aneurysms: correlation of MR and pathologic findings. Radiology 1987; 162:111–114.
40. Zimmerman RA, Atlas S, Bilaniuk LT, Hackney DB, Goldberg HI, Grossman RI. Magnetic resonance imaging of cerebral aneurysm. Acta Radiol Suppl 1986; 369:107–109.
41. Mills CM, Brant-Zawadzki M, Crooks LE, et al. Nuclear magnetic resonance: principles of blood flow imaging. AJR 1984; 142:165–170.
42. Bradley WG Jr, Waluch V. Blood flow: magnetic resonance imaging. Radiology 1985; 154:443–450.
43. Valk PE, Hale JD, Crooks LE, et al. MRI of blood flow: correlation of image appearance with spin-echo phase shift and signal intensity. AJR 1986; 146:931–939.
44. George GR, Jacobs G, Macintyre WJ, et al. Magnetic resonance signal intensity patterns obtained from continuous and pulsatile flow models. Radiology 1984; 151: 421–428.
45. Biondi A, Scialfa G, Scotti G. Intracranial aneurysms: MR imaging. Neuroradiology 1988; 30:214–218.
46. Schwaighofer BW, Klein MV, Lyden PD, Hesselink JR. MR imaging of vertebrobasilar vascular disease. J Comput Assist Tomogr 1990; 14:895–904.
47. Huber P, Robert F. Changes of saccular cerebral aneurysms: angiographic follow-up examination in conservatively treated saccular aneurysms. ROFO 1969; 111:184–195. [German]
48. Burleson AC, Turitto VT. Identification of quantifiable hemodynamic factors in the assessment of cerebral aneurysm behavior: on behalf of the Subcommittee on Biorheology of the Scientific and Standardization Committee of the ISTH. Thromb Haemost 1996; 76:118–123.
49. Burleson AC, Strother CM, Turitto VT. Computer modeling of intracranial saccular and lateral aneurysms for the study of their hemodynamics. Neurosurgery 1995; 37:774–784.
50. Fry DL. Acute vascular endothelial changes associated with increased blood velocity gradients. Circ Res 1968; 22:165–197.
51. O'Brien JR. Shear-induced platelet aggregation. Lancet 1990; 335:711–713.
52. Salar G, Mingrino S. Development of intracranial saccular aneurysms: report of two cases. Neurosurgery 1981; 8:462–465.
53. Yasargil MG, Fox JL. The microsurgical approach to intracranial aneurysms. Surg Neurol 1975; 3:7–14.
54. Servo A. Agenesis of the left internal carotid artery associated with an aneurysm on the right carotid syphon: case report. J Neurosurg 1977; 46:677–680.
55. Sachs A, Perret G, Locksley H, et al, eds. Intracranial aneurysms and subarachnoid hemorrhage: a cooperative study. Philadelphia, Pa: Lippincott, 1969; 38–52.
56. Tognetti F, Limoni P, Testa C. Aneurysm growth and hemodynamic stress. Surg Neurol 1983; 20:74–78.
57. Batjer H, Suss RA, Samson D. Intracranial arteriovenous malformations associated with aneurysms. Neurosurgery 1986; 18: 29–35.
58. Olsen WL, Kucharczyk W, Keyes WD, Norman D, Newton TH. Magnetic resonance characterization of non-flowing intravascular blood. Acta Radiol Suppl 1986; 369:63–66.
59. Kaufman L, Crooks LE, Sheldon PE, Rowan W, Miller T. Evaluation of NMR imaging for detection and quantification of obstructions in vessels. Invest Radiol 1982; 17:554–560.
60. Feinberg DA, Crooks LE, Sheldon P, Hoenninger JD, Watts J, Arakawa M. Magnetic resonance imaging of the velocity vector components of fluid flow. Magn Reson Med 1985; 2:555–566.

Guillain-Barré Syndrome: MR Imaging Findings of the Spine in Eight Patients[1]

Woo Mok Byun, MD
Won Kyu Park, MD
Bok Hwan Park, MD
Sang Ho Ahn, MD
Mi Soo Hwang, MD
Jay Chun Chang, MD

Index terms:
Neuritis, 35.24, 36.24
Spinal cord, abnormalities, 35.24, 36.24
Spinal cord, diseases, 35.24, 36.24
Spinal cord, MR, 35.12141, 35.12143, 36.12141, 36.12143

Radiology 1998; 208:137–141

Abbreviations:
AIDS = acquired immunodeficiency syndrome
CSF = cerebrospinal fluid

[1] From the Departments of Diagnostic Radiology (W.M.B., W.K.P., B.H.P., M.S.H., J.C.C.) and Rehabilitation (S.H.A.), College of Medicine, Yeungnam University, 317-1, Daemyung-dong, Namku, Taegu 705-717, South Korea. Received September 25, 1997; revision requested November 25; revision received February 5, 1998; accepted March 9. **Address reprint requests to** W.M.B.

Author contributions:
Guarantors of integrity of entire study, W.M.B., J.C.C.; study concepts, W.M.B., W.K.P.; study design, W.M.B., W.K.P., J.C.C.; definition of intellectual content, W.M.B., M.S.H., J.C.C.; literature research, W.M.B., W.K.P.; clinical studies, S.H.A.; data acquisition, W.M.B., W.K.P., S.H.A.; data analysis, W.M.B., S.H.A., B.H.P.; manuscript preparation, W.M.B., J.C.C.; manuscript editing, W.M.B., M.S.H.; manuscript review, W.M.B., B.H.P.

PURPOSE: To evaluate magnetic resonance (MR) imaging findings of the spine in patients with Guillain-Barré syndrome.

MATERIALS AND METHODS: MR imaging findings in eight patients (three male, five female; age range, 2–47 years) with Guillain-Barré syndrome were retrospectively reviewed. Guillain-Barré syndrome was diagnosed mainly on the basis of symptoms and also on the basis of supportive ancillary data, such as the results cerebrospinal fluid analysis and electrophysiologic evaluation. In addition, follow-up MR imaging was performed in three patients, who had slight clinical improvement.

RESULTS: All patients had thickening of the intrathecal spinal nerve roots and cauda equina, with varying degrees of enhancement on gadolinium-enhanced axial T1-weighted images. Two enhancement patterns were noted. One was enhancement of both the anterior and posterior spinal nerve roots ($n = 2$); the other was enhancement of the anterior spinal nerve roots only ($n = 6$). Follow-up MR imaging in the three patients with slight improvement of symptoms revealed that the thickening and the degree of enhancement of the spinal nerve roots were diminished.

CONCLUSION: Although the enhancement of the intrathecal spinal nerve roots is not specific to Guillain-Barré syndrome and can be seen in neoplasia and other inflammatory processes, the enhancement of only the anterior spinal nerve roots is strongly suggestive of Guillain-Barré syndrome.

Guillain-Barré syndrome is a clinical entity that exhibits an acute, predominantly demyelinating polyneuropathy. The diagnosis is usually established on the basis of symptoms and signs, aided by laboratory cerebrospinal fluid (CSF) findings and electrophysiologic criteria. Symptoms consist of symmetric, progressive motor weakness of more than one limb; hyporeflexia or areflexia; and little or no sensory change. Involvement of cranial nerves and autonomic dysfunction are common. Among the CSF laboratory findings, the most dependable are an elevated protein level and 10 or fewer mononuclear leukocytes per cubic millimeter (per microliter) (1,2). Although the precise cause of Guillain-Barré syndrome has to our knowledge not been determined, most evidence points to an immune-mediated phenomenon (3). At present, clinically, supportive measures are still the mainstay of therapy. Recently, however, plasmapheresis and infusion of immunoglobulin have gained recognition as playing important parts in clinical treatment (4–6).

Since the diagnosis of Guillain-Barré syndrome has been determined mainly on the basis of clinical findings, as well as on the basis of CSF laboratory findings and electrophysiologic results, to our knowledge, most of the radiologic studies used in Guillain-Barré syndrome cases have been performed to exclude conditions other than Guillain-Barré syndrome. Magnetic resonance (MR) imaging of the spine is known to be useful to define infiltrative or compressive causes of polyradiculopathy; however, this modality has not been used routinely in cases of Guillain-Barré syndrome.

We have found several reports on the MR imaging findings in Guillain-Barré syndrome. The authors of these reports concluded that there was good enhancement of the spinal nerve roots and that the diffuse enhancement of the spinal nerve roots was not specific to Guillain-Barré syndrome (7–9). Our purpose in this study was to evaluate MR imaging findings of the spine for the diagnosis of Guillain-Barré syndrome.

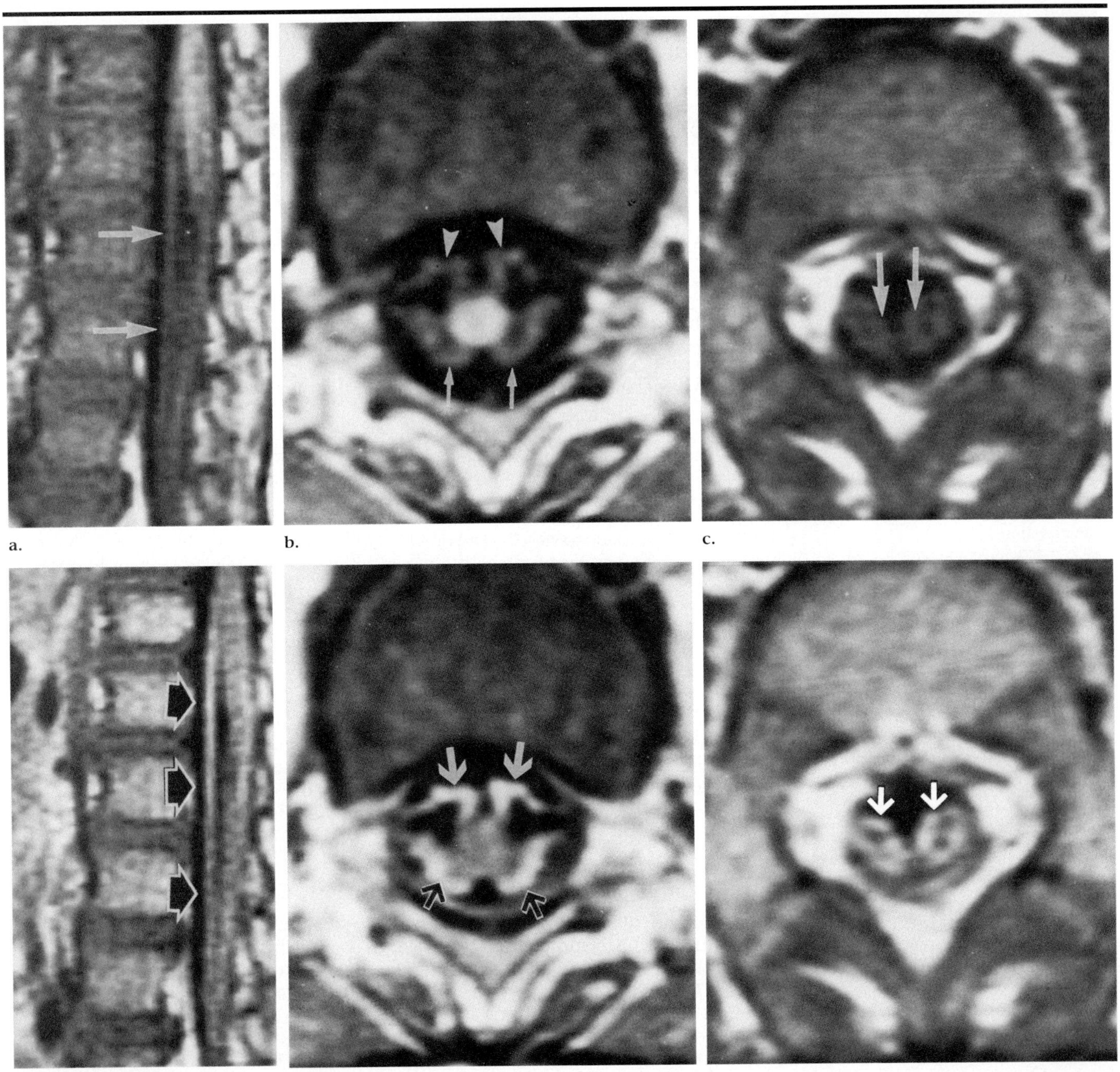

a. b. c. d. e. f.

Figure 1. Patient 1. (a–c) Precontrast (**a**) sagittal and (**b, c**) axial T1-weighted MR images (700/25) obtained (**b**) at the level of the L1 through L2 vertebrae and (**c**) at the level of the L4 vertebra show a diffusely thickened cauda equina (arrows in **a** and **c**) and both the anterior (arrowheads in **b**) and posterior (arrows in **b**) spinal nerve roots. (**d–f**) Postcontrast (**d**) sagittal and (**e, f**) axial T1-weighted MR images (700/25) obtained (**e**) at the level of the L1 through L2 vertebrae and (**f**) at the level of the L4 vertebra show strong enhancement in the cauda equina (arrows in **d** and **f**) and both the anterior (white arrows in **e**) and posterior (black arrows in **e**) spinal nerve roots.

MATERIALS AND METHODS

MR imaging findings in eight patients (three male, five female; age range, 2–47 years; mean age, 14 years) with a clinical diagnosis of Guillain-Barré syndrome were retrospectively reviewed. CSF and electrophysiologic studies were performed in all patients.

Originally, MR imaging was requested to exclude other possibilities, such as transverse myelitis or conditions that cause acute spinal cord compression. One of the eight patients examined had a clinical diagnosis of a Miller-Fisher variant of Guillain-Barré syndrome. In this patient, MR imaging was requested because of the clinical involvement of both the cranial nerves and the spinal nerve roots, which may be confused with other diffuse infiltrative and inflammatory conditions, such as leptomeningeal metastatic lesions or infectious polyneuropathy.

Initial MR imaging of the thoracolumbar spine was performed in all patients, and follow-up MR imaging was performed in three patients at 1, 2, or 8 months.

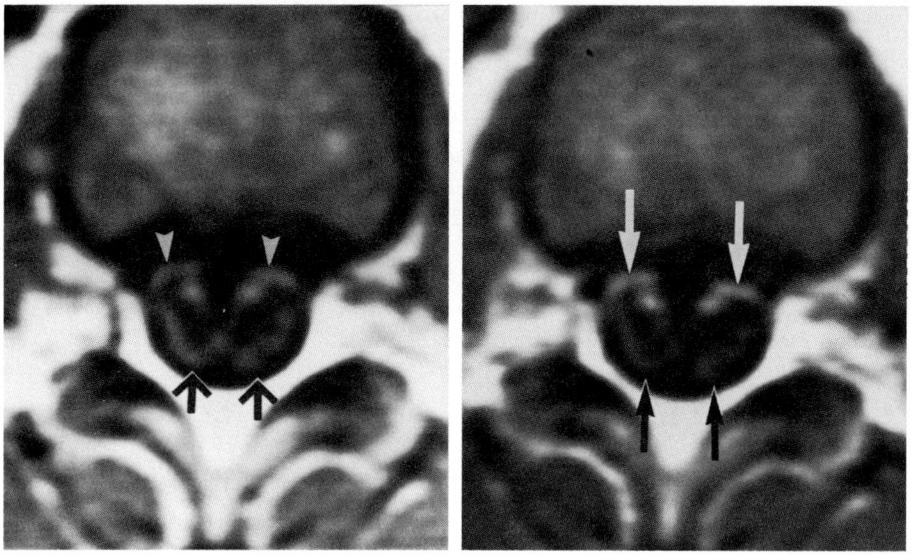

a. b.

Figure 2. Patient 3. Enhancement in the anterior spinal nerve roots only. (**a**) Precontrast and (**b**) postcontrast axial T1-weighted images (700/25). The anterior spinal nerve roots (arrowheads in **a**, white arrows in **b**) reveal slightly high signal intensity in **a** and good enhancement in **b**. The posterior spinal nerve roots (black arrows in **a** and **b**), however, are not enhanced.

MR imaging was performed with a 0.5-T (Gyroscan T5-II; Philips Medical Systems, Best, The Netherlands) or a 1.5-T (Vision; Siemens, Erlangen, Germany) imager. Axial and sagittal T1-weighted images (600–700/25–30 [repetition time msec/echo time msec]) were obtained before and after the administration of gadopentetate dimeglumine (Magnevist; Schering, Berlin, Germany; 0.1 mmol per kilogram of body weight); axial and sagittal T2*-weighted images (600/27) also were obtained before the administration of gadopentetate dimeglumine. MR imaging was performed 5–30 days after the onset of symptoms.

The change in the signal intensity and the thickening and enhancement patterns of the spinal nerve roots that surround the medullary cone and extend along the length of the cauda equina were evaluated. Enhancement of the spinal nerve roots was categorized as one of two patterns: enhancement of both the anterior and posterior nerve roots (pattern 1) and enhancement of the anterior spinal nerve roots only (pattern 2).

MR imaging findings were compared with symptoms and signs, laboratory findings of CSF analysis, and electrophysiologic findings.

Five radiologists (W.M.B., W.K.P., B.H.P., M.S.H., J.C.C.) were involved in the interpretation of all MR images; four interpreted the images blindly, without any clinical information or diagnosis given.

RESULTS

All eight patients showed motor weakness of the extremities, and hyporeflexia to areflexia. In addition, one patient showed sensory change. We were unable to evaluate sensory change in one patient because the patient was too young. Protein levels in the CSF were increased in all patients. The patient with the Miller-Fisher variant of Guillain-Barré syndrome had slowly progressive ptosis of the eyelids, ophthalmoplegia, facial palsy, weakness of back muscles, and mild weakness of limbs. Laboratory CSF findings showed mildly elevated protein levels (50 mg/dL [0.5 g/L]) without pleocytosis in the patient with the Miller-Fisher variant.

Axial and sagittal T1- and T2*-weighted images of the thoracic and lumbar vertebrae showed thickening of the nerve roots that surround the medullary cone and extend along the length of the cauda equina in all patients.

Enhancement of the thickened nerve roots on contrast material–enhanced T1-weighted images was demonstrated in all patients.

Two patients (25%) had enhancement pattern 1 (Fig 1), while the other six patients (75%) had enhancement pattern 2 (Fig 2).

In all cases, precontrast T1-weighted images showed slightly high signal intensity in the spinal nerve roots (Fig 2a), while T2*-weighted images showed no definite change in signal intensity.

We contrasted the relationship between the enhancement patterns of the spinal nerve roots with electrophysiologic findings, laboratory results of CSF analysis, and clinical signs and symptoms. Abnormal motor nerve conduction was noted in patients with pattern 1 enhancement and in patients with pattern 2 enhancement, while abnormal sensory nerve conduction was present in patients with pattern 1 enhancement but not in patients with pattern 2 enhancement.

In all patients, there was no relationship between patterns of nerve root enhancement and protein levels in the CSF and the time after the onset of symptoms that MR imaging was performed. Motor weakness of the extremities and sensory change, however, coincided with patterns of nerve root enhancement in all patients (Table).

Enhancement and thickening of the spinal nerve roots were slightly decreased at follow-up MR imaging (performed in three patients), and clinical findings and electrophysiologic findings showed minimal improvement (Fig 3).

DISCUSSION

The diagnosis of Guillain-Barré syndrome is established on the basis of the characteristic clinical signs and symptoms, along with laboratory and electrophysiologic results. The characteristic laboratory finding is an increased protein level without pleocytosis in the CSF. Electrophysiologic features supportive of Guillain-Barré syndrome include nerve-conduction slowing, conduction block, prolonged distal latencies, and prolonged or absent F waves. Typical symptoms and signs are symmetric, progressive motor weakness and hyporeflexia or areflexia (1,2).

Most patients clinically suspected to have Guillain-Barré syndrome do not undergo MR imaging. In patients with Guillain-Barré syndrome that is considered on the basis of clinical findings to be atypical, MR imaging is usually requested to exclude other possibilities, such as acute transverse myelitis, conditions that cause acute spinal cord compression, infantile poliomyelitis, and various infiltrative conditions that may have clinical findings similar to those of typical or atypical forms of Guillain-Barré syndrome (10–12). Also, MR imaging may provide supportive evidence of Guillain-Barré syndrome when results of electrophysiologic or CSF studies are equivocal.

Normally, the dorsal root ganglia and

Clinical, Electrophysiologic, and MR Imaging Findings in Eight Patients with Guillain-Barré Syndrome

Patient No./Age (y)/Sex	Motor Weakness	Sensory Change*	Duration of Symptoms (d)†	CSF Protein Level (g/L)	Motor Nerve Conduction Study Findings	Sensory Nerve Conduction Study Findings	MR Imaging Findings: Thickening of Nerve Roots	MR Imaging Findings: Enhancement of Nerve Roots on Contrast-enhanced T1-weighted Images: Anterior Roots	MR Imaging Findings: Enhancement of Nerve Roots on Contrast-enhanced T1-weighted Images: Posterior Roots
1/2/F	Yes	NA	7	1.79	Abnormal	Abnormal	Yes	Yes	Yes
2/6/F	Yes	Yes	7	0.60	Abnormal	Abnormal	Yes	Yes	Yes
3/7/M	Yes	No	6	0.55	Abnormal	Normal	Yes	Yes	No
4/4/M	Yes	No	5	0.70	Abnormal	Normal	Yes	Yes	No
5/8/M	Yes	No	10	1.76	Abnormal	Normal	Yes	Yes	No
6/47/F	Yes	No	30	1.49	Abnormal	Normal	Yes	Yes	No
7/11/F	No	No	17	1.16	Abnormal	Normal	Yes	Yes	No
8/25/F	Yes	No	13	0.50	Abnormal	Normal	Yes	Yes	No

* NA = not checked.
† Time from the onset of symptoms to MR imaging.

nerve roots are enhanced at MR imaging after they exit the theca; this is because of the absence of the blood-nerve barrier at these levels. Enhancement on MR images of the cauda equina with intrathecal ventral and dorsal nerve roots, however, is abnormal because of the presence of blood–nerve root barriers at these levels (13).

In Guillain-Barré syndrome, there is lymphocytic and macrophagic infiltration around endoneural vessels that is associated with demyelination of the affected nerves. Macrophages penetrate the basement membrane around the nerve fibers and strip the myelin away from the axons (14). The abnormal enhancement of intrathecal nerve roots in Guillain-Barré syndrome seen on MR images is suggestive of the breakdown of the blood-nerve barrier and is correlated with perivascular disease (13).

Nonspecific abnormal enhancement of nerve roots has been reported in patients with acquired immunodeficiency syndrome (AIDS)-related polyradiculopathy who also are affected with cytomegalovirus, arachnoiditis, sarcoidosis, or metastatic conditions. Patients with the human immunodeficiency virus, or HIV, may have progressive polyradiculopathy, which shares some of the clinical features of Guillain-Barré syndrome. Several reports on AIDS-related polyradiculopathy owing to cytomegalovirus infection have demonstrated diffuse enhancement of the cauda equina, which the authors of these reports considered to be nonspecific (15–19).

There are several reports on the MR imaging findings of Guillain-Barré syndrome. These reports note that there was marked enhancement of the thickened nerve roots, which was interpreted to be nonspecific. Authors of these reports also stated that MR imaging findings of Guillain-Barré syndrome should be differentiated from those of other pathologic conditions, such as AIDS-related polyradiculopathy with cytomegalovirus infection, arachnoiditis, and others (7–9,20,21).

Gorson et al (22) reported that there was a relationship between the degree of nerve-root enhancement and clinical findings. They mentioned that MR imaging was a sensitive but nonspecific examination in their cases of Guillain-Barré syndrome.

In our study, patients with Guillain-Barré syndrome demonstrated various degrees of gadolinium enhancement of the spinal nerve roots.

The descending spinal tracts and the anterior spinal nerve roots are concerned with somatic motor function, segmental reflexes, and modification of muscle tone; however, the ascending spinal tracts and posterior nerve roots transmit impulses concerned with specific sensations that reach consciousness (23).

Yanagihara et al (24) reported on one patient with Guillain-Barré syndrome who had abnormal enhancement in the anterior nerve roots on MR images that

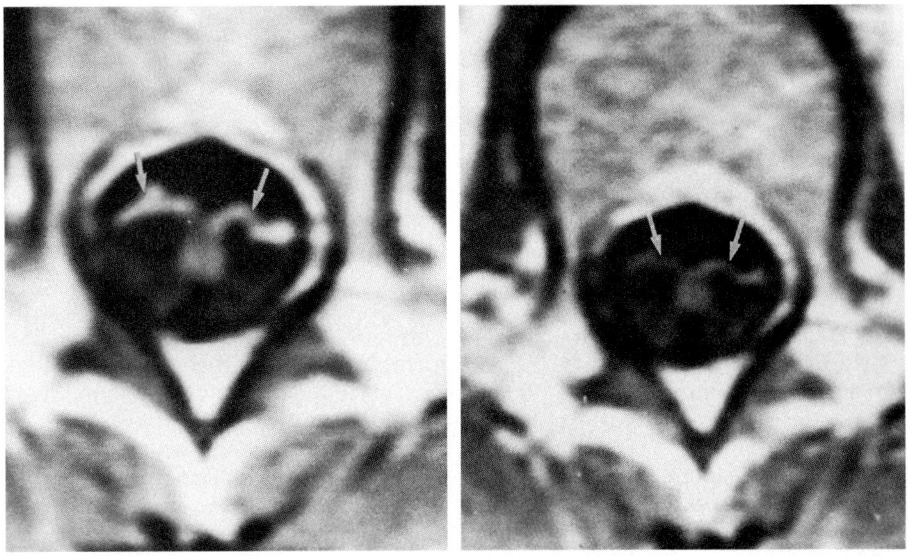

a. b.

Figure 3. Patient 7. **(a)** Initial axial contrast-enhanced T1-weighted image (680/25) shows marked enhancement and thickened anterior spinal nerve roots (arrows). **(b)** Follow-up axial contrast-enhanced T1-weighted image (680/25) obtained 2 months after **a** shows diminished enhancement and thickening of the anterior spinal nerve roots (arrows).

corresponded to the region of muscle weakness. The enhancement on MR images almost disappeared on the 89th day of illness, when symptoms had improved more. They (24) stated that enhanced spinal MR imaging is useful in revealing the involved nerve roots and the degree of illness in patients with Guillain-Barré syndrome.

All patients in our study had motor weakness of extremities and areflexia or hyporeflexia. Sensory change was noted among the patients with enhancement pattern 1; however, those patients with enhancement pattern 2 had no sensory change. Also, patients with pattern 2 had normal sensory nerve–conduction study findings. Abnormal motor conduction study findings were demonstrated in patients with pattern 1 and in patients with pattern 2 enhancement. Motor weakness and sensory change were correlated with patterns of nerve-root enhancement and nerve-conduction study findings in all patients. Six of the eight patients (pattern 2) had weakness of the lower limbs but no definite sensory change, which are correlated with enhancement of the anterior nerve roots only. Therefore, in Guillain-Barré syndrome, the most common site of enhancement on MR images of the spine may be the anterior nerve roots rather than the posterior nerve roots.

Guillain-Barré syndrome may be classified as typical or atypical. Patient 8 had the Miller-Fisher variant of Guillain-Barré syndrome. There was also localized enhancement in the anterior spinal nerve roots on postcontrast axial T1-weighted images in this patient. Nerve-root enhancement may be seen in both patients with typical and patients with atypical forms of Guillain-Barré syndrome. We need to evaluate more cases, however, to determine whether some variants of Guillain-Barré syndrome exhibit enhancement.

Follow-up MR imaging in the three patients with slight improvement of symptoms showed that the thickness and the degree of enhancement of the spinal nerve roots were diminished. Therefore, serial imaging may be useful in monitoring the response to therapy and assessing new treatment regimens. It may also yield a better understanding of the disease process.

In summary, MR imaging with gadopentetate dimeglumine is useful for diagnosing Guillain-Barré syndrome. And, although contrast material enhancement of the spinal nerve roots is a nonspecific finding that can be seen in neoplastic or other inflammatory processes, enhancement of only the anterior nerve roots is suggestive of Guillain-Barré syndrome. Further study of this pattern in more patients is needed.

Acknowledgments: We thank Jung Sang Ha, MD, and Han Gu Moon, MD, for clinical support and Kee Hyun Chang, MD, and Song Shik Choi, MD, for invaluable advice.

References

1. Asbury AK, Cornblath DR. Assessment of current diagnostic criteria for Guillain-Barré syndrome. Ann Neurol 1990; 27(suppl):21–24.
2. Asbury AK. Diagnostic consideration in Guillain-Barré syndrome. Ann Neurol 1981; 9(suppl):1–5.
3. McFarlin DE. Immunological parameters in Guillain-Barré syndrome. Ann Neurol 1990; 27(suppl):25–29.
4. Bril V, Ilse WK, Oearce R, Dhanani A, Sutton D, Kong K. Pilot trial of immunoglobulin versus plasma exchange in patients with Guillain-Barré syndrome. Neurology 1996; 46:100–103.
5. Korinthenberg R, Monting JS. Natural history and treatment effects in Guillain-Barré syndrome. Arch Dis Child 1996; 74:281–287.
6. McKhann GM. Guillain-Barré syndrome: clinical and therapeutic observations. Ann Neurol 1990; 27(suppl):13–16.
7. Perry JR, Fung A, Poon P, Bayer N. Magnetic resonance imaging of nerve root inflammation in the Guillain-Barré syndrome. Neuroradiology 1994; 36:139–140.
8. Crino PB, Zimmerman R, Laskowitz D, Rapes EC, Rostami AM. Magnetic resonance imaging of the cauda equina in Guillain-Barré syndrome. Neurology 1994; 44:1334–1336.
9. Georgy BA, Chong B, Chamberlain M, Hesselink JR, Cheung G. MR of the spine in Guillain-Barré syndrome. AJNR 1994; 15:300–301.
10. Ramsey KL, Kaseff LG. Role of magnetic resonance imaging in the diagnosis of bilateral facial paralysis. Am J Otol 1993; 14:605–609.
11. Jones HR. Childhood Guillain-Barré syndrome: clinical presentation, diagnosis, and therapy. J Child Neurol 1996; 11: 4–12.
12. Brody AJ, Sternbach G, Varon J. Octave landry: Guillain-Barré syndrome. J Emerg Med 1994; 12:833–837.
13. Sze G. Gadolinium-DTPA in spinal diseases. Radiol Clin North Am 1988; 26: 1009–1024.
14. Prineas LW. Pathology of the Guillain-Barré syndrome. Ann Neurol 1981; 9(suppl):6–9.
15. Johnson CE, Sze G. Benign lumbar arachnoiditis: MR imaging with gadopentetate dimeglumine. AJNR 1990; 11:763–770.
16. Sze G, Abramson A, Krol G, et al. Gadolinium-DTPA in the evaluation of intradural extramedullary spinal disease. AJR 1988; 150:911–921.
17. Bazan C III, Jackson C, Jinkins JR, Barohn RJ. Gadolinium-enhanced MRI in a case of cytomegalovirus polyradiculopathy. Neurology 1991; 41:1522–1523.
18. Talpos D, Tien RD, Hesselink JR. Magnetic resonance imaging of AIDS-related polyradiculopathy. Neurology 1991; 41:1995–1997.
19. Lim V, Sobel DF, Zyroff J. Spinal cord pial metastases: MR imaging with gadopentetate dimeglumine. AJNR 1990; 11:975–982.
20. Patel H, Garg BP, Edwards MK. MRI of Guillain-Barré syndrome. J Comput Assist Tomogr 1993; 17:651–652.
21. Baran GA, Sowell MK, Sharp GB, Glasier CM. MR findings in a child with Guillain-Barré syndrome. AJR 1993; 161:161–163.
22. Gorson KC, Ropper AH, Muriello MA, Blair R. Prospective evaluation of MRI lumbosacral nerve root enhancement in acute Guillain-Barré syndrome. Neurology 1996; 47:813–817.
23. Carpenter MB. Tracts of spinal cord. In: Satterfield TS, ed. Core text of neuroanatomy. 4th ed. Baltimore, Md: Williams & Wilkins, 1991; 83–114.
24. Yanagihara K, Imi K, Otani K, Futagi Y, Hishikawa M. Anterior nerve root enhancement on MRI in a case of Guillain-Barré syndrome. Clin Neurol 1995; 35: 1037–1039.

Book Review

Nuclear Medicine Physics: The Basics. 5th ed.
Ramesh Chandra, PhD
Baltimore, Md: Williams and Wilkins, 1998. ISBN 0-683-30092-X.
Softcover, $39.00; pp 182; 86 figures; tables.

This is the fifth edition of one of the most popular introductory books on nuclear medicine physics. The author is a medical physicist from the Department of Radiology, New York University Medical Center. Resident physicians in nuclear medicine and radiology will certainly find this book one of the best and most useful introductory textbooks on nuclear medicine physics. Nuclear medicine technicians and students of nuclear medicine technology will assuredly benefit from it as well.

The book is divided into 16 chapters that cover many important topics, ranging from basic physical foundations of nuclear medicine, radiopharmaceuticals, radiation dosimetry, and radiation protection to nuclear medicine instrumentation and imaging. Seven chapters and the references have been revised. The chapter on radiopharmaceuticals has been substantially enlarged to incorporate recent breakthroughs in nuclear pharmacy and address regulatory issues related to the misadministration of nuclear medicine drugs. The chapters on radiation dosimetry, detection of high-energy radiation, and scintillation camera have been updated and expanded. The chapter on emission tomography has been expanded and revised as well; it now covers such important topics as attenuation compensation, scatter correction, and high-energy single photon emission computed tomography. It also contains an expanded section on positron emission tomography and coincidence gamma camera. The updated and enlarged chapter on the biologic effects of radiation now includes many relevant topics, such as effective dose and committed equivalent dose.

Every chapter has been appended with a new "Key Points" section that succinctly describes and highlights crucial facts and ideas. The "Questions" sections, provided to facilitate understanding of the main concepts introduced in each chapter, have been enlarged, and this new edition now includes the answers to the problems. In addition, two very useful appendices have been added: "Radionuclides of Interest in Nuclear Medicine" and "Organ Masses of a Standard Man."

The book is well organized and easier to use than previous editions. This is due to its improved graphic design that includes a two-column page layout and clearly defined subsections. More than 80 figures and illustrations, many of them updated, enhance and clarify the text.

This is a very well balanced and well written book. It fully deserves to retain its place as one of the most popular introductory textbooks in nuclear medicine physics. This book is highly recommended to anyone who intends to work in the nuclear medicine field.

Reviewed by Andrzej Krol, PhD

Alan J. Holz, MD

The Sugarcoating Sign[1]

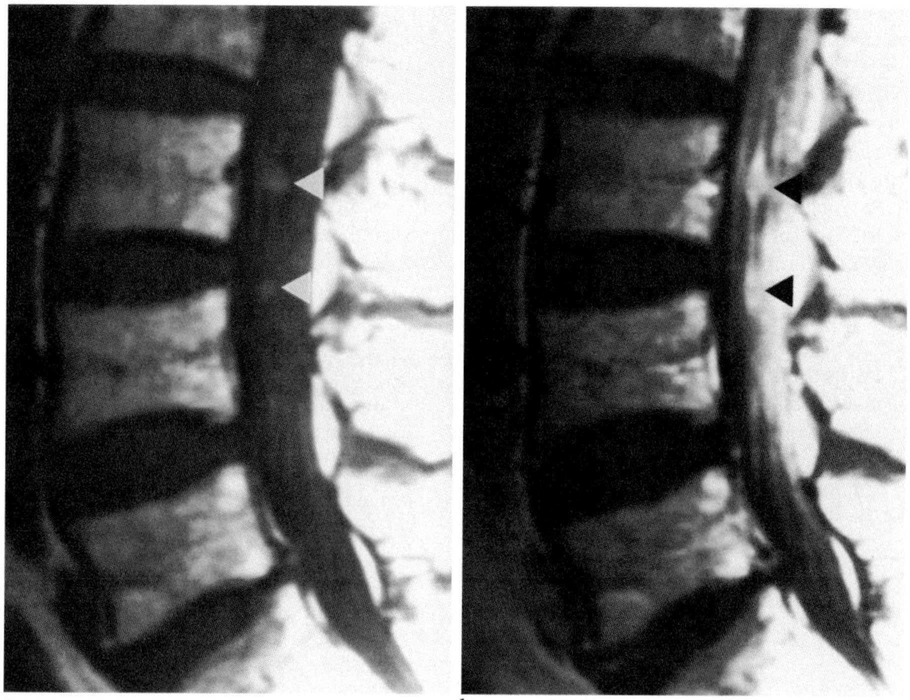
a. b.

(a) Sagittal T1-weighted precontrast MR image (500/10 [repetition time msec/echo time msec]) obtained in a patient with leptomeningeal carcinomatosis due to melanoma. Nodules are noted along the nerve roots (arrowheads). (b) Sagittal T1-weighted postcontrast MR image (500/10) in the same patient demonstrates a sheetlike enhancement along the surface of the cord and nerve roots that produces the sugarcoating appearance (arrowheads).

Index terms:
Spinal cord, MR, 36.12143
Spinal cord, neoplasms, 36.3634, 36.3636, 36.3637, 36.37
Spinal cord, radiography, 36.122

Radiology 1998; 208:143–144

Abbreviation:
CSF = cerebrospinal fluid

[1] From the Department of Radiology, North Shore University Hospital, 300 Community Dr, Manhasset, NY 11030. Received December 2, 1997; revision requested December 24; revision received February 9, 1998; accepted March 4. **Address reprint requests to** the author.

APPEARANCE

The "sugarcoating" (or "frosting") sign is a finding that may be seen on T1-weighted magnetic resonance (MR) images obtained after the administration of contrast material. It consists of diffuse linear and nodular areas of enhancement along the surface of the spinal cord and nerve roots (Figure).

EXPLANATION

The blood-brain barrier extends around the spinal cord and the intrathecal portion of the nerve roots. As a result, these structures usually do not enhance after the administration of contrast material (1). On the other hand, intradural (leptomeningeal) metastases, which adhere to the surface of the cord and nerve roots, typically demonstrate enhancement on postcontrast images (1–3). It is the striking contrast between nonenhancing neural tissue, sheetlike enhancing tumor implants, and dark cerebrospinal fluid (CSF) that produces the sugarcoating sign seen in patients with leptomeningeal carcinomatosis.

DISCUSSION

Leptomeningeal carcinomatosis has become more common as the longevity of patients with cancer has increased and as techniques for the identification of malignant cells in the CSF have improved. It predominates in the lumbosacral region, especially the cauda equina, likely because of the effects of gravity (2). Intradural metastases may spread hematogenously or through direct CSF seeding from brain lesions, in which case they are so-called drop metastases. Hematogenous spreading is most common and typically occurs with systemic tumors such as breast and lung carcinomas, melanoma, and non-Hodgkin lymphoma. Direct seeding of the CSF usually involves highly aggressive primary central nervous system neoplasms such as glioblastoma multiforme and those tumors with direct access to the ventricular system, including medulloblastoma, ependymoma, and choroid plexus carcinoma (2–4). Patients may present with lower extremity weakness, paresthesia, pain, or dysfunction of the bowel or bladder (2).

Although conventional radiography is useful in the evaluation of osseous metastases, it is not useful in the evaluation of intradural metastases. Computed tomographic (CT) scans may occasionally demonstrate thickening and irregularity of the cord and nerve roots. However, these findings are better seen at CT myelography, where nodular filling defects may be identified in the column of contrast material (3,4).

Because of its noninvasive nature, multiplanar capability, and superb soft-tissue contrast material enhancement, MR imaging is the best modality to use to evaluate the contents of the spinal canal. Routinely, sagittal T1- and T2-weighted images and axial T1-weighted images are obtained before the administration of contrast material, followed by postcontrast T1-weighted sagittal and axial images. Subarachnoid tumor implants manifest on non–contrast-enhanced images as nodular, thickened nerve roots. These are usually hyperintense to CSF on T1-weighted images and hypointense on T2-weighted images. Postcontrast T1-weighted images demonstrate diffuse linear and nodular areas of enhancement along the surface of the cord and nerve roots (2). This sugarcoating appearance is nonspecific and may be seen with any process that affects the meninges and disrupts the blood-brain barrier. A nodular enhancement pattern is said to be more typical of tumors than of infectious processes, which usually enhance in a more linear fashion. However, occasionally, nonneoplastic conditions such as granulomatous disease, arachnoiditis, and neurofibromatosis may produce nodular enhancement (2). As always, clinical information aids in narrowing the differential diagnosis.

Although the sugarcoating sign is highly suggestive of leptomeningeal tumor, its absence does not exclude neoplastic dissemination in the CSF. Because of the microscopic nature of the disease, only approximately 20%–25% of cases of proved leptomeningeal carcinomatosis will have positive imaging findings. CSF cytologic analysis is the most definitive test (2,3). It yields positive results in approximately 45%–55% of cases of leptomeningeal carcinomatosis. The yield may be further increased by performing serial lumbar punctures and may approach 95% after six consecutive taps (2).

References

1. Sze G. Gadolinium-DTPA in spinal disease. Radiol Clin North Am 1988; 26:1009–1024.
2. Sze G. Meningeal carcinomatosis. Presented at the Annual Meeting of the American Society of Neuroradiology, Seattle, Wash, June 21–27, 1996.
3. Zimmerman RA, Bilaniuk LT. Imaging of tumors of the spinal canal and cord. Radiol Clin North Am 1988; 26:965–1007.
4. Krol G, Sze G, Malkin M, Walker R. MR of cranial and spinal meningeal carcinomatosis: comparison with CT and myelography. AJNR 1988; 9:709–714.

John L. Doppman, MD
Monica C. Skarulis, MD
Richard Chang, MD
H. Richard Alexander, MD
David Bartlett, MD
Steven K. Libutti, MD
Stephen J. Marx, MD
Allen M. Spiegel, MD

Hypocalcemic Stimulation and Nonselective Venous Sampling for Localizing Parathyroid Adenomas: Work in Progress[1]

Index terms:
Angiography, 274.124, 90.1222, 94.1222
Iopamidol
Parathyroid, neoplasms, 274.363
Parathyroid, vascular studies, 274.124

Radiology 1998; 208:145–151

Abbreviations:
EDTA = ethylenediaminetetraacetic acid
PTH = parathyroid hormone
SVC = superior vena cava

[1] From the Diagnostic Radiology Department, Warren Grant Magnuson Clinical Center (J.L.D., R.C.), the Division of Intramural Research (M.C.S., A.M.S.) and the Metabolic Diseases Branch (S.J.M.), National Institute of Diabetes and Digestive and Kidney Diseases, and the Surgical Oncology Branch, Division of Cancer Treatment, National Cancer Institute (H.R.A., D.B., S.K.L.), National Institutes of Health, Bldg 10, Rm 1C660, Bethesda, MD 20892-1182. Received September 5, 1997; revision requested November 19; final revision received January 28, 1998; accepted March 8. **Address reprint requests to** J.L.D.

PURPOSE: To evaluate whether the release of parathyroid hormone (PTH) from parathyroid tumors during selective parathyroid arteriography can help localize the tumors.

MATERIALS AND METHODS: In 20 patients (six men, 14 women; age range, 24–72 years) with parathyroid tumors undergoing parathyroid arteriography after failed surgery, serial measurements of PTH were obtained during selective arteriography with nonionic contrast material. PTH levels were measured in the superior vena cava (SVC) before and at varying times from 20 to 120 seconds after arteriography.

RESULTS: A 1.4-fold increase in the PTH level of the postarteriographic SVC samples enabled correct prediction of the site of adenoma in 13 of the 20 patients (65%). Of nine patients with positive arteriograms, eight had positive results of postarteriographic sampling. Of 11 patients with negative arteriograms, five had positive results of postarteriographic sampling.

CONCLUSION: Sampling the SVC for PTH gradients after selective parathyroid arteriography correctly indicated the site of the adenoma in 13 of 20 patients (65%).

Intraarterial injection of a secretagogue at pancreatic arteriography with sampling in the right hepatic vein for hormonal response is the most sensitive preoperative test for localizing islet cell tumors. The specific secretagogue for gastrin-producing tumors is secretin (1–3), and the secretagogue for insulin-producing tumors is calcium (4–6). We have shown that these techniques are more sensitive than portal venous sampling and that they frequently help localize an adenoma to the distribution of a selectively injected artery in the absence of arteriographic depiction (2,6). In our practice, arterial stimulation with venous sampling has replaced portal venous sampling for the localization of functioning islet cell tumors.

For the past 2 years, we have been testing a similar technique for localizing parathyroid adenomas. The release of parathyroid hormone (PTH) at selective superior and inferior thyroid and internal mammary arteriography would help localize a hyperfunctioning parathyroid gland to the arterial distribution of the injected vessel and might, as in the case of islet cell tumors, prove more sensitive than angiographic depiction of the adenoma. The stimulus for the release of PTH from a normal, hyperplastic, or adenomatous parathyroid gland is a decrease in the level of calcium perfusing the gland, although hyperplastic and adenomatous glands may have a higher set-point (7). We initially experimented (7) with two hypocalcemic stimuli: (*a*) a 10-second perfusion of physiologic saline injected into the selectively catheterized artery at a rate that replaces blood flow, and (*b*) a standard arteriographic injection (4 mL/sec for 4 seconds) of a nonionic contrast material (iopamidol). We also considered two sampling sites: (*a*) a peripheral vein and (*b*) the superior vena cava (SVC) just below the confluence of the right and left innominate veins. On the basis of preliminary trials, we found that the simplest technique was to measure a transitory

Author contributions:
Guarantors of integrity of entire study, J.L.D., M.C.S.; study concepts, J.L.D., M.C.S., R.C.; study design, J.L.D., M.C.S.; definition of intellectual content, J.L.D., M.C.S., R.C., S.J.M., A.M.S.; literature research, J.L.D.; clinical studies, J.L.D., M.C.S., R.C., H.R.A., D.B., S.K.L., S.J.M., A.M.S.; data acquisition, J.L.D., M.C.S., R.C.; data analysis, J.L.D., M.C.S.; manuscript preparation, J.L.D., M.C.S.; manuscript editing and review, J.L.D.

TABLE 1
Summary of Study Results with a Diagnostic Gradient of 1.4-fold or Greater

Patient No./Sex/ Age (y)	No. of Previous Surgeries	Disease Status	Site of Adenoma Proved at Surgery or Angiographic Ablation*	Arterial Step-up	Increase	Time at Peak PTH Level (sec)	Result of Sampling
1/M/61	1	Cured	RTE groove	Right inferior thyroid†	1.7-fold	30	Positive
2/F/69	1	Cured	LTE groove	Left subclavian†	1.4-fold	30	Positive
3/F/39	1	Cured	Left side of lower neck	No gradient†	. . .	. . .	Nondiagnostic
4/F/38	1	Cured	Right hypopharynx	Right external carotid†,‡	1.5-fold	30	Positive
5/F/36	2	Cured	Within right thyroid lobe	No gradient†	. . .	. . .	Nondiagnositc
6/F/52	1	Cured	Right side of lower neck	No gradient†	. . .	. . .	Nondiagnostic
7/M/56	2	Cured	Right side of neck	No gradient†	. . .	. . .	Nondiagnostic
8/M/52	3	Cured	Right side of upper neck	Right thyrocervical trunk†	1.5-fold	60	Nondiagnostic
				Left thyrocervical trunk	1.4-fold	60	
9/F/43	2	Cured	Within right thyroid lobe	Right inferior thyroid†	1.4-fold	20	Positive
10/F/47	2	Cured	Aortopulmonary window	No gradient†	. . .	. . .	Nondiagnostic
11/F/56	1	Surgery refused	Right side of mediastinum	Right internal mammary‡	1.4-fold	60	Positive
12/F/24	1	Cured	Left side of mediastinum	Left internal mammary‡,§	2-fold	30	Positive
13/F/48	1	Cured	Right side of lower neck	Right inferior thyroid†,‡	4.3-fold	20	Positive
14/M/72	1	Cured	Left side of mediastinum	Left internal mammary‡,§	1.5-fold	40	Positive
15/F/38	3	Improved	Left deltoid muscle	Left circumflex humeral†,‡	1.8-fold	20	Positive
16/F/49	2	Cured	Right carotid sheath	Right inferior thyroid†	1.6-fold	60	Positive
				Right superior thryoid	1.4-fold	20	
17/F/58	4	Cured	Right side of neck	Right inferior thyroid†	1.5-fold	40	Positive
18/M/37	1	Cured	Right side of mediastinum	Right internal mammary‡,§	7.1-fold	60	Positive
				Left internal mammary	1.8-fold	60	
19/F/52	2	Cured	Left undescended gland	Left common carotid†,‡	1.5-fold	60	Nondiagnostic
				Left internal mammary	1.4-fold	20	
20/M/51	1	Cured	Aortopulmonary window	Bronchial†,‡	1.8-fold	60	Positive

* LTE = left tracheoesophageal groove, RTE = right tracheoesophageal groove.
† Tumor was surgically excised.
‡ Tumor was angiographically depicted.
§ Tumor was angiographically ablated.

increase in the PTH level in the SVC after routine selective arteriography of the internal mammary and inferior and superior thyroid arteries with the injection of nonionic contrast material.

We performed this study to evaluate whether the release of PTH from parathyroid tumors during selective parathyroid arteriography can help localize the tumors in patients undergoing parathyroid arteriography after initial failed surgical attempts at localization.

MATERIALS AND METHODS

Twenty patients with primary hyperparathyroidism and equivocal, contradictory, or negative noninvasive parathyroid localization studies (ultrasound, computed tomography [CT], magnetic resonance [MR] imaging, technetium-99m sestamibi scintigraphy) who had previously undergone unsuccessful exploratory surgery of the neck at least once underwent sampling in the SVC before and after selective injection of nonionic contrast material into the internal mammary and inferior and superior thyroid arteries. In one patient (patient 5 [Table 1]), who had an undescended right parathyroid adenoma, sampling was performed in the right internal jugular vein. In another patient (patient 17), who had parathyroid autografts in the left deltoid muscle, sampling was performed in the left subclavian vein. There were six men and 14 women aged 24–69 years. The study was carried out under a protocol approved by the Investigational Review Board of the National Institute of Diabetes and Digestive and Kidney Diseases, National Institutes of Health, Bethesda, Md. All patients were fully informed and gave written consent to undergo the procedure.

A 5-F pigtail catheter was inserted via a femoral vein and placed in the SVC just below the confluence of the right and left innominate veins. Selective arteriography of the internal mammary and inferior and superior thyroid arteries was performed bilaterally. The arteries of subclavian origin (internal mammary and inferior thyroid arteries) were catheterized first, and, if an adenoma was demonstrated, the superior thyroid arteries were not catheterized. In two patients, injection was performed in the carotid arteries (common carotid artery in one patient, external carotid artery in one patient) because the superior thyroid artery could not be catheterized. Nonionic contrast material (iopamidol [Isovue 300; Bracco Diagnostics, Princeton, NJ]) was injected into each internal mammary artery with an automatic injector at a rate of 4 mL/sec for 4 seconds. Ten to 12 milliliters of iopamidol were injected by hand into the superior and inferior thyroid arteries. The rate of manual injection was monitored with digitally subtracted images to minimize reflux and varied because many patients had previously undergone thyroid resection. The subclavian (one patient) or carotid (common carotid artery in one patient, external carotid artery in one patient) arteries were injected if the inferior or superior thyroid arteries could not be selectively catheterized. Tracker catheters (Target Therapeutics, Fremont, Calif) were used for selective injections in patients with very tortuous arteries. Elevated PTH levels after arteriography of the superior and inferior thyroid arteries on the same side helped localize the parathyroid adenoma to the ipsilateral neck.

Immediately before each arteriographic injection, a baseline sample was obtained in the SVC. In the initial six patients, arteriographic samples were obtained 30,

TABLE 2
Effect of Increasing Gradient Criteria on the Diagnostic Accuracy of Individual Arterial Injections

	Gradient			
Finding	≥1.2-fold	≥1.3-fold	≥1.4-fold	≥1.5-fold
Concordant*	26	23	21	14
Discordant*	8	4	2	1
No gradient	84	91	95	103

Note.—Data are from 118 arterial injections with venous sampling in 20 patients.
* With known anatomic location at surgery or arteriography.

TABLE 3
Effect of Increasing Gradient Criteria on the Diagnostic Accuracy of the Study

	Gradient			
Finding	≥1.2-fold	≥1.3-fold	≥1.4-fold	≥1.5-fold
Positive localization	13	13	13	11
Equivocal*	4	3	2	1
Nondiagnostic†	3	4	5	8

Note.—Data are number of patients (n = 20).
* Multiple gradients were found.
† No gradients were found.

60, and 120 seconds after the injection of contrast material. In two of these six patients, PTH levels were elevated only in the 30-second sample. The PTH levels in the 120-second samples always returned to baseline. To avoid missing a transient but diagnostic response, samples were obtained at 20, 40, and 60 seconds after injection of contrast material in the last 14 patients. Samples were processed and the PTH level was measured by using the Immulite Intact PTH assay (Diagnostic Products, Los Angeles, Calif).

All patients with nonvisualized adenomas underwent selective parathyroid venous sampling before surgery. Diagnostic accuracy was defined retrospectively after localization was confirmed at surgery. A gradient was determined as an increase in PTH level by 21% over baseline, which is three times the intraassay coefficient of variation for the PTH assay (7%).

RESULTS

Parathyroid adenomas were depicted arteriographically in nine patients: in the neck in three patients, in the anterior part of the mediastinum or aortopulmonary window in five patients, and at the site of a parathyroid autograft in the deltoid muscle in one patient. Of these nine patients, five had surgical confirmation of the anatomic location. Arteriographic ablation by staining the tumor with contrast material was attempted in four patients with mediastinal adenomas and was successful in three, all of whom are currently normocalcemic. Surgery is to be performed in one patient, who had only transient hypocalcemia in response to staining. Eleven patients with negative arteriograms underwent parathyroid venous sampling and surgery on the basis of these results. The anatomic location of the adenoma was determined surgically in all 11 patients. Table 1 summarizes the results.

One hundred eighteen arterial injections with venous sampling were performed in the 20 patients. In most cases, this was performed in both superior thyroid arteries, both thyrocervical trunks, and both internal mammary arteries. Other arteries were included when clinically indicated. The diagnostic accuracy of an individual injection was analyzed by means of increasing gradient criteria. The gradient criteria analyzed were 1.2-fold (representing three times the intraassay coefficient of variation for the PTH assay), 1.3-fold, 1.4-fold, and 1.5-fold over prearteriographic baseline PTH values. At each gradient criterion, the findings at venous sampling were concordant or discordant with a known anatomic lesion or there was no gradient. Table 2 shows the results of this analysis. The highest percentage of discordant findings occurred with a gradient of 1.2-fold, whereas the lowest percentage of concordant findings occurred with a gradient of 1.5-fold. The diagnostic accuracy of each study performed (n = 20) was assessed with gradients of 1.2-, 1.3-, 1.4, or 1.5-fold. Table 3 shows that a gradient of 1.4-fold yielded the highest number of positive studies (13 of 20 studies) and the fewest equivocal studies (two of 20 studies). Taken together, it appears that a gradient of 1.4-fold is likely to provide the greatest diagnostic accuracy with the fewest equivocal studies with current methods.

Table 1 shows summary data for the 20 patients with a diagnostic gradient of 1.4-fold. Five patients (patients 3, 5–7, 10) had no gradients, which resulted in nondiagnostic studies. Two of these five patients had incomplete sampling studies owing to ligation of a feeding vessel or because the tumor was in an unusual ectopic location. In patient 3, who had a left cervical parathyroid adenoma, the left inferior thyroid artery had been ligated at a previous surgery. In patient 10, who had an aortopulmonary window lesion, the bronchial artery was not injected. Two patients (patients 8 and 19) had second gradients that were discordant with the known anatomic location of the adenoma; this resulted in nondiagnostic studies.

Two additional patients had a second gradient, but the studies were considered diagnostic. Patient 16, who had an adenoma in the right carotid sheath, had diagnostic gradients in the right superior and inferior thyroid arteries. Patient 18, who had a right mediastinal adenoma, had a 7.1-fold gradient increase after right internal mammary arteriography and a 1.8-fold gradient increase after left internal mammary arteriography, probably because of cross circulation. Both studies were classified as diagnostic.

Localizing gradients resulted in a positive diagnostic study in 13 of the 20 patients (65%). Eight of these 13 patients (patients 4, 11–15, 18, 20) had a positive arteriogram. More important, in five of the 13 patients (patients 1, 2, 9, 16, 17) the adenomas were not depicted arteriographically. Localizing gradients in these five patients could have obviated venous sampling.

Figures 1–5 illustrate the findings in five patients.

DISCUSSION

The stimulus for the release of hormone from a normal parathyroid gland is a reduction in the level of serum calcium. Parathyroid adenomas and hyperplastic glands have higher set-points but respond to a decrease in the serum calcium level by releasing PTH (7). We initially investigated a 10-second injection of physiologic saline at a rate determined with arteriography to replace blood flow (spill-over phenomenon). However, because arteriography always preceded the saline injection, and because the response of an adenoma or hyperplastic gland to perfusion with a nonionic contrast material was unknown, we sampled immediately after selective arteriography in a few patients. We were also influenced by previous findings of striking elevations of PTH in peripheral veins during deliberate ablation of adenomas with contrast material staining (Doppman JL, unpublished data, 1980).

Preliminary results of this study show

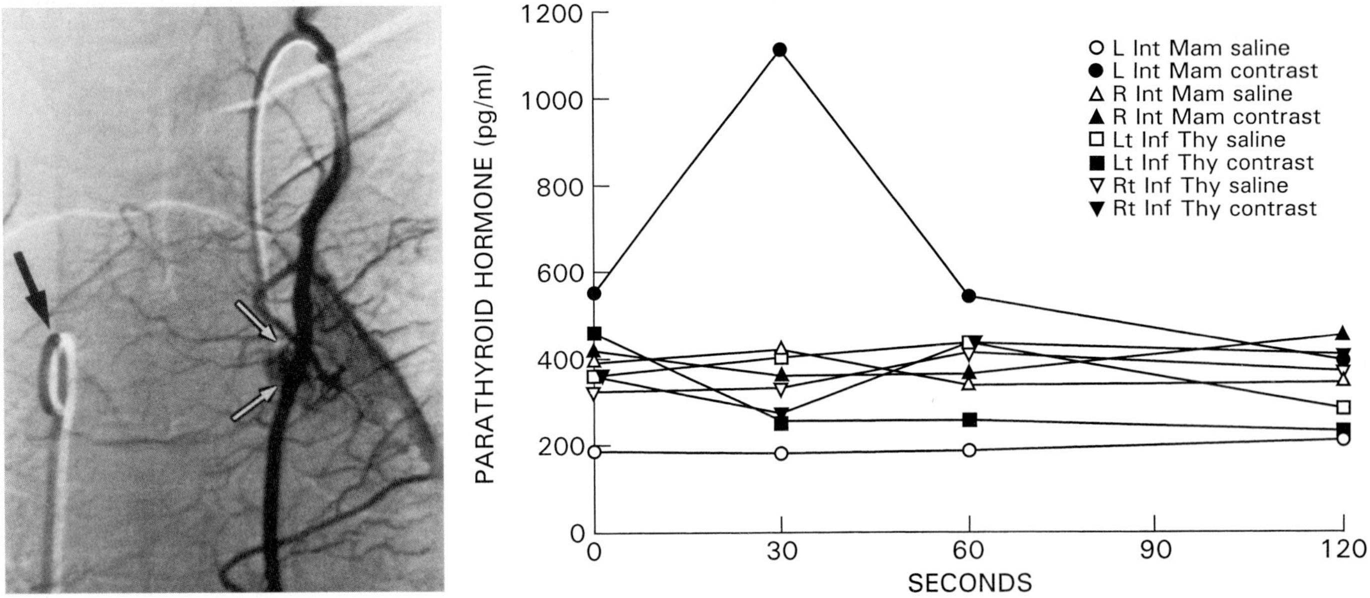

a. b.

Figure 1. Patient 12. **(a)** Selective left internal mammary arteriogram shows an anterior mediastinal adenoma (white arrows). The black arrow indicates the sampling pigtail catheter in the SVC. **(b)** Graph shows the PTH responses to arteriography. Note the elevated baseline PTH level (580 pg/mL [61 pmol/L]) at left internal mammary arteriography, which is presumably a response to the contrast material injected during placement of the catheter in the internal mammary artery. Also note the lack of response to the subsequent saline injection, which suggests depletion of PTH reserves in this small adenoma because of the preceding arteriogram. Sampling in this early study was performed 30, 60, and 120 seconds after arteriography. Only the 30-second sample showed a gradient; subsequently, sampling at 20, 40, and 60 seconds was initiated. *Contrast* = with contrast material injection, *L* = left, *Lt* = left, *Inf* = inferior, *Int* = internal, *Mam* = mammary arteriography, *R* = right, *Rt* = right, *Saline* = with saline injection, *Thy* = thyroid arteriography.

that nonionic contrast material is an effective stimulus for releasing PTH and simplifies the procedure by confining the imaging and sampling study to a single injection. At least one patient showed a positive response to contrast material and a negative response to the subsequent saline injection (Fig 1). In addition, the arteriographic distribution helps define the area in which the adenoma or hyperplastic gland is contained, which enables more precise localization than might a saline injection. We did not investigate the roles of ionic versus nonionic contrast material or more specific calcium-lowering agents such as citrate or ethylenediaminetetraacetic acid (EDTA), but, we based the test on the empiric observation that iopamidol appeared to cause PTH to be released from an adenoma. We also believed that the initial response of an adenoma to any stimulus might be greater than the response to a subsequent stimulus.

Intraarterial injection of contrast material lowers ionic calcium levels in the downstream vascular bed by means of four mechanisms (8–11). First, calcium-containing blood is replaced by the contrast material injected at a rate similar to that of the blood flow in the catheterized vessels. Second, dilution occurs owing to the hyperosmolarity of the contrast material, which draws interstitial fluid into the vessel. The hematocrit level of blood in the coronary sinus can decrease by as much as 17% after selective coronary arteriography with ionic contrast material (eg, diatrizoate sodium) or 13% with nonionic contrast material (eg, iopamidol) (9). Third, there is calcium binding by the dissociated anions of contrast material. This effect is greater with sodium than with meglumine salts and is seen only with ionic agents. Finally, the calcium level may be lowered by the chelators (eg, sodium calcium EDTA) present in all ionic and nonionic contrast media.

Sodium-containing ionic contrast media cause the greatest decrease in ionized calcium and hematocrit levels because of their hyperosmolarity and the greater dissociation of sodium as compared with methylglucamine salts. Mitsumori et al (9) showed that diatrizoate caused a 0.21 mmol/L decrease in the ionized calcium level in coronary sinus blood during coronary arteriography, as opposed to the 0.1 mmol/L decrease caused by iopamidol. The use of a sodium-containing ionic contrast material such as diatrizoate sodium might produce a more intense hypocalcemic stimulus and, consequently, a greater increase in the PTH level but at the expense of a more painful arteriographic examination. Ioxaglate sodium–ioxaglate meglumine (Hexabrix; Laboratoire Guerbet, Aulnay-sous-Bois, France) and diatrizoate meglumine–diatrizoate sodium (Urografin; Schering, Berlin, Germany) produce more prolonged decreases in the ionized calcium level in the coronary sinus than do nonionic contrast media such as iopamidol and iohexol. It is not known whether it is the magnitude or the duration of the hypocalcemic stimulus that is important in triggering PTH release. With all contrast media, ionic calcium levels in the coronary sinus return to normal 30 seconds after coronary arteriography; thus, the hypocalcemic stimulus is short-lived, regardless of the contrast material used.

In some cases, the baseline PTH value for the artery in which injection showed a positive response was higher than that for other arteries (Fig 2); this is known as baseline drift. To manipulate the catheter into any selected artery, small injections of contrast material are necessary, and, although an effort was made to keep those preliminary injections to a minimum, some effect on the baseline PTH

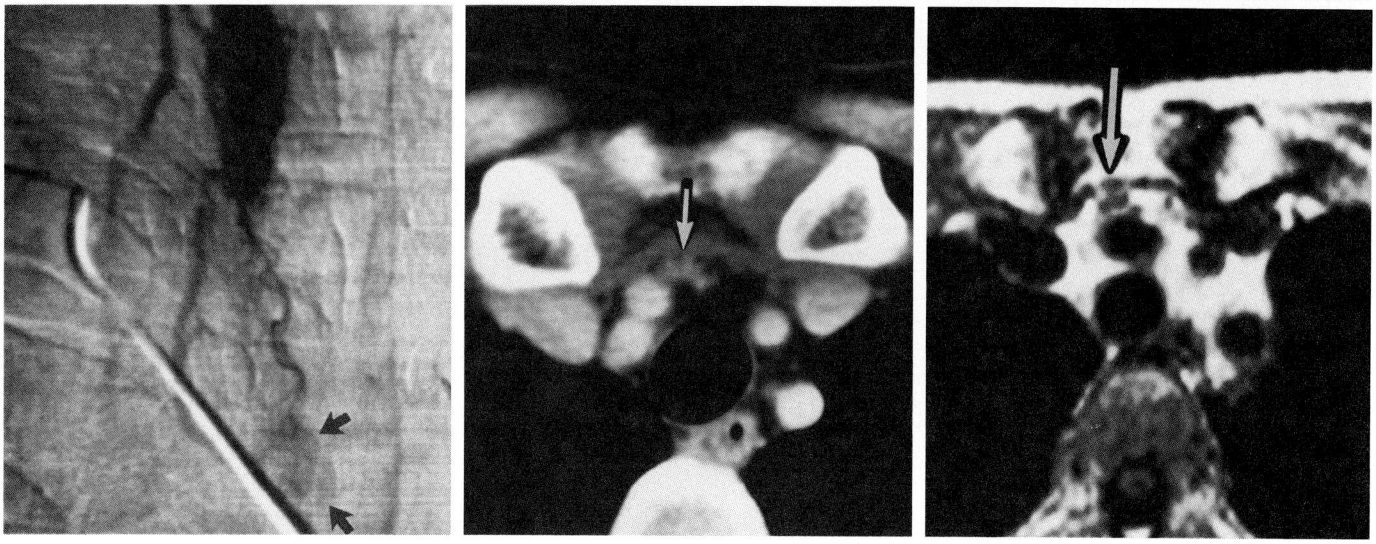

a. b. c.

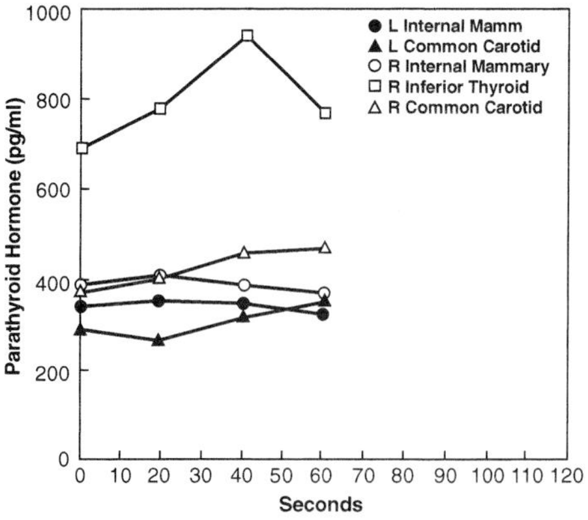

d.

Figure 2. Patient 13. (**a**) Arteriogram shows a faintly staining adenoma (arrows) supplied by a descending branch of the right inferior thyroid artery. This adenoma (arrow in **b** and **c**) was misinterpreted as a lymph node on (**b**) CT and (**c**) MR images because of its small size and irregular shape. Results of Tc-99m sestamibi scintigraphy were negative. (**d**) Graph shows the PTH response to arteriography. The response to right inferior thyroid arteriography confirmed the arteriographic suspicion and led to successful resection. Note the displaced baseline measurement obtained at right inferior thyroid arteriography owing to the effect of preliminary contrast material injection for catheter placement. *L* = left, *Mamm* = mammary arteriography, *R* = right.

level was seen. If one extrapolates the baseline PTH levels of the positive studies to control baseline values, many gradients are even higher.

The SVC just below the junction of the right and left innominate veins was selected as the site for venous sampling. The inferior thyroid veins drain into the left innominate vein. Both the right and left vertebral veins, which are frequent sites of positive venous samples from cervical adenomas when the inferior thyroid veins have been ligated, drain into the ipsilateral innominate veins. The right and left thymic veins draining the anterior part of the mediastinum also empty into the left innominate vein. Venous effluent from the lower neck and anterior part of the mediastinum, therefore, should be sampled with a catheter in the SVC. Less is known about the venous drainage from undescended cervical adenomas, but they most likely drain into the ipsilateral internal jugular veins (12). Adenomas in the aortopulmonary window receive their blood supply from the bronchial arteries, but little is known about their venous drainage (13).

Laminar streaming of the effluent from thyroid, vertebral, and thymic veins in the nonpulsatile, high-volume flow of the SVC may account for negative results in some patients. One of the advantages of hepatic vein sampling for insulinomas and gastrinomas is the mixing of portal venous blood that occurs during transit through the liver. Streaming is a problem when sampling the portal vein for insulin or gastrin levels (14), and there is no easy mechanism for inducing turbulence or complete mixing in such laminar high-flow venous channels. More complete mixing might occur in the right atrium, but then one must deal with increased dilution due to inflow from the inferior vena cava.

Early in our experience, one patient not included in this series showed an elevation in the PTH level in a peripheral vein that peaked 4–5 minutes after selective arteriography. This response was delayed compared with the response in the SVC, and peripheral sampling would prolong the study. Consequently, peripheral sampling was not evaluated further.

Patient 4, who had a right undescended adenoma, had no PTH level elevation in the SVC but did have diagnostic gradients in the right internal jugular vein after right external carotid arteriography. We are investigating the possibility that sampling in ipsilateral internal jugular veins rather than in the SVC during external carotid arteriography may be more sensitive for undescended parathyroid adenomas (12).

Patient 15, who had functioning parathyroid autografts in the deltoid muscle, showed no response to left subclavian arteriography when samples were obtained in the SVC but a definite response when the sampling catheter was positioned in the left subclavian vein. Sampling to evaluate autografts in the upper extremities should be performed in the subclavian veins. In addition, intraarterial hypocalcemic stimulation may prove to be more sensitive for evaluating the viability of a parathyroid autograft than unstimulated sampling of veins draining the graft site. In the presence of functioning remnant glands in the neck, patients with parathyroid hyperplasia or multiple

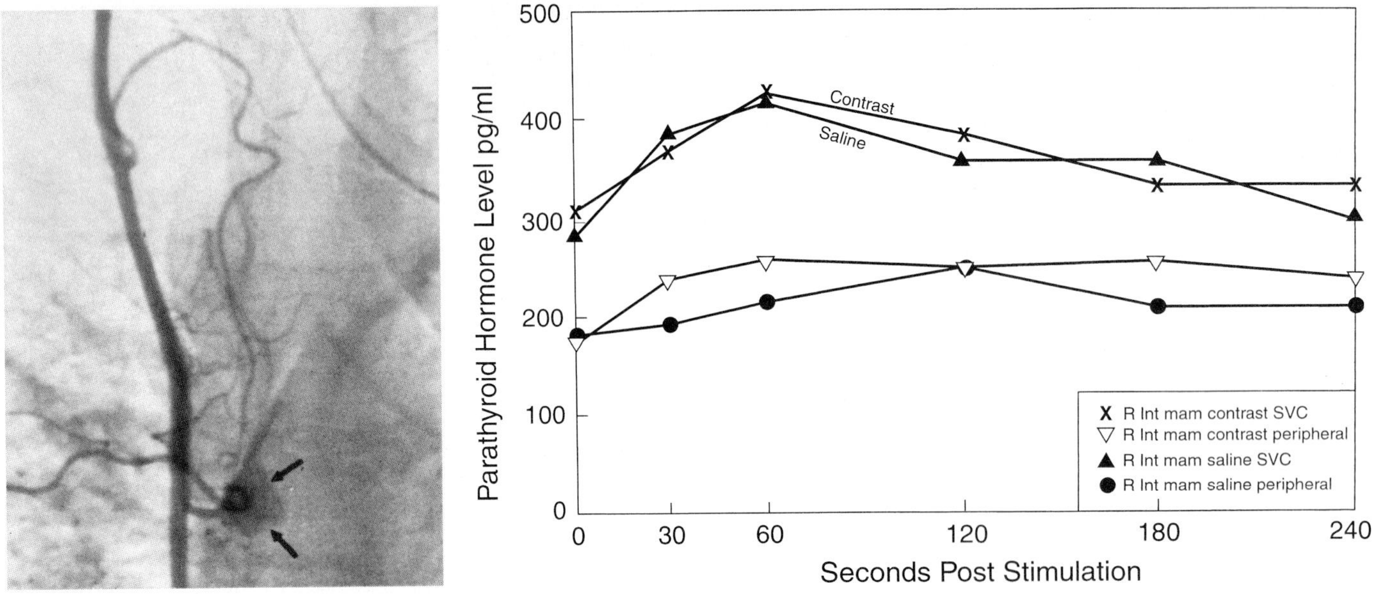

a. b.

Figure 3. Patient 11. **(a)** Selective right internal mammary arteriogram shows an adenoma (arrows) supplied by the thymic branch of the right internal mammary artery. **(b)** Graph of the PTH response to arteriography demonstrates that samples from the SVC and a peripheral vein showed a response to both contrast material and saline injections but that the gradients in the peripheral vein samples were smaller and delayed. An attempt at staining failed because of the length and tortuosity of the feeding thymic artery. This patient has refused to undergo sternotomy. *Int* = internal. *mam* = mammary arteriography, *R* = right.

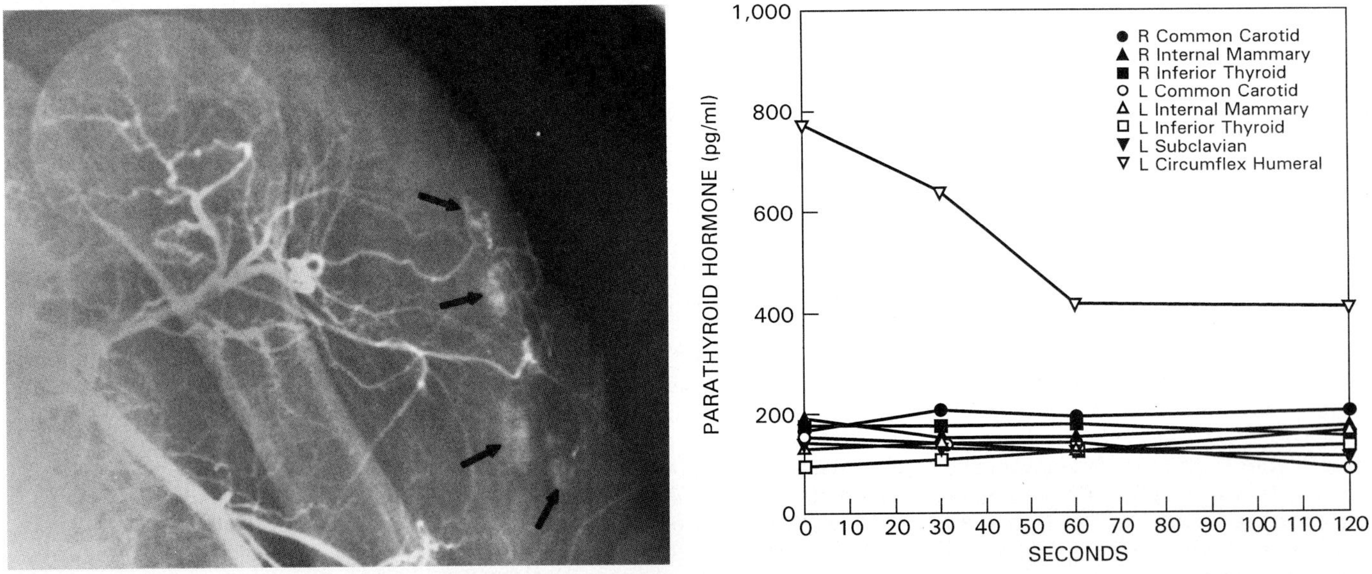

a. b.

Figure 4. Patient 15. **(a)** Arteriogram obtained in the left arm shows multiple enhancing parathyroid autografts (arrows) in this patient with multiple endocrine neoplasia I and recurrent hypercalcemia. Sampling after arteriography of the left circumflex humeral artery revealed an elevated baseline PTH level (800 pg/mL [84 pmol/L]) due to preliminary injection of contrast material for catheter placement. **(b)** Graph shows the PTH response to arteriography. A decrease in the PTH concentration suggests that the parathyroid autografts were depleted of PTH with the initial injection of contrast material. Negative responses to internal mammary and inferior thyroid arteriography are suggestive of an absence of functioning parathyroid tissue in the neck, which was substantiated by the hypocalcemia that followed resection of the autografts. *L* = left, *R* = right.

endocrine neoplasia syndrome may have viable but non–PTH-secreting autografts that are not detectable with brachial vein sampling but could be stimulated with a hypocalcemic injection.

The gradients of PTH after parathyroid arteriography are not as robust as those after arterial stimulation and venous sampling for insulinomas. Increased dilution and streaming in the SVC may partially account for these lesser gradients. It is possible that a more specific stimulant (eg, intraarterial EDTA or citrate) might evoke a stronger response. We are investigating these possibilities.

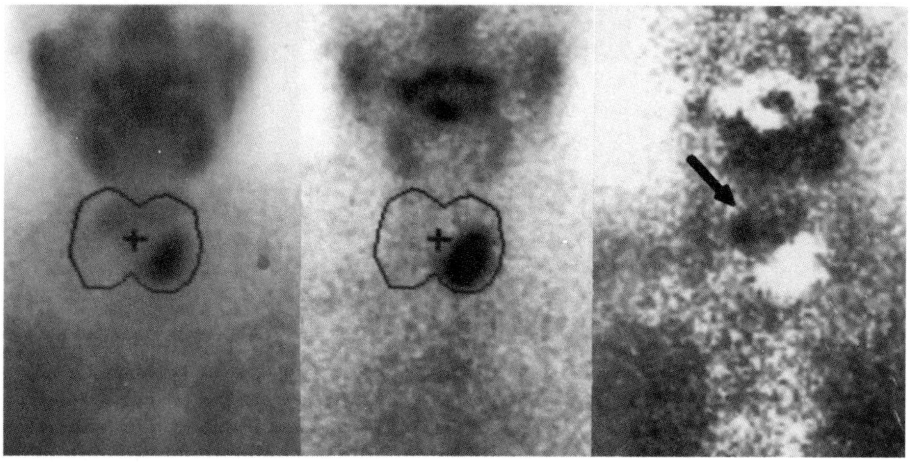

a.

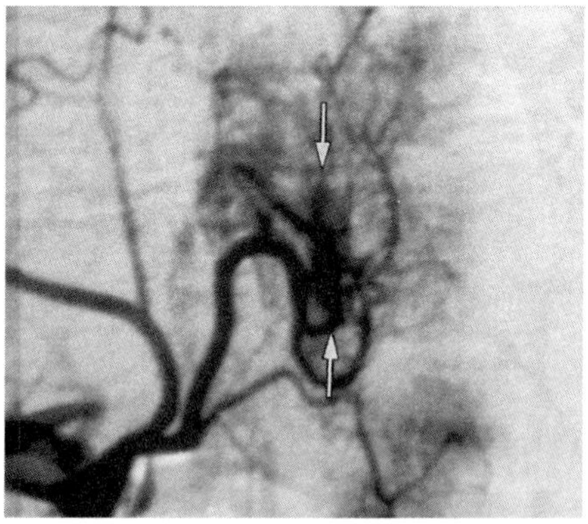

b.

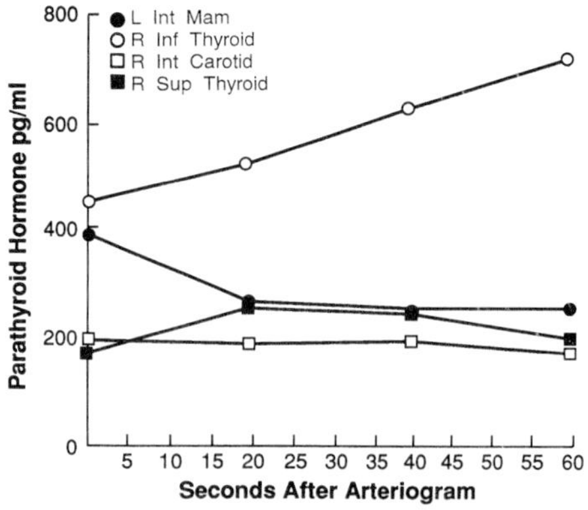

c.

Figure 5. Patient 16. This patient underwent two surgical explorations of the neck with negative results. Right thyroid lobectomy was performed at the second unsuccessful surgery. Sestamibi scintigraphy was performed after both procedures, with similar findings. **(a)** Sestamibi scan (left panel), technetium pertechnetate scan (middle panel), and subtraction study (right panel) show persistent activity (arrow, right panel) in the right side of the neck. **(b)** Right inferior thyroid arteriogram reveals an area of staining (arrows) that could represent parathyroid tissue or residual thyroid tissue. **(c)** Graph of PTH response to arteriography. The PTH level in SVC samples increased progressively after right inferior (*R Inf*) thyroid arteriography, thereby helping to identify the area of staining as parathyroid. At surgery, the adenoma was within the right carotid sheath. *L Int Mam* = left internal mammary artery, *R Inf thyroid* = right inferior thyroid artery, *R Int carotid* = right internal carotid artery, *R sup thyroid* = right superior thyroid artery.

There are a number of limitations to this preliminary study. The sensitivity of hypocalcemic stimulation with venous sampling for PTH cannot be determined from our experiences because parameters were changed during the accrual of this small group of patients. The selective catheterization of the internal mammary artery and inferior and superior thyroid arteries cannot always be accomplished in this 50–60-year-old, frequently hypertensive population, but diagnostic arteriography with positive venous gradients can be performed with Tracker catheters. The venous drainage pattern of the neck and anterior part of the mediastinum is not constant, particularly after unsuccessful neck surgery and transcervical thymic extractions. Nevertheless, SVC sampling after arterial stimulation is far simpler than parathyroid venous sampling, and arterial stimulation with venous sampling may provide information that obviates the latter.

References

1. Imamura M, Takahashi K, Adachi H, et al. Usefulness of selective arterial secretin injection tests for localization of gastrinomas in the Zollinger-Ellison syndrome. Ann Surg 1987; 205:230–239.
2. Doppman JL, Miller DL, Chang R, et al. Gastrinomas: localization by means of selective intraarterial injection of secretin. Radiology 1990; 174:25–29.
3. Thom AK, Norton JA, Doppman JL, Miller DL, Chang R, Jensen RT. Prospective study of the use of intraarterial secretin injection and portal venous sampling to localize duodenal gastrinomas. Surgery 1992; 112:1002–1009.
4. Doppman JL, Miller DL, Chang R, Shawker TH, Gorden P, Norton JA. Insulinomas: localization with selective intraarterial injection of calcium. Radiology 1991; 178: 237–241.
5. Doppman JL, Miller DL, Chang R, Gorden P, Eastman RC, Norton JA. Intraarterial calcium stimulation test for detection of insulinomas. World J Surg 1993; 17:439–443.
6. Doppman JL, Chang R, Fraker DL, et al. Localization of insulinomas to regions of the pancreas by intraarterial stimulation with calcium. Ann Intern Med 1995; 123: 269–273.
7. Brown EM, Wilson RE, Thatcher JG, Marynick SP. Abnormal calcium-regulated PTH release in normal parathyroid tissue from patients with adenoma. Am J Med 1981; 71:565–570.
8. Morris TW, Sahler LG, Violante M, Fischer HW. Reduction of calcium activity by radiopaque contrast media. Radiology 1983; 148:55–59.
9. Mitsumori M, Hayakawa K, Torizuka T, et al. Ionized calcium levels in coronary sinus blood during coronary angiography: effects of four contrast media. Radiology 1992; 183:159–161.
10. Hayakawa K, Okuno Y, Fujiwara K, Shimizu Y. Effect of iodinated contrast media on ionic calcium. Acta Radiol 1994; 35:83–87.
11. Pedersen HC. Electrolyte addition to nonionic contrast media. Acta Radiol Suppl 1996; 37:7–31.
12. Fraker DL, Doppman JL, Shawker TH, Marx SJ, Spiegel AM, Norton JA. Undescended parathyroid adenoma: an important etiology for failed operations for primary hyperparathyroidism. World J Surg 1990; 14:342–348.
13. Doppman JL, Skarulis MC, Chen CC, et al. Parathyroid adenomas of the aortopulmonary window. Radiology 1996; 201: 456–462.
14. Miller DL, Doppman JL, Metz DC, Maton PN, Norton JA, Jensen RT. Zollinger-Ellison syndrome: technique, results and complications of portal venous sampling. Radiology 1992; 182:235–241.

fu•ture, *n.*

1. *a:* time that is to come *b:* what is going to happen; **2.** an expectation of advancement or progressive development

RSNA Defines the Future of Radiology

In this era of rapid technologic advancement, the possibilities for radiology are wide open. RSNA recognizes that the road to the future is paved by improved clinical practice, innovative research, and excellence in teaching — all of which demand quality continuing medical education. Through the development and implementation of education-oriented innovations, RSNA is dedicated to helping radiologists and allied health professionals improve their radiologic skills and knowledge.

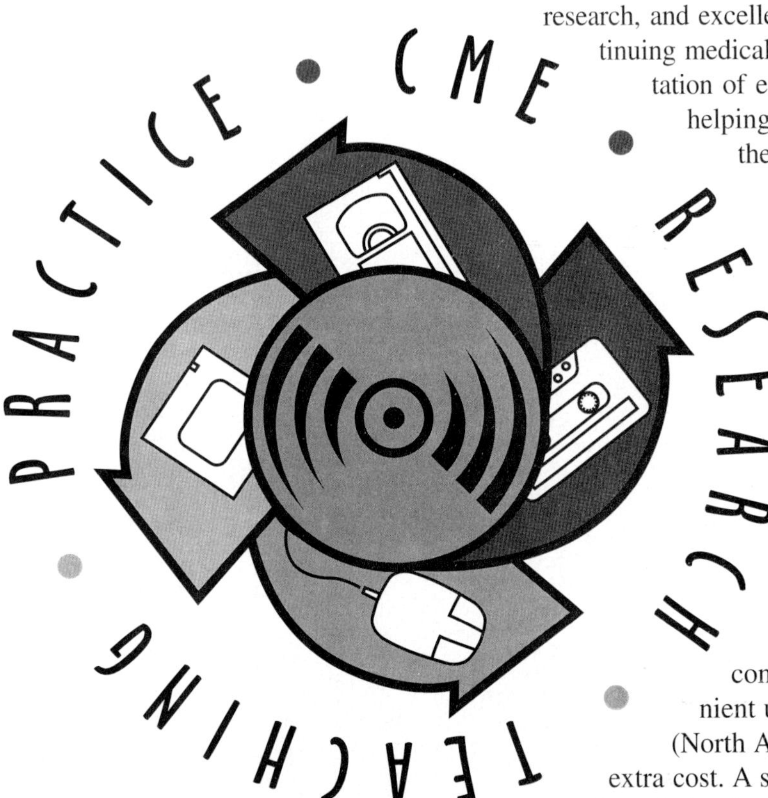

Learning Resources for the 21st Century

Leaders in radiology depend on RSNA Educational Resources recorded live during RSNA's Annual Scientific Assembly. Developed in partnership with the most highly regarded experts in their fields, these instructional materials feature specific, practical information that progressive radiologists can use every day to enhance the level of diagnostic and/or therapeutic care they deliver.

Available for purchase or rental, these programs come in slide/audiocassette and video formats for convenient use in the home or office. Videos are available in NTSC (North American), PAL and SECAM television standards at no extra cost. A selection of syllabi and scientific exhibits is also available on CD-ROM. All materials are developed by using advanced computer enhancements that offer program users the greatest instructional impact possible.

At the forefront of quality educational programs, this collection includes more than 200 courses in eleven clinical categories in all imaging modalities. All of these materials can be found in the Learning Center Resources Catalog, updated each year to ensure that the materials are relevant to current and future directions of radiology. RSNA Learning Resources are available for both Category 1 and Category 2 CME credit.

Order RSNA Educational Resources by calling 800/272-2920 (toll free in the U.S. and Canada). Net revenues from the sale of these educational materials go the RSNA Research and Education Fund in support of research and education in all radiologic subspecialties.

For more information on RSNA see our World Wide Web site: http://www.rsna.org

RSNA Radiological Society of North America Founded in 1915

Learning Center Resources Program

The Radiological Society of North America is accredited by the Accreditation Council for Continuing Medical Education to sponsor continuing medical education for physicians.

Dual-Helical CT for Detecting Aortic Atheromas as a Source of Stroke: Comparison with Transesophageal Echocardiography[1]

Alexander Tenenbaum, MD, PhD
Alexander Garniek, MD
Joseph Shemesh, MD
Enrique Z. Fisman, MD
Chaim I. Stroh, MD
Yacov Itzchak, MD, PhD
Zvi Vered, MD
Michael Motro, MD

Index terms:
Aorta, arteriosclerosis, 56.754, 94.72
Aorta, US, 56.12983, 94.12983
Brain, ischemia, 10.77
Computed tomography (CT), helical, 51.12115
Embolism, 10.77, 92.77
Extremities, embolism, 92.77

Radiology 1998; 208:153–158

Abbreviation:
TEE = transesophageal echocardiography

[1] From the Cardiac Rehabilitation Institute (A.T., J.S., E.Z.F., C.I.S., M.M.), the Department of Diagnostic Imaging (A.G., Y.I.), and the Heart Institute (Z.V.), Chaim Sheba Medical Center, 52621 Tel-Hashomer, Israel; and the Sackler Faculty of Medicine, Tel-Aviv University, Tel-Aviv, Israel (A.G., J.S., E.Z.F., Y.I., Z.V., M.M.). Received September 29, 1997; revision requested November 26; revision received February 5, 1998; accepted February 11. **Address reprint requests to** A.T.

PURPOSE: To investigate whether unenhanced dual-helical computed tomography (CT) is useful in the rapid, noninvasive detection of protruding aortic atheromas.

MATERIALS AND METHODS: Thirty-two consecutive patients at least 50 years of age who had recent ischemic stroke, systemic emboli, or both, underwent transesophageal echocardiography (TEE) and unenhanced dual-helical CT with thin sections (section thickness, 3.2 mm; reconstruction increment, 1.5 mm).

RESULTS: TEE demonstrated protruding aortic atheromas in 15 patients (47%); dual-helical CT depicted protruding aortic atheromas in 13 of those 15 patients (87%). Of the 17 patients without a protruding aortic atheroma at TEE, dual-helical CT helped confirm the absence in 14 (82%). Dual-helical CT yielded a sensitivity of 87%, a specificity of 82%, and an overall accuracy of 84%. Thirty-six protruding plaques were detected with TEE, of which 34 (94%) were correctly identified with dual-helical CT. Of those 34 plaques, 27 (79%) contained variable amounts of calcium and seven (21%) showed hypoattenuation suggestive of soft plaques and thrombi. In six patients, dual-helical CT depicted a protruding aortic atheroma between the distal ascending aorta and the proximal arch; these plaques were not included in the comparative statistics and were analyzed separately.

CONCLUSION: Unenhanced dual-helical CT with thin sections appears to be useful for the rapid, noninvasive detection of a protruding aortic atheroma, especially in areas not clearly visualized with TEE.

Ischemic stroke and peripheral embolic events are leading causes of serious disability in most industrialized countries (1). Systemic emboli from atheromas in the thoracic aorta were previously thought to be rare, but with the growing use of transesophageal echocardiography (TEE), they have been reported with increasing frequency (2–12). Moreover, recent studies have demonstrated that protruding aortic plaques may be an important source of iatrogenic stroke (eg, resulting from coronary angiography or coronary artery bypass grafting) and embolic events in the elderly (13–16). The single modality available at present for detecting aortic plaques is TEE, a semi-invasive method that usually requires topical anesthesia, sedation, or both and is not suitable for screening potentially high-risk subjects. Because of the interposition of the air column in the trachea and left bronchus, as well as arching of the aorta, TEE does not usually allow full visualization of the upper part of the ascending aorta and the proximal aortic arch. Therefore, TEE cannot help exclude the presence of plaques in these two regions (16,17).

Our study was undertaken to investigate whether unenhanced fast dual-helical computed tomography (CT) is useful for the rapid, noninvasive detection of protruding aortic atheromas.

Author contributions:
Guarantors of integrity of entire study, A.T., M.M.; study concepts, A.T., E.Z.F., M.M.; study design, J.S., Z.V.; definition of intellectual content, A.T., J.S., M.M.; literature research, A.T., J.S., E.Z.F.; clinical studies, C.I.S., Z.V., M.M.; data acquisition, A.G., Z.V., M.M.; data analysis, A.T., A.G., M.M.; statistical analysis, A.T.; manuscript preparation, E.Z.F.; manuscript editing and review, Y.I., Z.V., M.M.

MATERIALS AND METHODS

Patients

Over a period of 13 months (May 1995 through May 1996), 32 patients (19 men, 13 women) at least 50 years of age (mean age, 64 years ± 9 [standard deviation]) who had a recent ischemic stroke, systemic emboli, or both (emboli occurred within 15 days after the onset of the event) were enrolled in the study and underwent TEE and unenhanced dual-helical CT. Twenty-five patients had strokes, four had systemic emboli, and the remaining three had both. Informed consent for both procedures was obtained from all patients. The study protocol was approved by the institutional review board (Helsinki Committee).

TEE Examination

All TEE studies were performed with a Sonos 1000 or 1500 ultrasound system (Hewlett Packard, Andover, Mass) and 5-MHz multiplane transducers. Midazolam and lidocaine 10% topical spray were used for local anesthesia. All visible regions of the thoracic aorta were fully explored in every patient, including the proximal ascending aorta beginning from the aortic valve as seen on the vertical view of the heart. The descending aorta and the arch were visualized in multiplane projections, including both horizontal and vertical axes. All studies were recorded with a 6200 Super VHS tape recorder (Matsushita Electric, Osaka, Japan). The plaque thickness was measured perpendicular to the wall as the distance between the medial-adventitial border and the internal side of the lesion; protruding aortic atheromas were defined as plaques that protruded at least 4 mm into the aortic lumen. Measurements were made off-line from the recorded images. TEE preceded dual-helical CT in all cases.

Dual-Helical CT Protocol

Dual-helical CT studies were performed with a CT-Twin scanner (Elscint, Haifa, Israel). With the patient in the supine position, a posteroanterior scout image was obtained to determine the upper level of the aortic arch. A 25-second unenhanced helical scan was obtained at the upper border of the aortic arch and extended caudally during suspended respiration. During helical scanning with the tube rotating at 1 revolution per second and the table moving at 5 mm/sec with a 1:1 scanning pitch, images were obtained with an effective section thickness of 3.2 mm (a nominal section width of 2.5 mm) and a reconstruction increment of 1.5 mm (overlapping section method). Scanning was performed with 120 kVp and 210 mAs, standard resolution, and a 43-cm field of view. The total duration of the procedure was 10 minutes; the absorbed dose with this technique was about 18 mGy (1.8 rad).

Images of the ascending aorta, the arch, and the thoracic descending aorta were reconstructed in multiangular projections, allowing reception of transverse and longitudinal images similar to the short- and long-axis views obtained with TEE. All measurements were performed by using dual-helical CT hardware and software on an Omniview workstation (Elscint). The plaque thickness was measured in the transverse view as with TEE (ie, perpendicular to the aortic wall) as the distance between the aortic border and the point of greatest lesion protrusion.

A positive dual-helical CT scan was defined as the presence of at least one calcium deposit or clearly visualized area of hypoattenuation at least 4 mm thick adjacent to the aortic wall with both transverse and longitudinal projections. Plaques of such thickness found only on images obtained in one projection were not considered protruding aortic atheromas.

The thickness of atheromas at dual-helical CT was evaluated in all patients by two independent observers (A.T., A.G.), and by one of them on two different occasions (A.T.), by using intraclass correlation coefficients. Inter- and intraobserver variability were, respectively, 0.99 and 0.99 for calcified plaques, 0.89 and 0.93 for noncalcified plaques, and 0.96 and 0.97 for both types of plaques when pooled together.

Definition of Aortic Areas Not Clearly Visualized with TEE

The upper ascending aorta was defined as the distal third of the ascending aorta, and the proximal arch was defined as the first third of the arch. In all cases, these areas, which were not visualized with TEE and therefore not included in the comparative analysis, included the origin of the brachiocephalic and left common carotid arteries. The origin of the left subclavian artery, however, was clearly visualized with TEE in 12 patients and incorporated in the comparative analysis with dual-helical CT.

Data Analysis

Comparisons between findings at dual-helical CT and TEE were performed in three ways, as follows: (*a*) comparisons on the basis of patient-to-patient analysis, where the presence of at least one protruding aortic atheroma was defined as a positive study and the absence of a protruding aortic atheroma as a negative study (analyses of dual-helical CT and TEE scans were performed with the readers blinded to findings with other modalities); (*b*) comparisons on the basis of plaque-to-plaque analysis (these comparisons were performed after patient-to-patient analysis with knowledge of findings from the other study); and (*c*) dual-helical CT findings regarding the upper ascending aorta and proximal arch, which were analyzed separately.

Statistical analysis for intergroup comparisons was performed by using the Student *t* test. A *P* value less than .05 was considered statistically significant. The Pearson analysis was used to examine the correlation between the thickness of a given atheroma measured with TEE and dual-helical CT.

Comparison of TEE and Dual-Helical CT in the Detection of PAAs

Finding at TEE	Finding at Dual-Helical CT: PAA Present	Finding at Dual-Helical CT: PAA Absent
PAAs present		
Patient-to-patient comparison (n = 15)	13 (87)	2 (13)
Plaque-to-plaque comparison (n = 36)	34 (94)	2 (6)
PAAs absent		
Patient-to-patient comparison (n = 17)	3 (18)	14 (82)

Note.—PAA = protruding aortic atheroma. Numbers in parentheses are percentages.

RESULTS

Patient-to-Patient Analysis

TEE revealed the presence of a protruding aortic atheroma in 15 of the 32 patients (47%) enrolled in the study (positive TEE scan) and the absence in 17 patients (negative TEE scan) (Table). Dual-helical CT revealed the presence of protruding atheromas in 13 of the 15 patients with positive TEE scans (87%) (Fig 1); in the two remaining patients (13%), the dual-helical CT scans were negative. In patients without atheromas at TEE, dual-helical CT revealed the absence of atheromas (in areas defined as "visible" at TEE) in 14 patients (82%) and the presence of atheromas in three (18%). Dual-helical CT

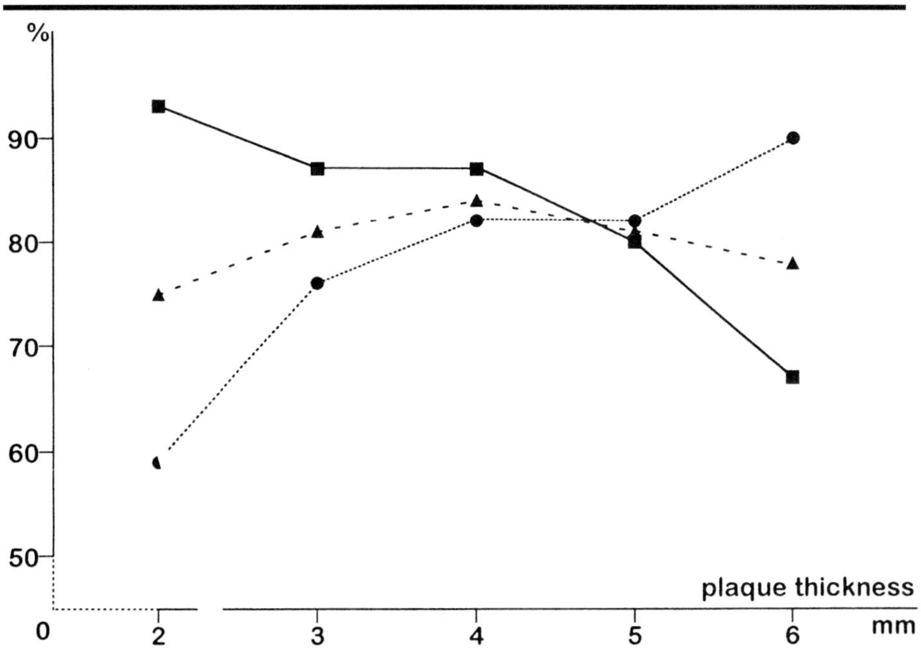

Figure 1. Sensitivity (■), specificity (●), and overall accuracy (▲) of dual-helical CT with use of different values of atheroma thickness as the criterion for protrusion. Note that the best balance between sensitivity and specificity was achieved by using a cutoff point of 4 mm.

yielded a sensitivity of 87%, a specificity of 82%, and an overall accuracy of 84%.

Figure 1 depicts the sensitivity, specificity, and overall accuracy of dual-helical CT with use of different values of atheroma thickness as the criteria for protrusion. The best balance between specificity and sensitivity was achieved by using a cutoff point of 4 mm. It should be noted that a shift of 2 mm upward to 6 mm or downward to 2 mm significantly reduced sensitivity and specificity, respectively.

Plaque-to-Plaque Analysis

Of the 36 protruding aortic atheromas depicted with TEE, 34 (94%) were correctly identified with dual-helical CT. Two noncalcified plaques (6%), which were located between the aortic arch and the descending aorta, remained undetected. Three nonprotruding aortic plaques depicted at TEE (thickness of more than 4 mm) were diagnosed as protruding atheromas at dual-helical CT.

Fourteen of the protruding atheromas (39%) found with TEE were located in the arch, and 22 (61%) were located in the descending aorta; none were located in the proximal part of the ascending aorta, although in five subjects intimal thickness and a number of nonprotruding plaques were disclosed in this region. From the 34 atheromas correctly identified with dual-helical CT, 13 (38%) were located in the arch and 21 (62%) in the descending aorta; 27 plaques represented calcified deposits, and seven plaques clearly demonstrated hypoattenuation (a CT finding suggestive of soft plaque and thrombus) (Fig 2).

The mean thickness of protruding atheromas was 5.6 mm ± 2.6 at TEE and 5.3 mm ± 2.5 at dual-helical CT (the difference was not statistically significant); the thickness measurements with both modalities showed good correlation ($r = .83$).

Dual-Helical CT Findings in the Upper Ascending Aorta and Proximal Arch

Six protruding aortic atheromas were found at dual-helical CT in six patients (one per patient) between the distal ascending aorta and the proximal arch (Fig 3); these atheromas were not included in the comparative analysis. Four patients in whom plaques were not seen at TEE had single plaques at dual-helical CT, and two patients had plaques accompanied by protruding atheromas in other regions. Four plaques represented large calcium deposits, and two plaques showed a clearly visualized area of hypoattenuation suggestive of thrombus (noncalcified plaques).

DISCUSSION

TEE has opened a new window for imaging of the thoracic aorta (16), enabling, for the first time, direct visualization of atherosclerotic plaque morphology in vivo and emphasizing the important role of these lesions as a source of stroke and systemic embolism. However, because of the limited visualization of the upper part of the ascending aorta and the proximal arch including the origin of the cervical arteries, the role of protruding aortic atheroma as a source of cerebral emboli is underestimated (18), both in epidemiologic studies and in the clinical evaluation of patients with stroke.

The high accuracy with unenhanced dual-helical CT (also called "fast dual-section spiral CT") in the detection of coronary calcification is well established (19–21). The main finding of the present study is the potential of this technique to enable detection of a protruding aortic atheroma, particularly in the ascending aorta and the arch. Images may be easily reconstructed in multiangular projections. The use of multiangular projections is the best way to determine the extension and degree of protrusion into the lumen of aortic atheromas. Aortic tortuosity may represent a diagnostic pitfall if a single transverse or longitudinal plane is employed, because thin-surfaced calcium deposits can mimic a protruding aortic atheroma. Although the routine use of multiangular reconstructions is still controversial (22,23), there is a consensus regarding their properties to achieve an improved display of the anatomy in confusing cases, especially those with pathologic lesions in the aortic arch or in areas of aortic tortuosities.

Data are sparse regarding the use of conventional contrast material–enhanced CT for detecting penetrating atherosclerotic ulcers of the aorta, differentiating them from aortic dissection, and evaluating morphologic changes of the aorta as a sign of atherosclerosis extension (24–26).

To our knowledge, ours is the first study in which unenhanced dual-helical CT was directly compared with TEE in the detection and evaluation of a protruding aortic atheroma as a source of stroke and systemic emboli. Dual-helical CT is very similar to the widely used single-section spiral (helical) CT; it differs only in the fact that acquisition of data is twice as fast owing to the two parallel arches of detectors simultaneously irradiated by a single anode. In our study, we elected to use an unenhanced rather than a contrast material–enhanced technique because the former is more suitable for screening studies. The latter technique should be used when the presence of a protruding aortic atheroma is already suspected.

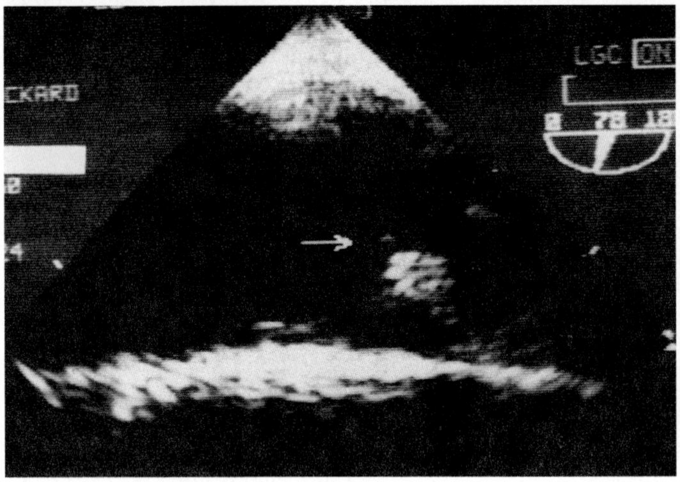

a.

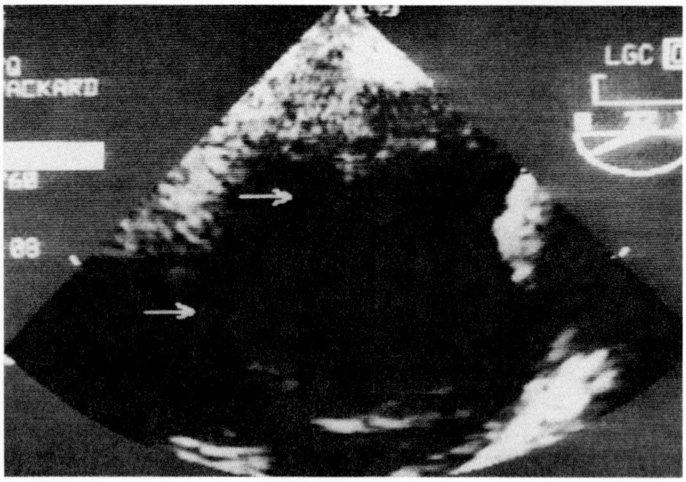

b.

Figure 2. Images in a 77-year-old man with stroke and peripheral emboli. (a) TEE scan shows a protruding atheroma with a small mobile component (arrow) in the area between the arch and the descending aorta. (b) TEE scan obtained with slight upward rotation of the transducer reveals a giant complicated atheroma (top and left side of the image) with large elongated mobile components representing thrombi (arrows). (c) Sagittal dual-helical CT scan (upper right panel, with magnified view [lower panel]). The lower panel demonstrates large extensive thrombotic masses in the arch and descending aorta (arrows), including the region not visible with TEE. The calcified protruding plaque is also seen (below *), and the mobile component is not visualized. An axial dual-helical CT scan is shown in the upper left panel.

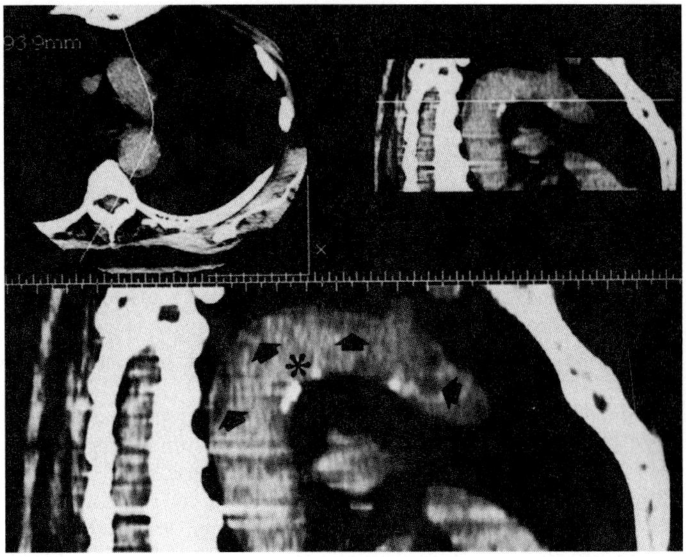

c.

Among the advantages of the newer fast CT studies—such as the various types of helical CT and electron-beam CT techniques—over conventional CT are an increased sensitivity and the possibility of better differentiation of aortic calcium deposits from other structures such as spine, cartilage, heart valves, and lymph nodes. Contrary to conventional CT, fast CT techniques enable examination of the ascending aorta and arch during a single breath hold, thus averting respiratory motion artifacts (27); this is essential for multiangular reconstruction, correct measurement of the atheroma thickness, and the decision regarding their protruding features. Because of the fast characteristics of dual-helical CT and the use of relatively thin sections (3 mm), detection of the soft aortic plaques and thrombotic masses became possible.

The advantages of dual-helical CT over TEE include its noninvasive character, the suitability for screening large populations, and the possibility of complete visualization of the ascending aorta and proximal arch with the origin of cervical arteries. This permits evaluation of the location (before or after the origin from the left subclavian, left common carotid, or brachiocephalic arteries) and extent of the plaque. In addition, dual-helical CT of the aorta and brain may be performed during the same session in patients undergoing evaluation for stroke. The technique also provides information about coronary calcification, and the presence of the physician during examination is unnecessary.

A protruding aortic atheroma may lead to vascular events in as many as one-third of patients in a single year (28). Several options have been suggested for the treatment of this condition and prevention of vascular complications (eg, warfarin, aspirin, heparin, ticlopidine hydrochloride, thrombolytic therapy, atherectomy, stent implantation, and resection by means of balloon or catheter). The accurate therapeutic approach for the management of a protruding aortic atheroma is not yet fully established; however, because patients with a protruding aortic atheroma are at an even greater risk for embolization during catheterization and heart surgery, comprehensive information regarding the condition of the aorta is of overwhelming importance in the decision-making process. The risk of embolization may be effectively reduced by avoiding invasive procedures or, alternatively, with modification of their technique (16,29).

Obvious disadvantages of unenhanced dual-helical CT compared with TEE include the inability with the former to detect intracardiac sources of emboli and mobile properties of the aortic lesions, as well as a reduced sensitivity for noncalcified plaques and thrombi detection. It should be noted that mural nonprotruding aortic calcification occurs so frequently in the elderly as to be almost

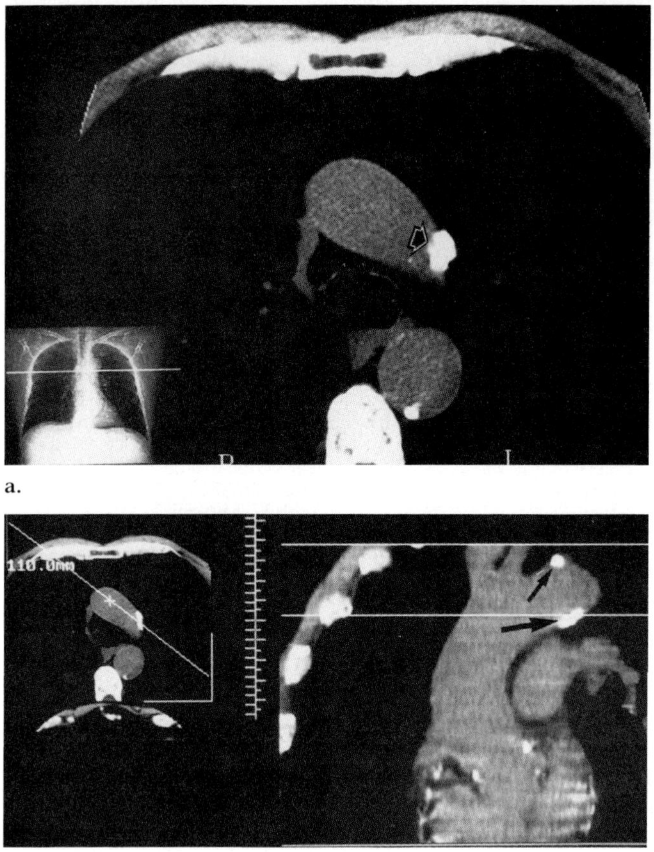

a.

b.

Figure 3. Images in a 74-year-old man who was hospitalized after recurrent ischemic stroke. Findings at TEE were negative. **(a)** Axial dual-helical CT scan shows a very large calcified protruding atheroma (arrow) in part of the arch. The left panel is a radiograph for guidance. **(b)** Sagittal dual-helical CT scan (right panel) shows the same plaque (lower arrow). Note an additional calcified plaque at the origin of the left subclavian artery (upper arrow). The left panel is an axial scan for guidance.

universal beyond the 7th decade. Consequently, the specificity of this finding with regard to plaque protrusion is low if a criterion is used that is less strict than 4 mm of atheroma thickness at both the transverse and longitudinal projections. Nevertheless, recent pathologic and TEE studies have shown that complicated aortic lesions (defined by the presence of mural thrombi, atheromatous debris, or ulceration) are well correlated with calcified lesions (30,31). In our opinion, a positive unenhanced dual-helical CT study should be followed by contrast material injection (enhanced dual-helical CT) or TEE.

Because of the relatively small number of patients in our study population, the data acquired regarding the sensitivity and specificity of dual-helical CT should be treated with caution. The dual-helical CT data regarding the presence of a protruding aortic atheroma in the upper ascending aorta and proximal arch were not confirmed with findings from any other modality (since no alternative techniques are currently clinically available). However, a good correlation between TEE and dual-helical CT findings in most portions of the thoracic aorta strongly supports the credibility of our observations. The use of unenhanced dual-helical CT may result in an underestimation of the amount of noncalcified thrombus, which is presumably at high risk of embolization. It also should be mentioned that it is possible that some patients—particularly those who have had a stroke recently—will not be able to hold their breath for 25 seconds as necessary to complete the protocol; this could be reflected in a suboptimal imaging examination of the distal part of the descending aorta.

Further studies should be performed to examine the feasibility of using dual-helical CT for detecting aortic sources of embolic events, especially regarding the use of contrast material after obtaining a positive unenhanced scan. Such a policy could help disclose additional undetected plaques. Moreover, the contrast-enhanced technique would be useful after a negative or equivocal unenhanced scan is obtained.

In conclusion, despite some limitations, unenhanced dual-helical CT with thin sections may become complementary, and occasionally even superior, to TEE in the rapid, noninvasive detection of protruding aortic atheromas in areas not well visualized with the latter technique.

References

1. Bornstein NM. Epidemiology of stroke. In: Daniel WG, Kronzon I, Mugge A, eds. Cardiogenic embolism. Baltimore, Md: Williams & Wilkins, 1996; 1–6.
2. Pop GP, Sutherland GR, Koudstaal PJ, Sit TW, Jong G, Roelandt J. Transesophageal echocardiography in the detection of the intracardiac embolic sources in patients with transient ischemic attacks. Stroke 1990; 21:560–565.
3. Tunick PA, Kronzon I. Protruding atherosclerotic plaque in the aortic arch of patients with systemic embolization: a new finding seen by transesophageal echocardiography. Am Heart J 1990; 120:658–660.
4. Karalis DG, Chandrasekaran K, Victor MF, Ross JJ, Mintz GS. The recognition and embolic potential of intracardiac atherosclerotic debris. J Am Coll Cardiol 1991; 17:73–78.
5. Amarenco P, Duyckaerts C, Tzourio C, Henin D, Bousser MG, Hauw JJ. Prevalence of ulcerated plaques in the aortic arch in patients with stroke. N Engl J Med 1992; 326:221–225.
6. Coy KM, Maurer G, Goodman D, Siegel RJ. Transesophageal echocardiographic detection of aortic atheromatosis may provide clues to occult renal dysfunction in the elderly. Am Heart J 1992; 123:1684–1686.
7. Horowitz DR, Tuhrim S, Budd J, Goldman ME. Aortic plaque in patients with brain ischemia: diagnosis by transesophageal echocardiography. Neurology 1992; 42: 1602–1604.
8. Bansal RC, Pauls GL, Shankel SW. Blue digit syndrome: transesophageal echocardiographic identification of thoracic aortic plaque–related thrombi and successful outcome with warfarin. J Am Soc Echocardiogr 1993; 6:319–323.
9. Nihoyannopoulos P, Joshi J, Athanasopoulos G, Oakley CM. Detection of atherosclerotic lesions in the aorta by transesophageal echocardiography. Am J Cardiol 1993; 71:1208–1212.
10. Amarenco P, Cohen A, Tzourio C, et al. Atherosclerotic disease of the aortic arch and the risk of ischemic stroke. N Engl J Med 1994; 331:1474–1479.
11. Davila-Roman VG, Barzilai B, Wareing TH, Murphy SF, Schechtman KB, Kouchoukos NT. Atherosclerosis of the ascending aorta: prevalence and role as an independent predictor of cerebrovascular events in cardiac patients. Stroke 1994; 25:2010–2016.
12. The French Study of Aortic Plaques in Stroke Group. Atherosclerotic disease of the aortic arch as a risk factor for recurrent ischemic stroke. N Engl J Med 1996; 334: 1216–1221.
13. Katz ES, Tunick PA, Rusinek H, Ribakove G, Spencer FC, Kronzon I. Protruding aortic atheromas predict stroke in elderly

patients undergoing cardiopulmonary bypass: a review of our experience with intraoperative transesophageal echocardiography. J Am Coll Cardiol 1992; 20:70–77.
14. Blauth CI, Cosgrove DM, Webb BW, et al. Atheroembolism from the ascending aorta: an emerging problem in cardiac surgery. J Thorac Cardiovasc Surg 1992; 103:1104–1112.
15. Tunick PA, Rosenzweig BP, Katz ES, Freeberg RS, Perez JL, Kronzon I. High risk for vascular events in patients with protruding aortic atheromas: a prospective study. J Am Coll Cardiol 1994; 23:1085–1090.
16. Kronzon I, Tunick PA. Aortic atheromas. In: Daniel WG, Kronzon I, Mugge A, eds. Cardiogenic embolism. Baltimore. Md: Williams & Wilkins, 1996; 177–187.
17. Joffe II, Jacobs LE, Lampert C, Kotler MN. Atherosclerotic disease of the aortic arch and the risk of ischemic stroke (letter). N Engl J Med 1995; 332:1237.
18. Amarenco P, Cohen A, Hommel M, Bousser MG. Atherosclerotic disease of the aortic arch and the risk of ischemic stroke: reply (letter). N Engl J Med 1995; 332:1237–1238.
19. Shemesh J, Apter S, Rozenman J, et al. Calcification of coronary arteries: detection and quantification with double-helix CT. Radiology 1995; 197:779–783.
20. Shemesh J, Tenenbaum A, Fisman EZ, et al. Coronary calcium as a reliable tool for differentiating ischemic from nonischemic cardiomyopathy. Am J Cardiol 1996; 77:191–194.
21. Broderick LS, Shemesh J, Wilensky RL, et al. Measurement of coronary artery calcium with dual-slice helical CT compared with coronary angiography: evaluation of CT scoring methods, interobserver variations, and reproducibility. AJR 1996; 167: 439–443.
22. Costello P, Ecker CP, Tello R, Hartnell GC. Assessment of the thoracic aorta by spiral CT. AJR 1992; 158:1127–1130.
23. Quint LE, Francis IR, Williams DM, et al. Evaluation of thoracic aortic disease with the use of helical CT and multiplanar reconstructions: comparison with clinical findings. Radiology 1996; 201:37–41.
24. Kazerooni EA, Bree RL, Williams DU. Penetrating atherosclerotic ulcers of the descending aorta: evaluation with CT and distinction from aortic dissection. Radiology 1992; 183:759–765.
25. Harris JA, Bis KG, Glover JL, Bendick PJ, Shetty A, Brown OW. Penetrating atherosclerotic ulcers of the aorta. J Vasc Surg 1994; 19:90–94.
26. Takasu J, Takanashi K, Naito S, et al. Evaluation of morphological changes of the atherosclerotic aorta by enhanced computed tomography. Atherosclerosis 1992; 97:107–121.
27. Shemesh J, Tenenbaum A, Fisman EZ, et al. Absence of coronary calcification on double-helical CT scans: predictor of angiographically normal coronary arteries in elderly women? Radiology 1996; 199: 665–668.
28. Kronzon I, Tunick PA. Atheromatous disease of the thoracic aorta: pathologic and clinical implications. Ann Intern Med 1997; 629–637.
29. Wareing TH, Davila-Roman VG, Barzilai BA, Murphy SF, Kouchoukos NT. Management of the severe atherosclerotic ascending aorta during cardiac operations: a strategy for detection and treatment. J Thorac Cardiovasc Surg 1992; 103:453–462.
30. Toyoda K, Yasaka M, Nagata S, Yamaguchi T. Aortogenic embolic stroke: a transesophageal echocardiographic approach. Stroke 1992; 23:1056–1061.
31. Khatibzadeh M, Mitusch R, Stierle U, Gromoll B, Sheikhzadeh A. Aortic atherosclerotic plaques as a source of systemic embolism. J Am Coll Cardiol 1996; 27:664–669.

Herman P. Wu, BA
Thomas M. Vesely, MD

Index terms:
Abscess, percutaneous drainage, 44.1263, 44.242, 45.1263, 45.242
Extremities, abscess, 44.201, 44.242, 44.243, 44.37, 44.454, 45.201, 45.242, 45.243, 45.37, 45.454
Extremities, neoplasms, 44.37, 45.37
Interventional procedures, 44.1263, 44.12986, 45.1263, 45.12986
Melanoma, 40.37

Radiology 1998; 208:159–165

Abbreviation:
WBC = white blood cell

[1] From the Mallinckrodt Institute of Radiology, Washington University School of Medicine, 510 S Kingshighway Blvd, St Louis, MO 63110. Received October 9, 1997; revision requested December 15; revision received January 20, 1998; accepted February 3. **Address reprint requests to** T.M.V.

Author contributions:
Guarantors of integrity of entire study, H.P.W., T.M.V.; study concepts and design, H.P.W., T.M.V.; definition of intellectual content, H.P.W., T.M.V.; literature research, H.P.W.; clinical studies, T.M.V.; data acquisition and analysis, H.P.W.; statistical analysis, H.P.W.; manuscript preparation, editing, and review, H.P.W., T.M.V.

Percutaneous Drainage of Fluid Collections in the Extremities[1]

PURPOSE: To analyze the results of percutaneous drainage of fluid collections in the extremities.

MATERIALS AND METHODS: From 1990–1997, 28 patients aged 14–90 years underwent percutaneous drainage of 33 fluid collections in the extremities; two patients underwent multiple drainages. Fluid collections were in the hip-groin area (n = 16), thighs (n = 6), buttocks (n = 6), knees (n = 3), calf (n = 1), and axilla (n = 1). Three intraarticular collections were included. The patients who had undergone prior procedures were eight who had undergone surgical drainage, 10 who had undergone needle aspiration, and one who had undergone surgical débridement. The two most common guidance methods of catheter placement were ultrasound localization and fluoroscopy.

RESULTS: The average drainage duration was 18.2 days (range, 1–93 days). The estimated cavity sizes were 4–733 cm^3. Purulent fluid was drained in 13 patients. *Staphylococcus aureus* was the most commonly identified organism (n = 9). Nine patients had postoperative lymphoceles; five of these patients underwent sclerotherapy. Two (7%) patients had two complications, one of which was major. Failure occurred in four (16%) of 25 patients; two needed repeat drainage for recurrence, and two needed subsequent surgery. Success could not be determined in three patients who were lost to follow-up.

CONCLUSION: Percutaneous drainage of fluid collections in the extremities is an effective alternative to open-incision drainage in inpatients and outpatients.

In recent years, the insertion of drainage catheters into abscesses for cure or for temporization has become an increasingly popular alternative to open-incision drainage (1–4). Such percutaneous drainages have been aided by ultrasound (US), fluoroscopic, or computed tomographic (CT) guidance (5,6). Previous reports (7–9) regarding the efficacy of drainage catheters in different intraabdominal fluid collections and in different clinical settings have been published. However, less attention has been devoted to the efficacy of similar drainages of fluid collections in the extremities (10,11). The purpose of this study was to analyze the results of percutaneous drainage of fluid collections in the extremities.

MATERIALS AND METHODS

Patient Characteristics

A computer search of the interventional radiology department's database revealed 28 patients who had undergone percutaneous drainage of a fluid collection in an extremity between 1990 and 1997. There were 11 male and 17 female patients, aged 14–90 years (mean age, 53 years). Ten patients were treated in the interventional radiology department as inpatients, and three were treated as outpatients. The remaining 15 patients were treated initially as inpatients and later as outpatients. The records of only those patients who had undergone insertion of a drainage catheter were reviewed; patients who had undergone radiologically guided needle aspiration were excluded from the study.

All but one of the patients had clinically relevant coexistent morbid conditions. The most common coexistent morbidities were melanoma (n = 7), paraplegia with chronic osteomyelitis and recurrent decubitus ulcers ($n = 3$), immunosuppression after renal transplantation ($n = 2$), coronary artery disease ($n = 2$), and problems after joint replacement (one knee, one hip). Other solid-tissue tumors were common also: There was one case each of active breast cancer, prostate cancer, meningioma, hepatocellular cancer, penile cancer, and sarcoma of the buttocks. There was one patient each with acquired immunodeficiency syndrome, chronic myelocytic leukemia treated with chemotherapy, Behçet disease treated with prednisone, sarcoidosis treated with prednisone, and a gunshot wound.

Coexistent morbidities were used to classify patients as either immunocompetent or immunocompromised. On the basis of the criteria established by Lambiase et al (7), a patient was immunocompromised when one or more of the following was present: absolute neutropenia; positive test results for the human immunodeficiency virus; active cancer requiring surgery, chemotherapy, irradiation, or all three; lymphoproliferative disorders; diabetes mellitus; chronic renal failure requiring hemodialysis; steroid or cyclosporine use; previous splenectomy; and severe alcohol abuse. According to these criteria, 19 (68%) of the 28 patients were immunocompromised.

Twelve patients had spontaneous appearance of a fluid collection, and 16 had postprocedural fluid collections. The most common procedure performed before the appearance of the fluid collection was inguinal node dissection for melanoma ($n = 7$) or penile cancer ($n = 1$), with the procedure leading to hip-groin lymphoceles. One patient, who had undergone radical gluteal resection for sarcoma of the buttocks, also had a postoperative lymphocele at presentation. Two of the three paraplegic patients had undergone Girdlestone resection for osteomyelitis before the appearance of hip-groin fluid collections. The patient with breast cancer had an abscess after axillary dissection. Of the two patients with coronary artery disease, one presented with a hip-groin hematoma after percutaneous transluminal coronary angioplasty; the other had a fluid collection at the site of saphenous vein harvesting for a coronary artery bypass graft. Both patients with joint replacements had fluid collections around their prostheses at presentation. Eleven of the patients with postprocedural fluid collections presented to the interventional radiology department within 1 month of the procedure. Four patients presented 2–5 months afterward, and one presented with an infected hip 15 years after undergoing total hip replacement.

Specific indications for percutaneous drainage were documented for each patient; the presence of a fluid collection at preprocedural imaging by itself was not sufficient for drainage catheter insertion. In eight patients, the indication was the presence of local symptoms such as pain or swelling; however, spontaneous fluid drainage from old surgical drain tracts or from wound dehiscence was seen also. In 16 patients, the fluid collections were associated with both local symptoms and evidence of infection (ie, body temperature > 38.3°C or white blood cell [WBC] count > 9.8×10^9/L). Three patients presented with vague or no local symptoms; they had an elevated temperature or an elevated WBC count, with a fluid collection that was localized with imaging. The remaining patient had a fluid collection in the buttocks that was localized incidentally with CT performed for abdominal pain; however, a Gram stain of the subsequent needle aspiration specimen revealed WBCs, and the culture yielded coagulase-negative *Staphylococcus* species. Of the 19 patients who had preprocedural elevations in temperature or WBC count, 12 had a temperature higher than 38.3°C (average, 38.9°C; maximum, 40.0°C) and 16 had a WBC count greater than 9.8×10^9/L (average, 17.4×10^9/L; maximum, 60.7×10^9/L).

In 19 patients, the attempts to resolve the fluid collection before percutaneous drainage were unsuccessful. Eight of these patients had previously inserted surgical drains in place, eight had undergone prior soft-tissue needle aspiration, two had undergone knee joint arthrocentesis, and one had undergone surgical incision and drainage.

Fluid Collection Characteristics

There were a total of 33 separate fluid collections in the 28 patients. In one patient, who had undergone bilateral inguinal node dissection, bilateral inguinal lymphoceles developed several months apart. In another patient, who was receiving prednisone for sarcoidosis, five separate, simultaneous thigh abscesses developed bilaterally. The fluid collections that recurred after catheter removal and required subsequent redrainage were not counted separately, because they were considered to be failures of the original drainage procedures. Similarly, catheter exchanges for the same fluid collection were not counted as separate procedures. In addition, the insertion of multiple drainage catheters into large fluid collections that crossed the midline (in two patients) or into apparently separate fluid collections that were proved only after contrast material injection to communicate (in two patients) were not counted separately.

The most common location for fluid collections was the hip-groin area (16 sites in 15 patients); the next most common area was the buttocks (in six patients). Fluid collections in the buttocks included unilateral collections as well as those that crossed the midline. Some patients had fluid collections that involved the superficial gluteus muscles, and some had collections in deeper muscles such as the piriform muscle. However, none of the collections involved the peritoneal cavity or communicated with the gastrointestinal tract. Two patients underwent drainage for fluid collections in the thighs, three underwent drainage of fluid around the knee, and one each underwent drainage in the axilla and in the calf.

Preprocedural imaging was performed in 23 of the 28 patients; the fluid collections in the remaining five patients were imaged initially during the percutaneous drainage procedure. Of the 23 patients, 11 underwent CT before the drainage procedure; three, magnetic resonance (MR) imaging; one, both CT and MR imaging; and eight, US.

By using both the preprocedural images and the percutaneous drainage notes, seven patients were deemed to have simple fluid collections and 17 were deemed to have complex ones. In four patients, there was insufficient radiologic information to characterize the fluid collections as simple or complex. A simple fluid collection was defined as a unilocular pocket of fluid with easily drainable contents. A complex fluid collection was defined as a collection with multiple loculations, communicating lobulations, or both, necessitating multiple-catheter placement. The character of the cavity borders and the presence of particulate debris were not considered in the differentiation between simple and complex fluid collections. Percutaneous drainage was allowed to proceed only if imaging enabled the detection of a discrete fluid collection as opposed to a solid region of inflammation.

The depth of the fluid collection was also noted. Fifteen patients had subcutaneous fluid collections, and six had fluid collections within the muscles or fluid collections dissecting between the muscles. Four patients had fluid collections that were adjacent to the bone, and three had intraarticular abscesses. Two of the intraarticular drainages were in the knee joint, and one was around an infected hip prosthesis.

The fluid collections were also subdivided by size. The most reliable determinant of size was the volume of the initial aspirate. Any fluid collection of 150 mL or more was arbitrarily deemed to be large. In the event that the initial aspirate volume was not available (n = 13), the cavity dimensions, as determined with preprocedural imaging (n = 6) or from the initial daily drainage records (n = 4), were used to estimate cavity size. The drainage records were found to have the lowest correlation with cavity size and were used only as a last resort. By using this method, 15 patients were determined to have small (<150-mL) fluid collections, and 10 were determined to have large fluid collections. The estimated cavity sizes were 4–733 cm^3 and could not be determined in three patients.

Patients with lymphoceles, hematomas, and abscesses, which encompassed both sterile and infected fluid collections, were included. Lymphoceles were defined as cysts with clear or yellow serous aspirates containing predominantly lymphocytes, while hematomas contained serosanguinous or sanguinous fluid. Abscesses were defined by the finding of purulent material. The criteria used to define an infected fluid collection were the same as those used by Lambiase et al (7): (*a*) a culture-positive aspirate, (*b*) a culture-negative but purulent aspirate, or (*c*) WBCs or bacteria on the initial Gram stained specimen.

Procedural Details

Before the drainage procedure, routine laboratory measurements, such as complete blood cell count, prothrombin time, and partial thromboplastin time, were obtained in each patient. Twenty-three patients were already being treated with intravenous antibiotics before undergoing drainage. Of the remaining patients, one inpatient was taking oral metronidazole (Flagyl; Searle Pharmaceuticals, Chicago, Ill) for colitis caused by infection with *Clostridium difficile*. Two patients were not being treated with antibiotics initially but later started to receive oral or intravenous antibiotics when cultures from their catheter drainages yielded bacteria. One outpatient underwent drainage for 8 days without antibiotics, while another outpatient was receiving oral dicloxacillin sodium during 37 days of drainage.

The guidance modalities that were used most commonly for percutaneous drainage were US and fluoroscopy; CT guidance was used in only one patient. In fifteen patients, both US guidance and fluoroscopic guidance were used. In seven patients, only fluoroscopic guidance was used, and in five, only US guidance was used. All of the patients were in conscious sedation, and catheters were inserted by using the Seldinger technique. The fluid collections were localized by using either US, physical examination, or anatomic landmarks identified on prior CT scans. An 18-gauge needle was then inserted. After initial aspiration of fluid to decrease intracavitary pressure and lessen the risk of bacteremia, fluoroscopic confirmation was typically performed by injecting a small amount of iodinated contrast material into the cavity. A guide wire was then inserted, with subsequent serial dilation of the tract before insertion of the drainage catheter.

Catheter size was 8.0–16.0 F, with the following size distribution: three 8.0-F, six 8.5-F, 18 10.0-F, seven 12.0-F, and three 16.0-F catheters. The majority (n = 32) of catheters were locking pigtail catheters; the remainder (n = 5) were straight catheters. All catheters were secured to the skin by using a 0-Prolene (Ethicon, Somerville, NJ) stitch. In 26 patients, the catheter was attached to a gravity drainage device, and in one patient each, the catheter was attached to a Hemovac wound drain reservoir (Baxter Healthcare, Deerfield, Ill) or a Jackson-Pratt silicone round drain (Baxter Healthcare).

All inpatients were seen daily by an interventional radiologist, with daily dressing changes and measurements of catheter output. Outpatients were instructed how to measure their drain outputs daily. There was no set protocol for obtaining follow-up images. Any subsequent decision to perform imaging, as well as the choice of imaging modality, was made individually on the basis of factors such as trends in drain output, the patient's clinical status, and the anatomic location of the fluid collection. Fourteen patients underwent imaging other than fluoroscopy of the fluid cavity to observe for decrease in cavity size. Follow-up CT was performed in 10 patients, US in three, and MR imaging in one. In addition, radionuclide studies (WBC scans [scintigraphy] or technetium-99m bone scans) were performed in two patients in whom there was a possibility of osteomyelitis. The time from catheter placement to follow-up imaging was 2 days to 4 months; six patients underwent multiple follow-up imaging procedures.

The decision to remove the catheter was also made on an individual basis, with consideration of not only the amount of drainage, but also the size of the cavity at subsequent radiologic examinations and resolution of clinical signs of infection.

For lymphoceles with persistent output and failure of cavity reduction (n = 5), sclerotherapy with absolute ethanol was performed either at the bedside or in the interventional radiology facility. Cavity volume was ascertained by injecting contrast material before injecting a smaller volume of absolute ethanol through the existing catheter. To maximize cavity exposure to the ethanol, injections were repeated three times for 3–5 minutes each, with the patient in the supine and right and left lateral decubitus positions. Sclerotherapy frequency was determined on an individual basis. Inpatients underwent sclerotherapy every day to every 3 days, while outpatients underwent the procedure weekly or biweekly. The end point for sclerotherapy was determined by decreased drainage output and cavity reduction at follow-up radiologic examinations.

Outcomes Assessment

Follow-up was performed by using several methods. The patients' hospital admission records were reviewed for any recurrence or long-term complications of the procedure. Outpatient clinic records and the interventional radiology department's outpatient procedure reports were reviewed also. Finally, telephone interviews in which patients were asked about the need for subsequent medical attention to the drainage site were conducted; in some cases, close relatives such as spouses or children were contacted if the patient was deceased. Of the 20 patients contacted by telephone, nine were able to be questioned.

In all cases, percutaneous drainage catheters were inserted initially for cure, not for temporization. Temporization was considered to be percutaneous drainage to stabilize the patient for subsequent surgical débridement or repair (4,7). Our definition of success is a modification of that used by Lambiase et al (7): the radiologic or clinical resolution of the primary acute medical problem, the fluid collection, at the time of catheter removal, with return of the patient to his or her previous state of health. Furthermore, we considered a procedure to be successful if, within 3 months of follow-up, no recurrence or delayed complications occurred.

In the Lambiase et al study (7), there was a 1-year follow-up; however, they noted that recurrences generally occurred within 2–3 months. In our study, death within the follow-up period did not affect the judgment of success, as long as the patient did not die of sepsis. In cases in which the patient died with the drainage catheter still in place, the effects of the percutaneous drainage on his or her clinical signs were used as measurements of success. Our definition of successful palliation also was modeled after that of Lambiase et al (7): relief of symptoms, with any fever resolved within 72 hours of the procedure. Inpatient deaths that were not attributable to sepsis did not affect the judgment of a successful drainage procedure.

A procedure was defined as failing if subsequent surgical intervention was needed, the fluid collection recurred, there were delayed complications within 3 months, or the patient's temperature or WBC count did not return to normal after drainage. In this series of patients, there were no instances of in-hospital deaths owing to sepsis. Among patients who required repeat percutaneous drainage, only the data from the initial drainage were considered in the statistical analysis, as any procedural failure served as the end point of data collection.

The analysis of success and complications was considered in terms of patients (n = 28) rather than in terms of separate fluid collections (n = 33). In our calculations, data on patients in whom success or failure could not be definitively ascertained because of a lack of follow-up (n = 3) were omitted. Furthermore, data on patients in whom the fluid collection size (n = 3) or complexity (n = 4) could not be ascertained were also not included in the calculations concerning fluid collection characteristics. Statistical analysis was performed by using either the Fisher exact probability test or the Student t test to correlate outcomes parameters (ie, success rate, complication rate, and duration of drainage) with certain preprocedural parameters (ie, sterile vs infected, fluid type, cavity size, simple vs complex collections, anatomic location of the fluid collection, and immune status).

RESULTS

At percutaneous drainage, purulent fluid was found in 13 patients. Clear or yellow fluid typical of lymphoceles was found in nine patients, and serosanguinous or old blood was found in six. Eleven patients had sterile fluid collections, and 17 had infected fluid collections; however, one sterile fluid collection later became infected with coagulase-negative *Staphylococcus* species while the drain was in place. The nine patients with sterile fluid collections consisted of four with hematomas and five with lymphoceles; none had any bacterial growth. Of the 17 patients with infected fluid collections, two had hematomas, four had lymphoceles, and 11 had abscesses.

The most common organism grown in culture was *S aureus* (in nine patients), with *Streptococcus* species being the next most common (in three patients). Four patients had no growth on cultures, but they had WBCs on Gram stained specimens; there was one patient each with *Candida* species, coagulase-negative *Staphylococcus* species, and polymicrobial growth (ie, *Escherichia coli, Bacteroides fragilis, Streptococcus viridans,* and *Enterococcus* species). None of the patients had tuberculous fluid collections. Three of the 19 patients had a recurrence of bacterial growth either before or after catheter removal; all of these recurrent bacterial infections involved *S aureus.*

Postprocedural Course

In the 12 patients who were febrile before percutaneous drainage (average temperature, 38.9°C), the average temperature the first day after the procedure decreased to 38.0°C. Seven patients had defervescence within 24 hours, while three had defervescence within 72 hours. One patient's temperature returned to normal after 5 days. A patient who continued to have temperature spikes for 11 days after the procedure was considered to have failed percutaneous drainage. Two patients who were afebrile at presentation developed an elevated temperature after the drainage; these fevers were most likely caused by bacteremia secondary to manipulation around the cavity. One of these patients had defervescence after 7 days, while another patient had only one temperature spike 2 days after the procedure.

In the 16 patients known to have an elevated WBC count (average count, $17.4 \times 10^9/L$) at presentation, the average WBC count decreased to $12.5 \times 10^9/L$ 1–3 days after catheter insertion. One patient continued to have steadily increasing WBC counts after the procedure (from $13.0 \times 10^9/L$ to $30.8 \times 10^9/L$); however, this elevation was later attributed to her worsening myeloproliferative disease.

The duration of percutaneous drainage was determined for 31 of the 37 catheters initially inserted; in most of the patients with multiple catheters in place, the catheters were removed at different times. The dates of catheter removal could not be determined in five patients. The average known duration of drainage was 18.2 days (range, 1–93 days). One patient with a chronically infected knee joint prosthesis had her catheter removed after 1 day, when only 13 mL of old blood was drained and it was ascertained that her symptoms were due to a solid-tissue infection.

The drainage procedures were associated with a 7% (two of 28 patients) complication rate. Three patients with postprocedural temperature spikes were not considered to have a complication, but rather a normal occurrence secondary to bacteremia from cavity manipulation. The patient with subsequent infection of an initially sterile lymphocele was considered to have a minor complication. Another patient had to be transferred to the surgical intensive care unit the day after percutaneous drainage because she had hypotension, tachypnea, continued fever, lethargy, and metabolic acidosis. Intubation was required; however, within 6 days, the patient was stable enough to be transferred back to the general medical ward. This patient was considered to have had a major complication, as her symptoms were consistent with sepsis, which, again, was most likely secondary to cavity manipulation. No patients had periprocedural or postprocedural bleeding problems, even though nine patients had abnormal coagulation profiles before.

Events such as the plugging of the catheter tube or the premature falling out of the catheter were not considered to be complications, but rather were noted as subsequent technical problems. Four patients experienced tube occlusions that necessitated a tube change. One of these cases involved an infected abscess; the other three involved sterile lymphoceles. Three of the occluded catheters were 10.0 F; the remaining one was an 8.5-F catheter. In two patients, the catheter fell out prematurely for unclear reasons; both of these patients noticed a foul-smelling output soon after, and the catheters were reinserted. One of these patients was readmitted because of a simultaneous central line infection; subsequent abscess cultures continued to grow *S aureus,* and the patient started to receive vancomycin again. The other patient's catheter was replaced in the outpatient setting, and she started a 10-day course of ciprofloxacin (chosen on the basis of past experience of what the most likely infecting organism would be in her situation).

Correlation of Outcomes with Patient and Fluid Collection Characteristics

Characteristic	No. of Patients with Complications	No. of Patients with Success
Patient		
Immunocompromised (n = 19)	2/19 (11)	16/19 (84)
Immunocompetent (n = 9)	0/9 (0)	5/6 (83)
Fluid collection		
Type		
Spontaneous (n = 12)	1/12 (8)	9/10 (90)*
Postoperative (n = 16)	1/16 (6)	12/15 (80)
Complexity		
Simple (n = 7)	0/7 (0)	6/7 (86)
Complex (n = 17)	2/17 (12)	12/14 (86)
Size		
Small (<150 mL) (n = 15)	1/15 (7)	11/13 (85)
Large (≥150 mL) (n = 10)	1/10 (10)	8/9 (89)
Fluid type		
Purulent (n = 13)	1/13 (8)	11/12 (92)†
Lymph and blood (n = 15)	1/15 (7)	10/13 (77)
Location		
Hip-groin (n = 15)	2/15 (13)	10/14 (71)‡
Non–hip-groin (n = 13)	0/13 (0)	11/11 (100)
Status of infection		
Sterile (n = 11)	1/11 (9)	8/9 (89)
Infected (n = 17)	1/17 (6)	13/16 (81)

Note.—Number in parentheses is the percentage.
* P = .62 (comparison of spontaneous vs postoperative collections).
† P = .60 (comparison of purulent vs lymph and blood fluid).
‡ P = .11 (comparison of hip-groin vs non–hip-groin collections).

Five of the nine patients with lymphoceles required subsequent sclerotherapy with absolute ethanol before the cysts resolved. Patients underwent an average of 3.8 sessions of sclerotherapy (range, 1–7 sessions); the interval between catheter placement and start of sclerotherapy was 2–31 days. After initial determination of the cavity size with iodinated contrast material, these five patients received 3–20 mL of absolute ethanol. The duration of sclerotherapy was 1–40 days. The average duration of drainage was 42.6 days for lymphoceles requiring sclerotherapy compared with 14 days for cases not requiring sclerotherapy.

Procedural Outcomes

Complete 3-month follow-up information was available in 25 patients through clinic chart review, radiology department outpatient report review, telephone interviews, or all three. Although three patients died within 3 months of the procedure, their follow-up information was still considered to be adequate. One of the patients died with the catheter still in place and, thus, was considered to be a palliative case. Three patients were lost to follow-up immediately after catheter insertion.

An overall failure rate of 16% (four of 25 patients) was seen. One patient, a 31-year-old woman who had undergone inguinal node dissection for melanoma, had a recurrent lymphocele that required simple aspiration about 2 months after drainage catheter removal. The second patient, a 57-year-old man who also had undergone inguinal node dissection for melanoma, had left groin swelling and nausea 70 days after removal of the initial catheter; the CT scan showed a recurrent fluid collection. He required 18 days of additional drainage along with sclerotherapy to expedite resolution of the fluid collection. The third patient was a 90-year-old man with an infected hip prosthesis that was managed with drainage because he did not desire surgery. However, the abscess recurred 23 days after catheter removal. A second percutaneous drainage was performed for temporization, with surgical removal of the prosthesis 6 days later. The last patient, a 36-year-old patient who had undergone renal transplantation and who had sclerosing cholangitis and non-A, non-B hepatitis, continued to have temperature spikes after placement of a drainage catheter in the hip area and required open-incision drainage 11 days after the initial drainage procedure.

Four other patients met the criteria for a successful cure, although they presented with continued problems around the site of drainage at follow-up examination. One patient with a hematoma that was drained from a chronically infected knee prosthesis continued to have recurrent soft-tissue infections; however, no drainable fluid collections were identified in the area. Two paraplegic patients with fluid collections around the hip continued to have chronic decubitus ulcers and soft-tissue inflammation, but they had no recurrence of an identifiable fluid collection. The last patient presented with recurrent local pain while his drainage tube was still in place. This patient's cultures again grew *S aureus;* however, his symptoms were controlled by administering antibiotics again.

Statistical Correlations

Statistical analysis was performed to identify any patient characteristics or fluid collection characteristics that could be used as reliable predictors of complications or procedural failures (Table). However, there was no statistically significant correlation of the success rate or the complication rate with any of the fluid collection characteristics examined. For three parameters (immune status, fluid collection complexity, and fluid collection size), the absence of a statistically significant difference, even with the small sample size, was sufficient to rule out any correlation with success rates. Fluid collections in the hip-groin area did demonstrate a 71% (10 of 14 collections) success rate compared with a 100% (11 of 11 collections) success rate in all other extremity locations combined (P = .11); this was the only correlation that approached statistical significance.

Immunocompromised patients were noted to have an average drainage duration of 19.8 days as opposed to 11.8 days in immunocompetent patients. A similar increase in drainage duration was seen in complex fluid collections as opposed to simple cavities. Neither of these associations, however, was statistically significant.

Percutaneous drainage of fluid collections in the extremities demonstrated an overall success rate of 84% (21 of 25 patients), with a 95% confidence interval of 64%, 95%; successes included both cures and palliations. For immunocompromised patients, there was a similar overall success rate of 84% (16 of 19 patients). The overall complication rate was 7% (two of 28 patients), with a 95% confidence interval of 0.8%, 24%.

DISCUSSION

The variety of percutaneous drainage procedures has expanded from drainage of simple unilocular cavities to include those of multiloculated, synchronous, or poorly defined fluid collections (3). Drainage catheters are inserted not only for simple cure of a fluid collection, but also in critically ill patients for clinical stabilization before definitive surgical intervention (4). Given the large amount of literature on percutaneous drainage of intraabdominal fluid collections in recent years, it is surprising that little attention has been given to the drainage of fluid collections in the extremities (10,11). Most fluid collections in the extremities are superficial, and one possible reason for the paucity of literature on this subject is that open-incision drainage still may be the primary method of management.

The results of this study of patients with fluid collections of varying size, depth, and complexity at presentation suggest that percutaneous drainage of fluid collections in the extremities is as effective as percutaneous drainage of abdominal or pelvic fluid. The overall failure rate in these patients was 16% (four of 25 patients), with a 95% confidence interval of 5%, 36%. This range overlaps with the 9% failure rate reported by Lambiase et al (7) in their large series of patients. The overall complication rate in our study was 7% (two of 28 patients), with a 95% confidence interval of 1%, 24%, which overlaps with the 10% complication rate seen by Lambiase et al (7).

The indications for percutaneous drainage in the extremities are the same as those for other drainage procedures: the presence of a fluid collection and evidence of infection or clinical symptoms. In this series, patient coexistent morbidities and immune status did not preclude drainage and were not statistically significant factors in the success or failure of the procedure. We found also that patients could be treated as outpatients or inpatients. Patients could be easily instructed how to record their drain output for follow-up appointments in the interventional radiology department, and ready treatment could be obtained if tubes became clogged or fell out prematurely. One patient's sclerotherapy was managed by a visiting home nurse on a set protocol.

Preprocedural imaging such as CT, MR imaging, or US is valuable in assessing not only the location but also the extent and complexity of any suspected fluid collection. However, our results suggest that fluid collection size and complexity are not strong predictors of final outcome, thus limiting the apparent usefulness of preprocedural imaging for diagnosis and localization. In contrast, Gerzof et al (3), in their study of intraabdominal collections, found that abscess complexity correlated with both increased complications and increased failures. One possible reason for this discrepancy is that the generally easier accessibility of extremity fluid collections tends to negate any difficulties posed by cavity size or complexity.

For fluid collections that are deeper in the subcutaneous tissue, preprocedural imaging is also important in planning the optimal route of drainage and the number of drainage catheters necessary. Doppler flow studies are helpful for preprocedural identification of suspected pseudoaneurysms. vanSonnenberg et al (10) stated that CT imaging was not necessary for guidance of catheter insertion into thigh abscesses. In our series, CT for procedural guidance was used in only one patient. However, CT scanning was actually the most common means of localizing fluid collections before the procedure.

There has been the claim that percutaneous drainage of spontaneously occurring fluid collections is less successful than surgical débridement because the underlying anatomic defect is not corrected (12). Moreover, a drainage catheter could not remove any necrotic tissue that could serve as a nidus for reinfection. However, the results of the study by Gerzof et al (3) suggested that postoperative and spontaneous intraabdominal abscesses had equal success rates of drainage. Our study results support those of Gerzof et al; again, a larger number of patients is needed to confirm this possible correlation.

Because it was thought that sterile fluid collections warranted a different therapeutic approach and a different assessment of outcomes, Lambiase et al (7) excluded them from their large series. However, the results of our series suggest that sterile and infected fluid collections in the extremities responded equally well to percutaneous drainage. With sterile fluid collections, there is the risk of introducing a de novo infection through the catheter, especially with prolonged drainage.

The only fluid collection characteristic that may correlate with successful outcome is anatomic location; drains placed in the hip-groin region seemed to be less successful than those placed elsewhere in the extremities. Thus, for fluid collections in this area, the decision to pursue percutaneous drainage versus open-incision drainage might be better reached on an individual basis in consultation with the surgeon. Percutaneous drainage still may be the ideal initial therapeutic choice; however, the threshold for subsequent surgical intervention may be lowered in such cases. More aggressive use of sclerotherapy with absolute ethanol also may be effective in preventing recurrence of groin lymphoceles. One should also be aware of the uncommon possibility that an abdominal pathologic condition may manifest as a fluid collection in the hip or upper thigh areas (13,14).

Intraarticular drains were shown to be a viable alternative to repeated arthrocentesis for treatment of septic arthritis. Both of the drainages of the knee joint in this series successfully resolved the infection, although one patient was lost to follow-up. However, a third patient, who underwent percutaneous drainage of the soft tissues around a knee prosthesis, did not fare so well. The drainage was labeled a success because the fluid collection did not recur, but the patient continued to have recurrent infections in the area, eventually requiring prosthesis removal. Another patient with an infected hip prosthesis had an unsuccessful percutaneous drainage, also requiring prosthesis removal. The presence of a foreign body, especially since it is a possible nidus for reinfection, seems to pose extra difficulty in intraarticular percutaneous drainage.

Even in patients in whom percutaneous drainage ultimately proves unsuccessful because of recurrence of fluid collection or because subsequent surgery is needed, the procedure is still an excellent means of providing relief of symptoms. In patients who had preprocedural elevations in temperature, WBC count, or both, percutaneous drainage quickly reduced these indicators of infection in most cases. Percutaneous drainage, then, can easily be extended to the setting of a debilitated patient with an extremity fluid collection in whom palliation or temporization is the goal. With use of only a local anesthetic and minimally invasive techniques, percutaneous drainage causes less physiologic stress than open-incision drainage. The only risk is the transient bacteremia that may result from catheter insertion, resulting in postprocedural temperature spikes or more serious signs of sepsis.

Catheter tube occlusions caused by particulate material were encountered in four patients. According to the study conducted by Gobien et al (15), use of catheters with lumens larger than 8.3 F was not associated with an improved success rate or a shorter drainage duration. They also proposed that the addition of more side holes is beneficial when tube occlusions are a problem. Other possible solutions to this technical problem are not only increasing the frequency of tube irrigation, but also changing from gravity drainage to suction drainage.

In summary, percutaneous drainage of fluid collections in the extremities demonstrates comparable efficacy to the more publicized percutaneous drainage of intraabdominal fluid collections. To our knowledge, at the time this article was written, there was no known prospective study comparing percutaneous drainage with open-incision drainage for fluid collections in the extremities. However, we believe that this method represents an effective alternative to open-incision drainage in both the inpatient setting and the outpatient setting. Intraarticular drainage provides a viable alternative to repeated arthrocentesis in patients with septic arthritis. The effectiveness of percutaneous drainage in relieving local symptoms and normalizing indexes of infection (eg, elevated body temperature and elevated WBC count) also makes it ideal for palliation or temporization in debilitated patients.

References

1. vanSonnenberg E, D'Agostino HB, Casola G, Halasz NA, Sanchez RB, Goodacre BW. Percutaneous abscess drainage: current concepts. Radiology 1991; 181:617–626.
2. Lambiase RE. Percutaneous abscess and fluid drainage: a critical review. Cardiovasc Intervent Radiol 1991; 14:143–157.
3. Gerzof SG, Johnson WC, Robbins AH, Nabseth DC. Expanded criteria for percutaneous abscess drainage. Arch Surg 1985; 120:227–232.
4. vanSonnenberg E, Wing VW, Casola G, et al. Temporizing effect of percutaneous drainage of complicated abscesses in critically ill patients. AJR 1984; 142:821–826.
5. Jeffrey RB, Wing VW, Laing FC. Real-time sonographic monitoring of percutaneous abscess drainage. AJR 1985; 144:469–470.
6. Porter JA, Loughry CW, Cook AJ. Use of the computerized tomographic scan in the diagnosis and treatment of abscesses. Am J Surg 1985; 150:257–262.
7. Lambiase RE, Deyoe L, Cronan JJ, Dorfman GS. Percutaneous drainage of 335 consecutive abscesses: results of primary drainage with 1-year follow-up. Radiology 1992; 184:167–179.
8. vanSonnenberg E, Mueller PR, Ferrucci JT Jr. Percutaneous drainage of 250 abdominal abscesses and fluid collections. I. Results, failures, and complications. Radiology 1984; 151:337–341.
9. Mueller PR, vanSonnenberg E, Ferrucci JT Jr. Percutaneous drainage of 250 abdominal abscesses and fluid collections. II. Current procedural concepts. Radiology 1984; 151:343–347.
10. vanSonnenberg E, Wittich GR, Casola G, Cabrera OA, Gosink BB, Resnick DL. Sonography of thigh abscess: detection, diagnosis, and drainage. AJR 1987; 149:769–772.
11. Sanders TR, Staple TW. Percutaneous catheter drainage of septic shoulder joint. Radiology 1983; 147:270–271.
12. Pruett TL, Simmons RL. Status of percutaneous catheter drainage of abscesses. Surg Clin North Am 1988; 68:89–105.
13. Rotstein OD, Pruett TL, Simmons RL. Thigh abscess: an uncommon presentation of intra-abdominal sepsis. Am J Surg 1986; 151:414–418.
14. Bohrer SP, Bodine J. Perforated cecal carcinoma presenting as thigh emphysema. Ann Emerg Med 1983; 12:42–44.
15. Gobien RP, Stanley JH, Schabel SI, et al. The effect of drainage tube size on adequacy of percutaneous abscess drainage. Cardiovasc Intervent Radiol 1985; 8:100–102.

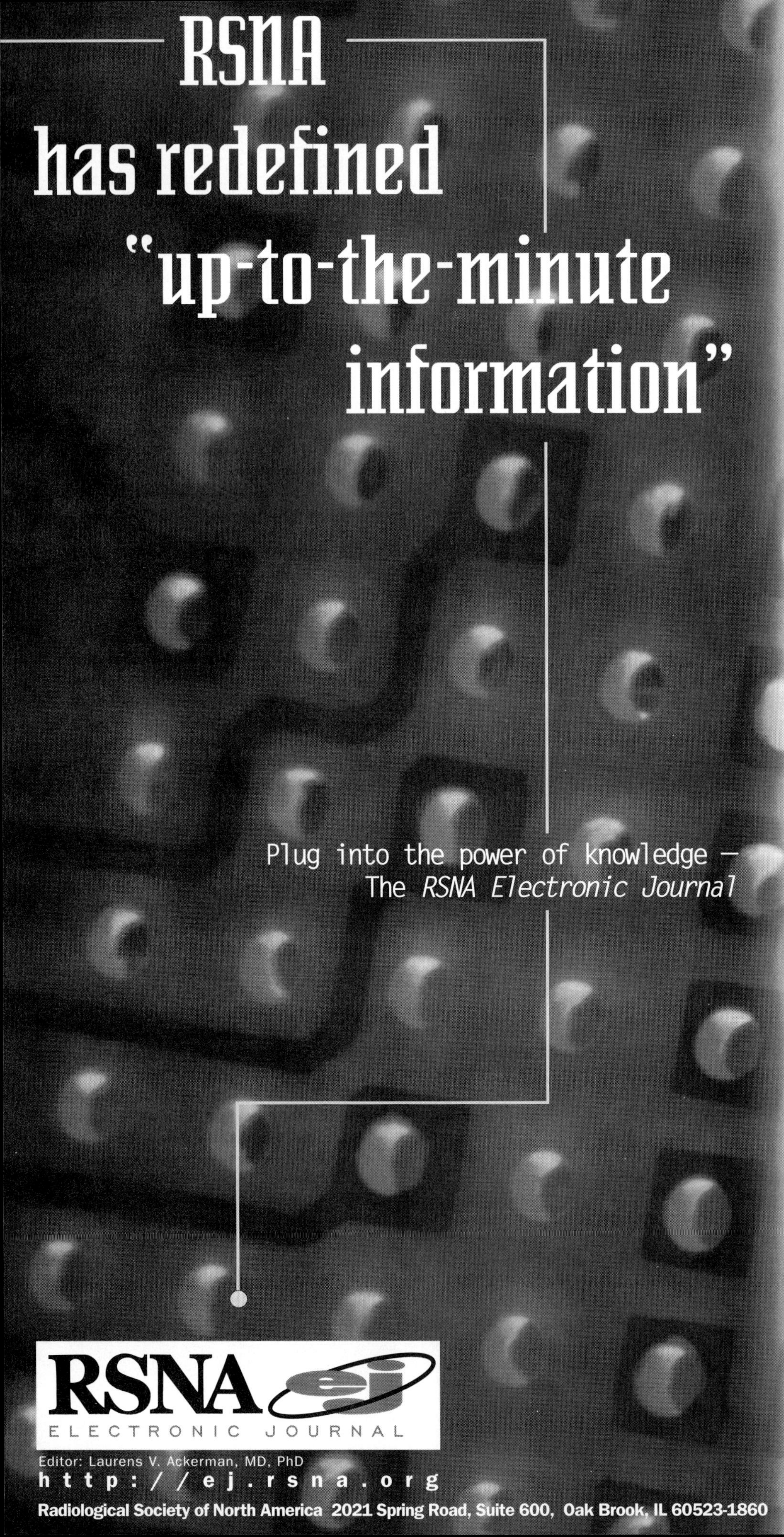
RSNA
has redefined
"up-to-the-minute
information"
Plug into the power of knowledge —
The RSNA Electronic Journal
RSNA ej
ELECTRONIC JOURNAL
Editor: Laurens V. Ackerman, MD, PhD
http://ej.rsna.org
Radiological Society of North America 2021 Spring Road, Suite 600, Oak Brook, IL 60523-1860

Coronary Artery Stenoses: Assessment with Contrast-enhanced Electron-Beam CT and Axial Reconstructions[1]

Gautham P. Reddy, MD, MPH
Daniel M. Chernoff, MD, PhD[2]
James R. Adams, MD
Charles B. Higgins, MD

Index terms:
Computed tomography (CT), electron beam, 54.12112, 54.12116, 54.12117, 54.12118, 54.12119
Coronary angiography, comparative studies, 54.1244
Coronary vessels, CT, 54.1211
Coronary vessels, stenosis or obstruction, 54.754

Radiology 1998; 208:167–172

Abbreviations:
LAD = left anterior descending coronary artery
LCX = left circumflex coronary artery
LMCA = left main coronary artery
MIP = maximum intensity projection
RCA = right coronary artery
STS = sliding thin slab

[1] From the Departments of Radiology (G.P.R., D.M.C., C.B.H.) and Medicine, Division of Cardiology (J.R.A.), University of California, San Francisco, 505 Parnassus Ave, Ste L308, San Francisco, CA 94143. From the 1997 RSNA scientific assembly. Received November 11, 1997; revision requested January 27, 1998; revision received February 10; accepted March 9. Supported in part by a grant from Imatron, South San Francisco, Calif. **Address reprint requests to** C.B.H.

[2] Current address: Department of Medical Imaging, Saint Mary's Hospital, Amsterdam, NY.

Author contributions:
Guarantors of integrity of entire study, G.P.R., D.M.C., C.B.H.; study concepts, G.P.R., D.M.C., C.B.H., J.R.A.; study design, G.P.R., D.M.C., C.B.H.; definition of intellectual content, G.P.R., D.M.C., C.B.H.; literature research, G.P.R.; clinical studies, J.R.A.; experimental studies, G.P.R., D.M.C., C.B.H.; data acquisition, G.P.R., D.M.C., C.B.H., J.R.A.; data analysis, G.P.R., C.B.H.; statistical analysis, G.P.R.; manuscript preparation, G.P.R.; manuscript editing, C.B.H.; manuscript review, D.M.C., C.B.H.

PURPOSE: To evaluate the usefulness of electron-beam computed tomography (CT) for identification of coronary artery stenoses.

MATERIALS AND METHODS: Coronary angiography and contrast material–enhanced, electrocardiographically triggered electron-beam CT of the heart were performed in 23 patients. With axial CT images and axial maximum intensity projection reconstructions, the coronary arteries were assessed by two observers blinded to the results of angiography.

RESULTS: Cardiac motion artifact (unsharpness) precluded evaluation of the right coronary artery (RCA) in six subjects and the left circumflex coronary artery (LCX) in one patient. With the vessels degraded by motion artifact eliminated from analysis, overall sensitivity of electron-beam CT for hemodynamically significant stenoses was 88%, and specificity was 79%. In the left anterior descending coronary artery (LAD), sensitivity was 93% and specificity was 63%; in the LCX, sensitivity was 100% and specificity was 67%; and in the RCA, sensitivity was 67% and specificity was 77%. The presence of coronary artery calcification did not have an effect on sensitivity for stenoses, but it did decrease specificity.

CONCLUSION: Electron-beam CT angiography can depict hemodynamically significant stenoses in the LAD and LCX with a sensitivity of more than 90%. The presence of coronary artery calcification resulted in decreased specificity but no appreciable change in sensitivity.

Coronary artery disease is a major health problem and the leading cause of death in the United States (1). Cardiac catheterization and conventional coronary angiography remain the definitive standard for evaluation of coronary artery disease. Because conventional angiography is an invasive procedure, attempts have been made to image the coronary arteries noninvasively with magnetic resonance (MR) imaging (2–7). Early results were encouraging (2,3), but some later studies indicated variable results (5–7). MR angiography is still limited by cardiac and respiratory motion artifacts and by a relatively long imaging time dictated by the need for multiple image acquisitions.

Electron-beam computed tomography (CT) has been used to detect coronary artery calcification as a sign of coronary artery disease in asymptomatic adults with coronary risk factors (8,9). Coronary calcium scores are closely associated with total atherosclerotic burden, but the presence and quantity of calcium do not always correlate with the location and severity of coronary arterial stenoses (9–12). A prior study assessed the performance characteristics of contrast material–enhanced electron-beam CT and showed that this technique can depict the lumen of long segments of the coronary arteries in healthy subjects (13). An early article about electrocardiographically triggered, contrast-enhanced electron-beam CT has shown the feasibility of this technique for visualization of coronary artery stenoses (14).

The present study was designed to compare electron-beam CT coronary angiography with conventional angiography in patients in whom coronary artery disease is suspected. The presence and location of stenoses in the four major coronary arteries were compared between the two examinations. No attempt was made to detect stenoses in branches of the major coronary arteries. The influence of coronary arterial calcification on the accuracy of detection of stenoses and the correlation of calcium score with the presence of coronary stenoses was also evaluated.

MATERIALS AND METHODS

Subjects

Twenty-three patients (17 men and six women; age range, 42–85 years; mean age, 59 years ± 12 [1 standard deviation]) in whom coronary artery disease was suspected underwent electron-beam CT angiography. Patients were enrolled in the study if they volunteered for CT angiography and if they had undergone clinically indicated conventional coronary angiography within 8 weeks of electron-beam CT. Patients with a history of reaction to contrast material, multiple drug allergies, unstable angina, or renal insufficiency were excluded from participation, as were women of childbearing age. The study was approved by the institutional committee on human research, and informed consent was obtained from all patients.

Electron-Beam CT

Electron-beam CT was performed with the C-150XP scanner (Imatron, South San Francisco, Calif). The matrix size was 512 × 512, and the field of view was 18 cm, yielding a pixel size of 0.34 × 0.34 mm.

Patients entered the scanner headfirst while supine. Subjects were instructed to breathe in the same way for each acquisition, first taking three deep breaths and then holding their breath in full inspiration when directed. The examination consisted of the acquisition of three series of scans, each obtained during a single breath hold with 3-mm section thickness, 100-msec acquisition time per section, and electrocardiographic triggering at 75% of the predicted R-R interval.

The first series was obtained without administration of contrast material (ie, the precontrast study). Thirty axial sections were imaged during a 25- to 40-second breath hold, starting just above the left sinus of Valsalva, with no gap or overlap of adjacent sections.

The second series determined the transit time of contrast media (also known as circulation time); it consisted of 10 images acquired at the level of the aortic root. A total of 12 mL of nonionic contrast material (iohexol, Omnipaque 350; Nycomed, Oslo, Norway) was injected at the rate of 4 mL/sec into an antecubital vein through a 20-gauge catheter. Starting 10 seconds after injection of contrast material, scanning was performed every second heartbeat for the first six images and every third heartbeat for the final four images. Transit time of contrast material was defined as the time from contrast material injection to peak luminal enhancement in the aortic root.

The final series was a contrast-enhanced volume acquisition (CT angiography), obtained after intravenous injection of 120–160 mL of iohexol at the rate of 4 mL/sec. Images were acquired after a delay equal to the contrast material transit time. Beginning just above the coronary sinus, 40 axial sections were scanned with 1-mm overlap. Breath-hold time was 30–50 seconds. Patients were instructed to hyperventilate before the start of the acquisition. They were advised that if they were unable to hold their breath for the entire duration of scanning, they should exhale slowly to minimize respiratory motion artifact. During the CT angiographic series, two of the subjects held their breath at less than the full degree of inspiration, resulting in exclusion of the left main coronary artery (LMCA) and proximal left anterior descending coronary artery (LAD) from the acquisition. These patients underwent immediate reinjection with 50 mL of iohexol to image the LMCA and proximal LAD.

Image Processing

The data from the third series (CT angiography) was transferred to a personal computer–based workstation with image reconstruction software (Accu-Image, Millbrae, Calif). Sliding thin slab (STS) maximum intensity projection (MIP) images were constructed with 6-mm section thickness.

Assessment of Electron-Beam CT Data and Comparison with Conventional Angiography

Each of the conventional coronary angiograms was interpreted as part of the clinical cardiac catheterization report by one of three cardiologists (J.R.A. and others) without knowledge of the electron-beam CT results. Angiographic results, including severity and location of stenoses, were extracted from the dictated catheterization reports.

The precontrast images were inspected for the presence and quantity of coronary artery calcification. Coronary artery calcium scores were calculated by using the Agatston method (8). Scores were obtained for each of the four major coronary arteries, and a total score was computed for each patient.

The contrast-enhanced electron-beam CT data were evaluated at the computer workstation by two independent observers (D.M.C., C.B.H.), both cardiac radiologists, who were blinded to the results of coronary angiography. By using the original axial postcontrast angiographic images and the STS-MIP reconstructions, the LMCA, LAD, left circumflex coronary artery (LCX), and right coronary artery (RCA) were appraised for stenoses. Each stenosis was assessed visually and graded for severity by use of the following scale: minimal (0%–25% reduction in luminal diameter), mild (25%–50%), moderate (50%–75%), severe (75%–99%), or occluded (100%). Stenoses with more than 50% narrowing of the luminal diameter were considered hemodynamically significant.

Specific landmarks were not used to define the segments of the major coronary arteries. The first 1–2 cm of each artery, however, was approximated as the proximal segment, the next 4–5 cm as the middle segment, and the remainder of the artery as the distal segment. After the images obtained in each subject were analyzed by the independent reviewers, any differences in the observers' assessments were resolved by means of consensus. Results at electron-beam CT were compared with those at conventional angiography by matching the stenoses on the basis of their location. After the observers had evaluated all arteries and were no longer blinded, they reevaluated the vessels to assess any discrepancies between the conventional angiographic and electron-beam CT findings.

Sensitivity and specificity were calculated for hemodynamically significant stenoses.

RESULTS

Electron-beam CT was successfully completed in all 23 subjects. No reactions to contrast material or adverse events occurred. Transit times of contrast material ranged from 18 to 26 seconds. Heart rates ranged from 46 to 86 beats per minute, resulting in an imaging time and breath-

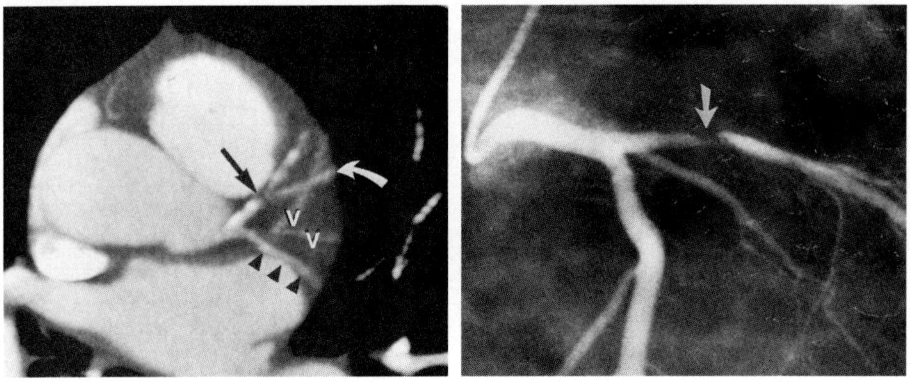

a. b.

Figure 1. (a) Axial STS-MIP image obtained in a 71-year-old man. Heavy calcification is noted in the LMCA and proximal LAD. Between the areas of calcification and just proximal to the origin of the first diagonal branch (curved arrow), a severe stenosis (straight arrow) can be identified in the LAD. The LCX (arrowheads) shows normal caliber. *V* = coronary veins. (b) Right anterior oblique coronary angiogram obtained in the same patient confirms a high-grade stenosis (arrow) in the proximal LAD.

TABLE 1
Segmental Distribution of Stenoses in Coronary Arteries at Coronary Angiography and CT

Vessel Segment	LAD			LCX			RCA			
	TP	FN	FP	TP	FN	FP	TP	FN	FP	M
Proximal	7	1	1	3	0	2	2	0	0	1
Middle	6	0	2	2	0	3	2	1	2	1
Distal	1	0	0	0	0	1	0	1	1	2

Note.—FN = false-negative, FP = false-positive, M = vessel not evaluated at CT because of cardiac motion artifact, TP = true-positive.

hold time between 30 and 50 seconds for the angiographic acquisition. By hyperventilating before acquisition of each series, all but three patients were able to hold their breath for the requisite period. When the three patients were no longer able to hold their breath, they exhaled slowly, as instructed. Because these patients exhaled during the final seconds of scanning, exhalation did not affect imaging of the proximal and middle segments of the major coronary arteries. In addition, the exhalation was slow enough that it did not cause substantial motion artifact (unsharpness) in the distal segments of the coronary arteries. All studies were performed in 30 minutes or less.

The RCA could not be adequately assessed in six subjects, and the LCX could not be evaluated in one patient, because of motion unsharpness caused by vessel movement during the heartbeat (also known as cardiac motion artifact). With conventional angiography as the standard of reference, electron-beam CT depicted 14 of 15 hemodynamically significant stenoses in the LAD (Fig 1), for a sensitivity of 93%. Specificity for the LAD was 63%. All five significant LCX stenoses were identified with electron-beam CT, yielding a sensitivity of 100%. Specificity was 67%. In the RCA, four of 10 significant stenoses were detected, for a sensitivity of 40%. Of the six hemodynamically significant RCA stenoses that were overlooked (false-negative findings), four were in vessels degraded by cardiac motion artifact. When these vessels were excluded from the analysis, sensitivity was 67% in the RCA. Specificity in the RCA was 77%. There were no significant stenoses in the LMCA, so sensitivity could not be calculated. Specificity for LMCA stenoses was 96% (one false-positive finding). For all vessels, overall sensitivity to hemodynamically significant stenoses was 77%, and specificity was 79%. When vessels degraded by cardiac motion artifact were excluded, overall sensitivity was 88%.

Of the 30 significant stenoses, 14 occurred in proximal segments, 12 in middle segments, and four in distal segments. The false-negative stenoses were in all three coronary artery segments (Table 1).

After observers were no longer blinded, the single stenosis missed in the LAD (proximal segment) was identified retrospectively at electron-beam CT, and two of the stenoses missed in the RCA (one middle segment, one distal) were retrospectively identified. None of these stenoses was obscured by arterial calcification. The remaining four hemodynamically significant stenoses missed in the RCA occurred in vessels where image quality was impaired by motion artifact at electron-beam CT. This retrospective analysis yielded sensitivity of 100% for the LAD and 60% for the RCA (100%, excluding vessels affected by artifact from cardiac motion).

Of the seven stenoses that were overlooked (false-negative findings), four were in vessels that were poorly evaluated owing to the presence of artifact from cardiac motion. None of the remaining three stenoses was associated with heavy calcification.

In 13 arteries without significant narrowing, the observers deemed that there were significant stenoses (false-positive findings). Ten of these 13 false-positive findings were in areas of heavy calcification.

Five of the 23 subjects had no significant coronary artery stenoses at conventional angiography. Their calcium scores ranged from 0 to 216 (mean, 63 ± 96). In three of these five patients, no coronary artery calcium was detected. The remaining 18 patients, all with at least one hemodynamically significant stenosis, had coronary calcium scores ranging from 88 to 2,657 (mean, 1,152 ± 772). The difference in calcium scores between these two groups of subjects was statistically significant ($P < .006$, Student *t* test).

Depending on the findings at electron-beam CT and coronary angiography, each of 85 vessels (excluding those degraded by motion artifact) was placed into one of four categories: true-positive, true-negative, false-positive, and false-negative. The mean calcium scores for each category are summarized in Table 2. The mean calcium score in the true-positive vessels (560 ± 365) was much higher than those in the other categories, with statistically significant differences between true-positive and true-negative vessels (mean, 74 ± 153; $P < .001$, Student *t* test) and between true-positive and false-negative vessels (mean, 145 ± 101; $P < .001$). In addition, false-positive vessels had a higher mean calcium score (283 ± 363) than true-negative vessels, although this difference was not statistically significant (P = .06). Because multiple comparisons were performed in this analysis, the level of statistical significance was set at P less than .01 (approximately equal to 0.05 divided by the number of comparisons), in accordance with the Bonferroni inequality (15).

TABLE 2
Calcium Scores in Individual Vessels by Category of Vessel

Finding	True-Positive	True-Negative	False-Positive	False-Negative
No. of vessels	23	46	13	3
Mean calcium score	560	74*	283	145*

* Statistically significant ($P < .001$) in comparison with true-positive findings (Student t test). Because multiple comparisons were performed, statistical significance was set at the level $P < .01$, in accordance with the Bonferroni inequality (15). All other comparisons were not statistically significant. Excludes seven vessels that were affected by substantial motion artifact.

DISCUSSION

Unenhanced electron-beam CT has been used to detect coronary artery calcification in asymptomatic subjects in an attempt to diagnose coronary artery disease and assess risk for coronary events (8–12). More recently, contrast-enhanced CT angiography has been proposed as a noninvasive means of directly imaging coronary artery stenoses. Thomas et al (16) first described an imaging protocol for electron-beam CT of the coronary arteries tested in a thorax phantom, in which the entire acquisition could be performed during a single breath hold. Chernoff et al (13) showed that electron-beam CT in healthy subjects imaged slightly longer segments of the LAD and LCX and approximately the same lengths of the LMCA and RCA compared with those reported for MR angiography. Initial studies of electron-beam CT coronary angiography in patients with coronary artery disease have produced promising results (14,17). These prior studies, however, used reconstruction techniques that are time-consuming, labor-intensive, and operator dependent. Moshage et al (14) used three-dimensional shaded surface display and two-dimensional MIP images, and Nakanishi et al (17) used multiplanar reformations.

STS-MIP reconstructions used in the current study have the advantage of being automatically created by the software program once the section thickness and overlap are specified. Thus, they require minimal time and skill to perform, and they are readily reproducible. Because the STS-MIP reconstructions are thicker than the original sections, a longer segment of each coronary artery is displayed in each image, but the contrast level is similar to that of the original 3-mm sections (18).

This study and prior reports (14,17) demonstrate that electron-beam CT angiography can readily image the coronary arteries and can depict coronary artery stenoses. Compared with those of previous reports, the sensitivities for detection of hemodynamically significant stenoses in the LAD and LCX were greater in the current study, but the specificities were lower. These findings may be a consequence of differences in subjective thresholds for identification of stenoses. In other words, the observers in the current study may have used a lower subjective threshold to locate stenoses, thereby increasing sensitivity at the expense of specificity. The difference in methods for image analysis, with use of STS-MIP reformations in this study, may also have contributed to the different results.

In contrast, the sensitivity for significant stenoses in the RCA was lower in this study than that in prior studies. This result can be explained in part by the degradation of RCA image quality by cardiac motion artifact in six of the 23 subjects in the current study. Of these six patients, an inordinately high proportion (67% [n = 4]) had significant stenoses that were obscured by cardiac motion artifact. Moshage et al (14) also described cardiac motion artifact in the RCA, but they were still able to identify most of the significant stenoses in the RCA. In addition, they reported low sensitivity in the LCX, attributed to cardiac motion artifact, small vessel size, and overlying venous structures. In the current study, cardiac motion artifact degraded the LCX in only one patient and overlying veins were not a substantial problem. Because no significant LMCA stenoses were present in our patients, sensitivity for LMCA stenoses could not be determined. The LMCA was clearly visualized in each patient, however, and significant stenoses can presumably be identified with a degree of certainty similar to that for the LAD.

When the observers were no longer blinded, the discrepancies between conventional angiography and electron-beam CT were reexamined. With the exclusion of patients whose RCA stenoses were obscured by cardiac motion artifact, retrospective analysis resulted in detection of all significant stenoses that were originally overlooked. These results indicate that the stenoses were depicted on the electron-beam CT images but were misinterpreted, perhaps because of inexperience with this technique. This possibility suggests the presence of a "learning curve": With greater familiarity with contrast-enhanced electron-beam CT, sensitivity for identification of hemodynamically significant stenoses should increase.

Proximal and middle segments of the coronary arteries were visualized equally well with contrast-enhanced electron-beam CT, and stenoses in these segments were detected with similar sensitivities. Because only a small number of vessels with distal stenoses were included in this study, it is difficult to draw definitive conclusions regarding evaluation of distal coronary artery stenoses. It is apparent that electron-beam CT can depict distal stenoses in at least some cases (Fig 2). Evaluation of distal coronary artery segments may be problematic, however, because these distal vessels are sometimes poorly opacified (13), are relatively small in caliber compared with the proximal and middle segments, are prone to be affected by respiratory motion artifact in patients who cannot hold their breath for the entire scan acquisition period, and in some cases may not be included in the examination because of the limited volume of acquisition achievable with current technology.

Influence of Coronary Artery Calcium

Results of the current study suggest that the presence of coronary artery calcification does not appreciably hinder detection of significant stenoses. Because calcium is much more dense than the intracoronary contrast media, it is difficult to misinterpret calcification as intraluminal contrast material on the original axial images or on the STS-MIP reconstructions (Fig 3). On the other hand, the presence of coronary calcification does seem to result in overestimation of the

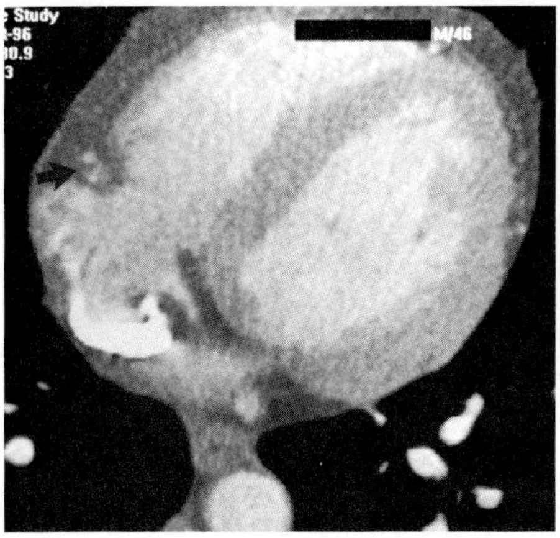

a.

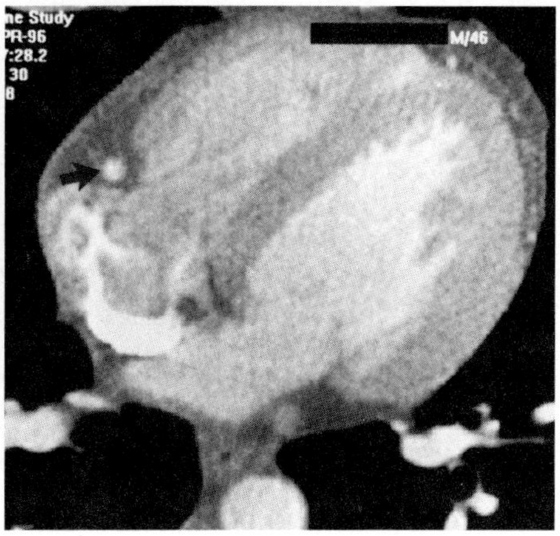

b.

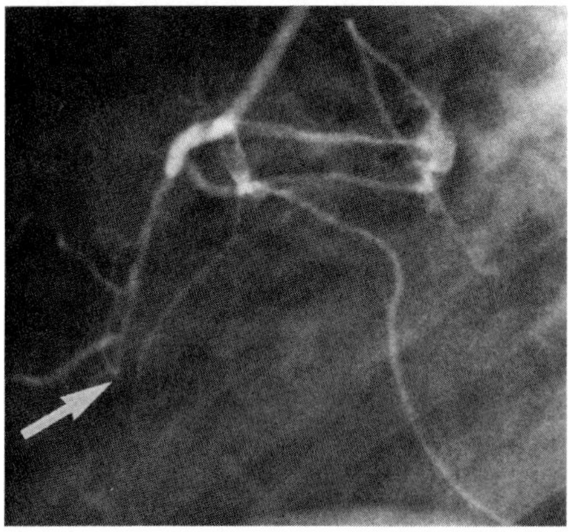

c.

Figure 2. Images obtained at the level of the distal right atrioventricular groove in a 46-year-old man. **(a)** Axial STS-MIP image shows the distal RCA (arrow) is severely narrowed. **(b)** Axial STS-MIP image obtained 6 mm below the level of **a** shows the RCA lumen (arrow) is filled with calcification and is occluded. **(c)** Right anterior oblique coronary angiogram demonstrates obstruction of the RCA (arrow).

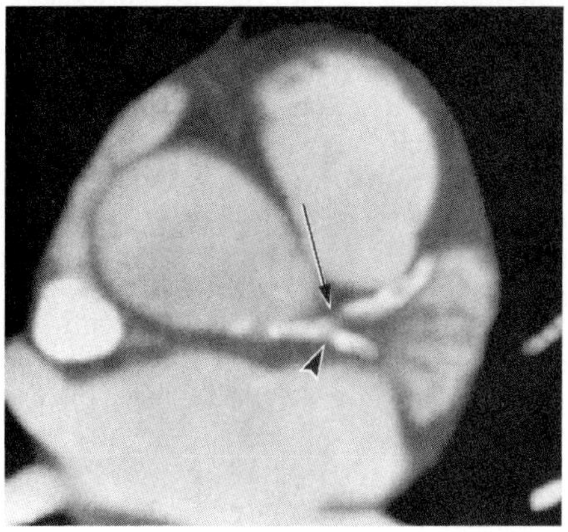

Figure 3. Axial STS-MIP image obtained in a 67-year-old woman shows heavy calcification in the LMCA, LAD, and LCX. A severe stenosis is present near the origin of the LAD (arrow). Mild narrowing can be seen at the origin of the LCX (arrowhead).

severity of luminal narrowing. Owing to partial volume averaging effects on electron-beam CT axial images and MIP reconstructions, mural calcification can sometimes cause the arterial lumen to appear narrower than it actually is. Coronary stenoses do not necessarily exist at sites of heavy arterial calcification (10,11,19), and this fact must be kept in mind during interpretation of CT coronary angiographic examinations.

In the present study, a lack of coronary artery calcification seems to correlate with absence of significant stenoses. All patients without detectable coronary artery calcium had angiographically normal coronary arteries, and all patients with one or more significant coronary artery stenosis had coronary artery calcification in the moderate to high range. The mean calcium scores in the groups of patients with no significant stenoses (63 ± 96) and those with significant stenoses (1,152 ± 772) were significantly different ($P < .006$). In this limited experience, lack of coronary artery calcification in a symptomatic patient indicates that the decision to proceed with coronary angiography or electron-beam CT angiography should be carefully considered. Significant coronary arterial stenoses, however, have been identified in patients, especially those aged less than 50 years, in the absence of coronary arterial calcification detectable at electron-beam CT (20).

A statistically significant difference ($P < .001$) was found in mean calcium scores between true-positive (560 ± 365) and true-negative (mean, 74 ± 153) vessels. This finding is in agreement with pathology studies that have shown coronary calcium scores correlate with atherosclerotic burden (10,11). There was also a significant difference ($P < .001$) in mean calcium score between true-positive and false-negative vessels (mean, 145 ± 101). In addition, the mean calcium score in false-positive vessels (283 ± 363) was much higher than the mean for true-negative vessels, although the difference was not statistically significant. These findings suggest that the observers were more likely to diagnose a stenosis in vessels containing large amounts of calcium than in those with little or no calcium.

With use of multiplanar reformations, Nakanishi et al (17) also reported false-positive readings when calcification was present at the site of stenosis, most commonly in the LAD. In contrast, Moshage et al (14) found that calcification did not substantially affect their results, although they described the theoretic possibility of underestimation of stenoses in calcified coronary artery segments when shaded surface display images are used.

In theory, it is possible to remove calcium from the electron-beam CT angiographic images by means of digital subtraction of the precontrast from the postcontrast data. Because of misregistration caused by differences in breath holding between the pre- and postcontrast acquisitions, however, calcium subtraction may be unreliable in practice.

Limitations of Electron-Beam CT Coronary Angiography

Cardiac motion artifact (unsharpness) limited evaluation of the RCA in six patients. Because the RCA courses in the atrioventricular groove, which has a considerable excursion during the cardiac cycle, the evaluation of this vessel seems to necessitate a shorter image acquisition time. In addition, artifact from cardiac motion can also hinder assessment of the LCX, although much less frequently than that of the RCA in this study. Decreasing imaging time from 100 msec to 50 msec or less should reduce cardiac motion artifact and substantially improve image quality and sensitivity, especially in the RCA.

Although most patients were able to hold their breath for the required 30–50 seconds during the angiographic acquisition, approximately one-fourth of the patients did not hold their breath for the entire period, and they slowly released their breath through their noses, as instructed, at the end of scanning. Because this exhalation was slow and occurred at the end of scanning, it did not cause substantial motion artifact in the proximal or middle areas of the coronary arteries, which are more important to evaluate than is the distal region of the coronary arteries. In the two patients who needed reinjection of contrast material, the LMCA and proximal LAD were well visualized at repeated scanning. These problems with patient breathing underscore the need to give each patient detailed breathing instructions before and during the examination. Other factors that can result in a suboptimal study are the presence of cardiac arrhythmia or premature ventricular contractions, although none of the subjects in this study had these conditions.

Comparison with Other Noninvasive Coronary Imaging Modalities

MR angiography has been extensively investigated as a noninvasive technique for imaging the coronary arteries. Although early studies with MR angiography yielded favorable results (2,3), subsequent articles have reported a wide range of diagnostic accuracies (5–7). The sensitivities and specificities reported for MR angiography in the detection of coronary artery stenoses are similar to those reported for CT angiography in this and prior studies. MR angiography appears to have greater diagnostic accuracy in the RCA and less in the LAD and LCX compared with electron-beam CT. MR angiography of the coronary arteries is still limited by respiratory and cardiac motion and by the relatively long imaging time needed to examine the coronary arteries in multiple oblique planes.

Transesophageal echocardiography has also been studied as a means of detecting coronary artery stenoses by imaging intraluminal atherosclerotic plaque (21,22). Color Doppler transesophageal echocardiography performed with use of intravenous ultrasound contrast agents has also been evaluated in the proximal LAD (23) and may provide more reliable identification of coronary artery stenoses than does standard transesophageal echocardiography. Both standard and contrast-enhanced transesophageal echocardiography, however, are limited by nonvisualization of middle and distal portions of the coronary arteries in the majority of subjects and by incomplete visualization of even proximal coronary arteries in some subjects. In addition, transesophageal echocardiography provides lower resolution and is a more invasive procedure than electron-beam CT angiography.

The major advantages of CT coronary angiography over MR angiography are the fast imaging time, use of a single breath hold for complete acquisition, and depiction of calcified plaques in the region of coronary artery stenoses. It is less invasive than transesophageal echocardiography and requires no sedation. Disadvantages of electron-beam CT compared with MR angiography and transesophageal echocardiography are the use of ionizing radiation and intravenous iodinated contrast material and perhaps decreased specificity in the presence of coronary artery calcium, as discussed earlier.

Clinical Importance

Although conventional angiography will remain the examination of choice for definitive evaluation of coronary artery disease for the foreseeable future, electron-beam CT potentially could be used as an initial imaging examination in patients in whom coronary artery disease is clinically suspected. In the future, patients with a moderate to high calcium score on an unenhanced study might benefit from undergoing contrast-enhanced CT. Electron-beam CT coronary angiography may also be effective for monitoring the morphology of stenoses after angioplasty (14).

References

1. American Heart Association. Heart and stroke facts. Dallas, Tex: American Heart Association, 1994; 1–2.
2. Manning WJ, Li W, Edelman RR. A preliminary report comparing magnetic resonance coronary angiography with conventional angiography. N Engl J Med 1993; 328:828–832.
3. Pennell DJ, Keegan J, Firmin DN, Gatehouse PD, Underwood SR, Longmore DB. Magnetic resonance imaging of coronary arteries: technique and preliminary results. Br Heart J 1993; 70:315–326.
4. Manning WJ, Li W, Boyle NG, Edelman RR. Fat-suppressed breath-hold magnetic resonance coronary angiography. Circulation 1993; 87:94–104.
5. Duerinckx AJ, Urman MK. Two-dimensional coronary MR angiography: analysis of initial clinical results. Radiology 1994; 193:731–738.
6. Hofman MBM, Paschal CB, Li D, Haacke EM, van Rossum AC, Sprenger M. MRI of coronary arteries: 2D breath-hold vs 3D respiratory-gated acquisition. J Comput Assist Tomogr 1995; 19:56–62.
7. Pennell DJ, Bogren HG, Keegan J, Firmin DN, Underwood SR. Assessment of coronary artery stenosis by magnetic resonance imaging. Heart 1996; 75:127–133.
8. Agatston AS, Janowitz WR, Hildner FJ, Zusmer NR, Viamonte M, Detrano R. Quantification of coronary artery calcium using ultrafast computed tomography. J Am Coll Cardiol 1990; 15:827–832.
9. Breen JF, Sheedy PF, Schwartz RS, et al. Coronary artery calcification detected with ultrafast CT as an indication of coronary artery disease. Radiology 1992; 185:435–439.
10. Simons DB, Schwartz RS, Edwards WD, Sheedy PF, Breen JF, Rumberger JA. Noninvasive definition of anatomic coronary artery disease by ultrafast computed tomographic scanning: quantitative pathologic comparison study. J Am Coll Cardiol 1992; 20:1118–1126.
11. Mautner SL, Mautner GC, Froehlich J, et al. Coronary artery calcification: assessment with electron beam CT and histomorphometric correlation. Radiology 1994; 192:619–623.
12. Agatston AS, Janowitz WR, Kaplan G, et al. Ultrafast computed tomography–detected coronary calcium reflects the angiographic extent of coronary arterial atherosclerosis. Am J Cardiol 1994; 74:1272–1274.
13. Chernoff DM, Ritchie CJ, Higgins CB. Evaluation of electron beam CT coronary angiography in healthy subjects. AJR 1997; 169:93–99.
14. Moshage WE, Achenbach S, Seese B, Bachmann K, Kirchgeorg M. Coronary artery stenoses: three-dimensional imaging with electrocardiographically triggered, contrast agent–enhanced, electron-beam CT. Radiology 1995; 196:707–714.
15. Ingelfinger JA, Mosteller F, Thibodeau LA, Ware JH. Biostatistics in clinical medicine. 2nd ed. New York, NY: MacMillan, 1987; 161.
16. Thomas PJ, McCollough CH, Ritman EL. An electron-beam CT approach for transvenous coronary arteriography. J Comput Assist Tomogr 1995; 19:383–389.
17. Nakanishi T, Ito K, Imazu M, Yamakido M. Evaluation of coronary artery stenoses using electron-beam CT and multiplanar reformation. J Comput Assist Tomogr 1997; 21:121–127.
18. Napel S, Rubin GD, Jeffrey RB. STS-MIP: a new reconstruction technique for CT of the chest. J Comput Assist Tomogr 1993; 17:832–838.
19. Bormann JL, Stanford W, Stenberg RG et al. Ultrafast computed tomographic detection of coronary artery calcification as an indicator of stenosis. Am J Cardiac Imaging 1992; 6:191–196.
20. Fallavollita JA, Brody AS, Bunnell IL, Kumar K, Canty JM. Fast computed tomography detection of coronary calcification in the diagnosis of coronary artery disease: comparison with angiography in patients <50 years old. Circulation 1994; 89:285–290.
21. Tardif JC, Vannan MA, Taylor K, Schwartz SL, Pandian NG. Delineation of extended lengths of coronary arteries by multiplane transesophageal echocardiography. J Am Coll Cardiol 1994; 24:909–919.
22. Memmola C, Iliceto S, Rizzon P. Detection of proximal stenosis of left coronary artery by digital transesophageal echocardiography: feasibility, sensitivity, and specificity. J Am Soc Echocardiogr 1993; 6:149–157.
23. Caiati C, Aragona P, Iliceto S, Rizzon P. Improved Doppler detection of proximal left anterior descending coronary artery stenosis after intravenous injection of a lung-crossing contrast agent: a transesophageal Doppler echocardiographic study. J Am Coll Cardiol 1996; 27:1413–1421.

Erich Minar, MD
Boris Pokrajac, MD
Ramazanali Ahmadi, MD
Thomas Maca, MD
Wolfgang Seitz, MD
Andreas Stümpflen, MD
Richard Pötter, MD
Herbert Ehringer, MD

Brachytherapy for Prophylaxis of Restenosis after Long-Segment Femoropopliteal Angioplasty: Pilot Study[1]

Index terms:
Arteries, femoral, 92.72, 92.7212
Arteries, stenosis or obstruction, 92.72, 92.7212
Arteries, transluminal angioplasty, 92.128
Therapeutic radiology, 92.1269

Radiology 1998; 208:173–179

Abbreviations:
ABI = ankle-brachial pressure index
PSV = peak systolic velocity
PTA = percutaneous transluminal angioplasty
PVR = peak velocity ratio

[1] From the Departments of Medical Angiology (E.M., R.A., T.M., A.S., H.E.) and Radiotherapy (B.P., W.S., R.P.), University Clinic Vienna, General Hospital Vienna, Waehringer Guertel 18-20, A-1097 Vienna, Austria. Received October 15, 1997; revision requested December 30; revision received February 5, 1998; accepted February 12. **Address reprint requests to** E.M.

PURPOSE: To evaluate in a pilot study the feasibility and efficacy of endovascular brachytherapy for prophylaxis of restenosis after femoropopliteal percutaneous transluminal angioplasty (PTA) without stent implantation in a group of patients with a high risk of restenosis.

MATERIALS AND METHODS: Ten patients (six women, four men; mean age, 68 years) with long-segment (mean length, 16 cm; range, 9–22 cm) restenosis underwent PTA followed by endovascular irradiation with high-dose-rate afterloading of an iridium-192 rod. A dose of 12 Gy was targeted to the inner intimal layer of the vessel. Follow-up examinations until 12 months after PTA included measurement of the ankle-brachial index, color duplex ultrasonography (US) with calculation of the peak velocity ratio, and intraarterial angiography when recurrence was suspected.

RESULTS: Irradiation was technically feasible in all patients without complications. In six patients, the dilated and irradiated segment remained widely patent at color US, with corresponding excellent hemodynamic and clinical results after 12 months. In four patients, clinical and laboratory findings indicated recurrence and arteriography demonstrated restenosis with a diameter reduction of 60%, 70%, 80%, or 90%.

CONCLUSION: Considering the negative selection of patients with a high risk of restenosis, the results of our pilot study are promising concerning the possibility of reduction of restenosis by means of endovascular brachytherapy after long-segment femoropopliteal PTA without stent implantation. The value of this approach should now be determined definitively in randomized trials.

Restenosis has remained until now a major limitation of the clinical usefulness of percutaneous transluminal angioplasty (PTA), and poor long-term results, especially after treatment of longer lesions in the femoropopliteal region, have been reported (1–5). Numerous pharmacologic (6) and mechanical (7–9) adjuncts have been tried with little success.

Over the past few years, there have been major advances in our understanding of the biology of the complex process leading to restenosis (10,11). The two primary phenomena that contribute to restenosis after successful angioplasty are chronic vessel constriction (remodeling) and neointimal hyperplasia by cell proliferation. Endovascular brachytherapy has shown strong potential in controlling this pathologic proliferation process in animal models of restenosis (12–15). Findings of recent clinical studies suggest a substantial reduction in the restenosis rate with intraluminal irradiation of coronary (16) and peripheral (17) arteries in conjunction with angioplasty and stent implantation.

Because, to our knowledge, there are no clinical data concerning postangioplasty irradiation without stent implantation, we performed this pilot study to evaluate the feasibility and efficacy

Author contributions:
Guarantor of integrity of entire study, E.M.; study concepts and design, E.M., B.P., W.S., R.P., H.E.; definition of intellectual content, E.M., B.P., R.P., H.E.; literature research, E.M., B.P.; clinical studies, E.M., R.A., T.M., A.S.; data acquisition, E.M., B.P., T.M., A.S.; data analysis, E.M., B.P., A.S.; manuscript preparation, E.M., B.P., A.S.; manuscript editing, E.M., A.S.; manuscript review, E.M., W.S., R.P., H.E.

TABLE 1
Baseline Patient Characteristics

Patient No./Sex/Age (y)	No. of Times PTA Performed Previously	Lesion		Length of Vessel in which PTA Performed (cm)	No. of Patent Crural Arteries	Coronary Heart Disease*	Diabetes Mellitus	Hypertension	Current Cigarette Smoker	Total Cholesterol Level (mg/dL)†	Low-Density Lipoprotein Cholesterol Level (mg/dL)†
		Kind	Percentage of Luminal Narrowing								
1/M/69	1	Stenosis	95	15	1	MI	Yes	Yes	No	236 (6.10)	154 (3.98)
2/F/78	1	Stenosis	99	16	0	AP	No	No	No	216 (5.58)	154 (3.98)
3/F/74	1	Occlusion	100	9	2	0	Yes	No	No	242 (6.26)	162 (4.19)
4/F/69	1	Stenosis	95	15	3	0	No	No	Yes	347 (8.97)	238 (6.15)
5/F/72	1	Stenosis	90	21	3	0	No	Yes	No	271 (7.01)	193 (4.99)
6/M/59	3	Stenosis	85	15	2	0	No	Yes	No	252 (6.52)	168 (4.34)
7/F/77	1	Occlusion	100	16	1	0	No	Yes	No	242 (6.26)	159 (4.11)
8/M/54	1	Stenosis	99	15	3	0	No	No	Yes	215 (5.56)	113 (2.92)
9/M/73	1	Stenosis	95	12	1	AP	No	Yes	No	247 (6.39)	165 (4.27)
10/F/53	1	Stenosis	90	22	2	0	No	No	Yes	233 (6.02)	173 (4.47)

* AP = angina pectoris, MI = prior myocardial infarction.
† Number in parentheses is the level in millimoles per liter.

TABLE 2
Hemodynamic Parameters and Clinical Category before and after Angioplasty and Brachytherapy

Patient No.	ABI*					PVR*					Clinical Category†			Angiographic Examination*		PTA*		Percentage of Restenosis at Intraarterial Angiography‡
	A	B	C	D	E	A	B	C	D	E	A	D	E	D	E	D	E	
1	0.59	1.00	1.08	0.89	1.03§	7.9	2.0	1.4	2.6	1.5§	3	2	0	Yes	No	Yes	No	60
2	0.24	0.50	0.52	0.35	0.64§	9.9	1.3	1.9	4.7	1.3§	5	5	1	Yes	No	Yes	No	90
3	0.54	1.07	1.00	0.95	0.96	NA	1.8	1.2	1.3	1.5	3	1	0	Yes	No	No	No	0
4	0.58	0.77	0.85	0.80	0.83	7.7	1.8	1.8	2.0	1.4	3	0	0	Yes	No	No	No	30
5	0.75	1.03	1.14	1.00	0.98	4.5	1.7	1.8	1.6	1.5	3	0	0	No	No	No	No	NP
6	0.75	0.86	1.09	1.09	0.88	4.2	1.8	1.2	1.2	3.2	3	0	2	No	Yes	No	Yes	70
7	0.22	0.66	0.68	0.55	0.46	NA	1.6	1.5	2.3	3.7	4	1	3	No	Yes	No	Yes	80
8	0.56	0.93	0.94	0.95	0.95	12.0	1.1	1.0	1.1	1.2	3	0	0	No	No	No	No	NP
9	0.52	0.80	0.74	0.77	0.75	6.0	1.1	1.2	1.1	1.1	3	1	1	No	No	No	No	NP
10	0.70	0.81	0.92	0.90	0.90	4.5	1.9	1.4	1.5	1.4	3	0	0	No	No	No	No	NP
Mean	0.55	0.84	0.90	0.83	0.84§	7.1	1.6	1.4	1.9	1.9§	NA	NA	NA	NA	NA	No	No	NA

* A = before PTA, B = 1 day after PTA, C = 3 months after PTA, D = 6 months after PTA, E = 12 months after PTA, NA = not available (because of occlusion in the case of PVR).
† Clinical category according to Rutherford (18). NA = not available.
‡ NA = not available, NP = not performed.
§ Value after further intervention not used to calculate the mean.

of endovascular brachytherapy for prophylaxis of restenosis after angioplasty without stent implantation in a group of patients with a high risk of restenosis, namely, patients with long-distance (>5-cm) recurrence after PTA in the femoropopliteal region.

MATERIALS AND METHODS

Patients

Between May and September 1996, a total of 59 consecutive patients who had been treated in our center with PTA for femoropopliteal lesions at least 6 months before were screened for entry into this pilot study. To be eligible, patients, with a minimum age of 50 years, had to have a recurrent lesion in the femoropopliteal region, with a minimal lesion length of 5 cm at least 10 cm after the femoral bifurcation (to prevent problems with anterograde recanalization). The primary screening examination was color duplex ultrasonography (US). Twelve patients were selected, but two had to be excluded after PTA because of failure to achieve an angiographically sufficient result.

The baseline characteristics of the 10 study patients (six women, four men; mean age, 68 years) are listed in Table 1. Eight patients presented with claudication; two patients had critical leg ischemia (see Table 2).

Each patient gave his or her written informed consent to participate in the study, which was approved by the hospital's ethics committee.

Angioplasty and Brachytherapy Procedure

An ipsilateral anterograde puncture and a 6-F introducer sheath (Cordis Europe, Roden, The Netherlands) were used in all procedures. Angioplasty was performed with 5- or 6-mm balloon catheters (Smash; Schneider Europe, Bülach, Switzerland). Uniplanar intraarterial digital subtraction angiography with a Bicor Medical System (Siemens, Erlangen, Germany) was performed in all patients immediately before and after the procedure. Postprocessing was used to achieve optimal mask-image combinations, and a hard copy was ob-

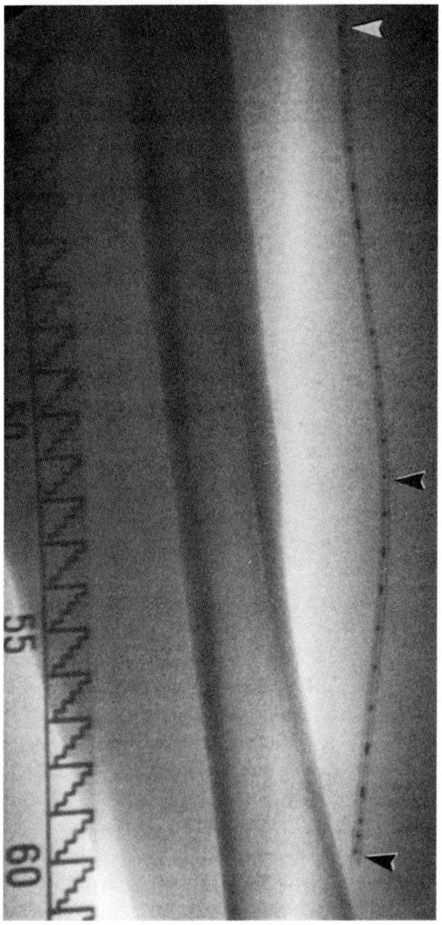

Figure 1. Radiograph demonstrates wire with markers (arrowheads) after insertion into a 5-F closed-tip catheter.

tained with a standard multiformat camera (X-Omat Processor M7B; Kodak, Rochester, NY). The degree of residual stenosis immediately after PTA, or the degree of recurrent stenosis in case of follow-up arteriography, was determined by comparing the width of the contrast material column at the point of maximal diameter reduction within the dilated segment to that of an unaffected arterial segment immediately proximal to the dilated segment. The measurements were done with a ruler. Technical success required angiographic patency with residual stenosis of less than 30% diameter reduction.

The region in which angioplasty was performed was marked with a radiopaque ruler, and movement of the table and angiographic unit was avoided to prevent parallax error. After successful recanalization, the angioplastic balloon was removed, the guide wire was left in place, and the standard sheath was exchanged for a 55-cm-long, 6-F sheath (Brite Tip; Cordis Europe), which was advanced until its tip was distal to the dilated segment. After placement of this sheath across the angioplastic site, a 5-F closed-tip applicator (Lumencath Applicator [Nucletron, Veenendaal, The Netherlands]; it accommodated the radiation source inserted during the afterloading procedure) was inserted and placed at 1 cm distal to the dilated segment. This catheter was equipped with a wire with markers at 1.0-cm intervals for exact measurement of the length of the angioplastic site (Fig 1). Then, the sheath and the applicator were fixed to the patient to prevent movement relative to the lesion during the transportation to the brachytherapy unit.

The dose distribution was calculated on the basis of post-PTA vessel diameter and length of the treated vessel segment, as well as the actual activity of the source, by using a computerized planning system. The reference dose of 12 Gy was prescribed to the inner intimal layer of the vessel, which corresponded to the area 2.5–3.0 mm from the source center (depending on the diameter of the angioplastic balloon used [5 or 6 mm]). We could not use a centering device for the source owing to the lack of such devices at the time this pilot study was performed. The length of the artery to be irradiated corresponded to the length of the angioplastic site with an additional 1 cm at each end.

The position of the 5-F delivery catheter and the marked wire in relation to the target volume was verified by means of radiography before starting the afterloading procedure. Then, the proximal end of the applicator was connected by means of a special 5-F adapter to the afterloader placed in a shielded room. To comply with standards established for high-dose-rate afterloading brachytherapy, only the patient was in the treatment room during radiation delivery; he or she was supervised by a television monitor and was able to communicate with the medical team. To ensure unimpeded placement of the active source (attached to a delivery cable), an inactive test wire ("dummy wire") was placed. Then, an iridium-192 source with a diameter of 1.1 mm was delivered by using a high-dose-rate afterloader (MicroSelectron; Nucletron). The source activity was 5–10 Ci (185–370 GBq). The radiation dose was controlled by using the computerized afterloading device to accurately adjust the source position and treatment time. This time was automatically corrected for the radioactive decay of the source. The afterloader monitored the delivered dose and automatically retracted the source after treatment. The mean irradiation time was 240 seconds (range, 160–600 seconds). The mean time for the total brachytherapy procedure (including transportation to the brachytherapeutic unit, radiographic verification of the applicator position, dose calibration, and irradiation) was 25 minutes.

The sheath was removed after brachytherapy, and the puncture site was manually compressed for 20 minutes. Duplex US was performed the next day to examine the puncture site as part of the routine protocol in all our patients.

Periinterventional Pharmacotherapy

Treatment with 100 mg of aspirin (Thrombo-ASS; Lannacher, Lannach, Austria) per day was initiated at least 2 weeks before the intervention and was prescribed as long-term treatment. After successful passage of the guide wire through the lesion, 5,000 IU of standard heparin (Liquemin; Hoffmann–La Roche, Basel, Switzerland) was administered through the sheath. Further continuous administration of heparin in a dosage of 1,000 IU/h was started before transportation to the brachytherapy unit (initially through the sheath and intravenously after removal of the sheath) and was continued until the next morning. Then, the patients received low-molecular-weight heparin (dalteparin sodium [Fragmin]; Pharmacia and Upjohn, Uppsala, Sweden) twice daily in a body weight–adjusted dose (100 IU/kg) for 2 additional days. In addition, all patients were treated with 2-hour infusions of 40 μg of alprostadil (Prostavasin; Gebro, Fieberbrunn, Austria) twice daily for 3 days (starting immediately after removal of the sheath and manual compression). The patients were hospitalized for 5 days, with the exception of the two patients with critical limb ischemia (hospitalized 10 and 14 days).

Follow-up

Follow-up examinations were performed the day after PTA and 1, 3, 6, and 12 months after the intervention. Follow-up examinations were assessment of symptoms, clinical examination (pulse palpation and auscultation of the treated vessel), noninvasive laboratory testing, pulse volume recording, and ankle-brachial arterial pressure measurement with Doppler US (the higher value of the ankle pressure measured at either the posterior tibial or dorsal pedal artery was used to

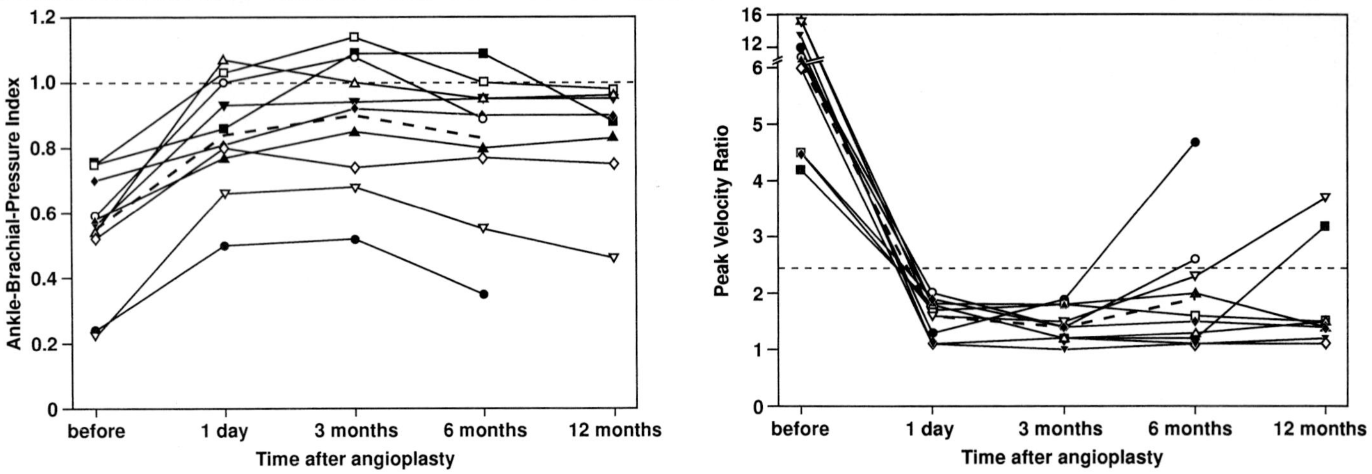

a. b.

Figure 2. Graphs show (a) ABI and (b) PVR versus time before and after angioplasty. Mean (bold dashed line) and individual values for the 10 patients are graphed. The dotted line at an ABI of 1.0 in **a** and the dotted line at a PVR of 2.4 in **b** are indicative of at least 50% stenosis. Values below the dotted lines are abnormal. In **a** and **b**, ○ = patient 1, ● = patient 2, △ = patient 3, ▲ = patient 4, □ = patient 5, ■ = patient 6, ▽ = patient 7, ▼ = patient 8, ◇ = patient 9, ◆ = patient 10.

calculate the ankle-brachial pressure index [ABI]); furthermore, color duplex US (5-MHz, linear-array color probe [model XP10; Acuson, Mountain View, Calif]) of the femoropopliteal segment was performed during each follow-up visit except for the visit at 1 month. The maximum peak systolic velocity (PSV) in the dilated region was determined and compared to the PSV in the preceding normal arterial segment. A focal increase in the PSV of at least 140% (corresponding to a peak velocity ratio [PVR] of ≥2.4) was considered indicative of a stenosis of greater than 50% at that site (19). If recurrent stenosis was suspected on the basis of clinical or laboratory findings (deterioration of the ABI by at least 0.15 from the maximum postprocedural level, a PVR in the dilated segment of at least 2.4, or both), intraarterial angiography was performed. Furthermore, arteriography was planned in patients with borderline PVR values (≥2) for angiographic documentation of the degree of stenosis. Restenosis was defined as an angiographically documented stenosis of greater than 50% narrowing of the luminal diameter compared with the diameters of normal segments of the vessel on the follow-up angiograms.

The follow-up was 12 months in all patients.

RESULTS

The mean degree of residual stenosis on postangioplasty angiograms was 15% (range, 0%–25%).

The irradiation procedure was technically feasible in all patients without complications. The patients experienced no adverse events. Transportation to the brachytherapy unit and the irradiation protocol prolonged the PTA procedure by about 30–45 minutes overall. The examination of the puncture site by means of duplex US the day after the intervention demonstrated no complications.

Complete follow-up information was obtained in all patients until 12 months after PTA. The hemodynamic parameters (ABI, PVR), the clinical category, and the angiographic data are listed in Table 2. Furthermore, the hemodynamic parameters also are graphed in Figure 2.

The mean ABI increased from 0.55 (range, 0.22–0.75) before PTA to 0.84 (range, 0.50–1.07) the day after PTA, and follow-up examinations demonstrated values of 0.90 (range, 0.52–1.14) after 3 months and 0.83 (range, 0.35–1.09) after 6 months. After 12 months, the mean ABI was 0.84 (range, 0.46–0.98) in the eight patients without further intervention.

The mean PVR decreased from 7.1 (range, 4.2–12.0) before PTA to 1.6 (range, 1.1–2.0) 1 day after PTA, and mean follow-up values were 1.4 (range, 1.0–1.9) after 3 months and 1.9 (range, 1.1–4.7) after 6 months. After 12 months, the mean PVR was 1.9 (range, 1.1–3.7) in the eight patients mentioned above.

After 3 months, no patient had restenosis according to clinical and hemodynamic criteria. Two patients (patients 1 and 2) had a PVR greater than 2.4 after 6 months (and a corresponding decrease in ABI from 1.08 to 0.89 and from 0.52 to 0.35), indicating restenosis, and intraarterial angiography demonstrated a diameter reduction of 60% (Fig 3) and 90%. Both patients underwent repeat PTA. In one (patient 4) of two patients (patients 4 and 7) with borderline PVR values (PVRs = 2.0 and 2.3), angiography demonstrated a non–clinically important diameter reduction (30%); the other patient (patient 7) refused angiography because of only mild claudication. After 12 months, with development of limiting claudication and a corresponding increase in the PVR to 3.7, a repeat interventional procedure was performed in patient 7 because of a short-segment 80% restenosis (Fig 4). Another patient (patient 6) with normal hemodynamic parameters after 6 months had an angiographically demonstrated short-segment 70% restenosis after 12 months. In six patients, the dilated and irradiated segment remained widely patent at color US, with corresponding excellent hemodynamic and clinical results after 12 months.

Arterial dilation or aneurysm formation was not observed in any of the patients during the 12-month follow-up. The tissue surrounding the irradiated artery demonstrated no morphologic abnormalities at US. Duplex US demonstrated no progression of atherosclerotic disease in the nontreated segments of the femoropopliteal arteries in the irradiated limbs.

DISCUSSION

The potential role of radiation in the prevention of restenosis after angioplasty

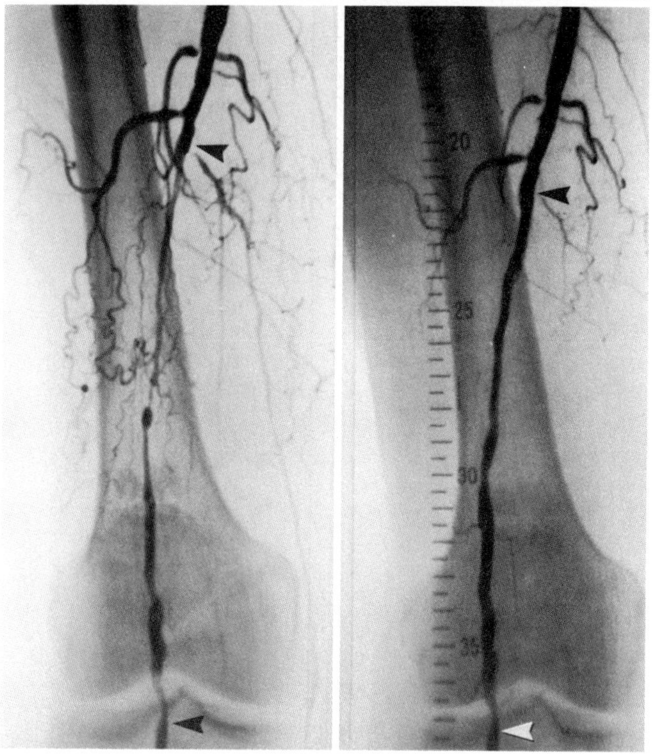

Figure 3. Patient 1. Left: Angiogram demonstrates long-segment restenosis 8 months after prior PTA. Right: Control angiogram demonstrates moderate (60%) restenosis 6 months after PTA and brachytherapy. The dilated segment is the segment between the arrowheads.

has generated much recent interest. Ionizing radiation inhibits cellular proliferation and has been used extensively in the treatment of neoplastic and nonneoplastic diseases such as keloid formation. The rationale in experimental studies to apply irradiation to prevent restenosis is that the latter is mediated at least in part by an uncontrolled proliferation of smooth muscle cells and abundant extracellular matrix synthesis (10,11). These processes are initiated by vascular injury. While the classic concept of restenosis suggests migration and proliferation of smooth muscle cells from the media (10,11), results of recent experiments demonstrate that mainly myofibroblasts in the adventitia proliferate during the first days after angioplasty and may migrate into the intima (20). This has implications for the brachytherapy protocol, because it is important to know definitively the target tissue. At this stage, to our knowledge, researchers are still uncertain whether the exact radiation target is the inner intimal layer of vessels, the media, or the outer adventitial layer. In our study, we prescribed the reference dose of 12 Gy to the inner intimal layer of the vessel, in accordance with the study by Böttcher et al (17).

Recent data indicate that vascular remodeling, as indicated by constriction of the external elastic lamina after angioplasty, is also an important mechanism for restenosis (21). The issue of whether intravascular radiation has an inhibitory effect on chronic recoil has not been adequately studied. Wilcox et al (22) suggested that both processes responsible for restenosis—cell proliferation and chronic vascular remodeling—can be affected by intravascular irradiation through its action on adventitial cells.

Extensive animal work (12–15) and recently published findings of studies in humans (16,17,23,24) have shown the feasibility of irradiation for the prevention of restenosis. Despite the use of different animal models, different arteries, and different isotopes with β or γ radiation, there is a remarkable consistency in the efficacy of endoluminal brachytherapy for inhibiting neointimal hyperplasia. However, there were some differences concerning the necessary dose to be applied in animal studies in which Ir-192 was used for irradiation after balloon overstretch injury in porcine coronary arteries (15,25). While Weinberger et al (25) observed a reduction of neointimal hyperplasia only with doses of 15 Gy and above, Waksman et al (15) also reported a statistically significant reduction in neointimal formation with doses of 7–14 Gy. The durability of the radiation effect at 6 months also was confirmed (15,26).

To our knowledge, Böttcher et al (17) were the first to present data showing endovascular irradiation is both feasible and safe in humans. This group, using the same high-dose-rate afterloading technique with an Ir-192 source as we did in our study, applied endovascular brachytherapy to prevent intimal hyperplasia after angioplasty of restenotic femoropopliteal lesions with stents. This group has used a dose of 12 Gy—applied to the inner intimal layer, as in our study—because of the long experience and positive results with this dose in the prevention of keloids and hypertrophic scars. Unlike in our study, they used postangioplasty irradiation only in segments with stents and shorter lesion lengths of 4.5–14.0 cm (mean, 6.7 cm) (27). The optimistic primary results have been confirmed recently by long-term results, with a range of follow-up of 4–68 months (27). They observed no recurrence in 22 of 30 patients. Furthermore, they observed no evidence of side effects, as investigated with magnetic resonance imaging, to the vessels, nerves, or soft tissue surrounding the femoral artery (27). With regard to potential induction of malignancy owing to irradiation, data from radiation therapy in benign and malignant diseases allow us to presume that the risk is extremely low for patients treated with intravascular brachytherapy (28).

Compared with the very limited number of studies with clinical data concerning the use of brachytherapy in the peripheral circulation, more studies have been initiated in which intracoronary radiation is used. Condado et al (23), performing an uncontrolled feasibility trial in 21 patients, have reported a 6-month angiography patency rate of 91% after coronary angioplasty and brachytherapy by using manually delivered Ir-192. Otherwise, Verin et al (24), using intracoronary β irradiation, observed a greater than 50%-diameter stenosis in six of 15 patients during 6 months of follow-up. Teirstein et al (16) have recently reported on a double-blind randomized trial in 55 patients who underwent catheter-based radiation therapy after coronary stent placement. The 6-month restenosis rate was 17% in 26 patients treated with irradiation and 54% in 29 patients treated with a nonradioactive placebo. Because of the great differences in outcome, the

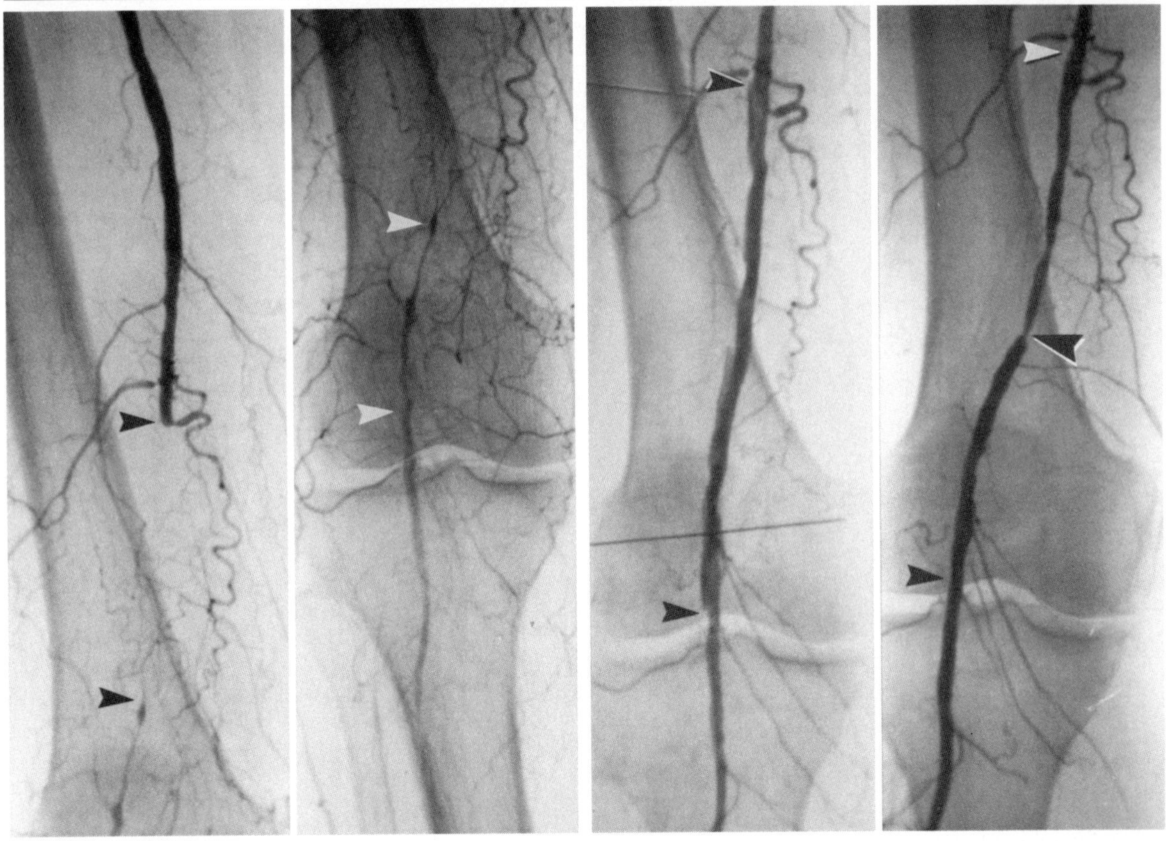

a. b.

Figure 4. Patient 7. **(a)** Angiograms demonstrate long-segment femoropopliteal recurrence after prior PTA (left: reocclusion seen between the arrowheads; right: restenosis of the reconstituted popliteal artery seen between the arrowheads). **(b)** Left: Angiogram of the femoropopliteal artery immediately after angioplasty (dilated segment is between the arrowheads). Right: Control angiogram obtained 12 months later in the same region (small arrowheads) demonstrates a short-segment 80% restenosis (large arrowhead).

committee monitoring data safety halted the trial before its completion.

A poor long-term patency rate after PTA of longer femoropopliteal lesions was repeatedly reported (1–5), and complex and longer areas of stenosis may have a 6-month patency rate as low as 23% (2). This well-known problem of late restenosis—occurring mainly within the first months after the intervention—constitutes the most important problem after successful angioplasty. Pharmacologic interventions have not decreased this restenosis rate (6), and in the femoropopliteal region newer interventional devices have not improved the long-term results (7–9). Therefore, angioplasty is not generally accepted for treatment of longer (>10 cm) femoropopliteal lesions by many interventional radiologists and especially by vascular surgeons, despite the increasing primary success rates due to experience and technical improvements (29,30).

Our study group consisted of patients at particular risk of restenosis because they have had at least one previous episode of restenosis. Morin et al (31) reported that angioplasty for recurrence after previous PTA has a further reduced long-term success rate, and—for all combinations of statistically significant variables—those patients who had previously undergone PTA had an approximately 20% lower long-term patency rate. Treiman et al (32) reported that recurrent femoral and popliteal stenoses treated with balloon angioplasty have a poor prognosis with a 1-year patency rate of 41% and a 3-year patency rate of only 11%. In contrast to a mean lesion length of 16 cm in our study, the lesion lengths in their study were mainly 1–5 cm. Therefore, they concluded that repeat PTA should be reserved for patients with limited life expectancy or with contraindications for surgery (32).

Considering the negative selection of patients with a high risk of restenosis, the results of our pilot study are promising with regard to the possibility of reduction of restenosis by means of endovascular brachytherapy after long-segment femoropopliteal PTA without stent implantation. However, we could not prevent restenosis in four of 10 patients. Restenosis in our study could be explained by different exposures of the vascular wall to the applied dose owing to a possible eccentric position of the source. Otherwise, the prescribed reference dose of 12 Gy could have been too low for inhibiting neointimal hyperplasia. The major problem facing intraluminal irradiation in peripheral vessels is the difficulty in delivering a uniform dose to the target tissue in large-diameter vessels owing to, to our knowledge, a current lack of good centering devices. The catheter can deviate from the ideal central position because of the configuration of the plaque material and the course of the vessel. Such poor centering of the source within the arterial lumen precludes homogeneous intramural dose delivery, which may result in areas of both relative underdosage and overdosage with respect to the prescribed dose. However, source centering for γ emitters, such as Ir-192, is not as critical as it is for β emitters. Böttcher et al (17), using a similar device as that used in our study, calculated that the dose applied to the vessel wall was 8–28 Gy.

New catheters with centering capability have been designed and will be used for this application in future clinical trials. However, even if the source is perfectly centered, dose asymmetries will result if the artery is not cylindric—as it often is not after angioplasty—or if irradiation is performed on a curved segment of artery.

A possible limitation of our study might be the surprisingly low number of patients with diabetes mellitus (two of 10 patients) and of smokers (three of 10 patients) in our study group of consecutive patients. While smoking was not related to long-term patency after femoropopliteal angioplasty in one of our previous studies (5), diabetes might negatively influence patency (1,3,5).

The antithrombotic regimen used in this study is part of our routine periinterventional pharmacotherapy. It proved useful in preventing early rethrombosis (33). Because of the proved efficacy of alprostadil in patients with critical limb ischemia (34) and because of its possible positive effect on early reocclusion (35), this drug has also been integrated into the routine periinterventional treatment in our department. However, we do not think that this intense periinterventional pharmacotherapy had any influence on our results, since none of these drugs has any proved effect on long-term patency (6).

Brachytherapy for the prevention of restenosis after angioplasty is still in its early stage, and there are still many issues to be resolved—such as the best radiation source, optimal dosing, and the most effective delivery method. Hall et al (36) have raised the question of whether irradiation might delay the restenosis kinetics. Therefore, it is important to have long-term follow-up.

In conclusion, γ irradiation with Ir-192 seems promising for the prevention of restenosis after femoropopliteal angioplasty without stent implantation. However, only randomized clinical studies can be used to definitively determine the value of this approach.

References

1. Gallino A, Mahler F, Probst P, Nachbur B. Percutaneous transluminal angioplasty of the arteries of the lower limbs: a 5-year follow-up. Circulation 1984; 70:619–623.
2. Murray RR Jr, Hewes RC, White RI Jr, et al. Long-segment femoropopliteal stenoses: is angioplasty a boon or a bust? Radiology 1987; 162:473–476.
3. Capek P, McLean GK, Berkowitz HD. Femoropopliteal angioplasty: factors influencing long-term success. Circulation 1991; 83(suppl 1):70–80.
4. Johnston KW. Femoral and popliteal arteries: reanalysis of results of balloon angioplasty. Radiology 1992; 183:767–771.
5. Minar E, Ahmadi A, Koppensteiner R, et al. Comparison of effects of high-dose and low-dose aspirin on restenosis after femoropopliteal percutaneous transluminal angioplasty. Circulation 1995; 91:2167–2173.
6. Boger RH, Bode-Boger SM, Alfke H. Restenosis after percutaneous transluminal angioplasty. II. Possibilities for pharmacologic intervention. Vasa 1996; 25:21–31.
7. Gray BH, Sullivan TM, Childs MB, Young JR, Olin JW. High incidence of restenosis/reocclusion of stents in the percutaneous treatment of long-segment superficial femoral artery disease after suboptimal angioplasty. J Vasc Surg 1997; 25:74–83.
8. Martin EC, Katzen BT, Benenati JF, et al. Multicenter trial of the Wallstent in the iliac and femoral arteries. JVIR 1995; 6:843–849.
9. Do DD, Triller J, Walpoth BH, Stirnemann P, Mahler F. A comparison study of self-expandable stents vs balloon angioplasty alone in femoropopliteal artery occlusions. Cardiovasc Intervent Radiol 1992; 15:306–312.
10. Falk E, Nobuyoshi M. Differences between atherosclerosis and restenosis. In: Fuster V, Ross R, Topol EJ, eds. Atherosclerosis and coronary artery disease. Philadelphia, Pa: Lippincott-Raven, 1996; 683–700.
11. Schwartz SM, Reidy MA. Restenosis: an assessment of factors important in arterial occlusion. In: Fuster V, Ross R, Topol EJ, eds. Atherosclerosis and coronary artery disease. Philadelphia, Pa: Lippincott-Raven, 1996; 701–714.
12. Mazur W, Ali NM, Dabaghi SF, et al. High dose rate intracoronary radiation suppresses neointimal proliferation in the stented and ballooned model of porcine restenosis (abstr). Circulation 1994; 90(suppl 1):652.
13. Wiedermann JG, Marboe C, Amols H, Schwartz A, Weinberger J. Intracoronary irradiation markedly reduces restenosis after balloon angioplasty in a porcine model. J Am Coll Cardiol 1994; 23:1491–1498.
14. Verin V, Popowski Y, Urban P, et al. Intraarterial beta irradiation prevents neointimal hyperplasia in a hypercholesterolemic rabbit restenosis model. Circulation 1995; 92:2284–2290.
15. Waksman R, Robinson KA, Crocker IR, Gravanis MB, Cipolla GD, King SB III. Endovascular low-dose irradiation inhibits neointima formation after coronary artery balloon injury in swine: a possible role for radiation therapy in restenosis prevention. Circulation 1995; 91:1533–1539.
16. Teirstein PS, Massullo V, Jani S, et al. Catheter-based radiotherapy to inhibit restenosis after coronary stenting. N Engl J Med 1997; 336:1697–1703.
17. Böttcher HD, Schopohl B, Liermann D, Kollath J, Adamietz IA. Endovascular irradiation: a new method to avoid recurrent stenosis after stent implantation in peripheral arteries—technique and preliminary results. Int J Radiat Oncol Biol Phys 1994; 29:183–186.
18. Rutherford RB. Standards for evaluating results of interventional therapy for peripheral vascular disease. Circulation 1991; 83(suppl 1):6–11.
19. Ranke C, Creutzig A, Alexander K. Duplex scanning of the peripheral arteries: correlation of the peak velocity ratio with angiographic diameter reduction. Ultrasound Med Biol 1992; 18:433–440.
20. Scott NA, Cipolla GD, Ross CE, et al. Identification of a potential role of the adventitia in vascular lesion formation after balloon overstretch injury of porcine coronary arteries. Circulation 1996; 93:2178–2187.
21. Mintz GS, Popma JJ, Pichard AD, et al. Arterial remodeling after coronary angioplasty: a serial intravascular ultrasound study. Circulation 1996; 94:35–43.
22. Wilcox JN, Waksman R, King SB, Scott NA. The role of the adventitia in the arterial response to angioplasty: the effect of intravascular radiation. Int J Radiat Oncol Biol Phys 1996; 36:789–796.
23. Condado JA, Gurdiel O, Espinoza R, et al. Long-term angiographic and clinical outcome following balloon angioplasty and intracoronary radiation therapy in humans (abstr). Circulation 1996; 94(suppl 1):209.
24. Verin V, Urban P, Popowski Y, et al. Feasibility of intracoronary beta-irradiation to reduce restenosis after balloon angioplasty: a clinical pilot study. Circulation 1997; 95:1138–1144.
25. Weinberger J, Amols H, Ennis RD, Schwartz A, Wiedermann JG, Marboe C. Intracoronary irradiation: dose response for the prevention of restenosis in swine. Int J Radiat Oncol Biol Phys 1996; 36:767–775.
26. Wiedermann JG, Marboe C, Amols H, Schwartz A, Weinberger J. Intracoronary irradiation markedly reduces neointimal proliferation after balloon angioplasty in swine: persistent benefit at 6-month follow-up. J Am Coll Cardiol 1995; 25:1451–1456.
27. Liermann DD, Bauernsachs R, Schopohl B, Böttcher HD. Intravascular irradiation therapy. In: Waksman R, King SB, Crocker IR, Mould SF, eds. Vascular brachytherapy. Veenendaal, The Netherlands: Nucletron, 1996; 279–290.
28. Wambersie A, Smeesters P, Fruhling J. Exposure to ionizing radiation: radiobiological effects and pathogenesis. Rev Med Brux 1996; 17:27–38.
29. Morgenstern BR, Getrajdman GI, Laffey KJ, Bixon R, Martin EC. Total occlusions of the femoropopliteal artery: high technical success rate of conventional balloon angioplasty. Radiology 1989; 172:937–940.
30. Murray JG, Apthorp LA, Wilkins RA. Long-segment (>10 cm) femoropopliteal angioplasty: improved technical success and long-term patency. Radiology 1995; 195:158–162.
31. Morin JF, Johnston KW, Wasserman L, Andrews D. Factors that determine the long-term results of percutaneous transluminal dilatation for peripheral arterial occlusive disease. J Vasc Surg 1986; 4:68–72.
32. Treiman GS, Ichikawa L, Treiman RL, et al. Treatment of recurrent femoral and popliteal artery stenosis after percutaneous transluminal angioplasty. J Vasc Surg 1994; 20:577–587.
33. Minar E, Ahmadi RA, Ehringer H, Marosi L, Czembirek H, Konecny U. Percutaneous transluminal angioplasty for iliac and femoropopliteal obstructions. Wien Klin Wochenschr 1986; 98:33–40.
34. European Working Group on Critical Leg Ischaemia. Second European consensus document on chronic critical leg ischemia. Circulation 1991; 84(suppl 4):1-26.
35. See J, Shell W, Matthews O, et al. Prostaglandin E1 infusion after angioplasty in humans inhibits abrupt occlusion and early restenosis. Adv Prostaglandin Thromboxane Leukot Res 1987; 17A:266–270.
36. Hall EJ, Miller RC, Brenner DJ. The basic radiobiology of intravascular irradiation. In: Waksman R, King SB, Crocker IR, Mould SF, eds. Vascular brachytherapy. Veenendaal, The Netherlands: Nucletron, 1996; 55–65.

Book Review

Radiotherapy of Ocular Disease

Edited by T. Wiegel, N. Bornfeld, M. H. Foerster, and W. Hinkelbein
Vol 30 in Frontiers of Radiation Therapy and Oncology series
Basel, Switzerland: S. Karger, 1997. ISBN 3-8055-6392-2.
Hardcover, $191.50; pp 310; 86 figures; tables.

Radiotherapy of Ocular Disease is the 30th volume of the long-running *Frontiers of Radiation Therapy and Oncology* series. It presents the results of the First International Symposium on Special Aspects of Radiotherapy held in Berlin, Germany, in May 1996. The four editors represent the fields of ophthalmology and radiation therapy. The majority of the 140 contributors are from institutions in Germany, with other contributors from the United States, Great Britain, Ireland, Hungary, and Switzerland. Thirty-one of the 34 chapters are multiauthored, and the contributors are well known in the fields of ophthalmologic oncology and radiation oncology. By bringing together so many contributors with special expertise, the editors achieve their goal of providing current information to the radiation therapy and ophthalmologic communities that will help them improve the results of treatment of ocular diseases with irradiation.

The book is divided into 11 sections and includes a thorough introduction. The diagnostic imaging section includes two chapters on magnetic resonance imaging, and the section on radiation therapy options includes four chapters that cover eye plaques and stereotactic irradiation—both linear accelerator and gamma knife. The treatment of retinoblastoma is discussed thoroughly by authors from four major centers, who provide an overview of treatment strategies, precision megavoltage external-beam irradiation, lens-sparing techniques, and chemoradiation therapy. Six chapters are devoted to uveal and conjunctival melanoma and two to choroidal metastases. Four chapters are devoted to orbital lymphomas and three to endocrine ophthalmopathy. The use of low-dose irradiation for age-related macular degeneration is presented in four chapters. Single chapters address postoperative irradiation for pterygia, hemangiomas of the choroid and retina, acute and late effects of irradiation, and side effects of proton-beam irradiation for melanoma. Surprisingly, rhabdomyosarcoma of the orbit was not discussed.

The editors have done a very good job of translating the original German text into very readable English and minimizing overlap, especially with regard to background information in various chapters. They provide an author index and an excellent subject index.

The treatment of ophthalmologic diseases with irradiation is a small but important part of radiation oncology and ophthalmology. There are few books that address this topic, and those physicians who employ radiation therapy in the treatment of ophthalmologic diseases are largely dependent on journal publications. In addition, most of these physicians gain experience and write about special topics such as benign diseases versus malignancies, adult malignancies versus those in children, brachytherapy techniques versus external-beam irradiation, and photon irradiation versus proton-beam irradiation. It is unusual for any one radiation oncologist to have extensive experience with each disease for which irradiation is employed. By combining up-to-date reviews of so many aspects of radiation therapy for ocular disease in a single volume, the editors have provided a great service to the community of radiation oncologists and ophthalmologists, to whom this volume is highly recommended. It should also be on the shelves of all radiation therapy and ophthalmology libraries as a source of information for practitioners and trainees, who will only occasionally see such patients.

Reviewed by Robert H. Sagerman, MD

Perry M. Gould, MD
James A. Bonner, MD
Timothy E. Sawyer, MD
Claude Deschamps, MD
Carla M. Lange, BS
Hongzhe Li, PhD

Bronchial Carcinoid Tumors: Importance of Prognostic Factors That Influence Patterns of Recurrence and Overall Survival[1]

Index terms:
Bronchi, neoplasms, 60.3111
Bronchi, therapeutic radiology, 60.3111
Lung neoplasms, therapeutic radiology, 60.3111

Radiology 1998; 208:181–185

[1] From the Division of Radiation Oncology (P.M.G., J.A.B., T.E.S.), Section of General Thoracic Surgery (C.D.), and Section of Biostatistics (C.M.L., H.L.), Mayo Clinic and Mayo Foundation, 200 First St SW, Rochester, MN 55905.
From the 1997 RSNA scientific assembly. Received December 18, 1997; accepted March 4, 1998.
Address reprint requests to J.A.B., Department of Radiation Oncology, University of Alabama in Birmingham, 619 S 19th St, WTI-105, Birmingham, AL 35233-6832.

PURPOSE: To analyze bronchial carcinoid characteristics that might influence patterns of disease recurrence and overall survival in patients with these tumors.

MATERIALS AND METHODS: In a retrospective review, the actuarial rates of local relapse, regional relapse, and overall survival were determined in patients who had undergone resection of bronchial carcinoid tumors. The evaluable files for 87 patients (50 male, 37 female; age range, 15–82 years) who underwent resection of bronchial carcinoid cancer at the authors' institution between 1980 and 1993 were reviewed for pathologic findings, extent of disease, and recurrence patterns after surgery.

RESULTS: The actuarial 4-year overall survival, local control, and regional control rates in the entire cohort of patients were 89%, 92%, and 94%, respectively. Univariate analyses revealed that an atypical histologic pattern was the only tumor-related factor that substantially affected local and regional control. Atypical histologic pattern and tumor size were among the multiple factors that independently affected overall survival.

CONCLUSION: Atypical histologic findings in patients who had undergone complete resection of bronchial carcinoid tumors were associated with increased local-regional disease recurrence and decreased survival compared with recurrence and survival in patients with typical histologic findings.

The patterns of recurrence and the clinical course in patients after resection of bronchial carcinoid tumors are not well defined, primarily because these tumors are rare. Fewer than 5% of patients with a primary thoracic neoplasm have had a histologic diagnosis of carcinoid tumor (1–3). In addition, although bronchial carcinoid tumors have a neuroectodermal stem cell in common with small-cell lung cancer (4–7), the potential for pulmonary malignancy arises from Kulchitsky cells within the bronchial tree.

Even though our understanding of the basic histologic features of this cancer has increased, much disagreement still exists with regard to what influence certain potential prognostic clinical and pathologic characteristics have on various patient outcomes (8–11). In most series (6,12–15) reported on, nodal involvement was associated with a worse outcome. The 5-year overall survival rates were 13%–59% in patients with nodal involvement but were 95%–98% in patients without nodal involvement. The influence of an atypical histologic pattern on patient outcome has also been a source of controversy. Barberis et al (13) found that patients who had bronchial carcinoid tumors with an atypical histologic appearance had a 5-year overall survival rate of 83%, which is similar to that in patients who had bronchial carcinoid tumors with a typical histologic appearance. Others (6,12,14–17), however, noted that the outcome was worse in patients with atypical histologic findings.

In the present study, we analyzed the patterns of disease recurrence and of long-term outcome in 87 patients after resection of localized bronchial carcinoid tumors. Because the

Author contributions:
Guarantors of integrity of entire study, P.M.G., J.A.B., T.E.S.; study concepts, P.M.G., J.A.B., T.E.S.; study design, P.M.G., J.A.B., T.E.S., C.M.L., H.L., C.D.; definition of intellectual content, P.M.G., J.A.B., T.E.S., C.D., C.M.L., H.L.; literature research, P.M.G., J.A.B.; clinical studies, P.M.G., J.A.B.; data acquisition, P.M.G., T.E.S.; data analysis, P.M.G., J.A.B., C.M.L., H.L.; statistical analysis, C.M.L., H.L.; manuscript preparation, editing, and review, P.M.G., J.A.B., T.E.S., C.D., C.M.L., H.L.

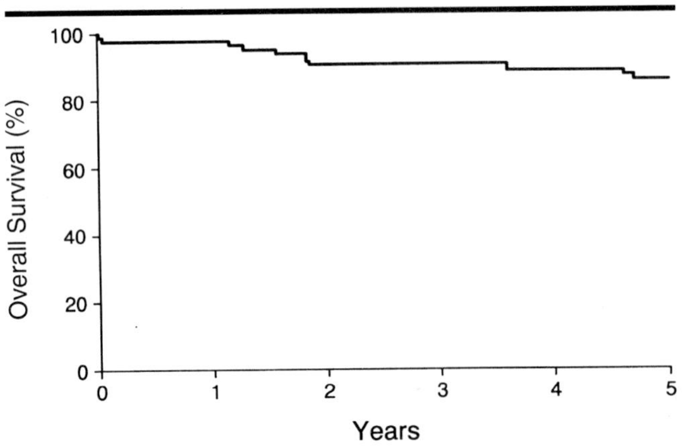

Figure 1. Graph of the actuarial overall survival rate versus years for the entire group of patients with bronchial carcinoid tumors (n = 87).

TABLE 1
Pretreatment Evaluation of Thoracic Tumors in 87 Patients

Pretreatment Study	No. of Patients
Chest radiography	87 (100)
Computed tomography of the chest and upper abdomen	42 (48)
Bronchoscopy	47 (54)
Mediastinoscopy	10 (11)

Note.—The numbers in parentheses are percentages.

TABLE 2
Tumor Characteristics in 87 Patients Who Underwent Complete Resection of Bronchial Carcinoid Tumors

Tumor Characteristic	No. of Patients*
Tumor size†	
≤3 cm	61 (70)
>3 cm	25 (29)
Unknown	1 (1)
Histologic findings	
Typical	64 (74)
Atypical	23 (26)
Nodal disease status	
Positive	23 (26)
Negative	64 (74)

* The numbers in parentheses are percentages.
† Size range, 0.1–12.0 cm; mean size ± Standard deviation, 2.5 cm ± 1.8.

factors affecting prognosis varied in previous reports, an effort was made to better define the influence of various tumor and patient characteristics that may alter patterns of recurrence and overall survival in these patients. A better understanding of the biologic characteristics of these tumors may lead to an improved ability to determine which patients may benefit from various possible surgical adjuvant treatments. This study was performed to analyze bronchial carcinoid characteristics that might influence recurrence of disease and overall survival in patients with these tumors.

MATERIALS AND METHODS

The medical records of all patients who underwent thoracotomy for lung cancer at the authors' institution between January 1, 1980, and December 31, 1993, were reviewed to identify the patients who had been treated for bronchial carcinoid tumor. Eighty-seven patients (50 male, 37 female; age range, 15–82 years; mean age ± standard deviation, 55 years ± 17) who had undergone complete resection of a histologically confirmed bronchial carcinoid tumor during this period were the subjects of this review. The following entities resulted in exclusion from the study: distant metastasis, residual disease after resection, and synchronous primary tumors. Surgical specimens were examined by pathologists in all cases. In addition, the records of these patients were analyzed for the following potential prognostic factors: tumor size, histologic findings (atypical, typical, or spindling), N2 nodal disease, and the presence of any regional nodal disease.

The pretreatment evaluation generally included a review of the patient history, a physical examination, a complete blood cell count, liver function tests, and a chest radiographic examination (Table 1). Other examinations, such as bronchoscopy, were performed if indicated.

Of the 87 patients with evaluable records who underwent complete resection, nine (10%) underwent resection of less than one lobe, six (7%) underwent pneumonectomy, 12 (14%) underwent bilobectomy, and 60 (69%) underwent lobectomy. All patients underwent complete mediastinal, hilar, and interlobar lymphadenectomy during surgery for staging purposes. No patient received adjuvant therapy.

The patterns of disease recurrence were assessed. Local recurrence was defined as tumor recurrence within the original tumor bed. Regional recurrence was defined as tumor recurrence within the ipsilateral hilum, mediastinum, or supraclavicular regions. Recurrences beyond these sites were deemed distant recurrences. The evaluated end points were freedom from local recurrence, freedom from regional recurrence, freedom from distant recurrence, disease-specific survival, and overall survival. The time to recurrence or death was measured from the date of surgical resection.

All survival distributions were estimated by using the actuarial Kaplan-Meier method (18), and the actuarial curves were compared by using the log-rank test (19). Multivariate analyses were performed by using the Cox proportional hazards model.

RESULTS

The tumor characteristics are outlined in Table 2. The median length of follow-up in the living patients at this analysis was 8.4 years. Of particular note is that 23 of the 87 patients had atypical bronchial carcinoid histologic findings and that the remainder of patients had typical histologic findings. Of the 23 patients with atypical histologic findings, 11 (48%) had regional nodal disease at thoracotomy. Twelve (19%) of the 64 patients with typical histologic findings had findings positive for nodal disease. Eight of the 23 patients with lymph node involvement had N2 nodal disease.

The actuarial 4-year overall survival rate for the entire group was 89% (Fig 1). The actuarial 4-year rate of freedom from local recurrence was 92%. The actuarial 4-year rate of freedom from regional recurrence and rate of freedom from distant recurrence were 94% and 96%, respectively.

The recurrence rates and salvage treatments in 13 patients are summarized in Table 3. In general, recurrent disease was difficult to control. Five patients received radiation therapy as a component of treatment for recurrent disease, and, in two of

TABLE 3
Recurrence and Salvage Treatment in 13 Patients after Resection of Bronchial Carcinoid Tumors

	Initial Disease					Recurrence				
Patient No.	Size of Tumor (cm)	Histologic Finding	Nodal Involvement	Initial Treatment	Diagnosis Date	Local	Regional	Distant	Salvage Treatment	Result
1	1.2	Typical	N0	Lobectomy	1/83	. . .	8/88, Ipsilateral hilum	. . .	Surgery	7/90, AWD
2	2.2	Typical	N0	Lobectomy	11/84	9/92, Lung	. . .	5/92, Bone and liver	Laser	10/95, AWD
3	1.2	Typical	N0	Lobectomy	11/87	. . .	10/91, Ipsilateral hilum	. . .	Surgery	9/95, AWOD
4	1.5	Atypical	N0	Segmentectomy	9/89	. . .	10/91, Contralateral hilum	. . .	Surgery	1/92, AWD
5	3.5	Typical	N0	Bilobectomy	7/88	. . .	9/90, Mediastinum and hilum	10/92, Diaphragm	RT and chemotherapy	12/93, AWD
6	0.4	Typical	N0	Lobectomy	6/92	7/94, Lung	. . .	7/94, Lung	Chemotherapy	12/95, AWD
7	3.5	Atypical	N1	Lobectomy	7/93	8/94, Beneath thoracotomy scar	. . .	. . .	RT	12/94, AWOD
8	7.0	Atypical	N2	Pneumonectomy	1/86	1/87, Lung	. . .	. . .	Supportive	8/87, DOD
9	1.5	Typical	N2	Pneumonectomy	5/86	. . .	3/91, Mediastinum	8/93, Lung and liver	Supportive	11/94, DOD
10	1.7	Atypical	N2	Pneumonectomy	8/87	8/92, Lung	8/92, Mediastinum	. . .	RT	4/93, DOD
11	1.5	Atypical	N0	Lobectomy	1/84	. . .	. . .	7/94, Bone	Chemotherapy	4/96, AWD
12	4.0	Atypical	N0	Lobectomy	9/88	. . .	. . .	1/89, Brain	RT	10/89, DOD
13	3.5	Atypical	N1	Pneumonectomy	7/90	. . .	. . .	10/90, Bone	RT	4/92, DOD

Note.—RT = radiation therapy, AWD = alive with disease, AWOD = alive without disease, DOD = died of disease.

these patients, radiation therapy was administered for a local-regional recurrence without distant metastasis. One of these patients was free of disease at 3 months after treatment of a recurrence at the previous thoracotomy scar (Table 3).

When the incidence of local recurrence was assessed in relation to tumor-related factors, an atypical histologic appearance was the only factor associated with increased local recurrence (Fig 2). Of the 64 patients with typical histologic findings, 60 (94%) were free of local recurrence at 4 years, whereas only 19 (83%) of the 23 patients with atypical bronchial carcinoid tumor findings were free of local recurrence. Neither the size of the primary lesion nor the nodal status adversely affected local control.

These same features were also assessed in relation to their effects on regional control. Again, the only factor that significantly contributed to regional disease recurrence was atypical histologic appearance (P = .003). One (2%) of the 64 patients with typical bronchial carcinoid tumors had regional disease recurrence at 4 years compared with four (17%) of the 23 patients with atypical tumors (Fig 3).

Although tumor size and regional nodal disease at thoracotomy did not adversely influence local or regional disease-free survival, these factors, along with atypical histologic findings, did affect the 4-year overall survival rate (Table 4). In fact, multivariate analysis revealed that tumors larger than 3 cm, N2 involvement, and atypical histologic findings all were independently associated with diminished overall survival.

DISCUSSION

Previous studies attempted to identify tumor and patient characteristics that influence patterns of recurrence (14,15,20,21) and overall survival (13–16,21,22) in patients who have undergone resection of bronchial carcinoid tumors. However, these studies showed conflicting results with regard to the influence potential prognostic factors such as tumor size, tumor histologic findings, and nodal involvement have on the study end points. The goal of the analyses we performed to identify the clinical and pathologic characteristics associated with patterns of recurrence and outcome in patients with bronchial carcinoid cancer was to find out whether certain subpopulations of patients are candidates for the investigation of various possible adjuvant surgical treatments.

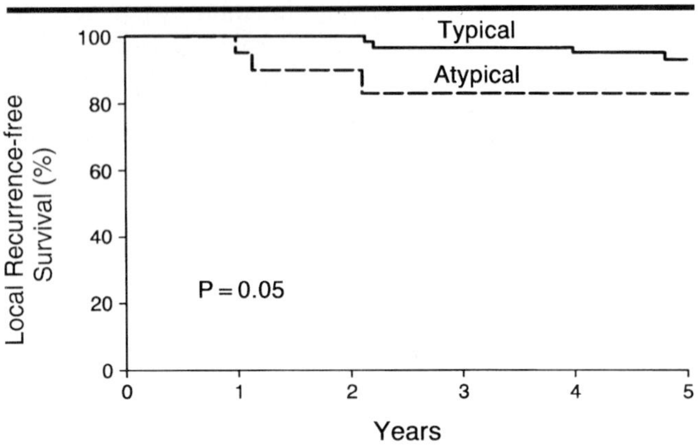

Figure 2. Graph of the local recurrence-free survival rate versus years in patients with typical and in patients with atypical histologic findings. Local control was substantially diminished in patients with atypical histologic findings.

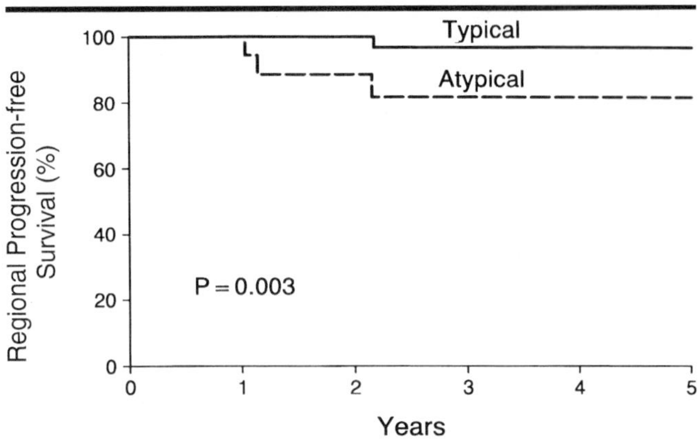

Figure 3. Graph of regional progression-free survival rate versus years in patients with typical and in patients with atypical histologic findings. Regional control was substantially diminished in patients with atypical histologic findings.

Our study results showed that patients with bronchial carcinoid tumors have a favorable outcome; this corroborates the work of others (13–16,21,22). The 4-year actuarial overall survival rate in patients in this study was 89%. There were relatively few recurrences, and 92%, 94%, and 96% of patients were free of local, regional, and distant recurrences, respectively, at 4 years.

The association between tumor size and outcome was assessed in this study. Some previous studies (6,15) have suggested that size does not adversely affect outcome. However, McCaughan et al (6) demonstrated a significantly increased recurrence rate in patients with tumors larger than 3 cm. In the present series, patients with primary tumors larger than 3 cm had a trend (P = .080) toward increased distant recurrence and a significant reduction in disease-specific and overall survival rates (P = .030 and P = .004, respectively). The overall survival rate at 4 years was 96% for patients with tumors smaller than 3 cm but only 69% for those with tumors larger than 3 cm.

TABLE 4
Factors Influencing 4-Year Overall Survival after Resection of Bronchial Carcinoid Tumors

Factor	4-Year Overall Survival Rate (%)	*P* Value*: Univariate Analysis	*P* Value*: Multivariate Analysis
Tumor size			
≤3 cm	96	.004	.010
>3 cm	69		
Histologic findings			
Typical	95	<.001	.001
Atypical	70		
Nodal disease status			
Negative	91	.030	>.050
Positive	80		

* Univariate analyses were performed by using the actuarial Kaplan-Meier method, and multivariate analyses were performed by using the Cox proportional hazards model.

Another area of controversy has been the effect of regional nodal involvement on recurrence and survival rates. Most reviews (6,12–15) have shown a correlation between regional nodal disease (at initial resection) and reduced overall survival. For example, Torre et al (15) found that the 5-year rate of overall survival was 97.6% in patients without nodal metastasis and 43% in those with nodal metastasis. Other authors (23,24), however, did not find this association between nodal involvement and survival. In our cohort of patients, initial nodal involvement did not significantly alter patterns of recurrence, although there was a trend toward increased regional disease recurrence after surgery (P = .100). Regional disease recurrence was noted in 10% of patients with lymph node involvement and in 4% of patients without such involvement. Nevertheless, nodal disease was associated with reduced outcome in these patients. The 4-year overall survival rate was 91% in patients without nodal metastasis compared with 80% in patients with nodal metastasis (P = .030).

Historically, the histologic subtype of bronchial carcinoid tumors has been considered to have the greatest effect on how well patients do after thoracotomy. Although a few previous studies (13,25) showed relatively good outcomes in patients with atypical tumors, many (6,12,14–17) noted reduced survival, with 11%–59% of patients alive at 5 years. In addition, atypical bronchial carcinoid cancer may have a propensity for metastasis to regional lymph nodes at presentation (6,14,15). This characteristic of atypical tumors was also found in the present review; 11 of 23 patients with atypical tumors but only 12 of 64 patients with typical tumors had nodal involvement at thoracotomy. Furthermore, atypical histologic findings substantially influenced both local and regional recurrence patterns. Seventeen percent of patients with atypical bronchial carcinoid tumors had local recurrence (4-year actuarial recurrence rate) compared with 3% of patients with typical tumors. The 4-year regional recurrence rate was 17% in patients with atypical bronchial carcinoid tumors and 2% in patients with typical bronchial carcinoid tumors. These increased rates of recurrence contributed to the lower 4-year overall survival rate in patients with atypical histologic findings (70%) compared with this rate in patients with typical tumors (95%).

In conclusion, atypical histologic findings were associated with higher rates of local recurrence and of regional recurrence than were typical histologic findings in this group of patients with bronchial carcinoid tumors. The patients with atypical tumors also had lower survival rates than did the patients with typical tumors. These results suggest that future investigations should explore the use of adjuvant local-regional irradiation in patients with atypical histologic findings. Although radiation therapy was used in too few patients to make any conclusion about its efficacy in this study, radiation therapy has been used in patients with nonresectable disease, and some responses have been noted in this group of patients with poor prognosis. For instance, Abrams et al (26) reported that 54% of malignant carcinoid tumors and the nonresectable or residual bronchial carcinoid disease in two of three patients had objective responses to local radiation therapy. Therefore, in patients with atypical histologic findings, who are most likely to have local-regional recurrence, local radiation therapy may be of benefit as an adjuvant treatment.

References

1. Churg A, Warnock ML. Pulmonary tumorlet: a form of peripheral carcinoid. Cancer 1976; 37:1469–1477.
2. Churg A. Large spindle cell variant of peripheral bronchial carcinoid tumor. Arch Pathol Lab Med 1977; 101:216–218.
3. Davila DG, Dunn WF, Tazelaar HD, Pairolero PC. Bronchial carcinoid tumors. Mayo Clin Proc 1993; 68:795–803.
4. Broers JL, Mijnheere EP, Rot MK, et al. Novel antigens characteristic of neuroendocrine malignancies. Cancer 1991; 67:619–633.
5. Gillespie JJ, Luger AM, Callaway LA. Peripheral spindled carcinoid tumor: a review of its ultrastructure, differential diagnosis, and biologic behavior. Hum Pathol 1979; 10:601–606.
6. McCaughan BC, Martini N, Bains MS. Bronchial carcinoids: review of 124 cases. J Thorac Cardiovasc Surg 1985; 89:8–17.
7. Warren WH, Gould VE, Faber LP, Kittle CF, Memoli VA. Neuroendocrine neoplasms of the bronchopulmonary tract: a classification of the spectrum of carcinoid to small cell carcinoma and intervening variants. J Thorac Cardiovasc Surg 1985; 89:819–825.
8. Greenberg RS, Baumgarten DA, Clark WS, Isacson P, McKeen K. Prognostic factors for gastrointestinal and bronchopulmonary carcinoid tumors. Cancer 1987; 60: 2476–2483.
9. Lequaglie C, Patriarca C, Cataldo I, Muscolino G, Preda F, Ravasi G. Prognosis of resected well-differentiated neuroendocrine carcinoma of the lung. Chest 1991; 100:1053–1056.
10. Okike N, Bernatz PE, Woolner LB. Carcinoid tumors of the lung. Ann Thorac Surg 1976; 22:270–277.
11. Vadasz P, Palffy G, Egervary M, Schaff Z. Diagnosis and treatment of bronchial carcinoid tumors: clinical and pathological review of 120 operated patients. Eur J Cardiothorac Surg 1993; 7:8–11.
12. Attar S, Miller JE, Hankins J, et al. Bronchial adenoma: a review of 51 patients. Ann Thorac Surg 1985; 40:126–132.
13. Barberis M, Valagussa E, Pieri Nerli F, Torre M, Borghini U. Carcinoid tumors of the lung: report of 66 cases. Pathologica 1983; 75:803–811.
14. Mills SE, Cooper PH, Walker AN, Kron IL. Atypical carcinoid tumor of the lung: a clinicopathologic study of 17 cases. Am J Surg Pathol 1982; 6:643–654.
15. Torre M, Barberis M, Barbieri B, Bonacina E, Belloni P. Typical and atypical bronchial carcinoids. Respir Med 1989; 83:305–308.
16. Akiba T, Naruke T, Kondo H, et al. Carcinoid tumor of the lung: clinicopathological study of 32 cases. Jpn J Clin Oncol 1992; 22:92–95.
17. Arrigoni MG, Woolner LB, Bernatz PE. Atypical carcinoid tumors of the lung. J Thorac Cardiovasc Surg 1972; 64:413–421.
18. Kaplan E, Meier P. Nonparametric estimation from incomplete observations. J Am Stat Assoc 1958; 53:457–481.
19. Mantel N. Evaluation of survival data and two new rank order statistics arising in its consideration. Cancer Chemother Rep 1966; 50:163–170.
20. Breederveld RS, Meijer S, Thunnissen FB, Stam J. Surgical treatment of bronchopulmonary carcinoid tumours. Neth J Surg 1989; 41:82–84.
21. Toledo J, Roca R, Anton JA, Martin de Nicolas JL, Varela G, Yuste P. Conservative and bronchoplastic resection for bronchial carcinoid tumours. Eur J Cardiothorac Surg 1989; 3:288–291.
22. Blondal T, Grimelius L, Nou E, Wilander E, Aberg T. Argyrophil carcinoid tumors of the lung: incidence, clinical study, and follow-up of 46 patients. Chest 1980; 78:840–844.
23. Brandt B III, Heintz SE, Rose EF, Ehrenhaft JL. Bronchial carcinoid tumors. Ann Thorac Surg 1984; 38:63–65.
24. Goldstraw P, Lamb D, McCormack RJ, Walbaum PR. The malignancy of bronchial adenoma. J Thorac Cardiovasc Surg 1976; 72:309–314.
25. Smith RA. Bronchial carcinoid tumours. Thorax 1969; 24:43–50.
26. Abrams RA, King D, Wilson JF. Objective response of malignant carcinoid to radiation therapy. Int J Radiat Oncol Biol Phys 1987; 13:869–873.

Jae-Woo Song, MD
Jung-Gi Im, MD
Young-Soo Shim, MD
Jae Hyung Park, MD
Kyung Mo Yeon, MD
Man Chung Han, MD

Index terms:
Arteries, bronchial, 569.79, 569.92
Bronchi, CT, 60.12111, 60.12115, 60.12116, 60.12118, 67.12111, 67.12115, 67.12116, 67.12118
Bronchiectasis, 60.26, 67.26
Computed tomography (CT), angiography, 56.12115, 56.12116

Radiology 1998; 208:187–191

[1] From the Department of Radiology, Seoul National University College of Medicine, and the Institute of Radiation Medicine, 28 Yongon-dong, Chongro-gu, Seoul 110-744, South Korea. Received September 23, 1997; revision requested November 25; revision received February 9, 1998; accepted March 10. J.G.I. was supported in part by grant 2-97-182 from the Seoul National University Hospital. **Address reprint requests to** J.G.I.

Author contributions:
Guarantors of integrity of entire study, J.G.I., K.M.Y., M.C.H.; study concepts, J.G.I., J.W.S., Y.S.S.; study design, J.G.I., Y.S.S., J.W.S.; definition of intellectual content, J.W.S., J.G.I., Y.S.S., J.H.P., K.M.Y., M.C.H.; literature research, J.W.S.; clinical studies, J.W.S., J.G.I., Y.S.S.; data acquisition, J.W.S.; data analysis, J.W.S., J.G.I.; manuscript preparation, J.W.S.; manuscript editing, J.W.S., J.G.I.; manuscript review, J.W.S., J.G.I., Y.S.S., J.H.P., K.M.Y., M.C.H.

Hypertrophied Bronchial Artery at Thin-Section CT in Patients with Bronchiectasis: Correlation with CT Angiographic Findings[1]

PURPOSE: To evaluate hypertrophied bronchial arteries on thin-section computed tomographic (CT) scans in patients with bronchiectasis by using CT angiographic correlation.

MATERIALS AND METHODS: Spiral CT angiography was performed prospectively in 14 patients (eight men, six women; age range, 34–71 years) with bronchiectasis who were suspected of having bronchial arterial hypertrophy at thin-section CT (performed without contrast medium). The inclusion criteria were tubular (in six patients) or nodular (in 14 patients) areas of soft-tissue attenuation that had an appearance unlike that of lymph nodes at thin-section CT and that were within the mediastinum and around the central airway. These findings were subsequently correlated with the spiral CT angiographic findings.

RESULTS: At comparative analysis of thin-section CT scans and CT angiograms, seven of the eight (88%) tubular lesions and 19 of the 36 (53%) nodular lesions in the mediastinal soft tissue were proved to be hypertrophied bronchial arteries. All of the six (100%) tubular and 19 of the 21 (90%) nodular lesions around the walls of the main (primary) and lobar bronchi were hypertrophied bronchial arteries. In eight (57%) patients, CT angiograms showed 11 intraluminal protrusions caused by hypertrophied bronchial arteries in the main bronchi, lobar bronchi, or both.

CONCLUSION: Nodular and tubular structures in the mediastinum and around the central airway on thin-section CT scans in the patients with bronchiectasis are suggestive of hypertrophied bronchial arteries. Recognition of the hypertrophied bronchial artery can be critical for the bronchoscopist.

The bronchial artery is the main source of blood for the bronchi. This blood supply normally constitutes 1% of the cardiac output. However, in various disease states, especially in cases of bronchiectasis, blood circulation in the bronchi can increase and represent as much as 30% of cardiac output (1). Enlarged bronchial arteries are commonly demonstrated in patients with bleeding bronchiectasis at bronchial arteriography performed for embolization. There are many articles (2–6) about the evaluation of bronchial arteries with contrast material–enhanced dynamic or spiral computed tomography (CT). However, although thin-section CT has been regarded as the imaging modality of choice in patients suspected of having bronchiectasis (7,8), the appearances of bronchial arteries at thin-section CT have seldom been described in the literature. One possible reason that the presence of an enlarged bronchial artery at thin-section CT has been overlooked is that contrast material is not administered with this imaging modality; thus, enlarged bronchial arteries cannot be differentiated from mediastinal lymph nodes or vessels.

Occasionally, we have encountered nodular or tubular structures within the mediastinal soft tissue and irregular or nodular thickening of the walls of the central airway on thin-section CT scans in patients with bronchiectasis. Assuming that these findings may represent hypertrophied bronchial arteries, we performed this study prospectively. The purpose of this study was to evaluate the hypertrophied bronchial artery on thin-section CT scans in patients with bronchiectasis by using CT angiographic correlation.

MATERIALS AND METHODS

Institutional review board approval and signed informed consent from all patients in our study were obtained. Spiral CT angiography was performed prospectively in 14 patients (eight men, six women; age range, 34–71 years; mean age, 52.5 years) who had bronchiectasis and were suspected of having bronchial arterial hypertrophy at thin-section CT performed without injection of contrast material. The inclusion criteria for suspected bronchial arterial hypertrophy at thin-section CT were tubular (in six patients) or 3–10-mm nodular (in 14 patients) areas of soft-tissue attenuation that were within the mediastinum and around the central airway and that had an appearance unlike that of lymph nodes because of their continuity with tubular shape and some tortuosity on contiguous scans.

In all patients, spiral CT angiography was performed immediately after or within 1 month after thin-section CT. The main clinical indications for performing thin-section CT examinations were to evaluate the cause of hemoptysis, to evaluate suspected bronchiectasis, or both. The main clinical indications for performing spiral CT angiography were hemoptysis and thin-section CT findings suggestive of hypertrophied bronchial arteries. The thin-section CT examination consisted of acquisition of a series of 1-mm–thick sections separated by 10-mm intersection spacing from the apex of the lung to 5 cm below the top of the diaphragm. A Somatom Plus S scanner (Siemens Medical Systems, Erlangen, Germany) was used. After thin-section CT scans were obtained, spiral CT angiography was performed with the same scanner by using the following parameters: 3-mm collimation, a 4-mm/sec table speed, and a 2-mm reconstruction interval. A mixture of 60 mL of ioxaglate meglumine (Rayvist 300, Schering, Berlin, Germany) and 40 mL of normal saline solution was injected at 4 mL/sec by using a power injector (Medrad, Pittsburgh, Pa), and scanning was performed 15 seconds after the start of the bolus injection. The area scanned covered from the top of the aortic arch to the origin of the right middle lobar bronchus. At first, we analyzed the tubular structures with or without some tortuosity within the mediastinal soft tissue and the nodular or tubular structures around the wall of the central airway on thin-section CT scans. Then, we compared and correlated the thin-section CT findings with the CT angiographic findings, with special attention to the thin-section CT findings that were suggestive of hypertrophied bronchial arteries. At spiral CT angiography, the origin, location, relationship with the bronchi, and size of the enlarged bronchial artery were analyzed.

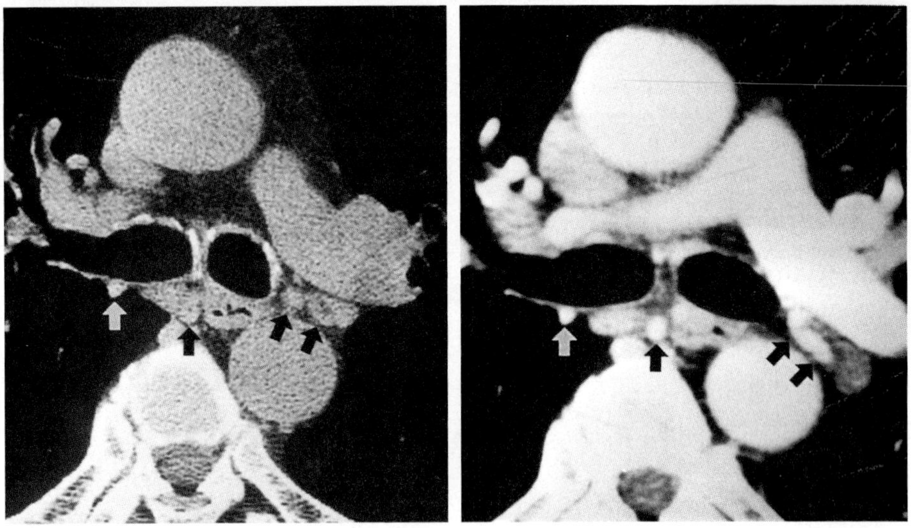

a. b.

Figure 1. Hypertrophied bronchial arteries within the mediastinal soft tissue in the right and left lungs in a 59-year-old man. **(a)** Thin-section CT scan shows tortuous tubular and nodular structures (black arrows in **a** and **b**) within the mediastinal and left perihilar soft tissues. **(b)** CT angiogram shows opaque vascular enhancement of the structures in **a**. We can also see the hypertrophied bronchial artery (white arrow in **a** and **b**) at the posterior wall of the right main bronchus.

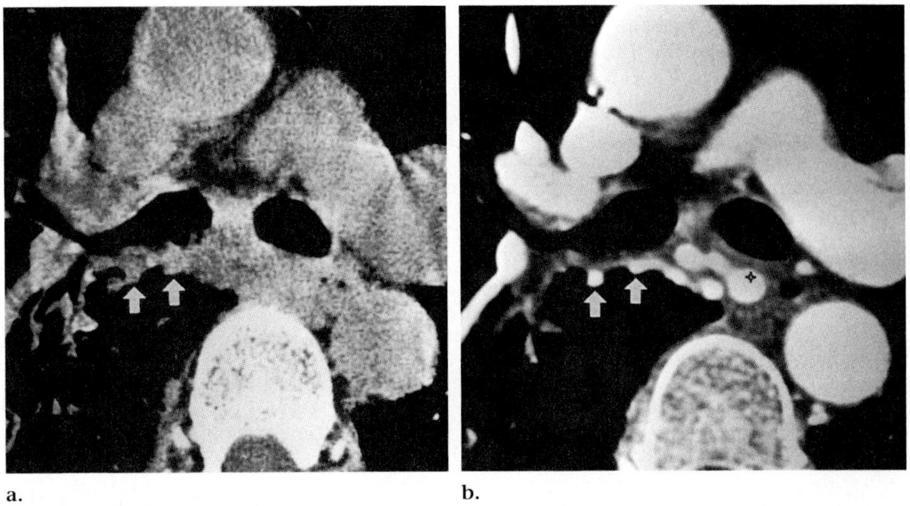

a. b.

Figure 2. Hypertrophied bronchial artery in the right lung near the central airway in a 69-year-old man. **(a)** Thin-section CT scan and **(b)** spiral CT angiogram show vascular-enhancing nodular and tubular structures (arrows) at the posterior wall of the right main bronchus and within the mediastinal soft tissue (cursor).

RESULTS

At comparative analysis of thin-section CT scans and CT angiograms, seven of the eight (88%) tubular lesions and 19 of the 36 (53%) nodular lesions within the mediastinal soft tissue were proved to be hypertrophied bronchial arteries (Fig 1). All of the six (100%)

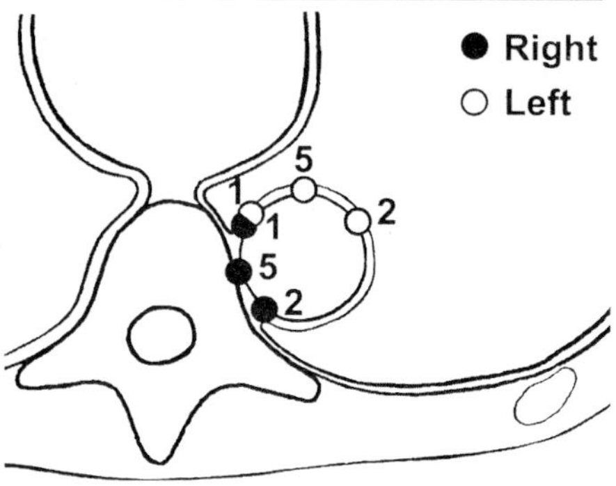

Figure 3. Diagram shows the origins of the bronchial arteries as they appeared on CT angiograms. CT angiography revealed the origin of the bronchial artery in eight patients. The numbers indicate the number of patients with each origin.

Major Locations of Hypertrophied Bronchial Arteries at CT Angiography

Location	No. of Patients (n = 14)
Retroesophageal area	11
Left main bronchus, posterior wall	11
Retrotracheal area	10
Right main bronchus, posterior wall	9
Left main bronchus, aorticopulmonary window	7
Bronchus intermedius, medial wall	6
Bronchus intermedius, posterior wall	5
Left main bronchus, anterior wall	4
Pretracheal area	3
Left main bronchus, lateral wall	3
Right main bronchus, medial wall	2

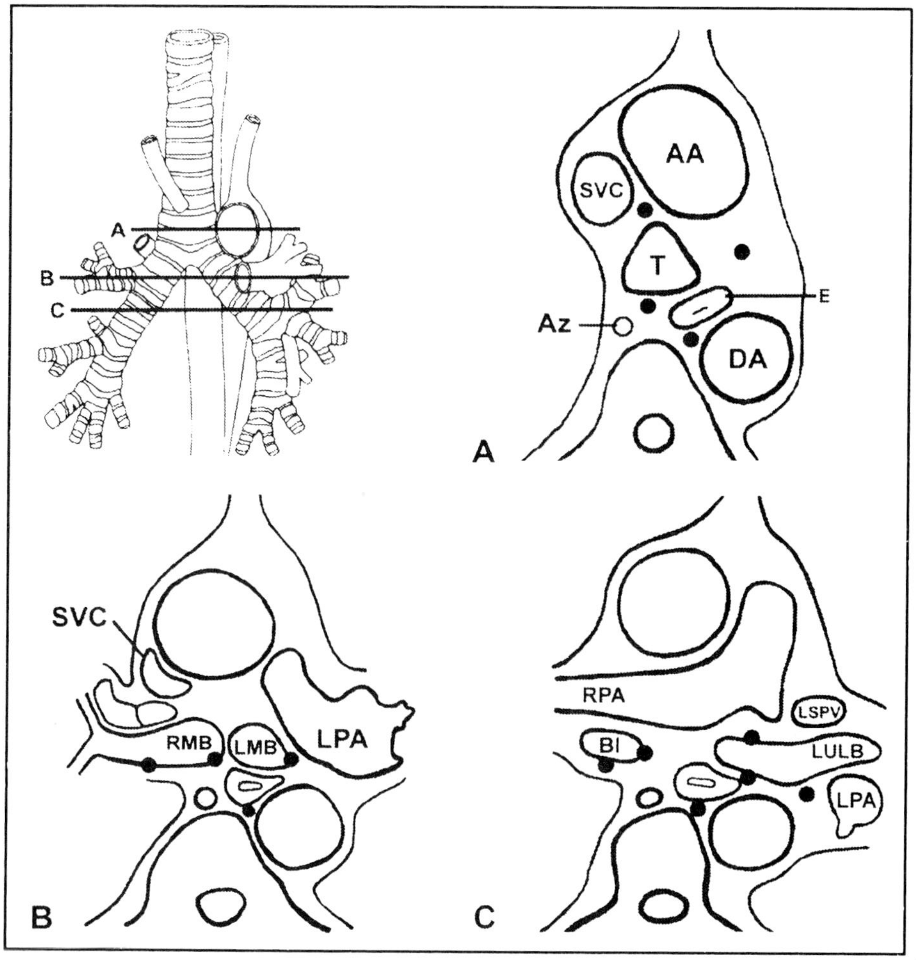

Figure 4. Schematic diagram of the major locations of hypertrophied bronchial arteries on CT angiograms at three levels: *A*, bronchial arteries at the level of the aorticopulmonary window; *B*, bronchial arteries at the level of the right main bronchus; and *C*, bronchial arteries at the level of the bronchus intermedius. The number of patients with bronchial arteries in each location is summarized in the Table. ● = bronchial artery, *AA* = ascending aorta, *Az* = azygos vein, *BI* = bronchus intermedius, *DA* = descending aorta, *E* = esophagus, *LMB* = left main bronchus, *LPA* = left pulmonary artery, *LSPV* = left superior pulmonary vein, *LULB* = left upper lobe bronchus, *RMB* = right main bronchus, *RPA* = right pulmonary artery, *SVC* = superior vena cava, and *T* = trachea.

tubular and 19 of the 21 (90%) nodular lesions around the walls of the main and lobar bronchi were hypertrophied bronchial arteries (Fig 2).

Spiral CT angiography revealed a hypertrophied bronchial artery in all 14 patients and the origin of the bronchial artery in eight patients (57%). The right bronchial artery arose in the medial (n = 5), posteromedial (n = 2), or anteromedial (n = 1) wall of the descending aorta at the level of or slightly lower than the tracheal carina (Fig 3). Hypertrophied right bronchial arteries were frequently found in retroesophageal and retrotracheal areas and in the posterior walls of the right main bronchus and the bronchus intermedius (Fig 4). The left bronchial artery arose at the anterior (n = 5), anterolateral (n = 2), or anteromedial (n = 1) wall of the descending aorta at the level of or slightly higher than the carina (Fig 3). Hypertrophied left bronchial arteries were frequently found in the aorticopulmonary window and the anterior and posterior walls of the left main bronchus (Fig 4). The number of patients with bronchial arteries in each location is summarized in the Table. In eight (57%) patients, highly enhancing intraluminal nodular protrusions, indicating hypertrophied bronchial arteries, were detected in the main bronchi, lobar bronchi, or both (Fig 5).

DISCUSSION

The normal bronchial artery is a small (≤2-mm-diameter) vessel that arises directly from the descending thoracic aorta and supplies blood to the airway up to the level of the nonrespiratory bronchioles, esophagus, and lymph nodes (6). The bronchial arteries become enlarged in various diseases, including acute or chronic pulmonary infections, pulmonary thromboembolism, and chronic obstructive pulmonary disease (9). Enlargement of the bronchial arteries is more prominent in bronchial disease than in bronchiolar or parenchymal lung disease (10). In bronchiectasis, enlargement of the bronchial vessels is associated with the development of granulation tissue during the course of the organizing pneumonitis that usually precedes bronchiectasis and with the metabolic demands of hypertrophied muscle and hypertrophied lymphoid tissue that are often observed (11).

Thin-section CT is the imaging method of choice after standard chest radiography for examining patients suspected of having bronchiectasis (7,8). When we read the thin-section CT scans or conventional contrast-enhanced chest CT scans in patients with bronchiectasis, occasionally we see abnormal tubular structures within the mediastinum that do not look like lymph nodes. We also occasionally see nodular structures around the wall of the central airway that mimic focal thickening of the bronchial wall.

Bronchial wall thickening can be observed in various disease processes such as pulmonary edema, bronchogenic carcinoma, lymphoma, metastasis, and the granulomatous diseases sarcoidosis and tuberculosis (12–15). In bronchiectasis, the bronchial walls may also be thickened with inflammatory cell infiltration and edema (16). As we observed in our cases, bronchial wall thickening in bronchiectasis may also be caused by hypertrophied bronchial arteries. Kim et al (17) also reported on a nodular structure attached to the posterior wall of the bronchus intermedius. This nodular structure was a branch of the pulmonary vein from the posterior segment of the right upper lobe or the superior segment of the right lower lobe.

By considering the normal anatomy and the course of the bronchial artery, we can anticipate the location of hypertrophied bronchial arteries on CT scans. The right intercostal artery-bronchial artery commonly takes an initial vertical or oblique course upward and to the right from the retroesophageal space within the mediastinum after arising from the aorta. The right bronchial artery often makes a hairpin turn at the level of the aortic arch and is directed caudad toward the right hilar area, while an intercostal artery continues its ascent prevertebrally and supplies peripheral branches to the corresponding rib. The left bronchial arteries usually originate from the anterior surface of the thoracic aorta or from the concavity of the aortic arch. Since most of the left bronchial arteries arise from the anterior surface of the aorta immediately behind the left main bronchus, they must pass anteriorly to meet the bronchus (6,18).

In our study, the most common locations of the hypertrophied bronchial artery were the retrotracheal area, the retroesophageal area, and the posterior wall of the main bronchus on the patient's right side and the aorticopulmonary window and the anterior and posterior walls of the main bronchus on the patient's left side (Fig 4). The locations seen in our study were the same as those in the study of Furuse et al (6), in which dynamic CT was performed.

In bronchiectasis or other chronic infectious diseases, a preexisting connection between the bronchial arteries and pulmonary arteries becomes functional at the precapillary and postcapillary levels. Fine networks of neovascularity supplied by the bronchial and intercostal arteries can also appear in inflammatory and neoplastic diseases. The enlarged bronchial vessels, which exist in the walls of the dilated bronchi, may be injured by infection, which is common. The blood under systemic pressure may pour into the respiratory tree, with serious or even fatal consequences (6,11). Hemoptysis is one of the major symptoms in patients with bronchiectasis. Hemoptysis frequently has an elusive cause and remains undiagnosed in approximately 50% of cases.

Fiberoptic bronchoscopy is of proved efficacy in examining patients with central endobronchial disease; definite diagnoses are made in more than 95% of cases of endoscopically visible primary malignancy (19). In addition to helping to identify central endobronchial disease, bronchoscopy has also proved valuable in the localization of bleeding sites before surgery, the removal of blood clots that may cause obstruction, and the removal of foreign bodies. On the other hand, CT has proved to be of considerable value in diagnosing peripheral airway disease—bronchiectasis, in particular—as well as radiographically occult parenchymal neoplasms. Thus, CT and bronchoscopy are not competitive but rather complementary modalities. CT cannot replace bronchoscopy, especially in the ability to help provide biopsy specimens for histologic or cytologic examination. In turn, bronchoscopy is limited in the ability to enable detection of peribronchial abnormalities and facilitate diagnosis of parenchymal disease, especially bronchiectasis (19,20).

CT is invaluable in providing a road map for bronchoscopists (19,21). This is especially true in patients for whom transbronchial needle aspiration, biopsy, or both, are planned. We have had several unfortunate episodes of accidental biopsy of hypertrophied bronchial arteries in patients with bronchiectasis and hemoptysis. Therefore, not only the presence of bronchiectasis but also the recognition of the hypertrophied bronchial artery can be valuable information to the bronchoscopist.

In summary, within the mediastinum and central airway, nodular and tubular structures with an appearance unlike that of lymph nodes or normal vessels on thin-section CT scans in patients with bronchiectasis can be suggestive of hypertrophied bronchial arteries. The presence of hypertrophied bronchial arteries that protrude from the lumen of the bronchi should alert the bronchoscopist.

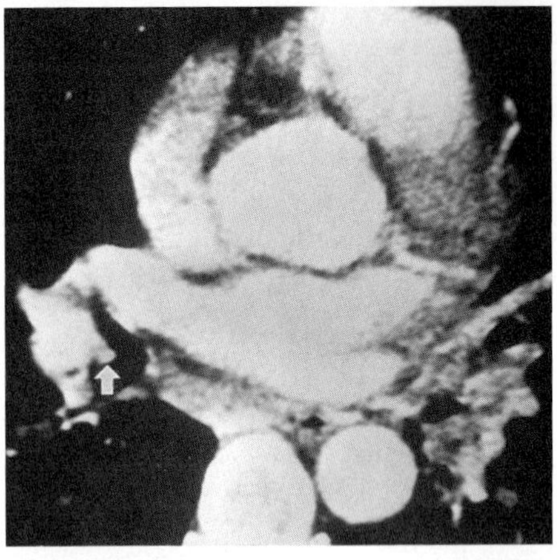

a.

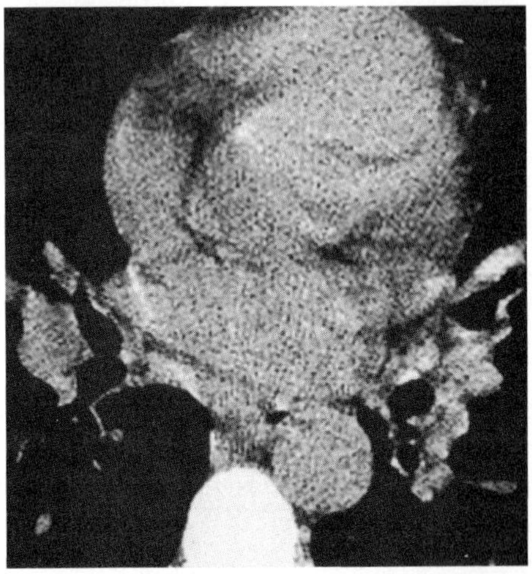

b.

Figure 5. Intraluminal protrusion of a hypertrophied bronchial artery in the right lung in a 41-year-old woman. **(a)** CT angiogram shows a high-attenuation nodular structure (arrow) around the wall of the central airway (bifurcation of the bronchus intermedius), which protrudes intraluminally. **(b)** Thin-section CT scan reveals that the high-attenuation structure in **a** is not calcified.

References

1. Defabach ME, Charan NB, Lakshiminarayan S, Butler J. The bronchial circulation: small but vital attribute of the lung. Am Rev Respir Dis 1987; 135:463–481.
2. Murayama S, Hashiguchi N, Murakami J, et al. Helical CT imaging of bronchial arteries with curved reformation technique in comparison with selective bronchial arteriography: preliminary report. J Comput Assist Tomogr 1996; 20:749–755.
3. Kauczor HU, Schwickert HC, Mayer E, Schweden F, Schild HH, Thelen M. Spiral CT of bronchial arteries in chronic thromboembolism. J Comput Assist Tomogr 1994; 18:855–861.

4. Schwickert HC, Kauczor HU, Schweden F, Schild HH. The anatomy of the bronchial arteries: their imaging with spiral CT. ROFO 1994; 160:506–512. [German]
5. Kauczor HU, Fischer B, Cagil H, Wilhelm K, Mildenberger P, Schild HH. Computed tomography of bronchial arteries before and after embolization. Pneumologie 1994; 48:395–399. [German]
6. Furuse M, Saito K, Kunieda E, et al. Bronchial arteries: CT demonstration with arteriographic correlation. Radiology 1987; 162:393–398.
7. McGuinness G, Naidich DP, Leitman BS, McCauley DI. Bronchiectasis: CT evaluation. AJR 1993; 160:253–259.
8. Grenier P, Maurice F, Musset D, Menu Y, Nahum H. Bronchiectasis: assessment by thin-section CT. Radiology 1986; 161: 95–99.
9. Boushy SF, North LB, Trics JA. The bronchial arteries in chronic obstructive pulmonary disease. Am J Med 1969; 46:506–515.
10. North LB, Boushy SF, Houk VN. Bronchial and intercostal arteriography in non-neoplastic pulmonary disease. AJR 1969; 107:328–342.
11. Liebow AA, Hales MR, Lindskog GE. Enlargement of the bronchial arteries and their anastomoses with the pulmonary arteries in bronchiectasis. Am J Pathol 1948; 25:211–231.
12. Webb WR, Hirji M, Gamsu G. Posterior wall of the bronchus intermedius: radiographic-CT correlation. AJR 1984; 141: 907–911.
13. Schnur MJ, Winkler B, Austin JHM. Thickening of the posterior wall of the bronchus intermedius: a sign on lateral chest radiographs of congestive heart failure, lymph node enlargement, and neoplastic infiltration. Radiology 1981; 139:551–559.
14. Webb WR, Gamsu G, Speckman JM. Computed tomography of pulmonary hilum in patients with bronchogenic carcinoma. J Comput Assist Tomogr 1983; 7:219–225.
15. Webb WR, Gamsu G, Glazer G. Computed tomography of the abnormal pulmonary hilum. J Comput Assist Tomogr 1981; 5:485–490.
16. McGuinness G, Naidich DP. Bronchiectasis: CT/clinical correlations. Semin Ultrasound CT MR 1995; 16:395–419.
17. Kim JS, Choi D, Lee KS. CT of the bronchus intermedius: frequency and cause of a nodule in the posterior wall on normal scans. AJR 1995; 165:1349–1352.
18. Cauldwell EW, Siekert RG, Lininger RE, et al. The bronchial arteries: an anatomic study of 150 human cadavers. Surg Gynecol Obstet 1948; 86:395–412.
19. McGuinness G, Beacher JR, Harkin TJ, et al. Hemoptysis: prospective high-resolution CT/bronchoscopic correlation. Chest 1994; 105:1155–1162.
20. Naidich DP, Funt S, Ettenger NA, Arranda C. Hemoptysis: CT-bronchoscopic correlations in 58 cases. Radiology 1990; 177: 357–362.
21. Millar AB, Boothroyd AE, Edwards D, Hertzel MR. The role of computed tomography in the investigation of unexplained hemoptysis. Respir Med 1992; 86:39–44.

Ventilator-associated Pneumonia in Patients with Adult Respiratory Distress Syndrome: CT Evaluation[1]

Helen T. Winer-Muram, MD
Robert M. Steiner, MD
Jud W. Gurney, MD
Rosita Shah, MD
S. Gregory Jennings, MD
Kristopher L. Arheart, EdD
Mahmoud A. Eltorky, MD
G. Umberto Meduri, MD

Index terms:
Lung, assisted ventilation
Lung, CT, 60.1211
Lung, infection, 60.21
Respiratory distress syndrome, adult (ARDS), 60.413

Radiology 1998; 208:193–199

Abbreviations:
ARDS = adult respiratory distress syndrome
PEEP = positive end-expiratory pressure
ROC = receiver operating characteristic

[1] From the Departments of Radiology (H.T.W.M.), Pathology (M.A.E.), and the Division of Pulmonary and Critical Care Medicine (S.G.J., G.U.M.), University of Tennessee, Memphis; the Department of Radiology, Thomas Jefferson University, Philadelphia, Pa (R.M.S.); the Department of Radiology, University of Nebraska, Omaha (J.W.G.); the Department of Radiology, Allegheny University of the Health Sciences, Medical College of Pennsylvania, Philadelphia (R.S.); and the Department of Biostatistics and Epidemiology, the Cleveland Clinic Foundation, Cleveland, Ohio (K.L.A.). Received August 5, 1997; revision requested October 23; revision received January 5, 1998; accepted February 2. **Address reprint requests to** H.T.W.M., Department of Radiology, New York Methodist Hospital, 506 6th St, Brooklyn, NY 11215-3609.

Author contributions:
Guarantors of integrity of entire study, H.T.W.M., S.G.J.; study concepts, H.T.W.M., S.G.J., G.U.M.; study design, H.T.W.M., S.G.J.; literature research, H.T.W.M.; clinical studies, G.U.M.; data acquisition, H.T.W.M., R.M.S., J.W.G., R.S., S.G.J., G.U.M.; data analysis, H.T.W.M., S.G.J., K.L.A.; statistical analysis, K.L.A.; manuscript preparation, H.T.W.M., S.G.J., K.L.A.; manuscript editing, H.T.W.M., R.M.S., J.W.G., S.G.J., K.L.A., M.A.E., G.U.M.; manuscript review, R.M.S., J.W.G., R.S., S.G.J., K.L.A., M.A.E., G.U.M.

PURPOSE: To determine the diagnostic accuracy of computed tomography (CT) for pneumonia in patients with adult respiratory distress syndrome (ARDS).

MATERIALS AND METHODS: CT scans were obtained within 1 week of bronchoscopic sampling in 31 patients receiving mechanical ventilation for ARDS for more than 48 hours. Of 11 patients with pneumonia, five developed symptoms less than 11 days after the onset of ARDS (early ARDS). CT scans were rated for pneumonia independently by four radiologists who were unaware of the clinical diagnosis. Diagnostic accuracy was defined by means of the area under the receiver operating characteristic curve, or A_z.

RESULTS: Diagnostic accuracy for pneumonia was fair ($A_z = 0.69 \pm 0.04$ [standard error]) owing to 70% true-negative ratings (vs 59% true-positive ratings). The generalizability coefficient was good (0.79). No single CT finding was significantly different for the presence of pneumonia. Nondependent opacities predominated in 10 (91%) of 11 patients with pneumonia and 12 (60%) of 20 without pneumonia. Nondependent opacities predominated in nine (56%) of 16 patients with early ARDS and 13 (87%) of 15 with late ARDS.

CONCLUSION: CT has fair diagnostic accuracy for ventilator-associated pneumonia in patients with ARDS owing primarily to identification of patients without pneumonia. No single CT sign was significantly different for pneumonia, but dependent atelectasis was more common in patients with early ARDS without pneumonia.

Adult respiratory distress syndrome (ARDS) refers to a clinical syndrome characterized by acute onset of dyspnea, diffuse pulmonary opacities, severe hypoxemia, and the rapid development of respiratory failure (1). Diffuse alveolar damage is the usual underlying pathologic manifestation owing to generalized inflammation of the lung parenchyma caused by a variety of precipitating factors (2). In patients with ARDS, the frequency of ventilator-associated pneumonia complicating the clinical course is as high as 70% (3). The mortality rate for ARDS patients with ventilator-associated pneumonia compared with that for ARDS patients without pneumonia is 67% and 23%, respectively (3). The chest computed tomographic (CT) features of ARDS have been described, but to our knowledge there has been no attempt to determine if the radiologic findings vary in patients with and those without pulmonary infection (4–9).

The purpose of this study was to determine the diagnostic accuracy of CT for the diagnosis of ventilator-associated pneumonia in patients with ARDS, by means of receiver operating characteristic (ROC) curve analysis. Chest radiography has been shown to be of limited value for the diagnosis of pneumonia in patients receiving mechanical ventilation; therefore, it is important to evaluate the utility of CT, an alternate imaging modality (10). To our knowledge, this has not been previously reported. We also determined if CT features permit discrimination between patients with and those without pulmonary infection.

MATERIALS AND METHODS

Study Process

The study was performed from July 1, 1989, to December 31, 1995, in the three Memphis hospitals of the University of Tennessee: the Regional Medical Center, the Veterans Affairs

Medical Center, and the William F. Bowld University of Tennessee Hospital. Medical records were reviewed retrospectively to identify patients with ARDS, as defined by Fowler et al (11), who had undergone chest CT within 7 days of lung sampling by means of either fiberoptic bronchoscopy or lung biopsy. These patients composed the study group. That lung sampling was called the index fiberoptic bronchoscopy.

In this review, the cases of 31 patients (17 men and 14 women) were identified. Median patient age was 41 years (age range, 17–69 years). Nineteen patients underwent index fiberoptic bronchoscopy a median 3 days (range, 1–7 days) before CT, and two 1 day before CT. Four patients underwent both procedures on the same day. Eight patients underwent index fiberoptic bronchoscopy ($n = 7$) or open lung biopsy ($n = 1$) a median 6 days (range, 1–7 days) after CT. Diagnoses at admission and clinical features the day of index fiberoptic bronchoscopy for these 31 patients are summarized in Table 1.

All 31 patients were receiving ventilatory support. Mechanical ventilation was initiated a median 1 day after hospital admission (range, 0–10 days). The median interval from the onset of assisted ventilation to index fiberoptic bronchoscopy was 11 days (range, 2–40 days). The median interval from hospital admission to index fiberoptic bronchoscopy was 13 days (range, 3–40 days).

Fiberoptic bronchoscopy was performed by one of eight experienced pulmonologists (G.U.M.). The pulmonary regions to be sampled were selected on the basis of findings on the most recent chest radiograph and at endoscopy during the procedure. The chest radiograph was used as a "road map" for sampling if focal abnormalities were present. When radiographic abnormalities were diffuse, specimens were obtained from the right middle lobe, the lingula, or both because recovery of lavage fluid from these areas is assisted by gravity in patients lying supine.

Pneumonia was diagnosed when specimens obtained at fiberoptic bronchoscopy yielded a sufficient concentration of organisms after quantitative culture: at least 10^5 colony-forming units per milliliter for bronchoalveolar lavage, 10^4 CFU/mL for protected bronchoalveolar lavage, and 10^3 CFU/mL for protected specimen brushing. For the patient who underwent open lung biopsy, results at histologic, cytologic, and microbiologic examinations were used to exclude pneumonia.

All medical records and procedure findings were reviewed in detail by one of the authors (S.G.J.). The majority of patients ($n = 28$) underwent multiple bronchoscopies (total procedures = 124). Repeat bronchoscopies were performed if the clinical course was suggestive of ongoing infection (eg, fever, elevated white blood cell count, purulent tracheal secretions). The index fiberoptic bronchoscopy was the first ($n = 8$), second ($n = 12$), third ($n = 7$), fourth ($n = 2$), or fifth ($n = 2$) bronchoscopy.

Of the 11 patients with pneumonia at index fiberoptic bronchoscopy, two had two pathogens isolated. Pathogens identified after specimen culture included *Pseudomonas aeruginosa* ($n = 5$), *Staphylococcus aureus* ($n = 4$), *Escherichia coli* ($n = 2$), *Proteus mirabilis* ($n = 1$), and diptheroid species ($n = 1$). Seven of the 31 patients had pneumonia demonstrated at previous fiberoptic bronchoscopy (Fig 1).

Seventeen (55%) of the 31 patients died during this hospital admission. Nine (82%) of the 11 patients with pneumonia at index fiberoptic bronchoscopy died, as did eight (40%) of the 20 patients with negative findings at index fiberoptic bronchoscopy.

In this study, four chest radiologists (H.T.W.M., R.M.S., J.W.G., R.S.) independently reviewed the CT scans obtained in each patient within 1 week of the index fiberoptic bronchoscopy. The radiologists were aware that all patients had a diagnosis of ARDS but were blinded to the presence or absence of pneumonia and to the clinical features of the cases.

Before the study began, the readers were instructed to base their ratings on the overall appearance of the CT scan rather than on the presence or absence of a single feature. For the purpose of this study, CT findings considered suggestive of pneumonia were agreed on by the readers before any scans were reviewed. These included asymmetry of air-space opacification with focal or multifocal opacities, low-attenuation consolidation, necrosis, cavitation, low-attenuation fluid bronchograms, and the split pleura sign. This approach was designed to reflect radiologic interpretation in clinical practice. The readers designated their level of certainty for the various conditions on the basis of these features and on their experience in interpreting CT scans.

The readers, without prior discussion, independently rated the CT images for the likelihood of pulmonary infection with a four-point scale (0 = not present, 1 = possibly present, 2 = probably present, and 3 = definitely present). The readers then reached a consensus for each patient about specific patterns of disease such as the type of opacification (air space, ground glass, interstitial, mixed), distribution of opacities (dependent or nondependent, unilateral or bilateral, focal or diffuse), and the presence of atelectasis, cavities, pleural disease, and barotrauma.

These CT studies were obtained on one of four scanners (model DR3 or model DRH, Siemens Medical Systems, Iselin, NJ; model 9800 or HiSpeed Advantage, GE Medical Systems, Milwaukee, Wis) Contiguous 7-mm-thick ($n = 1$), 8-mm-thick ($n = 19$), and 10-mm-thick ($n = 11$) scans were acquired from lung apices to bases with ($n = 17$) or without ($n = 24$) contrast material enhancement. Spiral CT was performed in seven patients. Additional thin-section CT scans were obtained in three patients.

TABLE 1
Admission Diagnoses and Clinical Features in 31 Patients with ARDS

Data	No. of Patients
Admission diagnosis	
Infectious	
Pneumonia*	4
Pneumonia, no organism	5
Pneumococcal meningitis	1
Sepsis†	3
Retropharyngeal abscess	1
Noninfectious	
Preeclampsia	1
Ectopic pregnancy	1
Intracranial hemorrhage	4
Seizure disorder	1
Renal failure	1
Ethanol withdrawal	1
Respiratory failure	1
Perforated ulcer	1
Gastrointestinal bleeding	1
Trauma	1
Sickle cell crisis	1
After vascular surgery	1
Pancreatitis	1
Coronary artery disease	1
Clinical features‡	
Temperature, >37.8°C	27
White blood cell count, >12 × 10^9/L	27
Purulent tracheal secretions	11
Antibiotic therapy earlier in this hospitalization	30
Antibiotics changed 24 h earlier	8
No antibiotic therapy 24 h earlier	5
Steroid therapy	9

* Patients with *Staphylococcus* species, coagulase-negative ($n = 1$); *Streptococcus pneumoniae* ($n = 1$); *Acinetobacter calcoaceticus* ($n = 1$); and *Varicellavirus* ($n = 1$) pneumonias.

† Patients with *Salmonella* ($n = 1$) and *Escherichia coli* ($n = 1$) sepsis.

‡ On the day of index fiberoptic bronchoscopy.

Previously Isolated Pathogens in Seven Patients

No Pneumonia at Index Fiberoptic Bronchoscopy* (n = 4)
Pseudomonas aeruginosa (n = 2)
Staphylococcus species
Staphylococcus aureus
Haemophilus influenzae
Streptococcus viridans
Streptococcus species

Pneumonia at Index Fiberoptic Bronchoscopy (n = 3)
Haemophilus parainfluenza
Diptheroid species
Enterobacter aerogenes
Acinetobacter calcoaceticus

*Index fiberoptic bronchoscopy was the first examination within 7 days of CT.

Figure 1. Previously isolated pathogens in seven patients obtained before or after CT.

Statistical Analyses

Demographic data are expressed as frequency and percentage for categorical variables and as median and range for continuous variables with nonnormal distributions. Statistical test differences with P values of .05 or less were considered statistically significant.

In this study, we defined diagnostic accuracy as the area under the ROC curve, or A_z, which represents the probability of correctly distinguishing patients who have a specific pathologic condition from those who do not. A_z values range between 0.0 and 1.0. An A_z value of 0.5 indicates random guessing (ie, the test is unable to distinguish between patients with and those without disease). An A_z value greater than 0.5 indicates increasing accuracy, with a value of 1.0 denoting perfect accuracy. An A_z value less than 0.5 indicates that the test criteria are incorrect (ie, absence of the criteria indicates the presence of disease). An A_z value of 0.0 indicates that the presence of disease can be perfectly distinguished from the absence of disease by reversing the test results. We defined the following categories to simplify the interpretation of the A_z values: excellent, $A_z \geq 0.80$; good, $0.70 \leq A_z \leq 0.79$; fair, $0.60 \leq A_z \leq 0.69$; poor, $0.50 \leq A_z \leq 0.59$.

To estimate the area under the ROC curve, we assumed that the ratings represented an underlying unidimensional variable with a binormal distribution and used the ROCFIT program to obtain a maximum likelihood fit of the data (12). The ROC curve parameters for each reader were averaged to produce a plot of the ROC curve as suggested by Metz (12).

The jackknife method given by Dorfman et al (13) was used to generalize the findings over patients and readers. In the jackknife method, the area under the ROC curve is calculated for each reader, first by using the ratings for all patients and then by deleting one patient at a time until all patients have been eliminated once. This latter step produces n areas based on a sample of $n - 1$ patients, where n is the number of patients. A set of n Quenouille-Tukey pseudovalues are then produced by using the first area computed for all n patients to adjust the other n areas. These pseudovalues are then used in analyses of variance to produce estimates of the area under the ROC curve, standard error, and 95% confidence limits and to estimate the reliability of the results.

The generalizability coefficient indicates the reliability of the estimated area under the ROC curve given by the average of the jackknife pseudovalues in this study (14). The generalizability coefficient indicates the likelihood of replication of the results of this study in a similar study with the average ROC areas of four readers randomly selected from a population of readers who interpret the findings in a random sample of patients with similar proportions of patients with and those without disease. The generalizability coefficient ranges from 0 to 1, with 1 indicating perfect reliability. We defined the following categories to simplify the interpretation of the generalizability coefficient (GC): excellent, GC $\geq$ 0.80; good, 0.60 $\leq$ GC $\leq$ 0.79; fair, 0.41 $\leq$ GC $\leq$ 0.59; poor, GC $\leq$ 0.40.

The true-positive, true-negative, false-positive, and false-negative fractions were computed to help explain the accuracy for some of the pathologic conditions. For these computations, the ratings were dichotomized into positive (ratings of 2 and 3) and negative (ratings of 0 and 1) and pooled over the readers.

The Fisher exact test was used to analyze the relationship between index bronchoscopic or biopsy diagnoses and specific radiologic features (on the basis of the consensus opinion of the readers). Differences with a P value of .05 or less were considered statistically significant.

RESULTS

The overall diagnostic accuracy for pneumonia was fair (A_z = 0.69 ± 0.04 [standard error]) (Fig 2, Table 2). The A_z values for the four readers ranged from 0.60 ± 0.15 to 0.76 ± 0.11. Fair diagnostic accuracy for pneumonia was primarily due to 70% true-negative ratings (vs 59% true-positive ratings) (Tables 2, 3). The interreader generalizability coefficient was good (0.79) (Table 2).

Table 4 demonstrates the relationship between consensus opinion of specific CT features and the presence of pneumonia. Although no single CT finding was significantly different for the presence of pneumonia, it is of interest that 10 (91%) of 11 patients with pneumonia and 12 (60%) of 20 patients without pneumonia had nondependent opacities.

Figure 3 demonstrates the relationship between dependence of opacities and duration of ARDS. Patients who underwent CT less than 11 days after the initial diagnosis of ARDS were considered to have early ARDS, whereas those who underwent CT later were considered to have late ARDS. On the basis of this definition, five of the 16 patients with early ARDS had pneumonia, and four (80%) of them had nondependent opacities (Figs 4, 5). All (100%) six patients with late ARDS and pneumonia had nondependent opacities.

Nondependent opacities predominated in both early ARDS (nine [56%] of 16 patients) and late ARDS (13 [87%] of 15 patients). Dependent opacities occurred primarily in early ARDS (seven [78%] of nine patients) (Figs 3, 6a).

DISCUSSION

In this series of 31 patients with ARDS, CT was fairly accurate (A_z = 0.69) and reliable (generalizability coefficient, 0.79) for ventilator-associated pneumonia. To our knowledge, no other reports have evaluated the role of CT for ventilator-associated pneumonia in patients with ARDS. In a previous series of 17 patients with ARDS, five of whom had pneumonia, the overall diagnostic accuracy of chest radiography for pneumonia was 0.42 on the basis of ROC curve analysis (10). Clearly, chest radiography cannot be used to discriminate patients with and those without infection. A recent report of 48 immunocompromised children, five of whom had bacterial pneumonia, described poor diagnostic accuracy of CT for bacterial pneumonia (A_z = 0.43) (15). In that study, improved reliability was achieved with CT rather than with chest radiography (0.51 vs 0.06, respectively).

In this study, the satisfactory accuracy with CT was based primarily on the ability of the readers to detect patients without pneumonia (specificity, 70%). Although this difference is not statistically significant, we assume that the absence of features of pneumonia in individual patients (ie, absence of asymmetric or low-attenuation consolidations, focal opacities, fluid bronchograms, cavitation, and empyema) probably accounted for the identification of patients without pneumonia. The frequency of pneumonia was similar in early ARDS (five [31%] of 16 patients) and late ARDS (six [40%] of 15 patients); therefore, knowledge of the patient's clinical time line would probably not have improved diagnostic accuracy.

We did not find a radiologic feature that was significantly different for the presence or absence of pneumonia. None of the combined radiologic features were significantly different for the presence or absence of pneumonia. Despite the small sample size, we performed a stepwise multiple logistic regression that included as candidate variables all features that were significantly different at the .20 level in the univariate analysis. In the final model, we kept only those predictors that were significantly different at the .10 level. None of the radiologic features was significantly different. However, when a pattern of nondependent opacification was present, patients were approximately seven times more likely to have pneumonia at index bronchoscopy (P = .097; odds ratio = 6.67; 90% confidence interval, 1.02, 43.75) (Figs 4, 5). Conversely, patients with a pattern of bilateral dependent opacities were approximately seven times more likely to not have pneumonia at index bronchoscopy (Fig 6a).

Only one patient with a pattern of dependent opacification had pneumonia. This feature was not significantly different, but findings in a larger series might prove it to be so. Because this feature has not been previously described, to our knowledge, it was not included in the guidelines for the readers. We retrospectively manipulated the data so that all patients with a pattern of bilateral dependent atelectasis received a hypothetical rating of 0 by all four readers, and the statistical analyses were recalculated. By altering the data in this way, A_z increased from 0.69 to 0.75, and specificity increased from 0.70 to 0.84 (Table 5).

Although nondependent opacities predominated in both early ARDS (56%) and late ARDS (87%), bilateral dependent opacities were visualized primarily in early ARDS. Seven (78%) of nine patients with bilateral dependent opacities had early ARDS. During the early phase, the increased lung weight due to increased edema and hyaline membrane formation causes collapse of the lung regions along the vertical axis by means of the transmission of hydrostatic forces (compression atelectasis) (Fig 6a). Thus, the lesions appear mainly in the dependent lung regions (1). Application of adequate PEEP has been shown to act as a counterforce, reopening previously collapsed pulmonary units and reducing the amount of nonaerated tissue (1).

Only 9% of patients with pneumonia demonstrated a pattern of dependent opacification. This may be due to multiple factors. In our study, 25 patients had PEEP values available from the day CT was performed. Patients with pneumonia received higher levels of PEEP than did those without pneumonia (median, 10 vs 5 cm of water, respectively). In patients with pneumonia, the increased airway pressure due to PEEP may have exceeded the compressive and adhesive forces that cause dependent atelectasis (4). Furthermore, Gattinoni et al (6) showed that the

TABLE 2
Accuracy and Interreader Reliability for Pneumonia

Diagnostic Accuracy*	95% Confidence Interval	Generalizability Coefficient	True-Positive Fraction	True-Negative Fraction	Sensitivity	Specificity
0.69 ± 0.04	0.60, 0.78	0.79	0.59	0.70	0.59	0.70

* Estimated area under the receiver operating characteristic curve (A_z ± standard error).

TABLE 3
Ratings for Pneumonia by Four Readers

Finding	n	0	1	2	3
Pneumonia (11 patients)	44	10	8	8	18
No pneumonia (20 patients)	80	31	25	11	13

Note.—Four-point scale for probability of pneumonia was used: 0 = not present, 1 = possibly present, 2 = probably present, 3 = definitely present. n = number of patients × four readers.

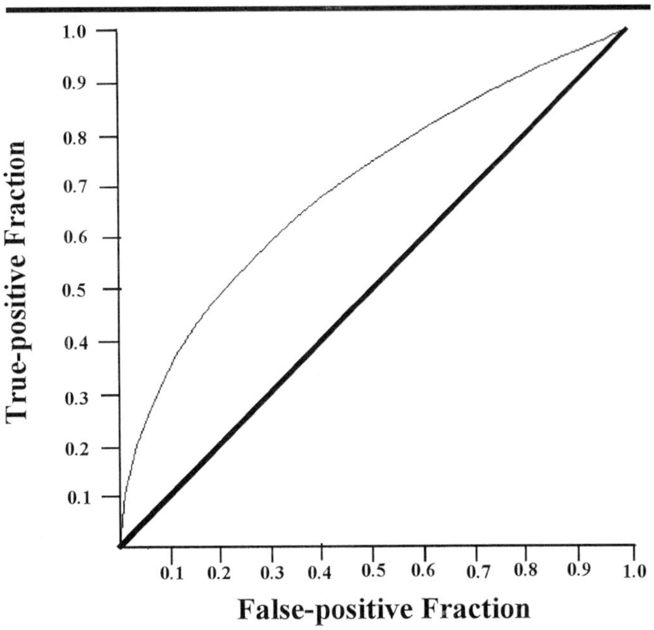

Figure 2. ROC curve for the diagnostic accuracy for pneumonia (A_z = 0.69 ± 0.04). The curve is based on maximum likelihood estimates of the curve intercept and slope parameters, which were averaged over the four readers. Thin line = pneumonia, thick line = no discrimination.

TABLE 4
CT Findings in 31 Patients with ARDS

CT Finding	No Pneumonia (*n* = 20)	Pneumonia (*n* = 11)
Opacities		
Bilateral dependent	8 (40)	1 (9)
Nondependent	12 (60)	10 (91)
Bilateral opacities	20 (100)	11 (100)
Focal pattern	1 (5)	2 (18)
Diffuse pattern only	5 (25)	2 (18)
Focal and diffuse patterns	14 (70)	7 (64)
Normal appearance	0 (0)	0 (0)
Disease		
Air-space disease only	8 (40)	5 (45)
Ground-glass opacities only	5 (25)	3 (27)
Interstitial disease only	0 (0)	0 (0)
Air-space and interstitial disease	3 (15)	1 (9)
Air-space disease and ground-glass opacities	3 (15)	1 (9)
Air-space and interstitial diseases and ground-glass opacities	0 (0)	1 (9)
Ground-glass opacities and interstitial disease	1 (5)	0 (0)
Other findings		
Air bronchograms	17 (85)	11 (100)
Fluid bronchograms	0 (0)	1 (9)
Atelectasis	6 (30)	4 (36)
Adenopathy	2 (10)	0 (0)
Spared lobules	3 (15)	1 (9)
Spared lobes	6 (30)	3 (27)
Spared subpleural region	2 (10)	1 (9)
Nodule(s)	5 (25)	3 (27)
Low-attenuation consolidation	2 (10)	1 (9)
Cavitation	3 (15)	0 (0)
Pneumatoceles or cysts	6 (30)	5 (45)
Pneumothorax	8 (40)	5 (45)
Pleural effusion	7 (35)	6 (54)
Pneumomediastinum	3 (15)	0 (0)
Emphysema	1 (5)	1 (9)

Note.—Data are numbers of patients. Numbers in parentheses are percentages.

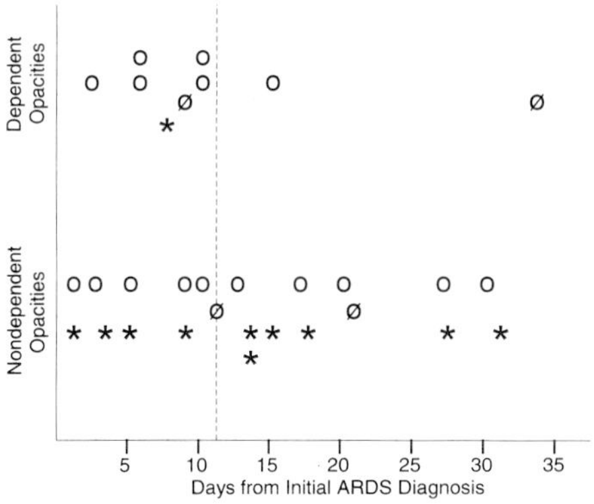

Figure 3. Relationship between dependence of opacities and duration of ARDS. ○ = No pneumonia at index fiberoptic bronchoscopy and no pneumonia at previous fiberoptic bronchoscopies. Ø = No pneumonia at index fiberoptic bronchoscopy but pneumonia at previous fiberoptic bronchoscopies performed more than 1 week before CT. ★ = Pneumonia at index fiberoptic bronchoscopy.

number of pulmonary units recruited with increasing PEEP in the lower lung is greater than that recruited in the middle and upper levels.

A statistical analysis comparing dependence of opacities with the level of PEEP administered proved that differences were not statistically significant ($P > .05$). For the 25 patients with PEEP values available the day CT was performed, 10 (56%) of 18 patients with nondependent opacities and four (57%) of seven patients with bilateral dependent opacities were receiving high levels of PEEP (>5 cm of water).

Thus, additional explanations as to why patients with pneumonia are more likely to have nondependent opacities must be considered. Opacification of nondependent lung with pneumonia may mask the dependent atelectasis (Fig 4). Finally, in late ARDS, lung fibrosis reduces the transmission of hydrostatic forces with a consequent decrease in the occurrence of dependent atelectasis (1). Fibroproliferation does not develop fully until 10–14 days after the onset of ARDS so the predominance of nondependent opacities in early ARDS is most likely due to other factors (16,17).

Tagliabue et al (8) found at CT that 86% of opacities in 74 patients with ARDS were gravity dependent. In the current study, only nine (29%) of the 31 patients had bilateral dependent opacities. Inclusion of more patients with late ARDS and more patients with higher levels of PEEP administered may account for a high percentage of nondependent opacities in our patients.

The typical features of pneumonia were used as a guide for the radiologic rating: asymmetry of air-space consolidation with focal or multifocal opacities, low-attenuation consolidation, necrosis, cavitation, low-attenuation fluid bronchograms, and the split pleura sign (10,15). In our study, focal or multifocal opacities were seen in 24 (77%) of the 31 patients. These opacities were seen in 15 (75%) of 20 patients without pneumonia and in nine (82%) of 11 with pneumonia; therefore, they cannot be used to distinguish patients with and those without infection (Fig 4). Similarly, Tagliabue et al (8) reported mixed or patchy opacities in 51 (71%) of 74 patients, but they did not identify patients with ventilator-associated pneumonia.

In patients with ARDS that is the result of focal lung disease such as trauma, pneumonia, or aspiration, inhomogeneity or asymmetry of pulmonary opacities is easily explained (Fig 4). In patients with ARDS caused by systemic problems, such as hypotension, sepsis, or toxic inhalation, the inhomogeneous pattern is less clear. Inhomogeneous delivery of blood-borne mediators may result from uneven perfusion of the lung caused by vasospasm, streaming of blood, or regional vascular occlusion (4,18). Inhalation of irritants may be uneven and cause varying amounts of damage to the alveolar epithelium (4,18). Preexisting lung disease may alter perfusion and ventilation and change the distribution of edema or atelectasis (4).

The presence of cavitation did not help identify patients with active infection. Lung cavities may represent bland residua from remote infection successfully treated with antibiotics (Fig 6b). Bland cavities may also occur as a result of parenchymal coagulative necrosis secondary to obliteration of large portions of the vascular bed by fibrin thrombi, a frequent occurrence in ARDS (19). Furthermore, the appearance of pneumatoceles and cavities may be similar radiologically. Findings of barotrauma (ie, pneumatoceles or cysts, pneumothorax, pneumomediastinum) did not help distinguish patients with and those without pneumonia.

A potential shortcoming of this study was the inclusion of patients who underwent CT as long as 7 days before or after the index bronchoscopy. We would have preferred to select only patients who un-

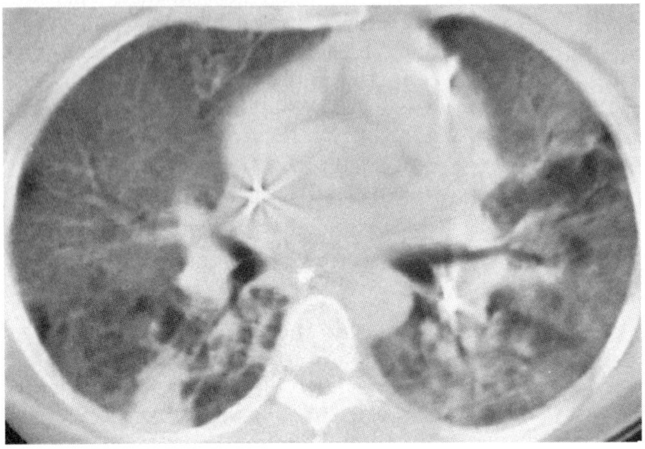

Figure 4. Findings in a 32-year-old pregnant woman admitted for suspected pneumonia and treated with mechanical ventilation from the day of admission. This CT scan was obtained after 6 days of mechanical ventilation, and the reader ratings for pneumonia were 1, 3, 2, 0. The scan depicts a pattern of nondependent diffuse ground glass opacification with focal air-space disease and air bronchograms posteriorly in the right lung. The positive end-expiratory pressure (PEEP) was 12 cm of water on the day the scan was obtained. Specimens from the second (index) bronchoscopy, performed 2 days after this CT scan was obtained, were positive for methicillin-resistant staphylococcus at the right middle lobe. Findings at the previous bronchoscopy were negative. The patient died after approximately 1 month of hospitalization.

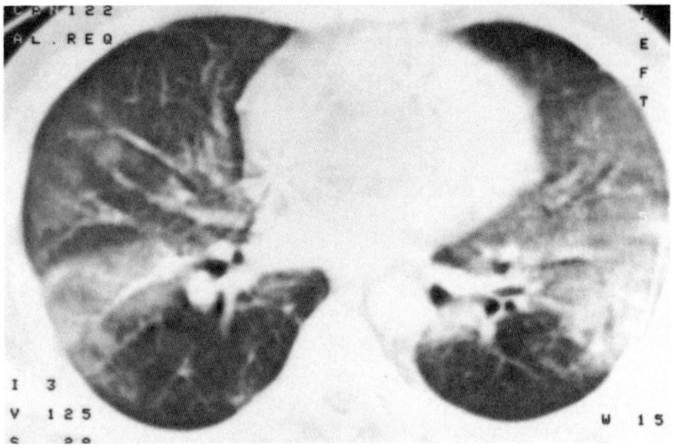

Figure 5. Findings in a 46-year-old man admitted with diarrhea and salmonella sepsis. Mechanical ventilation was begun 4 days after admission. This CT scan was obtained after 6 days of mechanical ventilation, and the reader ratings for pneumonia were 0, 0, 0, 0. The scan depicts a pattern of nondependent ground glass opacification with some areas of sparing of the lower lobes. PEEP was 7.5 cm of water on the day the scan was obtained. Specimens from the right middle lobe obtained at the first (index) bronchoscopy, performed 6 days after this CT scan was obtained, showed *Pseudomonas aeruginosa* pneumonia. The patient died after approximately 1 month of hospitalization.

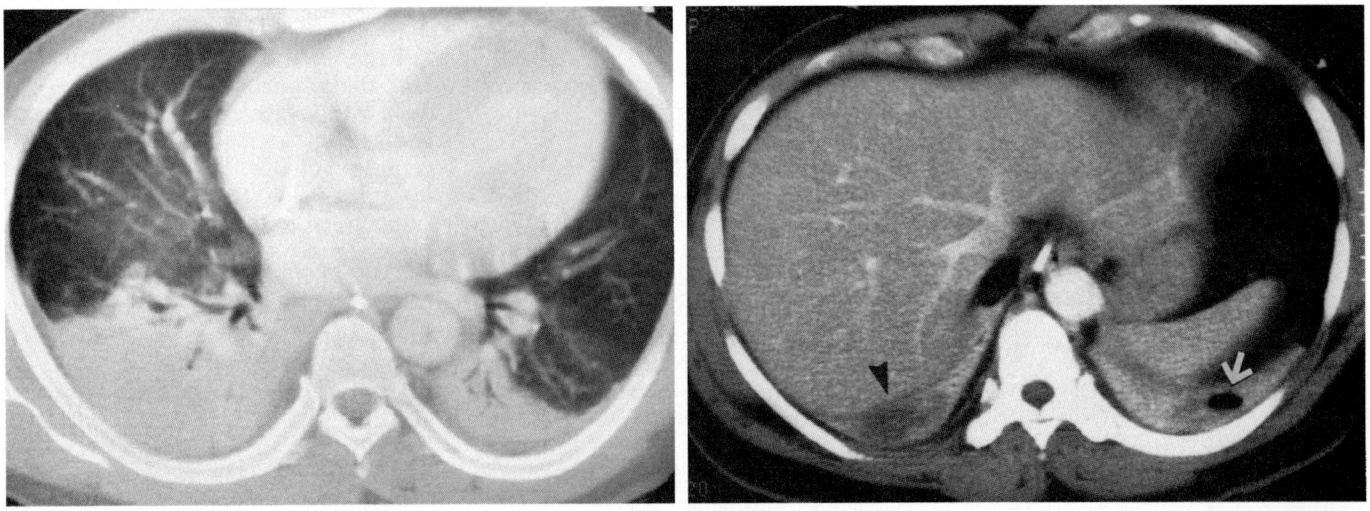

a. b.

Figure 6. Findings in a 34-year-old man admitted for an intracerebral hemorrhage. Mechanical ventilation was begun the day of admission. These CT scans were obtained after 8 days of mechanical ventilation, and the reader ratings for pneumonia were 3, 2, 2, 3. **(a)** Scan demonstrates a pattern of bilateral atelectasis or consolidation. **(b)** More inferiorly, scan depicts right lower lobe necrosis (arrowhead) and left lower lobe cavitation (arrow). PEEP was 5 cm of water the day **a** and **b** were obtained. Specimens from the second (index) bronchoscopy, performed the day after **a** and **b** were obtained, were negative for pneumonia. Specimens from the first bronchoscopy, performed 9 days before **a** and **b** were obtained, showed methicillin-sensitive *Staphylococcus aureus* and *Haemophilus influenzae* pneumonia in the right middle lobe. The patient was discharged from the hospital 40 days after admission.

derwent CT immediately before the index bronchoscopy. In addition, the study group includes two patients who underwent CT less than 24 hours after the index bronchoscopy. In these patients, the residual bronchoalveolar lavage fluid may have altered the pulmonary appearance (20). Four other patients underwent both procedures on the same day, but we were unable to retrospectively determine the sequence of procedures. Had we restricted our inclusion criteria further, however, we would have been unable to recruit a sufficient number of patients into the study. Despite these shortcomings, the diagnostic accuracy of CT for pneumonia was fair.

Clinicians and investigators have become increasingly aware of the lack of sensitivity and specificity of clinical and chest radiographic manifestations of ventilator-associated pneumonia. In a report

TABLE 5
Accuracy and Interreader Reliability after Hypothetical Adjustment of Data

Diagnostic Accuracy*	95% Confidence Interval	True-Positive Fraction	True-Negative Fraction	Sensitivity	Specificity
0.75 ± 0.04	0.67, 0.82	0.52	0.84	0.59	0.84

Note.—Dependent atelectasis is rated as no pneumonia (ie, rating of 0 or 1).
* Estimated area under the receiver operating characteristic curve (A_z ± standard error).

of the cases of 24 patients who died of ARDS and in whom results at histologic examination of the lungs were available, clinical predictions of the presence or absence of pneumonia were erroneous in nearly one-third of cases (21).

In a study reviewing 87 CT scans obtained in 56 patients in an intensive care unit, 70% of the CT studies were found to provide additional useful information, such as pneumonia, atelectasis, empyema, large pleural effusions, malpositioned tubes, pneumothoraces, lung abscesses or cysts, lung and extrapleural hematomas, bronchiectasis, and pericardial thickening and effusions (22).

On the basis of findings in our study, we have identified an additional role for CT in critically ill patients with ARDS. CT scans obtained in 16 (52%) of the 31 patients were interpreted as having no pneumonia present; these scans received ratings of 0 and 1 by at least three of the four readers. Results at bronchoscopy revealed that 13 (81%) of these 16 patients had no pulmonary infection, and the ratings by the readers were correct. In patients who are not deteriorating clinically, CT findings suggesting the absence of infection may delay or preclude invasive procedures so bronchoscopy may be reserved for patients who are more likely to have pneumonia.

Unfortunately, findings in this study have demonstrated that CT features are less useful in accurate identification of patients who have pneumonia. Eleven (35%) of our 31 patients had CT scans that were read as positive for pneumonia by at least three of the four readers (ratings of 2 and 3), and only seven (64%) of those 11 patients had bronchoscopically proved pneumonia. However, we have demonstrated improved performance when findings at CT are compared with those at chest radiography. In a previous study evaluating the diagnostic accuracy of chest radiography for pneumonia in patients with ARDS, the true-positive rate was 20% (three of 15 ratings) (10). In our study, we found that the true-positive rate for CT was 59% (26 of 44 ratings). When findings at CT are compared with those at chest radiography, CT improves the ability of the readers to identify patients who have pneumonia.

In summary, CT had fair accuracy (A_z = 0.69) for ventilator-associated pneumonia in patients with ARDS, and reliability was good (0.79). The fair diagnostic accuracy was primarily due to identification of patients who did not have pneumonia. Although no single radiologic sign was significantly different for the presence or absence of pneumonia, a pattern of dependent atelectasis was noted primarily in patients with early ARDS without pneumonia.

References

1. Pelosi P, Crotti S, Brazzi L, Gattinoni L. Computed tomography in adult respiratory distress syndrome: what has it taught us? Eur Respir J 1996; 9:1055–1062.
2. Petty TL, Asbaugh DG. The adult respiratory distress syndrome: clinical features, factors influencing prognosis and principles of management. Chest 1971; 60:233–239.
3. Leeper KV. Diagnosis and treatment of pulmonary infections in adult respiratory distress syndrome. New Horizons 1993; 1:550–562.
4. Goodman LR. Congestive heart failure and adult respiratory distress syndrome. Radiol Clin North Am 1996; 34:33–46.
5. Gattinoni L, Pesenti A, Bombino M, et al. Lung structure and function in different stages of severe adult respiratory distress syndrome. JAMA 1994; 271:1772–1779.
6. Gattinoni L, Pelosi P, Crotti S, Valenza F. Effects of positive end-expiratory pressure on regional distribution of tidal volume and recruitment in adult respiratory distress syndrome. Am J Crit Care 1995; 151:1807–1814.
7. Maunder RJ, Shuman WP, McHugh JW, Marglin SI, Butler J. Preservation of normal lung regions in the adult respiratory distress syndrome: analysis by computed tomography. JAMA 1986; 255:2463–2465.
8. Tagliabue M, Casella TC, Zincone GE, Fumagalli R, Salvini E. CT and chest radiography in the evaluation of adult respiratory distress syndrome. Acta Radiol 1994; 35:230–234.
9. Stark P, Greene R, Kott MM, Hall T, Vanderslice L. CT findings in ARDS. Radiologe 1987; 27:367–369.
10. Winer-Muram HT, Rubin SA, Ellis JV, et al. Pneumonia and ARDS in patients receiving mechanical ventilation: diagnostic accuracy of chest radiography. Radiology 1993; 188:479–485.
11. Fowler AA, Hamman RF, Zerbe GO, Benson KN, Hyers TM. Adult respiratory distress syndrome: prognosis after onset. Am Rev Respir Dis 1985; 132:472–478.
12. Metz CE. Some practical issues of experimental design and data analysis in radiological ROC studies. Invest Radiol 1989; 24:2334–2345.
13. Dorfman DD, Berbaum KS, Metz CE. Receiver-operating characteristic rating analysis: generalization to the population of readers and patients with the jackknife method. Invest Radiol 1992; 27:723–731.
14. Crocker L, Algina J. Introduction to classical and modern test theory. Fort Worth, Tex: Rhinehart & Winston, 1986; 157–191.
15. Winer-Muram HT, Arheart KL, Jennings SG, Rubin SA, Kauffman WM, Slobod KS. Pulmonary complications in children with hematologic malignancies: accuracy of diagnosis with chest radiography and CT. Radiology 1997; 204:643–649.
16. Katzenstein ALA, Askin FB. Surgical pathology of non-neoplastic lung disease. 3rd ed. Philadelphia, Pa: Saunders, 1997; 19.
17. Meduri GU, ElTorky M, Winer-Muram HT. The fibroproliferative phase of late ARDS. Semin Respir Infect 1995; 10:154–175.
18. Greene R, Putman CE, Goodman LR. Regional distribution of lung derangement in the adult respiratory distress syndrome. In: Potchen EJ, Grainger RG, Greene R, eds. Pulmonary radiology. Philadelphia, Pa: Saunders, 1993; 179.
19. Tomashefski JF Jr, Davies P, Boggis C, Greene R, Zapol WM, Reid LM. The pulmonary vascular lesions of the adult respiratory distress syndrome. Am J Pathol 1983; 112:112–126.
20. Gurney W, Sears K, Harrison WC, Robbins RA, Pobry CA, Rennard SI. Bronchoalveolar lavage: roentgenographic manifestations. Radiology 1987; 163:71–74.
21. Andrews PA, Coalson JJ, Smith JD, Johanson WG Jr. Diagnosis of bacterial nosocomial pneumonia in acute diffuse lung injury. Chest 1981; 80:254–258.
22. Mirvis SE, Tobin KD, Kostrubiak I, Belz H. Thoracic CT in detecting occult disease in critically ill patients. AJR 1987; 148:685–689.

Kavita Garg, MD
Carol H. Welsh, MD
Angela J. Feyerabend, MD
Stephen W. Subber, MD
Paul D. Russ, MD
Robert J. Johnston, MD
Janette D. Durham, MD
David A. Lynch, MD

Index terms:
Computed tomography (CT), comparative studies
Embolism, pulmonary, 60.72, 944.77
Lung, CT, 60.12112, 60.12115
Lung, radionuclide studies, 60.12171, 60.12176
Pulmonary arteries, CT, 944.12912, 944.12915
Radionuclide imaging, comparative studies, 60.72

Radiology 1998; 208:201–208

Abbreviations:
CI = confidence interval
PE = pulmonary embolism
PIOPED = Prospective Investigation of Pulmonary Embolism Diagnosis
V-P = ventilation-perfusion

[1] From the Department of Radiology (K.G., A.J.F., S.W.S., P.D.R., R.J.J., J.D.D., D.A.L.) and the Division of Pulmonary Medicine (C.H.W.), University of Colorado Health Sciences Center, 4200 E Ninth Ave, Denver, CO 80262, and the Department of Radiology, Imaging Service (114), Veterans Affairs Medical Center, Denver, Colo (K.G., C.H.W., S.W.S., R.J.J.). From the 1997 RSNA scientific assembly. Received October 13, 1997; revision requested December 11; revision received January 26, 1998; accepted March 3. **Address reprint requests to** K.G.

Author contributions:
Guarantors of integrity of entire study, K.G., C.H.W., A.J.F.; study concepts and design, K.G., C.H.W.; definition of intellectual content, K.G.; literature research, K.G.; clinical studies, C.H.W.; data acquisition, K.G., A.J.F., J.D.D., S.W.S., P.D.R.; data analysis, K.G., S.W.S., P.D.R., J.D.D., R.J.J.; manuscript preparation, K.G.; manuscript editing, K.G., C.H.W., J.D.D., D.A.L.

Pulmonary Embolism: Diagnosis with Spiral CT and Ventilation-Perfusion Scanning—Correlation with Pulmonary Angiographic Results or Clinical Outcome[1]

PURPOSE: To compare the accuracy of spiral computed tomography (CT) with that of ventilation-perfusion (V-P) scintigraphy in the diagnosis of pulmonary embolism (PE).

MATERIALS AND METHODS: Fifty-four patients in whom indeterminate V-P scans or discordant clinical and scintigraphic results were obtained underwent both V-P scanning and contrast material–enhanced spiral CT. The reference standard was pulmonary angiographic results in 26 patients (group I) or clinical outcome in 28 (group II).

RESULTS: Six (25%) of 24 group I patients had proved PE. The prospective sensitivity and specificity for segmental or subsegmental PE were 67% and 100%, respectively, and the positive and negative predictive values were 100% and 90%, respectively. In two group II patients, V-P scans had high probability for acute embolism, but spiral CT scans showed only chronic PE; in one patient, the V-P scan had low probability and the CT scan was positive for acute PE. An alternative CT diagnosis was established in four (31%) of 13 patients in whom a normal or low-probability V-P scan was obtained. Clinical outcome was consistent with spiral CT results in all cases.

CONCLUSION: Spiral CT has greater accuracy and specificity than V-P scanning in patients with an unresolved diagnosis and may be useful as the primary screening technique for PE.

Each year in the United States more than 600,000 patients have a symptom-producing pulmonary embolism (PE), and up to 50,000 patients die of acute PE (1,2). Although acute PE is found in 25%–30% of routine autopsies (3), this diagnosis is often elusive. Antemortem diagnosis of PE is made in less than one-third of patients who die of PE (2,3).

The initial diagnostic study in patients suspected of having PE often is ventilation-perfusion (V-P) scintigraphy. In the Prospective Investigation of Pulmonary Embolism Diagnosis (PIOPED) study (4), clinical assessment combined with a V-P scan helped establish or exclude the diagnosis of PE for only a minority of patients (174 [24.4%] of 713): those with clear and concordant clinical and V-P scan findings. Further imaging is indicated in patients with indeterminate V-P scans and in those with discrepancies between the results of a V-P study and those of the clinical assessment. Pulmonary angiography is then needed to help confirm or exclude PE. Even if available, however, pulmonary angiography is generally underused by physicians, because it is invasive and expensive (5–8).

An imaging modality that combines the noninvasive nature of V-P scanning with a high sensitivity and specificity and that enables direct visualization of the PE is desirable. Although a number of investigators (9–12) have demonstrated the high sensitivity and specificity of spiral computed tomography (CT) and electron-beam CT in the diagnosis of acute PE, at many institutions spiral CT is not yet included in the diagnostic algorithm for patients suspected of having PE (13). This is probably because spiral CT is not universally available, there is concern about the possibility that a peripheral PE may be overlooked, and, more important, clinicians control the referral of patients for diagnostic testing. In two recent studies (14,15), the role of spiral CT has been evaluated in patients with an unresolved diagnosis of PE. To our knowledge, there is only one study (16) in which spiral CT was prospectively compared with V-P scintigraphy.

The present prospective study was designed to compare V-P scanning with spiral CT in patients who had either an indeterminate V-P scan or a discordance between the clinical probability of PE and the V-P scan findings. The objectives of the study were to determine the accuracy of spiral CT in this selected group of patients and to determine if spiral CT findings could be used to establish a diagnosis of PE.

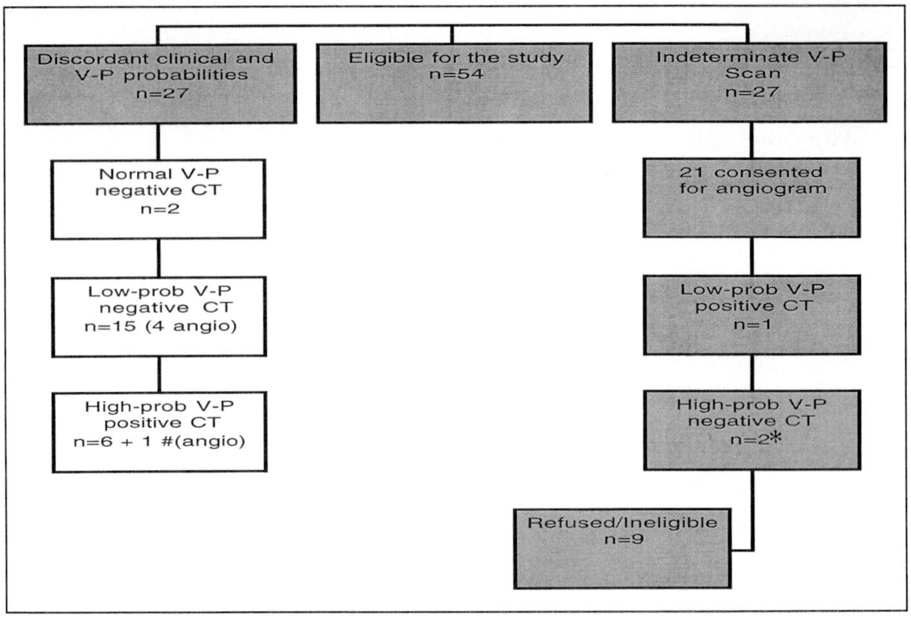

Figure 1. Flow chart shows the distribution of patients. Twenty-six patients (group I) underwent angiography (*angio*), and 28 patients (group II) did not. Unshaded boxes represent patients with concordant CT and V-P scan findings, who were therefore not required to undergo angiography, per our protocol. *angio* = angiogram, *High-prob* = high-probability, *low-prob* = low-probability, # = acute PE superimposed on chronic PE, * = chronic PE.

MATERIALS AND METHODS

Patients

Between November 7, 1996, and August 22, 1997, 185 patients, with or without a history of chronic PE, were evaluated for suspected acute PE by using V-P scanning at the University of Colorado Health Sciences Center. Patients with clinical findings suggestive of a low probability for PE and V-P scan findings suggestive of a normal to low probability for PE ($n = 52$) or clinical and V-P scan findings suggestive of a high probability for PE ($n = 31$) were not recruited. Other criteria for exclusion included (*a*) patients with a positive leg ultrasonographic (US) image obtained before the V-P scan ($n = 38$) and (*b*) a contraindication for the use of intravenous contrast material (renal failure [$n = 5$], history of allergy [$n = 2$], unstable hemodynamic status [$n = 2$]). One patient was excluded because he refused to undergo the ventilation part of the examination.

The remaining 54 patients with either discordant clinical and V-P scan findings ($n = 27$) or with an indeterminate V-P scan ($n = 27$) were eligible for the study (Fig 1). A clinical impression as to the likelihood of PE was recorded by the referring physician before the V-P scanning results were known. These impressions were formed on the basis of (*a*) clinical and laboratory information, including history, physical examination results, arterial blood gas analysis results, chest radiographs, and electrocardiograms ($n = 32$) or (*b*) the score from a questionnaire (17) about signs and symptoms known to correlate with the presence of PE ($n = 22$). The clinical estimate of the likelihood of PE was categorized as high, intermediate, or low.

Written informed consent for spiral CT was obtained from all 54 patients in accordance with a protocol approved by the hospital human subject committee and institutional review board. Our study protocol required the performance of angiography after CT in all patients with indeterminate V-P scans or with discordant CT and V-P findings. Nine patients did not undergo pulmonary angiography because they refused (n = 5) or were considered by their physicians to be ineligible for pulmonary angiography ($n = 4$). V-P scanning, spiral CT, and pulmonary angiography were performed in 26 patients (group I). We also analyzed clinical outcome in 28 patients who underwent V-P scanning and spiral CT (group II).

The study patients included 52 men and two women, aged 29–83 years (mean, 62.9 years). The majority had substantial coexistent morbid conditions, including malignancy ($n = 9$), respiratory insufficiency ($n = 6$), recent heart surgery ($n = 5$), abdominal surgery ($n = 3$), or orthopedic surgery ($n = 7$).

CT Evaluation

CT scans were obtained with a model 2000 CT unit (Picker International, Cleveland, Ohio). Routine examinations consisted of 1.5–2.0-mm-thick sections obtained without contrast material enhancement at 10-mm intervals. Patients underwent CT in the supine position, and scanning proceeded from the lung apex to the diaphragm to analyze airway and parenchymal changes. Lung images were reconstructed with a high-spatial-frequency algorithm and were photographed at a window width of 1,500 HU and level of −550 HU.

Thin-section CT was followed by spiral CT (200 mA; 130 kV; 1 second per rotation; mean z-axis coverage, 12 cm; pitch of 2; 17–23-second acquisition time; 3-mm collimation). Data were reconstructed with a 180° linear interpolation algorithm. In all patients, spiral CT was initiated at the middle of the aortic arch and extended inferiorly to at least the midventricular level to permit demonstration of the main, lobar, and segmental arteries of the upper, middle, and lower lobes. Three patients who could not sustain a breath hold due to ventilator use underwent CT during shallow breathing.

Iodinated contrast material was administered as a bolus with an automated injector (Medrad, Pittsburgh, Pa). The injection was carefully monitored by a registered nurse or a physician. A total of 100–140 mL of a dilute, 30% iopromide solution (Ultravist 300, Berlex Laboratories, Wayne, NJ); iothalamate meglumine (Conray 60; Mallinckrodt Medical, St Louis, Mo); or a dilute, 50% solution of iopromide (Ultravist 370; Berlex Laboratories) was injected at a rate of 4–5 mL/sec. The injection was performed through a 20-gauge intravenous catheter placed in the antecubital fossa, with a 7–15-second delay before scanning. In one patient, the contrast material was injected via an indwelling central catheter in the superior vena cava, with a 2-second delay before scanning.

The scanning delay was estimated on the basis of time-attenuation curves obtained in the first 23 patients and when indicated in subsequent patients; such indications included suspicion for subclavian venous or superior vena caval thrombosis and abnormal hemodynamic status. These curves were created by injecting 20 mL of a contrast agent and obtaining images every other second at the level of the central pulmonary arteries until peak contrast enhancement was achieved; imaging began at the start of the contrast material injection.

Pulmonary Angiography

Twenty-two patients were evaluated with selective right and left digital angiography ($n = 15$) or conventional angiography (recognized as the reference standard; $n = 7$); unilateral angiograms were obtained in another four patients. Multiple views of each lung were obtained in all of these 26 patients. V-P scans were available before angiography was performed in all 22 patients. Subselective catheter placement was performed and magnification views were obtained when indicated, at the discretion of the angiographer. Each angiographic series was performed with the administration of 30–50 mL of nonionic iopromide (Ultravist 300 or Ultravist 370; Berlex Laboratories), injected at a rate of 15–25 mL/sec. Digital subtraction angiograms were acquired at a rate of three or six frames per second; conventional angiograms were acquired at a rate of two images per second until the venous phase of the study. Standard angiographic criteria (18) were used for the diagnosis of the chronicity of PE.

CT was performed before angiography in 21 patients, and angiography was performed before CT in five patients, depending on the availability of the angiographic and CT equipment at the time of referral for suspected PE. CT and angiography were performed within 12 hours of each other in 16 patients, within 24 hours of each other in eight patients, and within 48 hours of each other in two patients.

V-P Scanning

V-P scans were obtained in all 54 patients. V-P scanning preceded spiral CT or angiography by less than 24 hours in 32 patients and by 24–48 hours in 22 patients. First, pulmonary perfusion imaging was performed after intravenous injection of 1–2 mCi (37–74 MBq) technetium-99m macroaggregated albumin. Images were recorded for 300,000 counts in eight views by using a large–field-of-view scintigraphy camera (Diacam; Siemens Gammasonics, Hoffman Estates, Ill) with a parallel-hole, low-energy, all-purpose collimator. Second, 4–5 mCi (148–185 MBq) Tc-99m diethylenetriaminepentaacetic acid aerosol was administered by using a commercial nebulizer (Medipart, Cary, Ill), and eight-view ventilation imaging was performed.

Clinical Follow-up and Outcome

Of the 28 patients who did not undergo pulmonary angiography, 25 were contacted by telephone and three were contacted by mail 5–42 weeks (mean, 24 weeks) after study entry. Medical records were reviewed in all 28 patients. Deaths, subsequent admission to a hospital, new symptoms, use of anticoagulant medication, and major bleeding complications were recorded.

Image Analysis

V-P scans, CT scans, and angiograms were independently evaluated. Each V-P scan was interpreted by a single nuclear medicine physician (A.J.F.), without knowledge of the CT findings. The V-P scans were classified as normal or low, intermediate, moderate, or high probability by using a modification of the diagnostic criteria of the PIOPED study (4). For the purposes of our analyses, intermediate- and moderate-probability V-P scans were considered to be indeterminate.

CT scans were interpreted independently by two of three radiologists (K.G., P.D.R., R.J.J.) experienced with chest CT. In all cases, the first reading of spiral CT scans was at the time of the examination, during the course of clinical work. All images were analyzed with mediastinal and lung window settings on the CT monitor and on hard copies. Multiple window and level settings were used while the images were viewed at a workstation, at the discretion of the reviewer. Discrepancies were resolved by consensus to establish the final interpretation. CT scans were evaluated in a blinded fashion, without knowledge of the findings from the V-P scans or angiograms.

Mediastinal images (window width, 350–400 HU; window level, 35–40 HU) were graded for the quality of vascular opacification. Image quality was considered to be poor when filling defects were depicted inadequately, satisfactory when the images were sufficient for analysis of pulmonary arteries (without a high degree of contrast enhancement), and good when a high degree of vascular opacification was demonstrated. Central and peripheral vascular zones, as described by Remy-Jardin et al (9), were evaluated in each lung for the presence of acute and chronic PE. An effort was made to assess subsegmental vessels. The CT appearance of PE and the criteria used for the diagnosis of acute and chronic PE have been previously described (9).

Pulmonary angiograms were scored independently by one of two angiographers (S.W.S., J.D.D.), without knowledge of the CT findings. Angiograms with motion artifacts were interpreted independently by the second reader. Angiograms and CT scans were compared on a vessel-by-vessel basis, and the results were recorded on a per patient and a per lung basis, to simplify reporting. When the CT and angiographic interpretations were in disagreement, a joint interpretation session was held between the CT scan and the angiogram reviewers.

The sensitivity, specificity, positive predictive value, and negative predictive value were determined for images obtained in group I patients only. Standard methods for proportions were used. For the group II patients, the concordance between spiral CT and V-P scans was used to help diagnose PE (positive CT scan, high-probability V-P scan) or exclude PE (negative CT scan, normal or low-probability V-P scan). PE was considered to be absent when the angiogram was negative for PE or, when a normal or low-probability V-P was scan acquired, the spiral CT scan was negative and when patients were discharged from the hospital with event-free clinical follow-up, without the administration of anticoagulant medication. PE was considered to be present when the pulmonary angiogram was positive, when the CT scan showed PE, or when a high-probability V-P scan and a positive spiral CT scan were obtained.

RESULTS

The results are summarized in Tables 1–3. CT demonstrated good or satisfactory

TABLE 1
Comparison of Results of V-P Scanning, Spiral CT and Pulmonary Angiography in 26 Patients (Group I)

Imaging Result	Angiographic Result Negative	Positive	Inconclusive
CT			
Negative	18	2*	0
Positive	0	4	1
Inconclusive	0	1	0
V-P			
Low probability	4	0	0
Indeterminate	14	7	0
High probability	0	0	1

* PE seen retrospectively in one patient.

TABLE 2
Comparison of Results of V-P Scanning and Spiral CT in 28 Patients (Group II)

V-P Result	CT Result Positive*	Negative†	Alternate or Additional Finding	Mean Clinical Follow-up (w)
Normal	0	2	0	32
Low probability	1	11	9	24
Indeterminate	0	6‡	6	24
High probability	6	2§	8	16

* Patients were treated with anticoagulant medication.
† Unless otherwise noted, patients were not treated with anticoagulant medication.
‡ One patient with chronic PE was treated with anticoagulant medication.
§ Both patients had chronic PE and were treated with anticoagulant medication.

opacification of pulmonary arteries in all patients except one. The only inconclusive study was obtained in a patient in the surgical intensive care unit with a documented patent foramen ovale. Additional findings at chest CT in this patient included a moderate-sized left pleural effusion and atelectasis of the left lower lobe and the lingula; lingular segmental and subsegmental PEs were detected on the angiogram in this patient. The technical quality of the CT scans was considered to be less than optimal in seven patients because of suboptimal opacification of upper lobe vessels secondary to initiation of scanning with inadequate delay after contrast material injection (time-attenuation curves were used in only two of the seven patients). In the majority of patients with normal-caliber vessels, only short portions of subsegmental vessels were visualized.

Group I Patients

Spiral CT allowed prospective identification of acute PE in five (20%) of the 25 patients with technically optimal CT scans (Table 1). The distribution of PEs visualized at CT is shown in Table 3. PEs were found in more than one location in the seven patients in each group who had PEs. Four patients were considered to have changes due to chronic PE: one patient with a central PE and three with a peripheral PE (not included in Table 3 and not considered in the statistical analysis); one patient had changes due to both acute and chronic PE (Fig 2).

There were two false-negative CT studies. In one case, PE in the superior lingular subsegmental vessels could not be demonstrated, even in retrospect (Fig 3). The other false-negative case was of PE in the anterior segmental artery of the right lower lobe, which was overlooked prospectively but could be seen in retrospect. One patient had acute segmental PE in the right lower lobe at CT and a high-probability V-P scan in addition to chronic changes in left lower lobe segmental arteries. The right lower lobe vessels were not well depicted on the angiogram owing to respiratory motion artifacts. Although unproved, this likely represents a false-negative angiogram.

Pulmonary angiograms were technically adequate in 25 of 26 patients. In four patients, there was excellent concordance between spiral CT and angiographic findings for both the occurrence and the location of acute PE. Changes suggestive of chronic PE were demonstrated at CT in five patients but were seen at angiography in only two of these patients with peripheral, chronic PE. In one case, mural thickening of central pulmonary arteries was exquisitely well depicted on the CT scan but was not evident on the angiogram. A "web" sign (a linear filling defect in a normal- to small-sized vessel), indicative of chronic PE, in a left lower lobe artery was shown only on the CT scan in a patient with a history of acute PE in this vessel 2 years before the CT study was obtained (Fig 2). Seven (33%) of 21 patients with indeterminate V-P scans had PE, which is comparable to the 32.6% prevalence found in the PIOPED study (4).

The prospective sensitivity of spiral CT, determined by including all vascular zones in 24 patients in whom technically satisfactory studies were obtained, was 67% (95% confidence interval [CI], 22%, 96%), and the specificity was 100% (95% CI, 81%, 100%). The positive predictive value was 100% (95% CI, 40%, 100%), and the negative predictive value was 90% (95% CI, 68%, 99%). The sensitivity, specificity, positive predictive value, and

TABLE 3
Distribution of PEs on CT Scans

Pulmonary Arterial System	Group I (n = 7)	Group II (n = 7)
Main	0	2
Interlobar	0	3
Lower lobe	1	3
Segmental	6	7
Subsegmental	7	7
Upper lobes	0	2
Middle lobe and lingula	2	2
Lower lobes	6	6

negative predictive value, calculated separately for 48 lungs, were 67% (95% CI, 22%, 96%), 100% (95% CI, 91%, 100%), 100% (95% CI, 40%, 100%), and 95% (95% CI, 84%, 99%), respectively. The sensitivity and specificity within the central vascular zones (main and lobar vessels) were each 100%.

Group II Patients

Seven (25%) of 28 patients in group II had acute PE (Table 2). There were more patients with central PE in group II than in group I (Table 3). Three patients subsequently underwent caval filter placement. Thirteen patients with a normal or low-probability V-P scan and a negative spiral CT scan had event-free survival (mean follow-up, 28 weeks) without the administration of anticoagulant medication. Only one patient in this group died, 9 weeks after entry into the study: This patient had prostate carcinoma with bone metastases and died of progressive hypoventilation. One patient, who had recently undergone hip surgery, developed a large thigh hematoma during empiric treatment with anticoagulant medication before the exclusion of PE.

In the nine patients who either refused to undergo angiography or were consid-

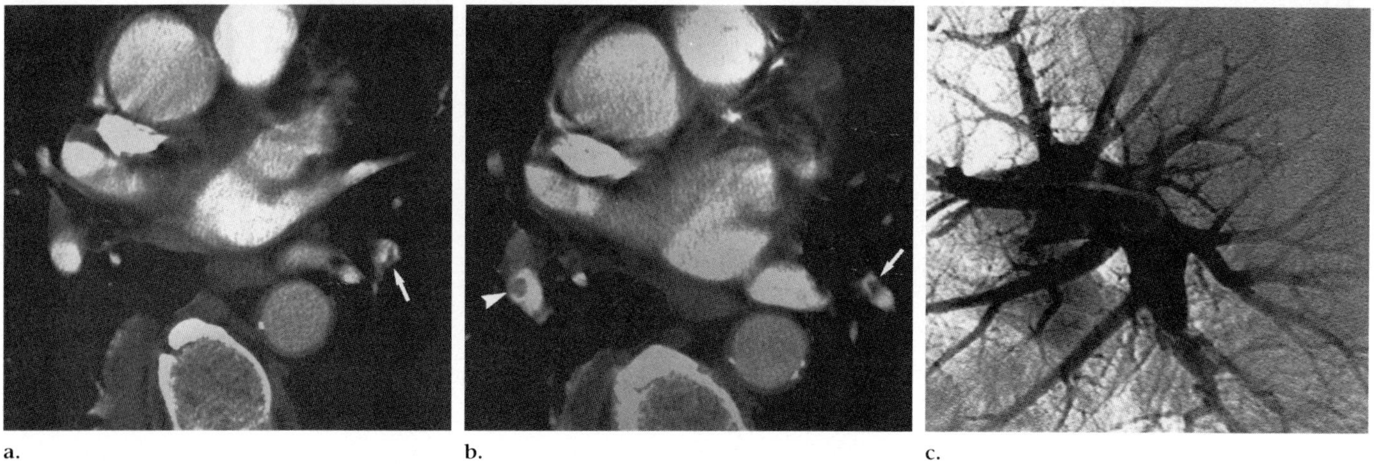

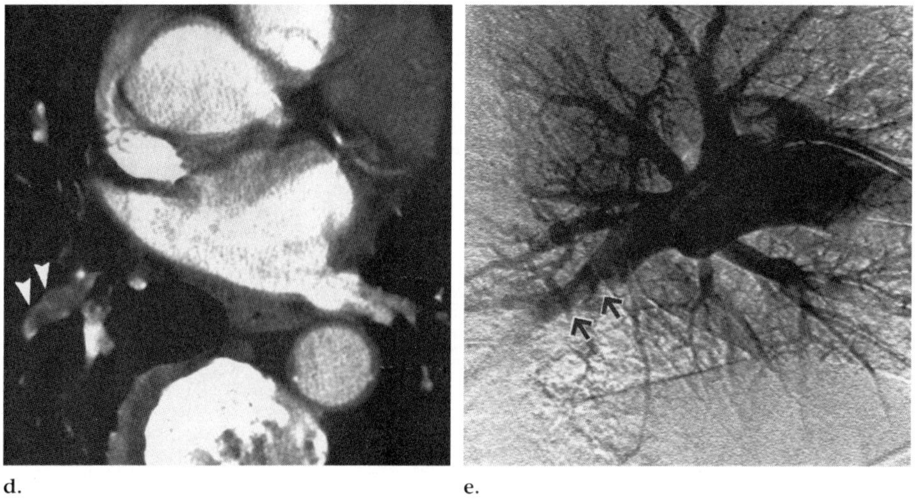

Figure 2. Acute and chronic PE in a 78-year-old man with a history of pulmonary hypertension and acute shortness of breath after total hip arthroplasty. (a, b) Spiral CT scans demonstrate a spiral linear filling defect (arrow) in a left lower lobe artery, indicative of a web. (c) Lateral projection of the left pulmonary angiogram was interpreted as normal. (b, d) Spiral CT scans show intraluminal filling defects in a right lower lobe artery (arrowhead in b) extending into the segmental vessels (arrowheads in d). (e) Lateral projection of the right pulmonary angiogram confirms these filling defects (arrows).

ered ineligible, CT scans were negative for PE in five of six patients in whom an indeterminate V-P scan was obtained. These five patients had event-free survival (mean follow-up, 24 weeks) without the administration of anticoagulant medication. One patient had chronic PE seen at CT in addition to bronchogenic carcinoma; this patient was treated with anticoagulant medication. Two patients in whom high-probability V-P scans were obtained had changes due to chronic PE on the spiral CT scan but no evidence of acute PE. Catheter placement in the right side of the heart in these two patients demonstrated a marked increase in pulmonary arterial and right atrial pressures. One patient in whom a low-probability V-P scan was obtained had segmental and subsegmental acute PE in the right lower lobe (Fig 4). Leg US findings obtained at the time of entry into the study were negative for deep venous thrombosis in this patient; however, repeated leg US, performed 7 days later, demonstrated peroneal and popliteal venous thrombosis. This patient was treated with anticoagulant medication.

Alternate Diagnoses and Additional Findings

In group II (Table 2), nine patients in whom a low-probability V-P scan was obtained had important additional findings, including esophageal cancer (n = 2), tumor that encased vessels (n = 2), and bone metastases (n = 1), all of which were previously known, and hypersensitivity pneumonitis (n = 1), aspiration pneumonia (n = 2), and extensive emphysema (n = 1), which were first found on CT scans obtained for the evaluation for PE. Additional findings in six patients in whom an indeterminate V-P scan was obtained included septic emboli (n = 1), thrombus in the residual right main pulmonary artery after a right pneumonectomy (n = 1), interstitial lung disease with honeycombing (n = 2), collateral vessels (n = 1), and bronchiolitis (n = 1), all but one of which were first found on the CT scan obtained for evaluation for PE; the case of interstitial lung disease was previously known. Additional findings in eight patients in whom a high-probability V-P scan was obtained included malignancy, enlarged pulmonary arteries, lung infarcts, and consolidation due to bronchiolitis obliterans with organized pneumonia, all of which, except the infarction, were previously known.

DISCUSSION

Our study included the most difficult to diagnose cases of PE: those with unresolved clinical and scintigraphic findings in elderly patients at high risk for PE, many with coexistent morbid conditions. Although we routinely used 3-mm collimation (to decrease volume averaging) and a pitch of 2 (to decrease motion artifacts and that helped cover an average of 12 cm of the thorax in a single breath hold), the prospective sensitivity for segmental or subsegmental PE was not significantly different from that reported by Goodman et al (14), who used 5-mm collimation and a 1:1 pitch. Recently, Remy-Jardin et al (19) reported marked improvement in the CT analysis of segmental and subsegmental vessels with 2-mm collimation at 75 seconds per revolution.

Hull et al (20) reported a 7.8% mortal-

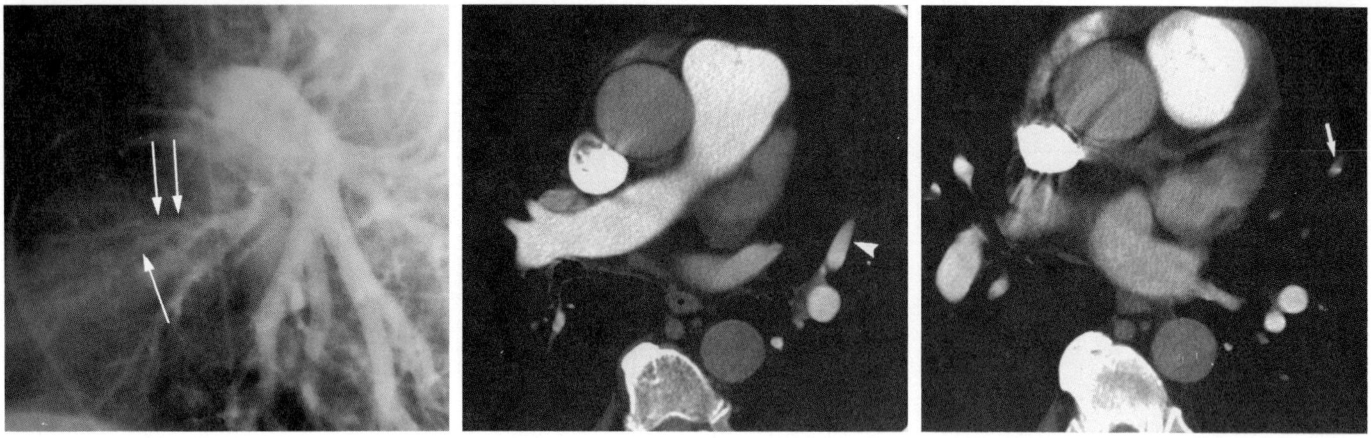

a. b. c.

Figure 3. Images in a 65-year-old man suspected of having acute PE, in whom an indeterminate V-P scan was obtained. (**a**) Magnified lateral view of the left pulmonary angiogram shows PEs (arrows) in the superior lingular subsegmental vessels. (**b, c**) On spiral CT scans, the PEs were not detected, even in retrospect: A normal superior lingular segmental artery (arrowhead in **b**) is shown, and subsegmental vessels (arrow in **c**) are poorly visualized.

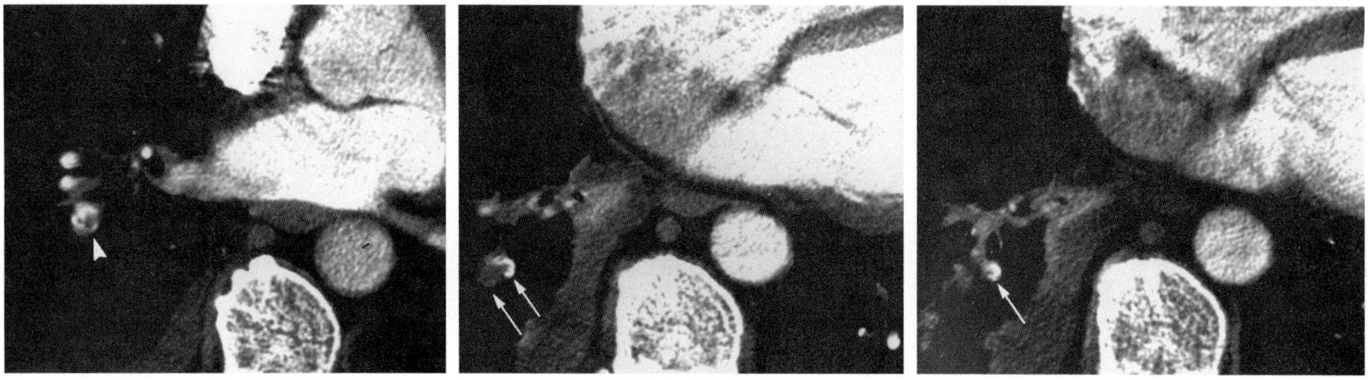

a. b. c.

Figure 4. Spiral CT scans in a 60-year-old man suspected of having acute PE, in whom a low-probability V-P scan was obtained. Intraluminal filling defects are seen in the (**a**) posterior basal segmental (arrowhead) and (**b, c**) subsegmental vessels (arrows in **b**, arrow in **c**) of the right lower lobe.

ity rate due to autopsy-proved PE in patients with inadequate cardiorespiratory reserve compared with a 0.14% mortality rate in patients with good cardiorespiratory reserve in whom low-probability lung scans had been obtained. Because many of our patients had coexistent cardiopulmonary diseases, which can potentially make isolated subsegmental clots clinically important (20), an attempt was made to evaluate the subsegmental vessels with care. However, only short portions of subsegmental vessels were demonstrated on the majority of negative CT scans (with normal-sized vessels), even with the use of 3-mm collimation. Longer portions of subsegmental vessels were seen in cases of acute PE with distended vessels (Fig 4). The prevalence in our series of isolated subsegmental clots (one [7%] patient) was within the reported (4,9,18) range of prevalence (5%–36%) in patients with acute PE. In our practice, patients with isolated subsegmental PEs are routinely treated with anticoagulant medication.

Confident evaluation with CT of nonvertical vessels (segmental arteries of the right middle lobe and the lingula, anterior segmental arteries of the right upper lobe and the left upper lobe, and apical segmental arteries of both lower lobes) remains a problem (9,11,14). In our study, two cases of lingular segmental and subsegmental PE were missed; in one case, this was due to a technically suboptimal study. In the later part of our study, we used time-attenuation curves to determine the scanning delay, but only in selected cases. Routine use of time-attenuation curves would increase the time of the examination but may help prevent an occasional case of suboptimal opacification (21).

Reformatting of images on a workstation was usually not helpful in our experience, even when meticulous data acquisition was performed. The failure in one of our cases to detect PE prospectively in the anterior basal segmental artery of the right lower lobe suggests that the false-negative rate should decrease as more experience is gained with interpretation of spiral CT studies.

Concordance between spiral CT and pulmonary angiographic findings was better for acute than for chronic PE in our study. CT is inherently better at depicting a nonoccluding PE or mural wall thickening (22). Because both sides of the chest are depicted on one CT image, a side-to-side comparison of segmental vessel size and opacification is easier with CT scans than with pulmonary angiograms. Disparities in the size of segmental vessels and mosaic patterns of lung attenuation were found to be useful for reliable differentiation of patients with chronic pulmonary thromboembolism from those with nonthromboembolic pulmonary arterial hypertension in a study with 67 patients by Bergin et al (23). Two patients in our study had focal bronchial dilatation in a region of small, poorly enhancing vessels; these findings are suggestive of chronic PE, as has been recently described (24). It is possible that CT may better demonstrate changes due to chronic PE than pulmonary angiography does.

The secondary objective of this study was a retrospective analysis of the CT results in 28 patients with clinical follow-up who did not undergo angiography (group II). The 100% positive predictive value suggests that a spiral CT scan that is unequivocally positive for acute PE obviates angiography. The lack of angiographic confirmation in patients with a negative spiral CT scan was a limitation of our study because the negative predictive value is known to be less than 100%. Event-free survival without the administration of anticoagulant medication is, however, a valid and important clinical outcome. None of the patients in whom a normal or low-probability V-P scan and a negative spiral CT scan were obtained developed clinically evident PE during the follow-up without anticoagulant medication, which indicates that important PE did not occur in this group. Clinical follow-up (mean, 28 weeks) was probably not long enough in some of our patients, but most deaths and recurrent emboli reported by Carson et al (25) occurred within 2 weeks of diagnosis. We plan to continue follow-up in these patients. Further studies with larger numbers of patients and a longer follow-up are needed to validate our results.

Although pulmonary angiography is associated with lower mortality (<1%) and morbidity (2%–5%) rates than empiric anticoagulant medication, it has not gained widespread acceptance and is invasive (5–8). Older patients experience a larger number of minor and major complications due to angiography, compared with younger patients (7). Thirty percent of the patients in our study either refused to undergo pulmonary angiography or were considered by their clinician to be ineligible for the procedure because of the perceived invasiveness.

In most cases, the decision to treat or not is made on the basis of the V-P scan findings and the clinical diagnosis (13), especially in small community hospitals where angiography is not readily available or offered. This probably results in many patients being either overtreated for PE that does not exist or, more important, undertreated when they do have PE. CT scans, like angiograms, are either positive or negative for PE in the majority of cases, whereas up to 73% of V-P scans are indeterminate for the diagnosis of PE (4). Direct visualization of PE on CT scans in seven patients in whom a high-probability V-P scan was obtained appeared to give "concrete" evidence to support a decision to administer anticoagulant medication. Direct visualization with CT of intraluminal PE and the vessels also may help in the assessment of the response to therapy or in the diagnosis of acute PE superimposed on chronic PE.

V-P scintigraphy provides only indirect evidence for PE and has poor spatial resolution. Negative CT scans in two patients in whom a normal V-P scan was obtained and in 11 patients in whom a low-probability V-P scan was obtained increased the confidence of clinicians to avoid treatment of these patients with anticoagulant medication. To further assist in the care of these patients, the CT scans provided an alternative (new) diagnosis in four (31%) of 13 patients. Four patients in whom a low-probability V-P scan and a negative spiral CT scan were obtained underwent pulmonary angiography during the initial part of our study, before the clinicians developed confidence in their ability to evaluate for PE by using CT scans. Pulmonary angiograms in all four patients confirmed the CT diagnosis. Our results support the criteria used by Mayo et al (16), namely, that a combination of normal or low-probability V-P scans and negative spiral CT scans is sufficient to exclude PE. In one patient in our study, a low-probability V-P scan and a positive spiral CT scan were obtained (Fig 4); this patient was treated with anticoagulant medication.

CT can potentially provide a reliable, noninvasive alternative to angiography, especially in patients who refuse to undergo angiography or who are at high risk for the development of angiography-related complications. Pulmonary angiography is indicated for patients with inconclusive or negative CT scans, especially for those in whom subsegmental PE may be clinically important. In our experience with patients who underwent both CT and pulmonary angiography within 48 hours of each other, the total contrast material load did not result in adverse reactions.

CT helped reduce the number of false-positive diagnoses in patients in whom a high-probability V-P scan was obtained: On CT scans in two such patients, there was no evidence of acute PE but there were changes due to chronic PE. Both of these patients had a history of PE. This is consistent with the fact that in the PIOPED study (4), only 14 (74%) of 19 patients with a history of PE in whom a high-probability V-P scan was obtained actually had PE, whereas 88 (91%) of 97 patients without a history of PE had PE.

The ability to differentiate acute from chronic PE on the basis of CT findings helped in the assessment of patients in whom there was a suspicion for acute PE superimposed on chronic PE—a situation where CT should be the primary screening examination. Further studies are necessary with larger numbers of patients to validate this recommendation.

In conclusion, in our subset of patients, the use of spiral CT yielded a more accurate and more specific diagnosis than V-P scanning did. CT findings can be used not only to exclude or demonstrate PE directly but also, in many cases, to provide an alternate diagnosis. Our results confirm the usefulness of spiral CT as a noninvasive screening examination for the diagnosis of PE.

Acknowledgment: We thank David N. Iklé, PhD, for help with statistical analyses.

References

1. National Institutes of Health Consensus Conference. Prevention of venous thrombosis and pulmonary embolism. JAMA 1986; 256:744–749.
2. Moser KM. Pulmonary embolism. In: Isselbacher KJ, Braunwald E, Wilson JD, Martin JB, Fauci AS, Kasper DL, eds. Harrison's principles of internal medicine. 13th ed. New York, NY: McGraw-Hill, 1994; 1214–1220.
3. Goldhaber SZ, Hennekens CH, Evans DA, Newton EC, Godleski JJ. Factors associated with correct antemortem diagnosis of major pulmonary embolism. Am J Med 1982; 73:822–826.
4. The PIOPED investigators. Value of the ventilation/perfusion scan in acute pulmonary embolism: results of the Prospective Investigation of Pulmonary Embolism Diagnosis (PIOPED). JAMA 1990; 263:2753–2759.
5. Henschke CI, Mateescu I, Yankelevitz DF. Changing practice patterns in the workup of pulmonary embolism. Chest 1995; 107: 940–945.
6. Sostman HD, Ravin CE, Sullivan DC, Mills SR, Glickman MG, Dorfman GS. Use of pulmonary angiography for suspected pulmonary embolism: influence of scintigraphic diagnosis. AJR 1982; 139:673–677.
7. Zukerman DA, Sterling KM, Oser RF. Safety of pulmonary angiography in the 1990s. JVIR 1996; 7:199–205.
8. Kelley MA, Carson JL, Palevsky HI, Schwartz JS. Diagnosing pulmonary embolism: new facts and strategies. Ann Intern Med 1991; 114:300–306.

9. Remy-Jardin M, Remy J, Deschildre F, et al. Diagnosis of pulmonary embolism with spiral CT: comparison with pulmonary angiography and scintigraphy. Radiology 1996: 200:699–706.
10. Teigen CL, Maus TP, Sheedy PF II, et al. Pulmonary embolism: diagnosis with contrast-enhanced electron-beam CT and comparison with pulmonary angiography. Radiology 1995; 194:313–319.
11. van Rossum AB, Pattynama PMT, Tjin A Ton ER, et al. Pulmonary embolism: validation of spiral CT angiography in 149 patients. Radiology 1996; 201:467–470.
12. Blum AG, Delfau F, Grignon B, et al. Spiral-computed tomography versus pulmonary angiography in the diagnosis of acute massive pulmonary embolism. Am J Cardiol 1994; 74:96–99.
13. Khorasani R, Gudas TF, Nikpoor N, Polak JF. Treatment of patients with suspected pulmonary embolism and intermediate-probability lung scans. AJR 1997; 169: 1355–1357.
14. Goodman LR, Curtin JJ, Mewissen MW, et al. Detection of pulmonary embolism in patients with unresolved clinical and scintigraphic diagnosis: helical CT versus angiography. AJR 1995; 164:1369–1374.
15. Ferretti GR, Bosson JL, Buffaz PD, et al. Acute pulmonary embolism: role of helical CT in 164 patients with intermediate probability at ventilation-perfusion scintigraphy and normal results at duplex US of the legs. Radiology 1997; 205:453–458.
16. Mayo JR, Remy-Jardin M, Muller NL, et al. Pulmonary embolism: prospective comparison of spiral CT with ventilation-perfusion scintigraphy. Radiology 1997; 205:447–452.
17. Hoellerich VL, Wigton RS. Diagnosing pulmonary embolism using clinical findings. Arch Intern Med 1986; 146:1699–1704.
18. Oser RF, Zuckerman DA, Guttierez FR, Brink JA. Anatomic distribution of pulmonary emboli at pulmonary arteriography: implications for cross-sectional imaging. Radiology 1996; 199:31–35.
19. Remy-Jardin M, Remy J, Artaud D, Deschildre F, Duhamel A. Peripheral pulmonary arteries: optimization of the spiral CT acquisition protocol. Radiology 1997; 204: 157–163.
20. Hull RD, Rascob GE, Pineo GF, Brant RF. The low-probability lung scan: a need for change in nomenclature. Arch Intern Med 1995; 155:1845–1851.
21. Kuzo RS, Goodman LR. CT evaluation of pulmonary embolism: technique and interpretation. AJR 1997; 169:959–965.
22. Bergin CJ, Sirlin CB, Hauschildt JP, et al. Chronic thromboembolism: diagnosis with helical CT and MR imaging with angiographic and surgical correlation. Radiology 1997; 204:695–702.
23. Bergin CJ, Rios G, King MA, Belezzuoli E, Luna J, Auger WR. Accuracy of high-resolution CT in identifying chronic pulmonary thromboembolic disease. AJR 1996; 166:1371–1377.
24. Remy-Jardin M, Remy J, Louvegny S, Artaud D, Deschildre F, Duhamel A. Airway changes in chronic pulmonary embolism: CT findings in 33 patients. Radiology 1997; 203:355–360.
25. Carson JL, Kelley MA, Duff A, et al. The clinical course of pulmonary embolism. N Engl J Med 1992; 326:1240–1245.

Mark V. Gosselin, MD[2]
Geoffrey D. Rubin, MD
Ann N. Leung, MD
Judy Huang, MD
Norman W. Rizk, MD

Index terms:
Computers, diagnostic aid
Embolism, pulmonary, 60.72, 944.77
Pulmonary arteries, CT, 944.12915
Pulmonary arteries, thrombosis, 944.77

Radiology 1998; 208:209–215

Abbreviations:
PE = pulmonary embolism
V-P = ventilation-perfusion

[1] From the Departments of Radiology (M.V.G., G.D.R., A.N.L.) and Medicine (J.H., N.W.R.), Stanford University School of Medicine, S-072B, Stanford, CA 94305-5105. Received November 5, 1997; revision requested December 11; revision received February 9, 1998; accepted March 9. **Address reprint requests to** G.D.R.

[2] Current address: Department of Radiology, University of Utah, Salt Lake City.

Unsuspected Pulmonary Embolism: Prospective Detection on Routine Helical CT Scans[1]

PURPOSE: To determine the prevalence of unsuspected pulmonary embolism (PE) on routine thoracic helical computed tomographic (CT) scans and to quantify the improvement in PE detection by using a cine-paging mode on a workstation instead of hard-copy review.

MATERIALS AND METHODS: Seven hundred eighty-five patients referred for routine contrast medium–enhanced thoracic CT within 9 months were prospectively recruited. Helical CT was performed. Studies were prospectively interpreted by four radiologists. Two radiologists performed routine, undirected, hard-copy consensus review for official interpretation; two of three thoracic radiologists independently performed a dedicated workstation-based search for PE. The presence of PE involving the main, lobar, or segmental pulmonary arteries was assigned a score of 1–5 (1 = definitely negative, 5 = definitely positive) by each independent reviewer. Patients with a score of 4 or 5 underwent lower-extremity ultrasound, ventilation-perfusion scintigraphy, or both, followed by pulmonary CT angiography if the findings were still equivocal.

RESULTS: Twelve (1.5%) of the 785 patients had unsuspected PE, with an inpatient prevalence of 5% (eight of 160) and an outpatient prevalence of 0.6% (four of 625). Of the 12 patients with unsuspected PE, 10 (83%) had cancer. Of the 81 inpatients with cancer, seven (9%) had unsuspected PE. A dedicated workstation-based search resulted in detection of PE in three more patients (25%) than did hard-copy interpretation.

CONCLUSION: The prevalence of unsuspected PE was highest among inpatients with cancer. A directed, workstation-based search can improve the PE detection rate over that with hard-copy review.

Approximately 500,000 cases of pulmonary embolism (PE) are documented each year in the United States (1); however, the reported incidence of PE is likely lower than the actual incidence, because of the prevalence of asymptomatic, or "silent," PE (2,3). The prevalence of PE detected at autopsy in hospitalized patients is 14%–26%, with approximately one-third representing unsuspected disease (4,5). Silent PE is most commonly detected in high-risk populations, including patients who have recently undergone major surgery (particularly orthopedic surgery), who have an underlying neoplasm, who have hypercoagulation, who have undergone trauma, who are immobilized, or who have congestive heart failure. Detection of unsuspected PE is important to prevent embolic recurrence, which is associated with substantial morbidity and mortality (1).

The advent of helical technology has improved the ability to use computed tomographic (CT) scanners to diagnose PE (6–11). To date, to our knowledge, there has been only one report of the prevalence of unsuspected PE detected at helical CT, which was retrospectively determined by means of an analysis of CT reports (12). We have performed a prospective, 8.5-month examination of all patients undergoing contrast medium–enhanced helical CT of the thorax at our institution to determine the frequency with which unsuspected PE is detected with routine, contrast-enhanced thoracic CT and the frequency with which potentially identifiable PEs are not detected during routine image interpretation.

Author contributions:
Guarantors of integrity of entire study, M.V.G., G.D.R.; study concepts, G.D.R.; study design, M.V.G., G.D.R., A.N.L., J.H., N.W.R.; literature research, M.V.G., J.H., N.W.R.; clinical studies, M.V.G., G.D.R., A.N.L., J.H.; data acquisition, M.V.G., G.D.R., A.N.L., J.H.; data analysis, M.V.G.; statistical analysis, G.D.R.; manuscript preparation, M.V.G., G.D.R., N.W.R.; manuscript editing, G.D.R.; manuscript review, A.N.L., J.H., N.W.R.

MATERIALS AND METHODS

All patients referred to our institution for routine contrast-enhanced thoracic CT scanning between July 22, 1996, and March 1, 1997, were entered into the study. The indications for CT included the staging or follow-up of neoplasms, evaluation to detect infection in immunocompromised hosts, trauma, and the characterization of tumors suspected because of chest radiographic abnormalities. All CT examinations performed for suspected PE and all CT angiograms of the thoracic aorta were excluded from the study. A total of 785 patients, 160 inpatients (20%) and 625 outpatients (80%), were enrolled, with a mean age of 54.9 years (age range, 18–96 years). Malignant neoplasia was present in 81 (51%) of 160 inpatients and in 507 (81%) of 625 outpatients.

Imaging

Helical CT scans were acquired cephalad to caudad from the thoracic inlet through the diaphragm by using a CT scanner (Somatom Plus 4, Siemens Medical Systems, Iselin, NJ; or HiSpeed CT/i, GE Medical Systems, Milwaukee, Wis.). All scans were obtained during a single 30-second breath hold unless patients were too dyspneic, in which case scans were obtained during quiet breathing. The first 50 examinations were performed with 7-mm (HiSpeed CT/i) or 8-mm (Somatom Plus 4) collimation and a pitch of 1.2–1.5; the remaining 735 examinations were performed with 5-mm collimation and a pitch of 1.7–2.0 (both scanners). Transverse sections were reconstructed with a bone reconstruction kernel every 7 or 8 mm for the first 50 examinations and every 2.5 mm for the subsequent 735 examinations by using 180° linear interpolation. Ninety to 100 mL of nonionic contrast medium (300 mg of iodine per milliliter of solution; iopamidol [Isovue 300; Bracco Diagnostics, Princeton, NJ] or iohexol [Omnipaque 300, Nycomed, Princeton, NJ]) was injected into a 22-gauge antecubital venous catheter at 2.0–2.5 mL/sec. Scanning delays were 20–30 seconds, depending on whether dedicated thoracic CT or thoracic CT in combination with abdominal CT was performed. Reconstructed sections were photographed at two window and level settings, (*a*) 400 HU and 40 HU and (*b*) 1,500 HU and −700 HU by using a laser camera. Twenty images were printed on each sheet of 14 × 17-inch film. Reconstructed sections were also transferred to one of two viewing computer workstations (MagicView, Siemens Medical Systems; or CT Independent Console, GE Medical Systems).

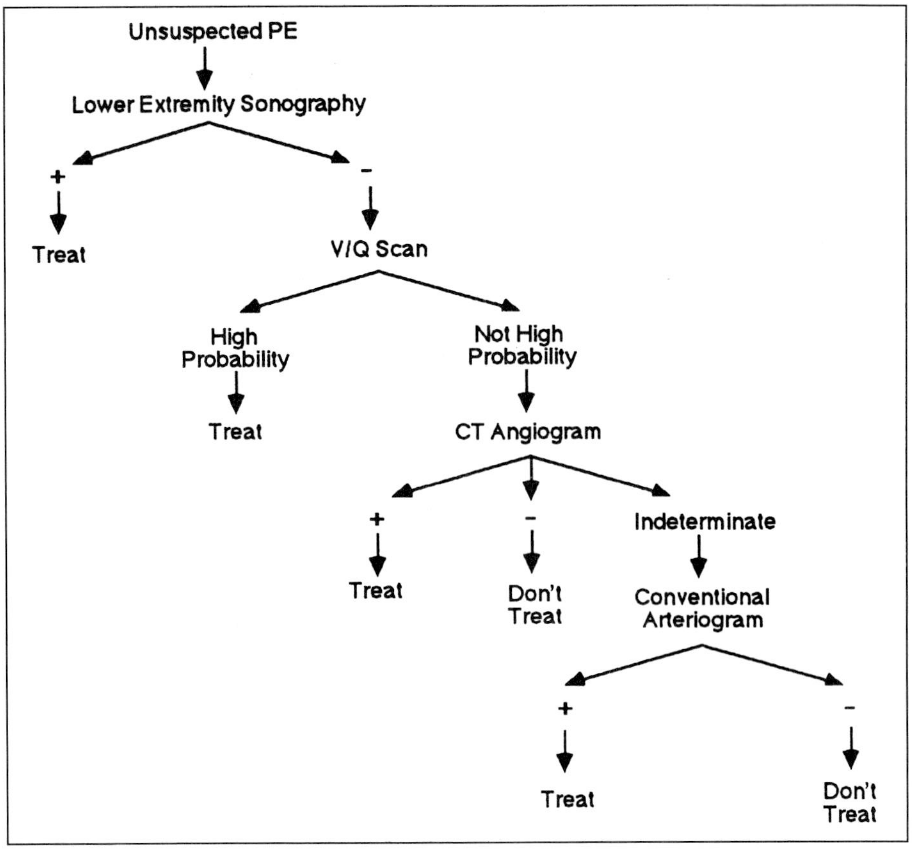

Figure 1. Flow chart provided to referring clinicians by the Division of Pulmonary Medicine within 24 hours of CT diagnosis of unsuspected PE.

Image Interpretation

All studies were prospectively interpreted in two ways: (*a*) routine, undirected, hard-copy consensus review performed by two thoracic or body imaging radiologists, and (*b*) dedicated workstation-based search for a PE by two of three independent thoracic radiologists (M.V.G., G.D.R., A.N.L.). For the latter interpretations, images were evaluated on a computer workstation within 72 hours of the study. The hard-copy consensus interpretations and the two independent workstation-based interpretations were blinded to each other. PEs were identified as present when either complete or partial filling defects within the main, lobar, or segmental pulmonary arteries were identified. For workstation-based interpretations, visualized emboli were localized to specific main, lobar, or segmental pulmonary artery branches, and a single, per patient confidence score of 1–5 (1 = findings definitely negative, 3 = findings indeterminate, 5 = findings definitely positive) was assigned by each reviewer, indicating the presence of at least one PE.

Patients in whom PE was diagnosed with a score of 4 or 5 by both reviewers underwent confirmatory imaging. When only one reviewer assigned a score a 4 or 5, a third thoracic radiologist evaluated the examination to render the deciding score. All patients with unsuspected PE diagnosed on thoracic CT scans were referred to the Division of Pulmonary Medicine to coordinate confirmation and follow-up. A recommended protocol for confirming the presence of PE on helical CT scans was provided to referring clinicians and is illustrated in Figure 1. Lower-extremity venous Doppler ultrasonography (US), ventilation-perfusion (V-P) scintigraphy, or both were performed. If findings were equivocal, further evaluation with pulmonary CT angiography was performed. Patients with equivocal CT angiograms were to undergo conventional angiography; however, this situation did not arise. Patients with positive examination findings were referred to the Division of Pulmonary Medicine for clinical evaluation, treatment coordination, and follow-up.

TABLE 1
Results in 15 Patients with Positive CT Scans

				Most Proximal Location of Filling Defect in Each Lung*			Correlative Studies†			CT Diagnosis‡			
Patient/ Sex/ Age (y)	Patient Status	Underlying Disease	Collimation (mm)	Main Arteries	Lobar Arteries	Segmental Arteries	Venous US	V-P	CT Angiography	Workstation	Hard Copy	Treatment§	Comments
1/M/81	Inpatient	Lung cancer	5	. . .	RL	. . .	NP	H	NP	TP	TP	AC	. . .
2/M/73	Inpatient	Laryngeal cancer	5	L	RU, RL	. . .	+	H	+	TP	TP	AC, F	. . .
3/M/86	Inpatient	Lung cancer	5	. . .	. . .	RL, LL	+	NP	NP	TP	TP	AC	. . .
4/M/56	Inpatient	Lung cancer	7	. . .	LL	. . .	−	H	+	TP	FN	AC	. . .
5/M/69	Outpatient	Paraplegia	5	. . .	RU, RL, LL	. . .	−	H	NP	TP	TP	AC	. . .
6/F/52	Inpatient	Non-Hodgkin lymphoma	5	R	LL	. . .	NP	NP	NP	TP	TP	AC	Obvious positive CT finding
7/M/48	Inpatient	Intravenous drug abuse, HIV	5	L	RL	. . .	−	H	NP	TP	TP	AC	. . .
8/M/89	Inpatient	Colon cancer	5	. . .	RU, RL	. . .	NP	H	NP	TP	TP	AC	. . .
9/F/51	Inpatient	Lymphoma	5	R	. . .	. . .	−	H	NP	TP	TP	AC	. . .
10/M/63	Outpatient	Leukemia	5	. . .	RL, LL	. . .	+	L	NP	TP	FN	None	Iliac vein clot on abdominal CT scan
11/M/68	Outpatient	Lymphoma	5	. . .	. . .	RL	+	H	NP	TP	FN	AC	. . .
12/F/51	Outpatient	Lymphoma	5	L	. . .	. . .	−	NP	NP	TP	TP	AC, F	Positive findings of pulmonary magnetic resonance (MR) angiography
13/M/45	Outpatient	Nasopharyngeal cancer	8	. . .	. . .	RL, LU	NP	NP	−	FP	TN	None	. . .
14/M/56	Outpatient	Lymphoma	8	. . .	. . .	RL, LU	−	−	NP	FP	TN	None	Negative findings of follow-up CT
15/F/72	Outpatient	Lymphoma	5	. . .	. . .	RL	−	−	NP	FP	TN	None	. . .

* L = left, LL = left lower, LU = left upper, R = right, RL = right lower, RU = right upper.
† H = high probability of PE, L = low probability of PE, NP = not performed, + = positive findings, − = negative findings.
‡ FN = false-negative, FP = false-positive, TN = true-negative, TP = true-positive.
§ AC = anticoagulation, F = inferior vena cava filtration.

An additional evaluation was performed to assess the relative segmental and lobar pulmonary arterial branch identification between the 7- and 5-mm collimation protocols. Every segmental and lobar branch in each of the first 35 patients undergoing each of the two acquisition protocols was scored as being identifiable or not.

Statistical Analysis

The association between the presence of unsuspected PE and (*a*) inpatient or outpatient status, (*b*) age, (*c*) sex, and (*d*) the presence of malignancy was determined and tested for significance by using the Student *t* test. True-positive CT studies were tabulated for each of the image-presentation methods, and the results were compared. Pulmonary arterial branch depiction was compared between the two acquisition protocols.

RESULTS

Fifteen of 785 patients had positive studies at dedicated workstation review by two thoracic radiologists. Correlative imaging findings in these 15 patients are presented in Table 1. Of these patients, three had false-positive studies, and 12 had true-positive studies. Therefore, the prevalence of unsuspected PE was 1.5% (12 of 785 patients). The prevalence of PE among inpatients was 5% (eight of 160), while the prevalence of PE among outpatients was 0.6% (four of 625; $P < .001$). The age range of these 12 patients was 48–89 years (mean age, 65.6 years). Unsuspected PE occurred in nine (1.9%) of 471 men and in three (1.0%) of 314 women ($P = .29$). Of the 12 patients with unsuspected PE, 10 (83%) had an underlying malignancy, one had paraplegia, and one had the human immunodeficiency virus, or HIV, and was an intravenous drug abuser.

Of the 81 inpatients with an underlying malignancy, seven (9%) had unsuspected PE. Of the 507 outpatients with malignancy, three (0.6%) had PE. The prevalence of malignancy as compared with the prevalence of benign disorders among patients with PE was significant ($P < .001$), and the prevalence of malignancy in inpatients was significantly greater than that in outpatients ($P < .001$). None of the 12 patients with unsuspected PE had recently undergone surgery.

In 10 (1.3%) of the 785 patients, PE was unsuspected by the referring physicians, while in two patients, incidental PEs were known to clinicians from previous imaging studies (V-P scintigraphy findings of high probability of PE in both) performed at other institutions. These results were unavailable to the radiologists interpreting the CT scans and were not cited in the clinical history that accompanied the examination request.

The proximal extent of the emboli involved the main pulmonary artery in one patient, a lobar artery in nine patients, and a segmental artery in two patients. All patients had PE in the lower lobe arteries. Multiple emboli were detected in nine patients; all of these emboli involved the lower lobes. Four of the nine patients had concurrent involvement of the upper lobes. The remaining three patients had single emboli in the lower lobe vessels (two in the right lung, one in the left lung).

Correlative imaging studies were obtained in 11 of the 12 patients with true-positive findings. These studies included eight US scans of the lower extremities (three were positive), one positive US scan of the upper extremities, nine V-P scans (eight had a high probability for PE), two positive CT angiograms, one gadolinium-enhanced three-dimensional pulmonary MR angiogram (which demonstrated a long left nonocclusive embolus that correlated exactly with the CT findings), and one abdominal CT scan, which demonstrated an iliac venous thrombus. All correlative imaging studies were obtained within 3 days of the initial CT scan. The remaining patient had a large occlusive PE in the right main artery. This represented a recurrent PE in a patient already receiving anticoagulation medication, which was subsequently determined to be subtherapeutic. The CT findings were so compelling that the clinicians elected to not perform correlative imaging (Fig 2). Although a protocol was provided to each referring physician, indicating a progression for obtaining confirmatory studies (Fig 1), some physicians selected confirmatory studies independently of the protocol.

Two of three false-positive CT studies were in patients who underwent imaging with 8-mm collimation. The first patient had an intersegmental lymph node that mimicked an eccentric mural thrombosis. The second patient had a contrast medium–blood mixing artifact. The third patient, who underwent imaging with 5-mm collimation, demonstrated a partial volume artifact in the right lower lobe superior segmental pulmonary artery. Follow-up studies (one CT angiogram, two V-P scans, and two lower-extremity US scans) in these three patients were unremarkable.

Routine hard-copy review resulted in the identification of PE in nine (75%) of the 12 patients; however, there were three (25%) false-negative findings at hard-copy review. In retrospect, these PEs were present on the hard copies. In two of the three patients, PEs were located in the lobar pulmonary arteries (Fig 3); in one of the three patients, a PE was located in a segmental branch of the left lower lobe artery (Fig 4).

All segmental pulmonary arterial branches were visualized in four of the 35 patients who underwent imaging with 7- or 8-mm collimation as compared with 25 of the 35 patients who underwent imaging with 5-mm collimation and reconstruction at 2.5-mm intervals (Table 2). Commonly excluded segments were arterial branches not perpendicular to the axis of table travel, such as the anterior and posterior segments of the upper lobes, the lingula, the right middle lobe, and the superior segments of the lower lobes (Fig 5).

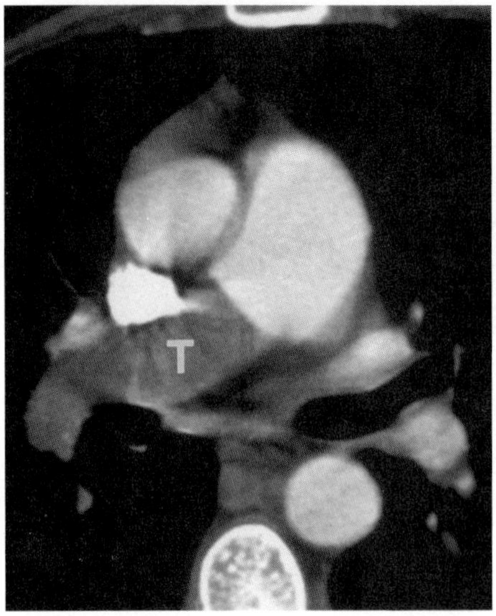

Figure 2. CT scan (5-mm collimation, 1.6 pitch) in a 52-year-old female inpatient after bone marrow transplantation for non-Hodgkin lymphoma demonstrates a completely occlusive filling defect (*T*) within the right pulmonary artery. The referring physician believed that the CT study was pathognomonic and elected to treat the patient with anticoagulation. Although confirmatory images were not obtained, the examination findings were considered positive.

Directed therapy with either systemic anticoagulation or an inferior vena caval filter was instituted in 11 of the 12 patients with true-positive findings at workstation review on the basis of positive correlative imaging studies in 10 and unequivocal PE demonstration on the CT scan in one patient. One patient was not treated despite a history of prior lower-extremity deep venous thrombosis, depiction of nonocclusive lobar and segmental pulmonary arterial thrombi with thoracic CT, subsequent documentation of an iliac venous thrombus with CT, and a partially occlusive thrombus in the lower-extremity deep venous system with US. A V-P scan in this patient was interpreted as having a low probability for PE.

Of the 11 patients in whom directed therapy was instituted, 10 were treated with anticoagulation and two received an inferior vena caval filter. Two patients undergoing long-term anticoagulation therapy were noted to have subtherapeutic clotting indexes after CT-documented recurrent emboli; their anticoagulation dose was increased.

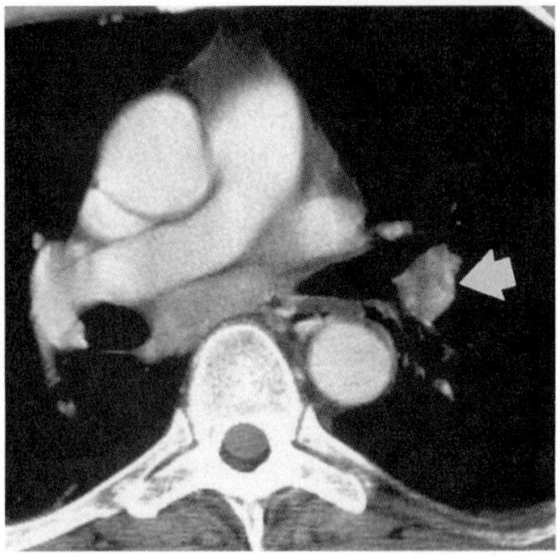

Figure 3. CT scan (7-mm collimation, 1.0 pitch) in a 56-year-old male inpatient with metastatic bronchogenic carcinoma demonstrates a completely occlusive thrombus (arrow) within the left hilar pulmonary artery. The finding was detected prospectively with workstation-based review only and was confirmed with a high-probability V-P scan. Findings of lower-extremity US were negative.

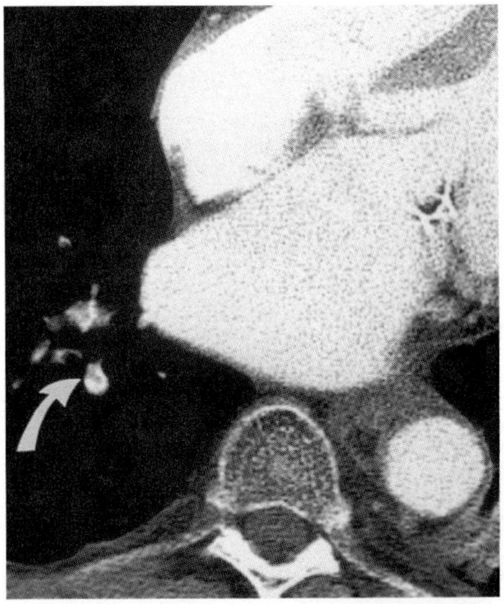

Figure 4. CT scan (5-mm collimation, 1.6 pitch) in a 68-year-old male outpatient with esophageal carcinoma demonstrates a filling defect (arrow) within the artery to the posterior basilar segment of the right lower lobe. The finding was detected prospectively with workstation-based review only and was confirmed with a high-probability V-P scan and positive findings of an upper-extremity venous US examination.

DISCUSSION

The occurrence of unsuspected PE is well recognized, but the actual prevalence has

TABLE 2
Segmental Pulmonary Arteries Visualized

Lobe	Scanning Collimation (mm): 7 or 8 (*n* = 35)	Scanning Collimation (mm): 5 (*n* = 35)	*P* Value*
Right upper			
Anterior	31 (89)	34 (97)	.170
Posterior	24 (69)	32 (91)	.020
Apical	35 (100)	35 (100)	.999
Left lower			
Apical posterior	19 (54)	34 (97)	<.001
Anterior	33 (94)	34 (97)	.560
Right middle and lingula	12 (34)	34 (97)	<.001
Right and left lower			
Superior	24 (69)	32 (91)	.020
Medial	22 (63)	32 (91)	<.004
Anterior	31 (89)	32 (91)	.700
Lateral	35 (100)	33 (94)	.160
Posterior	24 (97)	35 (100)	.320
All segments visualized	4 (11)	25 (71)	<.001

Note.—Numbers in parentheses are percentages.
* Two-tailed Student *t* test.

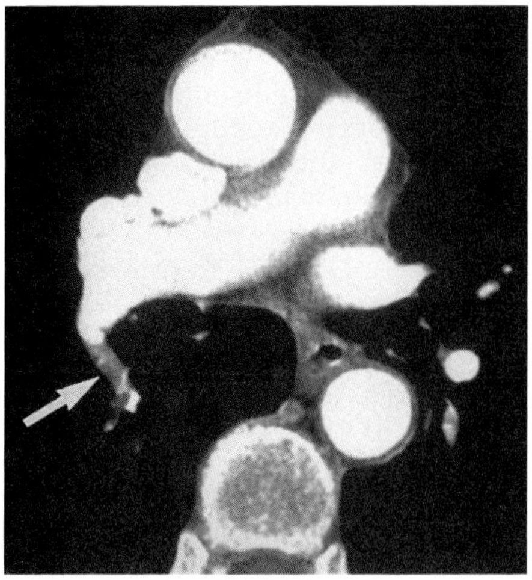

Figure 5. False-positive CT scan (5-mm collimation, 1.6 pitch) in a 72-year-old female outpatient with gastric carcinoma demonstrates an apparent filling defect (arrow) in the superior segmental artery to the right lower lobe. V-P scintigraphy demonstrated scattered subsegmental matched defects; findings of lower-extremity US were normal.

been difficult to quantify. Results of various autopsy studies have demonstrated rates of up to 7%–9% for incidental PE in highly select samples from predominately inpatient populations (4,5). The prevalence of patients with asymptomatic deep venous thrombosis above the knee but high-probability V-P scans has been reported to be 35%–50%, indicating in this very high-risk subset an extremely high rate of unsuspected emboli (2,3).

That such a high fraction of cases of PE in various clinical settings are asymptomatic raises the question of their clinical importance. Several lines of evidence indicate that these PEs probably are important. First, in a large autopsy series, PE was diagnosed before death in only 32% of the patients with fatal emboli (13). In fact, the diagnosis was considered before death in only half of the cases of fatal PE, and diagnostic tests directed at ruling in or out emboli were performed in only 22% (13). Last, as Prospective Investigation of Pulmonary Embolism Diagnosis, or PIOPED, data indicate that there is only an 8% recurrence rate and a 2.5% fatality rate in patients with this diagnosis who are treated conventionally (14), it follows that most of the problem resides in the undiagnosed and presumably unsuspected PEs, not in the largely successfully treated ones we do manage to diagnose.

However, one cannot conclude that the known fatality rate of 30% in patients with untreated symptomatic PEs (14) is equally high in patients with asymptomatic PEs. We can only postulate that some fraction of the unsuspected or asymptomatic PEs accounts for a major portion of the 70% of undiagnosed fatal cases (5). These considerations appear to reinforce the idea that asymptomatic PEs need to be treated; if a decision is made not to treat them, at the very least the potential source of PEs should be repetitively evaluated, since patients without thrombi in lower-extremity sites are known not to be at great risk for recurrent PEs (15).

Verschakelen and colleagues (16) found a 0.5% prevalence of incidental PE detected with conventional CT scanning, while Winston and co-workers (12) found a 1% prevalence of unsuspected PE in a retrospective analysis of helical CT scans reported to demonstrate PE. Helical acquisition in the latter study may have accounted for a higher prevalence owing to an improved detection rate. We found a 1.5% prevalence of detectable incidental PE (50% greater than that found by Winston et al [12] and 200% greater than that found by Verschakelen et al [16]). We attribute our higher detection rate primarily to a prospective, dedicated, workstation-based review of the CT scans. Had analysis of our study population been based solely on a retrospective review of radiology reports, similar to that in the study by Winston et al, PE would have been detected in 25% fewer patients and our overall detection rate would have decreased from 1.5% to 1.1%. Workstation review provides a flexible environment for varying window and level settings and for cine image presentation. We detected incidental PE in 25% more patients (three of 12 patients) who had incidental PE with a directed workstation review as compared with a hard-copy review. These included one inpatient (emboli in the left lobar artery) and two outpatients (emboli in lower lobar artery in one and lower lobe segmental artery in the other).

In both our study and the study by Winston et al (12), inpatients had a substantially higher prevalence of incidental PE (5% and 2%, respectively). Our population was composed of 20% inpatients versus 30% in the cohort of Winston and co-workers. This disparity in population composition might have resulted in a lower prevalence of unsuspected PE in our study, but our prevalence of unsuspected PE was found to be higher, even when those patients with PE detected only at dedicated workstation review were excluded. This greater prevalence may be attributable to greater detection with a helical acquisition and a narrower section thickness.

The prevalence of asymptomatic PE has been shown to be highest in patients with advanced age and an underlying problem such as neoplasia, recent surgery, trauma, hypercoagulation, immobilization, and long-term indwelling catheters (2,12,16,17). Evaluation of the pulmonary arteries on all contrast-enhanced thoracic CT scans should be routine, but we recommend a directed search for PE in these high-risk patients, particularly in inpatients with malignancy. In our cohort, seven (9%) of the 81 inpatients with an underlying neoplasm had incidental PE. The diagnosis is often not suspected by the referring physician, because other clinical conditions disguise the symptoms.

All three false-positive CT studies in our cohort occurred early in the study and were described only at workstation-based review. In retrospect, the first and second of these artifacts resulted from inexperience in interpreting pulmonary artery patency on helical CT scans, and one resulted from a previously unreported artifact. One patient had an enlarged intersegmental lymph node adjacent to the right lower lobe pulmonary artery that was mistaken for an eccentric mural thrombosis. The other patient had an apparent isolated filling defect in the right lower lobe superior segmental pulmonary artery but had a normal US scan and V-P scan. In retrospect, the isolated involvement of one transversely oriented vessel was interpreted as a volume-averaging artifact. Our subsequent experience was that apparent filling defects were common in transversely oriented vessels. Although this phenomenon was less prevalent with 5-mm collimation than with 7–8-mm collimation, assessment of transversely oriented vessels was still limited by volume averaging in many cases and remains a potential pitfall to diagnosing PE with routine helical CT.

The third false-positive PE manifested in a patient with central, low-attenuation "dot artifacts" in three lower lobe segmental arteries (Fig 6). The central dot extended 5–10 mm in length on the routine CT scans; however, a CT angiogram obtained the following day was normal. We believe that this artifact resulted from laminar contrast medium flow, which at the terminal phases of the bolus injection resulted in lower opacification of the central vessel than that of the peripheral regions. Clues to help differentiate this dot artifact from a PE include a lesser decrease in central opacification than occurs with a PE, similar involvement of other vessels on the same scan levels, and short (<1-cm) longitudinal extension. We observed this artifact on many subsequent scans but refrained from diagnosing PE.

Limitations of this study include the lack of pulmonary angiographic or autopsy confirmation. It was difficult to convince the referring physicians to proceed to pulmonary angiography in their asymptomatic patients on the basis of the incidental findings uncovered with the CT scan when correlative noninvasive studies were negative. Further, pulmonary arterial depiction and detection of PE will improve with scanning protocols that have a narrower effective section thickness (18). Our scanning protocol for this study was designed to balance minimal effective section thickness with a practical acquisition that could image the entire chest in a single breath hold for routine imaging. While we have demonstrated higher prevalence for unsuspected PE than, to our knowledge, have previous studies of CT scanning, we believe that the true prevalence of occult PE is higher and might be documented with a scanning protocol that provides higher longitudinal spatial resolution for the detection of isolated segmental and subsegmental PE.

In summary, among patients undergoing contrast-enhanced thoracic CT, the prevalence of incidental PE was 1.5%. This prevalence of incidental PE was six times higher in inpatients with underlying malignancy (9%). A directed, workstation-based evaluation for PE resulted in a 25% greater detection rate over that of routine hard-copy review. Interpretation of images in patients with a high risk of PE with a more directed PE search pattern on a workstation will likely improve detection of clinically important, unsuspected PE, leading to the institution of therapy to reduce recurrent embolic events.

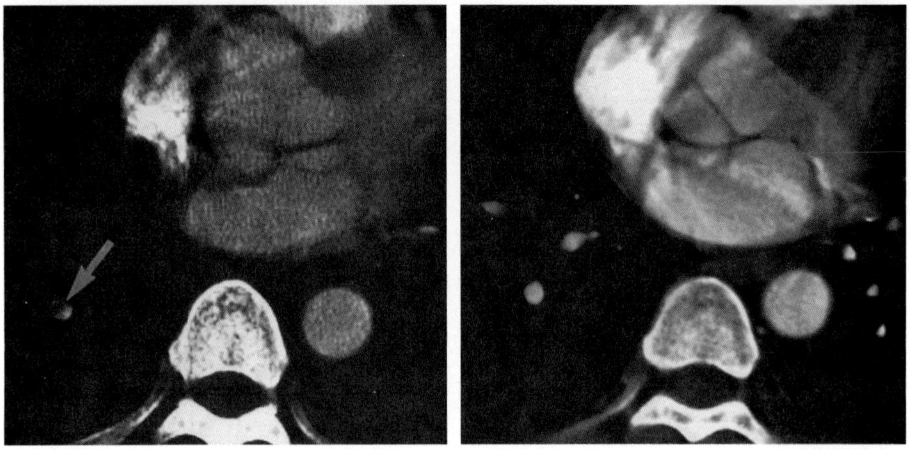

a. b.

Figure 6. (a) False-positive CT scan (8-mm collimation, 1.2 pitch) in a 45-year-old male outpatient with nasopharyngeal carcinoma. A central filling defect (arrow) is suggested in the posterior basilar segmental pulmonary artery to the right lower lobe, which was observed on two adjacent scans reconstructed at 8 mm apart. (b) Transverse CT angiogram (3-mm collimation, 2.0 pitch) obtained in the same patient as in **a** demonstrates that a filling defect is not present in this vessel. The artifact in **a** is likely caused by rapid inflow of unopacified blood into the central portion of the vessel during the terminal phase of the contrast medium injection. Contrast medium opacification in the vessel periphery persists because of slower flow near the vessel wall.

APPENDIX

V-P scintigraphy was performed after intravenous injection of 1.2-mCi (44.4-MBq) technetium-99m macroaggregates of human serum albumin followed by inhalation of krypton-81m gas. Anterior, posterior, left posterior oblique, right posterior oblique planar, and transverse single photon emission CT views were obtained by using a dual-isotope imaging technique with a MultiSPECT 3 or MultiSPECT 2 imager (Siemens Medical Systems).

US was performed with a 5-MHz linear-array transducer attached to a US imager (model 128XP; Acuson, Mountain View, Calif) or a 7-MHz linear-array transducer attached to a different US imager (model 140; Toshiba, Tustin, Calif). Graded-compression, B-mode, pulse-wave Doppler and color Doppler scanning from the inguinal ligament to the calf was performed.

CT angiography was performed from the inferior aspect of the aortic arch to a point 2 cm above the diaphragm during a single breath hold by using 3-mm collimation, 2.0 pitch, and image reconstruction every 2 mm. The scanning delay was determined from an initial 10-mL nonionic iodinated contrast medium injection at a rate of 4 mL/sec. After 4 seconds, 10 transverse sections were acquired through the main pulmonary artery every 2 seconds. A region of interest was placed in the pulmonary artery, and a time-attenuation curve was generated. The scanning delay was selected as the time to peak arterial opacification. CT angiography was performed with 120 mL of nonionic contrast medium injected at a rate of 4 mL/sec into a 20-gauge antecubital intravenous catheter. Images were viewed interactively with user-selected window and level settings on a computer workstation.

References

1. Moser EM. Venous thromboembolism. Am Rev Respir Dis 1990; 141:235–249.
2. Huisman MV, Buller HR, ten Cate JW, et al. Unexpected high prevalence of silent pulmonary embolism in patients with deep venous thrombosis. Chest 1989; 95: 498–502.
3. Dorfman GS, Cronan JJ, Tupper TB, et al. Occult pulmonary embolism: common occurrence in deep venous thrombosis. AJR 1989; 148:263–266.
4. Lindblad B, Sternby NH, Berqvist D. Incidence of venous thromboembolism verified by necropsy over 30 years. Br Med J 1991; 302:709–711.
5. Stein PD, Henry JW. Prevalence of acute pulmonary embolism among patients in a general hospital and at autopsy. Chest 1995; 108:978–981.
6. Remy-Jardin M, Remy J, Wattinne L, et al. Central pulmonary thromboembolism: diagnosis with spiral volumetric CT with the single-breath-hold technique—comparison with pulmonary angiography. Radiology 1992; 185:381–387.
7. Goodman LR, Curtin JJ, Mewissen MW, et al. Detection of pulmonary embolism in patients with unresolved clinical and scintigraphic diagnosis: helical CT versus angiography. AJR 1995; 164:1369–1374.
8. Goodman LR, Lipchik RJ. Diagnosis of acute pulmonary embolism: time for a new approach. Radiology 1996; 199:25–27.
9. Schwickert HC, Schweden F, Schild HH, et al. Chronic thromboembolic pulmonary artery obstruction: CT diagnosis and follow-up after thromboendarterectomy (abstr). Radiology 1993; 189(P):153.
10. Van Rossum AB, Treurniet FEE, Kieft GJ, et al. Role of spiral volumetric computed tomography scanning in the assessment of patients with clinical suspicion of pulmonary embolism and an abnormal ventilation-perfusion scan. Thorax 1996; 51: 23–28.
11. Remy-Jardin MJ, Remy J, Petyt L, et al. Diagnosis of acute pulmonary embolism with spiral CT: comparison with pulmonary angiography and scintigraphy. Radiology 1996; 200:699–706.
12. Winston CB, Wechsler RJ, Salazar AM, et al. Incidental pulmonary emboli detected at helical CT: effect on patient care. Radiology 1996; 201:23–27.
13. Morgenthaler T, Ryn JN. Clinical characteristics of fatal pulmonary embolism in a referral hospital. Mayo Clin Proc 1995; 70:417–424.
14. Carson JL, Kelley MA, Dutt A, et al. The clinical course of pulmonary embolism. N Engl J Med 1992; 326:1240–1245.
15. Hull RD, Raskob GE, Ginsberg JS, et al. A non-invasive strategy for the treatment of patients with suspected pulmonary embolism. Arch Intern Med 1994; 154:289–297.
16. Verschakelen JA, Vanwijck E, Bogaert J, et al. Detection of unsuspected central pulmonary embolism with conventional contrast-enhanced CT. Radiology 1993; 188: 847–850.
17. Gillum RF. Pulmonary embolism and thrombophlebitis in the United States, 1970-1985. Am Heart J 1987; 114:1262–1264.
18. Remy-Jardin M, Remy J, Artaud D, et al. Peripheral pulmonary arteries: optimization of the spiral CT acquisition protocol. Radiology 1997; 204:157–163.

Thomas J. Vogl, MD, PhD
Jörn O. Balzer, MD
Kai Dette, MD
Rainer Hintze, MD
Wassilios Pegios, MD
Jürgen Mäurer, MD, PhD
Heinrich Keck, MD
Peter Neuhaus, MD, PhD
Roland Felix, MD, PhD

Index terms:
Bile ducts, neoplasms, 76.321
Hepatic arteries, therapeutic blockade, 952.1264
Liver, CT, 76.12111, 76.12112, 76.12115
Liver, regeneration, 76.45
Liver, surgery, 76.45

Radiology 1998; 208:217–222

[1] From the Departments of Radiology (T.J.V., J.O.B., W.P., J.M., R.F.), Surgery (K.D., H.K., P.N.), and Gastroenterology (R.H.), University Hospital Charité, Campus Virchow, Humboldt University of Berlin, Augustenburger Platz 1, 13353 Berlin, Germany. Received September 2, 1997; revision requested November 13; final revision received February 16, 1998; accepted March 9. **Address reprint requests to** T.J.V.

Initially Unresectable Hilar Cholangiocarcinoma: Hepatic Regeneration after Transarterial Embolization[1]

PURPOSE: To assess with volumetric computed tomography (CT) the pattern and extent of hepatic regeneration induced with transarterial embolization of initially unresectable hilar cholangiocarcinoma (Klatskin tumor).

MATERIALS AND METHODS: In this prospective study, 13 patients (four men, nine women) with hilar cholangiocarcinoma, aged 43–74 years (mean ± 1 standard deviation, 59.9 years ± 9.6), underwent preoperative embolization of the right hepatic lobe. Embolization was performed transarterially by using four to 15 embolization coils. Volumetric measurements of the entire liver, left hepatic lobe, and spleen were performed with contrast material–enhanced and unenhanced helical CT before and after embolization in all patients.

RESULTS: After right lobe embolization, volumetric helical CT measurements revealed a 2%–33% decrease (mean, 10%) in the volume of the affected right hepatic lobe, an 11%–68% increase (mean, 37%) in the volume of left hepatic lobe parenchyma, and variations in splenic volume of −5% to +28% (mean, +11%). Nine patients underwent extended hepatectomy 27–75 days (mean, 44 days) after embolization. No patient had severe complications due to embolization.

CONCLUSION: In patients with an initially unresectable bilateral Klatskin tumor, right lobar arterial coil embolization results in enlargement of the left hepatic lobe (as verified with volumetric helical CT), thus allowing right hemihepatectomy.

At present, surgical resection offers the only hope for cure in patients with hilar cholangiocarcinoma, also known as Klatskin tumor (1–3). The limits of surgical treatment are determined on the basis of the amount of liver tissue that remains after removal of extensive portions of normal along with diseased liver parenchyma. Successful resection, with avoidance of the lethal posthepatectomy syndrome, is dependent on the volume and function of the future remnant liver tissue. Removal of more than 65% of the liver in adults greatly increases the risk of postoperative failure (4–6).

Various methods have been proposed to increase the regeneration and functional capacity of unaffected liver segments before surgery. In particular, venous and arterial embolizations have been performed, with variable results (7–9). Makuuchi et al (10) studied percutaneous portal venous embolization, which resulted in substantial parenchymal regeneration in noninvolved liver segments. The main differences between arterial and venous embolization of a liver segment are in the type of percutaneous approach used and the types of potential complications that arise from use of the two methods.

The purpose of this ongoing study was to evaluate the effectiveness of arterial embolization in the induction of liver regeneration. Volumetric helical computed tomography (CT) was used to measure liver parenchymal regeneration in preparation for hepatectomy in patients with initially unresectable Klatskin tumors. We used hepatic arterial branch embolization of the right hepatic lobe to stimulate parenchymal regeneration of the left hepatic lobe. Furthermore, we evaluated whether improved surgical resectability is achievable in patients with induced regeneration of the liver parenchyma.

Author contributions:
Guarantors of integrity of entire study, T.J.V., P.N., R.F.; study concepts, T.J.V., H.K., P.N.; study design, T.J.V., J.O.B.; definition of intellectual content, T.J.V., P.N., R.F.; literature research, W.P.; clinical studies, T.J.V., J.O.B., K.D., R.H.; data acquisition, T.J.V., J.O.B.; data analysis, J.O.B.; manuscript preparation, J.O.B.; manuscript editing, T.J.V., J.O.B.; manuscript review, T.J.V., J.M., W.P.

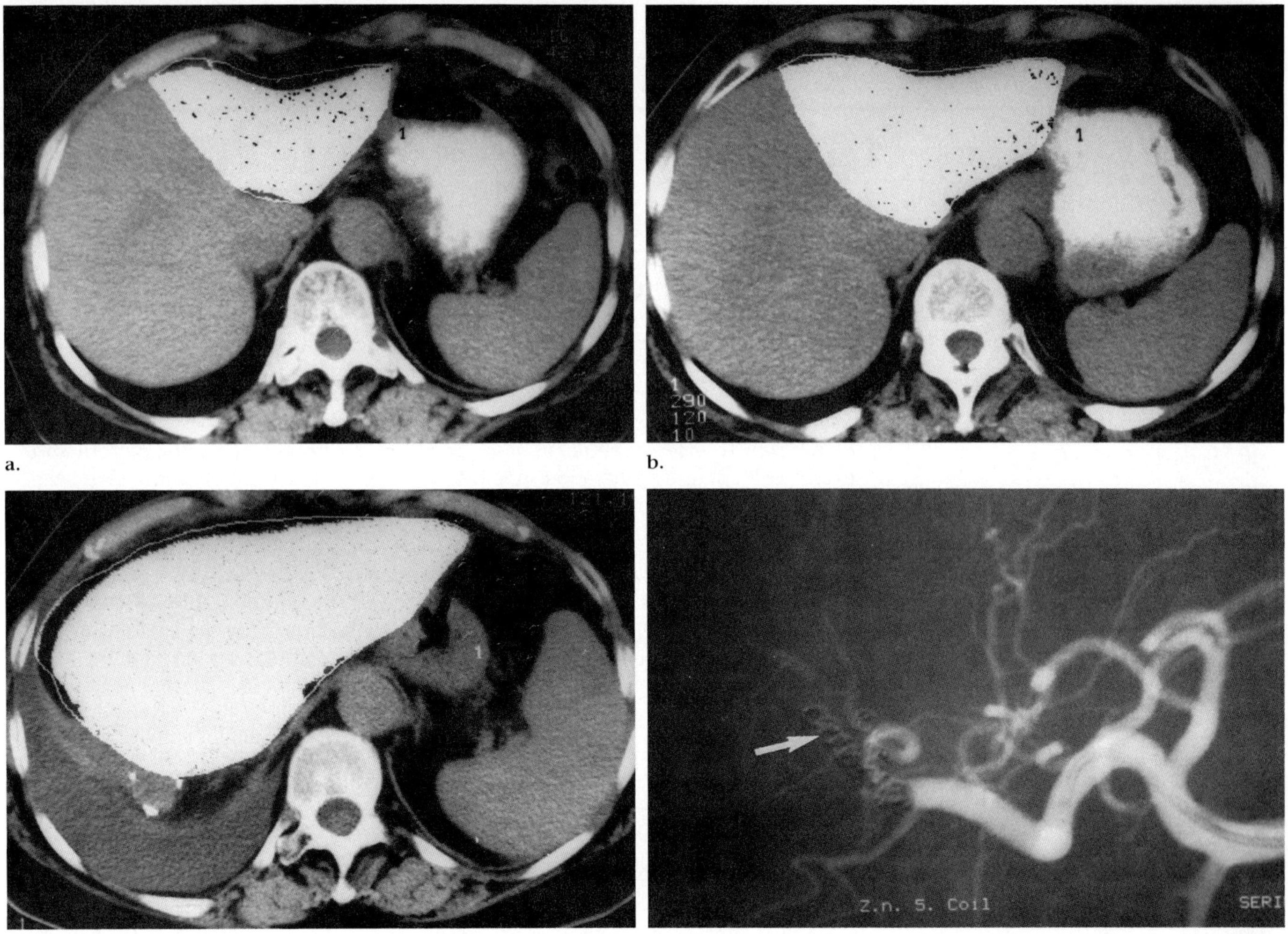

Figure 1. Patient 4. Cholangiocarcinoma in a 61-year-old woman. (a) Unenhanced axial CT scan is an example of the images used for volumetric measurement of the left hepatic lobe by means of the segmentation technique and area calculation before arterial embolization of the right hepatic lobe. (b) Unenhanced axial volumetric CT scan obtained 6 weeks after arterial embolization of the right hepatic lobe shows an increase in the volume of the left hepatic lobe in comparison with the initial measurement obtained with **a.** (c) Unenhanced axial volumetric CT scan obtained 1 week after hemihepatectomy shows a further increase in the volume of the remaining hepatic tissue. (d) Selective digital subtraction angiogram of the hepatic artery obtained in the anteroposterior projection immediately after embolization and placement of five coils (arrow) reveals reduced flow in the periphery of the right lobe, resulting in complete occlusion of the right lobar branches on digital subtraction angiograms obtained later (not shown). Disregard the *1* in **a–c.**

MATERIALS AND METHODS

Study Design

In this prospective study, 13 patients with initially unresectable bilateral Klatskin tumors of the liver underwent preoperative arterial embolization. All patients were referred to the Department of Radiology for localization and assessment of cholangiocarcinoma in the context of the overall liver morphology. Patients were selected for arterial embolization on the basis of (*a*) liver and tumor morphology as seen at initial helical CT, (*b*) liver function parameters, and (*c*) the consensus of a panel of radiologists and surgeons that the tumor was technically nonresectable in its present state.

Endoscopic retrograde cholangiographic studies helped to verify the CT diagnosis of Bismuth grade III tumors with bilateral involvement of the hepatic bile duct in all patients. For drainage of the dilated prestenotic bile ducts, a 10-F tube was placed, with endoscopic guidance, in the right hepatic duct in three patients and in the left hepatic duct in two patients. Preinterventional helical CT revealed the extension of the tumor and depicted a smaller volume or atrophy of the left hepatic lobe. Preoperative arterial embolization was performed after a normal portal venous blood supply to the future remnant liver could be confirmed angiographically. The study was approved by our clinical review board, and we obtained written informed consent from all patients.

Imaging and Embolization Protocols

All patients underwent helical CT (Somatom Plus; Siemens, Erlangen, Germany) without and with contrast material enhancement before and after embolization. Contiguous 10-mm-thick sections were acquired before the administration of nonionic contrast material (iopromide, Ultravist 370; Schering AG, Berlin, Germany). During intravenous administration of the iopromide (total volume, 205 mL), arterial and venous phase helical CT scans were obtained. For the arterial phase

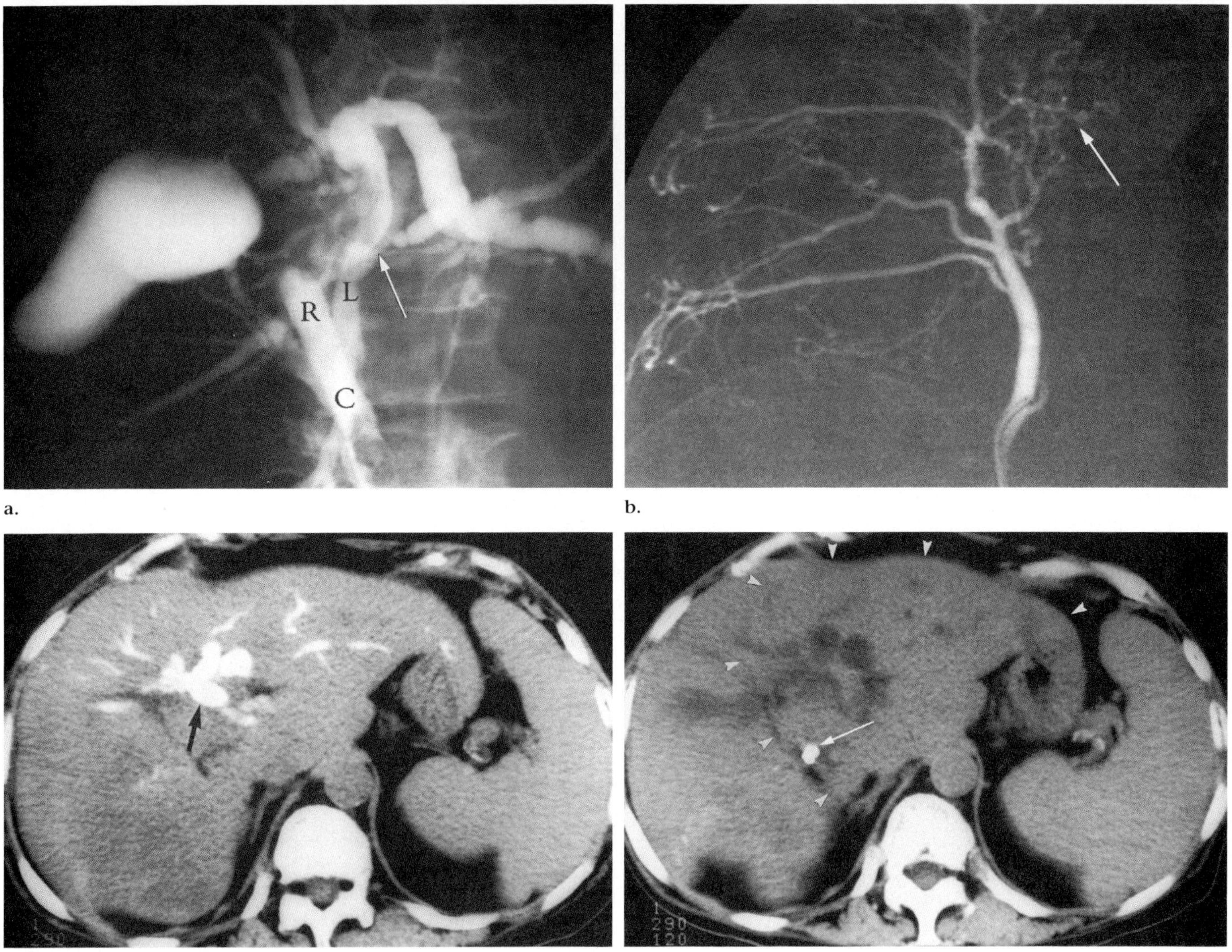

a. b. c. d.

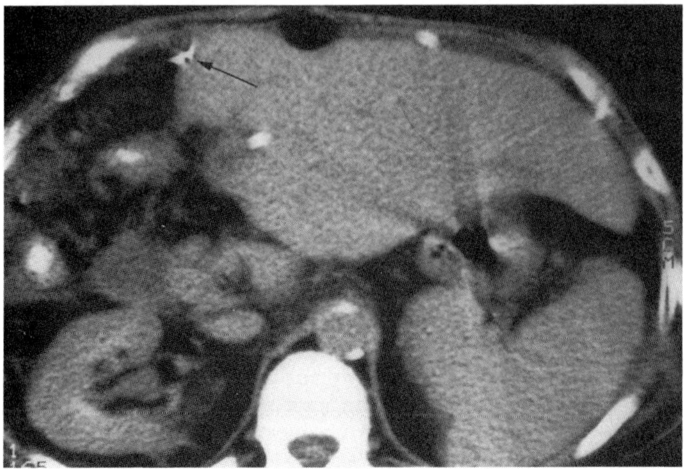

e.

Figure 2. Patient 12. Cholangiocarcinoma in a 61-year-old woman. **(a)** Conventional anteroposterior cholangiogram obtained after endoscopic placement of a catheter within the hepatic duct and administration of contrast material shows dilated intrahepatic bile ducts and proximal stenosis (arrow) of the left hepatic duct (*L*). *C* = common bile duct, *R* = right hepatic duct. **(b)** Selective digital subtraction angiogram of the hepatic artery obtained in the anteroposterior projection reveals tortuous intrahepatic vessels with increased vasculature (arrow) of the left hepatic lobe. **(c)** Unenhanced axial CT scan obtained after cholangiography and before embolization shows contrast material remaining within the bile ducts (arrow). **(d)** Unenhanced volumetric axial CT scan obtained 3 weeks after embolization reveals the still-dilated intrahepatic bile ducts, an increase in the volume of the left hepatic lobe (arrowheads), and shrinkage of the right hepatic lobe segments. The volume of the spleen is still increased in comparison with the initial measurement. Arrow = coils within the right hepatic artery. **(e)** Unenhanced axial CT scan obtained 2 weeks after successful right hemihepatectomy reveals a persistent increase in the volume of the left lobar parenchyma (356.32 cm^3), compared with initial measurements (249.25 cm^3). Arrow = artifact due to a surgical clip at the resection edge.

scans, a volume of 120 mL, a flow rate of 4 mL/sec, and a delay of 15 seconds after the iopromide injection were used; for the venous phase scans, a volume of 85 mL, a flow rate of 1 mL/sec, and a delay of 70 seconds were used. The arterial phase image reconstruction parameters were 5-mm/sec table feed, 5-mm section thickness, and 3-mm section increment; the venous phase image reconstruction parameters were 8-mm/sec table feed, 8-mm section thickness, and 8-mm section increment. Unenhanced follow-up CT examinations were performed during the 1st, 3rd, 5th, and 7th weeks after embolization.

Volumetric measurements.—Volumetric measurements of the entire liver, the left hepatic lobe, and the spleen were obtained by using an integrated workstation to calculate the area on all available unenhanced CT scans. The volume of each of these objects was determined by means of segmentation of the area of interest and calculation of the area from the unenhanced, contiguous 10-mm-thick CT sections. These measured areas were then summed and multiplied by the section thickness to arrive at the total organ volume (Fig 1). For each measurement, the lower limit of the segmentation interval was set to 0 HU, and the upper limit was set to 90 HU. In all patients, the attenuation of the liver parenchyma in this population varied from 25 to 75 HU. Therefore, only pixels with an attenuation value of 0–90 HU within the segmented area were considered for the volume calculation. Area calculation and segmentation were then performed by manually circling the region of interest. Each patient underwent initial volumetric helical CT before or immediately after embolization, and follow-up volumetric helical CT was performed after the 1st week, 2nd week, and 3rd–4th week and before surgery. Two patients (patients 6 and 11) underwent additional volumetric helical CT measurements during the 5th week after embolization.

Preoperative embolization.—In 13 patients, a 5-F pigtail catheter (Cook, Frankfurt, Germany) was used to perform preoperative embolization transarterially via the right femoral artery. Before embolization, an angiographic survey of the abdominal aorta was performed. After selective placement of a cobra catheter (Cook) in the common hepatic artery, the arterial blood supply to the individual liver segments was evaluated with angiography. The appropriate arteries were identified (Fig 2b), four to 15 embolization coils (Cook) with a diameter of 3 or 5 mm and of varying lengths (35–50 mm) were placed, and the vessels were occluded (Fig 1d). Embolization was considered to be successful when immediate angiographic follow-up demonstrated complete disappearance of arterial blood flow in the occluded vessel and in the supplied liver segments.

Patients

From January 1995 to August 1996, 13 consecutive patients (four men, nine women) with hilar bile duct carcinoma underwent preoperative embolization of the hepatic artery branch. The mean age ± 1 standard deviation of the patients was 59.9 years ± 9.6 (age range, 43–74 years). Only patients with no general contraindication for a surgical procedure were included in the study. In five patients with severe jaundice, bile was drained with endoscopically placed tubes (Fig 2a).

The appropriate time for each patient to undergo surgery was determined by a panel of radiologists and surgeons on the basis of frequent analyses of the helical CT follow-up studies and liver function test results. Criteria for surgery were an increase in the left hepatic volume and a return of the hepatic function values to near baseline values.

Twelve patients underwent laparotomy and one patient underwent laparoscopy 35–42 days after successful embolization. The surgeon judged the tumors in four patients as still unresectable at laparotomy, and palliative treatment was instituted. Among the remaining nine patients, hemihepatectomy (R0 resection [no evidence of tumor in the resection margins]) of the involved hepatic parenchyma was performed in four patients (Figs 1, 2), and liver-segment resection (R1 resection [microscopic evidence of tumor in the resection margin] or R2 resection [macroscopic evidence of tumor in the margin]) was performed in five. Two patients died of multiorgan failure after surgery.

At the time this article was written, follow-up examinations (CT, liver function tests, clinical examination) after arterial embolization over a period of 6 months and postoperative results were available in all remaining 11 patients.

Surgical, Imaging, and Volumetric Data in 13 Patients

Patient No.	Surgical Treatment	Time between First and Last CT (d)	Change in Volume (%)		
			Entire Liver	Left Lobe	Spleen
1	R0 resection	42	+7.02	+35.09	+0.68
2	R2 resection	33	+36.49	+40.20	+11.41
3	No resection	32	+18.19	+43.75	+13.76
4	R0 resection	37	+26.90	+46.26	+13.42
5	R1 resection	40	+16.52	+35.01	+28.21
6	R2 resection	47	+15.44	+16.99	+18.09
7	R0 resection	35	+22.39	+68.38	+7.96
8	No resection	39	+2.08	+11.34	−5.43
9	No resection	34	+7.98	+31.32	+12.09
10	No resection	44	+10.11	+29.56	−2.39
11	R0 resection	48	+22.71	+29.86	+11.23
12	R1 resection	37	+26.04	+42.96	+17.82
13	R1 resection	47	+14.05	+24.21	+5.59

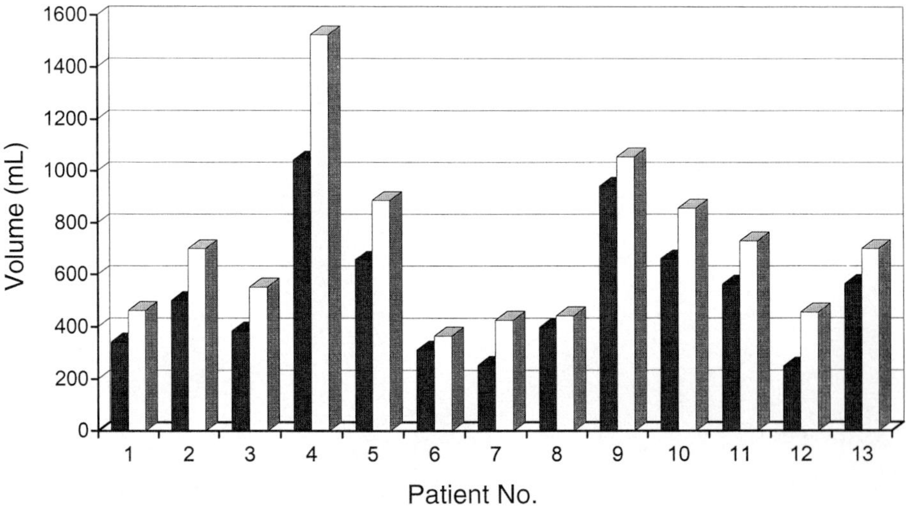

Figure 3. Graph shows comparison of volumetric data for the left hepatic lobe before and after successful embolization of the right hepatic lobe. Black bars = volume of the left lobe before embolization of the right lobe, white bars = volume of the left lobe after embolization of the right lobe.

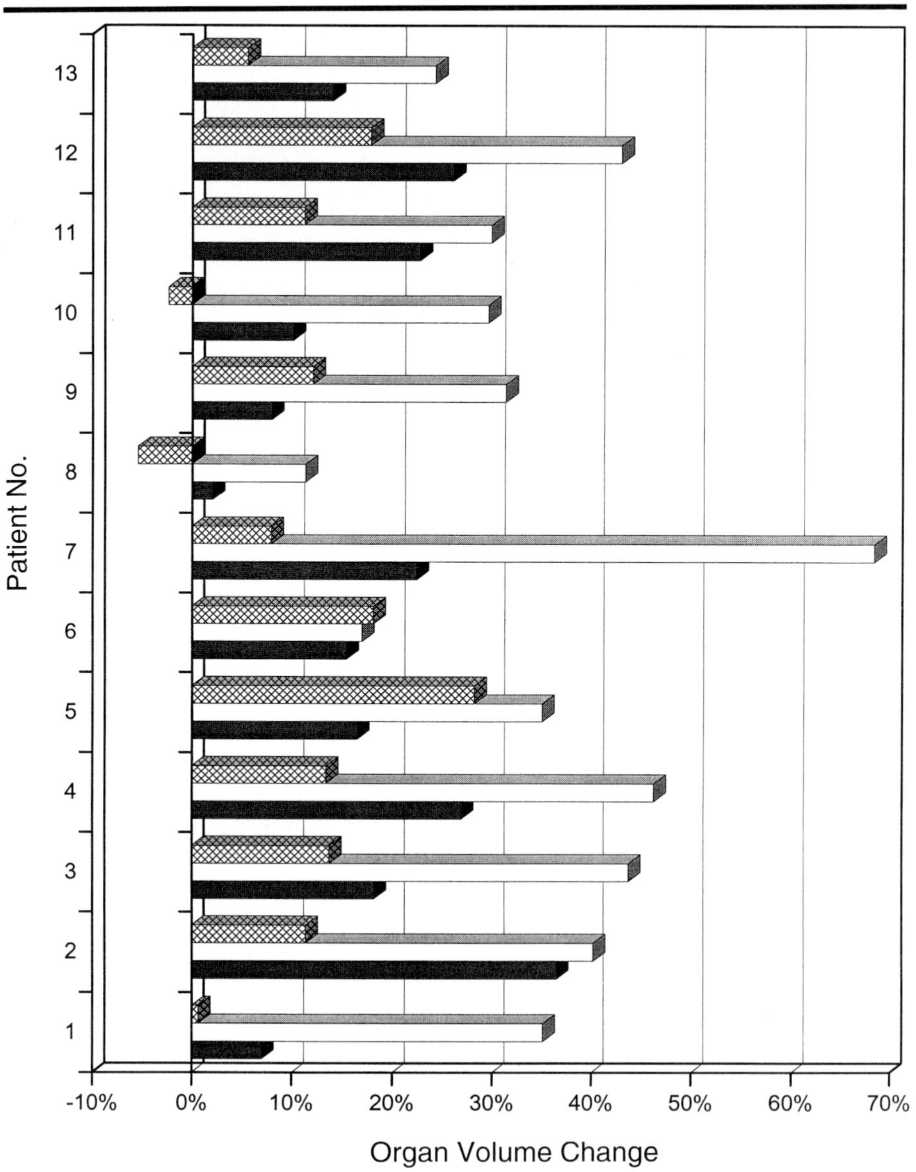

Figure 4. Graph shows the changes in organ volume after embolization of the right hepatic lobe, in comparison with initial volumetric measurements. Black bars = volume of the entire liver, white bars = volume of the left hepatic lobe, crosshatched bars = volume of the spleen.

RESULTS

In all patients, transarterial embolization of the hepatic artery branch was well tolerated, without major side effects. In six patients, we found a moderate increase in serum transaminase activity and bilirubin level, which returned to baseline values within 1 week.

Helical CT Findings

On unenhanced preinterventional CT scans, the Klatskin tumor was indistinguishable from dilated biliary ducts in both hepatic lobes in all patients. After administration of contrast material, the segmental and lobar hepatic arteries were markedly enhanced during the arterial phase. The tumor showed increased attenuation in five patients, which allowed assessment of the degree of tumor infiltration and differentiation from the dilated bile duct system, which had low attenuation. In seven patients, the extent of tumor infiltration could be identified on the arterial phase scans. During the portal venous phase, tumor tissue exhibited medium attenuation compared with the brighter portal venous vascular structures.

Volumetric Data

Before and after embolization, 67 measurements of the volumes of the entire liver, the left hepatic lobe, and the spleen were performed in all 13 patients. The volumetric data obtained from the immediately preoperative (postembolization) CT scans were compared with the initial pre-embolization values in all patients. The exact initial and preoperative volumetric measurements for each patient are given in the Table.

The volumetric measurements showed a 2%–36% decrease in the volume of the entire liver (mean decrease, 10%), an 11%–68% increase in the volume of the left hepatic lobe (mean increase, 37%), and variable changes in splenic volume of −5% to +28% (mean, +11%), compared with initial measurements. Of 13 patients, nine underwent hemihepatectomy 27–75 days (mean, 44 days) after successful embolization (Figs 3, 4). The increase in entire liver volume ranged from 27.91 cm^3 to 589.26 cm^3 (mean, 302.48 cm^3; median, 332.87 cm^3; 95% confidence interval, 208.72 cm^3, 396.24 cm^3). The increase in the left hepatic lobar volume ranged from 44.04 cm^3 to 480.99 cm^3 (mean, 182.26 cm^3; median, 144.02 cm^3; 95% confidence interval, 113.12 cm^3, 251.40 cm^3). Whereas a major increase in volume could be measured for the left hepatic lobe, there was also a minor increase in the volume of the right hepatic lobar segments. This was due mainly to an increase in the volume of the caudate lobe after embolization.

Treatment after Embolization

Eight of thirteen patients underwent extended right hepatectomy. One patient with infiltration of the connective tissue underwent extrahepatic bile duct resection; the other four patients could not undergo surgery because of advanced tumor progression, with peritoneal carcinosis. In these patients, palliative treatment was instituted.

Successful resection within the safety margins (R0 resection) could be achieved in four patients with initially inoperable tumors, and partially successful resection with remaining evidence of tumor tissue (either microscopically or macroscopically) within the resection margins (R1 or R2 resection) was performed in five patients.

The group of patients with an R0 resection had a mean volume increase in the left hepatic lobe of 44.9%, and the second group (R1 or R2 resection) had a mean volume increase in the left hepatic lobe of 31.9%. Of 13 patients, 11 were alive at 6-month and 1-year follow-up.

DISCUSSION

A variety of approaches have been used to stimulate regeneration of liver parenchyma in patients who undergo major liver resection for primary or secondary malignant liver lesions (4,6–10). The underlying principle is the well-known phenomenon of "atrophy and hypertrophy," which reflects the compensatory capacity of the structural and functional mechanisms of the liver.

For carcinoma of the hepatic hilum, hepatectomy with bile duct resection represents the only hope for cure (11,12). After extensive liver resection, however, the risk of hepatic failure is high because residual liver tissue is damaged by means of bile and usually lacks sufficient functional reserve if there has been no previous opportunity for compensatory enlargement. The clinical importance of compensatory hypertrophy of unoccluded liver segments after occlusion of some liver segments was observed as early as 1956 by Schalm et al (6). Since then, several techniques have been developed to increase the liver parenchymal reserve before the performance of hemihepatectomy. Two principal preoperative embolization techniques are used to accomplish this: the portal venous approach and the arterial approach (4,7,10,13). Results similar to ours were obtained by several groups who used portal venous embolization of tumor-bearing liver segments. In addition, several studies (2,7,13) have involved the use of coils.

The purpose of the present study was to assess induced liver regeneration with volumetric helical CT after transarterial embolization of the affected liver segments. Volumetric measurements from a CT data set proved to be accurate and reproducible, as repeated measurements in our patient series revealed. The benefits of this technique have been described previously by other groups (14,15) with similar results.

Our results show that after transarterial embolization there is a marked increase in the volume of the left hepatic lobe. We also noted, however, an increase in the volume of the right hepatic lobe. Our observations show that this increase was due to an increase in the volume of the caudate lobe, as well as to edema within the right hepatic lobe. These results are preliminary and must be validated by means of a study with a larger population and with histopathologic correlation.

In our study, arterial embolization proved to be fast and safe, with minimal overall examination and intervention times for the patient. By contrast, the portal venous procedure can be complicated because of hemobilia, arterioportal shunts, and portal thrombosis (8); these complications can be avoided with arterial embolization. In comparison with transarterial embolization, the entire procedure of preoperative portal venous embolization takes longer and is more invasive, although no major side effects, such as bleeding of biliary fistulas, were reported by Makuuchi et al (10) and de Baere et al (2). One advantage of portal venous embolization could be the avoidance of a sudden increase in portal pressure after hepatectomy.

A major disadvantage of the portal venous technique is the time it takes to regenerate liver parenchyma while the tumor continues to grow. Because the major blood supply to cholangiocarcinoma is arterial, we believe that our arterial approach may be advantageous in that it results in simultaneous reduction of tumor growth in the embolized right hepatic lobe.

In our study, extended right lobectomy was favored by the surgeon because of the position of the common bile duct on the right side of the hepatoduodenal ligament and because of easier reconstruction of the remaining left portal vein and bile drainage. In the near future, we expect to use and evaluate magnetic resonance (MR) imaging–compatible embolization coils, which would allow volumetric measurements with MR imaging and reduction of radiation exposure to the patient while providing increased information about soft tissues. Also, the outcomes in patients with unresectable tumors after embolization must be evaluated in greater depth in a long-term follow-up study.

In summary, the present data show that preoperative embolization of affected hepatic lobes results in a marked increase in the volume of noninvolved liver parenchyma. In some patients, stimulation of the unaffected hepatic lobe will allow reclassification of the case from an initially technically unresectable state to a resectable condition. The advantages of transcatheter arterial embolization in comparison with portal venous embolization still must be validated with a larger series of patients.

We highly recommend the use of preoperative hepatic arterial branch embolization in hilar bile duct carcinoma to initiate hypertrophy. The procedure should be performed approximately 4–8 weeks before surgery or when all liver function test results have returned to baseline levels and the increase in liver volume is evident on helical CT scans.

References

1. Klatskin G. Adenocarcinoma of the hepatic duct at its bifurcation within the porta hepatis. Am J Med 1965; 38:241–256.
2. de Baere T, Roche A, Vavasseur D, et al. Portal vein embolization: utility for inducing left hepatic lobe hypertrophy before surgery. Radiology 1993; 188:73–77.
3. Makuuchi M, Kosuge T, Lygidakis NJ. New possibilities for major liver surgery in patients with Klatskin tumors or primary hepatocellular carcinoma: an old problem revisited. Hepatogastroenterology 1991; 38:329–336.
4. Van der Heyde MN, Verbeek PCM, Lygidakis NJ. Decision-making in the treatment of patients with malignant proximal bile duct obstruction. Semin Liver Dis 1990; 10:145–148.
5. Nagasue N, Yukaya H, Ogawa Y, Kohno H, Nakamura T. Human liver regeneration after major hepatic resection. Ann Surg 1987; 7:30–39.
6. Schalm L, Bax HR, Mansens BJ. Atrophy of the liver after occlusion of the bile ducts or portal vein and compensatory hypertrophy of the unoccluded portion and its clinical importance. Gastroenterology 1956; 31:131–155.
7. Kanematsu T, Matsumata T, Shirabe K, et al. A comparative study of hepatic resection and transcatheter arterial embolization for the treatment of primary hepatocellular carcinoma. Cancer 1993; 71:2181–2186.
8. Nagino M, Nimura Y, Kamiya J, Kondo S, Kanai M. Selective percutaneous transhepatic embolization of the portal vein in preparation for extensive liver resection: the ipsilateral approach. Radiology 1996; 200:559–563.
9. Nagino M, Nimura Y, Kamiya J, et al. Changes in hepatic lobe volume in biliary tract cancer patients after right portal vein embolization. Hepatology 1995; 21:434–439.
10. Makuuchi M, Thai BL, Takayasu K, et al. Preoperative portal embolization to increase safety of major hepatectomy for hilar bile duct carcinoma: a preliminary report. Surgery 1990; 107:521–527.
11. Lorenz M, Hanisch E. Neue möglichkeiten der leberchirurgie bei patienten mit Klatskin oder primären hepatozellulären tumoren: ein altes problem aus neuer sicht. Z Gastroenterol 1993; 31:469–470.
12. Neuhaus P, Blumhardt G. Extended bile duct resection: a new oncological approach to the treatment of central bile duct carcinomas?—description of method and early results. Langenbecks Arch Chir 1994; 379:123–128.
13. Teng GJ, He SC, Guo JH, Cai XL, Gao GR. Preoperative transcatheter hepatic arterial embolization for hepatic malignancy. Invest Radiol 1993; 28:235–241.
14. Luomin G, Heath DG, Kuszyk BS, Fishman EK. Automatic liver segmentation technique for three-dimensional visualization of CT data. Radiology 1996; 201:359–364.
15. Okamoto E, Kyo A, Yamanaka N, Tanaka N, Kuwata K. Prediction of the safe limits of hepatectomy by combined volumetric and functional measurements in patients with impaired hepatic function. Surgery 1984; 95:586–591.

Gail S. Smith, MD[2]
Bernard A. Birnbaum, MD
Jill E. Jacobs, MD

Index terms:
Interventional procedures, complications, 761.458
Liver, blood supply , 95.72
Liver, CT, 761.1211, 761.12115
Liver, infarction, 761.795
Liver, surgery, 761.458

Radiology 1998; 208:223–229

Abbreviation:
GDA = gastroduodenal artery

[1] From the Department of Radiology, Hospital of the University of Pennsylvania, 3400 Spruce St, Philadelphia, PA 19104. Received April 20, 1997; revision requested October 27; revision received January 27, 1998; accepted February 11. **Address reprint requests to** B.A.B.

[2] Current address: Department of Radiology, Veterans Administration Clinic, Martinez, Calif.

Hepatic Infarction Secondary to Arterial Insufficiency in Native Livers: CT Findings in 10 Patients[1]

PURPOSE: To describe the computed tomographic (CT) appearance of hepatic infarcts resulting from arterial insufficiency in native livers.

MATERIALS AND METHODS: The authors retrospectively reviewed the clinical and imaging findings in 10 patients (five men, five women; age range, 28–70 years) with 14 hepatic infarcts seen over 3 years. CT scans were analyzed for infarct appearance, vessel patency, and evolution of infarct pattern over time.

RESULTS: Hepatic infarction resulted from hepatobiliary surgery (n = 6), radiologic intervention (n = 3), and celiac occlusion secondary to antiphospholipid syndrome (n = 1). All 14 infarcts were of low attenuation, peripheral, and wedge-shaped. Occluded arterial vessels were identified in eight patients. Follow-up CT revealed infarct diminution with parenchymal atrophy and scarring (n = 5), progressive liquefaction (n = 2), or both parenchymal atrophy and progressive liquefaction (n = 1).

CONCLUSION: Sudden interruption of hepatic arterial flow may cause acute native liver infarction. Patients at risk include those with underlying vascular disease who undergo complicated surgical procedures and those undergoing peripheral arterial embolization.

Hepatic infarction is thought to be relatively rare because of the liver's dual blood supply and extensive collateral pathways (1–5). When hepatic infarction does occur, it results from an insult either to the hepatic arterial supply or to both the hepatic arterial and portal venous systems, but not to the portal venous supply alone (6–10). The prevalence of hepatic infarction in several series of consecutive autopsies has ranged from 0.3% to 1.1%, suggesting that infarction is more common than typically realized (10–12). Reports of computed tomographic (CT) findings of hepatic infarction have been relatively rare (13–17) until a recent article by Holbert et al (18). Their series was composed of 18 patients, nearly all of whom had undergone liver transplantation. We have noted hepatic infarction in a number of patients who have not undergone liver transplantation or chemoembolization. We performed this study to describe the CT appearance of 14 hepatic infarcts detected in the native livers of 10 patients.

MATERIALS AND METHODS

A retrospective search of computerized reports dictated in January 1, 1993, to December 31, 1995, revealed a total of 21 patients with findings of hepatic infarction at CT. Patients who underwent liver transplantation or chemoembolization for hepatic metastases were excluded from this analysis, yielding a final study population of 10 patients. The study group consisted of five men and five women aged 28–70 years (mean age, 50 years).

A total of 28 CT scans were obtained and available for analysis. Twenty-six of these scans were acquired by using a helical CT scanner (HiSpeed Advantage; GE Medical Systems, Milwaukee, Wis). Scanning parameters were 7-mm collimation, a helical pitch of 1:1, a

Author contributions:
Guarantors of integrity of entire study, G.S.S., B.A.B., J.E.J.; study concepts, G.S.S., B.A.B., J.E.J.; study design, G.S.S., B.A.B.; definition of intellectual content, G.S.S., B.A.B.; literature research, G.S.S.; clinical studies, G.S.S., B.A.B., J.E.J.; data acquisition and analysis, G.S.S., B.A.B., J.E.J.; manuscript preparation, G.S.S.; manuscript editing, B.A.B., J.E.J.; manuscript review, G.S.S., B.A.B., J.E.J.

Summary of Patient Data

Patient No./Age (y)/Sex	Clinical History	Procedure	Vascular Injury	Peak Alanine Aminotransaminase Value Level (U/L)	Initial CT Findings	Interval between Initial and Follow-up CT and Follow-up CT Findings
1/70/M	Distal common bile duct cholangiocarcinoma	Whipple resection	GDA ligation, aortohepatic arterial bypass with saphenous vein graft	881	12-cm infarct in the medial and lateral segments, 6.3-cm infarct in the caudate segment	51 d; parenchymal atrophy in the left lobe, decreased infarct size
2/37/F	Common bile duct injury at laparoscopic cholecystectomy	Hepaticojejunostomy	Trauma to right hepatic artery during dissection in porta hepatis	1,863	10.5-cm infarct in the anterior and posterior segments	7 mo; parenchymal atrophy, decreased infarct size
3/65/F	Klatskin tumor	Hepaticojejunostomy	Right hepatic artery ligated	3,107	13-cm infarct in the medial, anterior, and posterior segments	NA
4/57/M	Gallbladder cancer extending to the right lobe of the liver	Gallbladder and adjacent liver resection	Right hepatic artery ligated with intraoperative repair	476	10.2-cm infarct in the anterior segment	15 wk; parenchymal atrophy and capsular retraction, decreased infarct size
5/66/M	Ampullary carcinoma invading the gallbladder	Hepaticojejunostomy, cholecystectomy	Ligation of the posterior branches of the right hepatic artery and portal vein	6,380	12-cm infarct in the anterior and posterior segments	25 d; progressive infarct liquefaction
6/63/F	Pancreatic carcinoma	Whipple resection	GDA ligation, preoperative celiac arterial stenosis with the hepatic artery fed by the GDA via the superior mesenteric artery	3,020	17.5-cm infarct in the medial and lateral segments, 4.3-cm infarct in the anterior segment, partial splenic infarct	27 d; parenchymal atrophy in the left lobe, decreased infarct size, evolving splenic infarct
7/28/F	Gardner syndrome, previous colectomy and Whipple resection, upper gastrointestinal tract bleeding	Pitressin tannate infusion therapy via the superior mesenteric artery	Thrombosed proximal celiac axis at angiography, prior GDA ligation	748	5.3-cm infarct in the medial segment, 4.5-cm infarct in the lateral segment, 4.2-cm infarct in the anterior segment, splenic infarct	10 mo; parenchymal atrophy in the left lobe, decreased infarct size, liquefied splenic infarct
8/43/F	Systemic lupus erythematosus and antiphospholipid syndrome, severe abdominal pain	None	Thrombosed celiac trunk at angiography	491	8.8-cm infarct in the anterior and posterior segments, gas within the liver infarct, splenic infarct	20 d; decreased size after percutaneous drainage of the infected infarct, evolving splenic infarct
9/38/M	Stab wound with extensive intraperitoneal hemorrhage	Embolization with gelatin sponges	Embolization of the medial branch of the left hepatic artery	NA	15-cm infarct in the medial and lateral segments	3 mo; initial liquefaction with subsequent decrease in infarct size
10/36/M	Right hepatic arterial pseudoaneurysm	Embolization with polyvinyl alcohol and coils	Embolization of the third-order branch of the right hepatic artery	345	5-cm infarct in the posterior segment	NA

Note.—GDA = gastroduodenal artery, NA = not available.

peak kilovoltage of 120 kVp, a tube current of 270–300 mA, and a 1-second scanning time. Two of the examinations were performed with conventional scanners by using an incremental dynamic scanning technique with contiguous 10-mm-thick sections, a 2-second scanning time, and a 6-second interscanning delay. All patients received 150 mL of the ionic intravenous contrast material iothalamate meglumine (Conray 60; Mallinckrodt Medical, St Louis, Mo). Contrast material was administered in a monophasic fashion with injection rates of 1.5–3.0 mL/sec by using calibrated power injectors (Liebel Flarsheim, Cincinnati, Ohio).

The initial CT scans were acquired within 3–10 days (mean, 7.3 days) of the hepatic insult. Follow-up CT scans were obtained in eight patients from 2.9–40 weeks (mean, 20 weeks) after hepatic infarction and ranged in number from 1 to 8 follow-up scans per patient (mean, 2.8 scans). Two patients did not undergo follow-up CT.

CT scans were analyzed by three readers (G.S.S., B.A.B., J.E.J.) in a combined

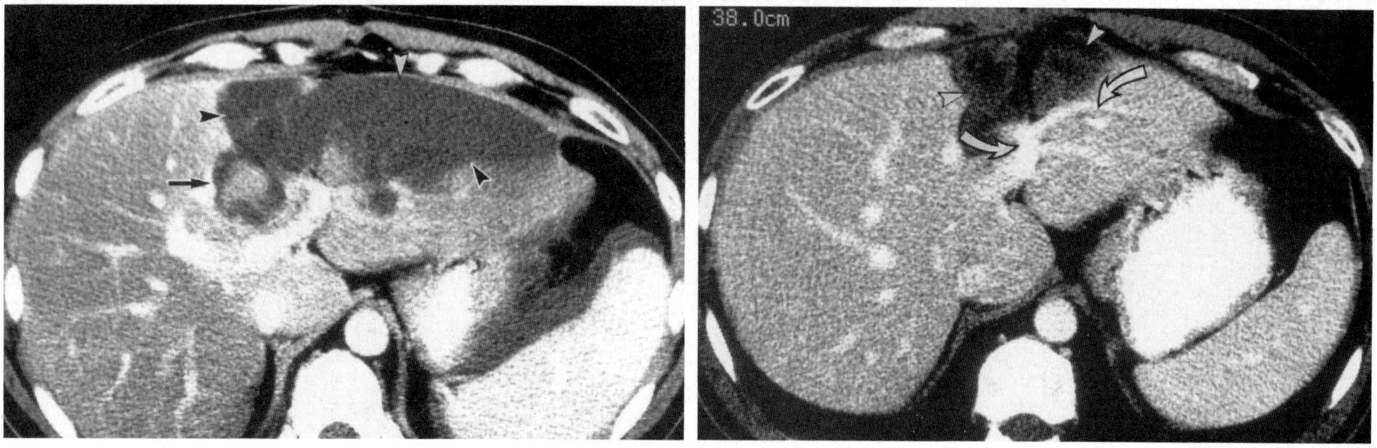

a. b.

Figure 1. Patient 9. Acute hepatic infarct in a 38-year-old man who underwent left hepatic artery branch embolization after a penetrating stab wound to the liver. **(a)** Contrast-enhanced CT scan reveals a peripheral, wedge-shaped low-attenuation defect (arrowheads) traversing the medial and lateral segments of the left lobe. A small intrahepatic hematoma (arrow), fatty liver, and perisplenic hemoperitoneum are also noted. **(b)** Contrast-enhanced CT scan obtained 3 months later shows that the infarct has decreased in size (arrowheads), with associated hepatic atrophy. The main portal vein and its left intrahepatic branches (arrows) appeared patent at both examinations.

review session with knowledge of patient history and the prospective study interpretation. Consensus agreement was reached in each case on the presence of geographic perfusion defects, infarct size (diameter), and patency of the hepatic arteries and portal veins. The findings were then correlated with surgical reports and angiograms when available. Follow-up CT scans were examined for changes in the appearance of the infarct over time.

The medical, surgical, laboratory, and radiologic records of these patients were reviewed. Proof of diagnosis of hepatic infarction was based on the coexistence of classic CT findings (geographic, low-attenuation perfusion defects without mass effect) seen in association with the following: acute increase in the serum alanine aminotransaminase level coinciding with the hepatic insult (elevated in all nine patients in whom this test was performed), normal CT ($n = 6$) or magnetic resonance ($n = 2$) image of the liver before the hepatic injury (eight patients), perfusion abnormality indicative of infarction on a liver-spleen sulfur colloid scintigraphic scan (one patient) or angiogram (three patients), autopsy findings (one patient), and follow-up CT scans demonstrating the expected pattern of infarct evolution (eight patients).

RESULTS

Cause of Infarction

Fourteen hepatic infarcts were identified in 10 patients. These occurred in six patients after a surgical procedure, in three patients after a radiologic interventional procedure, and in one patient with hypercoagulation secondary to antiphospholipid syndrome (Table).

The surgical procedures consisted of two Whipple resections, three hepaticojejunostomies, and one explorative resection of the gallbladder and adjacent liver for invasive gallbladder carcinoma that extended into the right lobe of the liver. Surgical reports revealed isolated ligation of the right hepatic artery in three patients, ligation of both the right portal vein and the right hepatic artery in one patient, and ligation of the GDA in two patients. Of note, both patients who underwent GDA ligation were at risk for hepatic ischemia because preoperative assessment in these patients demonstrated existing celiac arterial stenosis, with the hepatic artery being fed by the GDA via the superior mesenteric artery.

The interventional radiologic procedures that resulted in hepatic infarction were (*a*) gelatin sponge (Gelfoam; Upjohn, Kalamazoo, Mich) embolization of the medial branch of the left hepatic artery in a patient with a penetrating stab wound; (*b*) polyvinyl alcohol (Contour Embolization Particles; Target Therapeutics, Fremont, Calif) and coil embolization of a third-order branch of the right hepatic artery in a patient with a pseudoaneurysm secondary to biliary drainage catheter placement; and (*c*) infusion of pitressin tannate (Vasopressin; Fujisawa USA, Deerfield, Ill) via the superior mesenteric artery, which caused celiac arterial thrombosis in a patient with Gardner syndrome who had undergone multiple prior surgeries.

The patient with hypercoagulation had systemic lupus erythematosus with antiphospholipid syndrome. She presented with severe abdominal pain and was found to have a thrombosed celiac artery at angiography. This patient has been previously reported on in the literature (19).

Lesion Location and Appearance

The mean infarct diameter was 9.2 cm (range, 4.2–17.5 cm). Segmental infarcts occurred within the caudate segment ($n = 1$), the anterior segment ($n = 3$), the posterior segment ($n = 1$), the medial segment ($n = 1$), and the lateral segment ($n = 1$). Larger infarcts, encompassing multiple hepatic segments, occurred within both the anterior and posterior segments ($n = 3$), within both the medial and lateral segments ($n = 3$), and within the medial, lateral, and posterior segments ($n = 1$).

All infarcts appeared as peripheral wedge-shaped lesions that were easily identifiable as focal, well-demarcated areas of low attenuation relative to adjacent contrast material–enhanced liver parenchyma (Fig 1). Only one of the hepatic infarcts (in patient 8) had gas in it (Fig 2), and none demonstrated "bile lakes," findings that have previously been described in association with hepatic infarcts (18). Associated splenic infarcts were present in three patients. These were noted in a patient who underwent Whipple resection for pancreatic carcinoma (patient 6), a patient with celiac arterial thrombosis

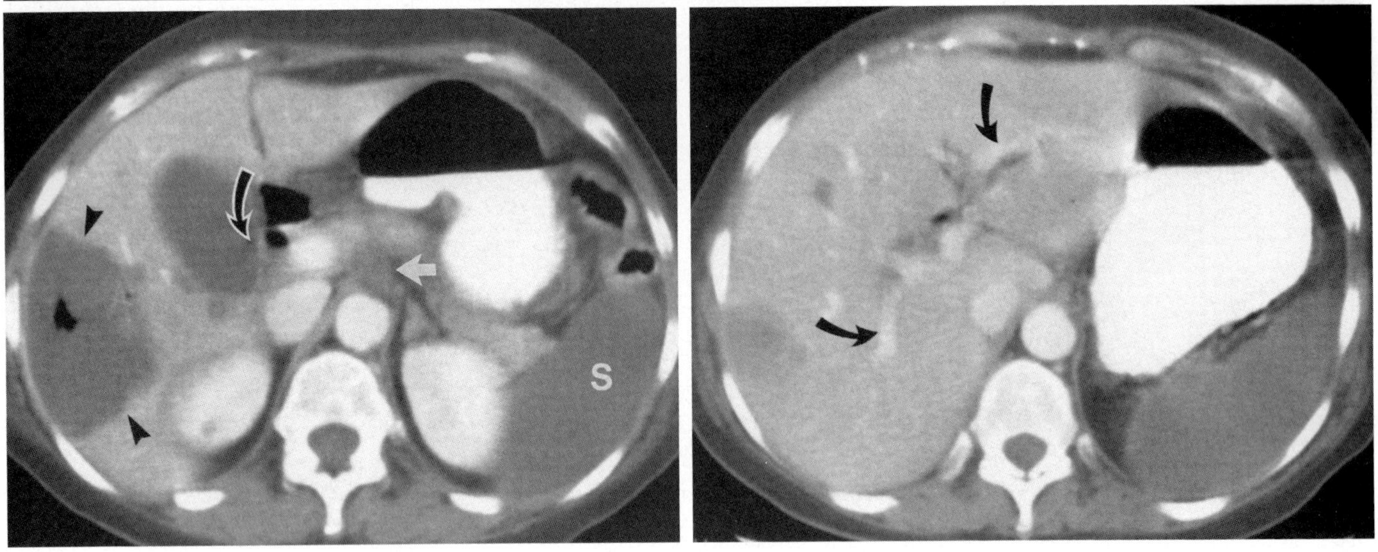

a. b.

Figure 2. Patient 8. Infected hepatic infarct in a 43-year-old woman with systemic lupus erythematosus who developed angiographically proved celiac axis thrombosis secondary to antiphospholipid syndrome. **(a)** Contrast-enhanced CT scan reveals the thrombosed celiac artery (straight arrow), a trapezoidal gas-containing infarct (arrowheads) in the right lobe of the liver, and a nonenhancing infarcted spleen (*S*). Contiguous images (not shown) revealed a classic wedge-shaped hepatic defect extending from the porta hepatis to the liver capsule. Gas in the gallbladder lumen (curved arrow) resulted from a prior endoscopic retrograde cholangiopancreatographic procedure. **(b)** Contrast-enhanced CT scan obtained at more cephalic level shows patent right and left intrahepatic portal vein branches (arrows) and central pneumobilia.

(patient 7), and a patient with antiphospholipid syndrome (patient 8).

Vessel Patency

An attempt was made to identify the hepatic artery and portal vein in all patients. Because congenital absence of hepatic vessels is rare, a vessel that was not visualized in its expected location was presumed to be occluded. The occluded hepatic artery or branch vessel was retrospectively detected in eight of the 10 patients. In two patients, the main hepatic artery and its right and left arterial branches appeared to be patent. In the first patient (patient 1), hepatic ischemia resulted after GDA ligation, necessitating aortohepatic arterial bypass grafting. Postoperatively, both the saphenous venous graft and the main hepatic artery appeared patent at CT. In the second patient (patient 6), the hepatic artery appeared patent despite the presence of celiac arterial thrombosis. The main, right, and left portal veins were definitely patent at CT in nine patients. In one patient (patient 5), the posterior branch of the right portal vein was not visualized, and, indeed, it had been ligated at surgery.

Lesion Evolution

Follow-up CT scans were available for review in eight patients (12 infarcts); these CT scans were obtained 20 days to 10 months after the initial vascular insult (Table). Nine of the 12 infarcts showed diminution with hepatic atrophy or scarring (Figs 3, 4). Three of the 12 infarcts showed evidence of liquefaction. One infarct contained gas and decreased in size after percutaneous drainage of a superimposed abscess (infected infarct) (Fig 2), one showed progressive liquefaction without size change, and one demonstrated decreased size at follow-up. Vessel patency and overall infarct shape did not change during the interval between initial and follow-up CT in any of the eight patients.

Clinical Course

Three patients died: One patient (patient 1) died after a complicated 3-month course of hepatic failure and sepsis, one patient (patient 7) died of coexistent bowel infarction, and one patient (patient 8) died of perforation of an ischemic gastric wall. A fourth patient (patient 5) had a complicated postoperative course as a result of hepatic necrosis. However, this patient recovered and was discharged from the hospital in satisfactory condition. The remaining six patients tolerated their infarcts well without serious clinical sequelae.

DISCUSSION

It is commonly believed that the liver's dual blood supply and extensive collateral pathways serve to protect this organ from ischemic insult (2,5–9). In fact, few reports of hepatic infarction exist in the radiology literature (13–18). This study is notable in that we report on 10 patients with hepatic infarction who did not undergo liver transplantation or chemoembolization, which are known risk factors for hepatic ischemia. Nine of our 10 patients developed infarcts after undergoing surgery or radiologic interventional procedures. Hepatic ischemia resulted from injury or thrombosis of the hepatic artery alone in nine patients. In one patient, ischemia resulted from coexistent hepatic arterial and segmental portal venous occlusion.

The liver's extensive collateral blood supply has been demonstrated in numerous studies during the past 90 years. As early as 1909, Gilbert and Villaret (20), using "visualizing material," demonstrated anastomoses between the hepatic arterial and portal venous branches as they passed through the interlobular spaces. Michels (2,21) dissected 200 cadavers and described both the tremendous anatomic variability in the liver's vascular supply and the presence of 26 possible collateral pathways. Subsequent reports described the most common collateral pathways that develop after the hepatic artery is ligated at various points along its course (5–7,22,23). After ligation of the

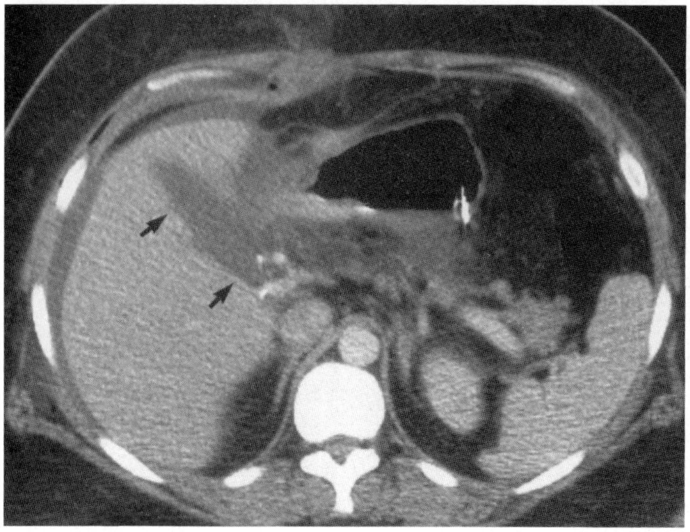

a.

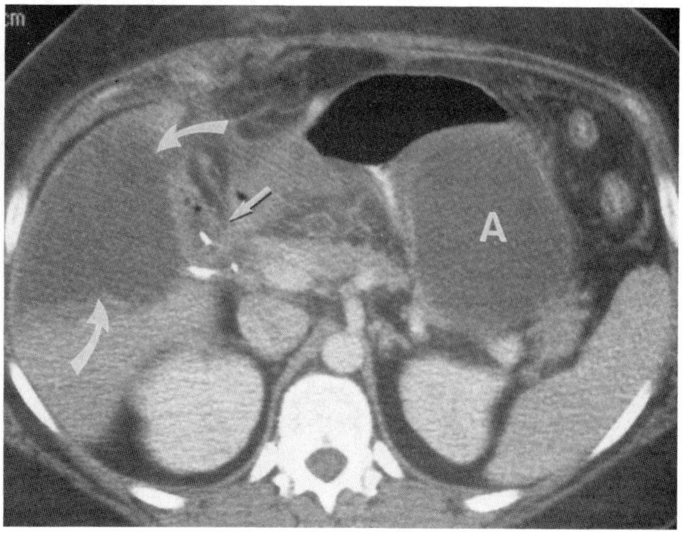

b.

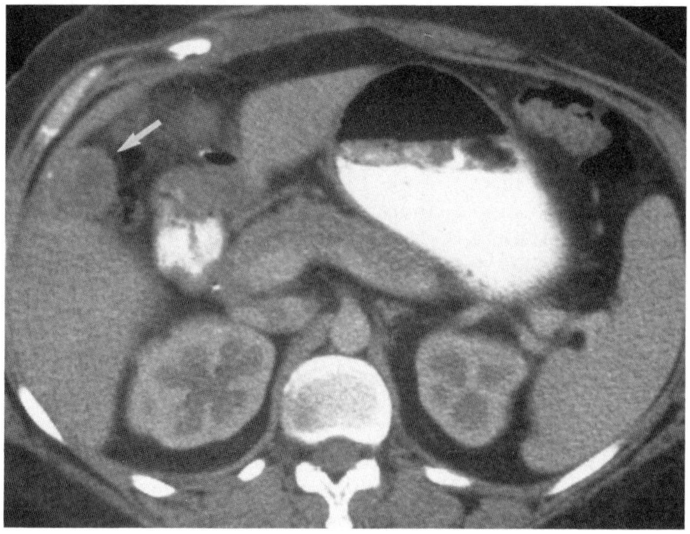

c.

Figure 3. Patient 2. Acute hepatic infarct in a 37-year-old woman who underwent biliary-enteric bypass after common bile duct injury. **(a)** Contrast-enhanced CT scan obtained after laparoscopic cholecystectomy reveals perihepatic ascites and fluid in the gallbladder fossa (arrows). Subsequent intraoperative cholangiogram (not shown) demonstrated transection of the common bile duct. Note the normal hepatic enhancement in the right lobe of the liver. **(b)** Contrast-enhanced CT scan obtained after hepaticojejunostomy shows a new, well-circumscribed, wedge-shaped perfusion defect (curved arrows) within the anterior and posterior segments of the right lobe. A perigastric abscess (*A*) is present. A surgical drain (straight arrow) lies within the jejunal limb of the biliary-enteric bypass. **(c)** Contrast-enhanced CT scan obtained 7 months later shows marked parenchymal atrophy of the right lobe of the liver. Note the new lateral location of the jejunal bypass loop (arrow) compared with the location seen on the immediate postoperative scan in **b**.

common hepatic artery, the pancreaticoduodenal artery and GDA serve as the major collateral pathways (5). Ligation of the proper hepatic artery results in the development of small collateral vessels in the hepatic ligaments and around the common bile duct (5). These collateral vessels may be noted immediately after temporary occlusion of hepatic arterial flow (5). If the right or left hepatic artery is ligated, collateral vessels may develop in both the hilus and subcapsular regions of the liver (5,23). Collateral arterial circulation may also arise from the inferior phrenic, intercostal, and gastric arteries (6,24,25).

The early surgical literature is replete with reports documenting the relative absence of major clinical sequelae after intentional or inadvertent ligation of the hepatic artery (26–30). The expendability of the hepatic artery was presumed to be due to the liver's dual blood supply and capacity for collateralization. In many of these reports, the authors noted the absence of risk factors that are believed to increase the likelihood of hepatic infarction, including decreased portal venous flow, sepsis, biliary obstruction, and inadequate oxygenation secondary to heart failure or chronic obstructive pulmonary disease (11,31). Nevertheless, isolated studies have found that hepatic infarction may result after sudden interruption of the hepatic arterial supply (7,18,26,29,32). These infarcts arose as complications of conventional and laparoscopic cholecystectomy in which the hepatic artery was inadvertently ligated. Serum alanine aminotransaminase levels have been shown to be a sensitive marker for hepatic dearterialization injuries (33–36). Surgeons now recognize the complication of hepatic ischemia when patients develop an elevation in their serum alanine aminotransaminase level after hepatic arterial ligation. This was the case at our institution, where most of the patients in our series were referred for CT evaluation of potential hepatic infarction after they developed an acute elevation in their serum alanine aminotransaminase level.

Given the fact that the liver possesses the ability to develop a rich collateral network, we must attempt to explain why our patients developed infarcts. Two patients (patients 1 and 6) had preoperative celiac arterial stenosis with collateral supply to the liver via the GDA, which was supplied by the superior mesenteric artery. In both of these patients, the GDA was ligated during surgery, which disrupted the predominant collateral supply to the liver. That infarction of the entire liver did not occur in these patients must

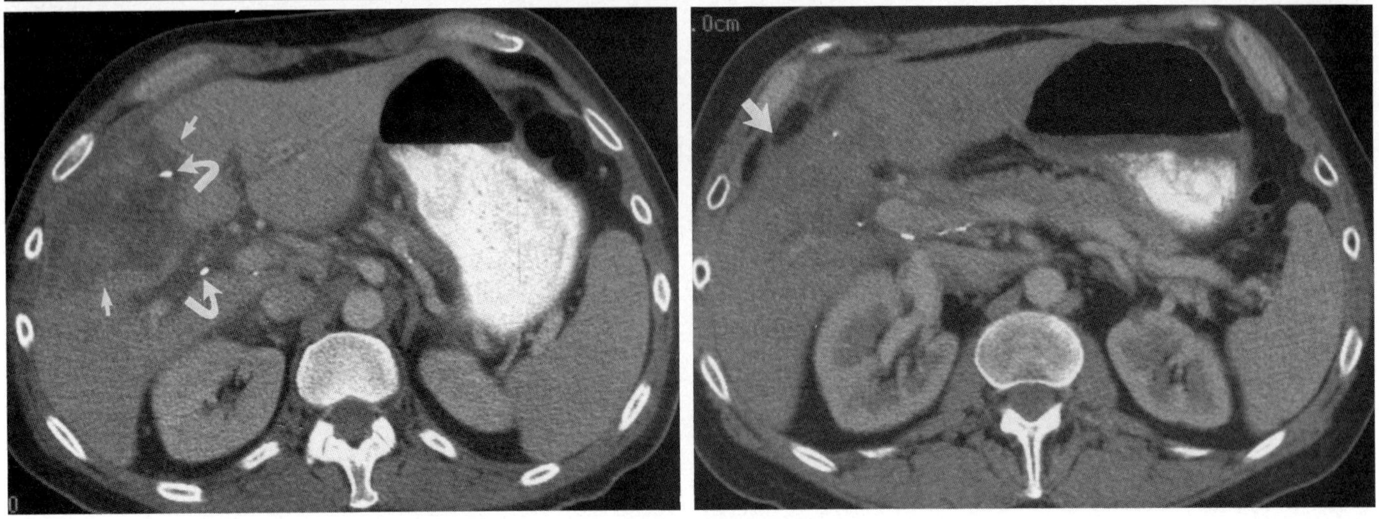

a. b.

Figure 4. Patient 4. Acute hepatic infarct in a 57-year-old man who underwent cholecystectomy and segmental hepatic resection for invasive gallbladder carcinoma. **(a)** Contrast-enhanced CT scan obtained to evaluate an acute postoperative increase in the peak alanine aminotransaminase level. A well-marginated, geographic, wedge-shaped low-attenuation defect (straight arrows) is present within the anterior segment of the right lobe of the liver. Surgical clips (curved arrows) are seen within and adjacent to the infarct. **(b)** CT scan obtained 1 year later shows diminished infarct size with parenchymal atrophy and capsular retraction (arrow).

be attributable to recruitment of other collateral pathways (eg, inferior phrenic arteries), which were presumably not disrupted at surgery.

Three patients (patients 2–4) underwent extensive dissection and manipulation of the porta hepatis. Although the surgical reports described ligation of only the right hepatic artery, several potential collateral pathways may also have been disrupted. In addition, two of these patients had preexisting biliary obstruction, which may increase the risk of hepatic infarction (11).

One patient (patient 5) underwent ligation of the posterior branches of both the right hepatic artery and the right portal vein. Results of the dog experiments performed by Popper et al (7) showed that hepatic ischemia did not occur after isolated ligation of either the portal vein or the common hepatic artery. Hepatic necrosis, however, resulted after simultaneous ligation of both the hepatic arterial and corresponding portal venous vessels. By extrapolation, this certainly explains the development of infarction in this patient.

Two patients (patients 7 and 8) had thrombosis of the celiac artery. In the first patient (patient 7), the GDA could not be recruited as a potential collateral pathway because the patient had undergone GDA ligation several years earlier, when she underwent a Whipple resection for ampullary carcinoma. The second patient (patient 8) had antiphospholipid syndrome and extensive thrombosis of the celiac, common hepatic, proper hepatic, and splenic arteries. She had infarction of the spleen and right lobe of the liver. We hypothesize that the left lobe was spared from ischemic injury owing to collateral pathway formation, which did not develop in the right lobe.

Two patients (patients 9 and 10) underwent embolization of hepatic arterial branches. Doppman et al (37) showed that gelatin sponge embolization of proximal hepatic arteries was associated with rapid collateral vessel formation and preservation of liver function, but silicone obstruction of peripheral vessels was accompanied by functional liver abnormalities and infarction. The results of their study suggested that peripheral hepatic arterial occlusion is more effective for preventing the development of collateral vessels and carries a greater risk of hepatic infarction. Stridbeck et al (38) showed that repetitive nondegradable microparticle embolization increases the likelihood of hepatic necrosis. Although gelatin sponge embolization was used in one of our patients (patient 9), it was introduced selectively into a branch vessel and was therefore considered "peripheral" embolization. In the other patient (patient 10), a peripheral vessel was embolized with both polyvinyl alcohol particles and 3- and 5-mm coils. Therefore, it is likely that collateral vessels did not develop in these patients owing to the presence of distal vessel obstruction.

All 14 hepatic infarcts in this study appeared as well-marginated, peripheral, wedge-shaped perfusion defects that extended to the liver capsule without mass effect. This appearance is similar to that described in the 10 previously reported cases of hepatic infarction arising in native livers (13–18). None of the infarcts in this series appeared as central round or oval perfusion defects, and none ran parallel to the bile ducts. These patterns appear to be more common when infarcts occur in transplanted livers (16,18), although Lev-Toaff et al (15) described central round infarcts in three patients with native livers. A potential study bias inherent in this investigation is that our patient selection criteria were dependent on the CT variables analyzed. As a result, a strong bias existed toward evaluating lesions that demonstrated a classic appearance of hepatic infarction, as previously described in the literature. Patients who demonstrated an atypical CT appearance of infarction (eg, nonperipheral rounded defect) may, therefore, have been excluded.

Nine of the 12 infarcts evaluated with follow-up CT demonstrated diminution with hepatic atrophy or scarring. Three infarcts demonstrated progressive liquefaction. These findings are similar to those reported by Holbert et al (18). Although Holbert et al reported that several peripheral wedge-shaped infarcts in their series changed shape over time to a more rounded appearance, all infarcts followed up in our series maintained their configuration and remained wedge-shaped.

One infarct in this study demonstrated gas formation at CT. Although in this case the gas was due to superinfection, there have been several cases reported in the literature describing the presence of gas in sterile infarctions. The distinction between a sterile or infected infarct can be made with percutaneous aspiration (15,18).

Helical contrast material–enhanced CT enables acquisition of volumetric data sets unencumbered by respiratory misregistration. This scanning method may help delineate vascular anatomy and demonstrate vessel occlusion to a greater degree than that achieved with conventional CT scanners. A limitation of this study was that the CT scanning parameters were not optimized to delineate small hepatic vessels, and the presence of vascular occlusion was inferred in cases where normal enhancing vessels were not visualized in their expected locations. We could not exclude the rare possibility that there may have been congenital absence of a hepatic vessel that could have caused an overestimation of the number of occluded vessels present in our study population.

In conclusion, hepatic infarction may occur in native livers despite the liver's dual blood supply and propensity to develop collateral blood flow. Patients at risk include those with preexisting vascular disease who undergo complicated surgical procedures with sudden hepatic arterial occlusion and those who undergo peripheral arterial embolization procedures. The clinical diagnosis may be suggested by acute elevation of serum alanine aminotransaminase levels. Contrast-enhanced CT is confirmatory when typical CT features of infarction are demonstrated.

References

1. Clarke JS. Hepatic necrosis following celiac artery ligation during gastric resection in man. Arch Surg 1955; 71:171–177.
2. Michels NA. Newer anatomy of liver: variant blood supply and collateral circulation. JAMA 1960; 172:106–112.
3. Kanter DM. Hepatic infarction. Arch Intern Med 1965; 115:479–481.
4. Temberg JL, Butcher HR. Blood flow relation between hepatic artery and portal vein. Science 1965; 150:1030–1031.
5. Redman HC, Stewart RR. Arterial collaterals in the liver hilus. Radiology 1970; 94:575–579.
6. Plengvanit U, Chearanai 0, Sindhvananda K, et al. Collateral arterial blood supply of the liver after hepatic artery ligation: angiographic study of twenty patients. Ann Surg 1972; 175:105–110.
7. Popper BL, Jefferson NC, Necheles H. Liver necrosis following complete interruption of hepatic artery and partial ligation of portal vein. Am J Surg 1953; 86:309–311.
8. Loeffler L. Factors determining necrosis or survival of liver tissue after ligation of hepatic artery. Arch Pathol 1936; 21:496–503.
9. Carrol R. Infarction of the human liver. J Clin Pathol 1963; 16:133–136.
10. Woolling KR, Baggenstoss AH, Weir JF. Infarcts of the liver. Gastroenterology 1951; 17:479–493.
11. Seely TT, Blumenfeld CM, Ikeda R, et al. Hepatic infarction. Hum Pathol 1972; 3:265–276.
12. Chen V, Hamilton J, Qizilbash A. Hepatic infarction. Arch Pathol Lab Med 1976; 100:32–36.
13. Damman HG, Hagemann MR, Kloppel G. In vivo diagnosis of massive hepatic infarction by CT. Dig Dis Sci 1982; 27:73–79.
14. Adler DD, Glazer GM, Silver TM. CT of liver infarction. AJR 1984; 142:315–318.
15. Lev-Toaff AS, Friedman AC, Cohen LM, et al. Hepatic infarcts; new observations by CT and sonography. AJR 1987; 149: 87–90.
16. Dupuy D, Costello P, Lewis D, et al. Abdominal CT findings after liver transplantation in 66 patients. AJR 1991; 156:1167–1170.
17. Wachsberg RH, Cho KC, Raina S. Liver infarction following unrecognized right hepatic artery ligation at laparoscopic cholecystectomy. Abdom Imaging 1994; 19: 53–54.
18. Holbert BL, Baron RL, Dodd GD III. Hepatic infarction caused by arterial insufficiency; spectrum and evolution of CT findings. AJR 1996; 166:815–820.
19. Insko EK, Haskal ZJ. Antiphospholipid syndrome: patterns of life-threatening and severe recurrent vascular complications. Radiology 1997; 202:319–326.
20. Gilbert A, Villaret M. Contribution à l'étude de la circulation portale: considérations sur la possibilité de l'expulsion transhépatic, a contre-courant, d'une injection poussée dans les veines sus-hépatiques. Compt Rend Soc Biol 1909; 67: 521.
21. Michels NA. Collateral arterial pathways to the liver after ligation of hepatic artery and removal of celiac axis. Cancer 1953; 6:708–724.
22. Mays ET, Wheeler CS. Demonstration of collateral arterial flow after interruption of hepatic arteries in man. N Engl J Med 1974; 290:993–996.
23. Mays ET. Lobar dearterialization for exsanguinating wounds of the liver. J Trauma 1972; 12:397–407.
24. Bengmark S, Rosengren K. Angiographic study of the collateral circulation to the liver after ligation of the hepatic artery in man. Am J Surg 1970; 19:620–624.
25. Ackerman NB, Lien WM, Silverman NA. The blood supply of experimental liver metastases: the effects of acute ligation of the hepatic artery or portal vein. Surgery 1972; 71:636–641.
26. Graham RR, Cannell D. Accidental ligation of the hepatic artery. Br J Surg 1933; 20:566–578.
27. Popper HL. Ligation of accidentally torn hepatic artery. Am J Surg 1953; 85:113–115.
28. Jefferson NC, Hassan MI, Popper HL, et al. Formation of effective collateral circulation following excision of hepatic artery. Am J Physiol 1956; 184:589–592.
29. Brittain RS, Marchioro TL, Hermann G, et al. Accidental hepatic artery ligation in humans. Am J Surg 1964; 107:822–831.
30. Cleveland JC. Inadvertent interruption of hepatic arterial flow. Am J Surg 1966; 111:573–574.
31. Tygstrup N, Winkler K, Mellemgaard K, et al. Determination of the hepatic arterial blood flow and oxygen supply in man by clamping the hepatic artery during surgery. J Clin Invest 1962; 41:447–453.
32. Halasz NA. Cholecystectomy and hepatic artery injuries. Arch Surg 1991; 126:137–138.
33. Wroblewski F, Ladue JS. SGOT activity as an index of liver cell injury: a preliminary report. Ann Intern Med 1955; 43:345–358.
34. Mason EE, Lee RA, Smith J, et al. A biochemical dissection of ischemic liver necrosis. Surgery 1959; 45:765–775.
35. Arturson G, Persson BH. Serum transaminase activity as an index of liver cell destruction. Acta Chir Scand 1959; 117: 221–229.
36. Almersjo O, Bengmark S, Engevik L, et al. Serum enzyme changes after hepatic dearterialization in man. Ann Surg 1968; 167: 9–17.
37. Doppman JL, Girton M, Kahn ER. Proximal versus peripheral hepatic artery embolization: experimental study in monkeys. Radiology 1978 128:577–588.
38. Stridbeck H, Lorelius LE, Reuter SR. Collateral circulation following repeated distal embolization of the hepatic artery in pigs. Invest Radiol 1984; 19:179–183.

Mucin-producing Pancreatic Tumors: Comparison of MR Cholangiopancreatography with Endoscopic Retrograde Cholangiopancreatography[1]

Kazumitsu Koito, MD, PhD
Tsutomu Namieno, MD, PhD
Takeshi Ichimura, MD
Naoya Yama, MD
Masato Hareyama, MD, PhD
Kazuo Morita, MD, PhD
Motoi Nishi, MD, PhD

Index terms:
Bile ducts, MR, 76.12117, 76.121411, 76.121419
Endoscopic retrograde cholangiopancreatography (ERCP), 76.1222, 77.1222
Pancreas, MR, 77.12117, 77.121411, 77.121419
Pancreas, neoplasms, 77.31222
Pancreatic ducts, MR, 77.12117, 77.121411, 77.121419

Radiology 1998; 208:231–237

Abbreviations:
ERCP = endoscopic retrograde cholangiopancreatography
MRCP = MR cholangiopancreatography
2D = two-dimensional
3D = three-dimensional

[1] From the Departments of Radiology (K.K., T.I., N.Y., M.H., K.M.) and Public Health (M.N.), Sapporo Medical University, S-1, W-17, Chuo-ku, Sapporo 060, Japan; and the First Department of Surgery, Hokkaido University School of Medicine, Sapporo, Japan (T.N.). Received September 5, 1997; revision requested November 19; final revision received February 16, 1998; accepted March 9. **Address reprint requests to** K.K.

Author contributions:
Guarantors of integrity of entire study, K.K., K.M.; study concepts, K.K., T.N.; study design, K.K., T.N.; definition of intellectual content, M.H.; literature research, T.I., N.Y.; clinical studies, K.K., T.N., T.I., N.Y.; data acquisition, K.K., T.N., T.I., N.Y.; data analysis, K.K., T.N.; statistical analysis, M.N.; manuscript preparation, K.K.; manuscript editing, T.N.; manuscript review, K.M.

PURPOSE: To compare magnetic resonance cholangiopancreatography (MRCP) with endoscopic retrograde cholangiopancreatography (ERCP) in the detection of mucin-producing pancreatic tumors.

MATERIALS AND METHODS: The authors retrospectively reviewed MRCP and ERCP images obtained in 28 patients with mucin-producing pancreatic tumors. Detectability of the pancreatic duct and its branches, intraductal cystic lesions, and intracystic nodules or septa was assessed.

RESULTS: MRCP depicted cystic dilated ductal branches significantly better than did ERCP ($P < .001$). The difference in the number of nodules or septa detected with MRCP compared with ERCP was not significant. MRCP, however, simultaneously showed not only the main pancreatic duct but also the cystic lesions; this was not always possible with ERCP.

CONCLUSION: MRCP appears to be more effective and less invasive than ERCP to evaluate changes in the size and extent of tumors and to determine if new lesions appear, as well as to follow up mucin-producing pancreatic tumors.

Mucin-producing pancreatic tumors have been described relatively recently (1,2). They are likely to originate from the main pancreatic duct or its collateral ducts (intraductal mucin-producing tumors) or from the peripheral ducts (mucinous cystadenocarcinoma and cystadenoma) of the pancreas. Mucinous cystadenocarcinoma and cystadenoma are malignant or premalignant tumors (3), so they should be surgically resected. Conversely, intraductal mucin-producing tumors have papillary hyperplastic, atypical, or overtly malignant epithelium (4). Some intraductal mucin-producing tumors (eg, papillary hyperplastic lesions) are not malignant and should be followed up instead of surgically resected (4).

Endoscopic retrograde cholangiopancreatography (ERCP) and endoscopic ultrasonography (US) are useful in the diagnosis of mucin-producing tumors, especially intraductal tumors (5,6). ERCP can show localized cystic dilatation of the ductal branches and filling defects, and endoscopic US can precisely display the internal architecture of the cysts (7). ERCP and endoscopic US, however, have some drawbacks: Acute pancreatitis occurs in 5% of all cases after ERCP (8–10), technical failure is a possibility (8,11), and some patients cannot tolerate an endoscopic examination.

Recently, magnetic resonance (MR) imaging technology has made it possible to visualize the pancreatic and bile ducts without the use of contrast material or endoscopy (12,13). Several studies have compared the usefulness of MR cholangiopancreatography (MRCP) and ERCP in the evaluation of biliary and pancreatic disorders (13–15). For example, the sensitivity of MRCP is 93%–100% for detection of biliary and pancreatic dilatation and strictures and 81%–89% for irregularities or defects of the main pancreatic duct (13,15). These authors suggest that MRCP will replace ERCP in the diagnosis of calculi of the biliary tract, cancers of the pancreatic and bile ducts and gallbladder, and chronic pancreatitis. To our

TABLE 1
Characteristics of the 28 Mucin-producing Pancreatic Tumors

Tumor Type	Pathologic Finding	Location						Total
		Head	Body	Tail	Head, Body, and Tail	Head and Body	Body and Tail	
Branch								
Solitary	Papillary adenocarcinoma	4	0	0	...	...	...	4
	Papillary adenoma	4	0	1	...	...	...	5
	Not proved*	5	0	1	...	...	...	6
Multiple	Papillary adenoma				1	0	1	2
	Not proved*				0	2	2	4
Peripheral								
	Mucinous cystadenocarcinoma	6	0	0	...	...	...	6
	Mucinous cystadenoma	0	0	1	...	...	...	1

* Diagnosis was made with endoscopic US.

knowledge, however, no studies have compared MRCP and ERCP in the diagnosis of mucin-producing tumors of the pancreas. The aim of this study was to compare the efficacies of MRCP and ERCP in the diagnosis of mucin-producing tumors of the pancreas.

MATERIALS AND METHODS

In our retrospective study, the ERCP images were reviewed by three radiologists (K.K., T.I., N.Y.), who agreed on image quality and lesion detectability. The MRCP images were analyzed retrospectively by the same radiologists without knowledge of any clinical data or ERCP findings. None of the radiologists had performed the MRCP examinations. When the interpretations differed, the interpreters reevaluated images and agreed on the diagnosis.

Patient Population

From April 1995 through June 1997, disease in 35 patients seen at our institutions was diagnosed as cystic lesions of the pancreas by means of US or computed tomography. Of those 35 patients, 28 (11 women, 17 men; mean age, 64 years; age range, 34–81 years) had mucin-producing pancreatic tumors. On the basis of the criteria of Nakazawa et al (1), 21 patients had branch-type (intraductal) tumors, seven had peripheral-type tumors (mucinous cystadenocarcinoma and cystadenoma), and none had "mucinous carcinomas" derived from adenocarcinomas. All patients successfully underwent ERCP, MRCP, and endoscopic US (7.5- and 12-MHz mechanical radial scanner [GF-UM3; Olympus, Tokyo, Japan]). The final diagnosis and the macroscopic appearance were determined on the basis of pathologic examination of the resected specimens in 18 patients (11 with branch-type tumors and seven with peripheral-type tumors) and endoscopic US findings in 10 (all with branch-type tumors). The criteria for endoscopic US diagnosis of mucin-producing tumors have been detailed previously (7) and include the following: (*a*) solid tumor of the cyst wall that protrudes into the cystic area from the cyst wall, (*b*) multiple thick septa (≥3 mm) in the cyst, and (*c*) macrocystic multilocular tumors with thick cystic walls. They have a thick wall, and multiple cysts are occasionally present in the tumor. In addition to the pathologic and endoscopic US examinations, we performed cytologic examination of the pancreatic fluid obtained during ERCP from the 21 intraductal tumors; no pancreatic fluid was obtained from peripheral tumors. In 15 of the 21 patients (71%) with intraductal tumors, a patulous orifice of the major papilla and mucinous fluid were observed. In these 21 patients with cytologic findings of adenocarcinoma or adenoma, surgical resection was performed in 11 and follow-up without surgery in 10. The pathologic characteristics of the 28 tumors are described in Table 1.

ERCP Examination

ERCP was performed in the morning or afternoon after the patients had fasted for at least 5 hours. In 11 patients, a 5-F balloon-tip cannula was used to allow more opacification of the branches of the pancreatic duct. In the remaining 17 patients, ERCP was performed by using a 5-F standard cannula. ERCP was successful in all patients. The contrast medium was 76% amidotrizoate sodium meglumine (76% Urographin; Schering, Osaka, Japan) in a volume of 8–25 mL (mean, 14 mL) with a model JF 1T-10 fiberscope (Olympus, Tokyo, Japan).

MRCP Examination

MRCP was performed with a 1.5-T unit (Visart Hyper; Toshiba, Tokyo, Japan), a surface body coil (spine quadrature coil), and commercially available software. MRCP images were obtained in the morning or afternoon, after the patients had fasted for 12 hours. MRCP was performed with breath-hold two-dimensional (2D) and three-dimensional (3D) half-Fourier fast spin-echo techniques with the patient supine. To restrain bowel motion, we routinely administered intramuscularly 10 mg of butylscopolamine bromide or 1 mg of glucagon for 2D and 3D imaging. In addition, 1,200 mg of ferric ammonium citrate (Otsuka Pharmaceutical, Tokyo, Japan) with 50 mL of water was administered orally to decrease the signal from the bowels.

All 28 patients underwent coronal or paracoronal (10°–30° left anterior oblique) 2D and 3D MRCP and axial 2D MRCP without supplemental oxygen. In 2D imaging, images were obtained during only one 90° pulse and then during 180° pulses for 160 times (repetition time msec/echo time msec = ∞/250), with echo train length of 180, field of view of 350 × 350 mm, matrix of 320 × 320, section thickness of 60 mm, 3-second breath hold, bandwidth of 83.3 kHz, echo spacing of 12.5 msec, acquisition time of 3 seconds, and fat suppression (inversion time, 170 msec). In 3D imaging (10,000/250), the pulse sequence included echo train length of 164, field of view of 350 × 350 mm, matrix of 288 × 384, section thickness of 2 mm and slab thickness of 60 mm (2-mm thickness × 30 sections) and no overlap, intermittent breath holds during each repetition time, bandwidth of 83.3 kHz, echo spacing of 12.5 msec, acquisition time of 5 minutes 30 seconds, and fat suppression (inversion time, 170 msec).

Postprocessing of 3D coronal images was performed with a maximum intensity projection algorithm by a radiologic

TABLE 2
Detectability of the Main Pancreatic Duct with MRCP and ERCP

Detectability Grade and Modality	Location		
	Head	Body	Tail
Excellent			
MRCP	26 (93)	26 (93)	23 (82)
ERCP	28 (100)	25 (89)	24 (86)
Moderate			
MRCP	2 (7)	2 (7)	4 (14)
ERCP	0	3 (11)	4 (14)
Poor			
MRCP	0	0	1 (4)
ERCP	0	0	0

Note.—Data are number of patients (n = 28) with finding. Numbers in parentheses are percentages.

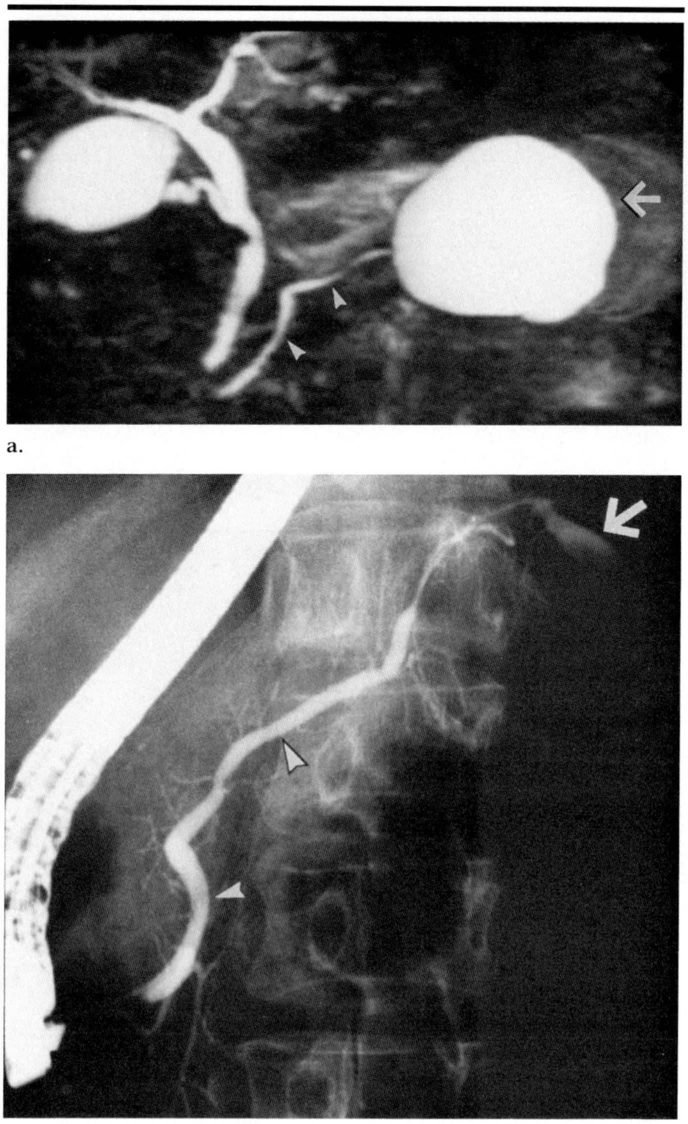

a. b.

Figure 1. Mucinous cystadenoma in the tail of the pancreas. Both the **(a)** coronal 3D MRCP image and **(b)** ERCP image clearly depict the main pancreatic duct (arrowheads). The branches of the pancreatic duct are clearly demonstrated in **b** but not in **a**. The cystic tumor (arrow) in the pancreatic tail is depicted entirely in **a** but only partially in **b**.

TABLE 3
Number of Normal Branches of the Pancreatic Duct Detected with MRCP and ERCP

Detectability Grade and Modality	Location		
	Head	Body	Tail
Excellent			
MRCP	3 (11)*	3 (7)*	0
ERCP	24 (86)*	20 (71)*	17 (61)
Moderate			
MRCP	2 (7)	2 (7)	8 (29)
ERCP	3 (11)	6 (21)	7 (25)
Poor			
MRCP	0	0	1 (4)
ERCP	1 (4)	2 (7)	4 (14)
Not shown			
MRCP	23 (82)	23 (82)	19 (68)
ERCP	0	0	0

Note.—Data are number of patients (n = 28) with finding. Numbers in parentheses are percentages.
* Difference between modalities was statistically significant ($P < .01$).

technician in 3–4 minutes per patient. The 3D images were reconstructed at 10° intervals.

Image Analysis

The three blinded radiologist readers evaluated the randomized MRCP images to assess the following: (*a*) detectability of the main pancreatic duct and its branches, (*b*) detectability of the intraductal cystic lesions in the branches, and (*c*) presence of intracystic nodules or septa. Detectability was graded as excellent (the whole anatomic part was seen), moderate (most of the anatomic part was seen), poor (the anatomic part was poorly seen), or not shown. Then, they evaluated the ERCP images on the basis of the same grading scale. In addition, they also compared findings on the 2D and 3D MRCP images. The 3D MRCP source images were used only to confirm the presence of intraductal cystic lesions and to rule out different sources of fluid signals such as hepatic and renal cysts and fluid in the gastrointestinal tract. When the interpretations differed, the readers reevaluated images and agreed on the diagnosis.

Statistical Analysis

The χ^2 test was used to compare detectability of the normal main pancreatic duct and its branches on MRCP and ERCP images and of the pancreatic ducts and lesions on 2D and 3D MRCP images. A paired Student t test was used to compare the number of cystic dilated branches detected in the pancreatic duct and the number of nodules or septa detected in the main pancreatic duct or its dilated branches with each of the two techniques. Differences with a P value of less than .05 were considered statistically significant.

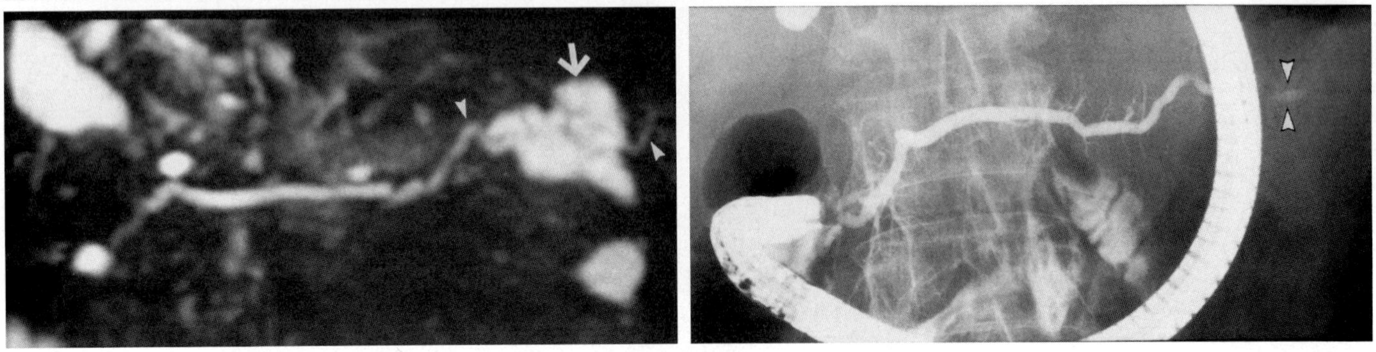

a. b.

Figure 2. Intraductal papillary adenoma (branch type) in the pancreatic tail. **(a)** Coronal 2D MRCP image clearly depicts the main pancreatic duct (arrowheads) and the cystic lesion (arrow) in the pancreatic tail. **(b)** ERCP image depicts the main pancreatic duct in the pancreatic tail (arrowheads) poorly and does not depict the cystic lesion. This is considered to be a result of mucin secretion in the main pancreatic duct and the cystic lesion.

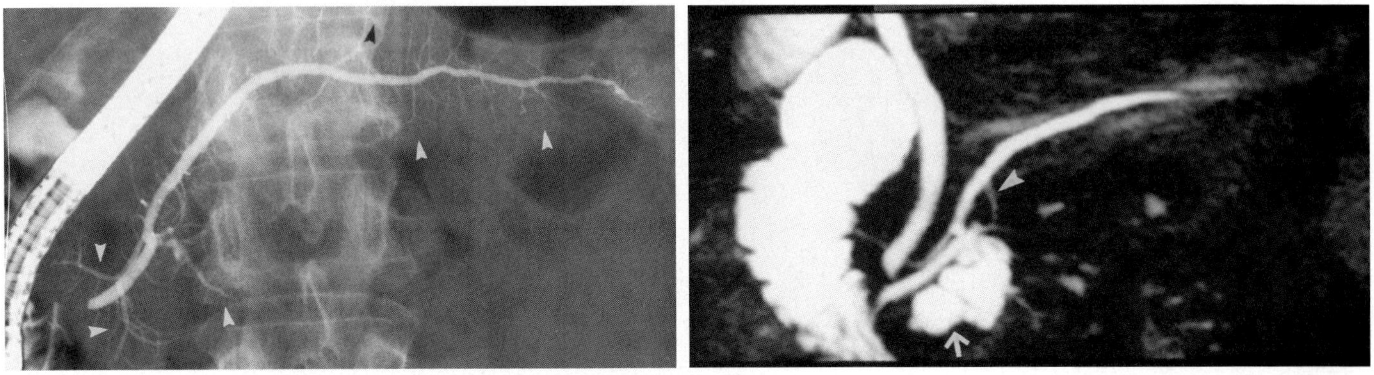

a. b.

Figure 3. Intraductal papillary adenoma (branch type) in the uncinate process. **(a)** ERCP image clearly depicts the branches of the pancreatic duct (arrowheads). **(b)** Coronal 3D MRCP image poorly depicts branches (arrowhead) but clearly depicts the cystic lesion with septa in the uncinate process (arrow), which is not depicted in **a**.

RESULTS

Tables 2 and 3 show the number of main pancreatic ducts and branches that were detected in the 28 patients on MRCP and ERCP images. In most cases, detectability of the main pancreatic duct was graded as excellent on both MRCP and ERCP images (Fig 1); there were no statistically significant differences between the two techniques. The main pancreatic duct in the pancreatic tail was only moderately detectable on ERCP images due to the presence of mucinous fluids in the duct (Fig 2). The number of normal branches with excellent detectability was significantly higher with ERCP than with MRCP ($P < .01$) (Figs 1, 3).

Table 4 shows the number of cystic dilated branches detected with MRCP and ERCP. Detection was significantly better with MRCP than with ERCP ($P < .001$) (Figs 3, 4).

Table 5 shows the number of nodules or septa detected in the dilated branches of the duct with MRCP and ERCP. Differences between modalities were not statistically significant. MRCP simultaneously depicted the main pancreatic duct and the cystic lesions in seven branch-type (Figs 3, 5) and all peripheral-type (Fig 1) mucin-producing tumors, but ERCP did not. ERCP depicted the normal main pancreatic duct and its branches better than did MRCP, but the latter depicted the diseased ducts more clearly than did the former.

Table 6 compares the detectability of the pancreatic duct and its branches and lesions on 2D and 3D MRCP images. Differences between the two techniques in the detection of the normal main pancreatic duct and its branches were not statistically significant, but 3D images depicted significantly more cystic dilated branches ($P < .01$) and nodules or septa in the dilated branches ($P < .05$) than did 2D imaging.

Finally, cytologic examination of the pancreatic fluid obtained from the intraductal lesions during ERCP showed that 11 of the 21 lesions (52%) were suspicious for adenocarcinoma or adenoma and 10 (48%) were suspicious for hyperplastic lesions. After the ERCP procedure, the serum amylase level was elevated (132–820 U/L; mean, 261 U/L) in eight of the 28 patients (29%), but no cases of clinically apparent pancreatitis were encountered.

DISCUSSION

Mucin-producing pancreatic tumors are a comparatively recently described entity (1,2). Of these tumors, intraductal mucin-producing pancreatic tumors have been reported by many Japanese researchers (1,2,5,6,16–21), as well as European and American researchers (22–25). In 1982, Ohhashi et al (16) defined mucin-hypersecreting pancreatic cancer at endoscopy

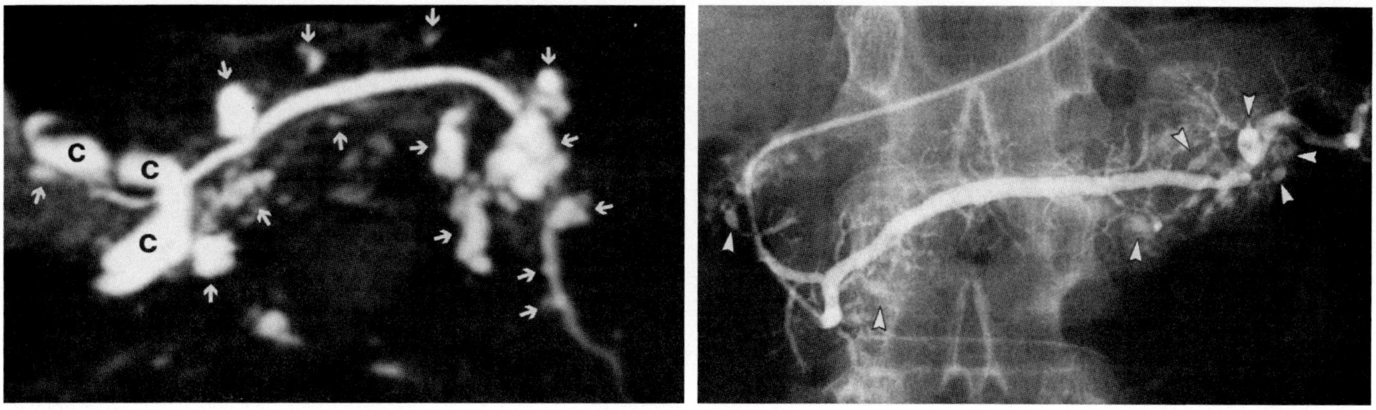

a. b.

Figure 4. Multiple intraductal papillary mucin-producing tumors in the head, body, and tail of the pancreas (nonsurgical case). **(a)** Axil 2D MRCP image depicts multiple cystic lesions (arrows) in the branches of the pancreatic duct. *C* = common bile duct. **(b)** ERCP image obtained with a 5-F balloon-tip cannula depicts some of the lesions (arrowheads) seen in **a**.

TABLE 4
Number of Cystic Dilated Branches of the Pancreatic Duct Detected with MRCP and ERCP

	Location		
Modality	Head (n = 35)	Body (n = 33)	Tail (n = 31)
MRCP	31	31	30
ERCP	17	20	15

Note.— Differences between modalities were statistically significant (P < .001).

TABLE 5
Number of Nodules or Septa in the Dilated Branches of the Pancreatic Duct Detected with MRCP and ERCP

	Location		
Modality	Head (n = 22)	Body (n = 5)	Tail (n = 7)
MRCP	13	4	4
ERCP	7	2	3

TABLE 6
Detectability of the Pancreatic Ducts and Its Branches and Lesions at 2D and 3D MRCP

Imaging Technique	No. of Main Pancreatic Ducts Detected	No. of Normal Branches with Excellent or Moderate Detectability			No. of Dilated Cystic Branches* (n = 99)	No. of Nodules or Septa in the Dilated Branches† (n = 34)
		Head	Body	Tail		
2D	26 (93)	3 (11)	2 (7)	5 (18)	75 (76)	12 (35)
3D	28 (100)	5 (18)	5 (18)	8 (29)	91 (92)	21 (62)

Note.—Numbers in parentheses are percentages.
* The difference between imaging techniques was statistically significant (P < .01).
† The difference between imaging techniques was statistically significant (P < .05).

as a tumor associated with hyperexcretion of the mucinous fluid through the patulous orifice of the papilla of Vater. They found dilation of the main pancreatic duct and/or its branches with filling defect(s) at pancreatography. Obara et al (17) also reported nine cases of mucin-hypersecreting pancreatic tumors, including cancer and adenoma. They found diffuse dilatation of the main pancreatic duct or its branches with nodules of mucin or tumors, as well as a better prognosis (range of postoperative follow-up, 3–41 months; mean follow-up, 21.8 months).

Kuroda (18), Nakazawa et al (1), and Yamada et al (2) proposed a new conceptual category, suggesting that mucin-hypersecreting pancreatic tumors and mucinous cystic tumors of the pancreas (mucinous cystadenocarcinoma and cystadenoma) belong to the same entity. Both tumors originate from the epithelium of the pancreatic duct, and they produce and excrete copious amounts of mucus. Tumors in the pancreatic duct or in cysts show papillary growth. Columnar, mucin-producing epithelium grows with papillary configuration. Malignant tumors typically contain extensive nonmalignant epithelium with a smaller amount of malignant epithelium. Thus, mucin-producing pancreatic tumors are composed of two morphologic features: One is the intraductal papillary tumors derived from the main pancreatic duct (main duct type) or its branches (branch type), and the other is the mucinous cystadenocarcinoma and cystadenoma that originate from the peripheral ducts (peripheral type).

As described previously, hyperplastic lesions that do not need to be surgically resected contain intraductal mucin-producing tumors (4). Therefore, a less invasive but precise technique to follow up those benign lesions instead of ERCP or endoscopic US is necessary. MRCP is a new technique for visualizing the biliary and pancreatic ducts and detecting various abnormalities such as cystic changes, stones, stenosis, dilatation, and nodules of the biliary or pancreatic ducts (12–15). MRCP does not require the use of contrast material or endoscopy, and the examination can be easily repeated.

In our study, the detection rate of the main pancreatic duct was equivalent for MRCP and ERCP, although the sensitivity of detecting the normal ductal branches with MRCP was less than that with ERCP. The most important finding in our study was that detectability of cystic dilatation of the branches and of nodules or septa in the cystic lesions was significantly better with MRCP than with ERCP (Figs 4, 5). We believe the reason MRCP was better at depicting the cystic lesions is that muci-

Figure 5. Intraductal papillary adenocarcinoma (branch type) in the pancreatic head. (a) Coronal 3D MRCP image depicts the cystic lobulations and septa of the tumor (arrow) more clearly than does (b) the ERCP image, which was obtained with a 5-F balloon-tip cannula. The poor depiction in b is probably a result of secretion of a large amount of mucin by the cystic tumor (arrow).

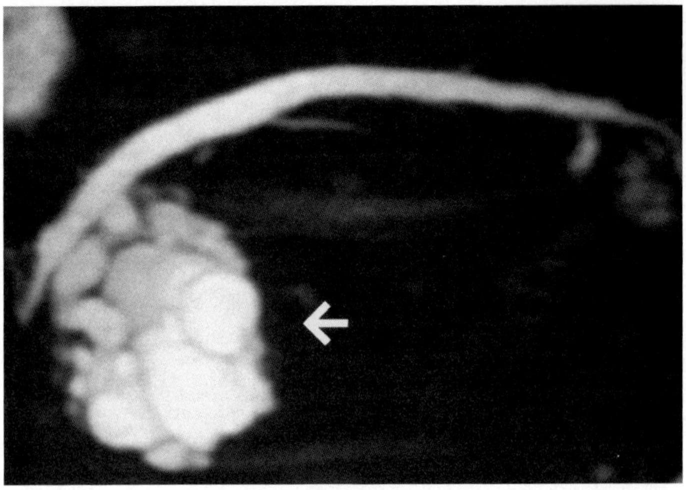

a.

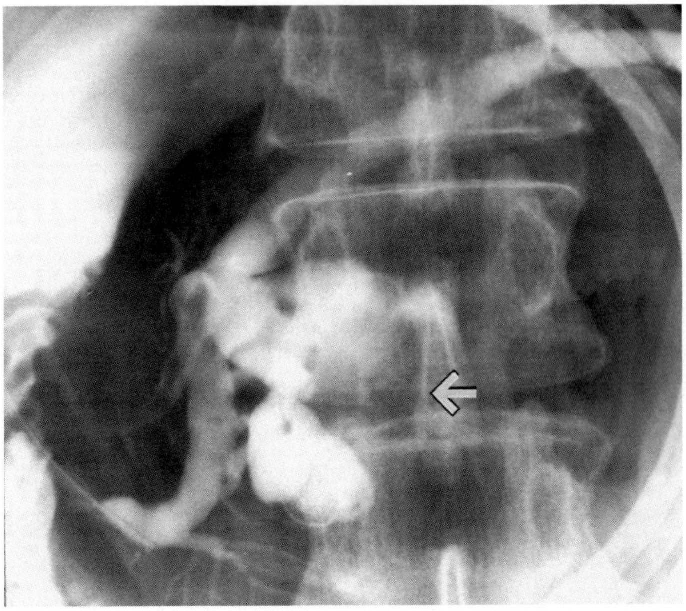

b.

nous fluid produced by the tumors or the tumors themselves inhibited adequate inflow of the contrast material into the cystic dilated branches. Thus, direct visualization of the fluid in the cystic lesions with MRCP was superior to that provided by opacifying the lesions with contrast material at ERCP. Most mucinous cystadenocarcinomas and cystadenomas are not connected to the main pancreatic duct or its branches; therefore, ERCP usually fails to depict their cystic appearance. In contrast, because MRCP can depict the fluid signal intensity, it is easily able to show both the cystic lesions and the ductal systems in the same plane (Fig 1). Conversely, MRCP does not offer any pathologic information for deciding whether the lesions are malignant. From this point of view, ERCP is superior to MRCP because pancreatic fluid sampling for cytologic examination and main pancreatic duct biopsy through the papilla are possible during ERCP. We believe, however, that MRCP is more useful and less invasive than is ERCP for follow-up to evaluate changes in the size and extent of tumors and to determine if new lesions appear.

In our study, 3D images enabled significantly better detection of cystic dilatation of the branches and of nodules or septa in the dilated branches than did 2D images (Table 6). This difference may be a result of differences in section thickness (2D imaging, 60 mm; 3D imaging, 2 mm). This means that 3D imaging is necessary to evaluate the extent of mucin-producing pancreatic tumors and to observe the relationships between the bile duct and the pancreatic duct and the pancreatic cystic lesions in the main pancreatic duct and its branches. Two-dimensional imaging can be used to provide an overview of the main pancreatic duct just before 3D imaging.

One of the drawbacks of MRCP is the poor detectability of normal pancreatic branches. Use of software developed to improve the detection of signal in the fine ducts and stimulation of the pancreatic fluid by means of secretin injection may help solve this problem. Nevertheless, we believe that MRCP is much more effective than ERCP in the follow-up of mucin-producing tumors of the pancreas because the pathophysiologic characteristics of the disorder is to induce mucin production, which leads to dilatation of the main pancreatic duct or its branches and causes dilated ducts as well as cystic tumors. These changes are easily detected with MRCP.

In conclusion, MRCP is more effective and less invasive than ERCP in the evaluation of the changes in size and extent of mucin-producing tumors of the pancreas, and the former may replace the latter in the evaluation of these tumors, for which follow-up is necessary.

Acknowledgment: The authors thank Tsutomu Tomita, who operated the MR imaging equipment and acquired the MRCP images.

References

1. Nakazawa S, Yamao K, Yamada M, et al. Study of the classification of mucin-producing cystic tumor of the pancreas. Jpn J Gastroenterol 1988; 85:924–932. [Japanese]
2. Yamada M, Kozuka S, Yamao K, Nakazawa S, Naitoh Y, Tsukamoto Y. Mucin-producing tumor of the pancreas. Cancer 1991; 68:159–168.
3. Compagno J, Oertel JE. Mucinous cystic neoplasms of the pancreas with overt and latent malignancy (cystadenocarcinoma and cystadenoma). Am J Clin Pathol 1978; 69:573–580.
4. Kimura W, Sasahira N, Hoshikawa T, Muto T, Makuuchi M. Duct-ectatic type of mucin producing tumor of the pancreas: new concept of pancreatic neoplasia. Hepatogastroenterology 1996; 43:692–709.
5. Itai Y, Ohhashi K, Nagai H, et al. "Ductectatic" mucinous cystadenoma and cystadenocarcinoma of the pancreas. Radiology 1986; 161:697–700.
6. Kobayashi G, Fujita N, Lee S, et al. Correlation between ultrasonographic findings and pathologic diagnosis of mucin produc-

ing tumor of the pancreas. Jpn J Gastroenterol 1990; 87:235–342. [Japanese]
7. Koito K, Namieno T, Nagakawa T, et al. Solitary cystic tumor of the pancreas: EUS-pathologic correlation. Gastrointest Endosc 1997; 45:268–276.
8. Bilbao MD, Dotter CT, Lee TG, Katon RM. Complications of endoscopic retrograde cholangiopancreatography (ERCP): a study of 10,000 cases. Gastroenterology 1976; 70:314–320.
9. Hamilton I, Lintott DJ, Rothwell J, Axon ATR. Acute pancreatitis following endoscopic retrograde cholangiopancreatography. Clin Radiol 1983; 34:543–546.
10. Thoeni RF, Fel SC, Goldberg HI. CT detection of asymptomatic pancreatitis following ERCP. Gastrointest Radiol 1990; 15: 291–295.
11. Silvis ES, Ansel HJ. Endoscopic retrograde cholangiography: application in biliary tract disease. In: Berk JE, ed. Gastroenterology. Philadelphia, Pa: Saunders, 1985; 3569–3579.
12. Takehara Y, Ichijo K, Tooyama N, et al. Breath-hold MR cholangiopancreatography with a long-echo-train fast spin-echo sequence and a surface coil in chronic pancreatitis. Radiology 1994; 192: 73–78.
13. Soto JA, Barish MA, Yucel EK, et al. Pancreatic duct: MR cholangiopancreatography with a three-dimensional fast spin-echo technique. Radiology 1995; 196:459–464.
14. Barish MA, Yucel EK, Chuttani R, Ferrucci JT. MR cholangiopancreatography: efficacy of three-dimensional turbo spin-echo technique. AJR 1995; 165:295–300.
15. Miyazaki T, Yamashita Y, Tsuchigame T, et al. MR cholangiopancreatography using HASTE (half-Fourier acquisition single-shot turbo spin-echo) sequences. AJR 1996; 166:1297–1303.
16. Ohhashi K, Murakami Y, Maruyama M, et al. Four cases of mucous secreting pancreatic cancer. Prog Dig Endosc 1982; 20:348–351. [Japanese]
17. Obara T, Maguchi H, Saitoh Y, et al. Mucin-producing tumor of the pancreas: a unique clinical entity. Am J Gastroenterol 1991; 86:1619–1625.
18. Kuroda A. Recent progress in clinicopathology of pancreatic tumors. Biliary Tract Pancreas 1988; 9:1459–1472. [Japanese]
19. Itai Y, Kokubo T, Atomi Y, Kuroda A, Haraguchi Y, Terano A. Mucin-hypersecreting carcinoma of the pancreas. Radiology 1987; 165:51–55.
20. Itho S, Ishiguchi T, Ishigaki T, Sakuma S, Maruyuama K, Senda K. Mucin-producing pancreatic tumor: CT findings and histopathologic correlation. Radiology 1992; 183:81–86.
21. Yamao K, Nakazawa S, Naito Y, et al. Clinicopathological study of the mucous producing pancreatic tumors. Jpn J Gastroenterol 1986; 83:2588–2597. [Japanese]
22. Agostini S, Choux R, Payan MJ, Satre B, Sashel J, Clement JP. Mucinous pancreatic duct ectasia in the body of the pancreas. Radiology 1989; 170:815–816.
23. Richaert F, Cremer M, Derviere J, et al. Intraductal mucin-hypersecreting neoplasms of the pancreas. Gastroenterology 1991; 101:512–519.
24. Tian F, Myules J, Howard JM. Mucinous pancreatic duct ectasia of latent malignancy: an emerging clinicopathologic entity. Surgery 1992; 6:109–113.
25. Procacci C, Grazing R, Bicego E, et al. Intraductal mucin-producing tumors of the pancreas: imaging findings. Radiology 1996; 198:249–257.

Charles C. Yoo, BS
Marc S. Levine, MD
Emma E. Furth, MD
Kevin E. Salhany, MD
Stephen E. Rubesin, MD
Igor Laufer, MD
Hans Herlinger, MD

Index terms:
Lymphoma, 72.349
Lymphoma, diagnosis, 72.123, 72.1261
Stomach, infection, 72.202
Stomach, neoplasms, 72.349

Radiology 1998; 208:239–243

Abbreviations:
GI = gastrointestinal
MALT = mucosa-associated lymphoid tissue

[1] From the Departments of Radiology (C.C.Y., M.S.L., S.E.R., I.L., H.H.) and Pathology and Laboratory Medicine (E.E.F., K.E.S.), Hospital of the University of Pennsylvania, 3400 Spruce St, Philadelphia, PA 19104. Received November 14, 1997; revision requested January 20, 1998; revision received January 30; accepted February 11. **Address reprint requests to** M.S.L.

Author contributions:
Guarantor of integrity of entire study, M.S.L.; study concepts, M.S.L., S.E.R., I.L.; study design, C.C.Y., M.S.L., S.E.R., I.L.; definition of intellectual content, M.S.L.; literature research, C.C.Y.; clinical studies, M.S.L., S.E.R., I.L., H.H.; data acquisition, C.C.Y., M.S.L., E.E.F., K.E.S.; data analysis, C.C.Y., M.S.L., S.E.R., I.L., E.E.F., K.E.S.; manuscript preparation, C.C.Y., M.S.L.; manuscript editing and review, E.E.F., K.E.S., S.E.R., I.L., H.H.

Gastric Mucosa-associated Lymphoid Tissue Lymphoma: Radiographic Findings in Six Patients[1]

PURPOSE: To determine the radiographic findings of low-grade gastric mucosa-associated lymphoid tissue (MALT) lymphoma on double-contrast upper gastrointestinal studies.

MATERIALS AND METHODS: Pathology records, double-contrast upper gastrointestinal studies, and medical records of six patients with gastric MALT lymphoma were retrospectively reviewed.

RESULTS: The most common clinical findings at presentation included epigastric pain ($n = 6$), dyspepsia ($n = 4$), and nausea and vomiting ($n = 4$). Double-contrast studies revealed rounded, often confluent nodules of varying size in four patients with low-grade MALT lymphoma. Nodularity was located in the gastric antrum ($n = 2$), body ($n = 1$), or body and fundus ($n = 1$). A fifth patient had a malignant-appearing 1-cm-diameter antral ulcer, and a sixth had a 10-cm-diameter polypoid, ulcerated mass in the gastric fundus. The latter patient was found to have high-grade MALT lymphoma with low-grade MALT lymphoma abutting the tumor. Five patients had associated *Helicobacter pylori* gastritis. Five patients had stage I disease, and one had stage IIB disease. At endoscopic follow-up ($n = 4$), marked regression of tumor occurred after treatment with antibiotics, chemotherapy, and/or radiation therapy.

CONCLUSION: When low-grade MALT lymphoma is suspected on the basis of barium study results, endoscopic biopsy specimens should be obtained for a definitive diagnosis so these patients can be treated before the development of high-grade gastric lymphoma.

Since the discovery of *Helicobacter pylori* by Warren and Marshall (1) in 1983, this organism has been recognized as a cause of gastritis, gastric and duodenal ulcers, gastric carcinoma, and, most recently, gastric lymphoma. In various studies (2–4), the prevalence of *H pylori* in patients with gastric lymphoma has ranged from 85% to 98%. The high frequency of *H pylori* gastritis in these patients might explain the seeming paradox of primary gastrointestinal (GI) lymphoma developing in an organ that is normally devoid of lymphoid tissue. It has been shown (5–7) that chronic infection of the stomach by *H pylori* is associated with the development of lymphoid follicles and aggregates in the lamina propria in 50%–70% of cases. Most low-grade primary gastric lymphomas are currently thought to arise from this mucosa-associated lymphoid tissue (MALT) and are therefore classified as gastric MALT lymphomas (2,3,8). Unlike high-grade gastric lymphomas, these low-grade MALT lymphomas may undergo complete regression after *H pylori* has been eradicated from the stomach with antibiotics (9–11). Thus, low-grade gastric MALT lymphomas are curable lesions.

To our knowledge, the English-language radiology literature contains only one report (12) of a gastric MALT lymphoma that was demonstrated on a double-contrast barium study as innumerable tiny nodules in the stomach. We had the opportunity to perform double-contrast studies in six patients with known gastric MALT lymphoma. These cases were reviewed retrospectively to determine the radiographic findings of gastric MALT lymphoma on double-contrast studies.

MATERIALS AND METHODS

A computer search of the pathology files at our institution revealed 32 patients with gastric lymphoma at our hospital during the 4 years between April 1993 and April 1997. In fifteen (47%) of those 32 patients, the lesions were classified at the time of diagnosis as gastric MALT lymphomas. A computer search of the radiology files revealed that six of those 15 patients underwent barium studies (all double-contrast) of the upper GI tract. One of those cases has been reported previously (12). The duration between the barium study and endoscopy was 1 day to 12 weeks (average, 3.7 weeks). These six patients formed our study group.

In all six cases, the final diagnosis was made on the basis of histopathologic examination results from multiple endoscopic biopsy specimens from the stomach. Five patients had varying degrees of lymphoplasmacytic infiltration of the lamina propria, focal lymphoepithelial lesions, and centrocyte differentiation compatible with low-grade gastric MALT lymphoma (Fig 1) (13). The remaining patient had high-grade MALT lymphoma (diffuse large cell type) in the gastric fundus with low-grade MALT lymphoma that adjoined the distal end of the lesion. Giemsa- or thiazine-stained endoscopic biopsy specimens were positive for *H pylori* in five of the six patients with gastric MALT lymphoma.

The double-contrast studies in the six patients with gastric MALT lymphoma were reviewed retrospectively to determine the appearance and location of the tumor. Finally, medical charts were reviewed to determine the clinical manifestation, treatment, and course of disease in the patients.

RESULTS

Clinical Examination Findings

Five patients with gastric MALT lymphomas were women, and one was a man. The average patient age was 66 years (age range, 61–76 years) at the time of diagnosis. All six patients had epigastric pain. Other symptoms at presentation included dyspepsia in four patients, nausea and vomiting in four, anorexia in two, and weight loss in two. The average duration of symptoms was 23 months (range, 1 week to 60 months).

Radiographic Findings

In four patients, double-contrast upper GI studies revealed multiple, rounded, often confluent nodules of varying size (2–7 mm in diameter) in the stomach (Figs 2–5). These nodules were located in the antrum in two patients, in the body in one, and in the body and fundus in one. One patient with nodularity in the antrum also had thickened, lobulated folds in the body and fundus (Fig 3b), and one patient with nodularity in the body and fundus had thickened, scalloped folds in the antrum. In all four patients, low-grade gastric MALT lymphoma was confirmed with results from endoscopic biopsy specimens from the region of the nodularity.

A fifth patient had a malignant-appearing ulcer (1 cm in diameter) on the anterior wall of the antrum (best seen on prone compression views), with thickened, lobulated folds that abutted the ulcer (Fig 6). Endoscopic biopsy specimens from the region of the ulcer also demonstrated low-grade gastric MALT lymphoma. The sixth patient had a 10-cm-diameter polypoid, ulcerated mass in the gastric fundus that extended into the distal esophagus (Fig 7). Endoscopic biopsy specimens of the mass demonstrated high-grade MALT lymphoma (diffuse large cell type) with low-grade MALT lymphoma that adjoined the distal end of the lesion.

Endoscopic Findings

In three patients with mucosal nodularity seen on barium studies, endoscopy demonstrated erythematous, edematous, and/or nodular mucosa in the same areas of the stomach. In the remaining patient with mucosal nodularity seen on the barium study, endoscopy demonstrated thickened folds in the fundus and body, with shallow areas of ulceration. In the patient with a malignant-appearing ulcer seen on the barium study, endoscopy demonstrated a shallow antral ulcer with disrupted, nodular folds that abutted the ulcer. In the patient with a polypoid mass in the gastric fundus seen on the barium study, endoscopic findings confirmed the presence of a bulky polypoid mass in the gastric fundus.

Treatment and Course of Disease

Five patients with gastric MALT lymphoma had disease confined to the stomach (stage I), and one had regional lymph node involvement (stage IIB). Two of the five patients with stage I disease were treated with antibiotics only; one was treated with antibiotics and radiation therapy; and two were treated with antibiotics, radiation therapy, and chemotherapy. Follow-up endoscopy in four patients demonstrated marked regression of tumor in the stomach. In one of those four patients, however, examination of follow-up endoscopic biopsy specimens from the gastroesophageal junction showed high-grade large cell lymphoma arising from a residual focus of low-grade MALT lymphoma. Three of the five patients became asymptomatic, but one with regression of tumor and one without endoscopic follow-up had recurrent epigastric pain and dyspepsia. In one patient with low-grade MALT lymphoma who had initial regression of

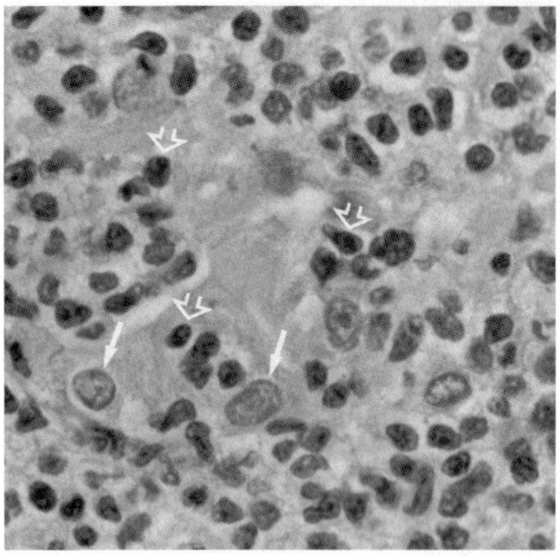

Figure 1. Photomicrograph of gastric biopsy specimen shows the typical lymphoepithelial lesions of low-grade MALT lymphoma, with destruction of gastric glands and infiltration by lymphoma cells (open arrows) with centrocyte differentiation. Solid arrows = epithelial cells of gastric glands. (Hematoxylin-eosin stain; original magnification, ×630.)

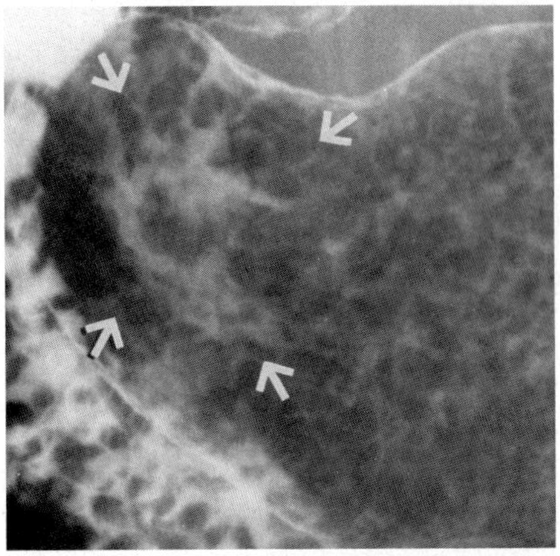

Figure 2. Low-grade gastric MALT lymphoma. Spot radiograph from double-contrast upper GI study shows multiple confluent nodules of varying sizes in the distal gastric antrum. Arrows = area of most severe involvement.

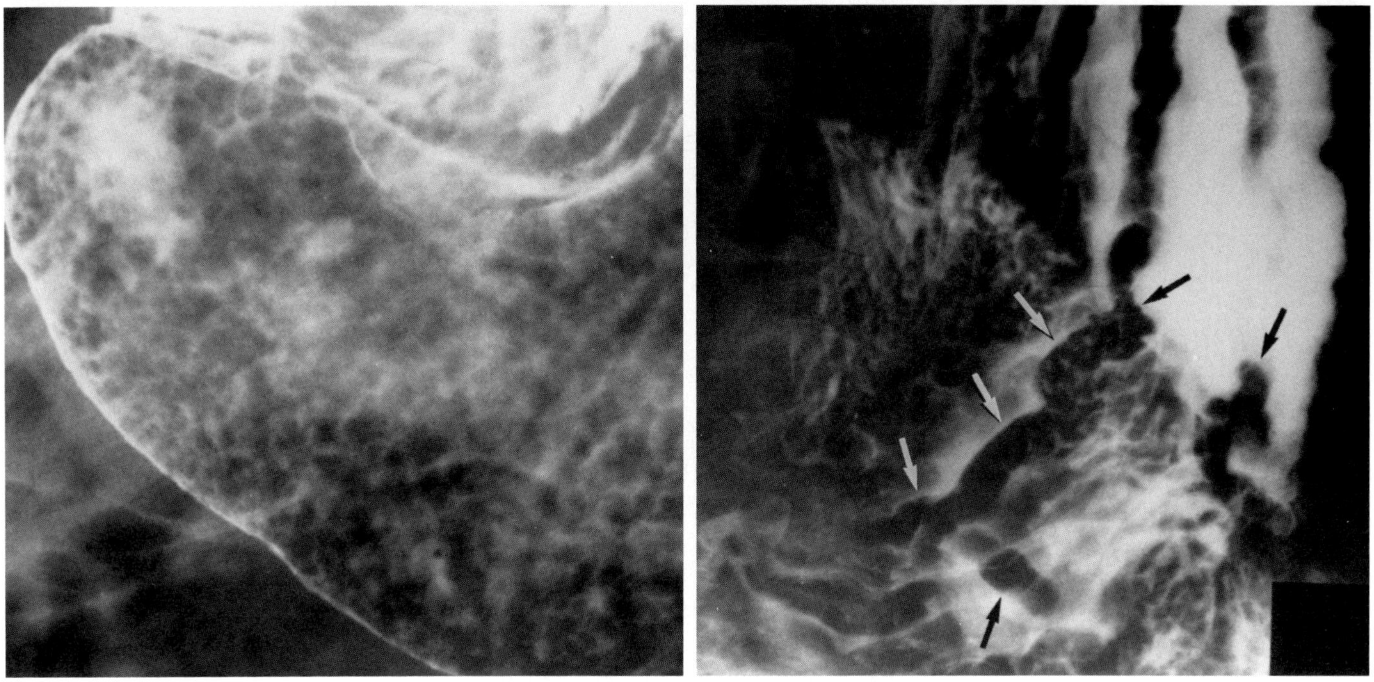

a. b.

Figure 3. Low-grade gastric MALT lymphoma. **(a)** Spot radiograph from double-contrast upper GI study shows antral nodules of varying sizes that could be mistaken for enlarged areae gastricae. **(b)** Another spot radiograph of the gastric body shows thickened, nodular folds (arrows) more proximally in stomach. Analysis of endoscopic biopsy specimens revealed low-grade MALT lymphoma in the antrum and body.

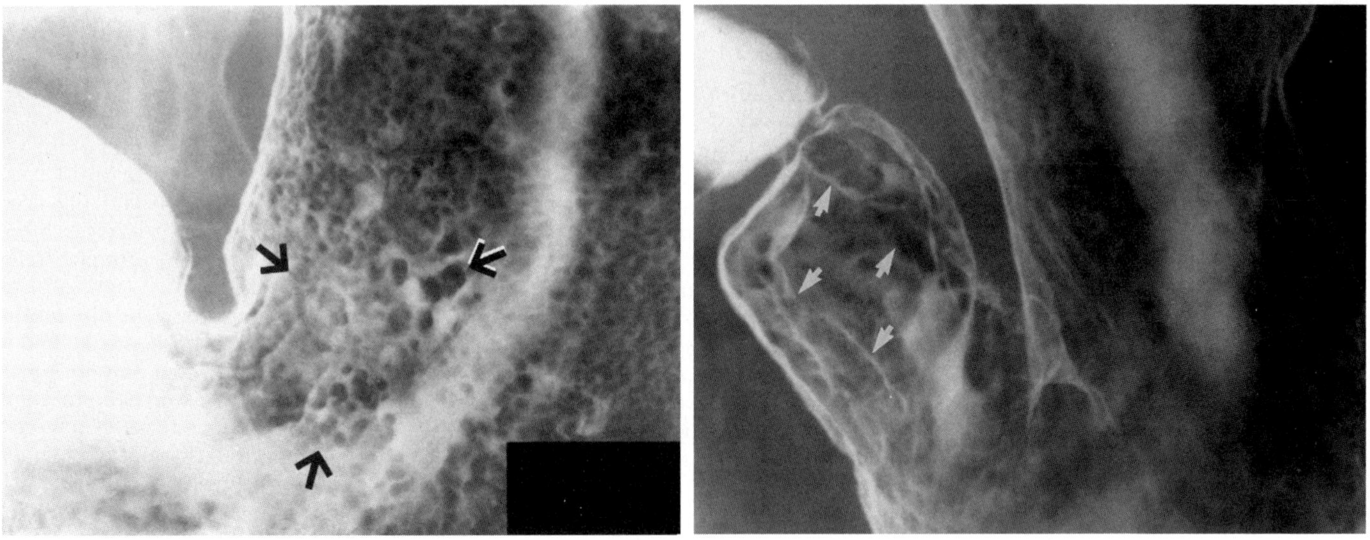

a. b.

Figure 4. Low-grade gastric MALT lymphoma. **(a)** Spot radiograph from double-contrast upper GI study shows confluent nodules of varying sizes in the gastric body. Arrows = area of most severe involvement. **(b)** Spot radiograph from follow-up double-contrast upper GI study obtained 2 years after **a** shows marked regression in comparison with the earlier study (even accounting for technical differences between the images), with minimal nodularity in the gastric body and scalloped folds (arrows) in the antrum.

tumor seen in endoscopic biopsy specimens, four follow-up double-contrast upper GI studies showed a marked decrease in the degree of mucosal nodularity over 2 years (Fig 4b). However, follow-up computed tomography, performed 2 years after the initial diagnosis, demonstrated mesenteric, right external iliac, and bilateral inguinal adenopathy that was presumed to represent disseminated lymphoma.

The remaining patient had concomitant low-grade MALT lymphoma and diffuse large cell lymphoma. In this case, endoscopic ultrasound demonstrated perigastric adenopathy (stage IIB). The patient underwent radiation therapy, and follow-up endoscopy demonstrated marked

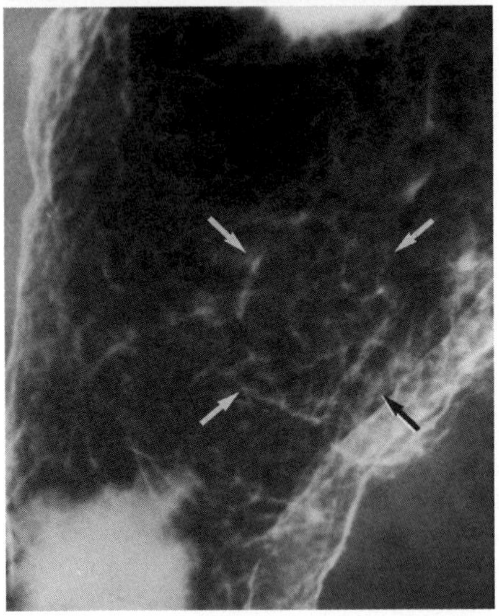

Figure 5. Low-grade gastric MALT lymphoma. Spot radiograph from double-contrast upper GI study shows a focal area of confluent nodularity (arrows) in the gastric body.

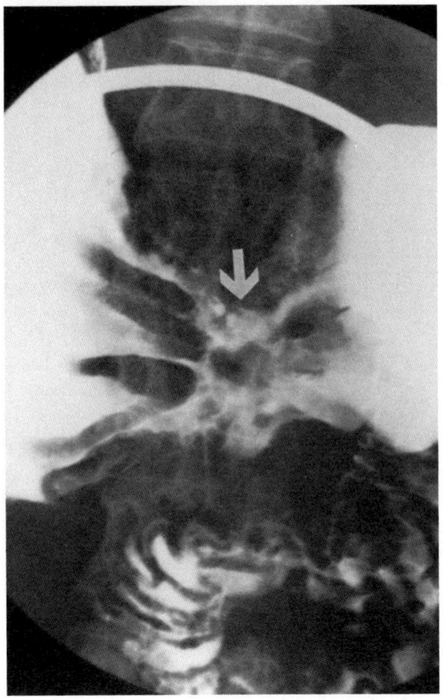

Figure 6. Low-grade gastric MALT lymphoma. Prone compression view from double-contrast upper GI study shows a malignant-appearing ulcer (arrow) on the anterior wall of antrum, with thickened, lobulated folds abutting the ulcer.

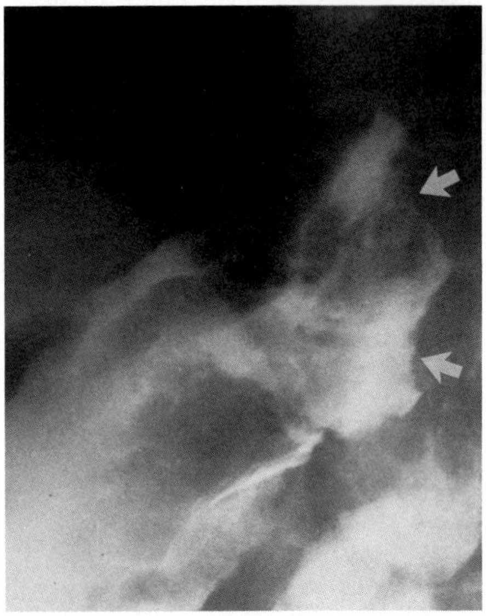

Figure 7. High-grade gastric MALT lymphoma (diffuse large cell type). Spot radiograph from single-contrast study shows a large polypoid mass in the gastric fundus, with irregular ulceration (arrows). Analysis of biopsy specimens from the mass revealed high-grade MALT lymphoma, but low-grade MALT lymphoma was observed in biopsy specimens that abutted the mass.

regression of tumor. This patient had no evidence of recurrent lymphoma after treatment.

DISCUSSION

It is well recognized that chronic *H pylori* gastritis is associated with the development of lymphoid tissue (ie, MALT) in the lamina propria of the stomach (5,6). This MALT is thought to be the precursor of low-grade B-cell gastric MALT lymphoma (2,3,8). In pathologic terms, low-grade MALT lymphoma is characterized by infiltration of the epithelium with small centrocyte-like cells, which give rise to the lymphoepithelial lesions that are characteristic of these tumors (Fig 1) (13). In previous series (14,15), low-grade MALT lymphomas have been found to constitute as many as 50%–72% of all primary gastric lymphomas. These data suggest that low-grade MALT lymphoma is a more common tumor than has previously been recognized.

Gastric MALT lymphoma may manifest at endoscopy as ulceration; polypoid masses; or erythematous, nodular mucosa (16,17). As a result, the endoscopic appearance may be difficult to differentiate from the appearance of benign ulcers or even severe gastritis (16). In a recent study (18), antral nodularity was reported at endoscopy in a series of patients with benign lymphoid hyperplasia due to *H pylori* gastritis, so the gross endoscopic findings in these tumors may closely resemble those in *H pylori* infection of the stomach. However, endoscopic biopsy specimens will demonstrate the characteristic pathologic findings of low-grade MALT lymphoma, thereby enabling differentiation from *H pylori* gastritis.

As in our study, patients with gastric MALT lymphoma usually present clinically with epigastric pain, dyspepsia, or both (11,16,17). As a result, the symptoms at presentation are indistinguishable from those caused by gastric or duodenal ulcers, gastritis, and duodenitis. Furthermore, the average duration of symptoms in our series was approximately 2 years; one patient had dyspepsia for as long as 5 years. We therefore suspect that some of our patients with low-grade MALT lymphoma may have presented because of their underlying *H pylori* gastritis and that the lymphoma was detected fortuitously in these cases. Whatever the explanation, it is important for radiologists to be aware of the findings associated with low-grade MALT lymphoma because of the opportunity to diagnose this curable form of gastric lymphoma with the aid of double-contrast studies.

To our knowledge, the English-language radiology literature contains only one report (12) of gastric MALT lymphoma in which a double-contrast upper GI series demonstrated multiple small nodules in the stomach. In four of the six patients in our study, gastric MALT lymphoma also manifested as variably sized (2–7 mm in diameter), rounded, often confluent nodules in the stomach (Figs 2–5).

Other considerations in the differential diagnosis include severe gastritis, leukemic infiltration, or even a polyposis syndrome involving the stomach. In some cases, this mucosal nodularity may also be difficult to differentiate from enlarged areae gastricae, a finding recently shown to be associated with *H pylori* gastritis (19). However, areae gastricae tend to be more uniform in size, producing a sharply marginated reticular network.

Endoscopy and biopsy should be performed for a definitive diagnosis when gastric MALT lymphoma is suspected on the basis of the radiographic findings. Although some patients may prove to have severe gastritis due to *H pylori* or other causes, it seems reasonable to accept a certain percentage of false-positive diagnoses because of the importance of the detection of low-grade MALT lymphoma at an early, curable stage. It is hoped that as experience with these tumors increases, the number of false-positive diagnoses will decrease and thereby result in fewer endoscopic examinations.

It is important to recognize that our study was limited by the small number of cases in our series. Furthermore, all six patients in our study were treated nonsurgically. As a result, no surgical specimens were available for radiologic-pathologic correlation. On the basis of results in the endoscopic biopsy specimens in our cases, however, we suspect that this nodularity results from focal infiltration and expansion of the lamina propria by the lymphoid infiltrate of gastric MALT lymphoma. In any case, further investigation is needed with a larger series of patients to better delineate the spectrum of radiographic findings associated with low-grade gastric MALT lymphoma.

One patient in our study was found to have a large, polypoid, ulcerated mass in the gastric fundus on the barium study (Fig 7). Endoscopic biopsy specimens in this case demonstrated diffuse large cell lymphoma arising from low-grade MALT lymphoma more distally in the stomach. This case is similar in gross morphology to the type of advanced gastric lymphoma that has been well described (20,21) in the radiology literature. Another patient had large cell lymphoma arising from a residual focus of low-grade MALT lymphoma at the gastroesophageal junction in follow-up endoscopic biopsy specimens after treatment. In a previous study by Chan et al (22), regions of low-grade MALT lymphoma were found at histopathologic examination in 10 (28%) of 36 of patients with high-grade gastric lymphoma. The findings from our study and from that by Chan et al support the concept that primary gastric lymphoma often originates as a low-grade MALT lymphoma, which subsequently undergoes transformation to intermediate or high-grade large cell lymphoma. Low-grade MALT lymphoma could, therefore, be considered to be a form of early gastric lymphoma. Indeed, patients with a low-grade gastric MALT lymphoma have a much better prognosis than do those with a high-grade MALT lymphoma; these low-grade tumors are associated with a 5-year survival rate of 75%–91% (14,16), whereas high-grade MALT lymphomas are associated with a 5-year survival rate of less than 50% (16).

The diagnosis of low-grade gastric MALT lymphoma also has important implications for patient treatment. Unlike high-grade lymphomas, which are treated with various combinations of chemotherapy, radiation therapy, and surgery, low-grade MALT lymphoma can often be successfully treated with antibiotics. In one study (7), complete regression of tumor occurred after treatment with antibiotics alone in five of six patients with gastric MALT lymphoma and concomitant *H pylori* gastritis. In other studies (10,11), partial or complete regression of tumor was reported in 60%–80% of patients treated with omeprazole and amoxicillin.

One theory is that *H pylori* may evoke an immunologic response that stimulates growth of the tumor. Eradication of *H pylori* from the stomach may therefore inhibit tumor growth, resulting in regression of the tumor (7). Whatever the explanation, eradication of *H pylori* from the stomach by using antibiotics appears to be a viable alternative to surgery, chemotherapy, or radiation therapy as the initial treatment for low-grade gastric MALT lymphomas.

In summary, low-grade gastric MALT lymphoma almost always occurs in the setting of chronic *H pylori* gastritis. This tumor may be manifested on double-contrast upper GI studies by variably sized, rounded, often confluent nodules in the stomach. When low-grade MALT lymphoma is suspected on the basis of barium study findings, endoscopic biopsy specimens should be obtained for a definitive diagnosis so these patients can be treated before the development of high-grade gastric lymphoma.

References

1. Warren JR, Marshall BJ. Unidentified curved bacilli on gastric epithelium in active chronic gastritis. Lancet 1983; 2:1273–1275.
2. Wotherspoon AC, Ortiz-Hidalgo C, Falzon MR, Isaacson PG. *Helicobacter pylori*–associated gastritis and primary B-cell gastric lymphoma. Lancet 1991; 338:1175–1176.
3. Eidt S, Stolte M, Fischer R. *Helicobacter pylori* gastritis and primary gastric non-Hodgkin's lymphomas. J Clin Pathol 1994; 47:436–439.
4. Parsonnet J, Hansen S, Rodriguez L, et al. *Helicobacter pylori* infection and gastric lymphoma. N Engl J Med 1994; 330:1267–1271.
5. Eidt S, Stolte M. Prevalence of lymphoid follicles and aggregates in *Helicobacter pylori* gastritis in antral and body mucosa. J Clin Pathol 1993; 46:832–835.
6. Genta RM, Hamner HW, Graham DY. Gastric lymphoid follicles in *Helicobacter pylori* infection: frequency, distribution, and response to triple therapy. Hum Pathol 1993; 24:577–583.
7. Stolte M, Eidt S. Lymphoid follicles in antral mucosa: immune response to *Campylobacter pylori?* J Clin Pathol 1989; 42: 1269–1271.
8. Isaacson P, Wright DH. Extranodal malignant lymphoma arising from mucosa-associated lymphoid tissue. Cancer 1984; 53:2515–2524.
9. Wotherspoon AC, Doglioni C, Diss TC, et al. Regression of primary low-grade B-cell gastric lymphoma of mucosa-associated lymphoid tissue type after eradication of *Helicobacter pylori*. Lancet 1993; 342:575–577.
10. Bayerdörffer E, Neubaeur A, Rudolph B, et al. Regression of primary gastric lymphoma of mucosa-associated lymphoid tissue type after cure of *Helicobacter pylori* infection. Lancet 1995; 345:1591–1594.
11. Roggero E, Zucca E, Pinotti G, et al. Eradication of *Helicobacter pylori* infection in primary low-grade gastric lymphoma of mucosa-associated lymphoid tissue. Ann Intern Med 1995; 122:767–769.
12. Levine MS, Elmas N, Furth EE, Rubesin SE, Goldwein MI. *Helicobacter pylori* and gastric MALT lymphoma. AJR 1996; 166:85–86.
13. Harris NL, Jaffe ES, Stern H, et al. A revised European-American classification of lymphoid neoplasms: a proposal from the International Lymphoma Study Group. Blood 1994; 84:1361–1392.
14. Cogliatti SB, Schmid U, Schumacher U, et al. Primary B-cell gastric lymphoma: a clinicopathological study of 145 patients. Gastroenterology 1991; 101:1159–1170.
15. Akaza K, Motoori T, Nakamura S, et al. Clinicopathologic study of primary gastric lymphoma of B cell phenotype with special reference to low-grade B cell lymphoma of mucosa-associated lymphoid tissue among the Japanese. Pathol Int 1995; 45:832–845.
16. Taal BG, Boot H, van Heerde P, de Jong D, Hart AAM, Burgers JMV. Primary non-Hodgkin lymphoma of the stomach: endoscopic pattern and prognosis in low versus high grade malignancy in relation to the MALT concept. Gut 1996; 39:556–561.
17. Seifert E, Schulte F, Weismüller J, de Mas CR, Stolte M. Endoscopic and bioptic diagnosis of malignant non-Hodgkin's lymphoma of the stomach. Endoscopy 1993; 25:497–501.
18. Sbeih F, Abdullah A, Sullivan S, Merenkov Z. Antral nodularity, gastric lymphoid hyperplasia, and *Helicobacter pylori* in adults. J Clin Gastroenterol 1996; 22:227–230.
19. Sohn J, Levine MS, Furth EE, et al. *Helicobacter pylori* gastritis: radiographic findings. Radiology 1995; 195:763–767.
20. Menuck LS. Gastric lymphoma: a radiologic diagnosis. Gastrointest Radiol 1976; 1:157-161.
21. Zornoza J, Dodd GD. Lymphoma of the gastrointestinal tract. Semin Roentgenol 1980; 15:272–287.
22. Chan JKC, Ng CS, Isaacson PG. Relationship between high-grade lymphoma and low-grade B-cell mucosa-associated lymphoid tissue lymphoma (MALToma) of the stomach. Am J Pathol 1990; 136:1153–1164.

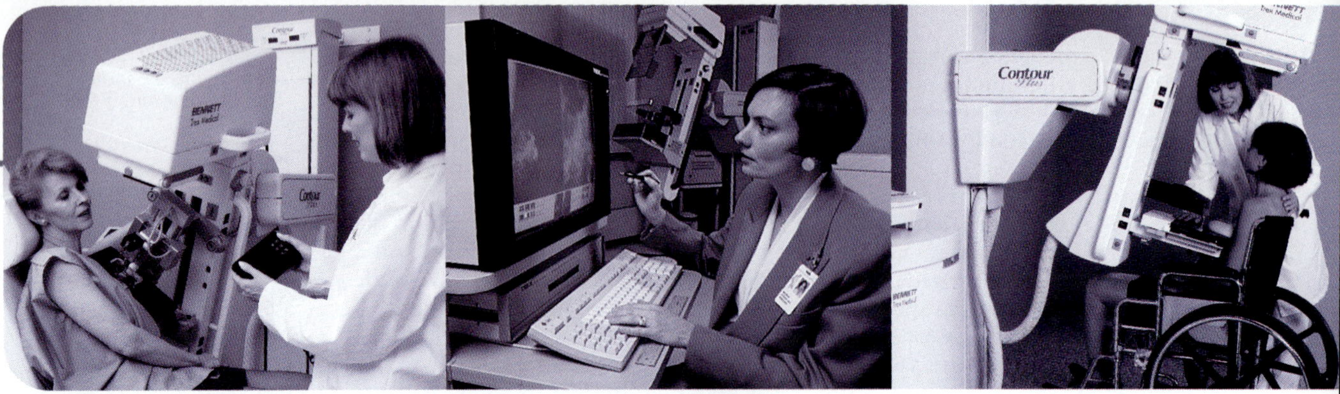

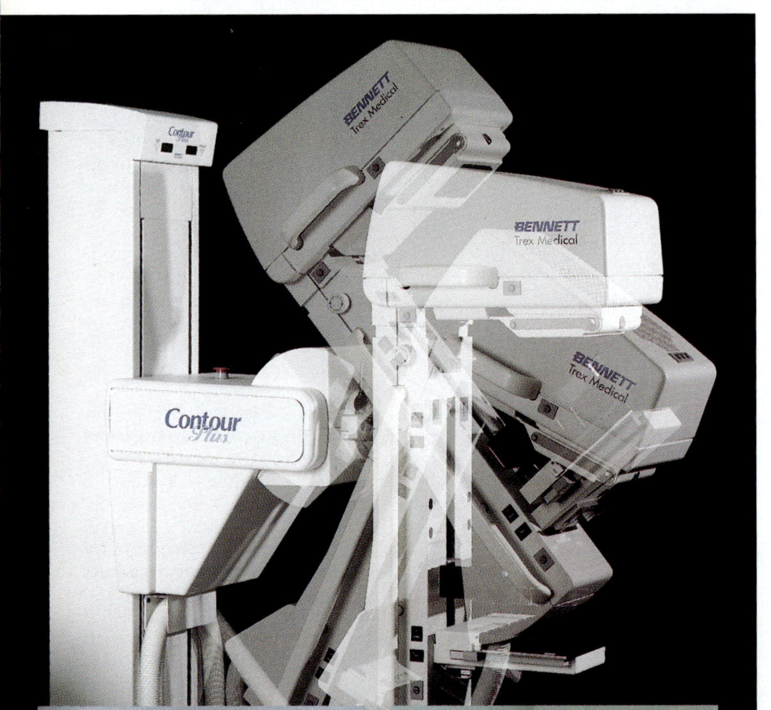

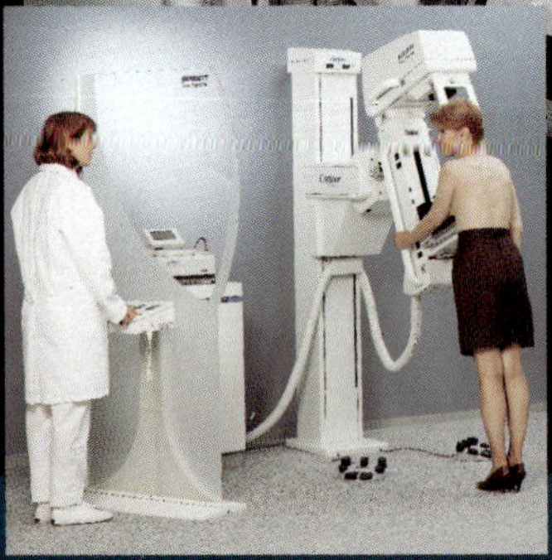

Contour Plus Mammography System

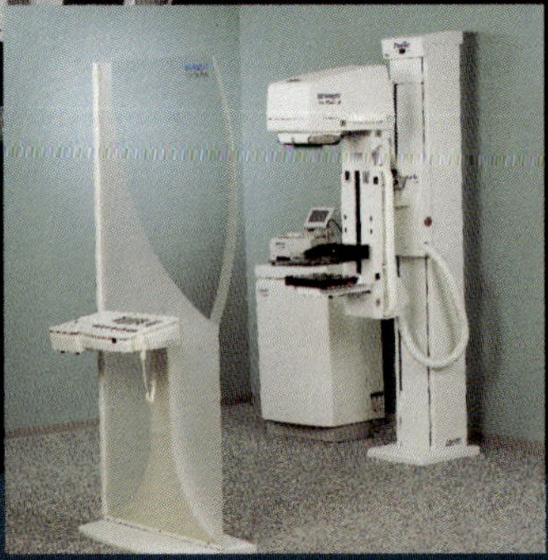

Profile Mammography System

Screening Behavior of Women after a False-Positive Mammogram[1]

Etta D. Pisano, MD
JoAnne Earp, ScD
Michael Schell, PhD
Kathryn Vokaty, MPH
Amy Denham, MPH

Index terms:
Breast radiography, utilization, 00.111
Cancer screening

Radiology 1998; 208:245–249

[1] From the School of Medicine, the Department of Radiology (E.D.P.), and the School of Public Health, the Departments of Health Behavior and Health Education (J.E., K.V., A.D.) and Biostatistics (M.S.), the University of North Carolina at Chapel Hill, 503 Old Infirmary Bldg CB7510, Chapel Hill, NC 27599-7510, and the University of North Carolina–Lineberger Comprehensive Cancer Center, Chapel Hill (E.D.P., J.E., M.S.). From the 1995 RSNA scientific assembly. Received October 2, 1997; revision requested October 27; revision received January 26, 1998; accepted March 4. Supported in part by a University of North Carolina–Lineberger Comprehensive Cancer Center small grant and by National Cancer Institute Specialized Program of Research Excellence (SPORE) developmental grant (National Institutes of Health grant CA-58223). **Address reprint requests to** E.D.P.

PURPOSE: To determine the effect of a false-positive mammogram that leads to open surgical biopsy on subsequent screening mammography behavior in women.

MATERIALS AND METHODS: This study was performed with a retrospective cohort design, and data were collected by means of telephone interview. All participants were women aged at least 50 years, with no history of breast cancer. Study patients (n = 43) were women who had an abnormal mammogram followed within 6 months by benign excisional breast biopsy. Control subjects (n = 136) were randomly selected: They included women with a normal mammogram who had not undergone biopsy, as well as women with an abnormal mammogram and the recommendation to undergo 6-month follow-up mammography.

RESULTS: Two differences between the study and control groups were statistically significant. Study patients were more likely than control patients to believe they had increased susceptibility to breast cancer (P = .039). Study patients were also more likely than control subjects to intend to undergo screening mammography annually in the future (P = .036).

CONCLUSION: A false-positive mammogram that leads to open surgical biopsy does not inhibit most women from undergoing subsequent screening mammography. In fact, such an experience may increase their intentions to undergo regular screening.

Both the acceptance of mammography and the number of women screened with mammography are increasing (1–5). One of the unintended consequences of this increase in the number of women screened is the growing number of women with abnormal mammograms. The proportion of mammograms interpreted as abnormal may be as high as 15%–20% (6,7). After a positive screening study that leads to biopsy, the likelihood of patients having cancer varies from 10% to 40% (8–14), and the remaining 60%–90% of patients have false-positive mammograms.

Little is known about how false-positive mammograms affect women's compliance with subsequent annual screening mammography. A survey of women in British Columbia, Canada, was performed to determine what variables encouraged compliance with return screening after the initial study; the women who returned annually for screening were more likely to have had a normal initial study than were "late compliers" and "noncompliers" (15). Whether women with false-positive mammograms are more or less likely to return for annual screening mammography in the future can clearly influence subsequent rates of morbidity and mortality from breast cancer.

To our knowledge, few studies have been performed to examine the psychologic and behavioral consequences of experiencing an abnormal screening mammogram. A negative psychologic effect of a false-positive mammogram may influence a woman's compliance with recommendations for subsequent annual screening mammography. Heightened perceived susceptibility to breast cancer has been found to be related to a reduced rate of breast self-examination among high-risk women (16). Anxiety and worry about cancer have also been associated with reduced participation in annual mammographic screening (1,2), as well as with longer delays in seeking care for possible cancer symptoms (10). However, the data regarding the relationship between breast cancer worry and breast cancer screening are variable, with studies showing no relationship, a positive relationship, and a negative relationship (17–25).

Author contributions:
Guarantor of integrity of entire study, E.D.P.; study concepts, E.D.P., J.E., K.V.; study design, E.D.P., J.E., K.V.; definition of intellectual content, E.D.P., J.E., K.V.; literature research, E.D.P., J.E., K.V., A.D.; experimental studies, K.V.; data acquisition, K.V.; data analysis, M.S.; statistical analysis, M.S.; manuscript preparation, E.D.P., A.D.; manuscript editing, E.D.P., J.E.; manuscript review, E.D.P., J.E., M.S., K.V., A.D.

In this study, we explored the relationship between a false-positive mammogram followed by benign excisional biopsy and subsequent compliance with recommendations to undergo annual screening mammography. We also examined the psychologic consequences of this experience.

MATERIALS AND METHODS

Study Design

The study was performed with a retrospective cohort design, and it was formally exempted from review by the human study board of our medical school. Cross-sectional data were collected by means of telephone interview to explore the relationship between an abnormal mammogram followed by benign breast biopsy and several outcomes. These outcomes included the intention to undergo screening mammography in the future and the patient actually undergoing future mammography after the biopsy. In the survey, questions were also included to help explain any relationships found. The survey was administered between January and August 1993.

The mammography database from our radiology department was used to identify all women meeting entry criteria. Participation in this study was limited to 57 women (*a*) with an abnormal mammogram obtained at the University of North Carolina Hospital or Mobile Mammography Service between January 1, 1989, and May 31, 1991, which was followed up within 6 months by a benign excisional breast biopsy at our hospital; (*b*) aged at least 50 years at the time of index mammography; and (*c*) with no history of breast cancer.

We also identified the cases of three control groups. All control subjects were aged at least 50 years at the time of index mammography and had no known prior history of breast cancer or benign breast biopsy. Control group 1 consisted of 94 women randomly selected from the 12,574 women with a normal mammogram obtained at our hospital or mobile mammography service between January 1, 1989, and May 31, 1991, and no biopsy within 6 months afterward. Control group 2 consisted of all 144 women with an abnormal mammogram obtained at our hospital or mobile mammography service between January 1, 1989 and May 31, 1991, and a recommendation to undergo a 6-month follow-up mammography. Initially, a third control group of women was also identified by cross referencing data from our pathology department with mammographic data from our radiology department (for age, mammography, and previous breast cancer). This group consisted of all 17 women with a normal mammogram obtained at our hospital or mobile mammography service during the same time who underwent surgical biopsy to evaluate palpable lesions.

Study and Control Groups

Of the 57 study patients, two were deceased at the time of the interview, three could not be located, and two were identified as ineligible by virtue of a subsequent diagnosis of breast cancer. Of the remaining 50 women, seven refused to participate or did not complete the telephone interview. Therefore, 43 (86%) of the 50 eligible study patients completed the interviews.

Of the 255 control subjects, six were deceased, 13 could not be located, and five had a subsequent diagnosis of breast cancer and were thus ineligible. Of the remaining 231 women, 58 either refused to be interviewed or did not complete the entire interview, yielding a total of 173 control subjects (response rate, 74.9% [173 of 231 control subjects]). Eight women in control group 1 and 22 women in control group 2 were excluded from analysis because they had undergone open surgical biopsy at our institution after their index mammographic study. Because only seven women in control group 3 met eligibility criteria and were willing or able to participate in this study, and because the experience of having a palpable lesion leading to biopsy is different from having a clinically occult lesion, this group was excluded from the analysis. The answers of these seven women were included in the analysis of the biopsy experience itself.

Thus, the comparisons between study patients and control subjects reported herein are based on the responses of the remaining 53 women in control group 1 and 83 women in control group 2, or a total of 136 control subjects. Results about the effects of the biopsy experience itself include the responses of all 73 women (43 study patients and 30 control subjects) who had undergone biopsy.

Telephone Interviews

A letter of introduction, signed by the study radiologist (E.D.P.), was sent to each participant approximately 1 week before an attempt was made to contact the woman by telephone. Repeated attempts were made to contact each woman. Those who could not be contacted by telephone after 15 or more attempts during various hours of the day and evening were sent certified letters with a return receipt requested. A postcard was enclosed for these women to indicate their current phone number and the best time to contact them. Finally, a written questionnaire of the telephone interview was mailed to women who still could not be contacted by telephone.

A structured questionnaire was designed specifically for this study on the basis of a preliminary, semistructured telephone interview that addressed these same research questions with a similar population (26). The questions themselves had been used previously in a large, National Cancer Institute–funded, random digit–dialed survey of black and white women in two North Carolina counties about compliance with breast cancer screening recommendations, as well as in the pilot study leading up to the present research (26,27). The questionnaire for this study contained seven sections and 98 items and required an average of 17 minutes to complete.

The major variables in the present study were the following: compliance with recommendations for screening mammography, intent to undergo screening mammography in the future, perceived barriers to undergoing screening, perceived benefits to undergoing screening, perceived negative effects of screening, perceived susceptibility to breast cancer, and perceived severity of breast cancer. The survey did not include questions that specifically assessed the prebiopsy screening mammography behavior of study patients and control subjects.

Interviews were conducted by one of three trained interviewers (K.V. and two others). In the telephone interview, a standard introduction was given to explain the study and ask for the woman's consent to be interviewed. Compliance was measured with one item, "When did you have your last mammogram?" A respondent was considered "compliant" if her last mammogram was obtained within the past year, "late" if it was obtained 1–2 years ago, and "noncompliant" if it was obtained more than 2 years ago. Behavioral intent was measured with two items: "How likely do you think you are to have a mammogram in the next year?" and "Do you intend to get a mammogram every year?" Responses to these two questions, which measured "immediate" and "long-term" behavioral intent, respectively, were combined so that respon-

Study Findings

Data	No. of Study Patients	No. of Control Group 1	No. of Control Group 2	*P*
Demographics				
Mean age (y)	63.26	63.51	65.66	.896
Black	18 of 43 (42)	16 of 53 (30)	29 of 83 (35)	.826
With ≤12 y education	32 of 43 (74)	28 of 53 (53)	57 of 83 (69)	.060
Married	19 of 43 (44)	32 of 52 (62)	47 of 83 (57)	.221
With income ≤$15,000/y	26 of 40 (65)	17 of 43 (40)	39 of 78 (50)	.066
With no insurance	19 of 42 (45)	3 of 53 (6)	11 of 83 (13)	.001*
Employed full or part time	16 of 43 (37)	22 of 52 (42)	30 of 53 (57)	.764
Breast cancer beliefs				
Believed annual mammography was necessary	39 of 41 (95)	46 of 50 (92)	66 of 75 (88)	.421
Reported barriers to undergoing mammography	9 of 43 (21)	19 of 53 (36)	30 of 82 (37)	.173
Reported high perceived benefit of mammography	31 of 41 (76)	26 of 48 (54)	46 of 77 (60)	.098
Reported negative effects of mammography	13 of 33 (39)	14 of 34 (41)	31 of 61 (51)	.485
High perceived susceptibility to breast cancer	5 of 40 (13)	1 of 50 (2)	2 of 72 (3)	.039*
High perceived severity of breast cancer	23 of 38 (61)	31 of 46 (67)	44 of 66 (67)	.769
Mammographic behaviors				
Likely to undergo mammography in the next year	39 of 41 (95)	48 of 49 (97)	72 of 79 (91)	.268
Intend to undergo mammography every year	41 of 42 (98)	44 of 49 (90)	63 of 77 (82)	.036*
Underwent mammography at least three times in the 3 y since index mammography	31 of 43 (72)	35 of 53 (66)	48 of 83 (58)	.263

Note.—Numbers in parentheses are percentages.

* Difference between study patients and control groups for this category was statistically significant.

dents were considered as strongly intending to undergo mammography in the next year if they had both high immediate and high long-term intent; all other combinations of the two items were coded as low intent to undergo screening in the next year.

Perceived barriers to undergoing mammography were evaluated with a group of seven psychosocial barriers (eg, not having the time, forgetting to go, trouble finding a ride, fear of finding out bad news) and six system barriers (eg, inconvenient clinic hours, having to wait too long, staff not helpful). These items were read to respondents one at a time and each was followed up with the question of whether this factor had kept the women from undergoing screening mammography "many times," "sometimes," or "never." Respondents were considered as perceiving serious barriers to screening mammography if they indicated that they were affected "sometimes" or "many times" by any of the 13 possible barriers or any additional barrier they were given an opportunity to add. Respondents received a score that ranged from 13 to 39, with a low score representing fewer barriers. The number of barriers reported "many times" were summed, and the percentages were compared for study patients and control subjects.

Perceived benefit of undergoing screening mammography was measured with two items: "Getting a mammogram every year will help find cancer at an early stage," and, "To find breast cancer early, would you say the one best method is checking your breasts yourself, having a doctor check your breasts, having a mammogram, or some other way?" Women were designated as perceiving screening mammography as strongly beneficial if they answered "strongly agree" (on a scale of strongly agree, agree, disagree, and strongly disagree) to the first item and if they mentioned mammograms (alone or in combination with clinical breast examinations or breast self-examinations) in response to the second question.

Respondents were considered to be reporting negative effects of mammography if they thought that mammography could be performed incorrectly and could cause breast cancer by bruising the breast or that the x rays at mammography could cause breast cancer.

Respondents were considered to have high perceived susceptibility to breast cancer if they considered their own chance of having breast cancer to be somewhat higher or a lot higher than that of other women their age and if they believed women their age (over 50 years) were at greater risk of breast cancer than women in other age groups.

Respondents were considered to have high perceived severity of breast cancer if they disagreed or strongly disagreed with the statement, "Finding breast cancer early helps a woman live longer," and if they agreed or strongly agreed with the statement, "Women can never be completely cured of breast cancer," and, "A woman will likely die of breast cancer is she gets it."

The questionnaire was pretested with nine women who met all criteria except age for inclusion as study patients. These women were aged 40–49 years rather than over 50 years. A few questions and the question order were subsequently modified.

Statistical Analysis

For analysis purposes, data were entered into a dBASE file and χ^2 tests of association were performed (SAS SYSTEM; SAS Institute, Cary, NC). Study patients were compared with only control groups 1 and 2 to represent all women after screening mammography. That is, after screening mammography, the recommendation is made to undergo biopsy (study patients), routine follow-up (control group 1), or short-term follow-up (control group 2). Women who had been identified as eligible for control group 2 but who were discovered during the telephone interview to have undergone breast biopsy after index mammography were excluded from all comparisons of study patients and control subjects. Their responses and those from control group 3, however, were included for queries regarding the effects of biopsy.

The Wilcoxon rank sum statistic was used to test the distribution of age across study patients and control groups 1 and 2. The χ^2 test of homogeneity or independence was used to perform other analyses.

RESULTS

The Table shows the demographic profile of the study patients and control subjects. No statistically significant differences were found between study patients and control subjects with respect to age, race, marital status, educational level, and income. We found a statistically significant difference between study patients and control subjects regarding their health insurance status: Significantly more study patients than control subjects were uninsured ($P = .001$).

The Table also presents the participants' beliefs and perceptions about breast cancer and mammography. Study patients and control subjects were similar regarding most variables, with a few notable exceptions. There was a nonsignificant tendency for study patients to report a high perceived benefit of mammography ($P = .098$), and study patients were significantly more likely than control subjects to perceive their susceptibility to breast cancer as high ($P = .039$).

As can be seen in the Table, differences between study patients and control subjects were not significant regarding– their intention to undergo screening mammography in the year after the survey, although significantly more study patients than control subjects intended to undergo routine screening on an annual basis ($P = .036$), as recommended in multiple published guidelines (28). Finally, study patients were no more likely than control subjects to have undergone annual mammography in the 3 years after index mammography.

When asked how worried they were immediately after the false-positive mammogram was obtained but before they underwent biopsy, 50% of the 57 study patients reported being very worried or somewhat worried. However, 97% reported that they were very satisfied that their questions about the procedure had been answered by the doctors and nurses involved, and 95% reported that the doctors and nurses had treated them well during the procedure.

Regarding the effect of the biopsy on the beliefs and fears of the 57 study patients, 58% did not experience increased awareness of their future risk of breast cancer, 84% did not fear needing another biopsy, and 93% did not worry about undergoing another mammographic examination. Only 3% thought they would ever need to undergo repeat breast biopsy in the future.

In contrast to the lack of psychologic sequelae reported by most of the patients who underwent biopsy, the majority of women who had this experience reported substantial physical morbidity. Of the 66 women who answered questions about the physical sequela of their biopsies, 92% reported they "had a lot of pain," "felt sick for more than 3 days after surgery," and/or "missed work for 3 days." Ninety-four percent reported they "experienced loss of arm motion for more than 7 days after the biopsy," and 80% recalled they "had less sexual feeling in their breast for more than 2 weeks."

DISCUSSION

It would appear that a false-positive mammogram that leads to open surgical biopsy does not inhibit most women from undergoing subsequent screening mammography, nor does it increase their fear of mammography or their worry about their future risk of breast cancer. In fact, such an experience appears to increase patients' intentions to undergo regular screening mammography.

Several researchers have suggested that the experience of a false-positive mammogram might be so traumatic to patients that screening mammography becomes of limited benefit, even for women over age 50 years, in whom the mortality benefit is clear (29). Some researchers have hypothesized that women who perceive their breast cancer risk as increased might be less likely to undergo screening because of feelings of anxiety and helplessness (30). Our results do not support these concerns: Our study patients had a higher perceived susceptibility to breast cancer than did control subjects, but they had similar screening mammography attendance records and greater intent to undergo mammography annually in the future. Although our survey contained no formal psychologic or psychiatric measures of depression or anxiety, our results suggest that the increased worry and physical morbidity that women report at the time of biopsy do not translate into increased fear of mammography and biopsy in the future. These findings confirm those in a recent meta-analysis of 19 studies to measure perceived risk in which women who felt vulnerable to breast cancer and women who had prior breast problems were found to be more likely to undergo screening mammography (31).

Significantly more study patients lacked health insurance than did control subjects, which would tend to predispose study patients to less screening behavior. Findings in multiple studies have confirmed that lack of health insurance reduces cancer screening behavior and intentions (32–34). The fact that our uninsured population was more likely to intend to undergo screening despite their lack of insurance supports the strong effect of the abnormal mammogram–biopsy experience on beliefs and behavior. We can only speculate about the effect of this event on other populations, but we believe our results probably underestimate the effect in women with private insurance or in a health maintenance organization.

The experience of a false-positive mammogram may serve as a "teachable moment" (35,36) for the patient. Health education research has emphasized the importance of timing in the increased motivation or readiness of an individual to learn. When a woman finds herself in a threatening situation or one that presents a certain degree of ambiguity, she may be more open to health education messages. In addition, individuals seem more ready to learn after they have taken an action consistent with what health care providers or educators want them to learn, which presents an opportunity to reinforce positive preventive behaviors (37).

In other words, a woman may be more open to hearing about the benefits of regular mammographic screening just after she has undergone mammography because the information gives her an opportunity to feel good about what she has just done. The event may suggest to a woman that abnormalities can be detected with a screening test when nothing is palpable by either her or her physician. In a survey of older women that compared screening participants with nonparticipants, women who understood that screening helped detection of asymptomatic cancers were found to be more likely to participate in screening (38). The experience of a false-positive mammogram followed by open surgical biopsy could represent just such a teachable moment in a woman's life, and it may give health care providers the opportunity to encourage patients who have not previously done so to initiate regular mammographic screening and compliance with national guidelines (1,39–42).

The results of this study must be interpreted with some limitations in mind. First, the survey did not contain as accurate a measure of mammography behavior *before* false-positive mammography as we would have wished. Because women were interviewed up to 3 years *after* index mammography, valid assessment of earlier screening behavior would have been difficult to obtain. Without such a measure, however, we could not compare the screening behaviors of study patients and control subjects at baseline.

Also, the study patients underwent open surgical biopsy to evaluate a mammographically detected lesion. We can only speculate on the effect after core needle biopsy to evaluate a nonpalpable lesion. As reported in a recent survey (43), the physical side effects after core biopsy are less serious than those after open surgical biopsy. Research about the psychosocial effects of core biopsy versus excisional biopsy is needed to determine their comparative consequences. The morbidity reported by our study patients supports the investigation of less invasive diagnostic strategies.

Women with a history of false-positive mammograms pose a special problem for radiologists, primary care physicians, and health educators. They need the same information about mammography and breast cancer that women in general need, but they also need special information to lessen their fear about biopsy without reducing their future compliance with screening guidelines. On the basis of our research, we conclude that future compliance with annual screening recommendations is not adversely affected in women with false-positive mammograms, although some such women may be at higher risk for noncompliance. Recommendations for an invasive procedure such as breast biopsy should be made with consideration for the possible impact on individual women.

Acknowledgments: The authors thank Tamara Gallant, Kristen Harris, Yuhua Lin, Edison Liu, Michael O'Malley, Michael Plankey, and Bonnie Yankaskas for their contributions to the completion of this study.

References

1. Lerman C, Rimer B, Trock B, Balshem A, Engstrom PF. Factors associated with repeat adherence to breast cancer screening. Prev Med 1990; 19:279–290.
2. Rimer BK, Keintz MK, Kessler HB, Engstrom PF, Rosan JR. Why women resist screening mammography: patient-related barriers. Radiology 1989; 172:243–246.
3. Zapka J, Stoddard AM, Costanza ME, Greene ML. Breast cancer screening by mammography utilization and associated factors. Am J Public Health 1989; 189: 1499–1502.
4. National Cancer Institute Breast Cancer Screening Consortium. Screening mammography: a missed clinical opportunity? results of the NCI Breast Cancer Screening Consortium and National Health Interview Survey studies. JAMA 1990; 264: 54–58.
5. Ackerman DP, Brackbill RM, Brewers BA, Cheal NE, Sanderson LM. Cancer screening behaviors among United States women: breast cancer, 1987–1989, and cervical cancer, 1988–1989. MMWR 1992; 41:17–34.
6. Winchester DP, Lasky HJ, Sylvester J, Maher ML. A television-promoted mammography screening pilot project in the Chicago metropolitan area. CA Cancer J Clin 1988; 38:291–309.
7. Bird RE. Low-cost screening mammography: report of finances and review of 21,716 consecutive cases. Radiology 1989; 171:87–90.
8. Schwartz G, Feig S, Patchefsky A. Significance and staging of nonpalpable carcinomas of the breast. Surg Gynecol Obstet 1988; 166:6–10.
9. Skinner M, Swain M, Simmon R. Nonpalpable breast lesions at biopsy. Ann Surg 1988; 208:203–208.
10. Landercasper J, Gunderson S, Gunderson A, et al. Needle localization and biopsy of nonpalpable lesions of the breast. Surg Gynecol Obstet 1982; 164:399–403.
11. Wright C. Breast cancer screening. Surgery 1986; 100:594–598.
12. U.S. Preventive Services Task Force. Guide to clinical preventive services: an assessment of the effectiveness of 169 interventions. Baltimore, Md: Williams & Wilkins, 1989; 39–62.
13. Houn F, Brown ML. Current practice of screening mammography in the United States: data from the national survey of mammography facilities. Radiology 1994; 190:209–215.
14. Kopans DB, Swann CA. Observations on mammographic screening and false positive mammograms. AJR 1988; 150:785–786.
15. Johnson MM, Hislop TG, Kan L, Coldman AJ, Lai A. Compliance with the screening mammography program of British Columbia: will she return? Can J Public Health 1996; 87:176–179.
16. Alagna SW, Morokoff PJ, Bevett JM, Reddy DM. Performance of breast self-examination by women at high risk for breast cancer. Women Health 1987; 12:29–46.
17. Lerman C, Trock B, Rimer BK, Jepson C, Brody D, Boyce A. Psychological side effects of breast cancer screening. Health Psychol 1991; 10:259–267.
18. Fuller SM, McDermott RJ, Roetzheim RG, Marty PJ. Breast cancer beliefs of women participating in a television-promoted mammography screening project. Public Health Rep 1992; 107:682–690.
19. Lerman C, Kash K, Stefanek M. Younger women at increased risk for breast cancer: perceived risk, psychological well-being and surveillance behavior. J Natl Cancer Inst Monogr 1994; 16:171–176.
20. McCaul KD, Reid PA, Rathge RW, Martinson B. Does concern about breast cancer inhibit or promote breast cancer screening? Basic Appl Soc Psychol 1996; 18:183–194.
21. Stefanek ME, Wilcox P. First degree relatives of breast cancer patients: screening practices and provision of risk information. Cancer Detect Prev 1991; 15:379–384.
22. Kash KM, Holland JC, Osborne MP, Miller DG. Psychological counseling strategies for women at risk of breast cancer. J Natl Cancer Inst Monogr 1995; 17:73–79.
23. Lerman C, Daly M, Sands C, et al. Mammography adherence and psychological distress among women at risk for breast cancer. J Natl Cancer Inst 1993; 85:1074–1080.
24. McCaul KD, Schroeder DM, Reid PA. Breast cancer worry and screening: some prospective data. Health Psychol 1996; 15: 430–433.
25. Lerman C, Trock B, Rimer BK, Boyce A, Jepson C, Engstrom PF. Psychological and behavioral implications of abnormal mammograms. Ann Intern Med 1991; 114:657–661.
26. Gallant T. Effects of a false positive mammogram and negative biopsy on subsequent mammogram screening behavior: a pilot study. Master paper. Department of Health Behavior and Health Education, School of Public Health, University of North Carolina–Chapel Hill, 1992.
27. Fletcher SW, Harris RP, Gonzalez JJ, et al. Increasing mammogram utilization: a controlled study. J Natl Cancer Inst 1983; 85:112–120.
28. American College of Physicians. Preventive care guidelines: 1991. Ann Intern Med 1991; 114:758–783.
29. Harris R, Leininger L. Clinical strategies for breast cancer screening: weighing and using the evidence. Ann Intern Med 1995; 122:539–547.
30. Kash KM, Holland JC, Halper MS, Miller DG. Psychological distress and surveillance behaviors of women with a family history of breast cancer. J Natl Cancer Inst 1992; 84:24–30.
31. McCaul KD, Branstetter AD, Schroeder DM. What is the relationship between breast cancer risk and mammography screening? a meta-analytic review. Health Psychol 1996; 15:423–429.
32. Kiefe CI, McKay SV, Halavey A, Brody BA. Is cost a barrier to screening mammography for low income women receiving Medicare benefits? a randomized trial. Arch Intern Med 1994; 154:1217–1224.
33. Blustein J. Medicare coverage, supplemental insurance, and the use of mammography by older women. N Engl J Med 1995; 332:1138–1143.
34. Makuc DM, Fried VM, Kleinman JC. National trends in the use of preventive care by women. Am J Public Health 1989; 79:21–26.
35. Earp JAL, Thomas RP, McCandless MW, Ory MG, Carr PA. An evaluation of an urban health department's prenatal education program. Appl Res Eval 1984; 5:5–23.
36. Nutting PA. Health promotion in primary medical care: problems and potential. Prev Med 1986; 15:537–548.
37. Hochbaum GM. Modern theories of communication. Children 1960; 7:13–18.
38. Taplin SH, Montano DE. Attitudes, age and participation in mammographic screening: a prospective analysis. J Am Board Fam Pract 1993; 6:13–23.
39. Zapka JG, Stoddard A, Maul L, Costanza ME. Interval adherence to mammography screening guidelines. Med Care 1991; 29:697–707.
40. Fox SA, Murata PJ, Stein JA. The impact of physician compliance on screening mammography for older women. Arch Intern Med 1991; 151:50–56.
41. Rimer BK. Understanding the acceptance of mammography by women. Ann Behav Med 1992; 14:197–203.
42. O'Malley MS, Earp JAL, Harris RP. Race and mammography use in two North Carolina counties. Am J Public Health 1997; 7:782–786.
43. Handy RB, Fajardo LL, Innis CA, Witzke DB, Hunter TB. Patient perception of stereotaxic large-core breast biopsy. Acad Radiol 1996; 3:1007–1011.

Expand Your Horizons with RSNA® International Programs

RSNA International Visiting Professor Program

RSNA is looking for dynamic, experienced radiology teachers interested in enhancing radiologic education in countries outside North America. Teach and travel in countries such as Chile, Ecuador, India, Jordan, Kenya, Malaysia and elsewhere. As an RSNA International Visiting Professor, you will teach in an active radiology training program and help educate those who will practice radiology for years to come.

Interested applicants willing to devote their time to teach overseas should contact the Committee on International Radiology Education for more information and an application form.

The deadline is August 31, 1998.

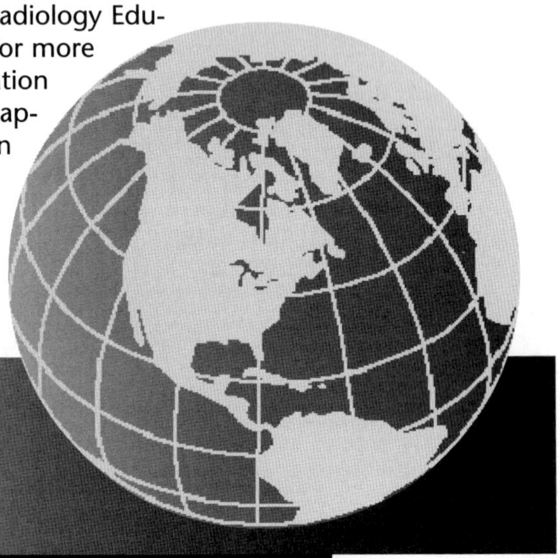

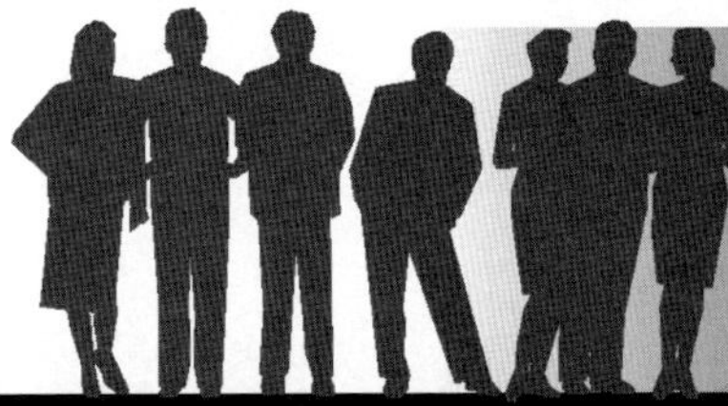

The RSNA Derek Harwood-Nash R&E Fund International Fellowship

RSNA is looking for promising scholars from outside North America who are embarking on a career in academic radiology and who wish to study at a North American institution for a minimum 6-week period. At appropriate host academic centers in North America, fellows will observe procedures and participate in conferences relating to their areas of special interest.

More information on this fellowship can be obtained from the article in the June issue of Radiology by Drs. Petasnick, Ferris, and Osborn ("The RSNA Derek Harwood-Nash R&E Fund International Fellowship." *Radiology* 1997; 203:630).

Interested scholars who can demonstrate that their specific educational goals would best be met by a course of study at a North American institution should contact the Committee on International Radiology Education for more information and an application form.

The deadline is July 1, 1998.

Anne G. Osborn, MD, *Chairman*
Committee on International Radiology Education
RSNA • 2021 Spring Road, Suite 600 • Oak Brook, IL 60523
(630) 368-3747 • FAX: (630) 571-7837 • e-mail: *glowacki@rsna.org*

Calcification Retrieval at Stereotactic, 11-gauge, Directional, Vacuum-assisted Breast Biopsy[1]

Laura Liberman, MD
Jennifer H. Smolkin, MD
D. David Dershaw, MD
Elizabeth A. Morris, MD
Andrea F. Abramson, MD
Paul Peter Rosen, MD

Index terms:
Breast, calcification, 00.81
Breast neoplasms, biopsy, 00.1261, 00.1267, 00.30
Breast neoplasms, diagnosis, 00.30
Breast neoplasms, radiography, 00.11, 00.128
Specimen, radiography, 00.128

Radiology 1998; 208:251–260

Abbreviations:
ADH = atypical ductal hyperplasia
BI-RADS = Breast Imaging Reporting and Data System
DCIS = ductal carcinoma in situ

[1] From the Departments of Radiology, Breast Imaging Section (L.L., J.H.S., D.D.D., E.A.M., A.F.A.), and Pathology (P.P.R.), Memorial Sloan-Kettering Cancer Center, 1275 York Ave, New York, NY 10021. Received November 3, 1997; revision requested December 24; revision received January 20, 1998; accepted February 12. **Address reprint requests to** L.L.

PURPOSE: To determine the frequencies of calcification retrieval and histologic underestimates at stereotactic, 11-gauge, directional, vacuum-assisted breast biopsy.

MATERIALS AND METHODS: Retrospective review of records revealed 112 calcific lesions in 80 women (aged 31–85 years) who underwent stereotactic, 11-gauge, directional, vacuum-assisted biopsy; a mean of 14 specimens per lesion were obtained. Calcification retrieval was defined as identification of calcifications on radiographs of specimens. Atypical ductal hyperplasia (ADH) underestimates were lesions that yielded ADH at stereotactic biopsy and carcinoma at surgery. Ductal carcinoma in situ (DCIS) underestimates were lesions that yielded DCIS at stereotactic biopsy and infiltrating carcinoma at surgery. Mammograms, stereotactic images, radiographs of specimens, and histologic findings were reviewed.

RESULTS: Stereotactic, 11-gauge, directional, vacuum-assisted biopsy removed all calcifications in 51 (46%) lesions, some calcifications in 55 (49%) lesions, and no calcifications in six (5%) lesions. Failure to retrieve calcifications was significantly more likely in lesions 5 mm or smaller (12% [five of 43] vs 1% [one of 69], $P = .03$), in calcifications with amorphous morphology (21% [three of 14] vs 3% [three of 98], $P < .03$), or if the probe was fired outside the breast (12% [five of 40] vs 1% [one of 72], $P = .02$). Surgery revealed DCIS in one (10%) of 10 lesions that yielded ADH at stereotactic biopsy. Surgery revealed infiltrating carcinoma in one (5%) of 21 lesions that yielded DCIS at stereotactic biopsy. No underestimation occurred when all calcifications were removed.

CONCLUSION: Stereotactic, 11-gauge, directional, vacuum-assisted biopsy resulted in successful calcification retrieval in 106 (95%) of 112 cases. Histologic underestimation was infrequent.

Stereotactic, 14-gauge, automated, large-core breast biopsy is an accurate and cost-effective alternative to surgical biopsy for the diagnosis of nonpalpable breast lesions (1–15); however, it has recognized limitations in the assessment of calcifications (16–21). The likelihood at automated, large-core biopsy of failing to sample the lesion (1–3,7–9,20,21), "underestimating" lesions containing atypical ductal hyperplasia (ADH) or ductal carcinoma in situ (DCIS) (6,16,17,20), or failing to spare the patient a surgical procedure (9,12,18–21) are higher for calcifications than for masses. The problems with automated large-core biopsy of calcifications reflect the geometric properties of calcifications, which provide a small and discontinuous target, and the histologic heterogeneity of these lesions (22), which may require a large volume of tissue for complete characterization.

Stereotactic, directional, vacuum-assisted breast biopsy is being used increasingly for the diagnosis of indeterminate or suspicious lesions identified at mammography (23–39). Previous work suggests that stereotactic, 14-gauge, directional, vacuum-assisted biopsy may provide better retrieval and characterization of calcifications than stereotactic, 14-gauge, automated, large-core biopsy (28–32). The improved performance of the directional, vacuum-assisted biopsy instrument in the assessment of calcifications is probably due to the larger size of each specimen and to the ability of the vacuum-assisted

Author contributions:
Guarantor of integrity of entire study, L.L.; study concepts and design, L.L.; definition of intellectual content, L.L., J.H.S., D.D.D., E.A.M., A.F.A., P.P.R.; literature research, L.L., J.H.S.; clinical studies, L.L., D.D.D., E.A.M., A.F.A., P.P.R.; data acquisition, L.L., J.H.S., D.D.D., E.A.M., A.F.A., P.P.R.; data analysis, L.L.; statistical analysis, L.L.; manuscript preparation, editing, and review, L.L., J.H.S., D.D.D., E.A.M., A.F.A., P.P.R.

device to acquire tissue outside of the line of fire, sample contiguously, suction blood from the biopsy cavity, and obtain multiple specimens with a single insertion.

The 14-gauge, directional, vacuum-assisted biopsy instrument has one important limitation: It does not enable accurate placement of a localizing marker (35). Complete removal of the mammographic lesion with stereotactic, 14-gauge, directional, vacuum-assisted biopsy has been reported in 13%–48% of all lesions and in 58%–93% of lesions 5 mm or smaller (27,29,30). If the mammographic lesion is completely removed, it is preferable to place a localizing marker at the biopsy site to facilitate accurate localization for subsequent surgical excision, if necessary (29,35,36). The importance of placing a localizing marker was illustrated in a recent study: Among 15 carcinomas in which the mammographic lesion was removed at directional, vacuum-assisted breast biopsy, surgery revealed residual carcinoma in 11 (73%) (40).

An 11-gauge probe is available for performing directional, vacuum-assisted breast biopsy. The 11-gauge probe is more expensive than the 14-gauge probe ($210 vs $135 [1997 list price, Biopsys–Ethicon Endo-surgery, Cincinnati, Ohio]) but enables accurate placement of a localizing marker at the biopsy site (35,36), obtains larger tissue specimens (27,34,39), and may decrease the frequency of histologic underestimates in lesions containing ADH and DCIS (38). Few data address the usefulness of 11-gauge, directional, vacuum-assisted biopsy in the evaluation of calcific lesions (37,38). This study was undertaken to determine the frequencies of calcification retrieval and histologic underestimates at stereotactic, 11-gauge, vacuum-assisted breast biopsy.

TABLE 1
Completeness of Excision of Calcifications versus Lesion Size

Lesion Size	All Calcifications Removed	Some Calcifications Removed	No Calcifications Removed
All (*n* = 112)	51 (46)	55 (49)	6 (5)
≤1 cm (*n* = 78)	50 (64)	22 (28)	6 (8)
≤5 mm (*n* = 43)	31 (72)	7 (16)	5 (12)

Note.—The numbers in parentheses are percentages.

TABLE 2
Features of Lesions in Which All, Some, or None of the Calcifications Were Removed

Feature	All Calcifications Removed (*n* = 51)	Some Calcifications Removed (*n* = 55)	No Calcifications Removed (*n* = 6)
No. of core specimens			
Median	13	13	14
Range	8–28	6–34	1–19
Lesion size (cm)			
Median	0.5	1.2	0.5
Range	0.2–1.4	0.2–10.0	0.4–1.0
Patient age (y)			
Median	60	55	64
Range	31–73	36–85	37–73
Calcifications seen at histologic analysis	51 (100)	53 (96)	3 (50)
Repeat biopsy recommended*	7 (14)†	8 (14)‡	4 (67)
ADH underestimates	0/5 (0)	1/5 (20)	. . .
DCIS underestimates	0/12 (0)	1/9 (11)	. . .

Note.—The numbers in parentheses are percentages.

* Refers to the number of cases in which repeat biopsy was recommended after stereotactic, vacuum-assisted biopsy.

† Surgical biopsy recommended owing to percutaneous biopsy findings of ADH in five, lobular carcinoma in situ and radial scar in one, and a mucocelelike lesion in one. The latter two lesions were benign at surgery; surgical histologic diagnoses in five lesions yielding ADH at percutaneous biopsy were benign in three and ADH in two.

‡ Surgical biopsy recommended owing to percutaneous biopsy findings of ADH in six, no calcifications at histopathologic analysis in one, and a mucocelelike lesion in one. The latter patient and one woman with ADH declined to undergo surgical biopsy; the lesion that yielded no calcifications at histopathologic analysis was benign at surgery. Surgical histopathologic diagnoses in five lesions yielding ADH at percutaneous biopsy were ADH in one, benign in three, and DCIS in one.

MATERIALS AND METHODS

Retrospective review of records was conducted in 180 consecutive lesions in which stereotactic, 11-gauge, directional, vacuum-assisted breast biopsy (Mammotome; Biopsys–Ethicon Endo-surgery) was performed from October 31, 1996, to September 15, 1997. Mammographic findings were an uncalcified mass in 58 lesions, a mass with calcifications in 10, and calcifications without mass in 112. The latter 112 lesions, which occurred in 80 women aged 31–85 years (median, 55 years), constitute the basis of this study.

The 112 mammographic lesions considered here measured 0.2–10.0 cm in greatest diameter (median, 0.7 cm). Calcification morphology was classified according to the American College of Radiology Breast Imaging Reporting and Data System (BI-RADS) lexicon (41) as pleomorphic in 90 lesions, amorphous in 14, and linear in eight. Lesions were located in the anterior third of the breast in 20 cases, the middle third in 57, and the posterior third in 35. Breast composition, as per the BI-RADS lexicon (41), was class 1 (fatty) in nine cases, class 2 (scattered fibroglandular densities) in 43, class 3 (heterogeneously dense) in 55, and class 4 (extremely dense) in five. The percutaneous biopsy specimens were determined to be benign in 67 (60%), ADH in 12 (11%), and malignant in 33 (29%) of the 112 lesions.

Biopsy was performed by one of four attending radiologists (L.L., D.D.D., E.A.M., A.F.A.) with a median of 6 years of experience in breast imaging at the outset of the study (individual radiologists' levels of experience were 1, 5, 6, and 15 years, respectively). Patients were prone on a dedicated table (StereoGuide with Digital Spot Mammography, LoRad, Danbury, Conn) during the biopsy. Scout and targeting stereotactic images were obtained in all lesions. Superficial anesthesia was ensured by means of injection of 1% lidocaine hydrochloride (Xylocaine; Astra USA, Westborough, Mass). In 85 (76%) of 112 lesions, deep anesthesia was ensured by using 1% lidocaine hydrochloride (10 mg/mL) with epinephrine (1:

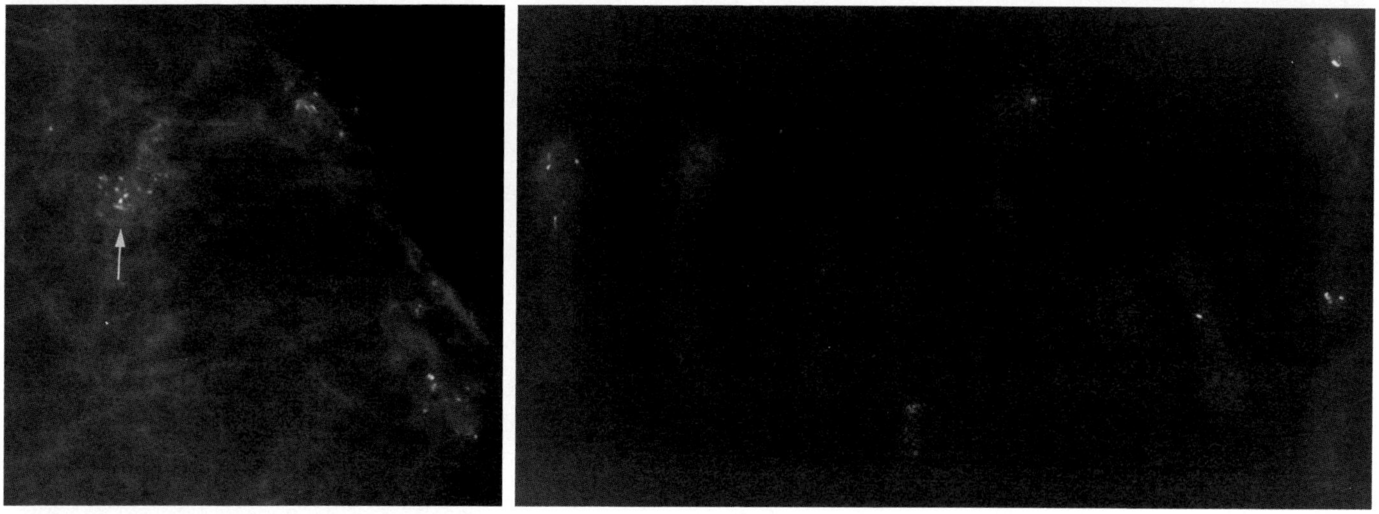

a. b.

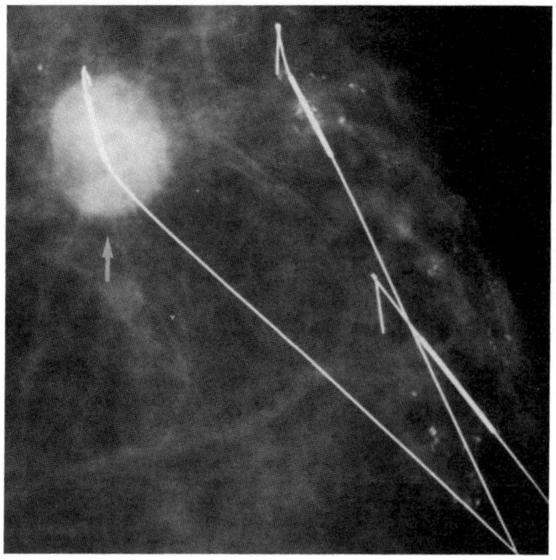

c.

Figure 1. **(a)** Craniocaudal mammogram of the right breast in a 66-year-old woman reveals three clusters of pleomorphic calcifications spanning 6.5 cm at the longest dimension. Stereotactic biopsy was performed in the most posterior cluster (arrow). **(b)** Radiographs of the stereotactic biopsy specimens reveal calcifications. Histologic analysis yielded ADH, focally bordering on DCIS. **(c)** Craniocaudal mammogram of the right breast obtained during needle localization 3 weeks after stereotactic biopsy shows three localizing wires. One marks the 1.5-cm hematoma (arrow) and a few residual calcifications at the biopsy site; the other two mark the additional areas of calcification in the retroareolar region. Surgical histologic analysis revealed solid and micropapillary DCIS adjacent to the biopsy site and in the retroareolar area.

100,000; 10 μg/mL epinephrine). Lidocaine hydrochloride with epinephrine was not given in patients with a history of cardiac disease. The median amount of anesthetic injected was 3 mL (range, 1–8 mL) of lidocaine hydrochloride and 3 mL (range, 0–15 mL) of lidocaine hydrochloride with epinephrine.

In 72 (64%) lesions, tissue was acquired after firing the probe inside the breast, with pre- and postfire stereotactic images documenting probe position for the first specimen. In 40 (36%) lesions, the probe was fired outside the breast and then placed in the appropriate postfire position, with one set of postfire stereotactic images obtained to document probe position. The reason for firing the probe outside the breast was that the lesion had a superficial location in 30 lesions (such that the collecting chamber or bowl of the probe would be partially outside the skin in the prefire position) and that thickness was inadequate to accommodate the excursion of the probe in 10 lesions. In the latter 40 cases, attempts at rolling and repositioning the breast before biopsy did not allow sufficient depth of lesion or thickness of tissue to allow internal firing.

Radiography of specimens was performed in all lesions evident as calcifications. Specimens were placed on a piece of x-ray film, moistened with saline solution, and radiographed by using magnification (×1.8) without compression at a kilovolt peak of 22 and 4 mAs. The median number of vacuum-assisted biopsy specimens obtained per lesion was 13, and the mean was 14 (range, 1-34 specimens); eight or more specimens were obtained in 108 (96%) of 112 cases. The planned protocol was to obtain a minimum of eight vacuum-assisted biopsy specimens by rotating the probe "around the clock" in 1.5-hour (45°) increments. Additional specimens were obtained at the discretion of the radiologist performing the biopsy on the basis of mammographic impression, stereotactic images obtained during biopsy, findings at radiography of the specimens, and findings at visual inspection of the tissue samples.

If stereotactic images obtained after tissue acquisition suggested that all of the calcifications had been removed, a localizing clip (MicroMark; Biopsys–Ethicon Endo-surgery) was placed through the 11-gauge probe to mark the biopsy site (35,36). The breast was compressed and ice was applied for approximately 30 minutes after biopsy; in three (3%) of the 112 lesions, compression for 60–90 minutes was necessary to achieve hemostasis. Postbiopsy craniocaudal and mediolateral oblique mammograms in the breast in which biopsy was performed were obtained in all cases.

Medical records, histologic findings, mammograms obtained before and those obtained after biopsy, images from the stereotactic biopsy procedure, and radiographs of the vacuum-assisted biopsy specimens were reviewed. Calcification retrieval was defined as the identification on radiographs of specimens of calcifica-

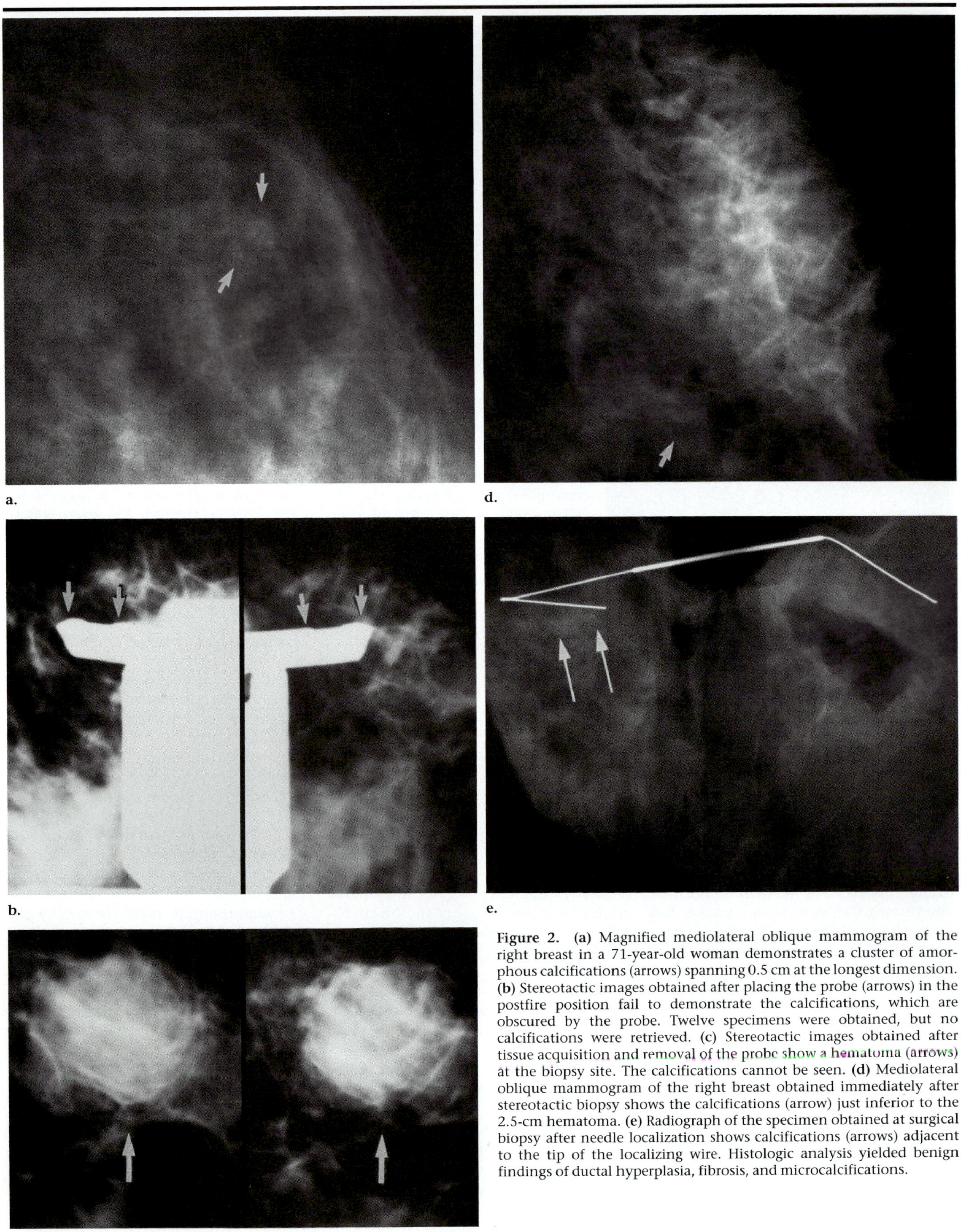

a. b. c. d. e.

Figure 2. (a) Magnified mediolateral oblique mammogram of the right breast in a 71-year-old woman demonstrates a cluster of amorphous calcifications (arrows) spanning 0.5 cm at the longest dimension. (b) Stereotactic images obtained after placing the probe (arrows) in the postfire position fail to demonstrate the calcifications, which are obscured by the probe. Twelve specimens were obtained, but no calcifications were retrieved. (c) Stereotactic images obtained after tissue acquisition and removal of the probe show a hematoma (arrows) at the biopsy site. The calcifications cannot be seen. (d) Mediolateral oblique mammogram of the right breast obtained immediately after stereotactic biopsy shows the calcifications (arrow) just inferior to the 2.5-cm hematoma. (e) Radiograph of the specimen obtained at surgical biopsy after needle localization shows calcifications (arrows) adjacent to the tip of the localizing wire. Histologic analysis yielded benign findings of ductal hyperplasia, fibrosis, and microcalcifications.

TABLE 3
Frequency of Failure to Retrieve Calcifications

Feature	No. of Lesions Yielding No Calcifications	*P* Value
Where probe was fired		
Outside breast	5/40 (12)*	.02
Inside breast	1/72 (1)	
Calcification morphology		
Amorphous	3/14 (21)	<.03†
Pleomorphic	3/90 (3)	
Linear	0/8 (0)	
Size of lesion (mm)		
≤5	5/43 (12)	.03
>5	1/69 (1)	
Radiologist‡		
A	3/37 (8)	.14
B	2/12 (17)	
C	1/39 (2)	
D	0/24 (0)	
Breast composition		
Dense (class 3 or 4)	5/60 (8)	.21
Fatty (class 1 or 2)	1/52 (2)	
BI-RADS category		
4	9/96 (9)	.35
5	0/16 (0)	
Breast lesion location		
Posterior part	3/35 (8)	.37
Middle or anterior part	3/77 (4)	
No. of lesions		
One	5/81 (6)	.99
Two	1/31 (3)	

Note.—The numbers in parentheses are percentages.
* In these five lesions, the probe was fired outside the breast owing to inadequate thickness to accommodate the excursion of the probe in three cases and owing to a superficial lesion in two cases.
† Comparison of the frequency of failure to retrieve calcifications with amorphous morphology with that to retrieve calcifications with all other morphologies.
‡ Listed in order of least experience (radiologist A) to most experience (radiologist D).

TABLE 4
Mean Specimen Weights with Different Percutaneous Biopsy Techniques

Study	Mean Specimen Weight with 14-gauge, Automated, Large-Core Breast Biopsy (mg)	Mean Specimen Weight with Directional, Vacuum-assisted Breast Biopsy (mg)	
		14-gauge	11-gauge
Berg et al (34)*	18	37	94
Burbank et al (27)†	17	34	. . .
Burbank (39)†	. . .	40	96

* In vitro data in a turkey breast parenchymal model.
† Data from clinical cases.

TABLE 5
Calcification Retrieval at Stereotactic Breast Biopsy

Study	No. of Lesions with Calcifications Retrieved at 14-gauge, Automated, Large-Core Breast Biopsy	No. of Lesions with Calcifications Retrieved at Directional, Vacuum-assisted Breast Biopsy	
		14-gauge	11-gauge
Liberman et al (5)	65/72 (90)	. . .	. . .
Lee et al (12)	133/151 (88)	. . .	. . .
Liberman et al (29)	. . .	50/55 (91)*	. . .
Meyer et al (32)	118/130 (91)	106/106 (100)†	. . .
Jackman et al (37)	1,122/1,196 (94)	1,195/1,209 (99)	720/723 (>99)‡

Note.—The numbers in parentheses are percentages.
* The frequency of calcification retrieval was 19/24 (79%) in the first half of the 8-month study and 31/31 (100%) in the second half.
† $P < .001$.
‡ The frequency of retrieving calcifications was significantly higher for 14-gauge, directional, vacuum-assisted biopsy than it was for 14-gauge, automated, large-core biopsy ($P < .001$) and was significantly higher for 11-gauge, directional, vacuum-assisted biopsy than it was for 14-gauge, automated, large-core biopsy ($P < .001$) but was not significantly different for 11- versus 14-gauge, directional, vacuum-assisted biopsy ($P = .15$).

tions consistent with those seen on the prebiopsy mammogram. The ADH underestimation frequency was defined as the percentage of lesions yielding ADH at percutaneous biopsy that had carcinoma at surgery (21,28,31). The DCIS underestimation frequency was defined as the percentage of lesions yielding DCIS at percutaneous biopsy that had infiltrating carcinoma at surgery (28). The χ^2 and Fisher exact tests were performed.

RESULTS

Stereotactic, 11-gauge, directional, vacuum-assisted biopsy resulted in removal of all calcifications in 51 (46%) of 112 lesions, some of the calcifications in 55 (49%) lesions, and no calcifications in six (5%) lesions (Table 1). All calcifications were removed in 50 (64%) of the 78 lesions 1 cm or smaller and in 31 (72%) of the 43 lesions 5 mm or smaller (Table 1).

The frequency of identifying calcifications histologically was significantly higher if at least some of the calcifications were retrieved than if none of the calcifications were retrieved (98% vs 50%, $P < .001$). No significant difference was observed in the frequency of identifying calcifications histologically when comparing retrieval of all versus some of the calcifications (100% vs 96%, $P = .5$). Repeat biopsy was recommended in 19 (17%) of 112 lesions (Table 2). A recommendation for repeat biopsy was made significantly more often if no calcifications were retrieved than if at least some of the calcifications were retrieved (67% vs 14%, $P = .007$). No significant difference was observed in the rate of recommending repeat biopsy when comparing retrieval of all versus retrieval of some of the calcifications (both 14%, $P = .87$).

Surgery revealed DCIS in one (10%) of 10 lesions yielding ADH at stereotactic, 11-gauge, directional, vacuum-assisted biopsy. This lesion consisted of calcifications that spanned approximately 6.5 cm at the longest dimension (Fig 1). Eighteen specimens were obtained at stereotactic biopsy and yielded ADH; subsequent needle localization and surgical excision yielded DCIS. Surgery revealed infiltrating carcinoma in one (5%) of 21 lesions yielding DCIS at 11-gauge, vacuum-assisted biopsy. This lesion consisted of calcifications that spanned 4.0 cm. Forty-three specimens were obtained from two separate sites within the lesion, yielding DCIS, comedo type; mastectomy revealed DCIS, comedo type, and a 1.0-cm infiltrating ductal carcinoma. There was no ADH or DCIS underestimation when all calcifications were removed. Retrieval of all as opposed to some calcifications resulted in lower frequencies of ADH underestimation

(0% vs 20%, $P = .99$) and of DCIS underestimation (0% vs 11%, $P = .43$) (Table 2).

No calcifications were retrieved in six lesions in six women (Fig 2). Failure to retrieve calcifications was significantly more frequent if the probe was fired outside rather than inside the breast (12% vs 1%, $P = .02$), if calcifications had amorphous morphology rather than pleomorphic or linear morphology (21% vs 3%, $P < .03$), and in lesions 5 mm or smaller rather than in lesions larger than 5 mm (12% vs 1%, $P = .03$) (Table 3). A higher frequency of failure was observed if the biopsy was performed by less experienced radiologists, in dense breasts, in lesions that were less suspicious according to the BI-RADS category (41), and in posterior lesions; however, these differences did not achieve statistical significance. The number of lesions in the same breast in which biopsy was performed did not affect the likelihood of retrieving calcifications.

In three of the six cases in which no calcifications were retrieved, the procedure was aborted before calcification retrieval owing to minor complications, which were bleeding ($n = 1$), vasovagal reaction ($n = 1$), and nausea ($n = 1$). The bleeding resolved with compression, and the other problems resolved without medical intervention. In one of the six instances of failure, the procedure was aborted owing to mechanical failure of the vacuum-assisted device after one specimen was obtained; 10 additional passes were performed with an automated needle, yielding no calcifications.

Repeat biopsy was performed in four of the six patients in whom no calcifications were retrieved at the initial procedure. Three women underwent needle localization and surgical biopsy, and one underwent repeat stereotactic biopsy. The histologic findings were benign in these four women. Short-term follow-up mammography was being performed in one woman who underwent stereotactic biopsy of two clusters of calcifications that were similar in morphology, one of which was successfully sampled with benign results. In the sixth patient, a mammogram obtained immediately after unsuccessful stereotactic biopsy demonstrated that the calcifications in question were located in the skin. In the latter patient, the dermal location of the calcifications was not initially appreciated owing to skin retraction from a previous lumpectomy.

TABLE 6
ADH and DCIS Underestimates at Stereotactic Breast Biopsy

Study	No. of Underestimated Cases with 14-gauge, Automated, Large-Core Breast Biopsy	No. of Underestimated Cases with Directional, Vacuum-assisted Breast Biopsy: 14-gauge	11-gauge
ADH underestimates			
Jackman et al (6)	9/16 (56)*	. . .	. . .
Liberman et al (17)	11/21 (51)†	. . .	. . .
Burbank (28)	8/18 (44)	0/8 (0)‡	. . .
Jackman et al (31, 38)	26/54 (48)§	13/74 (18)§	4/31 (13)§
This study	. . .	. . .	1/10 (10)‖
DCIS underestimates			
Jackman et al (6)	8/43 (19)*	. . .	. . .
Liberman et al (16)	3/15 (20)†	. . .	. . .
Burbank (28)	9/55 (16)#	0/32 (0)#	. . .
This study	. . .	. . .	1/21 (5)**

Note.—The numbers in parentheses are percentages.
* Mean of eight specimens per lesion.
† Mean of five specimens per lesion.
‡ $P = .03$. Mean of 17 specimens per lesion for 14-gauge, automated, large-core breast biopsy and mean of 27 specimens per lesion for 14-gauge, directional, vacuum-assisted breast biopsy.
§ The frequency of ADH underestimates was significantly lower for 14-gauge, directional, vacuum-assisted breast biopsy than it was for 14-gauge, automated, large-core breast biopsy ($P < .001$). It also was significantly lower for 11-gauge, directional, vacuum-assisted breast biopsy than it was for 14-gauge, automated, large-core breast biopsy ($P = .002$). A lower frequency of ADH underestimates was observed for 11-gauge versus 14-gauge, directional, vacuum-assisted breast biopsy; however, this difference was not statistically significant ($P = .76$). The mean numbers of specimens obtained per lesion were 10 for 14-gauge, automated, large-core breast biopsy; 16 for 14-gauge, directional, vacuum-assisted breast biopsy; and 14 for 11-gauge, directional, vacuum-assisted breast biopsy.
‖ Mean of 14 specimens per lesion. None of the five cases in which all calcifications were removed was underestimated.
\# $P = .02$. Mean of 19 specimens per lesion for 14-gauge, automated, large-core breast biopsy and a mean of 27 specimens per lesion for 14-gauge, directional, vacuum-assisted breast biopsy.
** Mean of 14 specimens per lesion. None of the 12 cases in which all calcifications were removed was underestimated.

DISCUSSION

The directional, vacuum-assisted biopsy device is advantageous for the evaluation of calcifications. In comparison with automated, large-core biopsy, directional, vacuum-assisted breast biopsy obtains larger tissue specimens (Table 4), has a higher rate of calcification retrieval (Table 5), and has a lower likelihood of ADH and DCIS underestimation (Table 6). For small mammographic lesions that may be completely excised at percutaneous biopsy, the 11-gauge, vacuum-assisted probe is preferable to the 14-gauge, vacuum-assisted probe, because it enables accurate placement of a localizing marker (35). In addition, the 11-gauge, directional, vacuum-assisted biopsy instrument may provide an incremental increase in diagnostic yield for calcific lesions as compared with the 14-gauge, vacuum-assisted device (38). Jackman et al (37,38) found comparable rates of calcification retrieval with 11- and 14-gauge, directional, vacuum-assisted biopsies (>99% vs 99%, $P = .15$) (37) and a slightly lower frequency of ADH underestimation with 11- rather than 14-gauge, directional, vacuum-assisted biopsy (13% vs 18%, $P = .76$) (38).

In our series, calcifications were retrieved in 106 (95%) of the 112 lesions in which stereotactic, 11-gauge, directional, vacuum-assisted biopsy was performed. The likelihood of identifying calcifications histologically and sparing the patient diagnostic surgical biopsy was significantly higher if calcifications were retrieved than if calcifications were not retrieved. The importance of repeat biopsy if no calcifications are retrieved has been emphasized by Dershaw et al (19), who reported that carcinoma was identified in four (57%) of seven women who underwent surgical biopsy after unsuccessful stereotactic, automated, large-core biopsy of calcifications.

Histologic underestimation occurred in two (2%) of the 112 lesions in this study: in one (10%) of the 10 lesions in which stereotactic, 11-gauge biopsy yielded ADH and in one (5%) of the 21 lesions in which stereotactic, 11-gauge biopsy yielded DCIS. No underestimation occurred when all calcifications were removed. Retrieval of all, rather than some, of the calcifications was associated with a

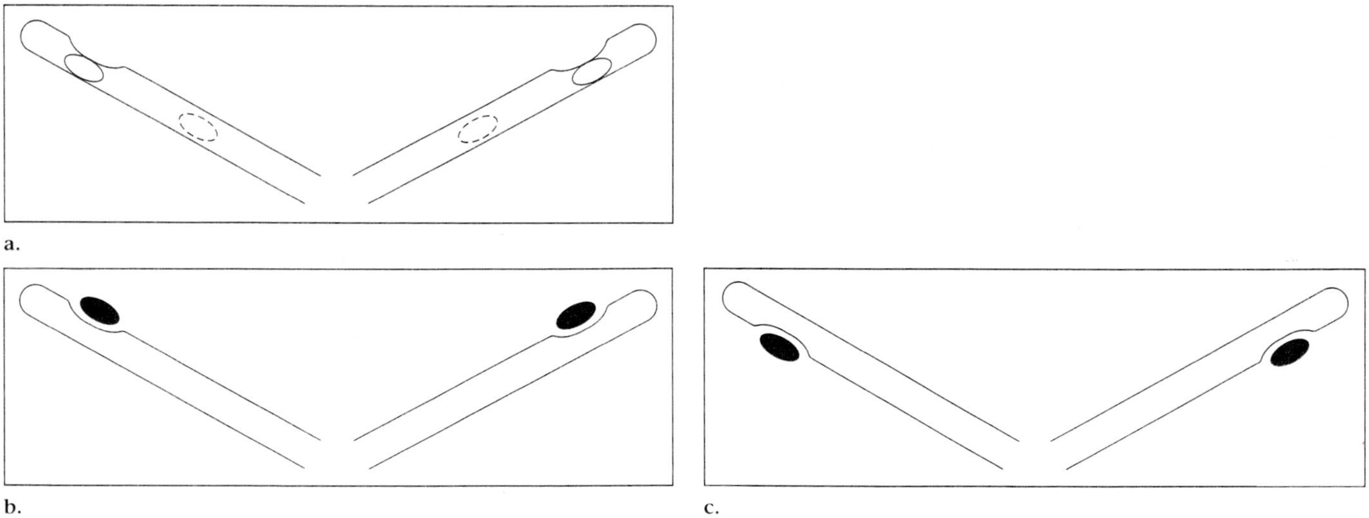

Figure 3. (a) Diagram demonstrates a suboptimal postfire position of the 11-gauge, directional, vacuum-assisted biopsy probe after firing the probe outside the breast as it appears on stereotactic images. If the probe obscures the lesion, it cannot be determined whether the lesion is immediately under the bowl (closed oval), which would be appropriate for tissue sampling, or under the shaft of the probe (dotted oval), which may not allow appropriate sampling. In addition, if the lesion is obscured by the probe, stereotactic images with the probe in place after tissue acquisition are not helpful in determining whether the mammographic lesion has been sampled. (b) Diagram demonstrates an acceptable postfire position of the 11-gauge probe as it appears on stereotactic images. The probe is low (toward the 6-o'clock position) with respect to the lesion (black oval). Tissue sampling should proceed from the 9-o'clock to the 3-o'clock axis superiorly (that is from the 9-o'clock position to a point halfway between the 10- and 11-o'clock positions, to the 12-o'clock position, to a point halfway between the 1- and 2-o'clock positions, and to the 3-o'clock position). (c) Diagram demonstrates an acceptable postfire position of the 11-gauge probe as it appears on stereotactic images. The probe is high (toward the 12-o'clock position) with respect to the lesion (black oval). Tissue sampling should proceed from the 3-o'clock to the 9-o'clock axis inferiorly (ie, from the 3-o'clock to a point halfway between the 4- and 5-o'clock positions, to the 6-o'clock position, to a point halfway between the 7- and 8-o'clock positions, and to the 9-o'clock position).

lower frequency of ADH and DCIS underestimation, but this difference did not achieve statistical significance. Because underestimation reflects sampling error, it is reasonable to expect that complete excision of small lesions and removal of a larger tissue volume from larger lesions provides more complete characterization of pleomorphic lesions and thereby a decrease in the frequency of underestimation. Although infrequent, underestimation may still occur in stereotactic, 11-gauge, directional, vacuum-assisted biopsy, particularly when sampling larger lesions (Fig 1). Obtaining tissue from more than one site within a larger lesion may be beneficial in such cases.

No calcifications were retrieved in six (5%) cases in this series. This frequency of failure to retrieve calcifications is comparable to that reported in a recent series of needle-localized surgical breast biopsy (42). In the latter study, needle-localized biopsy was successful in all of 94 masses and unsuccessful in seven (4%) of 186 calcific lesions. Small lesion size was associated with a significantly greater likelihood of failure to retrieve calcifications in our study of stereotactic, 11-gauge, vacuum-assisted biopsy and in Jackman and Marzoni's (42) study of needle-localized surgical breast biopsy. In our series, lesions 5 mm or smaller accounted for five (83%) of the six cases in which no calcifications were retrieved. Even among lesions 5 mm or smaller, which may not be suitable for 14-gauge, automated core or 14-gauge, directional, vacuum-assisted biopsy because of the unavailability of an accurate method to place a localizing marker with these techniques, 11-gauge, directional, vacuum-assisted biopsy resulted in retrieval of calcifications in 38 (88%) of 43 cases. A higher frequency of failure to retrieve calcifications with 11-gauge, vacuum-assisted biopsy was observed in calcifications with amorphous morphology rather than in calcifications with other morphologies, perhaps owing to difficulty in targeting faint calcifications on digital stereotactic images.

Failure to retrieve calcifications with 11-gauge, directional, vacuum-assisted biopsy was significantly more likely in lesions too superficial or in breasts too thin to accommodate the firing of the probe inside the breast. Superficial lesion location and inadequate tissue thickness are problematic for automated core biopsy, as well. In a study of 572 scheduled stereotactic biopsies by Philpotts et al (43), 89 (16%) were canceled; in 12 (13%) of the canceled cases, the reason for cancellation was posterior or superficial lesion location (n = 8 [9%]) or inadequate breast thickness (n = 4 [4%]). Firing the probe inside the breast is essential for tissue acquisition at automated core biopsy; if this cannot be accomplished, automated core biopsy cannot be performed.

Firing the probe outside the breast allows tissue acquisition at directional, vacuum-assisted biopsy but may pose two problems. First, when the probe is placed in the postfire position after being fired outside the breast, it may obscure a tiny lesion (Fig 3a). This problem can be alleviated by intentionally placing the probe "low" (toward the 6-o'clock position) or "high" (toward the 12-o'clock position) with respect to the lesion, so that both the lesion and the probe can be seen on the postfire stereotactic images, and then by acquiring tissue in the appropriate direction (Fig 3b, 3c).

Second, the lesion may be displaced, rather than pierced, by the biopsy probe when the probe is fired outside the breast and placed in the postfire position. Our experience with this differs from that reported by Parker and Klaus (33), who stated that firing the probe inside the breast is usually not necessary to perform directional, vacuum-assisted breast biopsy. The likelihood of displacing rather

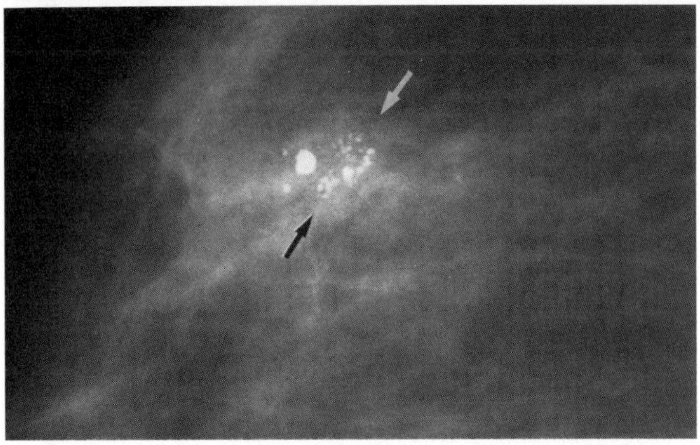

a.

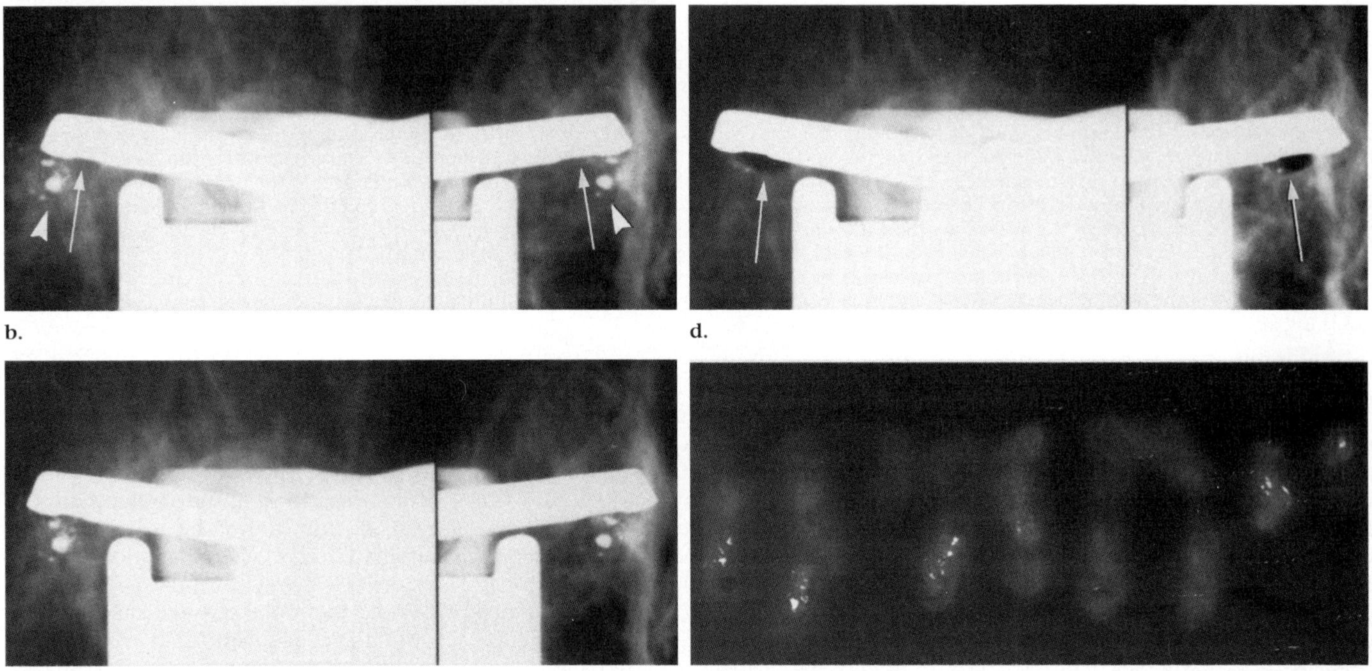

b. d.

c. e.

Figure 4. **(a)** Mediolateral oblique mammogram of the left breast in a 67-year-old woman demonstrates a superficial cluster of pleomorphic calcifications (arrows) spanning 0.9 cm at the longest dimension. **(b)** Stereotactic images obtained after placing the probe in the postfire position demonstrate that the calcifications (arrowheads) are slightly deep to the bowl (arrows) of the biopsy probe. **(c)** Stereotactic images obtained after advancing the probe an additional 8 mm show the calcifications adjacent to the bowl of the probe. The probe is high with respect to the lesion, and the bowl is directed toward the 6-o'clock position. **(d)** Stereotactic images obtained after tissue acquisition and suctioning demonstrate an air-filled biopsy cavity (arrows). The calcifications have decreased in number, which is consistent with interval sampling. **(e)** Radiographs of the stereotactic biopsy specimens confirm calcification retrieval. Histologic analysis yielded a fibroadenoma with calcification.

than piercing the lesion when placing the probe in the postfire position may depend on the equipment used. In the stereotactic table used by Parker and Klaus (Mammotest; Fischer Imaging, Denver, Colo), the depth is controlled by depressing a lever and manually advancing the probe driver; in the stereotactic table used in this study (LoRad StereoGuide), the depth is controlled by turning a dial. In some cases, the former approach may allow the force necessary to pierce the lesion, while the latter may not. Failure to pierce the lesion was also a factor associated with unsuccessful needle-localized surgical breast biopsy in the study of Jackman and Marzoni (42).

Several techniques may improve the diagnostic yield in cases in which the lesion is too superficial or the breasts are too thin to accommodate firing the probe inside the breast in the conventional fashion. First, in some thin breasts, one may have enough thickness to back the probe up a few millimeters from the ideal prefire position (z differential = −2 mm) and fire inside the breast. The lesion will not be in the center of the 19-mm bowl after firing, but at least part of the lesion should still be within the bowl and may be acquired with the vacuum-assisted device.

Second, the "air gap" technique may allow tissue acquisition even in thin breasts (25,26). In this method, in addition to the standard compression paddle with the aperture that overlies the lesion, a reversed compression paddle is placed between the far side of the breast and the breast support plate. The apertures of both compression paddles are aligned so that the probe, when placed to the postfire position, will displace breast tissue into the aperture on the far side of the breast rather than strike the paddle or plate.

Third, in superficial lesions, one may inject a generous amount of local anesthetic to form a large wheal, thereby increasing the thickness of compressed tissue at the skin surface, or one may use a 25-gauge needle as a hook to pull the skin over the proximal aspect of the aperture so that it is completely covered in the prefire position (33).

Finally, if one must fire outside the

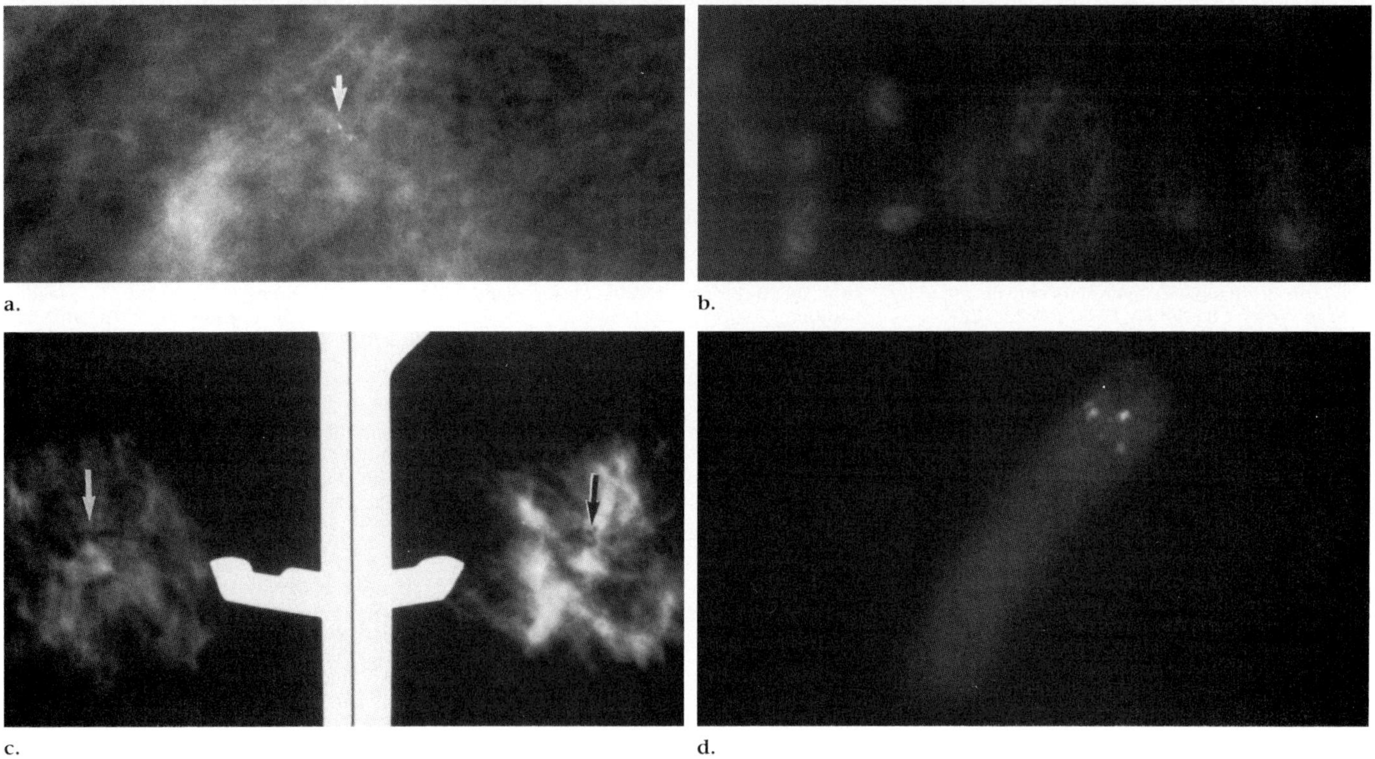

Figure 5. (a) Magnified mediolateral oblique mammogram of the left breast in a 57-year-old woman demonstrates a cluster of calcifications (arrow) spanning 0.3 cm at the longest dimension. (b) Radiographs of multiple specimens demonstrate no calcifications. (c) Stereotactic images obtained after removing the probe demonstrate that the calcifications are no longer evident at the biopsy site (arrows). (d) Radiograph of a small tissue fragment found in the probe after the probe was removed from the breast, inspected, and flushed demonstrates the calcifications (original magnification, ×4). A fibroadenoma with calcifications was found at histologic analysis.

breast, the likelihood of success may be increased by carefully monitoring the location of the lesion relative to the bowl of the probe on stereotactic images and by making appropriate adjustments until optimal positioning is achieved (Fig 4).

If multiple specimens have been obtained and no calcifications are observed on radiographs of specimens, it is helpful to obtain another pair of stereotactic images. If the calcifications are still present in the breast, one may retarget, reposition the probe, and continue tissue acquisition. If the stereotactic images suggest that the calcifications are no longer evident, the probe should be removed from the breast, carefully inspected, and flushed; on occasion, the calcifications may be present in a tissue fragment stuck in the probe (Fig 5).

Complications of directional, vacuum-assisted biopsy are infrequent. Liberman et al (29) reported clinical hematoma in one (1%) of 113 lesions in which 14-gauge, automated, large-core biopsy was performed versus clinical hematoma in four (4%) of 108 lesions in which 14-gauge, directional, vacuum-assisted breast biopsy was performed ($P = .20$); all bleeding resolved with compression. Burbank (39) reported approximately 1% complication rates for both 11-gauge and 14-gauge stereotactic directional vacuum-assisted breast biopsies. In the current series, complications led to termination of the 11-gauge, vacuum-assisted biopsy procedure in three (3%) of the 112 cases. Although the reported complication rates after core and vacuum-assisted biopsy are comparable, several investigators have instituted more aggressive measures to achieve hemostasis after vacuum-assisted biopsy, including the use of lidocaine hydrochloride with epinephrine for deep anesthesia with 14- and 11-gauge vacuum-assisted biopsies (27–29,39) and wrapping the chest with a 6-inch rubber elastic bandage for 24 hours after 11-gauge vacuum-assisted biopsy (39). Additional work is necessary to compare 11- with 14-gauge directional vacuum-assisted biopsy probes in terms of complication rates and diagnostic yield.

Our data show that stereotactic, 11-gauge, directional, vacuum-assisted breast biopsy resulted in successful calcification retrieval in 95% of cases. Failure to retrieve calcifications was significantly more likely in small lesions, amorphous calcifications, and when the probe was fired outside the breast. Use of special techniques for directional, vacuum-assisted biopsy in thin breasts and superficial lesions may increase the diagnostic yield in these cases. Underestimation of ADH and DCIS lesions was infrequent at stereotactic, 11-gauge, directional, vacuum-assisted biopsy. No significant diagnostic advantage was observed for removal of all as opposed to some of the calcifications; however, the diagnostic usefulness of percutaneous complete removal rather than sampling of the mammographic lesion deserves further investigation in a larger series of women.

Acknowledgments: The authors thank Lynda T. Zingaro, RT(R) (M), Youngduk Paik, RT(R) (M), and Cynthia M. Thornton, RT(R) (M), for expert technical support; Robert A. Field, MA, for his careful work with the illustrations; and David C. Perlman, MD, for invaluable assistance.

References

1. Parker SH, Lovin JD, Jobe WE, et al. Stereotactic breast biopsy with a biopsy gun. Radiology 1990; 176:741–747.
2. Parker SH, Lovin JD, Jobe WE, Burke BJ, Hopper KD, Yakes WF. Nonpalpable breast

lesions: stereotactic automated large-core biopsies. Radiology 1991; 180:403–407.
3. Elvecrog EL, Lechner MC, Nelson MT. Nonpalpable breast lesions: correlation of stereotaxic large-core needle biopsy and surgical biopsy results. Radiology 1993; 188:453–455.
4. Lindfors KK, Rosenquist CJ. Needle core biopsy guided with mammography: a study of cost effectiveness. Radiology 1994; 190:217–222.
5. Liberman L, Evans WP, Dershaw DD, et al. Specimen radiography of microcalcifications in stereotaxic mammary core biopsy specimens. Radiology 1994; 190:223–225.
6. Jackman RJ, Nowel KW, Shepard MJ, Finkelstein SI, Marzoni FA. Stereotaxic large-core needle biopsy of 450 nonpalpable breast lesions with surgical correlation in lesions with cancer or atypical hyperplasia. Radiology 1994; 193:91–95.
7. Gisvold JJ, Goellner JR, Grant CS, et al. Breast biopsy: a comparative study of stereotaxically guided core and excisional techniques. AJR 1994; 162:815–820.
8. Parker SH, Burbank F, Jackman RJ, et al. Percutaneous large-core breast biopsy: a multi-institutional study. Radiology 1994; 193:359–364.
9. Liberman L, Fahs MC, Dershaw DD, et al. Impact of stereotaxic core breast biopsy on cost of diagnosis. Radiology 1995; 195: 633–637.
10. Liberman L, Dershaw DD, Rosen PP, Cohen MA, Hann LE, Abramson AF. Stereotaxic core biopsy of impalpable spiculated breast masses. AJR 1995; 165:551–554.
11. Brenner RJ, Fajardo L, Fisher PR, et al. Percutaneous core biopsy of the breast: effect of operator experience and number of samples on diagnostic accuracy. AJR 1996; 166:341–346.
12. Lee CH, Egglin TK, Philpotts L, Mainiero MB, Tocino I. Cost-effectiveness of stereotactic core needle biopsy: analysis by means of mammographic findings. Radiology 1997; 202:849–854.
13. Liberman L, LaTrenta LR, Dershaw DD, et al. Impact of core biopsy on the surgical management of impalpable breast cancer. AJR 1997; 168:495–499.
14. Smith DN, Christian R, Meyer JE. Large-core needle biopsy of nonpalpable breast cancers: the impact on subsequent surgical excision. Arch Surg 1997; 132:256–259.
15. March DE, Raslavicus A, Coughlin BF, Klein SV, Makari-Judson G. Use of breast core biopsy in the United States: results of a national survey. AJR 1997; 169:697–701.
16. Liberman L, Dershaw DD, Rosen PP, et al. Stereotaxic core biopsy of breast carcinoma: accuracy at predicting invasion. Radiology 1995; 194:379–381.
17. Liberman L, Cohen MA, Dershaw DD, Abramson AF, Hann LE, Rosen PP. Atypical ductal hyperplasia diagnosed at stereotaxic core biopsy of breast lesions: an indication for surgical biopsy. AJR 1995; 164:1111–1113.
18. Berg WA. When is core breast biopsy or fine needle aspiration not enough? (editorial). Radiology 1996; 198:313–315.
19. Dershaw DD, Morris EA, Liberman L, Abramson AF. Nondiagnostic stereotaxic core breast biopsy: results of rebiopsy. Radiology 1996; 198:323–325.
20. Liberman L, Dershaw DD, Glassman JR, et al. Analysis of cancers not diagnosed at stereotactic core breast biopsy. Radiology 1997; 203:151–157.
21. Liberman L, LaTrenta L, Van Zee KJ, Morris EA, Abramson AF, Dershaw DD. Stereotactic core biopsy of calcifications highly suggestive of malignancy. Radiology 1997; 203:673–677.
22. Lennington WJ, Jensen RA, Dalton LW, Page DL. Ductal carcinoma in situ of the breast: heterogeneity of individual lesions. Cancer 1994; 73:118–124.
23. Parker SH, Stavros AT, Dennis MA. Needle biopsy techniques. Radiol Clin North Am 1995; 33:1171–1186.
24. Parker SH, Dennis MA, Stavros AT. Critical pathways in percutaneous breast intervention. RadioGraphics 1995; 15:946–950.
25. Parker SH, Burbank F. A practical approach to minimally invasive breast biopsy. Radiology 1996; 200:11–20.
26. Burbank F. Stereotactic breast biopsy: its history, its present, and its future. Am Surg 1996; 62:128–150.
27. Burbank F, Parker SH, Fogarty TJ. Stereotactic breast biopsy: improved tissue harvesting with the Mammotome. Am Surg 1996; 62:738–744.
28. Burbank F. Stereotactic breast biopsy of atypical ductal hyperplasia and ductal carcinoma in situ lesions: improved accuracy with directional, vacuum-assisted biopsy. Radiology 1997; 202:843–847.
29. Liberman L, Hann LE, Dershaw DD, Morris EA, Abramson AF, Rosen PP. Mammographic findings after stereotactic 14-gauge vacuum biopsy. Radiology 1997; 203:343–347.
30. Burbank F. Mammographic findings after 14-gauge automated needle and 14-gauge directional vacuum-assisted stereotactic breast biopsies. Radiology 1997; 204:153–156.
31. Jackman RJ, Burbank F, Parker SH, et al. Atypical ductal hyperplasia diagnosed at stereotactic breast biopsy: improved reliability with 14-gauge, directional, vacuum-assisted biopsy. Radiology 1997; 204:485–488.
32. Meyer JE, Smith DN, Dipiro PJ, et al. Stereotactic breast biopsy of clustered microcalcifications with a directional, vacuum-assisted device. Radiology 1997; 204:575–576.
33. Parker SH, Klaus AJ. Performing a breast biopsy with a directional, vacuum-assisted biopsy instrument. RadioGraphics 1997; 17:1233–1252.
34. Berg WA, Krebs TL, Campassi C, Magder LS, Sun CCJ. Evaluation of 14- and 11-gauge directional, vacuum-assisted biopsy probes and 14-gauge biopsy guns in a breast parenchymal model. Radiology 1997; 205:203–208.
35. Liberman L, Dershaw DD, Morris EA, Abramson AF, Thornton CM, Rosen PP. Clip placement after stereotactic vacuum-assisted breast biopsy. Radiology 1997; 205:417–422.
36. Burbank F, Forcier N. Tissue marking clip for stereotactic breast biopsy: initial placement accuracy, long-term stability, and usefulness as a guide for wire localization. Radiology 1997; 205:407–415.
37. Jackman RJ, Burbank FH, Parker SH, et al. Accuracy of sampling microcalcifications by three stereotactic breast biopsy methods (abstr). Radiology 1997; 205(P):325.
38. Jackman RJ, Burbank FH, Parker SH, et al. Atypical ductal hyperplasia diagnosed by 11-gauge, directional, vacuum-assisted breast biopsy: how often is carcinoma found at surgery? (abstr). Radiology 1997; 205(P):325.
39. Burbank F. Stereotactic breast biopsy: comparison of 14- and 11-gauge Mammotome probe performance and complication rates. Am Surg 1997; 63:988–995.
40. Liberman L, Dershaw DD, Rosen PP, Morris EA, Abramson AF, Borgen PI. Percutaneous removal of malignant mammographic lesions at stereotactic vacuum-assisted biopsy. Radiology 1998; 206:711–715.
41. American College of Radiology. Breast imaging reporting and data system (BI-RADS). 2nd ed. Reston, Va: American College of Radiology, 1995.
42. Jackman RJ, Marzoni FA. Needle-localized breast biopsy: why do we fail? Radiology 1997; 204:677–684.
43. Philpotts LE, Lee CH, Horvath LJ, Tocino I. Canceled stereotactic core-needle biopsy of the breast: analysis of 89 cases. Radiology 1997; 205:423–428.

Arno Martin
Reto J. Bale, MD
Michael Vogele
Andreas R. Gunkel, MD
Walter F. Thumfart, MD
Wolfgang Freysinger, PhD

Vogele-Bale-Hohner Mouthpiece: Registration Device for Frameless Stereotactic Surgery[1]

Index terms:
Computed tomography (CT), three-dimensional, 10.12117, 20.12117
Computers, examination control
Magnetic resonance, MR, three-dimensional, 10.1267, 20.1267
Stereotaxis, 10.1267, 20.1267

Radiology 1998; 208:261–265

Abbreviation:
VBH = Vogele-Bale-Hohner

[1] From the Departments of Ear, Nose, and Throat (A.M., M.V., A.R.G., W.F.T., W.F.) and Radiology I (R.J.B.), University of Innsbruck, Anichstrasse 35, A-6020 Innsbruck, Austria. From the 1997 RSNA scientific assembly. Received October 29, 1997; revision requested January 12, 1998; revision received February 12; accepted March 9. **Address reprint requests to** R.J.B.

Author contributions:
Guarantors of integrity of entire study, A.M., W.F.T; study concepts, R.J.B., A.M.; study design, R.J.B., A.M., W.F.; definition of intellectual content, R.J.B., M.V., A.M., W.F.; literature research, W.F., R.J.B., A.M.; clinical studies, A.R.G., W.F.T., A.M., W.F., R.J.B., M.V.; experimental studies, A.M., R.J.B., M.V., W.F.; data analysis, A.M., W.F.; statistical analysis, A.M., W.F.; manuscript preparation, A.M.; manuscript editing, A.M., W.F., R.J.B.; manuscript review, W.F., R.J.B., M.V., A.R.G.

The authors evaluated intraoperative accuracy of patient-image registration with the Vogele-Bale-Hohner mouthpiece during imaging-guided surgery. In 50 volunteers and 500 repositioning procedures, accuracy was within less than 1 mm in all cases. Use of the mouthpiece allows precise definition of spatial reference points relative to the patient's head.

Frameless stereotactic surgery, which evolved during the past decade, allows continuous spatial correspondence or registration between the head and a set of computed tomographic (CT) or magnetic resonance (MR) images by means of three-dimensional digitizers and computers (1). Use of intraoperative navigation systems may help reduce the risks of minimally invasive surgical techniques (2–4).

Accurate patient-image registration is the prerequisite for successful application of any navigation system. Specific well-suited points in the patient's three-dimensional CT or MR imaging data set ("virtual patient") are correlated with findings in the "real" patient. The availability of specifically defined points of reference, visible on the patient as well as in the data set (5,6), is the central requirement for patient-image registration in navigation systems. Ideally, these points should maintain their exact spatial position.

Use of marker systems screwed directly into the patient's skull helps attain the most accurate patient-image registration, but the implantation procedure is both cumbersome and invasive (7). We evaluated a patient-image registration device for frameless stereotactic surgical procedures in the ear, nose, and throat and neurosurgical regions that is a substantial part of the noninvasive Vogele-Bale-Hohner (VBH) head holder (8).

Materials and Methods

The VBH Mouthpiece

The VBH mouthpiece (Fig 1) consists of a vacuum dental impression of the maxillary teeth, a transverse plate, and two registration rods attached to the transverse plate by connecting elements.

The core of the VBH mouthpiece is the individualized vacuum dental impression, which allows precise repositioning and fixation of the registration device on the patient by means of underpressure between the mucosa of the hard palate and the dental impression. The dental impression tray is glued to the transverse plate, which is made of carbon fiber shaped to fit the impression tray. The registration rods are connected at right angles to the transverse plate by means of connecting cubes. Depending on the type of imaging, fiducial markers are mounted on the registration rods. We used radiopaque CT markers or MR imaging–compatible "donut" fiducial markers (ISG Technologies, Mississauga, Ontario, Canada). The connecting cubes allow variable positioning of the registration rods with respect to the transverse plate and the patient's head. They are adjusted bitemporally so the markers have an optimal spatial distribution in the field of surgery to allow maximum registration accuracy of the navigation system (9).

Production of an Individualized Vacuum Dental Impression of the Maxillary Teeth

The dental impression is made by filling an upper dental impression tray, into which a plastic tube has been securely placed, with a rapidly hardening, nonirritating, form-stable dental material (Impregum F; ESPE Dental-Medizin, Seefeld, Germany). A 1-mm-thick, self-adhesive rubber mat is pressed against the patient's hard palate, and the dental impression tray is inserted into the patient's mouth; after 3–5 minutes of hardening, it can be removed. The rubber mat (now on the dental impression) is peeled off to provide a space that serves as a vacuum chamber. The small tube becomes visible just under the vacuum chamber, and it is cut open with a scalpel. The mouthpiece is then reinserted, and the tube is connected to a vacuum pump with a minimal flow rate; ideally, the underpressure should reach about 0.25 atm between the hard palate and VBH mouthpiece.

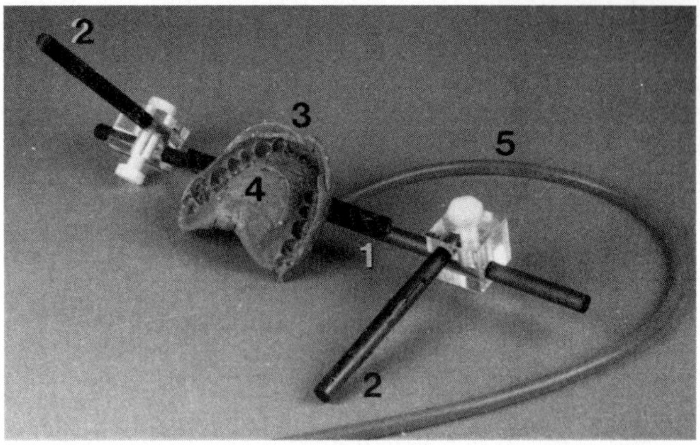

Figure 1. The VBH mouthpiece is composed of upper jaw transverse plate (*1*), registration rods (*2*), individual dental impression (*3*), vacuum area (*4*), and vacuum tube (*5*).

Repositioning Accuracy Test

We evaluated the repositioning accuracy of the VBH mouthpiece in 50 volunteers and 500 repositioning trials. Informed consent was obtained from all volunteers. All volunteers (31 men and 19 women, aged 19–26 years) were students at our institution who had stable dentition. The experimental study was performed after approval by our institutional review board.

A VBH mouthpiece was made for each volunteer. Each registration rod had two orthogonal needle guides at its end (Fig 2). Plexiglas plates covered with a layer of wax (average wax layer thickness, 0.21 mm) were mounted on the headband of headlamps commonly used in ear, nose, and throat surgeries. The volunteer wore this construction throughout all measurements. Measurements were performed by making a small impression in the wax layer with a needle inserted through the appropriate guide (Fig 2b). The measurements were taken bilaterally, in two orthogonal planes (Fig 2b), thereby allowing assessment of repositioning accuracy in craniocaudal, anteroposterior, and mediolateral directions. The VBH mouthpiece was removed, reinserted, and repositioned, and the needle impressions were repeated. This procedure was repeated 10 times. The accuracy test was performed for each volunteer within 30 minutes. The impressions on the wax layers were inspected microscopically (Fig 3), photographed, and evaluated to scale (10). Four investigators (A.M. R.J.B., M.V., W.F.T.) performed these experimental studies. Differences in their results were not statistically significant. Analysis of repositioning accuracy was based on the largest distance between the outer boundaries of needle imprints (Fig 3).

The measurements were performed on the ends of the registration rods, which were located a substantial distance from the actual site of repositioning; therefore, repositioning inaccuracies were magnified. To demonstrate the repositioning accuracy of the mouthpiece itself, the results were converted into the actual deviation at the level of the mouthpiece, with the geometric relations developed previously (10).

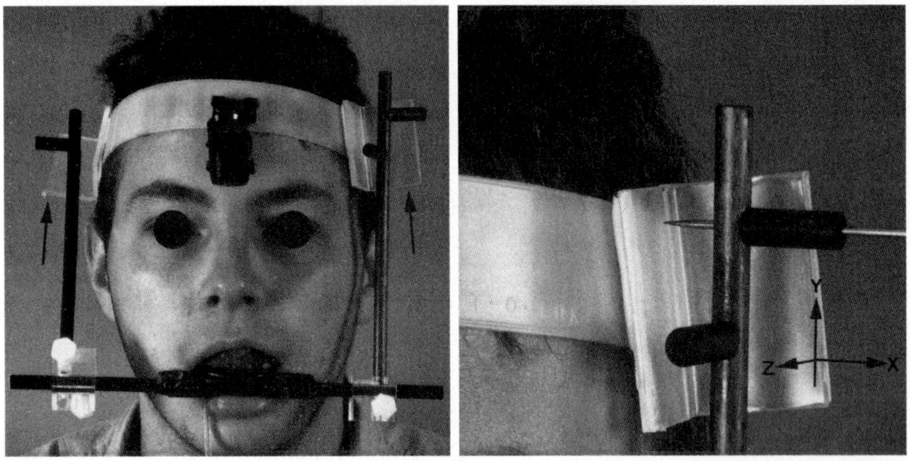

a. b.

Figure 2. Determination of repositioning accuracy with the VBH mouthpiece. **(a)** Setup. The mouthpiece is inserted, and the volunteer wears an ear, nose, and throat surgical headlamp to which waxed plastic plates (arrows) are attached. **(b)** Closeup of top right of **a** shows symbolic coordinate system with which to measure axial deviations. Needle guides define the principal axes relative to the patient's head: x = mediolateral, y = craniocaudal, z = anteroposterior.

In addition, we investigated intraoperative patient-image registration accuracy with the VBH mouthpiece during computer-assisted surgery in ear, nose, and throat regions (Fig 4). Frameless computer-assisted surgery was performed in 30 patients (13 men and 17 women, aged 28–65 years [including eight edentulous patients]) in the region of the paranasal sinuses and the anterior skull base, with the Viewing Wand navigation system (ISG Technologies). The indications for surgery included removal of nasal polyps in 15 patients, orbital decompression in five, tumor biopsy in the posterior and lateral aspects of the sphenoid sinus in three, and tumor resection in seven.

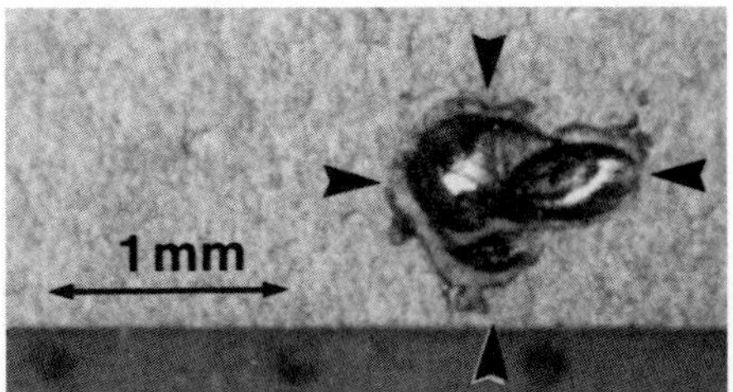

Figure 3. Typical magnified needle impression and scaled paper. Arrowheads indicate maximum diameters used for statistical analysis.

Results

Insertion of the VBH mouthpiece is easy and uncomplicated (8). A rigid and noninvasive connection between the registration device and the patient is real-

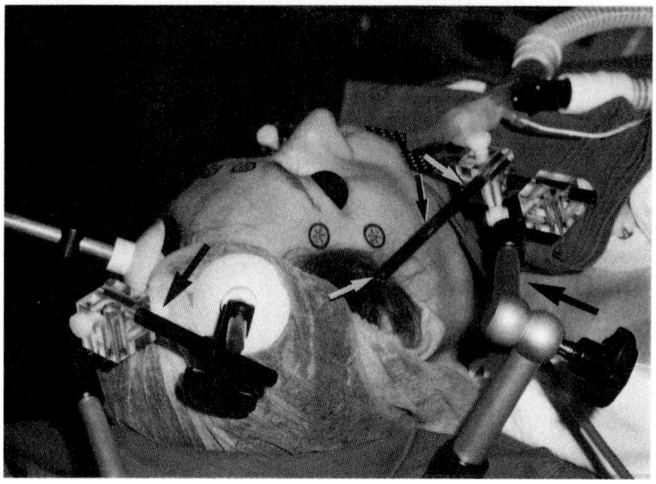

Figure 4. Preoperative setup. With rigid, noninvasive head fixation by means of the VBH head holder (long arrows), oral intubation is uncomplicated. To ensure accurate patient-image registration, the well-defined external points of reference on the VBH mouthpiece (short arrows) are used.

ized by means of the underpressure between the hard palate and the dental impression. To ensure this connection, precise production of the dental impression with its vacuum area is a prerequisite. The underpressure created by our vacuum pump caused no mucous membrane lesions on the hard palate even after long periods of application (up to 7 hours). The constant value of the underpressure can be reached only by means of exact repositioning of the VBH mouthpiece; therefore, maintenance of pressure with a vacuum pump monitored with a manometer is essential for control of repositioning. The size of the vacuum area determines the quality of adhesion between the hard palate and the dental impression. As a result of the underpressure, the entire mouthpiece clings to the upper jaw on its own. The VBH mouthpiece is easily removed from the patient's mouth by turning the vacuum pump off.

The accuracy of patient-image registration for computer-assisted surgery depends on the accuracy of mouthpiece repositioning onto the upper jaw. Repositioning accuracy was determined in the 50 volunteers with 500 measurements: Craniocaudal mean accuracy was 0.73 mm ± 0.45 (standard deviation); anteroposterior, 0.62 mm ± 0.44; mediolateral, 0.47 mm ± 0.33 (Fig 5a–c). Retrospective analysis showed that the deviations for volunteer 16 were caused by errors in the production of the dental impression: An air leak prevented optimal underpressure, fixation, and repositioning. The deviations for volunteer 37 were attributed to substantially deteriorated upper dentition; exact repositioning of the VBH mouthpiece was difficult, and the optimal underpressure of 0.25 atm was not always reached. Nonetheless, substantial deviations occurred in only one of the 10 repositioning trials. If the results of this one unsuccessful trial are omitted, mean accuracy values for this volunteer become the following: craniocaudal, 1.29 mm; anteroposterior, 0.5 mm; mediolateral, 0.66 mm; average, 0.82 mm.

After conversion of the measurement data set to reflect the repositioning accuracy of the dental impression itself, the following mean accuracy values were recorded: craniocaudal, 0.17 mm ± 0.11; anteroposterior, 0.15 mm ± 0.1; mediolateral, 0.17 mm ± 0.12.

Intraoperative repositioning accuracy of the VBH mouthpiece in the 30 patients was less than 1 mm (root mean square error, 0.96 mm ± 0.41) (Fig 5e). The root mean square is a measure of how consistently the registration points are mapped to the three-dimensional data set; it is not an absolute measure of error. Generally, a smaller number indicates a better patient-image registration, but not necessarily, and the accuracy of the registration has to be checked according to a special protocol (8). In all cases, the intraoperative registration evaluation yielded no discernible deviation between the calculated and actual position of the Viewing Wand probe.

Intraoperative registration of the patient's CT or MR imaging data set on the basis of anatomic landmarks led to average deviations of 2.5 mm. When skin markers were applied, the deviations were reduced to 1.5 mm depending on the extent of soft-tissue shift.

Discussion

Successful application of frameless stereotactic navigation depends primarily on the accuracy of patient-image registration. Various different registration methods for use in such computer-assisted three-dimensional surgery have been developed.

The simplest method is the use of anatomic landmarks (2), clearly defined locations accessible to the probe of the navigation system (ie, nasion, philtrum, supraorbital rim, inner and outer angle of the eye, mastoid process). It is not possible, however, to achieve submillimetric correlation of the anatomic landmarks by using the corresponding points on the CT or MR imaging data set, which leads to suboptimal accuracy of the patient-image registration.

The use of skin markers glued to the skin (5,6,8,11) can lead to patient-image registration inaccuracy due to soft-tissue shift when forces are exerted on the scalp. Owing to self-detachment of the skin markers, the stereotactic surgery must be conducted within 1–2 days after preoperative CT or MR imaging. Implanted fiducial markers allow temporal constancy, but they cause major patient discomfort and should not be left in place over an extended time (7).

The noninvasive stereotactic device of Oshio et al (12) allows creation of external points of reference to facilitate comparison of multiple MR studies. The device connects the nasion and external auditory canals, and reference points on the device can be used for patient-image registration. The system has a limited flexibility that may decrease patient-image registration accuracy (9), but to our knowledge this has not been investigated or applied clinically.

The stereoadapter of Laitinen (13) gives external points of reference and is mounted on the patient's head by means of two ear plugs, a nasion support, and a connector plate over the vertex. The repositioning accuracy of this stereoadapter depends on how tightly the support arms are braced between nasion, external auditory meatus, and vertex. Unfortunately, such rigid fixation devices exert pressure on the external auditory canals and can cause patient discomfort and pain. Furthermore, this prohibits its use in patients with an existing pathologic condition in an external auditory meatus.

The systems of Carini et al (14) and Hauser et al (6), the Gill-Thomas-Cosman localizer (15) (Radionics, Burlington, Mass), and the Banana Bar system (16) (a noninvasive, reattachable fiducial marker system that is not available commercially) are devices intended to create external points of correlation by using a dental impression for repositioning an element on the patient. The referencing system of Carini et al connects to the

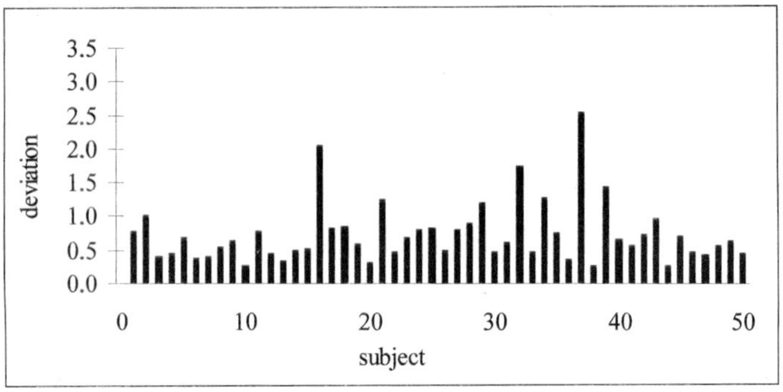

a.

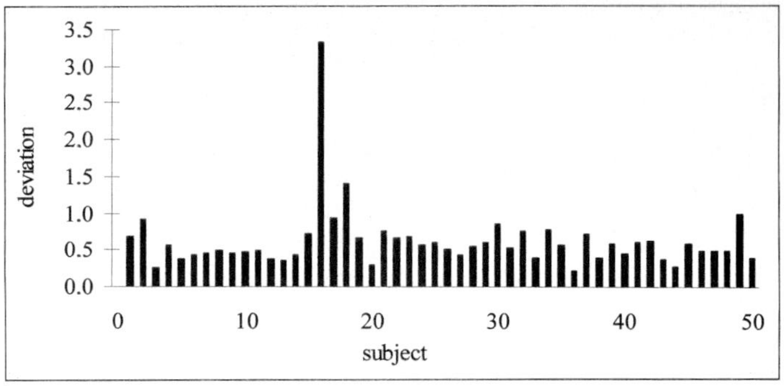

b.

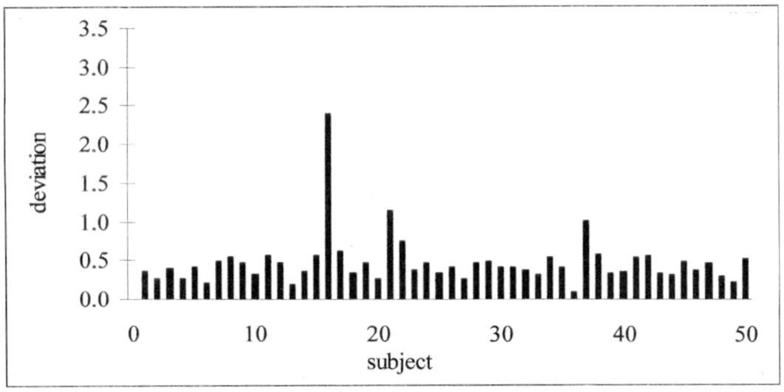

c.

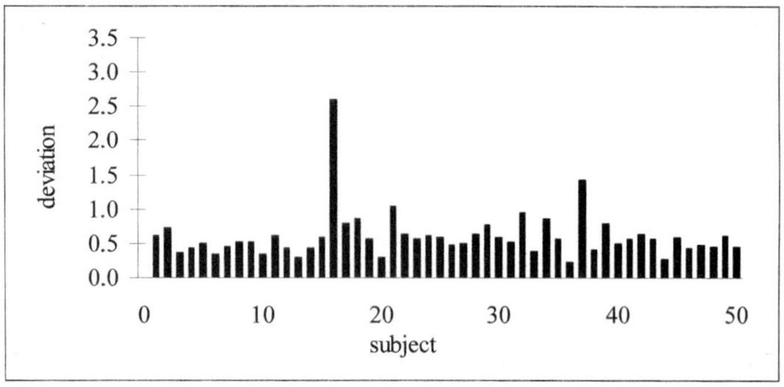

d.

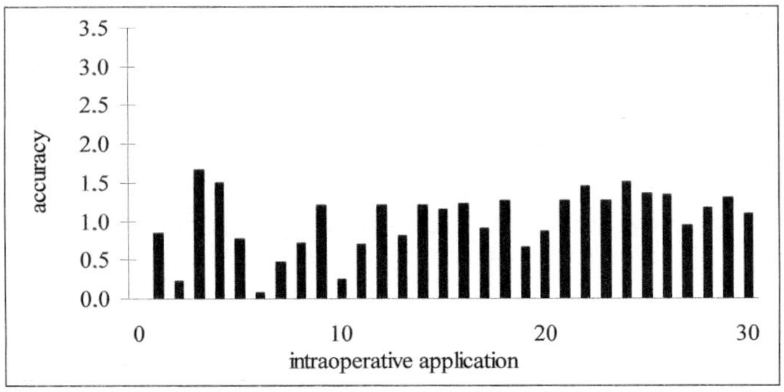

e.

Figure 5. **(a–c)** Maximum repositioning deviation of the VBH mouthpiece in each direction for each of the 50 volunteers: craniocaudal (0.73 mm ± 0.45), anteroposterior (0.62 mm ± 0.44), mediolateral (0.47 mm ± 0.33), respectively. **(d)** Average repositioning deviation of the VBH mouthpiece in all directions for each volunteer. **(e)** Intraoperative root mean square (0.96 mm ± 0.41) in the 30 patients. There is good correspondence between **d** and **e.** The two mean values are separated by less than the smaller standard deviation.

upper dentition by means of an orthodontic resin plate that is held in place by metallic hooks. The system weighs 0.35 kg and has been found to have repositioning deviations of up to 1.7 mm. It was designed for use during radiation therapy and is not suitable for use during surgery of the head and neck regions. The referencing system of Hauser et al is fixed on the patient by using an upper dental impression, nasion, and external auditory meatus. An attached N-shaped fiducial marker allows correction of movement artifacts that occur during imaging and creates external points of reference. The system has an average intraoperative repositioning error of 0.76–1.67 mm. It is well suited for use in endoscopic and transnasal surgeries but not in surgeries with other access routes in the head region. Use of the Gill-Thomas-Cosman localizer allows patient head fixation; registration rods connected to the base ring of the frame provide precisely defined correlation points. The somewhat bulky construction of this localizer can block many access routes for ear, nose, and throat surgery, and its use is not really an advantage for frameless stereotactic surgery. The Banana Bar consists of a symmetric U-shaped aluminum bar that sweeps backward bilaterally along the head. It is held in place by biting on a dental impression of both the maxillary and mandibular teeth. The fiducial markers can be attached to the two lateral arms. The bar is lightweight (97 g), provides reproducible marker repositioning, and is well tolerated, but it can be used only when the patient is awake and, most important, does not provide a means for intraoperative patient fixation. Patient cooperation may not be expected for longer than 30 minutes because of muscle fatigue, which is the limiting factor. In addition, its geometry cannot be changed to provide optimal three-dimensional patient-image registration (9) or to support various surgical access routes.

The VBH mouthpiece is a simple, noninvasive, rigid device that weighs about 100 g (including and depending on the size of the dental impression). Production of an entire mouthpiece takes about 20 minutes. Use of the form-stable impression material allows exact repositioning independent of the time the dental impression was produced. The possibility of this concept has been considered by other investigators in the field (6,14–16), but none of them used a vacuum system similar to the VBH mouthpiece, which allows repositioning and fixation of the dental impression on the patient with continuous monitoring of the accuracy of the reference points. Our repositioning results with the VBH mouthpiece show that the points of correlation on the mouthpiece are always in almost exact relation to the patient's head and are, thus, suitable for use in patient-image registration. The ex-

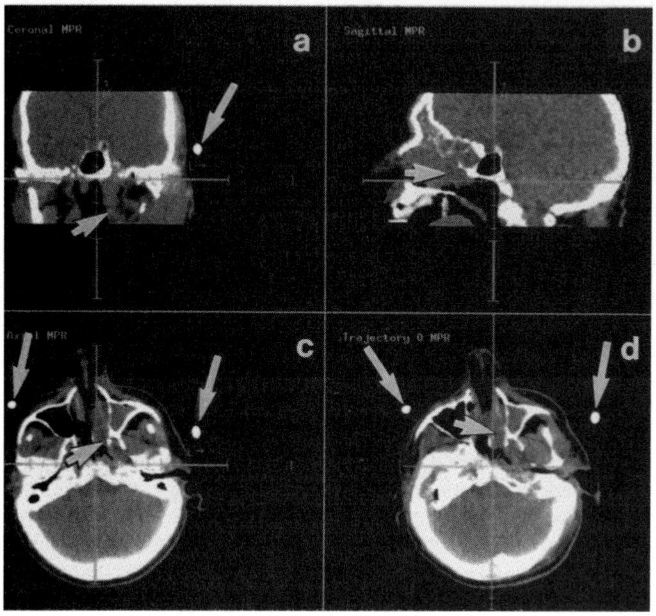

Figure 6. Intraoperative CT scans obtained in a patient with nasal and sinus polyposis during computer-assisted endoscopic revision. The crosshairs indicate the position of the measuring probe at one of the safe, routinely used intraoperative anatomic landmarks. Multiplanar reformatted scans (in *a*, *b*, and *d*) defined by the probe and its attachment to the position-sensitive arm depict the following views: *a*, coronal; *b*, sagittal; *c*, axial; *d*, trajectory 0 (in-line view shows the anatomic structures along the trajectory of the probe). The polyps (short arrows) and, bilaterally along the head, the registration rods (long arrows) can be seen.

cellent reproducibility also allows images to be acquired independently of the surgery schedule. With adequate markers, the VBH mouthpiece can be used at CT (Fig 6) as well as at MR imaging without artifact production (Vogele M, unpublished data, 1997). After the VBH mouthpiece has been used, only the dental impression material is discarded, so the average cost per patient is negligible (≈$10).

The quality of results for our repositioning accuracy tests depends on the spatially and temporally constant mounting of the Plexiglass plates on each volunteer's head. In the absence of other, better measurements, however, our approach is justified. Fiducial markers mounted on the VBH mouthpiece and the registration rods can be individually adjusted to the surgical field to allow maximum accuracy of patient-image registration (9). The VBH mouthpiece is held in position by means of underpressure of 0.25 atm. The constant underpressure serves as a permanent "measuring" tool to ensure repositioning accuracy of the VBH mouthpiece, which distinguishes this from any other concept. The VBH mouthpiece can be inserted during surgery with general anesthesia, and it does not interfere with oral intubation (Fig 4). The repositioning accuracy changes only with substantial changes in dentition (eg, tooth loss, dental work).

In combination with the VBH head holder (8), the VBH mouthpiece can be used for precise, reproducible, flexible, and noninvasive patient head fixation for computer-assisted surgery in ear, nose, and throat applications, neurosurgery, or frameless stereotactic interstitial brachytherapy (17). The patient-image registration device does not impede surgical access routes and may also be used in combination with other head fixation techniques (eg, Mayfield horseshoe or head clamp, tape fixation), and is particularly well suited for repeated frameless stereotactic procedures. The VBH mouthpiece is ideally designed to carry three-dimensional position sensors, which can be reproducibly mounted and thus be used to track patient movements intraoperatively.

We are currently working on an optimized design of the patient-image registration device to further reduce size and weight and on implementation of the device in CT, MR, and single photo emission CT image fusion.

In conclusion, the VBH mouthpiece is a device that offers precisely defined external correlation points for patient-image registration in computer-assisted frameless stereotactic surgeries with any three-dimensional navigation system. Clinical application and experimental repositioning in 50 volunteers confirm the submillimetric repositioning accuracy of the VBH mouthpiece. The VBH mouthpiece can be used in combination with various head holders and navigation systems that register patient head movement.

References

1. Guthrie BL. Graphic-interactive cranial surgery. Clin Neurosurg 1994; 41:489–516.
2. Anon JB, Lipman SP, Oppenheim D, Halt RA. Computer-assisted endoscopic sinus surgery. Laryngoscope 1994; 104:901–905.
3. Carrau RL, Snyderman CH, Curtin HB, Weissman JL. Computer-assisted frontal sinusotomy. Otolaryngol Head Neck Surg 1994; 111:727–732.
4. Golfinos JG, Fitzpatrick BC, Smith LR, Spetzler RF. Clinical use of a frameless stereotactic arm: results of 325 cases. J Neurosurg 1995; 83:197–205.
5. Zinreich SJ, Tebo SA, Long DM, et al. Frameless stereotaxic integration of CT imaging data: accuracy and initial applications. Radiology 1993; 188:735–742.
6. Hauser R, Westermann B, Reinhardt H, Probst R. Computerunterstützte chirurgie der nasennebenhöhlen mit einem optoelektronischen ortungssystem. Laryngorhinootologie 1996; 75:199–207.
7. Maciunas RJ, Fitzpatrick JM, Galloway RL, Allen GS. Beyond stereotaxy: extreme levels of application accuracy are provided by implantable fiducial markers for interactive image-guided neurosurgery. In: Maciunas RJ, ed. Interactive image-guided neurosurgery: neurosurgical topics. Park Ridge, Ill: American Association of Neurological Surgeons, 1993; 259–270.
8. Bale RJ, Vogele M, Freysinger W, et al. Minimally invasive head holder to improve the performance of frameless stereotactic surgery. Laryngoscope 1997; 107:373–377.
9. Vogele M, Freysinger W, Bale RJ, Gunkel AR, Thumfart WF. Einsatz der ISG Viewing Wand am felsenbein: eine modellstudie. HNO 1997; 45:74–80.
10. Martin A. A new method of registration for computer-assisted 3D surgery and the application in ear, nose, and throat surgery, radiotherapy and anaesthesiology. Thesis. University of Innsbruck, Innsbruck, Austria, 1998.
11. Laborde G, Gilsbach J, Harders A, Klimek L, Moesges R, Krybus W. Computer assisted localizer for planning of surgery and intra-operative orientation. Acta Neurochir Wien 1992; 119:166–170.
12. Oshio K, Panych LP, Guttmann CRG. A simple noninvasive stereotactic device for routine MR head examinations. J Comput Assist Tomogr 1996; 20:588–591.
13. Laitinen LV. Noninvasive multipurpose stereoadapter. Neurol Res 1987; 9:137–141.
14. Carini S, Calcagno E, Tortori-Donati P, Andreussi L. A new model for non-invasive, reproducible fixation of a stereotaxic frame using an orthodontic resin plate (technical note). Acta Neurochir Wien 1992; 118:159–161.
15. Kitchen ND, Thomas DG. Minimally invasive stereotaxy: clinical use of the Gill-Thomas-Cosman (GTC) repeat stereotactic localiser. Minim Invasive Neurosurg 1994; 37:61–63.
16. Howard MA, Dobbs MB, Simonson TM, LaVelle WE, Granner MA. A noninvasive, reattachable skull fiducial marker system (technical note). J Neurosurg 1995; 83:372–376.
17. Bale RJ, Vogele M, Martin A, et al. VBH head holder to improve frameless stereotactic brachytherapy of cranial tumors. Comput Aided Surg 1997; 2:286–291.

Letters to the Editor

Pneumothorax after Fine-Needle Aspiration Biopsy

From:
Piergiorgio Solli, MD,* Leonardo Cattelani, MD,* Michele Rusca, MD,* and Alessandra Ganzetti, MD†
Departments of General Thoracic and Vascular Surgery* and Radiological Science,† University of Parma
Via Gramsci 14, 43100 Parma, Italy

Editor:
We read with great interest the article by Dr Brown et al (1) in the October 1997 issue of *Radiology* regarding the management strategy of iatrogenic pneumothorax that develops after fine-needle aspiration biopsy (FNAB) of the lung.

Iatrogenic pneumothorax secondary to FNAB is a very common and well-recognized event, with a frequency of 36%–50%. However, as the authors rightly reported (1), only a minority of cases will usually require chest tube placement; the need for chest tube placement is related to the size of the pneumothorax (ie, pneumothorax >30% of the pleural cavity volume [2]) or to its tendency toward a symptomatic evolution.

Because, to our knowledge, computed tomographically guided FNAB is performed, at present, on an outpatient basis in the majority of institutions, we consider the proposal and the study of Brown et al stimulating.

However, our attitude toward iatrogenic pneumothorax after FNAB is different. We agree that the very common small asymptomatic pneumothorax (<20%–30% of the pleural cavity volume) that does not enlarge at imaging during the 2 hours after biopsy should not be regarded as a true complication and does not require any treatment other than telephone follow-up.

On the other hand, larger pneumothoraces (>30%–40% of the pleural cavity volume) deserve a different and careful approach. In our series of 119 consecutive FNAB cases, four (3.3%) patients required chest tube placement (3). It is not surprising that these were all high-risk cases of chronic obstructive pulmonary disease (eg, emphysema) and that the air leak did not show any self-limiting tendency within the first 18–24 hours after the procedure.

In the subset of patients with chronic obstructive pulmonary disease, precarious, deteriorated preoperative respiratory function can rapidly progress to a substantial and slowly self-limiting air leak, which causes severe impairment.

It is our perception that in such a circumstance, the outpatient criterion becomes secondary to patient treatment, and hospitalization of the patient is advisable to regain the preoperative respiratory status as soon as possible. This same rationale prompts us to favor routine use of larger chest tubes with suction treatment (20 mm Hg of negative pressure) with a caliber (24–28 F) adequate to compete with any air leak, allowing quick pulmonary reexpansion. In our experience, reexpansion has been rapidly attained, and the chest tubes have been removed within 24 hours without any further trouble.

This view is corroborated by the most frequent clinical and imaging patterns in patients who have been the subjects of such investigations. In fact, although indications for FNAB still vary, common indications are contralateral lung lesions in patients who have undergone previous major lung resection and a single pulmonary nodule of uncertain origin in patients unsuitable for surgery because of their respiratory status. In these cases, acute respiratory failure due to a large iatrogenic pneumothorax should be regarded as a life-threatening complication, and patients with this condition hardly will benefit from chest drainage with a small-caliber tube on an outpatient basis.

We congratulate Brown et al for their results in such a large series; the actual need to optimize the hospital costs is undeniable. Percutaneous fine-needle aspiration biopsy should be offered as an outpatient treatment in the majority of cases, with awareness that the rare complications will often require thoracostomy with normal-caliber tubes and hospital surveillance (usually no more than 24 hours with adjunctive costs that are not intolerable, taking into account the very low frequency) to avoid the dangerous progression of a modest complication in such high-risk patients.

References

1. Brown KT, Brody LA, Getrajdman GI, Napp TE. Outpatient treatment of iatrogenic pneumothorax after needle biopsy. Radiology 1997; 205:249–252.
2. Rhea JT, De Luca SA, Greene RE. Determining the size of pneumothorax in the upright patient. Radiology 1982; 144:733–739.
3. Cattelani L, Campodonico F, Rusca M, et al. CT-guided transthoracic needle biopsy in the diagnosis of chest tumors. J Cardiovasc Surg 1997; 38:539–542.

Dr Brown and colleagues respond:

We appreciate the interest of Dr Solli and colleagues in our article, "Outpatient Treatment of Iatrogenic Pneumothorax after Needle Biopsy" (1). We heartily agree with Solli et al that the safety of the patient is, of course, of the utmost importance. My colleagues and I sought to evaluate a different approach to the treatment of patients with a pneumothorax after FNAB, not to define a population of patients who should or should not undergo biopsy in the outpatient setting. We agree that there are certain patients, such as those with limited pulmonary reserve, those of advanced age, those who require long-term anticoagulant therapy, or those who are without companionship after biopsy, in whom it might be best to perform the biopsy in the inpatient setting. These clinical decisions obviously should be addressed with the referring physician before biopsy, without regard to cost.

As far as the size of the chest tube necessary to treat patients with symptomatic pneumothorax after FNAB, efficacious treatment with small-caliber chest tubes has been demonstrated in several studies (2–4). We have never had a patient in whom it was not possible to completely evacuate the pleural space with an appropriately positioned 8-F chest tube and who had successful treatment with a large-bore chest tube. We have seen patients treated with both 8- and 24-F chest tubes after needle injury have prolonged air leaks. All of these patients, however, were able to maintain complete expansion of the lung while on suction or water seal. Thus, there does not appear to be any advantage to using the larger tubes, and we see no reason to favor placing them.

References

1. Brown KT, Brody LA, Getrajdman GI, Napp TE. Outpatient treatment of iatrogenic pneumothorax after needle biopsy. Radiology 1997; 205:249–252.
2. Perlmutt LM, Braun SD, Newman GE, et al. Transthoracic needle aspiration: use of a small chest tube to treat pneumothorax. AJR; 148:849–851.
3. Casola G, vanSonnenberg E, Keightly A, et al. Pneumothorax: radiologic treatment with small catheters. Radiology 1988; 166:89–91.
4. Conces DJ, Tarver RD, Gray WC, et al. Treatment of pneumothoraces utilizing small caliber chest tubes. Chest 1988; 94:55–57.

Karen T. Brown, MD, Lynn A. Brody, MD, and George I. Getrajdman, MD
Department of Radiology, Vascular/Interventional Section, Memorial Sloan-Kettering Cancer Center
1275 York Avenue, New York, NY 10021

Liver Hemangioma: US-guided Core-Needle Biopsy

From:
Robert D. Harris, MD
Department of Radiology, Dartmouth Medical School, Dartmouth-Hitchcock Medical Center
One Medical Center Drive, Lebanon, NH 03756-0001

Editor:

The article by Drs Heilo and Stenwig (1) in the September 1997 issue of *Radiology* on core-needle biopsy of liver hemangioma was stimulating and thought-provoking. However, there are several points on which I feel compelled to comment. First, in the Materials and Methods section, it is stated that the authors' patients were sent to the cafeteria for 1 hour after biopsy before leaving the hospital. Socioeconomic and cultural differences between the United States and Norway aside, I do not think the cafeteria is a reasonable patient monitoring site, and in some hospitals in the United States, this location might lead to an aggravation of the patient's condition! I believe that these patients should be examined in a room that is physically close to the radiologist or nurse before being discharged from the hospital to see whether any subtle signs of bleeding or discomfort remain after the procedure.

Second, articles published in the premier English-language journal on radiology should strive for a higher standard with regard to the use of the English language. There are more acceptable medical phrases than jargon such as "indefinite metastases" and "white" ultrasound (US) appearance. I can only surmise that the reviewers, editor, or both must not have been totally attentive.

Finally, I believe that the authors were incorrect in stating "if the patient or the clinician does not trust the diagnosis at US, biopsy [of the liver] should also be performed (1)." The authors go on to say, "If the lesion is sonographically equivocal, no other imaging tests should be added, but US-guided biopsy should be performed" (1). This clearly goes against the experience in most, if not all, major North American medical centers, where the need for accurate noninvasive imaging of hemangiomas is clearly established, abundant, and well documented in the literature (2–6). Dynamic contrast material–enhanced computed tomography and gadolinium-enhanced magnetic resonance (MR) imaging, red blood cell scintigraphy, or even unenhanced MR imaging are well documented in their ability to enable noninvasive diagnosis in most cases. In my opinion, the authors are too quick to suggest that biopsy should be performed in hemangiomas in all equivocal cases. If it were my liver, I would want to exhaust all noninvasive methods before undergoing needle biopsy, regardless of the complication rates of the radiologists performing the biopsy. I am surprised the reviewers, or editor, allowed the authors to make these statements without referring to any of the exhaustive literature on the noninvasive diagnosis of hemangioma.

References

1. Heilo A, Stenwig AE. Liver hemangioma: US-guided 18-gauge core-needle biopsy. Radiology 1997; 204:719–722.
2. Nelson RC, Chezmar JL. Diagnostic approach to hepatic hemangioma. Radiology 1990; 176:11–13.
3. Whitney WS, Herfkens RJ, Jeffrey RB, et al. Dynamic breath-hold multiplanar spoiled gradient-recalled MR imaging with gadolinium enhancement for differentiating hepatic hemangiomas from malignancies at 1.5T. Radiology 1993; 189:863–870.
4. Semelka RC, Brown ED, Ascher SM, et al. Hepatic hemangiomas: a multi-institutional study of appearance on T2-weighted and serial gadolinium-enhanced gradient-echo MR images. Radiology 1994; 192:401–406.
5. Powers C, Ros PR, Stoupis C, Johnson WK, Segel KH. Primary liver neoplasms: MR imaging with pathologic correlation. RadioGraphics 1994; 14:459–482.
6. Semelka RC, Sofka CM. Hepatic hemangiomas. Magn Reson Imaging Clin North Am 1997; 5:241–253.

Dr Heilo responds:

I thank Dr Harris for his comments with regard to the use of core-needle biopsy in the diagnosis of hepatic hemangiomas. The algorithm we described reflects the experience gathered at the Norwegian Radium Hospital, Oslo, Norway. Over the years, we were able to document the efficacy and safety of the procedure, and our complication rate is very low. While the cafeteria does not appear to be an appropriate environment for monitoring patients, in our hospital the cafeteria is adjacent to the departmental waiting area. I believe that our patients are more comfortable spending the observation time in this friendlier environment. Because our complication rate has been exceedingly low, I believe that this is safe.

Clearly, there is a role for other imaging modalities in patients who are suspected of having hemangioma. However, the purpose of our article (1) was to describe an alternative that in our experience appears to be safe and cost-effective. Core-needle biopsy facilitates tissue diagnosis and thus has definite advantages in patients with malignant disease, in whom the presence of liver metastases alters treatment. By using our algorithm, we are able to ascertain the diagnosis without the delay and expense associated with the use of additional imaging studies.

Even in the United States, there are some radiologists who perform biopsy for hepatic hemangiomas (2–4), and perhaps with time, as the procedure becomes acceptable, more patients may benefit from it. I hope our article will encourage physicians giving treatment to consider this approach.

As for the comments on language use in our article, I admit that, as a Norwegian, it is difficult to use the correct English scientific terms. I hope that the editorial office will continue to assist foreign contributors in this regard. However, concerning one of the mentioned phrases, there are many different terms that describe a typical hemangioma: "hyperechoic," "homogeneous" (5), "well-developed hyperechoic" (6), "highly reflective" (7), "homogeneous echodense" (8), and other terms.

Again, I thank Dr Harris for his comments. I am pleased that he found the article stimulating and thought-provoking.

References

1. Heilo A, Stenwig AE. Liver hemangioma: US-guided 18-gauge core-needle biopsy. Radiology 1997; 204:719–722.
2. Cronan JJ, Esparza AR, Dorfman GS, Ridlen MS, Paolella LP. Cavernous hemangioma of the liver: role of percutaneous biopsy. Radiology 1988; 166:135–138.
3. Tung GA, Cronan JJ. Percutaneous needle biopsy of hepatic cavernous hemangioma. J Clin Gastroenterol 1993; 16:117–122.
4. Turlington BS, Charboneau JW, Reading CC, Goeliner JR. Percutaneous needle biopsy of hepatic cavernous hemangiomas (abstr). Radiology 1991; 181(P):224.
5. Bismuth H, Kunstlinger F, Castaing D. Ultrasonography and the diagnosis of space-occupying lesions of the liver. In: Bismuth H, Kunstlinger F, Castaing D. A text and atlas of liver ultrasound. Paris, France: Chapman & Hall Medical, 1991; 18–44.
6. Weill F. Primary tumors of the liver. In: Weill F, ed. Ultrasound diagnosis of digestive diseases. 4th ed. Berlin, Germany: Springer-Verlag, 1996; 157–177.
7. Grant EG. Liver. In: Mittelstaedt CA, ed. General ultrasound. New York, NY: Churchill Livingstone, 1992; 173–248.
8. Dewbury K. Benign focal liver lesions. In: Meire H, Cosgrove D, Dewbury K, eds. Abdominal and general ultrasound. New York, NY: Churchill Livingstone, 1993; 251–269.

Arne Heilo, MD
Department of Radiology, The Norwegian Radium Hospital
Ullernchausséen 70, N-0310 Oslo, Norway

A reviewer responds:

In Dr Harris's letter, there is criticism not only of the work by Dr Heilo and his colleague (1), but also of the peer-review process. As one of the reviewers of the manuscript, I was asked to respond to these objections. On accepting this assignment, the first thing I did was familiarize myself with the original reviews. You can imagine my amusement when I found the following statement in my own review: "The authors should be prepared to deal with the controversy that may result from this paper particularly related to their diagnostic algorithm." Nevertheless, all reviewers agreed that the article would be of value and interest to the readers of the journal with extensive revision and that it was worthy of publication. In addressing Dr Harris's disappointment in the reviewers for allowing this article (1) to be published, it is perhaps worthwhile to explore the purpose of the journal in the first place.

The overall purpose, as I see it, is to provide a platform for radiologists to learn from each other's experiences so that we can provide better service to our patients and referring clinicians. Is it necessary for me to agree with every detail published in the journal? Furthermore, is it necessary for me to incorporate into my practice every new technique described in the journal? The answer to these two questions is an emphatic "no." Is it necessary for me to evaluate data and concepts with objectivity and an open mind? The answer to this question is a resounding "yes!" Drs Heilo and Stenwig have reported their experience performing percutaneous biopsy of 47 hepatic hemangiomas by using an 18-gauge core needle. In doing so, they experienced a high diagnostic yield and very few complications. I agree with Dr Harris that the noninvasive imaging features must be emphasized when working up hepatic hemangiomas. However, there is some degree of overlap between malignant nodules (whether primary or metastatic) and hemangiomas. Furthermore, the imaging features are not always "classic." In these instances, it is conceivable that percutaneous biopsy may be requested as the most expeditious procedure, the most definitive procedure, or both. As an interventional radiologist who performs several hundred liver biopsies per year, I find it comforting to know that if I perform a biopsy of a hemangioma, whether purposely or inadvertently, with an 18-gauge core needle, the specimen is likely to be diagnostic and the complication rate is expected to be low.

I congratulate these interventional pioneers for their contribution to the radiology literature. As to Dr Harris's criticism that the reviewers were not "totally attentive" by allowing the authors to use jargon such as "indefinite metastases" and "white US appearance," it is my opinion that the reviewer is responsible mainly for evaluating the content of the manuscript, not the specific wording or typographic errors. Most reviewers, many who receive manuscripts from a number of different journals, prefer to leave this labor-intensive task to the copy editors.

Reference

1. Heilo A, Stenwig AE. Liver hemangioma: US-guided 18-gauge core-needle biopsy. Radiology 1997; 204:719–722.

A reviewer responds:

I agree with Dr Harris that the article by Heilo and Stenwig (1) was stimulating and thought-provoking. I also agree with him that there were many points to comment on with regard to this article, and I think that the message brought by this work was important. I agree with both the authors and with Dr Harris that, occasionally, the diagnosis of liver hemangioma cannot be ascertained by means of a combination of imaging modalities. As "it may at times be mandatory to have an absolute histologic diagnosis...especially in patients with a known malignancy" (1), the only option before the article by Heilo and Stenwig was that of an open surgical biopsy.

I, like Dr Harris, believe that the hemangioma can be diagnosed by using imaging (therefore, noninvasively) in the overwhelming majority of cases. However, we all have experienced situations where a lesion appears to be a hemangioma with one or several imaging modalities but not with others. I also agree with Drs Heilo and Stenwig that the results of fine-needle aspiration biopsy are nonconclusive, and that, in general, percutaneous biopsy of hemangioma has been considered unacceptable because of its risks. On the other hand, most experienced radiologists have performed biopsy in hemangiomas of the liver accidentally without complications. This makes sense since hemangioma, although tremendously vascular, is composed of vascular channels with low blood pressure, and, therefore, the risks of hemorrhage should be less than those in other hepatic neoplasms, such as hypercellular carcinoma, that have intramural shunting and high-pressure vessels. This is important since the potential dangers derived from performing biopsy in a hemangioma are secondary not to the vascular nature of the tumor but to the fact that a hemangioma is a lesion without inherent risks. Therefore, the cost-benefit ratio of performing biopsy in hemangiomas has to be carefully measured and reserved only for atypical cases or cases where a specific histologic diagnosis is needed.

I wholeheartedly agree with the first section of the discussion of this article, and I believe it was important to let the radiologic community know that 18-gauge core biopsy is diagnostic from a pathologic point of view and safe (only four cases of bleeding in almost 500 biopsies, with only one of these four cases involving major intraperitoneal bleeding that required transfusion).

In the last two sections of the discussion, the authors are trying to let the readership know the protocol in their particular center so this may be of help to other radiologists. The algorithms proposed are based on their experience and not directly related to the research presented in the article. I agree with Dr Harris that biopsy should not be performed in all cases of atypical US findings.

The real value of this article is to let us know that, in the cases in which histologic diagnosis of hemangioma is needed, we as radiologists can perform 18-gauge core biopsy safely without having the patient undergo a laparoscopic or open surgical biopsy. I would like to end by saying that if it were my liver, and if the imaging diagnostic methods were inconclusive for hemangioma, I would rather undergo percutaneous US-guided 18-gauge core-needle biopsy than surgical biopsy or fine-needle aspiration (which is too unspecific in the diagnosis of hemangioma).

Reference

1. Heilo A, Stenwig AE. Liver hemangioma: US-guided 18-gauge core-needle biopsy. Radiology 1997; 204:719–722.

Editor's response:

We thank Dr Harris for taking the time to share his concerns with regard to the article by Heilo and Stenwig (1). Both the authors and the reviewers have provided cogent responses to those concerns directed at them. With regard to Dr Harris's concern with the editorial process, as Editor of *Radiology,* I applaud the expertise of our manuscript editors and the high quality of their final product, namely, the edited articles. Nevertheless, we do appreciate and will respond to criticism that is constructive.

Reference

1. Heilo A, Stenwig AE. Liver hemangioma: US-guided 18-gauge core-needle biopsy. Radiology 1997; 204:719–722.

Anthony V. Proto, MD
Editor

Specimen Weights Obtained with 14- and 11-gauge Breast Biopsy Probes

From:

Fred Burbank, MD
30982 Steeplechase Drive
San Juan Capistrano, CA 92675

Editor:

I read with interest the article by Dr Berg and colleagues (1) in the October 1997 issue of *Radiology*. In their carefully performed, exhaustive comparison of 13 biopsy instruments, fresh turkey breasts at room temperature were used as the biopsy targets. By using the fresh turkey breast model, Berg and colleagues compared 11- and 14-gauge, directional, vacuum-assisted biopsy probes and concluded that 14-gauge probes are used to obtain an average of 36.8 mg per specimen, and 11-gauge probes are used to obtain an average of 94.4 mg per specimen.

Dr Forcier and I published articles (2,3) comparing the specimen weights obtained with these two vacuum-assisted probes during human breast biopsy. In our tissue-marking–clip article (2), the average weight of a specimen obtained with a 14-gauge probe was 44 mg; that of a specimen obtained with an 11-gauge probe was 105 mg. In the article (3) in which I compared the performances and complication rates of 14- and 11-gauge directional, vacuum-assisted probes (Mammotome; Biopsys Medical, Irvine, Calif), the average weights were 40 mg and 96 mg for 14- and 11-gauge probes, respectively. In these two studies, different patient populations were reviewed. Consequently, the average specimen weights varied slightly.

Overall, the weights reported by Berg and colleagues in their fresh turkey breast tissue model are very similar to the weights we obtained in human tissue during actual clinical breast biopsy. Specimens obtained with 11-gauge probes are approximately 2.5 times heavier than specimens obtained with 14-gauge probes. Furthermore, when a patient's breasts are wrapped with an elastic bandage for 24 hours after biopsy, complication rates (approximately 1%) are the same for the two probes (3).

Dr Burbank is a shareholder of Johnson & Johnson, whose division, Ethicon Endosurgery, owns Biopsys, the manufacturer of the Mammotome. He is the inventor of the Mammotome and founder of Biopsys.

References

1. Berg WA, Krebs TL, Campassi C, Magder LS, Sun CCJ. Evaluation of 14- and 11-gauge directional, vacuum-assisted biopsy probes and 14-gauge biopsy guns in a breast parenchymal model. Radiology 1997; 205:203–208.

2. Burbank F, Forcier N. Tissue marking clip for stereotactic breast biopsy: initial placement accuracy, long-term stability, and usefulness as a guide for wire localization. Radiology 1997; 205:407–415.
3. Burbank F. Stereotactic breast biopsy: comparison of 14- and 11-gauge Mammotome probe performance and complication rates. Am Surg 1997; 63:988–995.

Drs Berg and Krebs respond:

We are extremely gratified to see further verification of the results we obtained by using fresh turkey breast as a human breast parenchymal model to evaluate 14-gauge biopsy guns and 11- and 14-gauge, directional, vacuum-assisted probes (1). The two subsequently published reports of Dr Burbank (2) and Drs Burbank and Forcier (3) demonstrate the average weights of specimens obtained in patient biopsies with the 11-gauge, directional, vacuum-assisted probe to be similar to the weights we obtained in fresh turkey breast tissue and further validate the use of turkey breast as a breast parenchymal model. Our results in turkey breast are also similar to the clinical results of the study by Burbank and colleagues (4) in which the 14-gauge, directional, vacuum-assisted probe and 14-gauge Biopty gun (Bard, Covington, Ga) were used and to previously published results of our study (5) in which 14-gauge automated guns were used in human cadaveric breasts. As was nicely presented by Jackman and colleagues (6,7), the diagnostic accuracy of core-needle breast biopsy closely parallels the relative amount of tissue obtained with varying gun and gun-needle combinations. As we concluded in our article (1), manufacturers should be encouraged to evaluate the performance of any new biopsy guns or needle-gun combinations in breast parenchymal models (such as turkey breast) before marketing the devices for patient use. These recently published reports should provide benchmarks for further improvement.

References

1. Berg WA, Krebs TL, Campassi C, Magder LS, Sun CCJ. Evaluation of 14- and 11-gauge directional, vacuum-assisted biopsy probes and 14-gauge biopsy guns in a breast parenchymal model. Radiology 1997; 205:203–208.
2. Burbank F. Stereotactic breast biopsy: comparison of 14- and 11-gauge Mammotome probe performance and complication rates. Am Surg 1997; 63:988–995.
3. Burbank F, Forcier N. Tissue marking clip for stereotactic breast biopsy: initial placement accuracy, long-term stability, and usefulness as a guide for wire localization. Radiology 1997; 205:407–415.
4. Burbank F, Parker S, Fogarty T. Stereotactic breast biopsy: improved tissue harvesting with the Mammotome. Am Surg 1996; 62:728–744.
5. Krebs TL, Berg WA, Severson MJ, et al. Large-core biopsy guns: comparison for yield of breast tissue. Radiology 1996; 200:365–368.
6. Jackman RJ, Burbank FH, Parker SH, et al. Atypical ductal hyperplasia diagnosed by 11-gauge, directional, vacuum-assisted breast biopsy: how often is carcinoma found at surgery? (abstr). Radiology 1997; 205(P):325.
7. Jackman RJ, Burbank FH, Parker SH, et al. Accuracy of sampling microcalcifications by three stereotactic breast biopsy methods (abstr). Radiology 1997; 205(P):325.

Wendie A. Berg, MD, PhD, and Thorsten L. Krebs, MD
Department of Radiology, University of Maryland
22 South Greene Street, Baltimore, MD 21201

Hard- versus Soft-Copy Readings of Computed Radiographs

From:
Paula W. Brill, MD, and Patricia Winchester, MD
Department of Radiology, Division of Pediatric Radiology
New York Hospital–Cornell Medical Center
525 East 68th Street, New York, NY 10021

Editor:
We read with interest the important article by Dr Kundel et al (1) in the December 1997 issue of *Radiology* because of our similar interest in comparative studies of image display in patients in intensive care units (2,3). As Kundel et al noted, highly selected samples rather than samples representative of a clinical population have been used usually. We concur with the importance of the latter. We compared digital hard-copy interpretation versus 2.5K × 2K soft-copy interpretation of 1,104 sequential computed radiographs obtained in patients in neonatal and pediatric intensive care units (2). We found a high level of agreement between hard- and soft-copy interpretation of images obtained with computed radiography in this representative clinical sample.

Kundel et al (1) noted the value of studying abnormalities such as pneumothorax to test the fundamental limits of a method of diagnosis. In our study (2), there were 76 pneumothoraces. The κ statistic showed excellent agreement ($\kappa = 0.96 \pm 0.03$ [standard error]) in observations of pneumothorax between both methods of display. Our understanding of the article by Kundel et al is that 15 images obtained to rule out or follow up pneumothorax were included in the 95 cases selected for analysis. We would appreciate more information on the pneumothorax group. Were there 15 pneumothoraces, or were some cases in that group not pneumothoraces? Were any pneumothoraces detected as unexpected findings on images obtained for other reasons? Overall, were there sufficient data to draw conclusions with regard to the relative accuracy of soft-copy interpretations specifically for pneumothorax in this study?

References

1. Kundel HL, Gefter W, Aronchick J, et al. Accuracy of bedside chest hard-copy screen-film versus hard- and soft-copy computed radiographs in a medical intensive care unit: receiver operating characteristic analysis. Radiology 1997; 205:859–863.
2. Brill PW, Winchester P, Cahill P, et al. Computed radiography in neonatal and pediatric intensive care units: a comparison of 2.5K × 2K soft-copy vs digital hard copy film. Pediatr Radiol 1996; 26:333–336.
3. Brill PW, Winchester P. Computed radiography in neonatal and pediatric intensive care units: a comparison of 2.5K × 2K vs 1.6K × 1.2K monitor images (abstr). Radiology. 1997; 205(P):402.

Dr Kundel and colleagues respond:

We appreciate the interest of Drs Brill and Winchester in our study (1). We cannot make a specific statement about the comparative diagnostic accuracy of computed radiography and screen-film radiography in the evaluation of pneumothorax, because our study was designed to compare the performance of radiologists in the general spectrum of cases from the medical intensive care unit (MICU). Case selection was based on the clinical reason for requesting the examination by the MICU physicians and did not focus on specific diagnostic findings. Cases with and cases without pneumothorax were included in the rule-out or follow-up pneumothorax subset. Three of the 15 cases were in the computed radiography subset, and four were in the screen-film radiography subset. The cases without a pneumothorax are necessary for the receiver operating characteristic analysis, since diagnostic accuracy depends on the ability to recognize both the presence and the absence of the abnormality. The sets of cases that are selected to compare radiologists' performance in the evaluation of specific abnormalities frequently contain abnormal features that are difficult to detect and normal features that can be confused with abnormalities. These specially selected sets of cases are valuable "stress tests" for establishing the limits of performance and for screening for inadequate imaging systems; however, the results are difficult to apply to everyday clinical experience, because the cases are not representative. We attempted to get a more representative sample.

We cannot shed any light on the detection of "unsuspected" pneumothoraces, since there were none in either of the 95-case samples. This is not unusual, because the prevalence of pneumothorax is low in the MICU population. In the cohort of MICU patients from which the case samples were drawn, an unsuspected pneumothorax occurred in only one of 204 (0.5%) examinations requested to rule out or follow up pneumonia. A pneumothorax occurred in seven of 342 (2.0%) examinations requested to check the position of tubes and catheters. These numbers do not include pneumothoraces that were missed, but they do indicate that a very large sample is required to compare the number of unsuspected pneumothoraces missed at computed radiography and at screen-film radiography. We suspect that missing unsuspected pneumothoraces may be more a matter of human vigilance than a matter of radiologic technique.

Reference

1. Kundel HL, Gefter W, Aronchick J, et al. Accuracy of bedside chest hard-copy screen-film versus hard- and soft-copy computed radiographs in a medical intensive care unit: receiver operating characteristic analysis. Radiology 1997; 205:859–863.

Harold L. Kundel, MD, Wallace T. Miller Sr, MD, Wallace T. Miller Jr, MD, Judith Aronchick, MD, and Warren B. Gefter, MD

Department of Radiology, Pendergrass Diagnostic Research Laboratory, University of Pennsylvania Medical Center

308 Stemmler Hall, 36th and Hamilton Walk, Philadelphia, PA 19104-6086

Human Chorionic Gonadotropin Levels in the Evaluation of Ectopic Pregnancy

From:

Faye C. Laing, MD, and Douglas L. Brown, MD

Department of Radiology, Brigham and Women's Hospital

75 Francis Street, Boston, MA 02115

Editor:

We read with great interest the article in the November 1997 issue of *Radiology* by Dr Mehta and colleagues (1), who question whether 2,000 mIU/mL is a reasonable threshold for evaluating possible ectopic pregnancy. We have two reasons for writing this letter.

The first reason is to point out that, in the article by Mehta et al, 2,000 mIU/mL refers to a discriminatory level of human chorionic gonadotropin (hCG) as opposed to a threshold level. The distinction between these two terms has not always been clear, and there are other examples in the literature (2,3) in which these two words are confused. In early pregnancy, "threshold level" is best used to refer to the lowest hCG level at which an intrauterine gestational sac can be detected at ultrasonography (US), while "discriminatory level" refers to the lowest hCG level at which an intrauterine gestational sac should always be detected. With use of a vaginal transducer, the threshold level of hCG at which an early gestational sac can be detected is lower than the discriminatory level by a factor of approximately 10 (115 mIU/mL versus 1,000 mIU/mL, respectively [Second International Standard]) (3). The distinction between these two levels is important, because different clinical conclusions, based on whether the hCG level is below the threshold level or below the discriminatory level, will be reached if no gestational sac is seen.

The second reason for this letter is to emphasize that, in our opinion, despite the use of state-of-the-art US equipment and optimized scanning technique, it is not always possible to determine whether a small intrauterine fluid collection represents an early intrauterine pregnancy (IUP) or a pseudosac. In their article, Mehta et al (1) defined a normal IUP as a pregnancy in which there is an intradecidual sign, and they referred to the 91.7% sensitivity and 100% specificity of this sign for correct diagnosis of IUP that was reported by Yeh et al (4).

In our recently published study (5), which was in press when the article by Mehta et al was submitted, four independent observers reported a sensitivity of 34%–66% and a specificity of 55%–73% for diagnosing an IUP on the basis of the intradecidual sign. Therefore, we are not surprised that Mehta and colleagues (1, table 2), in their results, reported that 28 of 36 patients with presumed spontaneous abortion (14 patients) or IUP (14 patients) had initial hCG levels that exceeded the discriminatory level of 2,000 mIU/mL but did not have a clearly discernible IUP. Each of these patients was noted to have "endometrial fluid," but an incorrect diagnosis—that they did not have an IUP—was made, because the intrauterine fluid collection lacked either an intradecidual sign or other more definitive structures (eg, yolk sac or embryo) to confirm an IUP.

The findings reported by Mehta and colleagues confirm our own and emphasize that, in early pregnancy, it is often not possible to correctly interpret small intrauterine fluid collections that may be due to an IUP (normal or abnormal) or a pseudosac associated with an ectopic pregnancy. Our recommendations parallel the conclusions reached by Mehta et al. In a clinically stable patient, a follow-up US examination should be considered to look for a yolk sac or embryo. Serial hCG determinations may also be considered to look for a normal doubling pattern.

References

1. Mehta TS, Levine D, Beckwith B. Treatment of ectopic pregnancy: is a human chorionic gonadotropin level of 2000 mIU/mL a reasonable threshold? Radiology 1997; 205:569–573.
2. Cacciatore B, Tiitinen A, Stenman UH, Ylostalo P. Normal early pregnancy: serum hCG levels and vaginal ultrasonography findings. Br J Obstet Gynecol 1990; 97:899–903.
3. Nyberg DA, Mack LA, Laing FC, Jeffrey RB. Early pregnancy complications: endovaginal sonographic findings correlated with human choriogonadotropin levels. Radiology 1988; 167:619–622.
4. Yeh HC, Goodman JD, Carr L, Rabinowitz JG. Intradecidual sign: a US criterion of early intrauterine pregnancy. Radiology 1986; 161:463–467.
5. Laing FC, Brown DL, Price J, Teeger S, Wong M. Intradecidual sac sign: is it effective in diagnosis of an early intrauterine pregnancy? Radiology 1997; 204:655–660.

Drs Levine and Mehta respond:

We appreciate the comments of Drs Laing and Brown and agree that the diagnosis of ectopic pregnancy is most accurately described as having a discriminatory zone of values of β-hCG. However, according to *Taber's Cyclopedic Medical Dictionary* (1), a threshold is "the lowest value of the appropriate stimulus that will give the response." In our article (2), the stimulus value selected was a β-hCG level of 2,000 mIU/mL (International Reference Preparation), and the response was treatment for ectopic pregnancy. The impetus for writing the article was that clinicians at our institution were surprised that a normal IUP could be present when US examination findings were indeterminate for IUP and the β-hCG level was greater than 2,000 mIU/mL. Their policy was to treat individuals without an IUP but with a β-hCG level greater than 2,000 mIU/mL as patients with ectopic pregnancies. This absolute threshold for treatment is not realistic since there is a wide range of normal β-hCG values in early IUP.

References

1. Thomas CL. Taber's cyclopedic medical dictionary. Philadelphia, Pa: Davis, 1989.
2. Mehta TS, Levine D, Beckwith B. Treatment of ectopic pregnancy: is a human chorionic gonadotropin level of 2,000 mIU/mL a reasonable threshold? Radiology 1997; 205:569–573.

Deborah Levine, MD, and Teas S. Mehta, MD
Department of Radiology, Beth Israel Deaconess Medical Center
330 Brookline Avenue, Boston, MA 02215

In Memoriam

Dr B. Leonard Holman, chairman emeritus of the department of radiology at Brigham and Women's Hospital and Philip H. Cook Professor of Radiology at Harvard Medical School, both in Boston, Mass, died on February 1, 1998, after a long illness.

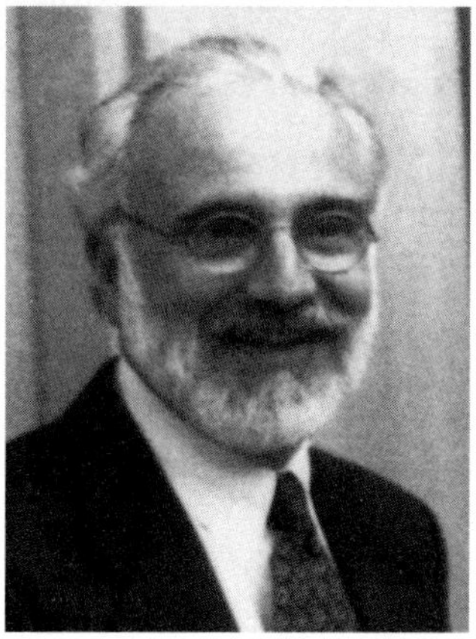

B. Leonard Holman, MD
1941–1998

He was born on June 26, 1941, in Sheboygan, Wis, to Max and Sophie Holman. He earned his BS degree from the University of Wisconsin–Madison and his MD degree from Washington University Medical School in St Louis, Mo, and completed his medical training at the Edward Mallinckrodt Institute of Radiology in St. Louis, Mo. In 1970, he joined (and later directed) the nuclear medicine department at the Peter Bent Brigham Hospital in Boston, Mass. In 1988, he assumed the chairmanship of the department of radiology at Brigham and Women's Hospital. He was a former president of the Society of Nuclear Medicine and of the Massachusetts Radiological Society, a trustee of the American Board of Radiology, the editor of major textbooks, and the author of over 300 reports.

Dr. Holman was recognized throughout his distinguished career with many awards and honors, such as the Herrman L. Blumgart Pioneer Award and the Distinguished Educator Award from the Society of Nuclear Medicine and the Gold Medal from the Association of University Radiologists. A professorship has been established in his name at Harvard Medical School.

His tenure as department chairman saw the growth of many new medical imaging technologies, and he fostered extraordinary innovation in the field of imaging-guided therapies and the use of the Internet for medical education. He ran the department with compassion and democracy and created a highly visible and respected department in the medical and academic communities. A strong advocate for patients, he was an early pioneer in departmental quality assurance. As a teacher and mentor, he helped train a whole generation of leaders in academic radiology.

In 1991, he developed and produced the video tape, *Cocaine and the Brain.* This educational video tape has received numerous awards, including the Freddie Award from the International Health and Medical Film Festival, and has become a major addition to drug education programs.

Throughout his career, his love and devotion to his family have been the paramount focus of his life. He is survived by his beloved wife, Dale; his cherished daughters, Amy and Allison; and his mother, Sophie.

—Steven E. Seltzer, MD

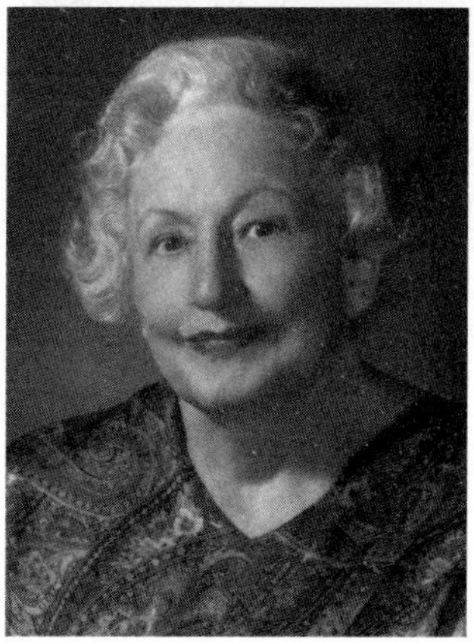

Lucy Frank Squire, MD
1915–1996

Dr Lucy Frank Squire died at her home in the Dakota Apartments in New York, NY, on September 15, 1996, at the age of 81 years.

Dr Squire was born on May 10, 1915. She received her MD degree in 1940 from the Women's Medical College of Pennsylvania (now the Medical College of Pennsylvania–Hahnemann/Allegheny General Hospital). She had difficulty in finding a residency in the era before the Second World War. Eventually, she entered a combined radiology and pathology residency at Massachusetts General Hospital in Boston; later, she entered the full radiology program because of the need for staffing during World War II. She finished her training at the New England Medical Center in Boston, Mass. She spent 2 years as chief of radiology at Syracuse General Hospital, NY, and then moved to the University of Rochester, NY, in 1950.

In 1966, she received her first appointment at the Health Science Center of the State University of New York, Brooklyn, and, other than a short hiatus in the late 1960s, was a faculty member there until her retirement in 1994. The university awarded her the title of Distinguished Teaching Professor.

She received the Gold Medal from the Radiological Society of North America for influence on the teaching of radiology, and the first Marie Curie Award from the American Association of Women Radiologists.

In 1964, with a grant from the Commonwealth Fund, *Fundamentals of Roentgenology* (Boston, Mass: Harvard University Press) was created. Subsequent editions from the same publisher, now named *Fundamentals of Radiology,* have been the standard resource for medical student radiology education all over the world, with translations into French, German, Greek, Spanish, and Japanese. In addition to *Fundamentals of Radiology,* she co-authored *Exercises in Diagnostic Radiology* (Philadelphia, Pa: Saunders).

During her tenure at the State University of New York, she became the proponent of small group teaching (later a most popular medical school curriculum under the "problem-based learning" designation). This evolved into the series of slides and tapes entitled "Seminars of Diagnostic Radiology."

The "nonphysician" Lucy Frank Squire was one of the most multifaceted individuals that one can have the privilege of knowing. We all love Lucy.

She is survived by her son, Gordon Squire, of Allentown, Pa.

—Joshua A. Becker, MD

Dr Cyrus Paul Klein passed away on June 6, 1997, after a long and distinguished medical career. He was 81 years old.

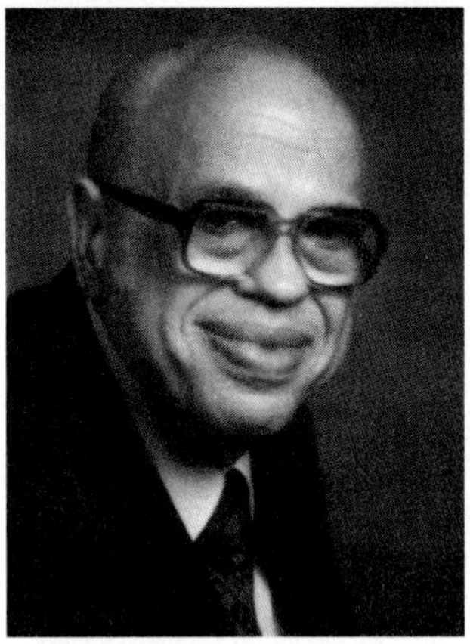

Cyrus Paul Klein, MD
1915–1997

Cy was born on October 27, 1915, in New York, NY. He was the son of Louis Klein, MD, who served for many years as medical director and product editor for Parke-Davis and later in the same capacities for Hoffman–La Roche.

He received his BA degree from the University of Michigan in Ann Arbor in 1937 and his MD degree from the Johns Hopkins University School of Medicine in Baltimore, Md, in 1941. He served a rotating internship at Harper Hospital in Detroit, Mich, and he had started a pediatrics residency at Children's Hospital of Michigan in Ann Arbor when he was called to active duty as a Second Lieutenant in the U.S. Army Medical Corps during World War II.

While in the service, a chance meeting with then Colonel Alfred A. deLorimier changed his life forever. Colonel deLorimier was head of the Army School of Roentgenology in Memphis, Tenn, and Cy soon found himself a member of this school. It was during this time that he developed a fascination with and a love for radiology that persisted throughout his entire life.

Cy retired as a Major at the end of World War II and immediately entered a radiology residency at the University of Texas at Galveston. He was certified in radiology in 1948. The war had substantially diminished the number of physicians across the land, and he was actively recruited to join Dr C. H. Frank, the only radiologist in Texarkana, a town on the border of Texas and Arkansas (population, approximately 40,000). Geography dictated that they also be licensed to practice in Louisiana and Oklahoma. Their practice flourished. Dr Frank retired after 10 years, but Cy never left.

He held memberships in the American Medical Association, the Texas Medical Association, the Radiological Society of North America, the American Roentgen Ray Society, and several smaller professional organizations. He was also a clinical professor of radiology at Louisiana State University Medical School in Shreveport. In 1970, he was honored by his colleagues with a fellowship in the American College of Radiology.

He was a pioneer in the private practice of small town radiology. He always maintained that as long as the radiologist kept up with the specialty, there was no reason for the large dichotomy, which had existed when Cy finished his residency, between the quality of radiology practiced in the small town and that practiced in the cities. He promoted this concept throughout his life, even to the extent of privately gifting such things as automatic film processing and image intensification equipment to small area hospitals before they were available in nearby cities. (He was chief radiologist at 10 area hospitals and three major clinics during his career.)

His sharp mind, his persistent intellectual curiosity, and his tremendous drive for excellence constantly drew him toward the academic. He formed friendships with future gold medalists Drs Isadore Meschan and Gil Brodgon while they were at the University of Arkansas at Little Rock. He would drive 300 miles round trip to meet and exchange ideas with this small "radiology club," which eventually formed the nucleus for the Arkansas chapter of the American College of Radiology. He served as president of this organization for two consecutive terms in 1971 and 1972.

He was in solo practice when I left academic radiology to join him in 1962. (Little did I realize that this was the beginning of a close professional and personal relationship that would last over 30 years.) We immediately set up an accredited school of x-ray technology because there was none within a 100-mile radius. The school is still in existence, and its graduates are always in popular demand.

His life was not without adversity. A childhood infection left him with a loss of hearing in his left ear; his older son, Robert, was killed at the age of 39 years; and when Cy was in his late 50s, he developed acromegaly. Such events would have shattered the average person, but Cy was a profoundly devoted Christian, and his deep religious feelings helped him stay the course without malice or self-pity. He served many terms as deacon and/or elder in the Presbyterian church and remained active in community affairs. He taught Sunday school and men's Bible classes until his death.

He never lost his warm friendly personality, his affable nature, or his witty sense of humor, nor did he ever retire from radiology. He was still practicing radiology with the latest modalities a half day a week at a 50-person multispecialty clinic at the time of his death. A devoted family man and true gentleman at all times, this remarkable man will be missed and long remembered by his colleagues and many friends. Our sympathy is extended to all the members of the family.

He is survived by his supportive and beloved wife of 53 years, Frances; a son, Dr Cordell L. Klein, a urologist, and his wife, Carolyn; a second daughter-in-law, Mary Flora Klein; a brother, Robert, and his wife, Lennie; a sister-in-law, Mary Whittington Steele; three grandsons; and two step-grandsons.

W. Richard Seibold, Jr, MD

Abstracts of Current Literature

Gastrointestinal System

Presacral Carcinoid Tumors: Report of Three Cases and Review of the Literature. Marcelo G. Horenstein, Robert A. Erlandson, Daniel M. Gonzalez-Cueto, et al. *Am J Surg Pathol* 1998; 22:251–255. (Juan Rosai, Department of Pathology, Memorial Sloan-Kettering Cancer Center, 1275 York Ave, New York, NY 10021)

The clinical, microscopic, immunohistochemical, and ultrastructural features of three carcinoid tumors of the presacral region are reviewed. All tumors occurred in young women and did not involve the rectum. The predominant microscopic pattern was trabecular. The differential diagnosis included paraganglioma and myxopapillary ependymoma. Immunohistochemically, neuroendocrine markers and low-molecular-weight cytokeratins were expressed in all cases. Neurosecretory granules were identified in the single case studied with electron microscopy. One case was associated with a tailgut cyst (retrorectal cystic hamartoma). Two patients were treated with complete local excision and are free of disease 3 and 4 years after surgery. One case metastasized to both breasts and recurred locally after an incomplete excision. This report expands the already long list of sites where carcinoid tumors can arise. The frequent association of these tumors with tailgut cysts and their histologic similarities to rectal carcinoid tumors suggest that the most likely derivation of presacral carcinoid tumors is from hindgut rests.
Authors' Abstract

Genitourinary System

Pseudotumors after Renal Parenchymal Sparing Surgery. Ashutosh V. Kshirsagar, Peter L. Choyke, W. Marston Linehan, et al. *J Urol* 1998; 159:1148–1151. (From the Urologic Oncology Branch and the Department of Radiology, National Cancer Institute, National Institutes of Health, Bethesda, Md)

Purpose: After renal parenchymal sparing surgery, residual defects may persist on imaging studies at the sites of resection. These "pseudotumors" may lead to confusion as to whether a lesion was removed or has recurred. The authors describe the imaging appearances and behavior of renal pseudotumors following renal parenchymal sparing surgery. *Materials and Methods:* From 1988 to 1997, 32 patients underwent 46 renal parenchymal sparing operations for removal of renal cancers, including von Hippel–Lindau disease in 27, hereditary papillary renal cancer in two, and sporadic disease in three. A median of 14 tumors (range, one to 114) were removed in each operation. A thrombin-soaked, absorbable gelatin sponge was placed in the tumor bed after resection to aid hemostasis. The authors reviewed all imaging studies performed after these operations to characterize these lesions and gain further understanding into the prevalence and etiology. *Results:* Nine patients had 13 pseudotumors on initial postoperative imaging studies, including von Hippel–Lindau disease in seven, hereditary papillary renal cancer in one, and sporadic renal cancer in one. Pseudotumors were observed after 10 of 46 operations (22%). All pseudotumors demonstrated round contours and enhancement after contrast media, simulating a tumor; yet, these lesions resolved in a mean of 13 months, leaving only small cortical scars. *Conclusions:* Renal pseudotumors are commonly seen after renal parenchymal sparing surgery and should not be confused with residual or recurrent disease. Enhancement is likely due to granulation tissue involving the lattice of an absorbable gelatin sponge. These lesions usually resolve within a year but can take longer to do so.
Authors' Abstract

The Fate of Patients with Locally Advanced Bladder Cancer Treated Conservatively with Neoadjuvant Chemotherapy, Extensive Transurethral Resection and Radiotherapy: 10-year Experience. Vincenzo Serretta, Giovanni Lo Greco, Carlo Pavone, et al. *J Urol* 1998; 159:1187–1191. (From the Department of Urology, Civic Hospital Benfratelli; the Department of Radiotherapy, Oncology Hospital M. Ascoli; and the Institute of Urology, University of Palermo, Italy)

Purpose: The authors assessed the results of bladder preservation for infiltrating bladder cancer. The potential for neoadjuvant chemotherapy followed by extensive transurethral resection and radiation therapy was evaluated in 40 patients with T2–T4a G2–G3 bladder carcinoma. *Materials and Methods:* From 1983 to 1995, 40 patients with bladder cancer underwent bladder-sparing treatment, consisting of neoadjuvant chemotherapy, extensive transurethral resection, and radiation therapy. Most patients had T3G3 cancer. A deep transurethral resection biopsy was performed before and after chemotherapy, and an extensive transurethral resection was repeated at the end of radiation therapy. Thirty patients received cisplatin and methotrexate, and 10 also received vinblastine. The total dose of radiation therapy was 60–65 Gy. Recurrent superficial tumors were treated transurethrally. Radical cystectomy was considered for persistent or recurrent invasive disease. *Results:* A complete response occurred after chemotherapy in 19 patients (47.5%) and after transurethral resection and radiation therapy in eight patients (67.5%). Within 10 years, eight responding patients (30%) had local recurrences and three underwent cystectomy. Fourteen (35%) patients are alive, including 13 with no evidence of disease (mean survival, 65 months), five died of unrelated disease, and 21 (52.5%) died of distant metastases (mean survival, 28 months). Of the 21 patients, 14 had residual tumor after radiation therapy, three presented with distant metastases after vesical infiltrating recurrence, and four had distant metastases in the absence of local-regional recurrence. In 22 patients (55%), the bladder was salvaged. Patients with complete response to chemotherapy had a low risk for recurrent infiltrating tumors and metastases. *Conclusions:* Complete tumor control was maintained at 5 years in more than 50% of the patients treated conservatively. Bladder salvage is feasible in select patients.
Authors' Abstract

Positron Emission Tomography in Urological Oncology. Carl K. Hoh, Marc A. Seltzer, John Franklin, et al. *J Urol* 1998; 159:347–356. (From the Department of Urology, University of California at Los Angeles School of Medicine)

Purpose: The authors provide scientists and clinicians with an introduction to the basic principles and methods of positron emission tomography (PET) and summarize the recent research and clinical applications of PET in the urologic field. Specifically, they introduce PET so that the reader can understand and objectively review current and future articles that involve this imaging technology. *Materials and Methods:* The recent applications of PET in urology in the published literature were searched and reviewed. *Results:* In prostate carcinoma, preliminary studies with the radio-isotope tracer 18-fluoro-2-deoxyglucose (FDG) demonstrated that PET cannot reliably be used to differentiate between primary prostate cancer and benign prostatic hyperplasia, and that PET is not as sensitive as bone scintigraphy for the detection of osseous metastases. However, PET may have a role in the detection of lymph node metastases in patients with prostate specific antigen relapse after primary local therapy. In renal cell carcinoma, recent studies have shown the ability of FDG PET to help detect primary and metastatic lesions and to help monitor response to therapy. In the staging of testicular cancer, FDG PET has been used to help differentiate viable carcinoma from benign teratomas and/or fibrotic or necrotic changes. *Conclusions:* Current developments in PET technology that allow accurate staging of the extent of tumor before surgery, as well as help monitor effectiveness or ineffectiveness of new or current therapies, may make PET a valuable tool in research and in the treatment of urologic diseases.
Authors' Abstract

Obstruction of the Renal Pelvis due to an Insoluble Blood Clot after Epsilon-Aminocaproic Acid Therapy: Resolution with Intraureteral Streptokinase Instillations. Leonard F. A. Wymenga, Wim J. V. van der Boon. *J Urol* 1998; 159:490–492. (From the Departments of Urology and Pharmacy, Nij Smellinghe Hospital, Drachten, The Netherlands)

Purpose: The authors demonstrate the effectiveness of intraureteral streptokinase instillations for the resolution of an insoluble

blood clot in the renal pelvis. *Materials and Methods:* A patient with renal adenocarcinoma had prolonged hematuria related to involvement of the "pyelum" by the tumor. An insoluble blood clot obstruction of the left renal collecting system developed as a consequence of ε-aminocaproic acid therapy, which was treated with low-dose streptokinase through a ureteral catheter. *Results:* Complete resolution of the clot and obstruction occurred within 3 days of therapy. *Conclusions:* This relatively simple approach should be used for the treatment of obstruction before radical surgery is performed.
Authors' Abstract

External Beam Radiotherapy for Stage T1/T2 Prostate Cancer: How Does It Stack Up? Alan Pollack, Gunar K. Zagars. *Urology* 1998; 51:258–264. (A.P., Department of Radiation Oncology [Box 97], University of Texas M. D. Anderson Cancer Center, 1515 Holcombe Blvd, Houston, TX 77030)

Objectives: To determine the impact of radiation dose on the response of stage T1/T2 prostate cancer to external-beam radiation therapy and to contrast the modern-day clinical and biochemical control rates to those seen after radical prostatectomy or permanent iodine-125 seed implants. *Methods:* The study cohort consisted of 643 patients with palpable stage T1/T2, NX/N0, M0 prostate cancer treated with external-beam radiation therapy between 1987 and 1995. No patient received neoadjuvant or adjuvant androgen ablation. The radiation therapy isocenter dose ranged from 60 to 78 Gy, with a mean of 67 Gy and a median of 66 Gy. The median follow-up was 43 months. The primary end point was freedom from relapse or rising prostate specific antigen (PSA) level. *Results:* The patients were divided into two dose groups, with the cut point based on the mean and median values and prior analyses. There were 354 patients treated to radiation doses of 67 Gy or less, and 289 treated to doses greater than 67 Gy. Those receiving the higher doses had a significantly greater 4-year freedom from failure rate (87% vs 67%; $P < .0001$). Multivariate Cox proportional hazards analyses revealed that isocenter dose was independent of Gleason score and pretreatment PSA level, which were the other significant covariates. *Conclusions:* Very high freedom from failure rates were achieved when the radiation dose to the prostate was above 67 Gy. These rates are promising when compared to published radical prostatectomy series and most permanent I-125 seed implant series in which patients were stratified by pretreatment PSA levels. Further follow-up is needed to confirm that these promising results are sustained.
Authors' Abstract

Transarterial Embolization and Ablation of Renal Arteriovenous Malformations: Efficacy and Damages in 30 Patients with Long-term Followup. Shigeo Takebayashi, Masahiko Hosaka, Yoshinobu Kubota, et al. *J Urol* 1998; 159:696–701. (S.T., Department of Radiology, Yokohama City University Hospital, 3-46 Urafune-cho, Minami-ku, Yokohama 232, Japan)

Purpose: The authors evaluate the long-term efficacy and side effects of transarterial embolization and ablation for renal arteriovenous malformations. *Materials and Methods:* Thirty patients with cirsoid arteriovenous malformations causing massive hematuria underwent 34 procedures of embolization or ablation. The authors confirmed the ratios of occluded arteriovenous malformation areas on angiograms and those of infarcted areas at computed tomography. All patients were followed up for 4.1–15.0 years (mean, 8.0 years ± 2.8) after the initial procedures. *Results:* Hematuria ceased in all patients after the initial procedures, including partial embolization or ablation of the arteriovenous malformations in eight. Massive hematuria recurred in four patients who had undergone absorbable gelatin sponge embolization (n = 2), combined alcohol and subselective absorbable gelatin sponge embolization (n = 1), and polyvinyl alcohol particles embolization (n = 1). In these four cases, total ablation of the arteriovenous malformations with alcohol was successful. In 29 patients, including the aforementioned four, no hematuria recurred after 5 years after total or partial ablation with alcohol. Large nontarget embolization with reflux of subselectively infused absorbable gelatin sponge caused a nonfunctioning kidney in one patient. The remaining 33 procedures caused 6.3%–48.0% (mean, 15.7% ± 6.9) areas of renal infarction. Polyvinyl alcohol embolization caused pulmonary embolism and renin-dependent hypertension. *Conclusions:* Partial or total transarterial ablation of arteriovenous malformations with alcohol proved effective for long-term cessation of hematuria. However, this procedure, as well as transarterial embolization, has the potential risk of nontarget infarction.
Authors' Abstract

Cardiovascular System

Concurrent Comparison of Endoluminal versus Open Repair in the Treatment of Abdominal Aortic Aneurysms: Analysis of 303 Patients by Life Table Method. James May, Geoffrey H. White, Weiyun Yu, et al. *J Vasc Surg* 1998; 27:213–221. (J.M., Department of Surgery, University of Sydney, D06, Sydney, New South Wales 2006, Australia)

Purpose: The aim of this study was to compare the outcome in consecutive patients with abdominal aortic aneurysm (AAA) treated by means of open operation versus endoluminal intervention, performed by the same surgeons during a defined interval. *Methods:* Between May 1992 and May 1996, 362 consecutive patients with AAA underwent repair. Fifty-three patients who underwent open operations for ruptured AAA plus two who underwent endoluminal repair of false AAA and four who underwent secondary endoluminal repair of AAA were excluded, leaving 303 patients who underwent elective repair of true AAA. The elective operations were conventional open repair in 195 patients (151 men, 44 women; mean age, 69 years) and endoluminal repair in 108 patients (100 men, eight women; mean age, 70 years). The decision to perform endoluminal repair was based on comorbidities that precluded open repair (n = 48) or patient choice (n = 60). The graft configuration in the open repair group was tubular (n = 180) or bifurcated (n = 15) and in the endoluminal repair group, tubular (n = 48), aortoiliac/femoral (n = 25), or bifurcated (n = 35). All procedures were performed in the operating department, and radiographic guidance was used in the endoluminal repair group. Follow-up was by means of interview, examination, and telephone. In addition, contrast material–enhanced computed tomography was performed within the first 10 days after operation, 6 months and 12 months after operation, and then annually thereafter in the endoluminal repair group. Outcome measures were successful exclusion of the aneurysm sac from the general circulation and survival. Data were analyzed by the life-table method. Other outcome measures were length of hospital stay, length of intensive care unit stay, and operative blood loss. *Results:* No significant difference was found between the perioperative mortality rate for open repair (11 deaths [5.6%] in 195 patients) and endoluminal repair (six deaths [5.6%] in 108 patients). Three of the six deaths in the latter group occurred in patients with successful endoluminal repair, and three occurred in 18 patients with failed endoluminal repair who were converted to open repair. Similarly, no significant difference was seen in the survival rate between the endoluminal repair and open repair groups according to log-rank analysis (P = .14). The rate of graft failure, however, was significantly higher in the endoluminal repair group than in the open repair group (Fisher exact test, $P < .001$). Success in the endoluminal repair group was defined as continuing graft function without endoleak or conversion to open repair. The Kaplan-Meier curve for graft failure times for the endoluminal group revealed a 3-year graft success probability of 70%. *Conclusions:* This study suggests that endoluminal repair is safe, sharing the same perioperative mortality risk as open repair despite 44% of the endoluminal repair group being rejected as unfit for open repair. Conventional open repair is the most reliable method of successfully managing AAA. The endoluminal method, however, results in shorter length of hospital stay, shorter length of intensive care unit stay, and less blood loss than the open method. Patients who opt for the endoluminal method of repair should be made aware that the minimally invasive technique carries the disadvantage of a higher failure rate.
Authors' Abstract

A Cost Comparison of Balloon Angioplasty and Stenting versus Endarterectomy for the Treatment of Carotid Artery Stenosis. William D. Jordan, Jr, G. Dean Roye, Wink S. Fisher III, et al. *J Vasc Surg* 1998; 27:16–24. (W.D.J.,

Section of Vascular Surgery, University of Alabama at Birmingham, 1922 7th Ave S, Kracke 431, Birmingham, AL 35294)

Purpose: Percutaneous transluminal angioplasty with stenting (PTAS) of the carotid artery has been advocated as an alternative treatment for high-grade stenosis. Rationales for this approach include less morbidity, shorter recovery, and lower cost when compared with carotid endarterectomy (CEA). *Methods:* The clinical results and hospital charges in patients who underwent elective treatment for carotid stenosis were reviewed. During a concurrent 14-month period, 218 patients were admitted 229 times for 234 procedures to treat 239 carotid bifurcation stenoses, 109 by means of PTAS and 130 by means of CEA. Hospital charges were reviewed for each hospitalization and were categorized according to radiology, operating room, cardiac catheterization laboratory, and all other hospital charges. *Results:* The combined incidence of postprocedure strokes and deaths were as follows: PTAS, eight strokes (7.7%) and one death (0.9%); and CEA, two strokes (1.5%) and two deaths (1.5%). Total hospital charges per admission for the two groups were $30,140 for PTAS and $21,670 for CEA. The average postprocedure length of stay for PTAS was 2.9 days (median, 2 days) and for CEA was 3.1 days (median, 3 days). Cardiac catheterization laboratory charges for the PTAS group were $12,968, whereas the operating room charges for the CEA group were $4,263. When hospitalizations that were extended because of complications were excluded, the average total charges for the PTAS group (n = 84) dropped to $24,848 (mean length of stay, 1.9 days) and for the CEA group (n = 111) to $19,247 (mean length of stay, 2.6 days). *Conclusions:* After evaluation of hospital charges, PTAS for the treatment of carotid stenosis cannot currently be justified on the basis of reduced costs alone. With future cost-containing measures, total hospital charges can be reduced in both groups.
Authors' Abstract

Musculoskeletal System

Use of P-31 Magnetic Resonance Spectroscopy to Detect Metabolic Abnormalities in Muscles of Patients with Fibromyalgia. Jane H. Park, Phomma Phothimat, Carolyn T. Oates, et al. *Arthritis Rheum* 1998; 41:406–413. (Nancy J. Olsen, Division of Rheumatology and Immunology, T3219 MCN, Vanderbilt University, Nashville, TN 37232-2681)

Objective: To investigate the metabolic and functional status of muscles of fibromyalgia patients by using phosphorus-31 magnetic resonance (MR) spectroscopy. *Methods:* Twelve patients with fibromyalgia and 11 healthy subjects were studied. Clinical status was assessed with a questionnaire. The biochemical status of muscle was evaluated with P-31 MR spectroscopy by determining concentrations of inorganic phosphate (Pi), phosphocreatine (PCr), adenosine triphosphate (ATP), and phosphodiesters during rest and exercise. Functional status was evaluated from the PCr/Pi ratio, phosphorylation potential (PP), and total oxidative capacity (V_{max}). *Results:* Patients with fibromyalgia reported greater difficulty in performing activities of daily living as well as increased pain, fatigue, and weakness compared with controls. MR spectroscopic measurements showed that patients had significantly lower than normal PCr and ATP levels ($P < .004$) and PCr/Pi ratios ($P < .04$) in the quadriceps muscles during rest. Values for PP and V_{max} were also substantially reduced during rest and exercise. *Conclusion:* P-31 MR spectroscopy provides objective evidence for metabolic abnormalities consistent with weakness and fatigue in patients with fibromyalgia. It may be useful in assessing clinical status and evaluating the effectiveness of treatment regimens in fibromyalgia.
Authors' Abstract

Orientation of Lumbar Pars Defects: Implications for Radiological Detection and Surgical Management. Asif Saifuddin, John White, Stewart Tucker, et al. *J Bone Joint Surg [Br]* 1998; 80:208–211. (A.S., Department of Radiology, Royal National Orthopaedic Hospital Trust, Brockley Hill, Stanmore, Middlesex HA7 4LP, England)

Lateral oblique radiographs are considered important for the identification of spondylolytic lesions, but these projections will give a clear view only when the radiologic beam is in the plane of the defect. The authors studied the variation in orientation of spondylolytic lesions on CT scans of 34 patients with 69 defects. There was a wide variation of angle: only 32% of defects were oriented within 15° of the 45° lateral oblique plane. Lateral oblique radiographs should not be considered as the definitive investigation for spondylolysis. The authors suggest that CT scans with reverse gantry angle are now more appropriate than oblique radiography for the assessment of spondylolysis. Variation in the angle of the defect may also need consideration when direct repair is being planned.
Authors' Abstract

Diagnostic Value of Intra-articular Anaesthetic in Primary Osteoarthritis of the Hip. R. W. Crawford, G. A. Gie, R. S. M. Ling, et al. *J Bone Joint Surg [Br]* 1998; 80:279–281. (R.W.C., Nuffield Orthopaedic Centre, Windmill Rd, Headington, Oxford OX3 7LD, England)

The authors investigated 42 patients who were being considered for primary total hip arthroplasty but in whom it was uncertain whether the hip was the source of their pain. They were given an injection of local anesthetic into the joint space. Of 33 patients who gained pain relief from their injection, 32 subsequently had successful total hip arthroplasty. The remaining patient has not had surgery. The intraarticular injection of local anesthetic is thus at least 96% sensitive. Of the nine patients who had no or only minimal pain relief from injection, one has had an unsuccessful total hip arthroplasty, three have been successfully treated for other conditions, and five have unresolved pain for which no organic basis has been established. The authors believe that the injection of local anesthetic into the hip is a reliable test, with low morbidity. In difficult cases, it will aid in the clarification of the cause of pain, which possibly arises from the hip.
Authors' Abstract

Hip Osteoarthritis Prevalence Estimates by Three Radiographic Scoring Systems. Rosemarie Hirsch, Richard J. Fernandes, Stanley R. Pillemer, et al. *Arthritis Rheum* 1998; 41:361–368. (R.H., National Arthritis and Musculoskeletal and Skin Diseases Information Clearinghouse, 1 AMS Circle, Bethesda, MD 20892-3675)

Objective: To estimate and compare the age- and sex-specific prevalence of radiographic hip osteoarthritis (RHOA) in a population-based study of the Pima Indians, by using three atlas-based methods for assessing features of RHOA. *Methods:* Pelvic radiographs from 755 Pima Indians aged 45 years and over enrolled in a population-based study were read by using the Kellgren/Lawrence (K/L) grading scale (grade 0–4) and two validated individual-radiographic-features (IRF) scales (grades 0–3 for narrowing and osteophytes). *Results:* The age- and sex-specific prevalence of RHOA among Pima Indians assessed with the K/L scale was less than 10% in all age and sex groups. The prevalence of osteophytes grade 2 or higher was similar for the two IRF scales in all age and sex groups. However, differences between the two IRF scoring systems were found for the prevalence of joint space narrowing grade 2 or higher. *Conclusion:* Pima Indians have an age- and sex-specific prevalence of RHOA similar to that found in the U.S. population. The authors' finding of different joint space narrowing prevalence with the two IRF grading scales supports the use of the same atlas-based case definitions for determining disease prevalence for comparative studies.
Authors' Abstract

Neurosciences

Herpes Simplex Encephalitis (HSE) and the Immunocompromised: A Clinical and Autopsy Study of HSE in the Settings of Cancer and Human Immunodeficiency Virus–Type 1 Infection. David Schiff, Marc K. Rosenblum. *Hum Pathol* 1998; 29:215–222. (M.K.R., Neuropathology and Autopsy Service, Department of Pathology, Memorial Sloan-Kettering Cancer Center, 1275 York Ave, New York, NY 10021)

Although herpes simplex encephalitis (HSE) is not regarded as an opportunistic infection, the occurrence of HSE in immunocompromised patients has been documented, and the suggestion has been made that unusual clinical and neuropathologic features

characterize the disorder in this population. To further characterize HSE as it affects the immunodeficient, the authors reviewed the clinical and pathologic findings in three immunocompromised patients with autopsy-proved HSE. Two patients had cancer (one lymphoma and one glioblastoma multiforme), one was known to be human immunodeficiency virus–type 1 (HIV-1) seropositive, and a second was suspected of harboring underlying HIV-1 infection. Two were receiving dexamethasone at the onset of HSE. All had fever, mental status changes, and new, focal neurologic deficits or worsening of established deficits. Cerebrospinal fluid (CSF) pleocytosis was absent or minimal, and head computed tomographic (CT) scans, obtained in all cases, were unrevealing. No patient was clinically suspected of having HSE, only one received acyclovir (for concurrent mucocutaneous herpes), and HSE played a major role in all deaths. Autopsy revealed an unusual form of HSE characterized by a noninflammatory, pseudoischemic, histologic presentation and the unexpected persistence of viral antigens in abundance despite survival beyond the clinical stage during which inflammatory responses usually peak and productive brain infection wanes. The incidence of HSE in the immunocompromised may be underestimated. Preexistent neurologic disease, a noninflammatory CSF profile, and a negative CT scan may confound the diagnosis in this population, a typical clinical presentation notwithstanding. Increased clinical suspicion, the use of magnetic resonance imaging, and polymerase chain reaction analysis of CSF for herpes simplex virus nucleic acid sequences may permit more rapid diagnosis and treatment. The absence of inflammatory infiltrates in some fatal cases of HSE suggests that an intact immune response is not requisite to the devastating neurologic injury characteristic of this disorder.
Authors' Abstract

Pathogen-free Granulomatous Diseases of the Central Nervous System. George Thomas, Sean Murphy, Hugh Staunton, et al. *Hum Pathol* 1998; 29:110–115. (Francesca M. Brett, Department of Neuropathology, Beaumont Hospital, Beaumont Road, Dublin 9, Ireland)

Pathogen-free granulomatous diseases of the central nervous system (CNS) are a group of disorders with protean clinical and pathologic findings. Failure to identify a causative organism leads to considerable diagnostic difficulty. The neuropathologic records between 1985 and 1995 were retrospectively reviewed, and the medical records were retrieved for all patients with a diagnosis of pathogen-free granulomatous diseases of the CNS. Patients in whom an infective agent was shown either by means of culture, special staining techniques, or immunohistochemical methods were excluded. The authors identified 11 patients (eight men, three women) who fulfilled the pathologic criteria for this condition. The average age at diagnosis was 38.7 years (range, 17–78 years). Neurologic symptoms were the presenting feature in nine patients. Neuroimaging findings included hydrocephalus (54.5%), meningeal enhancement (45.5%), and mass lesions (45.5%). Seven patients underwent antemortem CNS biopsies (brain/meninges, $n = 6$; spinal, $n = 1$), which showed noncaseating granulomas. Eight patients died (mortality rate, 72.7%). Postmortem examination showed granulomatous involvement of the leptomeninges and cerebral parenchyma in all cases, with systemic involvement in 50%, chiefly in the form of noncaseating granulomas of the hilar nodes. Six patients fulfilled the clinical, radiologic, and pathologic diagnostic criteria for neurosarcoidosis. The remaining five patients had an unclassifiable pathogen-free granulomatous disease of the CNS. Such diseases are associated with a poor prognosis. Although neurosarcoidosis may account for some of the cases, there remains an unclassifiable subgroup that continues to be a diagnostic and management challenge.
Authors' Abstract

HLA-DR–positive Dendritic Cells of the Normal Human Choroid Plexus: A Potential Reservoir of HIV in the Central Nervous System. Andrew Hanly, Carol Kaiser Petito. *Hum Pathol* 1998; 29:88–93. (C.K.P., Department of Pathology [Neuropathology], R5, University of Miami School of Medicine, Papanicolaou Building, Rm 417, 1550 NW 10th Ave, Miami, FL 33136)

In a previous study of the choroid plexus from patients with acquired immunodeficiency syndrome (AIDS), the authors found a population of stromal cells infected with the human immunodeficiency virus (HIV). To determine whether these represented antigen-presenting dendritic cells, the authors examined the phenotype of the normal human choroid plexus with light and electron microscopy and established the HIV-infected cell type with immunohistochemistry in patients with AIDS with an HIV-infected choroid plexus. Monoclonal antibodies were used to detect class II major histocompatibility antigens (MHCs), S-100 and S-100ß protein, lymphocytes, monocyte/macrophage markers, and HIV glycoprotein. A variable number of stromal cells had slightly elongated nuclei and long branching processes that were strongly immunoreactive for class II MHCs, rarely reactive for S-100 and S-100ß protein, and immunonegative for monocyte/macrophage markers. Phagocytic activity was absent, as indicated by electron microscopy and immunomarkers. They were numerous in the subepithelial region, and their processes occasionally extended toward the stromal capillaries or between the epithelial cells of the choroid plexus. The HIV-infected cells were intensely immunoreactive for class II MHC markers and often displayed a dendritic morphology. These results document the presence of dendritic cells in the normal human choroid plexus whose morphology and immunophenotype closely resemble those of dendritic cells elsewhere in the body. They also show that these immunoreactive MHC class II cells are the cell type infected by HIV. The authors suggest that the functional activity of the dendritic cells of the choroid plexus is similar to that of antigen-presenting dendritic cells elsewhere in the body. This includes the potential to harbor HIV during the prolonged period of clinical latency, acting as a central nervous system reservoir of infection before the onset of AIDS.
Authors' Abstract

Meningioma Grading: An Analysis of Histologic Parameters. Arie Perry, Scott L. Stafford, Bernd W. Scheithauer, et al. *Am J Surg Pathol* 1997; 21:1455–1465. (A.P., Department of Anatomic Pathology, Mayo Clinic, 200 First St SW, Rochester, MN 55905)

Histologic grading of meningiomas has prognostic and sometimes therapeutic implications, but diagnostic criteria for atypical meningioma are vague, and the importance of brain invasion in the determination of malignancy remains controversial. The authors reviewed their experience with 581 patients whose meningiomas were resected at the Mayo Clinic during the years 1978–1988. All patients were followed up until death or a median of 9.0 years. Ten histologic parameters were assessed and compared with recurrence-free survival. At univariate analysis, six variables were associated with recurrence, although most were statistically significant only in the subset of patients who underwent gross total tumor resection. With multivariate analyses, the most statistically significant parameters were histologic brain invasion (when assessable) and maximal mitotic rate of at least four per 10 high-power fields. Also significant were combinations of at least three of the following four parameters: hypercellularity, architectural sheeting, macronucleoli, and small cell formation. Proposed grading criteria based on these findings yielded 81% classic, 15% atypical, and 4% brain invasive meningiomas with respective 5-year recurrence rates of 12%, 41%, and 56%. There was no association between histologic grade and either extent of surgical resection or patient age. However, male sex was associated with high-grade (atypical, brain invasive) tumors. Too few frankly anaplastic meningiomas were encountered for statistical analysis. Brain invasion and an increased mitotic index (at least four per 10 high-power fields) are the most powerful histologic factors prognostic for recurrence in meningiomas. The authors propose an objective definition for atypical meningioma on the basis of their data. Because the difference in recurrence rates for brain invasive and atypical meningiomas was not statistically significant, it could not be determined whether brain invasion alone warrants a designation of malignancy. Likewise, the authors were unable to determine what constitutes histologic anaplasia, due to the rarity of such cases.
Authors' Abstract

Pediatrics

Prognosis in Perthes' Disease: A Comparison of Radiological Predictors. A. M. Ismail, M. F. Macnicol. *J Bone Joint Surg [Br]* 1998; 80:310–314. (M.F.M., Princess Margaret Rose Orthopaedic Hospital, 41-43 Frogston Rd W, Edinburgh EH10 TED, Scotland)

The authors compared the prognostic value of the Catterall grouping, the Salter-Thompson grading, the arthrographic shape of the femoral head, and the Herring lateral pillar grouping during the fragmentation stage of Perthes disease in 73 patients with 81 affected hips. Radiographs were available for study from the onset of the disease until skeletal maturity. The authors used the Stulberg classification to assess outcome. The Herring grade and arthrographic sphericity proved to be the best predictors of final outcome. Combining these two values further increased the predictive value. All but one patient in Herring group A achieved an excellent outcome. In Herring group B, the age of the child and the sphericity of the femoral head influenced the end result. If the child was less than 7 years old at the onset of symptoms, the prognosis was invariably good, and all spherical hips in group B had a good outcome with Stulberg grade 1 or 2. Moderately and severely deformed hips on arthrography resulted in Stulberg grade 3 or 4 hips. None of the hips in Herring group C had a normal appearance at maturity, and the outcome was not substantially influenced by the age at onset or the arthrographic appearance.

Authors' Abstract

Inhaled Nitric Oxide for the Early Treatment of Persistent Pulmonary Hypertension of the Term Newborn: A Randomized, Double-masked, Placebo-controlled, Dose-Response, Multicenter Study. Dennis Davidson, Elaine S. Barefield, John Kattwinkel, et al. *Pediatrics* 1998; 101:325–334. (D.D., Division of Neonatal-Perinatal Medicine, Schneider Children's Hospital, Long Island Jewish Medical Center, New Hyde Park, NY 11040)

Persistent pulmonary hypertension of the newborn (PPHN) is a syndrome of acute respiratory failure characterized by systemic hypoxemia associated with extrapulmonary shunting of venous blood and evidence of elevated levels of pulmonary artery pressure in the absence of congenital heart disease. The syndrome occurs more commonly in term infants who have underlying diseases such as meconium aspiration, respiratory distress syndrome, sepsis, or lung hypoplasia, or it may be idiopathic. The diagnosis of PPHN is usually made within 24 hours of birth. The objective of this trial was to determine if early inhaled nitric oxide therapy would reduce the overall mortality rate, the need for extracorporeal membrane oxygenation (ECMO), or the incidence of neurologic sequelae or bronchopulmonary dysplasia. Randomized, placebo-controlled, double-masked, dose-response clinical trials were undertaken at 25 tertiary centers. The primary end point was the PPHN major sequelae index, which includes the incidence of death, ECMO, neurologic complications, or bronchopulmonary dysplasia. The patients were maintained on a fraction of inspired oxygen of 1.0, a mean airway pressure of at least 100 mm H_2O on a conventional ventilator, and echocardiographic evidence of PPHN. Previous treatment with exogenous surfactant and concomitant high-frequency ventilation and lung hypoplasia were exclusion factors. The results indicated that efficacy was similar for different nitric oxide doses. By 30 minutes, the Pa_{O_2} for only the nitric oxide groups increased significantly from 64 mm Hg ± 39 to 109 mm Hg ± 78, and the systemic arterial pressure remained unchanged. There was a significant reduction in the baseline-adjusted time-weighted oxygenation index in the nitric oxide groups for the first 24 hours of treatment. The ECMO rate was 34% for control and 22% for the nitric oxide doses. Inhaled nitric oxide produced an acute and sustained improvement in oxygenation for 24 hours in a majority of term infants with early but moderately severe PPHN. Oxygenation appeared stabilized to a greater degree by nitric oxide, whether or not treatment was successful. The need for ECMO was reduced by 35%, similar to statistically proved reductions in other clinical trials.

Beverly P. Wood, MD
Childrens Hospital, Los Angeles, Calif

The Use of Albuterol in Hospitalized Infants With Bronchiolitis. Joseph V. Dobson, Susan M. Stephens-Groff, Shawn R. McMahon, et al. *Pediatrics* 1998; 101:361–368. (J.V.D., Department of Pediatrics, Maricopa Medical Center, 2601 E Roosevelt, Phoenix, AZ 85010)

Bronchiolitis is an acute inflammatory respiratory illness occurring in the first 2 years of life and clinically characterized by fever, rhinitis, tachypnea, expiratory wheezing, and increased respiratory effort. Bronchiolitis is seasonal, with peak incidence in the winter and spring months. Viral agents have been identified as respiratory syncytial virus (RSV), parainfluenza, adenovirus, influenza, and rhinovirus. RSV is the most prevalent. The incidence of bronchiolitis is as high as 11 cases per 100 children per year for both the first and second 6 months of life. The traditional approach to management of symptoms of bronchiolitis has been supportive care, with attention to oxygen therapy, hydration, and respiratory support as needed. The objective of this study was to determine whether the use of nebulized albuterol enhanced physiologic or clinical recovery in hospitalized infants with moderate bronchiolitis. This prospective, double-blinded, placebo-controlled, randomized clinical trial, performed from December 1995 to March 1996, included 52 patients younger than 24 months with a diagnosis of moderately severe acute viral bronchiolitis. The patients were assigned to receive nebulized albuterol or a normal saline placebo for 72 hours. The outcome measures were improvement in oxygen saturation during hospitalization and survival analysis to assess the time needed to reach preestablished discharge criteria on three measures. Oxygen saturation (Sa_{O_2}), accessory muscle use, and wheezing were assessed. The actual length of the hospital stay was also measured. Fifty-eight patients were initially randomly assigned to the study protocol. A unique feature of this study was the attempt to evaluate whether albuterol enhances overall clinical and physiologic recovery independent of short-term bronchodilator effects. There was no significant difference in mean Sa_{O_2} between albuterol and placebo at baseline or at 24 hours or in maximum Sa_{O_2} during hospitalization. Both groups showed substantial improvement in oxygen saturation over time. There was no difference in time to reach discharge criteria as defined by Sa_{O_2}, accessory muscle use, or wheezing. Nebulized albuterol therapy does not appear to enhance recovery or attenuate the severity of illness in infants hospitalized with acute moderate bronchiolitis.

Beverly P. Wood, MD
Childrens Hospital, Los Angeles, Calif

Idiopathic Dilated Cardiomyopathy in Children: Prognostic Indicators and Outcome. Anita Arola, Juhani Tuominen, Olli Ruuskanen, et al. *Pediatrics* 1998; 101:369–376. (A.A., Department of Pediatrics, University of Turku, MediCity Research Laboratory, Tykistökatu 6 A, Turku FIN-20520, Finland)

Dilated cardiomyopathy is a heterogeneous group of myocardial diseases characterized by cardiac dilatation and impaired contractility of the myocardium. The majority of cases are idiopathic in origin. The prognosis may be poor, with a reported 5-year mortality of up to 80% in children. In this study, Finnish children and adolescents with idiopathic dilated cardiomyopathy (IDCM) were followed up for outcome. Sixty-two children and adolescents were enrolled, with a median age of 13 months (age range, 1 day to 20 years). During a mean follow-up of 3.9 years, 10 (16%) patients recovered, 17 (27%) had residual disease, four (6.4%) underwent heart transplantation, and 31 (50%) died. The poorest outcome was in infants younger than 1 year and adolescent male patients older than 15 years with progressing symptoms of left ventricular failure. The study results confirm that the outcome of children with IDCM remains poor; however, a group of patients, mainly infants older than 1 year, make a full recovery. Adolescent male patients and infants suffering from endocardial fibroelastosis with persisting symptoms of congestive failure have the poorest outcome. The patients need careful follow-up at short intervals. When there is no response to medical treatment, with resulting failure to grow, urgent heart transplantation should be offered.

Beverly P. Wood, MD
Childrens Hospital, Los Angeles, Calif

Complicated Parapneumonic Effusions in Children Caused by Penicillin-Nonsusceptible *Streptococcus pneumoniae*. William D. Hardie, Nancy E. Roberts, Shirley F. Reising, et al. *Pediatrics* 1998; 101:388–392. (W.D.H., Department of Pulmonary Medicine, Children's Hospital Medical Center, 3333 Burnett Ave, Cincinnati, OH 45229-3039)

The etiology of complicated parapneumonic effusions (CPEs) in children seems to have come full circle in 60 years. *Streptococcus pneumoniae* was recovered in nearly two-thirds of all cases of CPE in the preantibiotic era, but this proportion declined with an increase in cases caused by *Staphylococcus aureus* in the late 1950s, at which time *S aureus* accounted for up to 92% of CPEs in children. That incidence has since declined with the introduction of penicillinase-resistant penicillins and other antimicrobials effective against *S aureus*. Recent reports now describe *S pneumoniae* as again the principal bacterial pathogen in CPE, accounting for more than 70% of identified cases. Children with parapneumonic effusions were identified retrospectively, their charts were reviewed for data obtained at the time of hospital admission, and the families of children were reviewed to identify specific risk factors. Sixty-four cases of CPE were identified, all secondary to community-acquired pneumonia. In 35 cases, the effusions were sterile, with contaminants present in three cases; in one case, one colony each of coagulase-negative *Staphylococcus* and *Haemophilus* species were found. In 26 cases, a bacterial pathogen was recovered, with *S pneumoniae* identified in 23 (88%). CPEs caused by penicillin-nonsusceptible *S pneumoniae* occurred in younger patients, compared with CPEs that were penicillin susceptible (2.1 vs 7.9 years). Nonsusceptible effusions also had a higher incidence of bacteremia than penicillin-susceptible effusions (100% vs 29%). There were no substantial differences between the two groups for duration of tube drainage, febrile days, oxygen use, and hospital stay. In this study, 88% of the cases of CPE with an identified bacterial pathogen were pneumococcal. This contrasted with the many studies in the 1970s and 1980s that identified *S aureus* and *Haemophilus influenzae* as the most frequent bacterial isolates in CPE. In this study, patients with CPE caused by penicillin-nonsusceptible *S pneumoniae* were substantially younger than those with penicillin-susceptible effusions. There were no objective differences in outcome measures between the groups of patients. Clinicians treating patients with complicated parapneumonic effusions must maintain a high index of suspicion for *S pneumoniae* not susceptible to penicillin, particularly in young children.

Beverly P. Wood, MD
Childrens Hospital, Los Angeles, Calif

Trampoline Injuries. Gary A. Smith. *Pediatrics* 1998; 101:406–412. (Department of Emergency Medicine, Children's Hospital, 700 Children's Dr, Columbus, OH 43205)

The trampoline was introduced in the United States by circus acrobat George Nissen in 1936. The use of trampolines became more popular among the civilian population in the United States and Europe during the 1950s and 1960s, with the first trampoline-related injuries reported in 1956 and 1960. Outcomes included quadriplegia and death. The current study is a retrospective analysis of data for children (≤18 years old) with an estimated 249,400 trampoline-related injuries. The number of injuries increased by 98% from 1990 to 1995. The median age was 10 years, and 50% of those injured were boys. Ninety-three percent of the injuries occurred at home; injuries to the extremities predominated. Upper-extremity injuries tended to be fractures or dislocations, whereas lower-extremity injuries tended to be soft-tissue injuries. Fractures and dislocations accounted for 64% of upper-extremity injuries, compared with 26% of lower-extremity injuries. There was a direct relationship between age and lower-extremity injuries and soft-tissue injuries and an inverse relationship between age and facial injuries, head and neck injuries, and lacerations. Fractures or dislocations accounted for 83% of injuries among admitted or transferred children. Among children released home from the emergency department, soft-tissue injuries accounted for 53%; fractures or dislocations, 30%; and lacerations, 14%. The conclusion indicates that injuries from trampolines are an important cause of pediatric morbidity. Children should not use trampolines at home, and the sale of trampolines for private recreational use should be stopped.

Beverly P. Wood, MD
Childrens Hospital, Los Angeles, Calif

Surgical Treatment of Gastroesophageal Reflux in Children: A Combined Hospital Study. Eric W. Fonkalsrud, Keith W. Ashcraft, Arnold G. Coran, et al. *Pediatrics* 1998; 101: 419–422. (E.W.F., Department of Surgery, UCLA School of Medicine, 10833 Le Conte, Los Angeles, CA 90095)

Gastroesophageal reflux is one of the most frequent symptomatic clinical disorders of the gastrointestinal tract in infants and children, as well as in adults. Gastroesophageal reflux has been recognized more frequently because of increased awareness of the condition and because of more sophisticated diagnostic techniques. Gastroesophageal fundoplication is currently one of the three most common major operations performed in infants and children in the United States. The present study was undertaken to provide a large clinical experience in the surgical treatment of gastroesophageal reflux by combining the clinical data from seven large children's surgery centers in the United States. The study included 7,467 patients who underwent anti-reflux operations. The most common symptoms in these children were failure to thrive (39.9%), feeding disorders (35.9%), respiratory symptoms (32.6%), and esophagitis (11.9%). An esophagram with an upper gastrointestinal series was the most frequently obtained diagnostic study in six of the hospitals, or 67.9% of the patients. The study was abnormal in 68.2% of the patients in whom it was obtained. Esophageal pH monitoring was performed in 54.2%, with abnormal findings in 94.5%. Esophagoscopy was performed in 25.6%, with esophagitis demonstrated in 70.1%. An isotope gastric emptying study was performed in 32%, with abnormal gastric emptying and more than 50% retention of the isotope meal at 90 minutes demonstrated in 58.8% of patients. Of the children undergoing fundoplication, 40% were under 12 months of age. The type of anti-reflux operation was Nissen fundoplication in 64%, Thal fundoplication in 34%, and Toupet fundoplication in 1.5%. Good to excellent results after fundoplication, as indicated by substantial clinical improvement in preoperative symptoms, were recorded in 94% of neurologically normal and 84.6% of neurologically impaired children. Major complications occurred in 4.2% and 12.8%, respectively. The most frequent complications were recurrent reflux, respiratory symptoms, gas bloating, and intestinal obstruction. The excellent results and low morbidity associated with gastroesophageal fundoplication, with or without a gastric emptying procedure, indicate that surgery should be used early for symptomatic gastroesophageal reflux in neurologically normal children and to facilitate enteral feedings and care in neurologically impaired children.

Beverly P. Wood, MD
Childrens Hospital, Los Angeles, Calif

Classified Services

POLICY

As a service to its readers, *Radiology* accepts classified advertising, and every effort is made to ensure that the ads are relevant to the practice of radiology. Acceptable categories include positions available, positions sought, fellowships, announcements of postgraduate courses or symposia, practices for sale, medical facilities for rent or sale, used radiologic equipment and apparatus for sale, medical employment bureau advertising, academic posts to be filled, available posts for interns and residents, and malpractice insurance. We retain the right to refuse any advertisement considered not relevant, and respondents are advised to investigate each offer since we cannot assume responsibility for the offers or claims of advertisers.

RATES (per insertion)

Line ads in *Radiology* (no agency commission)

50 words or less $90.00

51–100 words $135.00

Each word over 100—$1.00 per word.

Box Number—$30.00 additional per each insertion (this service is optional).

TERMS

Payment must accompany order.* Make checks payable to **Radiological Society of North America.** We accept American Express, VISA, Mastercard, and Diners Club for classified ads. Call for details. Send payment to:

RSNA, Radiology Classified Ad Department
Accounts Payable, 2021 Spring Road, Suite 600
Oak Brook, IL 60523-1860 USA.

*Purchase Order Numbers are accepted with prior approval.

Please mark each issue:

❒ Jan ❒ Feb ❒ Mar ❒ Apr ❒ May ❒ June
❒ July ❒ Aug ❒ Sept ❒ Oct ❒ Nov ❒ Dec

Send invoice and tearsheet to:

____
____
____
____

Advertisers who cancel ads will not receive refunds.

DEADLINE

Copy must be received by the **20th of the second month preceding issue.** Please submit copy typed and double-spaced. Initials or abbreviations equal one word. Telephone numbers with area code equal one word.

CLASSIFIED DISPLAY ADVERTISING

Black and white frequency rates are based on the total number of insertions used within a 12-month period from date of first insertion.

Ad Space	Size	1X	6X	12X
1 page	7" x 9-1/2"	$2250	2170	2090
2/3 pg vert	4-1/2" x 9-1/2"	$1900	1830	1760
1/2 pg horzt	7" x 4-1/2"	$1350	1300	1250
1/2 pg vert	3-3/8" x 9-1/2"	$1350	1300	1250
1/2 pg island	4-1/4" x 7-1/2"	$1350	1300	1250
1/3 pg vert	2-1/4" x 9-1/2"	$1085	1045	1005
1/3 pg square	4-1/2" x 4-1/2"	$1085	1045	1005
1/4 page	3-3/8" x 4-1/2"	$ 850	820	790
1/6 page	2-1/4" x 4-1/2"	$ 605	585	565
1/9 page	2-1/4" x 3"	$ 420	400	380

Preferred materials are composite negatives, right-reading, emulsion side down. (Conversion materials such as positive film, repro proofs, and camera-ready artworks are acceptable at additional charge.)

Customer supplied negative: cost as noted
Customer supplied mechanical: add 10%
Customer supplied copy to be set and ad prepared: add 20%

Call Production Department for additional information. Address for correspondence, insertion orders, copy, proofs, box number, and payment:

***Radiology* Advertising Production Office**
2021 Spring Road, Suite 600
Oak Brook, IL 60523-1860

To respond to a box number ad, send your CV and/or any other information to the above address; on the front of the envelope, please indicate the appropriate box number.

For further information:
Carissa Mucccianti, *Advertising Coordinator*
630.571.7817

Positions Available

INTERVENTIONAL RADIOLOGIST—Charlotte Radiology, a 42-member private, subspecialty based, radiology practice is seeking an ABR certified fellowship trained interventional radiologist with covered stent graft experience to join four other interventional radiologists. The practice covers all facets of interventional practice in a large level one trauma center and in three other acute care hospitals. Total beds covered are 1300. The hospital system has an active teaching program and an active multidisciplinary tumor program is in place. Send CV to A. Van Moore Jr, MD, c/o Diann McGuirt, Charlotte Radiology, PO Box 36937, Charlotte, NC 28236-6937.

DIAGNOSTIC RADIOLOGY—Neuro-interventionalist - Yale New Haven Medical Center, Yale University School of Medicine, is seeking a radiologist with fellowship training or significant experience in interventional neuroradiology. Academic rank depends on qualifications. Leadership of an active and growing neurointerventional service, in conjunction with outstanding colleagues in neurovascular surgery, neurology, neurosurgery, plastic surgery and ENT, is sought. The department emphasizes research and teaching and provides training and mentoring to faculty interested in developing careers in academic medicine. Applications from qualified women and members of minority groups are encouraged. Yale University is an equal opportunity/affirmative action employer. Please send inquiries along with curriculum vitae to Bruce L. McClennan, MD, Chair, Yale University School of Medicine, Department of

nity hospitals in beautiful western Montana. Full partnership track. Send CV with cover letter to Intercity Radiology, PC, 300 N Wilson, Suite 403D, Bozeman, MT 59715. Phone 406-587-8631, fax 406-587-1343.

BOARD CERTIFIED RADIOLOGISTS—Rapidly growing group in northeastern Pennsylvania seeks two aggressive Board certified radiologists with fellowship trainining in nuclear medicine and body imaging/MRI. State-of-the-art equipment including: GE LCA digital angio suite, GE Spiral CT with SUN workstation, two digital fluoroscopy suites, ATL HDI 5000 and Ultramark 9, Siemans Dual Head E Cam, fixed GE MRI, stereotactic breast. Outstanding opportunity to practice general radiology and to build the practice in your area of expertise. Excellent financial package with early partnership. Address inquiries to David Fontaine, MD, Chairman, 717-621-4420. Fax CV to 717-621-4582.

FACULTY - ULTRASOUND/ABDOMINAL IMAGING—The Department of Radiology, Beth Israel Deaconess Medical Center, Harvard Medical School is seeking applicants for a faculty position in the ultrasound section/abdominal imaging. We are seeking an individual with interest in clinical or basic research utilizing advanced ultrasound technology such as ultrasound contrast imaging, image reconstruction, outcomes analysis or ultrasound interventional techniques. Research should be focused on abdominal or general ultrasound categories. Additional responsibilities include clinical work in ultrasound (primarily abdominal and general ultrasound, but possibly including some OB/GYN) and other abdominal imaging including CT and fluoroscopy. Clinical responsibilities include teaching and supervision of residents, fellows, and medical students. Significant participation and contributions in ongoing or independently developed research is expected. The Ultrasound Section performs over 31,000 examinations per year, with active inpatient and outpatient clinical sites. State-of-the-art imaging equipment is available at all sites which are linked via an ALI PACS system, which is part of a larger GE PACS for all cross-sectional imaging. There are nine members of the ultrasound staff with research interests in abdominal, vascular, and OB/GYN ultrasound, and there are four abdominal imaging fellows and two women's imaging fellows. Applicants should be Board certified in diagnostic radiology, have fellowship training, and be eligible for licensure in the state of Massachusetts. Salary and academic rank will be commensurate with experience and qualifications. Interested applicants should send curriculum vitae to Robert A. Kane, MD, Associate Chief for Administration and Director of Ultrasound, Department of Radiology, Beth Israel Deaconess Medical Center, One Deaconess Rd, Boston, MA 02215. For further information contact Dr Kane at 617-754-2528, fax 617-754-2545, or e-mail *rkane@bidmc.harvard.edu*. Beth Israel Deaconess Medical Center is an EEO/AA employer. Visit our website at *www.bidmc.harvard.edu/radiology*.

RADIOLOGIST—Private progressive hospital based practice located in South central Kentucky is seeking Board certified. The practice has multiple hospital and outpatient locations, but is linked by teleradiography. The facilities offer state-of-the-art technology. The practice includes MRI, ultrasound, angiography, CT, mammography, nuclear medicine, and general radiology. The position offers an excellent compensation package. Please provide a curriculum vitae and names of references to Mona Wood, Physician Recruiter, 800 Park St, PO Box 9867, Bowling Green, KY 42102; fax 502-745-1518.

NUCLEAR MEDICINE STAFF POSITION—Candidate with strong interest in an academic career to join an active and well-equipped laboratory. Excellent research and clinical facilities are available and include all modern imaging modalities. Appointment will be at the rank of Assistant or Associate Professor in the clinician track depending on the years of experience and other qualifications. Candidates must be Board eligible or certified in nuclear medicine. For further information, please contact Abass Alavi, MD, Chief, Division of Nuclear Medicine, Hospital of the University of Pennsylvania, 3400 Spruce St, Philadelphia, PA 19104. AA/EOE.

ALLEGHENY UNIVERSITY OF THE HEALTH SCIENCES, ALLEGHENY GENERAL PITTSBURGH, PA; CHAIR, DIAGNOSTIC RADIOLOGY—Allegheny University Hospitals, Allegheny General, a 728-bed academic health center serving Pittsburgh and the surrounding five state area, is seeking a dynamic leader with strong clinical, administrative and academic skills to Chair a state-of-the-art, tertiary Department of Radiology staffed by 15 full-time radiologists performing approximately 250,000 examinations a year, including a full range of diagnostic and interventional procedures. The department oversees an ACGME accredited residency program, as well as a neuroradiology fellowship and a school of radiology technology. Appointment will be at the academic rank of Professor at the MCP Hahnemann School of Medicine, Allegheny University of the Health Sciences. Send CV to Jan F. Silverman, MD, Chairman, Department of Pathology, Allegheny University Hospitals, Allegheny General and Chair, Diagnostic Radiology Search Committee, Allegheny General, 320 E North Ave, Pittsburgh, PA 15212; telephone 412-359-6886 or fax 412-359-3598.

MUSCULOSKELETAL RADIOLOGISTS—The University of Pittsburgh School of Medicine is seeking a musculoskeletal radiologist at the Assistant Professor level for expansion of subspecialty service within our healthcare system. Candidates should have completed a musculoskeletal fellowship or equivalent, and be skilled in all aspects of musculoskeletal imaging including interventional procedures. Responsibilities include medical student, resident and fellow teaching, academic activities and patient care. The section enjoys a broad range of cases and close interaction with outstanding Departments of Orthopaedics, Emergency Medicine and Rheumatology. Send letters of inquiry and curriculum vitae to Jeffrey D. Towers, MD, Director of Musculoskeletal Imaging, University of Pittsburgh Medical Center, 200 Lothrop St, Pittsburgh, PA 15213. The University of Pittsburgh School of Medicine is an equal opportunity employer.

DUKE-AFFILIATED VETERAN AFFAIRS HOSPITAL—Is seeking a fellowship trained neuroradiologist interested in joining our academically oriented, clinical radiology practice. The successful applicant will spend 6/8ths of their time at the Durham VA Medical Center. Two-eights of their time will be spent as a neuroradiologist at the Duke University Medical Center which is adjacent to the VA Hospital. Candidates must have documented skills in all aspects of neuroimaging including neurorangiography, myelography, neuro CT and neuro MRI. Applicants willing and qualified to provide limited clinical service in body imaging (CT, ultrasound, MRI) will be given preference. Applicants must have sufficient experience in an academic radiology environment to excel in resident teaching, post-graduate education or limited writing of scientific papers. Successful candidates must meet criteria for academic appointment to Duke University Medical Center. Non-clinical time is regularly scheduled for the pursuit of academic projects and teaching preparation. The Durham VA is an integral site in the training of Duke radiology residents and, therefore, a strong commitment to resident teaching is required. All seven VA faculty members are experienced teachers, most with academic appointments at Duke. The position is ideal for applicants seeking an environment in which high quality clinical neuroradiology is practiced and opportunities for teaching and research are readily available. Benefits and salary are competitive. Applicants meeting all of the above criteria should submit their CVs to Dr Robert M. Vandemark, Chief of Radiology, Durham VA Medical Center, 508 Fulton St, Durham, NC 27705. EOE.

RADIATION ONCOLOGY DEPARTMENT CHAIR WANTED, UNIVERSITY OF MICHIGAN—The University of Michigan is seeking an academic leader to chair the Department of Radiation Oncology. Qualifications include an MD degree and Board certification in Radiation Oncology. Candidates should be recognized leaders in radiation oncology and have a record of scholarly achievement, including research in fundamental areas of radiation biology; clinical and management experience; and a commitment to excellence in medical and graduate medical education. Experience in conducting complex clinical and research programs in the setting of a large academic medical center with multi-institutional satellite facilities is highly desirable. Interested candidates should send a curriculum vitae by August 1, 1998 to Radiation Oncology Search Committee, c/o Linda Diebold, M7310 Med Sci I, University of Michigan Medical School, Ann Arbor, MI 48109-0624. The University of Michigan is a non-discriminatory, affirmative action employer. Women and minority candidates are encouraged to apply.

INTERVENTIONAL RADIOLOGIST—The Department of Diagnostic Radiology and Nuclear Medicine of Rush Medical College, Chicago, IL is seeking two vascular/interventional radiologists. The position will include teaching responsibilities at Rush-Presbyterian St. Luke's Medical Center, a 600-bed acute and tertiary care facility. The section performs approximately 6,000 vascular and non-vascular interventions per year. In this private practice group in an academic teaching hospital, CAQ eligibility is required. Interested parties should contact Terence A.S. Matalon, MD, Rush Presbyterian-St. Luke's Medical Center, 1653 W Congress Pkwy, Chicago, IL 60612. Rush-Presbyterian-St. Luke's Medical Center is an equal opportunity/affirmative action employer. Women and minority candidates are encouraged to apply.

PEDIATRIC RADIOLOGIST—KK Women's and Children's Hospital (KKH) of Singapore has an opening for a fellowship-trained pediatric radiologist to join four full-time faculty members. Requirements include a Board certification/FRCR or equivalent, and at least 1-year of pediatric radiology fellowship experience (the latter can be arranged). Compensation and rank will be commensurate with experience and qualifications. KKH is the newest (1997) and largest women's and children's hospital in Singapore, performing 75,000 examinations per year, using up to date facilities. Address inquiries to Anne Kendrick, MD, Diagnostic Imaging, KK Women's and Children's Hospital, 100 Bukit Timah Rd, Singapore 229899; fax 65-394-2254, e-mail *annetan@kkh.com.sg*.

TWO NEURORADIOLOGIST - CONNECTICUT—Fellowship-trained neuroradiologists with CAQ eligibility and fellowship trained body imaging specialists sought by growing, progressive, subspecialty-oriented group of 15 radiologists. Yale affiliated, community hospital-based private practice with residents and separate outpatient facilities. Position available now, but will wait for right person. Responsibilities divided between subspecialty area and general office and hospital radiology. Excellent opportunities with expectation for partnership. Send CV to Alan Kaye, MD, 777 Commerce Dr, Fairfield, CT 06432, or fax to 203-384-4363.

THE UNIVERSITY OF KENTUCKY—Is seeking a full-time, tenured line, open rank academic thoracic radiologist. Must be Board eligible; certification preferred. Duties would also include interpretation of film for evaluation of occupational lunch disease. Responsibilities include patient care, medical student and resident teaching, and regularly scheduled interdepartment conferences. Opportunity to pursue clinical research. Please mail or fax letter of interest and curriculum vitae to James C. Reed, MD, Chairman, Department of Radiology, HX304, UK Medical Center, Lexington, KY 40536-0084; fax 606-257-6014. UK is an equal opportunity employer.

ASSISTANT PROFESSOR - THREE POSITIONS—Temple University School of Medicine, Department of Diagnostic Imaging, three positions available at the rank of Assistant Professor to participate in clinical, teaching and research activities. Neuroradiology: Board certified with completed 2-year neuroradiology fellowship; CAQ certified or eligible; eligible for senior membership in ASNR; experience in pediatric neuroradiology would be advantageous. Clinical responsibilities in CT, MRI, special procedures, head and neck, and pediatric neuroradiology. Candidate's special interest in interventional neuroradiology can be accommodated. Abdominal imaging: Board certified and fellowship trained with primary interest in the areas of ultrasound and MRI. Vascular/Interventional radiology: Board certified, fellowship trained, CAQ certified or eligible. Position requires rotation with three current VIR faculty to provide additional clinical services and support for the ACGME accredited fellowship training program. Active clinical research work is being pursued in proton spectroscopy, diffusion/perfusion and functional MRI. Available equipment: two 1.5 GE Signa MRI scanners; two Picker spiral CT scanners; two Voxel-Q work stations for the three dimensional imaging and virtual endoscopy; seven ultrasound scanners; a CVIS system, for endoluminal and vascular ultrasound; CTA, MRA, and endovascular ultrasound. Imminent additions include an open MRI scanner, a PET scanner, and a biplane neuro/angio room. Filmless radiographic system is in place. Department converting to a fully digital format using an AGFA network. Applicants should forward a cover letter and curriculum vitae to Robert A. Gatenby, MD, Professor and Chairperson, Department of Diagnostic Imaging, Temple University School of Medicine, 3401 N. Broad St, Philadelphia, PA 19140. Temple University is an EEO/AA employer and strongly encourages applications from women and minorities.

RADIOLOGIST NEEDED—Linde Healthcare specializes in radiology locum tenens. We have openings for short and long-term assignments. Currently we are recruiting radiologists interested in working to improve their standard of living a manner that fits their lifestyle. Whether you want to work full-time, pick up extra hours on weekends and during vacation, or explore opportunities leading to permanent placement, we present opportunities leading to permanent placement, we present opportunities matching your specific needs. We provide competitive compensation, malpractice insurance, travel and lodging. You should be working with a company maintaining a high level of confidentiality with solid success history. Call Tammy Winters at 800-588-4343, fax your CV to 314-843-2262 or send e-mail to *Winters@lindehc.com.*

MRA AND FMRI ARE ESSENTIAL—Interest in research and teaching are important and opportunities exist to work with MS, alzeheimers disease, movement disorder, epilepsy, and stroke centers. Faculty rank dependent on publication and academic accomplishments. Send curriculum vitae to Michael S. Huckman, MD, Director of Neuroradiology, Rush-Presbyterian-St. Luke's Medical Center, 1653 W Congress Pkwy, Chicago, IL 60612. Phone 312-942-5781, fax 312-942-2114, e-mail *mhuckman@rush.edu.* RPSLMC is an AA/EOE employer.

THE UNIVERSITY OF KENTUCKY—Is seeking a full-time, tenured line academic neuroradiologist, with interventional neuroradiology expertise. Must be willing to cross cover in other areas. Responsibilities include patient care, medical student and resident teaching, and regularly scheduled interdepartment conferences. Must be CAQ certified or eligible for certification. Senior membership in the ASNR desired. Opportunity for research with nationally known Alzheimer's Research Center, with busy neurosurgery department. Please mail or fax letter of interest and curriculum vitae to James C. Reed, MD, Chairman, Department of Radiology, HX304, UK Medical Center, Lexington, KY 40536-0084; fax 606-257-6014. UK is an equal opportunity employer.

LOVELACE HEALTH SYSTEMS - ALBUQUERQUE, NM—A 300-physician multi-specialty practice, 14-member radiology department seeks two BC/BE radiologists: one interventional radiologist, CAQ preferred, and one fellowship trained body imaging radiologist. Comprehensive benefits package and state-of-the-art equipment. Contact Cheryl DeVita, 222 S Central Ave, Suite 400, St. Louis, MO 63105. Phone 800-678-7858, ID#5869RA, fax 314-726-0026, e-mail *cdevita@cejka.com.*

INTERVENTIONALIST NEEDED—Looking for young superstar interventionalist to earn his/her way into full partnership in the premier radiology group in the mid-Hudson Valley. Maintain skills in all aspects of imaging with state-of-the-art equipment and expert colleagues while helping to lead the interventional department of a 300-bed tertiary care hospital. Many outpatient offices also including multiple MRI/CT sites. Send CV or call V. Gaines, MD, Department Imaging, Vassar Brothers Hospital, Reade Place, Poughkeepsie, NY 12601; 914-431-5644.

THE DEPARTMENT OF RADIOLOGY, VIRGINIA COMMONWEALTH UNIVERSITY, MEDICAL COLLEGE OF VIRGINIA CAMPUS, RICHMOND, VA—Seeks candidates for several faculty positions in diagnostic radiology. These include positions in musculoskeletal/emergency radiology, angiography/interventional radiology, abdominal imaging. ABR certification or eligibility required. Fellowship training and interest in teaching and research are preferred. MCV Hospital is a 1,058-bed facility and a level I trauma center. Individuals should have experience working in a culturally diverse environment. Academic rank and salary commensurate with experience. For position description, or to submit CV, write or phone B.J. Manaster, MD, PhD, Department of Radiology, PO Box 980470, Richmond, VA 23298-0470; 804-828-6600, 804-823-6129 fax. VCU/MCV is an equal opportunity/affirmative action employer. Women, minorities, and persons with disabilities are encouraged to apply.

IMMEDIATE OPENING FOR TWO RADIOLOGISTS WITH CROSS-SECTIONAL IMAGING BACKGROUND, FELLOWSHIP PREFERRED BUT NOT A REQUIREMENT—Large progressive group near metropolitan Chicago in northwest Indiana. Covering four hospitals, several clinics and a free-standing imaging center, four MRIs, several CTs, state-of-the-art ultrasound and in-home PET scanner. Please send CV to Radiologic Associates of Northwest Indiana, Inc, 825 E. Lincolnway, Valparaiso, IN 46383 or call Dr James Forde at 219-464-4891.

BODY IMAGER - SEATTLE, WA—Radiology Consultants of Washington is an eight member outpatient private practice group that has an immediate opening for an ABR certified, fellowship trained body imager. Position will emphasize musculoskeletal and spinal MRI, helical CT, and ultrasound. Applicants should possess strong leadership skills and be comfortable with all aspects of outpatient radiology. Dynamic young group, competitive compensation and benefits, partnership track position, fabulous pacific northwest location. Please reply with CV to Randall K. Petersen, MD, Radiologist Consultants of Washington, 1041 116th Ave NE, Suite 101, Bellevue, WA 98004, or fax to 425-462-8309.

NUCLEAR MEDICINE RADIOLOGIST—A 14-person, expanding radiology group is seeking fellowship trained radiologist as division head. Highly competitive salary and fringe benefit package. Equal shareholder status and income after 1st-year if mutually agreeable. Practice located in the LeHigh of Pennsylvania. Hospital network includes three hospitals and three imaging centers; 200,000 examinations per year. Academic affiliation with major Philadelphia University, five residency programs, and a brand new level II trauma center. Call David W. Wilder, MD; 610-954-4808; fax CV 610-954-6455 or e-mail *dwilder@fast.net.*

NEURORADIOLOGIST - SEATTLE, WA—Growing eight member outpatient private practice group has an immediate opening for

Radiologist

Northwest Mississippi Regional Medical Center in Clarksdale, MS, a Health Management Associates, Inc. hospital, is seeking an experienced, general radiologist trained in all modalities with good interventional skills *(with or without a Fellowship in Interventional Radiology.)* Must be Board Certified in Radiology.

$300,000 income guaranteed.

Establish your practice in a comprehensive, newly renovated radiology department with state-of-the art equipment located in a rapidly expanding market serving a large rural area in the Mississippi Delta.

Wonderful small town quality of life with "Big City" culturally diverse amenities within a short drive. Excellent schools, team and outdoor sports, sportsman's paradise.

Please send CV to Clinton Eaves, Associate Executive Director, Northwest MS Regional Medical Center, P. O. Box 1218, Clarksdale, MS 38614. All replies will be handled confidentially.

Northwest MS Regional Medical Center is an Equal Opportunity Employer.

RADIOLOGIST

Gundersen Lutheran is seeking a board certified/board eligible Radiologist who has completed a fellowship in Magnetic Resonance Imaging to add to our rapidly expanding department. A new Siemens 1.5 T Vision unit and open system have just recently been installed.

Gundersen Lutheran is a large multi-specialty group practice with over 320 physicians located in La Crosse, WI. It's main campus is attached to a 402 bed acute care hospital. The Gundersen Lutheran system includes 36 regional community clinics based throughout western Wisconsin, eastern Minnesota and northeastern Iowa. Gundersen Lutheran is a modern state-of-the-art facility that has a service area for a population base of over 530,000. Gundersen Lutheran is also the designated western campus of the University of Wisconsin Medical School.

La Crosse, Wisconsin, nestled between towering bluffs, is located where the Mississippi, La Crosse, and Black Rivers merge. The area was untouched by the glaciers, leaving many hills and valleys. The metropolitan area of La Crosse, with its 100,000 people, offers exceptional year round opportunities for recreational activities. The area also offers outstanding public and private schools, low crime rates, and cultural activities.

We offer competitive salaries and excellent fringe benefits. Interested candidates should send a letter of application and curriculum vitae to Frank Perez-Guerra, Director, Recruitment, Retention, and Resource Planning, Gundersen Lutheran, 1836 South Avenue, La Crosse, WI 54601; or call 800-362-9567, Ext. 6325.

Equal Opportunity Employer

Gundersen Lutheran

a CAQ certified neuroradiologist. Position will emphasize spinal imaging and procedures; no angiography. Applicants should possess strong leadership skills and be comfortable with general outpatient radiology. Dynamic young group, competitive compensation and benefits, partnership track position, fabulous pacific northwest location. Please reply with CV to Randall K. Petersen, MD, Radiologist Consultants of Washington, 1041 116th Ave NE, Suite 101, Bellevue, WA 98004, or fax to 425-462-8309.

NEURORADIOLOGIST—Georgetown University has a unique opportunity to join an academic radiology group in Washington, DC. The neuroradiology section includes four faculty and four fellows. Excellent collaborative research opportunities exist with the Georgetown Imaging Science and Information Systems group, the Georgetown Institute for Cognitive and Computational Sciences, and the neighboring National Institutes of Health in Bethesda, MD. The candidate should exhibit special interest and knowledge in neuro MRI. Experience with non-anatomic or functional MRI and background in research are desirable. Working skills in traditional invasive techniques (diagnostic angiography, myelography, etc), Board certification, and a certificate of added qualification in neuroradiology (or eligibility) are required. The Department of Radiology operates two 1.5T Siemens magnets (Vision), three advanced GE CT scanners (two helical) and a new Siemens Neurostar angio/interventional suite. The position is expected to be filled on or before July 1, 1999. Interested parties should contact Michael J. Pentecost, MD, Professor and Chairman, Department of Radiology, Georgetown University Medical Center, 3800 Reservoir Rd, NW, Washington, DC, e-mail *pentecom@gunet.georgetown.edu*, fax 202-687-1804.

DIAGNOSTIC RADIOLOGIST, ISLAND OF GUAM—Immediate opening available in a recently opened private imaging office. GE spiral CT, Accuson sonography and general radiography support a full cancer treatment center as well as outpatient referrals. Opportunity for cross coverage with an affiliated Maui, HI based diagnostic radiology group. Partnership track, apartment and auto provided. Please send CV and direct inquiries ro Mr Nick Gladdis, Administrative Director, 221 Mahalani St, Wailuku, HI 96793; phone 808-242-2054, fax 808-242-1940, e-mail *mrc@maui.net*.

MAUI, HI—Hospital based radiology group seeks Board certified radiologist for evening and night coverage position. This 200-bed facility includes diagnostic radiology, interventional/angiography, nuclear medicine, computerized tomography, ultrasound and magnetic resonance. Basic angiography/interventional skills are a plus. As part of the interview process candidates will be required to spend a minimum of one week in locum tenens position in the hospital environment. Please send CV and direct inquiries to Mr Nick Gladdis, Administrative Director, 221 Mahalani St, Wailuku, HI 96793; phone 808-242-2054, fax 808-242-1940, e-mail *mrc@maui.net*.

NUCLEAR RADIOLOGIST—The Penn State Geisinger Health System is currently seeking a fellowship trained and licensed nuclear radiologist to join the Geisinger Medical Center in Danville, PA. The practice will combine general and nuclear radiology. Background and experience in nuclear medicine, MRI, CT, ultrasound and general diagnostic radiology is preferred. Call coverage is on a rotational basis with 12 other diagnostic radiologists. The position will include both clinical and teaching responsibilities in a 458-bed tertiary care hospital and level 1 trauma center with its own radiology program. Geisinger Medical Center supports a 40 county area throughout northeastern and

HSC

MUSCULOSKELETAL RADIOLOGIST

The Department of Radiology of SUNY, Health Science Center at Syracuse, University Hospital, is currently seeking a diagnostic radiologist with expertise in the following areas: musculoskeletal radiology including MRI and general diagnostic radiology. Fellowship training in musculoskeletal radiology is preferred but not mandatory. The candidate should be board certified, eligible for both academic appointment at the State University of New York and licensure in the state of New York. An interest and willingness to participate in a teaching program for residents and rotating medical students is required. The ability and willingness to cover more than one area in diagnostic radiology is preferred. Salary and academic rank are commensurate with experience. Applicants should forward a letter of interest along with his/her CV to:

Leonard S. Hojnowski, M.D.
Department of Radiology
University Hospital
750 E. Adams StreetSyracuse, NY 13210
Phone: 315/464-7487, Fax: 315/464-7458

MAYO CLINIC SCOTTSDALE

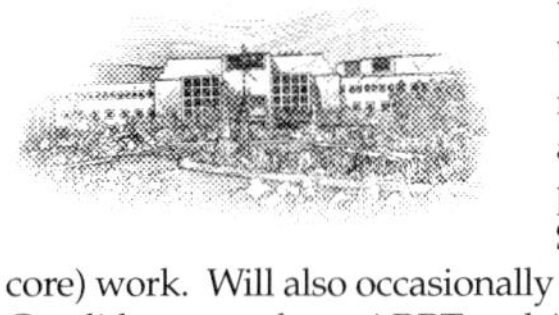

Mammographer

Will produce high-quality mammography images and assist with quality assurance programs, as well as perform Stereotactic/biopsy (needle core) work. Will also occasionally rotate into general radiology. Candidate must have ARRT and Arizona MRTBE license as well as mammography certification. Minimum 1 year of experience in mammography.

MAYO CLINIC SCOTTSDALE OFFERS AN EXCELLENT SALARY AND BENEFITS PACKAGE. RELOCATION ASSISTANCE AVAILABLE.

If you can imagine yourself contributing to the Mayo tradition of excellence, send your scannable resume, indicating position desired to: Mayo Clinic Scottsdale, Human Resources, 13400 E. Shea Blvd., Scottsdale, AZ 85259, or e-mail: staffing.arizona@mayo.edu; or call our 24-hour employment information line at 602-301-7678; or visit our website at www.mayo.edu

As an equal opportunity employer, we value diversity. Mayo Clinic Scottsdale conducts reference and background checks; drug testing is required of all new hires.

Mayo Clinic Scottsdale uses a computerized resume database. Resumes are accepted on a continuous basis for all positions. Individuals interested in other opportunities are encouraged to send a resume to Human Resources. Specific skills and education (i.e., RN, BSN, Word, Excel, PowerPoint) should be listed. For best results, please use a standard typeface (10-14 points recommended) and avoid using graphics and dark colored paper.

mayo

central Pennsylvania. We offer a competitive salary and excellent benefit package. For additional information regarding this opportunity please contact Kurt Scott, Penn State Geisinger Health System, Department of Professional Staffing and Credentialing (RAD-CT), 100 N Academy Ave, Danville, PA 17822-1528. Phone 800-845-7112. CVs can be faxed to 800-622-2515. EOE M/F/H/V.

TWO FULL-TIME RADIOLOGY POSITIONS—Available at LSUMC/University Medical Center in Lafayette, LA. Looking for hardworking radiologists for clinical work, teaching and research. Must be familiar with all imaging modalities. A 180-bed hospital with a separate radiology/oncology department, outpatient clinic, 25 technologists and eight clerical staff, performs 70,000 exams per year. State license required to practice but not to interview. Please send CV to Leonard R. Bok, MD, or Mark Gerscovich, MD, University Medical Center, 2390 W Congress, Lafayette, LA 70506; 318-261-6244. LSUMC is an EEO/AA employer.

SOUTHERN LOUISIANA—Growing community of 104,000 population is seeking a particular type of radiologist. We need a women's health specialist. Focus is to work at the Women's hospital. No MRI work involved. Primarily, breast biopsy, mammography, and CT. Call coverage 1:2 with a salary of $180,000 plus full benefits; 1-year to partnership! Great practice and community! Area has large university and metro amenities. Easy access to LSU and New Orleans! For details, call David at 800-677-7987 or fax CV to 800-440-2676; e-mail *dbgmsg@swbell.net*, website *www.medopps-hka.com*.

PITTSBURGH, VA-RADIOLOGY-NUCLEAR MEDICINE—Group of eight physicians is seeking a general radiologist. Advanced MRI musculoskeletal training desirable but not required. Our institution is the tertiary referral medical center among five VA centers in the western Pennsylvania and West Virginia, as well as for liver transplantation. It is close to and affiliated with the University of Pittsburgh School of Medicine. State-of-the-art equipment in all modalities. Please send CV to Herbert A. Klein, MD, PhD, Nuclear Medicine (132N-U), VA Pittsburgh Healthcare System, University Dr, Pittsburgh, PA 15240 or fax to 412-688-6907.

MEDICAL DIRECTOR RADIOLOGY SERVICES—Opportunity available for a Medical Director, Radiology Services in a Regional Medical Center located in the Pacific Northwest. Hospital and staff provide regional services in cancer, neurologic, rehabilitation, trauma, and all other medical specialty areas. The candidates should be capable of neuroaxial imaging and interventional radiology. State-of-the-art equipment includes CT, MRI, nuclear medicine, and digital an-

Radiology Opportunities in Virginia

Lexington, Virginia

Metro American Radiology, a Team Health affiliate, is seeking a radiologist to join our group in Lexington, Virginia. The position involves a commitment of approximately 35 weeks per year. Candidates must be board certified and well trained in all imaging modalities, including MRI.

Lexington is a 19th century college town located in the heart of the Shenandoah Valley of Virginia. The town is rich in history and is the home of Washington and Lee University and the Virginia Military Institute.

Richlands, Virginia

Metro American Radiology, a Team Health affiliate, is seeking a full-time radiologist for a two-physician practice in Richlands, Virginia. Candidates must be board certified and comfortable with all imaging modalities, including interventional procedures.

Richlands, rich in history, is located near the Tri-Cities area of Tennessee, which includes the cities of Bristol, Kingsport and Johnson City.

Full-time benefits include malpractice coverage, medical and life insurance, a 401k retirement plan and generous CME allowance. At Team Health, we offer practice opportunities designed to preserve physician incomes and maximize quality of life in today's rapidly changing healthcare environment.

For more information on these opportunities, please call Kathryn Watson at

(800) 662-6387

or fax your CV to David Forsberg, MD
(423) 693-4064
www.team-health.com

TEAM HEALTH®
Right Team, Right Now

CHIEF OF WOMEN'S IMAGING

The Department of Radiology of SUNY, Health Science Center at Syracuse, University Hospital, is currently seeking a Chief of Women's Imaging with expertise in the following areas: mammography, stereotactic breast biopsy and obstetrical ultrasound. Fellowship training and significant experience is preferred. The candidate should be board certified, eligible for both academic appointment at the State University of New York and licensure in the state of New York. An interest and willingness to participate in a teaching program for residents and rotating medical students is required. Salary and academic rank are commensurate with experience. Applicants should forward a letter of interest along with his/her CV to:

E. Robert Heitzman, M.D.
Department of Radiology
University Hospital
750 E. Adams Street
Syracuse, NY 13210
Phone: 315/464-7487, Fax: 315/464-7458

giography units. This position represents an opportunity to define the quality of general radiology, neuroradiology, and interventional radiology in the region. Business arrangements are flexible, depending upon the candidates capabilities and desires. Respond to Box R-074.

RADIOLOGIST-KITSAP PENINSULA, WA STATE—The Doctors Clinic of Bremerton, WA, a 55-provider, multi-specialty medical clinic, has an outstanding opportunity available for a BC radiologist. Experience is required in guiding the development of a radiology center with experience in a multi-specialty clinic preferred. The Kitsap area is regularly ranked as one of the top places to live and work in the U.S. and offers an abundance of outdoor and recreational opportunities with Seattle's cultural and sports events a short ferry ride away. We offer an excellent compensation package. Send CV to Human Resources, The Doctors Clinic, 2512 Wheaton Way, Bremerton, WA 98310. Fax 360-792-2716.

SPINE RADIOLOGIST—Unique opportunity for Board certified/eligible radiologist with fellowship in neuro or musculoskeletal CT and MRI, or special interest and expertise in spine imaging, to join well established subspecialty radiology group. Our expanding group owns and operates multiple outpatient imaging centers located in the upper midwest. This full-time position is immediately available, and is at the main imaging center location. State-of-the-art 1.5T MRI, spiral CT, and teleradiology equipment. Excellent salary and compensation package with many additional benefits. Please send CV and references to Box R-075.

UPPER MIDWEST—Established and expanding group, practicing in outpatient imaging centers, has immediate opening for musculoskeletal or neuro fellowship trained radiologist with spine expertise. Equipment includes current spiral CT, MRI, and conventional equipment. Generous starting salary, incentive plan, and benefit package. If interested, please send CV to Box R-076.

PUGET SOUND BASED RADIA MEDICAL IMAGING—A 32-member radiologist practice serving five hospitals, one large multispecialty clinic and various outpatient radiology sites, is seeking a Board certified general radiologist with cross-sectional imaging experience. Candidates with fellowship training are preferred. Implementation of 24-hour emergency services coverage via a teleradiology network and elevated exam volumes have increased the need for radiologists. If you are interested in working with a progressive practice, developing and promoting your area of subspecialization, sharing evenings and night work rotation, and living in an environment that allows access to a multitude of metropolitan and outdoor activities, please forward your curriculum vitae to Sanjiv Parikh, MD, Radia Medical Imaging, 3822 Colby Ave, Everett, WA 98201. Fax 425-339-8322.

A 20-PERSON RADIOLOGY GROUP IN MAJOR SOUTHWEST METROPOLITAN AREA—Seeks ABR certified diagnostic radiologist for part day time and part evening/ER coverage. A 750-bed hospital with approximately 55,000 ER visits per year. Familiarity with all diagnostic modalities, except interventional, required. State licensure not required for interview. Excellent back-up from progressive group, competitive salary. Address inquiries to H.C. Howerton, MD, 615-329-6385 or 615-284-5503.

FLORIDA - GENERAL RADIOLOGIST—Central Florida West Coast group seeks BE/BC radiologist. Interventional fellowship and/or body imaging fellowship desirable. Competitive compensation/benefits. CVs may be faxed to 813-898-4505.

RADIOLOGIST—We are seeking two Board certified radiologists to join a rapidly growing practice in Albert Lea, MN. The practice includes general radiology and all cross sectional imaging. The practice includes a busy outpatient practice and a 110-bed hospital. Albert Lea Medical Center is part of the Mayo Health System in southern Minnesota. For consideration, send a current CV to Jeffrey P. Lotts, MD, Medical Director, 1602 Fountain St, Albert Lea, MN, 56007 or fax 507-377-4826.

DIAGNOSTIC RADIOLOGIST—The University of Missouri-Columbia Health Sciences Center is seeking a radiologist with experience in all diagnostic radiology imaging modalities, including interventional radiology. Fellowship training in a sub-specialty is desirable. Board certification is required. Faculty rank commensurate with experience. Address inquiries to Robert Churchill, MD, University of Missouri Hospital & Clinics, One Hospital Dr, Columbia, MO 65212. An equal opportunity/affirmative action employer.

NEURORADIOLOGIST—The University of Missouri-Columbia Health Sciences Center is seeking a radiologist with expertise in neuroradiology and MRI. Interventional radiology experience is desirable. Board certification required. Fellowship training is desirable. Faculty rank to commensurate with experience. Address inquiries to Robert Churchill, MD, University of Missouri-Columbia Health Sciences Center, One Hospital Dr, Columbia, MO 65212. An equal opportunity/affirmative action employer.

DIAGNOSTIC RADIOLOGIST—To join seven member radiology group located one-hour from Pittsburgh. Job highlights include daytime hours, minimal call duty, and generous financial package. Necessary modalities are negotiable. Send CV to Mark Benson, MD, 15 Forest Rd, Wheeling, WV 26003. Daytime 304-243-3270, evenings 304-242-4077.

SOUTH FLORIDA, IMMEDIATE OPENINGS—Desirable private practice with two hospitals in need of fellowship trained MRI radiologist, fellowship trained interventional radiologist, and a fellowship trained pediatric radiologist. The successful candidates must be willing to do general radiology as well. Excellent positions for excellent individuals. Please send CVs to fax 561-488-8347.

STAFF RADIOLOGIST, CHEST SECTION—The Department of Radiology at the Brigham and Women's Hospital and Harvard Medical School is recruiting a full-time staff radiologist for a faculty position in its chest section. Radiology is a subspecialty oriented academic department with excellent programs in clinical service, research and teaching. Outstanding high technology equipment, including digital radiography, CT fluoroscopy and interventional MR is available. Candidates should be Board certified in diagnostic radiology, completed a fellowship in thoracic radiology and demonstrate competence in all clinical aspects of thoracic radiology. Faculty rank is expected to be Instructor or Assistant Professor level. Curriculum vitae and letter describing interest, background and qualifications should be sent to Steven E. Seltzer, MD, Chairman, Department of Radiology, Brigham and Women's Hospital, 75 Francis St, Boston, MA 02115. Brigham and Women's Hospital/Harvard Medical School is an affirmative action/equal opportunity educator and employer.

PUGET SOUND BASED RADIA MEDICAL IMAGING—A 32-member radiologist practice serving five hospitals, one large multispecialty clinic and various outpatient radiology sites, is seeking a Board certified general radiologist subspecializing in nuclear medicine with Board certification. Practice at a progressive 200-bed community hospital with state-of-the-art equipment. Practice involves developing and promoting nuclear medicine, working in other areas, sharing evening and night work rotation. Live in an environment that allows access to a multitude of metropolitan and outdoor activities, good schools and cultural diversity. Please forward your CV to Sanjiv Parikh, MD, c/o Cheryl West, Radia Medical Imaging, 3822 Colby Ave, Everett, WA 98201.

ALASKA - EXCITING OPPORTUNITY—Department of Veterans Affairs (VA) Medical and Regional Office Center is seeking Board certified radiologist for the position of Chief, Radiology Service. Excellent opportunity to work in state-of-the-art teleradiology hub. Anchorage is a cosmopolitan center within a pristine wilderness, which offers boundless cultural and recreational opportunities. No state income tax, plus tax-free COLA salary supplement, (COLA may be subject to change in the future). Travel and/or relocation expenses offered. U.S. citizenship is a condition of employment. Send CV with letter of interest to Christine Swink (11CP), VA Medical and Regional Office Center, 2925 Debarr Rd, Anchorage, AK 99508; 907-257-5485 or fax 907-257-3718. Position subject to drug testing. VA is an equal opportunity employer.

GENERAL DIAGNOSTIC RADIOLOGIST—Board certified or eligible, fellowship trained a plus. Partnership tract opportunity with a five person radiology group. Candidate will possess ability to provide quality radiology services including angiography, MRI, CT, US, nuclear, mammography and general radiology. Board certification required by 2nd-year. Group provides radiology services to a 300-bed Level 1 trauma center tertiary care hospital in Bismark, ND and several rural hospitals. Bismarck is a family-centered community with numerous outdoor recreational opportunities, located on the Missouri River. Excellent school system with both private and public schools. Generous benefit package, competitive starting salary and partnership opportunity. Please send CV to Douglas Peterson, MD, Central Dakota Radiologists, PC, 810 E Rosser Ave, Suite 201, Bismarck, ND 58501. Phone 701-224-7480; fax 701-224-8320; e-mail *Cendakrad@aol.com*.

RADIOLOGIST - METRO ATLANTA, PLUS OPENINGS IN SOUTH CAROLINA, NORTH CAROLINA, AND TEXAS—Community based outpatient imaging company needs BC radiologist for new state-of-the-art imaging centers, MRI and CT, Monday through Friday, excellent compensation and benefits. Send CV to Human Resource Manager, 3295 River Exchange Dr, Suite 275, Norcross, GA 30092.

LEXINGTON, KY—BC/BE diagnostic radiologist for salaried position in a six person radiology group. No weekend, on-call or holiday responsibilities. Expertise in general radiology, mammography, CT, nuclear medicine, and ultrasound required. Interest in women's imaging is a plus. MRI and angiography are a plus, but not required. Competitive salary and benefits. Please send CV to Scott Stevens, MD, Radiology, 1740 S Nicholasville Rd, Lexington, KY 40503.

DIAGNOSTIC RADIOLOGIST—With neuro fellowship (or equivalent with CAQ in neuro) plus interest in special procedures/interventional to complement existing angio/interventional and neuro specialists. Offering partnership track in our private practice group of nine Board certified radiologists with specialty interests in all imaging modalities including interventional, neuro and body MRI, MRA, stereotactic and FNA biopsies, SPECT, etc. Our main hospital is nearly fully digital. We are a primary teaching affiliate of University of Massachusetts Medical School with year round medical students and house staff in several departments. Our Berkshire mountains are a desirable destination for summer resort activities, foliage, downhill and cross-country skiing. Quality of our practice, hospitals, affiliated offices, and life style is superior. Please respond with CV to Robert Geehr, Chairman, Department of Radiology, Berkshire Medical Center, 725 North St, Pittsfield, MA 01201.

FIND YOUR NEXT JOB OR CANDIDATE ONLINE AT RADWORK.COM!—It has a new interactive database and other tools to help in your search. You'll also find areas for rad techs and radiology equipment. Point your browser to *http://www.radwork.com/* for a free and easy way to list or find a job.

GENERAL DIAGNOSTIC RADIOLOGIST—Full-time private practice opportunity is immediately available for one confident, Board certified diagnostic radiologist in a young, expanding, five-member group based in the greater Cincinnati area. This progressive, democratic practice provides essentially all diagnostic imaging services at two community hospitals and at two outpatient open MR imaging centers. Interested individuals must be competent in all areas of general diagnostic radiology including nuclear medicine and possess basic CVIR skills. Fellowship training or previous practice experience optimal but not required to apply for this partnership track position. The successful candidate will be motivated, hardworking and dedicated to the principles of small group practice. Submit CV with cover letter and references to John A. Botsford, MD, 8300 Eagle Ridge Dr, Cincinnati, OH 45243 or fax to 513-475-5258. For further information, call 513-559-2260.

PROGRAM DIRECTOR, CARDIOVASCULAR MRI—The Department of Radiology at Harvard Medical School, Brigham and Women's Hospital has an opening for a Director of its cardiovascular MRI program. Recent acquisition of new imaging technology, coupled with the core resources and expertise of an internationally recognized MRI program create an exciting opportunity to develop sophisticated cardiovascular MR clinical and research efforts. Candidates should have experience and expertise in developing and managing clinical and research programs, as well as technical and academic excellence in MRI. Opportunities will exist to develop interdisciplinary collaborative programs involving radiology, medicine and surgery. Interested candidates should send a letter of introduction and CV to Frank Jolesz, MD, Department of Radiology, Brigham and Women's Hospital, 75 Francis St, Boston, MA 02115. Brigham and Women's Hospital and Harvard Medical School are equal opportunity, affirmative action employers.

GRAND JUNCTION, CO VA MEDICAL CENTER—Seeks Board certified general radiologist to provide medical supervision for all imaging services including plain films and common special procedures, fluoroscopy, CT and ultrasound; 10,000 exams per year. Supportive hospital leadership and outstanding technical and clerical support. Up to date equipment. The radiologist plays an active collaborative role providing quality care in a team atmosphere. Unique primary care model with excellent professional staff. Spectacular setting with scenic views, unrivaled recreational pursuits, cultural opportunities. CV to Margo Cox, Personnel Management Specialist, 2121 North Ave, Grand Junction, CO 81501. Fax 970-244-7731; phone 970-242-0731 ext 2067. The Department of Veterans Affairs is an equal opportunity employer. U.S. citizens only, please.

ABR CERTIFIED RADIOLOGIST—Needed for nighthawk coverage in Raleigh, NC metropolitan area. Responsibilities include general, nuclear medicine, CT, ultrasound, and basic MR. Excellent salary, generous benefits and time off. Please send CV to William H. Johnson, Administrator at Wake Radiology, PO Box 19366, Raleigh, NC 27619.

A 14-MEMBER RADIOLOGY GROUP—Seeking two Board certified radiologists: one with

FACULTY POSITION
VASCULAR / INTERVENTIONAL IMAGING

The Department of Radiology of MetroHealth Medical Center, a Case Western Reserve University affiliated hospital, invites applications from interested, qualified radiologists for a faculty position in Vascular/Interventional Imaging. The ideal candidate will be ABR certified and have fellowship experience in vascular and interventional radiology. A faculty appointment will be made commensurate with candidate's experience and qualifications.

MHMC is a 746-bed trauma center providing tertiary care and general hospital services to the Cleveland metropolitan area. The medical center is committed to providing excellence in care with a highly qualified, interdisciplinary, hospital-based medical staff. The Department of Radiology is an active, expanding department, providing general and specialized services using state-of-the-art equipment, including new Picker Omnicon L and Picker Digicon angiographic units in a newly remodeled Angiography Suite.

The position provides an excellent opportunity for professional development, collaborative and/or individual research, as well as medical student and resident education.

Interested candidates should forward curriculum vitae and other pertinent information to:

Errol M. Bellon, MD, Chairman, Department of Radiology
MetroHealth Medical Center
2500 MetroHealth Drive • Cleveland, OH 44109-4020
Telephone: (216) 778-4020

MetroHealth Medical Center and Case Western Reserve University are Equal Opportunity Employers.

Position Sought

Fellowships

competitive. To receive more information, please contact Carlos J. Sivit, MD, Director, Pediatric Radiology, Rainbow Babies and Childrens Hospital of University Hospitals of Cleveland, 11100 Euclid Ave, Cleveland, OH 44106-5056. Telephone 216-844-1172; e-mail *sivit@uhrad.com*. EEO/AA.

FELLOWSHIP IN ABDOMINAL IMAGING AVAILABLE JULY, 1999—Department of Radiology, Louisiana State University Medical School at New Orleans. The Louisiana State University Department of Radiology has a 1-year position open for July, 1999. The division is staffed by eight radiologists with extensive specialization experience or fellowship training. Equipment includes two MRI scanners including a 1.5T GE Signa. Three Siemens Somatom Plus S CTs are in place with plans for at least two more CTs and upgrades in the near future. Nine ultrasound machines with color and power doppler capabilities are currently in use. One of the ultrasound departments is currently filmless and a hospital wide PACS is being implemented. All ultrasound and CT-guided procedures including chest procedures are performed by imaging fellows. Option for combination with musculoskeletal fellowship. Direct inquiries to Thomas R. Beidle, MD, RVT, LSU Radiology, Rm 308, 1542 Tulane Ave, New Orleans, LA 70112; e-mail *tbeidl@lsumc.edu*, phone 504-568-4968.

THE MAYO CLINIC DEPARTMENT OF RADIOLOGY—Rochester, MN, has an unanticipated opening for a fellowship beginning June 26, 1999. There is the potential for a fellowship position in the following areas: nuclear medicine, cross-sectional imaging (ultrasound, CT, MR), thoracic imaging and musculoskeletal imaging. Address correspondence to Thomas E. Hartman, MD, Department of Radiology, Mayo Clinic, Rochester, MN, 55905.

FELLOWSHIP IN NEURORADIOLOGY AVAILABLE 1998—Department of Radiology, Louisiana State University Medical Center. LSU neuroradiology section has one unexpected fellowship opening for 1998. This ACGME accredited program is staffed by four full-time academic neuroradiologist and one full-time neurointerventionalist and covers the 400-bed Charity Hospital of New Orleans as well as the adjacent 400-bed University Hospital. Candidate will get significant exposure to all aspects of neuroradiology, including low/high field MR, helical CT, myelography, diagnostic and interventional neuroangiography, and ENT radiology. Send CV to Albert Alexander, MD, LSU Medical School, Rm 212, 1542 Tulane Ave, New Orleans, LA 70112.

THORACIC RADIOLOGY FELLOWSHIP POSITION 1999—Department of Radiology, Louisiana State University Medical Center. The Louisiana State University School of Medicine program in New Orleans is offering a fellowship position beginning July of 1999. The fellow will rotate between two primary teaching hospitals; one being the major trauma center for the region. Both campuses are equipped with spiral CT, and one with digital radiography and PACS. A strong pulmonary medicine program and a large and varied case load contribute to the learning experience. Apply to Lisa Diethelm, MD, Department of Radiology, 1542 Tulane Ave, New Orleans, LA 70112.

FELLOWSHIPS IN RADIOLOGY, MEMORIAL SLOAN-KETTERING CANCER CENTER—The Department of Radiology at Memorial Sloan-Kettering Cancer Center offers fellowships beginning 7/1/00. Body Imaging - 1-year. Extensive clinical experience in body CT (25,000 cases/year), body MRI (1,800 cases/year) and ultrasound (5,000 cases/year). Equipment includes two GE HighSpeed (helical) Advantage CTs; two GE HiLite Advantage CTs; GE 1.5T Signa MRI; Picker 1.0T MRI; and three Acuson XP units with color doppler. Research is integral part of program. Director David Panicek, MD. Breast Imaging - 6 months (plus 6 months of body imaging). There are 60,000 mammograms, 500 preoperative needle localizations, 150 stereotaxic biopsies, and 1,400 breast sonograms and sonographically-guided breast biopsies performed yearly. Equipment includes nine dedicated mammography machines and a stereotactaxic biopsy table. Director David Dershaw, MD. Other fellowships include nuclear medicine (2-years; contact Steven Larson, MD at MSKCC), and combined New York Hospital/MSKCC fellowships in neuroradiology (2-years; contact Michael Deck, MD at NYH) and vascular/interventional radiology (1-year; contact Thomas Sos, MD, at NYH). Excellent opportunities for research exist at this Cornell University Medical College affiliate, with competitive salary and benefits. Request application from David Panicek, MD, Department of Radiology, Memorial Sloan-Kettering Cancer Center, 1275 York Ave, New York, NY 10021; *http://www.mskcc.org*. An equal opportunity employer.

UNEXPECTED CALIFORNIA INTERVENTIONAL FELLOWSHIP AVAILABLE 7/98—Interventional, MRI and cross-sectional imaging fellowship in tertiary care hospital, with 1.5T MRI, spiral CT and state-of-the-art digital angiography suite. Contact A.M. Levan, MD, at St. Mary Medical Center, 1050 Linden Ave, Long Beach, CA 90813 or call 562-491-9900.

NEURORADIOLOGY FELLOWSHIP—Unexpected opening has developed for a 2-year fellowship position starting July 1, 1999, with clinical, research and teaching duties. Also we have three openings for our 2-year fellowship program beginning July 1, 2000. Applicants must be Board certified and must have completed their residency in radiology by starting date. Interested candidates may contact Daniel K. Kido, MD, Neuroradiology Section, Mallinckrodt Institute of Radiology, Washington University School of Medicine, 510 S Kingshighway Blvd, St. Louis, MO 63110. Phone 314-362-5950; fax 314-362-4886.

THE UNIVERSITY OF MASSACHUSETTS MEDICAL CENTER—Offers fellowship positions in neuroradiology, vascular/interventional and body imaging/MRI. The University of Massachusetts includes a medical school and a 388-bed hospital and trauma center located 40 miles West of Boston. The radiology department performs approximately 170,000 exams per year. State-of-the-art equipment includes two vascular/interventional, two CT, and two 1.5 telsa MRI units. The positions include teaching of medical students and residents with opportunities for research and conference attendance. The neuroradiology and vascular/interventional fellowships are approved by ACGME. For information contact John Knorr, DO, for neuroradiogy. David Phillips, MD, for vascular/interventional. Ashley Davidoff, MD, for body imaging at University of Massachusetts Medical Center, Department of Radiology, 55 Lake Ave North, Worcester, MA 01655; 508-856-2215.

Announcements

COMPREHENSIVE TRAINING IN CENTRAL VENOUS ACCESS 1.5 DAY, JULY 23-24, OCTOBER 1-2, DECEMBER 7-8, 1998—The Section of Vascular & Interventional Radiology at the Cleveland Clinic Foundation offers a 1.5 day program in all aspects of central venous access (including chest port insertion). This experience consists of lectures, participation in animal laboratory device implantation, and live case demonstrations with simultaneous discussion during each case. We encourage attendance by a team of two, physician and assistant, but individual physicians may attend. This course has been approved for 11.5 hours in category 1 CME credit. For further information call 216-444-0617.

Practices for Sale

RADIOLOGIST RETIRING - OFFICE FOR SALE—At 666 Tyrone Blvd, St. Petersburg, FL 33710. Across from cathedral in junction of two main streets. Frontage 265, 3100 square ft, GE R-F. ATL sono, Siemens mammogram, plenty of room for expansion, gobs of parking; $600,000.

BOSTON—Medical imaging suite with radiography, mammography and ultrasound. Administrative offices. Located in Longwood medical area. Reply to Box R-079.

RSNA®
RSNA Executive Offices • 2021 Spring Road, Suite 600
Oak Brook, IL 60523 • (630) 571-2670

Bulletin Board

July 1998

✓ ***Radiology* Turns 75, Anniversary Content Planned**

✓ **RSNA Secretary-Treasurer Resigns**

✓ ***info*RAD and Scientific Exhibits to Be in Lakeside Center**

✓ **RSNA '98—A Smoke-Free Meeting**

■ 1998 marks the 75th anniversary of RSNA's premier journal *Radiology*. To help celebrate the milestone, special messages from presidents of numerous subspecialty imaging societies and commemorative advertisements are scheduled to appear throughout the year in the journal, which was first published as *Radiology* in 1923. Prior to 1923, the *Journal of Roentgenology* was published from 1918 to 1919 by the Western Roentgen Society, followed by the *Journal of Radiology*, published by the Radiological Society of North America from 1920 to 1923.

■ On March 17, Donald R. Kirks, MD, resigned his position as Secretary-Treasurer of the Radiological Society of North America, effective immediately.

Citing personal reasons for the decision, Dr Kirks, in his letter to RSNA President David B. Fraser, MD, noted, "The RSNA is an outstanding organization because of the excellence of its staff, the vision of its leadership, and the hard work and dedication of its many thousands of volunteers. I am certain that the RSNA, through its efforts in research and education, will continue to make many important contributions to improving the health care of our patients."

"Don Kirks has provided excellent service to the RSNA over the past 15 years, serving on the Scientific Program Committee and the Refresher Course Committee, in addition to his service on the Board of Directors," noted Dr Fraser. "The Board thanks him for his service and wishes him well in his new endeavors," he concluded.

At its June meeting, the RSNA Board of Directors will appoint an interim Secretary-Treasurer who will serve until a permanent Secretary-Treasurer is selected at the annual Business Session held during the 84th RSNA Scientific Assembly and Annual Meeting.

■ Attendees will be glad to see the promotion of RSNA '98 as a smoke-free meeting. While no-smoking regulations have existed in the past, they were difficult to enforce due to the sheer size of the meeting. This year, the only smoking areas will be outside of the building, and the no-smoking regulation will be strictly enforced. RSNA asks that exhibitors and attendees alike help enforce the no-smoking rule by directing persons who wish to smoke outside the building. These areas will be clearly marked for ease of use.

■ At RSNA '98, *info*RAD and Scientific Exhibits will occupy portions of McCormick Place's Lakeside Center (East Building). The newly remodeled Lakeside Center will provide more space for the exhibits and allow for a different configuration. Featured in the *info*RAD area in 1998 will be the basic, hands-on training in computers in radiology workshops and the Integrating the Healthcare Enterprise showcase exhibit, which will provide attendees with a technological look into the future of radiology.

*info*RAD
THE FUTURE IS HERE

■ The following is a list of applicants for RSNA membership, published as provided by the bylaws of the Society. Society members are asked to review these names. Should a member have a question concerning the eligibility of an applicant, within 30 days of the publication of this list, the member should request that the applicant's membership be withheld pending investigation and reconsideration by the Membership and Credentials Board. Please mark your signed letter of protest "Confidential" and address it to Secretary-Treasurer, RSNA, 2021 Spring Road, Suite 600, Oak Brook, IL 60523. Please note that listed here are only the locations in which the prospective members reside and the counselors for those areas.

ALABAMA
Counselor: Leon W. Bell III, MD
Angus T. Baird, MBChB, Birmingham

ARIZONA
Counselor: Pamela J. Lund, MD
Archana C. Lucchesi, MD, Phoenix

CALIFORNIA
Counselors: Deborah S. Ablin, MD
Gary R. Hansen, MD
Eric W. Olcott, MD
Zbigniew Petrovich, MD
Dolores H. Pretorius, MD
Morton Wexler, MD
Lincoln R. Davis, MD, Los Angeles
Thomas M. Bey, MD, Stockton
Jonathan H. Fish, MD, Piedmont

GEORGIA
Counselor: Robert F. Long, MD
James B. Edwards, MD, Savannah
Paula R. Greenfield, MD, Stone Mountain

ILLINOIS
Counselors: Boyd E. Nelson, MD
Steven M. Pinsky, MD
David S. Channin, MD, Chicago
Babak Yaghmai, MD, Chicago

INDIANA
Counselor: Smari Thordarson, MD
Brian A. Aronson, MD, Valparaiso
Robert R. Hasson, MD, Goshen
Mary L. Wolfe, MD, Greenfield

IOWA
Counselor: Charles N. Heggen, MD
Michael J. Geraghty, MD, Iowa City
Patrick P. Rheingans, MD, Ames

MICHIGAN
Counselors: Judith M. Bender, MD
Walter W. Laidlaw, MD
Won Chae, MD, Waterford
Randy D. Hicks, MD, Flint
Ming L. Hsieh, MD, Fenton

MISSISSIPPI
Counselor: Margaret T. Hatten, MD
Shaun W. Mckee, MD, Biloxi

MISSOURI
Counselors: David P. Diemer, MD
George D. Dixon, MD
William P. James, MD, Kirkwood
Eric S. Malden, MD, Saint Louis
James M. Milburn, MD, Town & Country

NEW JERSEY
Counselor: Karen L. Karlson, MD
Eugene C. Kennedy, MD, MBBCh, Summit

NEW YORK
Counselors: Mario A. Grosso, MD
David M. Panicek, MD
Arthur J. Segal, MD
Robert C. Greenbaum, MD, Mamaroneck

NORTH CAROLINA
Counselor: James A. Fagan, MD
Richard L. Webber, DDS, PhD, Winston-Salem

OHIO
Counselors: Michael A. Geisinger, MD
Jonathan S. Moulton, MD
John M. Grosel, MD, Marietta
Abraham Levitin, MD, University Heights

PENNSYLVANIA
Counselors: Nilima Dash, MD
Kathryn A. Evers, MD
John E. Madewell, MD
W. S. Enochs, MD, PhD, Wayne
Margarita L. Zuley, MD, Allison Park

TENNESSEE
Counselor: Joseph J. Busch, MD
Mary C. Soto, MD, Memphis

TEXAS
Counselors: Karl A. Glastad, MD
Franz J. Hallermann, MD
Timothy W. Lillick, MD
Henry J. Boehm III, MD, Waco
Douglas J. Swank, MD, San Antonio
Brian R. Turley, MD, Montgomery

WASHINGTON
Counselor: Robert A. Reiswig, MD
John J. Borsa, MD, Seattle

MEXICO
Counselors: Jose H. Arredondo, MD
Manuel A. Cabal, MD
Jose M. Cardoso, MD
Miguel A. Carrillo, MD
Ramon R. Ponte, MD
Francisco J. Reynaga-Garcia, MD
Soledad Cordova, MD, Mexico City

CANADA

ONTARIO
Counselor: Giles W. Stevenson, MD
Francis S. Marrocco, BSc, MD, Peterborough

QUEBEC
Counselors: Pierre M. Bourgouin, MD
Gilles Hudon, MD
Cuong N. Tran, MD, Cote St Luc

CORRESPONDING
Ali Akinci, MD, Turkey
Haluk Akman, MD, Turkey
Hector A. Camara, MD, Argentina
Vincent F. Cloots, MD, Belgium
Ludovico Dalla-Palma, Italy
Gurkan Ege, MD, Turkey
Sandra I. Ennis Caldera, MD, Colombia
Luiz C. Faria, MD, Brazil
Carlos H. Genro, Sr, MD, Brazil
Seppo V. Jauhola, MD, Finland
Jennifer L. Khoo, MB, BS, Hong Kong
Jarmo J. Lottonen, MD, Finland
Tomohiko Masumoto, MD, Japan
Reuben O. Obaro, MBBS, DMRD, United Kingdom
Raimundo S. Oliveira, MD, Brazil
Tanseli S. Ozer, MD, Turkey
Tom Pedersen, Sr, MD, Norway
Lucilo A. Pessoa, Jr, MD, Brazil
Stepheson N. Santana, MD, Brazil
Martti A. Soiva, MD, PhD, Finland
Takashi Sugiura, MD, Japan
Carla E. Tjon Pian Gi, MD, Netherlands
Kyo Tsuda, MD, Japan
Rolf M. Von Gumppenberg, MD, Germany
Masashi Yamashiro, MD, Japan
Yoshifumi Yasuhara, MD, Japan

NEW!

Cardiac MR Imaging *RSP 646*

Elliot R. McVeigh, PhD

Depiction of the heart and coronary vessels presents one of the greatest technical challenges in MR imaging. The daunting physiologic constraints make it imperative for the pulse-sequence designer to understand the physics of imaging moving objects and the methods available to eliminate the deleterious effects of motion. Cardiac imaging is an excellent application to illustrate the uses of real-time imaging techniques, gradient moment nulling, presaturation techniques, velocity imaging with phase, perfusion imaging, and angiography. *Learning objectives:* To understand (1) the constraints imposed by human physiology during cardiac imaging and (2) the MR techniques used to obtain optimal images within these constraints.

74 slides/audiotape *M$140, N$160*

VHS *M$140, N$160*

NEW!

Advanced Course in MR Angiography for Peripheral Vascular Disease *RSP 647*

Edgar Kent Yucel, MD

Richard Arthur Baum, MD

This program is intended for radiologists who wish to learn to perform peripheral MR angiography. It emphasizes the specific information required by vascular surgeons to manage patients and the complementary role of MR angiography in relation to noninvasive examination. An approach to complete and accurate peripheral MR angiography is provided. The authors explain how to integrate peripheral MR angiography into clinical practice, as well as how to use MR angiography to build and maintain an interventional radiology practice. *Learning objectives:* To learn the principles of MR angiography and strategies for complete clinical MR angiographic examination of the lower extremity. (E.K.Y. has received research support from Philips Medical Systems and is the medical director of EPIX Medical, Inc.)

109 slides/audiotape *M$205, N$225*

VHS *M$205, N$225*

NEW!

Diffusion and Perfusion with MR Imaging *RSP 648*

Denis J. LeBihan, MD, PhD

This presentation reviews molecular diffusion and the basic principles of diffusion MR imaging. An overview of the current and potential clinical applications is provided. Emphasis is given to difficulties of implementation. Concepts that led to perfusion imaging are introduced, as well as the bases of the main conventional methods used to evaluate tissue perfusion. The physical principles, limitations, and fields of applications of these techniques are presented. *Learning objectives:* (1) To become familiar with the concepts of diffusion and perfusion, (2) to understand the principles of diffusion and perfusion measurements with MR imaging, (3) to become familiar with the advantages and limitations of diffusion and perfusion MR imaging, and (4) to identify clinical conditions in which diffusion and perfusion imaging may be useful.

66 slides/audiotape *M$140, N$160*

VHS *M$140, N$160*

NEW!

Functional Neurologic MR Imaging *RSP 649*

Gary H. Glover, PhD

This course reviews the theory and techniques used to obtain MR images that depict neuronal response to cortical stimulation, including methods of data acquisition and analysis, stimuli techniques, and artifacts. Functional MR imaging (fMRI) techniques are based on changes in regional blood flow consequent to greater oxygen demand in the cortical parenchyma from neuronal activity. Blood oxygen level-dependent and inflow MR contrast mechanisms that exploit this process are reviewed. The technical requirements for fMRI acquisition and imaging strategies are discussed; the effects of physiologic motion and imaging artifacts are described and methods for their reduction are presented. Methods of statistical data analysis are described and examples of fMRI for sensorimotor and language mapping are presented. *Learning objectives:* To gain (1) understanding of the techniques for obtaining MR images of neuronal response to cortical stimulation and (2) exposure to examples of clinical applications of fMRI methods. (G.H.G. is a consultant to GE Medical Systems.)

88 slides/audiotape *M$140, N$160*

VHS *M$140, N$160*

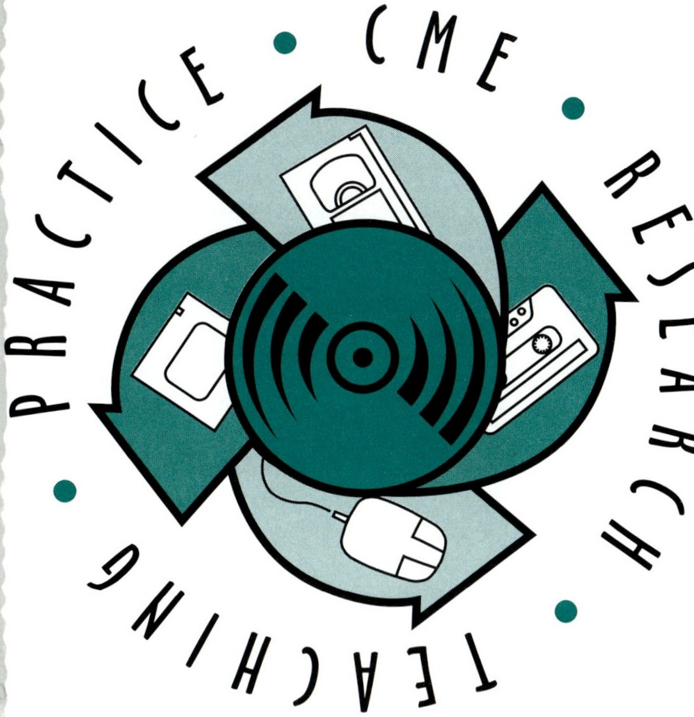

MR Imaging

Learning Center Resources

July 1998

RSNA® | Radiological Society of North America Founded in 1915

Featured Topics

- **Hardware and Coils for MR Imaging**
- **MR Angiography: General Principles**
- **Contrast-enhanced MR Angiography**
- **Real-Time Magnetic Resonance Imaging**

New Service

The entire 1997–1998 Learning Center Resources Catalog is now available on the RSNA Link, the Web site of the Radiological Society of North America, on the Internet.

You can reach us through the World Wide Web (WWW) by entering the uniform resource locator: http://www.rsna.org

We invite you to browse through the catalog, search for specific courses of interest, then simply order via our fax or 800 phone number.

Detach and store for your future use.

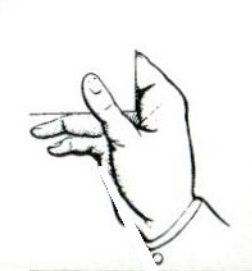

The following 9 MR Imaging titles are now available in the Learning Center Resources Library. All videotapes are available for purchase or rental (U.S., Canada, and Mexico). All video programs may be purchased in NTSC, PAL, and SECAM television standards. Slides and audiotapes are available for purchase only.

For more information, call or fax the RSNA Learning Center Resources at the numbers listed on the order form. To order by mail, use the form on the back.

NEW!

Spatial Encoding and k-Space *RSP 641*

Felix W. Wehrli, PhD

Unlike in other imaging modalities such as CT, the MR signal is sampled in spatial frequency (also denoted "k space") rather than in object space. Each k-space signal sample contains information from the entire excited portion of the object. Since most of the signal energy resides with the low spatial frequencies, the latter determine overall object shape and signal-to-noise ratio, whereas signals with higher frequency determine edge sharpness. *Learning objectives:* To understand the concept of the spatial frequency domain and how density, size, and scanning mode of k space determine the fundamental properties of the image.

VHS *M$140, N$160*

Not available in slide/audiotape

NEW!

Hardware and Coils for MR Imaging *RSP 642*

James R. MacFall, PhD

An MR system can be conveniently divided into two parts: (1) the computer, data storage and display system, which is much like that of digital medical imaging systems (CT, for example), and (2) the MR-specific components. This lecture focuses in depth on the MR-specific components: the magnet, gradient coil system, radiofrequency power system, spectrometer, and pulse programmer. *Learning objective:* To understand the functional performance requirements of the basic MR-specific components of an MR system.

59 slides/audiotape *M$140, N$160*

Not available on videotape

NEW!

MR Angiography: General Principles *RSP 643*

Dennis L. Parker, PhD

The most commonly used techniques of MR angiography (MRA) are based on the signal properties of moving blood. MRA methods include white blood techniques, such as time-of-flight and phase-contrast imaging, which enhance the signal from moving spins and suppress the signal from stationary spins, and black blood techniques, which suppress the signal from moving spins and enhance the signal from stationary tissue. *Learning objectives:* To understand the basic flow contrast mechanisms that are used in MRA, factors that affect vascular image quality, and sources of artifacts. Physics of these mechanisms are covered at a precalculus level. (D.L.P. has received funding from GE Medical Systems and has membership in an LLC related to MRA.)

VHS *M$140, N$160*

Not available in slide/audiotape

NEW!

Contrast-enhanced MR Angiography *RSP 644*

Frank R. Korosec, PhD

Contrast-enhanced MR angiographic techniques, when performed properly, provide high-quality MR angiograms. With these techniques, a T1-shortening contrast agent is injected into the blood stream. Imaging during the first pass of the contrast agent with an appropriate sequence permits acquisition of a high-contrast MR angiogram. Imaging parameters such as flip angle, repetition time, echo time, and image duration must be carefully chosen to achieve maximum contrast between blood vessels and stationary tissues. Total dose and injection rate also must be chosen properly to ensure optimal image quality. *Learning objectives:* To understand the fundamental principles of contrast-enhanced MR angiography well enough to obtain high-quality contrast-enhanced MR angiograms effectively and reproducibly.

VHS *M$140, N$160*

Not available in slide/audiotape

NEW!

Real-Time Magnetic Resonance Imaging *RSP 645*

Stephen J. Riederer, PhD

A real-time MR system ideally meets a number of technical specifications: (1) continuous data acquisition, (2) fast image reconstruction, and (3) real-time adjustment of imaging parameters. This program reviews and discusses approaches that have been developed to address each requirement, with emphasis on hardware developed for reconstruction and parameter alteration. It also discusses specific applications of real-time MR imaging. *Learning objectives:* (1) To understand the manner in which pulse sequences and hardware can be integrated to allow real-time interactive MR imaging, (2) to learn about specific applications of real-time MR imaging, and (3) to understand the technical challenges of real-time MR imaging. (S.J.R. has received a research grant from GE Medical Systems.)

VHS *M$140, N$160*

Not available in slide/audiotape

M/N = Member/Nonmember prices

To order call 800-272-2920 or FAX 708-409-9703

August 1998
Volume 208 • Number 2
RADLAX 208 (2) 281–560

1923–1998 75th ANNIVERSARY

Radiology

From the Editor	281
Subspecialty Society Messages	283
Perspectives	289
Editorials	293
Special Communication: Call to Meeting	300
How I Do It	303
Signs in Imaging	319
Thoracic Imaging	321
Diagnosis Please: Case 5	339
Case 1 Answer	341
Cardiac Imaging	345
Vascular and Interventional Radiology	353
Musculoskeletal Imaging	375
Health Policy and Practice	385
Technical Developments	393
Neuroradiology	417
Head and Neck Imaging	441
Ultrasound	453
Genitourinary Imaging	459
Breast Imaging	471
Experimental Studies	491
Nuclear Medicine	505
Radiation Oncology	511
Pediatric Imaging	521
Gastrointestinal Imaging	525
Letters to the Editor	549

THE RADIOLOGICAL SOCIETY • OF NORTH AMERICA

RSNA® **84th Scientific Assembly and Annual Meeting**
Chicago, November 29–December 4, 1998

Radiology

August 1998
Volume 208
Number 2

RSNA®
A monthly journal devoted to clinical radiology and allied sciences, owned and published by THE RADIOLOGICAL SOCIETY OF NORTH AMERICA, INC.

August 1998
Volume 208 • Number 2

Radiology

A monthly journal devoted to clinical radiology and allied sciences, owned and published by the Radiological Society of North America, Inc.

RSNA

From the Editor

281 *Radiology* 1998—Advertising and Our 75th Anniversary
Anthony V. Proto

Future Directions of Imaging Research: Subspecialty Society Messages

283 *The North American Society of Cardiac Imaging—*
Future Direction of Cardiovascular Research
Lawrence M. Boxt and Martin J. Lipton
The need to have radiology involved and, indeed, play an important role in the development, innovation, and application of all this exciting new imaging research will require a critical mass of adequately trained, creative radiologists who are interested in cardiovascular disease.

285 Commentary
Cardiac Imaging Research in the Next Century: A Commentary
Herbert L. Abrams
Our conception of cardiac imaging research for the next century is already rich in the scope of opportunities it offers; but, if history is any guide, we have not even dared to dream of the innovations that the next few decades will bring.

Perspectives

289 **A Compendium of Managed Care: Past, Present, and Hints of the Future—Part 1**
Richard M. Friedenberg
Managed care organizations have saved considerable sums by monitoring services, avoiding duplication of services, and avoiding obvious excesses.

Editorials

293 **A Promising Start on Overall Imaging Quality, but Far to Go on Costs**
Jonathan H. Sunshine
BlueCross BlueShield of Massachusetts has initiated a promising program for improving imaging quality that has yielded valuable information on where severe quality problems have been concentrated, but it has not made the same progress on getting the financial incentives right.

296 **Advances in Perfusion MR Imaging**
Peter Jezzard
The recently developed methods of arterial spin labeling for perfusion measurement offer the simplest and yet most powerful approach to perfusion MR mapping.

Special Communication

300 **The Radiological Society of North America 84th Scientific Assembly and Annual Meeting, Sunday, November 29 to Friday, December 4, 1998 McCormick Place, Chicago, Illinois**
David B. Fraser

How I Do It

303 **Technical Aspects of Needle Aspiration Lung Biopsy: A Personal Perspective**
Elizabeth H. Moore
The techniques in this article form a unified approach to lung biopsy, directed toward the pragmatic goals of maximizing specimen retrieval and minimizing complications.

Signs in Imaging

319 **The Luftsichel Sign**
Donna G. Blankenbaker
The sign manifests as a paraaortic crescent of hyperlucency with sharp margins that extend anywhere from the apex of the hemithorax to the left superior pulmonary vein and outline the medial aspect and sometimes the upper aspect of the opaque collapsed left upper lobe.

Thoracic Imaging

321 **Airway Hyperreactivity: Assessment with Helical Thin-Section CT**
Jonathan G. Goldin, Michael F. McNitt-Gray, Steven M. Sorenson, Timothy D. Johnson, Beth Dauphinee, Eric C. Kleerup, Donald P. Tashkin, and Denise R. Aberle
We designed a relatively robust technique that uses a combination of volumetric thin-section CT, classic flow-volume loops, and semiautomated postprocessing tools to assess regional lung function reproducibly and under varying physiologic conditions.

331 **Polypoid Lesions of Airways: Early Experience with Computer-assisted Detection by Using Virtual Bronchoscopy and Surface Curvature**
Ronald M. Summers, W. Scott Selbie, James D. Malley, Lynne M. Pusanik, Andrew J. Dwyer, Nikos A. Courcoutsakis, David J. Shaw, David E. Kleiner, Michael C. Sneller, Carol A. Langford, Steven M. Holland, and James H. Shelhamer
The results of this study suggest that a curvature-based algorithm may facilitate detection of polypoid airway lesions.

Diagnosis Please

339 **Case 5**
Jeremy J. Erasmus, H. Page McAdams, and Philip C. Goodman

341 **Case 1: Recurrent Pyogenic Cholangitis**
Ann S. Fulcher
Although the largest series of recurrent pyogenic cholangitis (RPC) has been reported in Asia, RPC is being identified with increasing frequency in the United States, primarily in Asian immigrants.

Cardiac Imaging

345 **Patency of Coronary Bypass Grafts: Assessment with Breath-hold Contrast-enhanced MR Angiography—Value of a Non–Electrocardiographically Triggered Technique**
Bernd J. Wintersperger, Markus G. Engelmann, Alexander von Smekal, Andreas Knez, Herbert V. Penzkofer, Berthold Höfling, Gerhard Laub, and Maximilian F. Reiser
Non–electrocardiographically triggered breath-hold contrast material–enhanced MR angiography is suitable for visualizing venous and arterial coronary bypass grafts and allows reliable assessment of graft patency.

Vascular and Interventional Radiology

353 **Breath-hold Gadolinium-enhanced MR Angiography of the Major Vessels at 1.0 T: Dose-Response Findings and Angiographic Correlation**
Markus G. Lentschig, Peter Reimer, Ursula L. Rausch-Lentschig, Thomas Allkemper, Michael Oelerich, and Gerhard Laub
The injected dose of gadolinium can be limited to 0.1 mmol/kg, which is sufficient for breath-hold gadolinium-enhanced MR angiography of larger vessels such as the aorta and its major branches.

Continued—

Radiology is published monthly by the Radiological Society of North America, Inc, 2021 Spring Rd, Suite 600, Oak Brook, IL 60523 (ISSN 0033-8419). Printed in USA. Periodical class postage paid at Oak Brook, Ill, and additional mailing offices. The nonmember subscription rate for the USA is $215.00 per year; for all other countries, $260.00 (includes postage). Information about subscription rates for residents is available on request. (Air freight is available; rates are furnished on request.) Single copies are $25.00 ($36.00 to a non-U.S. address). Notice of missing issues or change of address (include old mailing label and new address) should be sent to RSNA Subscriptions Department, 2021 Spring Rd, Suite 600, Oak Brook, IL 60523. Inquiries via e-mail should be directed to *subscrib@rsna.org*. POSTMASTER: Send address correction "changes" to: *Radiology*, RSNA, 2021 Spring Rd, Suite 600, Oak Brook, IL 60523.

Claims for copies lost in the mail are allowed within 90 days of the date of issue. Claims are not allowed for issues lost as a result of insufficient notice of change of address.

Membership in the Radiological Society of North America is by formal application. Membership information should be secured from the Executive Director, the Radiological Society of North America, Inc, 2021 Spring Rd, Suite 600, Oak Brook, IL 60523. Dues are payable annually in January. In accordance with U.S. postal regulations, $107.50 of active membership dues is allocated to a subscription to *Radiology*.

359 **Life-threatening Primary Postpartum Hemorrhage: Treatment with Emergency Selective Arterial Embolization**
Jean-Pierre Pelage, Olivier Le Dref, Joaquim Mateo, Philippe Soyer, Denis Jacob, Mourad Kardache, Henri Dahan, Danielle Repiquet, Didier Payen, Jean-Bernard Truc, Jean-Jacques Merland, and Roland Rymer
Selective arterial embolization should be the treatment of choice for severe primary postpartum hemorrhage in case of failure with conservative treatment.

363 **Spondylodiskitic Abscesses: CT-guided Percutaneous Catheter Drainage**
Gundula Staatz, Gerhard B. Adam, Peter Keulers, Dierk Vorwerk, and Rolf W. Günther
CT-guided percutaneous catheter drainage of spondylodiskitic abscesses seems to be an attractive alternative to surgical management.

369 **Aneurysmal Bone Cysts: Percutaneous Embolization with an Alcoholic Solution of Zein—Series of 18 Cases**
Laurent Guibaud, Denis Herbreteau, Josée Dubois, Noelle Stempfle, Jérome Bérard, Jean-Pierre Pracros, and Jean-Jacques Merland
Percutaneous embolization of aneurysmal bone cysts with alcoholic zein should be considered a reliable alternative to surgery, especially in cases with a difficult surgical approach or cases of postsurgical recurrence.

Musculoskeletal Imaging

375 **Glenohumeral Joint: Comparison of Shoulder Positions at MR Arthrography**
Sandy M. Kwak, Robert R. Brown, Debra Trudell, and Donald Resnick
MR arthrography of the glenohumeral joint with the shoulder in external rotation optimizes visualization of the biceps-labral complex, and abduction external rotation is the best position for evaluation of the inferior glenohumeral ligament and anterior capsular attachment.

381 **Anterior Interosseous Nerve Syndrome: Appearance at MR Imaging in Three Cases**
Andrew J. Grainger, Robert S. D. Campbell, and John Stothard
MR imaging is potentially useful and safe in the investigation of anterior interosseous nerve syndrome, excluding muscle and tendon trauma from the differential diagnosis and providing a good alternative to electromyography in the confirmation that the abnormality lies in the distribution of the anterior interosseous nerve.

Health Policy and Practice

385 **Design of a Privileging Program for Diagnostic Imaging: Costs and Implications for a Large Insurer in Massachusetts**
Diana K. Verrilli, Stephen M. Bloch, Jeanine Rousseau, Matthew E. Crozier, and Steven B. Yecies
Results from the technical privileging program, specifically from the site inspections, reveal compelling evidence that many providers own and operate equipment that they are not trained to use.

Technical Developments

393 **Tracheobronchial Tree: Assessment with Volume Rendering—Technical Aspects**
Martine Remy-Jardin, Jacques Remy, Dominique Artaud, Marc Fribourg, and Abdel Naili
The study findings suggest that this volume-rendering technique has the potential to create diagnostically useful images of the bronchial tree.

399 **Pulmonary Nodules: CT-guided Contrast Material Localization for Thoracoscopic Resection**
Byung Gil Choi, Hak Hee Kim, Bum-soo Kim, Ki Tae Kim, Kyung Sub Shinn, and Seok Whan Moon
CT-guided contrast material localization of pulmonary nodules is proved to be a simple and useful method for thoracoscopic resection.

402 **Brachial Plexus: Demonstration at US**
Declan G. Sheppard, Revathy B. Iyer, and Marc J. Fenstermacher
US of the brachial plexus is technically feasible although the entire brachial plexus cannot be demonstrated.

407 **Aneurysm Clips: Assessment of Magnetic Field Interaction Associated with a 0.2-T Extremity MR System**
Frank G. Shellock and John V. Crues
It is safe to perform MR imaging of patients with certain aneurysm clips in this 0.2-T extremity MR system.

410 **Multisection Cerebral Blood Flow MR Imaging with Continuous Arterial Spin Labeling**
David C. Alsop and John A. Detre
This strategy is highly effective at controlling for off-resonance effects and efficient at doubly inverting inflowing spins, thus retaining the signal advantages of continuous versus pulsed arterial spin labeling techniques.

Continued—

Neuroradiology

417 **Subarachnoid Space Disease: Diagnosis with Fluid-attenuated Inversion-Recovery MR Imaging and Comparison with Gadolinium-enhanced Spin-Echo MR Imaging—Blinded Reader Study**

Michael B. Singer, Scott W. Atlas, and Burton P. Drayer

Unenhanced fluid-attenuated inversion-recovery MR imaging is superior to contrast-enhanced T1-weighted MR imaging for the diagnosis of subarachnoid space disease processes.

423 **Subarachnoid Hemorrhage: Aneurysm Detection and Preoperative Evaluation with CT Angiography**

Birgitta K. Velthuis, Gabriël J. E. Rinkel, Lino M. P. Ramos, Theodoor D. Witkamp, Jan Willem Berkelbach van der Sprenkel, W. Peter Vandertop, and Maarten S. van Leeuwen

If CT angiography is to replace digital subtraction angiography, it must depict most true aneurysms, demonstrate no false-positive aneurysms as definitely present, and depict the parent artery of anterior communicating aneurysms; also, the CT angiographic display must be acceptable to neurosurgeons as preoperative work-up.

431 **Frontotemporal Dementia and Alzheimer Disease: Evaluation of Cortical Atrophy with Automated Hemispheric Surface Display Generated with MR Images**

Hajime Kitagaki, Etsuro Mori, Shigeru Yamaji, Kazunari Ishii, Nobutsugu Hirono, Syoji Kobashi, and Yutaka Hata

Automated hemispheric surface display and volumetry are complementary to tomographic MR images and are useful for the evaluation of focal cortical atrophy in degenerative dementias—especially frontotemporal dementia.

Head and Neck Imaging

441 **Anterior Facial Vein and Submandibular Gland Together: Predicting the Histology of Submandibular Masses with CT or MR Imaging**

Jane L. Weissman and Ricardo L. Carrau

The relationship between a submandibular mass, the anterior facial vein, and the submandibular gland will help predict whether the mass arose from or adjacent to the gland and, thus, the histology of the mass.

447 **Contrast-enhanced 3D MR DSA of the Carotid Artery Bifurcation: Preliminary Study of Comparison with Unenhanced 2D and 3D Time-of-Flight MR Angiography**

Donald S. Willig, Patrick A. Turski, Richard Frayne, Virgil B. Graves, Frank R. Korosec, J. Shannon Swan, Charles A. Mistretta, and Thomas M. Grist

Three-dimensional MR digital subtraction angiography is a robust technique that allows improved delineation of complex proximal internal carotid artery morphology after the bolus injection of intravenous contrast agent.

Ultrasound

453 **Doppler Perfusion Index: An Interobserver and Intraobserver Reproducibility Study**

Karen Oppo, Edward Leen, Wilson J. Angerson, Timothy G. Cooke, and Colin S. McArdle

The interobserver reproducibility of Doppler perfusion index measurements was clinically acceptable, which suggests that any dedicated sonologist, if specially trained, can perform this standardized technique.

Genitourinary Imaging

459 **Paraovarian Cystadenomas and Cystadenofibromas: Sonographic Characteristics in 14 Cases**

Craig D. Korbin, Douglas L. Brown, and William R. Welch

The majority of paraovarian cystadenomas contain one or more small nodular areas and occasionally have septations or appear as simple cysts at sonography.

463 **Dilated Fallopian Tubes: MR Imaging Characteristics**

Eric K. Outwater, Evan S. Siegelman, Peerapod Chiowanich, Alex M. Kilger, Charles J. Dunton, and Alexander Talerman

Findings in this study demonstrate that dilated fallopian tubes can be identified on MR images and distinguished from other adnexal masses.

Breast Imaging

471 **Findings at Mammographic Screening on Only One Standard Projection: Outcomes Analysis**

Edward A. Sickles

The great majority (>80%) of findings seen on only one standard projection can be correctly assessed as representing superimposition of normal breast structures, either without or with the aid of additional imaging studies.

Continued—

477 **Invasive Carcinomas and Fibroadenomas of the Breast: Comparison of Microvessel Distributions—Implications for Imaging Modalities**
Kirsten L. Weind, Cynthia F. Maier, Brian K. Rutt, and Madeleine Moussa
While further histologic studies are necessary to evaluate vascular patterns in nonpalpable lesions, such as in atypical hyperplasia and carcinoma in situ, the results reported here suggest that the additional information on spatial distributions of vessels and the ability to resolve vessel sizes may add valuable information to the diagnostic work-up of an indeterminate solid lesion.

485 **Effects of a Microbubble Contrast Agent on Breast Tumors: Computer-assisted Quantitative Assessment with Color Doppler US—Early Experience**
Sabine Huber, Thomas Helbich, Joachim Kettenbach, Wolfgang Dock, Ivan Zuna, and Stefan Delorme
The data presented support the subjective impression that benign and malignant tumors of the breast behave differently at US in both degree and dynamics of enhancement after the injection of a contrast agent.

Experimental Studies

491 **Benign Prostatic Hyperplasia: US-guided Transrectal Urethral Enlargement with Radio Frequency—Initial Results in a Canine Model**
S. Nahum Goldberg, Peter F. Hahn, Francis J. McGovern, Robert M. Fogle, Peter R. Mueller, and G. Scott Gazelle
Transrectal radio-frequency application offers the prospect of a minimally invasive, imaging-guided method for treating patients with benign prostatic hyperplasia.

499 **Effect of Insulin on Uptake of FDG by Experimental Mammary Carcinoma in Diabetic Rats**
Tatsuo Torizuka, Susan J. Fisher, Raya S. Brown, and Richard L. Wahl
Although insulin treatment markedly reduced tumor/muscle ratio of 2-[fluorine-18]fluoro-2-deoxy-D-glucose (FDG) uptake in diabetes, it may improve relative targeting of lung cancer and metastatic liver cancer with FDG because of increased tumor/lung and tumor/liver uptake ratios.

Nuclear Medicine

505 **Lymphoscintigraphic Identification of Sentinel Lymph Nodes: Clinical Evaluation of 0.22-µm Filtration of Tc-99m Sulfur Colloid**
Leonard R. Goldfarb, Naomi P. Alazraki, Dennis Eshima, Lorie A. Eshima, Stephen C. Herda, and Raghuveer K. Halkar
Lymphoscintigraphic imaging studies obtained with a modified preparation of technetium-99m sulfur colloid demonstrate that 0.22-µm filtration results in substantially more definitive sentinel lymph node identification and optimal studies.

Radiation Oncology

511 **Limited-Stage Small Cell Lung Cancer: Local Failure after Chemotherapy and Radiation Therapy**
Takuhito Tada, Kazuo Minakuchi, Mayuko Koda, Noriyuki Masuda, Kaoru Matsui, Ichiro Kawase, Toshifumi Nakajima, Masayuki Nishioka, Masahiro Fukuoka, and Takahiro Kozuka
Our results suggest that patients with N3 disease should undergo a protocol separate from that used in other patients and that the upper margin of the radiation field should be extended in patients with N2 or N3 disease.

517 **Choroidal Neovascular Membranes: Treatment with Reirradiation**
Charles S. Cathcart, Joshua N. Halpern, Christopher M. Seery, Ahmed Abdelsalam, and Marco A. Zarbin
Additional radiation therapy in selected patients with choroidal neovascularization who have failed to benefit from previous irradiation is well tolerated and appears to stabilize the disease process in a substantial proportion of these patients.

Pediatric Imaging

521 **Appropriate Imaging in Children with Skull Fractures and Suspicion of Abuse**
Kirsten I. Mogbo, Thomas L. Slovis, Alexa I. Canady, David J. Allasio, and Cynthia L. Arfken
We did not find any case for which, in the absence of neurologic signs or symptoms, head CT provided any information of clinical use or disclosed additional injuries for legal documentation.

Gastrointestinal Imaging

525 **Intraperitoneal Abscesses: Diagnostic Accuracy of and Appearances at MR Imaging**
Tara C. Noone, Richard C. Semelka, Suvipapun Worawattanakul, and Hani B. Marcos
MR imaging has high diagnostic accuracy in evaluation of suspected intraperitoneal abscesses.

529 **Fecal Incontinence in Scleroderma: Assessment of the Anal Sphincter with Thin Section Endoanal MR Imaging**
Nandita M. deSouza, Andreanna D. Williams, Helen J. Wilson, David J. Gilderdale, Glyn A. Coutts, and Carol M. Black
Endoanal MR imaging enables anatomic assessment of fecal incontinence by allowing evaluation of the bulk of the component muscles of the anal sphincter.

537 **Pancreatic Arterial Anatomy: Depiction with Dual-Phase Helical CT**
Maria Chong, Patrick C. Freeny, and Udo P. Schmiedl
Our results show that it is possible to delineate small pancreatic arteries on arterial phase helical CT scans by using the optimized techniques we have described.

543 **Atypical Small Hemangiomas of the Liver: "Bright Dot" Sign at Two-Phase Spiral CT**
Hyun-Jung Jang, Byung Ihn Choi, Tae Kyoung Kim, Eun Joo Yun, Kyoung Won Kim, Joon Koo Han, and Man Chung Han
Awareness of a tiny enhancing dot, which is likely to be overlooked, could lead to a correct diagnosis of atypical small hemangioma with two-phase spiral CT.

Letters to the Editor

549 **Intratumoral Blood Flow in Cavernous Hemangioma of the Liver: Radiologic-Pathologic Correlation**
Jeong-Sik Yu, Myeong-Jin Kim, and Ki Whang Kim

549 **Reply**
Yasuyuki Yamashita

550 **Three-dimensional MR Imaging of Neurovascular Compression in Trigeminal Neuralgia**
Karsten Papke, Georg Bongartz, Harald Masur, and Gerhard Schuierer

551 **Reply**
Charles B. L. M. Majoie, Frans-Jan H. Hulsmans, Jonas A. Castelijns, and Jacob Valk

552 **Reducing Artifacts in MR Imaging of the Shoulder**
H. Peter Higer

552 **Reply**
Kiaran P. McGee, Roger C. Grimm, Joel P. Felmlee, John R. Rydberg, Stephen J. Riederer, and Richard L. Ehman

552 **Mammographic Artifact due to Film**
Laurie Margolies

553 **Beware the Pseudo Guinea Worm!**
Shella Farooki, Leanne L. Seeger, and Richard H. Gold

554 **Cost of PACS and Computed Radiography in the United States**
André J. Duerinckx and Edward G. Grant

555 **Reply**
Curtis P. Langlotz, Steven C. Horii, Hugh M. Pratt, and Harold L. Kundel

Book Reviews

282 AIDS Imaging: A Practical Clinical Approach
374 Imaging in Musculoskeletal and Sports Medicine
440 Imaging of the Globe and Orbit: A Guide to Differential Diagnosis
452 Vascular Diagnosis with Ultrasound: Clinical References with Case Studies
470 Atlas of Breast Imaging
490 Radiographic Anatomy and Positioning: An Integrated Approach
490 Applications Manual for Radiographic Anatomy and Positioning
490 Competency Manual for Radiographic Anatomy and Positioning
490 Pocket Manual for Radiographic Anatomy and Positioning
510 Handbook of Health Physics and Radiological Health. 3rd ed.

Interludes

288 Ultrasound Scan Confirms the Diagnosis of the Patient's Ailment
330 Comet Hale-Bopp (C/1995 O1)
358 Bird in Flight

Departments

557 Abstracts of Current Literature
556 Erratum
16A Advertisers' Index
15A RSNA Quick Reference
39A *Radiology* Business Information
19A Announcements and Books, Audiovisual Materials, and Software Received
33A Continuing Medical Education
45A Publication Information for Authors
49A *Radiology* Manuscript Categorization Terms
44A Copyright and Certifications Agreement
51A Classified Services
65A RSNA Bulletin Board
520 Associated Sciences Workshop 1998

RSNA® Radiological Society of North America Founded in 1915

2021 Spring Road, Suite 600
Oak Brook, Illinois 60523
630/571-2670
FAX:630/571-7837

Quick Reference

RSNA PURPOSE

The purpose of the Radiological Society of North America is to promote and develop the highest standards of radiology and related sciences through education and research. The Society seeks to provide radiologists and allied health scientists with educational programs and materials of the highest quality, and to constantly improve the content and value of these educational activities. The Society seeks to foster closer fellowship among all radiologists and greater cooperation among radiologists and members of other branches of medicine and allied health care professionals.

RSNA OFFICERS FOR 1998

President, **David B. Fraser, MD**, Halifax, NS

President-Elect, **Seymour H. Levitt, MD**, Minneapolis, MN

First Vice-President, **Carol B. Stelling, MD**, Houston, TX

Second Vice-President, **Miguel E. Stoopen, MD**, Mexico City, Mexico

Third Vice-President, **Guy H. Simmons, Jr, PhD**, Lexington, KY

Historian, **William R. Eyler, MD**, Beverly Hills, MI

RSNA BOARD OF DIRECTORS FOR 1998

C. Douglas Maynard, MD, Chairman of the Board, Winston-Salem, NC

Jerry P. Petasnick, MD, Liaison for Education, Northbrook, IL

R. Nick Bryan, MD, PhD, Liaison for Publications, Baltimore, MD

Peggy J. Fritzsche, MD, Liaison for Annual Meeting Arrangements, Riverside, CA

Brian C. Lentle, MD, Liaison Designate for Education, Vancouver, BC

David B. Fraser, MD, President, Halifax, NS

Seymour H. Levitt, MD, President-Elect, Minneapolis, MN

Delmar J. Stauffer, Executive Director

RSNA IMPORTANT TELEPHONE NUMBERS

MAIN TELEPHONE	(630) 571-2670	MEMBERSHIP (630) 571-7873 e-mail:membersh@rsna.org	
FAX	(630) 571-7837	RESEARCH DEVELOPMENT	(630) 368-3756
ACCOUNTING	(630) 571-7812	PROGRAM SERVICES	(630) 571-7874
EXECUTIVE	(630) 571-7866	RESEARCH & EDUCATION FUND	(630) 571-7816
LEARNING CENTER	(630) 368-3753	ADVERTISING	(630) 571-7817
MARKETING COMMUNICATIONS	(630) 571-7830	CLASSIFIED ADVERTISING	(630) 571-7817
MEETINGS	(630) 571-7850	RSNA LINK	http://www.rsna.org
PERMISSIONS	(630) 571-7829	SUBSCRIPTIONS (630) 571-7873 e-mail: subscrib@rsna.org	

RSNA MEETING DATES AND LOCATIONS

1998 November 29 to December 4
McCormick Place, Chicago

1999 November 28 to December 3
McCormick Place, Chicago

2000 November 26 to December 1
McCormick Place, Chicago

RSNA YEAR-AT-A-GLANCE

September 1–2, 1998
R&E Fund Trustee Meeting

September 9–10, 1998
RSNA Board of Directors Meeting

September 15, 1998
Third Seed Grant Deadline

October 30, 1998
Deadline for Advance Registration Forms for RSNA Scientific Assembly

November 29 to December 4, 1998
RSNA 84th Scientific Assembly and Annual Meeting

January 1, 1999
Call for Scientific Papers, Scientific Exhibits, and *info*RAD Exhibits

January 9, 1999
Deadline for receipt of all RSNA R&E Fund Grant Materials

January 15, 1999
First Seed Grant Deadline

February 19–21, 1999
RSNA Board of Directors Meeting

March 1, 1999
Roentgen Centennial Fellow "Preliminary Letter of Interest" Deadline

March 23-24, 1999
R&E Fund Trustee Meeting

April 15, 1999
Deadline for Submission of Scientific Paper, Scientific Exhibit, and *info*RAD Applications

May 15, 1999
Second Seed Grant Deadline

June 16–20, 1999
RSNA Board of Directors Meeting

Advertisers' Index

RSNA Advertising Policy

According to the advertising policy of the Radiological Society of North America, the information describing radiological equipment, products, and services offered by vendors in their advertisements should be ethical, educational, professional, of value in furthering the radiologic evaluation and treatment of patients and furthering the education of the radiologists and allied scientists. The guidelines below should be followed for advertising in RSNA journals.

- All advertising must be directed to radiologic diagnosis, therapy, research, communication and/or to the professional and managerial roles of radiologists and allied scientists. Advertising material should be consistent with the highest standards of professionalism.

- RSNA reserves the right to reject copy which, in its opinion, is not in good taste, is unprofessional, or is inappropriate for a radiology publication, or offers products or services not in the best interest of the patient or the Society. Advertisements that are constructed to resemble the journal's editorial pages will not be accepted in that form.

- Acceptance of advertising does not mean endorsement by RSNA of the products or services advertised, the advertisers, or the claims made.

For media kits and questions about advertising ONLY, contact:
Jim Drew, *Director of Advertising*
RSNA Publications
2021 Spring Road, Suite 600
Oak Brook, IL 60523
(630) 571-2670
FAX (630) 571-7837

For all other RSNA department telephone numbers, see "RSNA Quick Reference"; consult "Departments" in the Table of Contents for page.

Able Software Company 34A

Bioscan 32A

Cejka & Company 59A
CompHealth 59A

Daniel & Yeager 53A
Diversified Diagnostic Products, Inc 13A, 24A, 41A

Fuji Medical Systems IFC

Gammex RMI 11A
GE Medical Systems 25A–28A, IBC–OBC
Gundersen Lutheran 56A, 64A

Hewlett-Packard 30A–31A
The Hospital for Sick Children 63A

InterAmerican Congress of Radiology 37A

Jackson & Coker 61A

Lippincott-Raven Publishers 7A
Locum Medical Group 55A

Marshfield Clinic 56A
Mayo Health System 57A
Medical Doctor Associates, Inc 57A

National University Hospital, Singapore 58A
Nationwide Medical Services, Inc 58A

NDC Health Information Services 21A
Northern Metropolitan Radiology Associates 61A
Nuclear Associates 9A

Osler Institute 32A

Picker 29A

Radiology 20A
Radiology Resources 55A
RADX 35A
Roswell Park Cancer Institute 59A
RSNA Associated Sciences 520
RSNA *EJ* 36A, 516
RSNA Learning Center 19A, 458, 476, 536, 67A–70A
RSNA *Link* 42A
RSNA Membership 43A
RSNA Online Journals 352
RSNA ORD 338
RSNA Research & Education Fund 22A–23A, 368
RSNA Resident Membership 17A–18A
RSNA Scientific Assembly and Annual Meeting 38A

Siemens Medical Systems, Inc 2A–3A

Team Health 58A
Toshiba 4A
Trex Medical 484

U.S. Army Reserve 32A

Vista Staffing Solutions 53A

Announcements and Books, Audiovisual Materials, and Software Received

Announcements

2nd Heidelberg Conference on Dynamic and Functional Radiological Imaging of the Brain

The Department of Radiology, University of Heidelberg Medical School, is sponsoring the 2nd Heidelberg Conference on Dynamic and Functional Radiological Imaging of the Brain on October 29–31, 1998, in Heidelberg, Germany. The conference will focus on radiologic techniques with regard to normal and abnormal cerebral physiology. Topics include dynamic and functional magnetic resonance imaging, dynamic spiral computed tomography, single photon emission computed tomography, positron-emission tomography, and magnetic source imaging. Fee: DM 350. For further information, contact Diana Brinkmann, Department of Neuroradiology, University of Heidelberg Medical School, Im Neuenheimer Feld 400, D-69120 Heidelberg, Germany; telephone 49 6221 567566; fax 49 6221 564673; e-mail *Diana_Brinkmann@ukl.uni-heidelberg.de*.

Books, Audiovisual Materials, and Software Received

Radiology carries a complete listing of all books, CD-ROMs, and other material received by the Radiological Society of North America. If the material is later reviewed, the reviews of books will be printed in *Radiology* and the reviews of CD-ROMs and electronic material will appear in *RadioGraphics*.

Send publications for review to Richard A. Szucs, MD, Book Review Editor, *Radiology* Editorial Office, 1001 E Broad St, Suite 310, Richmond, VA 23219.

Atlas of Human Anatomy. 2nd ed. Frank H. Netter, MD. Softcover, price not available; 596 pp, 525 illustrations. ISBN: 0-914168-81-9. Summit, NJ: Novartis Medical Education, 1997.

Basic Atlas of Sectional Anatomy with Correlated Imaging. 3rd ed. Walter J. Bo, PhD, Neil T. Wolfman, MD, Wayne A. Kreuger, PhD, Jeffrey Carr, MD, Robert L. Bowden, BA, Isadore Meschan, MD. Hardcover, $120.00; 512 pp, 829 illustrations. ISBN: 0-7216-3265-3. Philadelphia, Pa: Saunders, 1998.

Breast Imaging. 2nd ed. Edited by Daniel B. Kopans, MD, FACR. Hardcover, $165.00; 890 pp, 814 illustrations. ISBN: 0-397-51302-X. Philadelphia, Pa: Lippincott-Raven, 1997.

Current Radiation Oncology. Vol 3. Edited by Jeffrey S. Tobias, MD, FRCP, FRCR, Patrick R. M. Thomas, MB, FRCP, FRCR, FACR. Hardcover, $95.00; 420 pp, 99 illustrations. ISBN: 0-340-67739-2. New York, NY: Oxford University Press, 1997.

Fetal Echocardiography. Julia A. Drose, BA, RDMS, RDCS, RVT. Hardcover, $65.00; 314 pp, 280 illustrations. ISBN: 0-7216-6284-6. Philadelphia, Pa: Saunders, 1998.

Helical (Spiral) Computed Tomography: A Practical Approach to Clinical Protocols. Edited by Paul M. Silverman, MD. Softcover, $49.95; 286 pp, 86 illustrations. ISBN: 0-7817-1478-8. Philadelphia, Pa: Lippincott-Raven, 1998.

Understanding Helical Scanning. Cheryl Blanck. Softcover, $24.95; 94 pp, 43 illustrations. ISBN: 0-683-30304-X. Baltimore, Md: Williams & Wilkins, 1998.

Research Resident

Purpose –To provide educational opportunities for radiology residents to gain further insight into scientific investigation, or to develop competence in research and educational techniques and methods.

Amount –$30,000 grant for one year, payable to the department, to be used as stipend.

Requirements –Nominee should:
- possess an academic degree acceptable for the radiology residency, and
- at time of nomination, be in a residency program.

It is expected that the Research Resident will devote 90% of his or her time to the program outlined.

Seed Grant

Purpose –To assist young investigators in testing hypotheses and defining objectives before they apply for major grants from corporations, foundations, or government agencies.

Amount –One-year grant of $25,000 or less, payable to the department in equal installments.

Requirements –Applicant should hold full–time faculty position,
- have completed all advanced training, and
- have not served as principal investigator in a major ($50,000 or more) grant.

Any area of radiology–related research is eligible, including basic, clinical, developmental, health care planning and delivery, efficacy studies, and education.

Note: Applicant need not be citizen/resident of a North American country.

The Seed Grant Program will be offered three times each year. Deadlines are:
January 15 for July 1 start date
May 15 for November 1 start date
September 15 for March 1 start date

Roentgen Centennial Fellow Program

Purpose –To permit experienced practitioners the opportunity to explore and apply innovative solutions to key issues facing the radiology community. Such activity may include, but is not limited to: research studies, or program delivery focusing on topics such as health care policy/economics; educational methodology; evaluation methodology/outcomes research; basic or clinical research; rural health care delivery; or technology assessment.

Amount –This $100,000 award is designed to support a one–year program of study and/or research.

Requirements –Nominee should be beyond initial radiologic training and have several years of experience.

The individual who receives this award will devote a majority of his or her time to the proposed activity for a period of one year.

Application details differ for this program. Detailed letter of interest outlining applicant's innovative idea should be received at the Fund's office by March 1 each year.

Outstanding Researcher Award

Purpose –To honor one senior physician or radiology researcher who has made a career of significant contributions to the field of radiology or radiologic sciences through research.

Amount –$25,000 award payable to the recipient.

Requirements –Nominee must demonstrate a long–term commitment to radiology research.

Nomination packets must include:
- letter of nomination that addresses individual's appropriateness for award;
- corroborating letter of support; and
- nominee's CV, which includes a summary of candidate's grant support and research activities.

Nominations must be made by June 15. Nominee need not be a member of the RSNA.

Roentgen Resident/Fellow Research Award

Purpose –To recognize and encourage outstanding residents and fellows in radiologic research.

Recognition Award –Each participating residency program will receive an award plaque. Plaque includes place for additional names. Each year the Fund will provide a memento for the department to present to the selected resident or fellow.

Requirements –The director of the residency program or the department chair will identify an individual based on the following criteria:
- presentations or scientific papers at regional or national meetings,
- publication of scientific papers in peer-reviewed journals,
- receipt of a research grant, or
- other research activities.

The R&E Fund does not make the selections. Each department simply submits the name and address of the resident/fellow selected with a description of the individual's research activities. Nomination is to be submitted no later than April 1.

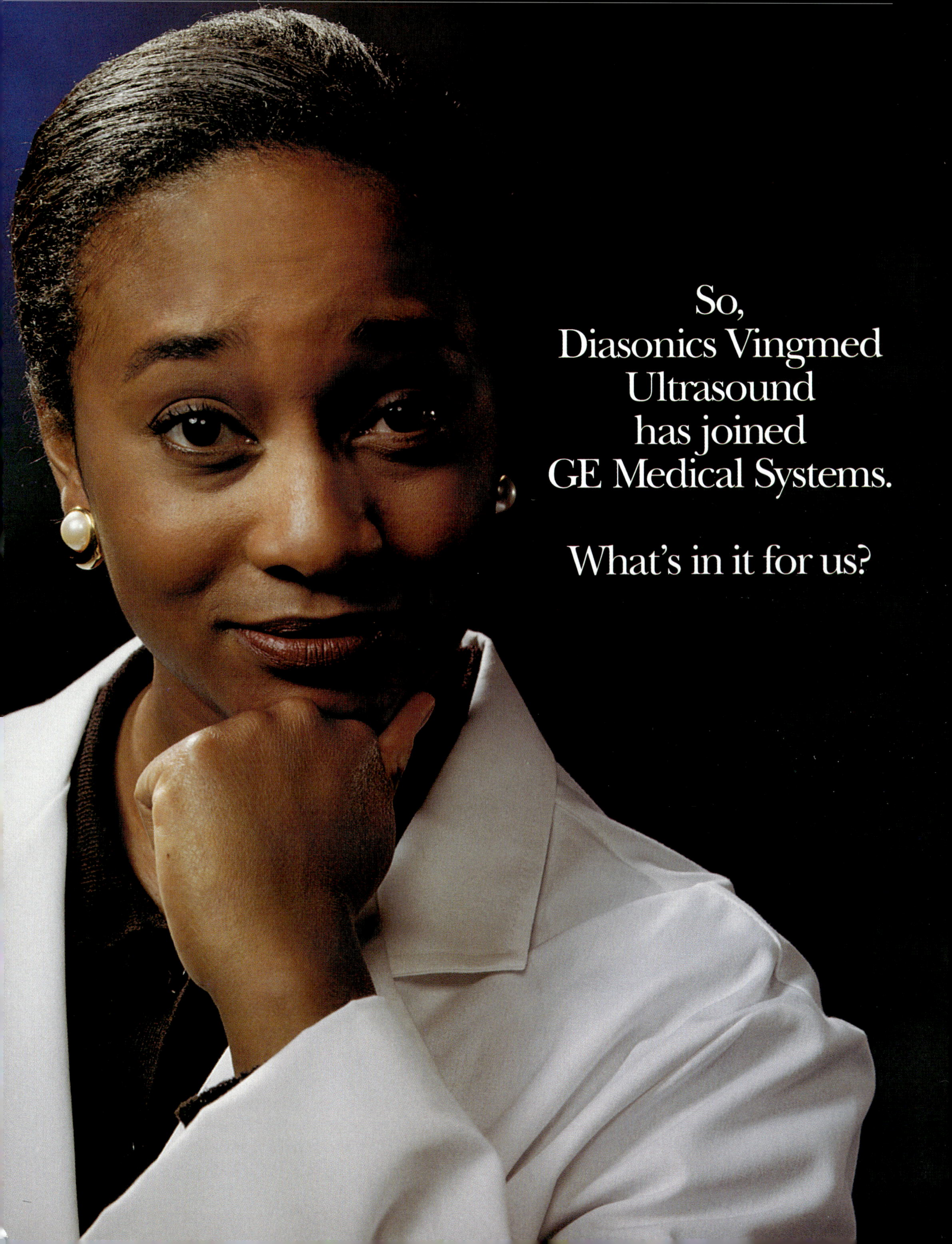
So,
Diasonics Vingmed
Ultrasound
has joined
GE Medical Systems.
What's in it for us?

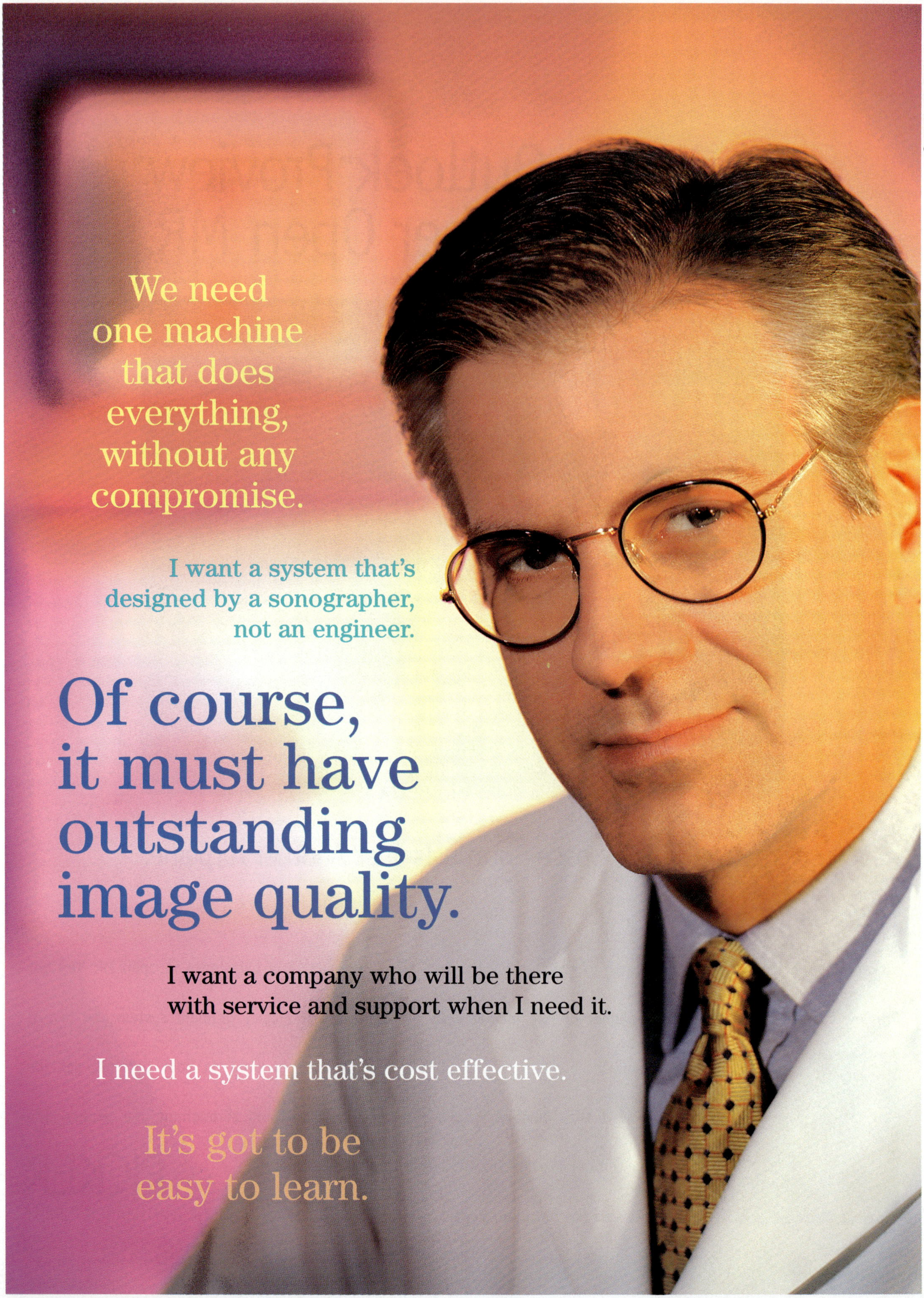
We need one machine that does everything, without any compromise.
I want a system that's designed by a sonographer, not an engineer.
Of course, it must have outstanding image quality.
I want a company who will be there with service and support when I need it.
I need a system that's cost effective.
It's got to be easy to learn.

Continuing Medical Education

NOTE: Notices of continuing medical education programs will be considered for publication in *Radiology* if the program is directly relevant to medical imaging and if the following information is included: (*a*) dates and location, (*b*) a brief description of the course, (*c*) a listing of local and visiting faculty, (*d*) fees, and (*e*) number of category 1 credits that are available. Such notices should be submitted *at least* 5 months before the meeting date. Announcements of CME programs we consider not pertinent will not be published. We assume no responsibility for the content of CME programs appearing here. **Address announcements to** Julie Pietryla, RSNA Publications, 2021 Spring Rd, Suite 600, Oak Brook, IL 60523.

Continuing medical education programs are listed according to diagnostic discipline; interdisciplinary programs are grouped under the predominant or first-listed specialty.

Diagnostic Imaging

General Radiology and Breast Imaging Review

The Department of Radiology, University of Kentucky College of Medicine, is sponsoring a "General Radiology and Breast Imaging Review" on October 10–11, 1998, at the Hyatt Regency Lexington, Lexington, Ky. This course is designed to provide radiologists with an update on current diagnostic techniques in general radiology using didactic lectures, panel discussions, and question-and-answer sessions with faculty members. Guest faculty: Brown, Mendelson. Local faculty: Buck, Fried, Kacki, Kriss, Lieber, Reed, Runge. Fee: $300 ($100 for technologists); 10 hours of category 1 credit will be available. For further information, contact Teresa McIver, conference coordinator, University of Kentucky, Kentucky Clinic L007, Lexington, KY 40536-0284; telephone (606) 323-5174; fax (606) 323-2008; *http://www.ukcme.org*.

Economics of Diagnostic Imaging

The "13th Annual Economics of Diagnostic Imaging 1998: National Symposium," sponsored by Educational Symposia, Inc, will be held on October 22–25, 1998, at the Hyatt Regency Washington, Washington, DC. Upon completion of this course, participants should be able to (*a*) implement strategies to help cope with the challenges of managed care, (*b*) discuss the practice implications of Medicare fraud and abuse, employer-employee relationships, and self-referral legislation, (*c*) prepare for the future of radiology by evaluating training, equipment, and information needs, (*d*) describe the impact of evolving economic changes on physicians, hospitals, and manufacturers, and (*e*) evaluate the impact of quality improvement and outcomes measures on the practice of radiology. Keynote speakers: Evens, Harris, Wilensky. Fee: $695; 27 hours of category 1 credit will be available. For further information, contact the program committee, Educational Symposia, Inc, 1527 S Dale Mabry Hwy, Tampa, FL 33629-5808; telephone (800) 338-5901 or (813) 254-4608; fax (800) 344-0668 or (813) 254-9773; e-mail *information@edusymp.com; http://www.edusymp.com*.

Pulmonary and Coronary MR and CT Angiography

The North American Society for Cardiac Imaging (NASCI) will hold its 26th annual meeting and scientific sessions on November 7, 1998, in Dallas, Tex. This meeting is co-sponsored by NASCI, University of California–Davis Health System Continuing Medical Education, and the American Heart Association. Topics include pulmonary magnetic resonance (MR) and computed tomographic (CT) angiography, coronary MR and CT angiography, and right ventricular dysplasia. Co-Chairmen: Bogren, Duerinckx. For further information, contact Joan Saluzzi, executive director, NASCI, PO Box 411106, San Francisco, CA 94141-1106; telephone (415) 487-9802; fax (415) 487-9803; e-mail *info@nasci.org; http://www.nasci.org*.

Breast Imaging

Breast Imaging Today and Tomorrow

The International Institute for Continuing Medical Education is sponsoring a course entitled "Breast Imaging Today and Tomorrow," to take place on November 2–5, 1998, at the Ritz-Carlton Resort Hotel, Naples, Fla. This course is designed for practicing diagnostic radiologists who have a basic knowledge of breast imaging. It covers aspects of mammographic interpretation, interventional procedures, screening controversies, MQSA, emerging technologies, and the self-audit. Faculty: Adler, Homer, Keda, Rubin. Fee: $650 ($450 for residents, fellows, and technologists); 26 hours of category 1 credit will be available. For further information, contact Ryals & Associates, Inc, PO Box 1925, Roswell, GA 30077-1925; telephone (770) 641-9773; fax (770) 552-9859; e-mail *webmaster@ryalsmeet.com; http://www.ryalsmeet.com*.

Interventional Radiology

Symposium on Peripheral Vascular Disease

The Brown University School of Medicine and Rhode Island Hospital are co-sponsoring the "8th Annual Symposium on Peripheral Vascular Disease" on August 14–16, 1998, at the Newport Doubletree Islander Hotel, Newport, RI. This program will utilize presentations and panel discussions to communicate the latest concepts, methodologies, and techniques in the surgical and percutaneous treatment of patients with peripheral vascular disease. Topics include arterial and venous occlusive disease, cerebrovascular disease, and dialysis graft maintenance. Faculty: Benenati, Bonn, Hobson, Matsumoto, Pomposelli, Waldman. Fee: $425 ($250 for residents, nurses, and technologists); 14 hours of category 1 credit will be available. For further information, contact Lifespan, CME Office, 593 Eddy St, Providence, RI 02903; telephone (401) 444-4260; fax (401) 444-4984; *http://www.mdpso.com/education/pvd.html*.

Advanced Interventional Techniques for Peripheral Vascular Disease

The "10th Annual Advanced Interventional Techniques for Peripheral Vascular Disease" course, sponsored by the Midwest Vascular Institute of Illinois, will be held on September 23–26, 1998, at the Hyatt Regency Oak Brook, Oak Brook, Ill. This course will present the latest developments and applications of interventional techniques through live demonstrations, video case presentations, lectures, and panel discussion. Topics include case selection, logical approaches, and technical aspects of interventional modalities. Course director: Motarjeme. Fee: $650 ($350 for residents, nurses, and technologists); 20 hours of category 1 credit will be available. For further information, contact the Midwest Vascular Institute of Illinois, 3825 S Highland Ave, Ste 306, Downers Grove, IL 60515; telephone (630) 963-0660; fax (630) 963-8348.

Interventional Radiology and Vascular Imaging 1998

The Department of Radiology, University of Pennsylvania, is sponsoring "Interventional Radiology and Vascular Imaging 1998," a course to be held on November 4–7, 1998, at the El Conquistador Resort, Fajardo, Puerto Rico. This course provides a thorough and intensive review of magnetic resonance angiography and interventional radiology throughout the body. Fundamentals of well-established procedures and the latest developments in new techniques will be reviewed by a faculty of nationally known experts. Course directors: Haskal, Soulen. Fee: $695 ($450 for residents and fellows); 24 hours of category 1 credit will be available. For further information, contact Janice Ford Benner, Department of Radiology, University of Pennsylvania Medical Center, 3400 Spruce St, 1 Founders Bldg, Philadelphia, PA 19104; telephone (215) 662-7825; fax (215) 349-5925.

Magnetic Resonance

Current Concepts of Magnetic Resonance

"Current Concepts of Magnetic Resonance," a course co-sponsored by the Stanford University School of Medicine and Duke University Medical Center, will take place on November 1–5, 1998, at the Monterey Plaza Hotel, Monterey, Calif. This course will present fundamental techniques and clinical applications of magnetic resonance (MR) imaging. Concepts are introduced through lectures and workshops and reinforced by clinical examples and applications. Although the basic aspects of MR are presented, the course is ideally suited to those with some knowledge of MR imaging. Topics include image formation, contrast manipulation mechanisms, vascular imaging, and fast imaging strategies. Course director: Pelc. Faculty: Bernstein, Butts, Daniel, Glover, Herfkens, Johnson, Lane, Li, Marks, Moseley, Napel, Norbash, Rubin, Sommer, Spielman. Fee: $650 until October 2, $700 thereafter ($450 [$500] for Stanford alumni and military personnel; $350 [$400] for residents, fellows, and technologists); 31.25 hours of category 1 credit will be available. For further information, contact Lorie Pelc, Department of Radiology, Stanford University School of Medicine, Lucas MRS Building, Mail Code 5488, Rte 8, Stanford, CA 94305; telephone (650) 723-8312; fax (650) 723-5795; e-mail *lrp@s-word.stanford.edu; http://www-radiology.stanford.edu/education/Monterey.html.*

Neuroradiology

AFIP Neuroradiology Course

The Armed Forces Institute of Pathology is sponsoring the "AFIP Neuroradiology Course" on August 22–23, 1998, at the Wyndham Emerald Plaza Hotel, San Diego, Calif. This course is designed to offer radiologists, neurologists, neurosurgeons, and pathologists a basic review and update of neuroradiology. The essential morphologic and physiologic principles that create the diagnostic image will be emphasized. Important radiologic-pathologic concepts will be illustrated by means of magnetic resonance imaging, computed tomography, and other conventional studies. Course director: Koeller. Faculty: Berger, Dowd, Gean, Kerber, Koeller, Osborn, Smirniotopoulos, Wong. Fee: $300 ($180 for residents; $75 for military personnel); 15 hours of category 1 credit will be available. For further information, contact the Department of Radiologic Pathology, Armed Forces Institute of Pathology, Washington, DC 20306-6000; telephone (202) 782-2438; fax (202) 782-8124.

Nuclear Medicine

Nuclear Cardiology Symposium and Workshop

The University of Wisconsin Medical School and the Heart Institute, Sinai Samaritan Medical Center, Milwaukee, Wis, are co-sponsoring a "Nuclear Cardiology Symposium and Workshop" on October 23–24, 1998, at the Grand Hotel, Milwaukee, Wis. This course is designed as a refresher course to prepare participants for certification. Fee: $490 ($285 for technologists); 14 hours of category 1 credit will be available. For further information, contact Sarah Aslakson, Continuing Medical Education, University of Wisconsin Medical School, 2715 Marshall Ct, Madison, WI 53705; telephone (608) 263-2856; fax (608) 262-8421; e-mail *aslakson @facstaff.wisc.edu; http://www.biostat.wisc.edu/cme/cme.html.*

Ultrasound

Focus on Ultrasound

"Focus on Ultrasound," a course sponsored by the University of Wisconsin Medical School, is taking place on October 29–30, 1998, at the Concourse Hotel, Madison, Wis. This course is designed to meet the educational needs of sonographers and practicing diagnostic radiologists. The focus is on the areas in which ultrasound has made the greatest inroads and on newly emerging areas. Topics include vascular imaging, peritoneal disease, musculoskeletal applications, the role of PACS, physics, the medicolegal system, and other specialties' view of the role of ultrasound in patient care. Planning committee: Propeck, Scanlan, Sterken. Fee: $365 ($285 for residents and technologists); 15 hours of category 1 credit will be available. For further information, contact Sarah Aslakson, Continuing Medical Education, University of Wisconsin Medical School, 2715 Marshall Ct, Madison, WI 53705; telephone (608) 263-2856; fax (608) 262-8421; e-mail *aslakson @facstaff.wisc.edu; http://www.biostat.wisc.edu/cme/cme.html.*

Obstetrical Ultrasound

"Obstetrical Ultrasound," a course sponsored by and being held at the Center for Medical Ultrasound, Wake Forest University School of Medicine, will take place on November 9–13, 1998. The course is devoted to the study of obstetrics and gynecology. About 15 hours are dedicated to lectures by experienced sonologists, with the remaining time spent in scanning laboratories with patients. Fee: $945; 30 hours of category 1 credit will be available. For further information, contact the Center for Medical Ultrasound, Wake Forest University School of Medicine, Medical Center Blvd, Winston-Salem, NC 27157-1039; telephone (800) 277-7654 or (336) 716-4505; fax (336) 716-4204; *http://www.wfubmc.edu/bgsm/ultrasound.*

Masters Symposium on Ultrasound in Obstetrics and Gynecology

The Institute for Advanced Medical Education is sponsoring its "Masters Symposium on Ultrasound in Obstetrics and Gynecology: The Best of the Big Apple" on November 13–15, 1998, at the Crowne Plaza, New York, NY. This program brings together leading speakers in Ob-Gyn and ultrasound. In addition to talks on the various clinical aspects of ultrasound, there will be presentations on newer imaging technologies and laboratory accreditation. Fee: $590; 18 hours of category 1 credit will be available. For further information, contact Penney Margeotes, Institute for Advanced Medical Education, 14 Elm Pl, Rye, NY 10580; telephone (914) 921-5700; fax (914) 921-6048; e-mail *info@iame.com.*

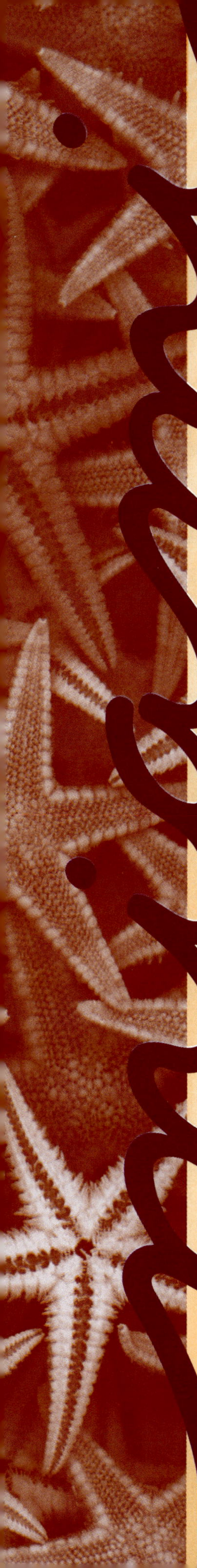

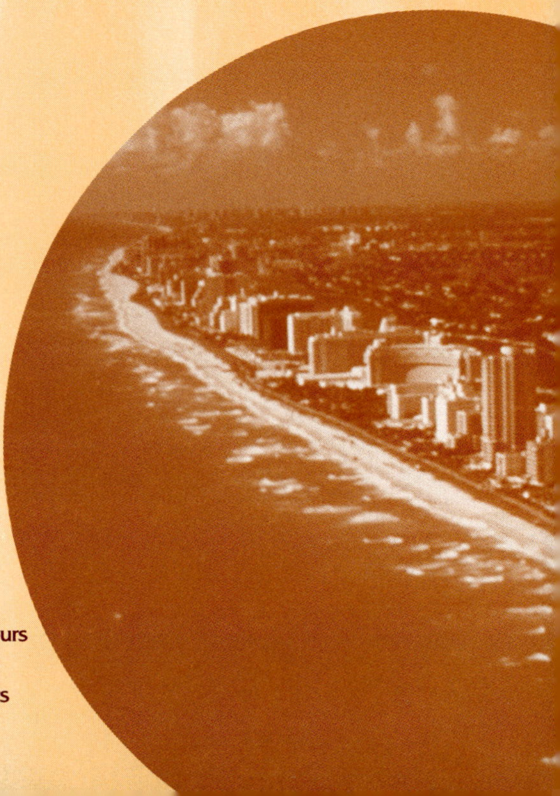

Radiology Business Information

Radiology, a monthly journal devoted to clinical radiology and allied sciences, is owned and published by

The Radiological Society of North America, Inc (RSNA)
2021 Spring Road, Suite 600
Oak Brook, IL 60523 USA
(630) 571-2670 • FAX (630) 571-7837
RSNA Link *http://www.rsna.org*

Delmar J. Stauffer, *Executive Director and Business Manager for Publications*

■ JOURNAL BUSINESS

Send new manuscripts to the address given in the Publication Information for Authors.

Correspondence concerning accepted or published material should be addressed to

Anthony V. Proto, MD–Editor, *Radiology*
Radiology Editorial Office • 1001 East Broad Street
Suite 310 • Richmond, VA 23219
(804) 644-5667 FAX (804) 644-5672
e-mail: *proto@rsna.org*

■ COPYRIGHT AND PERMISSIONS

Material printed in *Radiology* is covered by copyright. No part of this publication may be reproduced or transmitted in any form without written permission from RSNA, except under circumstances within "fair use" as defined by U.S. copyright law. Requests for permission to use previously published material must be **in writing** and mailed or faxed to the Permissions Coordinator, RSNA Publications, Oak Brook, IL (address above).

■ PHOTOCOPYING

Authorization to photocopy items for internal or personal use, or the internal or personal use of specific clients and educators, is granted by RSNA, provided that the appropriate fee is paid directly to Copyright Clearance Center, Inc (CCC), 222 Rosewood Dr, Danvers, MA 01923 (phone 978-750-8400; FAX 978-750-4744).

Consent for photocopying does not extend to copying for general distribution, resale, or advertising and promotional purposes, or for creating new collective works. Permission for the latter categories may be sought by writing to the Permissions Coordinator, RSNA Publications, Oak Brook, IL (address above).

■ SUBSCRIPTION INFORMATION

The nonmember subscription rate for the USA is $215.00 per year; for outside USA, $260.00 (includes postage). (Air freight is available; rates are furnished on request.) Residents who are members of the RSNA may subscribe to **both** *Radiology* and *RadioGraphics* for a special rate of $80.00 (for North American addresses; residents from outside North America, add $60.00 for postage). Single copies are $25.00 (air freight, $11.00). Orders for subscriptions, remittances, and questions about subscriptions should be sent to

RSNA Subscriptions Department
2021 Spring Road, Suite 600
Oak Brook, IL 60523 USA
(630) 571-7873
FAX (630) 571-7837
e-mail: *subscrib@rsna.org*

The page containing advertising information (Advertisers' Index) may be located by consulting the Departments section in the Table of Contents.

■ CHANGE OF ADDRESS

The Post Office will not forward your journal to a new address. To avoid missing any issues, you must notify us of a change in address. At least 5 weeks before you move, please send (*a*) your **new address**, with zip code, and (*b*) your **current mailing label** with your old address to the address above.

■ MISSING ISSUES AND BACK COPIES

Claims for copies lost in the mail are allowed within 90 days of issue. Claims are not allowed for issues lost as a result of insufficient notice of change of address. To replace a missing issue or order a back copy contact RSNA Subscriptions Department at the address above. Back copies cost $25.00 (air freight, $11.00).

■ REPRINTS

The first footnote on the first page of each *Radiology* article contains the name and address of the author who answers requests for reprints. For reprint orders of 100 or more, contact

(continued)

RSNA DEPARTMENT TELEPHONE NUMBERS

Accounting	(630) 571-7812
Advertising	(630) 571-7817
Copyrights and Permissions	(630) 571-7829
Executive	(630) 571-7866
Learning Center	(630) 368-3753
Meetings	(630) 571-7850
Membership	(630) 571-7873
Office of Research	(630) 368-3756
Permissions	(630) 571-7829
Program	(630) 571-7874
Research and Education Fund	(630) 571-7816
Reprints	(610) 250-7244
Subscriptions	(630) 571-7873
Syllabus sales	(800) 272-2920
Main telephone	(630) 571-2670
FAX	(630) 571-7837

Radiology Reprints
1991 Northampton St
Easton, PA 18042-3189 USA
(610) 250-7244

For reprints of advertisements, contact the Advertising Production Manager (address under Advertising).

■ MICROFORM

Radiology is available in microfilm and microfiche from

University Microforms International
300 N Zeeb Road
Ann Arbor, MI 48106 USA
(800) 521-3044

■ INDEXES

Radiology is included in the *RSNA Index to Imaging Literature,* a 3-year cumulative subject and author index of *Radiology* and 41 radiologic journals, available for $35.00 per copy (air freight, $11.00). Subscribers to the Journal receive the index free of charge. *Radiology* is indexed in *Current Contents/Clinical Medicine,* available from the Institute for Scientific Information, and *Index Medicus,* available from the National Library of Medicine.

■ BOOK REVIEWERS AND BOOKS FOR REVIEW

Any person who would like to help in reviewing books for *Radiology* should contact

Richard A. Szucs, MD, Book Review Editor
Radiology Editorial Office
1001 E Broad St
Suite 310
Richmond, VA 23219

Publishers wishing to have books reviewed should send them to the same address.

■ PUBLISHERS' ROW

As a service to readers and colleagues in medical publishing, *Radiology* publishes a list of current imaging publications of interest to radiologists and allied scientists. Complete addresses and phone numbers of participating publishers are included. Publishers' Row is featured quarterly, in the March, June, September, and December issues. For information on publishing a list, contact Mary Ann Morrissey at RSNA Publications (address under Journal Business).

■ ADVERTISING

The advertising policy appears on the Advertisers' Index of each issue. Questions about advertising and billing, advertising contracts, and insertion orders and requests for media kits should be addressed to

James F. Drew, *Director of Advertising*
RSNA Publications
2021 Spring Road, Suite 600
Oak Brook, IL 60523 USA
(630) 571-7819
FAX (630) 571-7837

Questions about advertising production should be addressed to:

Pat Hollingsworth, *Advertising Production Manager*
RSNA Advertising Department
2021 Spring Rd, Suite 600
Oak Brook, IL 60523 USA
(630) 571-7818
FAX (630) 571-7837

■ CLASSIFIED ADVERTISING

As a service to readers, *Radiology* accepts classified advertising, and every effort is made to ensure that the ads are relevant to the practice of radiology. For more details on the classified advertising policy and procedures, see the Classified Advertising section in each issue (consult the Departments section in the Table of Contents for page number) or contact the Advertising Production Manager (address under Advertising).

CHANGE OF ADDRESS FORM

Please allow 90 days for change to take effect

Name: ______________________________

Previous Address

Address: ______________________________

____

____

City/State/Zip: ______________________________

New Address

Address: ______________________________

____

____

City/State/Zip: ______________________________

Mail to:
RSNA Subscriptions Department • 2021 Spring Road • Suite 600 • Oak Brook, IL 60523 USA **FAX:** (630) 571-7837

Transfer of Copyright and Certifications Agreement

Manuscript No. (for Editorial Office use only)____________________

Complete copyright to the article entitled:

____

____

is hereby transferred to the Radiological Society of North America (for **U.S. government employees:** to the extent transferable), effective if and when the article is accepted for publication in ***Radiology,*** printed or electronic format. In the case of authors who are officers or employees of the U.S. government, the Radiological Society of North America recognizes that works prepared by them as part of their official government duties are in the public domain.

Authors reserve the following rights:

A. Other than copyright, all proprietary rights including patent rights relating to the subject matter of the article.
B. The license for personal use in lectures, lecture notes, and exhibits.

Please return this form as soon as possible. The signed statement **must** be received by the Editor **before** the manuscript can be processed for publication.

A. All authors certify that this material or similar material has not been and will not be submitted by them or by colleagues in their institution to any other publication prior to its appearance in ***Radiology.***

B. All authors certify that they have read the Publication Information for Authors found in the most recently published issue of ***Radiology*** at the time the manuscript is submitted. They further certify their compliance with the various requirements found therein.

C. All authors certify that they have submitted all required permissions and that all required statements have been inserted in the text where appropriate.

D. All authors certify that all individuals who have participated sufficiently in the conception and design of this work, in the analysis of the data, and in the writing of the manuscript have been listed as authors. All authors further certify that they have read the final version of the manuscript and approve it for submission for publication.

E. All authors certify that the Editor may correspond with the designated *corresponding author* regarding acceptance, rejection, revision of the manuscript and that the corresponding author is responsible for informing all other authors of the same.

F. All authors certify that responses, revisions received by the Editor from the designated *corresponding author* will be treated as if from all authors and that the corresponding author is responsible for informing all other authors of the same.

G. All authors certify that: **(must check one)**

- ❐ they have no direct or indirect financial interest in the products under investigation or subject matter discussed in this manuscript, or
- ❐ one or more (please name) authors do have a direct or indirect financial interest in the products under investigation or subject matter discussed in this manuscript. A separate statement is attached that details this proprietary interest, and the authors hereby grant permission to publish this information or an appropriate summary thereof with the manuscript if the manuscript is published.

TO BE SIGNED BY ALL AUTHORS:

Name (print) (First) ____________________ Signature ____________________

Name (print) ____________________ Signature ____________________

Name (print) ____________________ Signature ____________________

Name (print) ____________________ Signature ____________________

Name (print) ____________________ Signature ____________________

Name (print) ____________________ Signature ____________________

Use additional page if necessary.

This signed form (a photocopy is acceptable) must be submitted with all proffered works.

Radiology Publication Information for Authors

Radiology is published under the supervision of the Board of Directors of the Radiological Society of North America, Inc, which appoints the Editor who selects all material submitted for publication, including advertisements. No responsibility is accepted by the Board of Directors or the appointed Editor for the opinions expressed by the contributors. Please note that the instructions below are in accord with the *Uniform Requirements for Manuscripts Submitted to Biomedical Journals* (*Annals of Internal Medicine* 1997; 126:36-47). Although *Radiology* will receive material prepared and submitted according to these instructions, the right is reserved to introduce any changes necessary to make the contributions conform to the individual editorial standards of this Journal.

Full manuscripts should be addressed to:
Anthony V. Proto, MD—Editor, *Radiology*
Radiology Manuscripts • RSNA Publications
2021 Spring Road, Suite 600 • Oak Brook, IL 60523 USA
FAX (630) 571-7837

All other submissions and correspondence concerning accepted or published material should be addressed to:
Anthony V. Proto, MD—Editor, *Radiology*
Radiology Editorial Office • 1001 East Broad Street
Suite 310 • Richmond, VA 23219
(804) 644-5667 FAX (804) 644-5672
e-mail: *proto@rsna.org*

Assistant to the Editor: Deborah L. Hogan
Office Coordinator: Donna L. Schulze, Beth A. Stephenson

Inquiries about manuscript status and preparation, as well as letters to the editor, can be directed to *radiolog@ rsna.org*

The page containing advertising information (Advertisers' Index) may be located by consulting the Departments section in the Table of Contents.

TRANSFER OF COPYRIGHT AND CERTIFICATIONS AGREEMENT

Please send the copyright and certifications agreement with the initial submission of all proffered works. This may be accomplished by using a copy of the form that appears in this issue. **All** authors of any single composition must sign this agreement. In the case of officers or employees of the U.S. government, the Society recognizes that works prepared as part of their official government duties are in the public domain, but they must still sign the copyright and certifications agreement.

FINANCIAL INTEREST

Authors must describe any direct or indirect financial interest they may have in the subject matter of a submitted manuscript, and they must authorize the Society to publish this financial disclosure with the article if deemed appropriate. The Society's Financial Disclosure policy is as follows:

"Each author shall describe (*a*) any direct financial interest that author has in the subject matter discussed in the submitted manuscript, and (*b*) any affiliation or financial involvement that author has with or in any organization having a direct financial interest in the subject matter discussed in the submitted manuscript. Such information will be held in the confidence of the journal Editor during the review process. If necessary, in the Editor's view, this information may be shared with reviewers after discussion between the Editor and author. The submission of a manuscript to *Radiology* grants permission for RSNA to publish the financial information described above, or an appropriate summary thereof, with the manuscript if the manuscript is accepted for publication."

MANUSCRIPT PREPARATION

Original writings will be accepted only with the understanding that they are contributed solely to *Radiology*. Manuscripts should be typewritten and **double-spaced (all pages)** on only one side of the paper with at least 3-cm margins. Each manuscript component should begin on a **new page** in this order: title pages, abstract, text, acknowledgments, references, tables (each on a separate page), and captions for illustrations. The title pages and abstract page should not be numbered. Sequential numbering should begin with the text. To ensure anonymity in the review process, authors' names should appear on only the full title page; names of authors or the institution should **not** be given in the text or on the illustrations. **Three copies** of the manuscript and three complete sets of mounted illustrations should be submitted. The author should retain a complete copy of the manuscript, since accepted manuscripts will not be returned and only the illustrations of rejected manuscripts will be returned. All manuscripts are acknowledged; please allow 2-3 weeks from the time you mailed the manuscript for receipt of an acknowledgment.

TITLE PAGES, AUTHOR CONTRIBUTIONS

***Full Title Page*:** This page should include the title of the manuscript, the first and last names, middle initials, and degrees of all authors, the name and street address (not a postal box) of the institution from which the work originated, the telephone number, the FAX or Telex number, and the e-mail address (if available) of the **corresponding author**, and information concerning grants. The address for reprint requests should include

(continued)

the **complete** name, street address (not a postal box), and zip code. It is important to indicate on this title page whether your paper has been presented at an RSNA meeting (please give year) or has been accepted for presentation at a future meeting.

***Abbreviated Title Page*:** This page should include only the title of the manuscript so as to allow for anonymity during the review process.

Author Contributions: Authors are required to identify their manuscript contributions, for which they are responsible. The author(s) responsible for the integrity of the entire study should also be identified. Please list the following phrases on a separate page, to follow the *"Abbreviated Title Page,"* and beside each indicate the name(s) of the author(s) to whom these phrases apply:

- guarantor of integrity of entire study
- study concepts
- study design
- definition of intellectual content
- literature research
- clinical studies
- experimental studies
- data acquisition
- data analysis
- statistical analysis
- manuscript preparation
- manuscript editing
- manuscript review

For those phrases that do not apply, please list them and so indicate.

■ ABSTRACT, KEY WORDS, CATEGORIZATION TERMS, AND SUMMARY STATEMENT

An abstract of 200 words or less must be submitted with each manuscript of a major paper. The abstract must be divided into four paragraphs with the following headings.

Purpose: State the hypothesis being tested or the procedure being evaluated.

Materials and Methods: Briefly state what was done and what materials were used, including number of subjects. Also include the methods used to assess the data and to control bias.

RESULTS: Provide the findings of the study, including indicators of statistical significance. Include actual numbers, as well as percentages.

CONCLUSION: Summarize in one or two sentences the conclusion made on the basis of the findings.

Below the abstract, please list three to six key words as derived from the terms used in the most recent 3-year *RSNA Index to Imaging Literature.* Also, on the Manuscript Categorization Terms form provided at the end of these instructions, please select as many terms as are appropriate for your manuscript. It is important that you comply with this request, since the terms you select are utilized to match your manuscript with the appropriate reviewers.

On the reverse side of the Manuscript Categorization Terms form, the *author should reproduce from the text the one statement that best conveys or summarizes the message of the study.*

An abstract of 60 words or less must be submitted for each case report or Technical Developments paper. The abstract must state (*a*) what was done, (*b*) what was found, and (*c*) what was concluded.

■ TEXT

The text of observational and experimental studies is arranged in sections with the headings Introduction, Materials and Methods, Results, and Discussion. Lengthy papers may need subheadings within some sections to clarify their content, especially within the Results and Discussion sections.

Introduction: Clearly state the hypothesis or purpose of the study. Give only strictly pertinent references, and do not review the literature extensively.

Materials and Methods: Describe clearly the number and selection of the subjects studied (patients or experimental animals, including controls). Identify the methods, instrumentation (manufacturer's name and address in parentheses), and procedures in sufficient detail to allow other workers to reproduce the results. To ensure anonymity in the review process, do **not** include the name of the institution where the work was performed, either within the text or at the top of each manuscript page. Give references to established methods, including statistical methods that have been published but are not well known; describe new or substantially modified methods and give reasons for using these techniques. Include numbers of observations and the statistical significance of the findings when appropriate. Detailed statistical analyses, mathematical derivations, and the like should be presented in one or more appendixes.

Results: Present the results in logical sequence in the text, along with tables, and illustrations. Do not repeat in the text all the data in the tables and/or illustrations; summarize only important observations.

Discussion: Emphasize the new and important aspects of the study and conclusions that follow from them. Do not repeat in detail the data given in the Results section. Include in the Discussion the implications of the findings and their limitations, in particular with reference to the use of modified methods, statistical or otherwise. Relate the observations to other relevant studies. Link the conclusions with the goals of the study, but avoid unqualified statements and conclusions not supported completely by the data. Avoid claiming priority and alluding to work that has not been completed. State new hypotheses when warranted, but clearly label them as such. Recommendations, when appropriate, may be included.

For experimental studies, please describe the potential importance of your conclusions as they relate to future practical applications. Please identify this paragraph with the title "Practical Application(s)."

■ ACKNOWLEDGMENTS

List here those who have contributed substantially to the work reported in the manuscript, such as editorial and writing assistance, but who are not authors of the study. Authors are expected to obtain written permission of those acknowledged, and to submit the same, as readers might interpret that those acknowledged agree with the data and conclusions of the study.

■ REFERENCES

Number references consecutively in the order in which they are first mentioned. The abbreviations used for periodicals cited in the references should follow the style of *Index Medicus.* For journal articles, list surnames and initials of all authors when six or less, such as:

1. Stuart MJ, Elrad H, Graeber JE, Hakanson DO, Sunderji SG, Barvinchak MK. Increased synthesis of prostaglandin endoperoxides and platelet hyperfunction in infants of mothers with diabetes mellitus. J Lab Clin Med 1979; 94:12–26.

When seven or more authors are listed, only the first three names need to be identified, followed by "et al," such as:

1. Hibbard CT, Campbell S, Sabbagha RE, et al. Demonstration of tissue interfaces within the body by ultrasonic echo sounding. Br J Radiol 1961; 34:539–549.

Abstracts, editorials, and letters to the Editor should be noted as such. In the case of books, the authors of a chapter, title of the chapter, editor(s), title of the book, edition, city, publisher, year, and specific pages must be provided.

1. Brown M, Gray L. Indications for hematology. In: Wintrobe MM, ed. Clinical hematology. 3rd ed. Philadelphia, Pa: Lea & Febiger, 1975; 1146–1167.

It is the responsibility of the author(s) to ensure that all references are listed accurately.

■ TABLES

Tables should be numbered in Arabic numerals and should have a title. All abbreviations used in the table should be explained in a footnote.

Tables should be presented in the style used in recent issues of the Journal. No vertical lines or shading should be included. Avoid excessive use of horizontal lines within the table.

■ CAPTIONS FOR ILLUSTRATIONS

A caption must be supplied for each illustration, including drawings and graphs. It should not duplicate text material and should follow the style used in recent issues of the Journal. All captions should appear collectively on one or more pages separate from the text, and each caption should also appear below the corresponding illustration. It is essential that the caption describes all labels placed on the print of an illustration.

■ ILLUSTRATIONS

Illustrations should be limited to those required to show the essential features described in the manuscript. Space constraints prevent us from publishing redundant or excessive illustrations. Unretouched glossy prints no larger than 12.7 × 17.8 cm (5 × 7 inches) are desirable. Prints to be combined into one array, such as posteroanterior and lateral views, should be the same height or the same width to facilitate reproduction. They should correspond in appearance to the tonal relations of the original radiograph (ie, showing the bones white on a dark background, with the patient's right to the observer's left; computed tomograms and MR images should employ the "view from below"). If an image has been enhanced electronically, explain the alterations that have been made and send an original image along with the enhanced one. Drawings and charts should be rendered professionally in India ink on white paper. In computer-generated artwork, shading should be done in continuous tones (ie, solid black, solid gray, solid white): **Do not use dotted shadings.**

Since the size of the illustration printed in the Journal is typically smaller than that submitted by the author(s), it is essential that each submitted illustration show only the area(s) of interest with enough surrounding area for orientation puposes (e.g., to illustrate a cavity at the right lung apex, show only that area with enough surrounding area for orientation, rather than the entire chest).

All illustrations must be numbered and the top indicated on the back. For protection against loss or damage, each illustration should then be neatly attached to paper (one illustration per page), and the number and top should be reindicated on this page. For attachment, **avoid using glue, staples, or corner mounts.** Because it holds the illustration securely to the page without damage, we recommend Scotch Removable Magic Tape (3M, St Paul, Minn). **Please** do not add letters or numbers to the **face** of the illustration to identify the figure (such as 1A or 1B).

Arrows and other labels should be placed only on the final print, should be of professional quality, and should be **removable.** Professional artist service for such items is available to authors without charge. The desired additions may simply be indicated on tissue or a transparent overlay attached securely to the print.

Illustrations of accepted manuscripts become the property of the RSNA and will be stored for 2 years after publication. Illustrations will be returned only upon receipt of a written request from the corresponding author. We suggest that authors make and keep a set of illustrations in addition to the three sets submitted to the Journal.

■ UNITS AND ABBREVIATIONS

Radiation measurements and laboratory values should be given in the *International System of Units (SI)* (resources: SI Units in Radiation Protection and Measurements, NCRP Report no. 82 [August 1985]; "Now Read This: The SI Units Are Here," *JAMA* 1986; 255:2329–2339). Abbreviations should be spelled out when first used in the text, such as "cerebrospinal fluid (CSF)." Laboratory slang, clinical jargon, and uncommon abbreviations should be avoided.

■ INFORMED CONSENT

Manuscripts reporting the results of experimental studies on human subjects must include a statement in Materials and Methods to the effect that informed consent was obtained after the nature of the procedure(s) had been fully explained. In addition, a statement affirming approval of the appropriate institutional review board is required. If a review board does not exist, then the Declaration of Helsinki principles should be followed and a statement affirming the same should be made (41st World Medical Assembly. Declaration of Helsinki: recommendations guiding physicians in biomedical research involving human subjects. Bull Pan Am Health Organ 1990; 24: 606-609).

The maintenance and care of experimental animals to provide humane treatment and to ensure reliable results are described in the National Institutes of Health guidelines for use of laboratory animals. Authors must affirm compliance with these guidelines or approval of the appropriate institutional review board in the Materials and Methods section.

■ RIGHTS AND PERMISSIONS

Written permission (we require a copy) must be granted by the publisher and author to reproduce any previously published figures, including permission to reproduce in both print and electronic formats; any such material must be clearly noted and its source given in the manuscript. A signed letter of permission must be included with your manuscript for any individual who might be identified due to written descriptions, photographs (masking the eyes in photographs is not sufficient protection of anonymity), or otherwise. Informed consent, which requires that the individual be shown the manuscript, should be affirmed in the Materials and Methods section.

If reference is made in the text to personal communication (oral or written) as a source of information, a signed statement of permission is required from each such source.

AUTHOR RESPONSIBILITY

Authors must be certain that no manuscript on the same or similar material has been or will be submitted to another journal by themselves or others at their institution before their work appears in *Radiology*. The submission by authors of similar material to advertising media must be indicated at the time *Radiology* receives the manuscript.

ELECTRONIC SUBMISSION OF ACCEPTED MANUSCRIPTS

Manuscripts that have been **accepted** for publication must be submitted on computer disk (required for text, desirable for illustrations). A hard copy should accompany the disk and should match the disk file exactly. The disk should be labeled with its assigned manuscript number, the first author's last name, the word processing program used, and the file name.

Text File: Submit text on high-density 3½-inch disk prepared with an IBM- or Macintosh-compatible computer. Manuscripts should be prepared in WordPerfect 6.1 or Microsoft Word for PC (7.0) or Mac (5.0 or higher). Files prepared in any other word-processing program should be saved in an unformatted, text-only ASCII file and the program used should be indicated.

The entire article should be submitted as a single text file, with the elements in the standard order: title pages, abstract, text, acknowledgments, references, tables, captions. Only the final version of the article should be on the submitted disk. Keep the text file as free from formatting codes as possible: Do not use boldface, italic, underlining, strange fonts, codes for centering, unnecessary line spacing, etc. Use the default settings of the word-processing program; especially do not use right-justified margins. Use tabs to indent at the beginnings of paragraphs, and insert only one space after end punctuation marks. Use hard returns only at the ends of paragraphs or between sections of the manuscript; do not insert them mid-paragraph. Do not insert tabs in references; use only one hard return at the end of each reference.

Illustrations File: Although not required, submission of illustrations on 3½" disk, ZIP disk, or Syquest cartridge will improve image quality. For black and white images, we require that they be submitted in PC Tiff or PC eps format with a dot range of 5%–95% and resolution of 500 dpi. Four-color images should also be PC Tiff or PC eps format with a maximum of 280% total tonal density and resolution of 300 dpi. Each image file should be named, and with the disk or cartridge the following should be provided: a hard-copy inventory with specific information on the image, two sets of proofs obtained at 800–1,800 dpi, and one set of proofs obtained with a laser printer to be used as a reference set.

BOOK REVIEWERS

Any person who would like to help in reviewing books for *Radiology* should contact

Richard A. Szucs, MD, Book Review Editor
Radiology Editorial Office
1001 E Broad St
Suite 310
Richmond, VA 23219

BOOKS FOR REVIEW

Publishers wishing to have books reviewed should send them to the address above.

✔ Checklist of Requirements:

- ❐ 1. Send 3 copies of manuscript and 3 copies of illustrations.
- ❐ 2. Mount each illustration on a separate page, 8½ × 11 inches. Indicate figure number and top.
- ❐ 3. Double space all parts of manuscript.
- ❐ 4. Send copyright and certifications agreement with signatures of all authors.
- ❐ 5. Send institutional affiliation for each author and corresponding author's name, address, phone number, FAX or Telex number, and e-mail address.
- ❐ 6. Send a **brief** abstract: 200 words or less for regular articles, 60 words or less for case reports and Technical Developments papers.
- ❐ 7. Give SI units for radiation measurements and laboratory values.
- ❐ 8. Send copy of letter of permission to reprint any figure that was published previously or for any other reasons as noted in the instructions found above.
- ❐ 9. Send a completed copy of the Manuscript Categorization Terms form. Please remember to reproduce from the text the one statement that best conveys or summarizes the message of your study.

Radiology Manuscript Categorization Terms

Please PRINT your name: ______________________________

Please print the title of your manuscript ______________________________

____

For each section, please categorize your manuscript by checking off **as many terms as are appropriate.**

Modalities/Techniques

- ___ Absorptiometry/ Bone Densitometry
- ___ Angiography
- ___ Arthrography
- ___ Conventional Radiography
- ___ CT
- ___ CT-Angiography
- ___ CT-Electron Beam
- ___ CT-High Resolution
- ___ CT-Spiral
- ___ Dacryocystography
- ___ Defecography
- ___ Digital Radiography
- ___ Echocardiography
- ___ Fluoroscopy
- ___ Hysterosalpingography
- ___ Image Manipulation/ Reconstruction
- ___ Lymphography
- ___ MR-Angiography
- ___ MR-Diffusion/Perfusion
- ___ MR-Functional Imaging
- ___ MR-Imaging
- ___ MR-Spectroscopy
- ___ Neural Networks
- ___ PACS
- ___ PET
- ___ Radionuclide Studies
- ___ Sialography
- ___ SPECT
- ___ Ultrasound
- ___ Ultrasound-Color Doppler
- ___ Ultrasound-Doppler
- ___ Ultrasound-Power Doppler
- ___ Ultrasound-Spectral Doppler

Procedures

- ___ Angioplasty
- ___ Angioscopy
- ___ Balloon Insertions
- ___ Biopsy/Drainage
- ___ Dilation
- ___ Embolization
- ___ Endoscopy
- ___ Filter Insertions
- ___ Interventional Other ______________
- ___ Intraoperative
- ___ Laser
- ___ Lithotripsy
- ___ Localization
- ___ Myelography
- ___ Percutaneous
- ___ Radiation Therapy/Oncology
- ___ Radionuclide Therapy
- ___ Shunts
- ___ Stents
- ___ Thrombolysis

Areas/Systems

- ___ Abdomen
- ___ Biliary
- ___ Breast
- ___ Cardiac
- ___ CNS
- ___ Ear/Nose/Throat
- ___ Genital/Reproductive
- ___ GI
- ___ Head/Neck
- ___ Hematologic
- ___ Lymphatic
- ___ Muscular
- ___ Nervous-Peripheral
- ___ Skeletal-Appendicular
- ___ Skeletal-Axial
- ___ Soft Tissues/Skin
- ___ Thorax
- ___ Urinary
- ___ Vascular

Structures

- ___ Adrenal
- ___ Ankle
- ___ Anus
- ___ Aorta
- ___ Appendix
- ___ Arteries
- ___ Bile Ducts
- ___ Bladder
- ___ Brain/Brain Stem
- ___ Breast
- ___ Cervix
- ___ Diaphragm
- ___ Duodenum
- ___ Ear
- ___ Elbow
- ___ Esophagus
- ___ Extremities
- ___ Eye
- ___ Face
- ___ Fallopian Tubes
- ___ Foot
- ___ Gallbladder
- ___ Hand
- ___ Heart
- ___ Hip
- ___ Jaw
- ___ Joints
- ___ Kidney
- ___ Knee
- ___ Lacrimal Glands
- ___ Large Bowel
- ___ Larynx
- ___ Ligaments
- ___ Liver
- ___ Long Bones
- ___ Lung
- ___ Marrow
- ___ Mediastinum
- ___ Meninges
- ___ Mesentery
- ___ Omentum
- ___ Orbit
- ___ Ovaries
- ___ Pancreas
- ___ Paranasal Sinuses
- ___ Parathyroid
- ___ Pelvis
- ___ Pelvocalyceal
- ___ Penis
- ___ Pericardium
- ___ Peritoneum
- ___ Pharynx
- ___ Pineal
- ___ Pituitary
- ___ Pleura
- ___ Prostate
- ___ Pylorus
- ___ Rectum
- ___ Retina
- ___ Retroperitoneum
- ___ Ribs
- ___ Salivary Glands
- ___ Scrotum
- ___ Shoulder
- ___ Skull
- ___ Small Bowel
- ___ Spinal Cord
- ___ Spine-Cervical
- ___ Spine-Lumbar

Continued

Structures, continued

- ___ Spine-Sacrum/Coccyx
- ___ Spine-Thoracic
- ___ Spleen
- ___ Stomach
- ___ Tendons
- ___ Testes
- ___ Thymus
- ___ Thyroid
- ___ Tongue
- ___ Tracheobronchial Tree
- ___ Ureters
- ___ Urethra
- ___ Uterus
- ___ Vagina
- ___ Valves
- ___ Veins
- ___ Vena Cava
- ___ Wrist

Topics

- ___ Abscess
- ___ Acceptance Testing
- ___ Acute
- ___ Adults
- ___ AIDS
- ___ Anatomy
- ___ Aneurysms
- ___ Animal Investigations
- ___ Arteriosclerosis
- ___ Arthritides
- ___ Artifacts
- ___ Atelectasis
- ___ Athletic Injuries
- ___ AVM
- ___ Axilla
- ___ Biological Effects
- ___ Biostatistics
- ___ Blood
- ___ Calcifications/Calculi
- ___ Cardiac Assist Devices
- ___ Catheters
- ___ Cavitation
- ___ Cerebral Palsy
- ___ Chemistry
- ___ Chronic Obstructive Airways Disease
- ___ Cirrhosis
- ___ Comparative Studies
- ___ Complications
- ___ Computer Applications-3D
- ___ Computer Applications-Teleradiology
- ___ Computer Applications-Virtual Imaging
- ___ Computer Applications-Other___________
- ___ Congenital
- ___ Connective Tissue Disorders
- ___ Contrast Agents-Intravenous
- ___ Contrast Agents-Oral
- ___ Cost-effectiveness
- ___ CSF
- ___ Cysts
- ___ Dementia
- ___ Demineralization-Bone
- ___ Dilatation
- ___ Dissection
- ___ Diverticula
- ___ Dosimetry
- ___ Drugs/Reactions
- ___ Dysplasias
- ___ Eating Disorders
- ___ ECMO
- ___ Edema
- ___ Education
- ___ Efficacy Studies
- ___ Embolism
- ___ Endocrine Disorders
- ___ Equipment
- ___ Ethics
- ___ Experimental Investigations
- ___ Fetus
- ___ Fistula
- ___ Foreign Bodies
- ___ Forensics
- ___ Genetic Defects
- ___ Grafts
- ___ Health Policy and Practice
- ___ Hemangioma
- ___ Hematologic Diseases
- ___ Hemodynamics/Flow Dynamics
- ___ Hemorrhage
- ___ Hernia
- ___ History
- ___ Hyperplasia/Hypertrophy
- ___ Hypertension
- ___ Imaging Sequences
- ___ Infection
- ___ Inflammation
- ___ Instrumentation
- ___ Ischemia/Infarction
- ___ Laboratory Tests
- ___ Leukemia
- ___ Lymphoma
- ___ Medicolegal Issues
- ___ Metabolic Disorders
- ___ Metastases
- ___ Monoclonal Antibodies
- ___ Motility
- ___ Neoplasms-Primary
- ___ Normal Variants
- ___ Observer Performance
- ___ Obstetrics
- ___ Obstruction/Occlusion
- ___ Occupational/Environmental Hazards
- ___ Outcomes Analysis
- ___ Parasites
- ___ Pathology
- ___ Pediatric Population-Adolescents
- ___ Pediatric Population-Children
- ___ Pediatric Population-Infants
- ___ Pediatric Population-Neonates
- ___ Physics
- ___ Physiological Studies
- ___ Pregnancy
- ___ Prostheses
- ___ QA/QC
- ___ Radiation Effects
- ___ Radiation Safety
- ___ Radiobiology
- ___ Safety
- ___ Screening
- ___ Sedation
- ___ Seizure Disorders
- ___ Socioeconomic Issues
- ___ Speech Disorders
- ___ Staging
- ___ Statistics
- ___ Surgery
- ___ Technical Aspects
- ___ Technology Assessments
- ___ Tissue Characterization
- ___ Transplantation
- ___ Trauma
- ___ Treatment Effects
- ___ Tropical Diseases
- ___ Varices
- ___ Volvulus

Please reproduce here the **one sentence** from the text that best conveys or summarizes the message of your study.

____

____

Please provide author initials by appropriate author contribution category.

- _______ Guarantor of integrity of entire study
- _______ Study concepts
- _______ Study design
- _______ Definition of intellectual content
- _______ Literature research
- _______ Clinical studies
- _______ Experimental studies
- _______ Data acquisition
- _______ Data analysis
- _______ Statistical analysis
- _______ Manuscript preparation
- _______ Manuscript editing
- _______ Manuscript review

This form *must be* included with your manuscript submission.

From the Editor

Anthony V. Proto, MD

Radiology 1998—Advertising and Our 75th Anniversary

As you know, 1998 marks the 75th Anniversary of our Journal, *Radiology*. To celebrate this occasion, we introduced two features (1). The first is a series of subspecialty society messages that focus both on the direction of imaging research over the upcoming 5–10 years and on how the results of this research might change the way we currently image certain disease states or body areas. Each message is followed by a commentary from a noted, respected person in that subspecialty area. These messages and commentaries will continue through December 1998.

The second feature introduced for our 75th Anniversary celebration relates to advertising. Some companies have chosen to take the opportunity to publish ads featuring the past and present status of their imaging equipment, showing the major advances that have occurred during the intervening period. Others have responded to our invitation sent to all advertisers to display an ad in this issue of *Radiology*, which we have identified as a special advertising issue in recognition of our Diamond Anniversary. Those companies displaying such special ads and the pages on which the ads appear are the following:

- GE Medical Systems (IBC, OBC)
- Lippincott-Raven Publishers (p 7A)
- Nuclear Associates (p 9A)
- Siemens Medical Systems, Inc (pp 2A–3A)
- Toshiba America Medical Systems, Inc (p 4A)

Two of these five companies have shown additional support of *Radiology* and our 75th Anniversary celebration by placing special ads earlier this year—Siemens Medical Systems, Inc, in our January 1998 issue (pp 32A–33A) and GE Medical Systems in our May 1998 issue (IBC, OBC).

Companies that advertise in *Radiology* serve many important functions for the Journal. They provide financial support to help defray the costs associated with a journal that adheres to the highest standards throughout every facet of the production process, in particular image quality. They provide information for our readers regarding technologic advances in equipment, new products, services, and educational materials, all of which relate to research, practice, and teaching in our specialty. In return, *Radiology* provides our advertisers a wide circulation of their ads, reaching some 37,000 subscribers worldwide every month. Our readers read *Radiology* to learn of the newest advances in imaging science. Our readers also know that each issue offers them a wealth of information—a ready reference—regarding the latest products and services available from our advertisers.

As Editor of *Radiology*, I am privileged to acknowledge the support of those companies who have participated in our 75th Anniversary celebration. We trust our readers also value that support and find useful the information contained in their ads. On behalf of *Radiology*, thank you!

Index terms:
Editorials
Radiology (journal)

Radiology 1998; 208:281

Reference

1. Proto AV. *Radiology*—1998 and the future. Radiology 1998; 206:1.

Book Review

AIDS Imaging: A Practical Clinical Approach

Edited by Jacques W. A. J. Reeders, MD, PhD, and John R. Mathieson, MD, FRCPC

Philadelphia, Pa: Saunders, 1998. ISBN 0-7020-1904-6. Hardcover, $140.00, pp 342, 244 illustrations; tables.

In recent years, there has been a new sense of optimism in the battle against acquired immunodeficiency syndrome (AIDS), with advances in our understanding of the molecular biology of the human immunodeficiency virus (HIV) and the development of new and promising therapeutic agents. Despite this progress, the varied manifestations of the numerous infectious and neoplastic processes that affect these patients continue to present a diagnostic challenge to radiologists. To guide radiologists in the interpretation of imaging studies of AIDS patients, Drs Reeders and Mathieson, along with 40 international contributing authors, have constructed a comprehensive textbook on AIDS imaging with a distinctly practical approach.

The result of their collaborative efforts, *AIDS Imaging: A Practical Clinical Approach* is an up-to-date reference textbook that is broad in scope, clearly written, and beautifully illustrated. The book is well organized, and it is conveniently divided into three sections. The first section presents a multidisciplinary, general overview of AIDS that provides the reader with a solid background for the clinically oriented second and third sections. It includes brief chapters that succinctly review the history, the basic science, and the epidemiologic and pathologic aspects of AIDS. The second section presents an organ system–based review of the clinical and imaging features of AIDS. These chapters provide the reader with information regarding both the usual and unusual features of the various infectious and neoplastic processes that affect each major organ system. There are also separate chapters devoted to pediatric AIDS and women with AIDS. The third section comprises concise, easy-to-read reference tables that provide a convenient listing of the common disease processes that affect each major organ system, along with a succinct summary of their common radiologic features and relevant differential diagnoses. These tables will be easily referenced in daily practice.

One of the highlights of the book is its wealth of pertinent illustrations, which are of consistently superb quality. The text is complemented by numerous images obtained from a variety of radiologic studies and examples of gross pathologic and cytopathologic specimens, which clearly illustrate and enhance the written material. Moreover, the radiologic images in the gastrointestinal section are enhanced by the frequent appearance of correlative endoscopic images.

A minor criticism is the occasional repetition of material between the clinical and imaging chapters, which directly follow one another in the second section of the book. The editors acknowledge this repetition in their preface, and they state that the book is structured in this way so each chapter can be read individually without requiring reference to other chapters. When the book is read in its entirety, this is only a minor inconvenience to the reader, and it does not detract considerably from the book as a whole.

I recommend this textbook to both general radiologists and subspecialty radiologists who encounter AIDS patients in their practices. It will also make an invaluable addition to a diagnostic radiology library. It is well worth its price of $140.00.

AIDS Imaging: A Practical Clinical Approach is an up-to-date, comprehensive textbook on AIDS imaging. It provides a wealth of information to guide radiologists in interpreting diagnostic imaging studies of AIDS patients, and it will likely become the standard reference book for this purpose.

Reviewed by Phillip M. Boiselle, MD

Lawrence M. Boxt, MD ▮ Martin J. Lipton, MD

The North American Society of Cardiac Imaging

Future Direction of Cardiovascular Research[1]

Cardiac imaging research in the next 10 years will be driven by the vast number of patients with known or undiagnosed atherosclerotic cardiovascular disease, new developments in technology and computer science, and the need for online measurement of function as well as morphology. Moreover, imaging research will be performed in a different environment. Imaging research has become so dependent on hardware, and therefore on capital investment, that it will be tied to clinical practice and modified to meet the service needs of a diminishing number of academic centers. Cooperative studies among these centers, all using standardized imaging systems with the same analytical software packages, will provide studies with sufficient numbers of patients for meaningful analysis of subtle findings. In particular, large longitudinal studies of patients with different clinical syndromes of atherosclerotic disease will be studied in this manner, allowing insight into more subtle variants of atherosclerosis (1).

The diagnosis and medical management of atherosclerosis always have been fragmented and often have been performed in response to a specific clinical problem. Accordingly, atherosclerosis may be looked on as a systemic disease in which there is a race among various body organs for symptomatic manifestation. If a lower extremity vessel becomes obstructed, then the patient presents with intermittent claudication. Coronary artery occlusion may cause an acute myocardial infarction or sudden death. Carotid artery stenosis can result in a stroke. The aging of the baby-boomer generation reaching its 6th decade will drive research in the direction of early detection and successful treatment of silent atherosclerotic heart disease.

Research for increasing spatial and contrast resolution will be driven by the clinical need to identify smaller, more peripheral blood vessels and coronary arteries. Continued industry-based research in x-ray generation and detector technology probably will result in devices with higher sensitivity and speed and, we hope, lower radiation dose.

Advances in the application of noninvasive technologies, however, will provide the greatest changes in how medicine is practiced. Such developments may broaden the role of CT in clinical cardiovascular diagnosis. Strategies for alternative sampling of magnetic resonance (MR) imaging–acquired data will produce faster acquisition sequences and encourage more extensive angiography of the vascular tree. Furthermore, design and implementation of organ-specific surface coils will allow higher resolution of small body parts, including the coronary arteries. As new hardware and software are developed and begin to make their way into clinical practice, pressure will be felt to identify and implement new clinical protocols to acquire such information in a clinically relevant time frame. Clinical collaboration between multiple screening and diagnostic modalities will require radiologists, cardiologists, and vascular surgeons, as well as other specialists studying the metabolism of the arterial wall, to forge a more global approach to the general problems of atherosclerosis, including criteria for early screening and long-term management (2). Longitudinal follow-up of patients with atherosclerosis will evolve from an organ-based clinical practice to a more disease-based endeavor, setting the stage for outcome analysis studies of new imaging technologies, as well as medical and interventional therapy for this disease (3).

New contrast materials will be investigated. Gadolinium and other paramagnetic compounds with a special affinity for atherosclerotic plaques will be demonstrated. Imaging with high-field-strength MR equipment and the use of organ-specific intravascular and surface coils should provide an increased signal-to-noise ratio in quantitative information concerning plaque burden and change in plaque burden as a function of a specific medical intervention. More rapid acquisition of MR images will facilitate research on evaluation of whole-body atherosclerosis, screening for the disease, and evaluation of the effects of intervention.

MR studies of the coronary arteries will continue to be an important focus of research (4). The great difference in cost between conventional contrast material–enhanced coronary arteriography and noninvasive MR imaging will drive the development of clinically useful MR techniques for evaluating coronary arterial morphology and function, as well as the metabolic consequences of such changes in pathophysiology. The clinical need for a reliable, robust, and noninvasive tool for the diagnosis and characterization of disease and the follow-up of patients with coronary artery disease will stimulate the development of new pulse sequences, new coils for improved image quality, and innovative contrast agents for the characterization of myocardial stunning, infarction, and hibernation. Improvements in

Index terms:
Heart
Radiology and radiologists, research
Subspecialty society messages

Radiology 1998; 208:283–284

[1] From the Department of Radiology, University of Chicago, Box 429, 5841 S Maryland Ave, Chicago, IL 60637. Received December 16,1997; accepted February 23, 1998. **Address reprint requests to** M.J.L.

See also the article by Abrams (pp 285–287) in this issue.

spatial, contrast, and temporal resolutions of MR and computed tomographic (CT) machines, and no doubt in other modalities as well, will allow rapid acquisition of robust three-dimensional data sets, which will allow reconstruction of high–spatial resolution images of the coronary arteries, their major branches, and coronary artery bypass grafts.

The most dramatic cardiac research advances will be made in the development and application of new computer technology (5). During the past several years, the speed of the computer chip has doubled every 2–4 years while its price has halved. This trend will continue for several more years, enabling faster and faster acquisition and processing speeds of digital imaging data. The complex motion of the heart and the small caliber of the coronary arteries and their branches pose the greatest challenge to investigators in applying computer techniques. Development of high-speed data interfaces will allow production of high-speed imaging systems that use electronic, computer-based acquisition methods for the display, transfer, manipulation, analysis, and storage. Two- and three-dimensional displays using these systems will provide a basis for evaluating changes in the ventricular myocardium and systemic blood flow (6). Accurate evaluation of small temporal and regional changes in myocardial thickening, as well as the fate of intravenously administered contrast materials, will broaden our understanding of the short- and long-term physiologic effects of blood vessel stenosis. Correlation of morphologic and anatomic information with physiologic abnormalities should improve our understanding of subclinical and silent cardiac events. We can anticipate improved screening of populations with use of various techniques including, for example, electron-beam CT. Similarly, studies of lower extremity muscles will reveal insights into changes in regional water diffusion and water content, which are the results of chronic and acute peripheral atherosclerotic vascular change. Correlation of metabolic positron emission tomography (PET) studies with morphologically detailed MR images should provide important information concerning regional myocardial dysfunction and the fate of chronically ischemic myocardium. Three-dimensional models of a beating heart, created from CT scans and MR images, will become powerful tools for displaying and interpreting diagnostic information, as well as educational tools for training physicians and informing patients' families and the public. Segmentation techniques will allow identification of regions of interest for further computer-enhanced visualization, to answer questions not necessarily raised at the time of examination. Acquired in digital format, these studies will be made available in other areas of the hospital, as well as at other sites, by means of electronic transmission via the Internet and local area networks. Digital simulators will provide vastly improved training methods for many aspects of diagnosis, including interventional radiology, with a revolutionary impact much like that in the airline industry.

In summary, for the foreseeable future, high-speed acquisition will rely primarily on large-field-of-view devices—that is, area detectors, which are currently being used in cardiac catheterization and interventional radiology laboratories. Robust, three-dimensional imaging tools will be developed to provide accurate reconstruction of vessel lumina and cardiac structures and to produce dynamic three-dimensional images. Similar applications will dramatically enhance the information available from CT and MR imaging, providing greater spatial and temporal resolution. Vessel size will be measured from these data sets, with reproducible arterial blood flow measurements made in selected arteries. Methods for estimating and characterizing the entire vascular bed will enable global and regional myocardial perfusion to be calculated on an absolute, rather than relative, scale. Vessel and epicardial motion will also be measured, along with precise measurements of cardiac chamber walls, volumes, and myocardial contraction.

Some of these postprocessing tools are currently available for segmentation and three-dimensional rendering. At present, however, they are time-consuming and are dependent, to varying degrees, on operator experience and interaction. Furthermore, this approach is now being applied predominantly to CT and MR imaging data. Once digital imaging is extended to conventional x-ray systems, however, these techniques will be applied universally (7). Advances in the development and application of new contrast media will also be a major research area for investigation. Newer imaging methods for investigating transgenic mechanisms in congenital and acquired heart disease, including innovations such as the use of radiation to reduce vessel restenosis, will be fertile fields for cardiovascular research in the future.

The need to have radiology involved and, indeed, play an important role in the development, innovation, and application of all this exciting new imaging research will require a critical mass of adequately trained, creative radiologists who are interested in cardiovascular disease (8). Leaders in radiology as well as trainees will need to understand the pivotal role they must play if we are to reach our potential as a successful specialty and provide the knowledge base and added value for rendering and interpreting image data during the next millennium (9,10).

Acknowledgments: We thank those members of the Board of the North American Society of Cardiac Imaging who provided input and advice in preparation of this manuscript. We also thank Charles Metz, PhD, for his assistance in editing the text and Bernadette Brogan for secretarial support.

References

1. Eng J, Siegelman SS. Improving radiology research methods: what is being asked and who is being studied? Radiology 1997; 205:651–655.
2. Ellrodt G, Cook DJ, Lee J, Cho M, Hunt D, Weingarten S. Evidence-based disease management. JAMA 1997; 278:1687–1692.
3. Lipton MJ, Metz CE, Ranahan LA. Outcome and benefit analysis in MRI. In: Grant D, Harris RK, ed. Encyclopedia of nuclear magnetic resonance. London, England: Wiley, 1995; 3419–3425.
4. Duerinckx AJ, Lipton MJ. Noninvasive coronary artery imaging using MR or CT: is it almost ready for larger clinical trials? AJR 1998; 170:900–902.
5. Napel S, Marks MP, Rubin GD, et al. CT angiography with spiral CT and maximum intensity projection. Radiology 1992; 185:607–610.
6. Chen SYJ, Metz CE. Improved determination of biplane imaging geometry from two projection images and its application of 3D reconstruction of coronary arterial trees. Med Phys 1997; 24:633–654.
7. Fencil LE, Doi K, Chua KG, Hoffmann KR. Measurement of absolute flow rate in vessels using a stereoscopic DSA system. Phys Med Biol 1989; 34:659–671.
8. Hillman BJ, Putman CE. Fostering research by radiologists: recommendations of the 1991 summit meeting. Radiology 1992; 182:315–318.
9. Levin DC, Abrams HL, Castaneda-Zuniga WR, et al. Lessons from history: why radiologists lost coronary angiography and what can be done to prevent future similar losses. Invest Radiol 1994; 29:480–484.
10. Hillman BJ. Medical imaging in the 21st century. Lancet 1997; 350:731–733.

Herbert L. Abrams, MD

Commentary

Cardiac Imaging Research in the Next Century: A Commentary[1]

The century now ending embodied both the beginning of cardiac imaging and its extraordinary growth and development into a series of research and clinical methods of unusual power and sophistication. Looking back, we may enhance our perspective and broaden our vision of what the next millennium may bring (1).

If we divide the 20th century into 4 quarters, the astonishing rate of progress can be readily appreciated. During the 1st quarter, from 1900 to 1925, cardiac imaging was dominated by the widespread use of plain radiography and the analysis of topographic anatomy. The changes in overall heart size and in chamber size and configuration associated with valvular, congenital, and arteriosclerotic heart disease, as well as with pericardial disease, were depicted and analyzed, related to the underlying pathologic anatomy, and incorporated into the diagnostic armamentarium. Research was largely clinical and descriptive in character.

The period from 1925 to 1950 witnessed the introduction of many novel methods for studying the heart and blood vessels with use of contrast media to display the internal anatomy in normal and abnormal states. The demonstration by Forssman (2) in 1928 that cardiac catheterization was achievable was followed by a lag of almost 15 years before its application to sophisticated physiologic and clinical studies. Meanwhile, angiocardiography, thoracic and translumbar aortography, pulmonary and carotid angiography, peripheral arteriography, and venography were introduced and subjected to intensive investigation both in animals and in man. These advances moved gradually toward the threshold of clinical application, setting the stage for an era in which the new methods would have increasing application to aggressive palliative and curative surgical therapy. As with all areas of curative and palliative surgery—in the brain, lungs, kidneys, intestine, pelvic organs—so too with the heart: No radical surgical advance was feasible until a meaningful imaging infrastructure had been created to guide diagnosis and management. Research in this era was primarily in engineering, technology, gross morphology, and physiology, some in the experimental laboratory, some in human subjects.

During the 3rd quarter of the century from 1950 to 1975, angiocardiography and selective angiography moved rapidly ahead, propelled by the dramatic progress in image amplification, rapid film changers and cine technology, as well as the development of new catheter materials and safer contrast agents. Precurved catheters for percutaneous insertion and biplane image-amplified cine technology graduated from the experimental to the applied. The advances in imaging paved the way for the great progress in open heart surgery and vascular surgery, just as coronary arteriography provided a road map for coronary bypass surgery. Cardiovascular nuclear medicine was furnishing an array of blood flow studies and dynamic data, while its imaging aspects were slowly improving. Computed tomography (CT) and a more sophisticated cardiac ultrasonography (US) were on the way, and cross-sectional imaging of the heart would soon become a reality. It was a spectacular growth period for contrast material–enhanced studies of the heart and vessels, while the use of the catheter as a therapeutic tool—the angiographer as interventionalist—was opening new horizons.

In the final quarter of the century from 1975 to 2000, we have observed and participated in a continuation of the remarkable changes in cardiovascular imaging at a rate that no one could have imagined. Echocardiography surged ahead technically and became a true imaging method of great power rather than a useful but limited graphical trace. CT went through a striking series of improvements in quality and speed of data acquisition, with spiral CT and three-dimensional imaging defining a special niche in their capacity to replace conventional catheter angiography in many vascular beds. Positron emission tomography (PET), and single photon emission CT, or SPECT, afforded unusual opportunities for investigating some of the metabolic and perfusion abnormalities in diseases of the myocardium and central nervous system; their potential continues to be explored. In similar fashion, magnetic resonance (MR) imaging took off jet-propelled as a unique static and dynamic method of looking at the interior of the heart noninvasively and depicting anatomic detail exquisitely. With cine MR imaging, a host of functional applications became feasible. This was an era in which digital imaging—CT, MR imaging, radionuclide studies, digital angiography, even conventional radiography—came into its own, with the promise of more to come. Interventional radiology with use

Index terms:
Heart
Radiology and radiologists, research
Subspecialty society messages

Radiology 1998; 208:285–287

[1] From the Department of Radiology, Stanford University School of Medicine, Rm S-056, Stanford, CA 94305. Received January 29, 1998; accepted February 23. **Address reprint requests to** the author.

See also the article by Boxt and Lipton (pp 283–284) in this issue.

of the catheter to dilate stenosed cardiac valves, coronary arteries, and coarctation or to plug patent ductus arteriosus, place stents, close bleeding arteries, and drain abscesses expanded logarhythmically.

As the century ends, we can look back not only at progress in technology and clinical application, but also at a body of research in which the new imaging methods have been applied to clarifying the underlying nature of numerous facets of cardiovascular dynamics and pathophysiology. Without the investigative power of these tools, many fundamental problems could never have been addressed.

As the next millennium begins, is there anything left to do in cardiovascular imaging research? Should we anticipate a plateau as the natural and expected consequence of such a burst of innovation and the acquisition of new knowledge?

Boxt and Lipton (3) have responded to these questions in their article with a resounding "no"! They have indicated the need for and the likelihood of major technologic advances that will result in better resolution, better contrast agents, wider application of noninvasive approaches such as MR coronary angiography, greater usefulness of new computer developments in analyzing myocardial motion and in digital data acquisition and transmission, and correlative studies of metabolism and morphology by using PET and MR imaging to enhance our understanding of disease processes. They have painted an impressive canvas of considerable scope and opportunity.

For the most part, these forward steps extend the march of progress of the last half of the 20th century. Perhaps of necessity, they are incremental rather than radical, configured by the past of imaging rather than visions of dramatic change well beyond the end of the current pipelines. But the widened use of MR spectroscopy will propel us into areas of in vivo cellular and tissue characterization that should enable giant steps toward a heightened understanding of a host of disorders. Whereas the application to the brain and other solid organs will surely be profoundly rewarding, cardiac motion presents a special challenge that will be surmounted more slowly. Genetic and molecular tagging with use of innovative contrast agents and tissue-seeking molecules combined with radioisotopes will enable the identification of damaged myocardial cells, infarction, infection, tumors, amyloid, and atheroma in vivo at a level of definitiveness never before attainable. Distinctions between ischemic, injured, and dead myocardium will form the basis for more precise therapeutic regimens, whether medical or surgical. In this process, motion studies will be abetted by innovative analyses of shape changes with use of algorithms and computer-driven technology never before applied to clinical and physiologic assessments of cardiac muscle. Similar motion analyses applied to blood flow may well strengthen our understanding of atherogenesis and other aspects of vascular pathophysiology.

Freeman Dyson has suggested that while concept-driven science is clearly important to progress, genuine advance is even more closely related to "tool" revolution. He points out that the telescope enabled the Galileo revolution in astronomy, just as x-ray crystallography radically changed modern biology so that Rosalind Franklin's images of DNA—the first—were the real foundation behind the Watson-Crick discovery of the DNA molecule (although she never received the Nobel prize)(4). In cardiac imaging as well, tool revolutions (angiocardiography, coronary arteriography, CT, MR imaging, US) have triggered the astonishing increase in our capacity to derive information about gross morphology and physiology.

As the rapidity of information acquisition time changes in the next century, from tens of minutes, to minutes, to tens of seconds, to seconds, we will approach the magic moment when cardiac MR imaging and CT throughput are so radically increased that the 5-second morphologic, physiologic, and pathologic evaluation becomes a reality. Congenital and acquired abnormalities of the chambers and great vessels will be disclosed as part of a walk-through screening process, and instantaneous measurements and readouts of ventricular volumes, ejection fraction, cardiac output, myocardial wall thickness, and wall motion will be available before the patient has left the dressing room. The infarcted, or ischemic, or normal myocardium will stand out as a loud and distinct signal on the image, reflecting both past events and the hazardous present and future. Instead of two MR examinations per hour and 16 per day, 30 per hour and 250 per day will be feasible. Such a throughput will radically reduce the unit cost of examinations and permit baseline profiles of the normal as well as the abnormal on a routine basis. Furthermore, the interpretation of the images will be performed by the computer on the basis of a huge storage capacity and database for all known patterns of heart disease, so that the radiologist may well serve as the human agency whereby precision and accuracy are constantly monitored and updated.

Collateral angiogenic factors will be tagged so that the progress of neovascularization in the presence of coronary disease and ischemia can be assessed (5). The distribution of tissue-specific agents that deposit in large enough concentrations to enable a local therapeutic effect will be demonstrated with MR imaging or PET so as to guide the therapeutic process. Clearly, multiple research frontiers will challenge many of the best investigative minds in the field.

One of the most explosive advances in radiology has been the spread of interventionalism—the catheter as a tool for the radiologist to achieve therapeutic goals formerly in the province of the surgeon. These far less traumatic procedures, which avoid the massive insult to the organism that open thoracotomy or laparotomy constitute, are not simply a godsend for the patient, they also are an avenue to more expeditious, less costly, more efficient handling of complex therapeutic problems, and their scope will increase with every year that passes in the next decade. Many of these procedures have been created in the experimental laboratory, with subsequent technology transfer to human subjects successfully achieved, a pattern that will be repeated in the future.

Boxt and Lipton have indicated the likelihood of future technology assessment focused on a smaller number of centers, capable of rapid evaluation of sufficient numbers of subjects so as to prevent the diffusion of useless technologies, while permitting rapid application of important advances. Some years ago, we described a model "laboratory" to achieve exactly such goals with a modest investment in a limited number of well-equipped and carefully designed centers (6). It included representatives of each of the major clinical departments, with input as well from such disciplines as economics, sociology, statistics, epidemiology, engineering, and the basic sciences. Such a laboratory can work only with strong leadership and with the full support and collaboration of the administration of the medical center. The establishment of linked centers of technology assessment represents an important goal, still to be achieved, and one which will enable sophisticated clinical trials as new technologies emerge from the inventive minds of imaging scientists. It will simultaneously amplify the capacity to perform meaningful outcome studies that will clarify the true impact of new technologies on patient care.

Boxt and Lipton have alluded to the aging of the baby-boomer generation as a stimulus for research designed to detect "silent" coronary disease. The problem is larger. Imaging research in the future must respond broadly to the sociocultural changes that are altering the complexion of society. The Western world is in the middle of an explosion of the aging population. In the United States, life expectancy at birth in 1900 was 46 years; in 1997, 76 years. Thirty years have been added as this century has witnessed the creation of "old age" as a phenomenon rather than an anecdote, virtually a new segment of life to be addressed. Today, 12% of the population is over age 65 years; in 2030, this figure will reach a staggering 20% (7).

It is not that biologic life itself has been extended (although the cloning of the "immortality" gene and its insertion into healthy human cells raises many possibilities)(8). Rather, more people are living longer. The implications are clear: more heart disease, stroke, diabetes, vascular disease, cancer, pneumonia. A man aged 75–84 years is 17 times more likely to die of heart disease and 34 times more likely to die of stroke than one aged 45–54 years (9). Even though the death rates from heart disease and stroke have come down in the past decade, the absolute number of deaths per year has remained constant at almost 750,000 for the past 25 years because of the increased population and a higher proportion of elderly. There are 400,000 new cases of heart failure each year, largely due to coronary disease.

Hence, both the challenges and the opportunities for developing and evaluating new imaging technologies should follow "Sutton's Law." Willie Sutton robbed banks because that's where the money is, and imaging advances combined with therapeutic innovations should target the elderly in particular because that's where the lethal diseases are. Beyond the increased incidence of disease, there is the knowledge that a large percentage of those over age 80 and 85 years are more or less dependent and cannot function without assistance. Many are institutionalized and more will be so; those who remain in the community are most comfortable in familiar surroundings. For this huge part of the population now and so much greater in the future, we should be looking to their needs, their comforts, their quality of life. Nothing is more disorienting to them than to be transferred to the unfamiliar, often cold and distant walls of a hospital room; for many of them, their apprehension is based on their sense that it may be the end.

So we must think in terms of portability of MR imaging and CT, and perhaps of miniaturization, but most important of bringing the diagnostic armamentarium to the dependent and disabled, rather than vice versa. Our research should be at least partially designed to make certain before the fact that what truly troubles the elderly does indeed require their physical removal from their customary and everyday surroundings into a new and threatening world.

Finally, we can and should speculate on new directions as the 20th century ends. Our conception of cardiac imaging research for the next century is already rich in the scope of opportunities it offers; but, if history is any guide, we have not even dared to dream of the innovations that the next few decades will bring. Who would have thought in 1950 that the next half century could possibly have been as rich in discoveries and improvements in health care as it has proved to be? As it is, the agenda that confronts mature and younger investigators in cardiac imaging is full of bracing challenges for visionaries. They will find the 21st century a wonderful time to be alive, as those alert to human disease will have the chance to improve the quality of life for all.

References

1. Abrams HL. Cardiac radiology. In: Gagliardi RA, McClennan BL, eds. A history of the radiologic sciences: diagnosis. Radiol Centennial 1996; 10:255–269.
2. Forssman W. Uber kontrastardstellung der hohlen des lebenden rechten herzens un der lungenschlagader. Munch Med Wschr 1931; 78:489–492.
3. Boxt LM, Lipton MJ. The future direction of cardiovascular research. Radiology 1998; 208:283–284.
4. Dyson FJ. Science as a craft industry. Science 1998; 280:1014–1015.
5. Abrams HL. The collateral circulation: response to ischemia— Caldwell lecture. AJR 1983; 140:1051–1063.
6. Sox H, Stern S, Owens D, Abrams HL. Assessment of diagnostic technology in health care: rationale, methods, problems and directions. (Study sponsored by the Institute of Medicine.) Washington, DC: National Academy Press, 1989.
7. Bandon A. The age boom: a special issue. New York Times Magazine, 1977; Mar 8: 44–45.
8. Bodnar A, Ouellette M, Frolkis M, et al. Extension of life-span by introduction of telomerase into normal human cells. Science 1998; 279:349–352.
9. Calcualted from statistics in health, United States, 1994. DHHS Publication no. (PHS) 95-1232. Hyattsville, MD: US Department of Health and Human Services, Public Health Services, National Center for Health Statistics, 1995; 113–116.

Interlude

Ultrasound Scan Confirms the Diagnosis of the Patient's Ailment

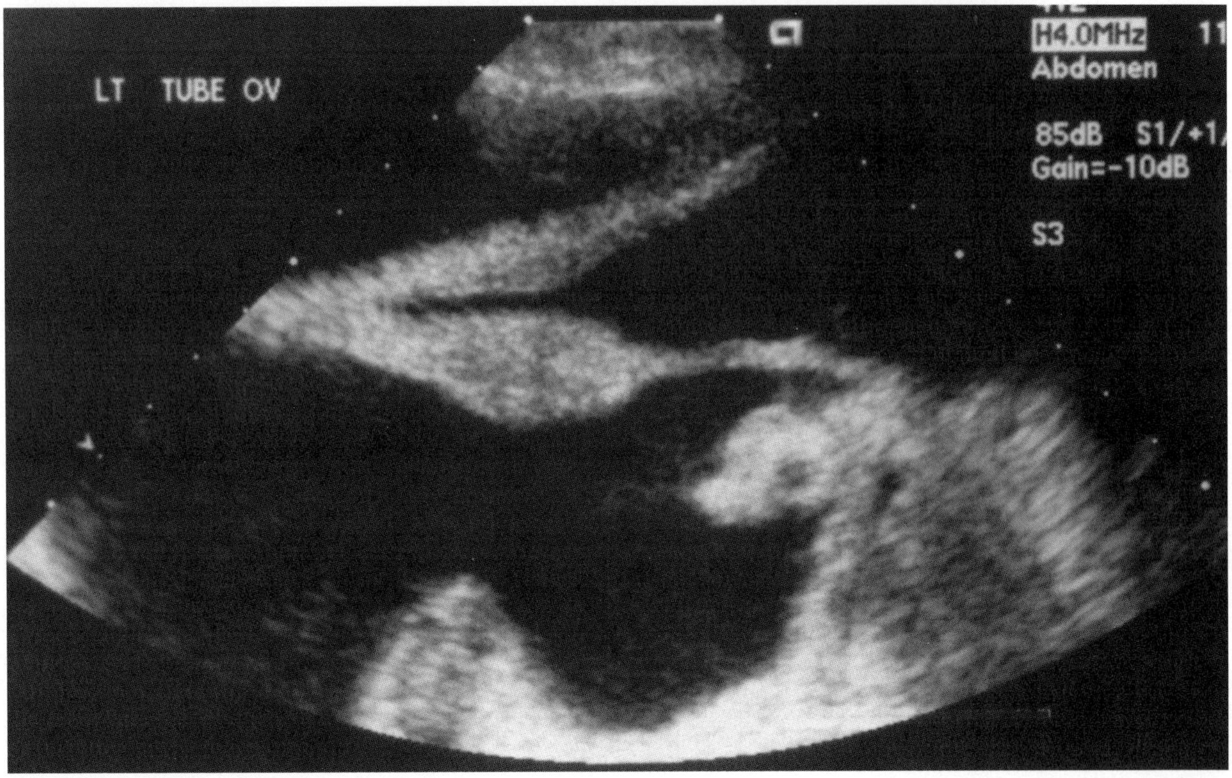

A snake is swimming in an ocean of ascites.

Courtesy of Monzer Abu-Yousef, MD, Iowa City, Iowa

Richard M. Friedenberg, MD

A Compendium of Managed Care: Past, Present, and Hints of the Future—Part I[1]

This is my attempt to write a personal compendium on managed care, reviewing the history, discussing the developments that have led to the present, and suggesting some future possibilities. For the historical aspects found below, I have borrowed liberally from two articles, one by Sam Shapiro (1) from the Johns Hopkins University School of Hygiene and Public Health, and the other by Douglas Scutchfield and colleagues (2) from the Center for Health Services, Research, Policy and Management of the University of Kentucky. I will divide this Perspective into two parts, since I believe that readers prefer that each Perspective be limited in length. The second part will appear in a subsequent issue of *Radiology.*

Managed care in the United States is not a new concept. In 1929, nearly 70 years ago in Elk City, Oklahoma, the first prepaid medical cooperative was established that provided medical care through group practice with prepayment through insurance policies. The purpose of this cooperative was to provide high-quality care affordably and economically. These early efforts were strongly opposed by organized medicine and ended in the depression of 1930–1931.

The next major managed care effort occurred in 1937 with the formation of the Group Health Association in Washington, DC, a cooperative for employees of the government and their families. In the late 1930s, at the beginning of World War II, Henry Kaiser with Dr Sidney Garfield started the Kaiser Permanente Medical Care Program for the employees of Kaiser Industries. When the war ended, the Permanente plan was opened to the community through contracts with industry and labor.

In 1947, the Health Insurance Plan of Greater New York, commonly called HIP, was formed as a health plan for city employees and their dependents. In the same year, the Group Health Cooperative of Puget Sound opened in the Pacific Northwest. HIP became a major player in the health field in New York, as did Kaiser and Puget Sound on the West Coast. Although these major plans thrived, they were strongly opposed by organized medicine, which considered them unethical and as practicing of inferior medicine (Table 1).

Overshadowing the managed care activities in the postwar period was the development of Blue Cross–Blue Shield plans, which were based on fee for service and were strongly supported by organized medicine and the bulk of the medical profession. As late as 1970, there were less than 30 prepaid medical plans offered in the United States.

About this time, the cost of health care was beginning to increase dramatically. The rapid development of new technologies was providing physicians with multiple types of examinations, which they used in increasing numbers to sift through differential diagnoses, thereby increasing both the individual's health care bill and the physician's income. The prevailing method of cost reimbursement by insurance companies allowed every hospital and doctor's office to duplicate expensive equipment, which was essentially paid for by the insurance companies—and once you had the equipment you had to make use of it. Hospitals, physicians, and medical societies did nothing to control health costs.

TABLE 1
Early History of Managed Care

Program	Year Established
Community Hospital Association, Oklahoma	1929
Ross Loos Medical Clinic, California	1929
Group Health Association, Washington, DC	1937
Kaiser Permanente Medical Care Program, California	1939
Health Insurance Plan of New York	1947
Group Health Cooperative of Puget Sound, Washington	1947

The government, unions, employers, insurance companies, and patients were concerned about costs and began to consider methods to control them. In 1970, a Minneapolis physician by the name of Paul Ellwood, Jr, at a meeting with federal officials, coined the term *health maintenance organization,* or *HMO,* as an alternative concept to the then-current fee-for-service system. The federal government, concerned over the rapidly increasing cost of Medicare and Medicaid, embraced this concept as a means of cost containment. Many of you may not realize that in 1971, President Nixon, in his health message to Congress, enthusiastically embraced the HMO concept and proposed legislation to allow Medicare patients to join such organizations. This led to the Health Maintenance Organization Act of 1973, which provided incentive grants to establish HMOs. From 1970 to approximately 1980, patient enrollment in HMOs increased from 3 million to 13 million (1). In 1985, enrollment was approxi-

Index terms:
Economics, medical
Perspectives
Radiology and radiologists, socioeconomic issues

Radiology 1998; 208:289–292

[1] From the Department of Radiological Sciences, University of California, Irvine Medical Center, 101 The City Dr, Orange, CA 92868-3298. Received and accepted April 20, 1998. **Address reprint requests to** the author.

mately 19 million, but by 1995 it had increased to 56 million, and HMOs were now a powerful force in American medicine and increasing at a rapid rate (Table 2) (1,3).

A major stimulus for the development of managed care was the rapid rise in the cost of health care for workers, which became a large part of industry's budget. By the early 1990s, it was obvious that something had to be done to stop the increased spiraling costs of health care. President Clinton proposed a fairly comprehensive health care system, but when this proposal was defeated in 1993 and the government backed off totally from involvement in structuring the health care system, entrepreneurs took over. Venture capitalists and other entrepreneurs quickly recognized managed care as a new major industry with potentially substantial profits. From that point on, health care was treated as a commodity, and, as such, it was subject to the constraints of reducing costs and obtaining profits.

It is interesting to speculate why the federal government removed itself completely from the health care scene. Politicians do not like to propose plans that will reduce benefits to citizens and that will, by decreasing patient satisfaction, produce a voter backlash. Politicians would rather allow these changes to happen by means of outside intervention and then be able to criticize the results that they indirectly fostered.

The simplest definition of managed care is a health care delivery and reimbursement system. There are a number of different arrangements that have evolved over the past several years, most with acronyms such as HMO and IPA, or independent practice association (Table 3) (5). The term *HMO* has no strict definition. Although a few individuals use it synonymously with *managed care,* it probably should be used only for capitation programs. An HMO combines insurance functions and health care delivery systems to offer a stated range of prepaid comprehensive health care for both hospital and physician services regardless of the number of services provided.

There are different subcategories of HMOs, although as modifications are being made the distinctions are becoming somewhat blurred. A staff model HMO employs physicians to provide services at its own facilities. The physician is salaried and has no financial risk. This HMO is usually within one edifice and therefore is more easily structured and supervised so that it has very efficient cost containment. However, because of its restrictive nature within a single geographic facility, the number of staff model HMOs has declined more than 50% (5). A group model HMO contracts with physician groups who are not its employees; therefore, these physicians may also provide services to non-HMO patients.

TABLE 2
HMO Enrollment

Year	No. of Patients Enrolled
1970	Three million
1980	13 million
1985	19 million
1996	68 million

Source.—Reference 4.

TABLE 3
Types of HMOs

HMO Type	Definition
Staff model	Salaried physicians supply services for facility owned by HMO
Group model	Contracts with physicians and physician groups who are not employees of the HMO and may treat non-HMO patients
IPA	Individual physicians and physician groups contract with the IPA, which contracts with an HMO
PHO*	Hospital and physicians form an HMO
Mixed models	Variations of HMOs that develop to enhance marketing

* PHO = physician hospital organization.

An IPA consists of physician groups and independent physicians who contract with the IPA, which then contracts with one or more HMOs. In the group and IPA models, in which the physician is in a capitation program, he or she bears some financial risk for the cost of utilization, making the gatekeeper role more critical. The IPA model can cover a large geographic area, since it utilizes physicians' offices as well as group practices, which is attractive to patients but more difficult to control and less efficient in cost containment.

To cope with patient demands and physician complaints, many HMOs have expanded services, altering the original provisions of the HMO. HMOs with such changes have been termed *mixed models.* Most group and IPA models and some staff HMOs now offer point-of-service or open-access privileges. With point of service, the patient has the right to see a physician outside of his or her HMO, perhaps for a second opinion, but must pay a substantial copayment, perhaps 50% of the physician's fee.

Open access allows patients to see specialists in the HMO without going through their gatekeeper physician. Open access may be limited to certain specialties, such as obstetrics, gynecology, and dermatology, or the HMO may charge an additional fee for the privilege of open access. As these options are added, the overall cost increases and premiums must increase. The most recent HMO model has been the PHO. A hospital with its staff physicians form an HMO and offer a continuum of services contained in one area. Most PHOs accept capitation and therefore share in the financial risk. Within the HMO group in managed care, the trend has been to pay physicians through capitation or salary (Table 4).

TABLE 4
Pay of Primary Care Physicians in HMOs

Type of Pay	1989	1994
Fee for service	36	24
Salary	23	26
Capitation	35	50
Unknown*	6	0

Sources.—References 6 (1989) and 7 (1994).
Note.—Data are percentages.
* Six percent of the responding HMOs that paid a contracting middleman rather than the individual physician did not know how the physician was paid.

Over the past few years, preferred provider organizations (PPOs) have become popular and are the fastest growing area in managed care. A PPO provides specified medical benefits at a negotiated reduced rate. This, in essence, is a modified fee-for-service plan and is more popular among physicians and patients because of its flexibility. As managed care expands outside of California, many communities are trying to avoid the restrictive type of managed care that developed in that state (Table 5).

The PPO is a preferred plan. The physician reduces his fees in return for an expected increased volume. There is no gatekeeper, and the patient has a wider range of choices. However, there is less control over procedures and referrals, and these plans are much less efficient in cost containment. In most PPOs, the patient

TABLE 5
Populations Receiving Care through PPOs

Year	Population (in millions of people)
1992	50.4
1993	60.0
1994	79.2
1995	91.0

Source.—Reference 8.

TABLE 6
Percentages of HMOs Reporting a Profit or Surplus

Year	Percentage of HMOs
1988	36
1990	83
1992	86
1993	89
1994	88
1995	61

Source.—Reference 4.

pays a small copayment each time he or she visits a physician.

To cope with the rise of managed care, indemnity insurance has modified its approach, attempting to obtain better control over costs. *Managed indemnity,* the new term, requires approval before elective hospitalization and for expensive procedures. Despite attempts at cost control, the costs of managed indemnity plans exceed those of managed care. The number of patients covered by indemnity insurance is decreasing rapidly throughout the United States, particularly in the metropolitan markets, where HMOs have their strongest hold.

As managed care entities acquire more and more of the health care market, they acquire more control over the practicing physicians in their areas. The fear that managed care might exclude some practicing physicians from participating has led more than half of the states to enact "any willing provider" laws. These laws prohibit discrimination between physicians who agree to the terms of the HMO. This primarily affects PPOs and has less effect on staff and group HMOs, in which physicians are paid on a capitation basis and the HMO decides on the number and type needed.

Another changing mode is in the gatekeeper role. Many group HMOs and IPAs pay their primary physicians on a capitation basis; these physicians are expected to be gatekeepers, control referrals, and pay specialists on a reduced fee for services. In California, because of patient resistance, less than half the plans now require the patient to see a gatekeeper. When people are healthy, they are willing to see a primary care physician, but when they are sick, they want access to a specialist.

There are several problems with the gatekeeper philosophy to which patients object. It is not uncommon for the income of the gatekeeper to be inversely proportional to the number of tests and consultations ordered. I personally find this unconscionable. A gatekeeper who orders diagnostic tests or consultations may be decreasing his income. In these cases, it may be the patient who is being penalized to protect the physician's income. There are other methods of quality control and physician review to see whether excess tests and consultations are being ordered by the individual physician. Many HMOs encourage primary care physicians to perform sigmoidoscopies and routine obstetric examinations for which the physicians may not be well qualified. Their capitation may increase with the number of procedures that they perform rather than refer.

In *JAMA,* Halm (9) reported that gatekeepers were effective in controlling costs and in preventing inappropriate or duplicate behavior, but they also decreased the quality of care and freedom in clinical decisions. Gatekeepers also had a negative effect on the physician-patient relationship. Some HMOs are combating patient resistance to gatekeepers by allowing more access to specialists but paying the specialists on a capitation basis to control costs. This makes it easier for the HMO to predict its costs and maintain relatively level premiums.

Although most polls of patients in managed care show that the majority of patients are satisfied with their service, these polls really represent the healthy individuals, who are the bulk of the enrollees. These patients are paying 20%–30% less for medical care and are receiving preventive medical care free. There are no major polls on the 10%–20% of patients who are chronically ill with regard to their degree of satisfaction. The implications are that many chronically ill patients are not happy with the difficulties they have in accessing health care.

In California, the mecca of managed care, there has been considerable interest in how managed care affects hospital costs. Robinson (10) has studied this situation and reported in *JAMA* that in hospitals in areas of high HMO penetration, costs grew 44% less rapidly because of reductions in occupancy, expensive tests performed, and the volumes of tests and consultations. Most diagnostic and therapeutic procedures that previously were performed in hospitals are now performed in outpatient clinics or surgicenters. In the United States, between 1983 and 1993, the number of community hospitals declined by 9%. In California, the number of community hospitals declined by 19%; of overall beds, by 10%; of inpatient days, by 21%; and of inpatient surgical procedures performed, by 33% (4). These decreases were due to better control and a massive shift of procedures and services from the inpatient setting to the outpatient setting.

The figures regarding bed utilization are dramatic. Indemnity plans may utilize 900–1,000 days per 1,000 beneficiaries per year. An efficient HMO may utilize 500–600 days per 1,000 patients per year. Similarly, a non-HMO Medicare plan might utilize 1,800 hospital days per 1,000 patients, while an HMO Medicare plan utilizes 1,000 days per 1,000 patients (10). There is evidence that when Medicare patients become ill, they tend to leave HMO Medicare groups and return to regular Medicare. This will be discussed in detail in the second part of the compendium. Also, it is not known whether the efficiency of HMOs is causing a reduction in the quality of care and whether the decrease in hospitalization is causing an increase in morbidity and mortality.

One of the major problems with managed care is the concern with reducing costs rather than with improving quality. Medicine is a profession and a business. The ethics of the profession make the physician the patient's advocate. The physician must be concerned with the patient's rights, including the access to quality care. Since under managed care the physician does not control the business of medicine, he or she must be a political advocate to the government to ensure the patient's rights. Because of this, I have always believed that managed care, which is the business of medicine, must be controlled by government regulation. Access to quality care is the right of our public no less than is clean water, clean air, or public safety.

Managed care organizations must be considered in a different category from other corporate entities and must accept regulation for the public good. When we see chief executive officers of managed care organizations using 20% of the premium for dividends and excessive salaries, the need for regulation becomes obvious (11). We cannot allow patient health to become secondary to corporate earnings. When managed care organizations refer to their loss ratio, they refer to the money they spent on health care. The public has always accepted that physicians in hospitals must be monitored. As long as managed care organizations affect the actions of physicians in hospitals, the organizations must be monitored as well. With the new obsessive focus on costs, we cannot allow quality to slide. There has been no substantial work in which the outcomes of managed care were compared with those of indemnity care. As you know, it is difficult to measure outcomes, but an assessment of outcomes in managed care is desperately needed if we are to maintain quality of care.

In 1993 and 1994, approximately 90% of HMOs reported a profit or surplus. In 1995, only 61% reported a profit or surplus, and this percentage may be less today (Table 6) (4). Those of you who follow the U.S. stock market probably have noticed that a majority of health plans have had major decreases in their stock prices. In 1996, HMO stocks as a group dropped 22%; this probably resulted from several different causes.

First, when HMOs initially started, they recruited primarily healthy individuals. Their major thrust was preventive medicine. To the healthy individual, receiving totally free care, including the necessary vaccinations for the children, annual physical examinations, mammography, Papanicolaou tests, and the like made the HMO very attractive. With healthy individuals, the expenses of the HMO were very moderate. More recently, the addition of chronically ill patients has increased HMO costs substantially.

Second, employers have formed purchasing groups, and, especially in high-density metropolitan areas where the majority of HMOs reside, these purchasing groups have created intense competition between various HMOs, reducing premiums to bare minimums.

Third, administrative expenses in most HMOs are high. In for-profit HMOs, administrative expenses average 14%, and in many, these expenses are as high as 18%–20% (12). This means that, on the average, only 86 cents of every dollar paid by beneficiaries goes toward medical care. In Kaiser, a non-profit HMO, over 90 cents of every dollar goes toward medical care. The reason for the high administrative costs of for-profit HMOs is that stock dividends as well as the multimillion dollar yearly salaries of the chief executive officers and administrators of major HMO plans must be paid.

Managed care organizations have saved considerable sums by monitoring services, avoiding duplication of services, and avoiding obvious excesses. Much of the above has already been trimmed to the bone. Managed care organizations are under considerable pressure not to increase their premiums substantially. How else can they save money? To save additional sums, medical care must be more severely budgeted, and as budgeting becomes tighter, it becomes rationing.

We must realize that managed care has altered our traditional approach, which was to do everything for the individual patient. Managed care attempts to provide the best care possible for the greatest number, which, by necessity, excludes a portion of the sick and chronically ill. We might restate this as the best medical care for the many and restricted medical care for the few. Some patients will lose extra years of life.

References

1. Shapiro S. A historical perspective on the roots of managed care. Curr Opin Pediatr 1996; 8:159–163.
2. Scutchfield FD, Lee J, Patton D. Managed care in the United States. J Public Health Med 1997; 19:251–254.
3. Berlin B. Whither managed care. N Engl J Med 1997; 94:27–30.
4. Hamer R, Van Antwerp S. Study results show decline in HMO operating margins. Health Care Fin Manage 1997; 51:78–80,82,84.
5. Offner E, Zacker HB. Understanding different models of health maintenance organizations. Curr Opin Pediatr 1996; 8:171–175.
6. Hillman AL, Welsh WP, Pauly MV. Contractual arrangements between HMOs and primary care physicians. Med Care 1992; 30:142.
7. Gabel J. Ten ways HMOs have changed during the 1990s. Health Aff 1997; 16:141.
8. de Guzman MM. Are specialists staging a comeback? Health Syst Leader 1997; 4:6.
9. Halm EA. Is gatekeeping better than traditional care? JAMA 1997; 278:1677–1681.
10. Robinson JC. Decline in hospital utilization and cost inflation under managed care in California. JAMA 1996; 276:1060–1064.
11. Bodenheimer T. The HMO backlash: righteous or reactionary? N Engl J Med 1996; 335:1601–1603.
12. Sachs MA. Managed care: the next generation. Front Health Serv Manage 1997; 14:3–26.

Jonathan H. Sunshine, PhD

A Promising Start on Overall Imaging Quality, but Far to Go on Costs[1]

For at least 3 decades, cost, quality, and access have been virtually a holy trinity by which those who think systematically about American health care evaluate it. For most of this time, cost drew by far the most attention, probably because the United States has spent substantially more of its total national output on health care than has any other country and because health care spending was nonetheless increasing rapidly. In contrast, quality received relatively little attention or empirical study, perhaps because of a conviction in the United States that "we have the best health care in the world." Recently, quality has been drawing more attention, possibly only for the negative reasons that (*a*) with the growth of health care spending greatly slowed in the past few years, it became easier to worry about other issues and (*b*) the rise of managed health care brought a major new actor onto the scene that is often attacked—sometimes unfairly—on grounds of quality.

In this issue of *Radiology,* we have a good example of this new focus on quality: In their article, Verrilli and colleagues (1) report on a large-scale quality improvement program of a type we are likely to see more of in the future, a project designed to improve the whole range of imaging in an entire state and simultaneously reduce costs by eliminating inappropriate services. The authors not only provide a description of the program and how it has—and has not—worked, but also provide important information on what the overall quality of imaging was, including imaging performed by nonradiologists, prior to the implementation of their program.

The quality improvement program that the authors' firm, Radiology Management Sciences, instituted at the behest of BlueCross BlueShield of Massachusetts (BCBSMA) is sensible in its broad outlines. As they point out, hospitals have had at least a basic quality assurance regimen through accreditation by the Joint Commission on Accreditation of Health Care Organizations for the accreditation and hospital privileging of physicians. No such systematic program was in existence for nonhospital care, and this care, therefore, is the focus of their program. There are two major types of participants in the imaging process: (*a*) facilities and (*b*) physicians and other providers; the authors' program covers both. For facilities, the program pursues the sound strategy of concentrating on major deficiencies and, at the same time, not ignoring lesser problems. As regards providers, the program addresses the first-order concern of assuring that the providers are trained in the types of imaging they perform and avoids more contentious issues and other matters that are more difficult to address.

However, a number of concerns about this program, or any like it, must be mentioned. For one, what is the whole scope of what Radiology Management Sciences and BCBSMA are undertaking? If part of their agenda is "care management" of the type physicians often feel is intrusive and arbitrary, they will encounter much more hostility than would a sensible quality assurance program by itself.

Second, the facilities portion of their program may, to some extent, be targeting form rather than substance. A generation ago, Avedis Donabedian, the father of systematic thinking about health care quality, pointed out that quality assurance programs could focus on structure, process, or outcome, but that such programs typically focused heavily on structure—although the real concern is outcomes—and secondarily on process—to the extent that process affects outcomes. The Radiology Management Sciences program seems to have focused on structure in that it often appears to be concerned about paperwork (eg, whether there is a shielding floor plan on-site) rather than about reality (whether adequate shielding is present). In like manner, another major criterion of the program described by Verrilli et al is the paperwork question of whether there is a record transfer policy in case the medical office shuts down.

Third, the program's privileging of physicians and other providers somewhat similarly omits a core issue. It is valuable to ensure that providers perform only the imaging procedures for which they have been trained, and the program does this. However, it is equally important to know if the providers can interpret the images with reasonable accuracy, although this is much more difficult to ascertain operationally. The program does not at all address accuracy.

Fourth, the response burden on facilities and providers is an important concern. The facility questionnaire had 100 items; that is a large number of questions. More important, if physicians and facilities must pass through a similar program a dozen times as each major insurer and managed care provider requires it of them,

Index terms:
Economics, medical
Editorials
Radiology and radiologists

Radiology 1998; 208:293–295

[1] From the Department of Research, American College of Radiology, 1891 Preston White Dr, Reston, VA 20191. Received May 15, 1998; accepted May 26. **Address reprint requests to** the author.

The views expressed herein are those of the author and not necessarily those of his employers.

See also the article by Verrilli et al (pp 385–392) in this issue.

the overall burden will be grossly excessive, although a single pass through a program is quite reasonable. BCBSMA is, I believe, by far the largest payer in Massachusetts, so their undertaking of such a program seems reasonable, but I would hope that other payers and managed health care plans will accept credentialing by BCBSMA. Unfortunately, this has not been the case. Moreover, I understand the National Committee for Quality Assurance, a major certifier of quality for managed health care organizations, has required each organization to credential its own providers, which virtually guarantees that physicians and facilities will be subjected to a large number of credentialing programs. An attractive solution would be for insurers and managed health care organizations to accept the credentialing programs being developed by professional societies, such as the American College of Radiology, much as they have long accepted board certification as an important credential.

Fifth, by concentrating primarily on eliminating substandard care, the Radiology Management Sciences program embodies a purportedly outdated approach to quality improvement. New thinking about quality, usually known as "total quality management" (TQM) or "continuous quality improvement" (CQI), disparages a concentration on substandard care because such care comprises only a small percentage of all health care. Instead, the purpose of TQM or CQI is to improve the quality of all care, including the vast majority that already is better than substandard. In fact, what really matters is what a program achieves, not the theoretic merits of its underlying concept.

The findings of Verrilli and associates are striking: "many providers own and operate equipment that they are not trained to use. Lack of knowledge about requirements for safety and equipment" is common. Thirty percent of facilities had at least one major deficiency; 10% had two or more fundamental, serious deficiencies. If this is the situation in Massachusetts, a heavily regulated state with many academic institutions, the overall national picture is probably worse. Indeed, the authors present preliminary findings indicating that the percentage of imaging performed outside the (generously defined) scope of competence of providers is much higher elsewhere than the 2% found in Massachusetts.

These extrapolations from Massachusetts, while tempting to undertake, call attention to one important consideration regarding this study. It is a study of only a single state, and until more studies have been conducted we cannot definitively conclude anything about the national quality situation or, for that matter, about how quality improvement programs work in practice. Despite this, the authors deserve praise for obtaining the information they have garnered. The quality of imaging performed by nonradiologists relative to that performed by radiologists is an important issue in the overall topic of self-referral, but it is one on which extremely little information has been available (2). Thus, Verrilli et al make a much-needed contribution to our knowledge.

Radiologists will be reassured to know that their performance is among the best. The highest rates of facility deficiencies are found among podiatrists and chiropractors and, to a lesser extent, among obstetricians and gynecologists and physicians in medical specialties other than cardiology or primary care. Previous studies (2) found broadly similar patterns, so we are, I think, beginning to obtain reasonably good empirical evidence on where the problems with quality lie.

The work of Verrilli and colleagues demonstrates a characteristic typical of studies performed by operational organizations. Because of limited research resources, some of the important and interesting questions are not answered. For example, Verrilli et al note that they do not know whether net savings actually resulted when BCBSMA limited the imaging procedures for which providers receive professional component reimbursement to each provider's defined area of competence. Providers may be compensating for the loss resulting from this limitation through increased imaging outside their field, which brings increased technical-component reimbursements to their facility (Hillman et al [3] found such behavior), or through more imaging in their defined field of competence. It would be desirable to know whether total costs were reduced; complex data analysis could probably provide an answer, but the authors did not have the necessary intensive analytic resources to perform such an analysis. Many health services researchers in academic settings would, I think, be strongly interested in "real world" applied projects like that described in this paper. Insurers, managed health care organizations, and others who undertake substantial projects would do well to invite such academic researchers to join their project teams so that more sophisticated analyses could be undertaken.

The BCBSMA program is strange in that providers' offices are paid for the technical component of imaging procedures outside the providers' approved scope of competence, although the professional-component payments for these procedures are denied. Elimination of this technical-component reimbursement would be logical and would remove what is probably an undesirable financial incentive.

However, with many payers and managed health care plans likely, in coming years, to undertake projects to improve the quality and moderate the cost of imaging, financial incentives should be considered not in light of BCBSMA's current arrangements, but from a broad perspective of what is desirable. From this perspective, it seems clear that the currently dominant pattern in the United States, in which treating physicians both order imaging and (generally) may perform it, provides excessive financial incentives for imaging. Hillman and colleagues (4,5) found that nonradiologists who performed their own imaging ("self-referrers") generated imaging expenditures per episode of care that were two to seven times as high as those of nonradiologists in the same specialties who examined patients with the same problems but who referred those patients to radiologists for imaging. A sizable literature (6–8) bears out this finding that financial self-interest is associated with more frequent imaging. Most observers would agree, on the other hand, that incentives are tilted toward underprovision of services if, at the opposite extreme, the treating physician's income is decreased by a substantial fraction of the charges for the imaging work he or she sends to radiologists (and for all other referral costs). (A few managed care plans use this arrangement.) The correct solution would seem to be a financially neutral system—that is, one in which treating physicians neither gain nor lose financially when they order imaging procedures.

The only arrangement that has the requisite financial neutrality is one in which, as now, treating physicians order imaging, but the imaging must be performed by a practitioner with no financial link to the referring physician. In general, in such an arrangement the practitioner who performs the imaging will be a radiologist, because radiology is the imaging specialty. I suggest that payers adopt this policy as the best strategy for achieving their twin goals of improving the quality and containing the cost of imaging. It is certainly a far less intrusive strategy than the developing "care management" routine of having to obtain preauthorization for each high-cost procedure. I would hope that some of the many payers seeking to improve health care while restraining costs will test this model and will do so with a researcher involved, so we can learn how it actually turns out.

BCBSMA has initiated a promising program for improving imaging quality that has yielded valuable information on where severe quality problems have been concentrated, but it has not made the same progress on getting the financial incentives right.

References

1. Verrilli DK, Bloch SM, Rousseau J, Crozier ME, Yecies SB. Design of a privileging program for diagnostic imaging: costs and implications for a large insurer in Massachusetts. Radiology 1998; 208:385–392.
2. Hopper KD, Rossetti GF, Edmiston RB, et al. Diagnostic radiology peer review: a method inclusive of all interpreters of radiographic examinations regardless of specialty. Radiology 1991; 180:557–561.
3. Hillman BJ, Olson GT, Colbert RW, Bernhardt LB. Responses to a payment policy denying professional charges for diagnostic imaging by nonradiologist physicians. JAMA 1995; 274:885–887.
4. Hillman BJ, Joseph CA, Mabry MR, Sunshine JH, Kennedy SD, Noether M. Frequency and costs of diagnostic imaging in office practice: comparison of self-referring and radiologists-referring physicians. N Engl J Med 1990; 323:1604–1608.
5. Hillman BJ, Olson GT, Griffith PE, et al. Physicians' utilization and charges for outpatient diagnostic imaging in a medicare population. JAMA 1992; 268:2050–2054.
6. Testimony before the Subcommittee on Health Care of the House of Representatives Committee on Ways and Means. 1st Sess (1993) (Testimony by J. L. Shikles, Director, Health Financing and Policy Issues, General Accounting Office).
7. The Subcommittee on Health Care of the House of Representatives Committee on Ways and Means. 2nd Sess (1994) (Letter by L. G. Aronovitz of the General Accounting Office).
8. Swedlow A, Johnson G, Smithline N, Milstein A. Increased costs and rates of use in the California workers' compensation system as a result of self-referral by physicians. N Engl J Med 1992; 327:1502–1506.

Peter Jezzard, PhD

Advances in Perfusion MR Imaging[1]

Magnetic resonance (MR) imaging offers unparalleled soft-tissue diagnostic specificity. In the near future, it is also likely to be useful for diagnostic functional imaging, yielding maps of a number of metabolic parameters. A functional parameter of particular clinical importance is tissue perfusion. Perfusion describes the rate at which nutrient-supplying blood passes through tissue. In an MR imaging experiment, the most common definition of perfusion is the volume of blood delivered to a unit mass (or volume) of tissue per unit time, and is usually stated as milliliters per 100 grams per minute. The ability to map this quantity by using MR imaging would allow the noninvasive, high-resolution evaluation of tissue viability and function. In turn, this would enhance the sensitivity and specificity of diagnosis in several areas, including degenerative and metabolic disorders, chronic vascular disease, and ischemia.

A decade ago, Villringer et al (1) proposed an MR imaging method for measuring regional cerebral blood volume and perfusion. This method uses a bolus of paramagnetic contrast agent, the concentration of which can be mapped as it passes through the tissue of interest. The contrast agent most commonly used, and indeed one of the only MR agents approved for clinical use in the United States, is the lanthanide chelate, gadolinium diethylenetriaminepentaacetic acid (DTPA). Depending on the tissue and application of interest, the contrast mechanism can be either the T1-enhancing properties of the unpaired electrons within the agent or the T2- or T2*-enhancing properties of the magnetic susceptibility difference between the agent and the surrounding tissue. In the case of more permeable tissue (such as myocardial tissue), in which the contrast agent can cross the capillary endothelium and enter the tissue, a T1-weighted spin-echo sequence is most effective because the contrast agent induces strong dipole-to-dipole T1 relaxation of the tissue water, rendering it bright on the image. In the case of the brain, however, the contrast agent (550–600 d for Gd-DTPA) cannot cross the intact blood-brain barrier and T2*-weighted gradient-echo sequences provide a better means of contrast. This is because the compartmentalized susceptibility differences in the blood pool create microscopic magnetic field gradients that extend into the tissue and enhance T2* dephasing, rendering the tissue dark.

For both the T1- and T2-weighted approaches, a bolus injection of contrast agent is given and a high-speed imaging technique (typically echo-planar or fast gradient-echo imaging) is used to track the passage of contrast agent through the tissue of interest. In the late 1980s and early 1990s, much work was done to characterize the relationship between the concentration of agent in the tissue and the change in image signal intensity (2,3). Studies during this period showed that the relevant relaxation rate change [$\Delta(1/T1)$ or $\Delta(1/T2^*)$] is roughly proportional to the concentration of the agent in the image voxel. This result allows application of the classic results of tracer kinetic theory to determine physiologic parameters of interest. Specifically, one can deduce relative regional cerebral blood volume by integrating under the concentration-time curve formed by the passage of the bolus of contrast agent through the tissue. This is most easily done by calculating the change in the relaxation rate (4) of the tissue versus time. It is also possible, but much more difficult, to measure an approximate tissue mean transit time for the passage of contrast agent through the tissue (5,6). To do this accurately, the effects of perfusion need to be deconvolved from the finite length and time course characteristics of the arterial input function. Techniques have been proposed to accomplish this with MR imaging (7), but they are difficult to apply. If the tissue mean transit time can be obtained, as well as absolute regional cerebral blood volume, then calculation of perfusion can be made (8) by means of the central volume theorem. This states that the regional blood flow is equal to the regional volume distribution of the contrast agent (eg, the regional blood volume in the case of an intravascular contrast agent) divided by the tissue mean transit time (9). In practice, though, it is almost impossible to obtain absolute flow, since accurate determination of the absolute regional cerebral blood volume is very difficult (10).

Despite considerable effort in applying MR bolus tracking methods clinically, they have remained largely qualitative: They are mostly restricted to obtaining relative rather than absolute regional blood volume maps and are rarely used to measure absolute perfusion. This emphasis on the qualitative stems from the difficulties of accurate estimation of the arterial input function and the tissue mean transit time. Until these difficulties can be overcome, it is unlikely that bolus tracking MR imaging methods will provide rigorously quantitative results.

An alternative technique—initially promising but ultimately problematic—is the concept of intravoxel incoherent motion proposed by LeBihan et al (11). By taking a macroscopic perspective, this method sees capillary perfusion as a summation of randomly oriented flow seg-

Index terms:
Cerebral blood vessels, flow dynamics
Editorials
Magnetic resonance (MR), echo planar, 17.121412
Magnetic resonance (MR), perfusion study, 17.121412
Magnetic resonance (MR), vascular studies, 17.121412

Radiology 1998; 208:296–299

[1] From the Department of Clinical Neurology, Functional Magnetic Resonance Imaging of the Brain (FMRIB) Centre, John Radcliffe Hospital, University of Oxford, Headington, Oxford OX3 9DU, England. Received May 15, 1998; accepted May 26. **Address reprint requests to** the author.

 See also the article by Alsop and Detre (pp 410–416) in this issue.

ments, in contrast to large vessel bulk flow. In this sense, perfusion can be likened to molecular self-diffusion. True self-diffusion of tissue water can be distinguished from the pseudodiffusion of intravoxel incoherent motion by means of the markedly different "diffusion" coefficients of the two processes (12). Practically, this is done by adding diffusion-sensitizing magnetic field gradients to the MR imaging sequence. A rapid decay occurs when signal intensity is plotted against increasing diffusion field gradient for low gradient values. This is followed by a slower decay of the signal as the diffusion field gradients are steadily increased. The rapid decay can be ascribed to the perfusion component. The slower decay belongs to the molecular self-diffusion of the tissue water. The advantage of this technique is that it requires no bolus injection of contrast agent, and, as such, it is totally noninvasive. Unfortunately, in practice, one obtains noticeable image artifacts from the diffusion-sensitizing gradients, and, even more troubling, the dynamic range of the technique is very low. This latter problem occurs because the signal relating to perfusion constitutes only a small fraction (typically 5%) of the total signal, even though the apparent diffusion coefficient of the perfusion component can be 10 times greater than that of the molecular diffusion component.

The most recent, and potentially the most promising, class of perfusion MR imaging techniques are those that magnetically label the proximal endogenous water in arterial blood (13) and then observe the effect of this water as it freely diffuses into the tissue. In the simplest form of these techniques, all arterial water spins are inverted (by using a radio-frequency inversion pulse) before they enter the brain section. When the inverted arterial water spins diffuse into the extracellular space and exchange with the unperturbed tissue spins, the net magnetization of the tissue is reduced, relative to a control condition in which the arterial spins are not inverted. For the resulting small difference in signal (1% or 2%) to be quantitatively related back to tissue perfusion, it is necessary to know the equilibrium partition coefficient for water concentration in blood versus tissue and the relevant T1 values for blood and tissue. The former can be taken from the literature, and the latter can be measured, although care must be taken that the correct T1 is being measured (14). The huge attractions of these methods of arterial spin labeling are that they require no exogenous contrast agent and they offer a way of obtaining quantitative perfusion values.

Since the original proposal by Williams et al (13), two complementary variants of the technique with arterial spin labeling have already evolved. First, the technique with continuous arterial spin labeling as originally described by Williams et al (in which arterial spins are continuously labeled and a steady-state condition is measured) has been supplemented with various schemes that compensate for imperfections in the quantitative measurement of perfusion. These include correction for unwanted effects of magnetization transfer contrast (13,15), suppression of macrovascular effects (16,17), and accurate estimates of the degree of arterial inversion (18). Second, a series of techniques with pulsed arterial spin labeling have been proposed that enable observation of the dynamic response to a transiently inverted arterial spin population (19–22). Although the latter are more difficult than the former to make quantitative, they do not require correction for unwanted effects of magnetization transfer contrast. They may also prove to be more useful at higher static magnetic field strengths, in which radio-frequency pulses must be limited to minimize energy deposition in the tissue.

The effect of magnetization transfer contrast has been a particular impediment to techniques with continuous arterial spin labeling, because thus far it has restricted their application to single-section protocols. This is because, to date, the compensation for magnetization transfer contrast has been an additional image in which the control radio-frequency "labeling" pulse is applied symmetrically distal to the section of interest. This second image causes no arterial labeling but mirrors the effects of magnetization transfer contrast. By making the control label symmetrically distal to the section, the large effect of magnetization transfer contrast of the continuous labeling pulse (typically 15% or more signal change) could be corrected to reveal the much smaller perfusion effect (1%–2%).

In this issue of *Radiology,* Alsop and Detre (23) present a solution to the single-section limitations by obtaining multiple sections in an experiment with continuous arterial spin labeling. With an entire, quantitative brain perfusion study obtained totally noninvasively in 10–15 minutes, perfusion measurements with arterial spin labeling are close to being a practical clinical reality. Clearly, a short examination time is desirable not only from the point of view of patient care (and cost) but also because all the perfusion MR techniques require correction for image misregistration problems if the examination time is long.

So much for the MR methods: What are the potential applications and current limitations?

Perfusion imaging has many potential clinical applications. Oxygen-15 positron emission tomography (PET) is probably the current standard of reference for measuring this parameter, followed by single photon emission computed tomography (SPECT) (for qualitative assessments) or xenon-enhanced CT. A major advantage of the new MR imaging methods over these established methods is that MR imaging can be performed without a contrast agent (and never requires use of a potentially damaging, complicated, and expensive ionizing radioisotope agent). MR imaging also enables the gathering of anatomic and functional information in the same study and a higher spatial resolution than either PET or SPECT. Finally, of course, MR technology is more widely available than either PET or SPECT technology and is usually well integrated into the clinical (vs research) environment. Various applications of perfusion MR imaging have already been described in the literature, including contrast agent (24) and preliminary spin labeling (25,26) studies in the heart; spin labeling studies in the renal system (27); and various studies in the brain, including stroke (28) and degenerative disorders such as Alzheimer disease (29).

An obvious application of quantitative perfusion MR imaging is the measurement of perfusion after stroke and assessment of the risk of early extension of the infarct, although it remains to be defined if such measurement is of practical prognostic use (30). In rat brain, studies have found that rates of perfusion to gray matter below approximately 15 mL/100 g/min indicate irreversible infarction (31) and perfusion rates below normal ranges would suggest tissue at risk of infarction. Findings in preliminary human studies suggest that similar thresholds may be defined in humans (32). A methodologic problem in the full realization of quantitative perfusion MR imaging of stroke, at least in regard to the techniques with arterial spin labeling, is that the transit time from the labeling volume to the section of interest can exceed the T1 relaxation time of the water spins considerably at low flow. Water T1 times in blood and tissue are on the order of 1 second, and the water spins must reach the tissue within approximately three or four T1 times for an effect to be detected. This transit time problem presents a challenge to MR physicists that must be solved before perfusion MR imaging with arterial spin labeling can find widespread application to stroke. Transit time can also cause problems in distinguishing adequate collateral flow from low flow (or no flow), since the "half life" of the tagging is so short. A combination of bolus tracking techniques (to obtain a map of time to peak effect) and methods of arterial spin labeling may help when characterizing forms of stroke and cerebrovascular disease.

Looking to the future, the fact that quantification is possible with arterial spin labeling techniques makes them useful in cases in which absolute perfusion values or absolute perfusion differences are required. For instance, pharmacologic stress tests in the heart with adenosine or dobutamine, or in the brain with acetazolamide, may yield information about perfusion reserve and could help in the early diagnosis of vascular disease (33). Certainly, perfusion MR imaging would lend itself to the development and monitoring of psychoactive drug treatments, and, in general, any longitudinal study that requires absolute quantification at each time point would benefit from techniques with arterial spin labeling. MR imaging with arterial spin labeling could also prove an important tool for investigating the presence and severity of perfusion deficits in hypoxic neonates, the question of whether perfusion abnormalities contribute to migraine, and a host of other ailments that are, or may be, related to perfusion.

Finally, there is increasing interest in the use of MR imaging in mapping flow and blood oxygenation changes for "activation" studies. Though quantitative perfusion measurements would not necessarily be needed to map brain function (eg, for presurgical mapping), the additional information obtained by mapping perfusion changes could enhance the evaluation of activation results, for example, by disentangling the effects of abnormal flow and abnormal neural firing on the activation signal. Comparisons of quantitative perfusion MR imaging measurements with PET results have shown that the data obtained are equivalent (34). Interest is also being shown in quantification of MR imaging blood oxygenation measurements (35). This presents the exciting possibility of being able to measure not only perfusion but also metabolic parameters, such as oxygen extraction fraction or the rate of oxygen consumption. Methods are also being developed that would enable the perfusion territory from a single arterial source to be examined, which may be of particular relevance in the characterization of border zone infarcts. These extensions could give MR imaging outstanding power in moving beyond anatomic and pathologic diagnosis to true functional mapping.

In summary, while it is probably premature to consider perfusion MR measurements as being wholly ready for widespread diagnostic use, they clearly now stand on the threshold of clinical applicability. The recently developed methods of arterial spin labeling for perfusion measurement offer the simplest and yet most powerful approach to perfusion MR mapping. Their immediate use in research and drug development is now possible.

Acknowledgments: I thank the scientists and clinicians at several sites who gave invaluable input into this editorial. In particular, I thank Alan C. McLaughlin, PhD, of the National Institutes of Health and Alex de Crespigny, PhD, of Stanford University for helpful discussions.

References

1. Villringer A, Rosen BR, Belliveau JW, et al. Dynamic imaging with lanthanide chelates in normal brain: contrast due to magnetic susceptibility effects. Magn Reson Med 1988; 6:164–174.
2. Strich G, Hagan PL, Gerber KH, Slutsky RA. Tissue distribution and magnetic resonance spin lattice relaxation effects of gadolinium-DTPA. Radiology 1985; 154: 723–726.
3. Fisel CR, Ackerman JL, Buxton RB, et al. MR contrast due to microscopically heterogeneous magnetic susceptibility: numerical simulations and applications to cerebral physiology. Magn Reson Med 1991; 17:336–347.
4. Rosen BR, Belliveau JW, Aronen HJ, et al. Susceptibility contrast imaging of cerebral blood volume: human experience. Magn Reson Med 1991; 22:293–299.
5. Axel L. Tissue mean transit time from dynamic computed tomography by a simple deconvolution technique. Invest Radiol 1983; 18:94–99.
6. Weisskoff RM, Chesler D, Boxerman JL, Rosen BR. Pitfalls in MR measurement of tissue blood flow with intravascular tracers: which mean transit time? Magn Reson Med 1993; 29:553–558.
7. Perman WH, Gado MH, Larson KB, Perlmutter JS. Simultaneous MR acquisition of arterial and brain signal-time curves. Magn Reson Med 1992; 28:74–83.
8. Remp KA, Brix G, Wenz F, Becker CR, Gückel F, Lorenz WJ. Quantification of regional cerebral blood flow and volume with dynamic susceptibility contrast-enhanced MR imaging. Radiology 1994; 193: 637–641.
9. Zierler KL. Theoretical basis of indicator-dilution methods for measuring flow and volume. Circ Res 1965; 16:393–407.
10. Ostergaard L, Sorensen AG, Kwong KK, Weisskoff RM, Gyldensted C, Rosen BR. High resolution measurement of cerebral blood flow using intravascular tracer bolus passages. II. Experimental comparison and preliminary results. Magn Reson Med 1996; 36:726–736.
11. LeBihan D, Breton E, Lallemand D, Grenier P, Cabanis EA, Laval-Jeantet M. MR imaging of intravoxel incoherent motions: application to diffusion and perfusion in neurologic disorders. Radiology 1986; 161:401–407.
12. LeBihan D, Breton E, Lallemand D, Aubin ML, Vignaud J, Laval-Jeantet M. Separation of diffusion and perfusion in intravoxel incoherent motion (IVIM) MR imaging. Radiology 1988; 168:497–505.
13. Williams DS, Detre JA, Leigh JS, Koretsky AP. Magnetic resonance imaging of perfusion using spin inversion of arterial water. Proc Natl Acad Sci USA 1992; 89:212–216.
14. McLaughlin AC, Ye FQ, Pekar JJ, Santha AKS, Frank JA. Effect of magnetization transfer on the measurement of cerebral blood flow using steady-state arterial spin tagging approaches: a theoretical investigation. Magn Reson Med 1997; 37:501–510.
15. Pekar J, Jezzard P, Roberts DA, Leigh JS Jr, Frank JA, McLaughlin AC. Perfusion imaging with compensation for asymmetric magnetization transfer effects. Magn Reson Med 1996; 35:70–79.
16. Alsop DC, Detre JA. Reduced transit-time sensitivity in noninvasive magnetic resonance imaging of human cerebral blood flow. J Cereb Blood Flow Metab 1996; 16:1236–1249.
17. Ye FQ, Mattay VS, Jezzard P, Frank JA, Weinberger DR, McLaughlin AC. Correction for vascular artifacts in cerebral blood flow values measured by using arterial spin tagging techniques. Magn Reson Med 1997; 37:226–235.
18. Maccotta L, Detre JA, Alsop DC. The efficiency of adiabatic inversion for perfusion imaging by arterial spin labeling. NMR Biomed 1997; 10:216–221.
19. Kwong KK, Belliveau JW, Chesler DA, et al. Dynamic magnetic resonance imaging of human brain activity during primary sensory stimulation. Proc Natl Acad Sci USA 1992; 89:5675–5679.
20. Kim SG. Quantification of relative cerebral blood flow change by flow-sensitive alternating inversion recovery (FAIR) technique: application to functional mapping. Magn Reson Med 1995; 34:293–301.
21. Edelman RR, Siewert B, Darby DG, et al. Qualitative mapping of cerebral blood flow and functional localization with echo-planar MR imaging and signal targeting with alternating radio frequency. Radiology 1994; 192:513–520.
22. Wong EC, Buxton RB, Frank LR. Implementation of quantitative perfusion imaging techniques for functional brain mapping using pulsed arterial spin labeling. NMR Biomed 1997; 10:237–249.
23. Alsop DC, Detre JA. Multisection cerebral blood flow MR imaging with continuous arterial spin labeling. Radiology 1998; 208: 410–416.
24. Atkinson DJ, Burstein D, Edelman RR. First-pass cardiac perfusion: evaluation with ultrafast MR imaging. Radiology 1990; 174:757–762.
25. Williams DS, Grandis DJ, Zhang W, Koretsky AP. Magnetic resonance imaging of perfusion in the isolated rat heart using

steady-state spin inversion of arterial water. Magn Reson Med 1993; 30:361–365.
26. Reeder SB, Atalay MK, McVeigh ER, Zerhouni EA, Forder JR. Quantitative cardiac perfusion: a noninvasive spin-labeling method that exploits coronary vessel geometry. Radiology 1996; 200:177–184.
27. Roberts DA, Detre JA, Bolinger L, et al. Renal perfusion in humans: MR imaging with spin tagging of arterial water. Radiology 1995; 196:281–286.
28. Warach S, Dashe JF, Edelman RR. Clinical outcome in ischemic stroke predicted by early diffusion-weighted and perfusion magnetic resonance imaging: a preliminary analysis. J Cereb Blood Flow Metab 1996; 16:53–59.
29. Alsop DC, Grossman M, Detre JA. Quantitative multi-slice perfusion imaging of patients diagnosed with Alzheimer's of frontal dementia (abstr). In: Proceedings of the Sixth Meeting of the International Society for Magnetic Resonance in Medicine. Berkeley, Calif: International Society for Magnetic Resonance in Medicine, 1998; 3:1587.
30. Powers WJ, Zivin J. Magnetic resonance imaging in acute stroke: not ready for prime time. Neurology 1998; 50:842–843.
31. Heiss WD, Rosner G. Functional recovery of cortical neurons as related to degree and duration of ischemia. Ann Neurol 1983; 14:294–301.
32. Heiss WD, Grond M, Thiel A, et al. The critical residual flow level for successful thrombolytic therapy (abstr). J Cereb Blood Flow Metab 1997; 17(suppl):S109.
33. Samuels OB, Detre JA, Alsop DC, Kasner SE, Teener JW, Raps EC. Evaluation of focal perfusion defects due to symptomatic middle cerebral artery stenosis using arterial spin labeling perfusion magnetic resonance imaging (abstr). Neurology 1998; 50(suppl):A77.
34. Ye FQ, Berman KF, Ellmore T, et al. $H_2{}^{15}O$ PET validation of arterial spin tagging measurements of cerebral blood flow in humans (abstr). In: Proceedings of the Fifth Meeting of the International Society for Magnetic Resonance in Medicine. Berkeley, Calif: International Society for Magnetic Resonance in Medicine, 1997; 1:87.
35. van Zijl PC, Eleff SM, Ulatowski JA, et al. Quantitative assessment of blood flow, blood volume and blood oxygenation effects in functional magnetic resonance imaging. Nature Med 1998; 4:159–167.

Special Communication

David B. Fraser, MD
President, Radiological Society of North America

The Radiological Society of North America 84th Scientific Assembly and Annual Meeting Sunday, November 29 to Friday, December 4, 1998 McCormick Place, Chicago, Illinois

Even after 83 years of experience, careful planning, and continuous improvement, the RSNA Scientific Assembly and Annual Meeting somehow still manages to improve each year. With the grand opening of the McCormick Place South Building in Chicago last year, it seems hard to believe that even more changes and improvements are in store for RSNA '98 attendees—but they are.

The theme of the 84th Annual Meeting is "Science to Practice." This theme reflects the interdependent relationship between science and practice. Just as science influences practice, the practice of radiology has a great impact on science. This close relationship will be more apparent this year as, for the first time, all of the exhibits will be presented on the same level (third) of the McCormick Place complex, allowing attendees to walk with ease from the "science" to the "practice" portions of the meeting.

Index term:
Radiological Society of North America, 84th scientific assembly and annual meeting

Radiology 1998; 208:300–302

In accordance with the bylaws of the Radiological Society of North America (section 6.12), the Board of Directors has appointed a Committee on Nominations. In 1998, the Committee on Nominations consists of Seymour H. Levitt, MD, Chairman, Minneapolis, MN; Michael A. Sullivan, MD, New Orleans, LA; and Ritsuko U. Komaki, MD, Houston, TX. Suggestions for nominations should be addressed to the Chairman.

Also new this year is a special section located in the Lakeside Center (formerly the East Building) near the *info*RAD area where leaders in the radiology equipment industry have reserved classroom space to conduct classes on their respective proprietary computer systems. The new section, **Hands-on Computer Workshops: Basic Training for Radiologists**, allows participating technical exhibitors to schedule sessions throughout the week to teach new and existing customers about the intricacies of their software programs and to provide training on software upgrades.

Besides all of the learning that takes place, the Annual Meeting also offers attendees a great networking opportunity and a chance to catch up with colleagues and friends from around the world.

The hallmarks of the RSNA Annual Meeting remain science and education. The exchange of scientific information is the most important reason radiology professionals from around the world regard the RSNA Annual Meeting as the No. 1 educational event in the field. Ultimately, it is the quality of the content of our meeting that draws such a large, varied, and influential group.

Again this year, we predict an excellent RSNA Annual Meeting. More than 27,000 of your peers will attend, ready to take advantage of the more than 1,700 scientific papers, 275 refresher courses, 1,000 scientific and *info*RAD exhibits, and 700 technical exhibits, in addition to the many demonstrations, workshops, and symposia.

The **Opening Session**, beginning at 8:30 AM on Sunday, November 29, will feature "Cardiac Imaging," moderated by Theresa C. McLoud, MD. That presentation will be preceded by my **President's Address.**

On Sunday afternoon, beginning at 3:30, O. Wayne Houser, MD, chairman of the Board of Trustees of the **RSNA Research and Education Fund**, will announce the RSNA Roentgen Centennial Fellow for 1999 and present other Fund news. Dr Houser's announcements will be followed by the always well-received **Sunday Image Interpretation Session**, moderated this year by James G. Smirniotopoulos, MD.

On Monday afternoon, beginning at 1:00, RSNA recognizes the contributions three individuals have made to radiology by awarding them **Honorary Membership** in the Society. Guozhen Li, MD, of Beijing, China; Roberto Passariello, MD, of Rome, Italy; and Ad E. Van Voorthuisen, MD, of Leiden, The Netherlands are being honored this year. After that presentation, C. Carl Jaffe, MD, will give the **Eugene P. Pendergrass New Horizons Lecture** on "Imaging and Information in the 21st Century."

The excitement continues on Tuesday with the 1:00 PM plenary session, which opens with the presentation of **RSNA Gold Medals** to Thomas S. Harle, MD, of Winston-Salem, NC; Eugene C. Klatte, MD, of Sun City, Ariz; and Carl J. Zylak, MD, of Detroit, Mich. The Gold Medal

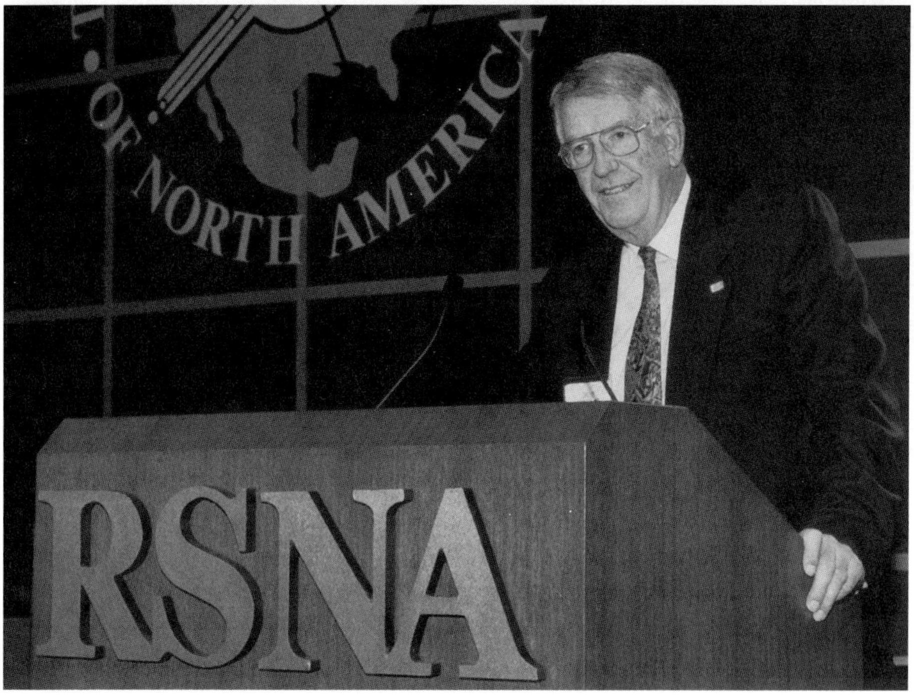

David B. Fraser, MD, President

ceremony will be followed by the **Annual Oration in Diagnostic Radiology**, featuring Giles W. Stevenson, MD, lecturing on "Colorectal Cancer: A Challenge for All Aspects of Medical Imaging."

Eight **Special Focus Sessions** will be presented at 4:00 PM on Tuesday, and another six will be presented at 4:15 PM on Thursday. Topics for the Tuesday sessions include "Child Abuse Revisited," moderated by Paul K. Kleinman, MD; "Breast Imaging: The MQSA Final Regulations—What You Should Do in the Next 5 Months," moderated by Lawrence W. Bassett, MD; "Gene Therapy: Opportunities for Radiology," moderated by Thomas J. Brady, MD, and Elias A. Zerhouni, MD; "Colorectal Cancer Screening: If We Build It, Will They Come?" moderated by David J. Vining, MD; "Prostate Imaging: How, What, Where, and When?" moderated by Matthew D. Rifkin, MD; "The Transition to an Outcomes-based Accreditation Process," moderated by Dennis S. O'Leary, MD; "Vascular Stents: Current Concepts and Controversies," moderated by Curtis W. Bakal, MD, PhD; and "Functional MR Imaging in Stroke," moderated by Bruce R. Rosen, MD, PhD.

The Wednesday afternoon plenary session begins at 1:00 with the announcement of the **Scientific Exhibit Awards**. After that presentation, J. Frank Wilson, MD, will give the **Annual Oration in Radiation Oncology** on "From Basic Discovery toward an Image-guided Methodology: One Hundred Years of Progress in Brachytherapy." At 4:00 PM Wednesday, Edward G. Shaw, MD, will moderate the **Oncodiagnosis Panel**, which will look at the "Central Nervous System."

The **RSNA/AAPM Symposium** is scheduled for Thursday afternoon and will focus on "Diffusion-Perfusion MR." The session will be moderated by Gary H. Glover, PhD, and will follow the 1:00 PM inauguration of the 1999 RSNA Board of Directors and introduction of 1998 AAPM officers and council chairs.

The second group of Special Focus Sessions begins at 4:15 PM on Thursday. The topics being presented are "You, Your Business, and Ethics: The Intersection of Business and Professional Ethics," moderated by Douglass F. Adams, MD; "Radiology of the Acute Abdomen: Old Problems, New Insights," moderated by Stephen R. Baker, MD; "Imaging Pulmonary Emboli: Is There a Choice?" moderated by Alexander Gottschalk, MD; "Osteoporosis: Controversies in Bone Densitometry—Techniques and Interpretation," moderated by Judith E. Adams, MD; "Ischemia and Infarction from Head to Toe," moderated by Melissa L. Rosado de Christenson, MD; and "Radiation Oncology in Pancreatic Cancer," moderated by Nora A. Janjan, MD.

On December 4, the final plenary session of the 1998 meeting, the **Friday Imaging Symposium**, is set to begin at 12:30 PM. The symposium will focus on "Acute Radiology—Where Minutes Count" and will be moderated by Frederick A. Mann, MD.

An integral part of the meeting is the **Refresher Course Program**, which is conducted throughout the week. RSNA '98 will feature over 275 courses, including 32 limited-attendance workshops. Two Categorical Courses and four Update Courses will be included in the Refresher Course program. The **Categorical Course in Diagnostic Radiology** will focus on vascular imaging and is being directed by Ernest J. Ferris, MD, Elliot R. Fishman, MD, Joseph F. Polak, MD, E. J. Potchen, MD, and Arthur C. Waltman, MD. The **Categorical Course in Physics** will feature cardiac catheterization imaging and will be directed by Edward L. Nickoloff, DSc, and Keith J. Strauss, MS. The **Update Courses** this year are "Technical Aspects of Breast Imaging," "Computers," "Brachytherapy Physics," and "The Basic Physics of MR Imaging." Syllabi will be available for purchase at the meeting for both of the Categorical Courses. In addition, a CD-ROM version of the syllabus for the vascular imaging course will be available for purchase and will offer CME credit.

Immediately before the official opening of the RSNA Scientific Assembly and Annual Meeting, the Associated Sciences Consortium will conduct its **Associated Sciences Workshop**, beginning at 10:15 AM on Saturday, November 28. The theme of the workshop will be "Integrating Science into Practice," and the keynote speaker will be Heinz U. Lemke, PhD.

Three joint AAPM/RSNA physics presentations are also being offered Saturday afternoon. The **AAPM/RSNA Physics Tutorial for Residents**, discussing "Basic Radiation Safety and Protection," was organized by Mark S. Rzeszotarski, PhD, and James G. Kereiakes, PhD, and will be held from 1:00 to 5:00 PM. The **AAPM/RSNA Tutorial on Equipment Selection**, featuring "Radiography and Fluoroscopy," was organized by Joel E. Gray, PhD, and Beth A. Schueler, PhD, and will be held from 2:00 to 5:00 PM. And, the **AAPM/RSNA Basic Physics Lecture for the Radiologic Technologist**, on "Vascular Imaging Physics," was organized by Gerald A. White, Jr, MS, and will be held from 3:00 to 4:30 PM.

The scientific assembly of the RSNA continues to grow and be successful because of the dedication and hard work of more than 2,000 volunteer committee members. I especially thank the Program

Committee, directed by Theresa C. McLoud, MD; the Refresher Course Committee, guided by Glenn S. Forbes, MD; the Scientific Exhibits Committee, chaired by Steven K. Teplick, MD; the Technical Exhibits Committee, headed by Alan E. Oestrich, MD; the Audiovisual Services Committee, directed by Susan A. Stafford, MD; and the Associated Sciences Committee, led by Samuel L. Hissong, MD.

The Program Subcommittee chairs are responsible for selecting the papers and organizing the sessions in their respective disciplines. The quantity of work they take on and the quality of the result are nothing short of amazing. The Subcommittee chairs are Robert M. Miller, MD, Cardiovascular Radiology; Lawrence R. Goodman, MD, Chest Radiology; Pablo R. Ros, MD, Gastrointestinal Radiology; Carl J. D'Orsi, MD; General Radiology/ Breast Imaging; Stanford M. Goldman, MD, Genitourinary Radiology; Mark D. Murphey, MD, Musculoskeletal Radiology; Allan J. Fox, MD, Neuroradiology/ Head and Neck Radiology; Gary L. Dillehay, MD, Nuclear Medicine; Joanna J. Seibert, MD, Pediatric Radiology; Stephen J. Riederer, PhD, Physics; Nora A. Janjan, MD, Radiation Oncology and Radiobiology; and Christopher B. Merritt, MD, Ultrasound. I give my many thanks to each subcommittee chair and member.

I look forward to seeing you at this year's Annual Meeting. The excitement and exchange of knowledge that will fill McCormick Place this year could not exist without your contribution.

Please join us in 1998.

Elizabeth H. Moore, MD

Index terms:
Biopsies, complications, 60.126
Lung, biopsy, 60.126
Radiology and radiologists, How I Do It

Radiology 1998; 208:303–318

Abbreviation:
AIDS = acquired immunodeficiency syndrome

[1] From the Department of Radiology, University of California, Davis Medical Center, 2516 Stockton Blvd, Sacramento, CA 95817. Received October 3, 1997; revision requested November 25; revision received March 3, 1998; accepted April 3. **Address reprint requests to** the author.

Technical Aspects of Needle Aspiration Lung Biopsy: A Personal Perspective[1]

Needle aspiration lung biopsy is a procedure often approached with trepidation. Even experienced operators vary substantially in both rates of retrieval of diagnostic specimens and rates of complication. Unfortunately, many aspects of lung biopsy have not been subjected to large controlled trials due to the length of time necessary to accumulate a large series, the difficulty of separating interrelated aspects of the procedure, and, from a personal perspective, ethical considerations related to depriving a control group of what is standard procedure at a particular institution.

The techniques included in this article form a unified approach to lung biopsy, directed toward the pragmatic goals of maximizing specimen retrieval and minimizing complications. They represent personal choices evolved from many years of clinical practice, observations from an in vitro model of lung biopsy, studies reported in the literature, and discussions with valued colleagues. Certain aspects may be viewed as controversial by some.

PREPARATION

Lung biopsy should be limited to cases that are both truly indicated and technically feasible and to those in which the possible benefits outweigh the risks. Results should potentially change the therapy or surgical approach; rarely, patient insistence may be an indication. Considerations include an assessment of the likelihood of a serious complication, the probability of successful needle placement, the likelihood of obtaining a diagnostic specimen, and the extent to which identification of the disease process is expected to affect management.

Review of the patient's computed tomographic (CT) scan and medical history is crucial. Information gained may influence the technical aspects of the procedure. For example, a CT scan that shows emphysema might lead to the use of a saline and lidocaine paraspinal infiltration to produce an extrapleural pathway to a mediastinal mass; however, the same approach in a patient with normal lungs but severe coronary artery disease might be unwise because of potential vagal stimulation.

The risk of a pneumothorax is heightened by the presence of emphysema or obstructive pulmonary disease (1–4). The unavoidable direct puncture of a superficial bulla will result in the rapid development of a pneumothorax in the majority of cases (4). There may be higher rates of biopsy-induced of pneumothorax in patients with acquired immunodeficiency syndrome (AIDS) (5). Patients with one lung can undergo biopsy successfully, but, as in any extremely high-risk patient, it is advisable to prepare the skin for drainage of a pneumothorax before the procedure and have the assembled drainage system and all necessary connectors on the table and ready for use.

The risk of pulmonary hemorrhage is heightened by abnormal clotting factors, factors that affect platelet function (thrombocytopenia, chronic renal failure, aspirin use), biopsy of inherently vascular lesions (chronic inflammatory cavities likely to have enlarged bronchial arterial vessels in the wall, carcinoid tumors, vascular metastases), the use of a cutting biopsy gun, central lesions, and pulmonary hypertension. When biopsy is necessary despite an increased risk of hemorrhage, a single pass into the lesion with a thin-gauge needle is recommended; cutting guns pose a substantial and usually unacceptable risk. Bronchoscopic backup to tamponade a bleeding site and personnel experienced in double-lumen intubation should be placed on standby. Biopsy is not advisable with an abnormal clotting function approaching therapeutic anticoagulation (eg, international normalized ratio greater than 1.3), a platelet count of less than 100,000/mL, or pulmonary hypertension.

Positive pressure ventilation may lead to pneumothorax or may aggravate a bronchove-

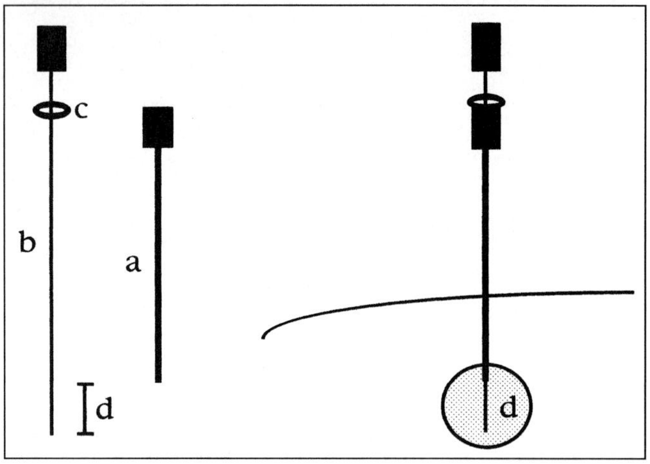

Figure 1. Diagram of outer (*a*) and inner (*b*) needles used in coaxial technique. The plastic ring (*c*) marks the desired depth of insertion of the inner needle into the outer needle and the resultant pass length (*d*). During sampling, the outer needle is placed in the peripheral portion of the nodule, while the inner needle is used to sample the majority of available nodule without extending into normal lung deep to the nodule.

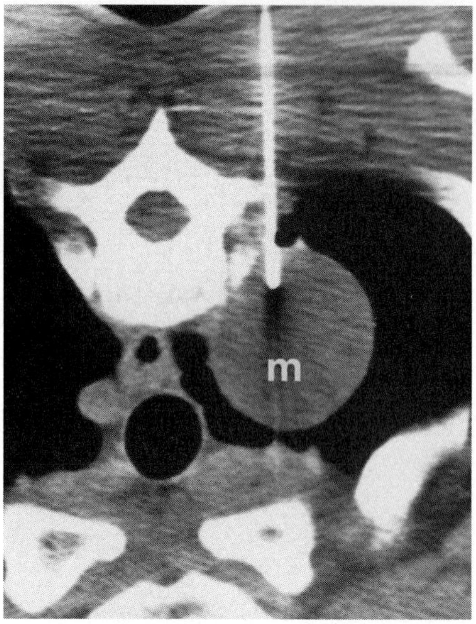

Figure 2. CT scan shows sampling of a well-circumscribed apical extrapleural mass (*m*) is accomplished with an extrapleural paraspinal approach. Because a neurogenic tumor was suspected, a detachable coaxial cutting gun was used. Initial aspirates obtained through the outer needle of the gun yielded no tissue, but core specimens enabled a diagnosis of schwannoma.

nous fistula and lead to air embolism. An uncooperative patient is at risk for a variety of complications, the most serious being air embolism due to inspiration when the needle is open to air should its tip be in a pulmonary vein. These conditions are therefore contraindications.

Most other contraindications to lung biopsy are relative; risk factors must be weighed against the dangers of alternative procedures and the risks of failing to promptly diagnose a pulmonary process. Rather than refuse to perform the procedure in higher-risk patients, the operator should tailor it to maximize the safety for each particular patient while anticipating and preparing for likely complications.

All patients should be outfitted with an electrocardiographic monitor, a blood pressure monitor, and an oxygen saturation monitor. I prefer to have a working intravenous line in all patients because of the rare (although occasionally dramatic) occurrence of vasovagal episodes, because any needed sedation or medications can be given immediately and without interrupting the procedure or moving the patient, and because lung biopsy patients often have serious coexistent medial problems such as heart disease. Oxygen, suction equipment, oral and nasal airways, an Ambu bag (Ambu International, Glostrup, Denmark), equipment for needle or catheter aspiration of a pneumothorax, small- and large-bore chest tubes, Pleur Evac materials (Atrium Medical, Hudson, NH), and appropriate connectors and tubing should be in the biopsy room. A resuscitation cart should be immediately available. Every physician performing needle aspiration lung biopsy should be able to place a small-bore chest tube quickly and reliably and should be familiar with the treatment for a severe vasovagal episode, marked hemoptysis, and air embolism.

THE PATIENT AS A BIOPSY PARTNER

It is important to spend time explaining the biopsy technique to the patient, emphasizing the patient's own role in a quick and successful procedure. Breathing instructions should be explained and practiced, and the potentially serious consequences of failure to follow instructions should be spelled out in lay terms. Phrases such as "tearing the skin of the lung causing air to leak out" and "sucking air into the bloodstream that could go to the head or the heart and cause stroke or a heart attack" can be well understood by most adults. Other aspects of the informed consent session with the patient should include a realistic assessment of the likelihood of pneumothorax, chest tube placement, and hemoptysis based on the performance statistics of the operator, smoking history of the patient, and any other special risk factors applicable to the patient. Preventive measures that will be used should be explained (eg, puncture-site-down positioning after the biopsy, placement of an occlusive blood patch at the puncture site), and the planned management of common complications should be addressed. If the patient is considered at extreme risk for a particular complication, a warning of the likely occurrence of that complication and the specific aspects of treatment will help the patient remain calm and able to cooperate regardless of the outcome.

Patient comfort is crucial for maintaining a designated position, which, in turn, is crucial for accurate needle placement. Supine patients are more comfortable with their arms at their sides, if possible, and with a wedge under their knees. Prone patients are most comfortable with their arms folded under their head and the head turned to one side. If it is necessary to move the scapula laterally for access, that arm may be placed at the patient's side, with the shoulder dropped forward. Decubitus positions are used only if absolutely needed because the patients tend to drift out of the chosen position over time, even if the hips and knees are bent for stability. Abundant pillows, blankets and wedges, and straps to rest the arms against if they are held medially will help the patient remain comfortable and motionless throughout the procedure.

In general, with use of adequate local anesthetics, lung biopsy is not a particularly painful procedure within the spec-

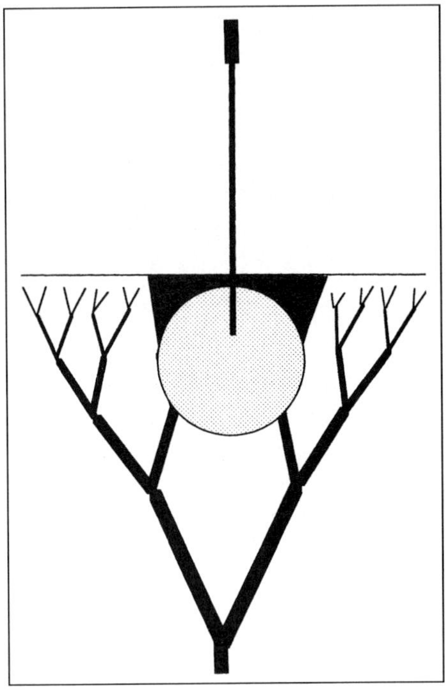

Figure 3. Diagram of bronchial structures in the region of a peripheral nodule. Theoretically, the bronchial air supply directly peripheral to a large lesion will be obstructed by the mass itself, and thus the shaded area will be collaterally ventilated. Massive air leakage from a pleural puncture in this region would be unlikely.

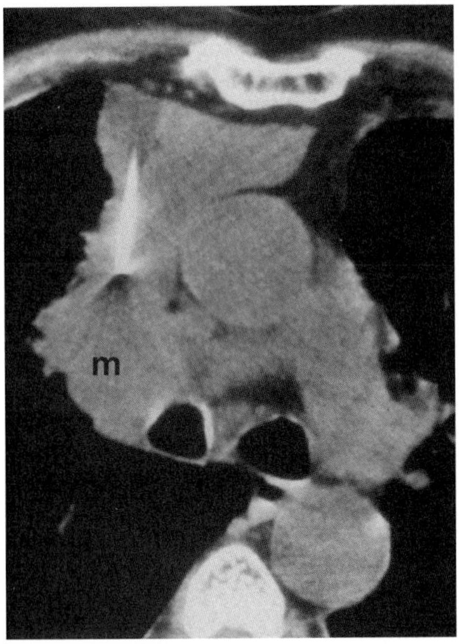

Figure 5. CT scan shows a biopsy of an obstructing hilar mass (*m*), diagnosed as small cell carcinoma, performed via collapsed portions of the right upper lobe.

trum of interventional radiologic procedures. Unlike many other procedures,

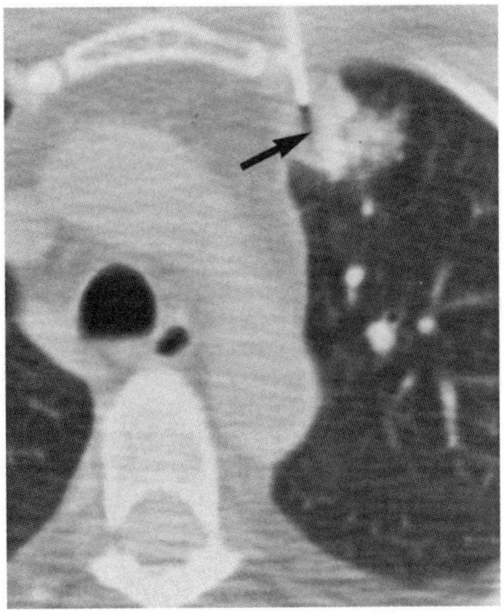

Figure 4. CT-guided direct puncture into this non–small cell carcinoma abutting the pleura (arrow) precludes the development of a pneumothorax.

lung biopsy requires the active participation of the patient. An unclouded sensorium will help the patient remain attentive during the procedure and reproduce the designated respiration more reliably. After the procedure, an alert patient will be in a better position to report any symptoms that may occur. I start the procedure without sedation or pain medication, advising the patient that it can be given if necessary. Most patients do not request it or require it, either for pain or anxiety, but there are certainly exceptions.

IMAGING MODALITY SELECTION

For a patient with normal lung parenchyma on a diagnostic CT scan and a lesion well visualized in two fluoroscopic projections, fluoroscopic guidance offers many advantages. It is faster, taking as little as 15 minutes; room time may be less costly. The operator can easily visualize ribs and adjust for patient movement if it occurs. If necessary, the needle may be advanced under direct visualization by holding it with a surgical clamp. Sampling may also be performed under direct visualization by using lateral fluoroscopy with appropriate collimation. The lesion may be "jiggled" with the needle, confirming needle placement. For a small but visible lesion in a less than cooperative patient, fluoroscopic guidance may offer the quickest route to accurate needle placement.

In general, however, I prefer CT guidance, despite longer procedure durations in the range of 30 minutes to 1 hour or more. It offers important advantages, including the opportunity to avoid hazards such as large vessels, fissures, bullae, and even small superficial blebs or areas of air trapping. It is the safest method for biopsy of central, hilar, and mediastinal lesions. Documentation of needle-tip location is best achieved with thin-section CT. Thin sections can also be used to identify and target the most worrisome parts of a mass, avoiding areas of necrosis or adjacent postobstructive pneumonitis. Traditionally, CT-guided procedures have been thought to have a higher complication rate than fluoroscopy-guided procedures; however, it is difficult to eliminate selection bias, since cases in which CT guidance is used are those with more technical difficulty. In my experience, switching for purely logistic reasons from fluoroscopy guidance primarily to CT guidance exclusively led to a slight reduction in the complication rate.

The advent of CT fluoroscopy combines certain advantages of the two techniques (6). Real-time imaging may permit rapid localization of smaller or more disadvantageously located lesions, even in less than cooperative patients. Image quality in the fluoroscopy mode, while inferior to the diagnostic mode, is more than adequate for needle placement, and CT fluoroscopy can be combined with conventional thin-section CT to localize the needle tip precisely if desired.

In certain pleura-based lesions, ultrasound may provide real-time biopsy imaging (7). A linear puncture probe with central channel guidance is preferable to the freehand technique for smaller lesions.

NEEDLE SELECTION

Single versus Coaxial

Currently, most lung biopsies performed in the United States involve use of a single-needle technique (8). In a large but non-necrotic lesion that is likely to be a carcinoma and be diagnosable with a single sampling, this technique saves a few dollars in needle costs. However, a coaxial technique of inserting a thinner sampling needle through a larger needle placed in the lesion (Fig 1) has numerous advantages. I believe these advantages make it preferable in most cases. A primary feature of a complication-reduction

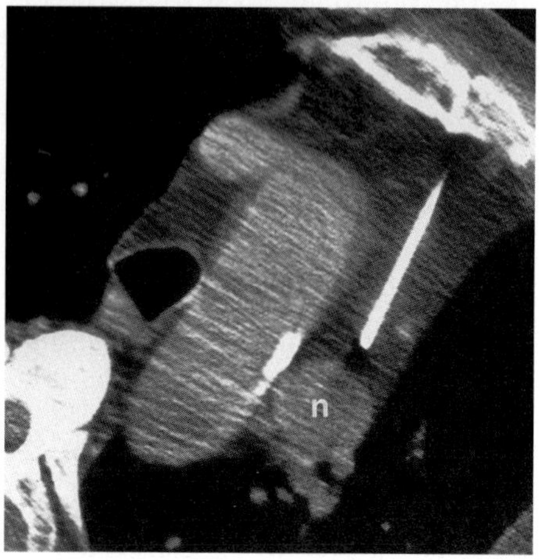

Figure 6. Abundant mediastinal fat allows direct access, with use of CT guidance, to this mediastinal nodal metastasis (*n*) from non–small cell carcinoma.

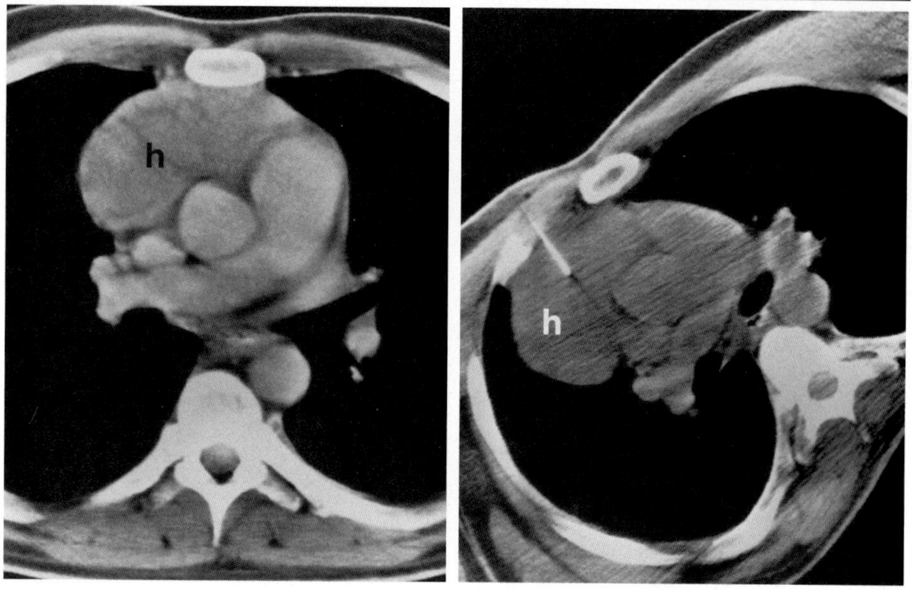

a. b.

Figure 7. CT images show that changing the patient from **(a)** a supine to **(b)** an oblique position makes use of mediastinal mobility to allow direct access to what proved to be a large organizing spontaneous hematoma (*h*) in a patient with hemophilia and AIDS.

program is to limit pleural punctures to one (9). Each puncture site has a unique and reproducible pressure above which air leakage will occur (discussed later). Even in punctures of normal lung, there is substantial variability in these "pop-off" pressures. Performing additional punctures increases the risk that one will leak at a relatively low intrathoracic pressure and cause a pneumothorax. With a coaxial technique, any number of samples can be obtained quickly through the outer needle, without positioning additional needles and without repuncturing the pleura. The depth of the sampling passes can be preplanned with precision. The outer needle is quite stiff, allowing substantial torque to be placed on the needle during manipulation without bending it. This makes redirection easier to achieve. It also allows for the outer needle to be angled during sampling, allowing correction of an imperfect puncture or sampling of various portions of the lesion during a single pass (discussed later). The outer needle usually prevents air leakage from the puncture site during the procedure, and at the end of the procedure it can be used to obtain a large-bore specimen, mark the lesion for thoracoscopic resection, or deliver an occlusive "blood patch."

Certain biopsy techniques should be avoided in the chest. If an outer needle is left in the chest wall and the pleura is coaxially punctured multiple times with needle inserts, high complication rates may result. There is no role in lung biopsy for tandem needle techniques, which also involve unnecessary pleural punctures. Coaxial techniques, in which the hub of the thin needle is removed to allow coaxial placement of a larger needle, offer no advantage over initial puncture with a larger needle, which is easier to manipulate in any case.

In selected cases, I use a single needle. For example, a tiny subpleural nodule in which a perpendicular direct puncture is planned may be approached with direct fluoroscopic visualization by holding the needle with a surgical clamp. After the lesion is transfixed and the needle is passed through it, the patient is allowed to breathe. Then, in a single breath hold and with lateral fluoroscopic guidance, the needle tip is pulled back to the center of the nodule, and the deep half of the nodule is repeatedly aspirated by using a pass length equal to the radius of the lesion. If a transcaval approach or puncture through a brachiocephalic vein cannot be avoided, use of thinner needles may be safer. In lesions known to have hemorrhaged or suspected to be at risk for hemorrhage, a single pass with a thin-gauge needle is used. If coaxial technique is selected in this situation, the outer needle is not placed within the lesion as is usual, but rather it is placed slightly outside the lesion.

Needle Design

Few studies have been performed to compare the pleural damage associated with the great variety of needles developed for lung biopsy. Available information is either in the form of anecdotal reports from colleagues or is from studies performed for other purposes. I know of no studies performed to examine the relative advantages of a single-bevel trocar, a triangular triple-bevel trocar, or a circumferentially tapered trocar similar to a sewing needle for pleural puncture. Similarly, the effects of architectural features of the needle shaft, such as side aspiration or cutting channels, have not been investigated. Any features that may start a linear tear are undesirable. With my colleagues, I have learned from our lung biopsy model that while a simple pinhole withstands a pressure challenge fairly well, any visible tearing of the pleura leads to air leakage at trivial pressures (10).

There is little clinical evidence that needle gauge affects complication rate within the size range of the smaller needles generally used for lung biopsy (11), although this issue has not been widely investigated in clinical practice. Our preliminary laboratory investigations confirm this. However, needles larger than 18 gauge are considered a risk for causing both bleeding and pneumothorax, and their use should be avoided.

Cutting Guns

A cutting gun should be easy to use and should reliably produce a core specimen suitable for histologic evaluation. New coaxial models with a detachable, thin-walled outer guide needle provide both

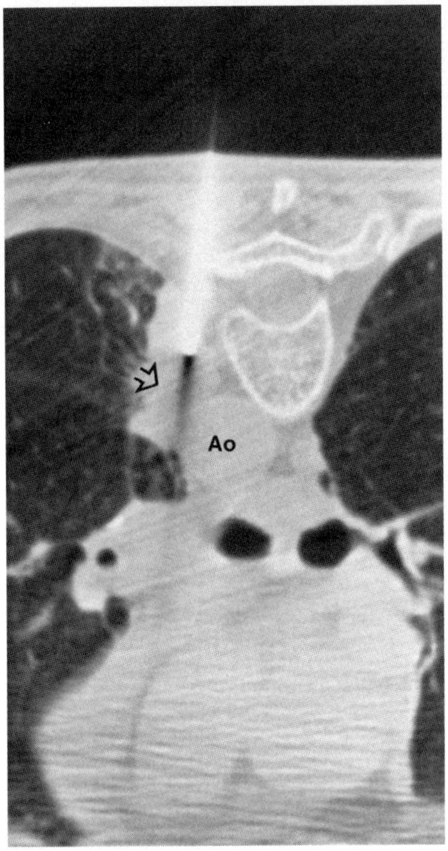

Figure 8. CT guidance facilitates a paraspinal approach and allows direct puncture of this non–small cell carcinoma (arrow) abutting the mediastinal pleura. A short pass length is necessary to avoid damage to the aorta (*Ao*).

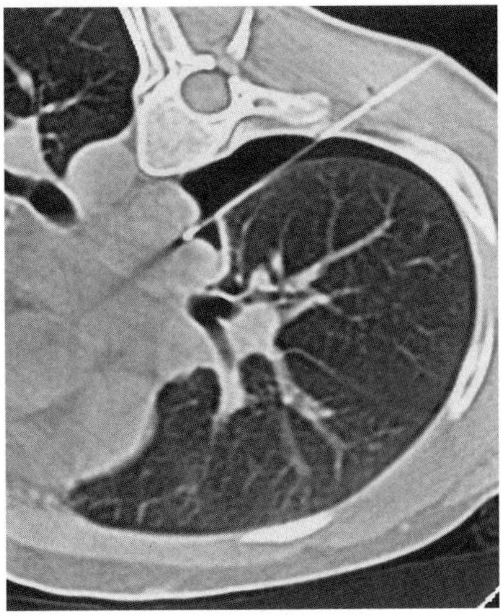

Figure 9. CT scan after instillation of oxygen into the pleural space demonstrates direct access to this subcarinal teratoma, which developed after chemotherapy for seminoma. After the lesion was sampled, the residual gas was aspirated by using the outer coaxial needle.

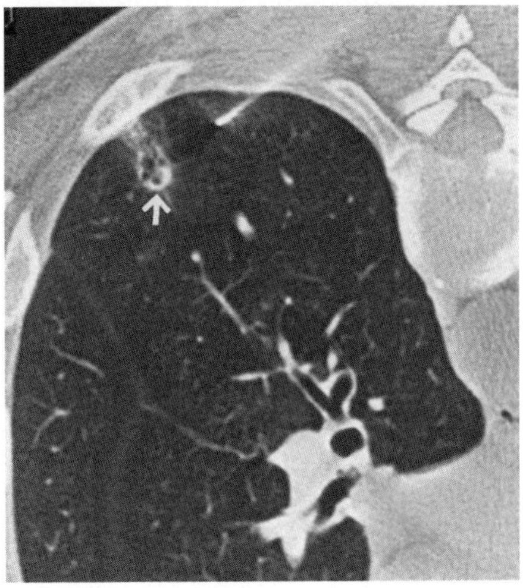

Figure 10. CT image shows a near tangential approach that allows ample distance for course correction, if necessary, before encountering this small, peripheral lung abscess (arrow).

the reliability of a gun and the ability to obtain numerous coaxial core specimens with only one pleural puncture of moderate gauge. A variety of throw lengths, or a variable throw option, is desirable to adapt to different biopsy circumstances, since adjacent normal lung should not be included in the sample. Use of a cutting gun increases risk of hemorrhage and probably also air embolism, but it improves accuracy of diagnosis in benign disease and certain malignancies such as lymphoma (12,13).

On review of the CT scan obtained before biopsy, some opinion is formed whether the lesion is likely to represent a carcinoma, in which case aspiration should be the first biopsy modality used. Guns should be reserved for situations in which a lesion other than carcinoma is suspected, or if aspiration does not produce a definitive diagnosis. In cases unlikely to represent primary or metastatic carcinoma, the outer guide needle from a coaxial cutting gun system can be used as the guide needle for coaxial aspiration, followed if necessary by coaxial core sampling; this offers flexibility yet averts a second pleural puncture (Fig 2).

FEASIBILITY OF THE BIOPSY TARGET: A FUNCTION OF SIZE AND LOCATION

Various principles can be used to predict the feasibility of a biopsy or to select the most suitable target if multiple lesions exist. Size and location should both be considered when assessing a target: A smaller lesion in a favorable location may be preferable to a larger lesion in a less desirable location. As a general rule, most lesions of 1 cm can be sampled for biopsy when they are in all but the most unfavorable locations. Even when innumerable lesions are present, a single nodule should be selected for biopsy; indiscriminate needle passes through the lung are not likely to yield diagnostic results.

The ideal larger target abuts the pleura, which allows direct puncture without traversal of aerated lung. If aerated lung is not violated, a pneumothorax will not occur. A 1-cm pleura-based lesion may be safely directly accessed in the upper lung zones in a cooperative patient because the upper lung zones move little with respiration. However, a 1-cm lesion would be an undesirable target for direct puncture in the lower lung zones because of the high likelihood of respiratory misregistration (in the absence of real-time imaging guidance) at the moment of pleural puncture.

If no pleura-based lesions are available for sampling, a larger, relatively peripheral lesion is preferable; a perpendicular puncture should be directed at the center of the lesion. Theoretically, the lung at the puncture site will be collaterally ventilated because the lesion itself will probably have obstructed the direct bronchial supply to portions of the lung immediately peripheral to the nodule (Fig 3). It is unlikely that substantial air leakage will occur from an area of collaterally ventilated lung. Biopsy of small, deep lesions has long been thought to be associated with an *increased* rate of complication (compared with larger and more peripheral lesions) due to longer procedures with more needle manipulations (14–16). I suspect instead that large peripheral lesions have a relatively *decreased* complication rate because leakage is less likely to occur from a collaterally ventilated puncture site. This possible relationship has never, to my knowledge, been examined, but certainly the data exist to do so.

The ideal location for a small nodule target is neither very peripheral nor central (allowing room for redirection after initial pleural puncture, but avoiding proximity to larger central vessels) and in the upper lung zone (because this part of the lung moves little with respiration). Unfavorably located small lesions are usually difficult to sample. Even with a near tangential approach (see Trajectories Passing through Lung), small subpleural lesions can be very challenging to sample.

Small lesions abutting the heart are unsuitable for biopsy (unless CT fluoroscopy is available) because marked cardiac motion makes accurate placement of the needle tip unreliable. Nodules in the superior portion of the right middle lobe, just under the dome-shaped minor fissure, can be difficult to access, even with an angled gantry. Small lesions deep in the costophrenic sulci are difficult to sample, since the lung moves a great deal and any respiratory misregistration may lead to puncture of the diaphragm or liver. Even when favorably located, lesions smaller than 5–7 mm in diameter are unlikely to yield diagnostic material, although nodules as small as 4 mm have been successfully sampled (17).

When a choice exists and if no fissures will be violated, a posterior approach is favored for several reasons. First, it is associated with a decreased pneumothorax rate (18). The reasons for this are not clear but may relate to the bucket-handle motion of the ribs (and chest wall) during respiration. Second, assuming the patient will be placed in puncture-site-down position after the procedure (see Positional Precautions and Follow-up Imaging) (19–21), it is easier for the patient to be supine rather than prone during initial follow-up. Finally, the prone patient does not have the opportunity to view the needles and other biopsy paraphernalia, thus diminishing apprehension. If the patient cannot be prone either during or after the procedure (eg, because of recent abdominal surgery), a lateral puncture is favored when a choice exists.

Previous thoracotomy substantially reduces the chance of a pneumothorax because the pleurae are usually adherent due to scarring. Thus, in a patient with multiple lesions, the side on which the surgery was performed should be selected for biopsy. The thoracotomy scar itself should be avoided, because it is hard, fibrous tissue that precludes easy needle manipulation.

When a single pulmonary nodule and enlarged nodes are present, diagnosis and staging of a lesion with node biopsy should be given strong consideration, particularly when treatment will be affected. Biopsy of hilar or mediastinal lesions must be preceded by good quality contrast material–enhanced CT to delineate vascular structures. It is imperative to avoid both systemic and pulmonary arteries (because of hemorrhage risk) and pulmonary veins (because of hemorrhage risk and, even more important, possible air embolism). Certain parts of the mediastinum may be inaccessible even with aggressive biopsy techniques. Smaller nodes in the precarinal area or interposed between the trachea and the transverse portion of the aortic arch generally cannot be accessed percutaneously.

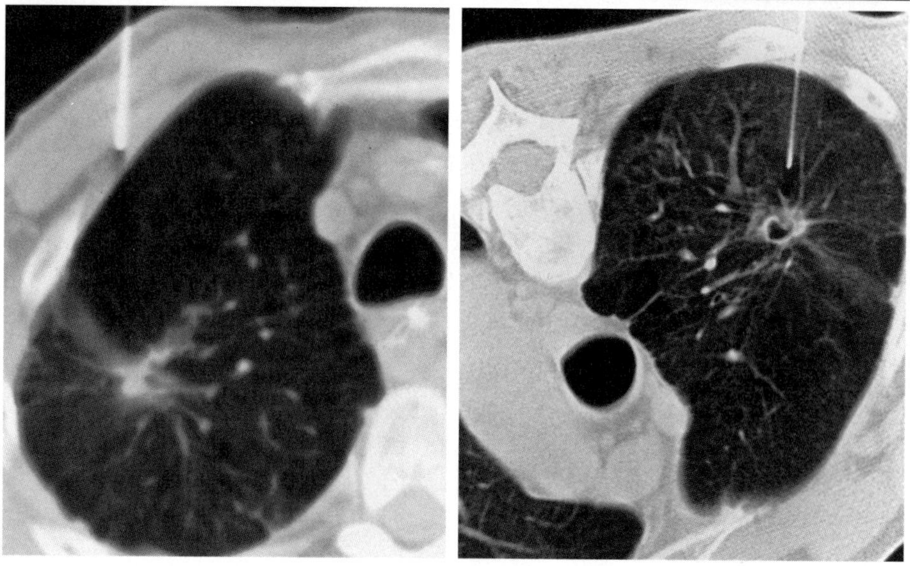

a. b.

Figure 11. **(a)** CT scan of a biopsy attempt. The operator used 10-mm sections. Although the needle has been appropriately brought to a position just outside the parietal pleura before this anterior pleural puncture, the lung in the region of the proposed puncture appears hyperinflated and probably emphysematous, although it is suboptimally visualized. The biopsy attempt resulted in a pneumothorax that required chest tube placement. **(b)** CT scan of repeat biopsy performed at a later date. Biopsy was performed by identifying an area of relatively normal lung with 2-mm sections. The normal grayish appearance of the lung at the posterior puncture site is visible even on this 5-mm needle localization image. No air leakage occurred. The diagnosis was granulomatous inflammation.

PLANNING A TRAJECTORY

Avoidance of Aerated Lung Altogether

If aerated lung is not violated, a pneumothorax will not occur. This rule can be used to good advantage by the direct puncture of pleura-based lesions large enough to ensure a direct hit on the first attempt (Fig 4). Other opportunities for avoiding aerated lung include passage through a collapsed or consolidated portion of lung (22) (Fig 5). If a central obstructing mass is to be sampled, examination of a contrast-enhanced CT scan of the region will help avoid sampling adjacent areas of postobstructive pneumonitis, often manifested by a branching pattern of enhancing vessels associated with dilated, fluid-filled bronchial structures.

Access to the mediastinum without transgression of the lung is particularly desirable. Because the mediastinum is very mobile, oblique positioning may allow the mediastinal fat (Fig 6) or the mass itself (Fig 7) to create a pathway into the mediastinum. Access to mediastinal lesions or lung lesions that abut the mediastinal pleura may be achieved with a paraspinal approach to avoid puncture of aerated lung (Figs 2, 8). If necessary, a saline-lidocaine mixture can be instilled into the paravertebral soft tissues to widen the extrapleural pathway (23). With ap-

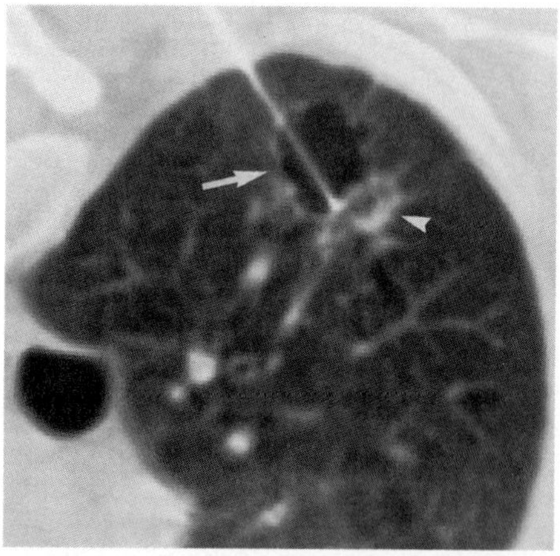

Figure 12. Because leakage occurs only at the pleural surface, a central bulla (arrow) seen on this CT image adjacent to this non–small cell carcinoma (arrowhead) can be punctured with impunity.

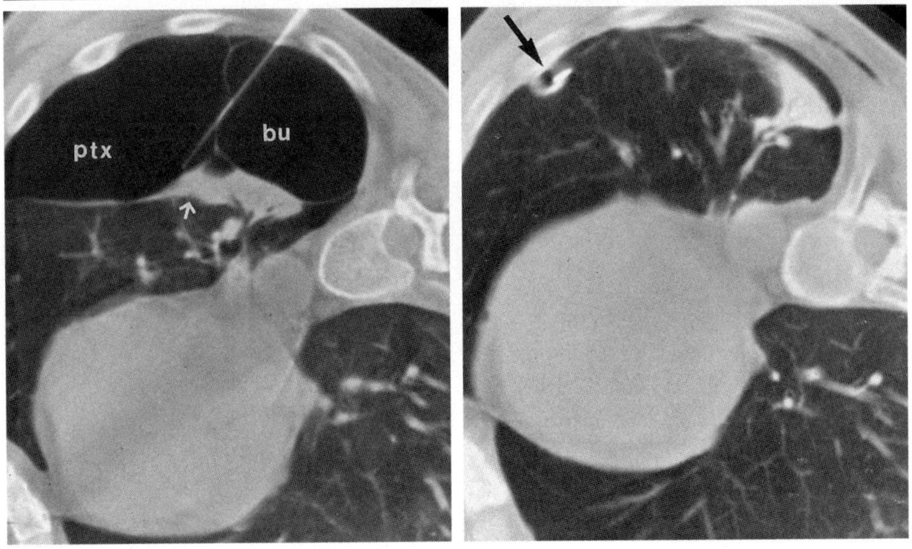

a. b.

Figure 13. CT scans. **(a)** Intentional needle lacerations of a peripheral bulla (*bu*) leads to an immediate large pneumothorax (*ptx*). Adjacent atelectatic lung (arrow) is present. **(b)** Although the bulla was successfully collapsed with a chest tube (arrow) and pleurodesis attempted, the bulla reappeared in a matter of weeks.

propriate positioning, any pleural fluid or pleural air present may be used to access the mediastinum. Alternatively, oxygen or room air may be injected into the pleural space by using the sharp and blunt trocars of the Hawkins-Akins needle (Cook, Bloomington, Ind) sequentially to pass through the chest wall and access the pleural space. The gas may be withdrawn at the end of the procedure (Fig 9). A test injection is important because accidental extrapleural injection of gas may produce vagal stimulation. Although the superior vena cava and brachiocephalic veins can be transgressed with a thin needle to access middle mediastinal nodes, this route may not be advisable in some patients, depending on risk factors. Access to the middle mediastinum via the thoracic inlet—which has been advocated by some authors (24,25)—is a technique likely to be associated with a substantial learning curve.

The particular risk factors of each patient should be considered when deciding to access the mediastinum through the lung or other routes. Saline-lidocaine instillation, oxygen instillation, and thoracic inlet access should not be used in the elderly, in patients with AIDS, or in patients with known cardiac disease because of the propensity to produce vagal stimulation resulting in hypotensive bradycardic episodes.

Trajectories Passing through Lung

If only one target is present, a variety of trajectories can be considered. Fissures should be avoided, since transgression results in three, rather than one, visceral pleural punctures. In general, it is desirable to puncture the pleura perpendicularly, both because the needle will not tend to slip over the pleura during entry and because of the aforementioned potential advantage of occlusion of the direct airway supplying the puncture site by the lesion itself. A direct perpendicular puncture is required if a biopsy is performed at the same time as localization for thoracoscopic resection with hook wire or methylene blue injection methods.

When a small lesion is in a subpleural or relatively peripheral location, a direct puncture may be unwise. If the puncture enters the lesion, all is well, but often, due to respiratory misregistration, an unsalvageable puncture results, and a second puncture is necessary. To avoid this situation in the case of a small peripheral lesion, one may use a near-tangential approach, assuming no fissures are transgressed (26). In this way, the needle enters the lung at some distance from the target, and there is plenty of room for course adjustment before encountering the lesion (Fig 10).

A course should be selected that passes over, not under, the adjacent rib, since the neurovascular bundle travels just below the rib. This is less of an issue in the anterior chest wall, since the intercostal arteries diminish in caliber as they travel anteriorly. The needle should also avoid direct contact with the rib, both because periosteal irritation may result in vagal stimulation and because if the needle directly contacts a rib it is difficult to manipulate later in the procedure. Although it is easy to avoid the inferior aspect of the ribs during fluoroscopically guided biopsies, it takes greater care with CT-guided biopsies. Precise localization of the ribs and interspaces is achieved by using thinner sections ($\leq$5 mm), which prevents the dense ribs from volume averaging into sections above and below their true positions. The ribs will appear as elongated ovals on CT images. Because the ribs spiral caudally as they progress anteriorly, the superior edge of the rib is the end of the oval the farthest away from the spine and the inferior edge of the rib, best avoided, is the portion of the oval nearest to the spine.

If a rib is in the way of a desired trajectory, the following techniques may help solve the problem: moving the patient's arms up or down, puncturing more medially or more laterally and adjusting the trajectory, rotating the patient into a slight decubitus position, using a near-tangential approach, puncturing from the opposite side (assuming no fissures will be transgressed), varying the designated respiration, or angling the fluoroscopy tube or CT gantry (27). I have never encountered a situation in which the transosseous approach, advocated by some, was necessary.

High-Resolution Interrogation of the Proposed Biopsy Site

The use of CT for needle aspiration lung biopsy has a unique advantage not enjoyed with conventional fluoroscopy: the ability to specifically examine the proposed pleural puncture site. In patients with any evidence of parenchymal lung disease, I routinely perform CT with the thinnest possible sections through the region, searching for the most normal feasible secondary pulmonary lobule for puncture. Blebs and bullae are carefully avoided, since puncture of these entities usually results in substantial air leakage. Some secondary pulmonary lobules may show air trapping, recognized with reduced CT attenuation, or fibrosis. Such areas are best avoided. Even in severely diseased lungs, there are usually a few more normal secondary pulmonary lobules that can be selected for puncture (Fig 11). Because only the puncture site leaks air and air does not track within the interstitium during or after biopsy, traversing bullae or other abnormal lung in deeper portions of the needle trajectory is not a risk factor (Fig 12).

Direct puncture of a bulla usually creates massive air leakage and an emergent situation (4) (Fig 13). If it is necessary to traverse a large superficial bulla, it is wise to preemptively position a non–sharp-tipped needle with a sharp trocar (eg, Hawkins-Akins, with the sharp stylet option) just outside the parietal pleura, ready to advance into the pleural space and connect to a suction trap if a pneumothorax occurs. A chest tube can then be placed in a less chaotic setting. Alternatively, the patient may be preemptively prepared for tube placement.

Phase of Respiration

The ideal respiratory volume for a biopsy is a small inspiration, within the range of normal, quiet breathing. Puncture during deep inspiration or full expiration places greater stress on the pleura at the puncture site if the needle is left in during normal breathing, increasing the likelihood of a pleural tear. During the sampling phase, the patient is asked to breath hold for 10–15 seconds. Patients are better able to maintain the breath hold in a degree of inspiration than in expiration. Also, if the patient fails to hold the breath, the tendency is to exhale if an inspiration is held but to inhale if an expiration is held, the latter being a far more dangerous situation from the perspective of the risk of air embolism.

PLACEMENT OF THE NEEDLE

Once the appropriate trajectory and designated breath hold are selected and a sterile field is established, 1% lidocaine is used for local anesthesia. The patient is instructed to hold the designated breath during administration of the anesthetic, and the planned trajectory of the needle is followed, delivering lidocaine to approach, but not transgress, the pleura. The biopsy needles should not be used to deliver local anesthetic, because the fluid dilutes the specimens and material will be lost during alcohol fixation before staining. After administration of lidocaine and confirmation of needle position by using the lidocaine needle as a guide, a small skin nick is placed to facilitate entry of the biopsy needle. Any undue bleeding noted at this point should redirect attention to the patient's clotting function, and the procedure should be reconsidered. The outer needle of a coaxial system is then introduced, just far enough to stand the needle upright at the appropriate angle in the soft tissues of the chest wall. In the thin and nonmuscular patient, approximately only 1 cm of soft tissue may be available; the needle may be maintained at the selected angle by forming a small supportive tepee shape out of gauze pads. If puncture at a steep angle is desired, the needle may be supported by forming a small sling with a bandage strip, resting the needle shaft on the nonsticky pad portion. Alternatively, the patient may also be angled obliquely so that the needle is vertically oriented during an oblique puncture.

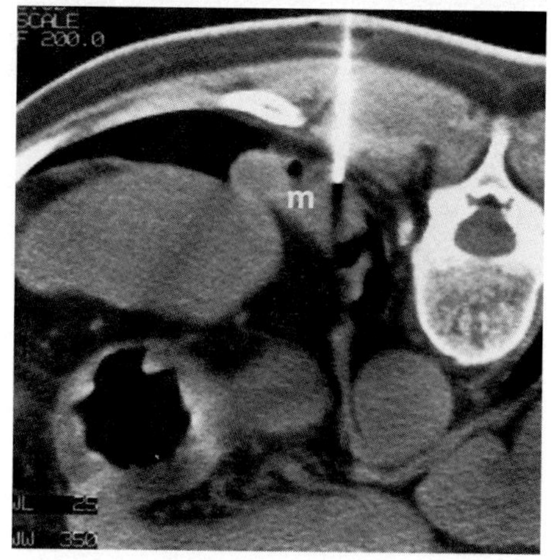

Figure 14. CT scan shows excessively peripheral needle placement in a lower lobe metastasis from colon carcinoma (*m*). The needle was dislodged into the pleural space by respiratory motion, which caused an immediate pneumothorax.

A careful and stepwise advancement of the needle, remaining within the plane of the gantry, to a position just outside the parietal pleura is crucial. Positioning the needle tip just outside the pleura reduces the sometimes disastrous effects of marked motion of the patient's chest wall musculature on attempted entry into the lung. With the needle just outside the pleura, directed at the lesion, the patient can be tested for reproducibility of the designated respiration, and appropriate coaching and retesting can be performed before entry into the lung. If the patient is unable to reproduce the appropriate respiration, another approach that is less sensitive to respiration accuracy may be considered, such as a near-tangential approach, described earlier. All needle manipulations, even those in the chest wall, should be performed with the patient in the designated breath hold because respiration moves the chest wall substantially. Needle placement in the chest wall should be in the plane of the gantry when the patient is holding the designated breath, a situation that cannot be achieved if manipulations are made without the appropriate breath hold.

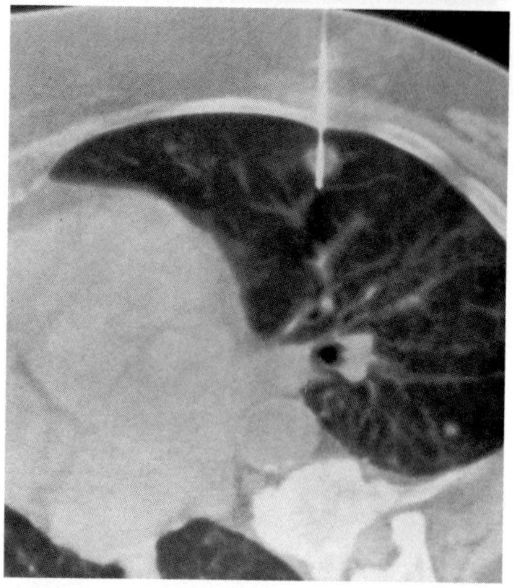

Figure 15. CT scan shows a desirable "resting position" for the outer coaxial needle between sampling passes of a peripheral nodule, one of numerous metastases from endometrial carcinoma. For sampling, the outer needle tip is withdrawn into the lesion, the trocar is removed, coaxial sampling is performed, the trocar is reinserted, and the needle is readvanced into the resting position, all in one breath hold. A relatively lateral puncture was selected in this patient, who recently underwent abdominal surgery and who could not tolerate the prone position either during or after the procedure. After the procedure, the patient was placed in the left lateral decubitus position (puncture site down).

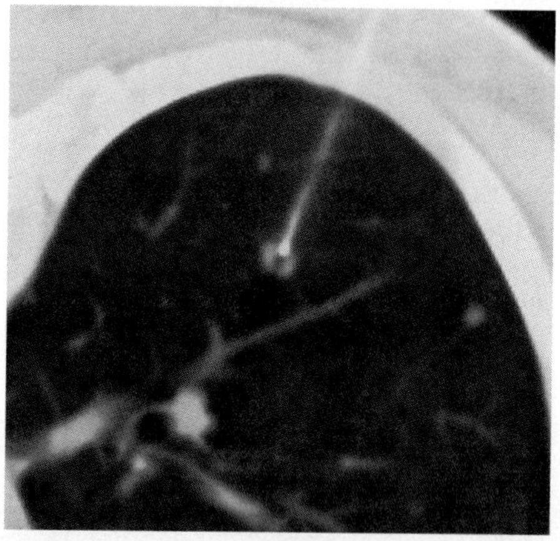

Figure 16. For coaxial biopsy, the outer needle should be positioned in the periphery of the nodule, as on this CT scan of a 6-mm metastasis from cervical carcinoma. This gives the outer needle some purchase on the nodule during sampling.

Entry into the lung causes momentary

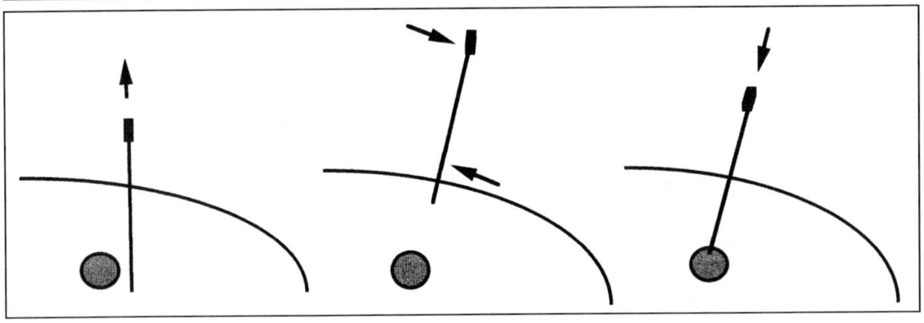

Figure 17. Correction of course can usually be achieved (left) by partial withdrawal of the outer needle, (middle) redirection by pushing the hub in the desired direction while applying fulcrumlike pressure at the skin surface, and (right) by readvancement of the needle while the desired angle is maintained. Arrows indicate direction of motion or applied pressure; curved lines represent chest wall.

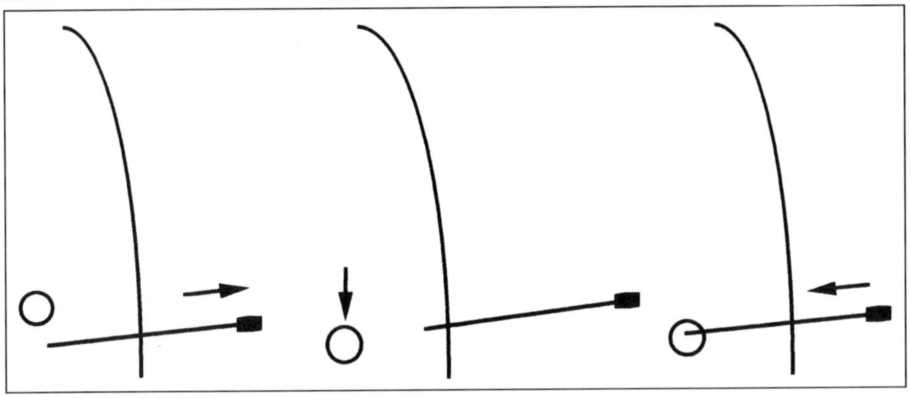

Figure 18. If the lesion is cephalic to the needle tip (left), partial needle withdrawal followed by a larger inspiration (middle) and needle readvancement (right) will correct position and make biopsy possible. Arrows indicate direction of motion; curved lines indicate chest wall.

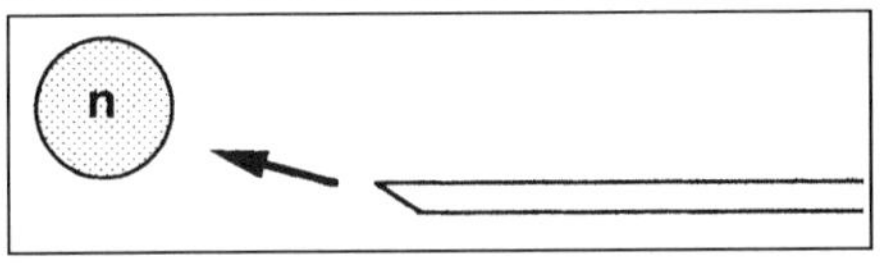

Figure 19. When passing through tissue, a single beveled needle will "steer" slightly in a direction away from the face of the bevel (arrow), which may be used to correct the course toward a nodule (*n*). The effect is less in lung than in soft tissue, so this technique should be used in concert with other methods of redirection.

pain, and therefore the patient should be warned to anticipate the pain and not react with a sudden inspiration, of particular importance with a smaller, peripheral target. After entry into the lung, the needle should not be touched except during the designated breath hold for manipulations. The needle should be allowed to rock freely during quiet breathing, to avoid excess stress on the puncture site.

When the needle is manipulated, the nondominant hand should grasp the needle close to the skin and the dominant hand should grip the hub of the needle like a thumbtack or pushpin, with the thumb on the hub of the trocar. This two-handed method allows tough tissues to be punctured without course deflection and without pushing the trocar out. A two-handed approach also facilitates redirection by using the nondominant hand positioned at the skin as a fulcrum.

On entry into the lung, the needle should be advanced into a resting position at least 1 cm into the lung, 1.5 cm in the lower lung zones, regardless of the depth of the target lesion. Because there is substantial movement of the lung during breathing, particularly in the lower lung zones, some degree of purchase on the lung is needed to prevent the needle from falling out into the pleural space during respiration, an event often associated with the development of a pneumothorax (Fig 14). Ideally, the outer needle should pass directly through a peripheral lesion (Fig 15). Coaxial sampling can then be performed by withdrawing the outer needle into the middle portion of the lesion, coaxially sampling the deep half of the lesion, and (after replacing the trocar) readvancing into the resting position, all within one breath hold. The coaxial pass length would be adjusted to a length equal to the radius of the lesion in this case.

For lesions deeper in the lung, the needle should be advanced in increments, depending on the size of the target and the necessity for course correction. Monitoring of the location of the needle tip between manipulations should be performed with use of 5-mm sections or 1–2-mm sections when approaching small targets. When using a coaxial technique, the outer needle is advanced to a position just puncturing the nodule or mass to allow purchase on the lesion during sampling (Fig 16). Occasionally, with a tiny lesion, the large outer needle pushes the lesion away, failing to puncture it. Puncture can usually be achieved with the thinner insert needle during sampling.

CORRECTION OF AN IMPERFECT PUNCTURE

Limiting pleural punctures to one is crucial in minimizing operator-controlled complications. Therefore, all corrective manipulations of the needle should be performed by partially withdrawing the needle (but not through the pleura) and readvancing (Fig 17). Rather severe apparent overangulation with two hands may be needed during redirection, especially in the patient with a thicker chest wall. An advantage of the outer needle in a coaxial system is that it is relatively stiff and much torque can be placed on it during redirection without bending the shaft by using the hand at the skin surface as a fulcrum. This may be difficult if the needle is buried to the hub, thus for deeper lesions in obese patients, a longer needle (15 rather than 10 cm) is used if it fits through the gantry during initial advancement through the chest wall.

In the obese patient, attempts to redirect the needle within the lung also may be difficult because the thick chest wall tends to keep the needle in the same trajectory. However, if the needle is misplaced cephalad or caudally, the needle may be withdrawn into a relatively peripheral position, expiration or inspiration (respectively) performed, and the needle readvanced (Fig 18). This constitutes an exception to the rule that biopsy

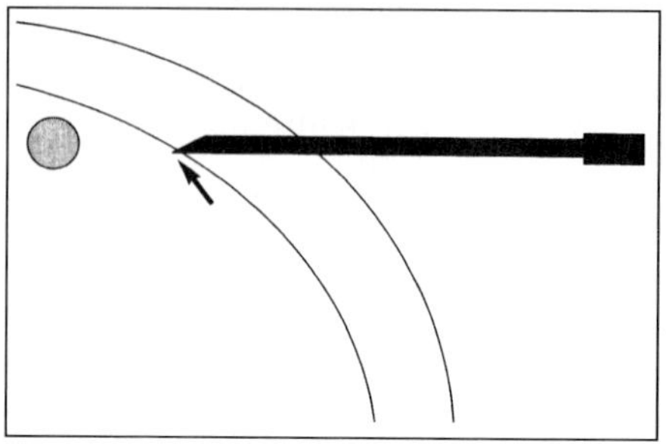

Figure 20. When the lung is entered at an oblique angle, the face of the bevel should be directed away from the pleural surface so that the point will "catch" on the pleura (arrow).

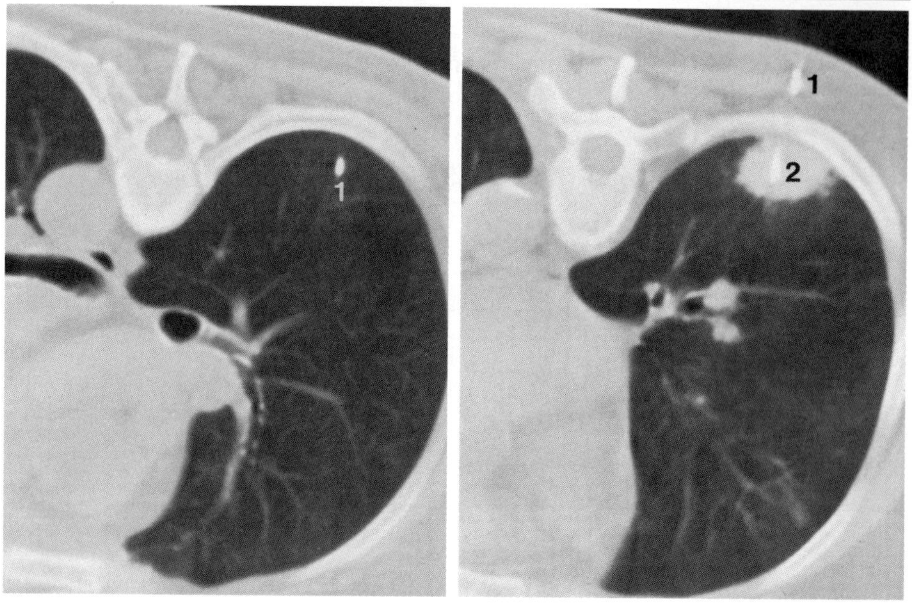

a. b.

Figure 21. CT scans. (a) After an irretrievably misdirected puncture, the errant needle (*1*) lies far cephalad to the lesion. (b) Leaving this needle (*1*) in place prevents air leakage from that site during the procedure and pins the lung in a relatively fixed position, making placement of a second needle (*2*) easier. The errant needle was used to place a blood patch at the site of the unusable pleural puncture on completion of the procedure.

should not be performed at high or low lung volume. This maneuver should be used in conjunction with standard redirection techniques.

If a needle with a single beveled tip is used, a minor amount of course correction can be achieved by "bevel steering" (28). In soft tissue, and much less so in lung, a needle tends to "pull" toward the direction of the pointed tip and away from the face of the bevel (Fig 19). This can and should be used at the same time as other means of course correction. Bevel position also can be used to advantage to ease passing over a rib or penetrating between a rib and a transverse process. Often a needle that catches on the edge of a bone can be freed if rotated into a different bevel orientation. The point of the needle also can be used to advantage to "catch" on the lung when entering at a near-tangential angle and prevent the needle from slipping into the pleural space (Fig 20). The operator should examine the needle before the procedure to note the relative position of the locking notch on the hub of the needle and the bevel and remain conscious of bevel position, adjusting it to advantage throughout the procedure.

In some cases, despite attempts, ideal positioning of the outer needle cannot be achieved. Fortunately, by pulling the needle tip back peripheral to the target, course correction can be achieved during the coaxial sampling process itself by canting the outer needle (discussed later). Most needle malpositions can be salvaged in this way, avoiding a second puncture.

Occasionally, initial needle placement is so far from the desired location that it cannot be corrected without repuncturing the pleura. This usually occurs due to failure to advance the needle to a position just outside the parietal pleura before puncture or to gross patient motion or respiratory misregistration. It is preferable to leave an unsalvageable needle in place until completion of the procedure (Fig 21). Its presence discourages leakage from that puncture site during the course of the procedure, it transfixes the lung making subsequent punctures less subject to respiratory variation, and it can be used to place a blood patch at the site of the unusable pleural puncture at the termination of the procedure.

SAMPLING

The length by which the needle insert extends out from the guide needle is preset before the procedure (Fig 1). After discarding the needle insert stylet and connecting the insert to a syringe, the insert is set for a particular pass length by inserting it into the outer needle until it protrudes the desired amount, marking the depth of insertion into the outer needle with a plastic guide. Later in the procedure, the pass length can be adjusted if necessary. It is not of any use diagnostically to obtain a biopsy sample in normal lung deep to the lesion; in fact, this increases the risk of hemorrhage. Other obstacles deep to the lesion, such as fissures or vessels, also may be avoided by limiting pass length. Presetting the needle pass length is of particular use when supervising an inexperienced trainee.

I favor constant suction during sampling with use of a 20-mL syringe. The syringe-needle combination can be held like an ice pick, and strong suction can be exerted by pushing the plunger up with the thumb. If some air enters the syringe, there is room to continue generating suction without pushing the plunger all the way out. It has been shown that the same amount of suction can be generated in this fashion as with a 10-mL syringe, despite the larger cross-sectional area of the 20-mL syringe (29). Suction of air into the syringe indicates that normal lung is being sampled or that there is a poor connection between the syringe and the needle.

Sampling requires both hands. The nondominant hand is used to stabilize the outer needle, which is grasped after the patient has taken the designated breath hold. The trocar is removed, and sampling is performed with the dominant hand. Short, forceful thrusts are used with elbow action, again very much like using an ice pick. Five rapid thrusts are made, fewer if blood appears in the syringe; if this occurs, further passes will further dilute the specimen with blood. After sampling, the trocar is replaced and the patient resumes normal shallow respiration.

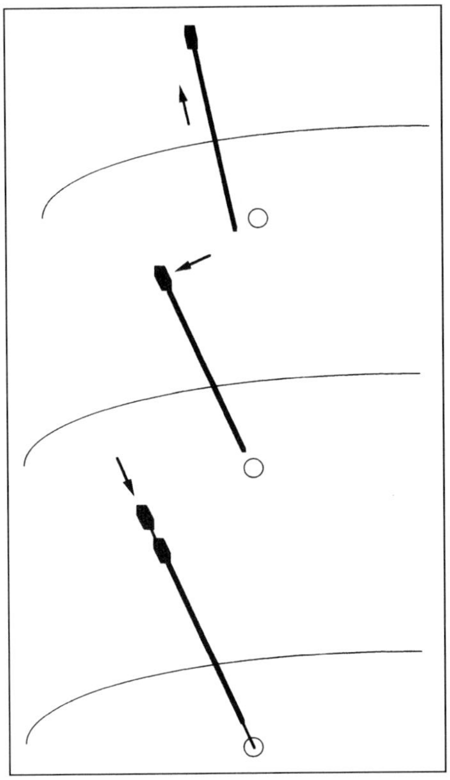

Figure 22. Substantial course correction can be achieved during sampling. The outer needle is withdrawn slightly (top) and, after appropriately lengthening the distance by which the insert will protrude from the outer needle, the outer needle is canted toward the lesion with the nondominant hand (middle) while the dominant hand samples the lesion with the insert (bottom). Arrows indicate the needle insert passing through the outer needle and into the lesion.

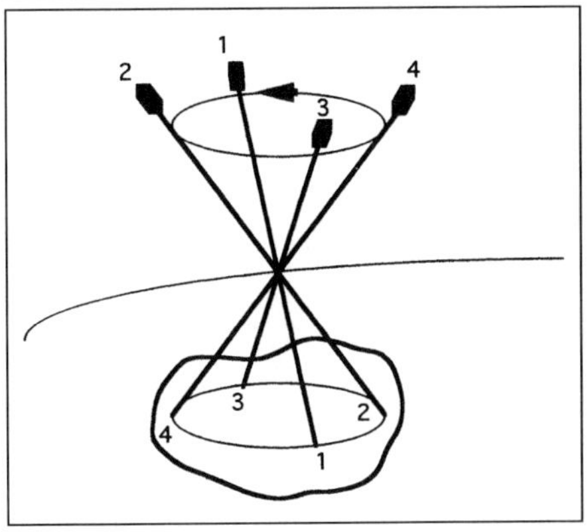

Figure 23. Multiple areas of a mass can be sampled by moving the outer needle with the nondominant hand while coaxial passes are being made with the dominant hand.

As indicated above, correction of an imperfect puncture can also be achieved at the time of sampling. The outer needle may be pulled back about 1 cm peripheral to the lesion (depending on available lung and degree of correction needed), and the insert pass is length adjusted to an appropriately longer distance. Then, during application of substantial torque on the hub to direct the passes in the desired direction, sampling may occur (Fig 22). Similarly, by moving the hub of the needle in a circular or random pattern during sampling, specimens can be obtained from various areas within a larger lesion (Fig 23). This technique is usually very effective. Alternatively, the needle insert tip can be curved slightly with the fingers to correct the course at the time of sampling. Use of a side-exit coaxial needle system will achieve much the same result as these maneuvers by redirecting the needle insert laterally.

Tactile sensation and the size of the specimen retrieved during sampling may give some information to the operator. The lesion may seem crunchy or firm, textures often associated with carcinomas. The operator may have the sensation that the lesion is being pushed away from, rather than being punctured by, the needle. Thinner needle inserts may be tried if the lesion is difficult to penetrate. In general, rock-hard or rubbery texture is a clue that the lesion is likely to require a core sample for diagnosis. Cutting guns easily penetrate most lesions. Similarly, if an aspirating needle does not yield any tissue after a few passes (assuming adequate positioning), the lesion may not be a carcinoma, since carcinomatous cells tend to be rather loosely adherent to each other and are easily aspirated. If appropriate, a cutting gun may then be used. An example of a lesion unlikely to be diagnosed with aspiration biopsy is a benign fibrous tumor of the pleura, often suspected on the basis of its smooth, rounded contour; peripheral location; and large size. If a lesion other than a carcinoma is suspected on the basis of CT appearance, the outer guide needle for a detachable coaxial gun may be first used for an aspiration; if these findings are not diagnostic, it may be used for a core biopsy (Fig 2). In this way, a second pleural puncture is avoided. Again, the throw of the cutting gun should not extend beyond the lesion into normal lung, if at all possible.

Since sampling may change the position of the outer needle, the needle and lesion should be reimaged after each coaxial pass while one waits for preliminary results of cytologic examination; this is a good use of otherwise wasted time. The needle may also be moved to a different location within the lesion or otherwise adjusted during this time. The resulting images will also give information about a developing pneumothorax or parenchymal hemorrhage.

With use of coaxial technique, many passes can be made quickly and without additional pleural punctures. This technique is of particular value when the procedure is not guided by cytologic examination or if there are long delays between sampling and preliminary results. Extra passes can easily be made, lessening the chance of an insufficient specimen. When coaxial technique is used, and assuming that a bleb has not been punctured, it is unusual to have a pneumothorax occur during even a prolonged procedure because the needle itself serves to obstruct the puncture site. If a pneumothorax does occur, the outer needle will usually remain lodged in the lesion, allowing further samples to be obtained. Aside from issues related to the clinical effects of a pneumothorax, the presence of a pneumothorax makes additional pleural punctures difficult if single-needle technique is used, because the lung is no longer fixed in position in the chest and may be balloted by, rather than accurately punctured by additional needles.

The biopsy will be terminated on acquisition of an adequate specimen, development of a symptomatic pneumothorax, or development of parenchymal hemorrhage with severe coughing or hemoptysis.

PRELIMINARY CYTOLOGIC RESULTS

Ideally, every lung biopsy should be directed by the feedback of on-site cytologic examination (30). A rapid stain technique, such as the toluidine blue stain, can give results in less than 1 minute. Acquisition of tumor tissue will stop the procedure with a minimum of potentially damaging manipulations or biopsy passes. Lack of cellular samples may suggest needle repositioning or a switch to a cutting-type needle. Acquisition of necrotic material will allow the needle to be repositioned into the periphery or into another area of the mass. Abundant inflammatory cells will indicate that specimens are required for culture, and the presence of multinucleated giant cells will indicate culture for mycobacterial disease. Some fungi can also be identified with quick stains, and appropriate cultures can be obtained. Gross visual inspection of a sample is completely inadequate, with the exception of core specimens. If a cytologist or technician is not available, the operator may wish to learn the basics of cytologic examination, including smear technique, fixation, quick staining, and identification of the general features of neoplasia, normal bronchial cells, and inflammatory cells. Even a tyro can determine if there is nothing but blood on the slide.

DAMAGE CONTROL

Blood-Patch Technique

The blood-patch technique involves use of the patient's own blood to prevent leakage from the pleural puncture (31–35). A blood patch cannot be placed with single-needle technique, but it is placed after a coaxial biopsy has been completed by injecting blood during withdrawal of the outer needle. If aerated lung has not been violated, a blood patch is not necessary and the outer needle can be used to obtain a larger bore specimen at the time of needle withdrawal. The original blood-patch technique described used clotted blood injected through the entire needle track. However, I use about 4 mL of freshly drawn patient blood, obtained through venipuncture or intravenous access, and I inject it only in the most peripheral 2 cm of the needle track as the needle is slowly withdrawn through the visceral pleura and into the chest wall (Fig 24). We have shown this to be as effective in stopping air leakage as the originally described method in a lung biopsy model (10). While all nonpatched punctures could be forced to leak by increasing the pressure in the lung specimen, one-fourth of the patched punctures could not be forced to leak at any achievable pressure. For patched punctures that did leak, the pressure at which leakage occurred was twice as high as for unpatched punctures. Obviously, a blood patch, like other methods of damage control, will not be effective when air leakage is caused by large lacerations of the pleura.

There are various potential advantages of using freshly drawn patient blood delivered only in the peripheral 2 cm of the needle track. Because only events at the pleural surface are relevant to leakage, injection of blood deep into the lung does not have any advantage and can even cause airway irritation and coughing. Central portions of the needle path may have transgressed larger pulmonary veins, so with track injection, some clot or perhaps some air from the hub of the needle might enter a larger pulmonary vein and embolize systemically. Intravascular injection would be unlikely to happen in the tiny vessels in the periphery of the lung. When clotted blood is used, clot will occasionally block the needle and prevent injection; if only serum is delivered, it will not clot in place. Use of freshly drawn, nonclotted blood has an additional potential advantage when combined with instantaneous puncture-site-down positioning after injection. Assisted by gravity, the mobile liquid blood may tend to collect in the subpleural periphery of the lung at the puncture site and clot in place there (Fig 25). Several studies published in the literature have addressed the clinical results of the blood-patch technique (with use of clotted blood) with mixed results (31–35). To our knowledge, however, no study has been performed to examine the effects of a freshly drawn blood patch in concert with immediate puncture-site-down positioning.

A similar pleural-patch technique has also been developed and involves the use of Gelfoam (Upjohn, Kalamazoo, Mich) (36).

Postprocedure Monitoring and Activity Restrictions

It is now known that postbiopsy care affects the development and the course of complications. The most crucial time for appropriate management is immediately after needle withdrawal, because most substantial air leakage and essentially all hemoptysis begin early in the course of follow-up. The patient should rest in a recumbent position and should be closely monitored for the development of symptoms. Vital signs should be recorded at least every 20 minutes, more frequently if symptoms ensue or the patient's condition becomes unstable. Oxygen saturation should be monitored. If a pneumothorax is known to be present, oxygen may be administered to improve oxygenation and to facilitate resorption of the existing pneumothorax and any further leakage (37,38). Unfortunately, the use of supplemental oxygen removes a relatively sensitive indicator to follow a pneumothorax, so its use should be carefully considered given the clinical situation.

Early recognition of complications is essential for avoiding morbidity and mortality. Even if they develop, the course of complications can be altered by means of aggressive management.

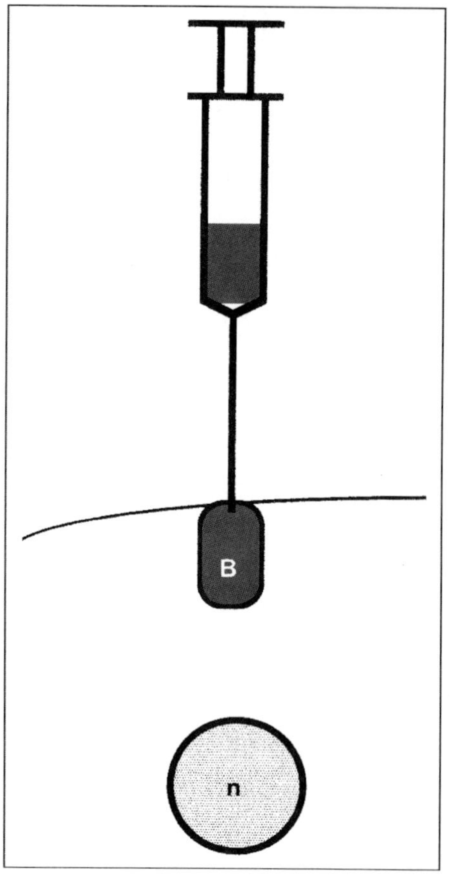

Figure 24. Modified blood-patch technique. Four milliliters of freshly drawn patient blood (*B*) is injected in the peripheral 2 cm of the needle track on withdrawal of the coaxial outer needle. The entire track to the nodule (*n*) need not be injected.

Pressure Precautions

An interesting ancillary body of information regarding pressure challenges to a puncture site was revealed by our lung biopsy model (10). This was of as much practical interest as the intended subject of the study, blood patches. It was learned that a particular puncture site will have a unique and very specific pressure above which leakage will reliably and repeatedly occur. Most small puncture wounds to the pleura tolerate pressure relatively well, leaking at 10–40 mm Hg, if at all. A coughing fit will generate pressure in excess of 100 mm Hg at which all nonpatched and probably most patched punctures would be expected to leak. However, any visible tearing of the pleura will allow leakage at pressure of 1–2 mm Hg, justifying care taken during the procedure to avoid pleural tears.

In patients with pleural punctures, it is therefore essential to strictly prevent all activities that may elevate intrathoracic pressure, such as coughing, excessive talk-

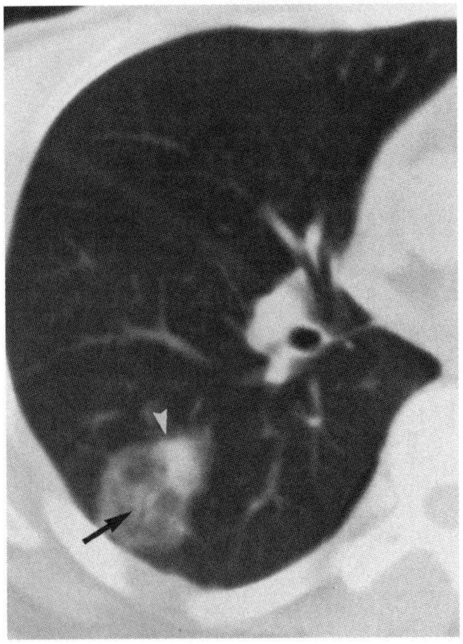

Figure 25. After completion of the biopsy depicted in Figure 16, a blood patch is injected and the patient is placed in the puncture-site-down position. The blood patch (arrow) can be seen peripheral to the target nodule (arrowhead).

ing, sitting up in bed without assistance, raising the head off the pillow, deep breathing, lifting, and straining. Delayed pneumothorax can be seen if pressure precautions are grossly violated. In my practice, examples of violations that have lead to late air leakage include severe straining in the bathroom related to constipation, a choking fit from soup aspiration, and rooting loudly at a Little League game (against medical advice!).

Positional Precautions and Follow-up Imaging

Immediately after blood-patch placement and needle removal, I roll the patient off the CT or fluoroscopy table into the puncture-site-down position. The patient should remain passive, with the rolling performed by many assistants to ensure that the patient does not strain or perform a Valsalva maneuver in any way while trying to assist. A Valsalva maneuver is less likely to occur if the roll is performed while the patient lets his or her breath out. The needle removal and the rolling should take no more than a few seconds.

Puncture-site-down positioning was first suggested by Zidulka and colleagues (19) and was tested in a canine model with promising results. When properly applied, the technique has met with good success in most studies, particularly in avoiding chest tube placement in patients with a pneumothorax (20,21). It probably works by diminishing aeration to the somewhat atelectatic periphery of the dependent lung, while also helping tamponade leakage from the puncture, since the weight of the lung itself ensures good visceral-parietal pleural apposition even if a pneumothorax is present. Were the puncture site up, leakage would be unimpeded into a pneumothorax.

To achieve the full effect of the technique, the patient must be placed in the puncture-site-down position immediately after the needle is withdrawn. For this reason, the technique can be appropriately applied only with coaxial technique or with a single puncture if single-needle technique is used. Some investigators have tried to use this technique in association with multiple pleural punctures. While a second, third, or fourth puncture is being performed, the earlier puncture sites are upward and potentially leaking into a pneumothorax. A similar situation occurs while waiting for cytologic results with the puncture site up after withdrawing a single needle. Such studies have shown the expected poor results for obvious reasons.

No chest radiograph is obtained immediately after the biopsy unless symptoms or a dropping oxygen saturation level suggest a pneumothorax may be present. The reason for this is that despite the best intentions of the technician, sitting the patient up for an upright, expiratory radiograph will probably entail at least some degree of straining or Valsalva maneuver. The puncture site is at its most tenuous immediately after needle withdrawal, which is not a good time to apply a pressure challenge. Oxygen saturation monitors provide enough clinical information to permit delayed acquisition of the first image.

Assuming that aerated lung has been violated at the pleural surface, the patient is left puncture site down for 1–2 hours. I use 2 hours for an extra margin of safety in the elderly and in any patient with lung disease or a smoking history (most patients are in these categories). Upright expiratory images are obtained at 1 hour and 2 hours after the procedure. If no air leakage has occurred after 2 hours with the patient in the puncture-site-down position, or if a pneumothorax present on the first image is unchanged, the patient is told to sit up and behave as he or she would at home for 1 hour. An additional image is then obtained at 3 hours after the procedure. If this image also shows no leakage, the patient is discharged to home.

I use a minimum of three follow-up images, all obtained with the patient upright and in full expiration. Images are obtained at 1 and 2 hours because therapy will change if there is leakage on the 1-hour image (oxygen will be applied, aspiration might be considered). On completion of the 2-hour image, two radiographs from different times will be available to assess the dynamics of air leakage, should this occur. In this protocol, patients lie puncture site down until they have had no leakage for at least an hour. In the absence of serial images, continuing leakage cannot be distinguished from leakage that occurred immediately after the procedure and then stopped. The third image confirms that no leakage is occurring when the patient is doing the activities he or she will be doing at home. If there is going to be a problem, it is best to know about it before discharge.

A potentially dangerous variation of the puncture-site-down technique is the practice of discharging patients after follow-up only in the puncture-site-down position. Unfortunately, this position may mask a small air leak, and thus one must be sure to obtain an image after an hour in the upright position.

MANAGING COMPLICATIONS

Pneumothorax

Many patients will experience pleuritic chest pain with even a relatively small pneumothorax. The size of pneumothorax necessary to cause shortness of breath is extremely variable and depends on the underlying condition of the lungs. In the absence of supplemental oxygen, oxygen saturation is useful in monitoring patients for substantial pneumothorax.

If air leakage occurs at any time during follow-up, an additional hour of puncture-site-down positioning is mandated, and images should be obtained hourly until leakage stops in this position. Then, an hour of upright positioning is tried, followed by discharge if no leakage occurs or another hour puncture-site-down positioning if leakage occurs; this continues until the patient can be discharged or requires pleura drainage due to symptoms, a pneumothorax exceeding about 30%, or an unremitting pattern of leakage. In general, when a pneumothorax begins to track down the lateral aspect of the chest, the likelihood increases that it will require drainage. Previous thoracotomy, radiation therapy, or pneumonia may influence the appearance of a pneumothorax; the lung may be tethered in some places and not collapse fully. Pneumothorax is, however, very rare in patients who have undergone a thoracotomy on that side.

Recently it has been demonstrated that aspiration of a pneumothorax may obviate chest tube placement in at least some patients with a substantial pneumothorax (39). Although this maneuver is unlikely to help patients with severe laceration of the pleura, it may be useful in patients with more normal lungs who have developed a pneumothorax due to breaks in technique such as multiple pleural punctures or coughing fits. Although use of plastic intravenous catheters has been recommended for aspiration of pneumothorax, these catheters may kink or collapse, particularly in the obese patient. A relatively large gauge, preferably nonsharp needle with a sharp trocar (eg, Hawkins-Akins needle) can be used for aspiration and hooked directly to a suction trap with the appropriate connectors. The needle tip is positioned just deep to the parietal pleura. A pneumothorax can be evacuated much more quickly with this technique than with a syringe and three-way stopcock system. Needle aspiration can also be used to temporize when a larger tube is needed, thus reexpanding the lung and allowing for a more permanent drainage catheter to be placed under nonemergent conditions. I keep the tubing and connectors for direct needle hub aspiration available in the biopsy room with a diagram instructing assistants in proper assembly. Should a pneumothorax occur during the procedure, aspiration can also be performed with the outer biopsy needle itself after placement of a blood patch (Fig 26).

When a longer-term drainage catheter is necessary, a small-gauge (eg, 9-F Teflon, Cook) pneumothorax catheter with a trocar can be placed (40,41). Although sites ranging from the second to sixth intercostal spaces have been recommended, I use the third intercostal space at the midclavicular line. A higher placement sometimes gives insufficient distance to bury all side ports within the pleural space before the tip of the catheter contacts the apex. This contact can be very painful for the patient. The third intercostal space is high enough to be well away from the heart on the left side. The distance from the skin to the pleural space can be determined by aspiration at the appropriate 45° angle to the chest wall with the anesthesia syringe. Knowing the distance prevents subpectoral placement of the tube, an occasional problem in the obese patient. Once the tip of the trocar enters the pleural space, the catheter is advanced slightly so that it leads, preventing the trocar from damaging the collapsed lung. After appropriate positioning, the catheter is fed off the trocar and stitched in place. If pleural fluid is present, a small-gauge drainage catheter is inappropriate because it can become clogged. In general, patients with tube drainage require hospital admission. Pleur Evac suction is preferable to a Heimlich valve in terms of maximizing pleural apposition and should be used if the patient is admitted to the hospital.

Hemoptysis

Hemoptysis related to lung biopsy is usually self-limiting. It occurs in about 5% of cases, probably double that when a cutting gun is utilized. However, it remains the most common cause of death in lung biopsy, as determined by a national survey (8). Although most cases of hemoptysis are probably caused by trauma to the pulmonary vessels, massive hemoptysis may be from enlarged bronchial artery branches associated with chronic cavities or bronchiectasis. Clues to the onset of hemoptysis are unusually bloody specimens, blood emerging from the hub out the outer coaxial needle, and the development of increasing amounts of ground-glass attenuation in the region of the biopsy on CT images (Fig 27). If these findings are present, less aggressive biopsy manipulations and the earliest possible termination of the procedure are recommended. Hemoptysis is often associated with a coughing fit due to airway irritation. Severe coughing is likely to tear the pleura and therefore is an indication for needle removal. Dramatic negative intrathoracic pressures occur during the large inspiration prior to the coughing, and high positive intrathoracic pressures occur during coughing. This places the patient at risk both for air embolism, should venous damage be responsible for the bleeding, and for pneumothorax.

The patient is placed in the decubitus position with the lung biopsy site down to prevent spillage of blood into the other lung. Oxygen is applied, if possible. Coughing helps clear blood from the airways and in any case cannot be prevented. Trendelenburg positioning may be added to the decubitus positioning to facilitate expectoration of blood. Intubation should be avoided, but if it is necessary it should be performed with a double-lumen tube. If the bleeding does not stop immediately, bronchoscopic tamponade of the lobar bronchus is recommended. The bronchoscope itself or a Fogarty catheter may be used. Other options, depending on the suspected source of the blood,

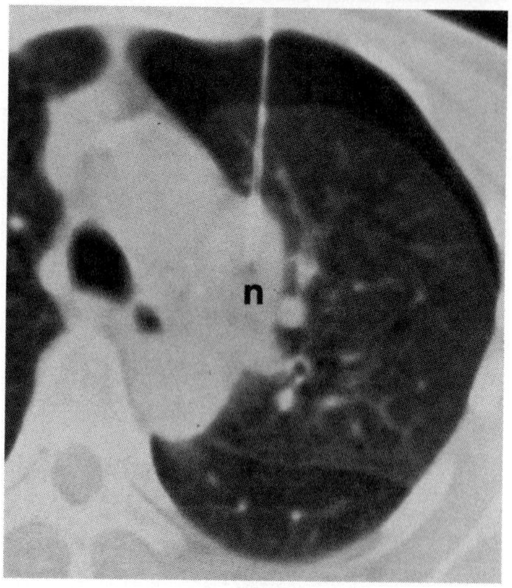

a.

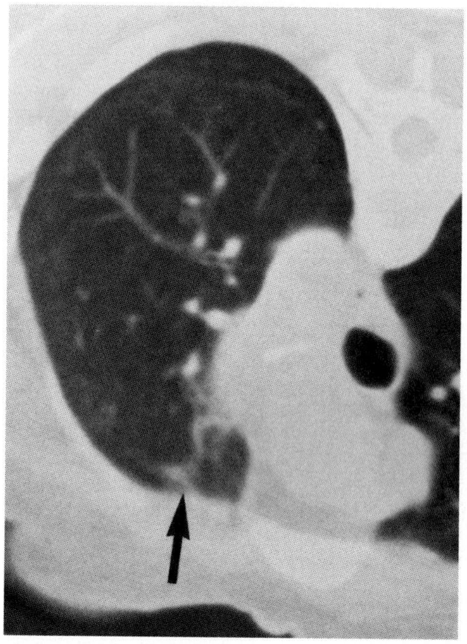

b.

Figure 26. CT scans. **(a)** During biopsy of a mediastinal node (*n*), a pneumothorax appears, an unusual event when a coaxial technique is used because the outer needle occludes the puncture site. **(b)** After blood-patch placement at the puncture site on withdrawal of the needle through the visceral pleura, the outer coaxial needle was connected to a suction trap and the pneumothorax was evacuated. Puncture-site-down positioning was instituted. A portion of the blood patch can be seen in a dependent position (arrow). No further air leakage occurred.

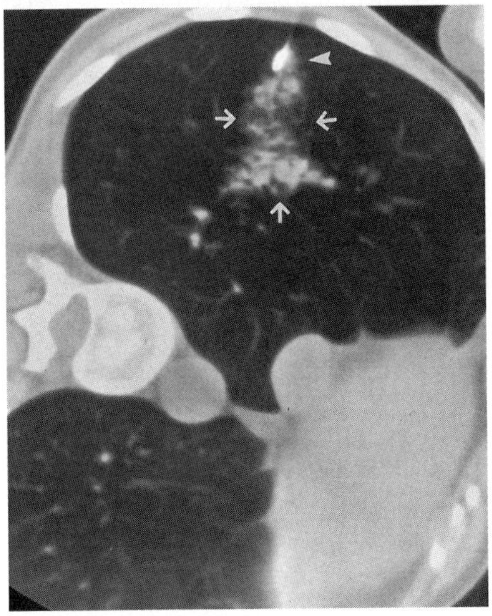

Figure 27. Extensive hemorrhage (arrows) developed after a single sampling from this small hamartoma (arrowhead). Surprisingly, no hemoptysis occurred.

include bronchial artery embolization, pulmonary artery embolization, and surgery. Prenotification of backup specialty services is crucial in high-risk cases.

Air Embolism

A particularly unfortunate complication of lung biopsy is air embolism, entry of air into the patient's pulmonary venous circulation with subsequent systemic embolization (42–44). Two causative mechanisms exist. Unauthorized inspiration by the patient when the trocar has been removed and the needle tip happens to be located in a pulmonary vein can draw air into the pulmonary venous system; this is sometimes appreciated by the operator as an audible sucking sound. The iatrogenic creation of a bronchovenous fistula by a needle or a cutting gun is another potential cause; air embolism often occurs immediately after the large inspiration that usually precedes an episode of hemoptysis. The patient may lose consciousness or show evidence of stroke or seizure. Immediate measures include delivery of 100% oxygen to facilitate absorption of the nitrogen bubbles and positioning in the left lateral decubitus and/or Trendelenburg position to prevent air from exiting the left atrium and to prevent bubbles from traveling to the cerebral circulation. If a bronchovenous fistula is suspected, intubation and positive pressure ventilation may aggravate the situation. Definitive therapy is transfer to a decompression chamber in concert with supportive care. CT of the head may show infarction or air. The condition is often fatal.

PATIENT DISCHARGE

In addition to a discussion of the success of the procedure, any complications, and recommendations for follow-up, I give patients written instructions to take home. Included are information about which lung was sampled for biopsy; whether a pneumothorax was present at discharge; and, if so, its width in centimeters at the lung apex on an upright, expiratory chest radiograph. (Better still, the patient can be given the last follow-up chest radiograph, should symptoms lead to a return visit to the hospital or emergency room.) Instructions should also include advice about activity (rest in bed or easy chair), diet (regular), bathing (yes), and worrisome level of hemoptysis (more than a teaspoon of pure fresh blood) and warnings to avoid lifting, raising the voice, straining in the bathroom, and all activities likely to generate a Valsalva maneuver. Symptoms of a pneumothorax should be listed, including shortness of breath and unilateral pleuritic chest pain, and the patient should be given specific instructions about what to do if these symptoms occur. The patient is advised not to take public transportation home, except taxicabs, and must spend the night with a family member or friend in attendance. If a substantial pneumothorax is present, the patient is warned not to fly or travel to high-altitude areas for several days, the length of time depending on the pneumothorax size. If any particular concerns are present, the patient may return for a follow-up radiograph the next day.

Naturally, the decision to discharge a patient, as opposed to admitting for observation or treatment, is dependent on the condition of the patient, home situation, and home location. Only those who could tolerate a larger pneumothorax, have a responsible family, and live reasonably close to a medical facility are candidates for discharge with other than a trivial pneumothorax.

I do not generally discuss the biopsy findings with the patient, because preliminary and final pathologic results are not always the same and because the primary physician has presumably built a long-term relationship with the patient and can more appropriately convey what is often bad news while at the same time propose a plan of treatment and answer questions. It is certainly important, however, for the radiologist to inform both patient and referring physician of any complications that occur, as well any factors, such as suboptimal needle placement, which affect the quality of the specimen and thus the reliability of the biopsy results.

CONCLUSION

Lung biopsy is a procedure with a distinct learning curve. I try new techniques and learn from mistakes on a daily basis. The above recommendations have been put together over many years and are meant to be used together as a unified program for lung biopsy. Some may be unnecessary. A few, when used together, may produce an effect greater than the sum of their parts. This program, applied to a mix of primarily parenchymal biopsies and occasional mediastinal biopsies in a patient population heavily weighted toward primary lung malignancy, consistently yields complication rates of approximately 12% pneumothorax, 1% chest tube placement, and 4%–5% hemoptysis. I suspect that a small further reduction in the pneumothorax rate may be possible with further improvements in needle configuration.

To summarize, in my opinion, the most important features of a lung biopsy program are anticipation of and preparation for complications, patient education and involvement, selection of the most normal puncture site possible with use of high-resolution CT, a single pleural puncture coaxial technique with a needle type appropriate for the suspected diagnosis, uncompromising needle-tip positioning within the lesion, immediate cytologic evaluation, blood patch placement, immediate postbiopsy puncture-site-down positioning, and pressure precautions. With the exception of on-site cytologic examination, none of these items contribute substantially to the cost of the procedure. Indeed, since complications requiring hospital admission are very expensive, use of this comprehensive program may result in overall cost savings.

References

1. Fish GD, Stanley JH, Miller KS, Schabel SI, Sutherland SE. Postbiopsy pneumothorax: estimating the risk by chest radiography and pulmonary function tests. AJR 1988; 150:71–74.
2. Quon D, Fong TC, Mellor J, Brandschwei FH, Desautels JEL. Pulmonary function testing in predicting complications from

percutaneous lung biopsy. J Can Assoc Radiol 1988; 39:267–269.
3. García-Río F, Pino JM, Casadevall J, et al. Use of spirometry to predict risk of pneumothorax in CT-guided needle biopsy of the lung. J Comput Assist Tomogr 1996; 20:20–23.
4. Kazerooni EA, Hartker FW, Whyte RI, Martinez FJ, Lynch JP. Transthoracic needle aspiration in patients with severe emphysema. Chest 1996; 109:616–619.
5. Wallace JM, Batra P, Gong H, Ovenfors C. Percutaneous needle lung aspiration for diagnosing pneumonitis in the patient with acquired immunodeficiency syndrome (AIDS). Am Rev Resir Dis 1985; 131:389–392.
6. Katada K, Kato R, Anno H, et al. Guidance with real-time CT fluoroscopy: early clinical experience. Radiology 1996; 200: 851–856.
7. Chen C, Hsu W, Huang C, Hsu J, Chiang C. Ultrasound-guided fine needle aspiration biopsy of small pulmonary nodules abutting to the chest wall. Chin Med J (Taipei) 1996; 57:106–111.
8. Protopapas Z, White CS, Miller BH, Miller DL, Westcott JL. Transthoracic needle biopsy practices: results of a nationwide survey (abstr). Radiology 1996; 201(P): 270–271.
9. Greene R. Transthoracic needle aspiration biopsy. In: Athanasoulis CA, ed. Interventional radiology. Philadelphia, Pa: Saunders, 1982; 587–634.
10. Moore EH, Shelton DK, Wisner ER, Richardson ML, Bishop DM, Brock JM. Needle aspiration lung biopsy: reevaluation of the blood patch technique in an equine model. Radiology 1995; 196:183–186.
11. Sinner WN. Complications of percutaneous transthoracic needle aspiration biopsy. Acta Radiol (Diagn)(Stockh) 1976; 17:813–828.
12. Klein JS, Salomon G, Stewart EA. Transthoracic needle biopsy with a coaxially placed 20-gauge automated cutting needle: results in 122 patients. Radiology 1996; 198:715–720.
13. Boiselle PM, Shepard JO, Mark EJ, Szyfelbein WM, Halpern EF, McLoud TC. Utility and safety of routine automated cutting needle core biopsy in thoracic lesions (abstr). Radiology 1996; 201(P):270.
14. Poe RH, Kallay MC, Wicks CM, Odoroff C. Predicting risk of pneumothorax in needle biopsy of the lung. Chest 1984; 85: 232–235.
15. Kazerooni EA, Lim FT, Mikhail A, Martinez FJ. Risk of pneumothorax in CT-guided transthoracic needle aspiration biopsy of the lung. Radiology 1996; 198: 371–375.
16. Miller KS, Fish GB, Stanley JH, Schabel SI. Prediction of pneumothorax rate in percutaneous needle aspiration of the lung. Chest 1988; 93:742–745.
17. Li H, Boiselle PM, Shepard JO, Trotman-Dickenson B, McLoud TC. Diagnostic accuracy and safety of CT-guided percutaneous needle aspiration biopsy of the lung: comparison of small and large pulmonary nodules. AJR 1996; 167:105–109.
18. de Geer G, Gamsu G, Klein JS. Pneumothorax rate following fine needle aspiration biopsy of the lung: influence of patient position (abstr). Radiology 1989; 173(P):277.
19. Zidulka A, Braidy TF, Rizzi M, Shiner RJ. Position may stop pneumothorax progression in dogs. Am Rev Respir Dis 1982; 126:51–53.
20. Moore EH, Shepard JO, McLoud TC, Templeton PA, Kosiuk JP. Positional precautions in needle aspiration lung biopsy. Radiology 1990; 175:733–735.
21. Moore EH, Leblanc J, Montesi SA, Richardson ML, Shepard JO, McLoud TC. Effect of patient positioning after needle aspiration lung biopsy. Radiology 1991; 181: 385–387.
22. Hamarti LB, Austin JHM. Complications after CT-guided needle biopsy through aerated versus nonaerated lung. Radiology 1991; 181:778.
23. Kandallu K, Grant TH, Stull MA, Chambliss JF Jr. Percutaneous needle biopsy of mediastinal and pulmonary masses with a CT guided extrapleural approach (abstr). Radiology 1996; 201(P):270.
24. Belfiore G, Camera L, Moggio G, Vetrani A, Fraioli G, Salvatore M. Middle mediastinum lesions: preliminary experience with CT-guided fine-needle aspiration biopsy with a suprasternal approach. Radiology 1997; 202:870–873.
25. Bressler EL, Kirkham JA. Mediastinal masses: alternative approaches to CT-guided needle biopsy. Radiology 1994; 191:391–396.
26. Tanaka J, Sonomura T, Shioyama Y, et al. "Oblique path": the optimal needle path for computed tomography–guided biopsy of small subpleural lesions. Cariovasc Intervent Radiol 1996; 19:332–334.
27. Stern EJ, Webb WR, Gamsu G. CT gantry tilt: utility in transthoracic fine-needle aspiration biopsy. Radiology 1993; 187: 873–874.
28. Yankelevitz DF, Davis SD, Chiarella D, Henschke CI. Needle tip repositioning during computed-tomography-guided transthoracic needle aspiration biopsy of small deep pulmonary lesions: minor adjustments make a big difference. J Thorac Imaging 1996; 11:279–282.
29. Yankelevitz DF, Hayt D, Henschke CI. Transthoracic needle biopsy: what size syringe? Clin Imaging 1995; 19:208–209.
30. Austin JHM, Cohen MB. Value of having a cytopathologist present during percutaneous fine-needle aspiration biopsy: report of 55 cancer patients and metaanalysis of the literature. AJR 1993; 160:175–177.
31. Vine HS, Kasdon EJ, Simon M. Percutaneous lung biopsy using the Lee needle and a track-obliterating technique. Radiology 1982; 144:921–922.
32. McCartney R, Tait D, Stilson M, Seidel GF. A technique for the prevention of pneumothorax in pulmonary aspiration biopsy. AJR 1974; 120:872–875.
33. Bourgouin PM, Shepard JO, McLoud TC, Spizarny DL, Dedrick CG. Transthoracic needle aspiration biopsy: evaluation of the blood patch technique. Radiology 1988; 166:93–95.
34. Suprenant EL. Transthoracic needle aspiration biopsy: evaluation of the blood patch technique (letter). Radiology 1988; 168:285.
35. Herman SJ, Weisbrod GL. Usefulness of the blood patch technique after transthoracic needle aspiration biopsy. Radiology 1990; 176:395–397.
36. Engeler CE, Hunter DW, Castaneda-Zuniga W, Tashjian JH, Yedlicka JW, Amplatz KA. Pneumothorax after lung biopsy: prevention with transpleural placement of compressed collagen foam plugs. Radiology 1992; 184:787–789.
37. Hill RC, DeCarlo DP, Hill JF, Beamer MS, Hill ML, Timberlake GA. Resolution of experimental pneumothorax in rabbits by oxygen therapy. Ann Thorac Surg 1995; 59:825–828.
38. Barr J, Lushkov G, Starinsky R, Klin B, Berkovitch M, Eshel G. Heliox therapy for pneumothorax: new indication for an old remedy. Ann Emerg Med 1997; 30: 159–161.
39. Yankelevitz DF, Davis SD, Henschke CI. Aspiration of a large pneumothorax resulting from transthoracic needle biopsy. Radiology 1996; 200:695–697.
40. Perlmutt LM, Braun SD, Newman GE, et al. Transthoracic needle aspiration: use of a small chest tube to treat pneumothorax. AJR 1987; 148:849–851.
41. Conces DJ, Tarver RD, Gray WC, Pearcy EA. Treatment of pneumothoraces utilizing small caliber chest tubes. Chest 1988; 94:55–57.
42. Aberle DR, Gamsu G, Golden J. Fatal systemic arterial air embolism following lung needle aspiration. Radiology 1987; 165:351–353.
43. Westcott JL. Air embolism complicating percutaneous needle biopsy of the lung. Chest 1973; 63:108–110.
44. Pereira P. A fatal case of cerebral artery gas embolism following fine needle biopsy of the lung. Med J Aust 1993; 159:755–757.

Donna G. Blankenbaker, MD

The Luftsichel Sign[1]

APPEARANCE

The luftsichel sign may be seen on posteroanterior chest radiographs obtained in patients with left upper lobe collapse (1). The sign manifests as a paraaortic crescent of hyperlucency with sharp margins that extend anywhere from the apex of the left hemithorax to the left superior pulmonary vein (Fig 1) and outline the medial aspect and sometimes the upper aspect of the opaque collapsed left upper lobe.

EXPLANATION

The luftsichel (*luft* is the German word for *air,* and *sichel* is that for *sickle*) sign represents the hyperexpanded superior segment of the left lower lobe interposed between the atelectatic left upper lobe and the aortic arch. The luftsichel sign is a clue to the diagnosis of left upper lobe collapse. As the left upper lobe collapses, it moves anteriorly and superiorly to lie against the anterior chest wall, with the hyperexpanded left lower lobe located behind the upper lobe (2) (Fig 2). The left pulmonary artery, left upper lobe bronchus, and left superior pulmonary vein anchor the collapsed lobe (3). The superior segment of the left lower lobe expands upward to the apex of the left hemithorax and is positioned medially between the mediastinum and the collapsed left upper lobe, thus producing the luftsichel sign. The appearance and extent of the luftsichel depend on the severity of the collapse. The inferior and medial extents of the luftsichel are delineated by the left superior pulmonary vein (2).

Computed tomographic (CT) scans of left upper lobe collapse show a homogeneous opacity that extends from the anterior chest wall to the mediastinum. The posterior margin of the collapsed lobe (major fissure) has a V-shaped contour extending from the apex of the collapsed lobe to the hilum (3). The hyperexpanded superior segment of the left lower lobe is positioned between the collapsed lobe and the aortic arch, explaining the luftsichel (3) (Fig 3).

Index terms:
Lung, collapse, 64.748
Lung, CT, 64.1211
Lung, radiography, 64.11

Radiology 1998; 208:319–320

[1] From the Department of Radiology, University of Wisconsin, 600 Highland Ave, Madison, WI 53792. Received December 12, 1997; revision requested January 20, 1998; revision received February 25; accepted April 6. **Address reprint requests to** the author.

DISCUSSION

The luftsichel is a well-documented radiographic sign seen on the images obtained in patients with collapse of the left upper lobe. This paraaortic area of hyperlucency was once thought to represent a herniated anterior part of the right lung that is compensating for the loss of volume in the left hemithorax. However, careful evaluation of the radiographic anatomy and correlation with bronchographic and CT findings clearly demonstrate that expansion of the superior segment of the left lower lobe accounts for this finding (3). The appearance of left upper lobe collapse is different from that of right upper lobe collapse, because the right lung is divided into three lobes and the left lung is divided into two. There is usually no minor fissure in the left lung.

The luftsichel sign can be right- or left-sided, but it is typically a left-sided phenomenon (1). In left upper lobe collapse, the major fissure is displaced anteriorly and parallels the anterior chest wall on the lateral radiograph. The left upper lobe collapses against the mediastinum anteromedially and can obliterate the left cardiac border on the posteroanterior chest radiograph. The volume loss in the left hemithorax results in posterior and leftward rotation of the heart. On the posteroanterior radiograph, the collapsed lobe produces a hazy opacification that is distributed about the hilar area and that fades superiorly, laterally, and inferiorly (2). The left hilum is elevated, and the left main bronchus has a nearly horizontal course.

This paraaortic area of hyperlucency should not be mistaken for a herniation of the right lung across the midline. When the right lung herniates, it does so anteriorly, behind the manubrium and body of the sternum. This results in a leftward displacement of the anterior junction line. Because of leftward displacement, the line does not contact the aortic arch (2). A medial pneumothorax should not be mistaken for a luftsichel sign when other associated signs of left upper lobe collapse are recognized.

Recognition of the luftsichel sign as a finding of left upper lobe collapse is important in the adult patient, because the

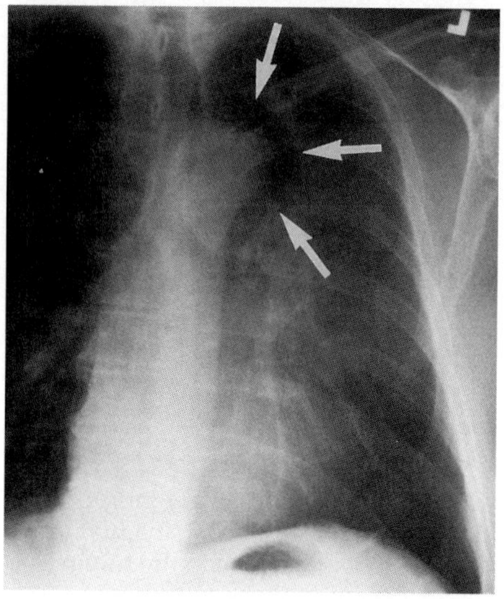

Figure 1. Posteroanterior chest radiograph obtained in a 67-year-old man shows left upper lobe collapse. The paraaortic area of hyperlucency, the luftsichel sign (arrows), represents the hyperexpanded superior segment of the left lower lobe, which is situated between the atelectatic left upper lobe and the aortic arch.

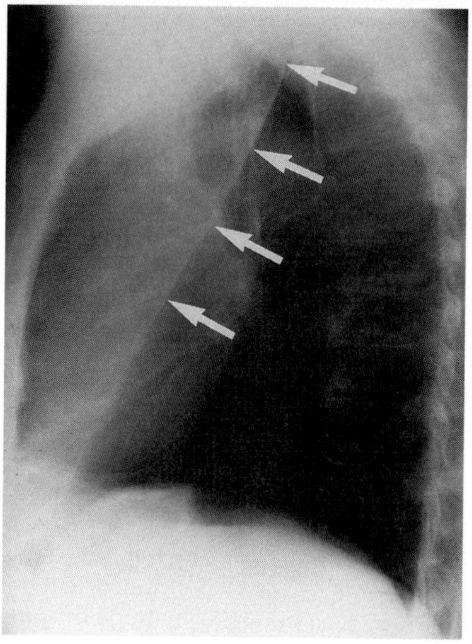

Figure 2. Lateral chest radiograph obtained in the same patient as in Figure 1 shows left upper lobe collapse, with anterior displacement of the major fissure (arrows) and retrosternal opacification. The hyperexpanded left lower lobe is located behind the upper lobe, and the superior segment of the lower lobe extends to the apex of the chest.

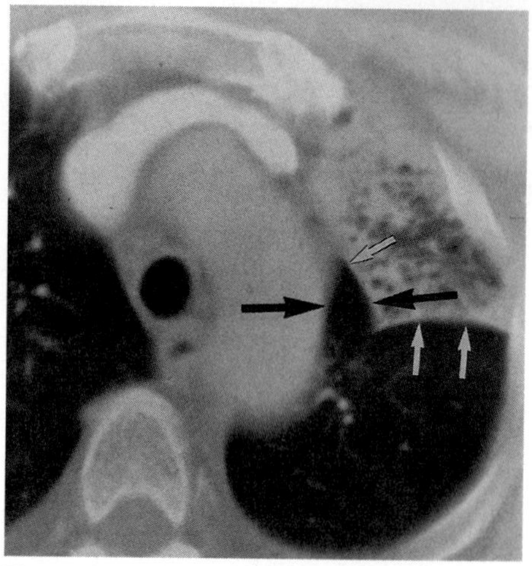

Figure 3. CT scan obtained in the same patient as in Figure 1 helps to confirm medial interposition of the hyperexpanded superior segment of the left lower lobe (black arrows) between the aortic arch and the collapsed left upper lobe. The white arrows outline the medial and posterior aspects of the opaque collapsed left upper lobe.

cause of the collapse may be due to an endobronchial neoplasm.

Acknowledgment: I wish to thank Jannette Collins, MD, MEd, for assistance in editing.

References

1. Webber M, Davies P. The luftsichel: an old sign in upper lobe collapse. Clin Radiol 1991; 32:271–275.
2. Proto AV, Tocino I. Radiographic manifestations of lobar collapse. Semin Roentgenol 1980; 15:117–173.
3. Khoury MB, Godwin D, Halvorson RA, Putman CE. CT of obstructive lobar collapse. Invest Radiol 1985; 20:708–716.

Airway Hyperreactivity: Assessment with Helical Thin-Section CT[1]

Jonathan G. Goldin, MD, PhD
Michael F. McNitt-Gray, PhD
Steven M. Sorenson, MD
Timothy D. Johnson, MS
Beth Dauphinee, RT
Eric C. Kleerup, MD
Donald P. Tashkin, MD
Denise R. Aberle, MD

Index terms:
Asthma, 67.754
Bronchi, CT, 67.12111, 67.12115, 67.12118
Bronchi, stenosis or obstruction, 67.55, 67.754
Computed tomography (CT), helical, 67.12115, 67.12118
Computed tomography (CT), thin-section, 67.12118

Radiology 1998; 208:321–329

Abbreviations:
FEV_1 = forced expiratory volume at 1 second
FEV_3 = forced expiratory volume at 3 seconds
FRC = functional residual capacity
RV = residual volume

[1] From the Depts of Radiological Sciences (J.G.G., M.F.M.G., S.M.S., T.D.J., D.R.A.) and Critical Care and Pulmonary Medicine (B.D., E.C.K., D.P.T.), UCLA School of Medicine, 10833 Le Conte Ave, B2-168 CHS, Los Angeles, CA 90095-1721. Received Sep 25, 1997; revision requested Nov 25; revision received Feb 17, 1998; accepted Apr 3. Supported by Cigarette and Tobacco Surtax Fund of State of California through Tobacco-Related Disease Research Program of University of California, grant 2RT0081; NCI grant PHS P01 CA-51198-06; and Kodak Research Fellowship, England. **Address reprint requests to** J.G.G.

Author contributions:
Guarantor of integrity of entire study, J.G.G.; study concepts, J.G.G., D.R.A.; study design, J.G.G., D.P.T., D.R.A.; definition of intellectual content, J.G.G., D.R.A.; literature research, J.G.G.; clinical studies, J.G.G., E.C.K., M.F.M.G., D.P.T., D.R.A.; data acquisition, J.G.G., M.F.M.G., S.M.S., B.D.; data analysis, J.G.G., T.D.J., M.F.M.G., D.R.A.; statistical analysis, J.G.G., T.D.J.; manuscript preparation, J.G.G., D.R.A.; manuscript editing and review, D.P.T., D.R.A.

PURPOSE: To determine the accuracy of helical computed tomography (CT) for assessing reversible changes in bronchial size and air trapping due to airway hyperreactivity.

MATERIALS AND METHODS: Spirometry and helical CT were performed in 15 patients with mild asthma and six healthy control subjects before and after bronchial provocation with methacholine chloride and after reversal of provocation with albuterol. CT was performed at suspended functional residual capacity and at residual volume in two lung regions (above and below the carina). Bronchial area and lung attenuation measurements were compared.

RESULTS: At baseline, lung attenuation frequency distribution curves were similar between the control and asthma groups. After methacholine, control subjects showed a decrease of less than 10% in the forced expiratory volume at 1 second (FEV_1) and no significant differences in lung attenuation curves. Patients with asthma showed a 20%–36% decrease in FEV_1, with significant decreases in the median and lowest 10th percentile regions of the attenuation curves and in the cross-sectional area of small (<5-mm^2) airways ($P < .001$ for all comparisons). After albuterol, control subjects showed no change in spirometric measurements, lung attenuation, or bronchial size, whereas all such parameters returned to baseline levels in patients with asthma.

CONCLUSION: Functional helical CT can accurately demonstrate reversible airflow obstruction resulting from airway hyperreactivity.

Airway reactivity refers to the degree of reversible constriction of airways in response to bronchial provocation. It is well known (1–9) that heightened airway reactivity can contribute substantially to the morbidity and mortality of obstructive airway diseases, including asthma, chronic bronchitis, emphysema, bronchiectasis, and cystic fibrosis. Airway hyperreactivity is a cardinal feature of asthma (5,10–13) and has been demonstrated in some cohorts before the clinical expression of asthma. Some data suggest that long-term bronchodilator therapy or other pharmacologic suppression of airway hyperreactivity may retard the decline of lung function in affected individuals (14–18), although conflicting results have more recently been published (7).

Airway reactivity can be assessed directly by measuring airflow obstruction induced by means of bronchial provocation or indirectly by measuring improvements in expiratory airflow obstruction after the use of a bronchodilator (11,16,17,19–21). The peak expiratory flow rate and forced expiratory volume in one second (FEV_1) are the most commonly performed measures of reversible expiratory airflow obstruction, but they primarily reflect the function of large airways. Measurements of small airways function, such as the forced expiratory flow over the middle half of the forced expiratory curve, or FEF_{25-75}, and the forced expiratory flow volume at 3 seconds (FEV_3), are also abnormal in patients with airflow obstruction; these measurements are highly variable, however, and their use is limited (22). Pulmonary function tests are also inconsistently related to symptoms in patients with fixed or reversible airflow obstruction (23). Moreover, virtually all measures of airway function derive from global tests reflecting the composite function of the lungs.

Such measures can neither express the regional heterogeneity of bronchial reactivity and airflow obstruction nor localize the distribution or the generations of airways involved. Finally, it may not be possible to use conventional pulmonary function tests to distinguish between the various physiologic aberrations contributing to expiratory airflow obstruction such as bronchial wall edema, mucous hypersecretion, and airway hyperreactivity.

Thin-section computed tomography (CT) is an established technique for the detailed evaluation of the lung parenchyma and can characterize individual anatomic details of the lung as small as 200–300 μm in size. With respect to the airways, this corresponds to bronchi with a wall thickness of roughly 200 μm and a diameter of 2 mm or larger, which represents the proximal seventh to ninth airway generations (24–27). Changes in airway morphology at the bronchiolar (microscopic) level cannot be directly visualized on thin-section CT scans; however, the air trapping that results from bronchiolar disease is indirectly reflected by abnormal decreases in lung attenuation (28), called the mosaic pattern of lung attenuation. In the context of the phase of respiration and the physiologic state of the patient, quantitative changes in bronchopulmonary morphology identified at thin-section CT may advance our understanding of the specific sites and various factors contributing to airflow obstruction (29).

The aim of this investigation was to determine the accuracy of helical thin-section CT studies acquired at standardized lung volumes and under defined physiologic conditions for the assessment of airway hyperreactivity in patients with asthma on the basis of measurable changes in airway diameters and lung attenuation.

MATERIALS AND METHODS

Twenty-one subjects, six of whom were healthy (six men; mean age, 35 years; age range, 34–36 years) and 15 of whom had a clinical diagnosis of mild asthma (13 men, two women; mean age, 38 years; age range, 18–42 years), were recruited from the Pulmonary Medicine Clinic at the University of California, Los Angeles. Subjects were classified according to established clinical and functional criteria (30–32). Only subjects in whom the course of disease had been stable for at least 1 year were eligible for participation. Healthy, age-matched volunteers without a history of asthma or other pulmonary disorders were recruited from the staff of the medical center at our institution to serve as control subjects. Informed consent was obtained from all participants according to the protocol approved by our institutional review board. The entire experimental protocol is summarized in Figure 1.

1) Questionnaire	- Demographic - Cardiorespiratory Symptom Screen - Adverse respiratory health exposure screen - Asthma severity grade		
2) Lung Function Tests	- Screening spirometry - Baseline Full Methacholine Challenge Test - Limited Methacholine Challenge During Functional Study		
3) Functional Imaging Protocol			
STATE	SEQUENCE*		LOCATION
Baseline	FRC**	Scout	
	FRC	3 mm pitch 1	upper† and lower‡
	RV**	Scout	
	RV	3 mm pitch 1	upper and lower
Post methacholine	FRC	Scout	
	FRC	3 mm pitch 1	upper and lower
	RV	Scout	
	RV	3 mm pitch 1	upper and lower
Post bronchodilator	RV	3 mm pitch 1	upper and lower

Figure 1. Chart shows the functional study protocol. For the CT sequences (*), lung volumes were determined with simultaneous flow-volume loops. The upper zone of scanning (†) was centered 2 cm above the carina and spanned 20 mm. The lower zone of scanning (‡) was centered 3 cm below the carina and spanned 30 mm. ** indicates that FRC = functional residual capacity and RV = residual volume.

All subjects completed a demographic and respiratory questionnaire modified from the American Thoracic Society Division of Lung Disease respiratory questionnaire (30). The questionnaire was completed in the presence of personnel experienced in its administration. Subjects were excluded if they were not lifelong nonsmokers, had adverse respiratory conditions other than asthma, or had one or more of the following: cancer, recent myocardial infarction, angina pectoris, systemic hypertension, insulin-dependent diabetes mellitus, acromegaly, pregnancy, or a history of excessive alcohol use (25 or more drinks per week).

Baseline spirometry and a standardized methacholine chloride challenge were performed in the Pulmonary Function Research Laboratory at our institution. Subjects were asked to omit short-acting inhaled medications on the morning of their tests and longer-acting oral or inhaled agents 24–48 hours before the tests. Timed spirometry during a forced expiratory maneuver from total lung capacity to residual volume (RV) was performed with a Pulmoscreen spirometer (S & M Instrument, Doylestown, Pa), with calculation of the forced vital capacity, FEV_1 and FEV_3. All maneuvers and equipment conformed to American Thoracic Society recommendations (33).

A standardized methacholine challenge test (16,34) was used to confirm the clinical diagnosis of asthma. The subjects and patients first inhaled nebulized 0.9% saline followed by incremental concentrations of methacholine chloride to a maximum concentration of 25 mg methacholine per milliliter (mg/mL) of solution. Spirometry was performed after the administration of saline and each concentration of methacholine. The test was stopped after inhalation of a maximum methacholine concentration of 25 mg/mL or after the lowest concentration that produced a decrease in the FEV_1 of 20% or greater from the post–saline inhalation baseline value (ie, the 20% provocation concentration). The 20% provocation concentration of methacholine was recorded for use in subsequent physiologic imaging tests.

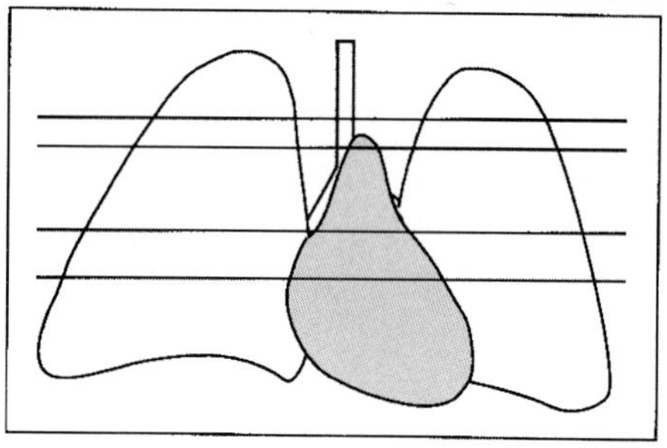

Figure 2. Schematic representation of the image location protocol. The upper zone (top pair of horizontal lines) was centered 2 cm above the carina and spanned 20 mm. The lower zone (bottom pair of horizontal lines) was centered 3 cm below the carina and spanned 30 mm.

Helical thin-section CT was performed within 24 hours of the pulmonary function tests by using a HiSpeed Advantage scanner (GE Medical Systems, Milwaukee, Wis) with a technique of 120 kVp, 300 mA, 3-mm beam collimation, and 3-mm/sec table increment (pitch of 1.0). Imaging sequences were performed at

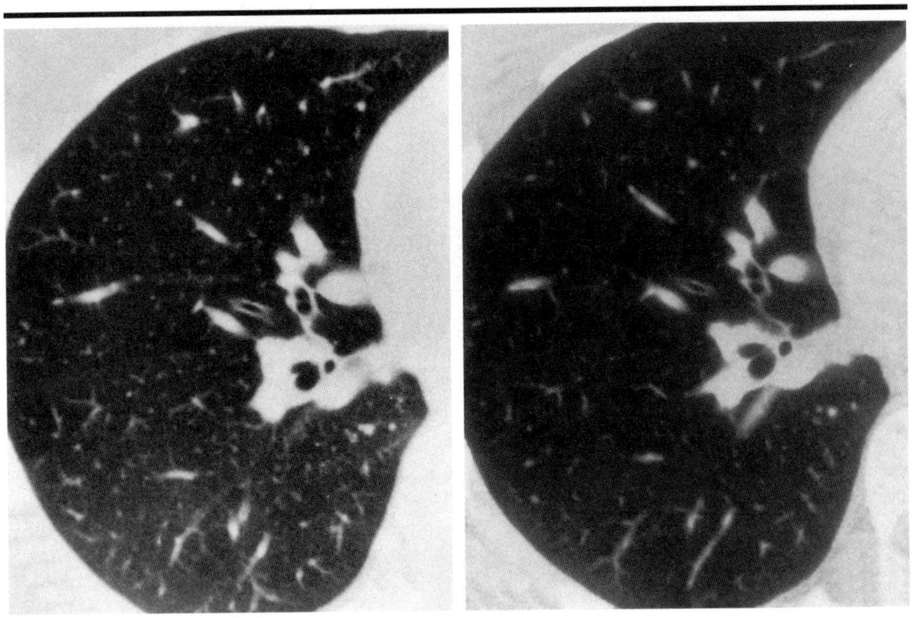

a. b.

Figure 3. CT images demonstrate bronchial segmentation through the visible airways of a patient with mild asthma (36-year-old man) at suspended functional RV **(a)** at baseline and **(b)** after the methacholine challenge. Thin-section images obtained at the same level (inferior bronchial veins) demonstrate a slight increase in airway diameter in **b** relative to the diameter in **a.** Bronchial areas and changes in bronchial areas between the baseline and bronchial provocation sequences are automatically calculated after semiautomated contouring.

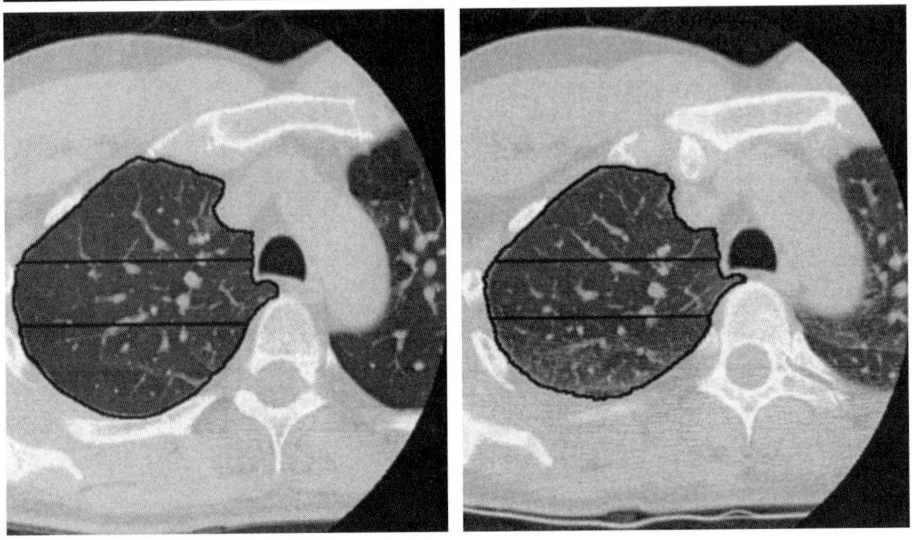

a. b.

Figure 4. In a healthy control subject (36-year-old man), **(a)** inspiratory and **(b)** expiratory CT images at the same anatomic level of the right upper lobe demonstrate relatively homogeneous, increasing lung attenuation from the nondependent to the dependent parts of the lung. Expiratory images exaggerate this gradient. By using a semiautomated segmentation program, the lung parenchyma was segmented and divided into three area-equivalent regions that corresponded to nondependent, middle, and dependent parenchyma. Lung attenuation measures from the entire cross section or from these individual zones provide the basis for the frequency distribution curves of lung attenuation.

two levels of breath hold corresponding to functional residual capacity (FRC) and RV. These levels were chosen to enable bronchial measurements made at the resting end-expired volume (ie, the FRC), at which time the elastic forces of the lung and chest wall are physiologically balanced and are at the optimal volume for the demonstration of air-trapping (ie, the RV). Images were acquired in single-volume data sets of 6–10 seconds through each of two anatomic regions of interest (Figs 1, 2). Digital scout views obtained at both FRC and RV were used to localize the two anatomic regions of interest, which were centered 2 cm above and 3 cm below the carina, respectively.

A limited methacholine challenge test was performed immediately after baseline imaging and consisted of the inhalation of 0.9% saline followed by either the predetermined methacholine 20% provocation concentration or a maximal concentration of 25 mg/mL, depending on the results of the initial standardized challenge test. Before and after the methacholine challenge, the participants underwent spirometry both while sitting and while supine. Immediately after the methacholine challenge, CT of the two anatomic sites was performed at suspended FRC and RV.

Methacholine-induced bronchoconstriction was reversed by means of an aerosolized bronchodilator administered as three inhalations from a metered-dose inhaler β_2 agonist (100 mg albuterol per inhalation; Dey Pharmaceutical, Napa, Calif), with the participant in the supine position. Supine spirometry was performed 15 minutes later to ensure reversal of bronchospasm. During the course of our study, institutional review board approval was obtained to acquire additional postbronchodilator sequences to assess the degree of reversibility. Two control subjects and eight patients with asthma completed postbronchodilator sequences at suspended RV for the optimal visualization of changes in lung attenuation.

From the volumetric data sets, original projection data were used to reconstruct images at 2-mm intervals to optimize the visual registration of anatomic regions between sequences. Images were reconstructed with the high-spatial-frequency bone algorithm by using the smallest field of view possible for the size of the subject and a 512 × 512 matrix. In addition, targeted reconstructions of the right lung were obtained (to limit the effects of cardiac motion); these consisted of (*a*) a 15-cm field of view centered on the central airways and (*b*) a 20–25-cm field of view to encompass the entire cross section of the right lung. All original and reconstructed image data were electronically archived.

Participants were extensively coached

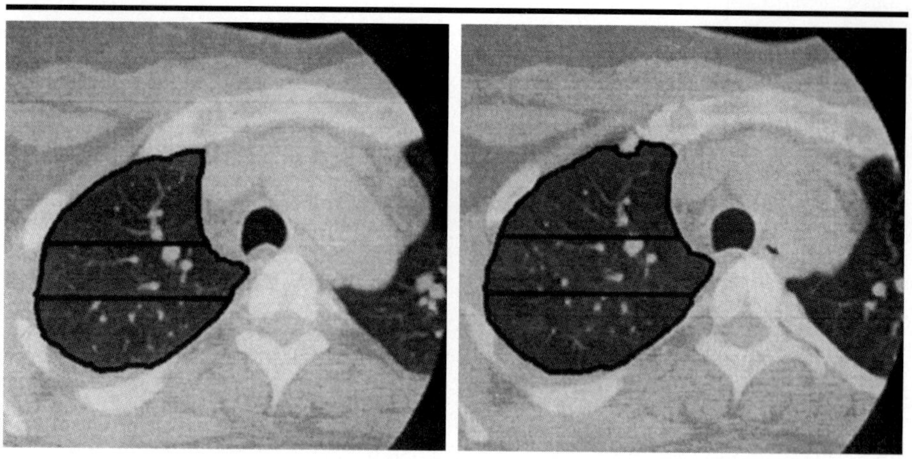

a. b.

Figure 5. Axial CT scans through the right upper lobe in a patient (38-year-old man) with mild asthma were obtained during suspended RV **(a)** at baseline and **(b)** after the methacholine challenge. Lung contouring isolates the right lung and automatically divides the lung into three area-equivalent zones for lung attenuation analysis. After bronchial provocation, there is a global decrease in lung attenuation, which is most obvious in the dependent lung zone. This is also reflected by a leftward shift of the frequency distribution of lung attenuation and is associated with expiratory airflow obstruction at simultaneous spirometry.

TABLE 1
Patient Demographic and Spirometric Data

		Mean Spirometric Value (% predicted)						
		Baseline			After Methacholine		After Bronchodilator*	
Group	Mean Age (y)†	FVC‡	FEV_1	FEV_3	FEV_1	FEV_3	FEV_1	FEV_3
Asthma (n = 15)§	38 (18–42)	90	90	90	67	68	87	89
Healthy (n = 6)‖	35 (34–36)	97	96	98	94	90	96	97

* Postbronchodilator spirometric sequences were performed in two healthy subjects and in eight subjects with asthma.
† Numbers in parentheses are the range.
‡ FVC = forced vital capacity.
§ Group included 13 men and two women.
‖ All subjects were men.

during all spirometric and imaging tests by an experienced pulmonary function technologist to reproduce the forced expiratory maneuver and breath hold at FRC and RV. The reproducibility of the breath-hold volume in all subjects was ensured by using either a computer-assisted inductive plethysmograph (Respitrace; Non-Invasive Monitoring Systems, Miami Beach, Fla) or a volumetric spirometer. Imaging was only completed in subjects able to reproduce spirometric maneuvers to within 10% or 100 mL of their best effort as measured during baseline pulmonary function tests. Subjects remained attached to the spirometer during imaging to detect leakage or a loss of the suspended breath hold.

Quantitative measures of internal airway dimensions and lung attenuation were obtained by using semiautomated image processing routines at a custom-developed Thoracic Radiology Image Analysis and Display, or TRIAD, workstation (35,36) (Figs 3, 4). Comparisons among the five physiologic sequences were made from identical anatomic regions on the basis of visual registration of bronchi and vessels. Bronchial measurements were performed on the targeted reconstructions with the 15-cm field of view of the right lung; lung attenuation measurements were performed on the targeted reconstructions with the 20–25-cm field of view.

Measurements of the internal bronchial area were limited to airways that had a roughly circular cross section on the baseline images (ratio of largest to smallest internal diameters ≤ 1.25). Measurements were recorded for each individual airway. In addition, mean dimensions ± 1 standard deviation were calculated for specific airway generations (lobar, segmental, and subsegmental or higher) and for three categories of macroscopic airway areas corresponding to large (>20-mm²), medium (6–20-mm²), and small (2–5-mm²) airways.

Variations in lung attenuation (as an indirect measure of air trapping) were characterized in two ways: median lung attenuation and the lowest 10th percentile of the frequency distribution. Lung attenuation was assessed on the first image of both the upper and lower anatomic regions obtained at each of the five physiologic conditions. In individuals, lung attenuation parameters were compared by using corresponding axial images from the different physiologic sequences (*a*) at baseline versus after methacholine challenge and (*b*) at baseline versus after bronchodilator use. Averages of the median and 10th percentile values for upper and lower lung regions were compared between the asthma and control groups under each physiologic condition, as were differences in the percentage change from baseline between physiologic conditions. Semiautomated routines divided axial right lung sections into three area-equivalent gravitational zones—anterior (nondependent), middle, and posterior (dependent)—which were intended to correspond roughly to West's (37) three physiologic zones (Fig 5). At any axial level, whole lung as well as regional (gravitational zone) measurements were obtained.

Statistical analysis was performed by using the S-PLUS software package (SAS Institute, Cary, NC). To assess the distribution and validity of the data, univariate analysis was performed to describe the data set and individual subgroups. Group comparisons of the airways were studied with the paired Student *t* test. Because the frequency distributions of lung attenuation were characterized as median values, lung attenuation distributions were analyzed with the Wilcoxon rank sum test (38).

RESULTS

There were no significant differences in age or height between participants in the asthma and control groups. All participants were lifelong nonsmokers and, except for the presence of mild asthma in the symptomatic group, all subjects were healthy (Table 1). No significant differences were found between the pa-

TABLE 2
Lung Attenuation Measures at Baseline and after Methacholine Challenge

Lung Attenuation and Breath-hold Volume	Healthy Group			Asthma Group		
	Baseline (HU)	After Methacholine (HU)	*P* Value*	Baseline (HU)	After Methacholine (HU)	*P* Value*
	Upper Lung Region					
Median lung attenuation						
FRC	−706 (−715 to −693)	−716 (−720 to −698)	.563	−737 (−748 to −725)	−786 (−802 to −744)	.003
RV	−575 (−588 to −559)	−606 (−640 to −581)	.063	−624 (−661 to −598)	−735 (−785 to −702)	.003
Least 10th percentile						
FRC	−789 (−795 to −787)	−800 (−804 to −788)	.536	−801 (−815 to −798)	−840 (−860 to −814)	.001
RV	−687 (−707 to −674)	−726 (−739 to −710)	.063	−735 (−756 to −716)	−811 (−843 to −781)	.007
	Lower Lung Region					
Median lung attenuation						
FRC	−723 (−735 to −710)	−753 (−763 to −729)	.125	−739 (−757 to −734)	−789 (−802 to −749)	.001
RV	−639 (−668 to −601)	−655 (−611 to −642)	.438	−686 (−696 to −644)	−740 (−798 to −718)	.002
Least 10th percentile						
FRC	−818 (−828 to −810)	−831 (−839 to −818)	.645	−837 (−847 to −832)	−837 (−847 to −832)	.010
RV	−760 (−769 to −742)	−759 (−765 to −755)	.688	−793 (−798 to −752)	−817 (−864 to −794)	.005

Note.—Numbers in parentheses are ranges.
* *P* values are for differences in lung attenuation between baseline and after methacholine challenge sequences. *P* values were determined with the one-sided Wilcoxon rank sum test.

TABLE 3
Mean Percentage Change from Baseline in Airway Areas

Size of Visible Airways	Healthy Group (n = 6)		Asthma Group (n = 15)	
	After Methoch####oline	After Bronchodilator	After Methacholine	After Bronchodilator
Small (2–5 mm²)	30*	10	95*	26
Medium (6–20 mm²)	10	10	28	10
Large (>20 mm²)	19	11	32	19

Note.—Measurements were obtained on images obtained at FRC. Numbers are the mean percentage change in bronchial areas of each airway size category from corresponding anatomic levels at baseline.
* Difference in percentage change between the healthy group and the asthma group was significant ($P < .001$).

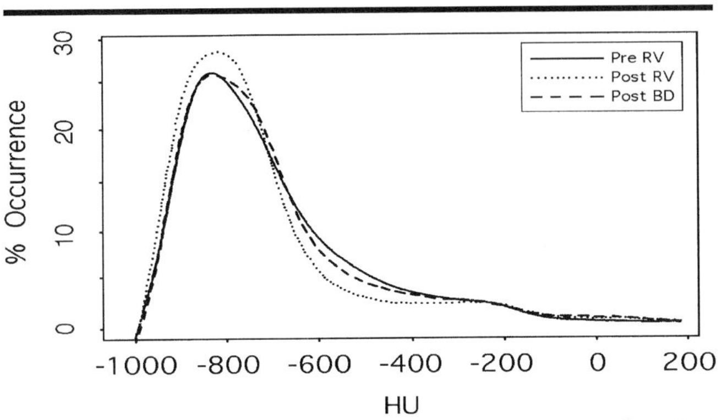

Figure 6. Frequency distribution of lung attenuation numbers in a healthy control subject (36-year-old man) at suspended RV. The data were obtained at baseline, after the methacholine challenge, and after administration of a β_2-agonist bronchodilator (*BD*). There are no statistically significant changes in the character of lung attenuation among the three physiologic states.

tients with asthma and the control subjects in baseline spirometric measures (Table 1). When comparing the median and least 10th percentile of lung attenuation at baseline, the asthma group demonstrated a consistent trend toward lower lung attenuation relative to the normal group, but these differences were not significant ($P > .05$) at either level of breath hold or in either lung region (Table 2).

After the methacholine challenge, the control subjects demonstrated slight, nonsignificant mean decreases of less than 10% in baseline measures of forced vital capacity, FEV_1, and FEV_3 (Table 1). These minor functional changes were associated with no significant change in bronchial areas for any of the three size categories (Table 3) and no demonstrable change in the frequency distributions of lung attenuation (Table 2, Fig 6).

After the methacholine challenge, the patients with asthma demonstrated a significant decrease in mean FEV_1 from 90% to 67% of predicted volume (26% decrease) and in mean FEV_3 from 90% to 68% of predicted volume (24% decrease) (Table 1). These spirometric declines were associated with a 95% decrease in the area of small visible airways relative to the areas at baseline, without significant decreases in the areas of medium or large visible airways. The difference in the percentage change from the baseline area of small airways was significant ($P < .001$) between the control and asthma groups (Table 3). In the patients with asthma, lung attenuation curves after the metha-

TABLE 4
Lung Attenuation Measurements at Baseline and after Bronchodilator Use in Healthy Subjects and Subjects with Asthma

Lung Attenuation and Breath-hold Volume	Asthma Group		Healthy Group	
	Baseline (HU)	After Bronchodilator (HU)	Baseline (HU)	After Bronchodilator (HU)
		Upper Lung		
Median				
FRC	−721 (−748 to −694)	Not applicable	−727 (−757 to −697)	Not applicable
RV	−657 (−678 to −636)	−662 (−680 to −644)	−613 (−632 to −594)	−601 (−621 to −581)
Lowest 10th percentile				
FRC	−806 (−825 to −787)	Not applicable	−809 (−824 to −794)	Not applicable
RV	−763 (−794 to −732)*	−794 (−797 to −791)*	−729 (−762 to −696)	−710 (−726 to −704)
		Lower Lung		
Median				
FRC	−736 (−760 to −712)	Not applicable	−732 (−755 to −709)	Not applicable
RV	−704 (−748 to −660)*	−732 (−761 to −703)*	−672 (−708 to −636)	−642 (−660 to −624)
Lowest 10th percentile				
FRC	−828 (−853 to −803)	Not applicable	−825 (−842 to −808)	Not applicable
RV	−801 (−821 to −781)	−823 (−848 to −798)	−779 (−793 to −765)	−756 (−768 to −744)

Note.—Data are means. Numbers in parentheses are ranges.
* Difference between baseline and after bronchodilator measurements approached significance ($P < .06$).

choline challenge exhibited a leftward shift to lower attenuation, with correspondingly significant ($P < .001$) decreases in both median and least-10th-percentile CT numbers in the upper and lower lung regions (Table 3, Fig 6). These attenuation changes after bronchial provocation were observed at both FRC and RV.

In eight patients with asthma and two control subjects, the bronchodilator was administered after the methacholine challenge, and the subjects were reevaluated with spirometry and imaging. After administration of the β_2 agonist, the control subjects showed no significant change relative to baseline spirometry, bronchial areas, or frequency distributions of lung attenuation (Tables 1, 3, 4). In the asthma group, spirometric measurements returned to nearly baseline values (Table 3), airway areas returned to within 20% of the baseline areas, and the frequency distributions of lung attenuation shifted back to higher attenuation numbers (Table 4). In neither control subjects nor patients with asthma were there significant differences between baseline and post-bronchodilator sequences in terms of spirometric measures, airway areas, or lung attenuation (Tables 3, 4).

DISCUSSION

The results of the present study show the ability of functional thin-section CT to demonstrate the reversible alterations due to airway hyperreactivity in humans. Control subjects and patients with asthma were chosen because they represent two ends of the clinical spectrum of reversible airflow limitation. By using customized image processing routines, alterations in the size of visible airways were directly observed, whereas bronchiolar obstruction and distal air trapping were indirectly assessed on the basis of alterations in lung attenuation.

After methacholine-induced bronchospasm, the greatest airflow obstruction occurred at the bronchiolar level, consistent with previous evidence of the small airways as the predominant site of obstruction in mild asthma (40); this was reflected by the abnormal decreases in lung attenuation. Significant changes in the area of macroscopic airways occurred only in the smallest visible airways. The effects of the reversal of methacholine-induced bronchoconstriction with a bronchodilator were also observed.

Changes in bronchial diameter as a measure of hyperreactivity were first observed at thin-section CT in animal models exposed to aerosolized bronchial stimulants (41–44). In sensitized dogs, considerable heterogeneity in airway reactivity occurred independently of the initial size or location of the airway (42), which underscored the presence of pathophysiologic changes not documented with global pulmonary function tests. More recently, three-dimensional histologic models have quantified differences in airway morphology between patients with airflow obstruction and healthy subjects (27). Unfortunately, these histologic techniques necessitate an invasive procedure to obtain microscopic, bronchiolar anatomic specimens (45–47).

With thin-section CT, only the macroscopic, proximal seventh to ninth airway generations are directly observable. Alterations of the bronchioles cannot be directly visualized, yet these peripheral airways are the major sites of airflow obstruction in asthma and chronic obstructive pulmonary disease (40,48,49). Premature bronchiolar closure has been correlated with alterations in lung attenuation numbers. The attenuation of the lung represents a composite of the individual components of air, soft tissue, and blood and will be affected by changes in any one or more of these components (50). In the interpretation of lung attenuation measurements, the confounding variables of the phase of respiration and lung volume, pulmonary blood volume, and the influence of gravity must be considered.

In the supine human, an increasing gradient of lung attenuation from the nondependent to the dependent lung regions is normally related to the relatively greater perfusion and smaller alveolar size of the dependent lung (51,52). With expiration, the normal lung exhibits increases in attenuation due to a relative decrease in air content within the volume (voxel) of lung tissue being imaged. In conditions of airflow obstruc-

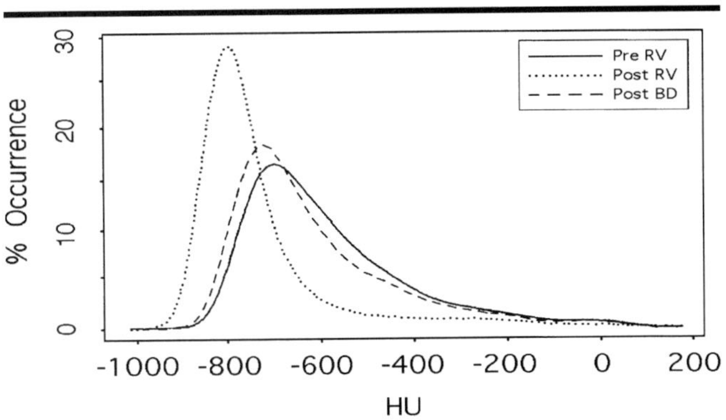

Figure 7. Frequency distributions of lung attenuation in a patient (38-year-old man) with mild asthma at suspended RV obtained during the three physiologic states. After the methacholine challenge, there is a dramatic leftward shift of the frequency distribution of lung attenuation numbers. After bronchodilator (*BD*) administration, the lung attenuation does not completely return to the baseline level.

tion, expiratory air trapping results from expiratory airway narrowing and premature closure. Regions of air trapping are reflected by abnormally low lung attenuation, as well as a failure to decrease in volume relative to normally emptying lung components. If air trapping occurs at the bronchiolar level, decreased lung attenuation may have a mosaic appearance, with alternating areas of normal lobular attenuation. Air trapping due to diffuse bronchiolar or more proximal airway disease may assume subsegmental, segmental, or lobar patterns. These attenuation patterns, particularly if lobular, are exaggerated on expiratory images. Because focal air trapping can be found in healthy subjects, it is the extent of air trapping and not simply its presence that is physiologically relevant (28).

Quantitative measures of air trapping have been shown to provide important information about both the status of the lung parenchyma and the behavior of airways. The distribution of CT numbers within an image can be represented in the form of a frequency distribution of lung attenuation (Figs 6, 7). Some investigators (50,53) have postulated that the area under the curve that represents attenuation of less than −900 HU correlates with intrathoracic gas (without lung tissue) and, when referenced to the specific phase of respiration, is the most sensitive measure of the extent of either emphysematous lung destruction or air trapping due to premature airways closure. The greater the leftward shift of the frequency distribution curve (ie, reflecting a greater proportion of low attenuation), the more extensive the lung destruction due to emphysema and/or air trapping secondary to expiratory airflow obstruction. This correlation is supported by the demonstration of a strong correlation between a threshold of −910 HU and a pathologic assessment of the severity of emphysema (54). Between −900 and −700 HU, strong correlations have been demonstrated with normal values for vital capacity, single-breath diffusing capacity for carbon monoxide, and arterial oxygen saturation during exercise (50).

A number of investigators (53,55–59) have used thin-section CT in vivo to characterize patients with asthma or chronic obstructive pulmonary disease. In patients with the latter disease, Lamers et al (53) used spirometrically gated CT to assess lung attenuation at 10% and 90% of suspended vital capacity. By using lung attenuation numbers and changes in attenuation at these breath-hold levels, they were able to differentiate patients with emphysema, those with chronic bronchitis, and healthy subjects. Similarly, in a prospective study of asymptomatic patients with asthma and nonsmoking healthy subjects, Newman et al (58) compared lung attenuation on conventional CT images with that on thin-section CT images obtained through the lung bases and found that the expiratory mean pixel index (percentage of pixels with attenuation < -900 HU) was significantly higher in patients with asthma. The mean pixel index correlated significantly with pulmonary function measures of airflow obstruction and air trapping, including FEV_1, RV, and FRC.

The accuracy of cross-sectional lung and bronchial measurements and the percentage change in these measurements under different physiologic conditions are key elements of a functional imaging analysis but are influenced by a number of technical factors. Functional observations must be made at the same anatomic location and at strictly specified lung volumes. These are challenging requirements: The same segment of lung can move as much as 2 cm or more in either the cephalocaudal or the transverse direction during the course of a forced expiratory maneuver. Moreover, a given lung region may not move in absolute synchrony with other regions at the same initial axial level. Cardiac position also varies with respiration (60), and cardiac motion can affect regional lung volumes by an amount equivalent to the tidal volume (47).

In the present study, we addressed a number of technical considerations designed to maximize spatial resolution, achieve valid coregistration of anatomy between sequences, and ensure the accuracy of the suspended breath-hold conditions. As in other published studies (25,61), we used visual registration to localize identical axial planes from the different physiologic sequences. A number of potential factors can introduce measurement error in studies of this type. Variations in anatomic registration between different physiologic conditions would be expected to bias results by influencing the calculations of the percentage change in airway areas or lung attenuation. Unless anatomic misregistration occurs systematically, however, such as when comparing lung or bronchial anatomy under a given physiologic condition at a consistently higher (or lower) level, variations might be expected to cancel one another out. Errors in the measure of bronchial size are greatest for airways with the smallest diameter. For this reason, all quantitative airway measures were performed on targeted axial reconstructions with a 15-cm field of view, in which spatial resolution was optimal (0.29×0.29 mm). Moreover, our results were stratified according to bronchial size to isolate potential measurement errors introduced in the measurement of smaller bronchi.

All cross-sectional imaging was registered with simultaneous flow-volume loops to ensure that the image data were a true reflection of the specific breath hold. Imaging at RV was only performed if subjects were able to reproduce their best expiratory effort to within 5%, as defined by the American Thoracic Society guidelines for the standardization of pulmonary function tests (33). Scanning at FRC was performed by using inductive plethysmography or spirometry as a guide to the achievement of the end-tidal expiratory lung volume. We chose suspended FRC for our measurements because this lung volume is more reproducible and requires less exertion than suspended total lung capacity; moreover, at that level, the net forces influencing airway diameter are balanced. Finally, subject training and encouragement by an experienced pulmonary function technologist using the flow-volume loop as visual feedback is essential for quality control in the performance of functional thin-section CT.

Helical CT images were obtained in a single breath hold to reduce motion unsharpness and intrasequence variations introduced by respiratory misregistration. We exploited the volumetric data sets to produce overlapping axial reconstructions that would optimize anatomic registration. Finally, our methods effectively used each subject as his or her own control. Specifically, all measurements obtained after bronchial provocation or bronchodilatation were made relative to baseline spirometric and image data. In this way, variations in absolute values across subjects were minimized. Moreover, the use of each subject and his or her flow-volume loops obtained during rigorously controlled conditions strengthened the premise that measurable differences in visible airways or lung attenuation are related to hyperreactivity and not to inadvertent variations in the level of the suspended breath hold. In our experience, this was critical to the reduction in errors due to breathing inconsistencies.

In conclusion, we designed a relatively robust technique that uses a combination of volumetric thin-section CT, classic flow-volume loops, and semiautomated post-processing tools to assess regional lung function reproducibly and under varying physiologic conditions. This technique provides a direct measure of the changes in macroscopic airways and an indirect measure of the function of regional small airways. Visual inspection of the frequency distribution curve for lung attenuation can be compared with that of the flow-volume loop; moreover, these frequency distribution curves provide information about lung function independent of absolute attenuation numbers.

Our validation of the method in two well-defined groups (healthy subjects and patients with asthma) provides a foundation for future physiologic imaging that may help (*a*) elucidate the separate contributions of physiologic airflow obstruction, structural abnormalities of bronchial morphology, and airway hyperreactivity in asthma and chronic obstructive pulmonary disease; (*b*) identify individuals with potentially important airway hyperreactivity who do not satisfy conventional diagnostic criteria for hyperreactive airways disease but who may benefit from therapeutic intervention; and (*c*) further explore a variety of unexplained phenomena in individuals with obstructive pulmonary disorders (62).

References

1. Ferguson GT, Cherniack RM. Management of chronic obstructive pulmonary disease. N Engl J Med 1993; 328:1017–1022.
2. McFadden ER. Airway responsitivity and chronic obstructive lung disease. In: Cherniack RM, ed. Chronic obstructive pulmonary disease. Philadelphia, Pa: Saunders, 1991; 90–96.
3. Pratter MR, Irwin RS. Is the demonstration of bronchial hyper-reactivity the sine qua non for diagnosing symptomatic bronchial asthma? Allergy Proc 1989; 10: 323–327.
4. Hopp RJ, Townley RG, Biven RE, et al. The presence of airway reactivity before the development of asthma. Am Rev Respir Dis 1990; 141:2–8.
5. Ransdell JW, Nachtwey FJ, Moser KM. Bronchial hyperreactivity in chronic obstructive bronchitis. Am Rev Respir Dis 1982; 128:829–836.
6. Ip M, Lam WK, So SY, et al. Analysis of factors associated with bronchial hyperreactivity to methacholine in bronchiectasis. Lung 1991; 169:43–51.
7. Tashkin DP, Altose MD, Connett JE, Kanner RE, Lee WW, Wise RA. The Lung Health Study Research Group: methacholine reactivity predicts changes in lung function over time in smokers with early COPD. Am J Respir Crit Care Med 1996; 153:1802–1811.
8. Sparrow D, O'Connor G, Weiss ST. The relationship of airway responsiveness and atrophy to the development of chronic obstructive lung disease. Epidemiol Rev 1989; 10:29–47.
9. Josephs LK, Gregg I, Mullee MA, Holgate ST. Nonspecific bronchial reactivity and its relationship to the clinical expression of asthma: a longitudinal study. Am Rev Respir Dis 1989; 140:350–357.
10. Bleecker ER. Airways reactivity and asthma: significance and treatment. J Allergy Clin Immunol 1985; 75:21–24.
11. Parker CD, Bilbo RE, Reed CE. Methacholine aerosol as test for bronchial asthma. Arch Intern Med 1965; 115:452–454.
12. Klein RC, Salvaggio JE. Nonspecificity of the bronchoconstricting effect of histamine and acetyl-beta-methacholine in patients with obstructive airways disease. J Allergy 1966; 37:158–163.
13. McFadden ER, Gilbert IA. Asthma. N Engl J Med 1992; 325:1928–1937.
14. Anthonisen NR, Wright EC. Response to inhaled bronchodilators in COPD. Chest 1987; 5(suppl 5):36S–39S.
15. Postma DS, DeVries K, Koeter GH, Sluiter HJ. Independent influence of reversibility of air-flow obstruction and nonspecific hyperreactivity of the long-term course of lung function in chronic air-flow obstruction. Am Rev Respir Dis 1986; 134:276–280.
16. Townley RG, Bewtra AK, Nair NM, et al. Methacholine inhalation challenge studies. J Allergy Clin Immunol 1979; 64:569–574.
17. Cockcroft DW, Killian DN, Mellon JA, Hargreave FE. Bronchial reactivity to inhaled histamine: a method and clinical survey. Clin Allergy 1977; 7:235–243.
18. James AL, Paré PD, Hogg JC. The mechanics of airway narrowing in asthma. Am Rev Respir Dis 1989; 139:242–246.
19. Jaeschke R, Guyatt GH, Willan A, Cook D, Harper S. Effect of increasing doses of beta agonists on spirometric parameters, exercise capacity, and quality of life in patients with chronic airflow limitation. Thorax 1994; 49:479–484.
20. Deltorre L, Melica EV, Deltorre M. Effectiveness of salmeterol in patients with emphysema. Curr Ther Res 1992; 52:888–898.
21. Palmeiro EM, Hopp RJ, Biven RE, Bewtra AK, Nair NN, Townley RG. Probability of asthma based on methacholine challenge. Chest 1992; 101:630–633.
22. Kamp DW. Physiologic evaluation of asthma. Chest 1992; 101(suppl 6):396S–400S.
23. Mahler DA, Weinberg DH, Wells CK, et al. The measurement of dyspnea: contents, interobserver agreement and physiologic correlates of two new clinical indexes. Chest 1984; 85:751–758.
24. Webb WR. High-resolution CT of the lung parenchyma. Radiol Clin North Am 1989; 27:1085–1097.
25. Klein J, Gamsu G. High-resolution computed tomography of diffuse lung disease. Invest Radiol 1989; 24:805–812.
26. Mathieson JR, Mayo JR, Staples CA, Müller NL. Chronic diffuse infiltrative lung disease: comparison of CT and chest radiography. RadioGraphics 1989; 171:111–116.
27. Murata K, Itoh H, Todo G, et al. Centrilobular lesions of the lung: demonstration by high-resolution CT and pathologic correlation. Radiology 1986; 161:641–645.
28. Stern EJ, Webb WR. Dynamic imaging of lung morphology with ultrafast high-resolution computed tomography. J Thorac Imaging 1993; 8:273–282.
29. Kalender WA, Fichte H, Bautz W, Skalej M. Semiautomatic evaluation procedures for quantitative CT of the lung. J Comput Assist Tomogr 1991; 15:248–255.
30. Ferris BG. Epidemiologic Standardization Project (American Thoracic Society). Am Rev Respir Dis 1978; 118(6 pt 2):1–88.
31. Hargreave FE, Ryan G, Thomson N, et al. Bronchial responsiveness to histamine and methacholine in asthma: measurement and clinical significance. J Allergy Clin Immunol 1981; 68:347–355.
32. Natural Asthma Education Congress. Expert panel report: guidelines for the diagnosis and management of asthma—National Heart, Lung, and Blood Institute. HHS publication no. 91-3042. Washington, DC: U.S. Department of Health and Human Services, 1991.
33. American Thoracic Society. Standardization of spirometry: 1994 update. Am J Respir Crit Care Med 1995; 152:1107–1136.
34. Chai H, Farr RS, Froehlich CA, et al. Standardization of bronchial inhalation challenge procedures. J Allergy Clin Immunol 1975; 56:323–327.
35. McNitt-Gray MF, Johnson TD, Aberle DR. TRIAD: a thoracic radiology image analy-

sis and display workstation. Med Phys 1994; 21:905–907.
36. McNitt-Gray MF, Goldin JG, Johnson TD, Tashkin DP, Aberle DR. Development and testing of image-processing methods for the quantitative assessment of airway hyperresponsiveness from high-resolution CT images. J Comput Assist Tomogr 1997; 21:939–947.
37. West JB. Ventilation/blood flow and gas exchange. 2nd ed. Philadelphia, Pa: Davis, 1970.
38. Lehman EL. Nonparametrics: statistical methods based on ranks. San Francisco, Calif: Holden Day, 1975.
39. Crapo RO, Morris AH, Gardner RM. Reference spirometric volumes using techniques and equipment that meet ATS recommendations. Am Rev Respir Dis 1981; 123:659–664.
40. Wagner EM, Liu MC, Weinmann GG, Permutt S, Bleecher ER. Peripheral lung resistance in normals and asthmatic subjects. Am Rev Respir Dis 1990; 181:584–588.
41. McNamara AE, Müller NL, Okazawa M, Arntorp J, Wiggs BR, Paré PD. Airway narrowing in excised canine lungs measured by high-resolution computed tomography. J Appl Physiol 1992; 73:307–316.
42. Herold CJ, Brown RH, Mitzner W, Links JM, Hirshman CA, Zerhouni EA. Assessment of pulmonary airway reactivity with HRCT. Radiology 1991; 181:368–374.
43. Brown RH, Zerhouni EA, Hirshman CA. Reversal of bronchoconstriction by inhaled nitric oxide: histamine versus methacholine. Am J Respir Crit Care Med 1994; 150:233–237.
44. Brown RH, Herold CJ, Hirshman CA, Zerhouni EA, Mitzner W. Individual airway constrictor response heterogeneity to histamine assessed by high-resolution computed tomography. J Appl Physiol 1993; 74:2615–2620.
45. Stern EJ, Webb WR, Golden JA, Gamsu G. Cystic lung disease associated with eosinophilic granuloma and tuberous sclerosis: air trapping at dynamic ultrafast high-resolution CT. Radiology 1992; 182:325–329.
46. Webb WR, Stern EJ, Kanth N, Gamsu G. Dynamic pulmonary CT: findings in healthy adult men. Radiology 1993; 186: 117–124.
47. Wei JH, Hoffman EA, Ritman EL, et al. Cardiogenic motion of right lung parenchyma in anaesthetized intact dogs. J Appl Physiol 1985; 58:384–391.
48. Macklem PT. Obstruction in small airways: a challenge to medicine. Am J Med 1972; 52:721–723.
49. Cosio MG, Hale KA, Niewoehnet DE. Morphologic and morphometic effects of prolonged cigarette smoking in small airways. Am Rev Respir Dis 1980; 122:265–271.
50. Rienmüller R, Behr J, Kalender WA, et al. Standardized quantitative high-resolution CT in lung diseases. J Comput Assist Tomogr 1991; 15:742–749.
51. Rosenblum LJ, Mauceri RA, Wellenstein DE. Density patterns in the normal lung as determined by computed tomography. Radiology 1980; 137:409–416.
52. Hoffman EA. Interactions of the heart and integrated lungs. In: Sideman S, Beyar R, eds. Interactive phenomena in the cardiac system. Advances in experimental medicine and biology, vol 346. New York, NY: Plenum, 1993; 347–366.
53. Lamers RJ, Thelissen GR, Kessels AG, Wouters EF, van Engelshoven JM. Chronic obstructive pulmonary disease: evaluation with spirometrically controlled CT lung densitometry. Radiology 1994; 193: 109–113.
54. Müller NL, Staples CA, Miller RR, Abboud RT. Density mask: an objective method to quantitate emphysema using computed tomography. Chest 1988; 94:782–787.
55. Aberle DR, Goldin JG, McNitt-Gray MF, Greaves SM, Kleerup E, Tashkin D. High-resolution computed tomography of airway reactivity in asthmatics after bronchoprovocation testing (abstr). Radiology 1994; 193(P):368.
56. Goldin JG, Aberle DR, Matthias PM, et al. Airway hyperreactivity (AHR) using helical HRCT following methacholine bronchoprovocation in asthmatics (abstr). Am Rev Respir Dis 1995; 151:673.
57. Kee ST, Chen D, Webb WR, Golden J. Use of expiratory high-resolution CT in assessing emphysema patients following single lung transplantation (abstr). Radiology 1995; 197(P):438.
58. Newman KB, Lynch DA, Newman LS, Ellegood D, Newell JD Jr. Quantitative computed tomography detects air trapping due to asthma. Chest 1994; 106:105–109.
59. Paganin F, Vignola AM, Seneterre E, Bruel JM, Chanez P, Bousquet J. Heterogeneity of airways obstruction in asthmatic patients using high-resolution computed tomography. Chest 1995; 107(suppl 3): 145S–147S.
60. Stern EJ, Graham CM, Webb WR, Gamsu G. Normal trachea during forced expiration: dynamic CT measurements. Radiology 1993; 187:27-31.
61. Kramer SS, Hoffman EA. Physiologic imaging of the lung with volumetric high-resolution CT. J Thorac Imaging 1995; 10:280–290.
62. Anthonisen NR. Lung Health Study. Am Rev Respir Disease 1989; 140:871–872.

Interlude

Comet Hale-Bopp (C/1995 O1)

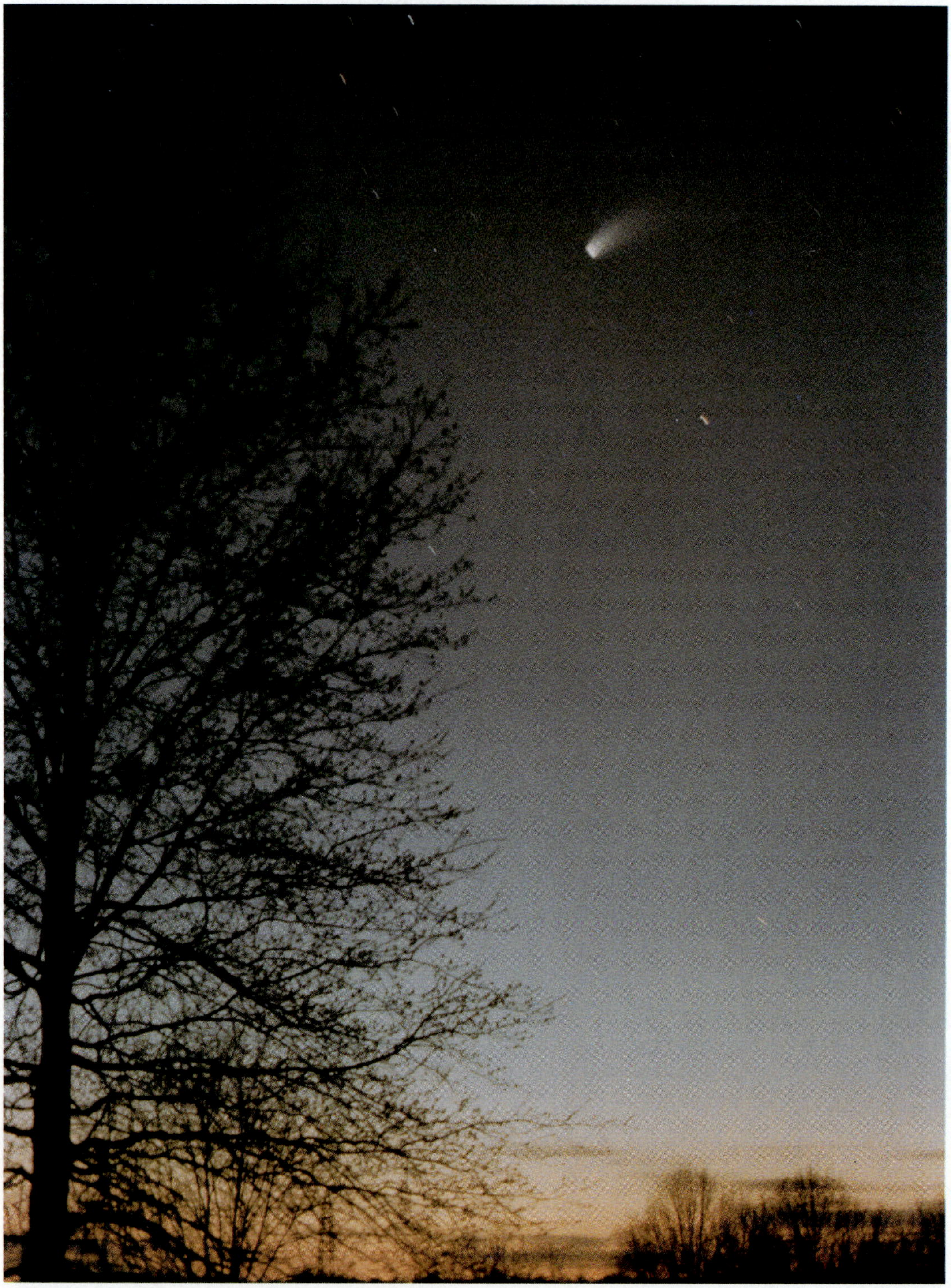

The beauty of the world and the orderly arrangement of everything celestial makes us confess that there is an excellent and eternal nature which ought to be worshiped and admired by all mankind.—Cicero

Photograph by Robert G. Levitt, MD, St Louis, Mo

Polypoid Lesions of Airways: Early Experience with Computer-assisted Detection by Using Virtual Bronchoscopy and Surface Curvature[1]

Ronald M. Summers, MD, PhD
W. Scott Selbie, PhD
James D. Malley, PhD
Lynne M. Pusanik, BSME, MEng
Andrew J. Dwyer, MD
Nikos A. Courcoutsakis, MD
David J. Shaw, MD
David E. Kleiner, MD
Michael C. Sneller, MD
Carol A. Langford, MD, MHS
Steven M. Holland, MD
James H. Shelhamer, MD

Index terms:
Bronchi, CT, 671.12115, 671.12117
Bronchi, neoplasms, 671.30
Computers, diagnostic aid

Radiology 1998; 208:331–337

Abbreviation:
VB = virtual bronchoscopy

[1] From the Diagnostic Radiology Department (R.M.S., L.M.P., A.J.D., N.A.C., D.J.S.) and the Division of Critical Care Medicine (J.H.S.), Warren Grant Magnuson Clinical Center; the Voice and Speech Section, National Institute on Deafness and Other Communication Disorders (W.S.S.), and the Office of the Assistant Director, Division of Computer Research and Technology (J.D.M.), the Laboratory of Pathology (D.E.K.), and the National Institute of Allergies and Infectious Diseases (M.C.S., C.A.L., S.M.H.), National Institutes of Health, Bldg 10, Rm 1C660, 10 Center Dr, MSC 1182, Bethesda, MD 20892-1182. Received September 19, 1997; revision requested November 19; revision received January 7, 1998; accepted February 11. **Address reprint requests to** R.M.S.

Author contributions:
Guarantor of integrity of entire study, R.M.S.; study concepts, R.M.S., W.S.S., J.D.M., A.J.D.; study design, R.M.S.; definition of intellectual content, R.M.S., W.S.S., J.D.M., L.M.P., A.J.D., N.A.C., D.J.S., D.E.K., M.C.S., C.A.L., S.M.H., J.H.S.; literature research, R.M.S., W.S.S.; clinical studies, R.M.S., M.C.S., C.A.L., S.M.H., J.H.S.; experimental studies, R.M.S., N.A.C., D.J.S., D.E.K.; data acquisition, R.M.S., N.A.C., D.J.S; data analysis, R.M.S., J.D.M., L.M.P.; statistical analysis, R.M.S., A.J.D.; manuscript preparation, R.M.S.; manuscript editing, R.M.S., A.J.D.; manuscript review, R.M.S., W.S.S., J.D.M., L.M.P., A.J.D., N.A.C., D.J.S., D.E.K., M.C.S., C.A.L., S.M.H., J.H.S.

PURPOSE: To test the application of a technique developed by the authors for the computer-assisted diagnosis of polypoid airway lesions from surface-rendered virtual bronchoscopic reconstructions.

MATERIALS AND METHODS: A computer algorithm was developed to detect polypoid airway lesions by means of segmentation of the bronchial surface with curvature classification. This method was tested with a bronchial phantom, five cadaveric lung specimens, and virtual bronchoscopic studies in 16 patients.

RESULTS: For the patient studies, the sensitivity and specificity of the method were 47%–88% and 58%–89%, respectively, depending on the value of an adjustable parameter (the mean curvature threshold). The sensitivity increased (by 20% to 34%) when only lesions larger than 5 mm in diameter were considered.

CONCLUSION: With this method, polypoid airway lesions can be detected automatically, although false-positive diagnoses present an important limitation.

Three-dimensional imaging is a well-established method in the diagnosis of diseases of the airway. In conjunction with fiberoptic bronchoscopy, three-dimensional imaging of the airways with computed tomography (CT) has proved to be useful in the detection of tumors, obstructions, strictures, and certain inflammatory lesions (1–4).

Recently, a display method for three-dimensional imaging of the airway has been devised. This method, called virtual bronchoscopy (VB), involves the use of perspective surface or volume rendering to allow endoscopic-like visualization of the airway (5–7). These reports suggest that this method may be useful for clinical diagnosis, for guidance during interventional procedures, and for medical education and training.

Evaluation of an entire VB examination is time-consuming, however, and lesions may be overlooked due to observer fatigue. We have therefore devised a method for computer-assisted diagnosis that allows automatic detection of polypoid lesions of the airway on surface-rendered VB studies. This method is based on a surface curvature classification, with detection of a mean curvature that is characteristic of polypoid lesions. Our purpose was to describe the method, determine its validity for simulated elemental surfaces, and apply it in an airway phantom, cadaveric specimens, and studies in patients.

MATERIALS AND METHODS

Background

When a radiologist examines the airways on a CT scan, he or she identifies potential lesions primarily on the basis of the shape of the lesion (other features that may also be important include attenuation or contrast material enhancement of the lesion, the appearance of surrounding tissues, or abnormalities of bronchial wall thickness). This approach is successful because the airway is composed of branching, cylindric tubes; structures that protrude into the lumen are distinctly abnormal.

Types of Surface Curvature

Class	Shape*	H	κ_{min} and κ_{max}	K
Elliptic	Peak, pit	<0, >0	Same sign	>0
Hyperbolic	Saddle point	Varies	Opposite sign	<0
Cylindric	Ridge, valley, plane	<0, >0, 0	One or both equal zero	0

Sources.—References 11, 19, and 20.
* The shapes are shown graphically in Figure A2.

The mathematic attribute corresponding to this perceived abnormality in the shape of the airway wall is called curvature. In numeric terms, the curvature of a surface at a point is equal to the reciprocal of the radius of a sphere that has the same slope as the surface at that point. The sign of the curvature depends on which side of the surface one could fit the sphere. A surface that curves away from a point has the opposite sign of a surface that curves toward a point. For surfaces that are not radially symmetric, the curvature at a point will vary as a function of direction. The smallest and largest curvatures at a point are called the minimum (κ_{min}) and maximum (κ_{max}) principal curvatures, which are oriented in the principal directions. Additional parameters, called the mean *(H)* and Gaussian *(K)* curvatures, are the average and product of the principal curvatures, respectively.

A practical example will prove illustrative. Imagine a hemispheric polypoid lesion protruding into the lumen. At a point on the tip of this polyp, an observer would see the walls of the polyp curve away from the lumen. Now imagine a hemispheric ulcer protruding into the airway wall. At a point at the base of the ulcer, an observer would see the walls of the ulcer curve toward the lumen. In curvature terminology, the surface near the tip of the polyp and near the base of the ulcer have "elliptic" curvature, which can be further subdivided on the basis of the sign of the curvature into "peak" (negative curvature) and "pit" (positive curvature) subtypes, respectively. We confine ourselves here to the detection of polypoid lesions and not ulcers. The mathematics of the computation and classification of curvature is described in the Appendix.

Algorithm and Implementation

The VB surface renderings were generated from helical CT images (HiSpeed Advantage; GE Medical Systems, Milwaukee, Wis) by using a previously described (7) region-growing and threshold-based segmentation algorithm. The VB surfaces were first smoothed with 50 iterations of smoothing (8). Next, a biparametric fourth-order b-spline patch was fitted to local neighborhoods with a 5-mm radius around each vertex (9). The first- and second-order partial derivatives of the fitted patch were determined for the center vertex of the patch (9). The curvatures for the center vertex were calculated from these partial derivatives (see the Appendix), and the vertex was then classified according to the scheme shown in the Table. Vertices in regions of hyperbolic and cylindric curvature were discarded. Only vertices in regions of elliptic curvature with a negative mean curvature (peak subtype) below a threshold (ϵ) were retained. This process was repeated for each vertex on the surface.

The processed vertices were filtered to discard isolated vertices or those that constituted lesions smaller than an arbitrarily minimum size of 30 vertices. Lesions were then defined as a cluster of connected vertices that shared the desired curvature classification and exceeded the minimum size. Vertex connectivity was determined by using a region-growing process that began with those local neighbors that formed a triangle and proceeded recursively until all neighbors with the appropriate curvature classification were found.

The surfaces were displayed and manipulated on a workstation (Indigo[2] Maximum Impact; Silicon Graphics, Mountain View, Calif) equipped with 320 Mbyte of memory and a 195-MHz R10000 central processing unit (10). Potential lesions classified with the methods described above were colored red to distinguish them from the background anatomy, which was colored a pink tone.

Our visualization software allowed movement of the viewpoint to each lesion in turn for further analysis. The position of the viewpoint was set by using a three-step process. First, the centroid of the lesion was determined by using the coordinates of each vertex that constituted the lesion. Second, the normal to the lesion was determined by averaging the normals of all the vertices that constituted the lesion. Third, the camera viewpoint was moved 1 cm from the centroid along the averaged normal and was set to point toward the centroid. Fine adjustments to the viewpoint could then be made interactively (eg, if the bronchus was smaller than 1 cm in diameter).

By using this software, lesion detections at sites of "segmentation leakage" (the undesired presence of surfaces in the VB model that are unrelated to the bronchial lumen; eg, those due to blood vessels, the outer wall of bronchi, the edge of the mediastinum, or fibrosis) could be readily identified and disregarded, because they were not within bronchial passages. For true lesions, this procedure placed the viewpoint inside the airway lumen pointing toward the lesion.

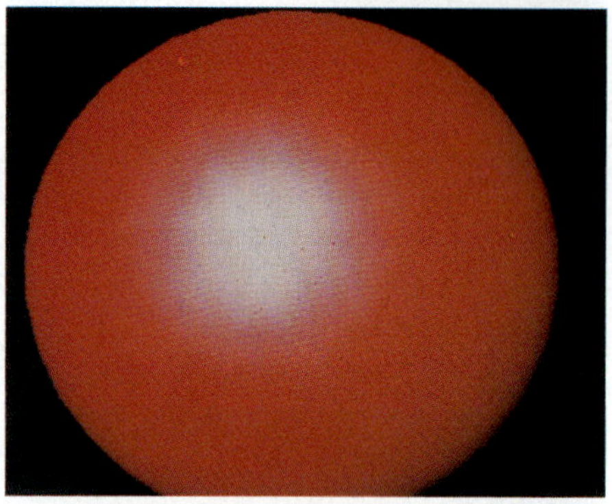

a.

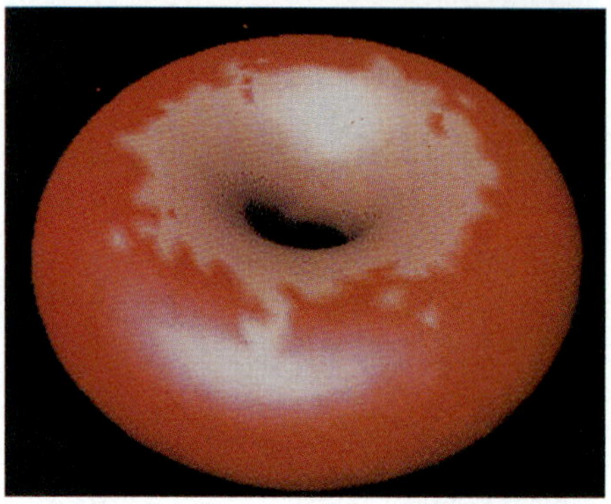

b.

Figure 1. Computer-generated images show the curvature classification for elemental surfaces. **(a)** The curvature of a sphere is uniformly of the elliptic peak type and is constant everywhere on its surface, as indicated by the smooth red coloring. **(b)** The curvature of a torus is of the elliptic peak type on its outer rim, as indicated by the red coloring.

Evaluation of the Technique

The method was tested with simulated elemental surfaces (sphere and torus), an

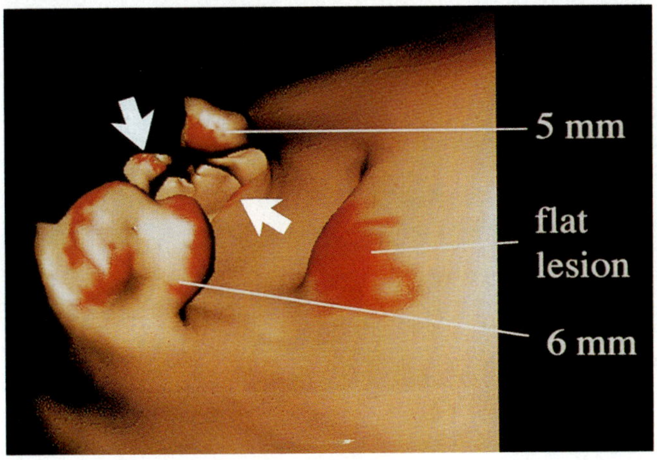

Figure 2. VB image of an airway phantom shows a close-up view of several lesions in a second-order bronchus. Spherical lesions with a diameter of 5 and 6 mm and a flat lesion are shown, with red shading to indicate the segmented surfaces of elliptic curvature of the peak type. The mean curvature threshold ϵ was 0. The mean curvatures of these lesions obtained by sampling six vertices within each lesion were -5.6 cm^{-1} $\pm$ 1.6 (5-mm spherical lesion), -8.2 cm^{-1} $\pm$ 2.8 (6-mm spherical lesion), and -1.8 cm^{-1} $\pm$ 0.4 (flat lesion). The 5-mm-diameter lesion is slightly flattened (a consequence of the pitch of 2 and of the smoothing function), which explains why its curvature value is intermediate to those of the flat and 6-mm-diameter lesions. Two false-positive detections (arrows) can be seen distally.

airway phantom fitted with simulated lesions, cadaveric lung specimens, and airway studies in patients. Each of the phantom, cadaveric, and patient studies was processed at three different thresholds for mean curvature ($\epsilon \leq 0$, $\epsilon \leq -1$, $\epsilon \leq -2$ cm^{-1}). The effect of changes in ϵ can be understood by means of reference to the spherical polyp analogy. For $\epsilon = 0$, all lesions are detected. As ϵ is made more negative, progressively more highly curved lesions (with smaller radii of curvature) are detected, and more gently curved, larger lesions are excluded. In practice, more gently curved areas ($\epsilon \sim 0$ cm^{-1}) tend to represent minor undulations in the bronchial wall rather than true lesions.

Tessellated surfaces that represented a sphere and a torus were created by generating isosurfaces of the corresponding implicit functions. The surface normals were set to point outward. A sphere has constant elliptic curvature, and its minimum and maximum principal curvatures are equal everywhere on its surface. A torus has curvature of all three types: elliptic curvature along the outer margin, hyperbolic curvature on the inside (the hole in the torus), and cylindric curvature at the junction between the two.

A latex airway phantom, used by our institution's department of critical care medicine for bronchoscopy training, was fitted with 17 simulated lesions that consisted of spherical plastic beads with a diameter that ranged from 3 to 10 mm (three 10-mm, three 6-mm, four 5-mm, three 4-mm, and four 3-mm beads). A simulated flat lesion composed of latex was also placed into the phantom. CT was performed once on the phantom, with 3-mm collimation, a pitch of 2, and a section index of 1 mm. Lesion detections determined automatically by the software were compared with the known lesion locations.

Intact human whole-lung specimens, including the central airways, were obtained from cadavers after approval was given by our institution's office of human subjects research. Specimens were scanned helically with the CT scanner within 3 hours of autopsy by using 3-mm collimation, a pitch of 1, and a section index of 1.0 or 1.5 mm; VB was then performed. Histopathologic analysis results served as the reference standard for lesion detection in cadaveric specimens.

VB in patients was performed by using helical CT scans of the chest obtained with 3-mm collimation, a pitch of 2, and a section index of 1 mm. The imaging protocol was approved by our institutional review board, and the studies were performed after written informed consent had been obtained. Eighteen studies were obtained in 16 patients.

The patients included both those with known or suspected airway disease and those with lung cavities in which airway disease was not suspected. Patients in the first category included four patients with Wegener granulomatosis and three with endobronchial masses due to a neoplasm (lymphoma, melanoma, renal adenocarcinoma). One patient with Wegener granulomatosis underwent CT three times during 4 months. Patients in the second category included nine with cavitary lung disease (five with Job syndrome, one with a *Mycobacterium avium-intracellulare* infection, one with multiple-drug–resistant tuberculosis, one with chronic granulomatous disease, one with an *Echinococcus* infection). The patients were aged 26–58 years (mean $\pm$ 1 standard deviation, 36 years $\pm$ 9). There were nine male and seven female patients.

The two-dimensional source CT images, recorded on hard copy with standard lung window settings (level, -550 HU; width, 2,000 HU), served as the reference standard for lesion detection among the VB studies. True lesion sites determined by analyzing the CT scans and lesion detections determined automatically with the software were recorded on an anatomic drawing of the airway for each specimen and patient study. True lesion size was measured from the CT images by using calipers.

A single radiologist (R.M.S.) experienced with chest CT and VB performed an unblinded evaluation of the studies. We attempted to limit bias by using the following procedure: After initial testing of the method with several VB studies that showed obvious polypoid lesions, all CT scans (including those in patients initially tested) were evaluated for the presence of polypoid lesions. The locations of any lesions were recorded on an anatomic diagram. The locations of lesions automatically detected at VB were recorded on the same diagram. Results of the two evaluations were reconciled to determine the cause of false-positive and false-negative results at VB. The VB examinations were not blinded, because the computer, not a human observer, performed the lesion detection.

Statistical Analysis

The sensitivity and specificity were computed only for the patient studies. Sensitivity (from the true-positive and false-negative results) was computed on the basis of lesions and airway segments. Specificity (from the true-negative and false-positive results) was computed on the basis of airway segments. The airway segment method was devised to determine specificity, because the potentially infinite number of true-negative lesion sites would yield a specificity of 1.

Five airway segments were defined: the trachea, the left and right main bronchi, and the left and right lobar and segmental bronchi. The data were further subdivided to analyze lesions smaller than 5 mm and those 5 mm or larger in diameter. The sensitivity and specificity for these segment data as a function of lesion size and mean curvature threshold (ϵ) were plotted as a receiver operating characteristic curve.

RESULTS

The curvatures of the sphere and torus were correctly classified with the method (Fig 1). The computed mean curvatures ± 1 standard deviation were -1.96 cm^{-1} ± 0.03 for the sphere and -0.10 cm^{-1} ± 0.01 for the outer edge of the torus, which agreed closely with the expected values (-2.0 and -0.10 cm^{-1}, respectively). The junction between elliptic and cylindric curvature on the torus was somewhat irregular. This finding was due to slight variations in the orientation and size of the biparametric spline patches and to a finite number of vertices in these areas of low curvature.

In the airway phantom experiment, the method was used to correctly detect 10 of 10 lesions with a diameter of 5 mm or larger (sensitivity, 100%) (Fig 2). None of five lesions smaller than 5 mm in diameter were detected (sensitivity, 0%). There were 17 false-positive lesion sites for $\epsilon = 0$ cm^{-1}, 12 for $\epsilon = -1$ cm^{-1}, and two for $\epsilon = -2$ cm^{-1}.

In the five cadaveric lung specimens with no endobronchial lesions, there were eight false-positive lesion sites for $\epsilon = 0$ cm^{-1}, two for $\epsilon = -1$ cm^{-1}, and none for $\epsilon = -2$ cm^{-1}. Six lesion sites in areas of segmentation leakage and 17 related to tubing used to inflate one specimen were easily disregarded.

There were 30 known lesions on the patient CT studies (Fig 3). Twenty-five lesions were in either the trachea or the main bronchi; four were in the lobar or segmental bronchi; and one straddled both regions. After 31, 19, and 13 detections at sites of segmentation leakage were disregarded, the curvature-based method allowed correct detection of 27 lesions for $\epsilon = 0$ cm^{-1}, 26 lesions for $\epsilon = -1$ cm^{-1}, and 15 lesions for $\epsilon = -2$ cm^{-1}, which yielded sensitivities of 90%, 87%, and 50%, respectively, when lesions of all sizes were considered. For lesions 5 mm or larger in diameter ($n = 16$), the sensitivities were 94%, 94%, and 63%, respectively. For lesions smaller than 5 mm in diameter ($n = 14$), the sensitivities were 86%, 86%, and 36%, respectively. There were 117, 51, and 14 false-positive lesion sites, respectively. On the basis of 90 airway segments, the specificity was 58%–89%, and the sensitivity was 47%–88% when lesions of all sizes were considered (Fig 4). As expected, the sensitivity was greater for lesions 5 mm or larger in diameter, with an increase of 20%–34%; the specificity remained similar, with increases of only 0%–3% (Fig 4).

The most frequent causes of false-positive detection were a posterior indentation of the proximal trachea due to the esophagus (eight of 90 segments) and an irregular bronchial wall (seven of 90 segments). Other, less frequent causes were artifacts due to breathing and beam hardening due to the presence of vascular clips, vascular impressions, mucus, and bronchial webs (each in less than five segments).

DISCUSSION

We developed an algorithm that allows automatic detection of polypoid airway lesions on surface-rendered VB images. In our application of the technique to a series of patient studies, the sensitivity was higher for lesions 5 mm or larger in diameter and was dependent on the choice of the threshold parameter ϵ. For the latter, there is a trade-off in that a more negative ϵ (greater mean curvature) yields fewer false-positive results but at the expense of some true-positive results and vice versa for a less negative ϵ.

None of the small (<5-mm-diameter) lesions in the airway phantom were detected, whereas lesions of similar size in the patient studies were detected. The reason for this discrepancy is that high curvature regions were poorly fit by the spline algorithm. The small simulated lesions in the airway phantom had uniformly high curvature values (because they were spherical). True lesions are not spherical, and their curvature spans a range of values that are more readily detected with our algorithm.

False-positive results were an important limitation of this computer-assisted technique. In our experience, false-positive results were caused by a posterior indentation of the proximal trachea due to the esophagus, an irregular bronchial wall, or the presence of various artifacts, vascular impressions, mucus, or bronchial webs. Although bronchial inflammation and edema are not polypoid lesions, they can cause irregularities of the bronchial wall and webs and therefore may be incorrectly classified as false-positive results with this technique.

False-positive sites occur in regions of segmentation leakage; it is therefore desirable to minimize such leakage. Segmentation leakage is a weakness of region-growing–based airway segmentation methods for VB; such leakage can be minimized but is sometimes difficult to completely eliminate. When leakage cannot be prevented during the segmentation process, false-positive sites in areas of segmentation leakage can be readily iden-

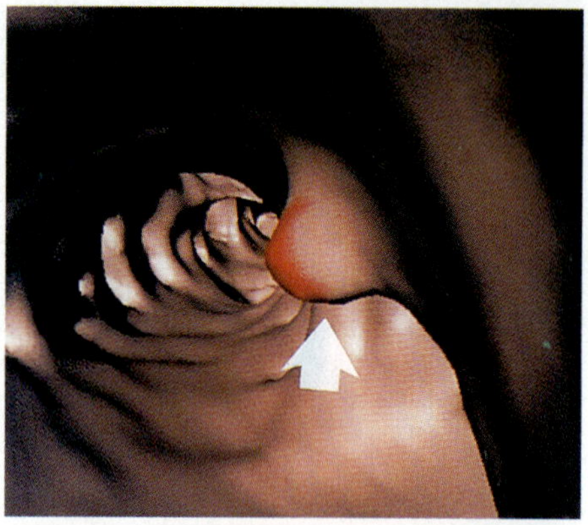

a.

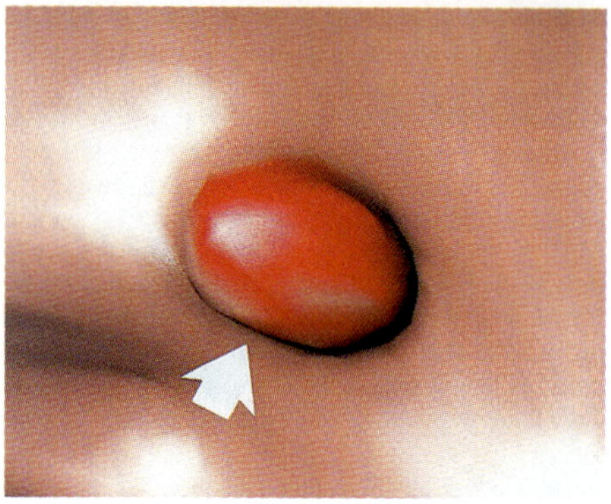

b.

Figure 3. VB images show a 4-mm-diameter lesion (arrow) in the right main stem bronchus of a 39-year-old man with Wegener granulomatosis. **(a)** Profile and **(b)** en face views of the lesion are shown with red shading to indicate the segmented surface with elliptic curvature of the peak type. The mean curvature threshold ϵ was 0. The mean curvature of this lesion, obtained by sampling six vertices within the lesion, was -8.4 cm^{-1} ± 3.5. The remainder of the bronchial mucosa has a pink tone, which indicates that it did not fit the curvature criteria for a polypoid lesion (elliptic curvature of the peak subtype).

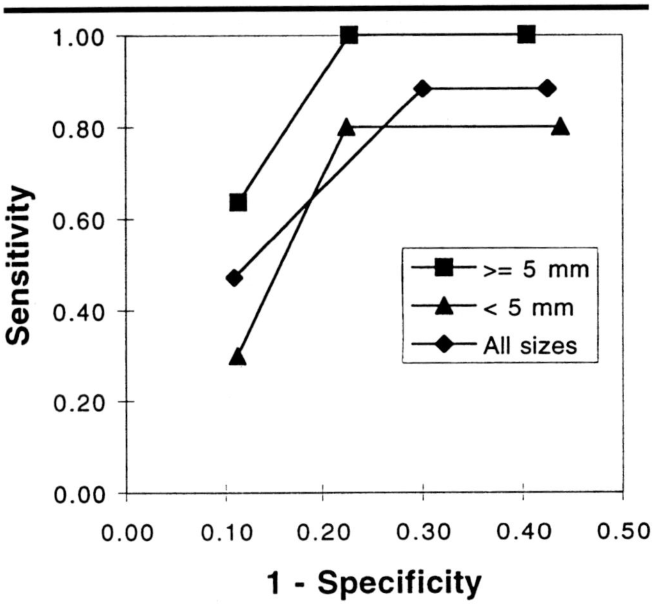

Figure 4. Receiver operating characteristics curve for airway lesions detected on 18 studies in 16 patients. Results for all lesions, for lesions smaller than 5 mm in diameter, and for lesions 5 mm or larger in diameter are shown. Each curve was constructed by using three different thresholds for mean curvature ($\epsilon = 0, -1$, and -2 cm^{-1}).

tified later by cross-referencing the "lesion" to the orthogonal two-dimensional source images (axial, coronal, and sagittal) and eliminating those that are not within a bronchus.

Classification of structures by using surface curvature analysis has been applied for shape analysis in computer vision systems and to identify sulci and gyri on reconstructions of the cortical surface of the brain obtained from magnetic resonance images (11,12). In our application of surface curvature analysis to the airways, we made a basic assumption that airway lesions have an elliptic curvature of the peak type. It is of interest to speculate whether this assumption is generally valid. To do so, a geometric anatomic ("geoanatomic") argument will be made. The airways consist of branching tubular structures that, in human beings, bifurcate at variable intervals. More proximal parts of the airways contain cartilage in their walls that ripples the wall like an accordion. More distal parts do not contain cartilage but are below the resolution of current CT scanners. Each generation of bronchi is progressively smaller in caliber, and individual bronchi tend to taper. On the basis of these characteristics, normal bronchi consist of surfaces of cylindric curvature, and the crotch at a bifurcation consists of a saddle-shaped set of points (hereafter, saddle points) of hyperbolic curvature, because the crotch is the junction of two intersecting tubular bronchi. Therefore, elliptic surfaces of the peak type are uncharacteristic of the normal airway.

Our method may also be applicable to tubular, hollow anatomic structures other than the airways for which a similar geometric taxonomy may be constructed. For example, blood vessels are also tubular branching structures but without rippling striations. Atherosclerotic plaque may modify curvature in this situation. A distended colon is a series of concave-walled chambers with elliptic curvature of the pit type (as seen from the lumen) interspersed with haustral folds that are saddle points with hyperbolic curvature. Colonic polyps, precursors of malignant lesions, may be plaquelike or may extend into the lumen, in which case their abnormal curvature may be detected.

Determination of wall thickness is another method of lesion detection at virtual endoscopy (13). This method is not ideal for the airways because the outer wall of the airway must be detected and can be easily misidentified. Detection of the outer edge of the airway wall is routinely difficult because juxtaposed structures with similar CT attenuation are common in the mediastinum and promote overestimation of the thickness of the wall.

Surface rendering was used to generate VB displays in our study. The alternative method of volume rendering is favored by some investigators because, with volume rendering, one can do away with the time-consuming preprocessing stage that reduces the volume data to a set of surface patches and normals; one can thus avoid certain artifacts due to the considerable information loss that this data reduction entails (5). The curvature-based lesion detection methods we used fundamentally require generation of a surface. By their very nature, these methods are not applicable to perspective volume rendering.

The results of this study suggest that a curvature-based algorithm may facilitate detection of polypoid airway lesions, but this work is still preliminary. A high rate of false-positive results is a major limitation of the technique, but this problem is inherent to any scheme of automatic computer-assisted detection due to the heterogeneity of lesions and the variability of normal anatomic structures. The number of false-positive results are manageable (an average of seven per patient in our study), however, and the sensitivity is high. With further optimization, it may be possible to further improve the sensitivity and specificity of the algorithm.

A potential limitation of this study was the use of axial CT scans as the reference standard for the determination of the sensitivity and specificity. Further investigation should be performed in which VB findings are correlated not only with axial CT findings but also with fiberoptic bronchoscopic findings. A larger patient population and a greater variety of airway lesions should be studied. The clinical usefulness for the radiologist should be evaluated to test for potential time-saving aspects and a reduction in incorrect diagnoses. The application of this method to other tubular structures, such as blood vessels and the colon, may also be explored.

APPENDIX

The study of the mathematic properties of smooth surfaces is encompassed by the field of differential geometry (14–18). A basic problem in differential geometry is the determination of geometric quantities that distinguish one shape (curve, surface, or higher dimensional analogue) from another (18).

In our particular case, we wish to distinguish lesion-bearing bronchial surfaces from lesion-free surfaces. To do this, we must determine appropriate quantities to distinguish these two situations. A brief over-

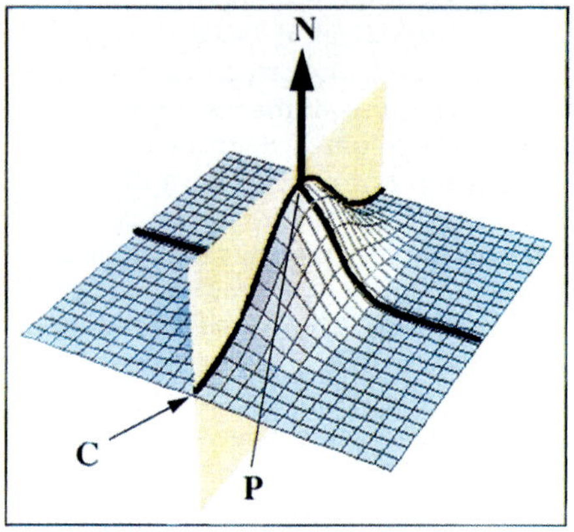

Figure A1. Graph shows the relationship of curvature terminology to the shape of polypoid lesions. The curvature at a point *P* on a surface (such as surfaces obtained at VB) is defined by consideration of the curve *C* formed by the intersection of a normal section at *P* with the surface. There is an infinite number of such curves formed by means of rotation of the normal section about the surface normal *N*, each with a curvature at *P*. The theory focuses on descriptors based on minimum and maximum curvatures, which are shown as heavy black lines. The Gaussian curvature is the product of these curvatures, and the mean is their average. In this example, the curvature of *C* at *P* is the minimum principal curvature. The curve with the maximum principal curvature at *P* is shown as a thick line perpendicular to *C*. In the algorithm described in this article, polyps are detected when these curvatures are always negative (which defines elliptic curvature of the "peak" subtype) for all normal sections within a local neighborhood of a specified size on the surface.

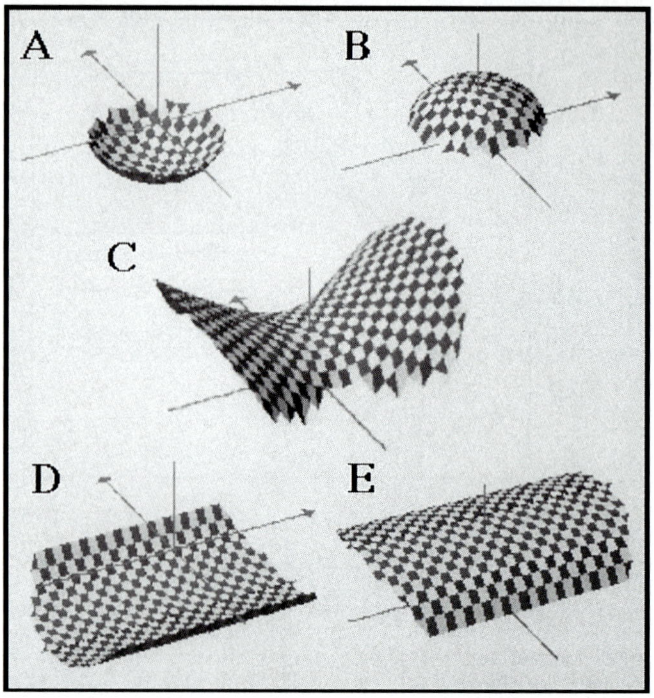

Figure A2. Drawing shows types of surface curvature. Elliptic curvature of the (*A*) pit and (*B*) peak types, (*C*) hyperbolic curvature (saddle point), and cylindric curvature of the (*D*) valley and (*E*) ridge types are shown. Analogous anatomic structures for these shapes are (*A*) ulceration and grooves between cartilaginous rings, (*B*) polypoid lesion, (*C*) bronchial bifurcation and cartilaginous rings, (*D*) smooth bronchial wall and grooves between cartilaginous rings, and (*E*) bronchial bifurcation.

view is given here. Further details can be found in differential geometry textbooks.

If we first consider a simple curve in a plane, we find that this curve is uniquely determined by two scalar quantities—curvature and torsion—which are functions of arc length (18). The concept of curvature can be extrapolated to surfaces as follows (Fig A1): Consider a point *P* on a surface. A normal section at *P* is defined as a plane containing *P* and its unit normal. Now consider the family of curves formed by the intersection of the surface with the normal section as the normal section is rotated about the unit normal. At point *P*, each of the curves in this family has a curvature value associated with it, called the normal curvature. The largest normal curvature value is called the maximum principal curvature (κ_{max}) and the smallest is called the minimum principal curvature (κ_{min}). From these principal curvatures, the important mean [$H = (\kappa_{min} + \kappa_{max})/2$] and Gaussian ($K = \kappa_{min} \cdot \kappa_{max}$) curvatures are easily derived.

Curvature has a number of properties that make it a good shape descriptor. Curvature is intrinsic to the surface and is not dependent, for example, on how a surface is illuminated. Gaussian and mean curvature are invariant to arbitrary transformations of the parameterization and to arbitrary rotations and translations. Thus, these curvature quantities are independent of the viewpoint, which is another important feature.

Rogers and Adams (19) and Dill (20) have shown that the mean and Gaussian curvatures can be computed from the following equations, which are functions of the vector **S**, which describes the parameterized surface and its partial derivatives:

$$A = \mathbf{Q} \cdot \mathbf{S}_{uu}, B = \mathbf{Q} \cdot \mathbf{S}_{uv}, C = \mathbf{Q} \cdot \mathbf{S}_{vv},$$

$$\mathbf{Q} = \mathbf{S}_u \times \mathbf{S}_v,$$

$$\mathrm{H} = \frac{A|\mathbf{S}_v|^2 - 2B\mathbf{S}_u \cdot \mathbf{S}_v + C|\mathbf{S}_u|^2}{2|\mathbf{Q}|^3},$$

$$K = \frac{AC - B^2}{|\mathbf{Q}|^4},$$

where *A, B,* and *C* are intermediate scalar values, **Q** is a vector parallel to the surface normal, and the subscript notation indicates partial differentiation, for example,

$$\mathbf{S}_u(u,v) = \frac{\partial \mathbf{S}}{\partial u}$$

and so on.

The principal curvatures can then be computed from

$$b = \sqrt{H^2 - K},$$

$$\kappa_{max} = H + b,$$

$$\kappa_{min} = H - b,$$

where *b* is an intermediate scalar value.

These curvatures are important because they can be used to classify a surface shape. The surface can be classified locally into three major shapes on the basis of the sign of K, κ_{min}, and κ_{max}: elliptic, hyperbolic, or cylindric (Table, Fig A2). The elliptic shape describes peaks or pits, the hyperbolic shape describes saddle points, and the cylindric shape describes ridges, valleys, or troughs (19,20). Normal (lesion-free) bronchial walls can be characterized in terms of surfaces of hyperbolic and cylindric shapes or of an elliptic shape of the pit subtype (Summers RM, Selbie WS, Malley JD, et al, unpublished observation, 1997). Polypoid lesions, which are of interest for this application, have elliptic curvature of the peak subtype. For example, a spherical polypoid lesion of radius r has elliptic curvature of the peak type and its mean and principal curvatures are identical, namely, $-1/r$ (this approach neglects the lesion edge, which may have higher curvature where it meets the bronchial wall). A spherical crater or ulceration of radius r has elliptic curvature of the pit type, and its mean and principal curvatures are $1/r$. The Gaussian curvature of both lesions is the same, namely, $1/r^2$.

Acknowledgments: We thank Peter Basser, PhD, for critical review of the manuscript and the CT technologists at the Clinical Center for their assistance in performing scanning in the patients.

References

1. McCarthy MJ, Rosado-de-Christenson ML. Tumors of the trachea. J Thorac Imaging 1995; 10:180–198.
2. Shepard JA. The bronchi: an imaging perspective. J Thorac Imaging 1995; 10:236–254.
3. Naidich DP, Gruden JF, McGuinness G, McCauley DI, Bhalla M. Volumetric (helical/spiral) CT (VCT) of the airways. J Thorac Imaging 1997; 12:11–28.
4. Quint LE, Whyte RI, Kazerooni EA, et al. Stenosis of the central airways: evaluation by using helical CT with multiplanar reconstructions. Radiology 1995; 194:871–877.
5. Rubin GD, Beaulieu CF, Argiro V, et al. Perspective volume rendering of CT and MR images: applications for endoscopic imaging. Radiology 1996; 199:321–330.
6. Vining DJ, Liu K, Choplin RH, Haponik EF. Virtual bronchoscopy: relationships of virtual reality endobronchial simulations to actual bronchoscopic findings. Chest 1996; 109:549–553.
7. Summers RM, Feng DF, Holland SM, Sneller MC, Shelhamer JH. Virtual bronchoscopy: segmentation method for real-time display. Radiology 1996; 200:857–862.
8. Taubin G. A signal processing approach to fair surface design. In: Cook R, ed. SIGGRAPH 95 conference proceedings. Reading, Mass: Addison-Wesley, 1995; 351–358.
9. Dierckx P. Curve and surface fitting with splines. Oxford, England: Clarendon, 1993.
10. Summers RM. Navigational aids for real-time virtual bronchoscopy. AJR 1997; 168: 1165–1170.
11. Besl PJ, Jain RC. Segmentation through variable-order surface fitting. IEEE Trans Pattern Analysis Machine Intell 1988; 10: 167–192.
12. Davatzikos C, Bryan RN. Using a deformable surface model to obtain a shape representation of the cortex. IEEE Trans Med Imaging 1996; 15:785–795.
13. Vining DJ, Stelts DR, Hunt G, Ahn D, Ge Y, Hemler PF. Technical improvements in virtual colonoscopy (abstr). Radiology 1996; 201(P):524–525.
14. Eisenhart LP. An introduction to differential geometry. Princeton, NJ: Princeton University Press, 1947.
15. Kreyszig E. Differential geometry. Toronto, Ontario, Canada: University of Toronto Press, 1959.
16. do Carmo MP. Differential geometry of curves and surfaces. Englewood Cliffs, NJ: Prentice-Hall, 1976.
17. Besl PJ. Surfaces in range image understanding. New York, NY: Springer-Verlag, 1988.
18. Lipschutz MM. Theory and problems of differential geometry. New York, NY: McGraw-Hill, 1969.
19. Rogers DF, Adams JA. Mathematical elements for computer graphics. 2nd ed. New York, NY: McGraw-Hill, 1990.
20. Dill JC. An application of color graphics to the display of surface curvature. Comput Graphics 1981; 15:153–161.

Diagnosis Please

Jeremy J. Erasmus, MD | H. Page McAdams, MD | Philip C. Goodman, MD

Case 5[1]

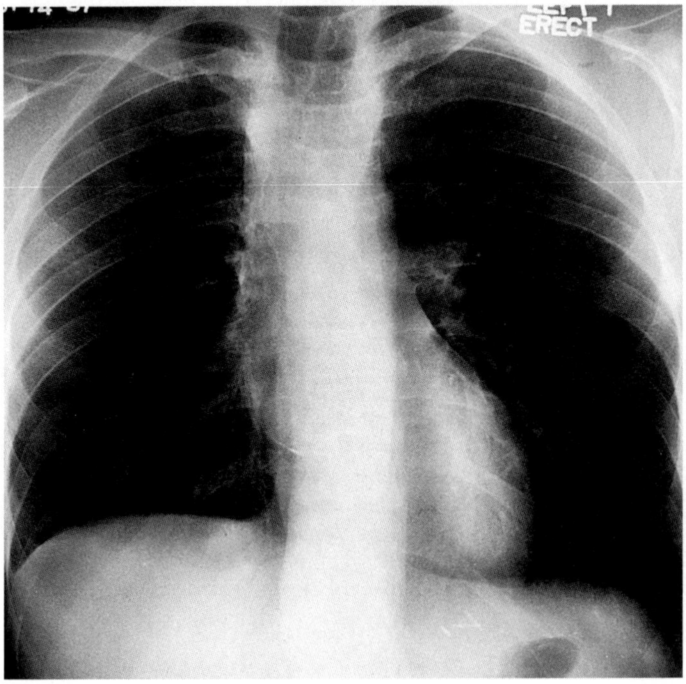

a.

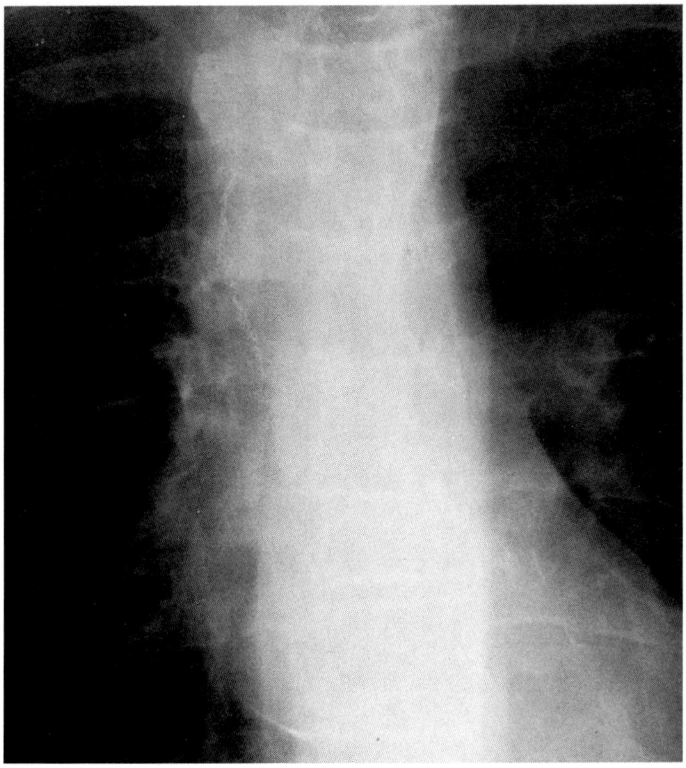

b.

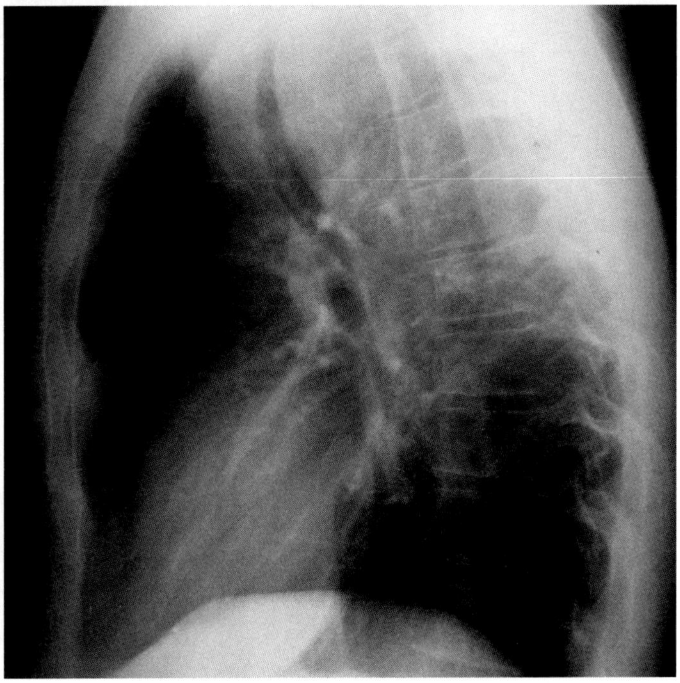

c.

Figure 1. **(a)** Posteroanterior chest radiograph. **(b)** Close-up photograph of posteroanterior chest radiograph. **(c)** Lateral chest radiograph.

(continued)

Submit the most likely diagnosis to *dxplease@rsna.org* (use ***only*** for submission of diagnosis). Include case number, your name (as you would want it to appear in the journal), address, phone and fax numbers. Multiple diagnoses, multiple submissions, submissions without a case number will not be considered. ***Deadline***: October 19, 1998. Answer will appear in the December issue. See also the editorial by Proto (p 1) in the April 1998 issue.

Index terms:
Diagnosis please

Radiology 1998; 208:339–340

[1] From the Department of Radiology, Duke University Medical Center, Box 3808, Durham, NC 27710. Received November 25, 1997; revision requested January 7, 1998; revision received January 27; accepted February 2. **Address reprint requests to** J.J.E.

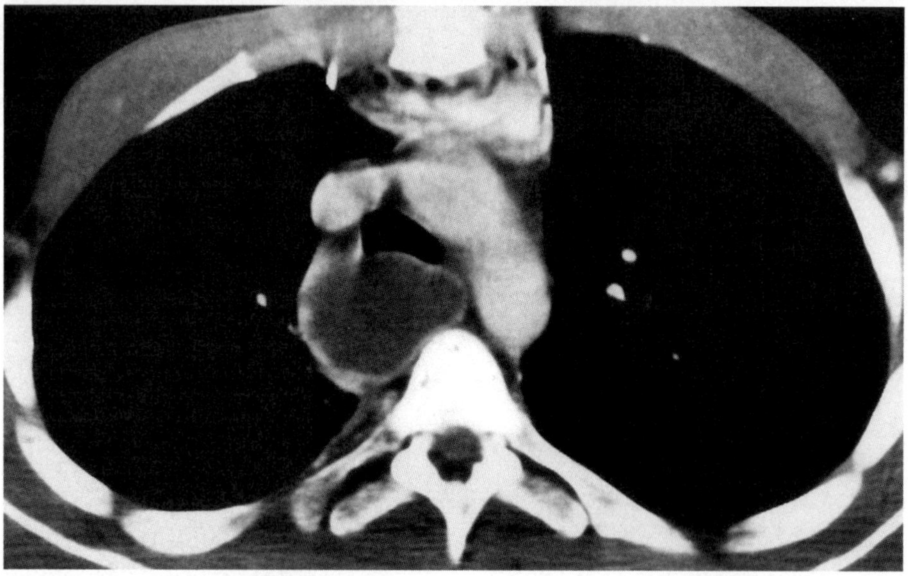

Figure 2. Contrast material–enhanced CT scan.

HISTORY

A 31-year-old man developed persistent postprandial vomiting and abdominal pain. He also complained of early satiety and weight loss. Three years earlier, he was treated with radiation therapy, chemotherapy, and palliative surgery for an esophageal malignancy.

At physical examination, his temperature, pulse, and blood pressure were normal. His abdomen was soft, nontender, and nondistended, with normal bowel sounds. There were no palpable masses or adenopathy. The results of laboratory tests that included red blood cell count, white blood cell count, serum bilirubin, and liver enzyme levels were normal.

Chest radiography (Fig 1) and computed tomography (CT) with contrast enhancement (Fig 2) were performed.

Ann S. Fulcher, MD

Case 1: Recurrent Pyogenic Cholangitis[1]

HISTORY

The patient is a 31-year-old Filipino woman with a 5-year history of intermittent jaundice and abdominal pain. She now presents with a 2-month history of worsening epigastric pain and pruritus.

IMAGING FINDINGS

A sagittal sonographic image of the liver demonstrates echogenic, shadowing calculi parallel to an intrahepatic branch of the right portal vein (Fig 1a). A transverse sonographic image of the porta hepatis reveals an echogenic, shadowing calculus in the dilated extrahepatic bile duct (Fig 1b). Axial computed tomographic (CT) images of the abdomen obtained without contrast material enhancement show high-attenuation calculi in the dilated intrahepatic and extrahepatic bile ducts (Fig 2). Axial CT images obtained with contrast material enhancement reveal the enhancing portal veins parallel to the dilated intrahepatic bile ducts (Fig 3a) and the dilated intrapancreatic common bile duct, which contains a calculus (Fig 3b). An intraoperative cholangiogram confirms the biliary ductal dilatation, the common bile duct calculus, and the calculi that formed castlike filling defects in the intrahepatic bile ducts (Fig 4).

DISCUSSION

Recurrent pyogenic cholangitis (RPC), also known as oriental cholangiohepatitis, recurrent pyogenic hepatitis, and intrahepatic pigment stone disease, is a common cause of abdominal pain and cholangitis in patients in Southeast Asia. In fact, in Hong Kong, it is the most common disease of the biliary tract that requires surgery (1). Although the largest series of RPC has been reported in Asia (2), RPC is being identified with increasing frequency in the United States, primarily in Asian immigrants (3). Clinically, RPC is characterized by recurrent abdominal pain, fever, chills, and jaundice. The natural course of RPC is that of chronic recurrent cholangitis resulting in a progressive, destructive cholangiopathy and liver failure (4). RPC

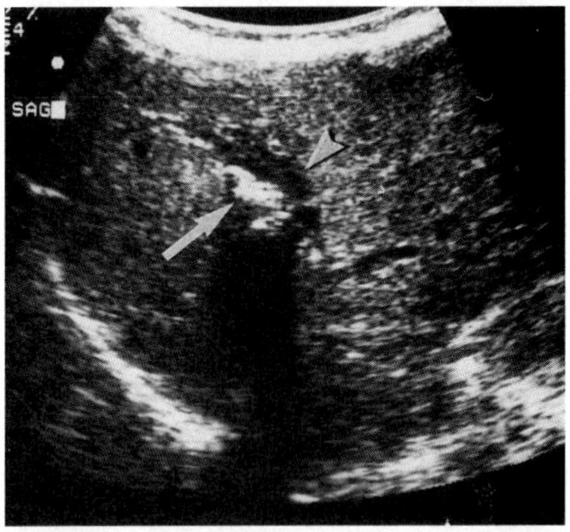

a.

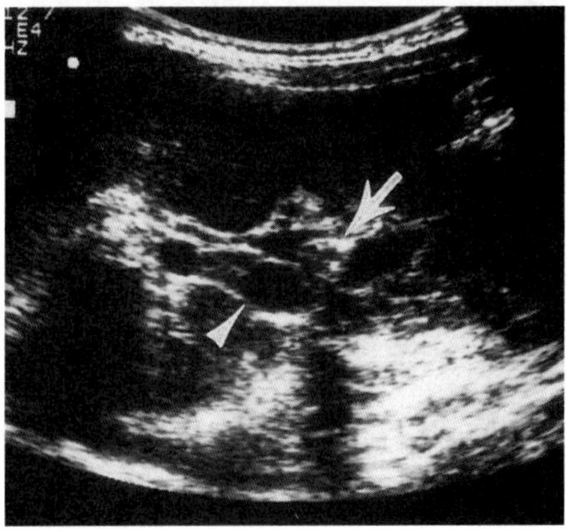

b.

Figure 1. **(a)** Sagittal sonographic image of the liver shows echogenic, shadowing calculi (arrow) that parallel a branch of the right portal vein (arrowhead). **(b)** Transverse sonographic image of the porta hepatis demonstrates an echogenic, shadowing calculus (arrow) in the dilated extrahepatic bile duct. The main portal vein (arrowhead) is noted posterior to the bile duct.

Index terms:
Diagnosis please
Cholangitis, 76.289

Radiology 1998; 208:341–344

[1] From the Department of Radiology, Medical College of Virginia of Virginia Commonwealth University, 401 N 12th St, Box 980615, Richmond, VA 23298-0615. Received September 30, 1997; revision requested December 9; revision received December 10; accepted December 11. **Address reprint requests to** the author.

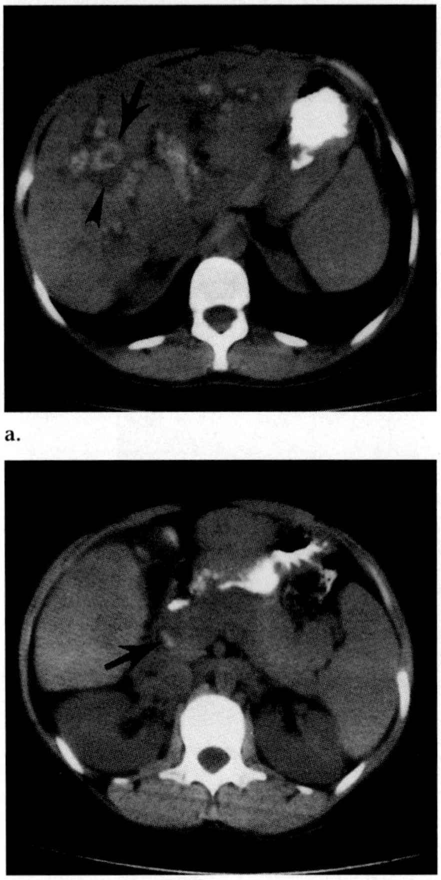

Figure 2. **(a)** Unenhanced axial CT image of the liver shows high-attenuation calculi (arrow) in the dilated intrahepatic bile ducts; the calculi lie adjacent to the unopacified portal vein branches (arrowhead). **(b)** Unenhanced axial CT image of the pancreas shows a high-attenuation calculus (arrow) in the dilated intrapancreatic bile duct.

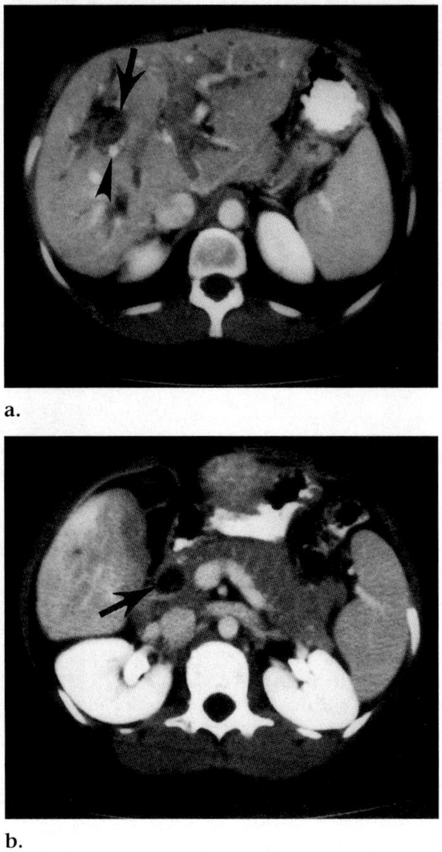

Figure 3. **(a)** Enhanced axial CT image of the liver reveals enhancing portal veins (arrowhead) that parallel the dilated intrahepatic bile ducts (arrow). **(b)** Enhanced axial CT image of the pancreas better demonstrates the dilated intrapancreatic bile duct (arrow). The intraductal calculus is barely perceptible.

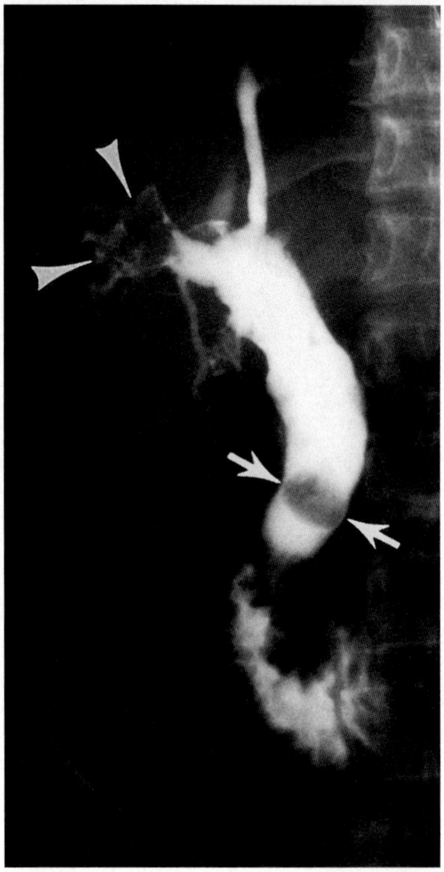

Figure 4. Intraoperative cholangiogram shows biliary ductal dilatation, a calculus in the intrapancreatic bile duct (arrows), and calculi filling an intrahepatic bile duct (arrowheads).

occurs most commonly in people aged 30–40 years; there is no sex predominance (5). Although bile cultures are nearly always positive for *Escherichia coli* and other enteric organisms and although parasites such as *Clonorchis sinensis* have been implicated as an inciting factor, the cause of RPC remains undetermined (1–3). Pathologic analysis of the liver reveals pericholangitis, periductal abscesses, fibrosis of the bile duct walls, heavy infiltration of the portal tracts by polymorphonuclear leukocytes, and intraductal bile pigment calculi (1,2,6).

The major imaging features of RPC include intrahepatic and extrahepatic bile duct dilatation and biliary calculi. In a series of 47 patients with RPC, Lim et al (7) noted that sonography demonstrated ductal dilatation in 96% and intraductal calculi in 98%. The ductal dilatation was noted both proximal and distal to the calculi. The majority were located in both the intrahepatic and extrahepatic bile ducts or within the extrahepatic duct only; 15% were confined to the intrahepatic ducts. In most cases, the stones were echogenic and resulted in shadowing. It should be noted, however, that sonography may not depict all calculi because of their small size, sludgelike consistency, hypoechogenicity, lack of shadowing, and associated pneumobilia (3,8). CT findings of RPC include biliary ductal dilatation with a predilection for the lateral segment of the left hepatic lobe, high-attenuation biliary calculi, pneumobilia, segmental atrophy of the liver, enhancement of the bile duct wall, and hepatic abscesses (5). Associated findings include gallstones, splenomegaly, and varices. Although endoscopic retrograde cholangiography and percutaneous transhepatic cholangiography provide high-resolution images, these procedures may induce sepsis due to the underlying infection of the biliary tract. In one series, worsening of cholangitis occurred as a complication of endoscopic retrograde cholangiography in 23% of RPC patients who did not receive antibiotics before the procedure (9).

The differential diagnosis of RPC is limited. Although Caroli disease is associated with biliary calculi, ductal dilatation, and hepatic abscesses, the saccular dilatation of the intrahepatic bile ducts characteristic of Caroli disease allows for its differentiation from RPC. Although biliary calculi occur in association with primary sclerosing cholangitis, primary sclerosing cholangitis is associated with bile duct dilatation that is focal and discontinuous, unlike that of RPC. Clonorchiasis must be considered in the differential diagnosis of RPC since it is endemic in Asia and results in biliary ductal dilatation. However, the ductal dilatation of clonorchiasis is typically limited to the intrahepatic bile ducts (10).

Whereas acute cholangitis due to RPC can be controlled with antibiotics, definitive treatment requires biliary drainage, which can be achieved surgically with procedures such as choledochoduodenostomy (2). More recently, percutaneous biliary procedures and endoscopic sphincterotomy have proved effective in establishing biliary drainage especially in patients with increased surgical risk and with stones predominating in the extrahepatic bile duct (11–15).

References

1. Stock FE, Fung JHY. Oriental cholangiohepatitis. Arch Surg 1962; 84:409–412.
2. Ong GB. A study of recurrent pyogenic cholangitis. Arch Surg 1962; 84:199–225.
3. Federle MP, Cello JP, Laing FC, Jeffrey RB Jr. Recurrent pyogenic cholangitis in Asian immigrants: use of sonography, computed tomography, and cholangiography. Radiology 1982; 143:151–156.
4. Khuroo MS, Dar MY, Yattoo GN, et al. Serial cholangiographic appearances in recurrent pyogenic cholangitis. Gastrointest Endosc 1993; 39:674–679.
5. Chan FL, Man SW, Leong LLY, Fan ST. Evaluation of recurrent pyogenic cholangitis with CT: analysis of 50 patients. Radiology 1989; 170:165–169.
6. Lim JH. Oriental cholangiohepatitis: pathologic, clinical, and radiologic features. AJR 1991; 157:1–8.
7. Lim JH, Ko YT, Lee DH, Hong KS. Oriental cholangiohepatitis: sonographic findings in 48 cases. AJR 1990; 155:511–514.
8. Itai Y, Araki T, Furui S, Tasaka A, Atomi Y, Kuroda A. Computed tomography and ultrasound in the diagnosis of intrahepatic calculi. Radiology 1980; 136:399–405.
9. Lam SK, Wong KP, Chan PKW, Ngan H, Ong GB. Recurrent pyogenic cholangitis: a study by endoscopic retrograde cholangiography. Gastroenterology 1978; 74:1196–1203.
10. Choi BI, Kim HJ, Han MC, Do YS, Han MH, Lee SH. CT findings of clonorchiasis. AJR 1989; 152:281–284.
11. vanSonnenberg E, Casola G, Cubberley DA, et al. Oriental cholangiohepatitis: diagnostic imaging and interventional management. AJR 1986; 146:327–331.
12. Kerlan RK Jr, Pogany AC, Goldberg HI, Ring EJ. Radiologic intervention in oriental cholangiohepatitis. AJR 1985; 145:809–813.
13. Lam SK. A study of endoscopic sphincterotomy in recurrent pyogenic cholangitis. Br J Surg 1984; 71:262–266.
14. Lai ECS, Mok FPT, Tan ESY, et al. Endoscopic biliary drainage for severe acute cholangitis. N Engl J Med 1992; 326:1582–1586.
15. Choi TK, Wong J. Endoscopic retrograde cholangiopancreatography and endoscopic papillotomy in recurrent pyogenic cholangitis. Clin Gastroenterol 1986; 15:393–415.

One hundred three individuals submitted the most likely diagnosis (recurrent pyogenic cholangitis) for Diagnosis Please, Case 1. We are listing the names of the following 103 individuals as submitted (some did not include their degrees).

Gholamali Afshang, MD, *Tinley Park, Ill*
Roger Antonelli, MD, *Dayton, Ohio*
Ronald Arams, MD, *Tenafly, NJ*
Ken Baliga, MD, *Rockford, Ill*
Zubin N. Balsara, MD, *Fort Smith, Ark*
Paulo M. B. Bernardes, *Rio de Janeiro, Brazil*
Lawrence R. Bigongiari, MD, *Little Rock, Ark*
Adrian P. Brady, FFRRCSI, *Cork, Ireland*
Larkin Breed, Jr, MD, *Pleasant Hill, Calif*
Eric L. Bressler, MD, *Minnetonka, Minn*
James A. Brink, MD, *New Haven, Conn*
Karen T. Brown, MD, *New York, NY*
Steven J. Burbidge, MD, *Minneapolis, Minn*
Manuel Cabal, MD, *Yucatan, Mexico*
Dennis Carlyle, MD, *Houston, Tex*
Royce A. Chrys, MD, *Castro Valley, Calif*
Timothy J. Clark, MD, *Greenville, NC*
Martin I. Cohen, MD, *Westlake Village, Calif*
Beatty Crawford, MD, *Sharon, Conn*
LeNine Cunha, *Porto Alegre, Brazil*
Manoel de Souza Rocha, *Sao Paulo, Brazil*
Peter Drescher, MD, *Milwaukee, Wis*
Peter English, FRACR, *Hong Kong, China*
Andy Fisher, MD, *St Louis, Mo*
Arnold C. Friedman, MD, *New York, NY*
Akira Furukawa, MD, *Shiga, Japan*
Douglas Gardner, MD, *Windsor, Ontario, Canada*
Ted A. Glass, MD, *Fredericksburg, Va*
Jacob A. Goldenberg, MD, *Fargo, ND*
Robert Greenstein, MD, *Evanston, Ill*
D. Joseph Grunz, MD, *Creve Coeur, Mo*
Flavius F. Guglielmo, MD, *Somerset, NJ*
Ferris Hall, MD, *Boston, Mass*
Richard Hasson, MD, *Cleveland, Ohio*
Harvey R. Hatch, MD, *Gold Beach, Ore*
Peter B. Hathaway, MD, *Seattle, Wash*
Helen T. Ho, MD, *Chicago, Ill*
Lowrey H. Holthaus, MD, *Richmond, Va*
Mindy M. Horrow, MD, *Wynnewood, Pa*
Paul D. Kamin, MD, *Los Alamitos, Calif*
Robert Kanterman, MD, *St Louis, Mo*
Douglas S. Katz, MD, *Mineola, NY*
Loren Ketai, MD, *Albuquerque, NM*
Richard Krauthamer, MD, *Torrance, Calif*
Jong Beum Lee, MD, *Seoul, Korea*
Ross Levatter, MD, *Phoenix, Ariz*
Jae Hoon Lim, MD, *Seoul, Korea*
Joachim Lotz, MD, *Hannover, Germany*
George Lyons, MD, *Denver, Colo*
António José Madureira, MD, *Matosinhos, Portugal*
K. Marsot-Dupuch, *Paris, France*
Mitesh Mehta, MD, *Toronto, Ontario, Canada*
Edward Menges, MD, *Aptos, Calif*
Michael P. Meyers, MD, FRCPC, *Winnipeg, Manitoba, Canada*
Mehran Midia, MD, *Ringfield, Ill*
Frank Miller, MD, *Chicago, Ill*
Robert E. Mindelzun, MD, *Stanford, Calif*
Ari Mintz, MD, *Northbrook, Ill*
Hidetoshi Miyake, MD, *Oita, Japan*
Sergio J. Moguillansky, MD, *Rio Negro, Argentina*
William B. Morrison, MD, *San Antonio, Tex*
Dana Murakami, MD, *Las Vegas, Nev*
Brian L. Murphy, MD, *Boston, Mass*
Levon N. Nazarian, MD, *Cherry Hill, NJ*
Michael Nelsen, MD, *Bellevue, Wash*
Michael Neuman, MD, *Wichita, Kan*
Al Nizzero, MD, FRCPC, *Worcester, Mass*
Ismail Oran, MD, *Izmir, Turkey*
David M. Panicek, MD, *New York, NY*
Ulisses C. Parente, MD, *Minas Gerais, Brazil*
Suresh Patel, MD, *Chicago, Ill*
Anthony Peduto, *Westmead, NSW, Australia*
Roberto E. Perez Gautrin, MD, *Sonora, Mexico*
Pedro J. S. Pinto, MD, *Gondomar, Portugal*

Jonathan Posin, MD, *Walnut Creek, Calif*
G. Lee Pride, Jr, MD, *Bedford, Tex*
George T. Puskar, MD, *Vero Beach, Fla*
Shawn P. Quillin, MD, *Charlotte, NC*
M. R. Ramakrishnan, MD, *Big Stone Gap, Va*
Lorenz (Larry) Ramseyer, MD, *Enid, Okla*
Lawrence N. Rappaport, MD, *Avon, Conn*
Douglas C. Riehle, MD, *Danville, Calif*
Derek J. Roebuck, FRCR, FRACR, *Hong Kong, China*
Fernando Roithmann, MD, *Porto Alegre, Brazil*
Michael Roossin, MD, *Newport Beach, Calif*
Stuart A. Royal, MS, MD, *Birmingham, Ala*
Nicholas C. Russo, MD, *Rochester, NY*
Steven M. Schultz, MD, *Forth Worth, Tex*
Michael C. Scruggs, MD, *Rutherfordton, NC*
Matt Shapiro, MD, *Boxborough, Mass*
L. H. Sie, MD, *Beverwijk, The Netherlands*
A. Michael Simon, MD, *Philadelphia, Pa*
Joanne B. Speigle, MD, *Richmond, Va*
Gary W. Swenson, MD, *APO, AE*
J. Keith Thompson, MD, *Richmond, Va*
John To, MD, *Kingsford, Mich*
Sibley N. Turner, MD, *Dothan, Ala*
Carlos Valls, MD, *Barcelona, Spain*
Angelo Vanzulli, MD, *Milan, Italy*
Jim Ver Steeg, MD, *Colorado Springs, Colo*
Andrew L. Wagner, MD, *Tampa, Fla*
Han Hyun Young, *Taejon, South Korea*
Marc Zins, MD, *Paris, France*

Patency of Coronary Bypass Grafts: Assessment with Breath-hold Contrast-enhanced MR Angiography—Value of a Non–Electrocardiographically Triggered Technique[1]

Bernd J. Wintersperger, MD
Markus G. Engelmann, MD
Alexander von Smekal, MD
Andreas Knez, MD
Herbert V. Penzkofer, PhD
Berthold Höfling, MD
Gerhard Laub, PhD
Maximilian F. Reiser, MD

Index terms:
Arteries, grafts and prostheses, 949.4529
Arteries, internal mammary, 949.4529
Arteries, internal thoracic, 949.4529
Coronary vessels, surgery, 54.4551
Magnetic resonance (MR), vascular studies, 54.12142
Veins, grafts and prostheses, 933.4521

Radiology 1998; 208:345–351

Abbreviations:
CI = confidence interval
ECG = electrocardiography
ITA = internal thoracic artery
LAD = left anterior descending
LCx = left circumflex
RCA = right coronary artery
SNR = signal-to-noise ratio
3D = three-dimensional

[1] From the Departments of Diagnostic Radiology (B.J.W., A.v.S., H.V.P., M.F.R.) and Cardiology (M.G.E., A.K., B.H.), Klinikum Grosshadern, Ludwig-Maximilians-University Munich, Marchioninistrasse 15, 81377 Munich, Germany; and Siemens Medical Systems, Erlangen, Germany (G.L.). From the 1997 RSNA scientific assembly. Received October 27, 1997; revision requested November 25; revision received February 6, 1998; accepted March 5. **Address reprint requests to** B.J.W.

Author contributions:
Guarantors of integrity of entire study, B.J.W., M.G.E.; study concepts, B.J.W., A.v.S., G.L.; study design, B.J.W., M.G.E., A.v.S.; definition of intellectual content, B.J.W.; literature research, B.J.W.; clinical studies, B.J.W., M.G.E., A.K., B.H.; data acquisition, B.J.W., A.K., B.H.; data analysis, B.J.W., A.v.S., M.G.E., A.K.; statistical analysis, H.V.P.; manuscript preparation, B.J.W., M.G.E.; manuscript editing, H.V.P., G.L.; manuscript review, M.F.R.

PURPOSE: To determine the value of non–electrocardiographically triggered contrast material–enhanced magnetic resonance (MR) angiography in assessing the patency of venous and internal thoracic artery (ITA) grafts after coronary bypass surgery.

MATERIALS AND METHODS: Twenty-seven patients with 76 coronary bypass grafts (48 venous, 28 ITA) were examined 26.5 months ± 5.8 after surgery with MR angiography and conventional angiography. MR angiography was performed with a three-dimensional gradient-echo sequence after automated injection of contrast material; contrast agent administration was based on measurement of the individual transit time of the agent. Results of MR angiography were interpreted by two independent observers and compared with results of conventional angiography.

RESULTS: The independent interpretations of the MR angiograms agreed with the results of conventional angiography in 96% and 91% of the grafts. After a final consensus reading, sensitivity was 95% for all grafts, 94% for venous grafts, and 96% for ITA grafts. Specificity was 85% for venous grafts and 67% for ITA grafts. Positive predictive value was 95% for all grafts, 94% for venous grafts, and 96% for ITA grafts.

CONCLUSION: Non–electrocardiographically triggered contrast-enhanced MR angiography allows reliable assessment of the patency of venous and arterial coronary bypass grafts.

Coronary bypass surgery is one of the most common revascularization procedures, especially in patients with multivessel ischemic heart disease (1). The clinical outcome of coronary bypass surgery depends mainly on the status of the graft (whether it is patent) (2). There are major differences in the occlusion rate between saphenous vein grafts (up to 20% in the 1st postoperative year) and internal thoracic artery (internal mammary artery) (ITA) grafts (up to 5% in the 1st postoperative year) (3,4). Although creation of ITA grafts does not improve clinical outcome in the 1st postoperative year (4), the superior long-term patency of ITA grafts leads to improved long-term survival (5). In patients with recurrent chest pain after bypass surgery, graft patency is routinely determined with conventional angiography. Although conventional angiography is the standard of reference in graft assessment, this modality has certain disadvantages, which include invasiveness and x-ray exposure.

Magnetic resonance (MR) imaging allows reliable, noninvasive assessment of the patency of saphenous vein grafts for coronary bypass and has been proposed as a useful screening procedure for assessment of graft patency (6,7). Current approaches to demonstrating graft patency primarily use electrocardiographically (ECG) triggered two-dimensional spin-echo or gradient-echo techniques with multiple data acquisitions and limited spatial resolution. Three-dimensional (3D) spoiled gradient-echo imaging in combination with paramagnetic contrast material can demonstrate the thoracic and abdominal aorta and the major aortic branches in a single breath hold (8–10). Preliminary results indicate that bypass graft patency can be determined with ECG-triggered contrast-enhanced MR angiography (11). However, this technique is not well established.

We performed a prospective study to determine the value of non–ECG-triggered contrast-enhanced 3D MR angiography in assessing the patency of venous and arterial coronary bypass grafts.

MATERIALS AND METHODS

Patients

We studied 27 patients (26 men, one woman) who had undergone coronary bypass graft surgery. Their mean age at MR imaging was 58.3 years ± 9.1 (standard deviation) (range, 42.6–75.8 years). The mean interval between surgery and MR imaging was 26.5 months ± 5.8 (range, 22.5–50.7 months). All patients were regularly scheduled for follow-up conventional angiography as part of another study protocol and gave written informed consent for that study and for MR angiography, both of which were approved by the review board of our hospital. MR angiography was performed before (n = 14) or after (n = 13) conventional angiography, with a mean interval between MR angiography and conventional angiography of 12.6 hours ± 10.5 (range, 1.5–40.6 hours).

A total of 76 grafts were created in these patients: 48 venous grafts (63%) and 28 ITA grafts (37%) (24 left sided, four right sided). Thirty-nine grafts (16 venous, 23 ITA) were attached to the left anterior descending (LAD) artery or diagonal branches of this artery. Twenty-four grafts (22 venous, two ITA) were attached to the left circumflex artery (LCx) or marginal branches of this artery. Thirteen grafts (10 venous, three ITA) were attached to the right coronary artery (RCA) or posterior descending artery (Table 1).

MR Angiography

MR angiography was performed with a 1.5-T whole-body system (Magnetom Vision; Siemens Medical Systems, Erlangen, Germany) equipped with 25 mT/m high-performance gradients that enabled a 600-μsec rise time. A four-element phased-array body coil was used to optimize signal detection. A 3D radio-frequency spoiled fast low-angle shot sequence without ECG triggering was used (repetition time msec/echo time msec = 5/2). The last 10 patients were examined with an upgraded version of the sequence (4.4/1.8). In both versions, a flip angle of 40° was used.

Sagittal and coronal data acquisitions were performed consecutively. The base matrix size in the readout direction was 512 (reduced to 70% in the phase-encoding direction) with a 500-mm field of view. The rectangular field of view was adapted to the patient's constitution and the imaging orientation and was 250–313 mm in the sagittal orientation and 250–375 mm in the coronal orientation. The 3D volume had a thickness of 96 mm and was subdivided into 26–40 partitions, which yielded a maximum acquisition time of approximately 30 seconds.

The mean section thickness was 2.8 mm ± 0.3 (range, 2.4–3.7 mm) for sagittal acquisitions and 3.3 mm ± 0.3 (range, 2.8–3.7 mm) for coronal acquisitions ($P <$ .001 [t test]) with an in-plane resolution of 1.37 mm² (0.98 × 1.40 mm). The mean acquisition time was 29.6 seconds ± 1.9 (range, 26.9–32.2 seconds) in the sagittal slab orientation and 30.9 seconds ± 1.7 (range, 26.9–35.5 seconds) in the coronal slab orientation (P = .001 [t test]).

Each data acquisition was enhanced with a 20-mL bolus of gadopentetate dimeglumine (Magnevist; Schering, Berlin, Germany). Contrast material was automatically administered with a 20-gauge needle and an MR-compatible power injector (Spectris; Medrad, Pittsburgh, Pa) into an antecubital vein at a constant flow rate of 2 mL/sec. Contrast agent administration was followed by flushing with 20 mL of saline. The mean patient weight was 79.8 kg ± 12.3 (range, 65–106 kg), which resulted in a mean gadolinium dose of 0.13 mmol/kg ± 0.02 (range, 0.09–0.15 mmol/kg).

To optimize contrast enhancement, the transit time of the contrast agent was evaluated with a sequential TurboFLASH (Siemens Medical Systems) (fast low-angle shot) sequence combined with a 2-mL bolus of contrast material and the same injection parameters (flow rate of 2 mL/sec, flushing with 20 mL of saline). After time-intensity analysis, the individual start delay to cover the central k-space acquisition with contrast material was calculated as follows: $T_d = T_t - (T_a/2) + 4$, where T_d is the delay (in seconds) between the start of contrast material injection and data acquisition, T_t is the transit time (in seconds) of the contrast agent between the injection site and the volume of interest, and T_a is the 3D data acquisition time (in seconds).

TABLE 1
Types of Bypass Grafts and Vessel Areas Supplied

Supplied Vessel Area	ITA Grafts	Venous Grafts	Total
LAD	23 (30)	16 (21)	39 (51)
LCx	2 (3)	22 (29)	24 (32)
RCA	3 (4)	10 (13)	13 (17)
Total	28 (37)	48 (63)	76 (100)

Note.—Values are numbers of patients; values in parentheses are percentages.

Graft patency was assessed independently by two radiologists experienced in MR (B.J.W., A.v.S.) who were blinded to the results of conventional angiography. In cases of disagreement about graft patency, a final consensus reading of the images was performed. Surgical notes were available in all patients, and images obtained in both orientations (sagittal and coronal) were read together to cover the whole volume of possible graft courses. Each graft was divided into three sections (proximal anastomosis or origin, course, and distal anastomosis), and each section was judged to be visible or nonvisible. Grafts were considered patent if the course was visible.

Contrast enhancement and image quality (ie, the presence of blurring or respiratory artifacts) were ranked subjectively with a three-step scale. Contrast enhancement was considered poor (grade 1) when insufficient for diagnosis of graft patency, good (grade 2) when sufficient for diagnosis of graft patency without excellent vascular opacification, and excellent (grade 3) in cases with a high degree of vascular opacification. Image quality was ranked as grade 1 when insufficient for diagnosis due to blurring or major artifacts, as grade 2 when sufficient for diagnosis with only minor blurring or artifacts, and as grade 3 when sufficient for diagnosis without blurring or artifacts.

Signal-to-noise ratio (SNR) was assessed for each data acquisition in the ascending aorta and the main pulmonary artery. SNR in the ascending aorta was measured to objectify differences between different grades of vascular opacification; the ratio of SNR in the ascending aorta to SNR in the pulmonary artery was used to esti-

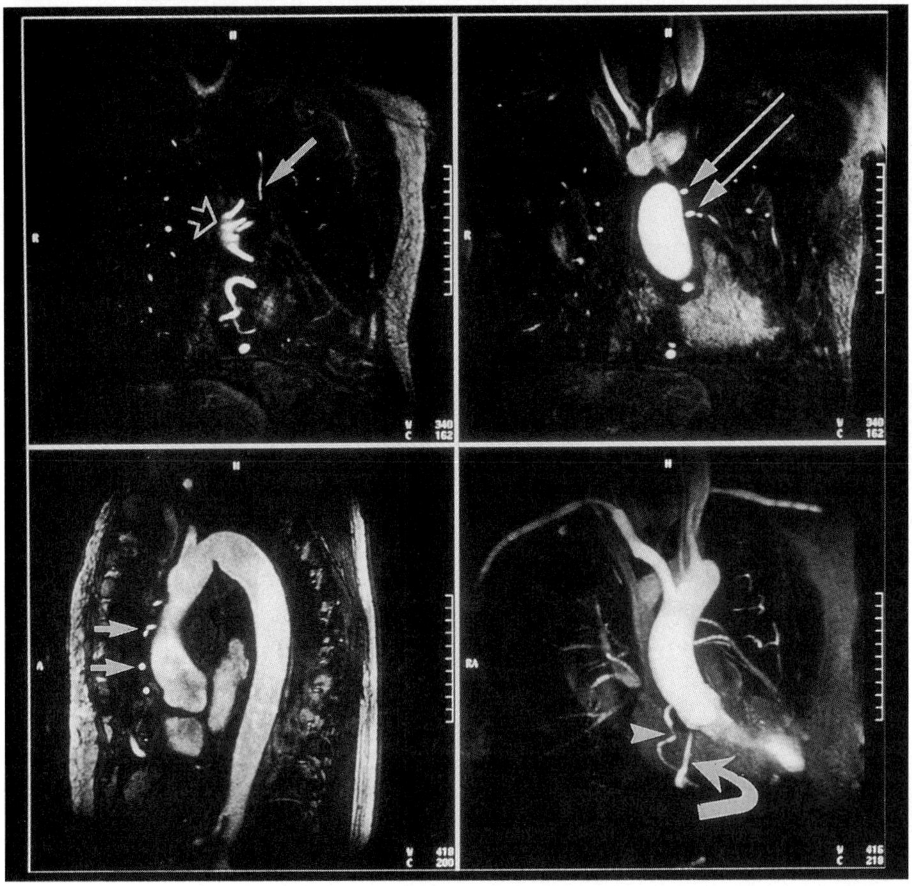

Figure 1. Top left: Coronal MR angiogram shows the aortic anastomosis site of five venous grafts (open arrow) and a middle portion of the course of a left-sided ITA graft (solid arrow). Top right: Coronal MR angiogram in the same patient shows parts of the courses of the venous grafts (arrows). Bottom left: Sagittal MR angiogram in the same patient shows the venous grafts (arrows) anterior to the ascending aorta. Bottom right: Coronal maximum intensity projection MR angiogram in the same patient shows a venous graft (arrow) to the RCA. A severe stenosis of the RCA (arrowhead) is also visible.

TABLE 2
SNRs according to Contrast Enhancement and Timing of Contrast Material Administration

Characteristic Evaluated	SNR by Type of Data Set: Sagittal	Coronal
Contrast enhancement*		
Grade 1	3.3, 3.6	NA
Grade 2	7.9 ± 2.3	9.8 ± 3.3
Grade 3	11.4 ± 2.2	12.4 ± 2.8
Timing of contrast material administration†		
Grade 1	0.3, 0.4	NA
Grade 2	1.8 ± 1.0	1.5 ± 0.5
Grade 3	2.6 ± 1.2	2.0 ± 0.6

Note.—NA = not applicable.
* SNR was measured in the ascending aorta.
† SNR in the ascending aorta was compared with SNR in the pulmonary artery.

mate the quality of the timing of contrast material administration in different degrees of subjective contrast grading. SNR was calculated as the ratio of the signal in the vessel of interest to the mean background signal (12).

Conventional Angiography

Biplane conventional angiography was performed with the Judkins technique. Before selective catheterization of the native coronary arteries and the bypass grafts, aortography and ventriculography were performed. The angiograms were analyzed by two experienced cardiologists (M.G.E., A.K.) who scored the grafts according to the classification used in the Thrombolysis in Myocardial Infarction trial (13). Grafts classified as grade 0 or 1 were considered occluded; all others were considered patent.

Statistical Analysis

The sensitivity, specificity, and positive predictive value of contrast-enhanced MR angiography in the assessment of graft patency were calculated, as well as 95% confidence intervals (CIs). Sensitivity was calculated as truly patent grafts/(truly patent grafts + falsely occluded grafts). Specificity was calculated as truly occluded grafts/(truly occluded grafts + falsely patent grafts). Positive predictive value was calculated as truly patent grafts/(truly patent grafts + falsely patent grafts). The results of conventional angiography served as the standard of reference.

The Cohen κ statistic was used to evaluate interobserver agreement and agreement between MR angiography and conventional angiography. The Fisher exact test was used to compare proportions (sensitivity, specificity, positive predictive value). The paired or unpaired Student *t* test was used to compare data acquisition parameters and SNRs. A P value less than .05 was considered to indicate a statistically significant difference.

RESULTS

Contrast Enhancement and Image Quality

In all but one patient, data acquisition could be performed in both orientations (Fig 1). One patient's examination was interrupted after sagittal data acquisition due to claustrophobia. Thus, contrast enhancement and image quality could be evaluated in 53 data sets (27 sagittal, 26 coronal).

Contrast enhancement was grade 3 in 23 data sets (43%), grade 2 in 28 (53%), and grade 1 in two (4%). Although the contrast enhancement was not of diagnostic value in two sagittal data sets, in both patients a final diagnosis could be made with the coronal data set, which had better, diagnostic contrast enhancement. Image quality was diagnostic in all data sets, with eight (15%) considered grade 3 (no artifacts) and 45 (85%) considered grade 2 (minor artifacts).

Mean SNR in the ascending aorta was 11.4 ± 2.2 (range, 8.3–15.6) for sagittal data sets with grade 3 contrast enhancement and 7.9 ± 2.3 (range, 4.4–11.8) for sagittal data sets with grade 2 contrast enhancement ($P < .001$ [*t* test]) (Table 2); the higher SNR indicates better vascular opacification. The two sagittal data sets with nondiagnostic contrast enhancement had SNRs in the ascending aorta of only 3.3 and 3.6.

The mean ratio of SNR in the ascending

aorta to SNR in the pulmonary artery was higher in sagittal data sets with grade 3 image quality than in those with grade 2 image quality (2.6 ± 1.2 vs 1.8 ± 1.0) (P = .128 [t test]). In the nondiagnostic data sets, this ratio was only 0.3 and 0.4, indicating inadequate timing of contrast material administration with better vascular opacification in the pulmonary artery than in the ascending aorta during acquisition of central k space.

Mean SNR in the ascending aorta was 12.4 ± 2.8 (range, 8.2–17.0) for coronal data sets with grade 3 contrast enhancement and 9.8 ± 3.3 (range, 4.7–16.0) for coronal data sets with grade 2 contrast enhancement (P = .045 [t test]). Contrary to the results in the sagittal data sets, the mean ratio of SNR in the ascending aorta to SNR in the pulmonary artery was significantly higher in coronal data sets with grade 3 image quality than in those with grade 2 image quality (2.0 ± 0.6 vs 1.5 ± 0.5) (P = .01 [t test]).

TABLE 3
Results of MR Angiography according to Graft Type

Type of Graft	Sensitivity (%)	Specificity (%)	Positive Predictive Value (%)
ITA (n = 28)	96 (89, 100)	67 (49, 84)	96 (89, 100)
Venous (n = 48)	94 (88, 100)	85 (74, 95)	94 (88, 100)
All grafts (n = 76)	95 (90, 100)	81 (72, 90)	95 (90, 100)

Note.—Values in parentheses are 95% CIs.

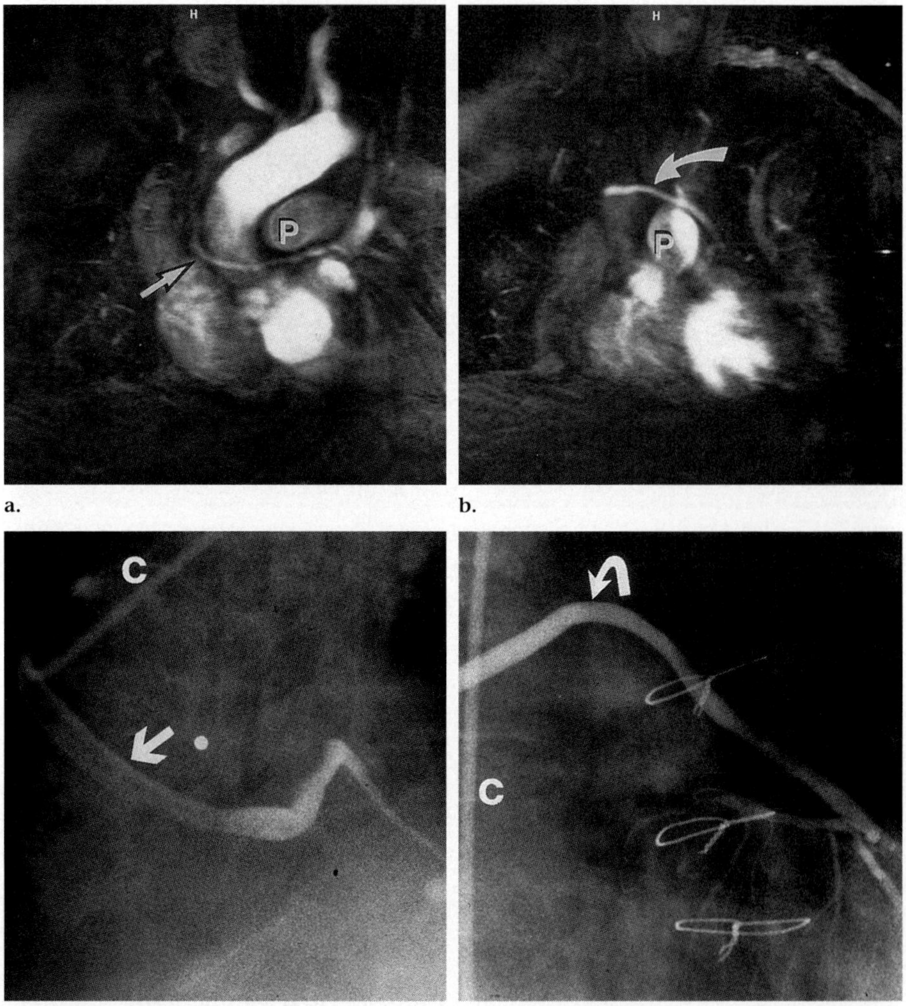

a. b. c. d.

Figure 2. **(a)** MR angiogram shows a patent venous graft (arrow) to the obtuse marginal branch of the LCx artery that courses through the transversal pericardial sinus. P = main pulmonary artery. **(b)** MR angiogram shows a patent venous graft (arrow) to the LAD artery that courses over the main pulmonary artery (P). **(c)** Corresponding conventional angiogram shows the patent venous graft (arrow) to the obtuse marginal branch of the LCx artery. C = catheter. **(d)** Corresponding conventional angiogram shows the patent venous graft (arrow) to the LAD artery. C = catheter.

Graft Patency

At conventional angiography, 79% of all grafts (60 of 76), 73% of venous grafts (35 of 48), and 89% of ITA grafts (25 of 28) were patent. There was interobserver agreement in 87% of all grafts (66 of 76) (κ = 0.65), 88% of venous grafts (42 of 48) (κ = 0.71), and 86% of ITA grafts (24 of 28) (κ = 0.44). One observer agreed with the results of conventional angiography in 96% of all grafts (73 of 76) (κ = 0.88); the other agreed with the results of conventional angiography in 91% (69 of 76) (κ = 0.75).

After final consensus reading of images of the 10 grafts (six venous, four ITA) with discrepant interpretations, 60 grafts (including three falsely patent grafts) were found to be patent at MR angiography, resulting in a sensitivity of 95% (95% CI = 90%, 100%) (Table 3). Of the 35 patent venous grafts at conventional angiography, 33 were truly patent and two falsely occluded at MR angiography (sensitivity, 94%; 95% CI = 88%, 100%) (Fig 2). Of the 25 patent ITA grafts at conventional angiography, 24 were correctly assessed at MR angiography (sensitivity, 96%; 95% CI = 89%, 100%) (Fig 3). There were no statistically significant differences between the sensitivities (P = 1.0 [Fisher exact test]).

Of 13 occluded venous grafts and three occluded ITA grafts at conventional angiography, two venous grafts and one ITA graft were falsely patent at MR angiography, resulting in a specificity of 85% (95% CI = 74%, 95%) for venous grafts and 67% (95% CI = 49%, 84%) for ITA grafts (P = .49 [Fisher exact test]). The specificity for all grafts was 81% (13 of 16; 95% CI = 72%, 90%) (Table 3). Exclusion of the false-positive ITA graft, which was clearly patent at MR angiography but was considered occluded at conventional angiography, would have resulted in a specificity of 100% (two of two) for ITA grafts and 87% (13 of 15) for all grafts.

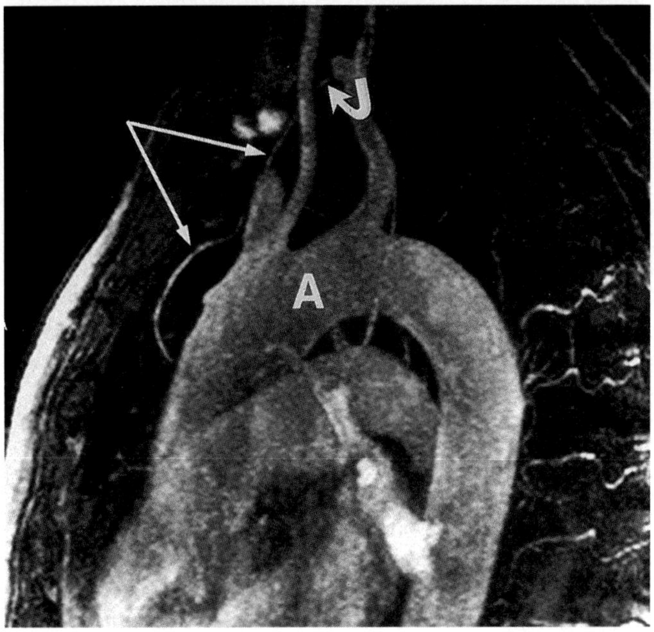

Figure 3. Sagittal maximum intensity projection MR angiogram shows a patent left-sided ITA graft (straight arrows) that originates (curved arrow) at the left subclavian artery. *A* = aorta.

TABLE 4
Results of MR Angiography according to Vessel Area Supplied

Supplied Vessel Area	Sensitivity (%)	Specificity (%)	Positive Predictive Value (%)
LAD (*n* = 39)	97 (92, 100)	100 (100, 100)	97 (92, 100)
LCx (*n* = 24)	87 (73, 100)	78 (61, 94)	87 (73, 100)
RCA (*n* = 13)	92 (77, 100)	50 (23, 77)	100 (100, 100)
All grafts (*n* = 76)	95 (90, 100)	81 (72, 90)	95 (90, 100)

Note.—Values in parentheses are 95% CIs.

The positive predictive value was 94% (95% CI = 88%, 100%) for venous grafts, 96% (95% CI = 89%, 100%) for ITA grafts, and 95% (95% CI = 90%, 100%) for all grafts (P = 1.0 [Fisher exact test]) (Table 3). Graft status was correctly assessed with MR angiography in 22 of 27 patients (81%); in five patients (19%), the status of at least one graft was incorrectly assessed.

The sensitivity of MR angiography varied according to the site of the distal anastomosis. Sensitivity was higher for LAD artery grafts (97%; 95% CI = 92%, 100%) than for LCx artery grafts (87%; 95% CI = 73%, 100%) or RCA grafts (92%; 95% CI = 77%, 100%) (P = .67 [Fisher exact test]) (Table 4). Specificity ranged from 50% (95% CI = 23%, 77%) for RCA grafts to 78% (95% CI = 61%, 94%) for LCx artery grafts to 100% (95% CI = 100%, 100%) for LAD artery grafts (P = .21 [Fisher exact test]). Exclusion of the false-positive ITA graft, which was clearly patent at MR angiography but was considered occluded at conventional angiography, would have resulted in a specificity of 100% for RCA grafts and 87% for all grafts.

The visibility of different graft sections in truly patent grafts varied. Because only grafts with visible courses were considered patent, the course could be visualized in all truly patent venous grafts (33 of 33) and ITA grafts (24 of 24). In all 33 truly patent venous grafts, the aortic anastomosis could be identified. Graft origin at the right or left subclavian artery could be seen in 21 of 24 ITA grafts (88%). None of the distal anastomoses at the level of the native coronary arteries could be identified; as a result, two stenoses of the distal anastomosis seen at conventional angiography were overlooked at MR angiography. In all 11 truly occluded venous grafts at MR angiography, an aortic stump could be seen at the proximal anastomosis.

DISCUSSION

In patients who have undergone coronary bypass surgery, chest pain occurs because of ischemic or nonischemic causes. Ischemic causes include severe graft stenosis, graft occlusion, and progressive atherosclerosis of the native coronary arteries. Knowledge of graft patency is required to distinguish nonischemic causes from problems with myocardial perfusion due to graft occlusion or worsening coronary artery status and to apply adequate therapeutic procedures. Assessment of graft patency is possible with direct or indirect imaging modalities (14,15). Indirect methods such as echocardiography, scintigraphy, and positron emission tomography allow graft patency to be inferred from regional myocardial perfusion or myocardial wall motion. In contrast, methods like helical computed tomography (CT), electron-beam CT, MR angiography, and conventional angiography allow direct visualization of patent vessels.

The standard of reference in graft diagnostics and assessment of graft patency is conventional angiography. However, conventional angiography is invasive and can be associated with minor or major complications such as bleeding, myocardial infarction, arrhythmia, or stroke. For these reasons, a reliable method of assessing graft patency that is noninvasive or minimally invasive would be preferable.

MR imaging of coronary bypass grafts was proposed by Herfkens et al (16) in 1983. Since that time, MR imaging studies of coronary bypass grafts have concentrated on use of noninvasive spin-echo or gradient-echo techniques. These techniques demonstrate patent bypass grafts with flow-related phenomena such as flow void in spin-echo imaging and flow-related enhancement or flow-induced phase shift in gradient-echo imaging.

Spin-echo imaging allows correct assessment of graft status in 78%–90% of venous grafts (6,17–19). This technique was quite promising from the beginning, even though investigators showed varying results, with an estimated sensitivity of 89%–98% at correlation with conventional angiography (6,17–19). Specificity ranged from 72% to 90% (6,17–19). At spin-echo imaging, grafts with normal flow appear dark because of the signal void due to movement of previous excited spins during the different pulses of the sequence. Accuracy limitations of spin-echo imaging are due to signal void produced by other factors: For example, metal artifacts along graft courses may mimic a patent graft or may obscure graft courses. The latter limitation especially affects ITA grafts along the inside of the thoracic wall.

In contrast, gradient-echo imaging involves flow-related enhancement due to inflowing spins without previous excitation. Therefore, patent grafts appear bright, whereas metal artifacts produce signal void. Special gradient applications in combination with gradient-echo techniques allow velocity and flow measurement. White et al (20) demonstrated the feasibility of gradient-echo imaging for graft assessment and reported a sensitivity and specificity of 93% and 86%, respectively. Other studies (21) showed different results, with sensitivity (88%) lower than specificity (100%). Initial evaluations of venous graft flow to verify graft function showed changes in graft flow during the cardiac cycle that may be helpful in quantification of graft stenosis and follow-up after interventional therapy (22–24).

On the basis of these results, MR imaging has been proposed as a useful screening procedure for assessing graft patency and function in postoperative pain syndromes (6,7). However, until now investigators have focused primarily on venous grafts. ITA grafts have been represented only minimally or excluded from statistical analysis, mostly because of obscuring metal artifacts. The presence of such artifacts and the exclusion from data analysis is a critical point because ITA grafts are widely used due to the positive effects on patients' long-term outcomes (5). To introduce MR imaging into the clinical routine as a screening method, reliable assessment of both venous and arterial graft patency is necessary.

Contrast-enhanced MR angiography, which involves T1 shortening of flow in vessels of interest by paramagnetic contrast agents, allows much faster acquisition of 3D data sets (25). Advances in hardware with high-performance gradients have led to data acquisition within a single breath hold (26). This technique extends the diagnostic usefulness of MR imaging in evaluating the thoracic and abdominal aorta and major aortic branches (8–10). With an optimized protocol for contrast agent administration, obscuring venous enhancement can be minimized and optimal image quality can be achieved (27).

A recent study (11) evaluated the use of ECG-triggered contrast-enhanced MR angiography for visualization of bypass grafts and assessment of graft patency. A large proportion of ITA grafts (36%) were included in that study. With graft occlusion regarded as a positive finding, the investigators achieved a sensitivity of 93% and specificity of 97%. Despite the different definitions of a positive finding, sensitivity was similar in our study (95% for all grafts and 96% for ITA grafts). However, there was a difference in overall specificity between the two studies; in particular, the specificity was only 67% for the ITA grafts in our study. The latter result may have been due to the small number of occluded ITA grafts in our study.

In our study, one ITA graft could not be selectively cannulated and was considered occluded at conventional angiography, even though it was clearly demonstrated at MR angiography. This case demonstrates potential problems in selective catheterization of ITA grafts that may lead to incorrect results. Exclusion of grafts incorrectly assessed with conventional angiography (as was done by Vrachliotis et al [11]) leads to a specificity of 100% for ITA grafts and 87% for all grafts in our study.

The proximal anastomosis could be visualized in 100% of truly patent venous grafts; in 88% of truly patent ITA grafts, the origin at the subclavian artery could be identified. In contrast to respiratory motion, rhythmic cardiac motion does not markedly affect visualization of proximal graft parts. Furthermore, respiratory motion can be easily avoided by means of breath holding. Conversely, distal graft parts are markedly affected by cardiac motion; therefore, none of the distal anastomoses could be visualized due to blurring caused by cardiac motion. Additional ECG triggering cannot improve identification of distal anastomoses because of the data acquisition window, which is too long to freeze cardiac motion (11).

Within the same acquisition time, spatial resolution can be improved by using a non–ECG-triggered technique. Vrachliotis et al (11) achieved a minimum pixel size of 2.0 × 1.6 mm, more than twice the pixel size in our study (1.4 × 1.0 mm). Smaller pixel size should result in improved graft visualization (especially for ITA grafts) and may be the basis for identification of graft stenosis. In addition, the timing of contrast agent administration is more complicated in ECG-triggered imaging than in non–ECG-triggered imaging (varying data acquisition times depending on the length of the cardiac cycle). Individual timing of contrast agent administration adapted to the patient's circulation improves enhancement of vessels of interest and the reproducibility of contrast-enhanced MR angiographic studies with a reasonable amount of contrast material. Our protocol for timing contrast agent administration provided diagnostic contrast enhancement with 0.09–0.15 mmol/kg of gadopentetate dimeglumine in 96% of data sets (51 of 53). The mean ratio of SNR in the ascending aorta versus SNR in the pulmonary artery was 1.5–2.6, which indicates adequate timing of contrast agent administration, with higher signal intensity in the ascending aorta than in the pulmonary artery. None of the falsely occluded grafts at MR angiography were misdiagnosed because of the presence of hemostatic clips, which represented a major problem with former techniques.

In contrast to most other investigations, we studied a homogeneous patient group with similar graft ages. Enrolling patients with no clinical reason for undergoing repeated conventional angiography enabled an objective comparison of MR angiography and conventional angiography without an increased pretest probability of graft occlusion. In addition, the high percentage of ITA grafts (37%) evaluated in our study reflects the current increase in use of ITA grafts in comparison to venous grafts.

The results of our study demonstrate that non–ECG-triggered breath-hold contrast-enhanced MR angiography is suitable for visualizing venous and arterial coronary bypass grafts and allows reliable assessment of graft patency. Identification of graft stenosis continues to be a problem, however, especially at the coronary artery anastomosis. Further improvement of spatial resolution and reduction of repetition time to minimize blurring due to rhythmic cardiac motion are possible means of overcoming this problem.

References

1. Angelini GD, Newby AC. The future of saphenous vein as a coronary artery bypass conduit. Eur Heart J 1989; 10:273–280.
2. Lipton MJ, Takaro T, Clayman J, Maley T. Factors associated with long-term graft patency after coronary bypass surgery. Prog Cardiovasc Dis 1986; 28:301–308.
3. van der Meer J, Hillege HL, Kootstra GJ, et al. Prevention of one-year vein-graft occlusion after aortocoronary-bypass surgery: a comparison of low-dose aspirin, low-dose aspirin plus dipyridamole, and oral anticoagulants. Lancet 1993; 342:257–264.
4. van der Meer J, Hillege HL, van Gilst WH, et al. A comparison of internal mammary artery and saphenous vein grafts after

coronary artery bypass surgery: no difference in 1-year occlusion rates and clinical outcome. Circulation 1994; 90:2367–2374.
5. Cameron A, Davis KB, Green G, Schaff HV. Coronary bypass surgery with internal-thoracic-artery grafts: effects on survival over a 15-year period. N Engl J Med 1996; 334:216–219.
6. Jenkins JP, Love HG, Foster CJ, Isherwood I, Rowlands DJ. Detection of coronary artery bypass graft patency as assessed by magnetic resonance imaging. Br J Radiol 1988; 61:2–4.
7. van Rossum AC, Galjee MA, Doesburg T, Hofman M, Valk J. The role of magnetic resonance in the evaluation of functional results after CABG/PTCA. Int J Card Imaging 1993; 9(suppl 1):59–69.
8. Prince MR, Narasimham DL, Stanley JC, et al. Breath-hold gadolinium-enhanced MR angiography of the abdominal aorta and its major branches. Radiology 1995; 197:785–792.
9. Holland GA, Dougherty L, Carpenter JP, Axel L. Breath-hold ultrafast three-dimensional gadolinium-enhanced MR angiography of the aorta and the renal and other visceral abdominal arteries. AJR 1996; 166: 971–981.
10. Snidow JJ, Johnson MS, Harris VJ, Trerotola SO. Three-dimensional gadolinium-enhanced MR angiography for aortoiliac inflow assessment plus renal artery screening in a single breath hold. Radiology 1996; 198:725–732.
11. Vrachliotis TG, Bis KG, Aliabadi D, Shetty AN, Safian R, Simonetti O. Contrast-enhanced breath-hold MR angiography for evaluating patency of coronary artery bypass grafts. AJR 1997; 168:1073–1080.
12. Kaufman L, Kramer DM, Crooks LE, Ortendahl DA. Measuring signal-to-noise ratios in MR imaging. Radiology 1989; 173:265–267.
13. Chesebro JH, Knatterud G, Roberts R, et al. Thrombolysis in Myocardial Infarction (TIMI) trial, phase I: a comparison between intravenous tissue plasminogen activator and intravenous streptokinase—clinical findings through hospital discharge. Circulation 1987; 76:142–154.
14. Stanford W, Galvin JR, Skorton DJ, Marcus ML. The evaluation of coronary bypass graft patency: direct and indirect techniques other than coronary angiography. AJR 1991; 156:15–22.
15. Stanford W, Galvin JR, Thompson BH, Grover-McKay M, Skorton DJ. Nonangiographic assessment of coronary artery bypass graft patency. Int J Card Imaging 1993; 9:77–86.
16. Herfkens RJ, Higgins CB, Hricak H, et al. Nuclear magnetic resonance imaging of the cardiovascular system: normal and pathologic findings. Radiology 1983; 147: 749–759.
17. White RD, Caputo GR, Mark AS, Modin GW, Higgins CB. Coronary artery bypass graft patency: noninvasive evaluation with MR imaging. Radiology 1987; 164: 681–686.
18. Rubinstein RI, Askenase AD, Thickman D, Feldman MS, Agarwal JB, Helfant RH. Magnetic resonance imaging to evaluate patency of aortocoronary bypass grafts. Circulation 1987; 76:786–791.
19. Frija G, Schouman-Claeys E, Lacombe P, Bismuth V, Ollivier JP. A study of coronary artery bypass graft patency using MR imaging. J Comput Assist Tomogr 1989; 13: 226–232.
20. White RD, Pflugfelder PW, Lipton MJ, Higgins CB. Coronary artery bypass grafts: evaluation of patency with cine MR imaging. AJR 1988; 150:1271–1274.
21. Aurigemma GP, Reichek N, Axel L, Schiebler M, Harris C, Kressel HY. Noninvasive determination of coronary artery bypass graft patency by cine magnetic resonance imaging. Circulation 1989; 80:1595–1602.
22. Hoogendoorn LI, Pattynama PM, Buis B, van der Geest RJ, van der Wall EE, de Roos A. Noninvasive evaluation of aortocoronary bypass grafts with magnetic resonance flow mapping. Am J Cardiol 1995; 75:845–848.
23. Galjee MA, van Rossum AC, Doesburg T, Hofman MB, Falke TH, Visser CA. Quantification of coronary artery bypass graft flow by magnetic resonance phase velocity mapping. Magn Reson Imaging 1996; 14:485–493.
24. Galjee MA, van Rossum AC, Doesburg T, van Eenige MJ, Visser CA. Value of magnetic resonance imaging in assessing patency and function of coronary artery bypass grafts: an angiographically controlled study. Circulation 1996; 93:660–666.
25. Prince MR. Gadolinium-enhanced MR aortography. Radiology 1994; 191:155–164.
26. Shetty AN, Shirkhoda A, Bis KG, Alcantara A. Contrast-enhanced three-dimensional MR angiography in a single breath-hold: a novel technique. AJR 1995; 165:1290–1292.
27. Hany TF, McKinnon GC, Leung DA, Pfammatter T, Debatin JF. Optimization of contrast timing for breath-hold three-dimensional MR angiography. JMRI 1997; 7:551–556.

Markus G. Lentschig, MD
Peter Reimer, MD
Ursula L. Rausch-Lentschig, MD
Thomas Allkemper, MD
Michael Oelerich, MD
Gerhard Laub, PhD

Index terms:
Angiography, comparative studies, 9*.121[2], 9*.12942
Aorta, MR, 9*.12942, 9*.12943
Aorta, stenosis or obstruction, 98.721, 94.721
Gadolinium
Magnetic resonance (MR), contrast enhancement, 9*.12943
Magnetic resonance (MR), vascular studies, 9*.12942, 9*.129416

Radiology 1998; 208:353–357

Abbreviations:
FLASH = fast low-angle shot
ROI = region of interest
TE = echo time
TR = repetition time
3D = three-dimensional

[1] From the Institute of Clinical Radiology, Westfalian Wilhelms-University, Albert-Schweitzer-Strasse 33, D-48129 Muenster, Germany (M.G.L., P.R., U.L.R.L., T.A., M.O.), and Siemens AG, Erlangen, Germany (G.L.). Received September 2, 1997; revision requested November 13; final revision received February 23, 1998; accepted March 4. **Address reprint requests to** M.G.L.

[2] 9* Vascular system, location unspecified

Author contributions:
Guarantor of integrity of entire study, M.G.L.; study concepts, M.G.L., P.R.; study design, M.G.L., P.R.; definition of intellectual content, M.G.L., P.R., G.L.; literature research, M.G.L., U.L.R.L.; clinical studies, M.G.L., T.A., M.O.; data acquisition, M.G.L., T.A., M.O.; data analysis, M.G.L., P.R., U.L.R.L.; statistical analysis, M.G.L., P.R.; manuscript preparation, M.G.L.; manuscript editing, P.R., U.L.R.L.; manuscript review, G.L.

Breath-hold Gadolinium-enhanced MR Angiography of the Major Vessels at 1.0 T: Dose-Response Findings and Angiographic Correlation[1]

PURPOSE: To find the appropriate contrast agent dose for gadolinium-enhanced magnetic resonance (MR) angiography by using individual measurements of contrast agent transit times in a randomized study.

MATERIALS AND METHODS: A total of 34 patients with disease of the aorta or its major branches or both were randomly assigned to receive a dose of 0.1, 0.2, or 0.3 mmol of gadopentetate dimeglumine per kilogram of body weight. Initially, contrast agent transit times were measured with use of a turbo fast-low-angle-shot sequence. Subsequently, a three-dimensional fast imaging with steady-state precession sequence (7.3-msec repetition time, 2.8-msec echo time) was used for breath-hold MR angiography. Gadopentetate dimeglumine was injected with an MR-compatible power injector. Efficacy was evaluated by measurement of vessel enhancement and by clinical correlation of MR angiograms with x-ray angiograms.

RESULTS: Evaluation of contrast agent transit time was possible in all patients with the test doses, which provided contrast-enhanced MR angiograms of constant quality. Neither vessel enhancement nor diagnostic information was significantly different across the three study groups.

CONCLUSION: The clinical gadolinium dose of 0.1 mmol/kg is sufficient for diagnostic assessment of the aorta and its major branches at contrast-enhanced MR angiography. High-dose studies appear not to be required for these large vessels.

Gadolinium-enhanced magnetic resonance (MR) angiography was introduced by Prince and co-workers (1–4), who used contrast material infusion techniques combined with non–breath-hold acquisitions. More recently, breath-hold MR angiography with acquisition times of 30 seconds or less have been developed by using high doses of gadolinium chelates (5,6). The latter approach uses fast bolus injection of gadolinium chelates at doses between 0.1 and 0.5 mmol/kg. However, doses greater than 0.1 mmol/kg have not been clinically approved. In addition, most studies have been performed at 1.5 T with ultrafast gradient capability (peak gradient strength between 16 and 25 mT/m).

Since the relaxivity of gadolinium chelates is independent of field strength from 0.2 to 1.5 T, gadolinium-enhanced MR angiography should also be feasible at a field strength of less than 1.5 T. Furthermore, optimized pulse sequences that use current gradient sets with short repetition times (TRs) and echo times (TEs) should allow breath-hold MR angiography with acquisition times of 30 seconds or less. We wished to demonstrate that breath-hold three-dimensional (3D) contrast material–enhanced MR angiography can be performed on a clinical 1.0-T system equipped with a regular gradient set by using such an optimized pulse sequence. The specific purpose of our study was to perform a randomized double-blind dose-response study with gadolinium ($\leq$0.3 mmol/kg) to determine the lowest effective dose for contrast-enhanced MR angiography of major vessels.

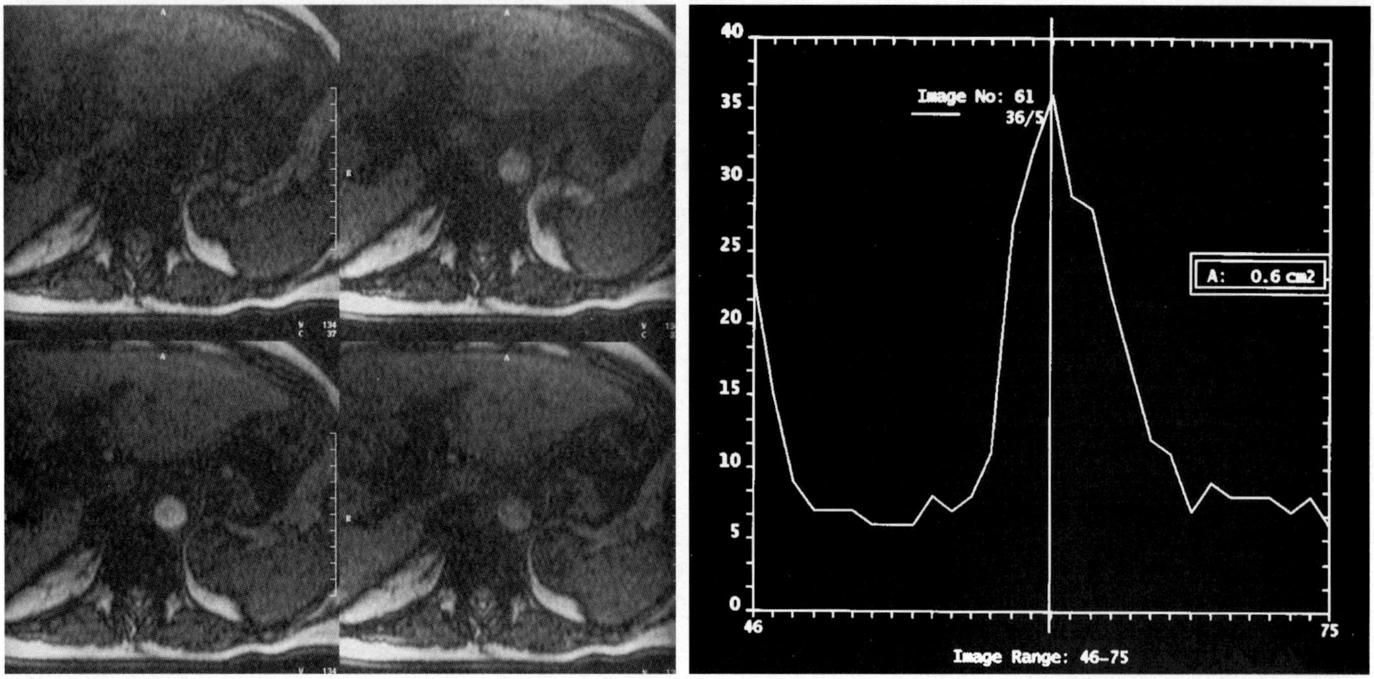

a. b.

Figure 1. Test examination performed with 1-mL bolus of gadopentetate dimeglumine and TurboFLASH sequence (8.5/4.0, 10° flip angle). **(a)** Sequential signal intensity measurement in an ROI (area, 0.6 cm^2) placed within the aorta (minimum signal intensity, 5; maximum signal intensity, 36). **(b)** Signal intensity–versus-time (46 = image number at 1st second, 75 = image number at 30th second) curve for calculating contrast agent transit time (image no. 61 − image no. 46, 15 seconds in this case).

MATERIALS AND METHODS

Patients

A total of 34 patients (13 women, 21 men; mean age, 54 years ± 17) underwent unenhanced and breath-hold gadolinium-enhanced ultrashort TE MR angiography of the thoracic or abdominal aorta and its major branches at 1.0 T (Magnetom Expert; Siemens, Erlangen, Germany). Informed consent was obtained from all patients, and approval from the Ethics Committee of our institution was also obtained. The study was performed in patients instead of volunteers to use the clinical diagnosis of vascular disease as one end point. Digital subtraction arteriography served as the imaging reference standard in 28 patients, and Doppler ultrasound (US) together with contrast-enhanced spiral computed tomography (CT) were available for the remaining patients, with availability of patient charts for all 34 patients. Patients were enrolled into the study over a period of 6 months, without any specific patient selection based on regular clinical referrals. Four patients had aortic aneurysms, two had aortic coarctation, 13 had atherosclerotic aortic disease, seven had thoracic outlet syndrome, four had atherosclerotic iliac disease, two had atherosclerotic carotid disease, and one each had stenosis of the mesenteric artery and the renal arteries.

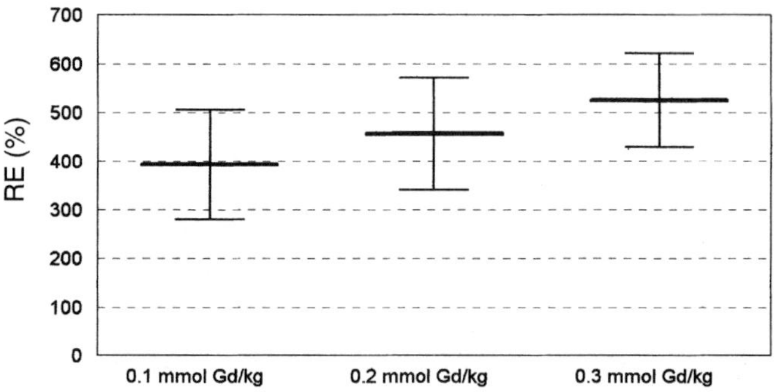

Figure 2. Relative vessel enhancement (*RE*) versus gadolinium dose per kilogram of body weight.

Contrast-enhanced MR Angiography

After the patient was positioned within a phased-array body coil, scout images were obtained to plan for measurements of individual contrast agent transit times into the region of interest (ROI). A test bolus of 1 mL of gadopentetate dimeglumine (Magnevist; Schering, Berlin, Germany) was injected by hand through an 18-gauge cubital intravenous line. The test bolus was flushed from the connecting intravenous line with 20 mL of saline within 4 seconds (5 mL/sec) after injection. A turbo fast-low-angle-shot (TurboFLASH; Siemens) sequence with a TR msec/TE msec/inversion time msec of 8.5/4.0/100, time delay of 84 msec, 10° flip angle, 96 (phase) × 256 (frequency) matrix, and 6/8 rectangular field of view of 350 × 400 mm was started simultaneously with contrast agent injection. A total of 60 axial images with a time resolution of 1,000 msec were acquired to calculate individual contrast agent transit times by means of sequential signal intensity measurements within an ROI placed in the aorta at the level of interest (Fig 1).

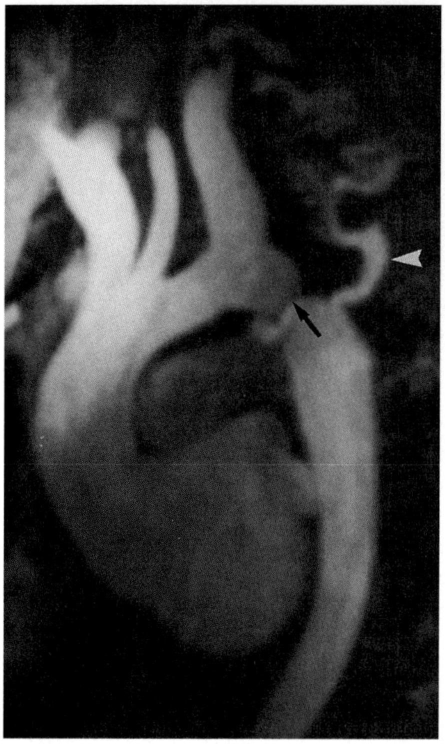

Figure 3. Breath-hold gadolinium-enhanced MR angiography at a dose of 0.1 mmol gadopentetate dimeglumine per kilogram of body weight. Maximum intensity projection image of the aortic arch (oblique image plane) shows postductal coarctation (arrow) of the thoracic aorta, with collateral vessels (arrowhead) originating from the left subclavian artery and draining into the descending aorta.

A nongated, 3D fast imaging with steady-state precession sequence (TR msec/TE msec = 7.3/2.8, 20° flip angle, 140 × 256 matrix, and 6/8 rectangular field of view of 350 × 400 mm) was used for breath-hold MR angiography. The coronal 3D slab was acquired with a slab thickness of 60–70 mm divided into 20 partitions, yielding an effective partition thickness of 3.0–3.5 mm and an acquisition time of 20 seconds. Prior to contrast agent injection, unenhanced 3D MR angiograms were acquired to quantitate signal intensity changes within vessels after contrast agent injection. Thereafter, the contrast-enhanced MR angiographic acquisition was timed to show peak inflow between 40% and 45% of k-space coverage with a standard k-space imaging scheme. A 3D gradient-echo sequence fill in k space linearly (phase-encoding direction) was used. Various parts of k space influence the appearance of the images in different ways. Because magnetic field gradients cause dephasing, the MR signal is strongest when the weakest phase-encoding gradients are applied. Data acquired from the center of k space, where image contrast is determined, are obtained with the weakest phase-encoding gradients. The weaker signals from the outer parts of k space (strongest phase-encoding gradients) contain high spatial frequencies that determine image detail. The central part of k space, with its low-spatial-frequency information and dominating image contrast, is acquired during the middle of the acquisition time. Therefore, it is generally necessary to achieve the optimal arterial gadolinium concentration just before the middle of the acquisition time to maximize vascular contrast. To achieve maximal arterial contrast in the middle of k-space data acquisition, we must subtract 40%–45% of the acquisition time from the calculated circulation time to obtain the delay time from bolus application to the start of the acquisition: Delay time (sec) = contrast agent transit time (sec) − (0.4 × acquisition time [sec]).

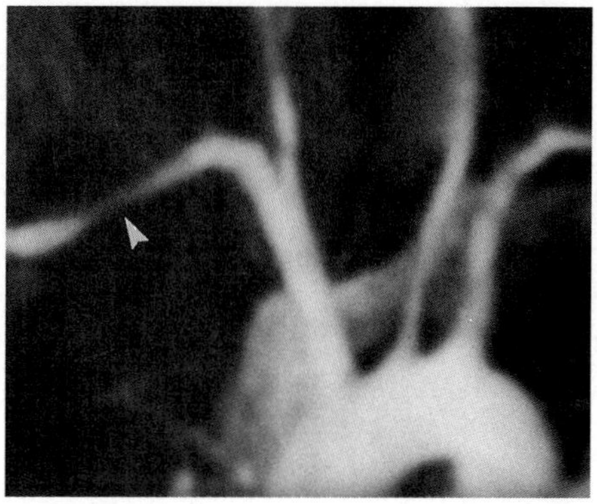

Figure 4. Breath-hold gadolinium-enhanced MR angiography at a contrast agent dose of 0.1 mmol/kg. Maximum intensity projection image of the supraaortic vessels (coronal image plane) shows thoracic outlet syndrome in a young female patient. Elevation of the right arm demonstrated a functional stenosis of the right subclavian artery (arrowhead).

Patients were randomly assigned to one of three dose groups: 0.1, 0.2, or 0.3 mmol of gadolinium per kilogram of body weight. Randomization and injection were monitored by two radiologists (T.A., M.O.) not involved in the image interpretation. Contrast agent administration was performed by means of automatic bolus injections with an MR-compatible power injector (Ulrich, Ulm, Germany), with a nominal flow rate of 5 mL/sec via an 18-gauge cubital intravenous line. The line was subsequently flushed with 20 mL saline, also injected with the power injector at the same flow rate. The contrast agent was not diluted to a fixed volume in order to keep the injected gadolinium concentration constant.

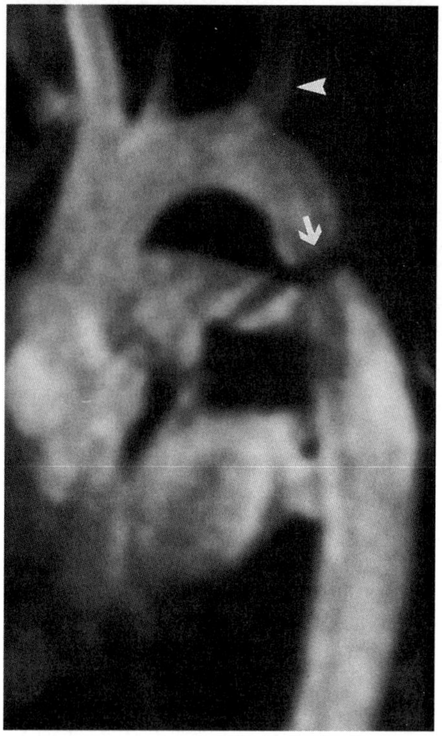

Figure 5. Breath-hold gadolinium-enhanced MR angiography at a contrast agent dose of 0.2 mmol/kg. Maximum intensity projection image of the aortic arch (oblique image plane) shows coarctation of the descending thoracic aorta (arrow). The relationship to the left subclavian artery (arrowhead) is clearly evident. The linear structure extending along the center of the aorta may be a ringing artifact; no aortic dissection is present.

Technical Efficacy Assessment

Quantitative image analysis was performed by a radiologist (M.G.L.) blinded to the injected dose. Signal intensity enhancement was calculated by measuring signal intensity within the aorta and its major branches in the anatomic ROI, as determined by the patient's disease, with the ROI technique. The same regions were used in both unenhanced and contrast-enhanced acquisitions. Measurements were obtained within the aorta (n = 19), the subclavian arteries (n = 7), the iliac arteries (n = 4), the carotid arteries (n = 2), the mesenteric artery (n = 1), and the renal artery (n = 1). Subsequently, the relative vessel enhancement and the signal-to-noise ratio within the aorta or its major branches were calculated as follows: RE = $[(SI_{pre} - SI_{post})/SI_{pre}] \times 100$, and SNR = (mean SI in vessel)/(standard deviation of background noise), where RE is relative vessel enhancement, SI is signal intensity, pre and post signify before and after administration of gadopentetate dimeglumine, and SNR is signal-to-noise ratio.

The nonparametric Kruskal-Wallis test was applied for statistical differences between the three different study groups. A P value less than or equal to .05 was considered significant (7).

Blinded Image Interpretation

Qualitative image analysis was performed by consensus by two radiologists (M.G.L, U.L.R.L.) blinded to the injected dose, without knowledge of x-ray angiography, spiral CT, or US results. Source images and maximum intensity projection images were assessed together for image quality (score 1–5 [1 = excellent, 2 = good, 3 = moderate, 4 = poor, 5 = nondiagnostic]) and the specific diagnosis and compared with results from x-ray angiography or spiral CT or both (no disease—mild stenosis—hemodynamically relevant stenosis [>50%]—occlusion—aneurysm). The criteria used for scoring image quality were vessel visibility, presence of venous overlap, and motion artifacts. The x-ray angiograms and spiral CT images were analyzed by the blinded readers at least 3 weeks after the MR image interpretation, with use of the same scale.

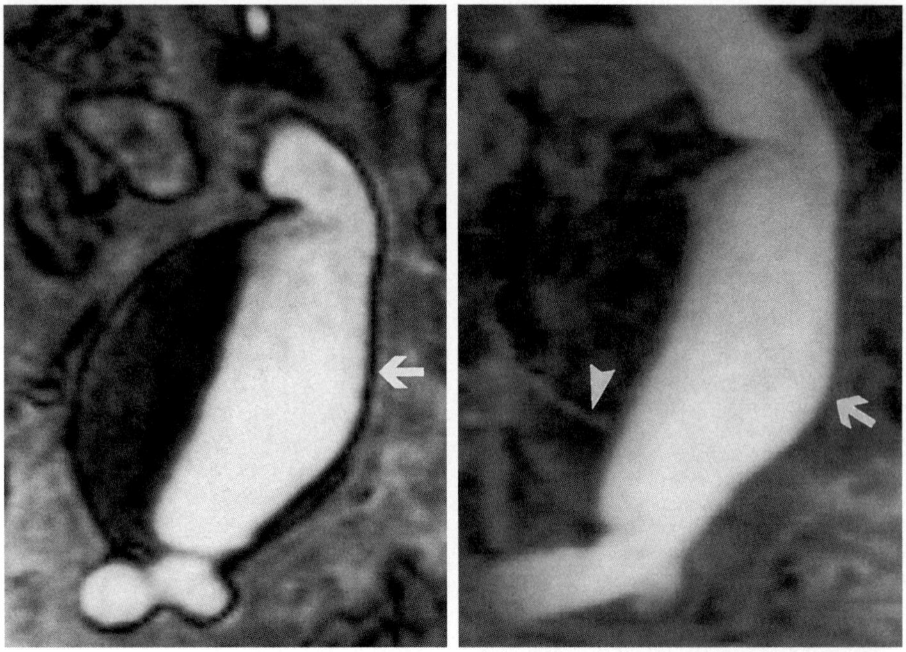

a. b.

Figure 6. Breath-hold gadolinium-enhanced MR angiography at a contrast agent dose of 0.2 mmol/kg. **(a)** Source image (60-mm coronal slab, 20 partitions, 3-mm effective partition thickness) and **(b)** maximum intensity projection image of the abdominal aorta (coronal image plane) show aneurysm of the infrarenal abdominal aorta (arrow in **a** and **b**), not extending into the iliac arteries. There is dystopia of the right kidney, and the small right renal artery (arrowhead in **b**) originates from the true lumen of the aneurysm. The false lumen is better visualized on the source image (relative signal void).

RESULTS

The contrast agent transit time in each of the 34 patients could be determined within 2 minutes and varied between 9 seconds and 30 seconds, with a mean of 17.6 seconds ± 5.8. The time delay from the start of contrast agent injection to the beginning of data acquisition varied between 1 and 22 seconds (Fig 1).

Relative vessel enhancement varied from 393% in the first group (0.1 mmol Gd/kg) to 525% in the third group (0.3 mmol Gd/kg). The overall signal-to-noise ratio was highest in the 0.3 mmol Gd/kg group (31.8 ± 6.4) and lowest in the 0.1 mmol Gd/kg group (26.2 ± 11.2), versus 28.5 ± 10.4 in the 0.2 mmol Gd/kg group. The differences in relative vessel enhancement across the three study groups were not statistically significant (P = .212). All MR angiograms allowed diagnosis, with prominent arterial enhancement and no or minimal venous enhancement (Figs 2–7).

The interpretation of the images by the two blinded radiologists showed no significant differences in diagnosis of vessel disease. In the 28 patients with x-ray angiographic correlation, 3D contrast-enhanced MR angiography resulted in the correct diagnosis in 27. One mild stenosis (<50%) of the right iliac artery was underestimated at 3D MR angiography (0.2 mmol Gd/kg) because of motion artifacts. The two readers classified image quality with the following scores: 2.1 for the 0.1 mmol Gd/kg group, 2.3 for the 0.2 mmol Gd/kg group, 1.9 for the 0.3 mmol Gd/kg group (no significant differences between these dose groups). The distribution of diseases among the three dose groups was even.

DISCUSSION

The results of the present study show that for large vessels such as the aorta or its major branches, a gadolinium dose of 0.1 mmol/kg is effective for the diagnosis of vascular disease.

The standard MR angiographic techniques for evaluating vascular structures have been time-of-flight and phase-contrast imaging. These techniques yield clinically useful results of diagnostic quality in normal vessels with normal flow patterns; however, clinically irregular flow patterns in diseased vessels cause turbulence in stenoses, in-plane saturation in tortuous vessels, and slow-flow saturation, all well-known reasons for signal loss (4,8,9).

Prince and co-authors demonstrated the value of a new MR angiographic technique that uses an MR contrast agent that may permit imaging of vessels with a contrast mechanism that is relatively independent of blood flow (1,2). Based on the intravenous administration of gadopentetate dimeglumine, a paramagnetic contrast material, the technique exploits the gadolinium-induced shortening of the T1 of blood. On the basis of these T1 relaxation differences, blood vessels can be sufficiently distinguished from surrounding tissues (1,2). Gadolinium-enhanced MR angiography improves image quality because it eliminates in-plane saturation and permits acquisition of the data set in the plane of the vessel of interest. Three-dimensional gradient-echo imaging can be used, providing high spatial resolution, high speed, and a high signal-to-noise ratio and permitting control of k-space effects over an entire imaging volume.

In the initial implementations of contrast-enhanced 3D sequences, the acquisi-

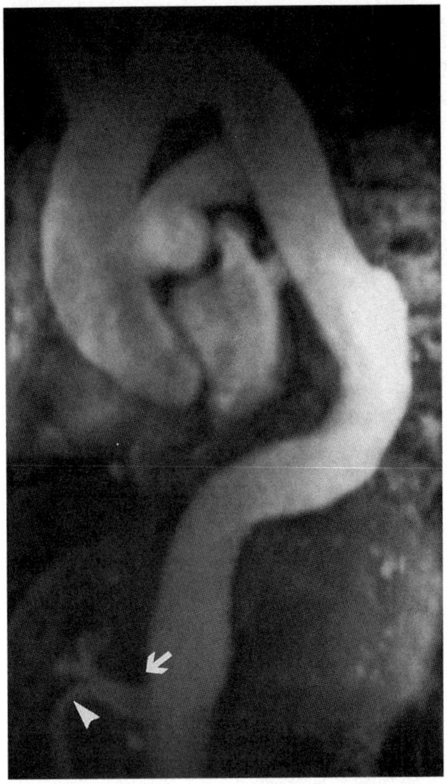

Figure 7. Breath-hold gadolinium-enhanced MR angiography at a contrast agent dose of 0.3 mmol/kg. Maximum intensity projection image of the aorta (oblique image plane) shows tortuous abdominal aorta with irregularities of the vessel diameter due to calcified and noncalcified plaques. Aneurysmal change in the aorta is excluded. The celiac trunk (arrow) and the superior mesenteric artery (arrowhead) are also visualized.

tion times ranged from 3 to 5 minutes (1,2). Strategies to reduce imaging time have recently been proposed. By reducing TR and TE and by using an asymmetric echo and flow compensation, it is possible to acquire a complete 3D data set in one breath hold (5,6,10–12). This results in an examination time of less than 30 seconds for the whole aorta and its major branches. Because of the short data acquisition time of these breath-hold gadolinium-enhanced MR angiographic studies, the quality of the examination depends more on optimal bolus timing than on data acquisition, as the central part of k space, with its low-spatial-frequency information and dominating image contrast, is acquired during the middle of the acquisition time (5,13).

The transit time, from the cubital vein to the aorta and its major branches, for the injected contrast agent demonstrates substantial differences from patient to patient. The transit time is typically shorter in young people with hypertension and longer in elderly patients, in patients with poor cardiac output, and in patients with aneurysmal disease with corresponding flow disturbances (5,14). To achieve a constant quality in clinical MR angiographic studies, an exact measurement of contrast agent transit time is necessary for each patient. This measurement is simple and requires less than 2 minutes.

We inject the contrast agent as a bolus and, to avoid a decrease in its concentration, do not dilute the volume, since the concentration of the injected formulation should be high to obtain a dense bolus during first-pass MR angiography. We speculate that if we had diluted the different doses in our study to a fixed volume, the concentration of the contrast agent would have decreased substantially in the lower-dose groups and biased the results toward higher doses.

When contrast-enhanced MR angiography first evolved, it was hypothesized that higher doses of gadolinium chelates, up to 0.5 mmol/kg, would be necessary to decrease T1 to the required range of about 80–100 msec. Our goal was to investigate whether these high doses are clinically necessary, and our data show that there was no significant difference in vessel enhancement and signal-to-noise ratio at gadolinium doses from 0.1 to 0.3 mmol/kg. The correct diagnosis can be made at a gadolinium dose of 0.1 mmol/kg for common vascular diseases.

The injected dose of gadolinium can be limited to 0.1 mmol/kg, which is sufficient for breath-hold gadolinium-enhanced MR angiography of larger vessels such as the aorta and its major branches. This approach is more cost-effective than high-dose strategies because no additional diagnostic information is obtained at a gadolinium dose of 0.2 or 0.3 mmol/kg (Figs 3–7). This dose can also be used clinically, since the bolus injection of a gadolinium dose of 0.1 mmol/kg has been approved by the U.S. Food and Drug Administration and been used in postapproval surveillance studies (15,16). To our knowledge, the safety of very large doses has not been studied, and the costs of the procedure increase substantially with dose ($70 per 20 mL of gadopentetate dimeglumine) (16). Although all recent studies have been performed at 1.5 T, gadolinium-enhanced ultrashort TE MR angiography is feasible at 1.0 T, which expands the clinical application of contrast-enhanced MR angiography to a much larger number of MR units.

Our results are valid, however, only for the aorta and its major branches. Additional studies are required to evaluate the dose response within abdominal organs, peripheral vessels, or the cervical arteries. Also, our results are valid only with the technical parameters used. If further reductions in TR and TE decrease the signal-to-noise ratio, a dose increase may be required to compensate for this decrease.

References

1. Prince MR, Yucel EK, Kaufmann JA, Harrison DC, Geller SC. Dynamic gadolinium-enhanced three-dimensional abdominal MR arteriography. JMRI 1993; 3:877–881.
2. Prince MR. Gadolinium-enhanced MR aortography. Radiology 1994; 191:155–164.
3. Prince MR, Narasimham DL, Stanley JC, et al. Gadolinium-enhanced magnetic resonance angiography of abdominal aortic aneurysms. J Vasc Surg 1995; 21:656–669.
4. Prince MR. Body MR angiography with gadolinium contrast agents. Magn Reson Imaging Clin N Am 1996: 4:11–24.
5. Prince MR, Narasimham DL, Stanley JC, et al. Breath-hold gadolinium-enhanced MR angiography of the abdominal aorta and its major branches. Radiology 1995; 197:785–792.
6. Shetty AN, Shirkoda A, Bis KG, Alcantara A. Contrast-enhanced three-dimensional MR angiography in a single breath hold: a novel technique. AJR 1995; 165:1290–1292.
7. Wassertheil-Smoller S. Biostatistics and epidemiology: a primer for health professionals. 2nd ed. New York, NY: Springer-Verlag, 1995.
8. Krinsky GA, Rofsky RM, Flyer M, et al. Gadolinium-enhanced three-dimensional MR angiography of acquired arch vessel disease. AJR 1996; 167:981–987.
9. Snidow JJ, Aisen AM, Harris VJ, et al. Iliac artery MR angiography: comparison of three-dimensional gadolinium-enhanced and two-dimensional time-of-flight techniques. Radiology 1995; 196:371–378.
10. Holland GA, Dougherty L, Carpenter JP, et al. Breath-hold ultrafast three-dimensional gadolinium-enhanced MR angiography of the aorta and the renal and other visceral abdominal arteries. AJR 1996; 166:971–981.
11. Leung DA, McKinnon GC, Davis CP, Pfammater T, Krestin GP, Debatin JF. Breath-hold, contrast-enhanced, three-dimensional MR angiography. Radiology 1996; 201:569–571.
12. Snidow JJ, Johnson MS, Harris VJ, et al. Three-dimensional gadolinium-enhanced MR angiography for aortoiliac inflow assessment plus renal artery screening in a single breath hold. Radiology 1996; 198:725–732.
13. Edelman RR, Wielopolski PA. Fast MRI. In: Edelman RR, Hesselink JR, Zlatkin MB, eds. Clinical magnetic resonance imaging. 2nd ed. Philadelphia, Pa: Saunders, 1996.
14. Earls JP, Rofsky NM, De Corato DR, et al. Breath-hold single-dose gadolinium-enhanced three-dimensional MR aortography: usefulness of a timing examination and MR power injector. Radiology 1996; 201:705–710.
15. Nelson KL, Gifford LM, Lauber-Huber C, Gross C, Lasser TA. Clinical safety of gadopentate dimeglumine. Radiology 1995; 196:439–443.
16. Rofsky NM, Johnson G, Adelman MA, Rosen RJ, Krinsky GA, Weinreb JC. Peripheral vascular disease evaluated with reduced-dose gadolinium-enhanced MR angiography. Radiology 1997; 205:163–169.

Bird in Flight

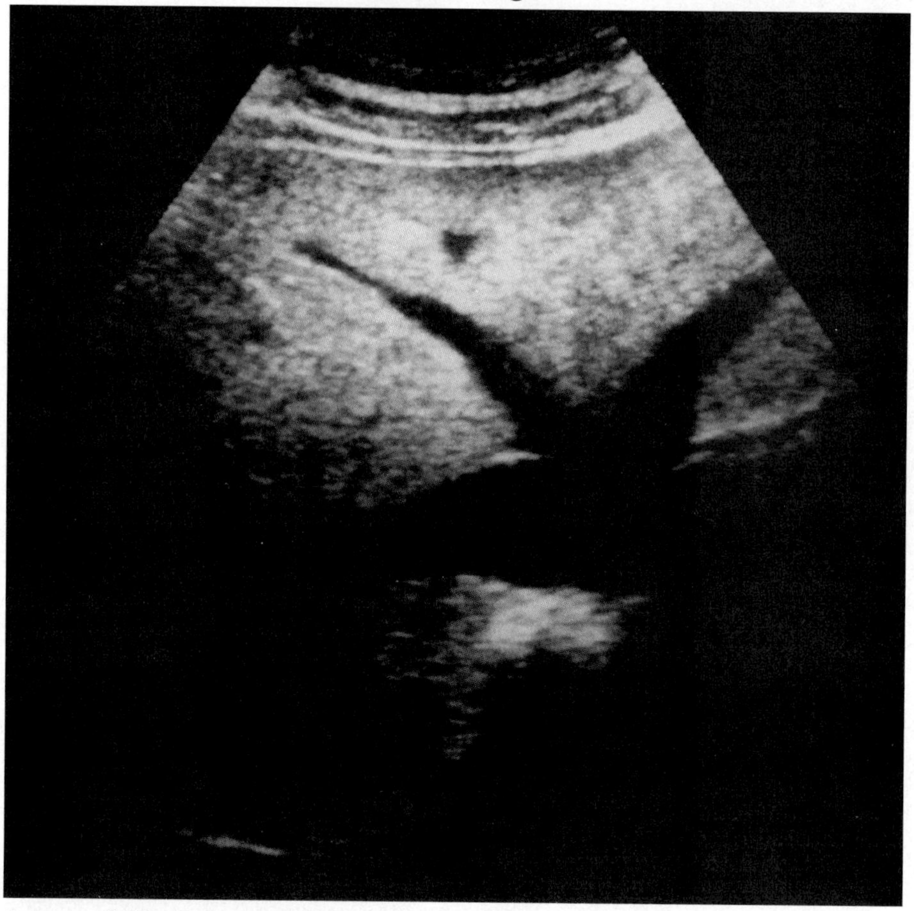

Courtesy of Akira Hokama, MD, PhD, Okinawa, Japan

Life-threatening Primary Postpartum Hemorrhage: Treatment with Emergency Selective Arterial Embolization[1]

Jean-Pierre Pelage, MD
Olivier Le Dref, MD
Joaquim Mateo, MD
Philippe Soyer, MD, PhD
Denis Jacob, MD
Mourad Kardache, MD
Henri Dahan, MD
Danielle Repiquet, MD
Didier Payen, MD, PhD
Jean-Bernard Truc, MD
Jean-Jacques Merland, MD
Roland Rymer, MD

Index terms:
Arteries, therapeutic blockade, 98.1264
Arteries, uterine, 98.1264
Pregnancy, complications, 854.82
Uterus, hemorrhage, 854.8269

Radiology 1998; 208:359–362

[1] From the Departments of Body and Vascular Imaging (J.P.P., O.L.D., P.S., M.K., H.D., J.J.M., R.R.), Obstetrics and Gynecology (D.J., D.R., J.B.T.), and Anesthesiology and Critical Care (J.M., D.P.), Hôpital Lariboisière, AP-HP, 2 rue Ambroise Parè, 75475 Paris 10, France. Received September 22, 1997; revision requested November 25; final revision received March 16, 1998; accepted March 27. **Address reprint requests to** J.P.P.

Author contributions:
Guarantors of integrity of entire study, J.P.P., R.R.; study concepts, J.P.P., O.L.D.; study design, J.P.P., P.S., R.R.; definition of intellectual content, J.P.P., O.L.D., J.B.T., D.P., J.J.M., R.R.; literature research, J.P.P., D.R., D.J.; clinical studies, J.P.P.; data acquisition, J.P.P., O.L.D., D.R., D.J., M.K., J.M.; data analysis, J.P.P., O.L.D., H.D., M.K.; manuscript preparation, J.P.P., O.L.D., D.R.; manuscript editing, J.P.P., P.S.; manuscript review, P.S., J.P.P., J.J.M.

PURPOSE: To prospectively evaluate the efficacy and safety of emergency selective arterial embolization in the management of intractable primary postpartum hemorrhage.

MATERIALS AND METHODS: Twenty-seven consecutively seen women with life-threatening primary postpartum hemorrhage underwent uterine embolization. In all cases, hemostatic embolization was performed because of intractable hemorrhage that could not be controlled with vaginal packing and administration of uterotonic drugs. The mean hemoglobin level before embolization was 7.48 g/dL ± 2.39 (74.8 g/L ± 23.9) (1 standard deviation). Hysterectomy performed in two patients before embolization failed to stop the bleeding.

RESULTS: Angiography revealed extravasation in nine patients and spasm of the branches of the internal iliac artery in five. The procedure consisted of embolization of uterine (n = 46), vaginal (n = 5), or ovarian (n = 2) arteries or anterior division of internal iliac arteries (n = 8). Immediate disappearance or dramatic diminution of external bleeding was observed in all cases. Two patients needed repeated embolization the next day. No major complication related to embolization was found. In one patient with placenta accreta, delayed hysterectomy was necessary. Normal menstruation resumed in all women except the two who underwent hysterectomy. One woman became pregnant after embolization.

CONCLUSION: Emergency arterial embolization is a safe and effective means of control of primary postpartum hemorrhage. The procedure obviates high-risk surgery and allows maintenance of reproductive ability.

Postpartum hemorrhage remains a major cause of maternal mortality throughout the world (1). The postpartum period is typically defined as 6 weeks after delivery of an infant (2,3). This obstetric complication may occur immediately or several hours or days after delivery. In most published studies about puerperal bleeding, immediate and late postpartum hemorrhage was treated in the aggregate when clinical presentation, causes, and maternal mortality are different (4). Primary postpartum hemorrhage is usually defined as excessive bleeding from the genital tract (ie, 500 mL or more during the first 24 hours after delivery) (2,3). The reported incidence of 3%–5% is probably underestimated because of difficulties in evaluation of blood loss by means of visual observation only (1,5,6).

Rapid identification of the source and control of bleeding are necessary because the situation is potentially life-threatening. In most cases, primary postpartum hemorrhage can be managed with conservative treatment involving vaginal packing and administration of uterotonic drugs. With persistent bleeding, vascular ligation or hysterectomy may be needed (3). Surgical treatment, however, sometimes may be technically difficult to perform and may fail to control hemorrhage. For these reasons, transcatheter embolization of the uterine arteries may represent an interesting alternate technique in the treatment of intractable bleeding, preserving future fertility. The goal of our study was to prospectively evaluate the efficacy and safety of emergency arterial embolization in the management of intractable primary postpartum hemorrhage.

MATERIALS AND METHODS

During a 30-month period, 27 consecutively seen women who had uncontrollable primary postpartum hemorrhage and were referred for emergency uterine angiography and treatment with selective arterial embolization were included in the study. The mean age of the women was 32.7 years ± 4.9 (1 standard deviation). Fourteen women (52%) were primiparas, and 13 (48%) were multiparas. There was one multiple pregnancy. Twenty-one women (78%) were transferred from another institution, and six delivered infants in our hospital. During the same period, 58 patients (including those who underwent embolotherapy) were referred to our institution for possible treatment with arterial embolization. Despite the severity of the condition of the patients, they had been transported to our institution for the following reasons: frequent impossibility to provide more efficient care in the initial hospital and the advantages offered by the French prehospital Service d'Aide Médicale Urgente, which include ambulances that always have a physician trained in medical resuscitation and emergency medicine, a nurse, and one or two specially trained ambulance drivers (7). Resuscitation of a patient can then be continuously performed during transportation. Thus, in our study, early transfer was possible in all patients.

In all cases, the protocol for treatment was determined by means of consensus among the anesthesiologist, obstetrician, and interventional radiologist available on a 24-hour basis in our institution. Initial evaluation and resuscitation were performed in the intensive care unit before the patient was transferred to the interventional radiology room. The evaluation was based on the clinical and hemodynamic status of the patient. The amount of blood loss was classified according to a subjective assessment made by the medical team. Evaluation of the seriousness of the hemorrhage was based on the quantity of drugs and fluids required to maintain hemodynamic parameters and biologic condition (2).

Medical treatment was aimed at three goals: correction of hypovolemic shock with intravenous administration of crystalloid or colloid substances and transfusion of specific blood units, treatment of disseminated intravascular coagulation with fresh-frozen plasma and with units of platelets or fibrinogen when needed, and management of uterine atony with pharmacologic measures and early introduction of intravenous oxytocin (Syntocinon; Laboratoires Sandoz, Rueil-Malmaison, France) and prostaglandin-E_2 analogue (sulprostone [Nalador]; Laboratoire Schering, Lys-Les-Lannoy, France) and with manual uterine massage. The decision to perform embolization was made on the basis of active, continuing hemorrhage despite the treatment just mentioned. The potential risks and benefits of the procedure were explained, and informed consent was obtained in all cases from the patient or her family.

Digital subtraction angiography was performed by a vascular radiologist (J.P.P., O.L.D., P.S., M.K., H.D.) on an emergency basis using a right-sided unifemoral approach. Contralateral internal iliac angiography and selective study of the anterior division were then performed in all cases with a 5-F cobra-type catheter (Cobra Radifocus; Terumo, Tokyo, Japan) and a hydrophilic polymer-coated 0.032-inch guide wire (Radifocus; Terumo) to analyze the uterine arteries. Superselective angiography of the uterine artery was attempted in all cases. Other anastomotic vessels, such as vaginal branches, were studied when necessary. The ipsilateral internal iliac artery and uterine artery were also catheterized by use of the same puncture site and the same cobra-type catheter. Pledgets of absorbable gelatin sponge (Gelfoam; Upjohn, Kalamazoo, Mich) in increasing sizes were freely introduced with fluoroscopic guidance. Polyvinyl alcohol dehydrated particles (Ivalon; Nycomed, Paris, France) with diameters of 300–600 μm were used during a period of a few weeks, before the nonbovine origin of the gelatin sponge was certified. Embolization was bilateral in all patients. Postembolization angiography was performed to ensure the complete occlusion of the vessels. All patients were transferred to the intensive care unit for further observation and coagulation studies with the arterial femoral introducer left in place until coagulation disorders were corrected.

RESULTS

The major clinical indication for transcatheter embolization was uterine atony (18 women [67%]), which was associated with uterine or cervical tears in five women and with retained portions of placenta in two women. Other causes of bleeding were a genital tract lesion (vaginal or cervical tears) without uterine atony in seven women and placenta accreta in two. All women delivered infants at 37–42 weeks of gestation. Six women (22%) delivered infants by means of cesarean section, and 21 women (78%) delivered infants vaginally. Twenty-seven children were in good health at the time of this writing. One full-term fetus died; the cause was unexplained.

At admission to our institution, all patients had a measured blood loss of more than 1,000 mL. The mean hemoglobin level was 7.48 g/dL ± 2.39 (74.8 g/L ± 23.9). The presence of disseminated intravascular coagulopathy was confirmed with laboratory tests showing thrombocytopenia (platelet count, 73,740/mm^3 ± 56,860 [73,740 × 10^9/L ± 56,860]), an elevated prothrombin time, and hypofibrinogenemia (fibrinogen level, 1.15 g/L ± 1.11). Coagulopathy was present in 20 patients (74%) before embolization.

Tracheal intubation and assisted ventilation were necessary in 12 women. Emergency management of cardiac arrest was necessary in four women. All patients needed blood transfusion because of hypovolemic shock. The average transfusion before embolization involved 12.1 units ± 7.3 of blood per patient. In patients with disseminated intravascular coagulopathy, fresh-frozen plasma (21 women), fibrinogen (four women), and platelet units (six women) were administered. Pharmacologic control or prevention of uterine atony consisted of intravenous administration of oxytocin alone in five patients, with a cumulative dose of 20 units, and in combination with prostaglandin-E_2 analogue in a total dosage of 1,000 μg (two injections of 500 μg each) in nine women. Sulprostone was used alone as a first-line therapy (one to three doses of 500 μg) in 11 women.

The obstetric procedure included manual exploration of the uterus in 19 women and manual uterine massage in 13 women. A subtotal hysterectomy was performed in two women before admission to our hospital but failed to control the bleeding.

Angiography showed no extravasation of contrast material in 18 patients (67%). Bleeding, shown in 11 arteries in nine patients, arose from the uterine artery in six (left in three and right in three) and from a vaginal branch in five. Spasms of the branches of the anterior division were observed in five patients.

Selective embolization of both uterine

arteries was performed in 23 women (85%), including the 18 patients without identifiable extravasation. In four women (15%), bilateral embolization of the anterior division of the internal iliac artery was performed. Five vaginal arteries were also selectively embolized because of active bleeding. Gelatin sponge was used as the embolic material in 23 women and was used in association with particles of polyvinyl alcohol in one woman. Polyvinyl alcohol alone was administered in four women. The embolization procedure lasted 60–110 minutes.

External bleeding disappeared in 25 women (92%) and decreased dramatically in two. Slight repeated bleeding was observed in three women. Two of them were referred for repeated angiography the next day, and the bleeding stopped spontaneously in the remaining, third woman. In one woman, the uterine artery was patent and repeated embolization stopped the hemorrhage. In the woman who had previously undergone hysterectomy, embolization was needed in both ovarian arteries that provided arterial flow to the bleeding site. Biologic coagulation disorders improved markedly within a few hours and without recurrence in all women. No subsequent transfusion was necessary in 22 patients. Five women needed only 2 units of blood after embolization.

Local complications included transient foot ischemia in one woman. In one woman, a hysterectomy was needed 5 days after embolization because of persistent hemorrhage due to placenta accreta. General complications were cardiogenic pulmonary edema related to hemorrhagic shock, vasoconstrictive drugs, and excessive fluid replacement in three women and death in one woman caused by cerebral hemorrhage due to severe eclampsia. This complication was not related to the embolization. The mean length of stay in the intensive care unit was 2.47 days ± 1.86. Women were discharged on the 10th day after embolization (9.63 days ± 4.72).

DISCUSSION

The widespread use of and recent improvements in angiographic catheters and embolic particles make it necessary to reassess the role of selective embolization of the uterine arteries in the management of primary postpartum hemorrhage. Multidisciplinary management is necessary to select patients for treatment with embolization techniques. Uterine atony, which accounts for 67% of our cases, is the main cause of primary postpartum hemorrhage (8,9). Other causes of bleeding include lower genital tract laceration or hematoma, retained placental tissue, and rupture of the uterine body (2,8,9). Secondary postpartum hemorrhage occurring more than 24 hours after delivery is mainly related to retained gestational products and tends to be associated with maternal morbidity rather than mortality (4).

Primary postpartum hemorrhage is usually controlled with specific surgical repair in case of vaginal or cervical tears, with curettage, and with vaginal packing (2). Atonic uterus is often managed satisfactorily with intravenous administration of oxytocin drugs as a first-line treatment and prostaglandin-E_2 analogues if oxytocin is ineffective in controlling hemorrhage (2,10). Prostaglandin-E_2 analogue (the most commonly used drug in Europe) is highly successful in the treatment of atony (10).

For patients whose condition continues to deteriorate, ligation of the internal iliac artery or its branches (11,12) or even hysterectomy is often the favored treatment (3,13). Ligation of the internal iliac artery, however, may fail to stop the bleeding in 50% of cases (11). The reason is that bilateral ligation of the proximal segment of the internal iliac artery reduces blood flow by only 48% and the average pressure by 24% (14). Surgical ligation is proximal so that collateral vessels can supply blood to the uterus, and the bleeding can recur (15). Ligation of uterine arteries seems to be efficient in cases of moderate bleeding if it is performed at the time of cesarean section (12).

Hysterectomy of a full-term gravid uterus carries with it a high operative risk and morbidity, including secondary bleeding due to edematous tissues and distorted anatomy (13). An extrauterine site of bleeding or inadequate arterial ligation may account for failure of hysterectomy to stop the bleeding. Finally, hysterectomy prevents future reproductive function. Because selective arterial embolization preserves the uterus, this technique should be considered first in cases of severe postpartum bleeding.

Transcatheter embolization has been used to control intractable bleeding associated with pelvic trauma (16) and tumors (17,18). Arterial embolization has also been successfully employed in short trials for the management of postoperative (19), postabortion (20), and postpartum (17,21–23) intractable bleeding. To our knowledge, Brown et al (24) reported the first case of embolization of the medial circumflex artery providing anastomotic flow to the internal pudendal artery in a patient who previously underwent bilateral hypogastric arterial ligation and hysterectomy for severe primary postpartum bleeding.

This case illustrates the advantages of selective embolization over surgery; selective embolization helps to localize the bleeding site by means of extravasation of contrast material outside the vascular space and is a less invasive procedure than surgery (24). If the bleeding is slow or intermittent or in case of atonic uterus, however, angiography may often fail to demonstrate active bleeding. Embolization should be performed as selectively as possible, either in the abnormal vessel or in the uterine artery even when no active bleeding is detected.

Thus, in our study, embolization of both uterine arteries in patients who had atonic uterus has proved the ability to stop external bleeding immediately and correct coagulopathy when medical treatment has failed. In case of severe vasoconstriction, however, embolization of the anterior division of the internal iliac artery (25), which maintains flow to the branches of the posterior division, is an alternative technique that permits a shorter procedure and reduces radiation exposure without any important complication. More studies are needed.

Pledgets of gelatin sponge, which provide a temporary occlusion, are particularly suitable because the injury and coagulopathy should be resolved in a relatively short period (17,21–23). We used polyvinyl alcohol particles in four patients in whom we feared transmission of Creutzfeldt-Jakob disease by means of gelatin sponge. Polyvinyl alcohol is also a short-term occlusive agent with a more limited potential for recanalization (18). The use of particles of large diameter to preserve the smaller branches and collateral vessels, however, has proved its value in our patients with no side effects. Steel coils may be useful in case of injury to the genital tract with identified extravasation (23).

Our success rate is comparable to the 85%–95% reported in previous, shorter studies (22,23). In our series, initial embolization failed in three women. In two women, repeated embolization was successful. In a third woman, however, surgical treatment was necessary because of placenta accreta. These causes of failure are similar to those reported in previous studies (22). Placenta accreta is one of the major causes of hysterectomy after embolization because of persistent bleeding (13). Failures are also likely to occur with unilateral treatment (19) and in patients who have undergone bilateral ligation of the hypogastric artery before embolization (17). Successful embolization via pelvic collateral vessels, however, has already been reported (17,24,26).

Although no complication was encountered in our series, arterial embolization is not free of side effects. Even if complications are minimal in skilled hands, the size and number of emboli, the location of the injection, and the material used for embolization may influence the safety of the procedure. Technical problems related to arterial catheterization should be virtually absent in young and healthy women. In addition, a high degree of flow to the uterine arteries tends to protect against unexpected reflux of the embolic material. Ischemic complications were found in two women with postpartum bleeding who underwent arterial embolization after ligation of the internal iliac artery was unsuccessful (17). Other reported complications after pelvic embolization were always found in elderly patients (27,28).

Embolization allows preservation of the mother's life and future reproductive function. Numerous cases of pregnancy after ligation of the internal iliac arteries have been reported (29). Likewise, after pelvic embolization, pregnancies are possible even though follow-up is shorter (17,30,31). In our study, all patients who did not undergo hysterectomy had normal resumption of menstruation after embolization (31). One woman had become pregnant by the time of this writing.

In conclusion, our study shows that selective arterial embolization should be the treatment of choice for severe primary postpartum hemorrhage in case of failure with conservative treatment. Multidisciplinary management for these patients should be realized in highly specialized centers open 24 hours a day to provide lower-risk conditions for the angiographer. Our experience confirms the usefulness of hemostatic embolotherapy to control intractable primary postpartum hemorrhage if it is applied early in the course of events. If our principles are adhered to, a high success rate with minimal morbidity and complications should follow, with maintenance of reproductive ability.

References

1. Gilbert L, Porter W, Brown VA. Postpartum haemorrhage: a continuing problem. Br J Obstet Gynecol 1987; 94:67–71.
2. Biehl DR. Antepartum and postpartum hemorrhage. In: Shnider SM, Levinson C. Anesthesia for obstetrics. 2nd ed. Baltimore, Md: Williams & Wilkins, 1987; 385–394.
3. Herbert WP, Afalo RC. Management of postpartum hemorrhage. Clin Obstet Gynecol 1984; 27:139–145.
4. King PA, Duthie SJ, Dong ZG, Ma HK. Secondary postpartum haemorrhage. Aust N Z J Obstet Gynaecol 1989; 29:394–398.
5. Ghares EE, Albert SN, Dodek SM. Intrapartum blood loss measured with Cr 51-tagged erythrocytes. Obstet Gynecol 1962; 19:455–462.
6. Newton M, Mosey LM, Egli GE, Gifford WB, Hull CT. Blood loss during and immediately after delivery. Obstet Gynecol 1961; 17:9–18.
7. Plaisance P, Adnet F, Vicaut E, et al. Benefit of active compression-decompression cardiopulmonary resuscitation as a prehospital advanced cardiac life support. Circulation 1997; 95:955–961.
8. Combs CA, Murphy EL, Laros RK. Factors associated with postpartum haemorrhage with vaginal birth. Obstet Gynecol 1991; 77:69–76.
9. Combs CA, Murphy EL, Laros RK. Factors associated with hemorrhage in cesarean deliveries. Obstet Gynecol 1991; 77:77–82.
10. Goffinet F, Haddad B, Carbonne B, Sebann E, Papiernik E, Cabrol D. Practical use of sulprostone for the treatment of postpartum hemorrhage. J Gynecol Obstet Biol Reprod (Paris) 1995; 24:209–216. [French]
11. Evans S, McShane P. The efficacy of internal iliac artery ligation in obstetric hemorrhage. Surg Gynecol Obstet 1985; 160: 250–253.
12. O'Leary JA. Stop obstetric hemorrhage with uterine ligation. Contemp Obstet Gynecol 1986; 28:13–16.
13. Zelop CM, Harlow BL, Frigoletto FD, Safon LE, Saltzman DH. Emergency peripartum hysterectomy. Am J Obstet Gynecol 1993; 168:1443–1448.
14. Burchell RC. Physiology of internal iliac artery ligation. J Obstet Gynaecol Br Commonw 1968; 75:642–651.
15. Chait A, Moltz A, Nelson JH. The collateral arterial circulation in the pelvis: an angiographic study. AJR 1968; 102:392–400.
16. Margolies MN, Ring EJ, Waltman AC, Kerr WS, Baum S. Arteriography in the management of hemorrhage from pelvic fractures. N Engl J Med 1972; 287:317–321.
17. Greenwood LH, Glickman MG, Schwartz PE, Morse SS, Denny DF. Obstetric and nonmalignant gynecologic bleeding: treatment with angiographic embolization. Radiology 1987; 164:155–159.
18. Lang EK. Transcatheter embolization of pelvic vessels for control of intractable hemorrhage. Radiology 1981; 140:331–339.
19. Rosenthal DM, Colapinto R. Angiographic arterial embolization in the management of post-operative vaginal hemorrhage. Am J Obstet Gynecol 1985; 151:227–231.
20. Haseltine FP, Glickman MG, Marchesi S, Spitz R, Dlugi A, DeCherney AA. Uterine embolization in a patient with postabortal hemorrhage. Obstet Gynecol 1984; 63(suppl):78S–80S.
21. Duvauferrier R, Priou G, Tasson D, Laurent MC, Ramée A. Emergency uterine artery embolization for immediate postpartum hemorrhage secondary to coagulation disorder. J Radiol 1984; 65:285–288. [French]
22. Mitty HA, Sterling KM, Alvarez M, Gendler R. Obstetric hemorrhage: prophylactic and emergency arterial catheterization and embolotherapy. Radiology 1993; 188: 183–187.
23. Yamashita Y, Harada M, Yamamoto H, et al. Transcatheter arterial embolization of obstetric and gynaecological bleeding: efficacy and clinical outcome. Br J Radiol 1994; 67:530–534.
24. Brown BJ, Heaston DK, Poulson AM, Gabert HA, Mineau DE, Miller FJ. Uncontrollable postpartum bleeding: a new approach to hemostasis through angiographic arterial embolization. Obstet Gynecol 1979; 54:361–365.
25. Alvarez M, Lockwood CJ, Ghidini A, Dottino P, Mitty HA, Berkowitz RL. Prophylactic and emergent arterial catheterization for selective embolization in obstetric hemorrhage. Am J Perinatol 1992; 9:441–444.
26. Collins CD, Jackson JE. Pelvic arterial embolization following hysterectomy and bilateral internal iliac artery ligation for intractable primary postpartum haemorrhage. Clin Radiol 1995; 50:710–714.
27. Braf ZF, Koontz WW. Gangrene of bladder: complication of hypogastric artery embolization. Urology 1977; 9:670–671.
28. Hare WS, Lond FR, Holland CJ. Paresis following internal iliac artery embolization. Radiology 1983; 146:47–51.
29. Mengert WF, Burchell RC, Blumstein RW, Daskal JL. Pregnancy after bilateral ligation of the internal iliac and ovarian arteries. Obstet Gynecol 1969; 34:664–666.
30. Poppe W, Van Assche FA, Wilms G, Favril A, Baert A. A pregnancy after transcatheter embolization of a uterine arteriovenous malformation. Am J Obstet Gynecol 1987; 156:1179–1180.
31. Stancato-Pasik A, Mitty HA, Richard HM, Eshkar N. Obstetric embolotherapy: effects on menses and pregnancy. Radiology 1997; 204:791–793.

Spondylodiskitic Abscesses: CT-guided Percutaneous Catheter Drainage[1]

Gundula Staatz, MD
Gerhard B. Adam, MD
Peter Keulers, MD
Dierk Vorwerk, MD
Rolf W. Günther, MD

Index terms:
Abscess, percutaneous drainage, 30.242
Interventional procedures, 30.1261, 30.1263, 30.1291
Spine, CT, 30.12111, 30.12112
Spine, intervertebral disks, 326.20, 336.20
Spine, MR, 30.121411, 30.12143
Spondylitis, 30.2012, 30.2013, 30.2021, 30.2023, 30.23, 30.242, 30.7813, 30.814

Radiology 1998; 208:363–367

[1] From the Department of Diagnostic Radiology, University-Hospital of the RWTH Aachen, Pauwelsstrasse 30, 52057 Aachen, Germany. From the 1997 RSNA scientific assembly. Received July 21, 1997; revision requested September 8; final revision received February 23, 1998; accepted April 3. **Address reprint requests to** G.S.

Author contributions:
Guarantors of integrity of entire study, G.S., G.B.A.; study concepts and design, G.S., G.B.A., R.W.G.; definition of intellectual content, G.S., G.B.A.; literature research, G.S.; clinical studies, G.S., G.B.A., P.K., D.V.; data acquisition, G.S., G.B.A.; data analysis, G.S., G.B.A.; manuscript preparation, G.S., G.B.A.; manuscript editing, G.S., G.B.A., R.W.G.; manuscript review, G.S., G.B.A., D.V.

PURPOSE: To determine whether computed tomographically (CT) guided percutaneous catheter drainage of spondylodiskitic abscesses is an appropriate and effective alternative to surgery.

MATERIALS AND METHODS: CT-guided percutaneous catheter drainage was performed in 21 patients (16 men, five women; age range, 24–81 years) with 33 spondylodiskitic abscesses. Nine intradiskal, 12 paravertebral, and 12 psoas abscesses were drained with 5.6–14.0-F catheters. In 29 cases, the catheter was inserted by using the Seldinger technique; in four cases, a trocar technique was used. All patients underwent follow-up CT or magnetic resonance imaging examinations for 6 months.

RESULTS: Successful placement of the drainage catheter was achieved in each patient without procedural complications. The duration of drainage was 4–56 days (average duration, 26.8 days). Three of 33 catheters were changed because of insufficient drainage; one of the 33 catheters had to be reinserted because of dislocation. Two patients underwent surgery for stabilization of the spine with the drainage catheter in place. In 16 of the 21 patients, specific organisms were isolated; thus, definitive medical therapy was possible. Complete evacuation of all abscesses was achieved initially, with no evidence of recurrence during the follow-up.

CONCLUSION: CT-guided percutaneous catheter drainage is an efficient and safe procedure in the management of spondylodiskitic abscesses.

Infectious spondylitis has been seen increasingly often in the past decade; it may involve osseous elements, disks, epidural space, or paraspinal soft tissues (1). Depending on the offending organism, specific spondylodiskitis (ie, that caused by *Mycobacterium tuberculosis* infection) and nonspecific spondylodiskitis (ie, that caused by *Staphylococcus aureus, Escherichia coli, Pseudomonas aeruginosa,* or other organisms) can be distinguished. Paraspinal abscess formations are observed in 70%–75% of cases and are most frequently seen with tuberculous spondylitis (2,3). Immediate treatment is necessary to prevent spinal deformation or neurologic damage. Conservative therapy is sufficient in cases detected early and in mild cases, whereas surgical intervention is required in cases of neurologic complication, epidural abscess, spinal cord compression, severe kyphotic deformity or spinal instability, or ineffective conservative treatment (4).

Abscess formation outside the spinal canal can be treated with computed tomographically (CT) guided percutaneous drainage, which has been well described for multiple organ systems (5–9). Percutaneous drainage of psoas abscesses secondary to vertebral osteomyelitis is an established procedure, but percutaneous drainage of paravertebral and especially intradiskal abscesses is rarely performed.

We report our experience with CT-guided percutaneous drainage of spondylodiskitic abscesses. We performed this study to determine whether CT-guided percutaneous catheter drainage of spondylodiskitic abscesses is an effective alternative to surgical treatment.

MATERIALS AND METHODS

From June 1989 to December 1996, 16 men and five women aged 24–81 years (mean age, 59.5 years) underwent percutaneous catheter drainage of a total of 33 spondylodiskitic abscesses. The diagnosis was established with CT (Somatom Plus; Siemens Medical Systems, Erlangen, Germany) in all patients. In six patients, the diagnosis had been previously established by using 1.5-T magnetic resonance (MR) imaging (Magnetom; Siemens Medical Systems). T2-weighted (2,000/90 [repetition time msec/echo time msec]) or T1-weighted (500–600/15), sagittal or axial spin-echo MR imaging was performed before and after the administration of gadopentetate dimeglumine (Magnevist; Schering, Berlin, Germany), which enabled us to exclude additional extradural or intrathecal abscess formations. For the CT examinations, we used a section thickness of 5 mm in 17 patients and of 8 mm in four patients.

CT scans were obtained after bolus injection of 75–100 mL of water-soluble contrast medium (Ultravist 370 [iopromide]; Schering) with the single-shot (in 18 patients) or spiral technique (in three patients).

The abscesses considered to be appropriate for percutaneous drainage were spondylodiskitis-associated abscesses larger than 1–2 cm that were located intradiskally, paravertebrally, or within the psoas muscle and that led to a marked increase in laboratory findings of inflammation. The criterion for excluding patients from CT-guided percutaneous abscess drainage was the finding of solid paravertebral or paraspinal granulation tissue associated with small, low-attenuating fluid collections. The excluded patients underwent CT-guided needle aspiration or biopsy with a side-cutting needle (Tru-Cut; Baxter Healthcare, Valencia, Calif) for microbiologic analysis and were treated conservatively with immobilization, antibiotic therapy, and chemotherapy. Patients who had an epidural or intrathecal abscess formation with compression of the spinal cord were also excluded and were immediately transferred to the Department of Neurosurgery.

For the drainage procedure, each of the 21 patients was placed in a prone (n = 19), supine (n = 1), or lateral (n = 1) position. After selecting the appropriate scanning section, we used CT guidance lights and skin marks to obtain depth, distance, and angle measurements, which were based on computer calculations performed at the CT scanner. For primary puncture of the abscess, we used an 18-gauge guiding cannula (William Cook Europe, Bjaeverskor, Denmark) in 23 cases and placed the needle tip in the most caudal part of the abscess cavity. In six cases, the intradiskal space was severely narrowed, so the primary puncture was performed with an 18-gauge side-cutting biopsy needle to attain stable guidance through the surrounding bone particles. After evacuation of the abscess fluid, 29 5.6–10.0-F pigtail catheters (Angiomed, Karlsruhe, Germany; three 5.6-F, four 6.0-F, 14 7.6-F, three 8.0-F, three 9.0-F, and two 10.0-F catheters) were inserted with an 0.035-inch, extrastiff guide wire (Amplatz; William Cook Europe) or superstiff guide wire (Lunderquist; William Cook Europe).

When larger catheters had to be placed, track predilation was performed with use of a suitable dilator first. In four paravertebral abscesses, a 14-F vanSonnenberg catheter was inserted with a trocar technique. A posterior approach was used in most (n = 32) cases, with the patient in a prone or lateral position; a lateroventral approach was used once to drain a psoas abscess in the pelvis, with the patient in a supine position. Eight milliliters to 510 mL of abscess fluid was evacuated after the initial catheter placement. To exclude fistula formation or perforation of the abscess membrane and to demonstrate correct drainage of the complete abscess cavity, we always performed sinography with diluted contrast media (one part contrast media, nine parts physiologic saline solution) in each patient.

All catheters were irrigated immediately with sterile saline solution until clear fluid was aspirated; this procedure was repeated daily during the whole drainage period. Furthermore, all patients were immobilized and received antibiotics; the choice of antibiotic depended on the organisms isolated from the abscess fluid.

The follow-up of all patients included clinical examinations and blood testing for inflammatory signs, as well as neurologic examinations, which were performed routinely for at least 6 months. The first follow-up CT examination was performed within 4–7 days, during which pre- and postcontrast scans were obtained in each patient. All further follow-up CT scans (an average of five per patient) were obtained during the next 1½–6 months. Seven patients underwent additional unenhanced and gadolinium-enhanced T1-weighted (500–600/15) and T2-weighted (2,000/90) spin-echo MR imaging of the spine 4–6 months after the drainage procedure.

All catheters were left in place as long as secretion was evident and irrigation of the catheters revealed purulent or turbid fluid. The drainage catheters were removed when follow-up CT examination findings demonstrated complete resolution of the abscess cavity and blood test results showed definitive retrogression of the inflammatory signs.

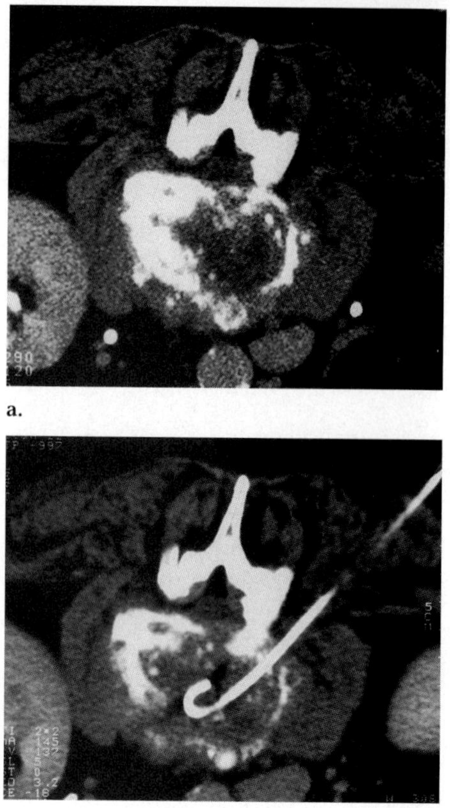

a.

b.

Figure 1. **(a)** CT image obtained in a 58-year-old man with spondylodiskitis of the lumbar spine and intradiskal abscess formation. **(b)** CT image in the same patient shows the exact placement from a dorsal approach of a 7.6-F pigtail catheter in the intradiskal space with the patient in the prone position.

RESULTS

The diagnosis of spondylodiskitis was assessed by using characteristic CT signs. Focal destruction of one or more vertebral bodies was visible in all patients; the location of the spinal lesion was thoracic in five, lumbar in 13, and thoracolumbar in three of the 21 patients. The involved segment was at the level of the T4 and T5 (n = 2), T7 and T8 (n = 1), T9 and T10 (n = 2), T12 and L1 (n = 3), L1 and L2 (n = 1), L2 and L3 (n = 6), L3 and L4 (n = 2), or L4 and L5 (n = 4) vertebrae. Two patients had a prolapse of inflammatory granulation tissue into the spinal canal; the tissue reached the myelon but did not compress it. An epidural abscess formation was excluded in each case by using MR imaging.

A total of 33 abscesses were depicted on

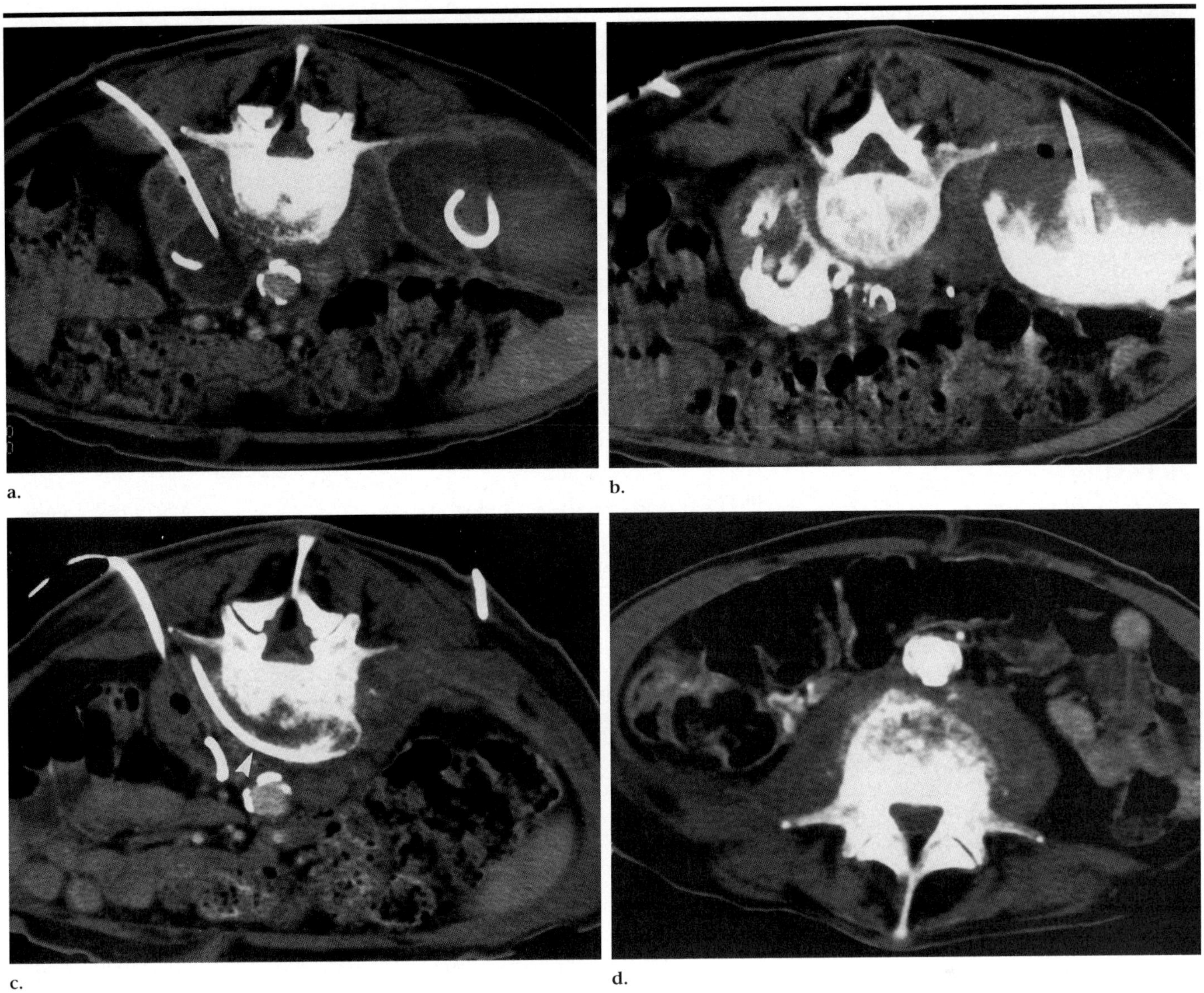

Figure 2. Bilateral spondylodiskitis-associated psoas abscesses in a 68-year-old man. **(a)** Postcontrast CT scan shows characteristic low-attenuating fluid collections with enhancing peripheral rims on both sides with pigtail catheters in place after percutaneous drainage. On the left side in **a**, diluted contrast medium is still visible after **(b)** a sinogram that was obtained with the patient in the prone position. **(c)** CT scan obtained after evacuation of the abscess fluid shows another pigtail catheter (arrowhead), which was inserted in the intradiskal space with the patient in the prone position. **(d)** Follow-up CT scan obtained 6 weeks after the drainage procedure and removal of all catheters, with complete evacuation of the former abscess cavities.

postcontrast CT scans obtained in 21 patients; the location was in the intradiskal space in nine (Fig 1a), was paravertebral in 12, and was in the psoas muscle in 12 of the 33 cases. Six patients had a single intradiskal abscess (Fig 1), three had either a combination of intradiskal and paravertebral abscesses or a combination of intradiskal and psoas abscesses (Fig 2), seven had paravertebral abscesses (Fig 3), and five had only psoas abscesses (Table 1).

Abscess drainage was successfully performed in each case, with no procedural complications. Twelve patients needed one drainage catheter, six needed two catheters, and three needed three drainage catheters (Table 1).

The drainage duration was 4–56 days, with an average duration of 26.8 days. In nine patients younger than 60 years, a total of 14 catheters were inserted and remained in place an average of 21.9 days. In 12 patients older than 60 years, a total of 19 drainage catheters were inserted and remained in place an average of 30.1 days.

Specific organisms were isolated in 16 of 21 patients (*M tuberculosis* in seven, *S aureus* in four, *Streptococcus* species in two, *P aeruginosa* in one, *E coli* in one, and *M morganii* in one), so an additional specific antibiotic treatment was possible. Most (14 of 33) catheters were placed in patients with tuberculosis and remained in place for an average of 31.1 days. The duration of drainage was the shortest (4 days) in a 40-year-old patient with a *P aeruginosa* infection and the longest (56 days) in a 68-year-old patient with tuberculous spondylitis (Table 2).

In all patients, the abscess cavity was initially completely evacuated (Fig 2c), and the patients had clinical improvement during the following days, with pain relief and retrogression of inflammatory signs. Three of 33 catheters were changed because of insufficient drainage caused by catheter leakage or obstruction; one drainage catheter (for a psoas abscess) had to be reinserted because of dislocation. Two patients (one with one paravertebral abscess and one with two paravertebral abscesses) underwent surgery for stabilization of the spine with the drainage catheter in place.

Treatment success during the drainage period was defined as the persistent complete evacuation of the former abscess cavity and the decrease in associated inflammatory soft-tissue swelling. After normalization of all laboratory findings and removal of all drainage catheters, no recurrence was visualized on follow-up CT or MR images in any patient.

DISCUSSION

Infectious spondylodiskitis is characterized by vertebral body destruction and collapse, disk space narrowing, extension into the spinal epidural space, and intraosseous or paraspinal abscess formations (2,9,10). MR imaging has been shown to improve visualization of the disease within the soft tissue and the spinal canal (2,11); thus, in six of our patients with neurologic symptoms, MR imaging was the first choice. Discovertebral lesions and paravertebral abscess formations are usually well assessed by using CT (2,10,12); spondylodiskitis-associated abscesses were correctly diagnosed in each of our patients with use of the typical sign, a low-attenuating fluid collection with an enhancing wall, on contrast-enhanced CT scans (10).

Although *S aureus* is the most common organism isolated in infectious osteomyelitis (13,14), abscess formations are most frequently seen in tuberculous spondylitis (1). Lindahl et al (2) examined 503 patients with tuberculosis and found spinal involvement in 63 patients, with paraspinal abscess formation in 74.9% of the 63 patients. In other series (3,15), tuberculous spinal abscesses were demonstrated in 71%–75% of cases; accordingly, most (14 of 33) drainage catheters were placed in tuberculous abscesses in our study.

Conservative treatment is generally accepted for mild and uncomplicated cases of infectious spondylitis and includes parenteral antibiotic therapy, immobilization, and physical therapy for several weeks or months (14,15). Malawski and Lukawski (13) reported on 295 conservatively treated patients, with good and satisfactory results in 98% of cases. In addition, small paraspinal abscess formations usually respond to nonsurgical treatment and should not be treated surgically unless they are clinically important (eg, associated with sepsis).

According to the literature (13), larger paraspinal abscess formations are usually treated surgically; satisfactory or good results are attained in up to 97% of cases. However, postsurgical complications, which include wound infections, sepsis, pneumonia, and pulmonary embolism, can occur at any point in the treatment course. Malawski and Lukawski (13) reported on four courses that

TABLE 1
Patient Characteristics, Catheter Sizes, Drainage Durations, and Microbiologic Findings

Patient No./Age (y)/Sex	Catheter Size (French)	Abscess Location*	Drainage Duration (d)	Isolated Organism
1/65/M	5.6	Intradiskal	12	*Streptococcus* species
2/77/M	5.6	Intradiskal	23	*E coli*
3/40/M	6.0	Intradiskal	4	*Pseudomonas* species
4/79/M	7.6	Intradiskal	7	. . .
5/58/M	7.6	Intradiskal	12	*S aureus*
6/73/F	9.0	Intradiskal	49	. . .
7/37/M	5.6	Paravertebral	9	*S aureus*
8/37/M	7.6	Paravertebral	20	*M tuberculosis*
9/24/M	7.6, 8.0	Paravertebral (2)	22, 22	*M tuberculosis*
10/74/M	9.0	Paravertebral	21	*M tuberculosis*
11/39/M	10.0	Paravertebral	21	. . .
12/38/F	14.0	Paravertebral (2)	33, 33	*M tuberculosis*
13/68/M	14.0	Paravertebral (2)	56, 56†	*M tuberculosis*
14/79/F	7.6	Psoas	20‡	*Morganella morganii*
15/81/M	8.0	Psoas	14	. . .
16/57/M	7.6	Psoas (2)	14, 39	*S aureus*
17/74/M	7.6	Psoas (2)	39, 41	*S aureus*
18/39/F	6.0	Psoas (3)	26, 26, 26	*M tuberculosis*
19/69/F	7.6	Intradiskal	47	*Streptococcus* species
	10.0	Psoas	50§	
20/68/M	7.6	Intradiskal	11	. . .
	8.0	Psoas	15	
	9.0	Psoas	17$^\|$	
21/73/M	7.6	Intradiskal	45	*M tuberculosis*
	7.6	Paravertebral	45	
	7.6	Paravertebral	5	

* The numbers in parentheses are the number of abscesses.
† Catheter changed on day 44 because of obstruction.
‡ Catheter reinserted on day 7 because of dislocation.
§ Catheter changed on day 21 because of leakage.
$^\|$ Catheter changed on day 4 because of obstruction.

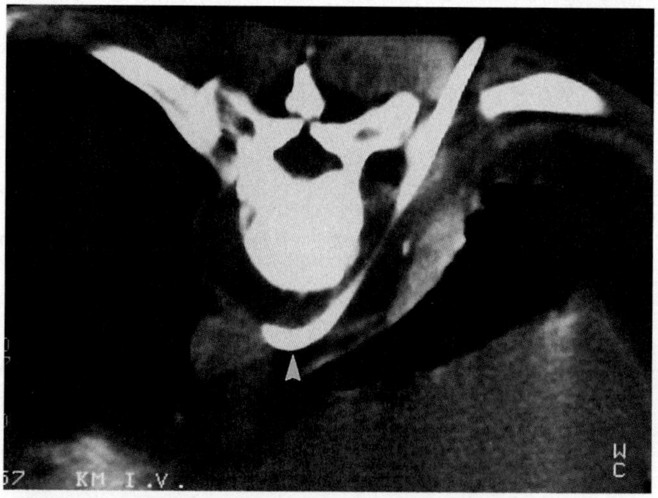

Figure 3. CT scan demonstrates thoracic spondylodiskitis with paravertebral abscess formation in a 68-year-old man. The 14-F vanSonnenberg catheter (arrowhead) is inserted by using a dorsal approach and is placed around the ventral side of the vertebral body, with the patient in the prone position.

TABLE 2
Drainage Catheters and Drainage Durations in Correlation to the Organisms Found in the Abscess Fluid

Isolated Organism	No. of Patients	Average Age (y)	No. of Catheters	Drainage Duration (d)		
				Minimum	Maximum	Average
P aeruginosa	1	40.0	1	4	4	4.0
None found	5	68.0	7	7	49	19.1
M morganii	1	79.0	1	20	20	20.0
E coli	1	77.0	1	23	23	23.0
S aureus	4	56.5	6	9	39	25.6
M tuberculosis	7	50.4	14	5	56	31.1
Streptococcus species	2	67.0	3	12	50	33.3

were lethal owing to cardiac or renal disease and secondary pneumonia in 147 surgically treated patients. To decrease the need for surgical intervention, CT-guided biopsy and drainage are performed in various organ systems (5,7,9,16), and percutaneous drainage of psoas abscesses is a recognized alternative to surgery (6,8,17–21).

As demonstrated in our study, paravertebral and even intradiskal abscess formations may be treated efficiently by using nonsurgical drainage, but the indications for this treatment protocol should be established properly. Surgical intervention cannot be avoided in cases of epidural abscess with neurologic compromise, of impingement on the spinal cord or cauda equina by collapsed osteomyelitic vertebral bodies, or when stabilization of the spine is indicated (14,22). Consequently, in our clinic, patients with these contraindications undergo surgery for removal of necrotic tissue, decompression of the spinal cord, drainage of combined abscesses, and fusion of the spine. In two of our patients, the inflammatory granulation tissue reached the spinal cord, but since there were no signs of spinal cord compression or neurologic damage, CT-guided percutaneous catheter drainage of the associated paravertebral spondylodiskitic abscesses was performed, without any complications noticed during follow-up. Another two patients required surgery for stabilization of the spine, but no surgical abscess drainage had to be performed.

For establishment of the final diagnosis and proper treatment of spondylodiskitis, verification of the spinal infection with histologic specimen analysis and isolation of the offending organism is essential (14). Precise localization of the biopsy site and of the needle tip (10,23) is a major advantage of CT-guided diagnostic and therapeutic procedures compared with MR imaging–guided procedures. Therefore, in our clinic, CT-guided side-cutting–needle or fine-needle aspiration biopsy of the vertebral disks or of the paravertebral solid granulation tissue are performed in all patients who are suspected of having spondylodiskitis. When abscess formations are visible, needle aspiration is performed first, followed by drainage.

Cultures of the disk specimen result in positive findings of germs more often than do blood cultures, but most authors report on negative culture findings in both instances in 50%–70% of patients (1). In our study, specific organisms were found in 16 (76%) of 21 patients, which is most likely due to the concentration of organisms in the microbiologically examined abscess fluid.

If side-cutting biopsy needles are used for primary puncture in cases of narrowed diskal space and for passing through bone particles caused by destruction of the adjacent vertebral bodies, the inner stylet can be removed and replaced with a suitable venous access needle. Aspiration of abscess fluid or irrigation of a small abscess with sterile saline solution can be performed easily with this technique. Because various catheters can be inserted with the Seldinger technique to complete the drainage, we prefer this technique whenever stable guidance for biopsy and drainage must be achieved. Insufficient drainage due to leakage or obstruction of the catheter was seen in three of 33 cases, but these catheters were easily exchanged with the Seldinger technique. One of 33 catheters had to be reinserted because of dislocation, which occurred when the abscess cavity collapsed.

All abscess cavities were drained successfully; no recurrence was seen during the follow-up. Nine of 21 patients needed two or three drainages; thus, the critically ill patients or patients who had a high risk of surgical or postsurgical complications with complicated large abscess formation could benefit from the avoidance of general anesthesia, laparotomy, and prolonged immobilization (17). In conclusion, CT-guided percutaneous catheter drainage of spondylodiskitic abscesses seems to be an attractive alternative to surgical management.

References

1. Sharif HS. Role of MR imaging in the management of spinal infections. AJR 1992; 158: 1333–1345.
2. Lindahl S, Nyman RS, Brismar J, Hugosson C, Lundstedt C. Imaging of tuberculosis: spinal manifestations in 63 patients. Acta Radiol 1996; 37:506–511.
3. Al-Mulhim FA, Ibrahim EM, El-Hassan AY, Moharram HM. Magnetic resonance imaging of tuberculous spondylitis. Spine 1995; 20: 2287–2292.
4. Calderone RR, Larsen JM. Overview and classification of spinal infections. Orthop Clin North Am 1996; 27:1–8.
5. Gobien RP, Stanley JH, Gobien BS, Vujic I, Pass HI. Percutaneous catheter aspiration and drainage of suspected mediastinal abscesses. Radiology 1984; 151:69–71.
6. Mueller PR, Ferrucci JT, Wittenberg J, Simeone JF, Butch RJ. Iliopsoas abscess: treatment by CT-guided percutaneous catheter drainage. AJR 1984; 142:359–362.
7. vanSonnenberg E, D'Agostino HB, Casola G, Wittich GR, Varney RR, Harker C. Lung abscess: CT-guided drainage. Radiology 1991; 178:347–351.
8. Pombo F, Martin-Egana R, Cela A, Diaz JL, Linares-Mondejar, P, Freire M. Percutaneous catheter drainage of tuberculous psoas abscess. Acta Radiol 1993; 34:366–368.
9. Langen HJ, Breiden-Langen CM, Klose KC. Ungewöhnliche manifestation einer spondylitis tuberculosa. Fortschr Röntgenstr 1990; 152:729–731.
10. Shanley DJ. Tuberculosis of the spine: imaging features. AJR 1995; 164:659–664.
11. Modic MT, Feiglin DH, Piraino DW, et al. Vertebral osteomyelitis: assessment using MR. Radiology 1985; 157:157–166.
12. Sartoris DJ, Moskowitz PS, Kaufman RA, Ziprkowski MN, Berger PE. Childhood discitis: computed tomographic findings. Radiology 1983; 149:701–707.
13. Malawski SK, Lukawski S. Pyogenic infection of the spine. Clin Orthop 1991; 272:58–66.
14. Ozuna RM, Delamarter RB. Pyogenic vertebral osteomyelitis and postsurgical disc space infections. Orthop Clin North Am 1996; 27:87–94.
15. Huang YC, Shih TT, Huang KM, Su CT. Infectious spondylitis: MRI characteristics. J Formos Med Assoc 1996; 95:458–463.
16. vanSonnenberg E, Mueller PR, Ferrucci JT. Percutaneous drainage of 250 abdominal abscesses and fluid collections. Radiology 1984; 151:337–341.
17. Ousehal A, Essodegui F, Abdelouafi A, Kadiri R. Ultrasonography in the diagnosis and treatment of psoas abscess: apropos of a study of 30 patients. J Radiol 1994; 75:629–634. [French]
18. Horvath G, Boda A, Repa I. CT-guided percutaneous drainage in the management of psoas abscesses. Orv Hetil 1994; 135:2597–2602.
19. Hoffer FA, Shamberger RC, Teele RL. Iliopsoas abscess: diagnosis and management. Pediatr Radiol 1987; 17:23–27.
20. Rieker O, Duber C, Godderz W. Spondylogenic psoas abscess: long term follow-up after percutaneous drainage. Aktuelle Radiol 1995; 5:112–114.
21. Thomas A, Albert AS, Bhat S, Sunil KR. Primary psoas abscess: diagnostic and therapeutic considerations. Br J Urol 1996; 78:358–360.
22. Broner FA, Garland DE, Zigler JE. Spinal infections in the immunocompromised host. Orthop Clin North Am 1996; 27:37–46.
23. Frager DH, Goldman MJ, Seimon LP, et al. Computed tomography guidance for skeletal biopsy. Skeletal Radiol 1987; 16:644–646.

Research & Education Fund

The RSNA R&E Fund's support of research and education in radiology and related scientific disciplines is made possible by your donations.

Scholar
Purpose — To support young faculty members by freeing at least one-half of their time to gain experience in research early in their academic careers.

Amount — $60,000 annually for two years, payable to the institution, to be used exclusively as stipend.

Research Resident
Purpose — To provide educational opportunities for radiology residents to gain further insight into scientific investigation, or to develop competence in research and educational techniques and methods.

Amount — $30,000 grant for one year, payable to the department, to be used as stipend.

Medical Student Departmental Award Program
Purpose — To provide opportunities for medical students to work as members of a research team.

Amount — $1,000 per month, payable to the department, to be matched by the department for a period of three or more months. These grants are designed to support medical students appointed to work with research mentors at their institution or another comparable research environment.

Medical Student/Scholar Assistant
Purpose — To provide promising medical students an opportunity to experience radiology research while assisting second year RSNA Scholars.

Amount — $5,000 payable to the institution.

Research Fellow
Purpose — To provide educational opportunities for young investigators not yet professionally established in the radiological sciences, to gain further insight into scientific investigation, or to develop competence in research and educational techniques and methods.

Amount — $35,000 Fellow stipend for one year, with opportunity to renew for a second year at $40,000. On request, $5,000 is given to the institution to be applied directly to expenses.

Seed
Purpose — To assist young investigators in testing hypotheses and defining objectives before they apply for major grants from corporations, foundations, or government agencies.

Amount — One-year grant of $25,000 or less, payable to the department in two equal installments. Applicants from any country in the world are eligible for this award.

Roentgen Centennial Fellow
Purpose — Designed to permit experienced practitioners the opportunity to explore and apply innovative solutions to key issues facing the radiological community.

Amount — $100,000 for a one year program of study and/or research.

Application details differ for this program. Detailed letter of interest outlining the applicant's innovative idea should be received by March 1 each year.

Awards, with the exception of the Seed Grant award, are restricted to citizens of North American countries and to individuals in the process of becoming citizens of the same.

Our gratitude to all those who contribute to the activities of the RSNA R&E Fund. We look forward to continued support.

RSNA® | Radiological Society of North America
Founded in 1915

2021 Spring Road, Suite 600
Oak Brook, Illinois 60523-1860
630/571-2670
FAX: 630/571-7837
www.rsna.org

RSNA Research and Education Fund

Laurent Guibaud, MD
Denis Herbreteau, MD
Josée Dubois, MD
Noelle Stempfle, MD
Jérome Bérard, MD
Jean-Pierre Pracros, MD
Jean-Jacques Merland, MD

Index terms:
Bones, cysts, 40.3183
Interventional procedures, in infants and children, 40.1269
Sclerotherapy, 40.1269

Radiology 1998; 208:369–373

[1] From the Departments of Pediatric Imaging (L.G., J.P.P.) and Pediatric Orthopedics (J.B.), Hôpital Debrousse, Université Lyon-Sud, 29 rue Soeur Bouvier, 69322 Lyon 05, France; the Department of Neuroradiology and Interventional Angiography, Hôpital Lariboisière, Paris, France (D.H., N.S., J.J.M.); and the Department of Imaging, Hôpital Sainte-Justine, Université de Montréal, Quebec, Canada (J.D.). Received November 4, 1997; revision requested January 20, 1998; revision received February 23; accepted April 3. **Address reprint requests to** L.G.

Aneurysmal Bone Cysts: Percutaneous Embolization with an Alcoholic Solution of Zein—Series of 18 Cases[1]

PURPOSE: To assess the efficacy of percutaneous embolization with an alcoholic solution of zein in the treatment of aneurysmal bone cysts.

MATERIALS AND METHODS: Eighteen patients with aneurysmal bone cysts were treated percutaneously with alcoholic zein. The cysts were in the lower limb ($n = 7$), upper limb ($n = 5$), pelvis ($n = 3$), cervical spine ($n = 2$), and mandible ($n = 1$). All patients were symptomatic; three had previously undergone surgery. Percutaneous embolization was performed with fluoroscopic or computed tomographic guidance with the patient under general anesthesia. Clinical and imaging follow-up lasted 18 months to 4 years.

RESULTS: Percutaneous embolization was performed in 16 cases. In two cases, cystograms showed marked venous drainage and thus embolization was not attempted. Six patients underwent repeat embolization. Complications consisted of a local transitory inflammatory reaction ($n = 5$), aseptic osteitis ($n = 1$), and a small pulmonary infarct without sequelae ($n = 1$). Relief of symptoms was achieved in all patients except one, who underwent surgery. At imaging, improvement was total in 13 cases (87%) and partial in two cases (13%). No recurrence was noted during follow-up.

CONCLUSION: Percutaneous embolization of aneurysmal bone cysts with alcoholic zein should be considered a reliable alternative to surgery, especially in cases with a difficult surgical approach or cases of postsurgical recurrence.

Conventional treatment of aneurysmal bone cysts is based on surgical curettage of the entire lesion with or without bone grafting. The recurrence rate after surgery is 10%–44% (1). Selective arterial embolization has been proposed to occlude vascular supply before surgery or as a definitive treatment (2,3). Adamsbaum et al (4) used percutaneous embolization with an alcoholic solution of zein in a small series of benign bone cysts with encouraging preliminary results. Alcoholic zein is used for renal artery embolization before nephrectomy or for occlusion of the pancreatic duct system after partial pancreatic resection; use of this agent for percutaneous sclerotherapy of soft-tissue vascular malformations has been proposed (5–7).

The histologic similarities between aneurysmal bone cysts and soft-tissue venous malformations led us to prospectively evaluate the use of alcoholic zein in percutaneous embolization of aneurysmal bone cysts.

Author contributions:
Guarantor of integrity of entire study, L.G.; study concepts, L.G., D.H., J.D., N.S.; study design, L.G.; definition of intellectual content, L.G.; literature research, L.G.; clinical studies, L.G., D.H., J.D., N.S., J.B., J.P.P., J.J.M.; data acquisition, L.G., D.H., J.D., N.S.; data analysis, L.G.; manuscript preparation, editing, and review, L.G.

MATERIALS AND METHODS

Between 1991 and 1995, 18 patients aged 4–15 years (mean, 10 years) underwent percutaneous embolization with an alcoholic solution of zein (Ethibloc; Ethnor Laboratories/Ethicon, Norderstedt, Germany) for aneurysmal bone cysts. The study was performed in accordance with institutional guidelines. Informed consent was obtained from all parents after the risks and benefits of treatment were fully explained. All patients had symptoms, which included pain and swelling related to bone expansion (Figs 1–3). In seven cases, the cysts were complicated by fractures. Seven lesions were in the lower extremity (two in the femur and one each in the fibula, talus, calcaneus, metatarsal, and phalanx), five in the upper extremity (four in the humerus and one in the radius), four in flat bones (three in the pelvis and one in the mandible), and two in the cervical spine (one in the odontoid and one in the posterior arch of C7). Five patients had previously undergone unsuccessful treatment: surgery (n = 3), local injection of steroids (n = 1), and local injection of calcitonin (n = 1). The mean interval between previous treatment and embolization with alcoholic zein was 16 months (range, 7–28 months). The diagnosis of aneurysmal bone cyst was established with percutaneous biopsy in five cases, open biopsy in 10 cases, and imaging (plain radiography, CT, and MR imaging) in three cases.

Percutaneous embolization was performed as follows: With the patient under general anesthesia, a standard needle (14–18 gauge according to cortical thickness) was inserted with fluoroscopic (n = 16) or CT (n = 2) guidance. Cyst fluid was aspirated and sent for cytologic analysis. Contrast medium was injected into the lesion to confirm good filling of the cyst and absence of leakage in surrounding soft tissue and to show the venous drainage. Assessment of venous drainage is less accurate with CT guidance than with fluoroscopic control. If only partial filling was achieved (Fig 2c), additional injections were performed to ensure complete filling. Reassessment of the venous drainage is mandatory after each additional injection and before each injection of alcoholic zein. Potential venous drainage was controlled with manual compression to prevent distal embolization of the venous draining system, then alcoholic zein was injected.

Alcoholic zein is available in sterilized 7.5-mL syringes. One milliliter of the solution contains 210 mg zein, 162 mg sodium-amidotrizoate-tetrahydrate, 145 mg oleum papaveris, 316 mg 96% ethanol, and 248 mg aqua ad injectabilia. The viscosity of this agent at 37°C is 200 cp versus 10 cp for a conventional water-soluble contrast medium. The solution is radiopaque and has a soft consistency per se. However, the radiopacity and solubility can be increased by adding iodized oil (Lipiodol; Andre Guerbet, Aulnay-sous-Bois, France) (2 mL per syringe of alcoholic zein) and ethanol (1 or 2 mL per syringe of alcoholic zein), respectively. If

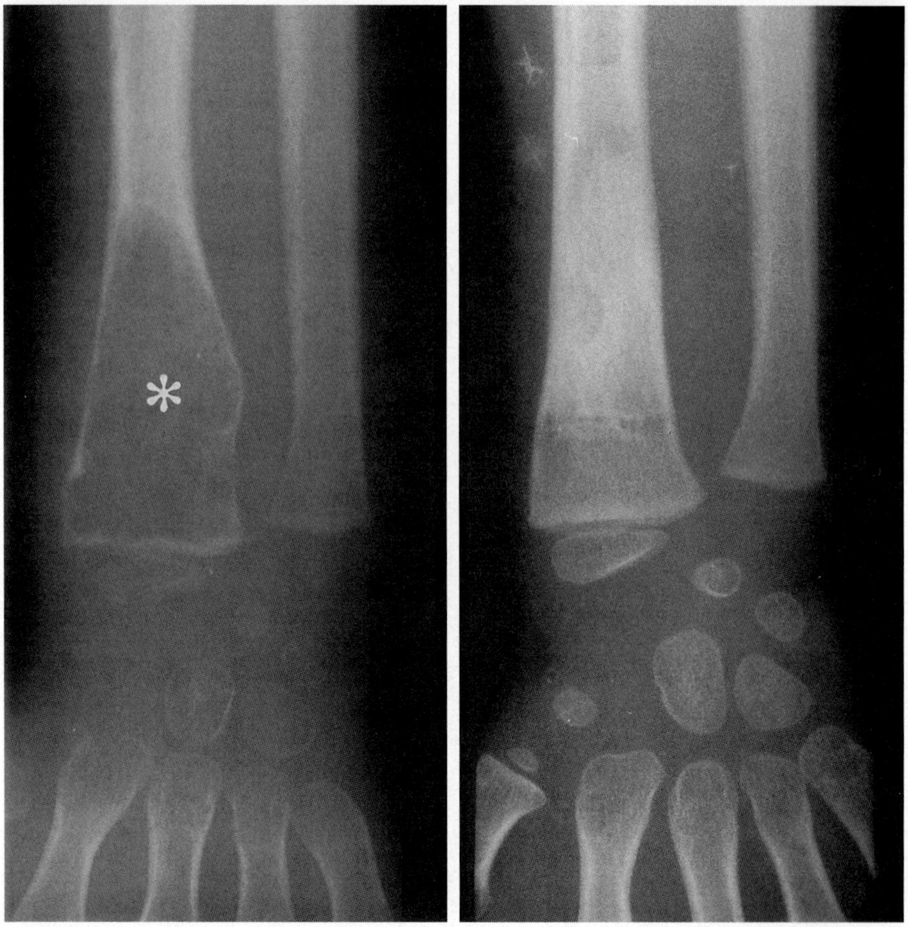

a. b.

Figure 1. Postsurgical recurrence of an aneurysmal bone cyst of the distal radius in a 4-year-old boy. **(a)** Initial plain radiograph shows an expansile, lucent lesion (*) with numerous septa in the distal end of the radius. **(b)** Follow-up plain radiograph obtained 5 months after percutaneous embolization with alcoholic zein shows complete reconstruction with normal bone volume and mineralization. The stellar areas of increased opacity projected on the soft tissue are film artifacts.

the cystogram shows poor venous drainage and limited diffusion of contrast medium into the lesion, ethanol can be added to increase diffusion of alcoholic zein. In cases of marked venous drainage, pure alcoholic zein is injected and additional injections are performed if cyst filling is partial.

The amount of alcoholic zein injected corresponded to the amount of contrast medium necessary to fully opacify the cyst. Fluoroscopic guidance ensured that the injection was confined to the cystic lesion. Manual compression, when required, lasted at least 10 minutes.

After the procedure, the patient was hospitalized for 24 hours to control occasional inflammatory reactions. Follow-up consisted of clinical and radiologic examination 3, 6, 12, and 18 months after the procedure. At imaging, bone reconstruction was assessed in terms of bone mineralization, cortical thickening, and normalization of bone volume. Reconstruction was graded as complete, partial (ie, residual cystic components and incomplete bone mineralization), or absent. Three-month radiologic follow-up involved only plain radiography to assess bone reconstruction. In cases of partial or complete reconstruction, plain radiography was performed at 6 months to check for complete healing. Lack of response to alcoholic zein was not assessed before 6 months because bone reconstruction can be a long process. If reconstruction was not seen at 6 months, repeat embolization with alcoholic zein or other treatment was considered. In cases of partial reconstruction, the lesion was reassessed at 12 months. If reconstruction remained partial, CT or MR imaging was performed to assess and localize residual cystic lesions before repeat embolization with

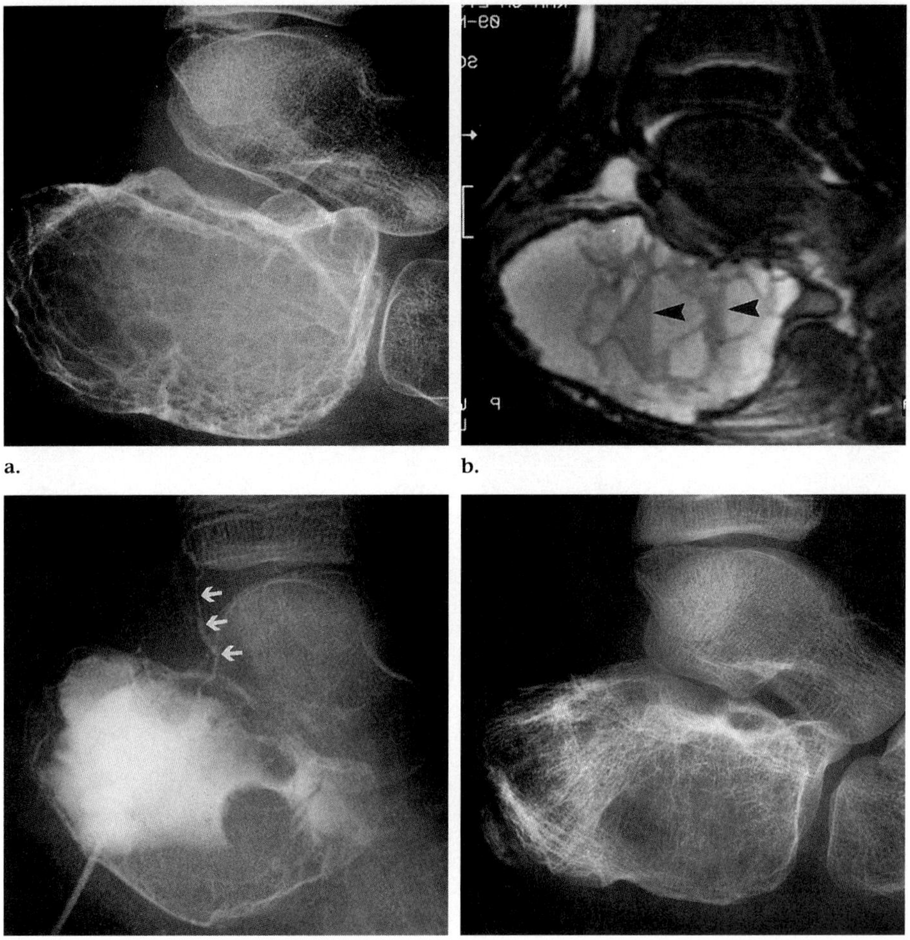

a. b. c. d.

Figure 2. Aneurysmal bone cyst of the calcaneus revealed by a fracture in a 10-year-old boy with recent enlargement of the heel. Imaging findings were highly suggestive of aneurysmal bone cyst; after a multidisciplinary discussion, we decided to perform percutaneous embolization with alcoholic zein due to difficulties in performing curettage and bone grafting. **(a)** Initial plain radiograph shows an expansile lesion with septa that involves the entire calcaneus. **(b)** Sagittal short inversion time inversion-recovery magnetic resonance (MR) image (repetition time msec/echo time msec/inversion time msec = 1,500/50/162) acquired with the patient supine shows typical fluid-fluid levels (arrowheads) involving the entire calcaneus. **(c)** Pretreatment cystogram shows the multiloculated cystic spaces of the lesion and the venous drainage (arrows). However, there was only partial filling of the cyst, and additional percutaneous injections were required. **(d)** Follow-up plain radiograph obtained 6 months after repeat embolization with alcoholic zein, which resulted in transitory aseptic osteitis, shows normal bone mineralization and normal osseous trabeculae.

alcoholic zein. In cases of total reconstruction, the lesion was reassessed 6 and 12 months after total healing.

RESULTS

In all 18 patients, needle insertion was successful and bloody fluid was aspirated. No atypical cells were found at cytologic analysis. However, percutaneous embolization with alcoholic zein was not performed in two cases because of high venous drainage, which could not be controlled in one case and was associated with major soft-tissue opacification in one case of a cervical lesion. Overall, 24 procedures were performed: Ten patients underwent one procedure, and six patients underwent two (n = 4) or three (n = 2) procedures. The interval between repeat procedures was 6–12 months.

Transitory local inflammatory reactions occurred in five patients and were controlled with an intravenously administered analgesic (acetaminophen [paracetamol]), orally administered nonsteroidal anti-inflammatory drugs, and immobilization. One patient who underwent three procedures had an inflammatory reaction only after the third procedure. In all cases, immobilization during the acute inflammatory phase was helpful in pain reduction (especially when the cyst involved an extremity). The pain was maximal during the first 48 hours and decreased during the 10 days after the procedure. Because this potential reaction necessitates at least 24 hours hospitalization for pain control, percutaneous embolization with alcoholic zein cannot be performed on an outpatient basis.

Two true complications occurred: Two months after an uneventful second procedure (performed 10 months after the first one) for incomplete bone reconstruction, a patient with a cyst that involved the entire calcaneus (Fig 2a) demonstrated severe bone destruction and leakage of alcoholic zein in soft tissue. The leakage resulted in local cellulitis. Bone destruction was assessed by comparing CT findings obtained before the second procedure with those obtained at the time of the leakage. The latter CT findings (bone demineralization and cortical disruptions) were suggestive of aseptic osteitis related to a markedly delayed inflammatory reaction. Treatment included both immobilization and surgical excision of alcoholic zein collected in soft tissue. After a few weeks, healing occurred with surprisingly complete bone reconstruction at imaging follow-up (Fig 2d). Another patient experienced thoracic pain with minimal pleural effusion a few days after a third procedure was performed under CT guidance. Scintigraphic results were consistent with a small pulmonary embolus; the symptoms disappeared in a few days.

After the initial procedure, bone reconstruction was complete in nine cases. Among the five cases in which reconstruction was partial, it became complete after a repeat procedure in three cases and after two repeat procedures in one case. In one patient, the reconstruction was improved by a repeat procedure but remained partial at the last follow-up. Two patients did not demonstrate any bone reconstruction after the initial procedure: One underwent surgery and the other two repeat procedures, which led to partial reconstruction. Thirteen of 15 patients treated only with alcoholic zein were completely healed (success rate of 87%); two had partial benefit at last follow-up. There were no recurrences during follow-up of 18 months to 4 years.

DISCUSSION

"The so-called ABC is neither a cyst nor a neoplasm; rather it is probably a periosteal or intraosseous vascular malformation" (10). This concept, initially suggested by Lichtenstein (8,9) and emphasized by Mirra (10), is based on histologic and radiologic similarities between aneurysmal bone cysts and soft-tissue vascular malformations. Histologic findings such as blood filling, anastomosis, and cavernous spaces separated by septa are characteristic of both aneurysmal bone cysts and soft-tissue venous malformations (11). MR imaging and angiography demonstrate similar findings in these entities: lobulated contours and internal septa, with low signal intensity on T1-weighted MR images and, in particular, very high signal intensity on T2-weighted MR images. Fluid-fluid levels often occur in both entities and reflect low intralesion blood flow, which allows differentiation between dependent and nondependent blood components (Fig 2b). Angiographic findings are typical in most cases of low intralesion blood flow, with no or discrete arterial hypervascularity but delayed and prolonged lesion staining in the venous phase with late opacification of variable venous drainage. Most aneurysmal bone cysts are similar to low-flow venous malformations, but a few are more suggestive of high-flow lesions, with substantial arterial supply and major venous drainage.

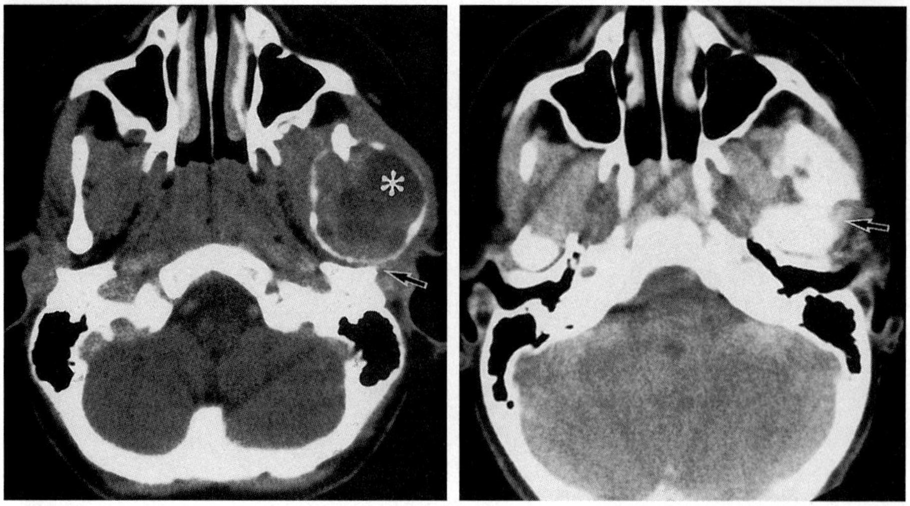

Figure 3. Histologically proved aneurysmal bone cyst of the neck of the mandible in an 8-year-old boy. **(a)** Initial computed tomographic (CT) scan shows an expansile lesion of the neck of the left mandible (*) close to the temporomandibular joint (arrow). Percutaneous embolization with alcoholic zein was chosen as the initial treatment because of the difficult surgical approach. **(b)** Follow-up plain radiograph obtained 14 months after two percutaneous embolization procedures shows complete regression of the cyst and good reossification of the neck of the left mandible (arrow).

Our study was based on these histologic and radiologic similarities and the good results reported for percutaneous embolization of venous soft-tissue malformations with alcoholic zein (6). Since Dubois et al (6) showed that percutaneous embolization with alcoholic zein is a safe alternative to surgery for treatment of soft-tissue venous malformations, with good to excellent results in 74% of cases, we have used this approach in aneurysmal bone cysts. Our hypothesis is that alcoholic zein should have the same efficacy in aneurysmal bone cysts as in soft-tissue venous malformations because these entities represent similar processes involving bone and soft tissue, respectively.

Alcoholic zein is a radiopaque alcoholic solution of corn protein. It is a biodegradable agent that induces intravascular thrombosis, marked local inflammation, and finally a fibrotic reaction (12,13). Inflammation and subsequent fibrosis may trigger the reparative process of mineralization by osteoblast stimulation. This reparative process, which results in bone reconstruction and bone volume normalization, lasts several months and even more than 1 year after percutaneous embolization with alcoholic zein. Therefore, one should wait at least 6 months to evaluate the efficacy of one procedure. Conversely, the initial inflammation is short-lived and limited to the injection site. The inflammatory reaction can induce local pain, which is well controlled by medication, as in percutaneous embolization of soft-tissue vascular malformations with alcoholic zein (5–7). However, the inflammation produced may overshoot the goal, as in one of our cases: Injection of alcoholic zein resulted in transient aggressive bone destruction suggestive of aseptic osteitis, which was followed by dramatic bone remineralization. One should be aware of the possibility of such a reaction, which resulted in serious concern in the acute phase of destruction.

The high viscosity of alcoholic zein allows excellent filling of the lesion with minimal risk of distal embolization of the draining venous system (6,14). However, injection should be performed carefully under fluoroscopic guidance. Although CT guidance is useful in the percutaneous approach to deep locations, such as in pelvic aneurysmal bone cysts, fluoroscopic control is recommended for injection of alcoholic zein to minimize the risk of migration. In retrospect, we should have used fluoroscopic guidance in the patient with a pelvic aneurysmal bone cyst that was treated exclusively under CT guidance and was complicated by a peripheral pulmonary infarct. Moreover, manual venous compression is mandatory as soon as cystograms show substantial venous drainage. High venous drainage that could not be controlled with compression precluded percutaneous embolization with alcoholic zein in two of our cases.

According to our experience, alcoholic zein is effective in the treatment of aneurysmal bone cysts. The total and partial regression rates in our series were 87% and 13%, respectively, with no recurrence at follow-up. These results led us to consider whether percutaneous embolization with alcoholic zein should be the treatment of choice for aneurysmal bone cysts. Because these cysts are considered to be tumor-induced anomalous vascular processes associated with underlying aggressive lesions, such as giant cell tumors or even osteosarcomas (1), we recommend percutaneous embolization with alcoholic zein only when the lesion is histologically proved and no associated aggressive lesion is found. Therefore, postsurgical recurrence of aneurysmal bone cyst, in which the histologic diagnosis is clearly proved, is a good indication for percutaneous embolization with alcoholic zein. Use of embolization with alcoholic zein as the initial treatment of aneurysmal bone cysts is a possibility in cases with a difficult surgical approach, such as a deep pelvic location or a flat bone of the face (in which case cosmetic sequelae should be considered). In such cases, a fluid-fluid level on MR images is highly suggestive of the diagnosis, even if this finding is not pathognomonic (1). In a review of six large studies of giant cell tumors that totaled approximately 1,300 cases, Abdelwahab et al (15) saw no mention of any tumor that contained fluid. Moreover, we have not noted an association of aneurysmal bone cysts with aggressive lesions when MR imaging showed typical fluid-fluid levels. However, use of percutaneous embolization with alcoholic zein as the initial treatment of aneurysmal bone cysts diagnosed exclusively with imaging should be limited to cases with a difficult surgical approach.

In summary, percutaneous embolization of aneurysmal bone cysts with alcoholic zein should be considered a reliable alternative to surgery, especially in cases with a difficult surgical approach or cases of postsurgical recurrence.

References

1. Kransdorf MJ, Sweet DE. Aneurysmal bone cyst: concept, controversy, clinical presentation, and imaging. AJR 1995; 164:573–580.
2. De Cristofaro R, Biagini R, Boriani S, et al. Selective arterial embolization in the treatment of aneurysmal bone cyst and angioma of bone. Skeletal Radiol 1992; 21: 523–527.
3. Konya A, Szendröi M. Aneurysmal bone cysts treated by superselective embolization. Skeletal Radiol 1992; 21:167–172.
4. Adamsbaum C, Kalifa G, Seringe R, Dubousset J. Direct Ethibloc injection in benign bone cysts: a preliminary report of four patients. Skeletal Radiol 1993; 22:317–320.
5. Dubois J, Garel L, Abel A, Laberge L, Yazbeck S. Lymphangiomas in children: percutaneous sclerotherapy with an alcoholic solution of zein. Radiology 1997; 204:651–654.
6. Dubois J, Sebag GH, De Prost Y, Teilac D, Chrétien B, Brunelle FO. Soft-tissue venous malformations in children: percutaneous sclerotherapy with Ethibloc. Radiology 1991; 180:195–198.
7. Herbreteau D, Riche MC, Enjolras O, et al. Percutaneous embolization with Ethibloc of lymphatic cystic malformations with a review of the experience in 70 patients. Int Angiol 1993; 12:34–39.
8. Lichtenstein L. Aneurysmal bone cysts: a pathological entity commonly mistaken for giant cell tumor and occasionally for hemangioma and osteogenic sarcoma. Cancer 1950; 3:279–289.
9. Lichtenstein L. Aneurysmal bone cysts: further observations. Cancer 1953; 6:1228–1237.
10. Mirra JM. Bone tumors: clinical, radiologic and pathologic correlations. Philadelphia, Pa: Lea & Febiger, 1989; 1233–1334.
11. Mulliken JB. Classification of vascular birthmarks. In: Mulliken JB, Young AE, eds. Vascular birthmarks. Philadelphia, Pa: Saunders, 1988; 24–37.
12. Kauffmann GW, Rasweller J, Richter G, Hauenstein KH, Rohrbach R, Friedburg H. Capillary embolization with Ethibloc: new embolization concept tested in dog kidneys. AJR 1981; 137:1163–1168.
13. Land W, Gebhardt C, Gall FP, Weitz H, Gokel MJ, Stolte M. Pancreatic duct obstruction with prolamine solution. Transplant Proc 1980; 12:72–75.
14. Kuhne D, Helmke K. Embolization with "Ethibloc" of vascular tumors and arteriovenous malformations in the head and neck. Neuroradiology 1982; 23:253–258.
15. Abdelwahab IF, Kenan S, Hermann G, Klein MJ, Lewis MM. Case report 845: fluid-filling giant cell tumor with an aneurysmal bone cyst component. Skeletal Radiol 1994; 23:317–319.

Book Review

Imaging in Musculoskeletal and Sports Medicine

Brian Halpern, MD, Stanley A. Herring, MD, David Altchek, MD, and Richard Herzog, MD

Malden, Mass: Blackwell Science, 1997. ISBN 0-86542-418-7.
Hardcover, $125.00; pp 288; 248 figures; tables.

Imaging in Musculoskeletal and Sports Medicine is a book written for a diverse audience whose common interest is sports medicine. The authors address primarily the imaging aspect of this growing field and offer concise, supporting clinical information. The book covers each topic systematically by providing an introduction to the topic, the clinical presentation, the imaging modalities best suited for diagnosis, and the management of each type of injury. This format, although at times repetitive, allows for a smooth flow of information, which makes the book an easy reference for general practitioners, orthopedic surgeons, and neurologists with a special interest in sports-related medical issues. Imaging specialists will benefit from the discussion of clinical background and treatment options, which are often lacking in the imaging literature.

Although the title suggests a book that addresses mainly imaging topics, the majority of the authors and contributors work in a variety of nonimaging specialties. This apparent incongruity does not seem to affect the quality of the up-to-date imaging information provided. The book addresses the most commonly encountered sports-related injuries; it is not an all-encompassing review of the subject.

The first two chapters are introductions to the epidemiologic aspects of sports injuries and the basics of the various medical imaging modalities. The ensuing chapters cover a spectrum of injuries beyond the musculoskeletal system, such as injuries to the head, soft tissue of the neck, and chest.

Although each chapter is written by different authors, the basic approach to each topic is consistent, which allows for better comprehension of the clinical and imaging factors discussed in the chapter. The photographs are up to date and are of excellent quality. The illustrations are mostly from the orthopedic literature and convey the clinical findings nicely. The text is well organized and printed on glossy paper.

Although this book is not an all-inclusive overview of imaging in sports medicine injuries, it does bridge the gap between the clinical and imaging literature. It is successful in offering an unbiased, up-to-date guide on the proper use of the various imaging modalities in this field. This success is not achieved through elaborate algorithms but a well-structured textbook that covers each topic adequately and conveys clinical data that enhance the reader's knowledge of sports medicine imaging.

Reviewed by Samy F. Saleeb, MD

Glenohumeral Joint: Comparison of Shoulder Positions at MR Arthrography[1]

Sandy M. Kwak, MD
Robert R. Brown, MD
Debra Trudell, RT
Donald Resnick, MD

Index terms:
Gadolinium
Shoulder, arthrography, 414.121411, 414.121412, 414.12143
Shoulder, injuries, 414.4819
Shoulder, MR, 414.121411, 414.121412, 414.12143

Radiology 1998; 208:375–380

[1] From the Department of Radiology, Veterans Administration Medical Center and University of California, San Diego. From the 1997 RSNA scientific assembly. Received September 22, 1997; revision requested October 27; revision received December 23; accepted March 3, 1998. Supported by Veterans Administration grant SA360.
Address reprint requests to S.M.K., Department of Radiology, University of Chicago Hospitals, 5841 S Maryland Ave, MC 2026, Chicago, IL 60637.

PURPOSE: To compare neutral, external rotation, and abduction external rotation positions of the glenohumeral joint during magnetic resonance (MR) arthrography in the assessment of the joint capsule, biceps-labral complex, and glenohumeral ligaments.

MATERIALS AND METHODS: MR imaging with intraarticular administration of gadopentetate dimeglumine was performed in 10 adult cadaveric glenohumeral joints. Fat-suppressed oblique coronal, oblique sagittal, and axial T1-weighted spin-echo imaging and axial three-dimensional spoiled gradient-recalled imaging were performed with each shoulder in the neutral, external rotation, and abduction external rotation positions. Shoulders were sectioned in the planes that yielded optimal MR images. Anatomic and MR imaging findings were correlated.

RESULTS: The biceps-labral complex was best visualized on oblique coronal and axial images obtained in external rotation. Oblique axial abduction external rotation imaging best delineated the inferior glenohumeral ligament but did not improve assessment of the superior and middle glenohumeral ligaments in comparison with findings in neutral and external rotation.

CONCLUSION: Although MR arthrography of the glenohumeral joint clearly delineates the biceps-labral complex and glenohumeral ligaments, external rotation of the shoulder optimizes visualization of the former structures. Abduction external rotation is the best position for evaluation of the inferior glenohumeral ligament and anterior capsular attachment.

Instability of the anterior glenohumeral joint and superior labral injuries can cause substantial disability. Imaging evaluation of these two conditions remains a diagnostic challenge. The radiology literature contains important discrepancies in the reported sensitivity and accuracy of magnetic resonance (MR) imaging for the evaluation of glenohumeral joint instability and superior labral tears (1–4).

MR arthrography has proved to be superior to other imaging techniques in the evaluation of many structures in the glenohumeral joint. The glenohumeral ligaments, labrum, and biceps-labral complex are better delineated in the presence of a joint effusion or intraarticular contrast material, principally because of joint distention (1,3,5–7). Furthermore, Tirman and associates (8) described positioning of the shoulder in external rotation to better assess the biceps anchor and in abduction and external rotation to evaluate suspected anterior labral tears. We designed a comprehensive MR arthrographic study to compare various shoulder positions with regard to optimal visualization of the labrocapsular ligamentous complex of the shoulder. We sought to determine which position and imaging plane best delineate the glenohumeral ligaments, labrum, biceps-labral complex, and anterior and posterior capsular insertions.

MATERIALS AND METHODS

Ten fresh frozen glenohumeral joints (five right, five left) from six cadavers (two female, four male) underwent MR arthrography. The age range at the time of death was 72–85 years (mean age, 77.3 years).

Author contributions:
Guarantors of integrity of entire study, S.M.K., D.R.; study concepts and design, S.M.K., D.R., R.R.B.; definition of intellectual content, S.M.K., D.R.; literature research, S.M.K.; experimental studies, S.M.K., R.R.B., D.T.; data acquisition, S.M.K., R.R.B., D.T.; data analysis, S.M.K., R.R.B., D.R.; manuscript preparation, S.M.K.; manuscript editing, D.R.; manuscript review, S.M.K., D.R., R.R.B., D.T.

TABLE 1
Arm Position and MR Imaging Sequence Best and Second Best for the Evaluation of Glenohumeral Joint Structures

Glenohumeral Joint Structure	Best		Second Best	
	Arm Position	MR Sequence	Arm Position	MR Sequence
Glenohumeral ligament				
Superior	Neutral	T1-weighted oblique sagittal	Neutral	Three-dimensional SPGR axial
Middle	Neutral	T1-weighted oblique sagittal	Neutral	Three-dimensional SPGR axial
Inferior				
Anterior band	ABER	T1-weighted oblique axial	Neutral and external rotation	T1-weighted oblique sagittal
Posterior band	ABER	T1-weighted oblique sagittal	ABER	T1-weighted oblique axial
Anterior labrum	Neutral, ABER, external rotation	T1-weighted and three-dimensional SPGR axial	Neutral, ABER, external rotation	T1-weighted oblique coronal
Posterior labrum	Neutral, ABER, external rotation	T1-weighted and three-dimensional SPGR axial	Neutral, ABER, external rotation	T1-weighted oblique coronal
Biceps-labral complex	External rotation	T1-weighted oblique coronal	Neutral	T1-weighted oblique coronal
Coracohumeral ligament	ABER	T1-weighted oblique sagittal	Neutral	Three-dimensional SPGR axial

Note.—ABER = 90° abduction external rotation, SPGR = spoiled gradient-recalled.

Once thawed, each cadaveric shoulder underwent arthrography. With fluoroscopic guidance, a 22-gauge spinal needle was directed into the glenohumeral joint from an anterolateral approach. One milliliter of iodinated contrast material (iothalamate meglumine, Conray 43%; Mallinckrodt Medical, St Louis, Mo) followed by 14 mL of gadolinium-saline solution (1 mL of gadopentetate dimeglumine [Magnevist; Berlex Laboratories, Wayne, NJ] in 250 mL of normal saline solution) was instilled in the joint (9). The shoulder was immediately imaged with a 1.5-T MR imager (Signa; GE Medical Systems, Milwaukee, Wis).

All 10 specimens were imaged in neutral and external rotation. Nine shoulders were studied with the shoulder in 90° abduction external rotation. One shoulder was imaged in 20° abduction external rotation. This position was eliminated because it did not contribute to better visualization of the biceps-labral complex. Two shoulders were initially imaged in internal rotation. This position was eliminated because there was no additional benefit in visualization of the glenohumeral ligaments or biceps-labral complex. Nine specimens were placed prone and imaged in each position. The prone position allowed better visualization of the glenohumeral ligaments because more of the contrast material collected in the anterior joint capsule, and artifact in the anterior aspect of the joint caused by small amounts of air introduced during arthrography was minimized.

Fat-suppressed T1-weighted spin-echo images were obtained in the axial, oblique coronal (parallel to the supraspinous tendon), and oblique sagittal planes with the shoulder in neutral and external rotation. Four cadaveric shoulders were also imaged in an oblique coronal plane that paralleled the origin of the tendon of the long head of the biceps brachii muscle and the bicipital groove. This plane was eliminated because it did not improve visualization of the biceps-labral complex. Three-dimensional Fourier-transform spoiled gradient-recalled images also were obtained in the axial plane. For the abduction external rotation position, T1-weighted spin-echo images were obtained in the axial oblique, sagittal oblique, and coronal oblique planes. The technical parameters were as follows: (*a*) for T1-weighted spin-echo sequences, 800/15 (repetition time msec/echo time msec), 14-cm field of view, 3-mm section thickness, 1-mm intersection gap, two signals acquired, and 256 × 128 image matrix with fat suppression; and (*b*) for three-dimensional spoiled gradient-recalled sequences, 58/10, 60° flip angle, 14-cm field of view, 1.5-cm section thickness, two signals acquired, and 256 × 128 image matrix with fat suppression.

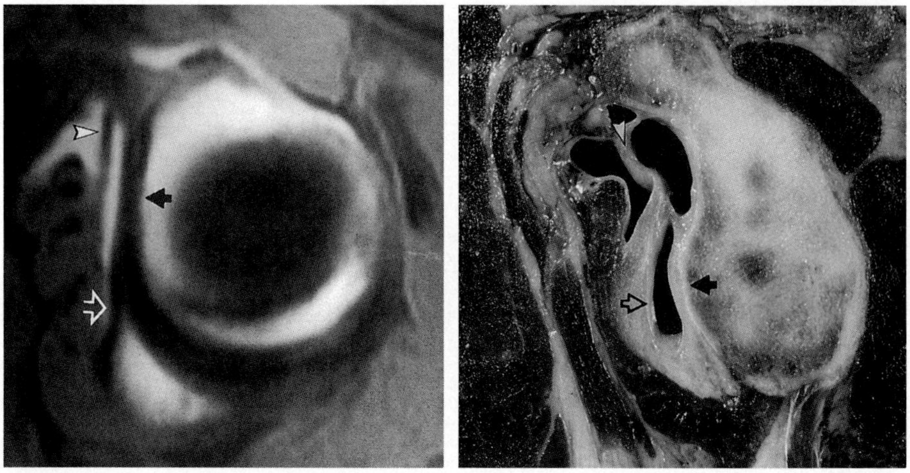

a. b.

Figure 1. (a) T1-weighted, fat-suppressed, oblique sagittal MR arthrogram (800/15) demonstrates the middle glenohumeral ligament (arrowhead in **a** and **b**), anterior band of the inferior glenohumeral ligament (open arrow in **a** and **b**), and anterior labrum (black arrow in **a** and **b**). There is excellent visualization of the entire middle glenohumeral ligament with the shoulder in neutral position. **(b)** Oblique sagittal anatomic slice just medial to the section in **a**.

After MR imaging, the shoulders were

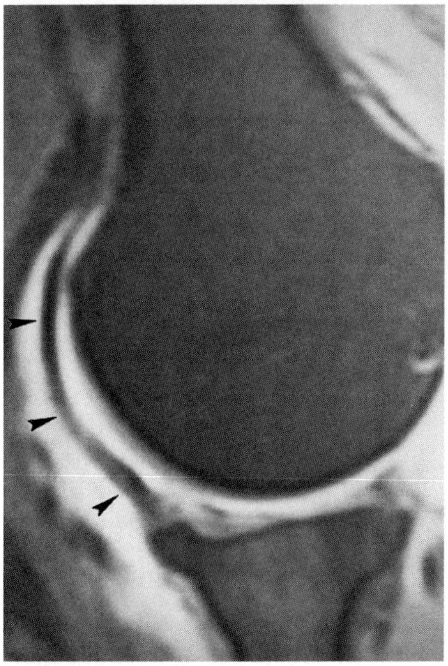

a.

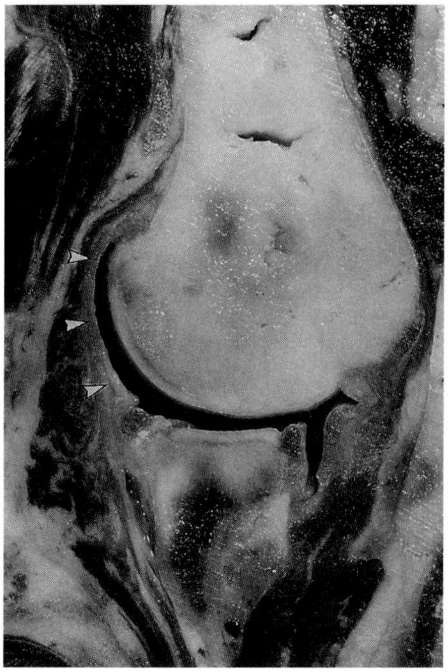

b.

Figure 2. **(a)** T1-weighted, fat-suppressed, axial MR arthrogram (800/15) shows excellent visualization of the anterior band of the inferior glenohumeral ligament (arrowheads in **a** and **b**) with the shoulder in abduction external rotation. The anterior band of the inferior glenohumeral ligament originates directly from the labrum and inserts into the proximal humerus. **(b)** Anatomic slice with the shoulder in abduction external rotation corresponds to the section in **a**.

frozen and sectioned in those planes that yielded optimal MR images. Three-millimeter-thick sections were obtained with a band saw. Findings on MR images were correlated with those in the anatomic sections.

The following structures of the glenohumeral joint were evaluated in consensus by two musculoskeletal radiologists (S.M.K., R.R.B): (*a*) superior glenohumeral ligament, (*b*) middle glenohumeral ligament, (*c*) anterior and posterior bands of the inferior glenohumeral ligament, (*d*) anterior and posterior portions of the labrum, (*e*) biceps-labral complex, and (*f*) coracohumeral ligament. A four-point rating system was used to document visualization of these structures (4 = excellent, 3 = good, 2 = poor, 1 = nonvisualization). An average score was obtained for each structure identified with each MR sequence in all three positions. Images of the three shoulder positions obtained with each MR imaging sequence were evaluated side by side. There were no substantial discrepancies between the two readers.

Anterior and posterior capsular insertions were assessed at the middle and inferior glenoid levels on the axial images and characterized according to the classification system of Moseley and Overgaard (10). A type 1 capsule was defined as the insertion of the anterior or posterior capsule on or at the labral base. A type 2 capsule was attached to the scapula within 1 cm of the labral base, and a type 3 capsule was attached to the scapula more than 1 cm medial to the labral base. The MR imaging capsular insertion classifications were correlated with anatomic findings in the five specimens sectioned in the axial plane.

RESULTS

Table 1 shows the best and second best shoulder positions and MR sequences for the evaluation of glenohumeral joint structures. All the structures were seen in all cadavers except the coracohumeral ligament, which was seen in only six specimens.

The superior glenohumeral ligament was best evaluated on the fat-suppressed, oblique sagittal, T1-weighted spin-echo images obtained with the shoulder in neutral position. Visualization of the superior glenohumeral ligament was excellent in eight of 10 shoulders and good in two.

The middle glenohumeral ligament was best demonstrated on the fat-suppressed, oblique sagittal, T1-weighted spin-echo images obtained with the shoulder in neutral position (Fig 1). The entire middle glenohumeral ligament could be assessed on a single image.

The anterior band of the inferior glenohumeral ligament was best assessed in abduction external rotation with the fat-suppressed, axial, T1-weighted spin-echo sequence (Fig 2). Among the nine shoulders that were imaged in abduction external rotation, visualization of the anterior band of the inferior glenohumeral ligament was excellent in six specimens and good in three.

The anterior and posterior portions of the labrum were best seen with the fat-suppressed, axial, T1-weighted spin-echo and three-dimensional spoiled gradient-recalled sequences. Shoulder position did not affect visualization of these portions of the labrum.

The biceps-labral complex includes the tendon of the long head of the biceps brachii muscle and the superior portion of the labrum. Visualization of the biceps-labral complex was excellent in all 10 shoulder specimens on the fat-suppressed, oblique coronal, T1-weighted images obtained with the shoulder in external rotation (Fig 3).

The coracohumeral ligament was not seen consistently with any of the MR sequences and shoulder positions used in this study. On the anatomic sections, the coracohumeral ligament was identified in six shoulder specimens and was approximately 2–3 mm thick.

The type of anterior capsular insertion varied substantially with shoulder position. The greatest discrepancy in the classification of the anterior and posterior capsular insertions occurred between the neutral and abduction external rotation positions (Fig 4). The anterior and posterior capsular insertions at the middle and inferior glenoid levels as assessed in the neutral, external rotation, and abduction external rotation positions are summarized in Table 2. In the two shoulders that also were imaged in the internal rotation position, a type 3 anterior capsular insertion was present at the middle glenoid level. In the same position at the inferior glenoid level, one shoulder had a type 3 and one a type 2 anterior capsular attachment. Two shoulders imaged in internal rotation had a type 1 posterior capsular attachment at the middle and inferior glenoid levels.

The anterior and posterior capsular insertions were evaluated on the axial anatomic sections in five shoulder specimens. The anatomic sections at the middle glenoid level demonstrated a type 1 anterior capsular insertion in four shoulders and a type 2 anterior capsular insertion in one shoulder. At the inferior glenoid level, the anatomic sections revealed a type 1 anterior capsular insertion in all five shoulders. These anatomic findings best correlated with the capsular findings seen in abduction external rotation. At the middle and inferior glenoid levels, a type 1 posterior capsular insertion was seen in the five specimens. These findings best correlated with capsular findings seen in the internal rotation and neutral positions.

DISCUSSION

That the glenohumeral joint is the most common site of dislocation and subluxation in the human body is related, in part, to the discrepancy in size between the relatively large articular surface of the humeral head and the smaller articular surface of the glenoid fossa. Stability of the glenohumeral joint is achieved by means of the anterior and posterior capsular mechanisms. The anterior capsular mechanism consists of the glenohumeral ligaments, anterior portion of the labrum, anterior joint capsule, scapular periosteum, synovial membrane and related recesses, and subscapular muscle, tendon, and bursa. The posterior capsular mechanism is composed of the posterior portion of the labrum, posterior joint capsule, scapular periosteum, synovial membrane and recesses, and the supraspinous, infraspinous, and teres minor muscles and tendons (10).

The structural abnormality predisposed to instability has been debated in the orthopedic and radiology literature. At present, it is believed that the inferior glenohumeral ligament is the most important structure in the maintenance of glenohumeral joint stability (5,11,12).

The superior glenohumeral ligament contributes little to the static stability of the glenohumeral joint (12,13). However, Schweitzer (14) indicated that the superior glenohumeral ligament may act as a secondary stabilizing force, especially in patients who are predisposed to inferior displacement of the humeral head. Coumas et al (15) reported that the superior glenohumeral ligament was best seen on axial images. In our study, the superior glenohumeral ligament was best seen in the oblique sagittal plane with the shoulder in neutral position.

The middle glenohumeral ligament is the most variable in size and site of origin (5,11,13,15–17). The middle glenohumeral ligament was best seen on the fat-suppressed, oblique sagittal, T1-weighted images obtained with the shoulder in neutral position. With the shoulder externally rotated, it was difficult to identify the middle glenohumeral ligament as a structure separate from the subscapular muscle and tendon. We believe this difficulty was due to apposition of the middle glenohumeral ligament and the subscapular muscle and tendon caused by the tension placed on the anterior joint capsule.

The inferior glenohumeral ligament serves as the primary restraint in the prevention of anterior and posterior dislocations (6,11,13,18). Our results confirm the finding reported by others (8,11) that the anterior band of the inferior glenohumeral ligament is best seen on abduction external rotation, oblique axial, T1-weighted images. In this position, traction is placed on the anterior band of the inferior glenohumeral ligament-labral complex, which allows complete evaluation of the inferior glenohumeral ligament and detection of subtle anteroinferior labral injuries that may be overlooked with the shoulder in neutral position.

Although the coracohumeral ligament is the most constant source of thickening of the glenohumeral capsule (13), this structure was the most difficult to see with MR arthrography. The coracohumeral ligament was best visualized in one shoulder with a full-thickness supraspinous tendon tear, as the contrast material that had passed from the joint to the subacromial bursa provided clear delineation of the coracohumeral ligament. Difficulty in delineation of this ligament on

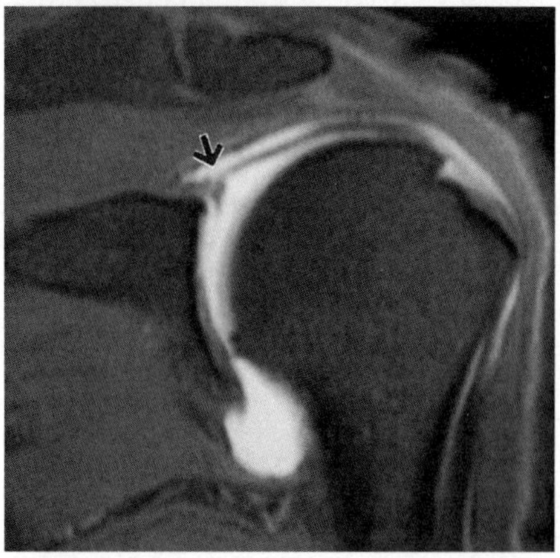

a.

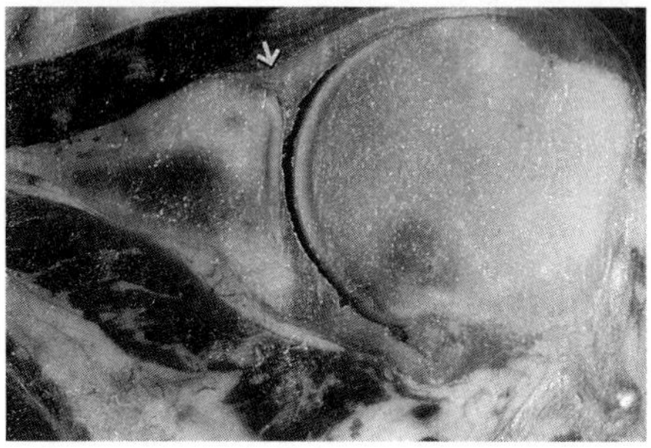

b.

Figure 3. **(a)** T1-weighted, fat-suppressed, oblique coronal MR arthrogram (800/15) delineates the biceps-labral complex (arrow in **a** and **b**). The tension on the biceps-labral complex that occurs with the shoulder in external rotation provides excellent visualization. **(b)** Oblique coronal anatomic slice corresponds to the section in **a**.

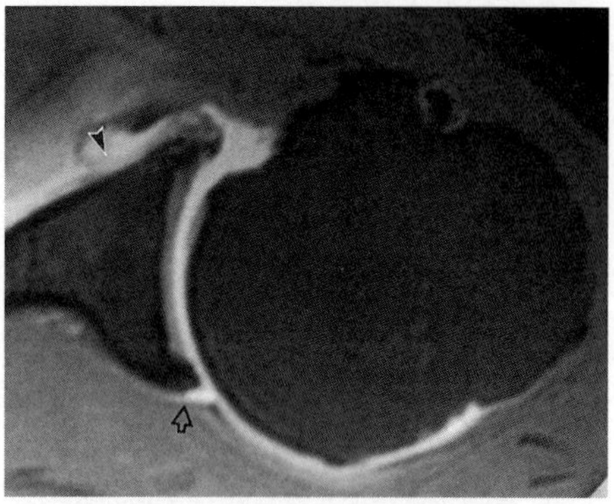

a.

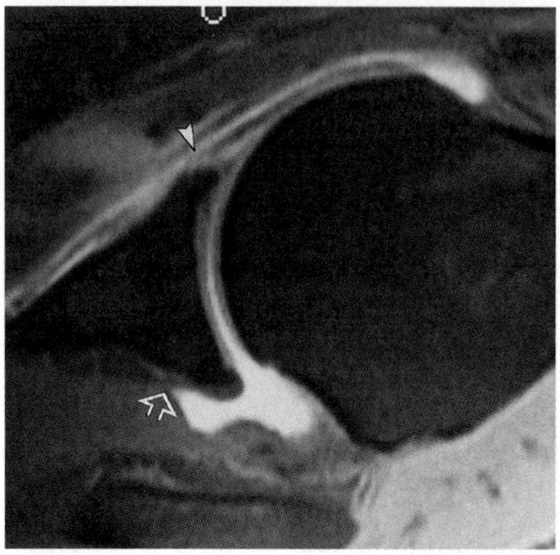

b.

Figure 4. T1-weighted, fat-suppressed, axial MR arthrograms (800/15) at the middle glenoid level demonstrate anterior (arrowhead in **a** and **b**) and posterior (arrow in **a** and **b**) capsular insertions that vary with change in shoulder position. **(a)** Type 3 anterior capsular insertion and type 1 posterior capsular insertion are seen with the shoulder in neutral position. The anterior capsular insertion type is overestimated, and assessment of the posterior capsular insertion is accurate. **(b)** Type 1 anterior capsular insertion and type 2 posterior capsular insertion are seen with the shoulder in abduction external rotation. Assessment of the anterior capsular insertion is accurate, and the posterior capsular insertion is overestimated when the shoulder is placed in abduction external rotation.

TABLE 2
Variability of Anterior and Posterior Capsular Insertion with Shoulder Position in 10 Cadaveric Shoulders

Type of Capsular Insertion	Middle Glenoid Level			Inferior Glenoid Level		
	Neutral	External Rotation	ABER	Neutral	External Rotation	ABER
Anterior capsule						
1	3	5	7	3	7	9
2	2	0	1	2	0	0
3	5	5	1	5	3	0
Posterior capsule						
1	9	7	0	10	9	3
2	1	3	3	0	1	4
3	0	0	6	0	0	2

Note.—ABER = 90° abduction external rotation (used in nine shoulders). Data are the number of shoulder specimens.

MR arthrograms, we believe, is related to its intimate position with regard to the superior aspect of the joint capsule.

The importance in determination of the type of anterior capsular insertion on MR arthrograms stems from the importance (albeit controversial) of a type 3 capsular insertion. Zlatkin (19) believes that a type 3 capsular insertion may predispose to shoulder instability. According to Resnick and Kang (13), it is not clear whether a type 3 anterior capsular insertion is a cause or result of anterior glenohumeral joint instability. Stoller (11) argues it is unlikely that a type 3 anterior capsular insertion predisposes to anterior humeral subluxation or dislocation. Our study showed dependence of the appearance of the anterior and posterior capsular insertions at the middle and inferior glenoid levels on the precise position of the shoulder. Oblique axial MR arthrograms obtained with the shoulder in abduction external rotation correlated best with the anatomic sections with regard to the anterior capsular insertion site. Because abduction external rotation places tension on the anterior capsule, evaluation of the anterior capsular insertion is more accurate when this position in used. With the shoulder in the internal rotation or neutral position, there is more laxity of the anterior joint capsule. This laxity results in redundancy of anterior capsular tissue and, thus, overestimation of the medial location of the capsular insertion. We found the opposite to be true for the evaluation of the pattern of posterior capsular insertion.

Typing of the anterior capsular insertion should not be performed at the superior glenoid level, because at this level a perceived type 3 anterior capsular attachment on MR arthrograms is related to contrast material filling the subscapular recess. In fact, Stoller (11) believes that the three types of anterior capsular insertions represent no more than variations in the size and morphology of the subscapular recess that are dependent on shoulder rotation. At the superior glenoid level and probably also at the middle glenoid level, variations in the perceived anterior capsular attachment sites evident in our specimens appeared to relate to differences in the degree of distention of the subscapular recess by the contrast material. The variations of anterior capsular attachment at the inferior glenoid level probably relate to the normal redundancy of the joint capsule in this location. With internal rotation, there is more contrast material in the subscapular recess and anterior aspect of the joint because the contrast material in the posterior aspect of the joint is pushed forward when the posterior joint capsule tightens.

In our study, the biceps-labral complex was most effectively imaged in the oblique coronal plane with the shoulder in external rotation. This shoulder position places tension on the biceps-labral complex and, when employed during MR arthrography, should allow better evaluation of injuries to the complex, which have been classified as superior labrum, anterior and posterior, or SLAP, lesions by Snyder and colleagues (20). Cartland and associates (4) suggested use of an oblique coronal plane parallel to a line that connects the bicipital groove of the proximal portion of the humerus and the anterior aspect of the superior part of the labrum to better visualize the biceps-labral complex, a plane that could be determined from the axial images. This protocol was used in four of our 10 shoulders in neutral, external, and abduction external rotation positions. We found, however, no difference in the clarity of visualization of the biceps-labral complex during comparison of those oblique coronal images parallel to the supraspinous tendon and those parallel to the course of the proximal portion of the biceps tendon.

There are several limitations to our study. Because we performed MR arthrography in cadaveric shoulders, mild anterior or posterior subluxation occurred in the majority of our shoulder specimens. Furthermore, the shoulders were derived from patients who were elderly at the time of death, and we cannot be certain that similar observations would have resulted from analysis of a younger population. Some investigators may consider that the prone position used here was a limitation to our study, because patients do not routinely undergo imaging in this position. We found no important difference in anatomic appearance between the specimen we imaged supine and the nine specimens imaged prone.

Our anatomic study was meant to investigate various positions that may yield better visualization of the glenohumeral joint structures. During clinical imaging, unintentional introduction of air during arthrography may limit the quality of the MR images. In this situation, we believe imaging in the prone position with addition of respiratory gating is superior to that in the routine supine position. We have tried this technique in several of our patients with successful results. Another drawback of our study was lack of pathologic examination. The purpose of our investigation, however, was to determine which position and MR imaging sequence best delineate the glenohumeral structures. Last, analysis of sites of capsular insertion was accomplished in only five of the 10 specimens; in the other five shoulders, sectioning in the oblique coronal or oblique sagittal planes prevented such analysis.

MR arthrography of the glenohumeral joint with the shoulder in external rotation optimizes visualization of the biceps-labral complex, and abduction external rotation is the best position for evaluation of the inferior glenohumeral ligament and anterior capsular attachment. On the basis of the results of this investigation, we recommend tailoring the MR arthrographic examination according to the clinical indications for the study. In patients with clinically suspected anterior instability of the glenohumeral joint, oblique axial images in abduction external rotation should be used as a supplementary technique or as a replacement for traditional axial images of the glenohumeral joint to allow evaluation of the anterior band of the inferior glenohumeral ligament and anteroinferior labral tears. If there is clinical concern about a superior labrum, anterior and posterior lesion, oblique coronal imaging with the shoulder in external rotation is suggested to fully evaluate the biceps-labral complex. We acknowledge that further research with patients is necessary to draw more accurate conclusions about the usefulness of the various shoulder positions used in our study.

References

1. Legan JM, Burkhard TK, Goff WB II, et al. Tears of the glenoid labrum: MR imaging of 88 arthroscopically confirmed cases. Radiology 1991; 179:241–246.
2. Garneau RA, Renfrew DL, Moore TE, El-Khoury GY, Nepola JV, Lemke JH. Glenoid labrum: evaluation with MR imaging. Radiology 1991; 179:519–522.
3. Hodler J, Kursunoglu-Brahme S, Flannigan B, Snyder SJ, Karzel RP, Resnick D. Injuries of the superior portion of the glenoid labrum involving the insertion of the biceps tendon: MR imaging findings in nine cases. AJR 1992; 159:565–568.
4. Cartland JP, Crues JV III, Stauffer A, Nottage W, Ryu RKN. MR imaging in the evaluation of SLAP injuries of the shoulder: findings in 10 patients. AJR 1992; 159:787–792.
5. Beltran J, Rosenberg ZS, Chandnani VP, Cuomo F, Beltran S, Rokito A. Glenohumeral instability: evaluation with MR arthrography. RadioGraphics 1997; 17:657–673.
6. Chandnani VJ, Gagliardi JA, Murnane TG, et al. Glenohumeral ligaments and shoulder capsular mechanism: evaluation with MR arthrography. Radiology 1995; 196:27–32.
7. Palmer WE, Brown JH, Rosenthal DI. Labral-ligamentous complex of the shoulder: evaluation with MR arthrography. Radiology 1994; 190:645–651.
8. Tirman PFJ, Applegate GR, Flannigan BD, Stauffer AE, Crues JV III. Magnetic resonance arthrography of the shoulder. Magn Reson Imaging Clin N Am 1993; 1:125–142.
9. Recht MP, Kramer J, Petersilge CA, et al. Distribution of normal and abnormal fluid collections in the glenohumeral joint: implications for MR arthrography. JMRI 1994; 4:173–177.
10. Moseley HF, Overgaard B. The anterior capsular mechanism in recurrent anterior dislocation of the shoulder. J Bone Joint Surg [Br] 1962; 44:913–927.
11. Stoller DW. MR arthrography of the glenohumeral joint. Radiol Clin North Am 1997; 35:97–115.
12. Massengill AD, Seeger LL, Yao L, et al. Labrocapsular ligamentous complex of the shoulder: normal anatomy, anatomic variation, and pitfalls of MR imaging and MR arthrography. RadioGraphics 1994; 14:1211–1223.
13. Resnick D, Kang HS. Shoulder. In: Resnick D, Kang HS, eds. Internal derangements of joints: emphasis on MR imaging. Philadelphia, Pa: Saunders, 1997; 163–333.
14. Schweitzer ME. MR arthrography of the labral-ligamentous complex of the shoulder. Radiology 1994; 190:641–643.
15. Coumas JM, Waite RJ, Goss TP, Ferrari DA, Kanzaria PK, Pappas AM. CT and MR evaluation of the labral capsular ligamentous complex of the shoulder. AJR 1992; 158:591–597.
16. Palmer WE, Caslowitz PL, Chew FS. MR arthrography of the shoulder: normal intra-articular structures and common abnormalities. AJR 1995; 164:141–146.
17. Palmer WE, Caslowitz PL. Anterior shoulder instability: diagnostic criteria determined from prospective analysis of 121 MR arthrograms. Radiology 1995; 197:819–825.
18. Turkel SJ, Panio MW, Marshall JL, Girgis FG. Stabilizing mechanisms preventing anterior dislocation of the glenohumeral joint. J Bone Joint Surg [Am] 1981; 63:1208–1217.
19. Zlatkin MB. MRI of the shoulder. New York, NY: Raven, 1991; 24–38.
20. Snyder SJ, Karzel RP, Del Pizzo W, Ferkel RD, Friedman MJ. SLAP lesions of the shoulder. Arthroscopy 1990; 6:274–279.

Anterior Interosseous Nerve Syndrome: Appearance at MR Imaging in Three Cases[1]

Andrew J. Grainger, FRCR
Robert S. D. Campbell, FRCR
John Stothard, MD, FRCS

Index terms:
Muscles, denervation, 42.209
Muscles, MR, 42.121411, 42.121413
Nerves, peripheral, 42.209

Radiology 1998; 208:381–384

Abbreviations:
EMG = electromyography
FDP = flexor digitorum profundus
FDP 1 = FDP of the index finger
FDP 2 = FDP of the middle finger
FPL = flexor pollicis longus
PQ = pronator quadratus
STIR = short inversion time inversion recovery

[1] From the Departments of Radiology (A.J.G., R.S.D.C.) and Orthopedic Surgery (J.S.), South Cleveland Hospital, Middlesbrough, TS4 3BW, England. Received October 17, 1997; revision requested December 12; revision received January 26, 1998; accepted March 26. **Address reprint requests to** R.S.D.C.

Author contributions:
Guarantor of integrity of entire study, R.S.D.C.; study concepts, R.S.D.C.; study design, R.S.D.C., A.J.G.; definition of intellectual content, R.S.D.C., A.J.G.; literature research, A.J.G.; clinical studies, R.S.D.C., A.J.G.; data acquisition, R.S.D.C., A.J.G; data analysis, R.S.D.C., A.J.G., J.S.; manuscript preparation, A.J.G.; manuscript editing, R.S.D.C.; manuscript review, J.S.

Three patients with symptoms attributable to anterior interosseous nerve syndrome underwent forearm magnetic resonance (MR) imaging. In all patients, short inversion time inversion-recovery, or STIR, images depicted increased signal intensity from some or all muscle groups innervated by the anterior interosseous nerve. In one patient, atrophy was depicted in these muscles. MR imaging may serve as a useful adjunct to electromyography in the investigation of anterior interosseous nerve syndrome.

The anterior interosseous nerve is one of the motor nerves of the anterior compartment of the forearm, arising 2–8 cm below the humeral medial epicondyle as a branch of the median nerve. It lies deep in the forearm, coursing along the anterior surface of the interosseous membrane. Usually, the nerve supplies three muscles of the forearm: the flexor pollicis longus (FPL), the flexor digitorum profundus (FDP) of the index finger (FDP 1) and middle finger (FDP 2), and the pronator quadratus (PQ) (1).

Isolated paralysis of the muscles supplied by the anterior interosseous nerve was described by Kiloh and Nevin in 1952 (2), and the condition is still referred to by their names. Since then, other descriptions of the anterior interosseous nerve syndrome have been presented (3–6). The condition is characterized by weakness of the muscles supplied by the anterior interosseous nerve in the presence of normal sensation.

Paralysis of muscles supplied by the anterior interosseous nerve may follow trauma due to laceration, penetrating injury, or fracture (6–8). It may also result from entrapment of the nerve by a number of structures, including the tendinous origin of the deep head of the pronator teres, enlarged bicipital bursae, and thrombosed ulnar collateral vessels (3–5,9). Many cases, however, occur spontaneously and resolve without intervention (4,9,10). These cases are thought to be a result of neuritis affecting the anterior interosseous nerve. Palsy of the anterior interosseous nerve is a syndrome with a variety of causes.

Patients with anterior interosseous nerve syndrome may not present with involvement of all expected muscles as a result of variants in innervation, which may lead to difficulty in diagnosis. One muscle (often the FPL) may be noticeably weaker than the others, and tendon rupture may be diagnosed. Electromyography (EMG) has been used to assist diagnosis of the syndrome (10–12).

We report the appearance of the affected forearm at magnetic resonance (MR) imaging in three patients with spontaneous, isolated palsy of the anterior interosseous nerve.

Materials and Methods

Patients

Case 1.—A 36-year-old man was referred with a 6-week inability to flex the distal interphalangeal joint of his left index finger. The episode was preceded by pain in his forearm. He experienced tenderness along the volar aspect of his forearm, as well as weakness of the FPL. He had no history of trauma. The provisional diagnosis was attritional rupture of the FDP 1 tendon due to a suspected bone spur at the scaphotrapezial joint. Concern was expressed that the weakness in the FPL was also a result of attenuation of this tendon. Anterior interosseous nerve syndrome was considered to be an alternative diagnosis. MR imaging was performed 3 months after the onset of symptoms.

Case 2.—A 44-year-old woman was referred with inability to flex her left thumb and the distal interphalangeal joint of the

Muscles Supplied by the Anterior Interosseous Nerve That Showed Increased Signal Intensity on STIR Images

Case	PQ	FPL	FDP 1	FDP 2
1	+	+	+	+
2	+	+	+	+
3	+	−	+	−

Note.—+ = increased signal intensity seen, − = no increased signal intensity seen.

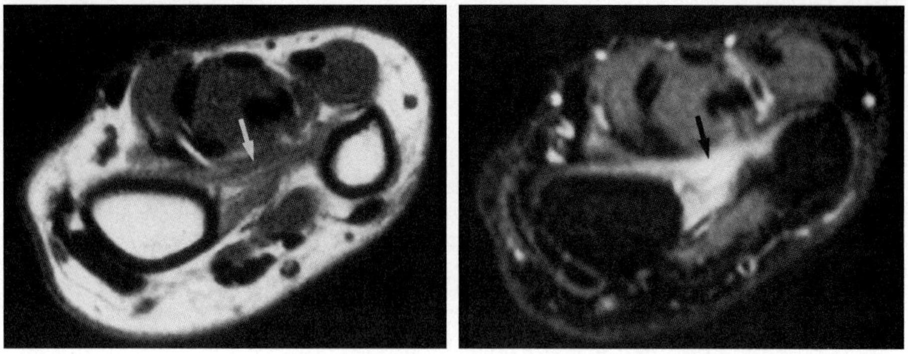

a. b.

Figure 1. **Case 2.** **(a)** T1-weighted spin-echo (440/12) and **(b)** fast STIR (5,300/30/150) axial images obtained through the distal forearm show increased signal intensity in the PQ muscle (arrow) in **b** compared with **a**. The muscle is atrophic.

left index finger for 8 weeks. She also reported pain that radiated down the volar aspect of her forearm. She had no history of trauma. Physical examination confirmed paralysis of the FDP 1 and FPL, and the PQ was believed to be weak. A provisional diagnosis of anterior interosseous nerve syndrome was made. EMG was attempted but was not helpful owing to difficulty in accurate placement of a needle in the affected muscles. The patient was referred for MR imaging when spontaneous improvement had not occurred 8 months after the onset of symptoms.

Case 3.—A 41-year-old man was referred with a 12-day history of inability to flex the distal interphalangeal joint of his right index finger. He had no definite history of trauma. At physical examination, other forearm muscles were found to be normal, but paralysis was found in the FDP 1. Isolated rupture of the FDP 1 was suspected, and surgical exploration of the tendon was arranged. At admission, however, considerable function was found to have been restored to the tendon, and plans for surgery were abandoned. The patient was subsequently referred for MR imaging 3 months after the onset of symptoms.

MR Imaging Technique

All images were acquired with a 1.0-T MR imaging unit (Impact; Siemens Medical Systems, Erlangen, Germany) and a dedicated quadrature transmit-receive extremity knee coil. Spin-echo axial T1-weighted imaging (440/12 [repetition time msec/echo time msec]; field of view, 75 × 100 mm; matrix, 192 × 256; section thickness, 7 mm) and fast short inversion time inversion-recovery (STIR) imaging (4,515–5,300/30/100–150 [inversion time msec]; echo train length, seven; field of view, 91 × 145 mm; matrix, 154 × 256; section thickness, 7 mm) were performed from the carpal tunnel to the elbow joint.

Results

MR Imaging Findings

In all cases, STIR images showed abnormally increased signal intensity from some or all of the muscles supplied by the anterior interosseous nerve (Table). The increase in signal intensity was seen diffusely throughout the affected muscle tissue. Signal intensity from the muscles was normal on the T1-weighted images.

In all cases, increased signal intensity was seen on the STIR images of the PQ (Fig 1) and FDP 1. In cases 1 and 2, findings were similar in the FPL and FDP 2 muscles (Fig 2a, 2b). In case 1, in addition to the four muscles usually supplied by the anterior interosseous nerve, the flexor carpi radialis muscle, which normally takes its nerve supply from the median nerve, also had increased signal intensity (Fig 2c).

In all cases, the tendons of the affected muscles were of uniformly low signal intensity without any discontinuity to suggest tear or rupture. The change in signal intensity observed in the muscles was diffuse, with no focal abnormality to indicate muscle tear.

The T1-weighted images showed no demonstrable abnormality in signal intensity characteristics of the muscles, tendons, and other structures of the forearm. In case 2, however, there was evidence of atrophy of all affected muscles, with loss of muscle bulk (Fig 1). There was no increased signal intensity on the T1-weighted images to indicate the presence of fatty infiltration.

In none of the three cases was the anterior interosseous nerve itself readily identified on any image. When it was identified, however, it was of normal size and signal intensity.

Patient Outcome

In cases 1 and 3, symptoms spontaneously resolved. In case 2, however, no such improvement was seen, and, after 9 months, surgical exploration was undertaken. The nerve had lost its normal glistening appearance, and no compression was identified. With use of a nerve stimulator, partial active flexion could be transmitted to the FDP 1, but no other transmission was possible. The median nerve was normal. In all three cases, findings were consistent with a spontaneous, isolated, neuritic palsy of the anterior interosseous nerve.

Discussion

Currently, the diagnosis of anterior interosseous nerve syndrome is based on the clinical findings of isolated involvement of the muscles supplied by the anterior interosseous nerve. Idiopathic neuritis frequently resolves spontaneously. In cases that do not resolve, surgical exploration is indicated to exclude nerve entrapment (as in case 2). For the clinician, the main differential diagnosis is rupture of the FPL or FDP tendons, a diagnosis that may be suggested by incomplete involvement of the muscles supplied by the anterior interosseous nerve. MR imaging undoubtedly has a role in the exclusion of tendon rupture from the diagnosis, but findings in our cases suggest it may also be useful in strengthening the clinical diagnosis of anterior interosseous nerve syndrome by indicating involvement of only those muscles supplied by the anterior interosseous nerve. Other studies have already shown MR imaging to be of use in the diagnosis and evaluation of a variety of other upper limb neuropathies, including carpal tun-

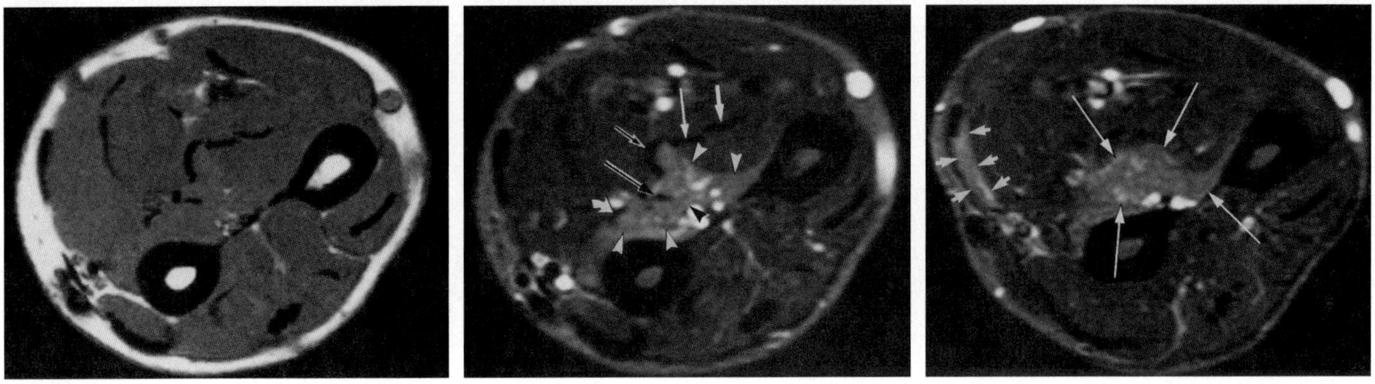

a. b. c.

Figure 2. Case 1. **(a)** T1-weighted spin-echo (440/12) and **(b)** fast STIR (4,515/30/100) axial images obtained through the middle of the forearm. In **a**, the signal intensity of the muscles is normal. In **b**, signal intensity is increased in the muscle (arrowheads) associated with the FPL tendon (curved arrow), FDP 1 tendon (long black arrow), and FDP 2 tendon (short black arrow). No such change is seen in the muscle associated with the tendons of the FDP of the third finger (long white arrow) and FDP of the little finger (short white arrow). **(c)** Fast STIR (4,515/30/100) axial image obtained proximal to the level in **a** and **b** shows unexpected involvement of the flexor carpi radialis muscle with increased signal intensity (small arrows). The increased signal intensity of the FPL and FDP muscles (long arrows) is also present.

nel syndrome, quadrilateral space syndrome, and suprascapular nerve entrapment (13–15).

We performed MR imaging with only two pulse sequences to minimize patient imaging time. T1-weighted spin-echo axial imaging provided excellent anatomic detail and helped particularly in the diagnosis of muscle atrophy. A fast STIR sequence was used because of its known sensitivity in the investigation of pathologic conditions in muscle (16–19).

The diffuse increase in signal intensity seen on STIR images of affected muscles in these patients accords with the changes, noted by other observers, in muscles affected by compartment syndromes in both the upper and lower limbs (20,21) and in muscles denervated owing to nerve transection or compressive and entrapment neuropathies (18,19). Prolongation of both T1 and T2 has been described experimentally in skeletal muscle after denervation (22); these changes are particularly well shown on STIR images. This finding is due not only to suppression of the signal from surrounding fat but also to prolonged T1 and T2, both of which result in an increase in signal intensity on STIR images. The basis of prolonged relaxation times in denervated muscle is not clear, but, experimentally, they correlate best with the increase in extracellular water seen in such muscles (22).

Atrophy is a feature that was clearly evident in only case 2 and is well recognized as a later finding in denervated muscle (17,18). It has been described in nerve entrapment neuropathies (14,15). As it is a later finding, it is not surprising that it was seen in case 2, in which imaging was performed 8 months after symptoms developed, as opposed to the other cases, in which imaging occurred at 3 months. It is difficult, however, to exclude lesser degrees of atrophy in cases 1 and 3 because comparative images of the contralateral nonsymptomatic side were not obtained.

While the cause of anterior interosseous nerve syndrome may vary, the underlying problem is with the innervation of the muscles normally supplied by the anterior interosseous nerve. In two of the cases, the PQ, FPL, FDP 1, and FDP 2 showed abnormality at MR imaging, as would be expected in this syndrome. In the third case, abnormality of the FPL and FDP 2 muscles was not seen. This finding concurred with the clinical findings of no weakness in either of these muscles. The other unexpected finding was the additional involvement of the flexor carpi radialis muscle in case 1. This muscle is normally innervated by the median nerve proximal to the origin of the anterior interosseous nerve (1). Anatomic variation in the nerve supply to the muscles of the forearm is well recognized, however, and may explain these unexpected findings (4).

One anatomic variation has been described in which the anterior interosseous nerve provides the motor supply to some of the intrinsic muscles of the hand, most often the first, second, and third dorsal interosseous muscles. This variant comes about as a result of a communication between the ulnar and anterior interosseous nerves, and patients with anterior interosseous nerve syndrome may experience weakness in these muscles (4). MR imaging in such cases would be expected to show changes in the dorsal interosseus muscles in the hand similar to those in the affected forearm muscles that we described. In none of our cases was weakness in the intrinsic hand muscles demonstrated at clinical examination. In case 1, imaging of the hand was also performed; review of these images showed no abnormality in any of the intrinsic muscles. In the other two cases, imaging of the hands was not performed distal to the carpal tunnel.

Although anterior interosseous nerve syndrome does not lead to sensory symptoms, because the anterior interosseous nerve has no cutaneous representation, it is not purely a motor nerve. Sensory fibers from the wrist joint travel in the anterior interosseous nerve, and injury to that nerve can be a source of dull aching volar wrist pain (23,24). Local block of the terminal anterior interosseous nerve has been diagnostic in this situation (23). Our patients in cases 1 and 2 reported pain in the volar aspect of their affected forearms.

Variation in the muscles supplied by the anterior interosseous nerve can lead to confusion in the diagnosis of anterior interosseous nerve syndrome. It is difficult to reliably test the PQ clinically, even with the elbow fully flexed to minimize action of the pronator teres. Indeed, Wertsch (12) describes a case of surgical removal of the PQ in which its absence was clinically undetected. Consequently, if either the FPL or FDP show isolated involvement, anterior interosseous nerve syndrome may not be suspected and another diagnosis (eg, tendon rupture) is more likely to be considered. This likelihood is well illustrated in case 3, in which involvement of only the FDP 1 and PQ was observed. MR imaging helped confirm the diagnosis of anterior interosseous nerve syndrome and exclusion of attrition rupture of the tendon.

This problem is well recognized, and EMG has been shown to help confirm diagnosis of anterior interosseous nerve syndrome (10–12). In case 2, however, such studies were not possible because of technical failure. EMG involves insertion of needle electrodes into the muscles of the forearm. Accurate positioning of these electrodes can be difficult, particularly in the PQ, which is a thin deep muscle (12). This problem is made worse in muscles that have started to atrophy, as in case 2.

Although the diagnosis of anterior interosseous nerve syndrome is made clinically, EMG may be requested to help confirm the diagnosis. Our findings suggest that MR imaging may prove useful in the investigation of anterior interosseous nerve syndrome. Compared with EMG, MR imaging is noninvasive and likely to be more acceptable to most patients. In our cases, STIR images showed increased signal intensity in the involved muscles, which in itself is a nonspecific response with a variety of possible causes, including myositis, delayed-onset muscle soreness, and muscle strain. As with anterior interosseous nerve syndrome, these conditions resolve spontaneously. It is the characteristic isolated involvement of muscles supplied by the anterior interosseous nerve, however, that indicates anterior interosseous nerve syndrome as the underlying cause.

As stated in the introduction, anterior interosseous nerve syndrome may be idiopathic but may arise from injury to the nerve. Further studies may address whether MR imaging can help discriminate between different causes of the syndrome. In our three cases, the anterior interosseous nerve itself appeared normal when it was demonstrated, although we observed macroscopic changes in the nerve in case 2 at surgery. Follow-up MR imaging to look for resolution of the findings has not yet been performed in our three patients, but it represents another area of study.

A potential advantage of MR imaging over EMG is in the evidence that increased signal intensity on STIR images is seen before changes in denervation become detectable at EMG. West et al (19) found that the first changes on STIR images were seen as early as 4 days after complete nerve injury, in contrast to changes seen at EMG, which are not detectable before 2–3 weeks. There is no certainty, however, that all neuropathies will give rise to muscle changes at similar times after the initial insult, and early imaging in patients with anterior interosseous nerve syndrome may show that changes at MR imaging have different times of onset, depending on the underlying cause.

In conclusion, MR imaging is potentially useful and safe in the investigation of anterior interosseous nerve syndrome, excluding muscle and tendon trauma from the differential diagnosis and providing a good alternative to EMG in the confirmation that the abnormality lies in the distribution of the anterior interosseous nerve. The radiologist needs to be aware that anatomic variation in the motor supply to the muscles of the forearm is common.

References

1. O'Brien M. Median nerve. In: Williams PL, Bannister LH, Berry MM, et al, eds. Anatomy of the human body. 38th ed. New York, NY: Churchill Livingstone, 1995; 1270–1271.
2. Kiloh LG, Nevin S. Isolated neuritis of the anterior interosseous nerve. Br Med J 1952; 1:850–851.
3. Fearn CBDA, Goodfellow JW. Anterior interosseous nerve palsy. J Bone Joint Surg [Br] 1965; 47:91–93.
4. Spinner M. The anterior interosseous nerve syndrome. J Bone Joint Surg [Am] 1970; 52:84–94.
5. Rask MR. Anterior interosseous nerve entrapment (Kiloh-Nevin syndrome). Clin Orthop 1979; 142:176–181.
6. Stern MB. Anterior interosseous nerve entrapment (Kiloh-Nevin syndrome). Clin Orthop 1984; 187:223–227.
7. Spinner M, Shreiber SN. Anterior interosseous nerve paralysis as a complication of supracondylar fractures of the humerus in children. J Bone Joint Surg [Am] 1969; 51:1584–1590.
8. Geutjens GG. Ischaemic anterior interosseous nerve injuries following supracondylar fractures of the humerus in children. Injury 1995; 26:343–344.
9. Spinner M, Spencer PS. Nerve compression lesions of the upper extremity. Clin Orthop 1974; 104:46–67.
10. Nakano KK, Lundergan C, Okihiro MM. Anterior interosseous nerve syndromes. Arch Neurol 1977; 34:477–480.
11. Gross PT, Royden Jones H Jr. Proximal median neuropathies: electromyographic and clinical correlation. Muscle Nerve 1992; 15:390–395.
12. Wertsch JJ. AAEM case report 25: anterior interosseous nerve syndrome. Muscle Nerve 1992; 15:977–983.
13. Mesgarzadeh M, Schneck CD, Bonakdarpour A, Mitra A, Conaway D. Carpal tunnel: MR imaging. II. Carpal tunnel syndrome. Radiology 1989; 171:749–754.
14. Linker CS, Helms CA, Fritz RC. Quadrilateral space syndrome: findings at MR imaging. Radiology 1993; 188:675–676.
15. Fritz RC, Helms CA, Steinbach LS, Genant HK. Suprascapular nerve entrapment: evaluation with MR imaging. Radiology 1992; 182:437–444.
16. Greco A, McNamara MT, Escher RMB, Trifilio G, Parienti J. Spin-echo and STIR MR imaging of sports-related muscle injuries at 1.5 T. J Comput Assist Tomogr 1991; 15:994–999.
17. Fleckenstein JL. Magnetic resonance imaging and computed tomography of skeletal muscle pathology. In: Bloom JL, Sartoris DJ, eds. MRI and CT of the musculoskeletal system—a text atlas. Baltimore, Md: Williams & Wilkins, 1992; 172–188.
18. Fleckenstein JL, Watumull D, Conner KE, et al. Denervated human skeletal muscle: MR imaging evaluation. Radiology 1993; 187:213–218.
19. West GA, Haynor DR, Goodkin R, et al. Magnetic resonance imaging signal changes in denervated muscles after peripheral nerve injury. Neurosurgery 1994; 35:1077–1086.
20. Ehman RL, Berquist TH. Magnetic resonance imaging of musculoskeletal trauma. Radiol Clin North Am 1986; 24:291–319.
21. Deutsch AL, Mink JH. Magnetic resonance imaging of musculoskeletal injuries. Radiol Clin North Am 1989; 27:983–1002.
22. Polak JF, Jolesz FA, Adams DF. Magnetic resonance imaging of skeletal muscle: prolongation of T1 and T2 subsequent to denervation. Invest Radiol 1988; 23:365–369.
23. Dellon AL, Mackinnon SE, Daneshvar A. Terminal branch of anterior interosseous nerve as a source of wrist pain. J Hand Surg 1984; 9:316–322.
24. Stern PJ, Kutz JE. An unusual variant of the anterior interosseous nerve syndrome: a case report and review of the literature. J Hand Surg 1980; 5:32–34.

Diana K. Verrilli, MS
Stephen M. Bloch, MD
Jeanine Rousseau, RT
Matthew E. Crozier, MM
Steven B. Yecies, JD, MBA

Index terms:
Economics, medical
Radiology and radiologists

Radiology 1998; 208:385–392

Abbreviations:
BCBSMA = BlueCross BlueShield of Massachusetts
CPT-4 = *Physicians' Current Procedural Terminology,* 4th edition
JCAHO = Joint Commission on Accreditation of Health Care Organizations

[1] From the Department of Research and Development, Radiology Management Sciences, 105-F Fremont Ave, Los Altos, CA 94022. Received August 18, 1997; revision requested November 13; final revision received March 25, 1998; accepted April 13. **Address reprint requests to** D.K.V.

Any opinions expressed are those of the authors and do not necessarily represent the opinions of BlueCross BlueShield of Massachusetts, an independent licensee of the BlueCross BlueShield Association.

The authors are employees of Radiology Management Sciences (Los Altos, Calif), which developed the program evaluated in this article.

Author contributions:
Guarantors of integrity of entire study, D.K.V., S.M.B., J.R., M.E.C., S.B.Y.; study concepts and design, S.M.B., J.R., S.B.Y., M.E.C.; definition of intellectual content, D.K.V., S.M.B.; literature research, D.K.V.; data acquisition, D.K.V., J.R.; data analysis, D.K.V.; statistical analysis, D.K.V.; manuscript preparation and review, D.K.V., S.M.B.; manuscript editing, D.K.V., S.M.B., M.E.C., S.B.Y., J.R.

Design of a Privileging Program for Diagnostic Imaging: Costs and Implications for a Large Insurer in Massachusetts[1]

PURPOSE: To evaluate the results of a privileging program aimed to ensure that health care providers and facilities adhere to standards of care.

MATERIALS AND METHODS: Technical and professional privileging applications were mailed to more than 1,800 diagnostic imaging facilities and more than 6,000 professional providers of services to members of a health care plan. Site inspections were used to determine whether facilities met standards of care. Specialty providers were assigned a range of current procedural terminology codes for which they had privileges to bill the payer.

RESULTS: Of 1,004 imaging sites inspected, 197 (20%) failed with the ability to remedy the violation, 106 (10%) failed with fundamental and serious deficiencies, and 701 (70%) passed. Site inspection pass rates varied substantially by specialty. Chiropractors and podiatrists were more likely to fail than medical and surgical specialists. A strong correlation was found between refusal to participate in the inspection and failure rate. Results suggest that reduction of the number of professional claims billed led to a 2% decline in total imaging expenditures, or a more than 10:1 return on the cost of implementing technical and professional privileging programs.

CONCLUSION: Health care plans can positively influence costs and quality by developing, monitoring, and enforcing their own quality standards for diagnostic imaging.

The rapid proliferation of imaging equipment into the outpatient setting, the lack of equipment standardization, and the increase in the performance of diagnostic imaging by nonradiologists in private offices pose difficult problems for quality assessment programs (1–7). This is due largely to the fact that, historically, most quality control and quality assessment and improvement methods (eg, those of the Joint Commission on Accreditation of Health Care Organizations [JCAHO]) have been implemented in hospital imaging settings. As a result, many outpatient imaging centers and medical offices have not established formal, comprehensive, and well-documented quality assessment and improvement programs.

Because purchasers of medical imaging services increasingly expect the same standard of care and quality monitoring activities in all treatment settings, quality of care concerns represent an important consideration in the development of affiliations and contracts with imaging providers (8). Further, with the standards set by regulatory agencies such as the Nuclear Regulatory Commission and state radiation control boards, the same consistency in quality evaluation programs is expected.

Organizations such as the JCAHO, the Agency for Health Care Policy Research, the National Committee for Quality Assurance, and numerous physician organizations have taken a lead in stressing improved quality of care, in developing standards of practice, and in setting up ways to measure and compare quality among providers (9–12). These efforts, however, have focused largely on ensuring that procedures and diagnostic tests are performed because of appropriate indications. Little attention has been devoted to the guarantee that physicians, chiropractors, and podiatrists are adequately trained and have proper credentials to perform procedures and diagnostic tests and that facilities providing services meet appropriate standards of care.

With the exception of mammography, which is heavily regulated by means of both state and federal initiatives, there is virtually no national mandatory certification process for providers who perform imaging services (13). Technologists are required to be licensed by a national body, but physicians, chiropractors, and podiatrists can obviate this requirement by performing studies themselves under their respective professional licenses. Some specialty societies require retesting or recertification (eg, the American Urological Association requires periodic board recertification), but most still have only voluntary requirements. The American College of Radiology has instituted a voluntary certification process to assess the clinical quality of imaging facilities and offers radiologists testing in specialty areas to certify special professional competence. Similarly, the American College of Cardiology offers cardiologists a voluntary test to certify competence in cardiac nuclear medicine.

It is difficult, however, to use one certifying body to define professional competence across specialties. Each specialty society wants to define its own criteria for professional and technical competence. Efforts by third parties to set criteria for imaging creates political "turf battles" that are not easily resolved. For example, the American Institute for Ultrasound in Medicine offers an ultrasound (US) accreditation program for which broad specialty consensus and representation was sought. Nevertheless, the American Urological Association sets its own performance standards for US and views board examination and board recertification, not American Institute for Ultrasound in Medicine accreditation, as the process to ensure professional competence. Similarly, the American College of Radiology has set up an alternative procedure to review US competence through its own accreditation program.

Whereas specialty societies tend to focus on developing and monitoring professional standards, state regulations to monitor imaging facilities focus on radiation safety, not clinical quality, and state regulatory bodies are frequently unable to inspect facilities to determine whether they are in compliance with established standards. Typically, this results from limited resources and staffing constraints, which are evident in most state regulatory agencies.

The results of recent investigations (1,14–16; Kurlantzick V, Bloschichak A, Rosetti G. Quality assurance of diagnostic x-rays in ambulatory settings. Camp Hill, Pa: Highmark Blue Cross Blue Shield, Center for Health Care Quality Information, 1996) of the performance and interpretation of diagnostic imaging studies have demonstrated deficiencies in both the technical performance and the physician interpretation of the studies. Professional and technical proficiency are critical components in the provision of high-quality diagnostic images. One way to ensure that providers adhere to high quality standards and to guarantee that patients have access to the highest quality service is to privilege providers (5). To address this issue directly, BlueCross BlueShield of Massachusetts (BCBSMA) retained Radiology Management Sciences to design and implement a diagnostic imaging privileging program to apply to all providers who submit professional and technical claims for diagnostic imaging services. The program was designed to establish minimum standards of care and to address substandard care as it relates to the provision of outpatient diagnostic imaging services and to the interpretation of images.

The program includes both a professional privileging program to qualify professional providers who interpret and report radiologic results and a technical privileging program to qualify facilities and equipment with which radiologic procedures are performed. This program affects thousands of imaging facilities, physicians, chiropractors, and podiatrists throughout the state of Massachusetts and covers all imaging modalities, including radiography, computed tomography (CT), magnetic resonance (MR) imaging, nuclear medicine, interventional radiology, and US.

BCBSMA operates in all areas of Massachusetts and, through numerous indemnity and managed health care services, has contracts or is affiliated with over 6,000 professional providers and over 1,800 facilities to provide imaging services to its enrollees. The largest percentage of imaging expenditures for BCBSMA patients are for services that include obstetrics, US, chest radiography, abdominal CT, and MR imaging of the back. These constitute more than half of all spending on imaging. Providers who bill for these services generally include radiologists, medical specialists (eg, cardiologists, internal medicine specialists), surgical specialists (eg, orthopedic surgeons, urologists), podiatrists, and chiropractors. More than half of all BCBSMA imaging expenditures are for services provided in medical offices or in outpatient imaging facilities, neither of which are subject to JCAHO regulations.

The objective of this study was to evaluate the results of this diagnostic imaging privileging program. First, we investigated whether the results of the site inspections of facilities that provide the technical component of imaging services vary according to provider specialty. Second, we examined common reasons for the failure to pass a site inspection. Third, we examined the professional privileging program that affects providers who render the professional component of imaging services, in terms of the potential cost savings obtained relative to the cost associated with program implementation. The results of these three analyses will illuminate how differences in provider training may affect the quality of diagnostic imaging delivered in non–JCAHO-approved facilities and shed light on the potential influence of quality assessment programs on improving the quality of imaging studies.

MATERIALS AND METHODS

Technical Privileging Program

The technical privileging program provides a mechanism for ensuring that providers who bill for the technical component of diagnostic imaging services maintain appropriate standards of care. All technical providers not affiliated with a JCAHO-approved facility were required to respond to the technical privileging application. This application sought to verify previously documented demographic information (eg, site location), to summarize the qualifications of the technologists at the facilities, and to provide details about the relevant equipment licensing requirements of the facilities. On the basis of this information, each facility was granted temporary privileges for the relevant diagnostic imaging modality it provided (eg, radiography, US, MR imaging, CT, nuclear medicine). After receipt of the application, each facility was subject to a site inspection by a quality assessment manager to determine whether the imaging site met appropriate standards of care. Each facility's privileging status was contingent on whether it passed the site inspection.

The quality assessment managers who conducted the site inspections were highly qualified, licensed radiologic technologists with over 15 years of training in most imaging modalities. In general, their expertise covered most modalities, but when a manager's expertise was limited or not current, he or she received additional training in that modality. This training involved work with specialists and technologists in the relevant modality. For example, one quality assessment manager with limited expertise in diagnostic US worked with physicians and technologists at a prominent US facility in Boston (Mass) to enhance her previous training.

During each site inspection, a detailed field instrument was completed. This instrument was prepared initially by quality assessment managers and physicians at Radiology Management Sciences and, before it was used in the field, was reviewed by the credentialing committee at BCBSMA and the staff at the American College of Radiology. The instrument was based largely on established standards of care developed by the American College of Radiology, the American Institute for Ultrasound in Medicine, the Mammography Quality Standards Act, the Nuclear Regulatory Commission, the Radiation Control Board of Massachusetts, the JCAHO, and the National Committee for Quality Assurance. The instrument included over 100 questions and focused on six dimensions designed to evaluate the quality of care, including (*a*) staff training and qualifications, (*b*) equipment specifications and performance, (*c*) quality control policies and procedures, (*d*) record management and storage, (*e*) facility safety, and (*f*) image audits.

Letters were sent to a random sample of over 1,223 facilities that responded to the technical privileging application to inform them that we would conduct a site inspection of their facility. Compliance was mandatory in that if they did not comply, their temporary privileging status would be suspended, and reimbursement for technical services billed to BCBSMA would be denied. In the packet of materials sent to each facility, we included a summary of the issues that would be addressed during the site visit, with a detailed list of the six dimensions we planned to evaluate and overall information about the technical privileging program. A member of our staff then contacted each facility to schedule an appointment for the site visit.

Field instruments were scored on the basis of responses to specific questions about each dimension. Facilities were required to receive a satisfactory score in all six categories to pass the inspection and maintain their privileging status. The response to each question was summed to yield three possible results: pass, failure with the ability to remedy the problem(s) identified, and failure with fundamental and serious deficiencies.

Each facility received a letter to inform them of the result of the inspection within 2 weeks of the site visit. Facilities that passed but failed to provide acceptable responses to some questions were sent a letter that included a list of suggestions to improve the standard of care rendered at the facility. Facilities that received a score that resulted in a failure because of a single serious violation had 30 days to submit proper documentation that indicated they had remedied the problem in question. Finally, facilities that failed the site inspection because of multiple serious violations had their ability to bill for the technical component suspended for 18 months, at which time they could apply for reinstatement. The results of the site inspection status decisions were reported to the remedial action committee and peer review department at BCBSMA for review and follow-up. Privileging status was then incorporated into the claims adjudication process, where technical claims for nonprivileging facilities are denied.

Professional Privileging Program

The objective of the professional privileging program is to ensure that providers who bill for the professional component of diagnostic imaging services have the appropriate background and training to interpret images. Professional claims would be denied if providers submitted claims to BCBSMA for any nonprivileged service. The privileging program consisted of a four-stage process: (*a*) verification of previously documented demographic information from providers (eg, practice location), specialty designation, and board certification or board-eligible status; (*b*) development of a list of appropriate codes from the *Physicians' Current Procedural Terminology,* 4th edition (CPT-4) (Kirschner CG, Burkett RC, Kotowicz GM, et al. Chicago, Ill: American Medical Association, 1997) that practitioners of each specialty would have privileges for billing; (*c*) provision of a list of these codes to each provider for comment; and (*d*) review of comments and consideration of appeals from providers who were seeking exceptions.

First, all providers who submitted professional claims to BCBSMA were mailed a professional privileging application to verify the demographic information available at BCBSMA. Second, to determine the appropriate codes for services that each physician, chiropractor, and podiatrist was trained to provide, a list was developed that specified the CPT-4 codes for services practitioners in each specialty would have privileges to provide.

The list of CPT-4 codes for services for which each specialty provider had privileges was developed on the basis of the following considerations: (*a*) Does the local specialty society recognize imaging as an integral part of the specialty's practice? (*b*) Is there a specific testing process, verifiable training regimen, or preceptorship process that all diplomates must undergo and pass? (*c*) Is supervised diagnostic imaging training available to all residents in the specialty, where reports are interpreted by the resident and formally reviewed by an expert? (*d*) Are providers in the specialty credentialed for specific diagnostic imaging procedures at local JCAHO facilities? After the development of each list, we asked numerous specialty societies and medical directors at BCBSMA to evaluate the list for completeness, accuracy, and appropriateness.

In addition, more specific privileging criteria were established in two key areas where practitioners in multiple specialties perform studies: US and cardiac nuclear imaging. For certification of professional competence in US, we required participating providers to become certified by one of the established specialty societies such as the American Institute for Ultrasound in Medicine, the American College of Radiology, the Intersocietal Commission for Accreditation of Vascular Laboratories, or the American Urological Association. For cardiac nuclear medicine accreditation, we jointly developed specific criteria in conjunction with the Massachusetts chapter of the American College of Cardiology. These criteria outlined a number of acceptable pathways to achieve professional accreditation, including verifiable nuclear medicine training beyond a cardiology fellowship, completion of additional course work and preceptorship, or passage of the American College of Cardiology's nuclear medicine test. For both US and nuclear medicine certification, we developed community and specialty consensus to ensure that our program would be accepted by the broad local medical community.

A final list of approved CPT-4 codes was developed for all specialty practices that submitted imaging claims to BCBSMA. This included 29 medical and surgical specialties and chiropractic medicine and podiatry. The range of approved CPT-4 codes varied substantially by specialty. For example, the list of approved codes for ophthalmology included six CPT-4 codes related to ophthalmic US (CPT-4 codes 76511–76529), whereas the list of approved codes for orthopedic surgery was much larger and included more than 75 CPT-4 codes related to musculoskeletal imaging. Some specialties, such as emergency medicine, did not have privileges to provide any professional diagnostic imaging services.

On the basis of preexistent criteria of the health care plan for which this program was designed, board eligibility was chosen as the minimum standard for consideration of a physician as a member of a given specialty. In other words, a physician who was board eligible was considered to be a member of a given specialty and, therefore, subject to the same privileging criteria. Few exceptions to board eligibility were made; any exceptions were on the basis of specific documentation of specialty training and were reviewed on a case-by-case basis by medical directors at BCBSMA.

Physicians, chiropractors, and podiatrists who responded to the professional privileging application were mailed a list of the CPT-4 codes for which BCBSMA would provide reimbursement. In a letter that accompanied this list, we explained to providers that payments for professional imaging services not included in this list would not be reimbursed. However, due to the sensitivity of the denial of payments, the program was not implemented until providers were given an opportunity to respond to the approved list of codes. In cases where providers requested privileges outside the normal boundaries of their specialty, they were asked to submit materials to document their additional diagnostic imaging training or geographic access needs that might prevent some patients from receiving necessary care. These requests were reviewed by Radiology Management Sciences medical directors on a case-by-case basis to determine if an exception was appropriate. Recommendations were then reviewed by the credentialing committee and the medical directors at BCBSMA for final determination.

Diagnostic Imaging Providers Included in the Technical Privileging Program

Type of Provider	No. of Facilities Selected	No. of Site Visits Completed	Response Rate (%)
Cardiology	41	33	80
Medical specialist	21	16	76
Primary care	109	84	77
Obstetrics and gynecology	49	40	82
Orthopedic surgery	148	130	88
Surgical specialist	55	45	82
Radiology	112	101	90
Mobile imaging unit	116	111	96
Chiropractor	337	265	79
Podiatry	235	179	76
Total	1,223	1,004	82

RESULTS

Technical Privileging

The Table provides a summary of the number of sites and the number of site inspections conducted, according to the type of provider, in the technical privileging program. Of the 2,545 applications mailed, we received 2,208 completed applications. Sites that did not respond were excluded from the study. It is plausible that these sites did not respond because an incorrect mailing address was used or the facility was not certain they would have passed the inspection. Owing to the quality of the demographic information available for each facility (address, practice size, etc), it is unfortunately not possible to evaluate thoroughly the characteristics of nonrespondents.

By using the complete pool of completed applications, we selected a sample of 1,223 facilities to participate in the site inspection component of the study. The types of providers included in the program were primary care physicians (n = 109), medical specialists (n = 21), cardiologists (n = 41), surgical specialists (n = 55), obstetricians and gynecologists (n = 49), mobile imaging units (n = 116), orthopedic surgeons (n = 148), radiologists (n = 112), chiropractors (n = 337) and podiatrists (n = 235). Medical specialties included allergy (n = 1), endocrinology (n = 2), neurology (n = 4), ophthalmology (n = 6), occupational medicine (n = 3), pulmonology (n = 1), and rheumatology (n = 4). Surgical specialties included general surgery (n = 3), hand surgery (n = 8), neurosurgery (n = 1), otolaryngology (n = 7), urology (n = 24), thoracic surgery (n = 1), and vascular surgery (n = 11). A number of facilities were not inspected because they refused or were unable to schedule a site visit. The 219 facilities that withdrew from the program were denied payment for technical claims submitted to BCBSMA.

Figure 1 shows a summary of the results of the site visit inspections and withdrawal rates according to specialty. Of 1,004 outpatient imaging sites inspected, 197 (20%) failed with the ability to remedy the violation cited; 106 (11%) failed with fundamental and serious deficiencies; and 701 (70%) passed.

The first category of failures typically included a single serious violation that could be addressed within a reasonable amount of time. For example, facilities often lacked a copy of the annual calibration report, or the image review showed evidence of processing problems. Each of these flaws could be remedied within a short amount of time. In addition, a number of sites used no dosimeter badges for monitoring of the radiation exposure to patients or staff. Each site in this category had an opportunity to address our concerns and convert their inspection status by providing documentation that showed the problem had been remedied. For example, we requested that facilities provide a copy of the calibration report, a service report on the processor, more images to verify that the problem was corrected, or a purchase order or bill to verify that dosimeter badges had been ordered. If the relevant sites did not comply within 30 days, they were called and encouraged to send us the information. Only five sites did not respond; thus, their site inspection status was converted to that of a failure with fundamental and serious deficiencies.

The second category of failures included those that had severe underlying problems that could not be easily remedied. This category of failures represented sites with serious violations that could not be addressed within a reasonable amount of time. The 106 sites in this

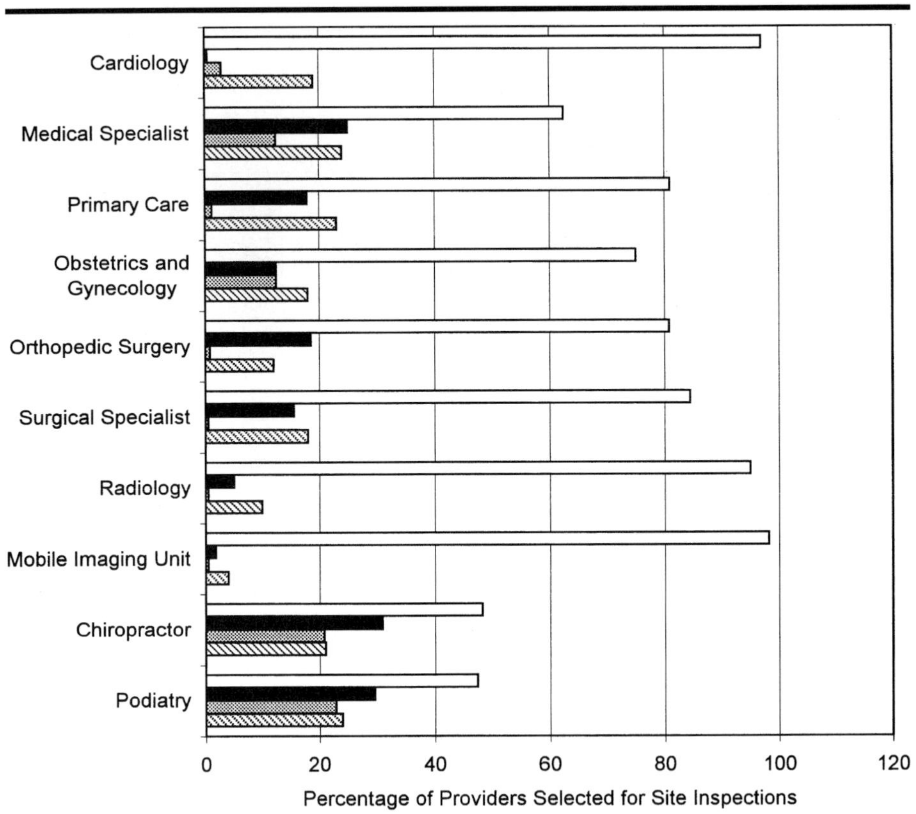

Figure 1. Facility site inspections by medical specialty. Bar graph depicts facility site inspection results according to whether the facility passed (white bars), failed with the ability to remedy (black bars), failed with fundamental and serious deficiencies (gray bars), or withdrew from the program (striped bars). The percentage of sites that withdrew is not included in the 100% total because that total is based on the entire sample and not on the sample of respondents only.

category group were suspended from billing BCBSMA for imaging services. These sites include 55 chiropractic, 41 podiatric, one orthopedic surgical, five obstetric and gynecologic, one primary care, two medical specialty, and one cardiology sites. One hundred of these facilities provide radiography services only, and six facilities provide US services only. Overall, these sites represent offices where providers were using imaging equipment for which they were not trained or certified to use. If any of these sites lacked a state certificate of registration for their equipment, they were reported to the state radiation control board.

As shown in Figure 1, there were large variations in the results of the site inspections according to provider type. For instance, pass rates ranged from a high of 98% (109 of 111) for mobile imaging units to a low of 47% (85 of 179) for podiatrists. Failure rates for facilities that had fundamental and serious violations were also large, ranging from a high of 23% (41 of 179) for podiatry facilities to a low of 0% (none of 111) for mobile imaging units, radiology facilities (none of 101), and surgical specialty facilities (none of 45). Finally, the rate of failure, with an ability to remedy the violation, ranged from a high of 31% (82 of 265) for chiropractic medicine to a low of 0% (none of 33) for cardiology.

The withdrawal rate provides an interesting insight into possible reasons why some facilities refused to participate in the inspection. Mobile imaging units had the highest pass rate and the lowest withdrawal rate. Surgical specialties had the second highest pass rate and one of the lowest withdrawal rates. This relationship suggests that specialties with few site inspection violations had a higher propensity to participate in the program. On the other hand, the specialties with the highest rate of failure with an ability to remedy the problem cited or the highest rate of failure with severe underlying problems were podiatry and chiropractic medicine. It is interesting that these two specialties also had the highest withdrawal rates. Across all 10 provider groups, we estimated a correlation coefficient of .96 ($P < .001$, one-tailed t test) between the rate of withdrawal and that of failure with fundamental and serious deficiencies. The correlation coefficient was .98 ($P < .001$, one-tailed t test) between the rate of withdrawal and that of failure with the ability to remedy. Thus, if specialties with particularly high withdrawal rates had participated in the study, it is likely the failure rate would have been even higher.

Figure 2 displays the most common reasons why sites failed with fundamental and serious deficiencies. Offenses ranged from practicing without a state certificate of radiation control to failure to maintain equipment properly. Whereas some of these reasons, considered alone, may not appear to be serious violations, in combination with other factors they reveal a serious inability to provide a prescribed level of care. Several violations related to image quality standards, including poor patient positioning, improper collimation, artifacts, scratches or chemical streaks on images, and improper exposure (eg, radiographs were either too light or too dark to provide bone detail). The quality issues relevant to the US sites that failed the inspection included improper positioning of the US probe, cursory or nonstandard studies, and inability to sterilize probes properly between internal examinations of different patients. Other violations related to quality control issues included failure to perform annual calibration of the imaging equipment and lack of an adequate quality control plan. Finally, some of the most serious offenses related to safety included the failure to post an "X-ray in use" or radiation exposure sign, failure to use adequate radiation monitoring devices (eg, dosimeter badges), failure to have a physicist review the shielding floor plan, or the lack of a shielding floor plan.

Professional Privileging

Professional privileging applications were mailed initially to 9,745 providers. Due to limitations in the accuracy and completeness of the address information and the inability to identify unique provider identification numbers easily, however, several mailings were necessary before all providers were contacted successfully. Thus, although we received 6,027 completed applications, data limitations precluded reliable estimates of a response rate to the application process. Further, it was not possible to analyze characteristics of nonrespondents that may influence response rates (eg, board certification status, practice size, years in practice since medical school graduation).

After receipt of the application, a list of approved, specialty-specific CPT-4 codes

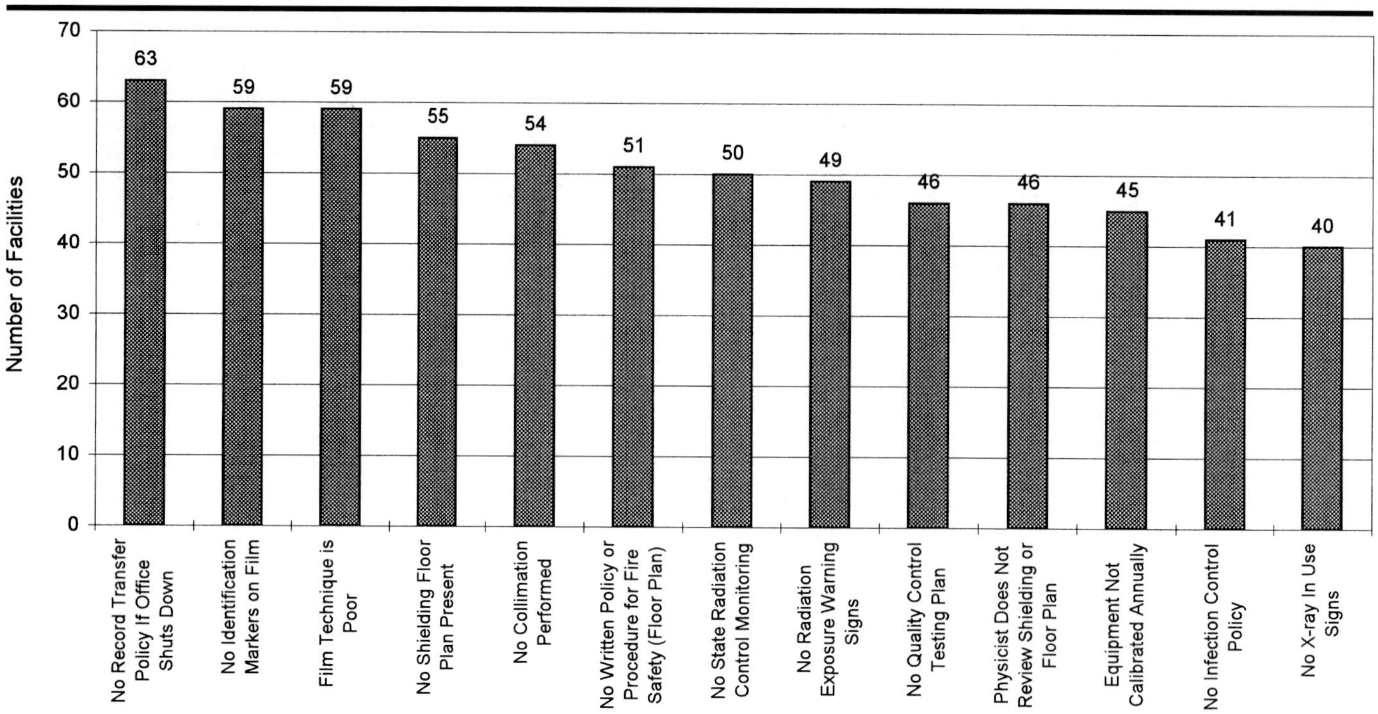

Figure 2. Common fundamental and serious deficiencies. Bar graph displays the number of sites that failed the site inspection due to specific deficiencies. The number above each bar is the number of sites.

was mailed to each provider. Four hundred eight providers submitted an appeals application to reverse the decision to deny reimbursement for services for which they were currently receiving reimbursement. The appeals process resulted in 70 denials and 338 exceptions. Applications that were denied included those from providers who sought an exception to provide and bill for services outside of their expertise (eg, they did not have adequate training to provide the service). The 338 exceptions primarily included providers who were granted a grace period to demonstrate specified certification or training and providers who sought to continue to provide vascular US or cardiac nuclear medicine services while applications for certification were pending with the Intersocietal Commission for the Accreditation of Vascular Laboratories or the American College of Cardiology. Approximately 10 exceptions were made on the basis of the demonstration of specific professional expertise in the absence of specialty board eligibility or on the basis of geographic access needs.

Some issues were resolved by making broader policy changes to entire specialty categories or by granting exceptions to individual providers with specific expertise in a given imaging technique. For instance, orthopedic surgeons and general surgeons were not initially permitted to bill for fluoroscopy. Because manipulation of fractures by orthopedic surgeons or central venous catheter placements by general surgeons may necessitate fluoroscopy, however, we created a policy revision to permit billing of the professional component of this procedure for these specialties.

Owing to the large number of appeals related to cardiac nuclear medicine and vascular US, we developed separate criteria for permitting exceptions for these services. We had initially required neurologists who perform carotid US and vascular surgeons who perform peripheral vascular US to become accredited by the Intersocietal Commission for the Accreditation of Vascular Laboratories. Initially, we had not permitted cardiologists to perform noncardiac US. Rather than engage in a "territorial battle" over peripheral vascular US, we allowed exceptions by requiring all cardiologists who perform vascular US to become certified within 18 months by the Intersocietal Commission for the Accreditation of Vascular Laboratories. For cardiac nuclear medicine accreditation, we jointly developed specific criteria in conjunction with the Massachusetts chapter of the American College of Cardiology. These criteria outlined a number of acceptable pathways to achieve professional accreditation, including verifiable nuclear medicine training beyond a cardiac fellowship, completion of additional course work and preceptorship, or passage of the American College of Cardiology's nuclear medicine test. For both US and nuclear medicine certification, we developed community and specialty consensus to ensure that our program would be accepted by the broad local medical community.

By using 1995 imaging expenditure data to estimate the potential cost savings of this program, we identified both claims for individual providers who were not privileged to bill BCBSMA and claims for specific combinations of CPT-4 codes and providers that would be denied under the program. By using these data, we estimated that overall imaging expenditures would decline approximately 2%, which would result in a return of more than 10:1 on the cost of the implementation of both privileging programs. Although implementation costs represent a one-time fee, we expect savings to be reaped annually, although such savings would be greater in the 1st year of implementation.

DISCUSSION

Professional and technical proficiency are critical components for the provision of high-quality diagnostic images. Given the rapid proliferation of imaging equipment in the outpatient setting, the qualifications of physicians interpreting and performing imaging studies needs to be monitored more rigorously. This issue of how best to review the use of diagnostic imaging studies becomes imperative in the absence of state and quality credentialing standards (eg, those of the National Committee for Quality Assurance), without detracting from patient care in the outpatient setting.

The program we have described provided an effective and straightforward means of addressing quality-of-care issues by ensuring that BCBSMA providers adhered to the highest quality standards while BCBSMA members were simultaneously guaranteed access to the highest quality services. Although it is premature to estimate the full cost savings attributable to the programs, initial estimates suggest that the limiting of radiology resource use to privileging providers and facilities only may be highly cost-effective for managed health care organizations. Investments in programs such as these are trivial, because the cost of implementation was more than recovered by the potential cost savings achieved in the 1st year from the professional privileging component of the program.

Increased cost savings might have been achieved had a less conservative implementation strategy been used. The objective of our implementation strategy was primarily to address the serious concerns we had about the professional competence of some specialists to perform imaging studies. This objective was balanced by the need to promote cooperation among providers and to minimize the number of territorial or political battles we would have to fight to achieve some success. Thus, the program was structured broadly enough so that it could be implemented easily and a process would be in place to narrow the scope of the privileging effort, if BCBSMA chose to pursue such a task. Thus, health plans interested in implementing tighter privileging standards may expect to obtain greater cost savings if fewer providers are granted privileges to perform diagnostic imaging services. However, because professional credentialing will always be controversial and have some degree of subjectivity, to respond adequately to the potential complaints (as we experienced in the implementation of these privileging programs) from both physicians who are affected by the policy and national physician organizations, health care organizations should carefully consider the trade-offs of the implementation of less versus more conservative strategies.

It should also be noted that the scope and financial effect of this privileging program was likely constrained by characteristics of the local health care market in Massachusetts. Hospitals and academic hospital–led networks dominate the delivery of health care in Massachusetts. Massachusetts health care is less entrepreneurial, more conservative, and more regulated than that in other parts of the country, with many physicians making use of their affiliated hospital for ancillary services (17,18). As a result, radiologists and other physicians in Massachusetts own fewer free-standing or office-based imaging facilities. A comparison of preliminary data we evaluated for a large health care plan in the metropolitan New York, NY, region revealed that a similarly applied privileging program could result in a savings of at least 10%, in contrast to the savings of 2% documented here. Thus, because relatively more nonradiologists bill for professional claims in this market compared with those in Massachusetts, more professional claims would be denied. Of interest, given the results from our Massachusetts study and the fact that more nonradiologists own and operate diagnostic imaging equipment in the metropolitan New York City market, if we applied the same technical privileging program to this health care market, pass rates may likely be even smaller than we observed in Massachusetts.

Of importance, as Hillman and colleagues (2) note in their evaluation of a payment policy designed in part to reduce imaging-related expenditures of nonradiologists, the denial of professional diagnostic imaging charges by all nonradiologists may not lead to cost savings. In fact, their results showed the opposite financial effect of the BCBSMA program: The program evaluated by Hillman and colleagues led to an increase in imaging expenditures. Given that providers continued to be reimbursed for their technical claims, nothing prevented them from increasing their billings of technical fees to offset revenues lost to the privileging program. Physicians' responses to changes in payment rates range from strong support for volume offsets (19) to refutation of their validity (20). As a result, there has been much disagreement about how physicians respond to reductions in payment rates. An important distinction between these two privileging programs is that the payment policy Hillman and colleagues evaluated denied payments for all professional claims submitted by nonradiologists. On the other hand, with the BCBSMA plan and its use of specialty-specific, approved lists of CPT-4 imaging codes, nonradiologists continue to bill for imaging services for which they have privileges. Differences in these payment policies may have important implications for the achievement of financial savings from professional privileging programs.

There are two reasons why it was not possible to inspect all of the approximately 1,900 imaging facilities that currently bill BCBSMA. First, it was not cost-effective to inspect each facility, and second, it was not logistically feasible to schedule a site inspection of each facility, especially those located in remote areas. As a result, unsatisfactory performance and quality standards may persist in noninspected sites.

The extent to which unsatisfactory performance standards persist in noninspected sites may be smaller than expected because the technical privileging program may have indirectly effected these facilities in two ways. First, the program was initially set up to include all diagnostic imaging programs. Thus, if a facility was not included in the first phase of site inspections, practitioners at the facility were under the impression that their facility would be included in the second phase of inspections. Second, after the initial site inspections, medical societies and other physician organizations contacted Radiology Management Sciences to discuss the results of the site inspections. As a result of this communication, uninspected providers were likely informed of the program and specific details of our site inspection protocol. We believe that widespread awareness of the program positively influenced the standards of care delivered at noninspected sites.

Whatever the uncertainties about savings, implementation of the privileging programs clearly resulted in important quality improvements. Results from the technical privileging program, specifically from the site inspections, reveal compelling evidence that many providers own and operate equipment that they are not trained to use. Lack of knowledge about requirements for safety and equipment, ignorance of the law with regard to licensing, and inability to distinguish between good and bad imaging techniques suggest the need for increased monitoring and education. Our findings substantiate the need for systematic assessment of imaging facilities and image quality. Voluntary programs such as those implemented by the American College of Radiology and the American Institute for Ultrasound in Medicine have been developed to address quality issues related to US and MR imaging. Mandatory programs to monitor quality and safety standards have been deemed essential to mammography and have been very successful. Consideration should be given to the implementation of similar quality assessment programs for other types of outpatient imaging.

Acknowledgments: The authors acknowledge the assistance provided by Lorraine Friestad, AA, Rekha Nigam, BA, and Christine Duh, BS. We also appreciate the administrative assistance of Jonni Hall, AA, and gratefully acknowledge the assistance of the numerous specialty societies, Meg Wallingford, and others at BCBSMA who were involved in the design and implementation of this program.

References

1. Levin DC. The practice of radiology by non-radiologists: cost quality and utilization issues. AJR 1994; 162:513–518.
2. Hillman BJ, Olson GT, Colbert RW, Bernhardt LB. Responses to a payment policy denying professional charges for diagnostic imaging by nonradiologist physicians. JAMA 1995; 274:885–887.
3. Hillman BJ, Joseph CA, Mabry MR, et al. Diagnostic imaging in office practice: a comparison of self-referring and radiologist referring physicians. N Engl J Med 1990; 323:1604–1608.
4. Thrall JH. Perspective: the radiologist in the 1990s—new practice expectations and management responsibilities. AJR 1994; 163:11–15.
5. Sunshine JH, Bansal S, Evens RG. Radiology performed by non-radiologists in the United States: who does what? AJR 1993; 161:419–429.
6. Hillman BJ, Olson GT, Griffith PE, et al. Physicians' utilization and charges for outpatient diagnostic imaging in a Medicare population. JAMA 1992; 268:2050–2054.
7. Rubin HR, Rogers WH, Kahn KL, et al. Watching the doctor watchers: how well do peer review organization methods detect hospital care quality problems? JAMA 1992; 267:2349–2354.
8. Kessler HB. Managed care and the radiologist: expectations and future trends. AJR 1994; 163:1–3.
9. AHCPR program note: clinical practice guideline development. Publication no. 93-0023. Washington, DC: Agency for Health Care Policy and Research, 1993.
10. American College of Radiology. Appropriateness criteria for imaging and treatment decisions. Reston, Va: American College of Radiology, 1995.
11. Iglehart JK. The National Committee for Quality Assurance. N Engl J Med 1996; 335:995–999.
12. McLelland R, Hendrick RE, Zinninger MD, et al. The American College of Radiology mammography accreditation program. AJR 1991; 157:473–479.
13. Nightingale SL. From the Food and Drug Administration: new mammography quality standards issued. JAMA 1994; 271:179.
14. Friedman DP, Rosetti GF, Flanders AK, et al. MR imaging: quality assessment method and ratings at 33 centers. Radiology 1995; 196:219–226.
15. Evan H. Doctors who perform fetal sonograms often lack sufficient training and skill. Wall Street Journal 1995; Jun 20:sect B:l.
16. Hooper KD, Rossetti GF, Edmiston RB, et al. Diagnostic radiology peer review: a method inclusive of all interpreters of radiographic examinations regardless of specialty. Radiology 1991; 180:557–561.
17. Seltzer SE, Holman BL, Thrall JH, Bramson RT, Roller W. Academic radiology in a networked environment. Acad Radiol 1996; 3:865–872.
18. Melnick GA, Zwanziger J. State health care expenditures under competition and regulation, 1980 through 1991. Am J Public Health 1995; 85:1391–1396.
19. Christensen S. Volume responses to exogenous changes in Medicare's payment policies. Health Serv Res 1993. 27:65–79.
20. Escarce J. Effects of lower surgical fees on the use of physician services under Medicare. JAMA 1993; 269:2513–2518.

Tracheobronchial Tree: Assessment with Volume Rendering—Technical Aspects[1]

Martine Remy-Jardin, MD, PhD
Jacques Remy, MD
Dominique Artaud, MD
Marc Fribourg, MD
Abdel Naili, RT

Index terms:
Bronchi, CT, 671.12117
Computed tomography (CT), technology, 671.12117
Computed tomography (CT), three-dimensional, 671.12117
Computed tomography (CT), volume rendering, 671.12117

Radiology 1998; 208:393–398

[1] From the Department of Radiology, Hôpital Calmette, Blvd Jules Leclerc, 59037 Lille, France. Received October 10, 1997; revision requested January 6, 1998; revision received January 22; accepted March 3. **Address reprint requests to** M.R.J.

A volume-rendering technique was applied at the level of normal airways. Two spiral computed tomographic data sets (central and peripheral bronchi) were selected to evaluate the influence of the technique parameters. Optimal bronchogram-like images were obtained with a continuous rim of peripheral voxels, a 70% opacity value, and the unshaded algorithm. Volume rendering allows creation of airway reconstructions that are very similar to conventional bronchograms.

Among the postprocessing techniques applicable to medical imaging, most attention has been focused on shaded surface display and maximum (or minimum) intensity projection with specific attention to their respective advantages and limitations. Surface rendering, widely available in commercial computed tomographic (CT) image processing packages, provides the most three-dimensionally intuitive images. However, two limitations are usually described with the use of this rendering technique. Each voxel is classified as either 100% or 0% of a tissue type, and it is not possible to integrate the voxels fractionally composed of the tissue of interest in the final image. Moreover, the resultant image is strongly dependent on the threshold chosen to display the organ of interest, which may interfere with the diagnostic information.

The second most frequently used rendering technique is maximum (or minimum) intensity projection, based on a two-dimensional display of the highest (or lowest) intensity voxels. Whereas the advantage of this technique is the ability to avoid any thresholding selection, its main drawback is the inability to maintain the three-dimensional structural relationships inherent in the data set.

With volume rendering, the third technique available for generating three-dimensional images, voxels are displayed according to the percentage of a given tissue of interest contained in each voxel. In addition to allowing selection of voxels that contain 100% of a tissue type, this technique allows the incorporation of voxels partially composed of that specific tissue. As recently described by Johnson et al (1), this voxel classification allows the inaccuracies posed by threshold selection in a binary algorithm as used in shaded surface display to be minimized. In addition, the volume-rendered images maintain the original anatomic spatial relationships of the CT data set, which are limited with maximum intensity projection. To our knowledge, this volume-rendering technique has been applied mainly to vascular imaging (2,3) since its introduction, and its use in evaluating the airways has not been explored as much (4). The purpose of this study was to evaluate the potential use of this volume-rendering technique in the creation of bronchogram-like (bronchographic) images and to determine the optimal image display parameters.

Materials and Methods

Patient Data Sets

From our database of spiral CT examinations of the airways, we selected data sets obtained in two different patients with normal airways to evaluate the influence of the parameters selected in the volume-rendering technique. We evaluated the quality of bronchographic images of the trachea and main stem bronchi (patient 1) and segmental and subsegmen-

Author contributions:
Guarantors of integrity of entire study, M.R.J., J.R.; study concepts, J.R.; study design, J.R., M.R.J.; definition of intellectual content, J.R., M.R.J.; literature research, J.R.; experimental studies, A.N.; data acquisition, M.R.J., J.R.; data analysis, M.R.J., J.R.; manuscript preparation, M.R.J., J.R.; manuscript editing, M.R.J.; manuscript review, D.A., M.F.

tal bronchi (patient 2). The clinical indications for the spiral CT examinations were to follow up bronchial anastomosis after left lung transplantation (patient 1) and suspicion for abnormal right hilum at chest radiography (patient 2). In every case, care was taken to select data sets obtained in strict apnea to ensure high-quality three-dimensional images. These examinations demonstrated an anastomotic shelf at the level of the left main bronchus and the absence of right hilar abnormality, respectively. The data set obtained to follow up left lung transplantation enabled creation of bronchographic images of central airways (ie, trachea, carina, and main bronchi), and the data set acquired at the level of the right hilum allowed creation of bronchographic images of more peripheral bronchi (ie, segmental and subsegmental bronchi of the right upper lobe).

CT Acquisition

The data sets were acquired with a Somatom Plus 4A scanner (Siemens Medical Systems, Erlangen, Germany) at 180 mA and 140 kV with a 0.75-second scanning time. The spiral CT examinations were obtained at deep inspiration without administration of contrast medium. The examinations consisted of a focal acquisition through the region of clinical interest with the following parameters: (*a*) patient 1 (left main stem bronchus), 5-mm collimation, 7 mm/sec table feed, pitch of 1.4, z-axis coverage of 80 mm (extending from 2 cm above the carina down to the left lower lobe bronchus), and 10-second breath hold; (*b*) patient 2 (right upper lobe bronchi), 1-mm collimation, 2 mm/sec table feed, pitch of 2, z-axis coverage of 65 mm (extending from 2 cm above the carina down to the right bronchus intermedius), and 26-second breath hold.

Volume-rendering Technique Reconstructions

To generate volume-rendering technique images, the first step was to reconstruct transverse CT scans at 1-mm intervals, by means of a soft-reconstruction kernel, after selecting a field of view of 110 mm for the patient 1 data set and 65 mm for the patient 2 data set. The next step consisted of manually drawing the contours of the airway(s) of interest on each CT scan to erase all the regions outside the defined area. This was performed by a technician (A.N.), who then transferred the edited images from the main console to a workstation (Magic View, Siemens Medical Systems) on which the bronchographic images were generated with the software.

With the volume-rendering technique, the voxels are classified according to the percentage of different materials present. Each probability curve is approximated by a function with trapezoidal shape (5). As in Figure 1, point *C* (the midpoint of segment *BD*) is the CT number most likely to exactly represent the material of interest. Points *B* and *D* represent the maximum variation acceptable from point *C* to ensure the voxel's attenuation number entirely represents this material. Points *A* and *E* represent the maximum and minimum CT numbers, respectively, of a voxel that is considered to contain none of the material.

The objective of the present study was to determine optimal selections for the following parameters to create bronchographic images. (*a*) The position of the trapezoid, which determines the attenuation of the voxels incorporated into the image. As emphasized by Johnson et al (2), the selection of this parameter consists of defining a window width and a window level, which determines the image sharpness of the bronchographic reconstruction. (*b*) The shape of the trapezoid, corresponding to the intersections between the sides of the trapezoid and the top, which modifies the airway wall homogeneity. (*c*) The opacity value, which determines the relative transparency of the voxels incorporated into the image, and thus the tracheobronchial transparency. (*d*) The shading option, which modifies the airway wall smoothness. The display is modified by directly manipulating the trapezoid (for position and shape) and/or by typing the selected value (for trapezoid position, trapezoid shape, opacity value, and shading option) on the corresponding menu.

Because four successive parameters had to be defined before a volume-rendered image could be generated, a truly independent evaluation of each parameter was not possible. Consequently, we used an empiric approach to define the a priori optimal parameters for generating images similar to conventional bronchograms. On a subjective basis, consensus was obtained among several chest radiologists (M.R.J., J.R., D.A., M.F.) for the following optimal parameters: triangular trapezoid shape, selection of voxels from −700 to −500 HU for the peripheral bronchi and from −550 to −350 HU for the central bronchi, 70% opacity value, and unshaded algorithm. Whenever we evaluated the influence of a given parameter selection on the final image quality, we preselected the remaining optimal parameters.

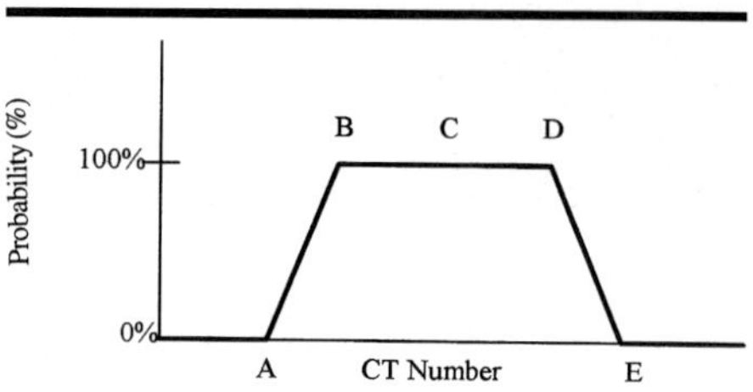

Figure 1. Graph demonstrates percentage classification for the presence of one material. Points *A* and *E* are the 0% levels. Points *B* and *D* are the boundaries of the 100% range. Point *C* is the nominal CT number for this material. (Adapted and reprinted, with permission, from reference 5.)

Selection of the Volume-rendering Technique Parameters

To generate bronchographic images, the trapezoid was positioned to select voxels located at the interface between the air column and the airway wall to allow creation of a sharp bronchographic reconstruction. The location of the voxels retained in the virtual image was depicted on a minimum intensity projection image of the edited data set (patient 1, anteroposterior views; patient 2, superoinferior views). Several trapezoid positions were manually selected for both data sets, which led to incorporation of a variable number of voxels in the final images. For the trachea and main stem bronchi (patient 1), window widths of 200 HU from −950 to −150 HU, in 200-HU steps, were successively selected. For the segmental and subsegmental bronchi (patient 2), window widths of 200 HU from −1,000 to −300 HU, in 100-HU steps, were successively selected.

Whenever the optimal trapezoid position was defined, namely the position that generated the sharpest image, airway wall homogeneity was evaluated on images generated with three different trapezoid shapes: rectangular, trapezoidal, and triangular. After the optimal parameters were selected, the next step was to evaluate the influence of the opacity value on the transparency of the tracheobronchial tree, in 20% steps from 10% to 90%. Next, the effect of the three shading algorithms (shaded, smooth, and unshaded) on the airway wall smoothness was evaluated. For each parameter, the following three-point scale was used to grade image quality after successive modi-

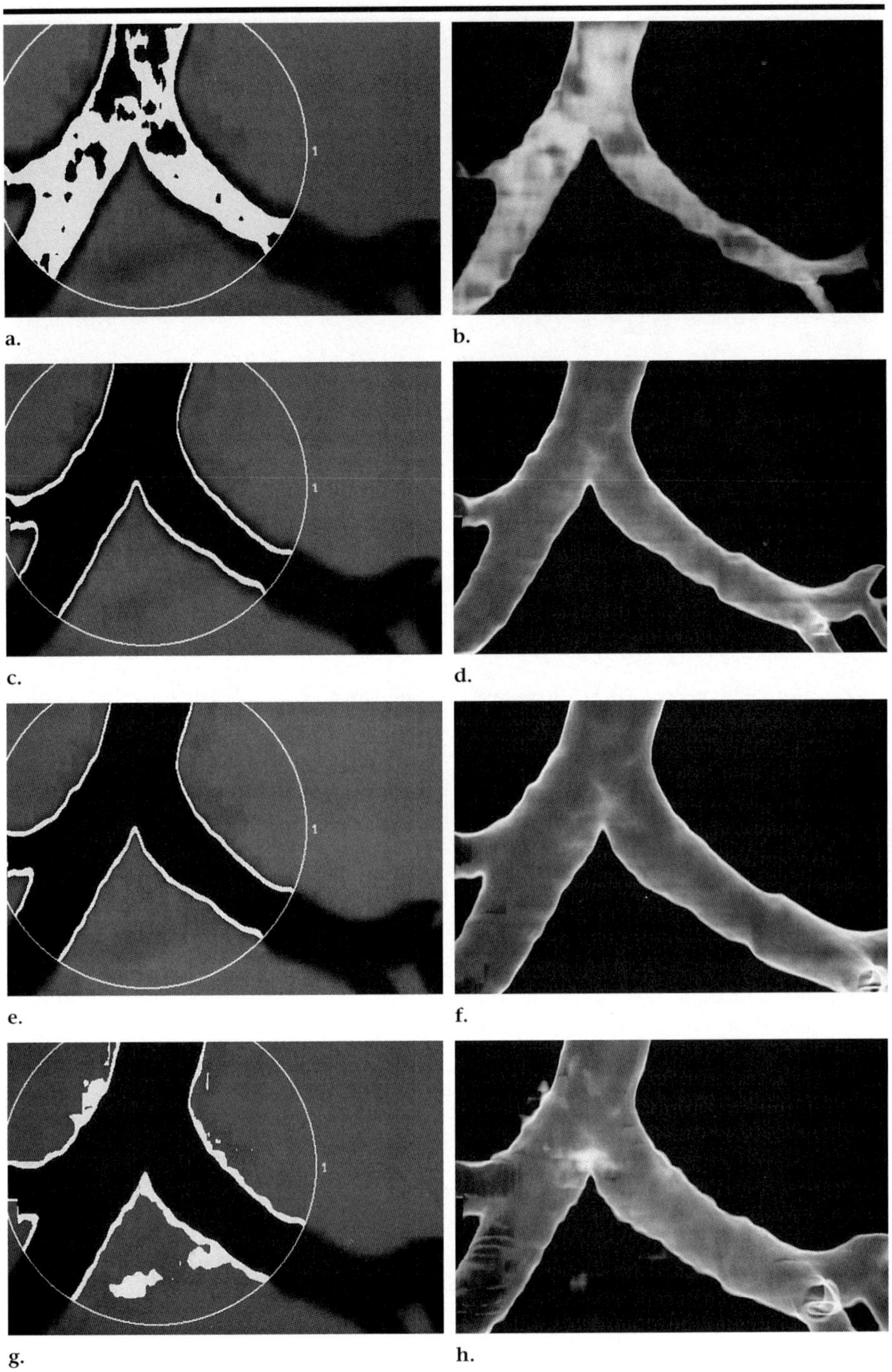

Figure 2. **Patient 1.** Adjustment of image sharpness for central airways. Boundaries of each trapezoid position are the following: **(a, b)** −950 HU, −750 HU; **(c, d)** −750 HU, −550 HU; **(e, f)** −550 HU, −350 HU; **(g, h)** −350 HU, −150 HU. **a**, **c**, **e**, and **g** are anteroposterior minimum intensity projection images on which the selected voxels are highlighted. **b**, **d**, **f**, and **h** are the corresponding bronchographic images.

fications on the basis of consensus among the four readers: 1 = poor, 2 = correct but not optimal, 3 = optimal.

No attempt was made to evaluate the influence of the gray percentage, the contrast on the final image, which is predetermined at 100% on the workstation. To avoid adding another variable in the analysis of virtual images, care was taken to select the same window settings for all virtual images: patient 1 (trachea and main stem bronchi), window width of 3,000 HU and window level of 900 HU; patient 2 (segmental and subsegmental bronchi), window width of 2,200 HU and window level of 650 HU.

Results

Adjustment of Image Sharpness

For volume images of the central airways (patient 1), the optimal trapezoid position resulted from the selection of a window width from −550 to −350 HU. This position enabled selection of a continuous rim of the most peripheral voxels, which resulted in a sharply defined bronchographic image (Fig 2e, 2f). This trapezoid position was considered more appropriate than that obtained with window width from −750 to −550 HU, which resulted in a thicker rim of peripheral voxels and, subsequently, a reduced airway diameter (Fig 2c, 2d). The remaining selections were considered suboptimal due to the following drawbacks: (*a*) Window width from −350 to −150 HU resulted in selection of voxels with high attenuation values, which led to the integration of numerous extraluminal voxels in the final image (Fig 2g, 2h). (*b*) Window width from −950 to −750 HU resulted in selection of too many intraluminal voxels, which resulted in acquisition of a positive "cast" of the air column rather than a bronchographic image (Fig 2a, 2b). For volume-rendered images of the peripheral airways (patient 2), the optimal trapezoid position was obtained with window width from −700 to −500 HU, which provided a sharp bronchographic image (Fig 3). Adjustments of the trapezoid position for both data sets were successively evaluated while the remaining parameters were preselected as follows: (*a*) triangular trapezoid shape, (*b*) 70% opacity, (*c*) unshaded algorithm.

Adjustment of Airway Wall Homogeneity

For the trachea and main stem bronchi (patient 1), selection of the triangular trapezoid shape enabled creation of a uniform bronchographic image (Fig 4a), whereas variable artifacts were observed with the rectangular and trapezoidal shapes (Fig 4b, 4c). Similar results were found at the level of the segmental and subsegmental bronchi (patient 2). The window levels for the triangular trapezoids were −450 and −600 HU, respectively. Adjustments of the trapezoid shape for both data sets were successively evaluated, while the remaining parameters were preselected as follows: (*a*) patient 1, window width from −550 to −350 HU, 70% opacity, unshaded algorithm; (*b*) pa-

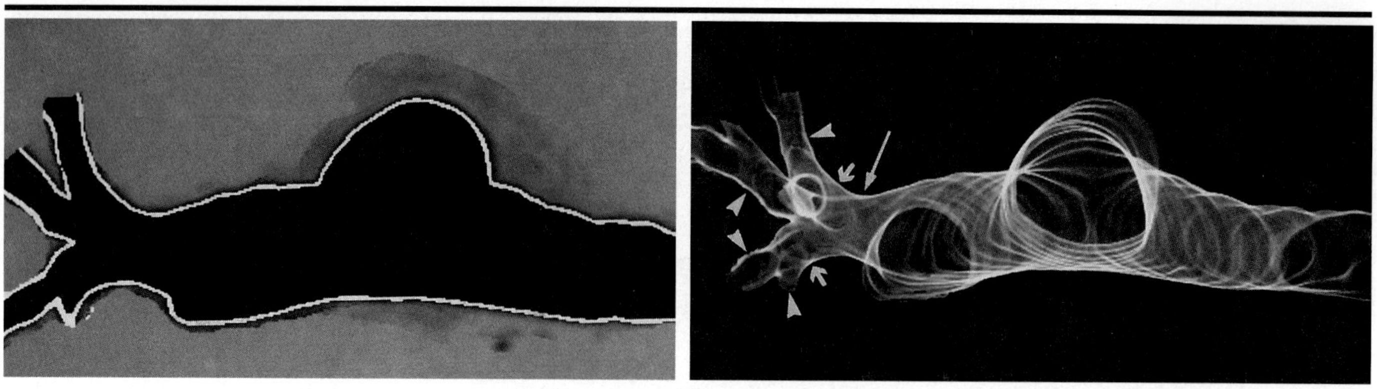

a. b.

Figure 3. Patient 2. Selection of trapezoid position for sharp reconstruction of peripheral airways. **(a)** Superoinferior minimum intensity projection image highlights the selected voxels. Boundaries of the trapezoid position are −700 HU, −500 HU. **(b)** Corresponding volume-rendered reconstruction provides sharp images of the right upper lobe bronchus (long arrow) as well as of the segmental (short arrows) and subsegmental (arrowheads) bronchi.

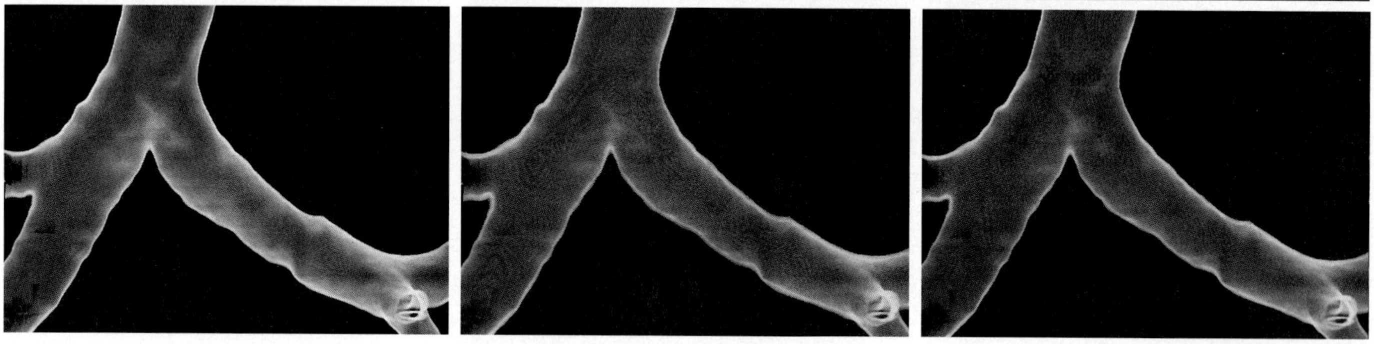

a. b. c.

Figure 4. Patient 1. Bronchographic images illustrate the adjustment of airway wall homogeneity for central airways: **(a)** triangular trapezoid, −550, −450, −350 HU; **(b)** rectangular trapezoid, −550, −550, −350, −350 HU; **(c)** trapezoidal shape, −550, −500, −400, −350 HU.

tient 2, window width from −700 to −500 HU, 70% opacity, unshaded algorithm.

Adjustment of Tracheobronchial Transparency

For both the central (patient 1) and peripheral (patient 2) bronchi, the subjectively optimal appearance of the bronchographic images was obtained with a 70% opacity value (Fig 2f). The influence of this parameter was found to be limited to the creation of bronchographic images varying from overly dark (opacity value of 10%) to overly bright (opacity value of 90%). Adjustments of the opacity value were successively evaluated while the remaining parameters were preselected as follows: (*a*) patient 1, window width from −550 to −350 HU, window level of −450 HU, triangular trapezoid shape, unshaded algorithm; (*b*) patient 2, window width from −700 to −500 HU, window level of −450 HU, triangular trapezoid shape, unshaded algorithm.

Adjustment of Airway Wall Smoothness

Bronchographic images were obtained with the shaded, unshaded, and smooth algorithms. For both the central and peripheral bronchi, the shaded algorithm resulted in a nonuniform rendering of the airway wall (Fig 5a); the smooth algorithm, a blurry image (Fig 5b); and the unshaded algorithm, a slightly heterogeneous airway wall (Fig 5c). For both data sets, the unshaded algorithm was thus considered optimal. Adjustments of the volume-rendering algorithm were successively evaluated while the remaining parameters were preselected as follows: (*a*) patient 1, window width from −550 to −350 HU, window level of −450 HU, triangular trapezoid shape, 70% opacity value; (*b*) patient 2, window width from −700 to −500 HU, window level of −450 HU, triangular trapezoid shape, 70% opacity value.

Discussion

This volume-rendering technique is based on the selection of voxels located at the interface between the airway wall and the air column. It appears well suited to the depiction of volume-averaged CT data that characterize bronchographic images. To generate these images, the first step consists of determining the range of Hounsfield unit values of the voxels of interest to define the image sharpness. With the percentage classification, the attenuation values of voxels that are assumed to contain a given tissue form a Gaussian distribution around a central value that theoretically represents a voxel composed of 100% of that tissue type. Above and below the ideal value are ranges of attenuation values in voxels with the probability of containing 0%–100% of the tissue of interest (6). To retain voxels in the final image that are partially composed of air and soft tissue, we empirically selected ranges of Houns-

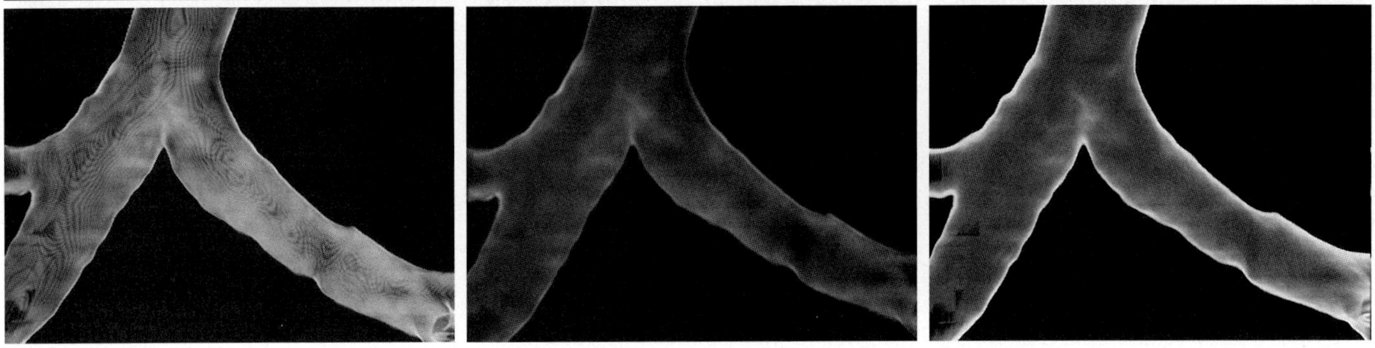

a. b. c.

Figure 5. Patient 1. Bronchographic images depict adjustment of the shading algorithm for central airways: **(a)** shaded, **(b)** smooth, **(c)** unshaded.

field units that corresponded to variable amounts of air and soft tissue within the selected voxels. At the level of the trachea and main stem bronchi, we found that a window width from −550 to −350 HU enabled selection of a continuous rim of voxels at the air and soft-tissue interface. When we selected voxels with lower attenuation values, the final image displayed an artificially narrowed air column; when we selected voxels with the highest attenuation value, the final image displayed a poorly defined and abnormally enlarged bronchographic view.

The voxels selected for the final rendering were highlighted on a minimum intensity projection image. For the trachea and main stem bronchi, the window level of the trapezoid was −450 HU (the average of +100 HU [the attenuation of bronchial wall] and −1,000 HU [the attenuation of air]), which corresponded to selection of voxels containing approximately one-half bronchial wall and one-half air (4). Theoretically, classification of more peripheral bronchi required selection of voxels with lower attenuation values to integrate more pronounced partial volume effects. At the level of the segmental and subsegmental bronchi, the bronchial wall is a thin structure with high attenuation, intermingled between two hypoattenuating regions (ie, the air column and the lung parenchyma). Ney et al (4,5) found that the smaller a structure, the closer its attenuation value is to that of air. We observed that a window width from −700 to −500 HU enabled optimal display of the segmental and subsegmental bronchi. The window level of −600 HU (the weighted average of +100 and −1,000 HU) in this trapezoid selection suggests that voxels containing approximately 20% bronchial wall and 80% air were retained in the final reconstruction.

The second parameter to be chosen at the console concerns the trapezoid shape, which influences the airway wall homogeneity. To evaluate the influence of this parameter on the overall image quality, the slope of the sides of the trapezoid was modified at the intersection of the sides of the trapezoid and the top, while the same threshold of Hounsfield units to be incorporated in the final image was maintained. Adjustment of the trapezoid shape was shown to minimally modify the quality of the bronchographic images. Nevertheless, we observed that use of a triangular trapezoid shape enabled creation of a homogeneous bronchographic image, but use of a rectangular or trapezoidal shape resulted in creation of an inhomogeneous bronchographic image.

The last two steps in generating volume-rendered images are selection of the opacity value and the shading option. The opacity index determines the relative transparency of the voxels incorporated into the image, and thus the tracheobronchial transparency. Johnson et al (1) found that modifications in opacity result in altered visualization of structures that are positioned posteriorly to other structures and can enable visualization of anatomic structures through more anteriorly positioned structures. Because our goal was to visualize airways exclusive of surrounding structures, modifications of this parameter did not interfere with the final rendering. Subjectively, we found that 70% opacity enabled optimal bronchographic appearance. Modifications in the shading option, which determines the airway wall smoothness, demonstrated that neither the shaded nor the smooth algorithms were suitable for use in the volume-rendering technique. For both central and peripheral bronchi, the shaded algorithm resulted in nonuniform rendering of the airway wall, and the smooth algorithm resulted in creation of blurry images. The unshaded algorithm resulted in creation of bronchographic images that were similar to conventional bronchograms, and this algorithm was considered optimal.

Unlike shaded surface display and maximum intensity projection options, which make use of approximately 10% of a data set, it is usually considered that this volume-rendering technique makes use of the entire data set (1,6). This assumption cannot be validated, however, as this technique is similar to the thresholding technique and excludes all but the voxels of interest, namely the voxels of the interface between air and airway wall. As in the reconstruction processes for shaded surface display and maximum intensity projection, the data set in the volume-rendering technique must be edited before the shading algorithm can be applied. Otherwise, all the air column voxels within the data set will be retained in the final reconstruction, resulting in depiction of not only the trachea and main bronchi but also of the intraparenchymal airways and the air located in the esophagus. Consequently, this volume-rendering technique is prone to inaccuracies potentially generated by manually drawing around the airway of interest. This is of minor importance at the level of the trachea and central airways but may be more important at the level of the peripheral airways, where the editing process requires cooperation between the technician and the radiologist at the console. Tracheal reconstructions can be obtained rapidly, but the creation of bronchographic images of the peripheral airways requires a time-consuming manual editing step.

The present implementation of the volume-rendering technique has obvious limitations. First, it does not allow active display of the three-dimensional data set and, thus, precludes rapid reorientation of the image on the workstation console to select the optimal projection. Moreover, the image display parameters could not be modified as quickly as is possible with real-time interactive rendering (1). After the editing step, the three-dimensional reconstruction was obtained within 5 minutes, but 1–2 minutes were needed to modify the display each time a parameter was modified. Graphics hardware accelerates real-time volume rendering and allows modification of the transfer function or rotation of the volume around any axis with results available within a fraction of a second (1). We attempted to evaluate the effect of each parameter of the virtual rendering technique on the final image, but this goal could be achieved only partially because four successive parameters had to be selected before a given reconstruction could be generated. To overcome this methodologic difficulty, we implemented a preliminary step to define the a priori optimal parameters. On the basis of a consensus reading, the following parameters were selected as optimal: selection of voxels from −700 to −300 HU, triangular trapezoid shape, 70% opacity value, and unshaded algorithm. We performed this study to validate each of these parameters by modifying each parameter separately while preselecting the remaining empirically selected optimal parameters.

In conclusion, our findings suggest that this volume-rendering technique has the potential to create diagnostically useful images of the bronchial tree. Unlike conventional bronchograms, these bronchographic images can depict airway anatomy in any orientation on the basis of a single data set obtained without administration of contrast medium. Despite a few technical limitations, the technique appears applicable in clinical practice, and the parameters can be adjusted easily by the radiologist at the workstation. The entire tracheobronchial tree cannot be depicted at thin-section spiral CT, but a region of interest can be focused on to find a compromise between z-axis coverage and spatial resolution. Future studies are needed to demonstrate whether this volume-rendering technique can be applied broadly in the evaluation of airway disorders and to rigorously compare results to those obtained with alternative reconstruction techniques.

References

1. Johnson PT, Heath DG, Bliss DF, Cabral B, Fishman EK. Three-dimensional CT: real-time interactive volume rendering. AJR 1996; 167:581–583.
2. Johnson PT, Heath DG, Kuszyk BS, Fishman EK. CT angiography with volume rendering: advantages and applications in splanchnic vascular imaging. Radiology 1996; 200:564–568.
3. Johnson PT, Heath DG, Kuszyk BS, Fishman EK. CT angiography: thoracic vascular imaging with interactive volume rendering. J Comput Assist Tomogr 1997; 21:110–114.
4. Ney DR, Kuhlman JE, Hruban RH, Ren H, Hutchins GM, Fishman EK. Three-dimensional CT volumetric reconstruction and display of the bronchial tree. Invest Radiol 1990; 25:736–742.
5. Ney DR, Fishman EK, Magid D. Volumetric rendering of computed tomography data: principles and techniques. Comput Graphics Appl 1990; 10:24–32.
6. Kuszyk BS, Heath DG, Bliss DF, Fishman EK. Skeletal 3-D CT: advantages of volume rendering over surface rendering. Skeletal Radiol 1996; 25:207–214.

Byung Gil Choi, MD
Hak Hee Kim, MD
Bum-soo Kim, MD
Ki Tae Kim, MD
Kyung Sub Shinn, MD
Seok Whan Moon, MD

Index terms:
Lung, biopsy, 60.126
Lung, nodule, 60.30, 60.3115
Lung neoplasms, surgery, 60.30

Radiology 1998; 208:399–401

[1] From the Department of Radiology, Kangnam Saint Mary's Hospital, 505 Banpo-Dong, Seocho-Ku, Seoul 137-701, South Korea (B.G.C., H.H.K., B.K., K.T.K., K.S.S.), and the Department of Radiology and Chest Surgery, College of Medicine, the Catholic University of Korea, Seoul (S.W.M.). Received October 30, 1997; revision requested January 6, 1998; revision received February 24; accepted March 27. Supported in part by the Clinical Research Fund of the College of Medicine, Catholic University of Korea. **Address reprint requests to** B.G.C.

Author contributions:
Guarantors of integrity of entire study, B.G.C., H.H.K.; study concepts, H.H.K., S.W.M.; study design, B.G.C., H.H.K.; definition of intellectual content, B.G.C.; literature research, B.G.C.; clinical studies, B.G.C., H.H.K., B.K., S.W.M.; data acquisition and analysis, B.G.C.; manuscript preparation and editing, B.G.C.; manuscript review, B.G.C., H.H.K., K.T.K., K.S.S.

Pulmonary Nodules: CT-guided Contrast Material Localization for Thoracoscopic Resection[1]

Fifteen patients underwent computed tomography (CT)–guided contrast material localization of pulmonary nodules, with barium and indigo carmine stain used in five patients, iodized oil and indigo carmine stain in five, and water-soluble contrast material and indigo carmine stain in five before fluoroscopy-assisted thoracoscopic resection. Contrast material localization was successful in all cases, and the surgeon confirmed accurate localization. CT-guided contrast material localization is simple and useful for thoracoscopic resection.

The rate of detection of small pulmonary lesions has recently increased owing to advances in radiologic technology. For small lesions, histopathologic diagnosis by means of transbronchial or percutaneous biopsy can be difficult. Development of endoscopic video and corresponding instrumentation has expanded the role of thoracoscopy, including that in the resection of peripheral pulmonary nodules (1). Identification of small or deep lesions is difficult during thoracoscopic surgery, however, because of inadequate palpation and the possibility of iatrogenic lung collapse.

Localization of pulmonary nodules with a percutaneous hook wire or a staining method with methylene blue and computed tomographic (CT) guidance has been previously reported (2–6). In our experience, the hook wire was dislodged during the thoracoscopic procedure. In some cases, the surgeon could not find the stained lesion because of extensive anthracotic pigmentation or a delay in the thoracoscopic procedure. For better localization, we present our experience with CT-guided contrast material localization of pulmonary nodules with contrast materials and indigo carmine stain before fluoroscopy-assisted thoracoscopic resection.

Materials and Methods

From December 1996 through August 1997, 15 consecutive patients (10 men and five women; age range, 22–74 years; mean age, 52.4 years) with questionable pulmonary nodules were included in this prospective study. All nodules were small or deep below the pleural surface, and results of transbronchial or percutaneous biopsy were not diagnostic because of insufficient material. The maximal diameter of the nodules ranged from 4 to 32 mm (mean ± 1 standard deviation, 14.2 mm ± 5.9). The distance from the visceral pleura to the nodule ranged from 5 to 30 mm (mean, 15.2 mm ± 8.4). All patients underwent plain chest radiography and CT followed by CT-guided contrast material localization for thoracoscopic resection. The study protocol was approved by our institutional review board, and written informed consent was obtained from each patient.

The patients were placed on the CT table in the supine, prone, or lateral decubitus position that allowed easy access to the nodule. The nodules were localized on 4- or 8-mm-thick axial CT sections obtained during inspiration. With use of alignment lights and a grid marker, the site for needle placement was selected. A 1% procaine hydrochloride solution was used for local anesthesia. A calibrated 20-gauge Chiba needle (Manan Medical Products, Northbrook, Ill) was advanced into the nodule. The needle position was confirmed at repeated CT. Approximately 2–3 mL of nonsoluble contrast material (barium or iodized oil [Lipiodol Ultra Fluide; Laboratoire Guerbet, Aulnay-sous-Bois, France]) or water-soluble contrast material (Optiray 320; Mallinckrodt Medical, Pointe Claire, Quebec, Canada) was injected within or near the nodule (Figure, parts a, b), and then 1 mL of indigo carmine stain (Inverin, Galway, Ireland) was injected through the needle pathway and visceral pleura while the needle was withdrawn.

All lesions were localized and marked, with barium and indigo carmine stain in five patients, iodized oil and indigo carmine stain in five, and water-soluble contrast material and indigo carmine stain in five. In the five cases of barium localization, 25–200 wt/vol thin barium (Solotop; Taejoon, Seoul, South Korea) was used. Barium powder was autoclaved with ethylene oxide gas, and saline solution was added. All but one of the patients underwent fluoroscopy-assisted thoracoscopic resection within 3–6 hours after localization.

Results

CT-guided contrast material localization was successful in all cases, and the surgeon confirmed accurate localization (Figure, parts c–e). The average time necessary for the localization procedure was 36 minutes (range, 25–47 minutes). Minor complications of this procedure included two cases of asymptomatic small pneumothorax and two cases of asymptomatic small pulmonary hemorrhage.

In a patient who underwent thoracoscopic resection 24 hours after localization, the injected water-soluble contrast material could not be identified during fluoroscopy-assisted thoracoscopy owing to dilution of the contrast material. In another patient, who was a chain-smoker, extreme anthracotic pigmentation interfered with the identification of injected indigo carmine stain. Well-defined staining of the lesion with contrast material, however, allowed thoracoscopic localization with fluoroscopic guidance. All lesions were completely excised with adequate safe margins and were histopathologically confirmed as two primary lung cancers (adenocarcinomas), seven metastases (three renal cell carcinomas, one peripheral primitive neuroectodermal tumor, one malignant round small cell tumor, one atypical carcinoid, and one adenocarcinoma), and six benign lesions (three cases of focal chronic inflammation, two hamartomas, and one case of tuberculosis).

Discussion

Recent developments in thoracic surgery have broadened the applications for thoracoscopy (7,8). Fluoroscopy-assisted thoracoscopic resection is a minimally invasive procedure used either as a therapeutic means or when findings at transbronchial or percutaneous needle aspiration biopsy fail to yield a diagnosis of benign disease in an indeterminate pulmonary nodule.

Because the thoracoscopic procedure is performed through three narrow access routes (or holes), the nodule cannot be palpated directly by hand. The surgeon should use an endoscopic grasping instrument (Endofinger; Ethicon Endo-Surgery, Cincinnati, Ohio) in a repeated groping manner to localize the nodule. After this time-consuming maneuver, wedge resection is performed. Currently, the major factor limiting the success of thoracoscopic resection is difficulty in localization of the pulmonary nodule when it is small and deep. To facilitate resection in such cases, percutaneous localization of pulmonary nodules with a hook wire or methylene blue stain has been performed (2–6). Several problems could occur with hook-wire localization: contamination due to cutting of the outer surface of the wire, pneumothorax, bleeding, and dislodgment of the hook wire from its proper position (3,4,6). Dislodgment has been due mostly to the traction maneuver during the surgical procedure or to movement of the patient. In two of our three cases, dislodgment of the hook wire was detected during thoracoscopy.

Identification of methylene blue staining could be difficult owing to anthracotic pigmentation or diffusion across the lung surface (5,6). In our patient who was a chain-smoker, anthracotic pigmentation and the indigo carmine–stained pulmonary surface could not be differentiated. Our combination methods allowed thoracoscopic localization with fluoroscopic guidance. With water-soluble contrast material, some diffusion to surrounding parenchyma and absorption occurred, as it did with methylene blue and indigo carmine stains. Because of easy diffusion and absorption of water-soluble contrast material, thoracoscopic localization was difficult. No difficulty, however, was encountered when barium or iodized oil were used. After 24 hours, no injected contrast material was identified at fluoroscopy in any case.

Thoracoscopic resection of the nodule is recommended soon after localization because water-soluble contrast material diffuses early. Barium and iodized oil tend to stay longer within the nodule. On the basis of our experience, thoracoscopy may be performed up to 6 hours after localization with barium or iodized oil. Among contrast materials, iodized oil is preferred because of early diffusion and absorption of water-soluble contrast material and difficulty in preparing thin, aseptic barium. Although minimal spread of contrast materials over the mass was noted in all cases during CT-guided localization, substantial obliteration of the mass was not observed.

In the patient with a 32-mm-diameter nodule, performance of thoracoscopic excision may not have been wise. It was possible, however, to remove the mass by means of additional incision of the skin after thoracoscopic wedge resection. The mass was 2.6 cm beneath the pleura, and previous percutaneous CT-guided biopsy failed to provide an adequate specimen.

Indigo carmine stain, barium, iodized oil, and water-soluble contrast material were nearly completely washed out during histologic preparation and we noticed no effect, such as denaturation of tissue, decoloration of staining, or uneven slicing of frozen or paraffin sections. Barium particles that remained within the nodule were too small to interfere with microscopic examination.

Advantages of our CT-guided contrast material localization include the following: (*a*) no major complications; (*b*) good visualization of the lesion during fluoroscopy-assisted thoracoscopic resection, especially with the use of barium or iodized oil; (*c*) confirmation of exact resection of the tissue containing contrast material by means of tissue radiography; (*d*) no dislodgment during the procedure or movement of the patient; (*e*) insurance of an adequately safe margin in case of suspected malignancy and of minimal excision in case of benignity; (f) reduction of surgical time; and (*g*) no need for an immediate thoracoscopic procedure after localization if barium or iodized oil is used, since there is less diffusion to surrounding tissue.

In summary, CT-guided contrast material localization of pulmonary nodules is proved to be a simple and useful method for thoracoscopic resection. The contrast material was correctly injected within or near the nodule, and subsequent thoracoscopic resection was successfully accomplished.

References

1. Mack MJ, Hazelrigg SR, Landreneau RJ, Acuff TE. Thoracoscopy for the diagnosis of the indeterminate solitary pulmonary nodule. Ann Thorac Surg 1993; 56:825–830.
2. Shah RM, Spirn PW, Salazar AM, et al. Localization of peripheral pulmonary nodules for thoracoscopic excision: value of CT-guided wire placement. AJR 1993; 161: 279–283.

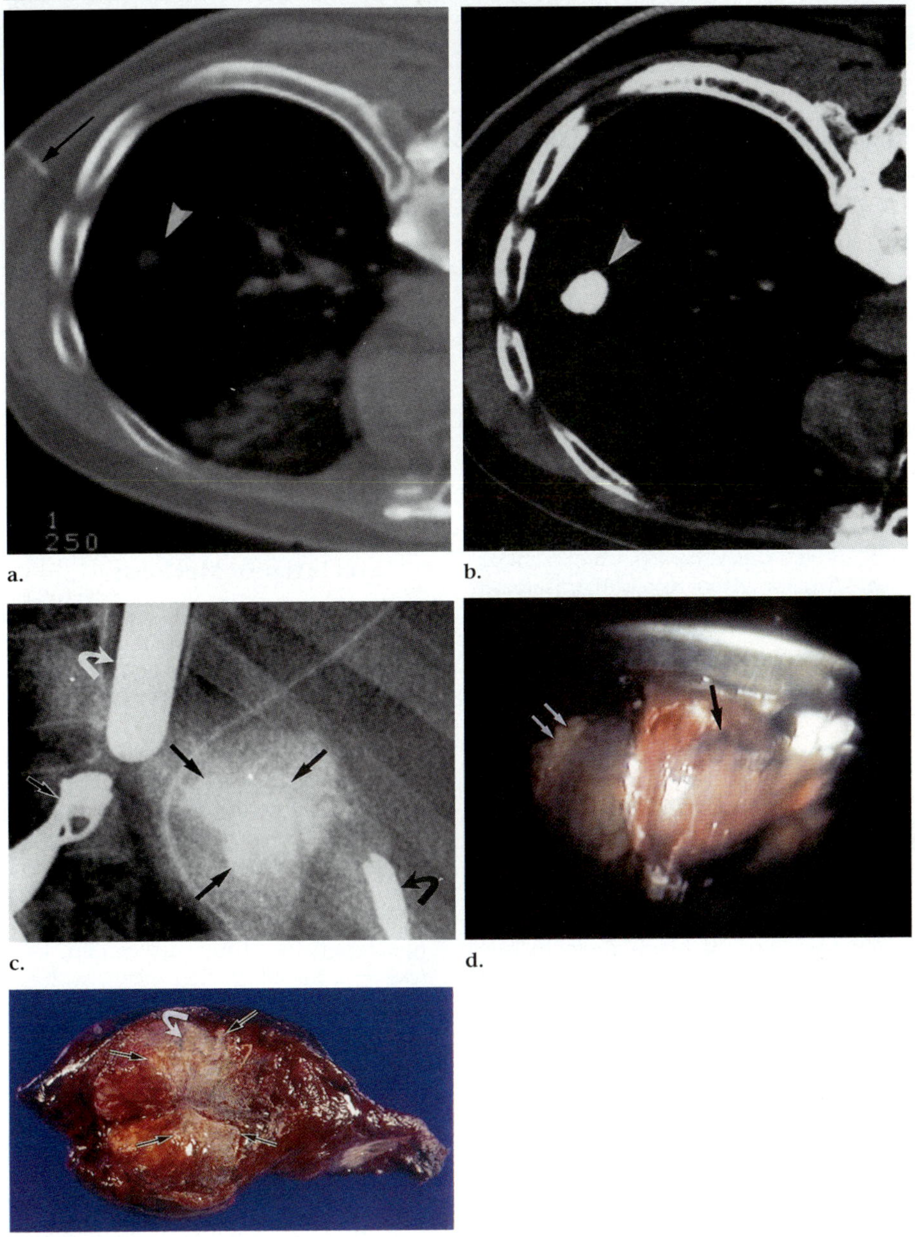

Pulmonary nodule in a 74-year-old man. **(a)** Axial CT scan obtained with the patient prone shows a 1-cm-diameter small pulmonary nodule (arrowhead) in the periphery of the right lower lobe. Pneumonic consolidation is seen in the right middle lobe. A biopsy needle (arrow) is seen in the thoracic wall. **(b)** Axial CT scan obtained at the same level as **a** after localization with barium and indigo carmine stain shows the nodule (arrowhead) as larger and with high attenuation as a result of barium staining. **(c)** Fluoroscopic spot radiograph obtained during thoracoscopic surgery shows a densely opacified pulmonary nodule (large arrows) approached with the thoracoscopic grasping instrument (small arrow), linear stapler cutter (black curved arrow), and thoracoscope (white curved arrow). An electrocardiographic lead is also seen across the midline. **(d)** Thoracoscopic video image demonstrates whitish area (white arrows) within the nodule, indicating barium. Dark blue staining by indigo carmine is also seen (black arrow). **(e)** Cut section of the surgical specimen reveals a barium-stained area (straight arrows) within the nodule. Dark blue staining by indigo carmine is also seen (curved arrow). Adenocarcinoma was confirmed histopathologically.

3. Plunkett MB, Peterson MS, Landreneau RJ, Ferson PF, Posner MC. Peripheral pulmonary nodules: preoperative percutaneous needle localization with CT guidance. Radiology 1992; 185:274–276.
4. Templeton PA, Krasna M. Localization of pulmonary nodules for thoracoscopic resection: use of needle/wire breast-biopsy system. AJR 1993; 160:761–762.
5. Wicky S, Mayor B, Cuttat JF, Schnyder P. CT-guided localizations of pulmonary nodules with methylene blue injections for thoracoscopic resections. Chest 1994; 106: 1326–1328.
6. Lenglinger FX, Schwarz CD, Artmann W. Localization of pulmonary nodules before thoracoscopic surgery: value of percutaneous staining with methylene blue. AJR 1994; 163:297–300.
7. Wakabayashi A. Expanded applications of diagnostic and therapeutic thoracoscopy. J Thorac Cardiovasc Surg 1991; 102:721–723.
8. Lewis RJ, Caccavale RJ, Sisler GE. Imaged thoracoscopic lung biopsy. Chest 1992; 102:60–62.

Declan G. Sheppard, FRCR
Revathy B. Iyer, MD
Marc J. Fenstermacher, MD

Brachial Plexus: Demonstration at US[1]

Index terms:
Brachial plexus, MR, 276.12141
Brachial plexus, US, 276.1298
Neck, US, 276.1298
Nervous system, US, 276.1298

Radiology 1998; 208:402–406

[1] From the Department of Diagnostic Radiology, University of Texas M.D. Anderson Cancer Center, Box 57, 1515 Holcombe Blvd, Houston, TX 77030. Received December 2, 1997; revision requested December 23; revision received February 17, 1998; accepted April 3. **Address reprint requests to** R.B.I.

Five healthy volunteers underwent ultrasonography (US) to determine the feasibility of visualizing the brachial plexus. The roots, trunks, and cords could be identified in the supraclavicular and infraclavicular regions. The roots within the neural foramina and the epidural space could not be evaluated. US may play a complementary role in the evaluation of patients with brachial plexopathy.

Magnetic resonance (MR) imaging is currently the technique of choice for imaging the brachial plexus because of the method's multiplanar capabilities and excellent soft-tissue contrast, which allow components of the brachial plexus to be visualized from their origin at the cervical spine roots to the trunks and cords as they traverse the supraclavicular and axillary regions. The MR imaging features of the normal and abnormal brachial plexus have been described elsewhere (1,2). However, MR imaging is expensive, time-consuming, and not readily available. Additionally, to our knowledge, there is little experience in MR-guided biopsy techniques, although there has been a recent report on the use of computed tomography–guided brachial plexus biopsy (3).

Conversely, ultrasonography (US), in experienced hands, is noninvasive, relatively inexpensive, and quick to perform, giving it distinct advantages over MR imaging. US is already routinely used to identify disease in the supraclavicular and axillary regions, and there is an established record for US-guided biopsy techniques.

Although US has been used for imaging of peripheral nerves (4–7), to our knowledge there are no reports in the radiology literature of its use in imaging of the brachial plexus. Additionally, there are only a few reports in the anesthesia and pain literature of the successful use of US to help identify the brachial plexus during examination with regional anesthesia (8–11). Our aims were to determine the feasibility of imaging the brachial plexus with US and to establish a standard examination technique.

Materials and Methods

Five healthy volunteers (one man, four women; mean age, 34 years) underwent MR imaging and US of the brachial plexus. Written informed consent was obtained from each.

MR imaging was performed at 1.5 T (GE Medical Systems; Milwaukee, Wis) with a body coil. Axial, axial oblique, sagittal, and coronal oblique T1-weighted images were obtained to cover the brachial plexus from the spine to the axilla. Sequence parameters included the following: repetition time msec/echo time msec = 400–500/9; field of view, 20–24 cm; section thickness, 5 mm; intersection gap, 1.0 mm; and reconstruction matrix, 256×192–256.

No specific subject preparation was required for the US examination. All studies (Sonoline Elegra; Siemens Medical Systems, Iselin, NJ) were performed by radiologists (D.G.S., R.B.I., M.J.F.). Because there was no established technique for the US examination of the brachial plexus, we used various linear and curvilinear transducers, ranging from 5 to 10 MHz and found that a linear transducer of at least 7.5 MHz yielded the best results. We used a coronal oblique plane, of approximately 30°, to identify the roots after they exited the cervical foramina (Figs 1–3). We were not able to examine the roots within the neural foramina because of shadowing from bone. Identification of the most cephalic and caudal roots was not always possible, even with meticulous technique. After they exited the neural foramina, the roots and trunks were followed up longitudinally and inferiorly to the clavicle and were again identified in the infraclavicular region. The cords were then followed up longitudinally in

Author contributions:
Guarantors of integrity of entire study, R.B.I., M.J.F.; study concepts, D.G.S.; study design, D.G.S., R.B.I., M.J.F.; definition of intellectual content, D.G.S., R.B.I., M.J.F.; literature research, D.G.S.; clinical studies, D.G.S., R.B.I., M.J.F.; data acquisition and analysis, D.G.S., R.B.I., M.J.F.; manuscript preparation, D.G.S.; manuscript editing, D.G.S., R.B.I., M.J.F.; manuscript review, R.B.I., M.J.F.

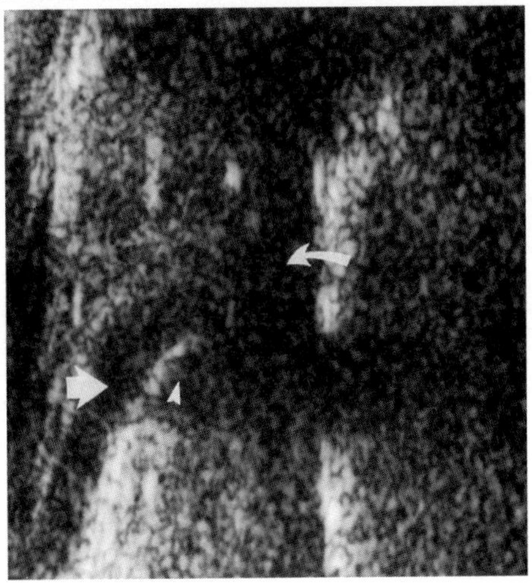

Figure 1. Coronal oblique US scan shows the roots (straight arrow) of the brachial plexus as they exit the neural foramina. Transverse processes (arrowhead) and the vertebral artery (curved arrow) are also demonstrated.

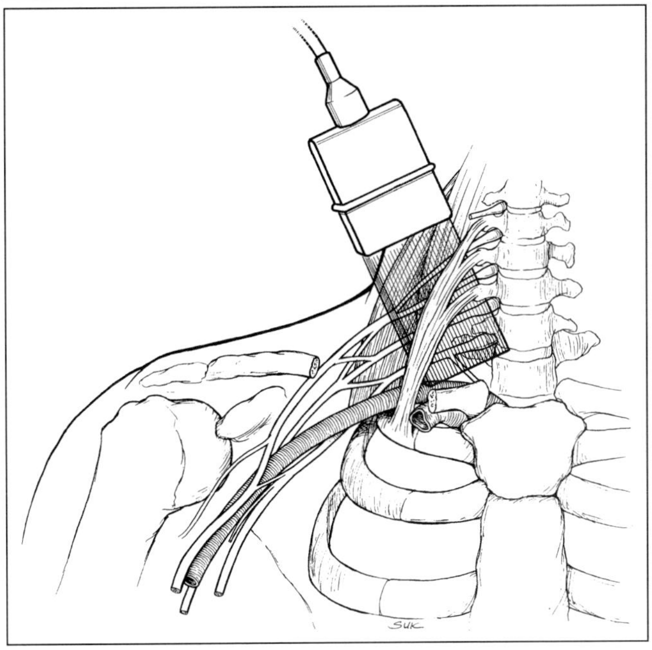

Figure 3. Diagram shows the position of the US probe in the coronal oblique plane to demonstrate the roots of the brachial plexus in longitudinal section as they exit the neural foramina.

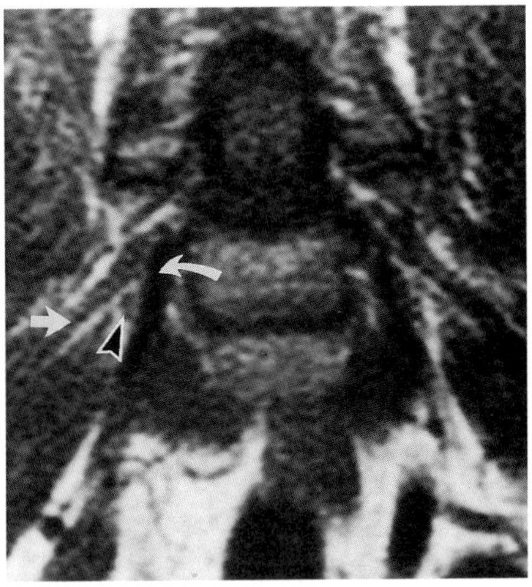

Figure 2. Coronal oblique T1-weighted MR image (400/9) shows the roots (straight arrow) of the brachial plexus as they exit the neural foramina. Transverse processes (arrowhead) and the vertebral artery (curved arrow) are also demonstrated.

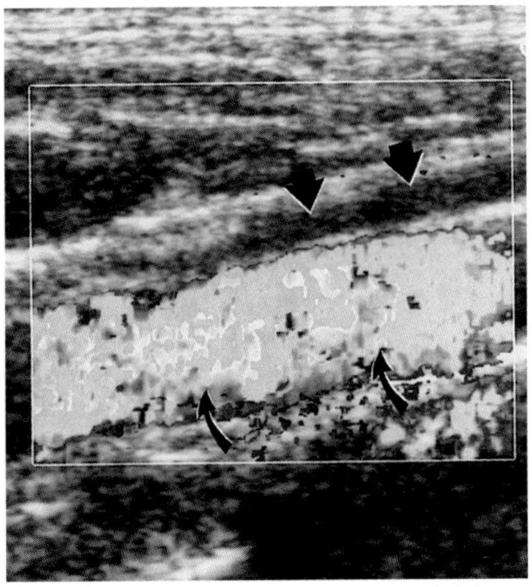

Figure 4. US scan of the infraclavicular fossa in a coronal oblique plane parallel to the axillary artery shows the cords (straight arrows) of the brachial plexus lying cephalad to the axillary artery (curved arrows).

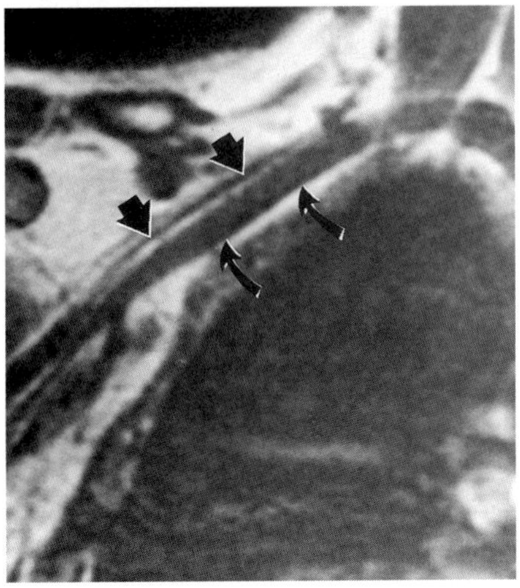

Figure 5. Coronal oblique T1-weighted MR image (400/9) of the infraclavicular fossa shows the cords (straight arrows) of the brachial plexus lying cephalad to the axillary artery (curved arrows).

relation to the subclavian and axillary arteries by using a plane running parallel to the vessels (Figs 4–6). Moving back to the immediate infraclavicular region, the probe was rotated through 90° into a plane at right angles to the vessels, and the trunks and cords were again followed up laterally into the axilla. After completing examination of the infraclavicular trunks and cords, we moved back into the supraclavicular region. The trunks were again identified posterior to the subclavian artery in a plane at right angles to the vessel (Figs 7–9). Moving cephalad up the neck as the trunks passed between the scalene muscles (Figs 10, 11), we converted the plane from sagittal or sagittal oblique (Fig 9) to axial oblique (Fig 12) and finally to axial. In the axial plane, the roots were then seen to dive deep toward the neural foramina.

The MR images were available at the time of the US studies and were used to confirm the identity of the components of the brachial plexus and the surrounding anatomy. We did not attempt, nor did we intend, to identify every component of the brachial plexus because these are not usually distinguished with conventional MR imaging. Our aims were instead to determine the normal US appearance of the brachial plexus, to identify its relationship to the surrounding anatomy, and to define a reproducible examination technique.

Results

Satisfactory US examinations were performed with the subjects in various scanning positions, from supine to lateral decubitus to seated upright. A semilateral decubitus position seemed optimal from the standpoint of subject and sonologist comfort. The brachial plexus was reliably identified in all five subjects, though subjects with long thin necks were more easily examined than those with shorter necks. Because the purpose of our study was to determine the feasibility and not the sensitivity or specificity of the technique, we deliberately chose subjects with a thin-to-average build.

The nerves appeared as hypoechoic structures with a thin hyperechoic rim. They appeared tubular on longitudinal scans and oval to round on transverse scans. The roots located centrally were larger than the trunks and cords located peripherally. An internal fascicular pattern was appreciated in the trunks and proximal cords, but it was not apparent in the roots.

In the supraclavicular region, we found that a plane at right angles to the subclavian artery (Figs 7–9) and an axial oblique plane (Figs 10–12) were the most reliable for accurate depiction of the anatomy, and the findings were the most reproducible. Careful technique must be used to follow up the individual roots in cross section because the roots are small and can be confused with muscle fascicles coursing in the same plane. It was difficult to follow up the roots in an axial plane as they passed deep toward the neural foramina. The technique was limited by the fact that we could not examine the epidural space and the C8 and T1 roots. US of the infraclavicular brachial plexus requires use of a combined approach at right angles or parallel to the subclavian and axillary arteries, although the plane parallel to the vessels is probably more useful. In addition, variable portions of the trunks behind the clavicle and in the infraclavicular region were difficult to follow up contiguously owing to problems of access.

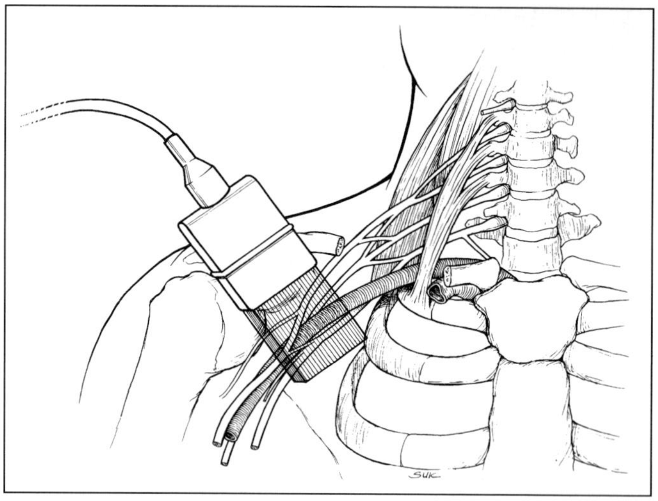

Figure 6. Diagram shows the position of the US probe in a plane parallel to the axillary artery to demonstrate the cords of the brachial plexus in longitudinal section in the infraclavicular fossa.

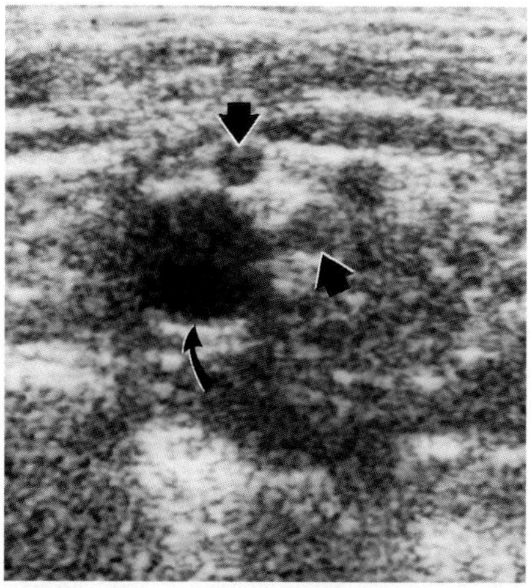

Figure 7. US scan of the supraclavicular fossa in a sagittal plane at right angles to the subclavian artery shows the trunks (straight arrows) of the brachial plexus lying posterior to the subclavian artery (curved arrow).

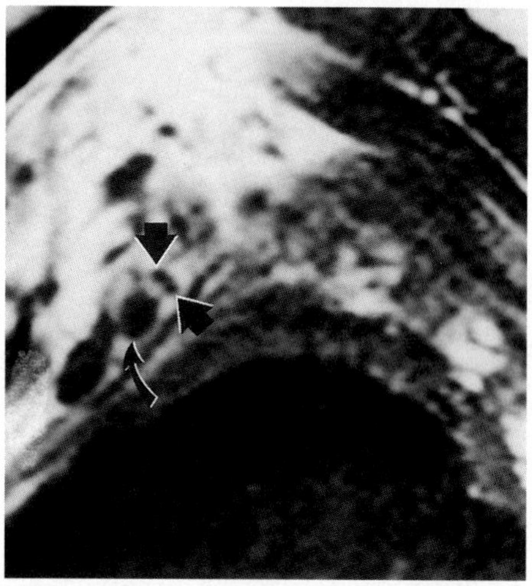

Figure 8. Sagittal T1-weighted MR image (400/9) of the supraclavicular fossa shows the trunks (straight arrows) of the brachial plexus lying posterior to the subclavian artery (curved arrow).

Discussion

The normal anatomy of the brachial plexus has been described previously (1,2), with considerable variation in the way in which the components of the brachial plexus are arranged and communicate with each other (Fig 13). Typically, the roots of the brachial plexus are formed by the union of the anterior rami from C5 to T1, with occasional contributions from C4 and T2. The exiting roots pass between the anterior and middle scalene muscles to form three trunks. As they pass beneath the clavicle, posterior and superior to the subclavian artery, they divide into anterior and posterior divisions, which subsequently unite to form three cords that surround or lie posterior to the axillary artery.

Normal peripheral nerves may appear as hypoechoic structures, which correspond to neuronal fascicles, separated by hyperechoic bands (4,5), or they may appear as echogenic fibrillar structures (6,7). A fascicular pattern has been identified in the median, ulnar, vagus, and sciatic nerves but not in the recurrent laryngeal nerve (5). Histologically, individual nerve fibers are grouped into fascicles surrounded by a thin perineurium. The entire nerve trunk is in turn surrounded by a thick epineurium, which is sonographically more echogenic (7). Our findings indicate that the brachial plexus has a hypoechoic fascicular pattern. Despite being thicker, the internal structure of the exiting roots (Fig 1) was not shown because of problems with resolution and the depth of the roots. As the trunks pass posterior to the subclavian artery (Fig 7) and between the anterior and middle

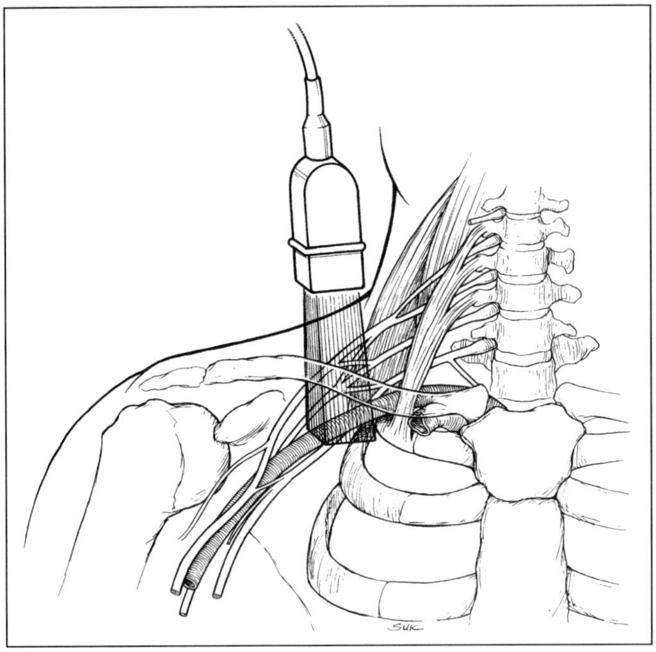

Figure 9. Diagram shows the position of the US probe in a plane at right angles to the subclavian artery to demonstrate the trunks of the brachial plexus in transverse section in the supraclavicular fossa.

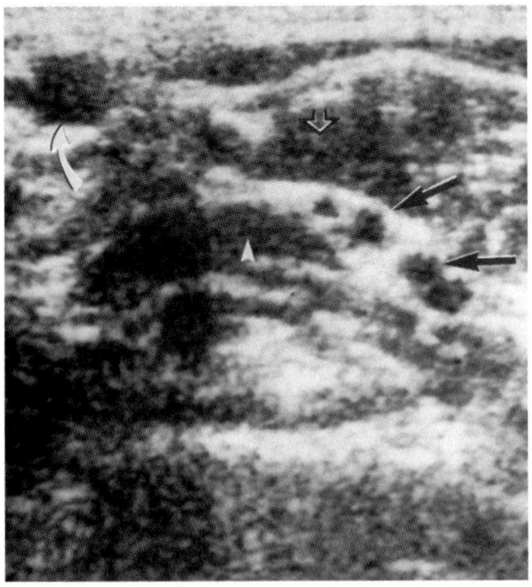

Figure 10. Axial oblique US scan shows the trunks (straight solid arrows) of the brachial plexus as they pass between the anterior (open arrow) and middle (arrowhead) scalene muscles. The external jugular vein (curved arrow) is also demonstrated.

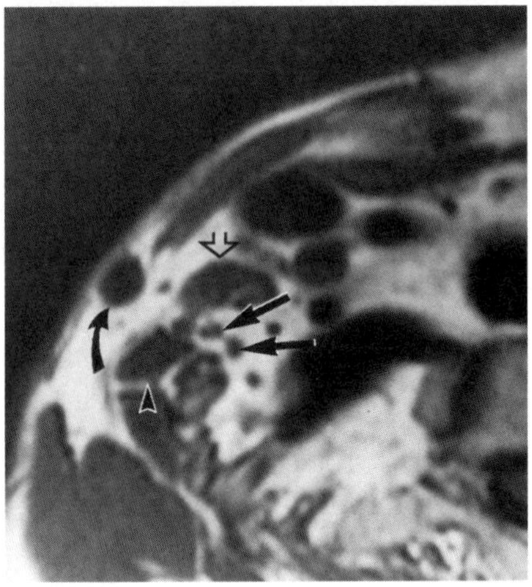

Figure 11. Axial oblique T1-weighted MR image (400/9) shows the trunks (straight solid arrows) of the brachial plexus as they pass between the anterior (open arrow) and middle (arrowhead) scalene muscles. The external jugular vein (curved arrow) is also demonstrated.

scalene muscles (Fig 10), it is possible to see the individual hypoechoic nerve fascicles. A thick, hyperechoic epineural layer was not apparent.

On the basis of our findings, we conclude that US examination of the brachial plexus is possible, although the technique has limitations. We have not proved that US depicts the brachial plexus as completely or as reliably as MR imaging. We found the MR studies very useful early on, given the nonstandard planes of examination. To this end, the availability of a good MR atlas would be of assistance and would allow most experienced sonologists to reproduce the technique. Whereas there is a learning curve, the technique can be learned in a few hours. Additionally, practicing of the technique in volunteers with thin necks makes identification of the normal anatomy and the components of the brachial plexus much easier. As the technique is likely to be requested in patients with additional cross-sectional imaging examinations, we believe the radiologist or sonologist should be actively involved in the performance of the study. As the entire brachial plexus cannot be visualized, each study will need to be tailored on the basis of the clinical and prior imaging findings. The use of color flow Doppler is essential. The nerves are small, are round on transverse scans and tubular on longitudinal scans, and can be easily mistaken for or confused with small vessels. After identification of the nerves, this is less of a problem provided the nerves are followed up contiguously.

Depending on the clinical indications, we believe that an acceptable study can be performed by identifying the trunks in the supraclavicular fossa posterior to the subclavian artery (Figs 7–9) by using a plane at right angles to the subclavian artery. The trunks can then be followed up cephalad as they pass between the scalene muscles (Figs 10–12) by using an axial oblique plane. The trunks lie posterior and lateral to carotid and internal jugular vessels and deep to the external jugular vein (Figs 10–11). The trunks and roots can be seen to dive deep toward the foramina by using an axial plane. A coronal oblique approach need be used only to confirm findings, to examine individual roots, and to identify the roots as they exit the foramina (Figs 1–3). By moving down to the infraclavicular region, the trunks and cords can be identified by using a plane parallel to the axillary artery (Figs 4–6).

US of the brachial plexus is technically feasible although the entire brachial plexus cannot be demonstrated. Ultimately the aim is to identify pathologic conditions, depicted as abnormal soft tissue or nodal disease impinging on the neurovascular bundle or as a distortion or loss of clarity of the neurovascular bundle as would be expected with radiation injury. Regardless of availability of MR imaging, we do not believe US will replace MR imaging as the primary diagnostic tool. Instead, US may play a complementary role in the evaluation of patients with brachial plexopathy by guiding percutaneous biopsy of areas shown to be abnormal at MR imaging or US. Additionally, with greater experience, an alternative diagnostic test may be available for use in patients unable to undergo MR imaging.

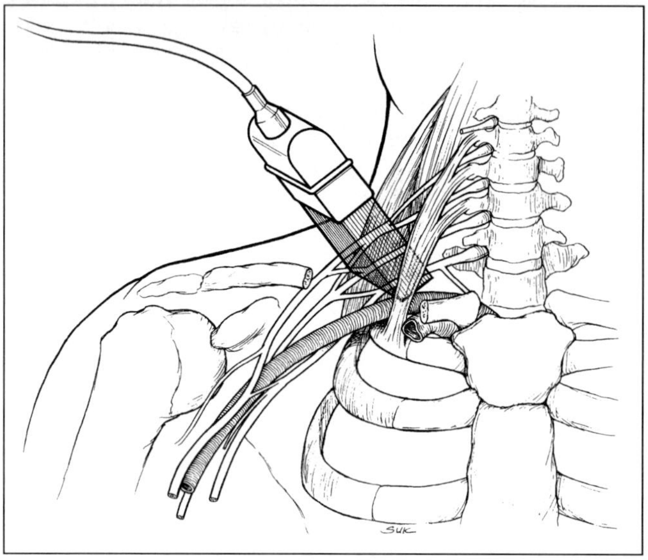

Figure 12. Diagram shows the position of the US probe in an axial oblique plane to demonstrate the trunks of the brachial plexus in transverse section as they pass between the anterior and middle scalene muscles.

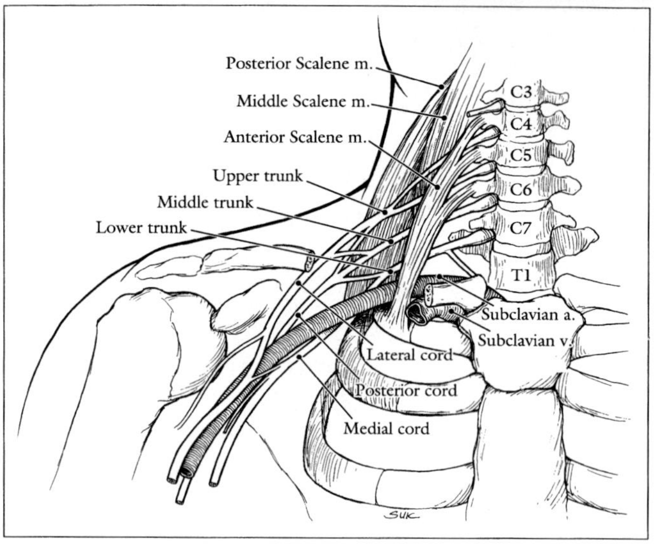

Figure 13. Diagram shows the idealized normal anatomy of the brachial plexus. *a* = artery, *m* = muscle, *v* = vein.

Acknowledgments: We thank the US and MR imaging technologists and Beth Notzon of Scientific Publications at our institution for their invaluable assistance. We also thank Ian Suk for his illustrations and Kelly Duggan and Bryan Gammon of Imaging Photography and Digital Services in the Department of Diagnostic Radiology at our institution.

References

1. Mukherji SK, Castillo M, Wagle AG. The brachial plexus. Semin Ultrasound CT MR 1996; 17:519–538.
2. Iyer RB, Fenstermacher MJ, Libshitz HI. MR imaging of the treated brachial plexus. AJR 1996; 167:225–229.
3. Cole JW, Quint DJ, McGillicuddy JE, Murphy KP. CT-guided brachial plexus biopsy. AJNR 1997; 18:1420–1422.
4. Solbiati L, De Pra L, Ierace T, Bellotti E, Derchi LE. High-resolution sonography of the recurrent laryngeal nerve: anatomical and pathological considerations. AJR 1985; 145:989–993.
5. Silvestri E, Martinoli C, Derchi LE, Bertolotto M, Chiaramondia M, Rosenberg I. Echotexture of peripheral nerves: correlation between US and histological findings and criteria to differentiate tendons. Radiology 1995; 197:291–296.
6. Graif M, Seton A, Nerubai J, Horoszowski H, Itzchak Y. Sciatic nerve: sonographic evaluation and anatomic-pathological considerations. Radiology 1991; 181:405–408.
7. Graif M. Peripheral nerves. In: Fornage BD, ed. Musculoskeletal ultrasound. New York, NY: Livingstone, 1995; 73–83.
8. Du P, La Grange P, Foster PA, Pretorius LK. Application of the Doppler ultrasound bloodflow detector in supraclavicular brachial plexus block. Br J Anaesth 1978; 50:965–967.
9. Ting PL, Sivagnanaratnam V. Ultrasonographic study of the spread of local anesthetic during axillary brachial plexus block. Br J Anaesth 1989; 63:326–329.
10. Friedl W, Fritz T. Ultrasound assisted brachial plexus anesthesia. Chirurg 1992; 63:759–760. [German]
11. Kapral S, Krafft P, Eibenberger K, Fitzgerald R, Gosch M, Weinstabl C. Ultrasound-guided supraclavicular approach for regional anesthesia of the brachial plexus. Anesth Analg 1994; 78:507–513.

Frank G. Shellock, PhD
John V. Crues, MD

Index terms:
Aneurysm, cerebral, 17.73
Extremities, MR, 40.1214
Head, MR, 10.1214
Magnetic resonance (MR), safety
Radiology and radiologists, iatrogenic injury

Radiology 1998; 208:407–409

Abbreviations:
ASTM = American Society for Testing and Materials
FDA = U.S. Food and Drug Administration

[1] From the Department of Radiology, School of Medicine, University of Southern California, Los Angeles (F.G.S.), and Radnet, Los Angeles, Calif (J.V.C.). From the 1997 RSNA scientific assembly. Received December 18, 1997; revision requested February 18, 1998; revision received March 2; accepted April 13. Supported in part by Lunar, Madison, Wis, and Esaote, Milan, Italy. **Address reprint requests to** F.G.S., 7511 McConnell Ave, Los Angeles, CA 90045.

Author contributions:
Guarantor of integrity of entire study, F.G.S.; study concepts, F.G.S., J.V.C.; study design, F.G.S., J.V.C.; definition of intellectual content, F.G.S., J.V.C.; literature research, F.G.S.; experimental studies, F.G.S.; data acquisition, F.G.S.; data analysis, F.G.S.; statistical analysis, F.G.S.; manuscript preparation, F.G.S.; manuscript editing, F.G.S.; manuscript review, F.G.S.; J.V.C.

Aneurysm Clips: Assessment of Magnetic Field Interaction Associated with a 0.2-T Extremity MR System[1]

Twenty-two different aneurysm clips were tested by means of the deflection angle test for magnetic field interaction associated with a 0.2-T extremity magnetic resonance (MR) system. At the opening of the magnet bore and 5 inches (13 cm) and 10 inches (25 cm) away from the magnet bore, respectively, deflection angles were 14°, 2°, and 0° for one clip and were 17°, 4°, and 0° for another, and were 0° for the remaining 20 clips. Because the patient's head does not enter the magnet bore, extremity MR imaging of patients with the aneurysm clips evaluated in this study should be safe.

Aneurysm clips are typically used for the surgical management of intracranial aneurysms and arteriovenous malformations (1). The presence of certain types of aneurysm clips represents a strict contraindication for magnetic resonance (MR) procedures because strong, magnetically induced forces can move or displace these implants and cause serious injuries or death (2–13). In contrast, patients with aneurysm clips that are nonferromagnetic or weakly ferromagnetic can safely undergo MR procedures (3–7,9–13).

In 1993, a specially designed, low-field-strength (0.2-T) MR system became available for MR imaging of the extremities (14–18). A major advantage of this extremity MR system is that it can be located in a relatively small space (eg, approximately 100 sq ft [9 m²]) without the need for a special power source, magnetic field shielding, or radio-frequency shielding (15,16). Currently, this is the only commercially available extremity MR system approved for use in the United States by the U.S. Food and Drug Administration (FDA). MR imaging with the extremity MR system has been demonstrated to provide a sensitive, accurate, and reliable assessment of various pathologic musculoskeletal conditions (14–18).

Because of the unique design features of the extremity MR system, which includes a low-field-strength static magnetic field with a relatively small fringe field, and in consideration of how patients are positioned for MR procedures with this device (ie, only the body part imaged is placed within the magnet bore while the rest of the body remains outside), it may be possible to safely perform imaging of patients with aneurysm clips, even if the clips are made of ferromagnetic materials. Therefore, the purpose of this investigation was to assess the magnetic field interaction for a variety of different aneurysm clips exposed to the 0.2-T extremity MR system.

Materials and Methods

Extremity MR System

A 0.2-T MR system (Artoscan; Lunar, Madison, Wis, and Esaote, Genoa, Italy) was used in this investigation (14–18). In this MR system, a small-bore permanent magnet is used to image extremities (eg, feet, ankles, knees, hands, forearms, wrists, and elbows). With the ergonomic design of the extremity MR system, the body part of interest is placed inside the magnet bore, with the patient positioned seated or supine, depending on the body part imaged. The entire MR system weighs approximately 800 kg and has a built-in radio-frequency shield, multiple body-part–specific extremity coils, and 10 mT/m magnetic gradients. The 5-G boundary line extends approximately 0.6 m from the opening of the magnet bore. Because of the unique aspects of the design, use, and magnetic field characteristics of this MR system, these data pertain to the magnetic field interaction for only the aneurysm clips and the extremity MR system used in this investigation.

Aneurysm Clips

Twenty-two different aneurysm clips were tested for magnetic field interactions associated with the 0.2-T extremity MR system. These aneurysm clips were selected because they represent the various types of aneurysm clips used in patients in the past and the present for temporary or permanent treatment of aneurysms or arteriovenous malformations. Owing to the reported variability in magnetic qualities for these implants (7), an effort was made to include aneurysm clips made from materials known to be nonferromagnetic or weakly ferromagnetic.

The following aneurysm clips were evaluated in this study:

1. Heifetz (17-7PH), 8-mm straight blade, Weck, Triangle Park, NJ.
2. McFadden Vari-Angle (MP35N), microclip, 9-mm straight blade, Codman, Johnson & Johnson Professional, Raynham, Mass).
3. McFadden Vari-Angle (MP35N), microclip, 9-mm straight fenestrated blade, Codman, Johnson & Johnson Professional.
4. Perneczky (stainless steel alloy), curved blade, Zeppelin Chirurgische Instruments, Pullach, Germany.
5. Sugita (Elgiloy), 8-mm straight blade, large aneurysm clip for permanent occlusion, Mizuho America, Beverly, Mass.
6. Sugita (Elgiloy), bent blade, mini aneurysm clip for temporary occlusion, Mizuho America.
7. Sugita (Elgiloy), bent blade, standard aneurysm clip for temporary occlusion, Mizuho America.
8. Sugita (Elgiloy), bent fenestrated blade, large aneurysm clip for permanent occlusion, Mizuho America.
9. Sugita (Elgiloy), sideward CVD bayonet, standard aneurysm clip for permanent occlusion, Mizuho America.
10. Sundt AVM Micro Clip (MP35N), 4-mm straight blade, Codman, Johnson & Johnson Professional.
11. Sundt Slim-Line Temporary Clip (MP35N), 10-mm straight blade, Codman, Johnson & Johnson Professional.
12. Sundt Slim-Line Graft Clip (MP35N), 8-mm straight blade, Codman, Johnson & Johnson Professional.
13. Sundt-Kees Slim-Line (MP35N), 9-mm fenestrated straight blade, Codman, Johnson & Johnson Professional.
14. Sundt-Kees Slim-Line (MP35N), 9-mm straight blade, Codman, Johnson & Johnson Professional.
15. Spetzler Titanium (commercially pure titanium), single turn, 9-mm straight blade, Elekta Instruments, Atlanta, Ga.
16. Spetzler Titanium (commercially pure titanium), double turn, 9-mm straight blade, Elekta Instruments.
17. Spetzler Titanium (commercially pure titanium), single turn, 13-mm straight blade, Elekta Instruments.
18. Spetzler Titanium (commercially pure titanium), double turn, 13-mm straight blade, Elekta Instruments.
19. Yasargil model FD (stainless steel alloy), 9-mm straight blade, Aesculap, South San Francisco, Calif.
20. Yasargil model FE (Phynox), 9-mm straight blade, Aesculap.
21. Yasargil model FE 750 (Phynox), 9-mm straight blade.
22. Yasargil model FE 780 (Phynox), 15-mm straight blade, Aesculap.

Assessment of Magnetic Field Attraction

Ex vivo testing was performed with the aneurysm clips to determine translational attraction to the 0.2-T static magnetic field (2,9,10,13). This procedure, called "the deflection angle test," was conducted with the aneurysm clips in three positions relative to the extremity MR system. These are representative of the possible positions for a patient's head during MR imaging under "worst case" conditions (eg, MR imaging of the elbow performed of a patient with a relatively short upper extremity). Testing was performed (*a*) at the opening of the magnet bore, (*b*) 5 inches (13 cm) from the opening of the magnet bore, and (*c*) 10 inches (25 cm) from the opening of the magnet bore.

Each aneurysm clip was suspended from a 20-cm-long piece of 4.0 silk thread attached to a plastic protractor to allow measurement of the angle of deflection (2,9,10,13). One observer (F.G.S.) performed the measurements. The accuracy of this testing apparatus is $\pm 1°$. For each aneurysm clip, the deflection angle was measured three times, and the results were averaged

Ex vivo evaluation of magnetic field interactions for metallic implants usually includes testing to determine the presence of magnet-related torque force (13). The Petri dish test is typically used for this purpose (13). The implant is placed in a Petri dish with a millimeter scale etched on the underside and then positioned in the center of the MR system, where the effect of torque force is known to be the greatest (13,19). Because it is not physically possible for a patient with an aneurysm clip to have his or her head placed in the center of the extremity MR system, this type of testing was not performed.

Results

At the opening of the 0.2-T magnet bore and 5 inches (13 cm) and 10 inches (25 cm) away from the magnet bore, deflection angles for the Heifetz aneurysm clip were 14°, 2°, and 0°, respectively, for the Yasargil model FD aneurysm clip were 17°, 4°, and 0°, respectively, and for the remaining 20 clips were 0°.

Discussion

In this study, ex vivo deflection angle testing was performed to determine magnetic field interaction for a variety of aneurysm clips during exposure to a 0.2-T extremity MR system. The deflection angle test, originally described by New et al (9), was used because it is considered to be an accurate, reliable, and reproducible test. It has been used for more than 12 years to assess magnetic field–induced translational forces for many metallic objects in the MR environment (2,9,10,13). Furthermore, the American Society for Testing and Materials (ASTM) issued a standard for the evaluation of aneurysm clips in 1994 that specifically indicated use of the deflection angle test (2). The FDA also issued a draft document (20) that suggests determining the magnetic characteristics of aneurysm clips by means of the deflection angle test. This document also indicates evaluation of torque-related force, which was not necessary in this study.

In the ASTM report (2), the following operational definition of a nonferromagnetic aneurysm clip at 1.5-T MR imaging is given: "The clip is suspended at the end of a string and held stationary in the vertical direction (that is, perpendicular to the ground) while it is placed in position at the portal of the imaging magnet. Following release of the clip, the deflection of the string from the vertical is then observed. The magnetic force is less than the gravitational force (that is, the clip's weight) if the deflection of the string with respect to the vertical is less than 45°. The clip is then judged to be non-ferromagnetic and suitable for implantation."

On the basis of the safety criteria of the ASTM (2), the Heifetz (17-7PH) and Yasargil model FD aneurysm clips are acceptable in patients referred to undergo 0.2-T MR imaging because the magnetic field–induced translational forces are relatively small. That is, there would be no risk to patients with respect to movement or dislodgement of these specific aneurysm clips in the magnetic environment associated with this extremity MR system. In contrast, various studies (3,5–7,9,10) have reported that patients with Heifetz (17-7PH) and Yasargil model FD aneurysm clips should not undergo MR imaging in systems with high-field-strength static magnetic fields because of the strong attraction shown by these aneurysm clips, which would pose a potential hazard to patients. Depending on where the clips were tested relative to a 1.5-T MR system (ie, at the magnet bore entrance or at the point of the highest spatial gradient field, which is usually 30–40 cm away from the entrance), the deflection angles for the Heifetz and Yasargil model FD clips may be as high as 90°.

We tested aneurysm clips made of metals known to be nonferromagnetic or weakly ferromagnetic (eg, Phynox, Elgiloy, stainless steel) because of the variable findings in the study by Kanal et al (7). In our study, however, none of these aneurysm clips exhibited a deflection angle greater than 0°; therefore, MR procedures with the extremity MR system would be safe in patients with these aneurysm clips.

In conclusion, results of this study indicate that it is safe to perform MR imaging of patients with certain aneurysm clips in the 0.2-T extremity MR system. Owing to the unique design features of this extremity MR system and to the way patients are positioned (ie, the head does not enter the magnet bore), none of the aneurysm clips tested displayed substantial magnetic field interaction. These findings support use of this important diagnostic imaging modality to evaluate the extremities of patients with implanted aneurysm clips who are suspected of having musculoskeletal abnormalities.

References

1. Dujovny M, Kossovsky N, Kossowsky R, et al. Vascular clips: an historic and biomedical perspective. In: Fein JN, Flamm E, eds. Cerebral vascular surgery. New York, NY: Springer-Verlag, 1985; 997–1046.
2. American Society for Testing and Materials. Standard specification for the requirements and disclosure of self-closing aneurysm clips. In: Annual Book of ASTM Standards, 1994. Philadelphia, Pa: American Society for Testing and Materials, 1994.
3. Barrafato D, Henkelman RM. Magnetic resonance imaging and surgical clips. Can J Surg 1984; 27:509–512.
4. Becker R, Norfray J, Teitelbaum G, et al. MR imaging in patients with intracranial aneurysm clips. AJNR 1988; 9:885–889.
5. Dujovny M, Gundamja NR, Misra M, Alp MS. Aneurysm clips. Crit Rev Neurosurg 1997; 7:169–175.
6. Dujovny M, Kossovsky N, Kossovsky R, et al. Aneurysm clip motion during magnetic resonance imaging: in vivo experimental study with metallurgical factor analysis. Neurosurgery 1985; 17:543–548.
7. Kanal E, Shellock FG, Lewin JS. Aneurysm clip testing for ferromagnetic properties: clip variability issues. Radiology 1996; 200: 576–578.
8. Klucznik R, Carrier D, Pyka R, Haid R. Placement of a ferromagnetic intracerebral aneurysm clip in a magnetic field with a fatal outcome. Radiology 1993; 187:855–856.
9. New PFJ, Rosen BR, Brady TJ, et al. Potential hazards and artifacts of ferromagnetic and nonferromagnetic surgical and dental materials and devices in nuclear magnetic resonance imaging. Radiology 1983; 147:139–148.
10. Shellock FG, Crues J. High-field strength MR imaging and metallic biomedical implants: an ex vivo evaluation of deflection forces. AJR 1988; 151:389–392.
11. Shellock FG. Pocket guide to MR procedures and metallic objects: update 1997. New York, NY: Raven, 1997.
12. Kato Y, Sano H, Katada K, et al. Effects of new titanium cerebral aneurysm clips on MRI and CT images. Minim Invasive Neurosurg 1996; 39:82–85.
13. Shellock FG, Shellock VJ. Spetzler titanium aneurysm clip: compatibility at MR imaging. Radiology 1998; 206:838–841.
14. Barile A, Masiocchi C, Mastantuono M, Passariello R, Satragno L. The use of a "dedicated" MRI system in the evaluation of knee joint diseases. Clin Magn Reson Imaging 1995; 5:79–82.
15. Peterfy CG, Roberts T, Genant HK. Dedicated extremity MR imaging: an emerging technology. Radiol Clin North Am 1997; 35:1–20.
16. Franklin PD, Lemon RA, Barden HS. Accuracy of imaging the menisci on an in-office, dedicated, magnetic resonance imaging extremity system. Am J Sports Med 1998; 25:382–388.
17. Masciocchi C, Barile A, Navarra F, et al. Clinical experience of osteoarticular MRI using a dedicated system. MAGMA 1994; 2:545–550.
18. Shellock FG, Stone K, Crues JV. Development and clinical applications of kinematic MRI of the patellofemoral joint using an extremity MR system. Med Sci Sports Exerc (in press).
19. Kagetsu N, Litt A. Important considerations in measurement of attractive force on metallic implants in MR imagers. Radiology 1991; 179:505–508.
20. U.S. Food and Drug Administration. Guidance for testing MR interaction with aneurysm clips (draft document). Rockville, Md: U.S. Department of Health and Human Services, Center for Devices and Radiological Health, 1996.

David C. Alsop, PhD
John A. Detre, MD

Index terms:
Cerebral blood vessels, flow dynamics
Cerebral blood vessels, MR, 17.121413, 17.121419
Magnetic resonance (MR), echo planar, 17.121419
Magnetic resonance (MR), vascular studies, 17.121419

Radiology 1998; 208:410–416

Abbreviations:
CBF = cerebral blood flow
RF = radio frequency

[1] From the Departments of Radiology (D.C.A., J.A.D.) and Neurology (J.A.D.), University of Pennsylvania Medical Center, 3400 Spruce St, Philadelphia, PA 19104-4283. Received September 3, 1997; revision requested November 19; revision received February 27, 1998; accepted April 10. Supported in part by National Institutes of Health grants P30-MG93880 and P50-NS08803. D.C.A. supported in part by a Biomedical Engineering Research Grant from the Whitaker Foundation. J.A.D. supported in part by the National Institutes of Health grant NS01668. **Address reprint requests to** D.C.A.

See also the editorial by Jezzard (pp 296–299) in this issue.

Author contributions:
Guarantor of integrity of entire study, D.C.A.; study concepts and design, D.C.A., J.A.D.; definition of intellectual content, D.C.A., J.A.D.; literature research, D.C.A., J.A.D.; experimental studies, D.C.A., J.A.D.; data acquisition, D.C.A., J.A.D.; data analysis, D.C.A.; statistical analysis, D.C.A.; manuscript preparation, D.C.A.; manuscript editing, D.C.A., J.A.D.

Multisection Cerebral Blood Flow MR Imaging with Continuous Arterial Spin Labeling[1]

A method was evaluated to control for off-resonance saturation in noninvasive magnetic resonance imaging with continuous arterial spin labeling of cerebral blood flow. In phantoms and humans, application of amplitude-modulated radio-frequency irradiation during the control image corrected for saturation across the whole brain and made possible cerebral blood flow imaging in multiple sections at arbitrary angles to the labeling plane.

Measurement of regional cerebral blood flow (CBF) provides useful information about both cerebrovascular sufficiency and regional brain metabolism because resting CBF and tissue metabolism are often strongly coupled (1). CBF imaging with single photon emission computed tomography (CT), or SPECT, positron emission tomography, or PET, and xenon-enhanced CT have been used to evaluate a multitude of cerebral disorders including stroke (2), dementia (3), epilepsy (4), trauma (5), and neoplasms (6). Positron emission tomography of CBF has also been an important tool for mapping task-induced brain activity in normal and pathologic states (7). For most central nervous system disorders, magnetic resonance (MR) imaging provides the greatest sensitivity to structural abnormalities. A robust MR imaging–based method for clinical imaging of CBF would allow both an anatomic and a functional assessment within the same examination. In addition to providing direct structure-function correlation, the higher spatial resolution of MR imaging compared with that of nuclear medicine methods might also lead to better image quality. MR imaging of CBF can be performed with either intravascular contrast agents (8,9) or arterial spin labeling (10,11). Instead of using an exogenous tracer, arterial spin labeling electromagnetically labels water proton spins in the feeding arteries before they flow into the tissue. Arterial spin labeling is attractive because it can help reduce the risk, complexity, and cost of a study. It is also more readily quantified and repeated than methods that involve use of contrast agents.

Arterial spin labeling techniques can be crudely divided into pulsed inversion techniques (eg, echo-planar imaging and signal targeting with alternating radio frequency, or EPISTAR [12]; flow-sensitive alternating inversion recovery, or FAIR [13,14]; and other variants) and techniques that employ continuous arterial spin labeling (11). Continuous arterial spin labeling produces more than twice the signal of pulsed inversion techniques (15). With both methods, multisection imaging is complicated by the effects of electromagnetic labeling on the signal intensity, as well as the relatively long time required for blood to flow from the arteries into the thick slab of tissue to be imaged.

The arterial spin labeling approach to MR imaging of CBF offers the potential for completely noninvasive, quantitative imaging of an important physiologic and diagnostic quantity. Practical implementations of arterial spin labeling in humans, however, have typically suffered from systematic errors and artifacts that have limited its applicability. Recently, the use of fast imaging methods and an increased understanding of the factors affecting quantification of CBF have led to the acquisition of single-section CBF images with sufficiently high quality to allow clinical and research applications to be explored (12,15,16). Unfortunately, most applications require greater section coverage, but the serial acquisition of

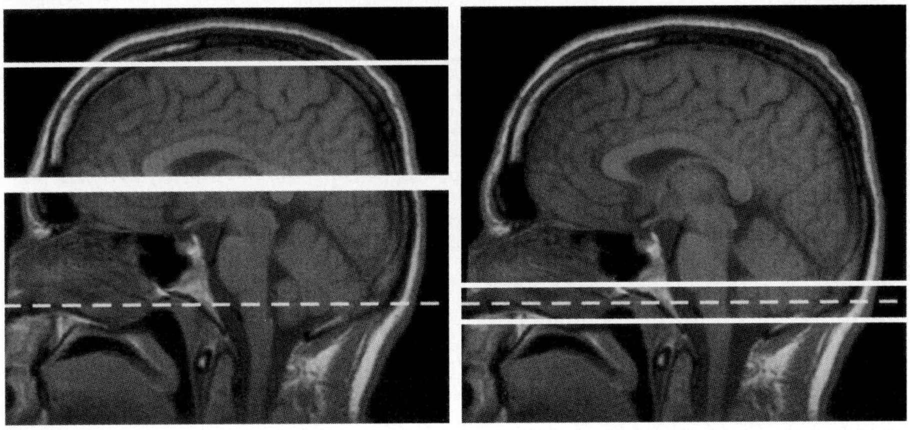

a. b.

Figure 1. Control methods for CBF imaging with continuous arterial spin labeling illustrated on sagittal T1-weighted spin-echo images. RF irradiation used to label inflowing blood as it crosses the labeling plane (dashed line in **a** and **b**) also causes direct effects on image intensity that vary with distance from the labeling plane. **(a)** In the single-section experiment, the control image is acquired with labeling (thin solid line) applied at an equal distance distal to the imaged section (thick solid line) to compensate for the spatially dependent off-resonance effects. **(b)** In the multisection experiment, amplitude-modulated irradiation applied for the control image creates two inversion planes (solid lines) close to the original labeling plane. Ideally, the inflowing spins are inverted twice as they flow through the planes, producing no net effect on arterial labeling, while the spatially dependent off-resonance effects of the RF irradiation are precisely reproduced.

many sections can be prohibitively time-consuming. Improved radio-frequency (RF) pulse shapes and sequence designs may make multisection pulsed arterial spin labeling techniques feasible (17). In this study, we evaluated a method for multisection imaging with continuous arterial spin labeling in which amplitude-modulated RF irradiation was used to control for the off-resonance effects of labeling. This method makes possible multisection imaging of CBF with good signal-to-noise ratio and arbitrary angles between imaging and labeling planes.

Materials and Methods

Amplitude-modulated Control

Continuous application of off-resonance RF power causes saturation of signal intensity as a result of the finite width of the water line and the transfer of saturated magnetization from water molecules adjacent to macromolecules, which have much broader lines (18). The off-resonance inversion power applied in continuous arterial spin labeling usually causes such saturation, and its presence complicates CBF imaging because the off-resonance effects may be large compared with the effects of blood flow. An approach to eliminating this saturation is the use of a second small RF coil for labeling that is far enough from the imaged section that the off-resonance power is negligible. This method has been used successfully to obtain multisection CBF images in rat brain (19), but it requires use of special RF hardware and a favorable geometry for the labeling, which limit its applicability. The alternative is to control for the saturation. Because CBF imaging with arterial spin labeling relies on the subtraction of the labeled image from a reference image obtained without labeling, achievement of equal off-resonance saturation in the reference image will control for the saturation effect.

The established method of controlling for off-resonance saturation with a single RF coil (11) is to apply an inversion distal to the section during acquisition of the control image (Fig 1a). If there are no noticeable background magnetic field gradients in the tissue, the off-resonance saturation is symmetric in frequency, and the labeling and control inversion are parallel to and equidistant from the image section, then the control image will experience equal off-resonance saturation. The requirement that the labeling and control inversion planes be parallel to and equidistant from the image section restricts the geometry of CBF imaging with arterial spin labeling and is not readily extended to use in a multisection examination. To overcome these limitations, use of an alternative control irradiation that mimics the frequency-dependent off-resonance effects of the labeling irradiation is required.

In this study, we evaluated application of an amplitude-modulated form of the labeling RF irradiation for the control. When a constant RF irradiation at a fixed frequency, f_0, is multiplied by a sine wave at frequency f_1, the signal produced is mathematically identical to continuous irradiation at two different frequencies, $f_0 + f_1$ and $f_0 - f_1$. If applied in the presence of a magnetic field gradient, each would separately perform an adiabatic inversion of inflowing arterial spins. When performed simultaneously, the combined effect is complicated because the equations governing spin evolution are not linear in the applied RF. However, the nature of resonance suggests that the effect of the first inversion on spins located near the plane of the second inversion should be small as long as the frequency spacing between the planes is large. In this case, the spins will be inverted twice after flowing through the two inversion planes (Fig 1b). Double inversion produces no net effect, so spins would not be labeled by the amplitude-modulated control. Because the average power and center frequency of the amplitude-modulated control are identical to those of the labeling RF irradiation, we hypothesized that the off-resonance effects of the control would be nearly identical to those of the labeling.

The performance of amplitude modulation of the RF irradiation as a control will depend on how perfectly the spins are doubly inverted, as well as on how well the off-resonance saturation of the labeling irradiation is matched. If the spins are partially labeled by the amplitude-modulated control, then the difference between the labeled and control images will decrease. This can be thought of as a loss of efficiency for labeling of blood flow. If the control does not perfectly match the off-resonance saturation of the labeling, then a difference between the images will occur even in the absence of blood flow. This would represent a systematic error in the blood flow measurement. We assessed both of these properties of the control experimentally.

MR Imaging

All studies were performed on a 1.5-T clinical imager (Signa; GE Medical Systems, Milwaukee, Wis) equipped with a prototypic gradient system for echo-planar imaging. Gradient-echo echo-planar images were obtained with a field of view of 24 (frequency) × 15 (phase) cm and an acquisition matrix of 64 × 40. Acquisition bandwidth of ±62.5 kHz al-

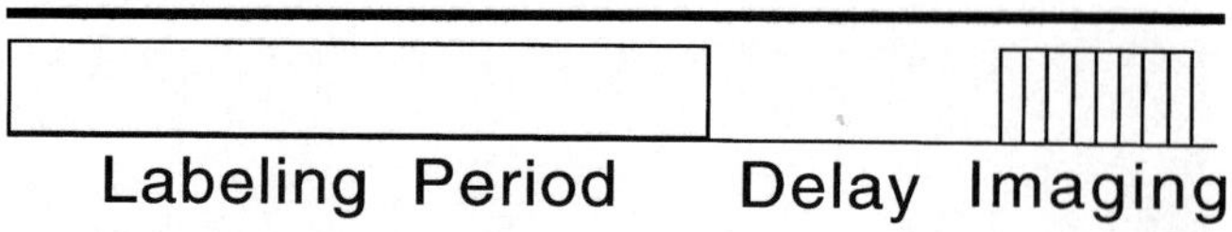

Figure 2. Pulse sequence timing diagram. Labeling RF and gradients are applied during the labeling period. A postlabeling delay is inserted between labeling and imaging to provide insensitivity to transit time. Finally, rapid gradient-echo echo-planar imaging is performed to acquire images in eight sections.

lowed an effective echo time of 22 msec and an image acquisition time of 45 msec. Multisection image acquisition was performed without pausing between sections; therefore, eight sections could be acquired in less than 400 msec. Section thickness was 6–10 mm and intersection gaps were 2 mm to minimize potential interference between sections.

Spin labeling was performed as previously reported for single-section CBF imaging (15) except for the amplitude-modulated control and the acquisition of more than one section. Specifically, a repetition time of 4,000 msec, temporal interleaving of labeled and control images, and a postlabeling delay were employed. The postlabeling delay reduces the sensitivity of the CBF image to the transit time from the labeling plane, attenuates the signal from intraluminal arterial spins, and decreases the off-resonance saturation of the signal intensity by the labeling RF (15). The postlabeling delay also allows time for all of the labeled blood to enter the tissue before imaging so that saturation of labeled spins by the imaging excitation pulses need not be considered. The duration of the labeling irradiation was determined on the basis of the postlabeling delay, the imaging time, and the repetition time. For a postlabeling delay of 1.2 seconds, the irradiation was applied for 2.3 seconds. A timing diagram for the entire sequence is shown in Figure 2.

Multisection versions of previously described echo-planar T1 mapping images (15) were obtained in addition to the CBF image. The T1 maps are needed to quantify the CBF images. Unlike in the single-section implementation, the labeling gradient had to be left on during T1 mapping to accurately measure the T1 shortening effect of the off-resonance saturation. In all other ways, the protocol was identical. The entire T1 mapping protocol required 3 minutes for all sections.

All raw echo amplitudes were saved and transferred to a workstation for processing. Custom software written within the Instructive Data Language (IDL; Research Systems, Boulder, Co) environment was used to reconstruct the images. Correction for image distortion and alternate k-space line errors was performed on each image on the basis of data acquired during phase-encoded reference imaging (20). Correction for distortion involves measurement of magnetic field nonuniformity throughout the image. A side effect of this correction is that image regions are set to zero in which insufficient MR signal is present to allow accurate measurement of the magnetic field. Magnitude images were then averaged, and CBF-weighted images were calculated by subtracting labeled images from control images. An algorithm to remove subtle motion artifacts from the images (21) was performed on the individual images before averaging to allow more accurate evaluation of the performance of the control.

Phantom Studies

Before evaluation in human subjects, the sequence was tested and calibrated on a uniform phantom consisting of 2% agarose by weight in distilled H_2O. Use of a phantom with noticeable magnetization transfer was necessary to fully test the control. The magnetization transfer properties of agarose are well studied (22), but they are considerably different from those of most human tissues (23). We hoped that the control would be accurate across a wide range of tissue types and that the agarose phantom would serve as an extreme case. The phantom consisted of a cylindric plastic container, 10 cm in diameter and 20 cm long, filled with the gelatinous mixture. The phantom was placed in the standard head coil of the imager with its axis parallel to that of the magnet. Single-section images obtained with the CBF labeling strategy were acquired in a plane perpendicular to the axis of the phantom. Labeling RF irradiation of 35 mG and a labeling gradient of 0.25 G/cm applied along the frequency direction of the image were used. Images were acquired with amplitude modulation frequencies of 125, 250, and 500 Hz. Off-resonance saturation was analyzed by averaging the images across the phase direction so that plots of off-resonance saturation as a function of frequency could be generated.

During evaluation of the sequence, we found that weak saturation of signal at the labeling plane occurred even when the RF amplitude was set to zero in the software. This indicated that a small amount of RF was leaking past the modulator. The saturation could be eliminated by setting the RF amplitude to a small negative value corresponding to 2% of the RF amplitude used for labeling. A constant value of 2% of the labeling amplitude was subtracted from the software values of all labeling-related RF amplitudes to compensate for this carrier leakage. Failure to correct for this leakage causes systematic error in the CBF measurement. Because the leakage is a subject-independent phenomenon, it can be calibrated with phantom measurements and need never be measured in subjects. The leakage on our imager has remained stable for more than 1 year.

Human Studies

All human studies were conducted on the basis of a protocol approved by our institutional review board. Written informed consent was obtained from 11 healthy volunteers. Three different studies were performed.

In one study, the amplitude-modulated control method was tested for systematic offset due to imperfect matching of the off-resonance saturation for label and control. Two subjects underwent MR imaging with control modulation frequency of 250 Hz, RF irradiation amplitude of 35 mG, postlabeling delay of 1.2 seconds, and 0.25 G/cm labeling gradient. Images of eight 8-mm-thick sections were obtained in both subjects when the labeling was applied to the carotid and vertebral arteries at the pontomedullary junction, to generate CBF images, and also when the labeling was applied distal to the imaging section at the top of the brain, which should produce no flow-related signal intensity in the absence of systematic error. One of the subjects underwent axial MR imaging and the other underwent coronal MR imaging to emphasize the flexibility of section geometry possible with use of amplitude-modulated control.

In a second study, the efficiency of multisection versus single-section CBF measurement was compared. In nine sub-

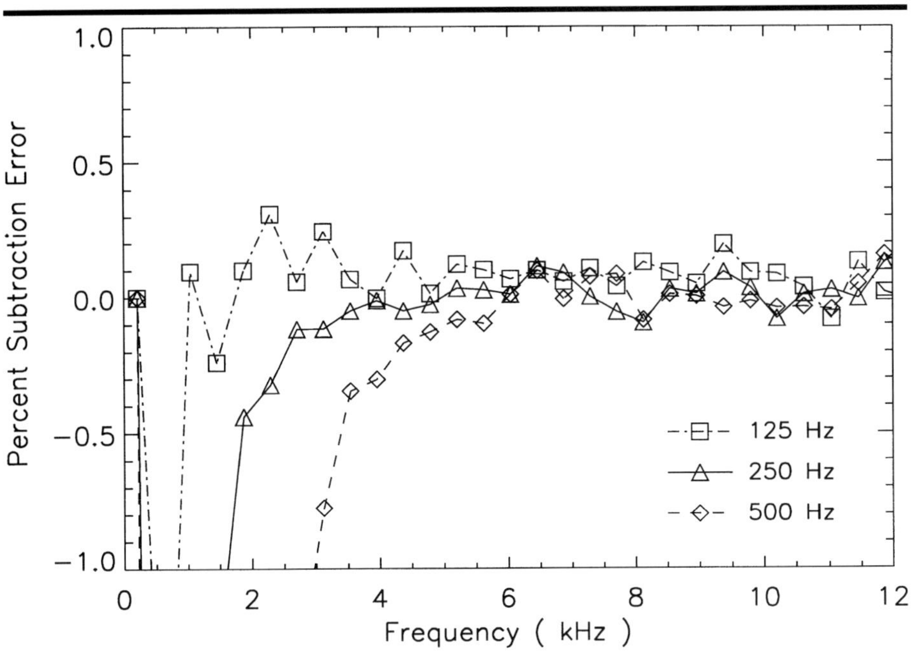

Figure 3. Graph depicts percentage difference between labeled and control images of the phantom as a function of frequency. Results for three different amplitude-modulation frequencies are shown.

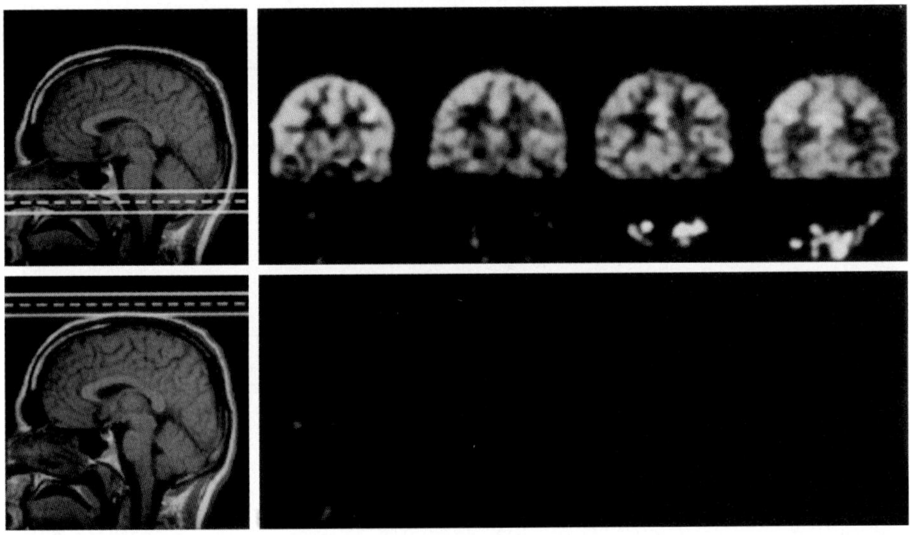

Figure 4. Evaluation of the amplitude-modulated control in a healthy subject. Left: Coronal echo-planar images (4,000/22 [effective]) were acquired with label and control placed at the pontomedullary junction (top) and above the brain (bottom) as indicated on the sagittal T1-weighted images. Right: Multisection subtraction images acquired with proximal labeling (top) demonstrate signal intensity from CBF. Images acquired with distal labeling (bottom) show no noticeable signal intensity.

jects, CBF images were acquired in a single axial section through the basal ganglia and thalamus. Images were acquired with both the single-section method, in which control labeling is distal to the section, and the multisection method. All subjects were studied with 0.25 G/cm labeling gradient, RF irradiation amplitude of 35 mG, control modulation frequency of 250 Hz, postlabeling delay of 1.2 seconds, and labeling plane offset of 4–8 cm from the section. From 15 to 45 pairs of labeled and control images were obtained in each subject for every combination of experimental parameters. In three of these subjects, the single-section and multisection methods were also compared at RF amplitudes of 30 and 20 mG. In three other subjects, the methods were also compared with modulation frequencies of 62.5, 100, 125, 200, and 500 Hz.

In the final human study in four subjects, multisection CBF images and T1 maps were obtained with 250-Hz modulation and 35-mG RF amplitude for quantitative analysis of CBF with use of previously presented methods (15). The entire CBF imaging sequence required 9 minutes including T1 mapping and acquisition of 45 pairs of labeled and control images. The efficiency value for multisection labeling measured in the first study was used for quantification.

Results

Phantom Study

Matching of frequency-dependent off-resonance saturation effects between the labeling and amplitude-modulated control was excellent at all three frequencies, as shown in Figure 3. Though both types of irradiation produced off-resonance saturation of greater than 15% of the unsaturated signal, the difference between the two was less than 0.1% except very close to the labeling plane. The frequency at which the difference between the labeled and control frequencies became noticeable was smaller for amplitude modulation at lower frequency. This suggests that labeling can be performed closer to the most inferior region to be imaged when slower amplitude modulation is used.

Human Studies

Excellent matching between the labeling and control off-resonance saturation in the phantom was also reproduced in the in vivo studies. Figure 4 shows the coronal subtracted images obtained with labeling 2 cm above the top of the brain and at the pontomedullary junction. The images with the pontomedullary junction label show strong CBF signal intensity in all distal regions of the brain, but those with the label above the brain show no noticeable signal intensity. To further quantify residual subtraction errors caused by imperfect matching of off-resonance saturation, the signal intensity was averaged across the section and phase directions, similar to the phantom analysis, and the results are plotted in Figure 5. CBF produces a signal intensity change of less than 1% on the proximal labeled images, whereas residual subtraction error for frequencies above 2 kHz as measured on the distal labeled images is consistent with noise and is always less than 0.05%. The average of the subtracted signal intensity across frequency from 2 to 10 kHz is less than 0.007% of the control signal intensity. Because the CBF images were acquired in a plane perpendicular to the labeling plane, their uniformity is also a direct indicator of the accuracy of the control. Errors in subtraction are apparent in the perfusion signal intensity (Fig 5) very near the labeling plane at offset frequencies below 2 kHz. The subtraction error produces a shift to a negative signal intensity; this finding is consistent with the phantom results (Fig 3). A comparable level of matching was observed on axial images acquired in another subject (not shown).

The mean efficiency ratio of the multisection and single-section methods was 61.6% ± 6.7 (standard deviation) across the nine subjects with a modulation frequency of 250 Hz. This efficiency was found to drop rapidly when the RF amplitude was lowered; efficiency at 30 mG was 58% and at 20 mG was only 35%. The efficiency at 36-mG amplitude improved to 75% when the modulation frequency was lowered (Fig 6). This suggests that a modulation frequency of 62.5 Hz is more desirable than 250 Hz.

Quantification of the CBF images was performed with use of methods described previously for single-section imaging. The averaged labeled images were first subtracted from the averaged control images and then divided by the signal intensity on an image obtained in the absence of off-resonance saturation. This ratio was then multiplied by a calibration factor (Eq [9] in reference 15), which is a function of the calculated T1 images, the transit times to the tissue from the labeling plane, and the postlabeling delay for each section. Because the transit time to the tissue was not measured, an assumed value of 1.5 seconds was employed for quantification. The long postlabeling delay minimized sensitivity of the calibration factor to differences between the assumed and actual transit times. Images were corrected for inefficiency of labeling by dividing by an efficiency value of 58.5%. This value was based on an efficiency value of 95% for the single-section experiment (24) and the ratio between multisection and single-section efficiency measured in this study, 61.6%. Calculated images from one of the subjects are in Figure 7. These images are not corrected for spatial variations in the blood-brain partition coefficient. Quantitative CBF values were derived by segmenting the tissue into gray and white matter on the basis of the T1 maps and by using partition coefficients of 0.98 for gray matter and 0.82 for white matter (25). Our measured CBF values (Table) are consistent with those obtained previously with single-section methods (15,26) and with other measurements of CBF (27).

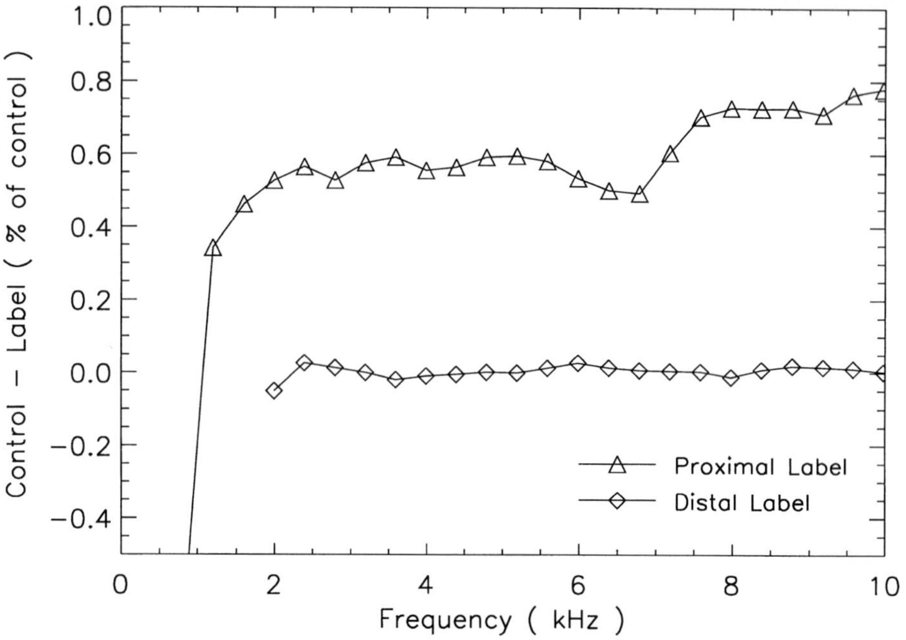

Figure 5. Graph depicts the mean difference in signal intensity obtained by averaging the images in Figure 4 across the anteroposterior and right-left directions. For plotting, distance from the labeling plane was converted into frequency offset. Proximal labeling at the pontomedullary junction produced a small but very noticeable change in the signal intensity due to CBF. Distal labeling above the brain produced no noticeable signal intensity change; this finding is consistent with negligible off-resonance errors for offset frequencies above 2 kHz.

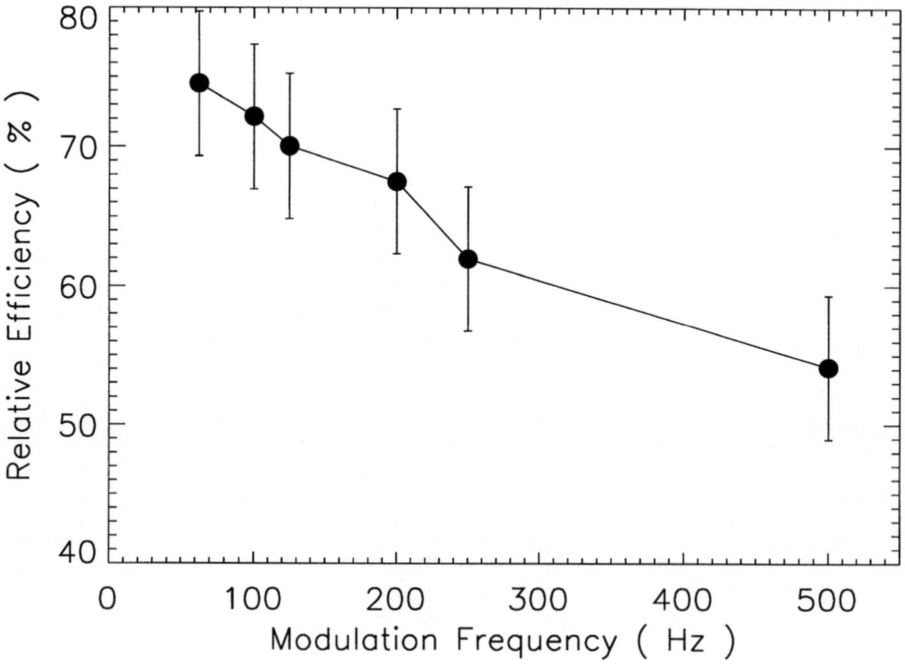

Figure 6. Graph depicts efficiency of spin labeling with the amplitude-modulated control as a function of modulation frequency relative to single-section labeling with 36-mG irradiation.

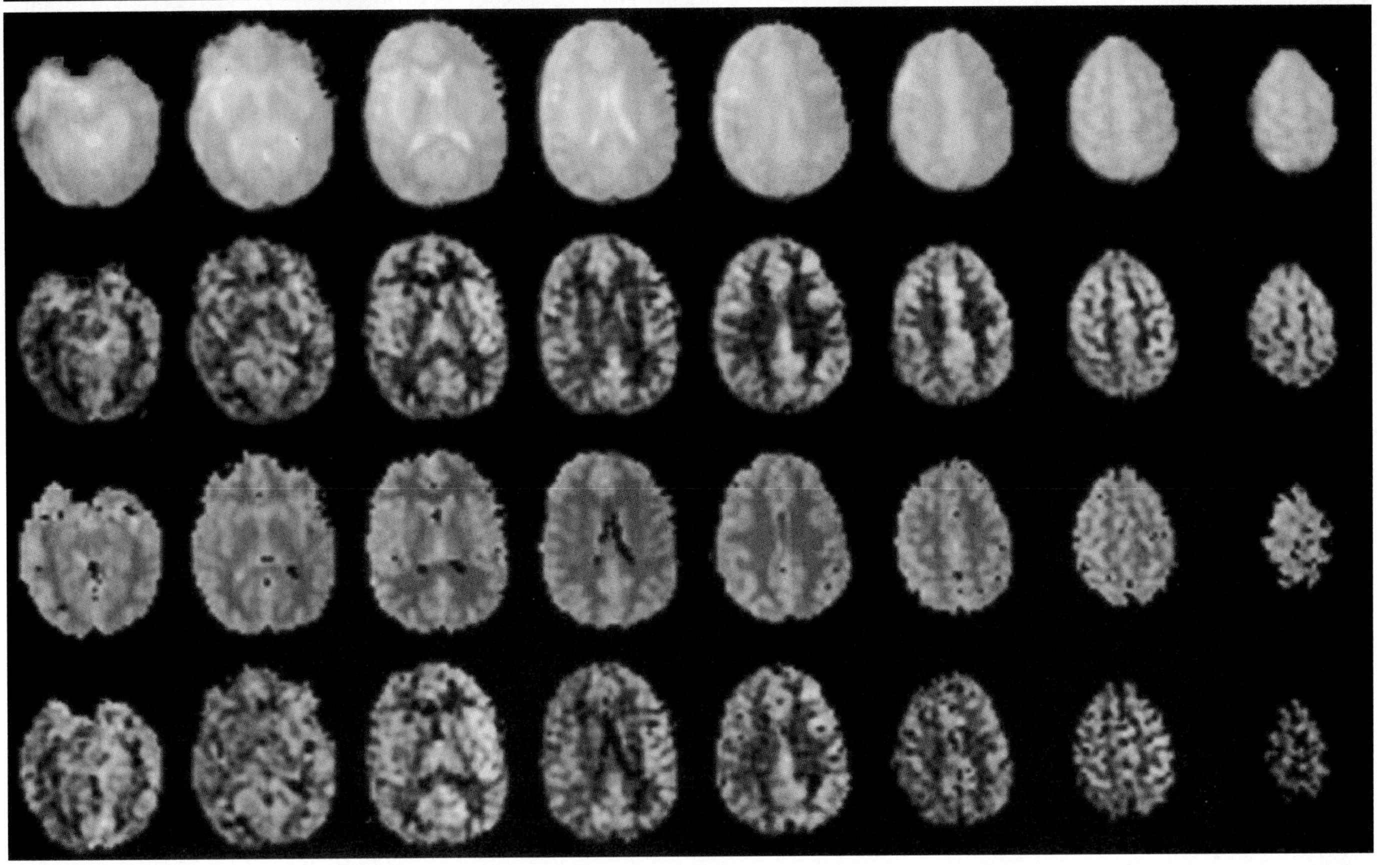

Figure 7. Multisection images acquired in a healthy volunteer. Echo-planar images (4,000/22 [effective]) from eight axial sections (top row) were used to generate CBF-sensitive images (second row). On the basis of the T1 maps (third row) also acquired, quantitative CBF images (bottom row) can be generated.

Discussion

We have presented a method for multisection CBF imaging using continuous arterial spin labeling with an amplitude-modulated control. This strategy is highly effective at controlling for off-resonance effects and efficient at doubly inverting inflowing spins, thus retaining the signal advantages of continuous versus pulsed arterial spin labeling techniques. The method is readily implemented with standard hardware, is effective in both gray and white matter, and allows flexible selection of the imaging and labeling planes. Because the control method is applied at the same location as the labeling and gives equal effect across a wide range of frequencies, there should be no errors associated with static magnetic field inhomogeneity or asymmetry in the off-resonance spectrum (28). The labeling method is therefore desirable for even single-section CBF imaging applications. This approach should also be applicable to blood flow measurements in organs other than the brain. Although these studies were carried out in eight sections, the number of sections is limited only by the image acquisition time and T1 of blood and tissue.

The highest efficiency was measured for the lowest modulation frequency in this study, 62.5 Hz. This was contrary to our initial intuition that the two inversion planes would start to interfere as they became closer. We have implemented numeric simulations of the control by using methods similar to those published for single-section labeling (24). These simulations suggest that inefficiency results primarily from nonlinear interactions between the two inversion planes rather than from T1 decay between the two planes. The simulation results did not faithfully reproduce the experimental behavior, however, so we report only the experimental results. Further study of the factors affecting efficiency, which we have already performed for the single-section method, are clearly necessary.

In this study, use of gradient-echo echo-planar imaging with a moderately long echo time caused signal loss in parts of the inferior frontal and temporal lobes because of nonuniform magnetic fields near bones and sinuses. Spin-echo echo-planar imaging was avoided because it would have increased the duration of image acquisition. Fractional k-space acquisition, which was not supported by our analysis software, could have enabled gradient-echo imaging with much shorter effective echo time or spin-echo echo-planar imaging with acquisition times comparable to or shorter than those in our sequence. If necessary for imaging speed or image quality, other methods such as interleaved echo-planar imaging (29) or rapid acquisition with relaxation enhancement, or RARE (30), might be employed as long as they do not unacceptably increase motion artifact.

Spin-labeled perfusion images clearly reflect CBF and its spatial and temporal variation, but further work is required to test and validate the quantitative values obtained with this technique. To our knowledge, validation of the technique only in rats with use of microspheres has been published (31). It is likely that such

Quantitative CBF in Four Healthy Volunteers

Subject No./ Age (y)*/ Sex	CBF (mL · 100 g^{-1} · min^{-1}) Gray Matter	White Matter	Mean
1/24/M	70.5	27.1	53.7
2/25/M	71.4	28.5	54.8
3/32/M	61.7	32.5	50.4
4/21/F	85.9	49.7	71.9
Mean†	72.4 ± 10	34.5 ± 10	57.7 ± 10

* Mean age, 25.5 years ± 5 (1 standard deviation).

† Data are the mean ± standard deviation.

studies will lead to refinements of the measurements and the equations for quantifying flow, but we are confident that reliable quantitative flow measurements can be obtained with the spin-labeling approach and that values obtained with the present technique are not far from correct.

The extension of CBF imaging with continuous arterial spin labeling to a multisection modality overcomes a major obstacle to clinical applications. We have already applied this approach successfully in patients with cerebrovascular disease (32). CBF measurements obtained with this approach are also likely to provide a sensitive and quantitative measurement of cerebrovascular reserve when performed in conjunction with administration of acetazolamide or CO_2 inhalation. Numerous other potential clinical applications can be envisioned, including differential diagnosis of dementing disorders and cerebral neoplasms. In addition, quantitative CBF measurements have applications in clinical and basic neuroscience, for imaging regional CBF changes during sensorimotor or cognitive tasks or after pharmacologic challenges, and for population-based studies of changes in regional CBF and metabolism.

References

1. Frackowiak RSJ, Pozzilli C, Legg NJ, et al. Regional cerebral oxygen supply and utilization in dementia. Brain 1981; 104:753–778.
2. Yudd AP, VanHeertum RL, Masdeu JC. Interventions and functional brain imaging. Semin Nucl Med 1991; 21:153–158.
3. Waldemar G. Functional brain imaging with SPECT in normal aging and dementia. Cerebrovasc Brain Metab Rev 1995; 7:89–130.
4. Spencer SS. The relative contributions of MRI, SPECT, and PET imaging in epilepsy. Epilepsia 1994; 35(suppl):S72–S89.
5. Jacobs A, Put E, Ingels M, Bossuyt A. Prospective evaluation of technetium-99m–HMPAO SPECT in mild and moderate traumatic brain injury. J Nucl Med 1994; 35:942–947.
6. Leenders KL. PET: blood flow and oxygen consumption in brain tumors. J Neurooncol 1994; 22:269–273.
7. Posner MI, Petersen SE, Fox PT, Raichle ME. Localization of cognitive operations in the human brain. Science 1988; 240: 1627–1631.
8. Belliveau JW, Rosen BR, Kantor HL, et al. Functional cerebral imaging by susceptibility contrast. Magn Reson Med 1990; 14: 538–546.
9. Ostergaard L, Sorensen AG, Kwong KK, Weisskoff RM, Gyldensted C, Rosen BR. High resolution measurement of cerebral blood flow using intravascular tracer bolus passages. II. Experimental comparison and preliminary results. Magn Reson Med 1996; 36:726–736.
10. Detre JA, Leigh JS, Williams DS, Koretsky AP. Perfusion imaging. Magn Reson Med 1992; 23:37–45.
11. Williams DS, Detre JA, Leigh JS, Koretsky AP. Magnetic resonance imaging of perfusion using spin inversion of arterial water. Proc Natl Acad Sci USA 1992; 89:212–216.
12. Edelman RR, Siewert B, Darby DG, et al. Qualitative mapping of cerebral blood flow and functional localization with echo-planar MR imaging and signal targeting with alternating radio frequency. Radiology 1994; 192:513–520.
13. Kwong KK, Chesler DA, Weisskoff RM, et al. MR perfusion studies with T1-weighted echo planar imaging. Magn Reson Med 1995; 34:878–887.
14. Kim SG. Quantification of relative cerebral blood flow change by flow-sensitive alternating inversion recovery (FAIR) technique: application to functional mapping. Magn Reson Med 1995; 34:293–301.
15. Alsop DC, Detre JA. Reduced transit-time sensitivity in non-invasive magnetic resonance imaging of human cerebral blood flow. J Cereb Blood Flow Metab 1996; 16:1236–1249.
16. Buxton RB, Frank LR, Siewert B, Warach S, Edelman RR. A quantitative model for EPISTAR perfusion imaging (abstr). In: Proceedings of the Third Meeting of the International Society for Magnetic Resonance in Medicine. Berkeley, Calif: International Society for Magnetic Resonance in Medicine, 1995; 132.
17. Wong EC, Frank LR, Buxton RB. Quantitative multislice perfusion imaging using QUIPSS II, EPISTAR, FAIR and PICORE (abstr). In: Proceedings of the Fifth Meeting of the International Society for Magnetic Resonance in Medicine. Berkeley, Calif: International Society for Magnetic Resonance in Medicine, 1997; 85.
18. Wolff SD, Balaban RS. Magnetization transfer contrast (MTC) and tissue water proton relaxation in vivo. Magn Reson Med 1989; 10:135–144.
19. Silva AC, Zhang W, Williams DS, Koretsky AP. Multislice MRI of rat brain perfusion during amphetamine stimulation using arterial spin labeling. Magn Reson Med 1995; 33:209–214.
20. Alsop DC. Correction of ghost artifacts and distortion in echo-planar MR imaging with an iterative image reconstruction technique (abstr.) Radiology 1995; 197(P):388.
21. Alsop DC, Detre JA. Reduction of excess noise in fMRI using noise image templates (abstr). In: Proceedings of the Fifth Meeting of the International Society for Magnetic Resonance in Medicine. Berkeley, Calif: International Society for Magnetic Resonance in Medicine, 1997; 1687.
22. Henkelman RM, Huang X, Xiang QS, Stanisz GJ, Swanson SD, Bronskill MJ. Quantitative interpretation of magnetization transfer. Magn Reson Med 1993; 29: 759–766.
23. Morrison C, Henkelman RM. A model for magnetization transfer in tissues. Magn Reson Med 1995; 33:475–482.
24. Maccotta L, Detre JA, Alsop DC. The efficiency of adiabatic inversion for perfusion imaging by arterial spin labeling. NMR Biomed 1997; 10:216–221.
25. Herscovitch P, Raichle ME. What is the correct value for the brain-blood partition coefficient for water. J Cereb Blood Flow Metab 1985; 5:65–69.
26. Ye FQ, Pekar JJ, Jezzard P, Duyn J, Frank JA, McLaughlin AC. Perfusion imaging of the human brain at 1.5 T using a single-shot EPI spin tagging approach. Magn Reson Med 1996; 36:217–224.
27. Matthew E, Andreason P, Carson RE, et al. Reproducibility of resting cerebral blood flow measurements with $H_2{}^{15}O$ positron emission tomography in humans. J Cereb Blood Flow Metab 1993; 13:748–754.
28. Pekar J, Jezzard P, Roberts DA, Leigh JS, Frank JA, McLaughlin AC. Perfusion imaging with compensation for asymmetric magnetization transfer effects. Magn Reson Med 1996; 35:70–79.
29. McKinnon GC. Ultrafast interleaved gradient echo planar imaging on a standard scanner. Magn Reson Med 1993; 30:609–616.
30. Hennig J, Nauerth A, Friedburg H. RARE imaging: a fast imaging method for clinical MR. Magn Reson Med 1986; 3:823–833.
31. Walsh EG, Minematsu K, Leppo J, Moore SC. Radioactive microsphere validation of a volume localized continuous saturation perfusion measurement. Magn Reson Med 1994; 31:147–153.
32. Detre JA, Alsop DC, Vives LR, Maccotta L, Teener JW, Raps EC. Noninvasive MRI evaluation of cerebral blood flow in cerebrovascular disease. Neurology 1998; 50: 633–641.

Michael B. Singer, MD
Scott W. Atlas, MD
Burton P. Drayer, MD

Subarachnoid Space Disease: Diagnosis with Fluid-attenuated Inversion-Recovery MR Imaging and Comparison with Gadolinium-enhanced Spin-Echo MR Imaging—Blinded Reader Study[1]

Index terms:
Brain, hemorrhage, 136.2521, 136.298, 139.2521, 139.298, 167.2521, 167.298
Brain neoplasms, MR, 139.36, 139.38
Encephalitis, 136.20, 136.253, 136.298, 139.20, 139.253, 139.298
Gadolinium, 136.12143, 139.12143, 167.12143
Magnetic resonance (MR), pulse sequences, 136.121411, 136.121413, 136.12143, 139.121411, 139.121413, 139.12143, 167.121411, 167.121413, 167.12143
Meningitis, 139.251, 139.36, 139.38

Radiology 1998; 208:417–422

Abbreviations:
CSF = cerebrospinal fluid
FLAIR = fluid-attenuated inversion recovery
HIV = human immunodeficiency virus
SAH = subarachnoid hemorrhage
SAS = subarachnoid space

[1] From the Department of Radiology, Mount Sinai School of Medicine, One Gustave L Levy Place, New York, NY 10029. From the 1997 RSNA scientific assembly. Received December 16, 1997; revision requested February 25, 1998; revision received March 11; accepted March 30. **Address reprint requests to** S.W.A.

Author contributions:
Guarantor of integrity of entire study, S.W.A.; study concepts and design, S.W.A.; definition of intellectual content, S.W.A.; literature research, M.B.S., S.W.A.; clinical studies, M.B.S.; data acquisition, S.W.A., B.P.D., M.B.S.; statistical analysis, M.B.S.; manuscript preparation, M.B.S., S.W.A.; manuscript editing and review, S.W.A., B.P.D.

PURPOSE: To evaluate fluid-attenuated inversion-recovery (FLAIR) magnetic resonance (MR) imaging in a blinded reader study for the detection of proved subarachnoid space (SAS) disease.

MATERIALS AND METHODS: FLAIR MR imaging was performed in 62 patients (21 with proved SAS or meningeal disease) and 41 control patients. A subset of 24 patients (eight patients with proved SAS disease and 16 control patients) also underwent gadolinium-enhanced T1-weighted MR imaging. FLAIR images were interpreted blindly and independently by two neuroradiologists.

RESULTS: For SAS disease, the overall sensitivity, specificity, and accuracy of FLAIR for both readers were 85%, 93%, and 90%. In the 15 patients with inflammatory or neoplastic meningitis only (six patients with acute subarachnoid hemorrhage [SAH] excluded), the sensitivity, specificity, and accuracy of FLAIR for both readers were 82%, 93%, and 90%. All six acute SAH cases were interpreted as abnormal on FLAIR images by both readers. In the 24 patients who underwent both FLAIR and gadolinium-enhanced T1-weighted MR imaging, the sensitivity, specificity, and accuracy of FLAIR imaging were 86%, 91%, and 89%; the sensitivity, specificity, and accuracy of gadolinium-enhanced T1-weighted imaging were 43%, 88%, and 74%.

CONCLUSION: FLAIR is highly sensitive and specific for the diagnosis of SAS disease. Unenhanced FLAIR is superior to gadolinium-enhanced T1-weighted MR imaging for the diagnosis of SAS disease. These data have important implications, because FLAIR is performed without the costs and inherent risks of intravenous contrast agents. FLAIR also appears to be highly sensitive but nonspecific for acute SAH.

The diagnosis of subarachnoid space (SAS) abnormalities has been a mainstay of neuroradiology since the advent of computed tomography (CT), particularly for the diagnosis of acute subarachnoid hemorrhage (SAH). More recently, despite the lack of blinded reader studies, it has become generally accepted that contrast agent–enhanced magnetic resonance (MR) imaging has the highest, although suboptimal, diagnostic yield for SAS and leptomeningeal abnormalities. To our knowledge, the single and important exception to the superiority of MR imaging over CT has been in the evaluation of acute SAH (1–3).

In fluid-attenuated inversion-recovery (FLAIR) MR imaging, an inversion-recovery pulse sequence is used with an inversion time that effectively nulls the high signal intensity of the cerebrospinal fluid (CSF). A long echo time is used to produce a heavily T2-weighted sequence, but without the high signal intensity typically associated with the CSF on

T2-weighted images. Several studies (4–8) have compared FLAIR MR imaging with conventional spin-echo MR imaging in the detection and characterization of brain parenchymal lesions. These studies have uniformly described the high sensitivity of FLAIR for parenchymal disease but have not uniformly advocated the routine use of FLAIR (9) because of the already high sensitivity of conventional MR imaging for such disease. Other preliminary study findings on FLAIR imaging have suggested that this sequence may be more sensitive than other MR sequences for the detection of acute, subacute, and chronic SAH (10,11). It has also been shown that the signal intensity of CSF on FLAIR images changes with protein concentration (12).

The purpose of our study was to evaluate FLAIR in a blinded reader study for the detection of proved disease processes of the SAS. We hypothesized that the nulling of CSF signal in the SAS with FLAIR would result in high sensitivity for diseases that affect the SAS. We also hypothesized that FLAIR without intravenously administered contrast agents would have a higher sensitivity than contrast-enhanced T1-weighted imaging in inflammatory and neoplastic leptomeningeal and SAS diseases. If true, the replacement of contrast-enhanced MR imaging with FLAIR MR imaging would be safer, less invasive, faster, and more cost-effective.

TABLE 1
Proof of Diagnosis in Patients with SAS Disease

Proof of Diagnosis	FLAIR and Contrast-enhanced MR Imaging (*n* = 8)	FLAIR MR Imaging Only (*n* = 13)
CSF analysis	8	10
CT*	0	3
Clinical history and hospital course	0	0

* CT findings were considered to be proof of diagnosis in patients with acute SAH.

TABLE 2
Causes of SAS Disease in 21 Proved Cases

Diagnosis	FLAIR and Contrast-enhanced MR Imaging (*n* = 8)	FLAIR MR Imaging Only (*n* = 13)	Total (*n* = 21)
Acute SAH	1	5	6
Inflammatory disorders	6	7	13
Carcinomatous meningitis	1	1	2

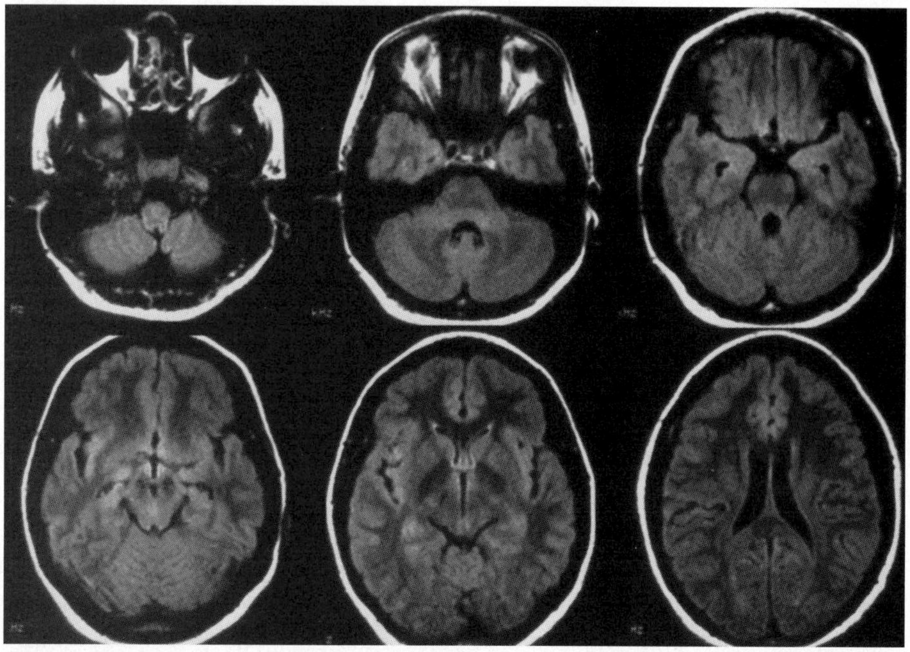

Figure 1. FLAIR images (10,000/147/2,200) obtained in a control patient show a normal SAS, inferior to superior. Serial axial FLAIR MR images from the foramen magnum cephalad to the level of the bodies of the lateral ventricles demonstrate markedly hypointense SASs, including basal cisterns, sulci, and ventricles. Suppression of the signal intensity of the normal CSF in all of these regions is essential for the accurate detection of abnormalities of the SAS or leptomeninges.

MATERIALS AND METHODS

Patient Population

FLAIR MR imaging studies were performed at 1.5 T (Signa; GE Medical Systems, Milwaukee, Wis) in 62 patients aged 2–71 years. Twenty-one of the 62 patients had a proved disease process in the SAS or meninges (Tables 1, 2). Of the 21 patients with a proved leptomeningeal or SAS disease process, 13 had acute inflammatory meningitis or meningoencephalitis, two had carcinomatous meningitis, and six had acute SAH. Of the 13 patients with inflammatory disorders, three patients had viral causes. Of the six patients with acute SAH, four were posttraumatic, and two had an aneurysm or arteriovenous malformation. All patients with acute SAH underwent MR imaging within 12 hours of CT or CSF retrieval.

Images obtained in 41 control patients also were included in the blinded readings. The control patients underwent FLAIR MR imaging but did not harbor leptomeningeal or SAS disease. The exclusion of such disease in this control group was based on findings of a combination of clinical history, physical and clinical course (ie, clinical diagnosis), CSF analysis, and (for the purposes of detecting acute SAH) CT. The clinical symptoms in the 41 control patients were as follows: focal neurologic deficit, 25 patients; headache, nine patients; psychiatric symptoms, six patients; and musculoskeletal pain, one patient. Leptomeningeal or SAS disease was excluded in these 41 control patients by means of the following methods: CSF analysis with clinical findings, nine patients; clinical findings with CT but no CSF analysis, eight patients; clinical findings, CSF analysis, and CT, four patients; and clinical findings alone, 20 patients. The detailed list of clinical settings in each of these subgroups of control patients in whom leptomeningeal or SAS disease was excluded is in Table 3.

It should be noted that no patient in whom the clinician suspected meningitis or any disease of the SAS or leptomeninges was cleared of harboring disease in the SAS or leptomeninges by means of CT alone, since it is well known that CSF analysis is the standard of reference; indeed, CSF analysis is necessary to exclude menin-

TABLE 3
Methods of Exclusion of SAS Disease in 41 Control Patients

Method of Exclusion of SAS Disease	Focal Neurologic Deficits	Headaches	Musculoskeletal Pain	Psychiatric Symptoms
Clinical findings alone	15	0	0	5
Clinical and CT findings	6	0	1	1
CSF analysis and clinical and CT findings	2	2	0	0
CSF analysis with clinical findings	2	7	0	0

Note.—All patients underwent MR imaging for clinical work-up.

TABLE 4
FLAIR in Patients with SAS Disease

Reader	Sensitivity (%)	Specificity (%)	Accuracy (%)
1	90 (19 of 21)	93 (38 of 41)	92 (57 of 62)
2	81 (17 of 21)	93 (38 of 41)	89 (55 of 62)
Average	85	93	90

TABLE 5
FLAIR in Patients with Nonhemorrhagic SAS Disease

Reader	Sensitivity (%)	Specificity (%)	Accuracy (%)
1	93 (13 of 14)	93 (38 of 41)	93 (51 of 55)
2	71 (10 of 14)	93 (38 of 41)	87 (48 of 55)
Average	82	93	90

gitis, and, in practice, normal CSF analysis results do indeed exclude meningitis.

CT was used to evaluate possible acute SAH (it was also used to detect a focal intraparenchymal lesion in some of these cases). In all nine control patients with a headache in whom meningitis was originally considered a diagnostic possibility by the clinician, CSF analysis was undertaken. CSF analysis in control patients without the human immunodeficiency virus (HIV) consisted of the following tests: cell count and differential, protein analysis, glucose analysis, cultures (eg, bacterial, acid-fast bacilli, fungal cultures), Gram staining, india ink capsule staining, and the VDRL test. In the CSF of control patients with HIV, the following additional tests also were performed: *Cryptococcus* antigen test, toxoplasmosis antibody titer, herpes simplex virus culture, and cytomegalovirus culture. No patients were included in the control group who had a possibility of harboring leptomeningeal metastases, since it is well known that routine sampling of CSF is not highly sensitive for such disease.

For the purposes of this analysis, these patients were then divided into subgroups as follows: Group 1 comprised patients who underwent FLAIR MR imaging and T1-weighted MR imaging after the intravenous administration of a contrast agent, while group 2 comprised patients who underwent FLAIR imaging but not contrast-enhanced T1-weighted MR imaging. Group 1 consisted of 24 patients. Eight patients within this group had documented evidence of a SAS disease process (Table 1). Proof of diagnosis was CSF analysis results in all eight of these patients. Group 2 consisted of 38 patients. Thirteen patients within this group had proved SAS disease (Table 2). Proof of diagnosis was CSF analysis results in 10 patients (Table 1). In three of the patients who had acute SAH, proof was CT findings positive for acute SAH.

MR Imaging Sequences and Interpretation

All patients underwent FLAIR imaging, which was performed by using a fast FLAIR sequence with 10,000/147/2,200 (repetition time msec/echo time [effective] msec/inversion time msec) and a 16-kHz bandwidth (acquisition time, 4 minutes 20 seconds). FLAIR images were interpreted randomly and independently by each of two experienced neuroradiologists (S.W.A., B.P.D.) without knowledge of specific clinical or laboratory data except for a history of "rule out SAS disease." The SAS was determined to be abnormal on FLAIR images if the reader detected abnormal hyperintensity in ventricles, cisterns, sulci, or any combination of these, since these regions are markedly hypointense in normal cases (Fig 1).

Contrast-enhanced MR images were obtained only in those patients in whom MR imaging was requested by the referring physician. Standard T1-weighted images were obtained (600/10 [repetition time msec/echo time msec], 192 × 256 matrix, 10.7-kHz bandwidth, 2-minute 4-second acquisition time). Flow compensation was not used. T1-weighted imaging was performed immediately after a bolus injection of a standard dose (0.1 mmol per kilogram of body weight) of gadopentetate dimeglumine (Magnevist; Berlex, Wayne, NJ). A single reader, reader 1 (S.W.A.), evaluated the contrast-enhanced T1-weighted MR images while blinded to patient identification and history and also to other MR imaging findings at a separate session from the FLAIR study interpretations.

To quantify the results of the blinded readings, standard statistical analysis was performed to calculate sensitivity, specificity, and accuracy.

RESULTS

Overall results for both groups 1 (patients who underwent both FLAIR and contrast-enhanced T1-weighted imaging) and 2 (FLAIR but no contrast-enhanced T1-weighted imaging), which includes all cases for the two readers, are shown in Table 4. The sensitivity and specificity for reader 1 in this group were 90% (19 of 21) and 93% (38 of 41), and the accuracy was 92% (57 of 62). Reader 2 (B.P.D.) had a sensitivity of 81% (17 of 21), a specificity of 93% (38 of 41), and an accuracy of 89% (55 of 62).

Results in both group 1 and group 2 patients with inflammatory or neoplastic meningitis only (ie, six patients with acute SAH excluded) for the two readers are shown in Table 5. The sensitivity and specificity for reader 1 in this group were 93% (13 of 14) and 93% (38 of 41). The accuracy for reader 1 was 93% (51 of 55). Reader 2 had a sensitivity of 71% (10 of 14), a specificity of 93% (38 of 41), and an accuracy of 87% (48 of 55).

The six patients with acute SAH all had abnormal FLAIR findings owing to areas of increased signal intensity in the SAS.

To compare the accuracy of FLAIR with that of contrast-enhanced T1-weighted MR imaging for SAS disease processes, we further separated group 1 patients from the patient cohort (Tables 6, 7). Group 1 consisted of 24 patients: eight patients with SAS disease, one of whom had acute SAH, and 16 control patients. The sensitivity and specificity of reader 1 in this group were 88% (seven of eight) and 94% (15 of 16). The accuracy of reader 1 was 92% (22 of 24). Reader 2 had a sensitivity of 88% (seven of eight) and a specificity of 88% (14 of 16). The accuracy was 88% (21 of 24). This subset of 24 patients also underwent gadolinium-enhanced T1-weighted MR imaging. The sensitivity, specificity, and accuracy of the contrast-enhanced MR studies were 50% (four of eight), 88% (14 of 16), and 75% (18 of 24).

To compare the accuracies of FLAIR and contrast-enhanced T1-weighted MR imaging for SAS disease processes exclusive of acute SAH (since cases of acute SAH are not routinely imaged with contrast-enhanced MR imaging and would not be expected to show abnormal contrast agent enhancement), we excluded the one case of acute SAH from this cohort (Table 7). The sensitivity and specificity for reader 1 in this group were 86% (six of seven) and 94% (15 of 16). The accuracy for reader 1 was 91% (21 of 23). Reader 2 had a sensitivity of 86% (six of seven) and a specificity of 88% (14 of 16). The accuracy was 87% (20 of 23). The sensitivity, specificity, and accuracy of the readings of contrast-enhanced MR studies were 43% (three of seven), 88% (14 of 16), and 74% (17 of 23).

Group 2 consisted of 38 patients in whom no contrast-enhanced T1-weighted images were obtained. Thirteen of these patients had a proved SAS disease process, five of whom were patients with acute SAH, and 25 others were included as control patients. The sensitivity and specificity for reader 1 in this group were 92% (12 of 13) and 92% (23 of 25). The accuracy for reader 1 was 92% (35 of 38). Reader 2 had a sensitivity of 77% (10 of 13), a specificity of 96% (24 of 25), and an accuracy of 89% (34 of 38). We again excluded the patients with acute SAH from this cohort (five patients) to evaluate the accuracy of FLAIR for SAS processes exclusive of acute SAH. The sensitivity and specificity for reader 1 in this group were 88% (seven of eight) and 92% (23 of 25). The accuracy for reader 1 was 91% (30 of 33). Reader 2 had a sensitivity of 62% (five of eight) and a specificity of 96% (24 of 25). The accuracy was 91% (29 of 33).

TABLE 6
FLAIR versus Gadolinium-enhanced T1-weighted MR Imaging in Patients with SAS Disease

Sequence	Sensitivity (%)	Specificity (%)	Accuracy (%)
FLAIR*	88 (7 of 8 for reader 1, 7 of 8 for reader 2)	91 (15 of 16 for reader 1, 14 of 16 for reader 2)	90 (22 of 24 for reader 1, 21 of 24 for reader 2)
Gadolinium-enhanced T1-weighted	50 (4 of 8)	88 (14 of 16)	75 (18 of 24)

* Data averaged for two readers.

TABLE 7
FLAIR versus Gadolinium-enhanced T1-weighted MR Imaging in Patients with Nonhemorrhagic SAS Disease

Sequence	Sensitivity (%)	Specificity (%)	Accuracy (%)
FLAIR*	86 (6 of 7 for reader 1, 6 of 7 for reader 2)	91 (15 of 16 for reader 1, 14 of 16 for reader 2)	89 (21 of 23 for reader 1, 20 of 23 for reader 2)
Gadolinium-enhanced T1-weighted	43 (3 of 7)	88 (14 of 16)	74 (17 of 23)

* Data averaged for two readers.

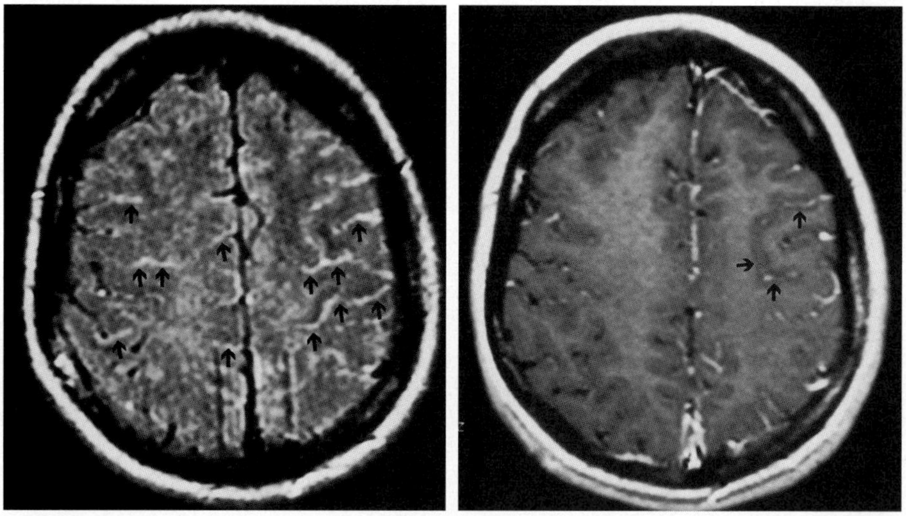

a. b.

Figure 2. MR images obtained in a 33-year-old woman with herpes meningoencephalitis. **(a)** FLAIR image (10,000/147/2,200) demonstrates extensive areas of increased signal intensity (arrows) within the SAS bilaterally. **(b)** Gadolinium-enhanced T1-weighted image (600/10) shows a smaller region of abnormal leptomeningeal enhancement (arrows) isolated in the left hemisphere. Both **a** and **b** were interpreted as positive for SAS disease.

DISCUSSION

MR imaging is widely regarded as being highly sensitive for nearly all disorders that involve the brain parenchyma, and continued development of software and hardware has further heightened its sensitivity and specificity for disease processes. FLAIR, an inversion-recovery pulse sequence that combines T2 weighting with CSF signal suppression, has been shown to be a highly sensitive sequence for the detection of parenchymal lesions (4–8).

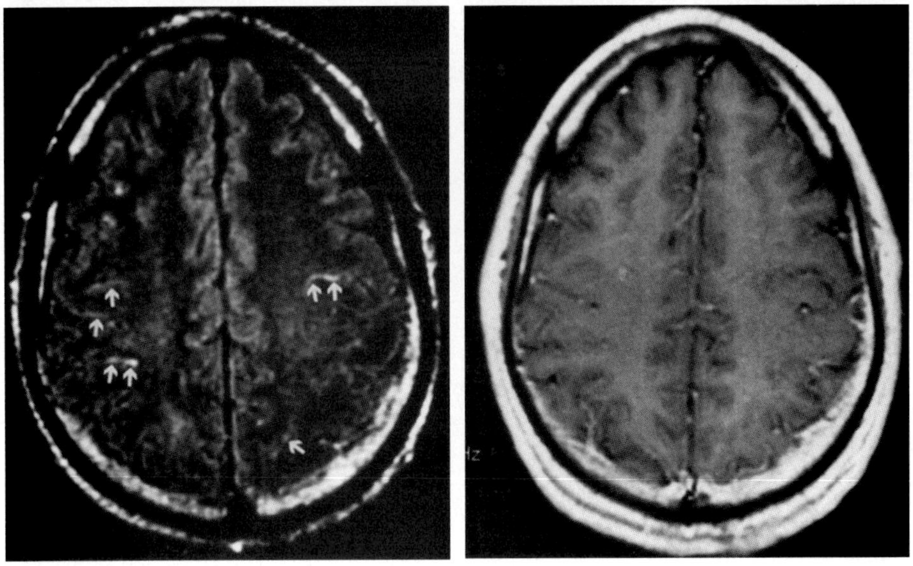

a. b.

Figure 3. MR images obtained in a 32-year-old man with HIV and cryptococcal meningitis. **(a)** FLAIR image (10,000/147/2,200) demonstrates bilateral areas of increased signal intensity (arrows) within the SAS, reported as abnormal by both blinded readers. **(b)** Gadolinium-enhanced T1-weighted image (600/10) shows no abnormal enhancement and was interpreted as normal.

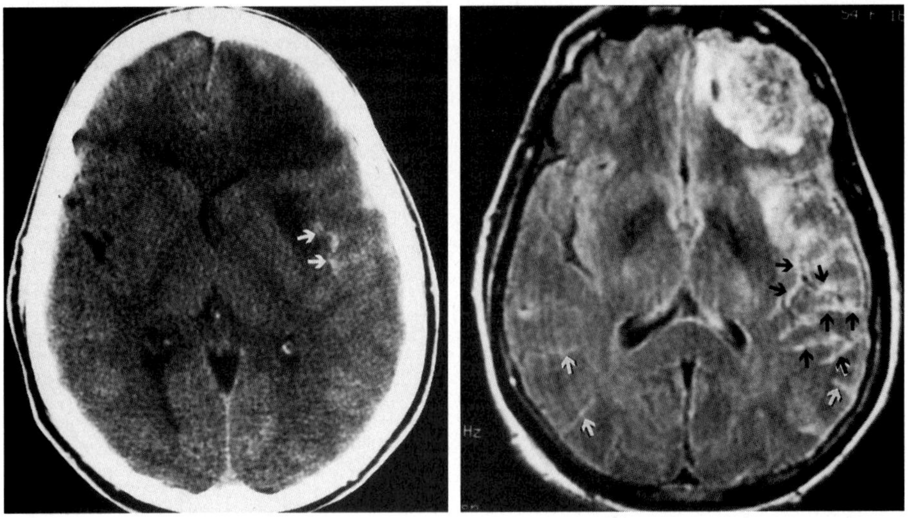

a. b.

Figure 4. Images obtained in a 54-year-old woman with acute SAH. **(a)** CT scan demonstrates acute SAH (arrows) in the region of the left sylvian fissure. Also note the large low-attenuation region in the left frontal lobe, which represents a contusion. **(b)** FLAIR image (10,000/147/2,200) demonstrates more extensive areas of increased signal intensity (arrows) within the left sylvian fissure and in the left and right temporal and parietal regions, reported as abnormal by both blinded readers. A left frontal lobe contusion is also clearly seen.

Since conventional MR imaging sequences are already sensitive to parenchymal lesions, the added value of FLAIR over that of conventional fast spin-echo sequences and therefore its precise role in routine imaging is still subject to debate (9). Notwithstanding this issue, many radiologists have incorporated FLAIR as an adjunct into brain MR imaging protocols, particularly for defining parenchymal lesions adjacent to the ventricles or sulci.

For the detection of inflammatory and neoplastic disease processes that affect the SAS or leptomeninges, contrast-enhanced conventional MR imaging has been widely regarded as the most sensitive imaging study and has thus become the standard method of imaging in these patients. For both animal models (13) and human studies of inflammatory disease, the superiority of contrast-enhanced MR over contrast-enhanced CT has been described in several nonblinded, side-by-side comparison studies.

However, even with the use of intravenous contrast agents, MR imaging has substantial limitations that have been repeatedly documented in the literature. The radiology literature states that abnormal contrast agent enhancement is noted in only 55%–70% of patients with proved infectious meningitis on contrast-enhanced MR images (14,15). It has also been noted that contrast-enhanced MR imaging is particularly insensitive to viral meningitis (14,16). For neoplastic leptomeningeal or SAS disease, abnormal MR findings are present in only 36%–71% of patients with proved carcinomatous meningitis (17,18). Despite this apparent overall lack of high sensitivity for either inflammatory or neoplastic leptomeningeal or SAS disease, MR imaging with contrast agent enhancement has become the de facto standard imaging technique.

The diagnosis of acute SAH at CT scanning is well established in clinical practice (19–21), where the sensitivity for acute SAH is thought to approach 100%. Chakeres and Bryan (22), who used an in vitro model, reported that theoretically MR should be more sensitive to acute SAH than CT. Although some clinical studies have claimed that conventional MR imaging has high sensitivity and therefore is a reliable imaging technique for acute SAH (23–25), these findings have been highly controversial (3). Despite in vitro relaxation rate changes and scattered clinical reports, it has been generally accepted that the use of conventional MR to evaluate acute SAH is limited and certainly suboptimal when compared with CT. It has been suggested from findings of in vitro experiments (26) that the cause of the insensitivity of conventional MR imaging to acute SAH is the relatively oxygen-saturated hemoglobin present in the SAS. Additional factors that have been invoked to explain the insensitivity of MR imaging for acute SAH include the lack of hemoconcentration and clot retraction in diffuse SAH, the confounding motion (circulation) of SAS contents, and brain and vascular pulsations during the cardiac cycle.

More recently, FLAIR imaging has been used in preliminary studies to evaluate acute, subacute, and chronic SAH. Noguchi et al (10) examined a group of 20 patients with acute SAH by using FLAIR imaging at 0.5 T in a blinded reader study. The accuracy of FLAIR in that study was 100%. Noguchi et al (11) also published a study in 14 patients with subacute or chronic SAH, in which FLAIR was again 100% sensitive and superior to conventional MR imaging.

In our blinded reader study reported on here, we compared the diagnostic yields of FLAIR and of contrast-enhanced T1-weighted MR imaging for the diagnosis of leptomeningeal or SAS disease processes, including acute SAH and inflammatory and neoplastic disorders. In our study, the data demonstrate that FLAIR is highly sensitive (Figs 2–4) and specific for leptomeningeal or SAS abnormalities (Tables 4, 5). Findings from the analysis of cases in which both FLAIR and contrast-enhanced T1-weighted imaging were performed (Tables 6, 7) show that contrast-enhanced T1-weighted MR imaging was equally specific but was far less sensitive then FLAIR in the inflammatory and neoplastic cases (see Table 7) (we separated out the acute SAH cases from this comparison, since contrast-enhanced T1-weighted MR imaging is not generally used for that diagnosis).

Since intravenous contrast agents by necessity are more costly, time-consuming, cause patient discomfort, and have some additional associated risks of morbidity, the data indicate that FLAIR could and even should be used instead of contrast-enhanced T1-weighted MR imaging in the search for leptomeningeal or SAS disorders of inflammatory or neoplastic causes. This is particularly relevant in those cases in which the diagnosis of isolated SAS disease is sought, since many patients with a suspected leptomeningeal or SAS abnormality also are undergoing imaging for parenchymal disease of the brain. In this latter group, it is likely that contrast-enhanced images of the brain parenchyma are desired in addition to the search for SAS and leptomeningeal enhancement.

Moreover, although we included only six patients with proved acute SAH in our study, our data do indicate the potential use of FLAIR imaging in that clinical setting and do confirm the data reported previously (10). We found FLAIR to have 100% sensitivity for the presence of acute SAH. In our small study group, there were no cases in which CT demonstrated SAH and FLAIR did not, and, in one case, FLAIR findings were abnormal whereas CT findings were normal (the diagnosis was proved by means of lumbar puncture). In some cases, the extent of the abnormality was clearly (albeit subjectively) more extensive on the FLAIR images than on the CT images. Although we did not design our study to assess the specificity of FLAIR for acute SAH, in retrospect, all cases of leptomeningeal or SAS disease, whether inflammatory, neoplastic, or hemorrhagic, appear identical at FLAIR: hyperintensity within the SASs. In our cases, FLAIR was nonspecific in its ability to differentiate SAS abnormalities related to blood from those related to neoplasm or from those related to inflammation.

In conclusion, FLAIR is highly sensitive and specific in the diagnosis of leptomeningeal or SAS disease. Furthermore, while contrast-enhanced T1-weighted MR imaging has become the standard method of evaluating such disease states, our blinded reader data suggest that contrast-enhanced imaging is actually not particularly sensitive in the clinical settings of either inflammatory or neoplastic meningitis. Unenhanced FLAIR is superior to contrast-enhanced T1-weighted MR imaging for the diagnosis of SAS disease processes. These data have important implications because FLAIR is performed without the costs and inherent risks of intravenous contrast agents. Although our sample size was small, FLAIR appears highly sensitive but nonspecific for acute SAH.

References

1. Bydder GM, Steiner RE, Young IR, Hall AS, Thomas DJ, Marshall J. Clinical NMR imaging of the brain: 140 cases. AJR 1982; 139:215–236.
2. Zimmerman RD, Heier LA, Snow RB, Liu DPC, Kelly AB, Deck MDF. Acute intracranial hemorrhage: intensity changes on sequential MR scans at 0.5T. AJNR 1988; 9:47–57.
3. Atlas SW. MR imaging is highly sensitive for acute subarachnoid hemorrhage . . . not! Radiology 1993; 186:319–322.
4. Hajnal JV, Bryant DJ, Kasuboski L, et al. Use of fluid attenuated inversion recovery (FLAIR) pulse sequences in MRI of the brain. J Comput Assist Tomogr 1992; 16: 841–844.
5. De Coene B, Hajnal J, Gatehouse P, et al. MR of the brain using fluid-attenuated inversion recovery (FLAIR) pulse sequences. AJNR 1992; 13:1555–1564.
6. Brant-Zawadzki M, Atkinson D, Detrick M, Bradley W, Scidmore G. Fluid-attenuated inversion recovery (FLAIR) for assessment of cerebral infarction. Stroke 1996; 27:1187–1191.
7. Tsuchiya K, Inaoka S, Mizutani Y, Hachiya J. Fast fluid-attenuated inversion-recovery MR of intracranial infections. AJNR 1997; 18:909–913.
8. Rydberg J, Hammond C, Grimm R, et al. Initial clinical experience in MR imaging of the brain with a fast fluid-attenuated inversion recovery pulse sequence. Radiology 1994; 193:173–180.
9. Amaral L, Fredriksson L, Atlas S. Fast FLAIR MRI in ischemic white matter lesions: quantitative comparison with fast SE imaging (abstr). Radiology 1996; 201(P): 308.
10. Noguchi N, Ogawa T, Inugami A, et al. Acute subarachnoid hemorrhage: MR imaging with fluid-attenuated inversion recovery pulse sequences. Radiology 1995; 196:773–777.
11. Noguchi N, Ogawa T, Seto H, et al. Subacute and chronic subarachnoid hemorrhage: diagnosis with fluid-attenuated inversion-recovery MR imaging. Radiology 1997; 203:257–262.
12. Melhem E, Jara H, Eustace S. Fluid-attenuated inversion recovery MR imaging: identification of protein concentration thresholds for CSF hyperintensity. AJR 1997; 169:859–862.
13. Mathews VP, Kuharik MA, Edwards MK, et al. Gd-DTPA enhanced MR imaging of experimental bacterial meningitis: evaluation and comparison with CT. AJNR 1988; 9:1045–1050.
14. Chang K, Han M, Kim I, Han M, Kim CW. Gd-DTPA enhanced MR imaging of the brain in patients with meningitis: comparison with CT. AJNR 1990; 11:69–76.
15. Ginsberg L. Contrast enhancement in meningeal and extra-axial disease. Neuroimaging Clin North Am 1994; 4:133–152.
16. Phillips M, Ryals T, Kambhu S, Yuh W. Neoplastic vs inflammatory meningeal enhancement with Gd-DTPA. J Comput Assist Tomogr 1990; 14:536–541.
17. Sze G, Soletsky S, Bronen R, Krol G. MR imaging of the cranial meninges with emphasis on contrast enhancement and meningeal carcinomatosis. AJNR 1989; 10:965–975.
18. Yousem D, Patrone P, Grossman R. Leptomeningeal metastases: MR evaluation. J Comput Assist Tomogr 1990; 14:255–261.
19. Scotti G, Ethier R, Melancon D, Terbrugge K, Tchang S. Computed tomography in the evaluation of intracranial aneurysms and subarachnoid hemorrhage. Radiology 1977; 123:85–90.
20. New PFJ, Aronow S. Attenuation measurements of whole blood and blood fractions in computed tomography. Radiology 1976; 121:635–640.
21. Norman D, Price D, Boyd D, Fishman R, Newton T. Quantitative aspects of computed tomography of blood and cerebrospinal fluid. Radiology 1977; 133:335–338.
22. Chakeres DW, Bryan RN. Acute subarachnoid hemorrhage: in vitro comparison of magnetic resonance with computed tomography. AJNR 1986; 7:223–228.
23. Satoh S, Kadoya S. Magnetic resonance imaging of subarachnoid hemorrhage. Neuroradiology 1988; 30:361–366.
24. Ogawa T, Inugami A, Shimosegawa E, et al. Subarachnoid hemorrhage: evaluation with MR imaging. Radiology 1993; 186: 345–351.
25. Ogawa T, Uemura K. MR imaging is highly sensitive for acute subarachnoid hemorrhage . . . not! reply. Radiology 1993; 186: 323.
26. Grossman RI, Kemp SS, Ip C, et al. The importance of oxygenation in the appearance of acute subarachnoid hemorrhage on high-field magnetic resonance imaging. Acta Radiol Suppl 1986; 369:56–58.

Subarachnoid Hemorrhage: Aneurysm Detection and Preoperative Evaluation with CT Angiography[1]

Birgitta K. Velthuis, MD
Gabriel J. E. Rinkel, MD
Lino M. P. Ramos, MD
Theodoor D. Witkamp, MD
Jan Willem Berkelbach van der Sprenkel, MD
W. Peter Vandertop, MD
Maarten S. van Leeuwen, MD

Index terms:
Aneurysm, intracranial, 17.73
Aneurysm, rupture, 17.73
Computed tomography (CT), angiography, 17.12116
Computed tomography (CT), clinical effectiveness
Computed tomography (CT), comparative studies, 17.12116, 17.12493
Digital subtraction angiography, comparative studies, 17.12116, 17.1219

Radiology 1998; 208:423–430

Abbreviations:
DSA = digital subtraction angiography
MIP = maximum intensity projection
PICA = posterior inferior cerebellar artery
SAH = subarachnoid hemorrhage

[1] From the Departments of Radiology (B.K.V., L.M.P.R., T.D.W., M.S.v.L.), Neurology (G.J.E.R.), and Neurosurgery (J.W.B.v.d.S., W.P.V.), Utrecht University Hospital, Rm E01.132, Heidelberglaan 100, 3584 CX Utrecht, The Netherlands. Received September 16, 1997; revision requested November 24; revision received February 2, 1998; accepted March 26. **Address reprint requests to** B.K.V.

Author contributions:
Guarantors of integrity of entire study, B.K.V., G.J.E.R., M.S.v.L.; study concepts, B.K.V., G.J.E.R., M.S.v.L.; study design, B.K.V., G.J.E.R., M.S.v.L., L.M.P.R., T.D.W., J.W.B.v.d.S., W.P.V.; definition of intellectual content, B.K.V., G.J.E.R., M.S.v.L.; literature research, B.K.V., G.J.E.R., M.S.v.L.; clinical studies, B.K.V., G.J.E.R., M.S.v.L., L.M.P.R., T.D.W., J.W.B.v.d.S., W.P.V.; data acquisition, B.K.V., L.M.P.R., T.D.W., J.W.B.v.d.S., W.P.V.; data analysis, B.K.V., G.J.E.R., M.S.v.L.; statistical analysis, B.K.V., G.J.E.R., M.S.v.L.; manuscript preparation and editing, B.K.V., G.J.E.R., M.S.v.L.; manuscript review, B.K.V., G.J.E.R., M.S.v.L., L.M.P.R., T.D.W., J.W.B.v.d.S., W.P.V.

PURPOSE: To evaluate if computed tomographic (CT) angiography can replace digital subtraction angiography (DSA) for aneurysm detection and as preoperative work-up in patients with subarachnoid hemorrhage (SAH).

MATERIALS AND METHODS: Prospectively, 100 patients with SAH underwent CT angiography; 80 also underwent DSA. Two observers independently evaluated CT angiographic source images and maximum intensity projection slabs. Neurosurgeons compared CT angiograms and DSA images for presurgical evaluation.

RESULTS: On CT angiograms, the observers detected 73 and 70 of 75 symptomatic aneurysms; 96% of the detected aneurysms were classified as definitely present. Of 16 incidental aneurysms, 12 and 10 were detected by the observers. With adequate CT angiographic quality, parent artery side of anterior communicating aneurysms was correctly predicted in 100% (95% confidence interval [CI]: 87%, 100%). Neurosurgeons assessed CT angiography as equal or superior to DSA in 83% (95% CI: 73%, 90%) of 87 aneurysms, and in 74% (95% CI: 63%, 82%) operation might have been based on CT angiographic findings alone.

CONCLUSION: CT angiography depicted 90% of all aneurysms, and 90% were classified as definitely present. CT angiography must be of high quality with adequate depiction of the aneurysm and the parent artery for surgery to be performed on the basis of CT angiographic findings alone.

Subarachnoid hemorrhage (SAH) from a ruptured aneurysm carries a poor prognosis, with a case fatality rate of approximately 45% worldwide (1). In patients who survive the initial hemorrhage, rebleeding is an important cause of mortality and morbidity. Surgical intervention is aimed at prevention of rebleeding, and since the frequency of rebleeding is highest in the first 24–48 hours after the initial hemorrhage (2,3), surgery should be performed as soon as possible. Conventional angiography, usually selective intraarterial digital subtraction angiography (DSA), is the method of choice for detection of aneurysms before surgery, but it is invasive, can be time-consuming, and carries a 1% complication risk with a 0.5% rate of persistent neurologic deficit (4). Moreover, angiography performed within the first 6 hours after the initial bleeding incident has been associated with an increased rebleeding rate (3,5). Alternative imaging modalities are magnetic resonance (MR) angiography and computed tomographic (CT) angiography. MR angiography is safe but less suitable for patients with SAH in the acute stage, because they are often restless or need extensive monitoring (6).

CT angiography seems very suitable in the acute stage after SAH; it does not require intraarterial catheterization, scanning time is only 1 minute, and it can immediately follow the initial unenhanced CT examination. After data acquisition, postprocessing techniques (7–23), such as shaded-surface display (7–15,22,23) or maximum intensity projection (MIP) (15–23), are required to produce angiographic-like display. In a pilot study, we found that cine review of the axial source images combined with MIP of a limited volume of interest (slab-MIP) was most practical for daily use in patients with SAH (22).

The purpose of this study was to prospectively evaluate CT angiography for detection and localization of aneurysms in patients with SAH and to determine in which patients surgery might have been based on CT angiographic findings alone.

MATERIALS AND METHODS

From July 1995 through October 1996, we prospectively evaluated 121 consecutive patients admitted with the diagnosis of SAH to the Utrecht University Hospital. Inclusion criteria for enrollment was the diagnosis of SAH on the basis of the presence of subarachnoid blood on unenhanced CT scans or xanthochromia (presence of old blood pigments) in cerebrospinal fluid at lumbar puncture in patients who did not have evidence of hemorrhage on unenhanced CT scans. Fifteen patients who had already undergone DSA at another hospital were not included in this study. Of the 106 patients enrolled, six were excluded because they were too restless or their condition was too critical for them to undergo CT angiography. The study population therefore comprised 100 patients (71 women, 29 men; age range, 24–78 years; mean age, 51.7 years). The study was approved by the institutional review board. When possible, informed consent was obtained from patients or relatives. Implied consent was obtained from the neurologist in comatose patients who were not accompanied by relatives.

CT angiography was performed in all 100 patients. Scanning was performed on the day the SAH occurred (day 0) in 40 patients, within 1–3 days in 39 patients, within 4–14 days in 19 patients, and 24 and 36 days after SAH in two patients. Eighty of the 100 patients also underwent DSA. DSA was performed between 0 and 14 days (median, 1 day) after SAH in 77 patients (96%) and after 25, 37, and 67 days, respectively, in three patients (4%). Among the 80 patients, CT angiography and DSA were performed on the same day in 16 patients (20%), within 1–3 days in 44 patients (55%), and within 4–10 days in 19 patients (24%); in one patient DSA was performed 67 days after CT angiography. In 77 patients (96%), CT angiography was performed before DSA. In the other 20 of the 100 patients, DSA was not performed because 18 patients died before the investigation could be performed and two patients underwent emergency surgery for evacuation of a temporal lobe hemorrhage. Autopsy was performed in two of the 18 patients who died.

TABLE 1
Aneurysm Detection according to Site and Size in 91 Confirmed Aneurysms

Site* and Detection by Observer	Aneurysm Size (mm) <5	5–10	11–15	16–25	Total	Detection with CT Angiography Observer 1	Observer 2
Anterior communicating artery	12	17	4	0	33	33	31
Pericallosal artery	2	0	0	0	2	2	2
ICA bifurcation	0	1	0	0	1	1	1
Ophthalmic artery	1	0	0	0	1	1	0
Other ICA locations	0	2	0	0	2	1	1
Posterior communicating artery	6	11	2	1	20	17	15
M1 segment	3	0	0	0	3	2	2
M1-M2	6	11	3	0	20	20	20
Top of basilar artery	2	1	0	1	4	4	4
Superior cerebellar artery	0	1	0	0	1	1	1
Vertebral artery or PICA	0	2	0	0	2	2	2
Distal PICA	1	1	0	0	2	1	1
Total	32	48	9	2	91	85	80
Detection with CT angiography							
Observer 1	28	46	9	2	. . .	85	. . .
Observer 2	24	45	9	2	. . .	. . .	80

Note.—Data are number of aneurysms.
* ICA = internal carotid artery, M1-M2 = bifurcation or trifurcation of middle cerebral artery.

TABLE 2
Analysis of Aneurysm Detection with CT Angiography

Parameter	Observer 1	95% CI*	Observer 2	95% CI*
Symptomatic aneurysms ($n = 75$)				
Sensitivity†	97% (73/75)	91%, 100%	93% (70/75)	85%, 98%
No. classified as definite	70/73	. . .	67/70	. . .
Incidental aneurysms ($n = 16$)				
No. detected	12	. . .	10	. . .
No. classified as definite	8/12	. . .	3/10	. . .
False-positive readings	1	. . .	1	. . .
PPV‡ for all detected aneurysms	99%	94%, 100%	99%	93%, 100%

* CI = confidence interval.
† Numbers in parentheses are number of aneurysms.
‡ PPV = positive predictive value.

CT Angiographic Acquistion

CT angiography was performed on a spiral CT scanner (Tomoscan SR 7000; Philips Medical Systems, Best, The Netherlands). The gantry was angled to the orbitomeatal line starting just above the posterior arch of C1, with 40 1-second rotations of 1.5-mm collimation and a table speed of 1.5 mm (pitch: 1). The 60-mm coverage with angled scan was sufficient to include the circle of Willis, the posterior inferior cerebellar arteries (PICAs), and the pericallosal arteries. Using this gantry angulation, we did not observe marked beam-hardening artifacts, which might be expected with an unangled scan. An 18-gauge needle was inserted into a cubital vein for injection of 140 mL of nonionic contrast material (iopromide, Ultravist [300 mg of iodine per milliliter]; Schering, Berlin, Germany), with use of a power injector (CT 9000 Digital Injection System; Liebel Flarsheim, Cincinatti, Ohio), at a rate of 3 mL/sec and with a 25-second delay before scanning. Other parameters were a 512 × 512 matrix, 140 kV, 125 mA, 16-cm field of view, and a reconstruction index of 1 mm. All parameters were consistent for each patient. In five instances, CT angiography was repeated within 48 hours because of image degradation due to patient motion or technical error. The source images of each scan were transferred to an off-line computer workstation (Easy Vision; Philips Medical Systems) for viewing and postprocessing.

CT Angiographic Postprocessing

MIP images were created by using a 2-cm-thick slab that was angled and rotated to evaluate the carotid and the vertebrobasilar circulation separately. The slab was angled above the anterior fossa to the carotid circulation (anterior circula-

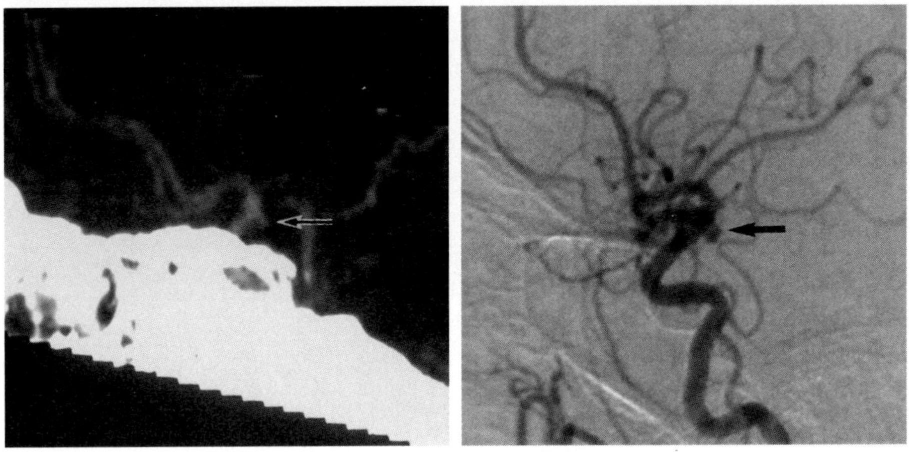

a. b.

Figure 1. On a CT angiogram of suboptimal quality **(a)**, a symptomatic right posterior communicating artery aneurysm (not shown) was detected as definitely present by both observers. A small, incidental left posterior communicating artery aneurysm (arrow) shown on the lateral **(a)** slab-MIP CT angiogram and **(b)** DSA image of the left internal carotid artery was judged by both observers as more likely an infundibulum on the CT angiogram. No posterior communicating vessel is seen on either the CT angiogram or the DSA image, making it difficult to differentiate an infundibulum from a small aneurysm.

tion) and rotated in two directions: 180° in 18 steps around the right-to-left axis and 90° in nine steps around the anteroposterior axis. Subsequently, the slab was angled parallel and just behind the clivus to the basilar artery (posterior circulation) and also rotated in two directions: 45° in nine steps around the right-to-left axis and 90° in nine steps around the craniocaudal axis. Last, midsagittal and sagittal views of both internal carotid arteries was made. On average, it took 3 minutes of operator time and 12 minutes of computer time to generate the slab-MIP images.

CT Angiographic Evaluation

CT angiograms were evaluated prospectively by two of three independent observers (B.K.V., L.M.P.R., T.D.W.) without knowledge of the results of DSA if performed before CT angiography. The first observer (B.K.V.) examined all 100 patients. The second observer was one of two neuroradiologists (L.M.P.R., T.D.W.) who had not seen the patient's images during the daily clinical consultation. The initial unenhanced CT scan was made available for the observers when evaluating the CT angiograms. First, the axial source CT angiograms were viewed in a cine loop on the workstation, and the presence of aneurysms was determined by using a five-point scale of confidence: 1, definitely present; 2, probably present; 3, possibly present; 4, probably not present; 0, definitely not present. The location of the aneurysm was also noted. Subsequently, the observers assessed the slab-MIP rotations on the workstation and determined, with use of the information from the source images and the slab-MIP images, the presence of aneurysms by using the same confidence scale. If more than one aneurysm was detected, the observers indicated which one caused the SAH, on the basis of subarachnoid blood distribution and the location of a possible intracerebral hemorrhage on the unenhanced CT scan. In the presence of anterior communicating artery aneurysms, the observers predicted the parent artery side of the aneurysm on the basis of anterior cerebral artery A1 segment asymmetry, asymmetric aneurysm location, or both. To categorize the size of the aneurysms, the greatest extent of each lesion was measured on the workstation. The quality of the CT angiograms was graded as good, suboptimal but adequate, or poor.

DSA Acquisition

Sixty-six (83%) of the 80 patients underwent standard, selective three- or four-vessel DSA with anteroposterior, lateral, and oblique views. The remaining 14 patients underwent only a Towne cerebral view with the catheter in the aortic arch and selective angiography of both common carotid arteries. No further catheterization of the vertebral arteries was done because a symptomatic aneurysm had been found on the anterior circulation and because these patients were older than 65 years. With this strategy, small, asymptomatic aneurysms may have been missed in the posterior circulation, but in our hospital we do not treat such aneurysms in patients older than 65 years. The field of view for cerebral angiography was usually 20 cm, and the matrix size was 1,024 × 1,024. In the 77 patients who underwent CT angiography before DSA, the CT angiogram was available for the angiography technologist.

Determination of the Reference Standard

For providing the standard of reference with respect to the number and location of aneurysms in the patients of this study, the findings of DSA, surgery, and autopsy were used. The DSA studies were first viewed independently by the same two observers who viewed the CT angiograms, at least 1 month after CT angiography and blinded to results of CT angiography. In cases of disagreement, a consensus opinion was obtained in a second session with all three observers. Sixty-seven of the 80 patients who underwent DSA also had surgical confirmation.

In the 20 patients who did not undergo DSA, two patients had surgical confirmation of the ruptured aneurysm and an additional two had autopsy confirmation of the ruptured aneurysm. In the remaining 16 patients who died without undergoing DSA, surgery, or autopsy, no reference standard was available.

In nine of the 84 patients who had a reference standard, no aneurysms were found. In the remaining 75 patients, 91 aneurysms were found: 75 symptomatic and 16 incidental aneurysms. In the 13 patients with multiple aneurysms, the symptomatic aneurysm was defined as the aneurysm that caused the SAH according to findings at surgery, pattern of hemorrhage, and site and size of the aneurysm.

Determination of Preoperative Value of CT Angiography

To determine whether surgery might have been based on CT angiographic findings alone, the CT angiograms were evaluated by one of two neurosurgeons (J.W.B.v.d.S., W.P.V.) between 3 and 6 months after surgery. For this part of the study, only the 71 patients who had undergone DSA and who had one or more aneurysms were included. In patients with multiple aneurysms, each aneurysm was assessed separately. In each case, the source and slab-MIP images of the CT angiographic study were shown to the neurosurgeon as if in a clinical demonstration. The neurosurgeon was then asked if surgery could be based on CT angiographic findings alone. If additional DSA was required, the reasons were noted. Subsequently, the DSA images were demonstrated, and the neurosurgeon was asked whether DSA provided additional information that was essential for surgery; if so, this information was recorded. Finally, the CT angiograms and DSA images were compared side by side, and the neurosurgeon determined whether CT angiograms, from a surgical standpoint, were superior, equal, or inferior to DSA images with respect to depiction of location, shape, orientation, neck, and parent artery of the aneurysm. Location included relationship to adjacent arterial branches, such as middle cerebral artery bifurcation or trifurcation, posterior communicating or anterior choroidal arteries, and so forth. Shape included the number of lobes of the aneurysm.

Data Analysis

Definitely, probably, and possibly present aneurysms were grouped as positive findings, and probably not or definitely not present aneurysms were grouped as negative findings. For analysis, we divided the aneurysms into two groups: symptomatic and incidental aneurysms. Sensitivity was calculated for detection of symptomatic aneurysms on CT angiograms, and positive predictive values were determined for the detection of all aneurysms and for the prediction of parent artery side of anterior communicating aneurysms on CT angiograms. Observer agreement for aneurysm detection was calculated for CT angiography by using κ statistics (24). The level of agreement was regarded as poor if κ was between 0.41 and 0.60, good if κ was between 0.61 and 0.80, and excellent if κ was between 0.81 and 1.0.

The neurosurgeon's assessment if aneurysm surgery could be based on CT angiographic findings alone was expressed in percentages and as a positive predictive value.

RESULTS

The quality of the CT angiograms was good in 76 of the 100 patients, suboptimal but adequate in 16, and poor in eight. The reasons for unsatisfactory CT angiographic quality were patient movement in six patients, vasospasm in three (as seen on DSA performed in the same period), technical error in seven (resulting in a prolonged delay between injection of contrast material and scanning), technician error (320 matrix instead of 512) in one, and unknown in seven patients. There were no patients in our study in whom dense subarachnoid blood interfered with maximum intensity projection for the detection of aneurysms. CT angiography was repeated in five of the patients with poor quality CT angiograms.

CT Angiographic Detection of Aneurysms

The results of detection of aneurysms with CT angiography are given in Tables 1 and 2. On CT angiograms, observer 1 (B.K.V.) detected 73 and observer 2 (L.M.P.R. or T.D.W.) found 70 of 75 symptomatic aneurysms. Both observers missed a small symptomatic PICA aneurysm located behind the fourth ventricle and an infraclinoid carotid aneurysm. Observer 2 missed three other symptomatic aneurysms: a 2-mm and a 6-mm aneurysm originating from the posterior communicating artery and a 3-mm aneurysm of the anterior communicating artery. Observer 1 detected 12 and observer 2 10 of the 16 incidental aneurysms. Both observers mistook two small posterior communicating aneurysms for infundibula (Fig 1), missed another small main trunk middle cerebral artery aneurysm, and recognized only one of two right-sided infraclinoid carotid aneurysms in one patient. In addi-

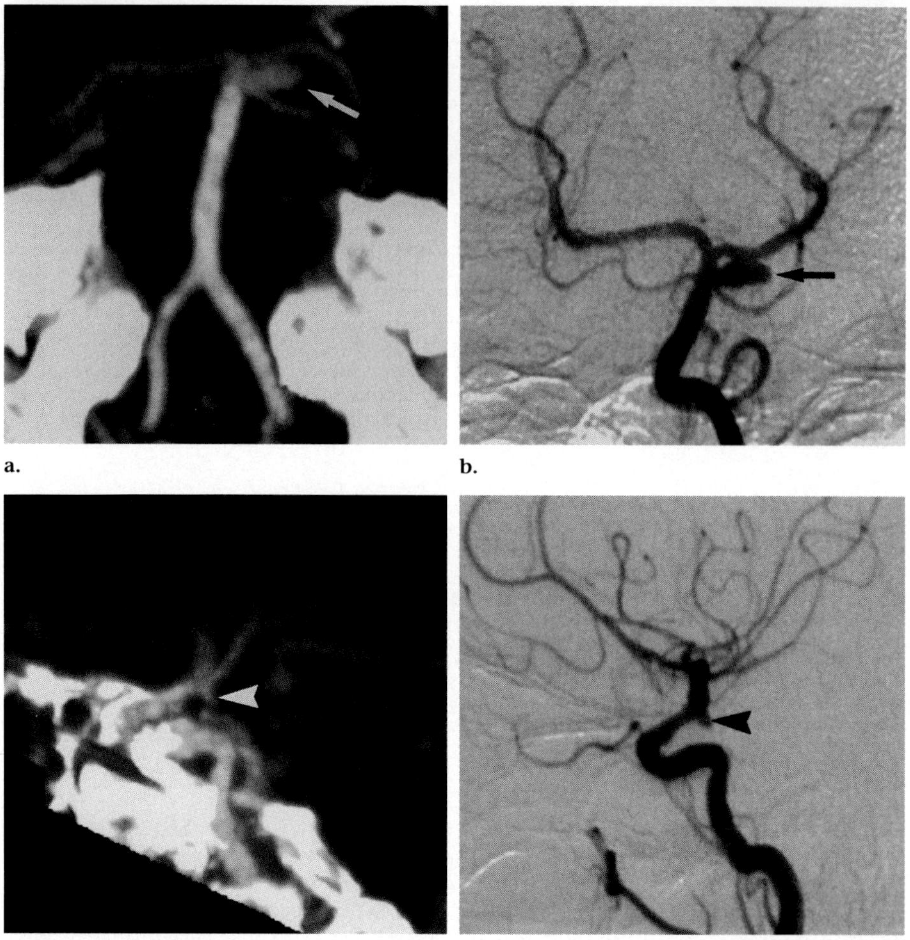

a. b. c. d.

Figure 2. Case of a patient with a symptomatic left superior cerebellar aneurysm (arrow in **a** and **b**) well demonstrated on frontal **(a)** slab-MIP CT angiogram and **(b)** DSA image of the vertebrobasilar circulation who was suspected of having an incidental left posterior communicating aneurysm (arrowhead in **c** and **d**) as shown on lateral **(c)** slab-MIP CT angiogram and **(d)** DSA image of the left internal carotid artery. As in Figure 1, no left posterior communicating artery is seen on either the CT angiogram or the DSA image. Surgical exploration revealed a posterior communicating artery infundibulum but no aneurysm.

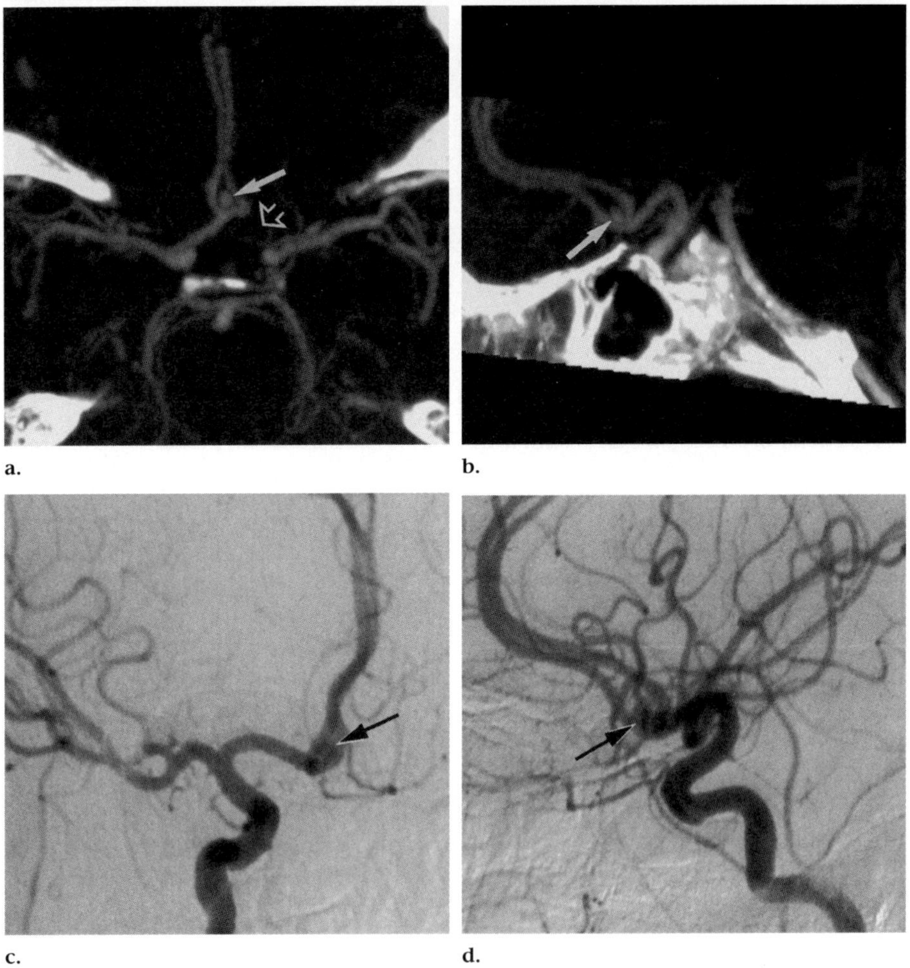

Figure 3. **(a)** Base and **(b)** lateral slab-MIP CT angiograms show an anterior communicating artery aneurysm (solid arrow). The parent artery was predicted as right-sided on the base CT angiogram because of the aplastic left A1 segment (open arrow). **(c)** Frontal oblique and **(d)** lateral DSA images of the right internal carotid artery confirm the presence of the aneurysm (arrow) and the right-sided parent artery. A left internal carotid artery with aplastic A1 segment is not shown. The neurosurgeon judged CT angiography better than DSA for all characteristics.

tion, observer 2 missed a 3-mm anterior communicating aneurysm and a 2-mm ophthalmic aneurysm.

Observer 1 diagnosed one false-positive incidental aneurysm on CT angiograms, classified as possibly present in a patient with a detected symptomatic aneurysm (Fig 2). In the nine patients with no aneurysm, observer 1 found no aneurysms on CT angiograms, and observer 2 diagnosed one false-positive aneurysm on CT angiograms, classified as possibly present. Of these nine patients with no aneurysm, five had patterns of SAH compatible with perimesencephalic hemorrhage (25). On CT angiograms, both observers found 96% of the detected aneurysms on source images (82 of 85 and 77 of 80, respectively). At subsequent slab-MIP viewing, the detection rate was increased by 4% and the level of certainty was raised in 7% of detected aneurysms. The level of agreement between observers for aneurysm detection with CT angiography was good for detection of all aneurysms ($\kappa = 0.79$) and also for detection of only symptomatic aneurysms ($\kappa = 0.79$).

In 15 of 16 patients with CT angiograms but without a reference of DSA, surgery, or autopsy, both observers found a symptomatic aneurysm, classified as certain. In one patient, a possible aneurysm was diagnosed by both observers.

Of the 33 anterior communicating artery aneurysms, observer 1 detected 33 aneurysms on CT angiograms and observer 2 found 31. In four patients, the parent artery could not be determined on CT angiograms because of poor quality. Among the remaining detected anterior communicating artery aneurysms, both observers correctly predicted the parent artery side in all patients on the basis of asymmetric A1 size (18 aneurysms [62%]), asymmetric aneurysm location (four aneurysms [14%]), or both (seven aneurysms [24%]) (Figs 3, 4). Thus, with good CT angiographic quality, the positive predictive value for parent artery side of anterior communicating aneurysms was 100% for observer 1 (95% confidence interval: 88%, 100%) and also 100% for observer 2 (95% confidence interval: 87%, 100%).

Determination of Preoperative Value of CT Angiography

When viewing CT angiograms alone, 64 (74%; 95% confidence interval: 63%, 82%) of the 87 aneurysms were assessed to be amenable for surgery. For these 64 aneurysms, subsequent review of the DSA images provided no essential extra information; thus, the positive predictive value of CT angiographic assessment for which surgery of the aneurysms could be performed on the basis of CT angiographic findings alone was 100% (95% confidence interval: 94%, 100%)(Fig 5).

The neurosurgeons requested DSA for 23 aneurysms. One reason for requiring DSA was the uncertain presence of 11 aneurysms, for which subsequent DSA assessment provided no extra information in nine. Other reasons for requesting DSA were (*a*) difficult location in three aneurysms (one distal PICA aneurysm, one PICA aneurysm with coexistent arteriovenous malformation, and one large basilar artery aneurysm with a wide neck), (*b*) the need for extra anatomic information in one middle cerebral artery aneurysm with unclear trifurcation, (*c*) uncertainty of the parent artery in four (two anterior communicating aneurysms, one pericallosal aneurysm, and one aneurysm at the junction of the posterior communicating artery with the posterior cerebral artery [Fig 6]), and (*d*) insufficient quality in four. In eight of these 12 cases, DSA provided the required additional information.

The results of the neurosurgeon's evaluation with respect to the five aneurysm characteristics on CT angiograms and DSA images are shown on the bar chart in Figure 7. CT angiography was superior or equal to DSA for all five characteristics in 72 (83%) of the 87 aneurysms, was inferior for all five characteristics in four (4%), and varied in 11 (13%).

DISCUSSION

The advantages of CT angiography for patients with SAH are that it is easily

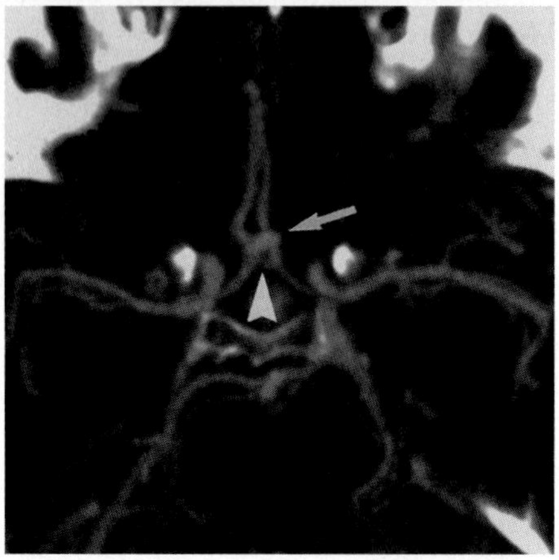

a.

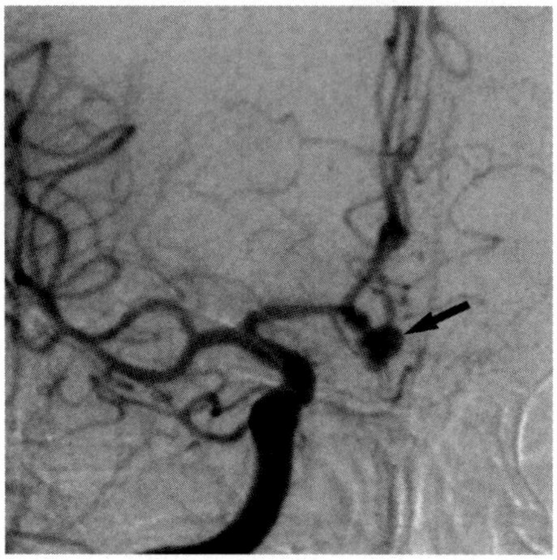

b.

Figure 4. **(a)** Slab-MIP CT angiogram in base view shows the asymmetric location of an anterior communicating artery aneurysm (arrow) on the right side of the anterior communicating artery (arrowhead). **(b)** Frontal DSA image of the right carotid artery confirms the predicted right-sided parent artery and demonstrates the aneurysm (arrow) of the anterior communicating artery. There was no filling of the aneurysm by the left carotid artery (not shown). The advantage of the slab-MIP CT angiographic base view with rotations resulted in a better judgment of CT angiography over DSA for determination of precise location and neck of the aneurysm by the neurosurgeon.

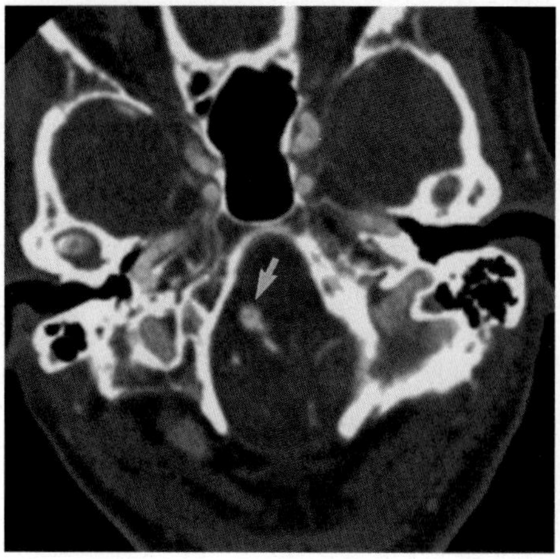

a.

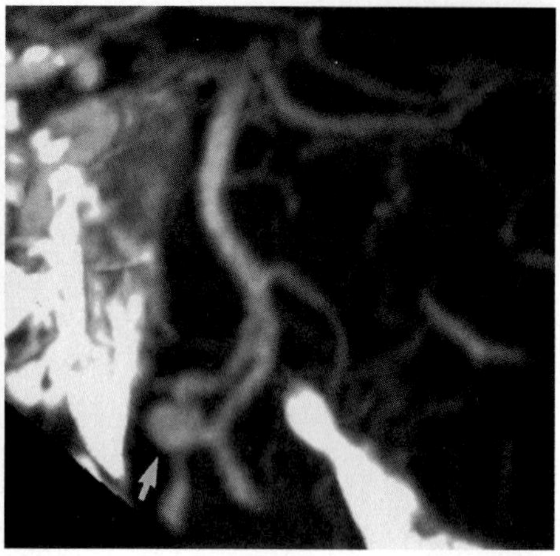

b.

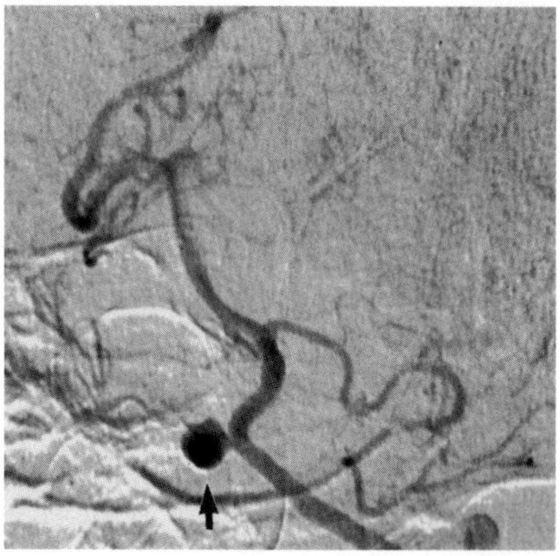

c.

Figure 5. **(a)** Axial CT source image, **(b)** slab-MIP CT angiogram, and **(c)** DSA image of the left vertebral artery demonstrate an aneurysm (arrow) of a tortuous left vertebral artery. The CT angiogram and DSA image are rotated views, which best demonstrate the aneurysm neck, and no left posterior inferior cerebellar artery is seen on either the CT angiogram or DSA image. The neurosurgeons judged CT angiography equal to DSA for all aneurysm characteristics, and DSA was considered unnecessary for surgery.

obtained immediately after unenhanced CT has demonstrated SAH, that it is minimally invasive, and that any desired projection can retrospectively be created from the CT angiographic data set. A disadvantage of CT angiography is that postprocessing is required for angiographic-like display, while the source images still need to be carefully examined for certain aneurysm locations. If CT angiography is to replace DSA, it must depict most true aneurysms, demonstrate no false-positive aneurysms as definitely present, and depict the parent artery of anterior communicating aneurysms; also, the CT angiographic display must be acceptable to neurosurgeons as preoperative work-up. In our study, CT angiography depicted 95% of the 75 symptomatic aneurysms and 90% of all 91 aneurysms, and 90% of all detected aneurysms (n = 165) were classified as definitely present. In addition, there were only two false-positive readings, and neither was classified as definitely present. Prediction of parent artery side of anterior communicating aneurysms was always correct on CT angiograms of adequate quality. According to a neurosurgeon's retrospective assessment, CT angiography obviated DSA for 64 (74%) of 87 aneurysms.

Most of the detected aneurysms (96%) were found on CT angiographic source images, confirming the results of the study by Schmid et al (26) of a 93% aneurysm detection rate on source images, with only multiplanar reconstruction images available. The added value of MIP over source images for aneurysm detection in our current study was limited, but MIP is helpful for clinical demonstration and preoperative planning. Some projections, such as a base view or a possible surgical view, are easily obtained with CT angiography but are difficult with DSA. The advantages of the slab-MIP images we used are the avoidance of time-consuming bone removal and the usefulness of the remaining bony landmarks for the neurosurgeon's preoperative planning (12). Also, MIP, unlike shaded-surface display, enables differentiation of vascular structures from bone (22). Disadvantages of the 2-cm slab-MIP images are that rotation of the slab is necessary to show all the vessels free of bone and that only limited volumes of interest are visible. For aneurysms located peripherally and at the skull base, careful examination of the source images in cine view is vital.

The factor most frequently involved in our false-negative readings was suboptimal or poor quality of the CT angiograms. In the instances with poor quality CT angiograms, several factors in the data acquisition may have played a role. First, we chose a standard 25-second delay for practical purposes, but individual delays with use of bolus timing may be preferable for optimization of contrast material enhancement (23). Second, at the time of the study, 125 mA was the upper limit on our CT scanner, with a small focus. Higher milliamperes are mentioned in the literature, probably with a large focus, and this might result in a better signal-to-noise ratio at the expense of lower spatial resolution. Third, we did not sedate restless patients, and in some patients, CT angiographic quality was hampered by motion artifacts. Finally, a technical error resulting in a prolonged delay between injection of contrast material and scanning was encountered only during the first part of the study and was rectified.

Other factors associated with false-negative readings are site and size of the aneurysm: Most undetected aneurysms were smaller than 5 mm, and most were located at the posterior communicating, ophthalmic, and infraclinoid carotid arteries, which have close proximity to bony structures of the skull base. A last factor associated with both false-negative and false-positive readings is differentiation of a posterior communicating artery infundibulum from a small aneurysm if the posterior communicating artery is not visualized. This could be due to the poorer spatial resolution of CT angiography in comparison with that of DSA; however, in the two false-negative readings and one false-positive reading of CT angiograms in our study, no posterior communicating arteries were visualized on DSA images either (Figs 1, 2).

In our study, we could not compare the sensitivity of CT angiography with that of DSA, because first, we did not have a reference standard for all DSA examinations, and second, the angiography technologist tailored his DSA examination according to the results of the CT angiographic examination, which may have increased the sensitivity of DSA. The combined data of seven studies of patients with SAH and angiograms negative for aneurysm revealed that 145 repeat angiograms demonstrated no less than 22 aneurysms (27). If one takes into account that patients with a perimesencephalic hemorrhage (who constituted two-thirds of patients without an aneurysm on the initial angiogram) were not excluded from these series, the yield of follow-up angiograms in patients with diffuse or anteriorly located hemorrhage on unenhanced CT scans must be even higher. We therefore think that the sensitivity for detection of aneurysms by means of CT angiography is comparable to that of DSA. Spatial and contrast resolution of both CT angiography and DSA are continuously improving, and three-dimensional rotational angiography is a promising new technique. A future study could perhaps compare CT angiography with three-dimensional rotational angiography.

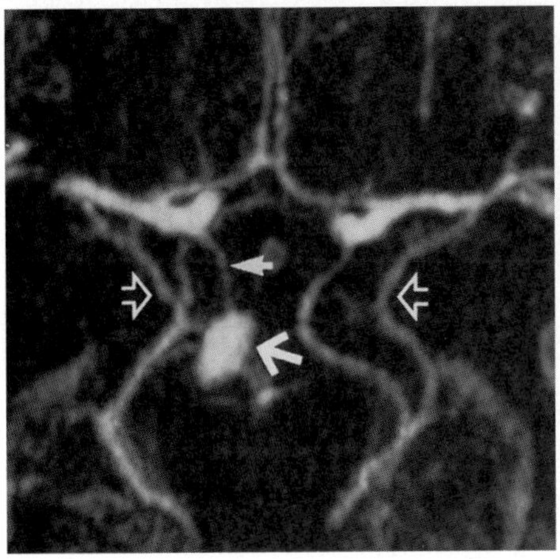

a.

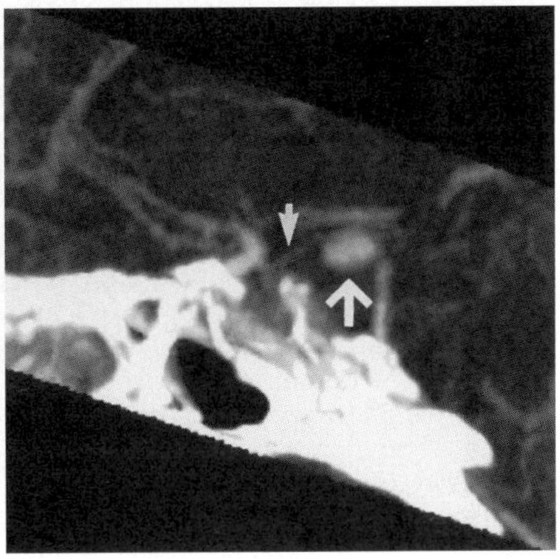

b.

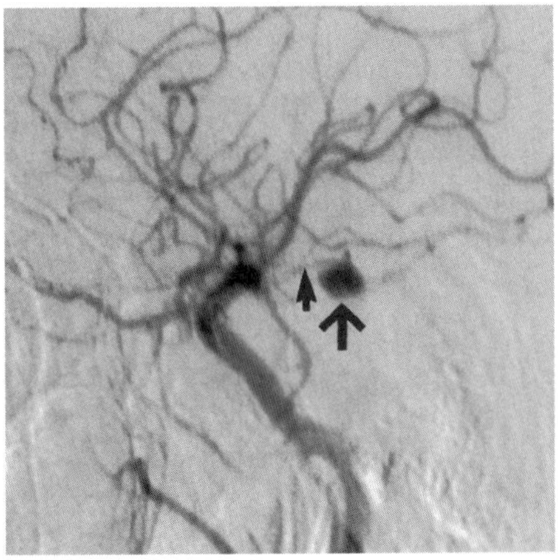

c.

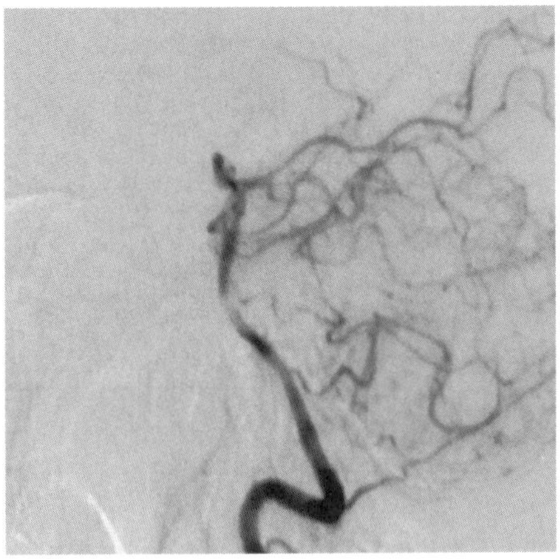

d.

Figure 6. **(a, b)** An unusual aneurysm (large arrow) at the junction of the right posterior communicating artery (small arrow) with the posterior cerebral artery was adequately demonstrated with **(a)** base and **(b)** lateral slab-MIP CT angiograms. The neurosurgeon, however, required DSA because of the unusual location and for determining the parent artery. **(c)** Lateral DSA image of the right internal carotid artery and **(d)** lateral DSA image of the vertebrobasilar circulation clearly demonstrate only the posterior communicating artery (small arrow in **c**) supplying the aneurysm (large arrow in **c**). Also note that venous structures such as the basal veins of Rosenthal (open arrows in **a**) on the CT angiograms, if recognized, do not interfere with detection of the aneurysm.

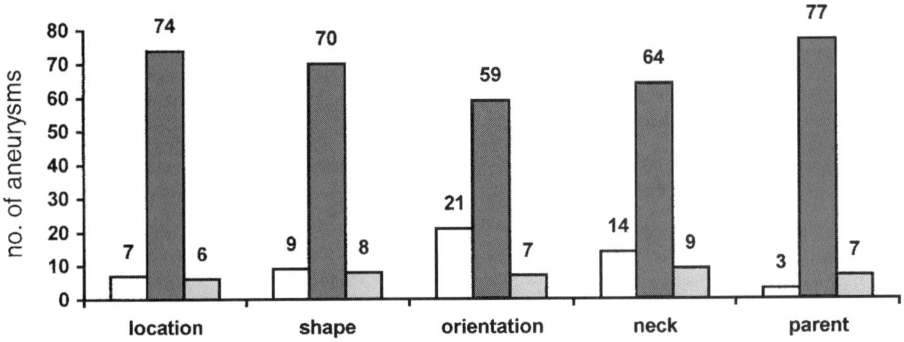

Figure 7. Bar chart with neurosurgeon's judgment of CT angiography versus DSA for 87 aneurysms. The neurosurgeon assessed if CT angiography was superior (white bars), equal (dark gray bars), or inferior (light gray bars) to DSA on the basis of five characteristics: location, shape, orientation, neck, and parent artery.

Anderson et al (23) also correctly predicted the filling side of the anterior communicating aneurysm, with asymmetric A1 segment and neck location on the anterior communicating artery. One aneurysm with symmetric A1 size and neck location on the middle of the anterior communicating artery was filled by both internal carotid arteries. They concluded that, in the setting of SAH with clear CT and CT angiographic results, no DSA is necessary for emergency surgery.

Although in this study the neurosurgeon's judgment was without clinical consequences for patient care, our results show that, with detected aneurysms classified as definitely present and with a certain parent artery, surgery could have been based on CT angiographic findings alone for most aneurysms. There were no false-positive readings classified as definitely present on CT angiograms, and the neurosurgeon's judgment for possible surgery on the basis of CT angiographic findings alone was never revoked with subsequent viewing of the DSA images. This is important if neurosurgeons are to base their decision for either surgery or additional DSA on CT angiographic findings alone. Our finding that CT angiography is superior or equal to DSA in most instances (83% [72 of 87 aneurysms]) is in accordance with that of Liang et al (10), who reported that neurosurgeons rated CT angiography as superior or equal to DSA in 12 (80%) of 15 aneurysms.

Recently, endovascular therapy of cerebral aneurysms is increasingly being used as an alternative to neurosurgery, but we have chosen to use neurosurgical evaluation of CT angiography, as this is still the standard method of treatment. We do not expect that CT angiography will become superfluous if endovascular therapy develops into the standard treatment, because CT angiography is easily performed directly after the initial unenhanced CT examination, and anesthesia is still necessary for endovascular treatment. Before giving the patient an anesthetic, CT angiography can demonstrate the presence and location of an aneurysm. Future studies are needed to assess if CT angiography enables prediction of whether the aneurysm is suitable for endovascular treatment. A limitation of our study was that the neurosurgeons judged the CT angiogram and DSA images after surgery, with no surgical consequences linked to their decision. Consequently, our findings that 74% of aneurysms could have undergone surgery without additional DSA will have to be validated prospectively.

In conclusion, CT angiography is minimally invasive and can be easily performed directly after unenhanced CT has demonstrated SAH. Most aneurysms are detected with certainty on CT angiograms and most aneurysms could have been operated on with only CT angiography as the preoperative work-up. CT angiograms must be of high quality with adequate depiction of both the aneurysm and the parent artery to perform surgery on the CT angiographic findings alone. Any uncertainty requires DSA.

Acknowledgments: We thank Eduard E. de Lange, MD, for critical review of the manuscript and Jan de Groot and Marcel Metselaar of the photography department for all their help.

References

1. Hop JW, Rinkel GJE, Algra A, van Gijn J. Case fatality rates and functional outcome after subarachnoid hemorrhage: a systematic review. Stroke 1997; 28:660–664.
2. Inagawa T, Kamiya K, Ogasawara H, Yano T. Rebleeding of ruptured intracranial aneurysms in the acute stage. Surg Neurol 1987; 28:93–99.
3. Inagawa T. Ultra-early rebleeding within six hours after aneurysmal rupture. Surg Neurol 1994; 42:130–134.
4. Heiserman JE, Dean BL, Hodak JA, et al. Neurologic complications of cerebral angiography. AJNR 1994; 15:1401–1407.
5. Saitoh H, Hayakawa K, Nishimura K, et al. Rerupture of cerebral aneurysms during angiography. AJNR 1995; 16:539–542.
6. Anzalone N, Triulzi F, Scotti G. Acute subarachnoid hemorrhage: three-dimensional time-of-flight MR angiography versus intra-arterial digital angiography. Neuroradiology 1995; 37:257–261.
7. Aoki S, Sasaki Y, Machida T, Ohkubo T, Minami M, Sasaki Y. Cerebral aneurysms: detection and delineation using 3D CT angiography. AJNR 1992; 13:1115–1120.
8. Dorsch NWC, Young N, Kingston RJ, Compton JS. Early experience with spiral CT in the diagnosis of intracranial aneurysms. Neurosurgery 1995; 36:230–238.
9. Harbaugh RE, Schlusselberg DS, Jeffrey R, et al. Three-dimensional computed tomographic angiography in the preoperative evaluation of cerebrovascular lesions. Neurosurgery 1995; 36:320–327.
10. Liang EY, Chan M, Hsiang JHK, et al. Detection and assessment of intracranial aneurysms: value of CT angiography with shaded-surface display. AJR 1995; 165:1497–1502.
11. Tampieri D, Leblanc R, Oleszek J, Pokrupa R, Melançon D. Three-dimensional computed tomographic angiography of cerebral aneurysms. Neurosurgery 1995; 36:749–755.
12. Vieco PT, Shuman WP, Alsofrom GF, Gross CE. Detection of circle of Willis aneurysms in patients with acute subarachnoid hemorrhage: a comparison of CT angiography and digital subtraction angiography. AJR 1995; 165:425–430.
13. Ogawa T, Okudera T, Noguchi K, et al. Cerebral aneurysms: evaluation with three-dimensional CT angiography. AJNR 1996; 17:447–454.
14. Rieger J, Hosten N, Neumann K, et al. Initial clinical experience with spiral CT and 3D arterial reconstruction in intracranial aneurysms and arteriovenous malformations. Neuroradiology 1996; 38:245–251.
15. Hope JKA, Wilson JL, Thomson FJ. Three-dimensional CT angiography in the detection and characterization of intracranial berry aneurysms. AJNR 1996; 17:439–445.
16. Napel S, Marks MP, Rubin GD, et al. CT angiography with spiral CT and maximum intensity projection. Radiology 1992; 185:607–610.
17. Schwartz RB, Tice HM, Hooten SM, Hsu L, Stieg PE. Evaluation of cerebral aneurysms with helical CT: correlation with conventional angiography and MR angiography. Radiology 1994; 192:717–722.
18. Katz DA, Marks MP, Napel SA, Bracci PM, Roberts SL. Circle of Willis: evaluation with spiral CT angiography, MR angiography, and conventional angiography. Radiology 1995; 195:445–449.
19. Alberico RA, Patel M, Casey S, Jacobs B, Maguire W, Decker R. Evaluation of the circle of Willis with three-dimensional CT angiography in patients with suspected intracranial aneurysms. AJNR 1995; 16:1571–1578.
20. Wilms G, Guffens M, Gryspeerdt S, et al. Spiral CT of intracranial aneurysms: correlation with digital subtraction and magnetic resonance angiography. Neuroradiology 1996; 38:S20–S25.
21. Zouaoui A, Sahel M, Marro B, et al. Three-dimensional computed tomographic angiography in detection of cerebral aneurysms in acute subarachnoid hemorrhage. Neurosurgery 1997; 41:125–130.
22. Velthuis BK, van Leeuwen MS, Witkamp TD, Boomstra S, Ramos LMP, Rinkel GJE. CT angiography: source images and postprocessing techniques in the detection of cerebral aneurysms. AJR 1997; 169:1411–1417.
23. Anderson GB, Findlay JM, Steinke DE, Ashforth R. Experience with computed tomographic angiography for the detection of intracranial aneurysms in the setting of acute subarachnoid hemorrhage. Neurosurgery 1997; 41:522–528.
24. Landis JR, Koch GG. The measurement of observer agreement for categorical data. Biometrics 1977; 33:159–174.
25. Rinkel GJE, van Wijdicks EFM, Vermeulen M, et al. Nonaneurysmal perimesencephalic subarachnoid hemorrhage: CT and MR patterns that differ from aneurysmal rupture. AJR 1991; 157:1325–1330.
26. Schmid UD, Steiger HJ, Huber P. Accuracy of high-resolution computed tomography in direct diagnosis of cerebral aneurysms. Neuroradiology 1987; 29:152–159.
27. Rinkel GJE, van Wijdicks EFM. Handbook of subarachnoid hemorrhage. Yanagihara T, Piepgras DG, eds. New York, NY: Dekker, 1997; 139–158.

Hajime Kitagaki, MD
Etsuro Mori, MD
Shigeru Yamaji, MD
Kazunari Ishii, MD
Nobutsugu Hirono, MD
Syoji Kobashi, MS
Yutaka Hata, PhD

Index terms:
Brain, atrophy, 13.83
Brain, emission CT (ECT), 10.12163
Brain, MR, 10.121411, 10.121412, 10.121419
Dementia, 13.83
Magnetic resonance (MR), image processing, 10.12144, 10.12149
Magnetic resonance (MR), three-dimensional, 10.121419

Radiology 1998; 208:431–439

Abbreviations:
AD = Alzheimer disease
FDG = 2-[fluorine-18]fluoro-2-deoxy-D-glucose
FTD = frontotemporal dementia
3D = three-dimensional

[1] From the Neuroimaging Research/Radiology Service (H.K., S.Y., K.I.) and Clinical Neurosciences/Neurology and Neurorehabilitation Services (E.M., N.H.), Hyogo Institute for Aging Brain and Cognitive Disorders, 520, Saisho-Ko, Himeji 670, Japan, and the Department of Computer Engineering, Himeji Institute of Technology (S.K., Y.H.), Japan. Received September 26, 1997; revision requested November 26; revision received January 30, 1998; accepted March 26. **Address reprint requests to** H.K.

Author contributions:
Guarantors of integrity of entire study, H.K., E.M.; study concepts, H.K., E.M., S.K., Y.H.; study design, H.K., E.M.; definition of intellectual content, H.K., E.M.; literature research, H.K.; clinical studies, E.M., H.K., N.H.; experimental device, S.K., Y.H.; data acquisition, H.K., S.Y., K.I.; data analysis, E.M., H.K., S.Y., K.I.; statistical analysis, N.H.; manuscript preparation, H.K.; manuscript editing and review, E.M.

Frontotemporal Dementia and Alzheimer Disease: Evaluation of Cortical Atrophy with Automated Hemispheric Surface Display Generated with MR Images[1]

PURPOSE: To determine the features of cortical atrophy in frontotemporal dementia (FTD) and Alzheimer disease by using a hemispheric surface display generated with magnetic resonance (MR) images.

MATERIALS AND METHODS: The extent of cortical atrophy was evaluated with automated MR hemispheric surface display and volumetry in 18 patients with FTD and in 18 matched patients with Alzheimer disease. Results were compared with those in 18 healthy, matched control subjects.

RESULTS: Most cortical regions were significantly atrophic in FTD and Alzheimer disease. The frontal and anterior temporal lobes were significantly more atrophic in FTD than in Alzheimer disease. The mean hemispheric-to-intracranial volume ratio in patients with FTD (56.2%) and those with Alzheimer disease (58.4%) was significantly smaller than the ratio in the control subjects (66.0%). Asymmetry of hemispheric volume was significantly larger in the FTD group than in the Alzheimer disease and control groups.

CONCLUSION: Cortical atrophy in FTD is more widespread than was previously thought. Asymmetric frontal and anterior temporal atrophy is a distinctive feature of FTD and distinguishes it from Alzheimer disease. Hemispheric surface display is a useful complement to tomographic images and is useful for the evaluation of focal cortical atrophy in degenerative dementias, especially FTD.

Although two-dimensional tomographic images from computed tomography (CT) and magnetic resonance (MR) imaging have brought great improvements in diagnostic effectiveness (1,2), they do not allow the inspection of the surface of an undissected organ, which is essential for a pathologic examination. External inspection may be helpful for a better understanding of the anatomy and anatomic location of lesions (3,4). Such inspection is especially important for the precise identification of gyri in terms of the relationship between brain anatomy and function. In three-dimensional (3D) images, identification of gyri and sulci is easy and accurate (3,4). Techniques for 3D volume rendering with MR images have been developed (5) and used in fields such as computer-aided surgery (6,7).

Hemispheric surface display with MR images consists of two major processes: segmentation of the brain (or a part of it) from two-dimensional tomographic head images and volume rendering of the segmented objects (3,4). Volume calculation of the objects is also attainable with the former process. The main obstacle to wide use of this technique is the former process, which usually involves laborious manual operations that are subject to the operator's expertise (3,4,8). We have developed software that automatically segments the brain matter from thin-section coronal MR images (9). This software simultaneously generates volumes and 3D volume-rendered images of the cerebral hemisphere, brain stem, cerebellum, and calvaria. Elimination of the factors of operator expertise and subjectivity makes possible the highly reliable evaluation of a large number of patients.

Frontotemporal dementia (FTD) is a non–Alzheimer disease (AD) type of degenerative dementia characterized by a peculiar behavioral disorder, with changes in personality and social conduct due to frontotemporal involvement (10). This disorder is an important and probably the second most frequent cause of degenerative dementia, particularly dementia of presenile onset. Although described for more than a century, FTD often goes undiagnosed or is mistaken for AD or a psychiatric disorder.

In 1994, the Lund and Manchester Groups (11) proposed consensus clinical and pathologic criteria for FTD. At least three types of histologic changes (Pick type, frontal lobe degeneration, and frontal lobe degeneration with motor neuron disease) underlie the atrophy and share an identical anatomic distribution in the frontal and temporal lobes. The most common histologic pattern consists of a severe, extensive loss of pyramidal neurons in the upper layers of the cerebral cortex of the frontotemporal area, with microvacuolation (spongiosis) and mild superficial gliosis. There may be severe gliosis within the gray and white matter, swollen achromatic neurons, and tau- and ubiquitin-staining neuronal inclusion bodies (Pick bodies). These features are never seen in AD. The advantage of this grouping of histopathologic entities with Pick disease and nonspecific FTD under the single heading of FTD is to increase awareness of these conditions and to distinguish them from AD (12), although controversy remains about the nomenclature and concept of FTD (13–15). The designation of FTD is now recognized both internationally and among different disciplines (12) . In several large families with FTD, there is evidence that the disease is linked to chromosome 17 (16).

With the development of neuroimaging, an abnormality of the frontal and temporal areas of the brain has been increasingly recognized in vivo. The neuroimaging findings of frontotemporal involvement (lobar atrophy on MR images and hypoperfusion and hypometabolism on radionuclide studies) now constitute a reliable and indispensable diagnostic approach as regards FTD (10). Differential patterns of cerebral degeneration in FTD and AD have been studied by using MR imaging or spectroscopy (17–20). However, an investigation focusing on features of cortical atrophy is lacking. The purpose of this study was to determine the features of cortical atrophy in patients with FTD and AD by using surface images of the cerebral hemisphere and automated volumetry. To our knowledge, this is the first study of this type. We also discuss the usefulness and limitations of this method for the evaluation of cortical atrophy in dementias.

MATERIALS AND METHODS

All procedures used in this study were performed strictly according to the clinical study guidelines of the ethics committee of our institution and were approved by the internal review board. After a complete description of the study was provided to all participants and their relatives, written informed consent was obtained.

Subjects

Patients who were admitted to the infirmary of the Hyogo Institute for Aging Brain and Cognitive Disorders (Himeji, Japan) from July 1, 1993, to December 31, 1996, because of cognitive disorders were examined comprehensively by both neurologists and psychiatrists (including E.M., N.H.). The patients underwent routine laboratory tests, electroencephalography, and standardized neuropsychologic examinations that included the Mini-Mental State Examination (21) and the Alzheimer's Disease Assessment Scale (22). Neuroimaging included MR imaging of the brain and MR angiography of the neck and head. In addition, cerebral glucose metabolism or cerebral blood flow images were obtained with positron emission tomography (PET) with 2-[fluorine-18]fluoro-2-deoxy-D-glucose (FDG) or the carbon-15 dioxide steady-state method or with single photon emission CT (SPECT) with iodine-123 iodoamphetamine or technitium-99m ethyl cysteinate dimer.

Patients with FTD.—We included 18 patients with FTD who fulfilled the following criteria: (*a*) International Classification of Diseases, or ICD-10 (23), diagnostic criteria for dementia; (*b*) the core diagnostic (behavioral, affective, speech, spatial orientation and/or praxis, physical, investigational) features of the Lund-Manchester clinical criteria for FTD (11), with special emphasis on the symptoms (loss of personal awareness, hyperorality,

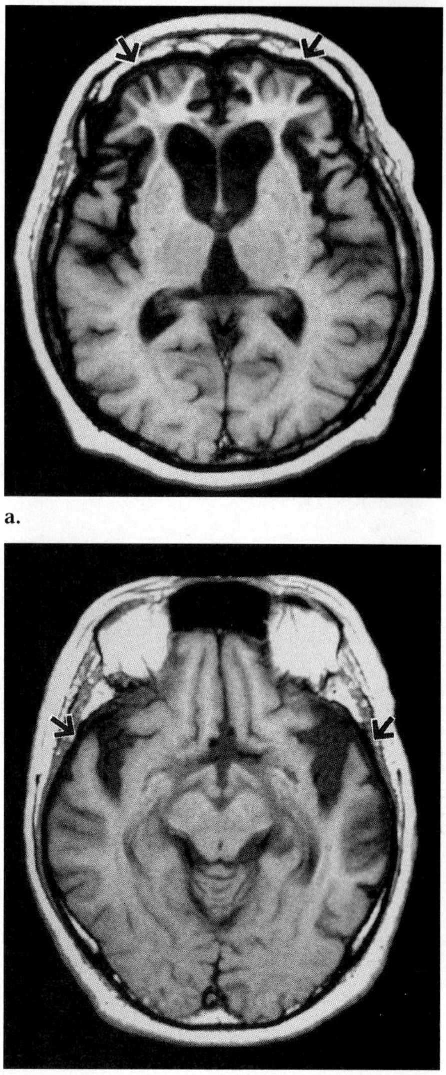

a.

b.

Figure 1. Axial T1-weighted MR images (500/15) in two patients with FTD show **(a)** bilateral frontal lobe atrophy (arrows) in a 58-year-old woman and **(b)** bilateral temporal lobe atrophy (arrows) in a 56-year-old man.

stereotyped and perseverative behavior, progressive reduction of speech, and preserved spatial orientation) described by Miller et al (24); (*c*) frontal lobe dysfunction on the Frontal Dysfunction Battery (the Luria fist-edge-palm test, the red-green test, the two-one tapping test, the Stroop color-word test, and the color-form sorting test) (25); and (*d*) frontal, temporal, or frontotemporal hypoperfusion or hypometabolism and relative sparing of parietal and occipital lobes at SPECT or PET (26,27). The exclusion criteria were (*a*) diagnostic exclusion features of the Lund-Manchester clinical criteria for FTD (11), and (*b*) an advanced stage of FTD, with severe deficits or behavioral

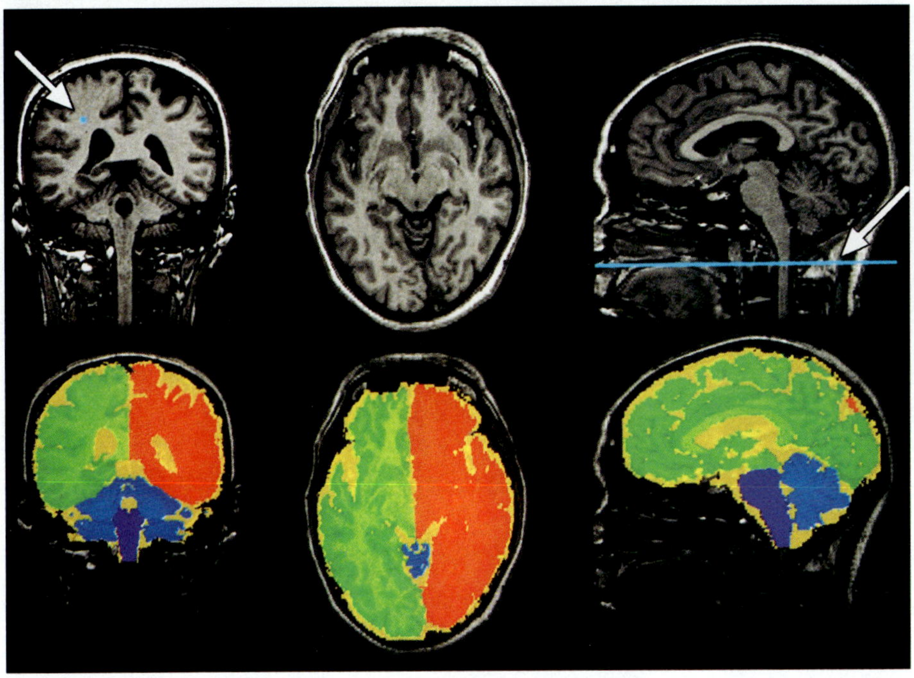

Figure 2. Automated brain segmentation generated with spoiled gradient-recalled echo MR images (14/3, 20° flip angle). The starting point of brain segmentation (left arrow) and the craniocervical boundary (right arrow), which were determined by means of interactive manual operations, are shown. Segmented objects were overlaid with color. Yellow = cerebrospinal fluid space, orange = left hemisphere, green = right hemisphere, blue = cerebellum, violet = brain stem.

disorders that would make assessment difficult.

The mean age ± 1 standard deviation was 65 years ± 7 (age range, 52–75 years) for the 13 women and five men in the FTD group, and the mean duration of illness was 4.0 years ± 2.5. The mean Mini-Mental State Examination score was 15.9 ± 6.5, and the mean Alzheimer's Disease Assessment Scale score was 33.7 ± 10.9. One patient had accompanying motor neuron disease. Fifteen patients had three or more of the symptoms mentioned above, and the rest had a progressive reduction in speech and preserved spatial orientation. All patients showed impaired performance in one or more of the domains of the Frontal Dysfunction Battery.

Frontotemporal hypoperfusion and hypometabolism were apparent in all patients at FDG PET (n = 15) and I-123 iodoamphetamine SPECT (n = 3). A bilateral frontotemporal abnormality was present in nine patients; a bilateral temporal abnormality, in four; a unilateral temporal abnormality, in three; and a unilateral frontal abnormality, in one.

In 14 patients, moderate to severe frontotemporal atrophy was noted on the routine MR images, which included axial spin-echo T1-weighted (repetition time msec/echo time msec, 550/15 [effective]; four signals acquired), fast spin-echo T2-weighted (3,000/105 [effective], four signals acquired), and fast spin-echo proton-density–weighted (3,000/35, four signals acquired) MR images. Predominant cortical atrophy was seen bilaterally (n = 5) or unilaterally (n = 2) in the frontal lobes and bilaterally (n = 2) or unilaterally (n = 5) in the temporal lobes (Fig 1). The amygdalohippocampal region was atrophic in 14 patients bilaterally and in two patients unilaterally. White matter signal hyperintensity, representative of subcortical gliosis (17), was noted in 13 patients in the frontal (n = 4) or temporal (n = 5) lobes or in the frontotemporal region (n = 4). In no patient were occlusive lesions in the major cerebrocervical arteries seen at MR angiography.

Patients with AD.—Eighteen patients with probable AD were randomly selected from the same cohort of patients who were admitted to our hospital for evaluation; they were matched for sex, age, and dementia severity (Mini-Mental State Examination score). The inclusion criteria were (*a*) probable AD, according to the criteria of the National Institute of Neurological Disease and Stroke and the Alzheimer's Disease and Related Disorders Association (28), and (*b*) hypoperfusion in the parietal lobe, the medial temporal lobe, or both, at PET or SPECT (29). Exclusion criteria were complications due to another neurologic disease.

All patients with AD underwent examinations similar to those undergone by the FTD group. The mean age was 65.3 years ± 6.5 (age range, 53–75 years) for the 13 women and five men, and the mean duration of illness was 3.1 years ± 1.9. The mean Mini-Mental State Examination score was 16.6 ± 5.5, and the mean Alzheimer's Disease Assessment Scale score was 26.1 ± 13.0. Temporoparietal hypoperfusion or hypometabolism was noted in all patients at FDG PET (n = 6), C-15–O_2 steady-state PET (n = 4), I-123 iodoamphetamine SPECT (n = 6), or Tc-99m ethyl cysteinate dimer SPECT (n = 2): bilateral temporoparietal abnormality in seven patients, bilateral frontotemporoparietal abnormality in six, bilateral parietal abnormality in three, bilateral temporal abnormality in one, and unilateral parietal abnormality in one. On the routine MR images, bilateral amygdalohippocampal atrophy was seen in 16 patients, and moderate to severe, almost symmetric cortical atrophy was noted in the parietal lobe (n = 2), in the parietal and frontal lobes (n = 2), in the temporal lobe (n = 2), in the frontal lobe (n = 1), or in the parietal, temporal, and frontal lobes (n = 1). Head and neck MR angiograms were normal in all patients.

Healthy control subjects.—Eighteen sex- and age-matched volunteers with normal cognitive findings were recruited from the community. Normal physical and neurologic examination results were obtained in all control subjects, none of whom had a history of psychiatric or neurologic disorders. No abnormal findings were seen on MR images in these subjects, and all scored 28 or higher on the Mini-Mental State Examination. The mean age was 65.4 years ± 6.2 (age range, 54–75) for the 13 women and five men.

MR Image Acquisition, Processing, and Surface Display

All studies were obtained with a 1.5-T MR unit (Signa Advantage 5; GE Medical Systems, Milwaukee, Wis). A circularly polarized head coil was used as both transmitter and receiver. Coronal 3D spoiled gradient-recalled echo images (14/3; flip angle, 20°; field of view, 220 mm; matrix, 256 × 256; 124 1.5-mm-thick sections) that covered the whole

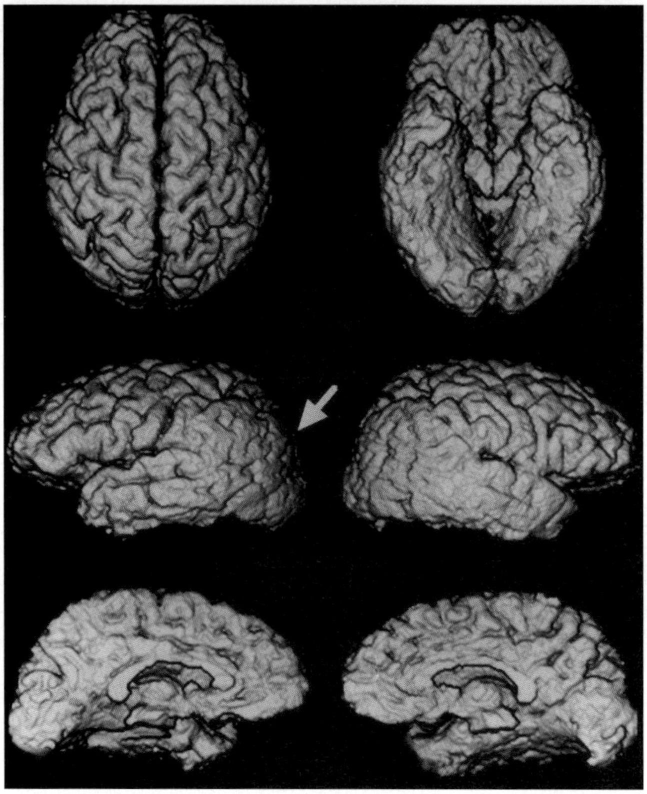

Figure 3. Hemispheric surface displays generated from MR images of the brain in a healthy 73-year-old female control subject. All gyri are clearly visible. The gyri in the posterior temporal, inferior parietal, and occipital lobes (arrow) appear rather packed in comparison with those in the other lobes. Top: left, view from above; right, view from below. Middle: left, left lateral view; right, right lateral view. Bottom (bisected brain): left, left inner surface; right, right inner surface.

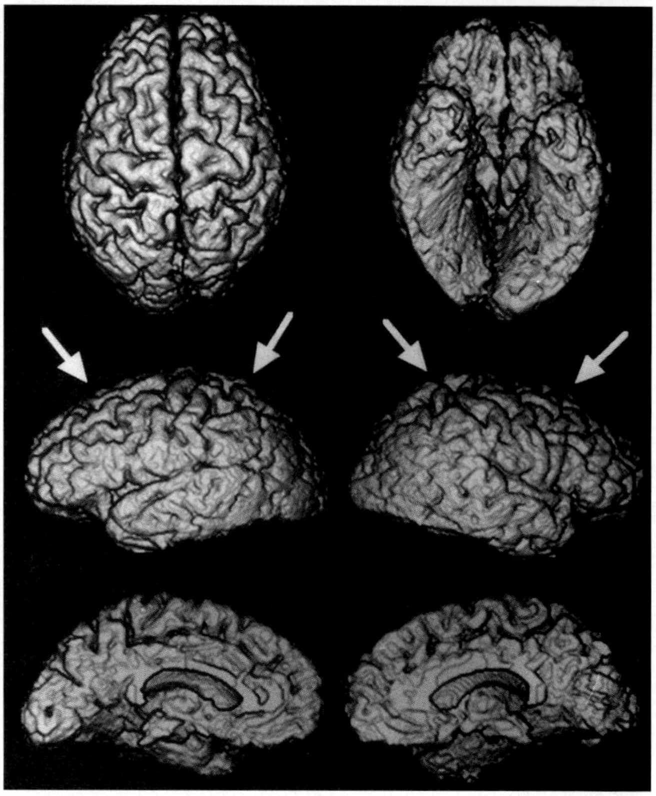

Figure 4. Hemispheric surface displays generated from MR images of the brain in a healthy 69-year-old male control subject. Mild cortical atrophy (arrows) is visible in the lateral frontoparietal cortex. (Tomographic MR images in this subject are shown in Figure 2.) Top: left, view from above; right, view from below. Middle: left, left lateral view; right, right lateral view. Bottom (bisected brain): left, left inner surface; right, right inner surface.

calvaria were the source data. The voxel size was 1.1 mm^3 ([220/256]^2 × 1.5).

The data sets of the spoiled gradient-recalled echo images were directly transmitted to a workstation (Indigo^2 Hi-Impact; Silicon Graphics, Mountain View, Calif) from the MR unit and were analyzed by using 3D MR image processing software developed by Kobashi et al (9). The software makes use of a combination of gray-scale (3D expansion with the region-growing method) and edge-detection algorithms (3D expansion with Sobel filtering) and some a priori knowledge by which a computer may perform an unsupervised identification of a given structure (eg, cerebral hemisphere, brain stem, cerebellum, calvaria) with a series of contiguous MR images (Fig 2). For each structure, the software can generate a 3D volume-rendered image, a two-dimensional reconstruction with optional angles, and volumetric measurements. This method is reliable and less complicated than current manual or semiautomated techniques such as tracing and thresholding, which involve extensive, time-consuming human interaction that is subject to inter- and intraoperator variation.

With this software, the whole brain was segmented by detecting the boundary between the cerebrospinal fluid and the gray matter, and the calvaria was segmented by detecting the outer surface of the dura mater. The volume of each structure was automatically calculated by multiplying the number of voxels in the segmented region by the voxel size. The caudal end of the whole brain and calvaria was manually set at the plane that intersects the occipitoatlantal junction (Fig 2), which is the only supervised operation necessary. The whole procedure takes approximately 5 minutes.

Assessment of Cortical Atrophy

A 3D volume-rendered image of each cerebral hemisphere was displayed on a high-resolution color monitor. One neuroradiologist (H.K.), blinded to the clinical data and diagnosis, used a mouse cursor to rotate the image and rate the regional cortical atrophy for each of 66 cortical regions of the medial and lateral hemispheric surfaces. There were five categories of atrophy: normal (nadir of the sulcus invisible, with stacked gyri), minimal (nadir of the sulcus visible), mild (bottom of the sulcus widened), moderate (gyrus thinner than the sulcus), and severe (very shrunken gyrus with a "knife-blade" appearance [17]). The regions included the orbitofrontal cortex, superior frontal gyrus (rostral and caudal for lateral and medial), middle frontal gyrus (rostral and caudal), inferior frontal gyrus (rostral and caudal), cingulate gyrus (rostral and caudal), precentral gyrus (superomedial and inferolateral), postcentral gyrus (superomedial and inferolateral), superior parietal lobule (rostral and caudal for lateral and medial), inferior parietal lobule (rostral and caudal), superior temporal gyrus (rostral and caudal), middle temporal gyrus (rostral and caudal), inferior temporal gyrus (rostral and

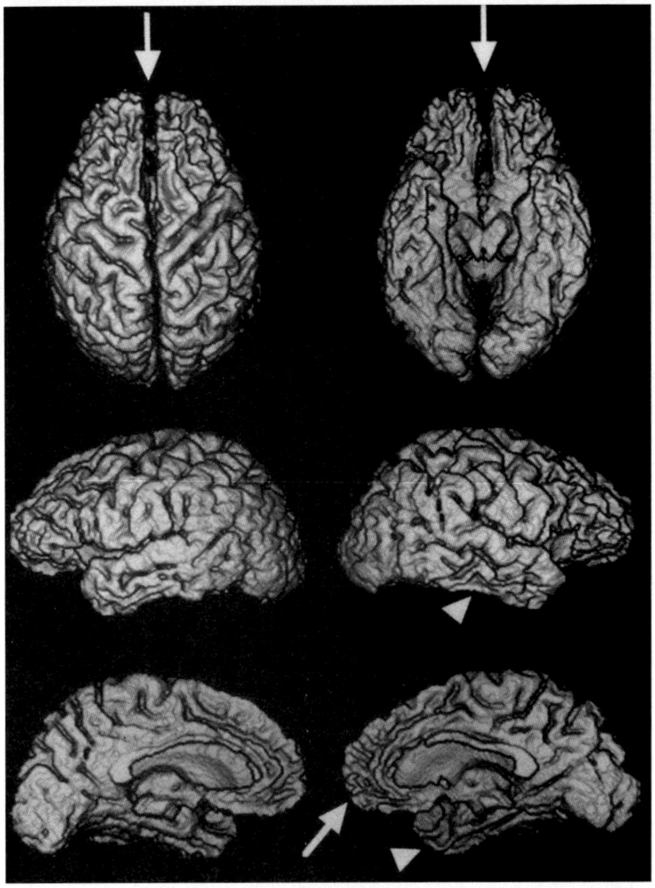

Figure 5. Hemispheric surface displays generated from MR images show severe frontotemporal atrophy in a 58-year-old woman with FTD. Knife-blade configurations of the gyri in the right frontal (arrows) and temporal lobes (arrowheads) are apparent. (Axial MR image in this patient is shown in Fig 1a.) Top: left, view from above; right, view from below. Middle: left, left lateral view; right, right lateral view. Bottom (bisected brain): left, left inner surface; right, right inner surface.

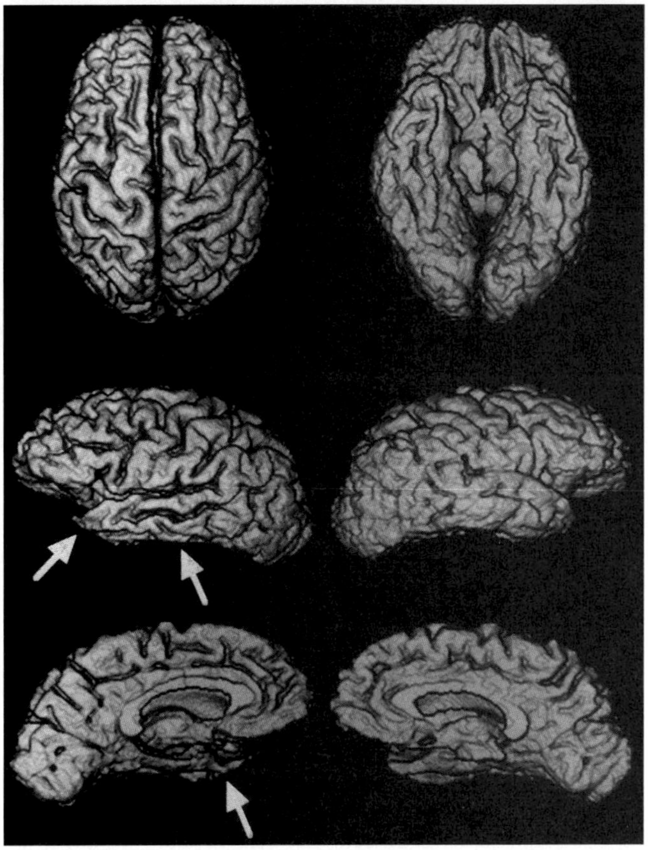

Figure 6. Hemispheric surface displays generated from MR images show severe temporal lobe atrophy in a 56-year-old man with FTD. The anterior portion of the left temporal lobe is severely atrophic (arrows) in contrast to the right temporal lobe. (Axial MR image in this patient is shown in Fig 1b.) Top: left, view from above; right, view from below. Middle: left, left lateral view; right, right lateral view. Bottom (bisected brain): left, left inner surface; right, right inner surface.

caudal), parahippocampal gyrus (rostral and caudal), and occipital gyri (rostral and caudal for lateral and medial) of each hemisphere. The score from the more affected side was used in each region, because the involved regions are frequently unilateral in FTD and more or less asymmetric in AD.

In addition, the volumes of the right and left cerebral hemispheres, the total cerebral volume (automatically separated at the level between the superior and inferior colliculi of the midbrain), and the total intracranial volume were determined. The interoperator reliability of the volume measurement, which was expressed as an intraclass correlation coefficient derived from repeated measurements in 20 randomly selected patients, was greater than .999 for both total intracranial and hemispheric volumes.

Statistical Analyses

The test-retest reliability of the visual inspection was assessed by calculating the intraclass correlation coefficients of two separate experimental ratings in 15 subjects who were randomly selected from the three groups. Differences among the groups were analyzed by using the Kruskal-Wallis one-way analysis of variance followed by the post hoc Tukey studentized range honestly-significant-difference test with the Dunn joint ranking for nonparametric ordinal data (atrophy rating) (30). The one-way analysis of variance and post hoc Tukey analysis were used for numeric data (volume). All statistical analyses were performed with a statistical software package (STATISTICA version 4.1; StatSoft, Evanston, Ill). The level of statistical significance was set at *P* less than .05.

RESULTS

In the experiment to determine the reliability of the atrophy rating, the intraclass coefficients ranged from 0.49 to 1.00, with a mean value of 0.75 ± 0.14. The test-retest reliability was fairly good (coefficient > .6) in most of the regions except the central cortices, superior parietal lobule, and occipital lobe, where severe atrophy is unlikely to be present.

On hemispheric surface images in the healthy control subjects, all gyri and sulci were clearly identified. The gyri in the posterior temporal, inferior parietal, and occipital lobes appeared rather packed in comparison with those in the other lobes (Fig 3). Although the medial frontal lobe, postcentral gyrus, and superior parietal lobule appeared mildly atrophic in half of the healthy subjects, the rest of the brain regions were largely intact (Fig 4).

In patients with FTD, focal atrophy that affected the frontal and temporal lobes was apparent on hemispheric surface images (Figs 5, 6). Atrophy in the lateral, ventral, and medial surfaces of the frontal lobe was clearly observed. A mild atrophy of the precentral gyrus was noted in half the patients. Atrophy of the temporal lobes was also apparent and was accentuated in the anterior portions. In the parietal lobe, mild to moderate atrophy was noted in the inferior parietal lobule and in the medial aspect of the superior parietal lobule. The occipital lobes appeared largely spared. In half the patients, knife-blade–shaped gyri were apparent (Table 1). Knife-blade atrophy was observed most often in the anterior part of the superior temporal gyrus. Clear-cut boundaries between severely atrophic and normal-appearing gyri were observed at the precentral sulcus or between the anterior and posterior parts of the temporal lobe in some patients. These features were present exclusively in FTD.

In patients with AD, on the other hand, mild to moderate cortical atrophy was observed in the frontal, temporal, and parietal association cortices in almost proportionately identical amounts (Fig 7). A mild atrophy of the occipital lobes was noted in half the patients. Knife-blade atrophy was never observed. The central areas were largely normal. The distribution of cortical atrophy was similar to that seen in normal aging, although the degree was more intense.

The regions where cortical atrophy was significantly different among the three groups (FTD vs control groups, AD vs control groups, FTD vs AD groups) are illustrated in Figure 8. In patients with FTD, 27 cortical regions, including the frontal lobe, temporal lobe, cingulate gyrus, part of the lateral and medial parietal lobe, and part of the occipital lobe, were significantly atrophic compared with the same regions in the control subjects. On the statistical maps (Fig 8), it can be seen that cortical atrophy was widespread in the frontoparietotemporal region. It is also apparent that atrophy affected the lower part of the primary sensorimotor cortices. In patients with AD, 19 cortical regions, including parts of the frontal lobe, lateral temporal lobe, parietal lobe, and occipital lobe, were significantly atrophic compared with the same regions in control subjects. In addition to atrophy in the inferoposterior temporal and inferior parietal lobes, some involvement in the prefrontal and limbic frontal regions was apparent on the statistical maps. A comparison of the FTD and AD groups revealed that seven regions in the frontal and temporal lobes were significantly atrophic in the patients with FTD compared with the same lobes in the patients with AD. Atrophy in the anterior temporal and medial frontal lobes was characteristic of FTD. There was no significant difference in the parietal lobe atrophy between the FTD and AD groups.

Table 2 shows the mean values and standard deviations of the total intracranial volume, hemispheric volume, ratio

TABLE 1
Cortical Atrophy in Frontotemporoparietal Regions

Region	FTD Group (n = 18)	AD Group (n = 18)	Control Group (n = 18)
Anterior cingulate	4/3	0/3	0/0
Orbital	3/2	0/1	0/0
Anterolateral superior frontal	3/4	0/0	0/0
Posterolateral superior frontal	6/2	0/1	0/0
Anteromedial superior frontal	4/3	0/3	0/0
Posteromedial superior frontal	2/5	0/3	0/0
Anterior middle frontal	2/3	0/1	0/0
Posterior middle frontal	1/5	0/1	0/0
Anterior inferior frontal	2/2	0/1	0/0
Posterior inferior frontal	2/3	0/1	0/0
Anterior superior temporal	8/5	0/2	0/0
Posterior superior temporal	0/0	0/0	0/0
Anterior middle temporal	3/5	0/0	0/0
Posterior middle temporal	0/7	0/0	0/0
Anterior inferior temporal	2/6	0/1	0/0
Posterior inferior temporal	0/3	0/0	0/0
Anterolateral superior parietal	0/2	0/5	0/0
Posterolateral superior parietal	0/1	0/3	0/0
Anteromedial superior parietal	0/1	0/6	0/0
Posteromedial superior parietal	0/3	0/2	0/0
Anterior inferior parietal	0/0	0/0	0/0
Posterior inferior parietal	0/0	0/0	0/0

Note.—Data are number of individuals with severe atrophy/number with moderate atrophy.

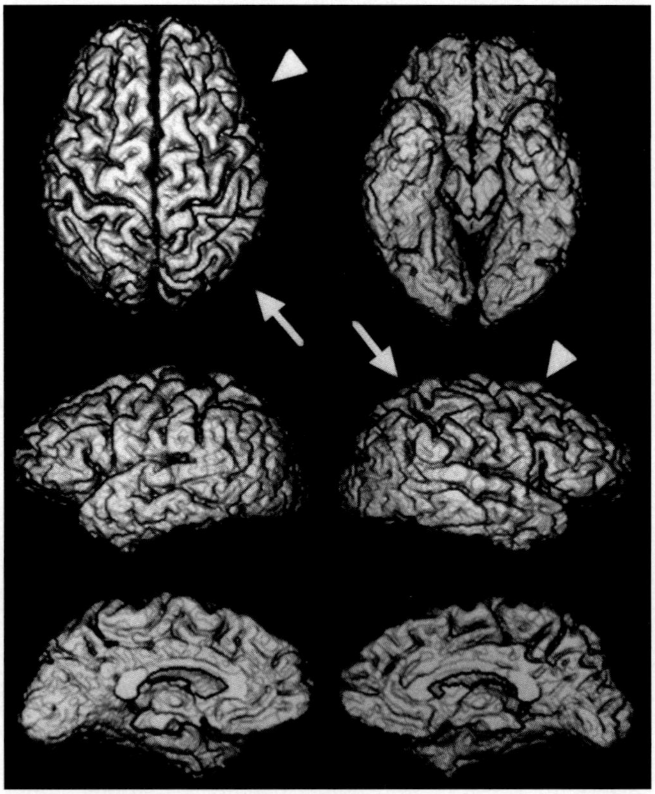

Figure 7. Hemispheric surface displays generated from MR images show diffuse cortical atrophy in a 58-year-old woman with AD. The parietotemporal association cortices show moderate atrophy (arrows), and the frontal association cortices show mild atrophy (arrowheads). Top: left, view from above; right, view from below. Middle: left, left lateral view; right, right lateral view. Bottom (bisected brain): left, left inner surface; right, right inner surface.

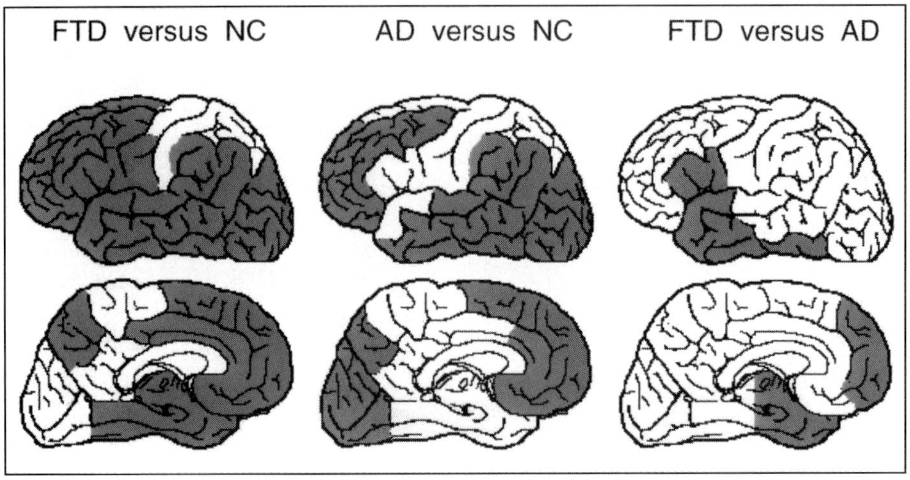

Figure 8. Statistical maps. Gray areas represent regions where the atrophy rating was significantly different between groups ($P < .05$). Left: atrophy was more profound in the FTD group than in the control group (*NC*). Middle: atrophy was more profound in the AD group than in the control group. Right: atrophy was more profound in the FTD group than in the AD group. Top: left lateral surface. Bottom (bisected brain): left inner surface.

TABLE 2
Volumetric Data

Parameter	FTD Group	AD Group	Control Group
Total intracranial volume (cm^3)	1,300 ± 87	1,345 ± 102	1,324 ± 99
Whole hemispheric volume (cm^3)*	731 ± 72	784 ± 77	876 ± 105
Ratio of total intracranial volume to whole hemispheric volume (%)†	56.2 ± 3.5	58.4 ± 5.2	66.0 ± 4.6
Left hemispheric volume (cm^3)‡	365 ± 35	390 ± 44	436 ± 51
Right hemispheric volume (cm^3)‡	375 ± 42	394 ± 35	440 ± 54
Laterality index (%)§	1.95 ± 1.10	0.96 ± 0.78	0.36 ± 0.26

Note.—Data are values ± 1 standard deviation.
* Significant differences were found among groups ($P < .001$), between FTD and control groups ($P < .001$), and between AD and control groups ($P < .007$).
† Significant differences were found among groups, between FTD and control groups, and between AD and control groups ($P < .001$ for all comparisons).
‡ Significant differences were found among groups ($P < .001$), between FTD and control groups ($P < .001$), and between AD and control groups ($P < .009$).
§ Significant differences were found among groups, between FTD and control groups, and between FTD and AD groups ($P < .001$ for all comparisons).

of hemispheric volume to total intracranial volume, and asymmetry index. The mean total intracranial volume was comparable among groups. Both the mean hemispheric volume and the mean ratio in the FTD group and those in the AD group were significantly smaller than those in the control group. There was no significant difference between the FTD and AD groups in either the mean hemispheric volume or the mean ratio. The asymmetry of the hemispheric volume was significantly larger in the FTD group than in the AD and control groups. There was no significant difference in the asymmetry index between the AD group and the control group.

DISCUSSION

Hemispheric surface images generated with our fully automated system allowed successful evaluation of cortical atrophy in patients with a degenerative dementia. Every gyrus could be identified, and atrophic changes could be rated for each gyrus. Automated hemispheric volumetry helped quantifiably detect cerebral atrophy in dementias.

In the absence of neuropathologic data, we used radionuclide studies to maximize the specificity of the clinical diagnosis. Frontotemporal hypoperfusion and hypometabolism is one of the items in the Lund-Manchester diagnostic criteria for FTD, and is now considered to be an important diagnostic standard (18,24,31). The specificity of the diagnosis of AD solely on the basis of the clinical criteria of the National Institute of Neurological Disease and Stroke and the Alzheimer's Disease and Related Disorders Association is reported (32) to be more than 80%, and that of the diagnosis of FTD solely on the basis of behavioral changes is also reported (24,33) to be high. Furthermore, in this study, other than the results of the screening examinations (MR imaging, MR angiography, and laboratory tests to exclude other causes of dementia), we used stringent criteria for the selection of subjects; our criteria combined clinical and radionuclide imaging information. Despite a lack of confirmatory histopathologic data, we expect that our diagnostic accuracy in both dementia groups was quite high.

Although cortical involvement that is accentuated in the frontal and anterior temporal lobes has been stressed in many pathologic (11) and neuroimaging (17,34) studies of FTD, our results indicate that atrophy was more widespread in the hemisphere that affects the primary sensorimotor cortex and in the parietal lobe. Parietal lobe involvement has been recognized in postmortem studies of advanced FTD (10,35,36) and is rarely predominant in patients with Pick disease (37,38); also, the precentral gyrus was involved in FTD with motor neuron disease (10). Central and parietal atrophy reflects the changes that may occur earlier and more commonly in patients with FTD. Nevertheless, knife-blade gyral atrophy, which was seen in half the patients, was restricted to the frontal and anterior temporal lobes. Our in vivo volumetric study clearly demonstrated an asymmetric hemispheric involvement in patients with FTD, which is consistent with gross postmortem findings (39). On the other hand, atrophy of the frontotemporoparietal association cortices in patients with AD was also appreciable on the surface images. All these features, especially the anterior temporal and medial frontal atrophy, are useful for distinguishing FTD from AD. In addition, FTD is often mistaken clinically for psychiatric disorders, as well as for AD. It should be stressed that the peculiar atrophic pattern in FTD is useful for the differentiation of FTD from psychiatric disorders.

The surface display of the hemispheres rendered with MR images is useful for the evaluation of the extent of the cortical area affected by atrophy in FTD. In our review of the routine MR images, atrophy accentuated in the temporal lobe was recorded in one-third of the patients with FTD, and atrophy that affected the frontal lobe was recorded in one-third of those with AD. This indicates the need to specify the exact location of the atrophy: in the frontal lobe or in the temporal lobe. Frisoni et al (20) used planiometric measurement on routine MR images and demonstrated that greater atrophy of the frontal lobe and preservation of the medial temporal lobe are of value for the rough distinction of FTD from AD. They did not, however, identify the specific structures affected in either disease. Anatomic identification on routine MR images is achievable, and one can apply our findings to such images, but the procedure may be fairly perplexing. The MR hemispheric surface display has obvious advantages over the routine MR images in the evaluation of cortical atrophy in patients with dementias. Because the diagnosis of dementia requires a multidisciplinary approach, the evaluation of cortical atrophy on the hemispheric surface display should provide additional diagnostic clues.

Other than the need for hardware and software postprocessing of the MR images, several limitations and disadvantages of the hemispheric surface display method should be raised. It has been pointed out that atrophy in the amygdalohippocampal region is the most useful sign for the diagnosis of AD (40,41), although the role of neuroimaging in the diagnosis of FTD remains unsettled (20). In any event, hemispheric surface displays are not suitable for the observation of these structures. An inability to evaluate atrophic changes that are not related to the gyral configuration is another limitation of surface displays. Visual inspection from the outside of the hemisphere would not allow correct evaluation of cortical atrophy in patients with concentric cerebral atrophy and a large subarachnoid or subdural space. In patients with hydrocephalus, where sulci and fissures are flattened owing to pressure from the expanded ventricles, surface images would likewise not be useful.

In conclusion, although volume rendering of the brain previously necessitated laborious manual operations that were subject to the operator's expertise, routine use of this technique has now been realized, owing to advances in computer technology. Automated hemispheric surface display and volumetry are complementary to tomographic MR images and are useful for the evaluation of focal cortical atrophy in degenerative dementias—especially FTD. They may facilitate the study of brain-behavior relationships and the differential diagnosis of dementia.

Acknowledgments: We thank Tatsuo Shimomura, MD, Yoshitaka Ikejiri, MD, Mamoru Hashimoto, MD, Manabu Ikeda, MD, Toru Imamura, MD, and Hikari Yamashita, MA, (Clinical Neurosciences, Hyogo Institute for Aging Brain and Cognitive Disorders) for providing clinical data on the patients examined in this study.

References

1. Bragg DG. Advances in diagnostic radiology: problems and prospects. Cancer 1977; 40(suppl 1):500–508.
2. Brant-Zawadzki M. MR imaging of the brain. Radiology 1988; 166:1–10.
3. Jack CR Jr, Marsh WR, Hirschorn KA, et al. EEG scalp electrode projection onto three-dimensional surface rendered images of the brain. Radiology 1990; 176:413–418.
4. Levin DN, Hu XP, Tan KK, Galhotra S. Surface of the brain: three-dimensional MR images created with volume rendering. Radiology 1989; 171:277–280.
5. Cline HE, Dumoulin CL, Hart HR Jr, Lorensen WE, Ludke S. 3D reconstruction of the brain from magnetic resonance images using a connectivity algorithm. Magn Reson Imaging 1987; 5:345–352.
6. Vannier MW, Marsh JL, Warren JO. Three-dimensional CT reconstruction images for craniofacial surgical planning and evaluation. Radiology 1984; 150:179–184.
7. Hu XP, Tan KK, Levin DN, et al. Three-dimensional magnetic resonance images of the brain: application to neurosurgical planning. J Neurosurg 1990; 72:433–440.
8. Mori E, Hirono N, Yamashita H, et al. Premorbid brain size as a determinant of reserve capacity against intellectual decline in Alzheimer's disease. Am J Psychiatry 1997; 154:18–24.
9. Kobashi S, Kamiura N, Hata Y, Yamato K. 3D automatic extraction method of the brain regions aided by fuzzy matching techniques. In: Asian fuzzy systems symposium: soft computing in intelligent systems and information processing. Piscataway, NJ: Institute of Electrical and Electronics Engineers, 1996; 164–175.
10. Snowden JS, Neary D, Mann DMA. Fronto-temporal lobar degeneration: fronto-temporal dementia, progressive aphasia, semantic dementia. New York, NY: Livingstone, 1996.
11. The Lund and Manchester Groups. Clinical and neuropathological criteria for frontotemporal dementia. J Neurol Neurosurg Psychiatry 1994; 57:416–418.
12. Pasquier F, Petit H. Frontotemporal dementia: its rediscovery. Eur Neurol 1997; 38:1–6.
13. Neary D. Frontotemporal degeneration, Pick disease, and corticobasal degeneration: one entity or 3? 3. Arch Neurol 1997; 54:1425–1427.
14. Kertesz A. Frontotemporal dementia, Pick disease, and corticobasal degeneration: one entity or 3? 1. Arch Neurol 1997; 54:1427–1429.
15. Hachinski V. Frontotemporal degeneration, Pick disease, and corticobasal degeneration: three entities or 1? Arch Neurol 1997; 54:1429.
16. Foster NL, Wilhelmsen K, Sima AA, Jones MZ, D'Amato CJ, Gilman S. Frontotemporal dementia and Parkinsonism linked to chromosome 17: a consensus conference—conference participants. Ann Neurol 1997; 41:706–715.
17. Kitagaki H, Mori E, Hirono N, et al. Alteration of white matter MRI signal intensity in frontotemporal dementia. AJNR 1997; 18:367–378.
18. Ernst T, Chang L, Melchor R, Mehringer CM. Frontotemporal dementia and early Alzheimer disease: differentiation with frontal lobe H-1 MR spectroscopy. Radiology 1997; 203:829–836.
19. Kaufer DI, Miller BL, Itti L, et al. Midline cerebral morphometry distinguishes frontotemporal dementia and Alzheimer's disease. Neurology 1997; 48:978–985.
20. Frisoni GB, Beltramello A, Geroldi C, Weiss C, Bianchetti A, Trabucchi M. Brain atrophy in frontotemporal dementia. J Neurol Neurosurg Psychiatry 1996; 61:157–165.
21. Mori E, Mitani Y, Yamadori A. Usefulness of Japanese version of the Mini-Mental State test in neurological patients. Jpn J Neuropsychol 1985; 1:82–90.
22. Mohs RC, Rosen WG, Davis KL. The Alzheimer's Disease Assessment Scale: an instrument for assessing treatment efficacy. Psychopharmacol Bull 1983; 19:448–450.
23. World Health Organization. ICD-10 classification of mental and behavioural disorders: clinical descriptions and diagnostic guidelines. Geneva, Switzerland: World Health Organization, 1992.
24. Miller BL, Ikonte C, Ponton M, et al. A study of the Lund-Manchester research criteria for frontotemporal dementia: clinical and single-photon emission CT correlations. Neurology 1997; 48:937–942.
25. Lezak M. Neuropsychological assessment. 2nd ed. New York, NY: Oxford University Press, 1983.
26. Ishii K, Sakamoto S, Sasaki M, et al. Cerebral glucose metabolism in patients with frontotemporal dementia. J Nucl Med (in press).
27. Starkstein SE, Migliorelli R, Teson A, et al. Specificity of changes in cerebral blood flow in patients with frontal lobe dementia. J Neurol Neurosurg Psychiatry 1994; 57:790–796.
28. McKhann G, Drachman D, Folstein M, Katzman R, Price D, Stadlan E. Clinical diagnosis of Alzheimer's disease: report of the NINCDS-ADRDA Work Group under the auspices of the Department of Health and Human Services Task Force on Alzheimer's Disease. Neurology 1984; 34:939–944.

29. Ishii K, Kitagaki H, Kono M, Mori E. Decreased medial temporal oxygen metabolism in Alzheimer's disease shown by positron emission tomography. J Nucl Med 1996; 37:1159–1165.
30. Dunn OJ. Multiple comparisons using rank sums. Technometrics 1964; 6:241–252.
31. Edwards-Lee T, Miller BL, Benson DF, et al. The temporal variant of frontotemporal dementia. Brain 1997; 120:1027–1040.
32. Blacker D, Albert MS, Basset SS, et al. Reliability and validity of NINCDS-ADRDA criteria for Alzheimer's disease. Arch Neurol 1994; 51:1198–1204.
33. Mendez M, Selwood A, Mastri A, Frey W II. Pick's disease versus Alzheimer's disease: a comparison of clinical characteristics. Neurology 1993; 43: 289–292.
34. Knopman DS, Christensen KJ, Schut LJ, et al. The spectrum of imaging and neuropsychological findings in Pick's disease. Neurology 1989; 39:362–368.
35. Mann DMA, South PW. The topographic distribution of brain atrophy in frontal lobe dementia. Acta Neuropathol (Berl) 1993; 85:334–340.
36. Mann DMA, South PW, Snowden JS, Neary D. Dementia of frontal lobe type: neuropathology and immunohistochemistry. J Neurol Neurosurg Psychiatry 1993; 56:605–614.
37. Lang AE, Bergeron C, Pollanen MS, Ashby P. Parietal Pick's disease mimicking cortical–basal ganglionic degeneration. Neurology 1994; 44:1436–1440.
38. Fukui T, Sugita K, Kawamura M, Shiota J, Nakano I. Primary progressive apraxia in Pick's disease: a clinicopathologic study. Neurology 1996; 47:467–473.
39. Cummings JL, Benson DF. Dementia: a clinical approach. 2nd ed. Boston, Mass: Butterworth, 1983; 3:81–82.
40. Jack CR, Petersen RC, O'Brien PC, et al. MR-based hippocampal volumetry in the diagnosis of Alzheimer's disease. Neurology 1992; 42:183–188.
41. Mori E, Yoneda Y, Yamashita H, et al. Medial temporal structures relate to memory impairment in Alzheimer's disease: a MRI volumetric study. J Neurol Neurosurg Psychiatry 1997; 63:214–221.

Book Review

Imaging of the Globe and Orbit: A Guide to Differential Diagnosis

Norbert Hosten, MD, and Norbert Bornfield, MD
Stuttgart, Germany: Georg Thieme Verlag, 1998. ISBN: 3-13-108181-3.
Hardcover, DM 168; pp 208; 137 figures; tables.

Although the orbit spans the customary territory of both the neuroradiologist and the head and neck specialist, it is an area with which many radiologists are uncomfortable. This is in part related to the large number of disease entities, most of which are seen exceedingly rarely in daily practice. In addition, while a compartmental approach is easiest to work with, there are many trans-spatial lesions that do not fit neatly into any purely anatomic scheme. Most radiologists who interpret the results of these examinations thus welcome new attempts at presenting this large volume of information in a clear and systematic fashion.

This is the goal achieved by the authors of this English translation of the German monograph originally published in 1995. While they believe their book, which is organized according to anatomic compartments, has utility for the practicing radiologist, they think it has exceptional value to the trainee, particularly one who is preparing for board examinations. Contributors include both radiologists and ophthalmologists, a strategy used successfully in other areas to provide full clinical context for the information provided.

The table of contents, on the inside cover page, does not list page numbers. Each chapter is represented by a line drawing of the area of interest, which is present on each page of the corresponding section. This emphasizes the compartmental approach employed by the authors, but it proves somewhat cumbersome to the reader. A useful chapter at the end on examination technique is not listed in the contents and is easily overlooked. The book covers the classic intraconal, extraconal, optic nerve, and globe segments, as well as additional chapters on the orbital apex/cavernous sinus and lacrimal gland and ducts. Each well-organized chapter starts with a brief differential diagnosis for the region, followed by sections on anatomy, examination technique, normal findings, and clinical entities.

Unfortunately, although the book provides a fairly exhaustive listing of entities encountered in the orbit, the individual discussions are lacking due to widely varying depth of treatment. For example, while multiple sclerosis is covered extensively, there is only a brief and superficial discussion of cavernous-carotid fistulae. In addition, some of the sentences are difficult to understand, as a result of the globally awkward and frequently confusing translation. Readers will find themselves re-reading paragraphs frequently in an attempt to decipher the meaning.

While the diagrams and line drawings are both informative and aesthetically pleasing, the radiologic images are of lesser quality than that of today's images. The welcome exception to this is the revised section on the globe, in which magnetic resonance images obtained with a custom surface coil are quite spectacular. The captions are too frequently inaccurate; there are instances in which the same image is used with different captions and others in which incorrect descriptions of the sequence parameters are used. This could prove especially confusing to trainees who may not be confident enough in their interpretive skills to attribute the lack of correspondence between the image and the caption to editing error.

Although this book has many good features, specifically its clear organization and some lovely images, it is too uneven and difficult to read to represent the ideal tool for the trainee or practicing radiologist. A more coherent and precise book based on the "bones" of this book could indeed prove very useful to anyone involved in imaging the orbit.

Reviewed by Deborah R. Shatzkes, MD

Anterior Facial Vein and Submandibular Gland Together: Predicting the Histology of Submandibular Masses with CT or MR Imaging[1]

Jane L. Weissman, MD
Ricardo L. Carrau, MD

Index terms:
Head and neck neoplasms, CT, 2642.12112
Head and neck neoplasms, diagnosis, 2642.30
Head and neck neoplasms, MR, 2642.12143
Salivary glands, diseases, 2642.2472
Salivary glands, neoplasms, 2642.373, 2642.375
Veins, facial, 907.92

Radiology 1998; 208:441–446

[1] From the Departments of Radiology (J.L.W.) and Otolaryngology (J.L.W., R.L.C.), University of Pittsburgh Medical Center, Rm D-132 Presbyterian University Hospital, 200 Lothrop St, Pittsburgh, PA 15213. From the 1997 RSNA scientific assembly. Received January 14, 1998; revision requested February 25; revision received March 13; accepted April 13. **Address reprint requests to** J.L.W.

PURPOSE: To test the hypothesis that the relationship of the anterior facial vein to the submandibular salivary gland and a mass in the submandibular fossa could help identify the origin of the mass at computed tomography (CT) or magnetic resonance (MR) imaging.

MATERIALS AND METHODS: Thirteen patients with 14 palpable submandibular masses, surgical and histologic confirmation, and contrast material–enhanced CT images (12 patients) or MR images (one patient) that showed the anterior facial vein were identified with review of files from 1985 to 1997. Six patients had submandibular gland disease: three with primary neoplasms, two with metastatic tumor invading the gland, and one with chronic sialoadenitis. Eight patients had masses arising outside the gland (seven with lymphadenopathy, one with a plexiform neurofibroma).

RESULTS: The anterior facial vein did not separate primary tumors, tumors invading the gland, or lobulations of the enlarged gland from the body of the gland. The vein was identified between enlarged lymph nodes and the gland. The vein did not separate the gland from the neurofibroma, but this tumor was medial to the gland; the vein runs lateral to the gland.

CONCLUSION: The anterior facial vein is a useful landmark in determining the origin of a submandibular mass. Primary disease of the gland is never separated from the gland by the vein. The vein does separate lymphadenopathy from the gland and, theoretically, separates the gland from soft-tissue tumors lateral to the gland.

A palpable submandibular mass in an adult may be an enlarged submandibular gland, submandibular lymph nodes, or a rare tumor adjacent to the gland (1–6). The most frequent causes of an enlarged submandibular gland are inflammation or a benign or malignant neoplasm. Submandibular lymphadenopathy is most often metastatic squamous cell carcinoma, lymphoma, or inflammation or infection. Soft-tissue tumors that arise adjacent to the gland, such as lipomas and neurofibromas, are rare. The surgical approach to a submandibular mass will depend on the origin and extent of the mass.

A fat plane between the mass and the gland on all computed tomographic (CT) or magnetic resonance (MR) images is strong evidence that the mass arises outside the gland. However, a large mass may compress the fat so that the origin of the mass cannot be determined.

The anterior facial vein sweeps around the lateral aspect of the submandibular gland (7) before emptying into the internal jugular vein (7,8). This study was designed to test the hypothesis that a tumor that arises from the gland should displace the vein away from the gland but that the vein will run between the gland and a submandibular node. The relationship between a submandibular mass, the anterior facial vein, and the submandibular gland will help predict whether the mass arose from or adjacent to the gland and, thus, the histology of the mass.

Author contributions:
Guarantor of integrity of entire study, J.L.W.; study concepts, J.L.W., R.L.C.; study design, J.L.W.; definition of intellectual content, J.L.W., R.L.C.; literature research, J.L.W.; clinical studies, J.L.W., R.L.C.; data acquisition, R.L.C., J.L.W.; data analysis, J.L.W.; manuscript preparation, J.L.W.; manuscript editing and review, J.L.W., R.L.C.

MATERIALS AND METHODS

The computerized clinical files of the Departments of Radiology, Otolaryngology, and Surgical Pathology from 1985 to 1997 were searched to identify patients with clinically palpable submandibular masses who had undergone surgical removal and histologic examination of the mass. For inclusion in this retrospective study, each patient had to have available for review a preoperative CT or MR study on which the anterior facial vein could be confidently identified. On each imaging study, the vein was verified by following the vein from the level of the mandible to the internal or external jugular vein.

Thirteen patients had disease that involved 14 submandibular fossae. There were five men and eight women aged 22–80 years at the time of imaging. Six patients had disease arising from or invading the submandibular gland: One had chronic sialoadenitis, three had primary neoplasms of the submandibular gland (one with pleomorphic adenoma, one with adenoid cystic carcinoma, and one with mucosa-associated lymphoid tumor), and two had squamous cell carcinoma invading the gland. Eight patients had masses arising outside the gland. One patient had a plexiform neurofibroma. Seven patients had neoplastic lymph nodes (five with metastatic squamous cell carcinomas, one with metastatic sinonasal undifferentiated carcinoma, and one with Hodgkin disease). One of these, a woman with metastatic squamous cell carcinoma, also had metastatic adenopathy invading the contralateral gland.

Twelve patients had CT studies, and one had an MR study. Ten CT studies were obtained with a 3-mm section thickness, two were obtained with a 5-mm section thickness, and all were obtained with the intravenous administration of contrast material (Optiray [ioversol]; Mallinckrodt Medical, St Louis, Mo) and use of a model 9800 Advantage scanner (GE Medical Systems, Milwaukee, Wis). The MR study included axial T1-weighted MR images (600/16 [repetition time msec/echo time msec]) 4 mm thick obtained with a 1-mm intersection gap before the administration of gadopentetate dimeglumine (Magnevist; Berlex Laboratories, Wayne, NJ) and with fat suppression (600/16) after the intravenous administration of a gadopentetate dimeglumine, with use of a Signa 1.5-T imager (GE Medical Systems). Fat-suppressed coronal images (683/15) 3 mm thick were obtained with a 1-mm intersection gap after gadopentetate dimeglumine administration.

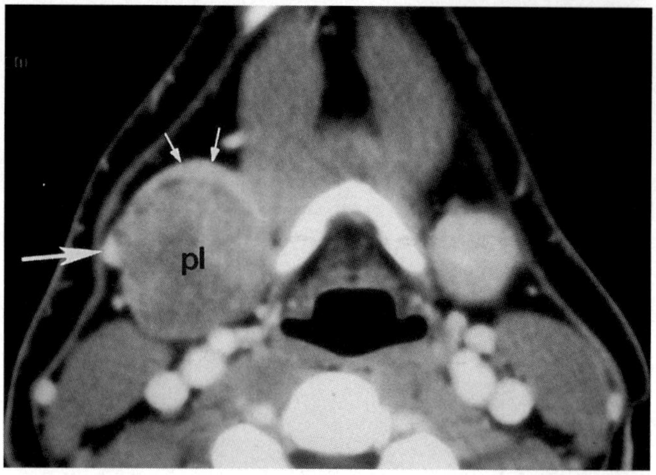

Figure 1. Contrast-enhanced CT image obtained in a 26-year-old man. A large pleomorphic adenoma (*pl*) arising from the submandibular gland (small arrows) displaces the anterior facial vein (large arrow) away from the gland. The gland is of higher attenuation than the tumor.

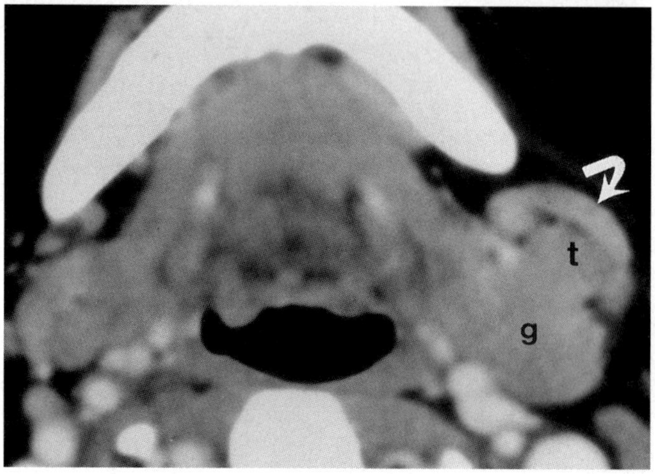

Figure 2. Contrast-enhanced CT image obtained in a 55-year-old woman. An exophytic tumor (*t*) arises from the submandibular gland (*g*). The anterior facial vein (arrow) is draped over both the tumor and the gland.

The relationship between the mass and the submandibular gland was evaluated by using two criteria, an intact fat plane and the anterior facial vein. If a fat plane separated the mass from the gland on all images, the mass could be considered to arise from outside the gland. If this plane was not present on all images, it was not possible to determine (by using this criterion) whether the mass arose outside the gland. The relationship of the anterior facial vein to the mass and the gland was also evaluated.

RESULTS

In all six patients with submandibular gland disease, a fat plane did not separate the mass from the gland on every image. The anterior facial vein was draped over the submandibular gland or over the gland and the mass (Figs 1, 2). In these patients, the vein did not separate the tumor from the gland (Fig 1) or lobulations of the enlarged gland from the body of the gland (Fig 2).

In all eight patients with extraglandular lymphadenopathy, the anterior facial vein separated enlarged lymph nodes from the gland (Figs 3, 4). This was seen both when the nodes were anterior or lateral to the gland (submandibular, or zone I, nodes) (Fig 3) and when the nodes were posterior to the gland (jugulodigastric, or zone II, nodes) (Fig 4).

One patient had metastatic lymphadenopathy on the right side, with the anterior facial vein clearly seen between the submandibular gland and the node (Fig 3). On the left side, however, she had what appeared to be a necrotic node that was not separated from the gland by the vein or by an intact fat plane. At surgery, both masses were lymph nodes containing squamous cell carcinoma. However, with extraglandular disease, there was at least one image on which an intact fat plane could not be identified between the mass and the gland (Figs 6, 7).

DISCUSSION

The submandibular fossa, or submandibular triangle, lies deep to the platysma muscle, between the mandible (above it) and the hyoid bone (below it) (7) (Fig 8). The largest structure in the submandibular fossa is the submandibular gland (7). The fossa also contains three to eight lymph nodes, lymphatic vessels, blood vessels, and fat (7,9).

The submandibular lymph nodes receive lymphatic drainage from "structures from above" (9), especially the floor of the mouth, the tongue, lips, gingiva, and nose (1,7,9). Submandibular lymph nodes also receive lymphatic drainage from the adjacent sublingual nodes (7,9).

Most of the venous drainage of the face converges on the anterior facial vein (7). The anterior facial vein begins as the angular vein, which crosses the body of the mandible and continues as the anterior facial vein, passing over the lateral surface of the submandibular gland (7) (Fig 8). The anterior facial vein then either empties into the internal jugular vein or joins the posterior facial (retromandibular) vein to form the common facial vein, which empties into the internal jugular vein at the level of the hyoid bone (7) (Fig 8).

Clinically, it may be difficult or impossible to differentiate a submandibular gland enlarged by tumor or chronic obstruction from a mass arising adjacent to the gland. All of these entities may be painless (10). Most of the time, CT or MR studies can help make the distinction. However, an exophytic tumor arising from the submandibular salivary gland can mimic an extraglandular mass or lymph node on imaging studies. Similarly, adenopathy or other masses arising outside the gland may not be clearly separated from the gland by an intact fat plane (Figs 6, 7a). Therefore, even with imaging studies, it has not always been possible to determine the origin of a submandibular mass.

The current study findings demonstrate the usefulness of the anterior facial vein in evaluating masses of the submandibular fossa. The vein is a relatively constant landmark. Primary submandibular gland disease displaces the vein away from the gland. If a tumor arises from the gland, no normal structure, not even the

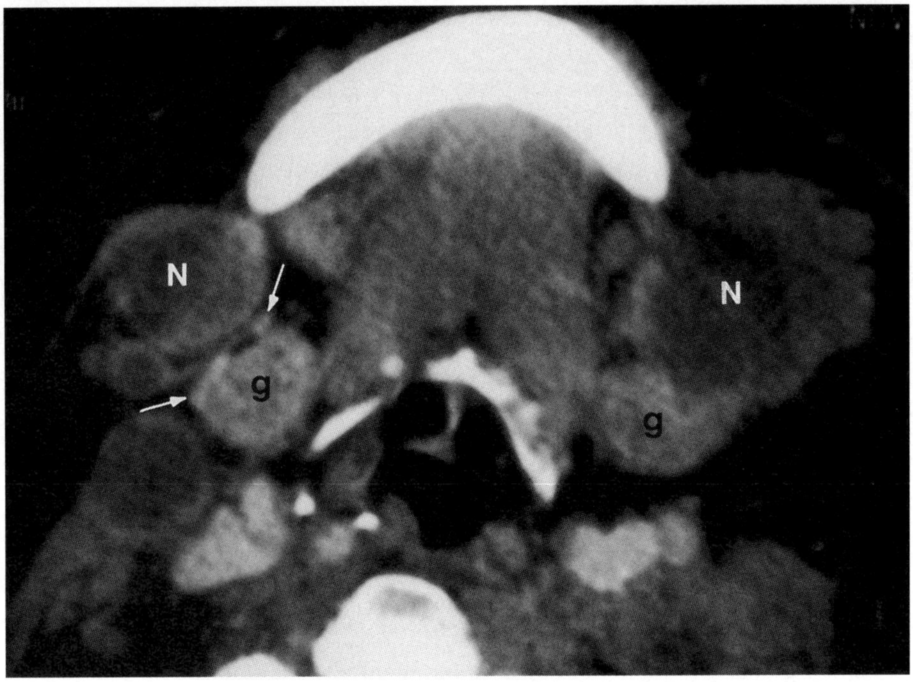

Figure 3. Contrast-enhanced CT image obtained in an 76-year-old woman shows bilateral necrotic submandibular lymph nodes (*N*). On the right side, the anterior facial vein (arrows) separates the node from the submandibular gland (*g*). However, on the left side, the vein does not separate the node from the gland. At histologic analysis, both nodes contained metastatic squamous cell carcinoma, but the tumor in the lymph node on the left invaded the submandibular gland.

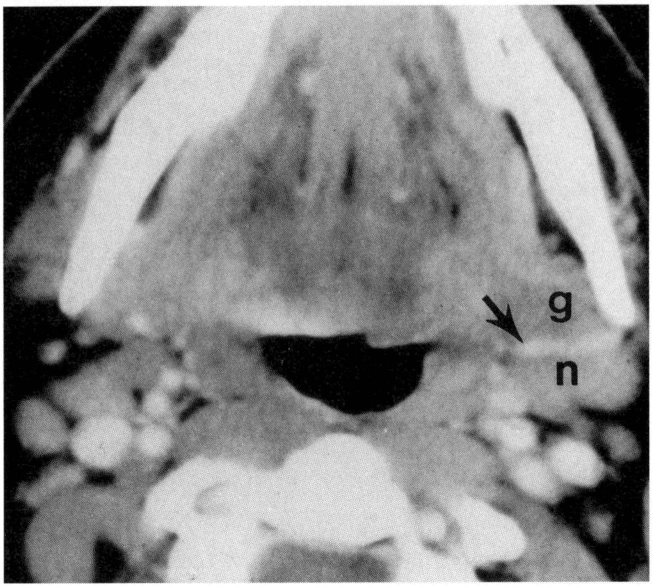

Figure 4. Contrast-enhanced CT image obtained in an 37-year-old man. The anterior facial vein (arrow) separates the submandibular gland (*g*) from the jugulodigastric lymph nodes (*n*).

extracapsular spread of tumor from the node on the left had invaded the submandibular gland.

One patient had a plexiform neurofibroma medial to and inseparable from the submandibular gland (Fig 5). The vein, which was lateral to the gland, therefore did not separate the tumor from the gland.

In only one of the eight patients with extraglandular disease did a fat plane separate the mass (non-Hodgkin lymphoma) from the gland on all images. In each of the remaining seven patients vein, separates the tumor from the gland (Figs 1, 2). In comparison, the vein does pass between the gland and an extraglandular mass (Figs 3, 4, 6b).

The anterior facial vein is a landmark that helps distinguish between submandibular gland disease and an extraglandular mass, but this useful landmark has several important limitations. First, it is not possible to rely on the vein if it is not possible to see the vein. The anterior facial vein may be small, poorly opacified at CT, or occluded. Second, because it follows a curving path, the vein may not be seen on every axial image through the submandibular fossa (Fig 6). Third, nameless small vessels in and around the submandibular gland can be mistaken for the anterior facial vein.

Another limitation is that the vein runs over the lateral surface of the gland. A tumor medial to the gland will therefore not be separated from the gland by the vein. This was seen on the images of the plexiform neurofibroma (Fig 5). Failure to identify the vein between the gland and the mass was, in this case, not evidence that the tumor arose from the gland.

It is possible to see the vein between the gland and an apparent extraglandular mass on some (Fig 6b) but not all (Fig 6a) images. This would be true with an exophytic tumor of the gland or a lobulated, inflamed gland. For this reason, it is important to obtain sections 3–4 mm thick with a 0–1-mm intersection gap and to look at all of the images through the submandibular fossa before making a diagnosis. MR imaging may prove better than CT in the identification of a thin residual fat plane between a mass and the gland. The sagittal and coronal images readily available with MR studies may show fat not seen well on axial images.

The ability to identify the origin of a submandibular mass helps to narrow the differential diagnosis for the mass (1,2). The submandibular gland enlarges because of benign and malignant salivary gland neoplasms, infection, and obstruction. Lymph node metastases, lymphoma, infection, and inflammation cause submandibular lymphadenopathy. Lipomas, schwannomas, lymphangiomas, hemangiomas, and other rare soft-tissue tumors also occur in the submandibular fossa separate from the gland (1,4–6).

Knowledge of the origin of a submandibular mass helps the surgeon with surgical planning and preoperative patient counseling. Needle biopsy findings may not be diagnostic if the specimen is inadequate or if a trained cytologist is not available to interpret the material (1), which necessitates excisional biopsy of the lymph node. If imaging studies demonstrate that a mass of the submandibular fossa is adenopathy, careful clinical and radiologic examination of the upper aerodigestive tract (upper respiratory and digestive tracts) may help identify the primary tumor. Squamous cell carcinomas of the floor of the mouth, the tongue, the tonsil, and the retromolar trigone have a predilection for submandibular lymph node metastases (9). Identification of the primary tumor may make biopsy of the submandibular node unnecessary. Hodgkin disease tends to involve contiguous chains of lymph nodes, whereas non-Hodgkin lymphoma may affect widely separated chains of nodes (11,12). This pattern can suggest the diagnosis, but histologic confirmation is necessary.

A submandibular lymph node or mass

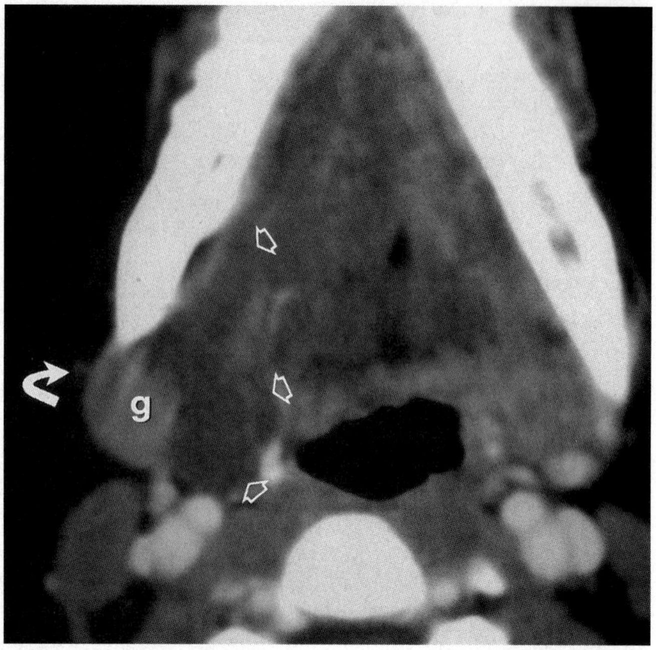

Figure 5. Contrast-enhanced CT image obtained in a 22-year-old woman. A low-attenuation plexiform neurofibroma (open arrows) is medial to the submandibular gland (*g*). The anterior facial vein (curved arrow), small and poorly opacified, is lateral to the gland. The vein, which is lateral, does not separate the gland from even a completely extraglandular tumor medial to the gland.

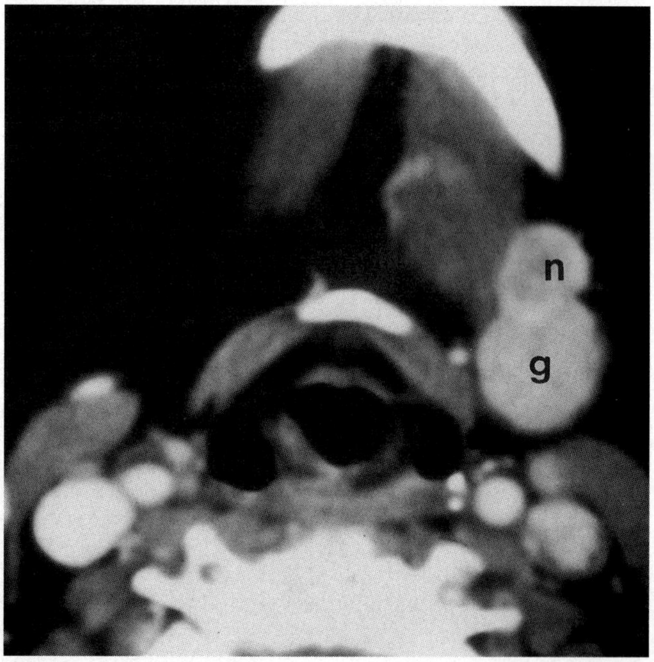

Figure 6. Contrast-enhanced CT image obtained in a 61-year-old woman. A lymph node containing metastatic squamous cell carcinoma (*n*) is inseparable from the submandibular gland (*g*). The fat plane between the gland and the node was compressed, but the tumor did not invade the gland. On this single image, the anterior facial vein is not seen. Adjacent images clearly showed the vein separating the node from the gland, emphasizing the importance of looking at all images obtained through the submandibular fossa.

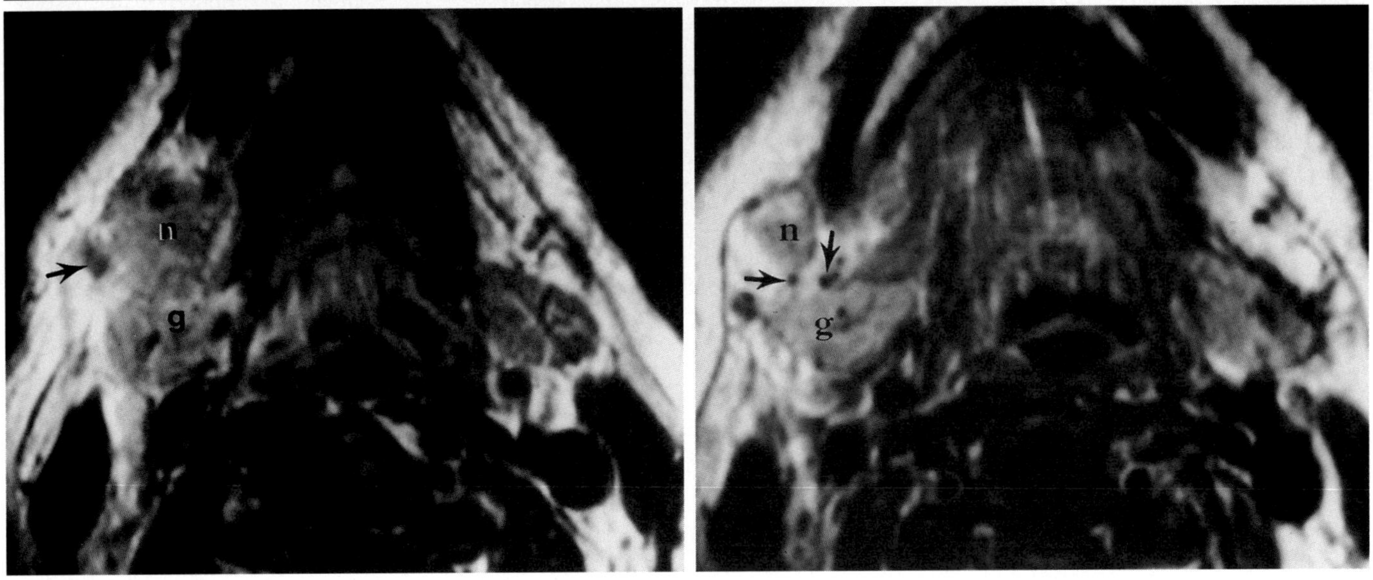

a. b.

Figure 7. **(a)** T1-weighted MR image (600/16) of metastatic submandibular lymphadenopathy in a 57-year-old man. On this image, there is no fat plane separating the lymph node (*n*) from the submandibular gland (*g*). The anterior facial vein (arrow) is lateral to both. **(b)** T1-weighted MR image (600/16) obtained at a slightly lower level demonstrates that loops of the anterior facial vein (arrows) separate the lymph node (*n*) from the submandibular gland (*g*). It is important to look at all images obtained through the submandibular fossa to determine whether a mass arises from the gland.

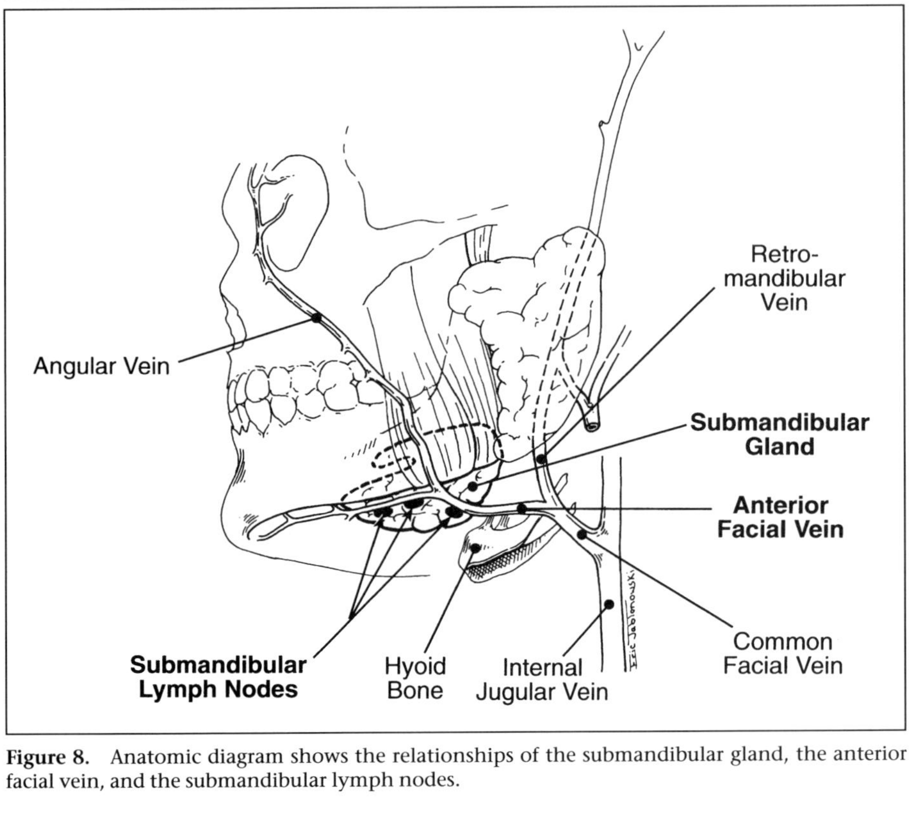

Figure 8. Anatomic diagram shows the relationships of the submandibular gland, the anterior facial vein, and the submandibular lymph nodes.

that is separate from the gland can usually be removed without removing the gland. However, the surgical approach to the gland necessitates identification of the marginal mandibular nerve, or the ramus mandibularis. This branch of the facial nerve is superficial to the anterior facial vein (1,10). With benign pathologic conditions of the submandibular gland, the nerve is preserved; with malignant disease, the nerve is often resected with the gland (12). These issues must be discussed with the patient during preoperative counseling. If biopsy is performed because the histologic diagnosis is not known, the surgeon usually preserves the nerve.

The anterior facial vein did not completely separate a primary submandibular gland mass or inflamed lobulation of the gland from the gland itself. The anterior facial vein did run between the submandibular gland and the adjacent lymph nodes. This information can influence preoperative planning and patient counseling.

Acknowledgments: The authors are grateful to Sabrina L. Jennings for her expert preparation of the manuscript and to Eric Jablonowski, AS, for his expert artwork.

References

1. Suen JY, Stern SJ. Cancer of the neck. In: Myers EN, Suen JY, eds. Cancer of the head and neck. 2nd ed. Philadelphia, Pa: Saunders, 1996; 462–484.
2. Meiselman F, Cuttino CL. Clinicopathologic conference: a large submandibular space mass. Oral Maxillofac Surg 1990; 8:63–67.
3. Correll RW, DeBoom GW, Jensen JL. Slowly enlarging, nontender mass in the right submandibular region. J Am Dent Assoc 1986; 113:667–668.
4. Sutay S, Tekinsoy B, Ceryan K, Aksu Y. Submaxillary hypoglossal neurilemmoma. J Laryngol Otol 1993; 107:953–954.

5. Amsberry JK, Witiak D, Rao VM, Pribitkin EA. Imaging case study of the month: lipoma masquerading as a submandibular mass. Ann Otol Rhinol Laryngol 1995; 104:585–586.
6. Bochlogyros PN, Kanakis P, Tsikou-Papafrangou N, Chase D. Clinicopathologic conference: a large, painless mass in the submandibular space. J Oral Maxillofac Surg 1992; 50:1213–1216.
7. Hollinshead WH. Anatomy for surgeons: the head and neck. 3rd ed. Philadelphia, Pa: Lippincott, 1982.
8. Osborne AG. Introduction to cerebral angiography. Philadelphia, Pa: Harper & Row, 1980.
9. Sessions RB, Hudkins CP. Malignant cervical adenopathy. In: Cummings CW, Fredrickson JM, Harker LA, Krause CJ, Schuller DE, eds. Otolaryngology: head and neck surgery. 2nd ed. St Louis, Mo: Mosby–Year Book, 1993; 1605–1625.
10. Saunders JR, Hirata RM, Jaques DA. Salivary glands. Surg Clin North Am 1986; 66:59–81.
11. Rodriguez MA, Hong WK. Diagnosis and management of lymphomas of the head and neck. In: Myers EN, Suen JY, eds. Cancer of the head and neck. 2nd ed. Philadelphia, Pa: Saunders, 1996; 670–678.
12. Alvi A, Myers EN, Carrau R. Malignant tumors of the salivary glands. In: Myers EN, Suen JY, eds. Cancer of the head and neck. 2nd ed. Philadelphia, Pa: Saunders, 1996; 525–561.

Contrast-enhanced 3D MR DSA of the Carotid Artery Bifurcation: Preliminary Study of Comparison with Unenhanced 2D and 3D Time-of-Flight MR Angiography[1]

Donald S. Willig, MD
Patrick A. Turski, MD
Richard Frayne, PhD
Virgil B. Graves, MD
Frank R. Korosec, PhD
J. Shannon Swan, MD
Charles A. Mistretta, PhD
Thomas M. Grist, MD

Index terms:
Carotid arteries, MR, 172.12142, 172.14143, 172.127
Carotid arteries, stenosis or obstruction, 172.721, 172.76
Gadolinium
Magnetic resonance (MR), comparative studies, 172.12142, 172.12143, 172.127
Magnetic resonance (MR), contrast enhancement, 172.12143
Magnetic resonance (MR), three-dimensional, 172.12142, 172.12143, 172.127

Radiology 1998; 208:447–451

Abbreviations:
DSA = digital subtraction angiography
MIP = maximum intensity projection
TOF = time of flight
2D = two-dimensional
3D = three-dimensional

[1] From the Depts. of Radiology (D.S.W., P.A.T., R.F., V.B.G., F.R.K., J.S.S., C.A.M., T.M.G.) and Medical Physics (R.F., F.R.K., C.A.M., T.M.G.), University of Wisconsin, 600 Highland Ave, Madison, WI 53792.
From the 1996 RSNA scientific assembly. Received Oct 31, 1997; revision requested Jan 7, 1998; revision received Mar 13; accepted Apr 10. Supported in part by Nycomed Pharmaceuticals and NIH grant R29 HL57501. R.F. supported by Heart and Stroke Foundation of Canada and the National Science and Engineering Research Council of Canada. T.M.G. by NIH grant K08 HL02848.
Address reprint requests to P.A.T.

Author contributions:
Guarantor of integrity of entire study, P.A.T.; study concepts, D.S.W., P.A.T., R.F., V.B.G., F.R.K., J.S.S., C.A.M., T.M.G.; study design, D.S.W., R.F., T.M.G.; definition of intellectual content, D.S.W., P.A.T., R.F., V.B.G., F.R.K., J.S.S., C.A.M., T.M.G.; literature research, D.S.W.; clinical studies, D.S.W.; data acquisition, D.S.W.; data analysis, D.S.W., P.A.T., V.B.G.; statistical analysis, D.S.W., T.M.G.; manuscript preparation and editing, D.S.W., R.F.; manuscript review, R.F.

PURPOSE: To compare the delineation of stenosis at the carotid artery bifurcation on three-dimensional (3D) magnetic resonance (MR) digital subtraction angiographic (DSA) images with that on two-dimensional (2D) and 3D time-of-flight (TOF) MR angiographic images.

MATERIALS AND METHODS: Twenty-six patients with 29 carotid artery bifurcations and symptoms of cerebral ischemia underwent 3D MR DSA. A time-resolved series was generated with 3D MR DSA after the bolus injection of gadodiamide. The resolution for a carotid artery examination was 0.4 × 0.4 × 1.0 mm, with volumes reconstructed at 4.5-second intervals. The 3D MR DSA images were compared with contemporaneously acquired unenhanced 2D and 3D TOF images. Two observers ranked the 2D and 3D TOF MR angiographic and 3D MR DSA images according to the following: (*a*) stenosis delineation, (*b*) internal carotid artery delineation, (*c*) intravascular signal intensity, and (*d*) diagnostic confidence.

RESULTS: The mean ranking for diagnostic confidence was 1.10 (1 = best technique, 3 = worst technique) for 3D MR DSA. Compared with the pooled 2D TOF and 3D TOF ranks, the 3D MR DSA rank was significantly better ($P < .01$). Similar levels of statistical significance were found for the other criteria.

CONCLUSION: Three-dimensional MR DSA improves the delineation of carotid arterial stenosis by virtually eliminating saturation effects and reducing intravoxel dephasing. Surface morphology and nearly occluded vessels ("string sign") were easily identified. Confidence in identifying carotid arterial occlusions was also very high with this technique.

Noninvasive imaging of the carotid artery bifurcation and the proximal internal carotid artery has become a focus of great clinical interest owing to the clear association between proximal internal carotid arterial stenosis and increased risk of stroke (1). Investigators in the North American Symptomatic Carotid Endarterectomy Trial (2) concluded that the risk of stroke could be reduced by performing carotid endarterectomy in patients with a stenosis of greater than 70% as measured with well-defined diameter criteria. Investigators in the Asymptomatic Carotid Atherosclerosis Study (3) also concluded that asymptomatic patients benefit from carotid endarterectomy, with some benefit realized even with a stenosis of 60%. These study findings emphasize the clinical importance of accurate delineation of the morphologies of the carotid artery bifurcation and the proximal internal carotid artery.

The clinical outcome for patients undergoing endarterectomy is a function of the complication rates of the surgery and the preceding conventional arteriogram. Surgical complication rates vary from 1% to 2%, and cerebral angiographic complication rates are reported to range from 0.7% to 1% (4). Thus, reducing the risk related to cerebral angiography would have a positive effect on patient outcome. Doppler ultrasound (US) has been advocated by some investigators (5) as a method for examining patients before carotid endarterectomy. Doppler US, however, is limited in its ability to help define the morphology of the carotid artery bifurcation and does not effectively help exclude tandem lesions of the carotid siphon. Doppler US also is compromised in its ability to help identify the nearly occluded carotid artery with extremely slow flow (6).

An approach that is rapidly gaining acceptance combines Doppler US and non–contrast agent–enhanced magnetic resonance (MR) angiography (7). The MR angiographic examination typically includes both two-dimensional (2D) time-of-flight (TOF) and three-dimensional (3D) TOF studies. The 2D TOF method has the advantage of improved sensitivity to slow flow (8). The 3D TOF method is more accurate in defining the morphology of proximal internal carotid arterial stenosis.

Both MR angiographic techniques, however, have substantial limitations. With 2D TOF imaging, there may be signal intensity loss related to in-plane saturation or to spin dephasing secondary to complex flow patterns. Another limitation of 2D TOF MR angiography is misregistration of the image sections. This misregistration can obscure regions of stenosis and distort carotid arterial anatomy. The 3D TOF technique typically involves thin sections, smaller voxels, and shorter echo times, which results in less signal intensity loss from spin dephasing (9). However, in the region of the stenosis, where flow conditions can be complex, there is frequently loss of signal intensity to a degree that compromises the accurate measurement of the stenotic segment. Several investigators (9,10) have demonstrated that the accuracy of measurement can be improved by using source images or reformatted source images. Even when using this approach, however, there are instances where measurement of the stenosis can be difficult (11).

One method to overcome these limitations is to administer a contrast agent to substantially shorten the T1 of blood (12,13); thus, saturation effects are minimized (14). Several authors have proposed combining very short 3D TOF acquisitions performed with echo times of less than 5 msec and repetition times of less than 11 msec with intravenous contrast agent enhancement to improve the delineation of the abdominal and peripheral vessels (15,16). Initial applications of these techniques to imaging of the carotid artery bifurcation were compromised by the overlap of venous structures and the enhancement of soft tissue caused by incorrect bolus timing (17,18).

To overcome this bolus timing limitation, we have developed a time-resolved 3D acquisition technique (19,20) in which several innovative methods are used to repeatedly image the vessels of interest during the passage of the contrast agent. This technique has been termed 3D MR DSA because of its similarities with conventional DSA. The technique allows reconstruction of 3D data sets with a temporal resolution of one frame every 2–6 seconds, which results in the creation of an angiographic series analogous to that of conventional DSA.

The acquisition process begins before the injection of contrast agent, allowing for the acquisition of a precontrast mask that can be subtracted from subsequent time frames to improve vessel conspicuity. This effectively eliminates background signal and allows multiple injec-

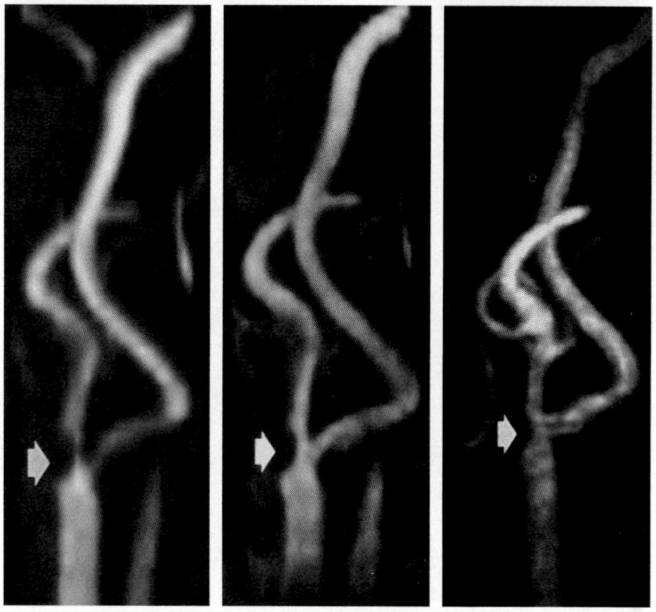

a. b. c.

Figure 1. Minimal stenosis (arrow) at the carotid artery bifurcation. **(a)** Two-dimensional TOF MIP image of the carotid artery bifurcation shows how a stenosis at the distal common carotid artery causes signal intensity loss. **(b)** Three-dimensional TOF MIP image of the carotid artery bifurcation shows how the 3D TOF technique recovers some of the signal intensity loss. **(c)** Three-dimensional MR DSA MIP image of the same region clearly delineates the lumen and demonstrates a 20% stenosis.

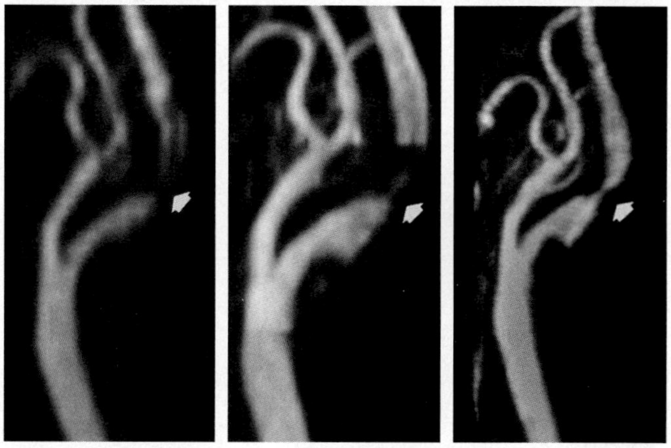

a. b. c.

Figure 2. Severe stenosis (arrow) of the proximal internal carotid artery. **(a)** A 2D TOF MIP image shows that complex flow limits the diameter of the lumen distal to the stenosis. **(b)** A 3D TOF MIP image shows saturation at the superior portion of the slab that is recovered at the inferior portion of a successive contiguous slab. **(c)** A 3D MR DSA MIP image of the carotid artery bifurcation shows the entire lumen, including the poststenotic region.

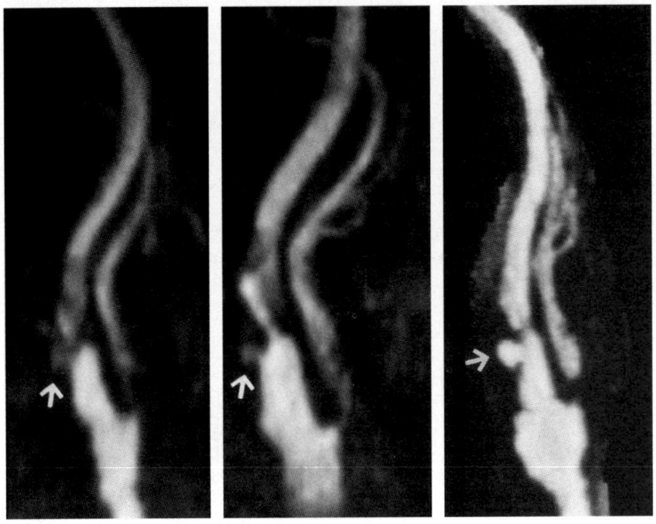

a. b. c.

Figure 3. Complex postoperative morphology on **(a)** 2D TOF MIP, **(b)** 3D TOF MIP, and **(c)** 3D MR DSA MIP images. The patient had undergone multiple previous surgeries, and the complex anatomy is best delineated in **c**. On close inspection, the outpouching (arrow; a probable pseudoaneurysm) is actually demonstrated on **a** and **b**; however, diagnostic confidence is not high. **c** clearly shows the outpouching (arrow) and achieves the best diagnostic confidence rank in this series of images.

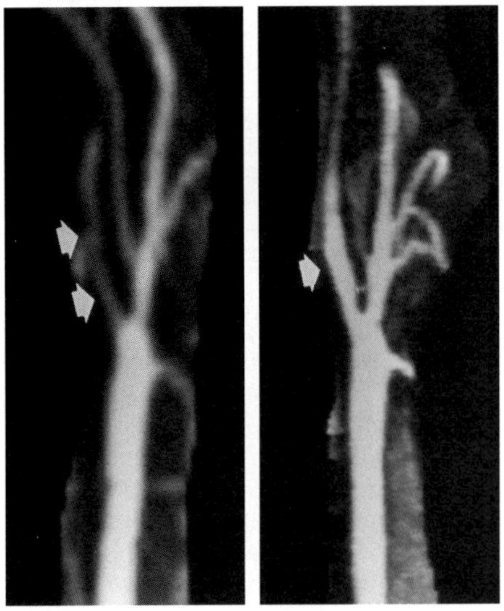

a. b.

Figure 4. Reduced flow volume within the internal carotid artery secondary to a cavernous carotid arterial stenosis. **(a)** Two-dimensional TOF MIP image shows that the lumen of the internal carotid artery (arrows) is collapsed. **(b)** Three-dimensional MR DSA MIP image shows the carotid bulb contour (arrow), although it is diminished in diameter. This bulb configuration is not appreciated in **a**.

tions of contrast agent in the same session. In the technique, variable-rate k-space sampling is used, and elements of k space are shared between image sets. With this technique, it is possible to depict the passage of contrast agent, first through the arteries, and then through the veins. The technique has the advantages of minimal sensitivity to the timing of the contrast agent injection and allows retrospective postprocessing of the volume images, such as image reprojection. Coordinating the exact arrival time of the bolus in the region of interest is less critical, because image acquisition begins before the injection and continues throughout the arterial and venous phases.

This study was performed to compare the delineation of stenosis at the carotid artery bifurcation on 3D MR DSA images with that on 2D and 3D TOF MR angiographic images.

MATERIALS AND METHODS

Twenty-nine carotid artery bifurcations in 26 patients were imaged with a 1.5-T system (Signa Horizon; GE Medical Systems, Milwaukee, Wis). Informed consent was obtained from all patients before the procedure. The 2D and 3D TOF MR images were obtained by using standard clinical protocols. The 2D TOF images were acquired with 40/8.7 (repetition time msec/echo time msec), a flip angle of 60°, 60–80 1.8-mm sections, a matrix of 192 × 256, and a field of view of 20 cm. The 3D TOF images were acquired by using a technique in which four sections were obtained per slab and that covered 32 mm with a 30% overlap, a flip angle of 20°–30°, 30/6.9, a section thickness of 1 mm, a matrix of 256 × 192, and a field of view of 20 cm.

The 3D MR DSA imaging protocol included a flip angle of 60°, 11/2.1, 24–32 1-mm sections, a 512 × 256 matrix, and a 20 × 10-cm field of view. Data were acquired for approximately 2 minutes. Approximately 20 seconds after the start of scanning, gadodiamide (Omniscan; Nycomed, Princeton, NJ; dose, 0.1–0.2 mmol/kg) was injected for 10 seconds by using a power injector (Spectris; Medrad, Pittsburgh, Pa). The images were reconstructed by means of offline image processing on a workstation (Solid Impact; Silicon Graphics, Mountain View, Calif). Data were zero filled to 512 × 512, and volume images were reconstructed to demonstrate a temporal resolution of one frame every 4.5 seconds. Volume images also were generated by using the first volume as a mask.

Patient motion resulted in minor image degradation in two 2D TOF examinations, one 3D TOF examination, and one 3D MR DSA examination. Six maximum intensity projection (MIP) images that profiled the stenosis were generated for each bifurcation from the 2D TOF angiographic, 3D TOF angiographic, and 3D MR DSA data sets. In the 3D MR DSA examination, the peak arterial time frame was chosen from the time series of volume images. The three sets of MIP images were presented to the two observers (P.A.T., V.B.G.) in a random order. The observers were asked to rank the three image sets on the basis of the following criteria: (*a*) delineation of the stenotic segment, (*b*) delineation of the morphology of the proximal internal carotid artery intimal surface, (*c*) intravascular signal intensity, and (*d*) diagnostic confidence. Identical projections from each of the three techniques were presented to the observers. The observers also were asked to rank their diagnostic confidence between the combination of 2D and 3D TOF MIP images and the 3D MR DSA MIP images.

Statistical tests were performed on the data to assess the statistical significance of our results. A Friedman two-way analysis of variance test (21) was used to determine whether there were statistically significant differences in the ranking of 3D MR DSA, 3D TOF MR angiography, and 2D TOF MR angiography. A Wilcoxon sign rank test (21) was used to assess statistical significance between the 3D MR DSA and the pooled TOF rankings. Both are nonparametric tests and are, therefore, appropriate for analyzing ranked data with an unknown distribution.

RESULTS

Figures 1–4 are examples of 2D TOF MR angiographic, 3D TOF MR angiographic, and 3D MR DSA images of the carotid bifurcation in patients with a variety of diseases. Figure 1 shows a bifurcation with minimal stenosis. In this case, the degree of stenosis was overestimated on both the 2D and the 3D TOF MR angiographic images compared with the degree of stenosis on the 3D MR DSA image.

A severe proximal internal carotid arterial stenosis is shown in Figure 2. Only the 3D MR DSA image clearly depicts the residual lumen. Both the 2D and the 3D TOF MR angiographic images show marked signal intensity loss at and downstream from the stenosis.

Figure 3 shows 2D TOF angiographic, 3D TOF angiographic, and 3D MR DSA images obtained in a patient with complex postoperative morphology. The 3D MR DSA image clearly depicts the anatomy, including an outpouching of the internal carotid artery. This outpouching is not clearly depicted on either the 2D or the 3D TOF MR angiographic images.

The effect of saturation in regions of slow flow, even in a 2D TOF examination, are shown in Figure 4. In this case, a cavernous carotid arterial stenosis restricted flow through the internal carotid artery, resulting in signal saturation (arrows in Fig 4a). This artifact was not observed on the 3D MR DSA images.

The following lesions were identified by means of 3D MR DSA measurements made by using North American Symptomatic Carotid Endarterectomy Trial criteria on the 29 3D MR DSA studies: eight 0%–49% stenoses, 10 50%–69% stenoses, 10 70%-99% stenoses, and one occlusion.

Table 1 summarizes the mean ranks for the three imaging techniques for each of the four criteria. For all criteria, the 3D MR DSA image was consistently ranked ahead of the 2D and the 3D TOF MR angiographic images. Friedman two-way analysis of variance test (21) results showed that the 3D MR DSA rank was best ($P < .005$) for each criterion. The same statistical test was applied to the ranks for each observer; results also demonstrated that the median ranks for each technique were not statistically equivalent ($P < .005$).

Table 2 summarizes the mean ranks for the comparison between the unenhanced 2D and 3D TOF MR angiographic images and the contrast-enhanced 3D MR DSA images. Observers ranked the diagnostic confidence of the 3D MR DSA images higher than that of the combination of 2D and 3D TOF MR angiographic images. Wilcoxon sign rank test (21) results indicated that this difference was statistically significant ($P < .01$).

TABLE 1
Mean Ranks for 3D MR DSA Images, 2D TOF MR Images, and 3D TOF MR Images

Criterion	3D MR DSA	2D TOF	3D TOF
Delineation of stenosis	1.14	2.48	2.38
Delineation of internal carotid artery	1.14	2.47	2.40
Intravascular signal intensity	1.14	2.43	2.43
Diagnostic confidence	1.14	2.47	2.40

Note.—For each criterion, the ranks for the three techniques were significantly different ($P < .005$, Friedman two-way analysis of variance [21]). This level of statistical significance was the same for both observers.

DISCUSSION

In light of the North American Symptomatic Carotid Endarterectomy Trial and Asymptomatic Carotid Atherosclerosis Study findings, there is little question that accurate measurement of internal carotid arterial stenosis is a critical step in the examination of patients before carotid endarterectomy. Current unenhanced MR angiographic techniques are useful and have been shown to be efficacious, particularly when used in combination with Doppler US. There are, however, many known limitations to unenhanced angiography, including saturation of slow flow (Fig 4a) and loss of signal intensity owing to intravoxel dephasing (Figs 2a, 2b, 3a, 3b). These limitations can be overcome with the use of contrast agent enhancement, which reduces the T1 of blood and virtually eliminates the effects of saturation (Figs 2c, 3c, 4b). Short echo times of less than 3 msec also greatly reduce the signal intensity loss that is related to complex and turbulent flow. When combined, short blood T1 and a short echo time result in marked improvement in the delineation of proximal internal carotid arterial stenosis. In practice, even regions of very slow flow along the edge of the vessel can be easily identified, and the measurement of internal carotid arterial stenosis can be accomplished by using techniques similar to DSA.

Three-dimensional MR DSA appears to have statistically significant advantages over unenhanced methods. Perhaps the most important feature is its ability to help identify very slow flow in narrowly occluded internal carotid arteries, such as in the case shown in Figure 4. This is most apparent in nearly occluded carotid arteries in which flow is markedly reduced (the carotid string), where saturation effects with conventional MR angiography may totally eliminate the signal from the vessel, resulting in an incorrect diagnosis of carotid arterial occlusion. Another major feature is the ability to retain blood signal intensity in regions of disturbed flow distal to the stenosis (Fig 2).

TABLE 2
Mean Ranks for Diagnostic Confidence in Interpreting Unenhanced Images and Contrast-enhanced Images

Observer	Contrast-enhanced Images*	Unenhanced Images†
A	1.03	1.97
B	1.17	1.83
Mean	1.10	1.90

Note.—The images were evaluated by two observers for diagnostic confidence. All differences were statistically significant ($P < .01$, Wilcoxon sign rank test [21]).
* 3D MR DSA images.
† Pooled 2D TOF and 3D TOF images.

Three-dimensional MR DSA minimizes the difficulty in delineating regions with stenoses of 50%–75%. This is beneficial because patients with stenoses in this range may have marginal benefit from carotid endarterectomy, and clear delineation is required before surgical planning. Findings of the preliminary investigation indicate that contrast agent enhancement improves diagnostic confidence and is preferred to unenhanced techniques for delineation of the stenosis of the proximal internal carotid artery. Our experience indicates that 3D MR DSA is a robust technique that allows improved delineation of complex proximal internal carotid artery morphology after the intravenous bolus injection of contrast agent. The images are not degraded by saturation effects, and the effects of intravoxel dephasing are reduced. These features provide images that are of improved diagnostic quality and that are preferred over unenhanced images for delineation of pathologic conditions of the proximal internal carotid artery. Continued validation of the technique with a standard of reference such as conventional angiography is needed. Nonetheless, findings of this preliminary investigation suggest that 3D MR DSA will assume a prominent role in the evaluation of carotid arterial stenosis.

The continued improvement and refinement of noninvasive diagnostic evaluation, as compared with diagnostic catheter angiography, of the carotid artery bifurcation region will have a positive effect on treatment by reducing cost and minimizing risk to the patient. In this preliminary study, we were able to demonstrate improvement over current 2D and 3D TOF MR angiographic methods by using a contrast agent with the 3D MR DSA technique. This method offers an alternative to catheter angiography in cases in which MR angiography and Doppler US findings are disparate. To develop this technique more thoroughly, additional questions must be answered. These questions include "What is the optimal dose and rate of gadolinium-based contrast agent injection?" and "What are the optimal imaging spacing and matrix required for proper delineation of carotid arterial stenosis?" Finally, a comparison with a standard of reference such as rotational catheter angiography should be made.

References

1. Warlow C, Peto R, Richards S, et al. MRC European carotid surgery trial: interim results for symptomatic patients with severe (70%–99%) or with mild (0%–29%) carotid stenosis. Lancet 1991; 337:1235–1243.
2. Taylor DW, Barnett HJM, Haynes RB, et al. Beneficial effects of carotid endarterectomy in symptomatic patients with high-grade carotid stenosis. N Engl J Med 1991; 325:445–453.
3. Executive Committee for the Asymptomatic Carotid Atherosclerosis Study. Endarterectomy for asymptomatic carotid artery stenosis. JAMA 1995; 273:1421–1428.
4. Kuntz KM, Skillman JJ, Whittemore AD, Kent KC. Carotid endarterectomy in asymptomatic patients: is contrast angiography necessary? a morbidity analysis. J Vasc Surg 1995; 22:706–716.
5. Wasserman BA, Haacke EM, Li D. Carotid plaque formation and its evaluation with angiography, ultrasound, and MR angiography. JMRI 1994; 4:515–527.
6. Steinke W, Kloetzsch C, Hennerici M. Carotid artery disease assessed by color Doppler flow imaging: correlation with standard Doppler sonography and angiography. AJR 1990; 154:1061–1068.
7. Patel MR, Kuntz KM, Klufas RA, et al. Preoperative assessment of the carotid bifurcation: can magnetic resonance angiography and duplex ultrasonography replace contrast arteriography? Stroke 1995; 26:1753–1758.
8. Bosmans H, Marchal G, Lukito G, et al. Time-of-flight MR angiography of the brain: comparison of acquisition techniques in healthy volunteers. AJR 1995; 164:161–167.
9. Masaryk TJ, Obuchowski NA. Noninvasive carotid imaging: caveat emptor. Radiology 1993; 186:325–331.
10. Anderson CM, Saloner D, Lee RE, et al. Assessment of carotid artery stenosis by MR angiography: comparison with x-ray angiography and color-coded Doppler ultrasound. AJNR 1992; 13:989–1003.
11. Bowen BC, Quencer RM, Margosian P, Pattany PM. MR angiography of occlusive disease of the arteries in the head and neck: current concepts. AJR 1994; 162: 9–18.
12. Prince MR, Yucel EK, Kaufman JA, Harrison DC, Geller SC. Dynamic gadolinium-enhanced three-dimensional abdominal MR arteriography. JMRI 1993; 3:877–881.
13. Prince MR. Gadolinium-enhanced MR arteriography. Radiology 1994; 191:155–164.
14. Runge VM, Kirsch JE, Lee C. Contrast-enhanced MR angiography. JMRI 1993; 3:233–239.
15. Lossef SV, Ragan SS, Pratt RH, et al. Gadolinium-enhanced magnitude contrast MR angiography of popliteal and tibial arteries. Radiology 1992; 184:349–355.
16. Petersen MJ, Cambria RP, Kaufman JA, et al. Magnetic resonance angiography in the preoperative evaluation of abdominal aortic aneurysms. J Vasc Surg 1995; 21: 891–899.
17. Levy RA, Prince MR. Arterial-phase three-dimensional contrast-enhanced MR angiography of the carotid arteries. AJR 1996; 167:211–215.
18. Cloft HJ, Murphy KJ, Prince MR, Brunberg JA. 3D gadolinium-enhanced MR angiography of the carotid arteries. Magn Reson Imaging 1996; 14:593–600.
19. Korosec FR, Frayne R, Grist TM, Mistretta CA. Time-resolved contrast-enhanced 3D MR angiography. Magn Reson Med 1996; 36:345–351.
20. Frayne R, Grist TM, Korosec FR, et al. MR angiography with three-dimensional MR digital subtraction angiography. Top Magn Reson Imaging 1996; 8:366–388.
21. Daniel WW. Biostatistics: a foundation for analysis in the health sciences. 4th ed. New York, NY: Wiley, 1987; 586–619.

Book Review

Vascular Diagnosis with Ultrasound: Clinical References with Case Studies

Michael Hennerici, MD, and Doris Neuerburg-Heusler, MD
Stuttgart, Germany: Georg Thieme Verlag, 1998. ISBN 3-13-103831-4.
Hardcover, DM 268; pp 518; 327 figures; 57 tables.

This book is a translation of the successful 2nd edition, published in 1995 in Germany, but I found it to be more than a translation. Numerous references from 1996 and 1997 were added. The latter references were inserted after the publication of the 2nd edition, which would effectively make this the 3rd edition. The intended audience for this book ranges from medical students to attending physicians in various specialties. It is an all-inclusive book, covering both neurologic and body applications.

The book is organized into 12 chapters. The first chapter, "Ultrasound Procedures," covers physics, equipment, and new developments. The next eight chapters cover various anatomic parts (extracranial cerebral arteries, intracranial cerebral arteries, cerebral veins, peripheral arteries, peripheral veins, abdominal arteries, abdominal veins, and vasculature of the male genitalia). The next chapter covers tumor vascularization and is a new addition. The next-to-last chapter, which accounts for one-fourth of the book, is devoted to extensive case histories that drive home principles discussed earlier in the book. The final chapter is a glossary.

The book is very well written. Information is presented clearly, and important points are often repeated, allowing the reader to build from one chapter to the next. The text—including printing, paper, figures, and tables—is of excellent quality, and the figures and tables clarify points made in the text. The only confusion I had with this book was the way the publisher laid out some of the pages with horizontal dividers. This caused me occasionally to skip to an incorrect paragraph. There are no major errors or omissions. On the contrary, this book is very comprehensive.

Vascular Diagnosis with Ultrasound: Clinical References with Case Studies certainly fills a need for a vascular ultrasound book that covers both body and neurologic applications; similar books are not as comprehensive as this one. Topics not usually covered in other books—but covered here—include cerebral veins, abdominal veins, vasculature of male genitalia, and tumor vascularization. This book is suitable for those in specialties such as radiology, internal medicine, neurology, and vascular surgery, and it serves its purpose well. It is reasonably priced, and I find that it would be a welcome addition to anyone's library.

Reviewed by Richard E. Rosenthal, DO

Karen Oppo, PhD
Edward Leen, MD
Wilson J. Angerson, PhD
Timothy G. Cooke, MD, FRCS
Colin S. McArdle, MD, FRCS

Index terms:
Hepatic arteries, US, 952.12983
Liver neoplasms, 761.32, 761.33
Portal vein, flow dynamics, 957.12983
Portal vein, US, 957.12983
Ultrasound (US), Doppler studies, 9*.12983[2]

Radiology 1998; 208:453–457

Abbreviations:
CV = coefficient of variation
DPI = Doppler perfusion index
SD = standard deviation

[1] From the University Department of Surgery (K.O., W.J.A., T.G.C., C.S.M.) and the Department of Radiology (E.L.), Royal Infirmary, Queen Elizabeth Bldg, 8-16 Alexandra Parade, G31 2ER Glasgow, Scotland. From the 1997 RSNA scientific assembly. Received October 29, 1997; revision requested January 20, 1998; revision received February 25; accepted April 3. Supported in part by the Scottish Home and Health Department. **Address reprint requests to** K.O.

[2] 9* Vascular system, location unspecified

Author contributions:
Guarantors of integrity of entire study, K.O., E.L.; study concepts, E.L., C.S.M.; study design, K.O., E.L.; definition of intellectual content, E.L., C.S.M.; literature research, K.O.; clinical studies, K.O., E.L.; data acquisition, K.O., E.L.; data analysis, K.O.; statistical analysis, K.O., W.J.A.; manuscript preparation, K.O., E.L.; manuscript editing, E.L., C.S.M.; manuscript review, W.J.A., T.G.C.

Doppler Perfusion Index: An Interobserver and Intraobserver Reproducibility Study[1]

PURPOSE: To assess the potential of Doppler perfusion index (DPI) measurement as a routine diagnostic tool in the detection of occult colorectal liver metastases.

MATERIALS AND METHODS: By using color Doppler ultrasound, two independent sonologists performed DPI measurements blindly in 20 patients aged 30–82 years; interobserver reproducibility was assessed. A second group of 20 patients aged 37–88 years were examined to assess the level of intraobserver reproducibility of DPI measurements attained by one sonologist. For each patient in this group, the DPI was measured three times in succession, and the variability between measurements was analyzed. Calculations of the intraclass correlation coefficient and the coefficient of variation (CV) were used to determine the levels of reproducibility. The data were also analyzed by using the Student paired *t* test, with significance established at *P* less than .05.

RESULTS: The interobserver CV and intraobserver CV were 20% and 16%, respectively. The two sonologists who examined the first group of patients agreed independently on the DPI status in 18 of 20 (90%) patients.

CONCLUSION: In this study, both the intraobserver reproducibility and the interobserver reproducibility of DPI measurements were clinically acceptable.

Colorectal cancer is the second most common cause of cancer-related death in the United States and in Western Europe (1). Less than 50% of patients undergoing apparently curative surgery for primary colorectal cancer will survive 5 years after the surgery; the majority die of disseminated disease within the first 2 years (2). It has been shown that up to 30% of these patients harbor occult liver metastases at the time of initial presentation (3). Despite continuing technologic improvements, current imaging modalities are limited in their ability to enable identification of these occult tumors, because there is a size threshold below which differentiation between normal and abnormal tissue is impossible.

In previous studies (4,5) in which we used color Doppler ultrasound (US), we showed that the Doppler perfusion index (DPI), the ratio of hepatic arterial blood flow to total liver blood flow, is abnormally elevated in the presence of overt or occult liver metastases. In a study (5) of 80 patients with colorectal cancer who underwent apparently curative surgery, 31 patients had a normal DPI, whereas 49 had an abnormal DPI. On the basis of 2-year follow-up data, Leen and colleagues (5) showed that 100% of patients with a normal DPI remained disease-free, while 75% of those with an abnormal DPI developed hepatic metastases. This technique would allow the administration of adjuvant chemotherapy on a selective basis, that is, those with an abnormally elevated DPI can be treated while those with a normal DPI can be spared inappropriate treatment and unnecessary morbidity. So far, the results described have been obtained by an experienced radiologist in a research environment. If the DPI technique is to be successfully implemented as a clinical diagnostic tool, its reproducibility has to be confirmed by other sonologists in a more realistic clinical setting.

We performed this study to assess the interobserver reproducibility and intraobserver reproducibility of DPI measurements and the potential of DPI measurement as a routine diagnostic tool in the detection of occult colorectal liver metastases.

MATERIALS AND METHODS

Operators

DPI measurements were performed by two sonologists: a dedicated radiologist (E.L.) with 10 years of experience in Doppler US who developed the DPI technique and a physicist (K.O.) who had no previous experience in Doppler US and no knowledge of abdominal anatomy and was specially trained in 5 months to measure the DPI.

Patient Groups

Approval from the hospital ethics committee to perform this study and informed consent from all subjects were obtained. Two subject groups were examined after they had fasted for 12 hours. The first group (10 men and 10 women; age range, 30–82 years) were examined to calculate the level of interobserver variability between two observers (E.L., K.O.) and consisted of eight patients with colorectal cancer, one with gastric cancer, one with esophageal cancer, two with breast cancer, four with hepatitis C, and four who did not have cancer and had been referred to the US clinic for routine abdominal examination. Obtaining DPI measurements can be very time-consuming (approximately 20 minutes), and because of the limited time available in the US clinics, for 2 months, one patient per clinic was recruited into this study. By using color Doppler US, hepatic arterial blood flow and portal venous blood flow were measured blindly in the 20 patients by two observers consecutively under the same conditions. Each patient was independently examined by one sonologist and then examined immediately afterward by the second sonologist.

The second group of subjects was examined to assess the intraobserver variability of DPI measurements performed by one sonologist (K.O.). This group of 20 patients (eight men and 12 women; age range, 37–88 years) consisted of six healthy control subjects, four patients with esophageal cancer, nine patients with colorectal cancer, and one patient with gastric cancer. Twelve patients with cancer had apparently disease-free livers, and two had overt liver metastases. This subject group was recruited to test the DPI technique for the entire range of possible blood velocities and blood vessel cross-sectional areas. For each subject, the series of DPI blood flow measurements was performed three times in succession; between each measurement, the US probe was removed from the patient, and the vessel was relocated.

For both groups, the only strict inclusion criteria were that the common hepatic artery could be visualized at sonography and that it arose from the celiac axis. At no time during this study did a subject present with altered arterial anatomy, such as a hepatic artery that arose from the superior mesenteric artery. Doppler flow measurements could not be completed in two subjects because of the appearance of abdominal gas; these subjects were therefore not included in this study.

DPI Measurement Technique

Blood flow measurements were performed in all subjects by using an ATL 3000 scanner (Advanced Technology Limited, Seattle, Wash) with color Doppler US functions and a 3.5-MHz curvilinear probe. All subjects were examined while in the supine position.

A transverse scan was obtained at the epigastrium to locate the common hepatic artery on its longitudinal axis. The Doppler cursor was placed over the lumen of the artery, as near to the origin as possible, at the point where the artery first becomes horizontally straight. The Doppler sample volume and the beam angle were adjusted, and the time-averaged velocity was calculated over four cardiac cycles. The cross-sectional area of the artery was measured at the same point where the velocity was measured, at right angles to the vessel during the systolic phase of the cardiac cycle. The cross-sectional area of the vessel was measured by mapping the perimeter of the vessel lumen with the "tracker ball." The arterial flow was measured in the common hepatic artery instead of in the hepatic artery proper to standardize for all anatomic configurations and thereby improve the reproducibility of the measurements.

In subjects with normal arterial anatomy, the common hepatic artery becomes the hepatic artery proper after the right gastric artery branch. Unfortunately, the right gastric artery is rarely visualized on US images; therefore, it is difficult to ensure accurate flow measurements from the hepatic artery proper. The fasting of all subjects before Doppler US examination ensured that blood flow through the right gastric and gastroduodenal arteries was minimized.

For the portal vein, the time-averaged velocity was measured while viewing the vessel on its longitudinal axis with a right lateral intercostal approach to achieve a more acute angle for Doppler measurement. Care was taken to ensure that the velocity was measured at the point where the portal vein becomes intrahepatic and before it branches into the left and right portal trunks. The cross-sectional area of the portal vein was measured by using a right subcostal approach, with the patient in suspended inspiration for optimal visualization. The cross-sectional area was calculated automatically by mapping the perimeter of the vessel lumen.

All velocity measurements were performed while the subject held his or her breath to allow optimal visualization of the vessels and to eliminate the abdominal pressure changes that affect portal flow. Each measurement was performed repeatedly until the most satisfactory spectral patterns were attained; that is, no spectral broadening or aliasing was seen. Doppler evaluation of both the hepatic artery and the portal vein was adequate in all subjects. The mean of the three values obtained for the time-averaged velocity and cross-sectional area in each vessel was calculated. Blood flow was calculated as the product of the time-averaged velocity in and the cross-sectional area of the vessel. The DPI was calculated as the ratio of the hepatic arterial flow to the sum of the hepatic arterial and portal venous blood flows. On the basis of previous results (4) in patients with overt liver metastases and in healthy control subjects, a DPI value of 0.30 or greater was abnormal.

Data Analysis

Interobserver bias for all measured and calculated variables was assessed by using the Student paired *t* test. Significance was established at *P* less than .05.

Interobserver reproducibility and intraobserver reproducibility were quantified by using the intraclass correlation coefficient R_i (6,7). This statistic overcomes a major drawback of the conventional Pearson product-moment correlation coefficient, which is a measure of linear association rather than of agreement. A high product-moment correlation coefficient does not necessarily imply close agreement; for example, there may be a consistent additive or multiplicative bias between the observers. In contrast, the R_i is a true index of agreement between observers' measurements. The following criteria for clinically relevant agreement were used: poor, R_i less than .40; fair, R_i greater than or equal to .40 but less than or equal to .59; good, R_i greater than or equal to

TABLE 1
Blood Flow Parameters Measured by Two Sonologists

Parameter	Observer 1	Observer 2
Hepatic artery		
Cross-sectional area (cm^2)	0.22 ± 0.10	0.25 ± 0.13
Time-averaged mean velocity (cm/sec)	26.3 ± 8.9	24.3 ± 10.4
Blood flow (mL/min)	361 ± 267	367 ± 254
Beam angle (degrees)	58.1 ± 8.0	58.1 ± 8.7
Portal vein		
Cross-sectional area (cm^2)	1.24 ± 0.30	1.36 ± 0.30
Time-averaged mean velocity (cm/sec)	13.7 ± 5.0	13.1 ± 4.4
Blood flow (mL/min)	1,005 ± 407	1,052 ± 403
Beam angle (degrees)	44.1 ± 18.3	46.0 ± 11.7
Total liver blood flow (mL/min)	1,367 ± 520	1,419 ± 476
DPI	0.26 ± 0.12	0.25 ± 0.12

Note.—All data are given as the mean ± SD.

TABLE 2
Intraclass Correlation Coefficients for Doppler Measurements

Parameter	Interobserver R_i	Intraobserver R_i
Hepatic artery		
Cross-sectional area*	.83	.55
Time-averaged mean velocity†	.49	.67
Blood flow‡	.85	.89
Portal vein		
Cross-sectional area*	.53	.90
Time-averaged mean velocity†	.65	.50
Blood flow‡	.39	.72
Total liver blood flow‡	.44	.74
DPI	.86	.88

Note.—Poor = $R_i < .40$, fair = $.40 \le R_i \le .59$, good = $.60 \le R_i \le .74$, and excellent = $R_i \ge .75$.
* In square centimeters.
† In centimeters per second.
‡ In milliliters per minute.

.60 but less than or equal to .74; and excellent, R_i greater than or equal to .75. The R_i is derived from a two-way analysis of variance, with observers and subjects as factors. The formula used to calculate the R_i was (MSS − MSE)/MSS + (k − 1) MSE + k/n(MSO − MSE), where MSS is the mean squared variation between subjects; MSO, the mean squared variation between observers (or repeated measurements); MSE, the residual mean squared; k, the number of observations; and n, the number of subjects.

Both the interobserver variability and the intraobserver variability were quantified also, by using the coefficient of variation (CV): 100% × standard deviation (SD)/mean.

To further assess the clinical importance of the differences between the two observers' DPI measurements, the parameter of primary clinical interest, the method proposed by Bland and Altman (8), was used. The difference between the two measurements was plotted against their mean for the entire patient population. The mean difference d was the bias, and the SD of the differences s enabled us to calculate the maximum difference that was likely to arise between the two observers. The limits of agreement were calculated as $d - 2s$ and $d + 2s$, and 95% of the differences were expected to lie between these limits.

RESULTS

Cross-sectional Area

There was no significant difference between the values obtained by the two observers for the cross-sectional area of the common hepatic artery (P = .06) and that of the portal vein (P = .08) (Table 1).

The level of interobserver reproducibility was fair for portal venous area measurements and excellent for hepatic arterial area measurements (Table 2). In contrast, the level of intraobserver reproducibility was fair for hepatic arterial measurements and excellent for portal venous measurements (Table 2).

The interobserver CV was approximately the same for both the common hepatic artery (17%) and the portal vein (18%) (Table 3). The intraobserver CV was 11% and 9% for the hepatic artery and the portal vein, respectively.

Time-averaged Velocity

There was no significant difference between the values obtained by the two observers for time-averaged velocity in both the common hepatic artery (P = .37) and the portal vein (P = .52) (Table 1).

The level of interobserver reproducibility was fair for hepatic arterial time-averaged velocity measurements and good for portal venous time-averaged velocity measurements (Table 2). The level of intraobserver reproducibility was good for hepatic arterial measurements and fair for portal venous measurements (Table 2).

The interobserver CV was higher in the common hepatic artery (30%) than in the portal vein (21%), whereas the intraobserver CV was 16% in both the hepatic artery and the portal vein (Table 3).

Beam Angle

For common hepatic arterial time-averaged velocity measurements, the angle of insonation was 40°–68°, and analysis showed there was no significant difference in the overall beam angle used by the two observers (P = .99) (Table 1). For portal venous time-averaged velocity measurements, the angle of insonation was 28°–60°; there was also no significant difference in the overall beam angle (P = .67) (Table 1).

Blood Flow

There was no significant difference between the blood flow measurements obtained by the two observers in both the common hepatic artery (P = .86) and the portal vein (P = .65) (Table 1).

The level of interobserver reproducibility was excellent for blood flow measurements in the hepatic artery but poor for blood flow measurements in the portal vein (Table 2). In contrast, the level of intraobserver reproducibility was excellent for both hepatic arterial and portal venous blood flow measurements.

The interobserver CV for blood flow measurements was comparable to the interobserver CV for time-averaged velocity measurements; the interobserver CV for blood flow measurements was 28% and 33% for the common hepatic artery and the portal vein, respectively (Table 3). The intraobserver CV for blood flow measurements was calculated to be 17% and 20% for the hepatic artery and the portal vein, respectively.

Doppler Perfusion Index

There was no significant difference in the overall DPI values obtained by the two observers (P = .60) (Table 1). The levels of interobserver reproducibility and intraobserver reproducibility were excellent (Table 2). The interobserver CV and

TABLE 3
Coefficients of Variation for Doppler Measurements

Parameter	Inter-observer Variability (%)	Intra-observer Variability (%)
Hepatic artery		
Cross-sectional area*	17	11
Time-averaged mean velocity†	30	16
Blood flow‡	28	17
Portal vein		
Cross-sectional area*	18	9
Time-averaged mean velocity†	21	16
Blood flow‡	33	20
Total liver blood flow	30	16
DPI	20	16

* In square centimeters.
† In centimeters per second.
‡ In milliliters per minute.

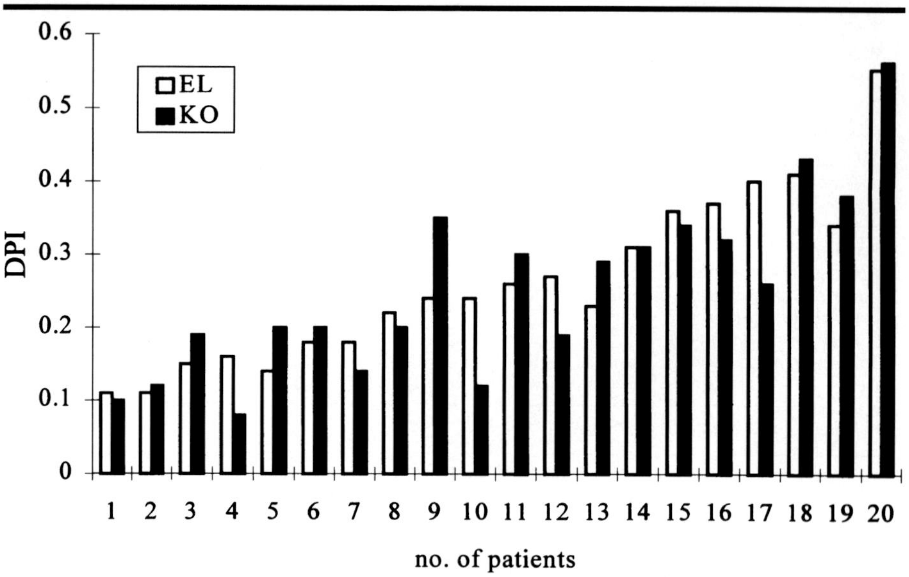

Figure 1. DPI measurements recorded for 20 patients by two independent sonologists.

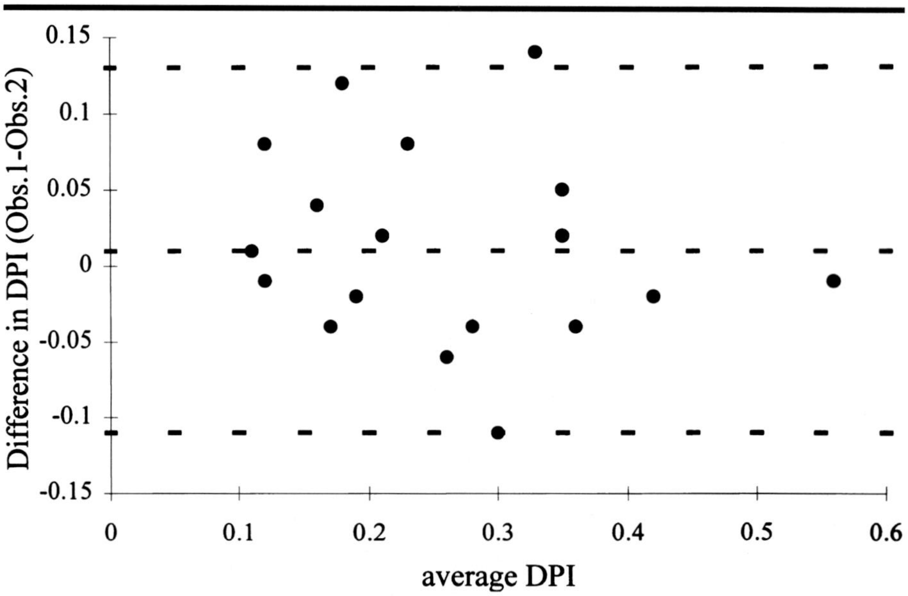

Figure 2. Bland-Altman plot for the difference in DPI measurements obtained by two sonologists. ● = difference in DPI measurements (the value obtained by observer 1 [E.L.] minus the value obtained by observer 2 [K.O.]). The middle dotted line is the mean difference in DPI measurements between the two observers. The upper and lower dotted lines are ± 2 SDs. *Obs.* = observer.

intraobserver CV for the DPI were 20% and 16%, respectively (Table 3).

The actual DPI values obtained by the two observers for each patient in the first group are shown in Figure 1, which illustrates the absolute variation in DPI values between the two sonologists.

A Bland-Altman plot of the DPI values obtained by the two observers was made to further analyze the spread of differences obtained (Fig 2). The mean difference ± SD was 0.01 ± 0.06, giving limits of agreement of −0.11 and 0.13. Although the mean difference was positive, indicating a slight tendency for observer 1 (E.L.) to have higher measurements than observer 2 (K.O.), this bias was not significant.

DISCUSSION

It is well known that velocity and area measurements obtained by using Doppler US are subject to systematic and random errors. Systematic errors such as those caused by observer variability and machine calibration can be minimized; however, random errors pose a more difficult problem. For the hepatic artery and the portal vein, measurement during respiratory suspension is required for optimal acquisition of the Doppler spectral waveform, which requires good patient cooperation. Our patient population tends to be elderly, and they often have a limited capacity to cooperate. This may lead to compromise, with measurements taken while the patient is breathing shallowly. However, during this study all subjects cooperated adequately.

In this study, the cross-sectional areas of the vessels were measured by mapping the perimeter of the vessel with the tracker ball; the area was automatically calculated by the US scanner onboard computer software. It has been shown previously (9) that a 1-mm uncertainty in the diameter of a 10-mm blood vessel can lead to a 20% error in the area measurement. The interobserver reproducibility of cross-sectional area measurements was excellent for the hepatic artery; this is because this vessel is smaller, and thus it is easier to obtain a cross section truly perpendicular to its longitudinal axis. In contrast, the portal vein—even its intrahepatic portion—is much larger and elliptical; thus, it may be difficult to obtain a cross section truly perpendicular to its longitudinal axis because of the ribs or costal cartilage overlying the region. In this instance, discrimination between the echogenic wall and the anechoic lumen may not be as clear-cut. Therefore, care must be taken in placing the cursors around the vessel lumen. This may explain the fair level of interobserver reproducibility of cross-sectional area measurements in the portal vein. The R_i and CV values obtained in this study are, however, comparable to those obtained in studies (10,11) in which the reproducibility of portal venous flow measurements has been investigated.

In velocity measurements, differences in insonation angle and position along the vessel may lead to errors and variability in the values obtained. For the common hepatic artery, the interobserver reproducibility was fair; this may be because this vessel is more tortuous and tapers distally. It is well known that velocities measured at different points along the artery will be different. Velocity measurements are therefore unlikely to be comparable unless both observers measure at exactly the same point. To standardize the technique and minimize such systematic errors, both of the observers made every attempt to measure the velocity as close as possible to the artery's origin from the celiac axis, where the arterial segment is straightest. However, that segment is also usually perpendicular to the ultrasound beam axis, which makes it difficult to obtain a more acute angle for accurate Doppler US measurements, especially when a relatively large curvilinear probe is used.

Angulation is not much of a problem in the portal vein, because an acute insonation angle is achievable when the vessel is viewed in the right intercostal position. However, care had to be taken to ensure that the main portal trunk—not the right portal branch—was sampled, and the measurements were taken during suspended expiration because of flow variation during respiration. In addition, the portal vein is much straighter than the hepatic artery. The interobserver reproducibility of time-averaged velocity measurements in the portal vein was, as expected, good. Again, the R_i and CV values we obtained are comparable to those obtained in similar reproducibility studies (11,12).

Although the hepatic arterial time-averaged velocity and portal venous cross-sectional area measurements had fair interobserver reproducibility, this was balanced to some degree by the excellent and good interobserver reproducibility of hepatic arterial cross-sectional area and portal venous velocity measurements, respectively. The interobserver reproducibility of hepatic arterial blood flow measurements was excellent, but that of portal venous blood flow measurements was poor. This is explained solely by the two observers' difficulty in measuring the portal venous cross-sectional area in the same way.

After analyzing the liver blood flow measurements, the two sonologists independently assigned each patient a DPI status. Although the DPI technique has been used primarily to detect the presence of occult colorectal liver metastases, it also has been shown to be sensitive in the detection of liver metastases arising from other primary carcinomas (13). The actual DPI values obtained by the two observers for each patient are shown in Figure 1. Although there appears to be a large variation between the actual DPI values obtained in several patients, the majority of patients were assigned the same DPI status by both sonologists (normal, <0.30; abnormal, ≥ 0.30). Among 20 patients, the interobserver variation was clinically important in two, patients 9 and 17, who were assigned a different DPI status. Patient 9 did not have cancer and was referred for US to check for renal failure, and patient 17 had colorectal cancer.

For this study, 0.30 was the cutoff point between normal and abnormal liver blood flow. In reality, there will be a diagnostic gray area of 0.25–0.35 owing to intraobserver variability, and patients with DPI values in this range should undergo repeat scanning on a different day to confirm their DPI status. Patients 9 and 17 both had one DPI value in this area of uncertainty.

Overall, the intraobserver reproducibility and interobserver reproducibility of the DPI technique were excellent. Ninety percent of the patients examined were given the same DPI status by both observers independently. This is in keeping with the use of a standardized technique in which systematic errors are minimized. The DPI may therefore be used clinically as a diagnostic tool in the early detection of colorectal liver metastases. The excellent level of intraobserver reproducibility also means that the DPI can be used in postoperative follow-up examinations.

The differences in the expertise and scientific backgrounds of the two observers might have been another source of degradation in the overall level of reproducibility that was achievable. The first observer (E.L.) is a consultant radiologist who has more than 10 years of Doppler US experience and first developed the DPI technique, whereas the second observer (K.O.) is a physicist who has had 5 months of specialized training in DPI measurement and no previous Doppler US scanning experience or knowledge of abdominal anatomy. Despite the differences in experience and expertise between the two observers in this study, the interobserver reproducibility of DPI measurements was clinically acceptable, which suggests that any dedicated sonologist, if specially trained, can perform this standardized technique.

It has been reported (7) that the reproducibility of Doppler flow measurements is only deemed acceptable within the clinical context when R_i is equal to or greater than .60 (7). Taking this viewpoint into account, both the interobserver reproducibility and the intraobserver reproducibility of the DPI technique in this study were clinically acceptable (R_i = .86 and .88, respectively).

References

1. O'Brien M. Cancer of the colon and rectum: current concepts of aetiology and pathogenesis. Br J Med Sci 1988; 157:5–15.
2. Slaney G. Results of treatment of carcinoma of the colon and rectum. In: Irvine WT, ed. Modern trends in surgery. 3rd ed. London, England: Butterworths, 1971; 69–89.
3. Finlay IG, McArdle CS. Occult hepatic metastases in colorectal carcinoma. Br J Surg 1986; 73:732–735.
4. Leen E, Goldberg JA, Robertson J, et al. Early detection of "occult" colorectal liver metastases using duplex/colour Doppler sonography. Br J Surg 1993; 80:1249–1251.
5. Leen E, Angerson WJ, Moule B, Cooke TG, McArdle CS. Prognostic power of Doppler perfusion index in colorectal cancer: correlation with survival. Ann Surg 1996; 223:199–203.
6. Bartko JJ, Carpenter WT. On the methods and theory of reliability. J Nerv Ment Dis 1976; 163:307–317.
7. Cichetti DV, Sparrow SS. Developing criteria for establishing interrater reliability of specific items: application to assessment of adaptive behaviour. Am J Ment Deficiency 1981; 86:127–137.
8. Bland JM, Altman DG. Statistical methods for assessing agreement between two methods of clinical measurement. Lancet 1986; 8:307–310.
9. Burns PN, Jaffe CC. Quantitative flow measurements with Doppler ultrasound: techniques, accuracy and limitations. Radiol Clin North Am 1985; 23:641–657.
10. Iwao T, Toyanaga A, Shigemori H, et al. Echo-Doppler measurements of portal vein and superior mesenteric artery blood flow in humans: inter- and intra-observer short term reproducibility. J Gastroenterol Hepatol 1996; 11:40–46.
11. Sabba C, Weltin GG, Cichetti DV, et al. Observer variability in echo-Doppler measurements of portal flow in cirrhotic patients and healthy volunteers. Gastroenterology 1990; 98:1603–1611.
12. de Vries PJ, van Huttum J, Hoekstra JBL, de Hooge P. Duplex Doppler measurements of portal venous flow in normal subjects: intra- and inter-observer variability. J Hepatol 1991; 13:358–363.
13. Leen E, Goldberg JA, Robertson J, et al. Detection of hepatic metastases using duplex/colour Doppler sonography. Ann Surg 1991; 214:599–604.

Paraovarian Cystadenomas and Cystadenofibromas: Sonographic Characteristics in 14 Cases[1]

Craig D. Korbin, MD
Douglas L. Brown, MD
William R. Welch, MD

Index terms:
Ovary, cysts, 852.3111, 852.3113, 852.315, 852.3172
Ovary, neoplasms, 852.3111, 852.3119, 852.315, 852.3172
Ovary, US, 852.12984, 852.12989
Pelvic organs, neoplasms, 852.3111, 852.3119, 852.31179, 852.3172, 85.318
Pelvic organs, US, 85.1298, 852.1298, 852.12981

Radiology 1998; 208:459–462

[1] From the Departments of Radiology (C.D.K., D.L.B.) and Pathology (W.R.W.), Brigham and Women's Hospital, Harvard Medical School, 75 Francis St, Boston, MA 02115. From the 1997 RSNA scientific assembly. Received October 28, 1997; revision requested January 6, 1998; revision received February 27; accepted April 10. **Address reprint requests to** D.L.B.

Author contributions:
Guarantors of integrity of entire study, C.D.K., D.L.B.; study concepts, C.D.K., D.L.B.; study design, C.D.K., D.L.B., W.R.W.; definition of intellectual content, C.D.K., D.L.B.; literature research, D.L.B.; data acquisition and analysis, C.D.K., D.L.B., W.R.W.; statistical analysis, C.D.K., D.L.B.; manuscript preparation, C.D.K., D.L.B.; manuscript editing and review, C.D.K., D.L.B., W.R.W.

PURPOSE: To describe the sonographic features of paraovarian cystadenomas.

MATERIALS AND METHODS: We searched the computerized pathology and radiology databases for cases of histopathologically proved paraovarian cystadenomas from January 1993 through December 1996 in which preoperative sonography had also been performed. Fourteen paraovarian cystadenomas or cystadenofibromas were identified in 14 patients aged 20–57 years. Sonographic and pathologic findings were correlated.

RESULTS: Three of the masses appeared as simple cysts sonographically. Of the remaining 11 masses, nine had solid nodular areas within the cyst; three had septations; and four had a thick wall, an irregular wall, or both at sonography. At sonography, four masses were thought to arise outside the ovary, four were erroneously thought to arise in the ovary, and the location was uncertain in six.

CONCLUSION: Paraovarian cystadenomas are cystic masses that usually contain one or more small solid nodules and occasionally contain septations.

The majority of paraovarian cysts appear as simple cysts at sonography (1–5); the diagnosis is generally straightforward if one recognizes their paraovarian location. It is unusual, however, to identify a paraovarian cyst that contains a solid nodular component. When one encounters an ovarian cystic mass with a solid nodular component, neoplasm is generally a strong consideration, but interpretation of an extraovarian adnexal cyst that contains a solid nodule may be problematic. Having encountered a few such cases that were proved to be paraovarian cystadenomas, we sought to describe the sonographic characteristics of these cystic masses.

MATERIALS AND METHODS

We searched the computerized pathology and radiology databases for histopathologically proved paraovarian cystadenomas or cystadenofibromas from January 1993 through December 1996 in which preoperative sonography had been performed. We first searched the pathology database for adnexal cystadenomas or cystadenofibromas.

The diagnosis of a cystadenoma was based on the histologic finding of a müllerian epithelial lining of the cyst wall, and the organization of the database was such that we were likely to primarily identify masses with a serous (ciliated) epithelial lining. Variable amounts of fibrous tissue may have also been present in the cyst wall, and when a substantial fibrous component was present (determined on the basis of subjective assessment), cystadenofibroma was diagnosed.

The surgical notes and pathologic findings were then reviewed to identify those masses that arose in a paraovarian location, thus excluding ovarian cystadenomas or cystadenofibromas.

The radiology database was then checked to identify those patients who had undergone preoperative sonography. We identified 14 cases of paraovarian cystadenoma or cystadenofibroma in which preoperative sonography had been performed. Fourteen patients aged 20–57 years (average age ± standard deviation, 39.1 years ± 10.9) were identified. The indications for sonography were pain (n = 7), a palpable adnexal mass (n = 2), suspected fibroids (n = 2), follow-up of a mass seen on a sonogram obtained at another facility (n = 1), infertility (n = 1), and a family history of ovarian cancer (n = 1).

All of the sonograms had been obtained, interpreted, or both, by physicians with 5 or more years of experience in gynecologic sonography. On the basis of the demographic data, original reports, and review of the images, several features were assessed: mass size (average of the largest diameter and the two orthogonal diameters), scanning method (ie, transvaginal, transabdominal, or both), and several gray-scale sonographic findings. If Doppler sonographic evaluation had been performed, those results were recorded also.

The sonographic findings included both the location of the mass relative to the ovary and the features of the mass itself. The sonographic location in reference to the ovary was recorded as "extraovarian," "intraovarian," or "uncertain." The location was recorded as extraovarian or intraovarian if it was stated as such in the original report or if the recorded images demonstrated such a location but the original report did not. The location was recorded as uncertain when it was stated as such in the original report or when the report did not specify the location and the location could not be determined from review of the images.

The sonographic findings of the mass that were evaluated were the presence or absence of the following: a simple cyst (ie, an anechoic cyst with a smooth, thin wall and distal acoustic enhancement), septations, a focal solid component (without septations), a diffusely thick wall (greater than 2 mm), or an irregular wall (considered present when the inner wall of the cyst was not smooth but was not frankly nodular). The sonographic findings were correlated with the pathologic findings.

RESULTS

All of the masses were benign, and none was complicated by torsion, rupture, or internal hemorrhage. The histopathologic diagnosis was serous cystadenoma in six cases and serous cystadenofibroma in eight cases (including one in which the solid nodule, which was a papillary adenofibroma, had been separated from the cystic portion of the mass during surgery).

Transvaginal sonography alone had been performed in five, transabdominal sonography alone had been performed in two, and both had been performed in seven patients. The mass size was 2.0–9.7 cm (average size ± standard deviation, 4.9 cm ± 2.3). At sonography, four masses were thought to arise outside the ovary, four were erroneously thought to arise in the ovary, and six had a location that was uncertain.

Sonographically, all of the masses were predominantly cystic. Three of the masses appeared to be simple cysts, and the remaining eleven appeared to be complex; that is, they had a solid component (Fig 1), wall thickening (Fig 2), an irregular wall (Fig 3), or septations (Fig 4). In nine (64%) of the 14 masses, one or more small (<1-cm) solid nodules were identified by using sonography; a single nodule was present in seven of the nine masses. At sonography, septations were seen in three cases, the wall was irregular in three cases, and the wall was thick in one case.

The nine nodules seen at sonography were confirmed with pathologic inspection. Of the five masses in which no nodularity was seen on the sonogram, three were simple cysts at sonography. Of these three masses, two had no nodularity at pathologic examination, although one had a smooth, focal area of wall thickening and one had a trabecular inner surface. A small nodule was present at pathologic examination in the third simple-appearing cyst, but it was missed at sonography. Review of the images in this case suggested that the mass was far away from the transvaginal transducer and was not optimally imaged.

Of the other two masses in which no nodularity was seen on the sonogram, one had an irregular wall at sonography and tiny (1-mm) nodules at pathologic examination. The other mass had several septations at sonography; two small (3-mm) nodular areas were present at pathologic examination but had not been seen sonographically. This mass had a mean diameter of 8 cm, it was not fully imaged at transvaginal scanning, and the nodules were not seen at transabdominal scanning. Hence, at pathologic examination, 12 (86%) of the 14 masses had a solid nodular component. Septations were confirmed pathologically in the three cases in which they had been seen sonographically.

Because Doppler sonographic evaluation had been performed in only three cases, we cannot reliably assess Doppler sonographic findings in paraovarian cystadenomas. In all three cases, the only recorded waveforms were very peripheral in the mass and appeared to be within the wall. Each mass had relatively high-resistance arterial flow; the lowest resistive indexes for each mass were 0.75, 0.82, and 0.88.

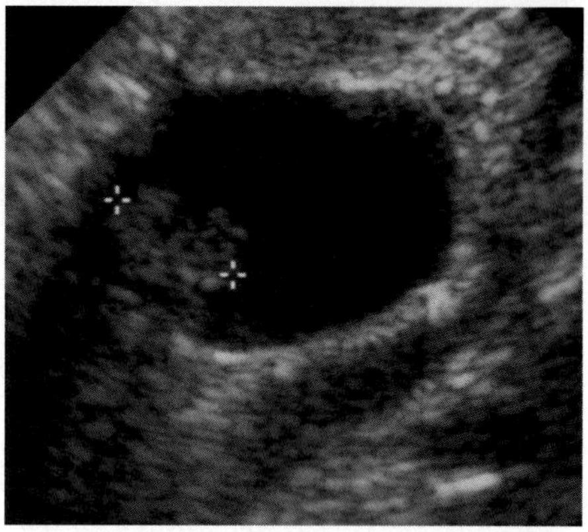

Figure 1. Transvaginal sonogram of a paraovarian serous cystadenofibroma. The cystic mass contains a small, nodular solid component (cursors).

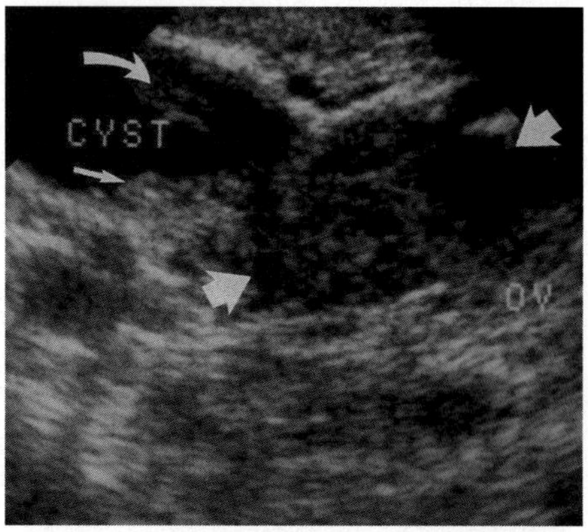

Figure 2. Transvaginal sonogram of a paraovarian serous cystadenofibroma. The cystic mass has focal wall thickening (small straight arrow). This image demonstrates that the mass (large straight arrows) is located outside the ipsilateral ovary (*ov*); the upper large straight arrow points to a normal follicle. In this image, it was uncertain whether the area indicated by the curved arrow was a true nodule or just a reverberation artifact; however, a distinct true nodule was seen along the far wall of the cystic mass on other images.

DISCUSSION

Paraovarian cysts are occasional findings both at surgery and at sonography. Larger paraovarian cysts may cause pelvic pain

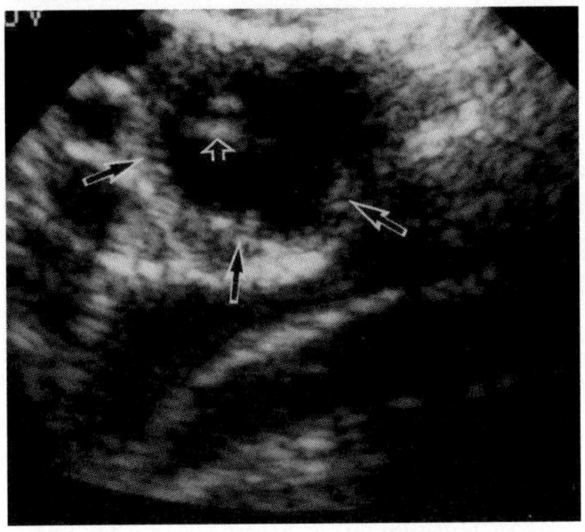

Figure 3. Transvaginal sonogram of a paraovarian cystadenoma. This cystic mass, incorrectly reported as arising from the ovary, has an irregular wall (solid arrows). Small distinct nodules were seen elsewhere in the mass on other images. The two short echogenic lines (open arrow) were thought to represent a reverberation artifact.

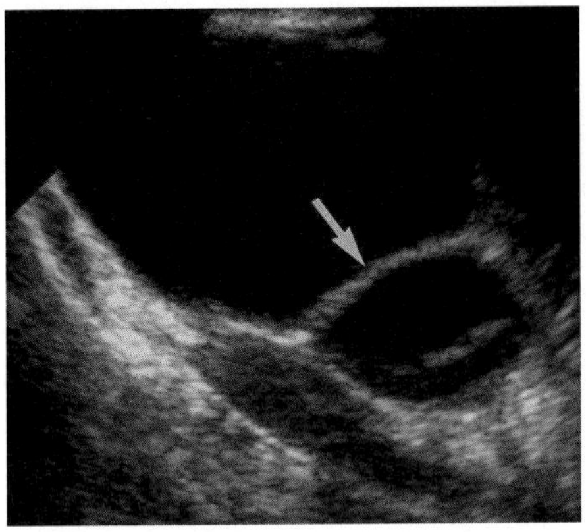

Figure 4. Transvaginal sonogram of a paraovarian cystadenoma. This cystadenoma contained a septation (arrow), but no wall thickening or nodularity was evident.

(2,4), but many paraovarian cysts are small and are incidental findings. Internal hemorrhage, torsion, or rupture of paraovarian cysts occurs rarely (2,4,5). Cystadenomas of paraovarian origin, however, are uncommon, and their cause is unknown (6). Malignancy has been reported in 2%–3% of paraovarian cystic masses studied by using histopathology (6,7), but it seems to be even less frequent in masses smaller than 5 cm (8). Paraovarian cystadenomas are typically unilateral (9) and have one or more small nodules along an otherwise smooth inner wall (6,7). In a few instances, paraovarian cystadenomas have been associated with von Hippel-Lindau disease (10,11).

Paraovarian cysts have been previously described in the imaging literature (1–4,12), and the majority are simple cysts at sonography. As opposed to most of these previously described paraovarian cysts, which have a thin, smooth inner wall (1–4,12), paraovarian cystadenomas tend to have a small nodular component along the wall. Paraovarian cystadenomas, however, are an infrequent finding in sonographic series of paraovarian cysts (2,3,5), and the specific sonographic appearance of paraovarian cystadenomas has received little attention. Misdiagnosis is likely if one is unaware of the entity of paraovarian cystadenomas and of their typical sonographic appearance and extraovarian location. While an adnexal cystic mass that contains a nodule, septation, or thick wall and that is recognized as paraovarian will probably still be removed surgically, the concern for malignancy is likely to be lower than that in a similar-appearing mass of ovarian origin, perhaps allowing for less invasive surgery.

Variable success in recognizing the extraovarian location of paraovarian cysts at sonography has been reported (1,3,5). The extraovarian location of the cystic masses in this study was correctly recognized in only four cases. The reason for the erroneous report of an intraovarian location in four other cases in this retrospective study is uncertain. It may have been due to a true difficulty in determining the location of the mass or because the mass was reported as ovarian on the basis of a presumption that an adnexal cyst is most likely to be ovarian.

Uncertainty as to whether the mass is ovarian or extraovarian is likely to occur when the ipsilateral ovary is not seen, which is probably more likely when the cyst is large. It may also be difficult to determine the origin of a mass that is at the extreme periphery of the ovary. Recognition that an adnexal mass is extraovarian is probably more likely if one actively attempts to distinguish an ovarian origin from an extraovarian origin. Applying gentle pressure, either with the hand on the abdominal wall or with the transvaginal transducer, may help to separate the mass from the ovary and thereby help to confirm an extraovarian location (3,4). We speculate that transvaginal scanning, alone or in combination with transabdominal scanning, generally might be more helpful than transabdominal scanning alone in identifying the extraovarian location of paraovarian cystadenomas. Transvaginal scanning also might be more reliable than transabdominal scanning in identifying small intracystic nodules.

As opposed to most paraovarian cysts, which are simple cysts at sonography, the majority of paraovarian cystadenomas in our series had nodular areas within them, and a minority had septations. Pathologic findings showed that 12 (86%) of the 14 masses had nodularity. In a few cases, the nodules were not seen sonographically, because they were tiny or the mass was not optimally imaged. Therefore, a paraovarian cystadenoma should be a consideration when one encounters an extraovarian cystic mass with a single small nodule or septation or, occasionally, several small nodules or septations.

Most other extraovarian masses are unlikely to be confused with paraovarian cystadenomas at sonography. A hydrosalpinx may appear as an extraovarian cystic mass, but it is more likely to have a tubular shape and often has a folded configuration or short echogenic lines protruding into the lumen (13). Pedunculated fibroids are generally solid, but even those with cystic degeneration usually do not contain as large an anechoic component as do most paraovarian cystadenomas. An extraovarian mass is also a key feature in diagnosing tubal pregnancy (14), but the clinical setting (eg, a positive pregnancy test result) is generally different, and again, the mass usually does not contain as large an anechoic component as do most paraovarian cystadenomas. Peritoneal inclusion cysts tend to surround much of the ovary and usually occur in women with a history of prior surgery or pelvic inflammatory disease (15). Cystic neoplasms of the fallopian tube are rare and might be difficult to distinguish, but they generally seem to have more of a solid component (16) than do paraovarian cystadenomas. A paraovarian cyst containing a solid nodular area due to hemorrhage (2) might be most likely to appear to be similar to a paraovarian cystadenoma. A follow-up sonogram that shows resolution of the clot or the evolving appearance of the hemorrhage might be helpful in such cases. In addition, if a complex ovarian cystic mass were exophytic, it might be difficult to distinguish from a paraovarian cystadenoma.

In summary, the majority of paraovarian cystadenomas contain one or more small nodular areas and occasionally have septations or appear as simple cysts at sonography. The paraovarian location of these cysts was not often recognized in this retrospective series, but it is hoped that increased awareness of paraovarian cystadenomas will prompt more careful assessment of their potential paraovarian location and contribute to more accurate sonographic diagnosis.

References

1. Athey PA, Cooper NB. Sonographic features of parovarian cysts. AJR 1985; 144: 83–86.
2. Alpern MB, Sandler MA, Madrazo BL. Sonographic features of parovarian cysts and their complications. AJR 1984; 143:157–160.
3. Barloon TJ, Brown BP, Abu-Yousef MM, Warnock NG. Paraovarian and paratubal cysts: preoperative diagnosis using transabdominal and transvaginal sonography. JCU 1996; 24:117–122.
4. Grant EG. Benign conditions of the ovaries. In: Nyberg DA, Hill LM, Bohm-Velez M, Mendelson EB, eds. Transvaginal ultrasound. St Louis, Mo: Mosby–Year Book, 1992; 199.
5. Kim JS, Woo SK, Suh SJ, Morettin LB. Sonographic diagnosis of paraovarian cysts: value of detecting a separate ipsilateral ovary. AJR 1995; 164:1441–1444.
6. Honore L, O'Hare K. Serous papillary neoplasms arising in paramesonephric parovarian cysts. Acta Obstet Gynecol Scand 1980; 59:525–528.
7. Genadry R, Parmley T, Woodruff JD. The origin and clinical behavior of the parovarian tumor. Am J Obstet Gynecol 1977; 129:873–880.
8. Stein AL, Koonings PP, Schlaerth JB, Grimes DA, d'Ablaing G. Relative frequency of malignant parovarian tumors: should parovarian tumors be aspirated? Obstet Gynecol 1990; 75:1029–1031.
9. Aslani M, Ahn GH, Scully RE. Serous papillary cystadenoma of borderline malignancy of broad ligament: a report of 25 cases. Int J Gynecol Pathol 1988; 7:131–138.
10. Korn WT, Schatzki SC, DiSciullo AJ, Scully RE. Papillary cystadenoma of the broad ligament in von Hippel-Lindau disease. Am J Obstet Gynecol 1990; 163:596–598.
11. Funk KC, Heiken JP. Papillary cystadenoma of the broad ligament in a patient with von Hippel-Lindau disease. AJR 1989; 153:527–528.
12. Reuter KL, Meyer RN. Unusual features of parovarian cysts: a report of two cases. J Reprod Med 1987; 32:371–374.
13. Tessler FN, Perrella RR, Fleischer AC, Grant EG. Endovaginal sonographic diagnosis of dilated fallopian tubes. AJR 1989; 153: 523–525.
14. Brown DL, Doubilet PM. Transvaginal sonography for diagnosing ectopic pregnancy: positivity criteria and performance characteristics. J Ultrasound Med 1994; 13:259–266.
15. Kim JS, Lee HJ, Woo SK, Lee TS. Peritoneal inclusion cysts and their relationship to the ovaries: evaluation with sonography. Radiology 1997; 204:481–484.
16. Slanetz PJ, Whitman GJ, Halpern EF, Hall DA, McCarthy KA, Simeone JF. Imaging of fallopian tube tumors. AJR 1997; 169: 1321–1324.

Eric K. Outwater, MD
Evan S. Siegelman, MD
Peerapod Chiowanich, MD
Alex M. Kilger, RN
Charles J. Dunton, MD
Alexander Talerman, MD

Index term:
Endometriosis, 853.3192
Fallopian tubes, 853.2172
Fallopian tubes, abscess, 853.2173
Fallopian tubes, MR, 853.121411

Radiology 1998; 208:463–469

Abbreviation:
SE = spin echo

[1] From the Departments of Radiology (E.K.O., P.C.), Obstetrics and Gynecology (C.J.D.), and Pathology (A.T.), Thomas Jefferson University Hospital, 132 S 10th St, 1096 Main, Philadelphia, PA 19107-5244, and the Department of Radiology, University of Pennsylvania Medical Center, Philadelphia (E.S.S., A.M.K.). Received November 28, 1997; revision requested February 18, 1998; revision received March 19; accepted April 13. **Address reprint requests to** E.K.O.

Author contributions:
Guarantor of integrity of entire study, E.K.O.; study concepts and design, E.K.O.; definition of intellectual content, E.K.O.; literature research, E.K.O.; clinical studies, E.K.O., E.S.S., P.C.; experimental studies, E.K.O., C.J.D., A.T.; data acquisition, E.K.O., E.S.S., P.C., A.M.K.; data analysis, E.K.O.; statistical analysis, E.K.O.; manuscript preparation, E.K.O.; manuscript editing, E.K.O., E.S.S., C.J.D., A.T.; manuscript review, E.K.O., E.S.S., C.J.D., A.T.

Dilated Fallopian Tubes: MR Imaging Characteristics[1]

PURPOSE: To determine the magnetic resonance (MR) imaging characteristics of hydrosalpinx and the accuracy of MR imaging for distinguishing hydrosalpinx from other adnexal masses.

MATERIALS AND METHODS: Cross-referencing of pathologic records and MR studies from two institutions disclosed 41 study patients with surgically proved dilated fallopian tubes. A set of 38 patients with surgically evaluated adnexal masses, but no hydrosalpinx, were randomly chosen as control subjects. All MR examinations included T1-weighted spin-echo and T2-weighted fast spin-echo imaging in multiple planes with a phased-array multicoil. Two blinded readers scored each adnexa for the presence of a dilated fallopian tube or thickened tubal wall and mucosal folds and the signal intensity of the intratubal fluid. Blinded readings were compared with surgical findings of dilated fallopian tube, endometriosis, and salpingitis. Radiologic-pathologic correlation was performed with adnexal specimens imaged in vitro in three study patients.

RESULTS: On a per patient basis, the blinded readers correctly identified dilated fallopian tubes in 31 of 41 study patients and correctly excluded dilated tubes in a mean 34 of 38 control subjects. On T1-weighted images, hyperintense tubal fluid was significantly correlated with the presence of endometriosis in the pelvis at surgery ($P < .002$, χ^2).

CONCLUSION: MR imaging can depict most dilated fallopian tubes and differentiate them from other adnexal masses on the basis of morphologic features. On T1-weighted images, high signal intensity is correlated with the presence of endometriosis affecting the tube.

Dilated fallopian tubes are a common cause for an adnexal mass and a common component of complex adnexal masses, which may include tubo-ovarian abscesses, endometriomas, and neoplasms. Distinguishing dilated fallopian tubes from other adnexal masses is important in the differentiation of benign from malignant adnexal disease. Overall, magnetic resonance (MR) imaging is an accurate technique with which to distinguish benign from malignant adnexal masses and may be superior to transvaginal ultrasonography (US) (1,2).

To our knowledge, the MR imaging characteristics of dilated fallopian tubes have not been examined in systematic studies. Furthermore, the importance of the MR imaging features of dilated fallopian tubes, such as the signal intensity of the luminal contents, has not been evaluated. The purposes of this study were to assess the accuracy of blinded readers in the distinction of dilated fallopian tubes from other adnexal masses and to determine the relevance of signal intensity of the intraluminal contents.

MATERIALS AND METHODS

The MR imaging and surgical records from our institutions were cross-referenced from 1992 to 1997 for patients who underwent MR imaging examination and subsequent surgical exploration in the pelvis ($N = 352$ [studies obtained in patients enrolled in the Radiology Diagnostic Oncology Group study of adnexal masses had been excluded]). All patients with surgical proof of a dilated fallopian tube ($n = 41$) were selected as the study patients in this blinded reader study. Proof of the dilated fallopian tube relied on the gynecologic surgeon's

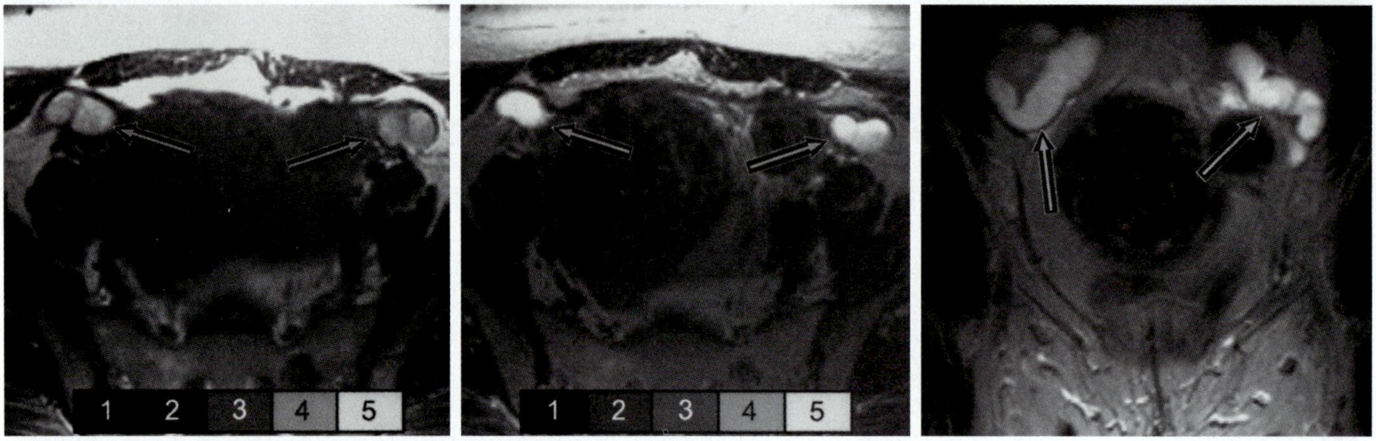

a. b. c.

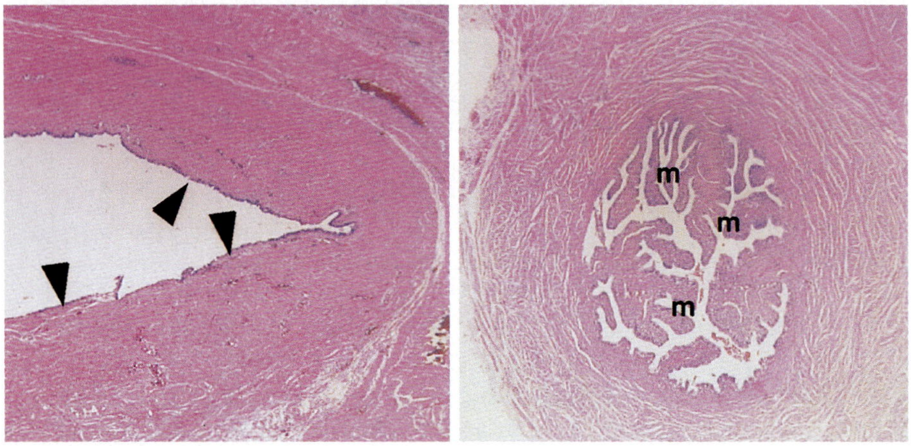

d. e.

Figure 1. Hydrosalpinx in a 50-year-old woman with endometriosis. **(a)** Axial T1-weighted image (550/16) and **(b)** axial T2-weighted fast SE image (3,600/119 [effective]) show bilateral hydrosalpinx (arrows). The gray scale shows the rating scale used by the blinded readers to rate signal intensity. **(c)** Coronal T2-weighted image (6,000/119 [effective]) depicts tubal morphology (arrows) most clearly. **(d)** Photomicrograph of histologic section from the left tube shows the effaced mucosa (arrowheads). (Hematoxylin-eosin stain; original magnification, ×40.) **(e)** Photomicrograph of histologic section from a normal tube allows comparison with normally infolded mucosa (*m*). (Hematoxylin-eosin stain; original magnification, ×40.)

impression as to whether the tube was abnormally dilated, rather than on measurements. Thirty-eight patients with adnexal mass(es) were randomly selected to serve as control subjects by using a random number generator. "Adnexal mass" was defined as any adnexal mass, including cysts greater than 2 cm in diameter. The clinical characteristics of the study patients and the control subjects are given in Table 1.

Clinical records, surgical reports, and pathologic records of the 79 patients were reviewed for the presence of dilated fallopian tubes, associated adnexal disease, presence of endometriosis in the pelvis, histologic evidence of chronic or acute salpingitis, and menopausal status.

MR Imaging Examinations

MR imaging examinations in the 79 patients were performed with 1.5-T magnet systems (GE Medical Systems, Milwaukee, Wis) and phased-array multicoils for

TABLE 1
Clinical and Pathologic Characteristics of 41 Study Patients with Surgically Proved Hydrosalpinx and 38 Control Subjects with Other Adnexal Pathologic Conditions

Characteristic	No. of Study Patients	No. of Control Subjects	*P* Value*
No.	41	38	NM
Age (y)†	43 ± 11	45 ± 15	.6266
Menopausal status			
Premenopausal	29	24	NM
Postmenopausal	6	11	.12
Hysterectomy	3	2	.71
Unknown	3	1	.34
No. of weeks to surgery†	7 ± 7	9 ± 11	.2273
Primary diagnosis‡			
Endometriosis	14	7	NM
Benign ovarian neoplasm	4	11	NM
Malignancy	2	5	NM
Cyst	3	4	NM
Uterine	2	8	NM
Other§	0	3	NM
Tubo-ovarian abscess	5	0	NM
Hydrosalpinx only	11	0	NM

* NM = comparison not made.
† Data are the mean ± standard deviation.
‡ Primary diagnosis is the postoperative diagnosis and indication for surgery.
§ Castleman disease, one patient; pseudocysts, two patients.

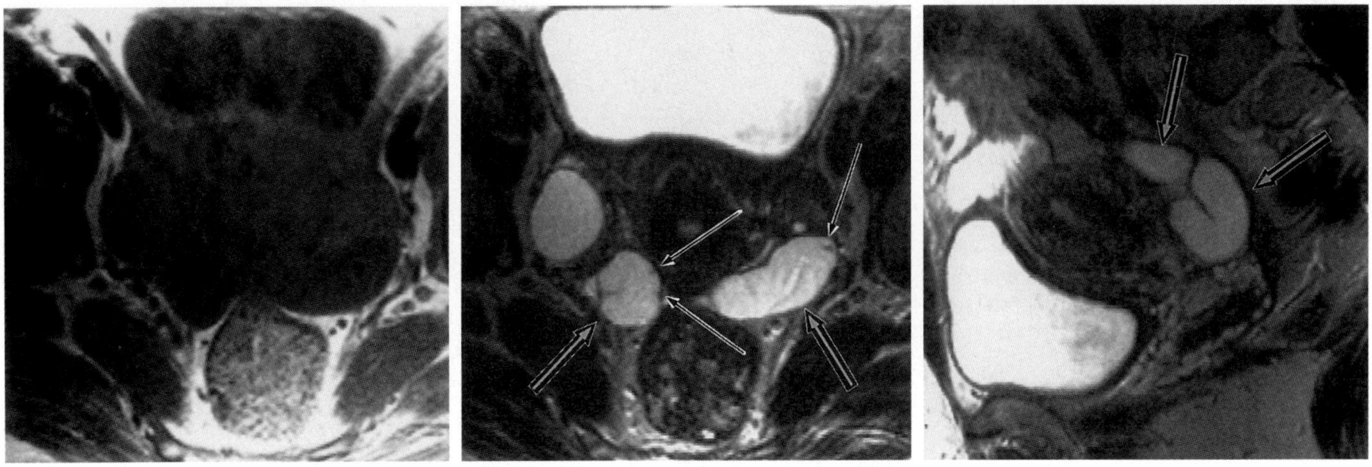

a. b. c.

Figure 2. Hydrosalpinx in a 49-year-old woman. **(a)** Axial T1-weighted image (800/16) and **(b)** axial T2-weighted fast SE image (3,983/119 [effective]) show bilateral hydrosalpinx (thick arrows in **b**). Thin mucosal plicae (thin arrows) are seen in both tubes. **(c)** Sagittal T2-weighted fast SE image (3,567/126 [effective]) shows tubal configuration of the right tube (arrows).

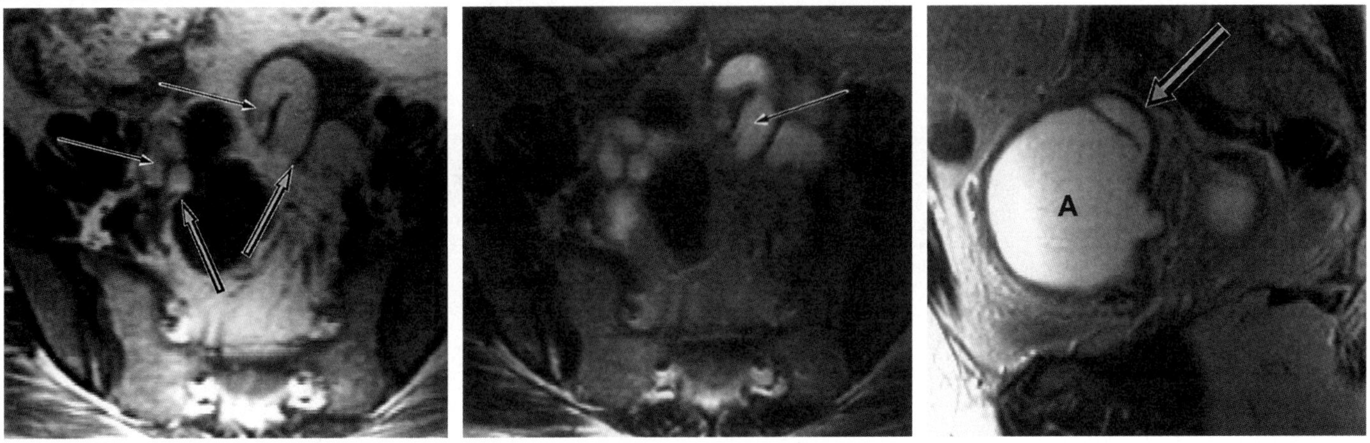

a. b. c.

Figure 3. Bilateral hydrosalpinx with mucosal plicae in a 40-year-old woman with endometriosis. **(a)** Axial T1-weighted image (600/10) and **(b)** axial T2-weighted fast SE image (5,000/102 [effective]) show bilateral hydrosalpinx (thick arrows in **a**). Thin longitudinal plicae (thin arrows) are seen in both tubes and were scored as positive by both readers. **(c)** Sagittal T2-weighted fast SE image (4,000/102 [effective]) shows continuity of the left tube isthmus (arrow) with a grossly dilated ampullary end of the tube (*A*).

TABLE 2
Performance of Two Blinded Readers for Detection of Fallopian Tubes in 79 Patients

		No. Detected		False-Negative		False-Positive		True-Negative	
Finding	*N*	Reader 1	Reader 2	Reader 1	Reader 2	Reader 1	Reader 2	Reader 1	Reader 2
Right side	79	15	17	5	3	1	5	58	54
Left side	79	22	23	11	11	2	5	44	46
Patients	79	31	31	10	10	3	6	35	32

pelvic imaging. All patients underwent axial T1-weighted spin-echo (SE) imaging (repetition time msec/echo time msec = 366–800/8–17, one to two signals acquired, 18–28-cm field of view) and axial T2-weighted fast SE imaging (3,000–8,000/72–144 [effective]; one to two signals acquired, 18–28-cm field of view). The acquisition matrix for the fast SE images was 256 × 256 with a 4–6-mm section thickness and 0–2-mm intersection gap. Echo train length was 16. In addition to axial T2-weighted fast SE images, T2-weighted images were obtained in the sagittal and/or coronal planes with similar parameters. Glucagon (1 mg) was injected intramuscularly before imaging to suppress bowel peristalsis.

Adnexal Specimens

Four surgically excised adnexal specimens containing dilated fallopian tubes were imaged with high-resolution specimen imaging prior to histopathologic processing. The study was approved by the institutional review board at Thomas Jefferson University Hospital. The specimens were removed for clinical indications from patients aged 43–89 years (mean, 63 years). Three were postmenopausal, and one was premenopausal.

The specimens were imaged fresh at room temperature with the 1.5-T system. A whole-volume transmit-receive coil designed for imaging the wrist (Medrad, Pittsburgh, Pa) was used. The T1-weighted SE images (400/20) were obtained with 8-cm field of view, 256 × 256 matrix, 3-mm interleaved sections, and one signal acquired. The T2-weighted fast SE images (3,000/110 [effective]) were obtained with 256 × 256 matrix, two signals acquired, and 8-cm field of view. Contiguous interleaved sections (3-mm thick) were obtained through the adnexa. After MR imaging, the specimens were sectioned and stained with hematoxylin-eosin after fixation.

Image Analysis

The MR studies from the study patients and control subjects were randomly sorted and presented to two blinded radiologists from two institutions (E.S.S., P.C.). One reader was an attending, body MR radiologist, and the other was a body MR imaging fellow. The blinded readers scored each adnexa for the presence or absence of a dilated fallopian tube. If a dilated fallopian tube was believed to be present, then the signal intensity of the tubal fluid was rated according to a five-point scale, as previously described (3). Signal intensity of the fluid was rated subjectively relative to the signal intensity of the myometrium on T1- and T2-weighted images. A five-point scale of signal intensity ranged from 1 (low signal intensity equivalent to that of urine on T1-weighted images or muscle on T2-weighted images) to 5 (very high signal intensity equivalent to that of urine on T2-weighted images and fat on non–fat-saturated T1-weighted images). Intermediate signal intensity (grade 3) was equivalent to that of normal outer myometrium on T1- and T2-weighted images. Grades 2 and 4 were intermediate levels of signal intensity that were determined subjectively and did not have a strict normal-signal-intensity counterpart. The scale as shown to the readers is displayed in Figure 1.

The readers scored each tube for the presence of thin longitudinally oriented folds along the interior of the tube and the presence of tubal wall thickening producing a multilayered appearance to the tube wall. Finally, the readers determined if there was evidence of endometriosis outside the tubes in the pelvis. Evidence of endometriosis was defined as a cyst with shading (low signal intensity) on T2-weighted images (4), multiple cysts with high signal intensity on T1-weighted images (4), or implants (5).

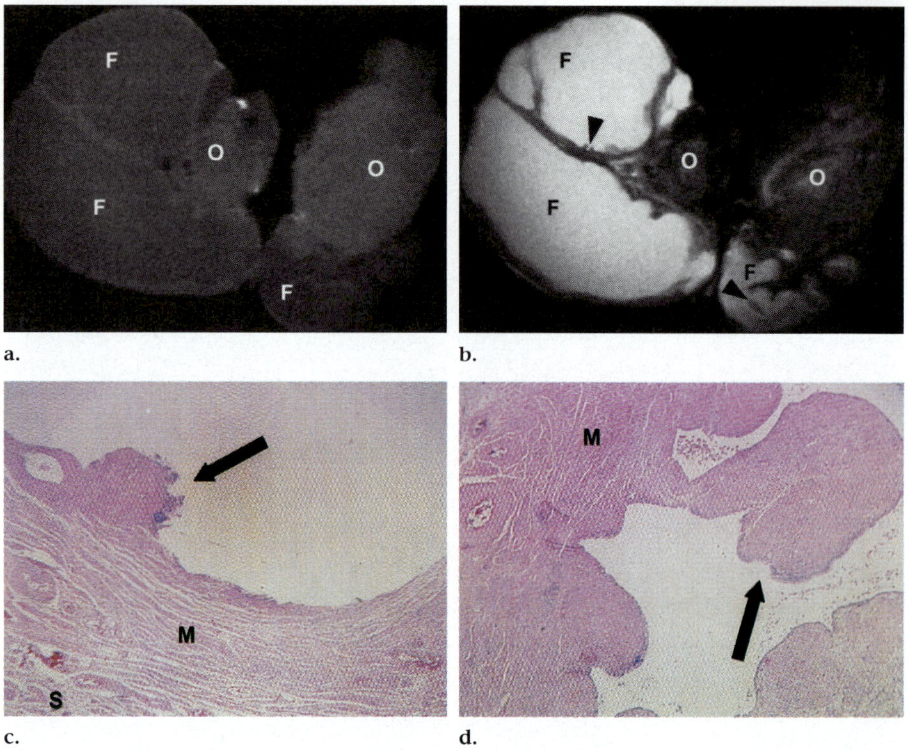

Figure 4. Hydrosalpinx ex vivo. **(a)** T1-weighted image (400/20) and **(b)** T2-weighted fast SE image (3,000/125 [effective]) obtained with an 8-cm field of view show bilateral postmenopausal ovaries (*O*) and bilateral hydrosalpinx (dilated fallopian tube, *F*). The dilated tubes show a discrete wall with blunted mucosal folds (arrowheads in **b**). **(c, d)** Photomicrographs of histologic sections from the right and left tubes, respectively, show the blunted mucosal plicae (arrow) and the muscularis (*M*) and serosa (*S* in **c**) of the tubes. (Hematoxylin-eosin stain; original magnification, ×40.)

Statistical Analysis

Comparisons between the clinical parameters in Table 1 were computed with the Student two-tailed *t* test. Associations between tubal signal intensity and surgical findings were made with χ^2 analysis. Because the right and left adnexal MR findings are not necessarily statistically independent, statistical correlations were made on a per patient basis, as well as a per adnexa basis, by considering the right and left sides separately.

RESULTS

Diagnostic performance for differentiation of hydrosalpinx from other adnexal masses is given in Table 2 for the two readers. On a per patient basis, both readers correctly detected fallopian tubes in 31 study patients and correctly rated 32 (reader 1) or 35 (reader 2) control patients as having no hydrosalpinx. Diagnoses were false-negative in 10 study patients. Fallopian tubes were depicted as fluid-filled tubular structures folded on themselves to form a C or S shape (Fig 1). Frequently, imaging in multiple planes was necessary to demonstrate the folded tubal structure of the dilated fallopian tube (Fig 2).

Longitudinal mucosal folds (plicae) (Fig 3) were seen in 37 of 53 dilated fallopian tubes by reader 1 and in 20 of 53 tubes by reader 2. The finding of plicae was specific for dilated tubes, however, with only two false-positive diagnoses for reader 1 and three for reader 2. Pathologic correlation for the specimens imaged in vitro showed that these longitudinal structures represented incompletely effaced mucosal plicae of the fallopian tube (Fig 4). A discrete wall in these specimens was depicted with low signal intensity on T2-weighted images, which represented the muscularis of the tube.

The signal intensity of the tubes on T1-weighted images correlated with the

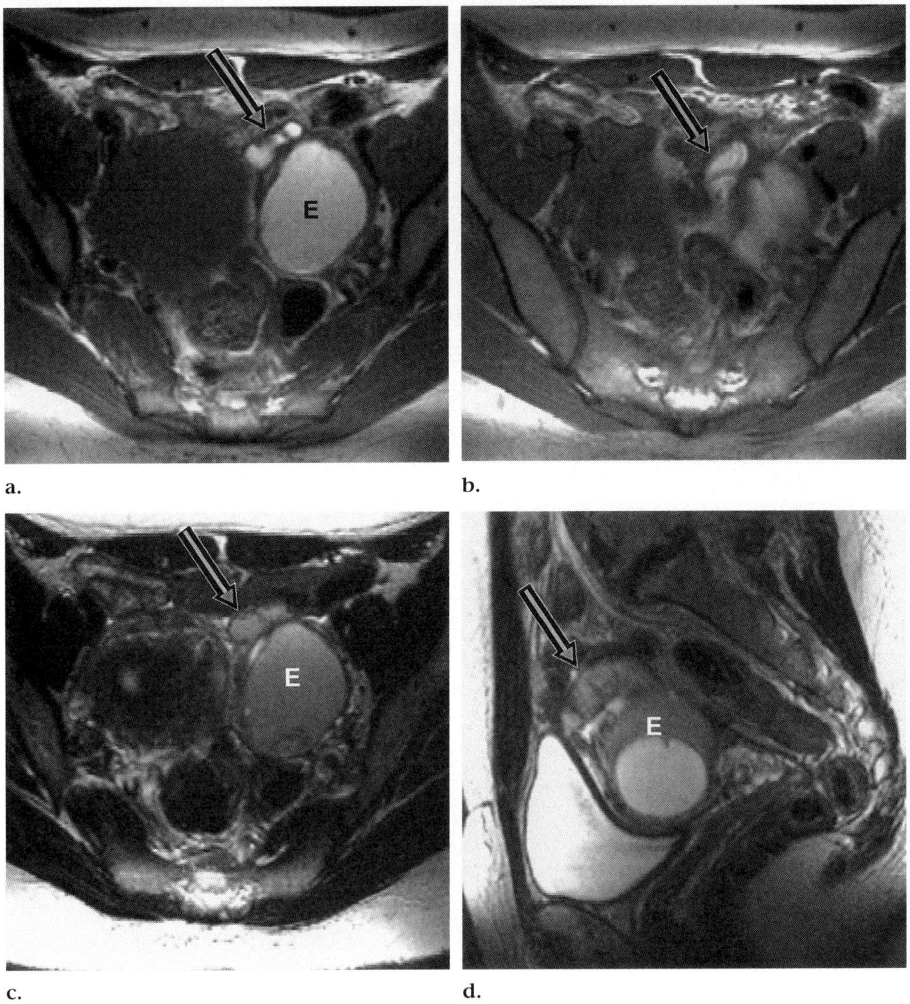

Figure 5. Hydrosalpinx in a 41-year-old woman with endometriosis. **(a, b)** Axial T1-weighted images (616/16) obtained at two positions show a hyperintense endometrioma (*E* in **a**) in the left ovary and a hematosalpinx anteriorly (arrow) with thin mucosal plicae. **(c)** Axial T2-weighted fast SE image (5,716/119 [effective]) shows low signal intensity in both the endometrioma (*E*) and hematosalpinx (arrow). **(d)** Sagittal T2-weighted fast SE image (6,000/119 [effective]) shows the tube (arrow) longitudinally anterior to the endometrioma (*E*).

TABLE 3
Signal Intensity of Tubal Fluid on T1-weighted SE Images Correlated with Pelvic Endometriosis or Histologic Findings of Salpingitis

		Endometriosis			Salpingitis		
Reader	Hyperintensity*	Present	Absent	*P*	Present	Absent	*P*
1	Present	10	4	.002	4	9	.37
	Absent	18	47	NP	8	34	NP
2	Present	12	4	.0002	5	9	.15
	Absent	16	47	NP	7	34	NP

Note.—Numbers do not total 79 patients because histologic examination of the tube was not performed in all patients. NP = comparison not performed.
* Signal intensity score, >3.

cause of the tubal pathologic condition (Fig 5). Specifically, high signal intensity on T1-weighted images (signal intensity score, >3) correlated with the presence of endometriosis in the pelvis at surgery (Table 3). Statistical analysis of findings on each side showed a statistically significant association for reader 1 on one side (right, P = .2; left, P = .002) and for reader 2 on both sides (right, P = .04; left, P = .0006). Both readers identified hyperintense dilated tubes on T1-weighted images in four study patients without other MR imaging evidence of endometriosis. In these study patients, endometriosis was documented at surgery.

T2-weighted signal intensity of the dilated tubes was scored as very high (signal intensity score, 5) for most tubes. Lower signal intensity was not significantly associated with endometriosis (P = .36 for reader 1, P = .44 for reader 2). Shortening of T2 consistent with shading was seen in four of 12 study patients identified with dilated tubes and endometriosis by reader 1 and three of 16 identified by reader 2.

The signal intensity of the fluid in the tubes was not associated with the presence of acute or chronic salpingitis, as determined by means of comparison with histologic findings in the adnexal specimen (Table 3). T1-weighted signal intensity was not correlated with salpingitis on the right or left side for either reader (P = .3 and .4, respectively, for reader 1; P = .06 and .15 for reader 2). Thickening of the tubal wall with a double-layered wall occurred in study patients with histologically proved acute or chronic salpingitis (Fig 6). This finding was statistically significant for both readers (reader 1, P = .007; reader 2, P =.05). There was no association of this sign with endometriosis on either side for either reader.

Interobserver agreement for the various findings was high. For the diagnosis of dilated fallopian tube, agreement was 87% on the right side and 94% on the left side. For the finding of tubal plicae, agreement was 86% on both sides; for thickened walls, agreement was 89% on the right and 91% on the left.

DISCUSSION

Findings in this study demonstrate that dilated fallopian tubes can be identified on MR images and distinguished from other adnexal masses. In general, the blinded readers had moderate detection rates and low false-positive rates for the diagnosis of hydrosalpinx. Fallopian tubes could be distinguished from adnexal masses of other origins and as a separate component of complex adnexal pathologic conditions that included both hydrosalpinx and other masses in the same adnexa.

Hydrosalpinx can also be diagnosed at US. Atri et al (6) reported a sensitivity of

34% for diagnosis at transvaginal US in 414 study patients who subsequently underwent hysterosalpingography, and this sensitivity was also reported by others (7). Other authors have reported higher rates of detection (8,9). Although simple hydrosalpinx is usually a straightforward diagnosis at US, a complex picture results when it occurs with other adnexal masses. The finding of mucosal plicae in hydrosalpinx was reported at US (8,10). These mucosal plicae may result from effacement of the mucosa and submucosa by the dilating tube or by blunting of the mucosal folds caused by chronic salpingitis (11).

The signal intensity of the tubal fluid was associated with tubal pathologic conditions. Specifically, high signal intensity on T1-weighted images was significantly correlated with endometriosis in the pelvis and tubes. The signal intensity within the fallopian tubes on T2-weighted images was generally very high, in contrast to the typical signal intensity of an endometrioma, which demonstrates moderate to marked T2 shortening in the form of shading (4). Therefore, in the proper clinical context, hematosalpinx may be an indicator of pelvic endometriosis; for both readers in this study, it was the only MR finding of endometriosis in some study patients. Hematosalpinx may be present in patients with endometriosis and should not be assumed solely to represent other pathologic conditions such as ectopic pregnancy (12).

The cause of the high signal intensity of the dilated tubes in study patients with endometriosis is not known. Tubal dilatation may be associated with endometriosis (13). Endometriosis implants on the serosal surface of fallopian tubes are common, although transmural or mucosal involvement is less common (14). In this study, transmural involvement was noted infrequently at histologic examination, although this determination depends on the thoroughness of sampling. Approximately 28% of women with endometriosis have tubal abnormalities depicted at hysterosalpingography (13), and a similar frequency of intratubal abnormalities is seen in women with endometriosis and infertility (15).

In our study, the signal intensity of the tubal fluid did not correlate with the presence of salpingitis, that is, the study patients with chronic or acute salpingitis did not show characteristic tubal changes. Findings of a thickened wall of a dilated fallopian tube with tubal contents of lower signal intensity have been reported on T2-weighted images in acute salpingitis (16). Although we noted wall thickening producing the double-wall sign in some study patients with acute salpingitis, this did not appear to be a strong predictor of the condition.

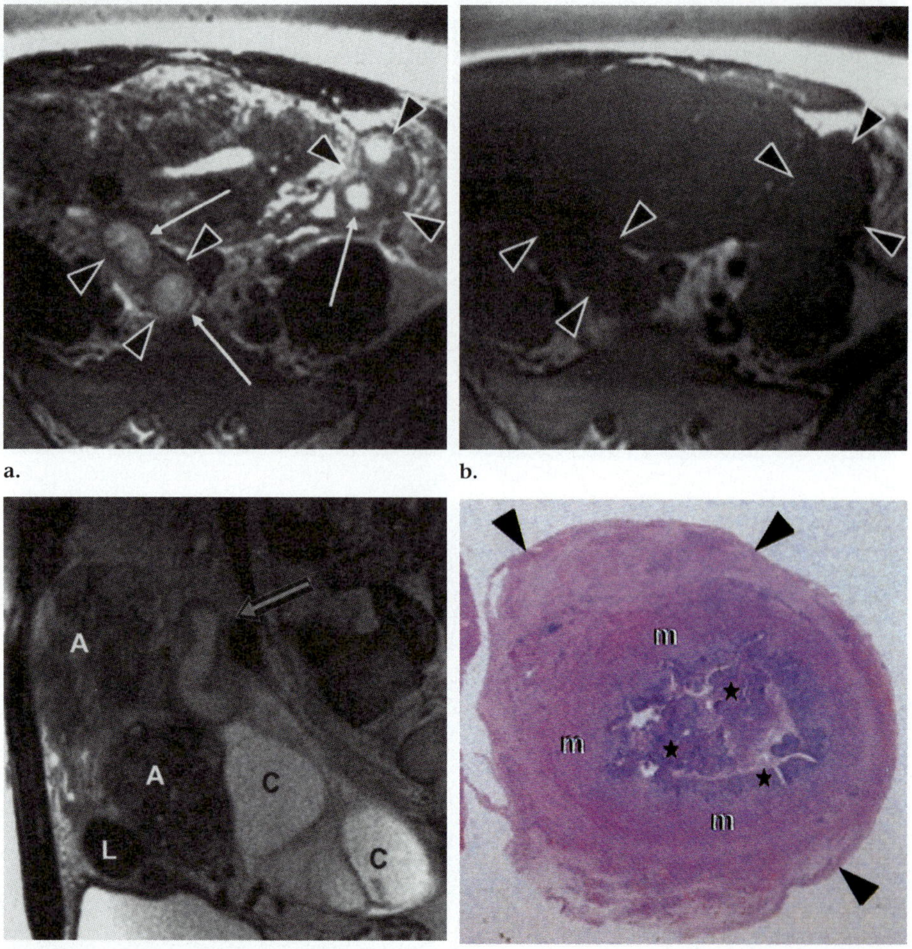

Figure 6. Bilateral hydrosalpinx with thickened wall in a 52-year-old woman with acute salpingitis. **(a)** Axial T2-weighted fast SE image (4,200/128 [effective]) shows bilateral pyosalpinx. The thickened wall of the tubes consists of an inner low-signal-intensity ring (arrows) around the distended lumen of the tube surrounded by higher signal intensity tissue (arrowheads). **(b)** Axial T1-weighted image (433/10) shows intermediate signal intensity (arrowheads) in both the tubal lumina and walls. **(c)** Sagittal T2-weighted fast SE image (5,000/119 [effective]) shows the right tube longitudinally (arrow). Adenomyoses (*A*), leiomyoma (*L*), and borderline serous tumors (*C*) of the right ovary are also shown. **(d)** Photomicrograph of a histologic section from the right tube shows the muscularis (*m*) surrounded by subserosal edema (arrowheads) and inflammation. The mucosa and lumen show inflammatory infiltrates (★). (Hematoxylin-eosin stain; original magnification, ×6.5.)

In summary, dilated fallopian tubes can be recognized at MR imaging, and they usually have a folded configuration. Longitudinal structures adjacent to the tubal wall represent incompletely effaced mucosal and submucosal folds. High signal intensity in dilated tubes on T1-weighted images correlates with the presence of pelvic endometriosis and may be the only MR imaging finding that indicates endometriosis.

References

1. Komatsu T, Konishi I, Mandai M, et al. Adnexal masses: transvaginal US and gadolinium-enhanced MR imaging assessment of intratumoral structure. Radiology 1996; 198:109–115.
2. Yamashita Y, Torashima M, Hatanaka Y, et al. Adnexal masses: accuracy of characterization with transvaginal US and precontrast and postcontrast MR imaging. Radiology 1995; 194:557–565.
3. Outwater EK, Mitchell DG. Normal ovaries and functional cysts: MR appearance. Radiology 1996; 198:397–402.
4. Togashi K, Nishimura K, Kimura I, et al. Endometrial cysts: diagnosis with MR imaging. Radiology 1991; 180:73–78.
5. Siegelman ES, Outwater EK, Wang T, Mitchell DG. Solid enhancing masses in

endometriosis: MR imaging observations. AJR 1994; 163:357–361.
6. Atri M, Tran CN, Bret PM, Aldis AE, Kintzen GM. Accuracy of endovaginal sonography for the detection of fallopian tube blockage. J Ultrasound Med 1994; 13:429–434.
7. Boardman LA, Peipert JF, Brody JM, Cooper AS, Sung J. Endovaginal sonography for the diagnosis of upper genital tract infection. Obstet Gynecol 1997; 90:54–57.
8. Tessler FN, Perrella RR, Fleischer AC, Grant EG. Endovaginal sonographic diagnosis of dilated fallopian tubes. AJR 1989; 153: 523–525.
9. Cacciatore B, Leminen A, Ingman-Friberg S, Ylostalo P, Paavonen J. Transvaginal sonographic findings in ambulatory patients with suspected pelvic inflammatory disease. Obstet Gynecol 1992; 80:912–916.
10. Timor-Tritsch IE, Rottem S. Transvaginal ultrasonographic study of the fallopian tube. Obstet Gynecol 1987; 70:424–428.
11. Wheeler JE. Diseases of the fallopian tube. In: Kurman RJ, ed. Blaustein's pathology of the female genital tract. 4th ed. New York, NY: Springer-Verlag, 1994; 529–561.
12. Atri M, Leduc C, Gillett P, et al. Role of endovaginal sonography in the diagnosis and management of ectopic pregnancy. RadioGraphics 1996; 16:755–775.
13. Ott DJ, Fayez JA. Tubal and adnexal abnormalities. In: Ott DJ, Fayez JA, eds. Hysterosalpingography: a text and atlas. Baltimore, Md: Urban & Schwarzenberg, 1991; 103–125.
14. Clement PB. Diseases of the peritoneum. In: Kurman RJ, ed. Blaustein's pathology of the female genital tract. 4th ed. New York, NY: Springer-Verlag, 1994; 647–703.
15. Bowman MC, Cooke ID. Comparison of fallopian tube intraluminal pathology as assessed by salpingoscopy with pelvic adhesions. Fertil Steril 1994; 61:464–469.
16. Rowling SE, Ramchandani P. Imaging of the fallopian tubes. Semin Roentgenol 1996; 31:299–311.

Book Review

Atlas of Breast Imaging

Carla K. Jones, MD, JD
Malden, Mass: Blackwell Science, 1997. ISBN 0-63204-303-2.
Hardcover, $95.00; pp 262; 194 figures.

This succinct, well-illustrated book was originally written as a section of a larger comprehensive textbook on women's imaging: *Gynecologic, Obstetric and Breast Radiology* (Cambridge, Mass: Blackwell Science, 1996). It is a primer of breast imaging practice with a brief review and update of breast imaging and interventions. The book is oriented toward the imaging professional who may already have a background in the fundamentals of breast anatomy, pathology, and imaging techniques, but radiology residents and physicians from backgrounds other than radiology may find it useful as an introduction to breast imaging. Also, it could serve as a supplement for those seeking certification or recertification in mammography.

The book is organized into eight chapters. The first chapter is brief and focuses on past and present literature on breast cancer screening and the controversies surrounding the issue of screening asymptomatic women. It also discusses counseling the high-risk patient and the risks of mammographic screening. The second chapter is much longer and deals with mammography. It contains an appropriately short discussion of findings on characteristically benign processes and is followed by 102 pages of copious illustrations and text on mammographic signs that may be related to malignancy. The chapter describes problems encountered in interpreting mammographic abnormalities and practical approaches to these problems, and it includes appropriate literature citations. The third chapter, on ancillary breast imaging modalities, is brief and discusses appropriate utilization of ultrasound, magnetic resonance imaging, and scintigraphy in breast imaging.

Chapters 4 and 5 focus on special imaging situations in the symptomatic patient and in the postsurgical breast. The chapters are well illustrated, appropriate references are given, and practical approaches to common imaging problems are reviewed. Chapters 6 and 7 cover diagnostic and therapeutic procedures and image-guided breast biopsy. They are also well illustrated and contain many examples of common pitfalls and problems, such as those related to the interventional equipment used and the type of abnormality or the position of the abnormality in the breast.

The last chapter, on medicolegal aspects of breast imaging, reviews information regarding breast cancer–related malpractice settlements and the failure to diagnose breast cancer. It includes discussions of legal responsibilities and duties related to clinical evaluation, breast imaging, and follow-up.

Atlas of Breast Imaging is intended for the practitioner and is clearly and concisely written. As the title implies, it is rich with well-placed illustrations and numerous examples. It is also well referenced, and landmark articles are frequently cited. I recommend it to anyone beginning to learn about breast imaging or those with a background in breast imaging who require an update and brief review.

Reviewed by Suzanne Mastin, MD

Findings at Mammographic Screening on Only One Standard Projection: Outcomes Analysis[1]

Edward A. Sickles, MD

Index terms:
Breast, calcification, 00.81
Breast, diseases, 00.30
Breast neoplasms, 00.30
Breast neoplasms, diagnosis, 00.11, 00.30
Breast radiography, 00.11
Breast radiography, technology, 00.11

Radiology 1998; 208:471–475

Abbreviations:
CC = craniocaudal
DCIS = ductal carcinoma in situ
IDC = invasive ductal carcinoma
ILC = invasive lobular carcinoma
MLO = mediolateral oblique

[1] From the Department of Radiology, University of California School of Medicine, Box 1667, San Francisco, CA 94143-1667. From the 1997 RSNA scientific assembly. Received November 11, 1997; revision requested January 29, 1998; revision received February 20; accepted April 10. **Address reprint requests to** the author.

Author contribution:
Guarantor of integrity of entire study, E.A.S.

PURPOSE: To determine the radiographic and clinical outcomes of findings seen at mammographic screening on only one standard projection.

MATERIALS AND METHODS: To identify prospectively marked benign-appearing and abnormal findings that were seen on only one standard projection, 63,836 consecutive two-view mammographic screening studies were reviewed. Subsequent outcomes analysis included determination of the frequency of occurrence, mammographic features, work-up performed, and final imaging assessment. For imaging findings that prompted tissue sampling, histopathologic diagnosis was recorded. To identify breast cancers among the remaining findings, screening cases were linked with a regional tumor registry.

RESULTS: Of the 61,273 screening studies available for review, 2,023 (3.3%) involved prospectively identified findings seen on only one standard projection. One thousand eighty-six (53.7%) studies with one-view-only findings were judged to represent superimposition of normal breast structures (summation artifact) simply from the standard projections obtained at screening; findings in an additional 587 (29.0%) studies were characterized as representing superimposition of normal structures after recall for further diagnostic imaging. None of these 1,673 cases was subsequently found to be cancer. Cancers were identified in 36 one-view-only studies; six involved ductal carcinoma in situ; 18, invasive ductal carcinoma; and 12, invasive lobular carcinoma (a large percentage [33%], since only 10% of all cancers are invasive lobular carcinoma).

CONCLUSION: Findings seen on only one standard projection are common among lesions identified at mammographic screening. More than 80% can be correctly assessed as representing superimposition of normal structures, either without or with the aid of additional imaging studies. Among those findings that truly are cancer, a disproportionately high percentage are invasive lobular carcinoma.

Not infrequently, potentially abnormal findings are identified at mammographic screening on only one of the two standard-projection images. Many of these findings represent superimposition of normal structures (summation artifact), while others are real lesions. Several imaging approaches have been described to distinguish summation artifacts from real lesions for findings seen on only one standard view (1–5). However, there is very little information on the mammographic and clinical outcomes for these one-view-only findings, except for the relatively few lesions that ultimately are found to be malignant (6–8). This study was undertaken to catalog the frequency of occurrence, mammographic features, work-up performed, final imaging assessment, and results of tissue diagnosis for a large series of consecutive screening examinations with one-view-only findings.

MATERIALS AND METHODS

The study population involved the 63,836 consecutive examinations performed in my institution's mammographic screening practice from April 1985 through December 1993.

TABLE 1
Mammographic Features of Findings Identified on Only One of Two Standard Mammographic Screening Views

Feature	No. of Cases (*n* = 2,023)
Density	1,716 (84.8)
Architectural distortion	217 (10.7)
Calcifications	83 (4.1)
Combinations	7 (0.3)

Note.—Number in parentheses is the percentage.

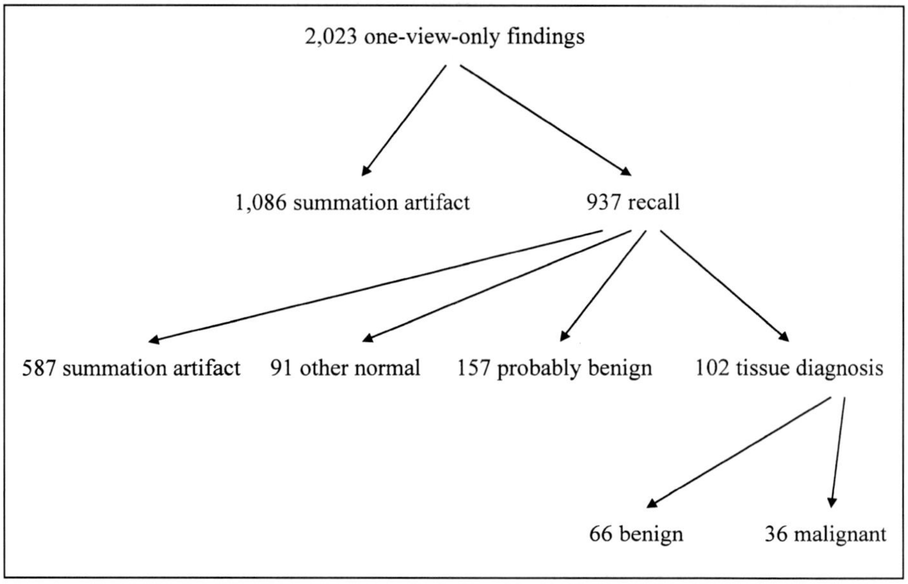

Figure 1. Diagram shows data on subsequent work-up and imaging assessment of findings identified on only one of two standard mammographic screening views.

During image interpretation, the radiologists in our practice routinely draw wax-crayon circles around a variety of mammographic findings that attract our attention, ranging from those we judge so likely to be benign that further imaging is not necessary to those that require prompt recall for additional imaging assessment (9). We may or may not choose to describe in the mammographic report those circled findings for which we render a normal screening interpretation; however, the circles remain, so that when the woman returns for subsequent screening, we are prompted to look in the same area to ensure stability. We always describe the nature and location of findings for which recall imaging is recommended, whether or not wax-crayon circles are drawn.

From the entire group of studies with prospectively circled or described findings (identified retrospectively by reviewing available images and mammographic reports), I selected for study those for which a finding was present on only one of the two standard screening views. I then cataloged the frequency of occurrence of examinations with one-view-only findings, the mammographic features of the findings, whether recall for additional imaging work-up was recommended, and the final assessment after imaging was complete. For cases with screening-detected findings in which tissue sampling was performed, the histopathologic diagnosis was recorded. Cancer was defined as ductal carcinoma in situ (DCIS), invasive ductal carcinoma (IDC), or invasive lobular carcinoma (ILC).

To identify breast cancers among the remaining studies with one-view-only findings, computer linkage was performed of our screening cases with the data stored in our regional tumor registry, the linkage taking place a minimum of 2 years after screening was done. Past experience has shown that such linkage, in combination with my institution's computer-based outcomes tracking system, helps identify more than 95% of breast cancer cases in our service area (9). Part of the outcomes tracking system involves an ongoing listing of all breast cancers detected at mammographic screening in my institution. Therefore, as a further means to identify cancer cases among the study population, an additional computer linkage was performed of all screening-detected cancers (as of October 1997, 3¾ years after the last study examination) with those studies having one-view-only findings for which no tissue diagnosis was obtained.

RESULTS

There were 61,273 screening examinations for which both the images and mammographic reports were available for review, composing 96.0% of the examinations performed. One-view-only findings were identified in 2,023 cases, representing 3.3% of the reviewed cases. Mammographic features of these findings are listed in Table 1; the great majority are noncalcified densities.

The subsequent work-up and assessment of the 2,023 studies with one-view-only findings are outlined in Figure 1. My colleagues and I interpreted 1,086 (53.7%) of the findings as representing superimposition of normal structures simply on the basis of the standard two-view screening examination findings (Fig 2). Each of these cases manifested as a noncalcified density or architectural distortion at mammographic screening. Of the remaining 937 cases, for which recall imaging was requested and performed, an additional 587 cases (also noncalcified densities or architectural distortions) were found to represent superimposition of normal structures (Fig 3). Thus, summation artifacts accounted for 1,673 (82.7%) of the 2,023 one-view-only findings. These assessments indicating the presence of summation artifacts indeed were highly accurate, despite the lack of confirmation by means of tissue diagnosis, because none of the cases was eventually found to involve breast carcinoma, either at subsequent routine mammographic screening (if performed) or by means of linkage with our regional tumor registry.

Of the remaining cases recalled for further imaging work-up, 91 others also were assessed as normal or benign, requiring nothing more than routine mammographic screening. These included 53 cases of simple cysts for which definitive diagnosis was made at ultrasonography or by means of aspiration. Also included were 38 cases diagnosed as benign at subsequent mammography and that involved skin calcification, arterial calcification, milk of calcium within tiny benign cysts, intramammary lymph node, a raised skin lesion, and suspected calcification found to represent artifactual opacities.

There also were 157 one-view-only lesions ultimately assessed as probably benign that required periodic mammographic surveillance (10,11). The great

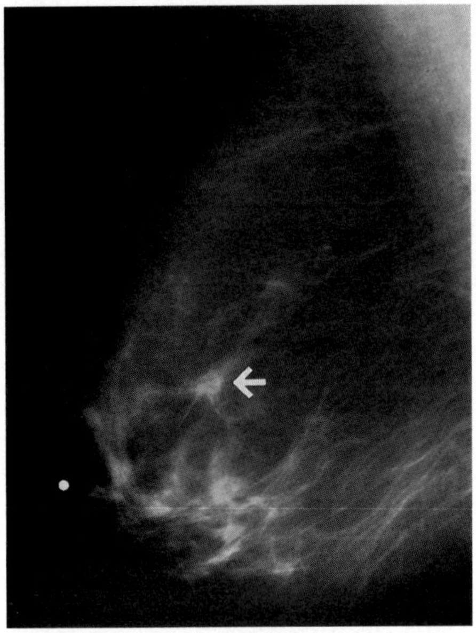

a.

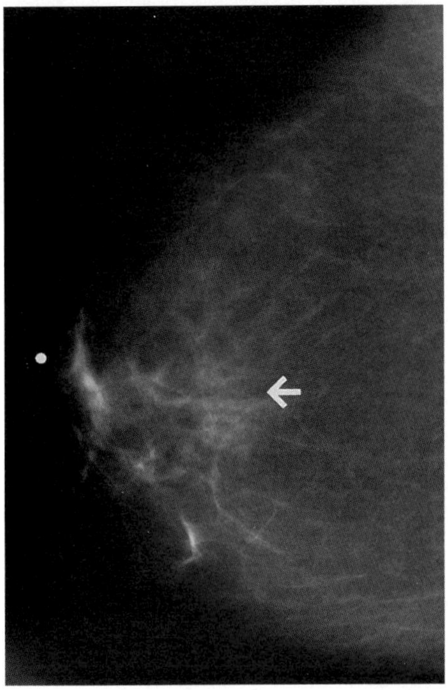

b.

Figure 2. Making the diagnosis of summation artifact on standard mediolateral oblique (MLO) and craniocaudal (CC) views only. **(a)** Baseline MLO projection mammogram in a 61-year-old asymptomatic woman demonstrates a 10-mm irregular spiculated density (arrow) in the superior aspect of the breast. The measured straight-line distance from the nipple (dot) to this finding is 5.9 cm (original magnification). **(b)** Standard CC view mammogram from this examination does not show a similar finding. Note that the measured distance from the nipple (dot) to the back edge of the CC film is 11.3 cm (original magnification), indicating that the MLO finding surely is included within the CC image. At a depth approximately 5.9 cm from the nipple on the CC view, there are no areas of fibroglandular tissue that are dense enough to obscure the MLO finding. This combination of mammographic features is sufficient to establish the mammographic diagnosis of summation artifact, but in this case there is even more convincing evidence to support the diagnosis: In **b**, at a depth of approximately 5.9 cm from the nipple in the central aspect of the breast, there is a much larger, less dense, and more vaguely defined nonspiculated area of benign-appearing fibroglandular tissue (arrow), interspersed with fat, which easily could have superimposed to create the more dense, irregular finding seen in **a**. No further work-up was recommended for this woman, a normal interpretation was made, and she was advised to undergo routine mammographic screening in 1 year. Repeat examination at that time also had normal findings; the summation artifact seen previously in **a** was no longer present.

majority (136 cases [86.6%]) were cases of focal asymmetric density or circumscribed mass, the remainder involving isolated clusters of round microcalcifications. Almost all of these cases demonstrated stability during the course of mammographic surveillance. Tissue diagnosis was performed in the four lesions that enlarged during follow-up, with benign results in each case.

Finally, after full imaging work-up, 102 one-view-only lesions were judged to be sufficiently suspicious for malignancy to require prompt tissue diagnosis (fine-needle aspiration, core biopsy, or surgical biopsy). Of these, 66 were found to be benign, including seven cases of atypical hyperplasia or lobular carcinoma in situ. There were 36 cases of malignancy, representing 1.8% of the 2,023 one-view-only findings identified at mammographic screening. Among these cancers, six were DCIS, 18 were IDC, and 12 were ILC.

DISCUSSION

This large series of consecutive mammographic screening studies indicates the imaging and clinical outcomes for cases in which potentially abnormal findings are identified prospectively on only one of two standard-projection images. Such one-view-only findings are detected with considerable frequency, having been seen in 2,023 (3.3%) of our 61,273 screening studies available for review. This amounts to one in approximately every 30 studies, so that a moderately busy mammographic screening practice can expect to encounter one-view-only findings on a daily basis.

The current study also demonstrates that the great majority (n = 1,673 [82.7%]) of one-view-only findings represent superimposition of normal breast structures rather than true lesions, so it is imperative for radiologists to learn to correctly characterize such summation artifacts. As further shown in this study, it is possible to recognize the majority of summation artifacts simply by means of careful analysis of the two standard-projection screening images (Fig 2); 1,086 (64.9%) cases involving superimposition were correctly assessed without the need for recall imaging. However, had these cases been recalled instead, the total number of recalls during the study would have increased from 3,224 to 4,310, thereby increasing our recall rate by slightly more than one-third, from 5.1% to 6.8%.

It also is important for radiologists to develop sufficient skills to diagnose summation artifact by using additional imaging after recall from screening (Fig 3). Indeed, to this end, there are several problem-solving approaches that are both accurate and readily performed (1–5). In the current study, had tissue diagnosis (fine-needle aspiration biopsy, core biopsy, or surgical biopsy) been performed in all 1,673 cases interpreted as summation artifacts, the number of biopsies during the study would have increased from 932 to 2,605, without any substantive increase in the 328 cancers discovered, thereby decreasing our positive predictive value for tissue diagnosis from 35.2% to approximately 12.6%.

Results of the current study also provide insight into the imaging and clinical outcomes of those cases with one-view-only findings not interpreted as summation artifacts. In general, such cases with one-view-only findings had similar outcomes as the overall group of cases recalled for additional imaging during the study, a group composed primarily of abnormalities seen on both standard screening views. The subset of cases with one-view-only findings in fact accounted for approximately 11% (350 of 3,224) of all recalled cases, 11% (102 of 932) of all cases undergoing tissue diagnosis, and 11% (36 of 328) of all cancer cases.

However, there also were several notable differences between the one-view-only cancers and the overall group of cancer cases. Table 2 shows the distribution of screening-detected cases of DCIS, IDC, and ILC as a function of whether the cancer was seen at screening on one or both standard views. Results for ILC are strikingly different than those for IDC and DCIS. A disproportionately high percentage of ILC cases manifested as one-

TABLE 2
Visibility of Screening-detected Cancers on Standard Mammographic Views

View	DCIS (n = 91)	IDC (n = 203)	ILC (n = 34)
CC only	0 (0)	5 (2.5)	8 (24)
MLO only	6 (7)	13 (6.4)	4 (12)
Both CC and MLO	85 (93)	185 (91.1)	22 (65)

Note.—Number in parentheses is the percentage.

view-only findings. Whereas 35% (12 of 34) of ILC cases were seen at initial screening on only one view, only 8% (24 of 294) of IDC and DCIS cases were identified initially on only one view. Furthermore, a disproportionately high percentage of one-view-only cancer cases were ILC cases. Whereas 33% (12 of 36) of one-view-only cancer cases were ILC cases, only 10% (34 of 328) of all cancer cases were ILC cases. Similar results have been observed by Newstead et al (8).

The tendency of ILC to be seen at mammography on only one standard view is likely due to its inherent pattern of growth. Rather than forming a cohesive mass of tumor cells, which would be readily visible as a mass on several mammographic projections, ILC cells generally grow in narrow rows, often single file, diffusely infiltrating surrounding tissues without disrupting glandular and ductal anatomy or inciting substantial connective tissue reaction (6,7,12,13). These features, coupled with the propensity of ILC to grow in multicentric foci separated by areas of normal tissue, reduce tumor opacity as seen at mammography, thereby limiting lesion visibility on any given mammographic view and increasing the likelihood that a tumor will be seen on only one standard view (6,7,12,14).

One expects most one-view-only cancers to be seen on an MLO projection, since the MLO view includes more fibroglandular tissue than does the CC view, especially in the upper outer quadrant, where most cancers develop. This is indeed the case for IDC and DCIS (Table 2), for which nonvisualization usually occurs when a lesion close to the chest wall is excluded from the image field. However, a disproportionately high percentage of ILC cases are seen only on a CC view, an observation made not only in this study (Table 2) but also in three previous investigations (6,8,15). A majority of our one-view-only ILC cases were not located close to the chest wall, so exclusion of lesions from the image field is not a satisfactory explanation for predominantly CC-view-only visualization. A more sensible explanation is that the

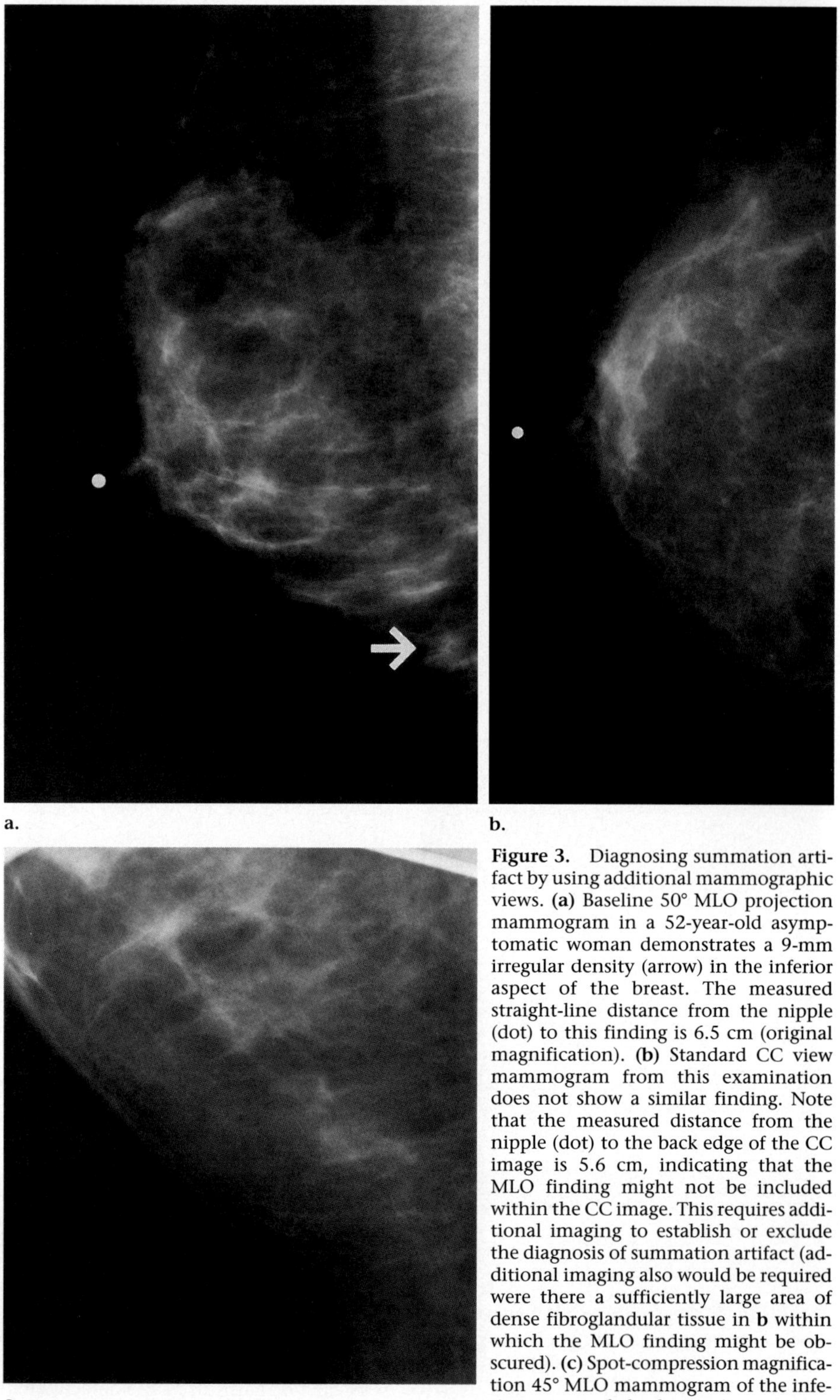

Figure 3. Diagnosing summation artifact by using additional mammographic views. **(a)** Baseline 50° MLO projection mammogram in a 52-year-old asymptomatic woman demonstrates a 9-mm irregular density (arrow) in the inferior aspect of the breast. The measured straight-line distance from the nipple (dot) to this finding is 6.5 cm (original magnification). **(b)** Standard CC view mammogram from this examination does not show a similar finding. Note that the measured distance from the nipple (dot) to the back edge of the CC image is 5.6 cm, indicating that the MLO finding might not be included within the CC image. This requires additional imaging to establish or exclude the diagnosis of summation artifact (additional imaging also would be required were there a sufficiently large area of dense fibroglandular tissue in **b** within which the MLO finding might be obscured). **(c)** Spot-compression magnification 45° MLO mammogram of the inferior aspect of the breast (a projection only 5° different in obliquity than **a**), in which the MLO finding is no longer apparent, thereby establishing the diagnosis of summation artifact. Other potentially successful imaging approaches include 5°-off-initial-projection imaging by using rolled view, spot-compression imaging alone, and 90° lateral projection imaging.

inherently low opacity of ILC makes the mammographic visibility of these insidiously growing tumors (noncalcified ill-defined densities, areas of architectural distortion) especially dependent on vigorous breast compression, which usually is applied more effectively on the CC view than on the MLO view (15). Note that the substantial thickness of pectoral muscle that is compressed during MLO-view exposure can reduce the compressive force applied to the (relatively thinner) anterior and middle portions of the breast, impairing the visibility of subtle lesions (5).

In conclusion, findings seen on only one standard projection are common among lesions detected at mammographic screening. The great majority (>80%) can be correctly assessed as representing superimposition of normal breast structures, either without or with the aid of additional imaging studies. Those one-view-only findings that are not interpreted as being summation artifacts generally have similar imaging and clinical outcomes as the overall group of screening-detected lesions recalled for additional assessment. However, among one-view-only cancers, a disproportionately high percentage are ILC, an insidiously growing malignancy that often displays subtle mammographic features more readily seen on a CC view than on an MLO view.

References

1. Sickles EA. Practical solutions to common mammographic problems: tailoring the examination. AJR 1988; 151:31–39.
2. Sickles EA. Tailoring the mammogram: problem solving and special views. In: Thrall JH, ed. Current practice of radiology. St Louis, Mo: Dekker/Mosby–Year Book, 1993; 393–402.
3. Feig SA. The importance of supplementary mammographic views to diagnostic accuracy (commentary). AJR 1988; 151:40–41.
4. Logan WW, Janus J. Use of special mammographic views to maximize radiographic information. Radiol Clin North Am 1987; 25:953–959.
5. Eklund GW, Cardenosa G. The art of mammographic positioning. Radiol Clin North Am 1992; 30:21–53.
6. Hilleren DJ, Andersson IT, Lindholm K, Linnell FS. Invasive lobular carcinoma: mammographic findings in a 10-year experience. Radiology 1991; 178:149–154.
7. Sickles EA. The subtle and atypical mammographic features of invasive lobular carcinoma (editorial). Radiology 1991; 178:25–26.
8. Newstead GM, Baute PB, Toth HK. Invasive lobular and ductal carcinoma: mammographic findings and stage at diagnosis. Radiology 1992; 184:623–627.
9. Wolverton DE, Sickles EA. Clinical outcome of doubtful mammographic findings. AJR 1996; 167:1041–1045.
10. Sickles EA. Periodic mammographic follow-up of probably benign lesions: results in 3,184 consecutive cases. Radiology 1991; 179:463–468.
11. Sickles EA. Nonpalpable, circumscribed, noncalcified solid breast masses: likelihood of malignancy based on lesion size and age of patient. Radiology 1994; 192:439–442.
12. Holland R, Hendriks JH, Mravunac M. Mammographically occult breast cancer. Cancer 1983; 52:1810–1819.
13. Linell F, Ljungberg O. Carcinomas. In: Atlas of breast pathology. Copenhagen, Denmark: Munksgaard, 1984; 200–214.
14. Gump FE, Shikora S, Habif DV, Kister S, Logerfo P, Estabrook A. The extent and distribution of cancer in breasts with palpable primary tumors. Ann Surg 1986; 204:384–388.
15. Helvie MA, Paramagul C, Oberman HA, Adler DD. Invasive lobular carcinoma: imaging features and clinical detection. Invest Radiol 1993; 28:202–207.

Kirsten L. Weind, BSc
Cynthia F. Maier, PhD
Brian K. Rutt, PhD
Madeleine Moussa, MD

Index terms:
Breast neoplasms, diagnosis, 00.31, 00.324
Breast neoplasms, MR, 00.12141
Breast neoplasms, US, 00.12983
Fibroadenoma, 00.31
Neoplasms, blood supply, 00.31, 00.324

Radiology 1998; 208:477–483

[1] From the Departments of Medical Biophysics and Diagnostic Radiology, University of Western Ontario, London, Canada (K.L.W., C.F.M., B.K.R.); the Tom Lawson Family Imaging Research Laboratories, John P. Robarts Research Institute, 100 Perth Dr, London, Ontario, N6A 5A5, Canada (K.L.W., C.F.M., B.K.R.); and the Department of Pathology, London Health Sciences Centre, Ontario, (M.M.). Received October 19, 1997; revision requested December 19; revision received February 20, 1998; accepted March 27. Supported in part by the National Cancer Institute of Canada Breast Cancer Research Initiative and the Breast Cancer Society of Canada. C.F.M. was supported by a U.S. Army breast cancer predoctoral fellowship. **Address reprint requests to** B.K.R.

Author contributions:
Guarantor of integrity of entire study, C.F.M.; study concepts and design, K.L.W., C.F.M., B.K.R., M.M.; definition of intellectual content, K.L.W., C.F.M.; literature research, K.L.W., C.F.M.; data acquisition, M.M.; data analysis, K.L.W., C.F.M.; statistical analysis, K.L.W.; manuscript preparation, K.L.W., C.F.M.; manuscript editing and review, K.L.W., C.F.M., B.K.R., M.M.

Invasive Carcinomas and Fibroadenomas of the Breast: Comparison of Microvessel Distributions—Implications for Imaging Modalities[1]

PURPOSE: To compare spatial patterns of blood vessels between invasive breast carcinomas and fibroadenomas to improve the diagnostic specificity of noninvasive vascular magnetic resonance imaging and color Doppler ultrasound.

MATERIALS AND METHODS: Nineteen invasive ductal carcinomas and 20 fibroadenomas from 39 patients were stained for factor VIII–related antigen. Vessels smaller than 40 μm were counted in ×200 fields defined in peripheral and central areas of the tumor and in normal tissue adjacent to fibroadenomas. Significant differences in vessel density were determined with Student *t* tests and one-way analyses of variance. Distributions of vessels 40 μm or larger were qualitatively evaluated.

RESULTS: There were 9–105 vessels (mean, 31.4 vessels) smaller than 40 μm per ×200 peripheral and 4–57 vessels (mean, 20.1 vessels) smaller than 40 μm per ×200 central carcinoma field. There was no significant difference in vessel density between the two groups. Peripheral microvessel density was significantly higher ($P < .01$) than central microvessel density in 15 (79%) of the 19 carcinomas and in three (16%) of 19 fibroadenomas. (A Student t test could not be performed in one case of fibroadenoma; size permitted only one countable field according to the authors' criteria.) The 18 cases with normal tissue had 21–229 vessels (mean, 80.5 vessels) per field; in 16 (89%) of the 18 cases, these vessel counts were significantly higher ($P < .01$) than those in the fibroadenoma cases. Vessels 40 μm or larger were found mainly in the periphery of carcinomas and were more uniformly distributed in fibroadenomas.

CONCLUSION: Evaluation of the spatial distribution of vessels and the ability to resolve vessel sizes may add valuable information to the imaging-based diagnostic work-up of indeterminate solid breast lesions.

At present, the primary method of the detection and diagnosis of breast disease is conventional mammography, which has a proved sensitivity of 85%–95% (1,2). However, specificity with this modality is substantially lower, and additional diagnostic procedures are often necessary (3,4). A definitive diagnosis is sometimes possible with noninvasive techniques, but, for most lesions, biopsy is necessary to obtain reliable results (5–8). In the majority of cases, breast lesions progressing to biopsy are benign (3,9,10). Surgical biopsy in these cases has served only to provide a diagnosis, since it is not necessary to remove a benign lesion unless it is causing pain (11,12). This has led to the evaluation of imaging methods such as magnetic resonance (MR) imaging and color Doppler ultrasound (US) as adjunctive noninvasive diagnostic examinations (13,14).

Both these modalities rely on the principle that an increase in the number of blood vessels, increased vascular permeability, or both around malignant lesions result from tumor angiogenesis and create characteristic, identifiable patterns that can be distinguished from those associated with benign lesions. Although early contrast material–enhanced MR imaging and color Doppler US studies were reported to have extremely high

TABLE 1
Invasive Ductal Breast Carcinomas: Clinical Data and Vessel Counts

Case No./Patient Age (y)	Tumor Diameter (cm)	Tumor Grade	Lymph Node Status	Vessel Count per Field: Mean ± Standard Deviation		Vessel Count per Field: Range		Ratio of Mean in Periphery to Mean in Center
				Periphery	Center	Periphery	Center	
1/44	1.5	II	Negative	13.0 ± 2.20	8.00 ± 2.20	9–16	5–12	1.63
2/66	0.7	II	Negative	20.8 ± 4.40	11.4 ± 2.10	16–26	9–14	1.82
3/74	2.0	I	Not known	25.1 ± 6.80	17.3 ± 3.70	17–38	13–23	1.45
4/47	1.7	II	Positive	32.0 ± 10.5	15.6 ± 5.50	20–53	8–25	2.05
5/75	3.0	II	Not known	19.8 ± 3.20	10.8 ± 2.40	16–24	7–15	1.83
6/70	2.5	III	Positive	19.8 ± 2.40	7.70 ± 1.80	16–22	5–10	2.57
7/54	2.5	II	Positive	24.5 ± 4.40	10.8 ± 4.70	17–30	4–17	2.27
8/55	1.5	II	Negative	29.1 ± 10.3	28.8 ± 4.30	14–49	23–35	1.01
9/49	2.2	III	Positive	29.0 ± 3.30	21.1 ± 7.00	25–32	14–32	1.37
10/30	1.8	III	Positive	71.0 ± 18.1	33.9 ± 10.8	54–105	24–57	2.09
11/80	2.5	III	Not known	30.2 ± 6.60	16.6 ± 3.20	22–43	13–23	1.82
12/31	2.0	III	Positive	23.4 ± 4.60	18.0 ± 4.90	16–30	10–27	1.30
13/52	1.3	II	Negative	35.4 ± 13.0	17.2 ± 3.90	17–55	9–22	2.06
14/57	1.0	I	Negative	21.6 ± 5.60	22.8 ± 4.30	16–31	18–29	0.95
15/79	2.0	I	Not known	41.6 ± 7.50	35.6 ± 9.50	28–54	24–51	1.17
16/46	5.0	II	Positive	23.6 ± 3.00	19.7 ± 2.60	17–27	16–24	1.20
17/49	2.5	II	Negative	30.1 ± 7.60	18.2 ± 3.30	20–45	13–22	1.65
18/47	1.5	I	Negative	52.5 ± 14.9	42.5 ± 6.30	39–88	36–57	1.24
19/61	0.4	II	Not known	55.1 ± 12.8	25.9 ± 6.40	35–72	18–40	2.13

diagnostic specificity (15–17), further studies with larger sample sizes did not achieve the same accurate delineation of breast carcinomas. In particular, a substantial fraction of fibroadenomas were indistinguishable from malignant lesions (13,18–20). The inability to accurately identify fibroadenomas is a considerable flaw for a potential adjunctive modality, because these lesions often resemble solid carcinomas at both mammography and clinical presentation (21,22) and account for 30%–50% of biopsies of benign lesions (23).

Recently, several MR groups have observed a pattern of heightened contrast material enhancement around the periphery of a lesion in 15%–30% of malignant lesions (24,25). This "positive rim sign" (18) has also been observed by using color Doppler US. It has been suggested that this criterion could aid in separating malignant from benign lesions.

Several researchers (25–27) have also compared MR contrast material enhancement parameters with numbers of blood vessels observed at histologic analysis. In these studies, vessels were counted in areas of highest vascularity or "hot spots," potentially valuable prognostic indicators for invasive carcinomas (28). Two of the three researchers (25,26) found a statistically significant correlation between the degree of enhancement and microvessel density in hot spots. Unfortunately, researchers in none of these studies attempted to evaluate the spatial distribution of vascularity over entire lesions. In addition, no data are available on the comparison of color Doppler results with histologic confirmation of the presence of larger vessels.

To use vascular imaging techniques effectively, it is necessary to first identify a difference in the vascular pattern between malignant and benign lesions that is prominent enough to allow differentiation of these lesions. In addition, the study of the differences, similarities, or both between vascular distribution and density in malignant and benign breast lesions could serve to illuminate the unique mechanisms contributing to the formation of a microcirculatory network in a malignant tumor and its subsequent role in tumor metastasis. With these objectives in mind, we have evaluated spatial patterns of blood vessel distribution and quantitatively assessed microvessel density in invasive ductal carcinomas and fibroadenomas.

MATERIALS AND METHODS

Routinely processed, formalin-fixed, paraffin-embedded tissue from 39 lumpectomies in 19 patients with 19 invasive ductal carcinomas and in 20 patients with 20 fibroadenomas was retrieved from the files of the Department of Pathology at London Health Sciences Centre, London, Ontario, Canada. Patients with carcinoma ranged in age from 30 to 80 years and patients with fibroadenomas ranged in age from 19 to 49 years. Immunohistochemical studies to detect factor VIII–related antigen (rabbit polyclonal antibody; Dimension Labs, Mississauga, Ontario, Canada; 1:100 dilution) were performed on 4 μm-thick recut sections by using the avidin-biotin peroxidase technique. All tissues were counterstained with hematoxylin. A standard hematoxylin-eosin slide was also prepared from an adjacent slice of the fibroadenomas for classification purposes.

Fibroadenomas were classified by one of the investigators (M.M.) by using the three categories defined by Ohtani and Sasano (29)—myxoid, fibrocellular, and sclerosed—with the addition of two categories: mixed lesions containing both myxoid and fibrous characteristics (fibromyxoid) and lesions showing only cellular characteristics (cellular). Patient age, tumor diameter, tumor grade (Scarff-Bloom-Richardson criteria) (30), and lymph node status were obtained from the surgical pathology consultation report.

To evaluate the spatial distribution of capillaries and smaller arterioles and venules, microvessels smaller than 40 μm in diameter (31) were counted by using light microscopy on ×200 fields (×20 objective lens, ×10 ocular lens) by one of the investigators (M.M.). Vessel identification was performed according to the criteria used by Weidner et al (28). Any brown-staining, freestanding endothelial cell or group of endothelial cells was counted as a vessel.

Ten fields were chosen at random in both the central and peripheral regions of each tumor (provided there was sufficient

TABLE 2
Fibroadenomas: Clinical Data and Vessel Counts

Case No./Patient Age (y)	Tumor Diameter (cm)	Tumor Classification	Vessel Count per Field						Ratio of Mean in Periphery to Mean in Center
			Mean ± Standard Deviation			Range			
			Periphery	Center	Normal	Periphery	Center	Normal	
20/41	1.0	Fibromyxoid	34.9 ± 13.2	25.3 ± 5.68	43.6 ± 9.02	15–57	17–35	32–55	1.42
21/47	1.4	Fibromyxoid	33.1 ± 7.34	36.7 ± 10.0	79.6 ± 16.5	24–44	19–58	54–92	0.9
22/43	1.0	Cellular	112 ± 29.8	95.6 ± 24.4	133 ± 58.2	54–157	76–137	75–200	1.17
23/19	3.5	Cellular	35.2 ± 11.9	17.0 ± 4.81	55.0 ± 6.82	20–57	7–25	43–60	2.07
24/44	1.0	Fibrocellular	48.5 ± 13.0	53.4 ± 10.4	75.6 ± 13.3	29–68	40–67	60–96	0.91
25/27	0.6	Sclerosed	47.9 ± 9.75	40.8 ± 5.26	46.8 ± 5.93	31–65	32–46	37–52	1.17
26/38	0.6	Myxoid	51.7 ± 9.04	68.0 ± 19.8	98.2 ± 32.1	41–70	54–82	65–151	0.76
27/43	2.0	Cellular	39.3 ± 13.1	45.7 ± 12.6	110 ± 26.2	20–60	25–71	85–144	0.86
28/31	1.5	Sclerosed	39.1 ± 7.23	27.3 ± 8.96	75.7 ± 16.6	26–47	14–39	57–89	1.43
29/39	2.5	Fibrocellular	29.1 ± 11.0	18.0 ± 6.02	39.6 ± 8.85	15–50	7–27	28–51	1.62
30/49	1.0	Myxoid	40.4 ± 11.0	24.0 ± 9.90	99.2 ± 58.5	27–58	17–31	39–167	1.68
31/22	2.7	Cellular	24.7 ± 6.93	15.0 ± 0.0	53.2 ± 37.2	14–34	15	21–113	1.64
32/34	1.7	Fibromyxoid	30.7 ± 15.8	34.4 ± 12.3	59.2 ± 12.0	14–59	11–51	45–71	0.89
33/35	2.0	Sclerosed	37.4 ± 8.28	30.6 ± 14.1	0	22–50	15–58	0	1.22
34/21	1.1	Fibromyxoid	64.9 ± 12.0	64.6 ± 12.2	0	47–78	46–88	0	1.0
35/27	1.4	Myxoid	51.2 ± 8.89	45.8 ± 10.4	100 ± 49.2	41–65	29–63	54–152	1.12
36/37	1.2	Myxoid	50.8 ± 14.9	52.6 ± 11.5	50.5 ± 24.8	33–77	34–71	33–68	0.97
37/20	2.5	Fibromyxoid	37.0 ± 9.57	21.8 ± 8.47	96.8 ± 25.0	23–55	11–40	66–130	1.7
38/37	1.2	Myxoid	46.0 ± 18.0	30.8 ± 6.58	86.8 ± 19.8	23–75	19–38	55–102	1.49
39/47	1.2	Myxoid	65.0 ± 14.4	66.2 ± 13.9	146 ± 77.9	48–90	48–81	66–229	0.98

tissue). A peripheral field was defined as a field inside the tumor boundary (ie, an imaginary line connecting the most peripheral nests was considered the leading edge of invading cells in the case of invasive carcinomas) with the microscopic field circumference touching the boundary. A central field was defined as a microscopic field inside the tumor at least one ×200 field of view away from the boundary. Central fields were not defined in necrotic, avascular regions of the carcinomas; however, tumors containing necrosis were noted. For fibroadenomas, up to five fields of normal tissue adjacent to the lesion were also evaluated (provided there was sufficient normal tissue within the slide limits).

No tissue present on a carcinoma slide, regardless of histologic appearance, was considered normal (normal-appearing lobules from cancerous breasts have shown an angiogenic up-regulation when compared with lobules from noncancerous breasts [32]). Microvessels 40 μm or larger in diameter were also qualitatively evaluated on each slide.

Student *t* tests were performed for individual lesions to determine whether there was a statistically significant difference between the vessel density in the periphery and that in the lesion center. (A Student *t* test could not be performed on one fibroadenoma [case 31]; size permitted only one countable central field according to our criteria.) Ratios of mean peripheral to mean central vessel counts were calculated for each lesion, and *t* tests were performed to assess differences in vessel counts or in this ratio between invasive carcinomas and fibroadenomas and between carcinomas with lymph node involvement and carcinomas without lymph node involvement. One-way analyses of variance were performed to evaluate differences in vessel counts between the five categories of fibroadenomas and also between the three grades of invasive carcinomas (Scarff-Bloom-Richardson criteria [30]). In all cases, a significant difference was defined at P less than .01.

RESULTS

Mean vessel counts (vessel density within a ×200 field) and their standard deviations and ranges are shown in Tables 1 and 2 for invasive ductal carcinomas and fibroadenomas, respectively. Invasive ductal carcinomas ranged in diameter from 0.4 to 5.0 cm, while fibroadenomas ranged in diameter from 0.6 to 3.5 cm. The invasive ductal carcinomas could be categorized as follows: four (21%) grade I carcinomas, two without lymph node involvement and two in which no lymph node dissection was performed; 10 (53%) grade II carcinomas, five without lymph node involvement, three with lymph node involvement, and two in which no lymph node dissection was performed; and five (26%) grade III carcinomas, all with lymph node involvement. Classification of the fibroadenomas yielded six (30%) myxoid, five (25%) fibromyxoid, four (20%) cellular, two (10%) fibrocellular, and three (15%) sclerosed lesions. Large necrotic centers (ie, >30%–40% of the lesion was necrotic) were evident in two (10%) of 19 carcinomas (cases 7 and 10). In one of these tumors (case 10), the area of necrosis was surrounded by a prominent ring of small blood vessels. Smaller areas of partial necrosis (approximately 10%–15% of the lesion was necrotic) were observed within the lesion center in an additional eight (42%) of the 19 invasive ductal carcinomas.

The number of vessels in a ×200 field for the invasive ductal carcinomas ranged between 9 and 105 (mean, 31.4) for the peripheral and 4 and 57 (mean, 20.1) for the central fields. In previous vessel density studies, only areas of highest vascularization within the tumor (tumor hot spots) were selected for vessel counting (28,33,34). Maximum vessel counts for invasive ductal carcinomas in our study were within these reported ranges. For fibroadenomas, the range of vessel densities for the peripheral fields was 14–157 vessels (mean, 46.0 vessels) and that for the central fields was 7–137 vessels (mean, 40.7 vessels). Normal tissue surrounding the fibroadenomas (present in 18 of the 20 cases) had a range of 21–229 vessels (mean, 80.5 vessels) per field. In 16 (89%) of the 18 cases, vessel counts in normal tissue were significantly higher than those in fibroadenomas. It is interesting to note that the highest normal tissue vessel counts were found in three women aged 43–49 years, while the mean age of patients with fibroadenomas was 35 years. For these three women, the normal breast tissue was noticeably more vascular than that in other patients and was predominantly composed of dense lobular and ductal tissue, with little fatty tissue present.

Vessel counts for invasive ductal carcinomas are shown in Figure 1a; those for fibroadenomas are shown in Figure 1b (cases have been arranged on the x axis in order of increasing tumor diameter). Microvessel density was significantly higher ($P < .01$) in the tumor periphery than it was in the tumor center in 15 (79%) of the 19 invasive ductal carcinomas and in three (16%) of 19 fibroadenomas.

Figure 2 shows high magnification fields in the periphery (Fig 2a) and center (Fig 2b) of a typical invasive ductal carcinoma (case 13). In one of the four carcinomas in which no significant difference was found between peripheral and central vessel densities (case 18), the carcinoma consisted of many nests of carcinoma cells with distinctive rings of small vessels surrounding each of the nests. The mean ratio of peripheral to central vessel counts was 1.66 ± 0.46 (standard deviation; range, 0.95–2.57) and 1.25 ± 0.36 (range, 0.76–2.07) in invasive ductal carcinomas and fibroadenomas, respectively, and the ratios of peripheral to central vessel counts was significantly different between these groups ($P < .01$).

The individual peripheral versus central vessel density ratios for both groups of lesions are compared in Figure 3. No correlation was observed between mean peripheral counts, mean central counts, maximum peripheral counts, maximum central counts, or in the peripheral versus central vessel density ratios with carcinoma grade or lymph node status.

One-way analyses of variance performed between the maximum peripheral, maximum central, mean peripheral, and mean central counts of the fibroadenomas yielded no statistically significant difference ($P < .01$) in vessel densities between the five classifications. All three sclerosed fibroadenomas in our study had numerous blood vessels, comparable even to the number of vessels observed for the cellular and myxoid groups. An example of a sclerosed but highly vascularized fibroadenoma (case 28) is shown in Figure 4, and a typical cellular fibroadenoma (case 22) is shown in Figure 5 for comparison. There was also no correlation of any vascular parameters with patient age or tumor size for either fibroadenomas or carcinomas.

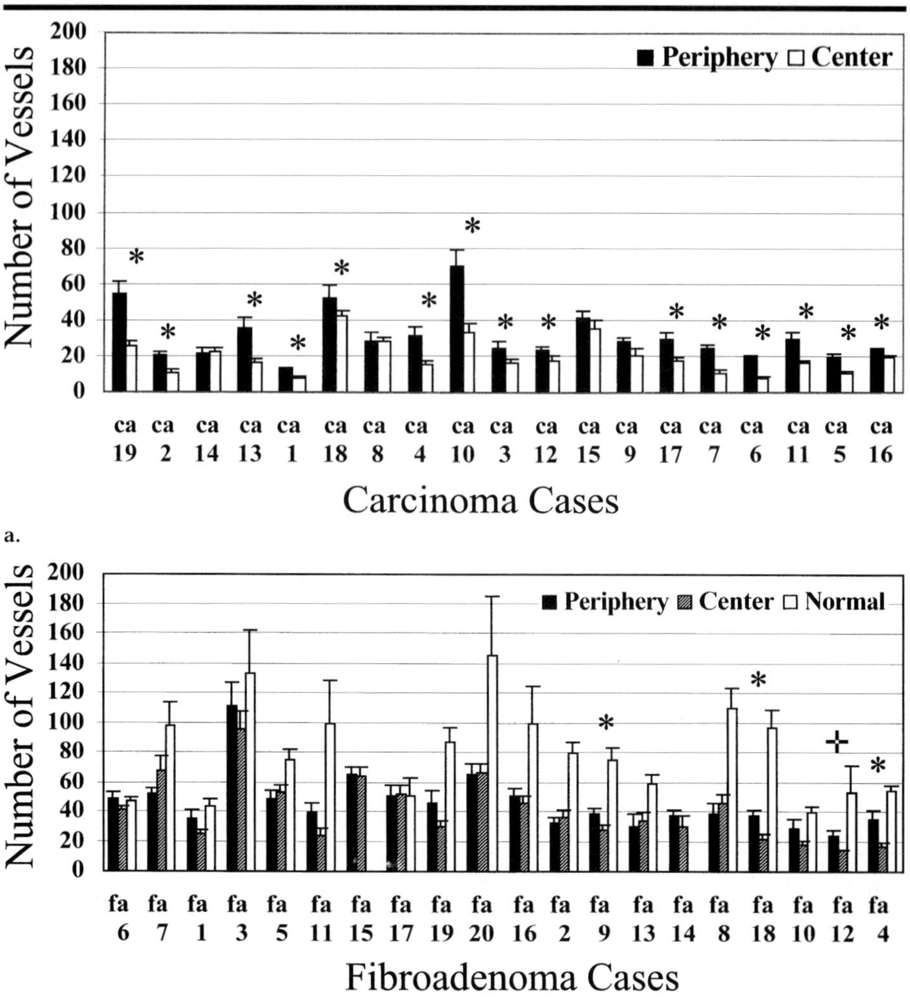

Figure 1. Mean vessel counts of lesions arranged in order of increasing tumor diameter. * = those cases in which the vessel density in the periphery was significantly greater than that in the center ($P < .01$). **(a)** Graph shows mean vessel counts in the peripheral and central fields of invasive ductal carcinomas (*ca*). **(b)** Graph shows mean vessel counts in the peripheral and central fields of fibroadenomas (*fa*) and mean vessel counts in the surrounding normal tissue. + = the fibroadenoma case in which only one central field was present and no statistical analysis could be performed. Fibroadenoma cases 1–20 correlate with cases 20–39 in Table 2 (eg, *fa* 1 = case 20 in Table 2, *fa* 2 = case 21).

In eight (42%) of the 19 invasive ductal carcinomas, vessels 40 μm or larger in diameter were observed just outside the leading edge of the tumor (Fig 6). In four (21%) of these cases, larger vessels could also be seen immediately inside the invading boundary. In five additional carcinomas (26%), a patch of larger vessels was observed within a peripheral field of a tumor. Larger vessels were not observed within the centers of any of the carcinomas in our study. In 10 (50%) of the 20 fibroadenomas, the presence of larger vessels was also noted. In six of these cases (30%), there were several large vessels present in the periphery of the lesion; while in two cases (10%), larger vessels in the periphery were abundant. In the remaining two fibroadenomas (10%), many large vessels were uniformly distributed throughout the lesion. These vessels were easily observed with low magnification.

DISCUSSION

We identified statistically significant overlap in microvessel counts between the invasive ductal carcinomas and fibroadenomas in our study. This finding may help explain the overlap in enhancement characteristics between invasive breast carcinomas and some fibroadenomas on contrast-enhanced MR imaging studies.

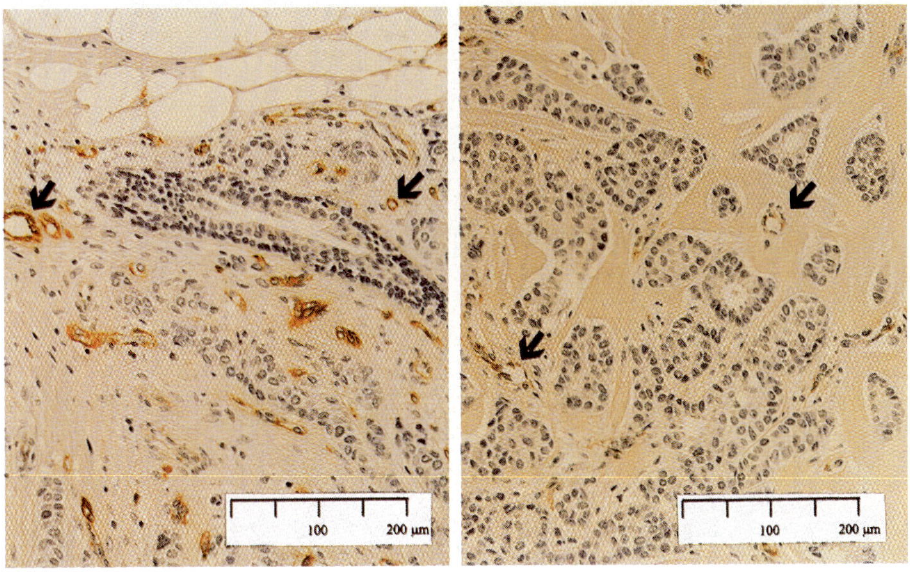

a. b.

Figure 2. Case 13. Typical invasive ductal carcinoma. **(a, b)** Pathologic slices show carcinoma in the **(a)** periphery and **(b)** center. (Stained for factor VIII–related antigen and counterstained with hematoxylin; original magnification, ×200.) In **a** and **b**, arrows show vessels outlined in brown (factor VIII–related antigen causes endothelial cells that line the lumen of the blood vessels to stain brown).

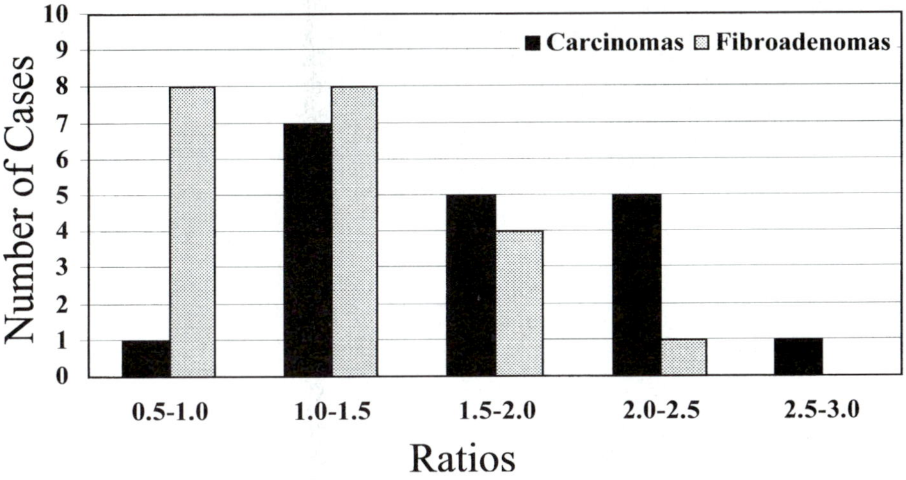

Figure 3. Histogram shows the distribution of mean peripheral versus mean central vessel count ratios for invasive ductal carcinomas and fibroadenomas.

Enhancement characteristics on a contrast-enhanced MR image reflect blood volume (microvessel density), blood flow, and vessel permeability, which are all vasculature characteristics that have been linked to tumor angiogenesis. The observed overlap in MR imaging enhancement curves and in microvessel density between carcinomas and fibroadenomas implies that the same processes may be controlling the vascular development in both of these classes of lesions.

It is possible that the numerous small vessels we observed in fibroadenomas may be the result of angiogenic stimulation initiated by the fibroadenoma. This hypothesis is also supported by the increased number of vessels 40 μm or larger observed in the periphery of the fibroadenomas, similar to the pattern of peripheral blood vessels known to be associated with angiogenesis in carcinomas (35). It is well known that premalignant lesions can induce angiogenesis, and it has been shown that benign breast tissue removed from a location distal to a carcinoma but within the same breast can induce new blood vessel formation in a rabbit corneal model (32,36). Therefore, it is not unrealistic to suggest that other benign breast diseases may also achieve an angiogenic state.

Our results support the observation that microvessel density is higher in the active tumor periphery of invasive ductal carcinomas than in the tumor center. These findings are consistent with contrast-enhanced MR imaging findings of rim enhancement in carcinomas. In the study by Buadu et al (25), rim-enhancing carcinomas were observed to have varying degrees of central desmoplasia, associated with lower vessel density. In the work of Orel et al (24), rim enhancement was observed in five of 16 carcinomas, but none of the rim-enhancing carcinomas exhibited central necrosis.

In our group of lesions, a significantly higher microvessel density was observed in the lesion periphery in 15 (79%) of the 19 invasive ductal carcinomas. Only two of these cases (cases 7 and 10) had well-defined necrotic cores, and, moreover, central fields were not defined within these avascular regions; rather, they were limited to areas of viable tumor. An additional eight cases had small necrotic regions within the tumor; however, only five of these had significantly higher peripheral vessel counts than central vessel counts. Although the mean microvessel density was significantly higher in peripheral fields than in central fields in most carcinomas in our sample, there was still considerable overlap between peripheral field counts and central field counts within each lesion. This may explain why the percentage of carcinomas reported to exhibit rim enhancement on MR images is much smaller than the percentage of lesions we found to have increased peripheral vessel density (24,25).

Vessel density in fibroadenomas was more uniform throughout the tumor than it was in carcinomas, with no statistically significant difference between periphery and center in 16 (84%) of 19 cases. Areas of increased vessel density did exist within fibroadenomas; however, these areas usually corresponded to a single or several lobules, within which a uniformly elevated distribution of blood vessels was observed. These results are in accord with the homogeneous MR imaging contrast-enhancement patterns observed for fibroadenomas and are suggestive of possible improvements in specificity that may result from the addition of the evaluation of morphologic features to an MR imaging examination (25,37,38).

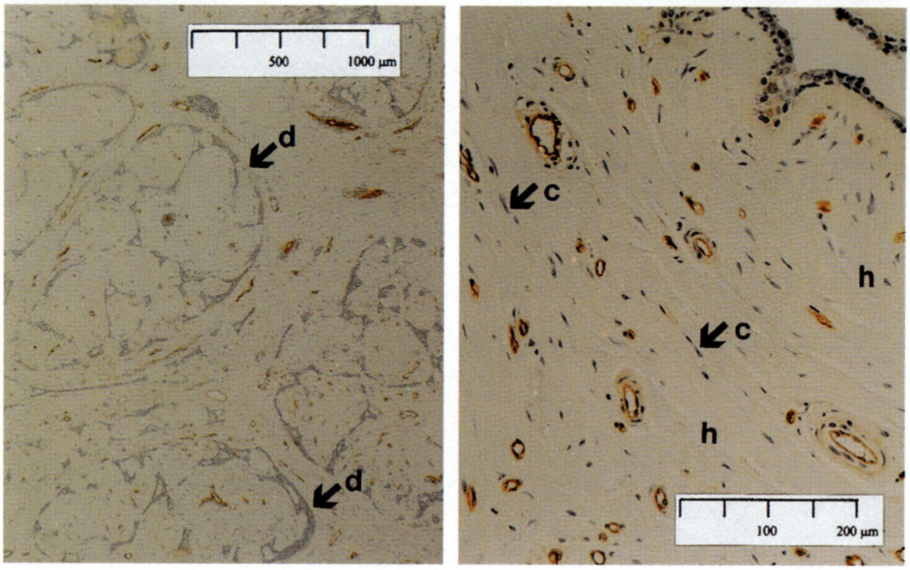

a. b.

Figure 4. Case 28. Pathologic slices show a sclerosed but highly vascularized fibroadenoma stained for factor VIII–related antigen and counterstained with hematoxylin. **(a)** Pathologic slice at ×40 magnification. **(b)** Part of a ×200 field in a pathologic slice. Salient features of this fibroadenoma stage are few stromal cells (*c* in **b**), hyalinized collagen fibers (*h* in **b**), and compressed ducts (*d* in **a**).

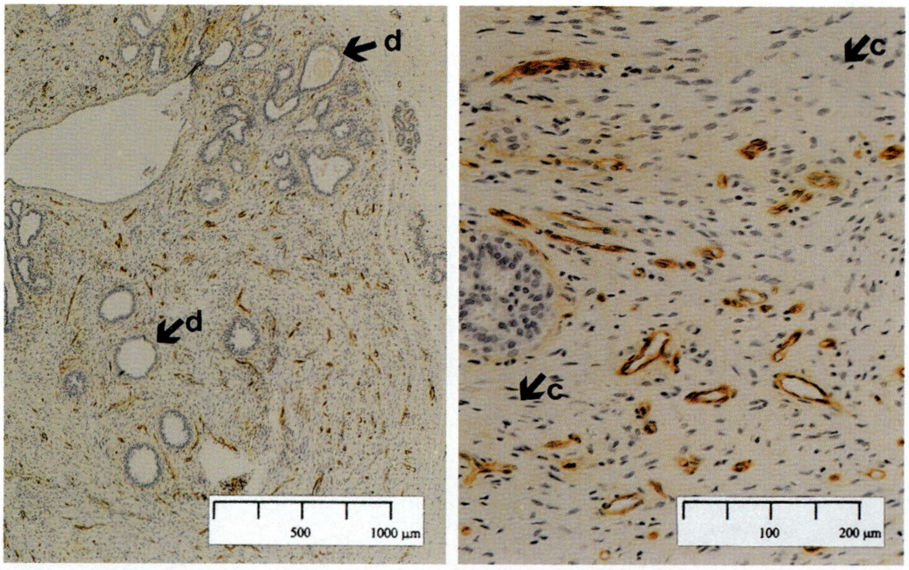

a. b.

Figure 5. Case 22. Pathologic slices show a typical cellular fibroadenoma stained for factor VIII–related antigen and counterstained with hematoxylin. **(a)** Pathologic slice at ×40 magnification. **(b)** Part of a ×200 field in a pathologic slice. Salient features of this fibroadenoma stage are high numbers of stromal cells (*c* in **b**) and open ducts (*d* in **a**).

Two authors (24,39) have compared contrast-enhancement characteristics with histologic findings in an attempt to explain the rapid, marked contrast material enhancement observed in some fibroadenomas. In these studies (24,39), nonsclerosed fibroadenomas enhanced strongly, but the enhancement of sclerosed fibroadenomas was highly variable, with some sclerotic lesions also exhibiting statistically significant rapid signal intensity increases. This finding was contrary to the expectation that sclerotic lesions, being acellular, would have fewer blood vessels than myxoid or cellular lesions. In the group of fibroadenomas in our study, no statistically significant decrease in the number of microvessels was observed in the three sclerotic lesions as compared to the number of microvessels in the cellular or myxoid category. Lesions in all these groups contained areas of low microvessel density and areas of high microvessel density, with no general trend observable with category; however, the number of fibroadenomas in each of our categories was small, and further investigation is required before any definite conclusions can be drawn.

Our observation of larger microvessels in the periphery of both carcinomas and fibroadenomas is consistent with the color Doppler US study by Kubek et al (18), in which a preponderance of detected blood flow near the peripheries of both malignant lesions and fibroadenomas was reported. This finding is not inconsistent with the fact that MR imaging rim enhancement is observed only in malignant lesions, since color Doppler US is sensitive to much larger vessels than is contrast-enhanced MR imaging, and our findings show that the spatial distribution of these larger vessels is different from that of smaller vessels. Two investigators (18,19) have reported that the number of vessels observed by using color Doppler US in fibroadenomas is increased with increasing lesion size. We have not noted any correlation between the number of vessels 40 µm or larger and fibroadenoma size. Very few vessels larger than 200 µm could be observed on a single slide; it was therefore not possible to conclude anything about the spatial distributions of Doppler-detectable vessels in our study.

Numerous investigators have established microvessel density in hot spots as an important prognostic indicator in breast carcinoma (28,40). Several authors have compared MR contrast-enhancement patterns with vessel density in hot spots; these investigations have been more directly relevant to assessing the applicability of MR to predicting disease outcome rather than to determining whether a lesion is malignant or benign. We have evaluated microvessel density over entire tumors to provide more pertinent information for using these noninvasive techniques for diagnostic applications. While most recent work in which US has been used to image breast carcinoma has focused on color Doppler US, substantial improvements in vessel detectability are expected with the use of intravenous US contrast material, and it is possible that sensitivity will be increased

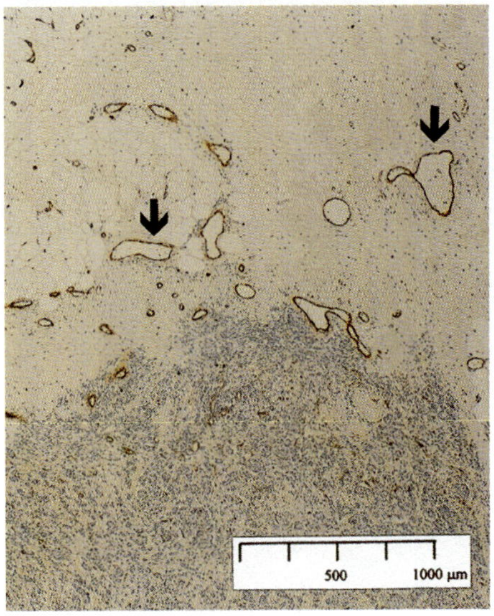

Figure 6. Case 7. Pathologic slice of an invasive carcinoma at ×40 magnification (stained for factor VIII–related antigen and counterstained with hematoxylin). Note the abundance of larger vessels (>200 μm; arrows) around the periphery.

to a level at which capillaries and other small microvessels will be visualized. Further gains in spatial resolution and vessel detectability with Doppler US and MR imaging will increase the potential for using these imaging modalities to identify tumor hot spots and noninvasively measure microvessel density.

While further histologic studies are necessary to evaluate vascular patterns in nonpalpable lesions, such as in atypical hyperplasia and carcinoma in situ, the results reported here suggest that the additional information on the spatial distribution of vessels and the ability to resolve vessel size may add valuable information to the diagnostic work-up of an indeterminate solid lesion. These examinations have important implications for younger women with palpable lesions, since diagnosis by using mammography is particularly unreliable in this age group and fibroadenomas are common.

Acknowledgment: The authors thank Elaine Hunter for assistance with photography.

References

1. Schmitt EL, Threatt B. Characteristics of breast cancer in an incident cancer population. AJR 1984; 143:402–406.
2. Xenophon L. Imaging techniques for breast disease. Clin Obstet Gynecol 1994; 37:933–943.
3. Baker LH. Breast cancer detection demonstration project: five-year summary report. CA Cancer J Clin 1982; 32:194–225.
4. Verbeek AL, Hendriks JH, Holland R, Mravunac M, Sturmans F, Day NE. Reduction of breast cancer mortality through mass screening with modern mammography: first results of the Nijmegen project, 1975-1981. Lancet 1984; 1:1222–1224.
5. Bassett LW, Kimme-Smith C. Breast sonography. AJR 1991; 156:449–453.
6. Jackson VP. The role of ultrasound in breast imaging. Radiology 1990; 177:305–309.
7. Jackman RJ, Nowels KW, Shepard MJ, Finkelstein SI, Marzoni FA. Stereotaxic large-core needle biopsy of 450 nonpalpable breast lesions with surgical correlation in lesions with cancer or atypical hyperplasia. Radiology 1994; 193:91–95.
8. Kopans DB. Caution on core. Radiology 1994; 193:325–328.
9. Williams SM, Kaplan PA, Petersen JC, Lieberman RP. Mammography in women under age 30: is there clinical benefit? Radiology 1986; 161:49–51.
10. Ciatto S, Cataliotti L, Distante V. Nonpalpable lesions detected with mammography: review of 512 consecutive cases. Radiology 1987; 165:99–102.
11. Furnival CM, Irwin JR, Gray GM. Breast disease in young women: when is biopsy indicated? Med J Aust 1983; 2:167–169.
12. Cant PJ, Madden MV, Coleman MG, Dent DM. Non-operative management of breast masses diagnosed as fibroadenoma. Br J Surg 1995; 82:792–794.
13. Heywang SH, Wolf A, Pruss E, Hilbertz T, Eiermann W, Permanetter W. MRI of the breast with Gd-DTPA: use and limitations. Radiology 1989; 171:95–103.
14. Burns PN, Halliwell M, Wells PN, Webb AJ. Ultrasonic Doppler studies of the breast. Ultrasound Med Biol 1982; 8:127–143.
15. Cosgrove DO, Bamber JC, Davey JB, McKinna JA, Sinnett HD. Color Doppler signals from breast tumors: work in progress. Radiology 1990; 176:175–180.
16. Dixon JM, Walsh J, Paterson D, Chetty U. Colour Doppler ultrasonography studies of benign and malignant breast lesions. Br J Surg 1992; 79:259–260.
17. Kaiser WA, Zeitler E. MRI of the breast: fast imaging sequences with and without Gd-DTPA—preliminary observations. Radiology 1989; 170:681–686.
18. Kubek KA, Chan L, Frazier TG. Color Doppler flow as an indicator of nodal metastasis in solid breast masses. J Ultrasound Med 1996; 15:835–841.
19. Holcombe C, Pugh N, Lyons K, Douglas-Jones A, Mansel RE, Horgan K. Blood flow in breast cancer and fibroadenoma estimated by colour Doppler ultrasonography. Br J Surg 1995; 82:787–788.
20. Flickinger FW, Allison JD, Sherry RM, Wright JC. Differentiation of benign from malignant breast masses by time-intensity evaluation of contrast enhanced MRI. Magn Reson Imaging 1993; 11:617–620.
21. Fearon ER, Vogelstein B. A genetic model for colorectal tumorigenesis. Cell 1990; 61:759–767.
22. Sato T, Akiyama F, Sakamoto G, Kasumi F, Nakamura Y. Accumulation of genetic alterations and progression of primary breast cancer. Cancer Res 1991; 51:5794–5799.
23. Dent DM, Cant PJ. Fibroadenoma. World J Surg 1989; 13:706–710.
24. Orel SG, Schnall MD, LiVolsi VA, Troupin RH. Suspicious breast lesions: MRI with radiologic-pathologic correlation. Radiology 1994; 190:485–493.
25. Buadu LD, Murakami J, Murayama S, et al. Breast lesions: correlation of contrast medium enhancement patterns on MR images with histopathologic findings and tumor angiogenesis. Radiology 1996; 200:639–649.
26. Frouge C, Guinebretiere JM, Contesso G, Di Paola R, Blery M. Correlation between contrast enhancement in dynamic magnetic resonance imaging of the breast and tumor angiogenesis. Invest Radiol 1994; 29:1043–1049.
27. Hulka CA, Smith BL, Sgroi DC, et al. Benign and malignant breast lesions: differentiation with echo-planar MR imaging. Radiology 1995; 197:33–38.
28. Weidner N, Semple JP, Welch WR, Folkman J. Tumor angiogenesis and metastasis: correlation in invasive breast carcinoma. N Engl J Med 1991; 324:1–7.
29. Ohtani H, Sasano N. Stromal cells of the fibroadenoma of the human breast. Virchows Arch 1984; 404:7–16.
30. Le Doussal V, Tubiana-Hulin M, Friedman S, Hacene K, Spyratos F, Brunet M. Prognostic value of histologic grade nuclear components of Scarff-Bloom-Richardson (SBR): an improved score modification based on a multivariate analysis of 1262 invasive ductal breast carcinomas. Cancer 1989; 64:1914–1921.
31. Less JR, Skalak TC, Sevick EM, Jain RK. Microvascular architecture in a mammary carcinoma: branching patterns and vessel dimensions. Cancer Res 1991; 51:263–273.
32. Jensen HM, Chen I, DeVault MR, Lewis AE. Angiogenesis induced by "normal" human breast tissue: a probable marker for precancer. Science 1982; 218:293–295.
33. Bosari S, Lee AKC, DeLellis RA, Wiley BD, Heatley GJ, Silverman ML. Microvessel quantitation and prognosis in invasive breast carcinoma. Hum Pathol 1992; 3:755–761.
34. Toi M, Kashitani J, Tominaga T. Tumour angiogenesis is an independent prognostic indicator in primary breast carcinoma. Int J Cancer 1993; 55:371–374.
35. Warren BA. The vascular morphology of tumors. In: Peterson HI, ed. Tumor blood circulation: angiogenesis, vascular morphology and blood flow of experimental and human tumors. Boca Raton, Fla: CRC, 1979; 1–48.
36. Ziche M, Gullino PM. Angiogenesis and neoplastic progression in vitro. J Natl Cancer Inst 1982; 69:483–487.
37. Brinck U, Fischer U, Korabiowska M, Jutrowski M, Schauer A, Grabbe E. The variability of fibroadenoma in contrast-enhanced dynamic MR mammography. AJR 1997; 168:1331–1334.
38. Nunes LW, Schnall MD, Orel SG, et al. Breast MR imaging: interpretation model. Radiology 1997; 202:833–841.
39. Heywang-Kobrunner SH, Haustein J, Pohl C, et al. Contrast-enhanced MR imaging of the breast: comparison of two different doses of gadopentetate dimeglumine. Radiology 1994; 191:639–646.
40. Gasparini G, Harris AL. Clinical importance of the determination of tumor angiogenesis in breast carcinoma: much more than a new prognostic tool. J Clin Oncol 1995; 13:765–782.

Sabine Huber, MD
Thomas Helbich, MD
Joachim Kettenbach, MD
Wolfgang Dock, MD
Ivan Zuna, PhD
Stefan Delorme, MD

Index terms:
Breast neoplasms, diagnosis, 00.30
Breast neoplasms, US, 00.12983
Computers, diagnostic aid
Microbubbles, 00.12988
Ultrasound (US), contrast media, 00.12988
Ultrasound (US), Doppler studies, 00.12983

Radiology 1998; 208:485–489

Abbreviations:
CPD = color pixel density
MCV = mean color value

[1] From the Department of Radiology, Lainz Hospital, Wolkersbergenstrasse 1, 1130 Vienna, Austria (S.H.); the Department of Radiology, University Hospital, Vienna, Austria (T.H., J.K., W.D.); and the Department of Oncologic Diagnostics and Therapy, German Cancer Research Center, Heidelberg, Germany (I.Z., S.D.). From the 1997 RSNA scientific assembly. Received October 7, 1997; revision requested December 16; revision received February 12, 1998; accepted March 27. Supported in part by Fond zur Foerderung der wissenschaftlichen Forschung grant no. J01280-MED and by the Ludwig Boltzmann Institute for Radiologic Tumor Research. **Address reprint requests to** S.H.

Author contributions:
Guarantors of integrity of entire study, S.H., S.D.; study concepts, S.H., S.D.; study design, S.H.; definition of intellectual content, S.D.; literature research, S.H.; clinical studies, S.H., J.K., T.H., W.D.; data acquisition, S.H., J.K.; data analysis, S.D.; statistical analysis, I.Z.; manuscript preparation, S.H.; manuscript editing, S.D.; manuscript review, S.H., T.H., J.K., W.D., I.Z., S.D.

Effects of a Microbubble Contrast Agent on Breast Tumors: Computer-assisted Quantitative Assessment with Color Doppler US—Early Experience[1]

PURPOSE: To evaluate objectively the effects of a microbubble contrast agent on the color Doppler ultrasound (US) examination of breast lesions.

MATERIALS AND METHODS: Forty-seven patients aged 23–71 years underwent color Doppler US before and after intravenous injection of a microbubble contrast agent. A 3-minute computer-assisted assessment of the color pixel density (CPD) was used to evaluate objectively the increase in the number of color Doppler US signals, the transit time of the microbubble bolus, and the potential additional differential diagnostic information.

RESULTS: Peak CPD at contrast agent–enhanced color Doppler US was 14.3% ± 8.1 (mean ± 1 standard deviation) for carcinomas and 9.3% ± 4.9 for benign lesions (P = .04). The time to peak enhancement was shorter in carcinomas (38 seconds ± 20) than in benign tumors (71 seconds ± 48, P = .02). Final CPD was close or equal to baseline values. With the median of 13% for peak CPD as a threshold, the sensitivity for this parameter was 55%, the specificity was 79%, and the accuracy was 62% (P = .04). For a median time to peak of 50 seconds, the sensitivity was 84%, the specificity was 57%, and the accuracy was 76%.

CONCLUSION: After microbubble contrast agent injection, carcinomas and benign lesions behave differently in degree, onset, and duration of Doppler US enhancement. High interindividual variability and temporal variations in the Doppler US signal still limit the value of these criteria for prospective diagnosis.

Findings in previous investigations have indicated that color Doppler ultrasound (US) can be used to demonstrate the characteristic features of neovascularization in malignant lesions (1–6). In cases in which signals are difficult to detect either because of small vessel size or inadequate equipment, intravascular contrast agents improve the detection of low-volume blood flow by increasing the signal-to-noise ratio. A recently developed galactose-based US contrast agent, SH U 508A (Levovist; Schering, Berlin, Germany), which contains microbubbles that are maintained during passage through the pulmonary vascular system, therefore providing systemic enhancement, has proved effective (7). The quantification of the increase in color Doppler US signals after the administration of SH U 508A in the cited study, however, relied only on descriptive criteria defined by the investigator, resulting in a subjective scoring system. Owing to the complexity of information contained in the color Doppler US image, objective quantification of enhancement dynamics is difficult, imprecise, and of unreliable reproducibility.

In this study, we attempted to quantify contrast agent enhancement by using image-based, computer-assisted analysis that has already proved useful in the assessment of unenhanced Doppler US studies of breast tumors (8). With this method, color pixel density (CPD) in a selected region of interest is quantified, and theoretic local flow velocities (mean

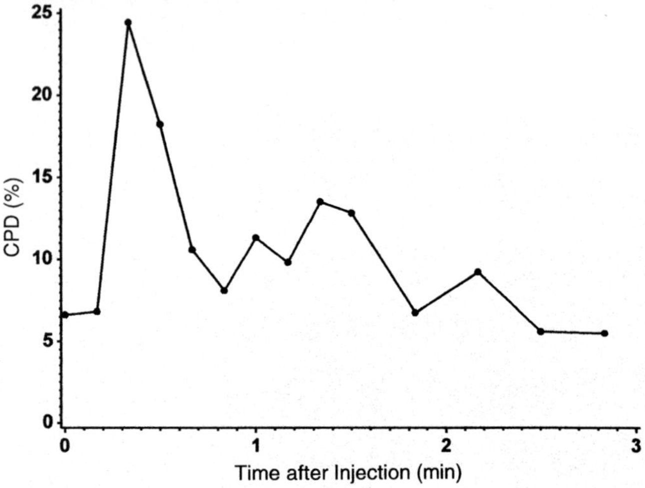

Figure 1. Graph of a typical time-CPD curve for a breast carcinoma shows an early, marked peak and early tapering.

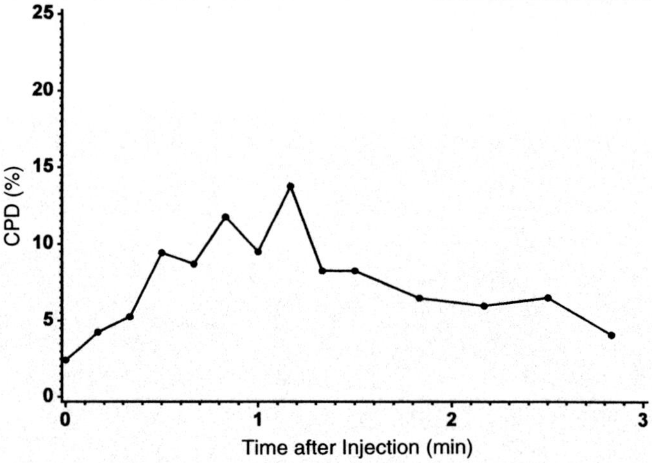

Figure 2. Graph of a typical time-CPD curve for a fibroadenoma shows weak and sluggish enhancement and slow decline in CPD.

color value [MCV]) are recalculated. Our intention was to determine whether the difference in enhancement between benign and malignant lesions reported by other authors (7) can be reproduced with an objective quantification tool. We therefore investigated (*a*) whether contrast agent–enhanced images are diagnostically more valuable than unenhanced images and (*b*) whether the enhancement kinetics in themselves carry additional information.

MATERIALS AND METHODS

Patients

Forty-seven patients aged 23–71 years who had palpable breast masses or suspicious mammographic findings at presentation were referred for Doppler US. Carcinomas were histologically confirmed in 31 patients aged 28–71 years (ductal invasive carcinoma in 28 patients, lobular invasive carcinoma in three), and benign disease was histologically confirmed in 16 patients aged 23–39 years (fibroadenoma in nine patients, suspicious areas of fibrocystic disease in seven). Histologic proof was obtained in all cases by means of excisional biopsy for all carcinomas, two fibrocystic breast changes, and three fibroadenomas. For the other benign lesions (six fibroadenomas and five fibrocystic disease cases), histologic proof was obtained by means of core biopsy. The diameter of lesions was 0.9–3.2 cm in carcinomas and 1.2–3.9 cm in benign lesions. All patients gave written informed consent, as approved by the hospital's research ethics committee.

US Unit

The mass or suspicious region was scanned by using a 7-MHz linear ATL Ultramark 9 scanner (Advanced Technology Laboratories, Bothell, Wash) that was operated at 5 MHz in the color Doppler US mode. Standard machine settings were used for color Doppler imaging to optimize the sensitivity to low-velocity and low-volume blood flow (wall filter, 50 Hz; dynamic range, 55 dB; spatial peak temporal averaged Doppler intensity, 43 mW/cm^2; persistence, 7; pulse repetition frequency, 1,000 Hz). The acquisition of color Doppler US data was limited to a region of interest (colored box) containing the tumor or suspicious region. Peripheral infiltration zones visible as hyperechoic rims were included, if present.

US Examination Procedure

All examinations were performed by two experienced examiners (S.H., J.K.). The breast was first scanned in B mode. The tumor or suspicious region was then studied with color Doppler US. Since no online frame-grabbing facility was available, images had to be recorded on super video home service, or S-VHS, videotapes. These tapes were mailed to our study cooperator (I.Z.) for frame grabbing and processing. At this facility, the selected video frame was grabbed and stored in a custom-developed digital format (9,10). Only frames apparently showing the systolic peak were selected. The frame-to-frame interval was approximately 10 seconds during the 1st minute and 20 seconds during the following minutes.

The transducer was attached to a tripod to maintain a constant probe position. Furthermore, the probe position was controlled by means of observation at the monitor. This method proved to be suitable for undisturbed color Doppler US examination and apparently was not affected by slight respiratory motion. The ultimate position, that which showed the most prominent vessels and color Doppler US signals, was selected after careful assessment of the whole tumor and adjacent tissue.

Before intravenous injection of the contrast agent, the tumor or suspicious region was assessed with color Doppler US and recorded for 10 seconds to obtain color Doppler US signals at the systolic maximum. We used the recommended dose of 10 mL of contrast agent at a concentration of 300 mg of galactose per milliliter, which was injected as a bolus at approximately 2 mL/sec by means of an 18-gauge plastic cannula inserted into a brachial vein and flushed with 10 mL of saline solution. For evaluation of the effects of the contrast agent, the video recording was started before injection and continued for 3 minutes (a time within which the intensity of the color Doppler US signals was judged subjectively to begin to return to the baseline level in all patients).

Image Acquisition and Evaluation, Statistical Analysis, and Definition of Parameters

We used a previously described method of computerized image capture and analysis (8–10). The red-green-blue output of the US scanner was frame-grabbed with an ITEX 768 CFG frame grabber (Imaging

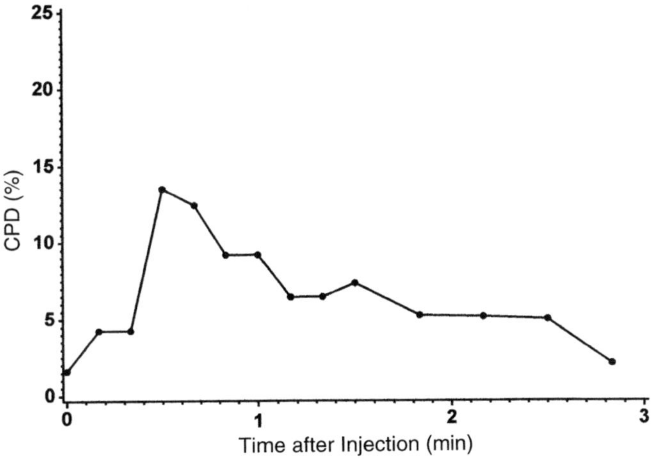

Figure 3. Graph of a typical time-CPD curve for a ductal invasive breast carcinoma. In contrast to that in Figure 1, the peak is early but less marked.

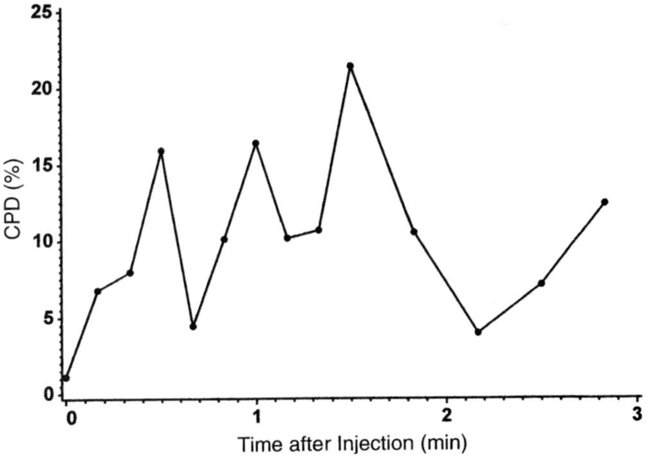

Figure 4. Graph of a typical time-CPD curve for fibrocystic disease. After the injection of the contrast agent, there are marked oscillations of the CPD; the ultimate peak is reached after approximately 100 seconds. It is apparent that one of the preceding smaller peaks might well have overridden the last one, thus determining the time of maximal CPD to approximately 30 seconds after injection.

Technology, Woburn, Mass) and digitized with an IBM-compatible personal computer. By matching the red and blue video levels of each image pixel with a color look-up table derived from the palette bar, color pixels of the stored image were identified and attributed to a corresponding flow velocity (assuming $\phi = 0°$ and neglecting the flow direction; velocity measured in centimeters per second), which is referred to as a "color value." In other words, the color value is the theoretic flow velocity in a given pixel, as determined by the position of its color on the color palette bar displayed with the image. The entire image was automatically scanned, and each pixel was classified as either gray-scale or color. Thereafter, it was stored in a modified format, with each color pixel characterized by its color value. For evaluation, the stored image was displayed on the screen, and a region of interest containing the tumor and excluding extratumoral vessels was defined. The percentage of color pixels in the region, or CPD, and the MCV were calculated for each region of interest.

In other terms, the system provides two parameters for quantitative assessment of the color Doppler US features of the lesion: How much color there is in the cross section and which color hues it contains. The amount of color is expressed by the percentage of the region of interest area occupied by color pixels (CPD) and is meant to describe the in vivo density of detectable vessels. The color hues are characterized by numeric descriptors (color values) for single pixels and by the MCV for the entire region of interest:

$$\mathrm{MCV} = \frac{1}{N}\sum_{i=1}^{N} |\mathrm{CV}_i|,$$

with CV as the color value in a given pixel and N as the number of color pixels in the region of interest. Since the color value of a pixel is defined as the flow velocity encoded by its color, the MCV is a parameter to globally express the flow velocities found in a cross section of a tumor. Since the Doppler angle cannot be accounted for, and, for example, aliasing and interpolation algorithms influence the color displayed, the MCV is a parameter not equivalent to, but determined by, flow velocities. It has been shown in phantom studies that the MCV is linearly correlated with flow velocities within a range mainly determined by the pulse repetition frequency used (9).

An almost identical method of automated semiquantitative evaluation of color Doppler US signals has been reported by Kedar et al (11). Calculation of the MCV in previous studies was performed with images grabbed from a three-channel red-green-blue video output (8–10). Since for this study we had to rely on videotape storage of images (which uses the single-channel output), only the CPD was available for analysis. The single-channel video signal quality is generally insufficient to ensure reliable color hue recognition and would cause flawed MCV measurements. The segmentation of the image, that is, the simple recognition of the presence of color, however, has in our experience proved to be reliable enough to calculate the CPD.

For each lesion, the mean and standard deviation of maximally achieved CPD and the time of maximum CPD and of CPD after 3 minutes were determined, and transit time curves were constructed. We also recorded the peak CPD, the lag between injection and peak, and the CPD at the end of recording (at 3 minutes) for each lesion. To assess sensitivity and specificity, the patient group was split by using the median value of the parameter in question as a threshold. To determine significance, we used the χ^2 test.

RESULTS

In carcinomas, there was typically early and marked enhancement, followed by a marked decline in CPD (Fig 1). Fibroadenomas (Fig 2) and fibrocystic disease showed markedly later enhancement, the peak CPD in fibroadenomas being lower than that in fibrocystic disease. In all cases, the CPD decreased at the end of recording. With regard to the shape of the time-CPD curve, however, deviations from these typical shapes described were noted as consisting, for example, of a more sluggish and weak enhancement in carcinomas (Fig 3) or in considerable variations in the measured value from frame to frame (Fig 4).

At baseline, the CPD did not differ significantly between carcinomas and benign lesions (Table). Peak CPD at contrast-enhanced color Doppler US was 14.3% ± 8.1 (mean ± 1 standard deviation) for carcinomas and therefore higher than that in all benign lesions, where only

9.3% ± 4.9 was reached (P = .04). The results were 8.4% ± 3.9 for fibroadenomas and 10.9% ± 6.6 for fibrocystic foci. The time elapsed to peak after injection was shorter in carcinomas (38 seconds ± 20) than in benign lesions (71 seconds ± 48, P = .02). At the end of the registration of color Doppler signals, the CPD was close to (in carcinomas and fibrocystic lesions) or equal to baseline values.

The median was 13% for the peak CPD. With all lesions with a peak CPD above median classified as malignant and all others as benign, the sensitivity for this parameter was 55% (55 of 100), the specificity was 79% (79 of 100), and the accuracy was 62% (62 of 100, P = .04). For the time to peak, the median was 50 seconds; thus, the sensitivity (all lesions below the median classified as malignant) was 84% (84 of 100), the specificity was 57% (57 of 100), and the accuracy was 76% (76 of 100). Neither baseline CPD, peak CPD, nor time to peak was correlated with patient age, tumor diameter, or tumor volume (calculated by means of a modified ellipsoid formula [8]).

Mean Baseline CPD, Peak CPD, and Time to Peak after Injection of Contrast Agent

Neoplasm	Baseline CPD (%)	Peak CPD (%)	Final CPD (%)	Time to Peak (sec)
Carcinoma	4.7 ± 6.6	14.3 ± 8.1	6.3 ± 7.6	38 ± 20
All benign lesions	2.7 ± 2.4	9.3 ± 4.9	3.4 ± 3.2	71 ± 48
Fibroadenoma	2.5 ± 1.1	8.4 ± 3.9	2.5 ± 2.1	73 ± 48
Fibrocystic disease	3.1 ± 4.0	10.9 ± 6.6	5.0 ± 4.5	68 ± 52

Note.—Values are expressed as the mean ± 1 standard deviation.

DISCUSSION

Findings of previous investigations with contrast-enhanced US of solid breast lesions indicate that microbubble contrast agents improve the detection of characteristic neovascular morphologic features by enhancing the signal strength in small vessels (7). The related investigations were reliant on the subjective assessment of tape-recorded examinations. Timing the transit of a bolus of contrast agent forms a new category of dynamic features for US. In a variety of examinations, however, we found it difficult to determine reliably the time to peak signal enhancement and the time of the decline of signal enhancement solely by reviewing the tapes. In our experience, the estimation by different readers may differ by as much as 60 seconds (S.D., unpublished observations, 1997). Therefore, we decided to use a method of computer-assisted quantification of color Doppler US signals to evaluate objectively the increase in the CPD and the transit time of the microbubble bolus. This method has already proved useful in unenhanced color Doppler studies (8).

Because of the known mechanism of SH U 508A, the amount of color, expressed as CPD, should increase in vascularized lesions. Color values, however, should remain grossly unchanged because the arrival of contrast agent will not affect the flow velocities in the lesion. Although the MCV might be of even higher diagnostic value than the CPD (8), this parameter was unfortunately not available for sensible analysis, owing to the mode of data transfer (see Materials and Methods). All examinations were performed in conventional Doppler mode because power Doppler mode was not available on the platform.

We found that at baseline, the in vivo vessel density displayed with color Doppler US, as expressed in terms of CPD, did not differ between benign and malignant lesions. After the injection of contrast agent, however, the peak CPD proved to be higher in malignant than in benign tumors. After injection, the peak was reached earlier in carcinomas than in fibroadenomas or fibrocystic disease. Definite pathophysiologic conclusions related to tumor hemodynamics are difficult to draw from these data for a variety of factors that influence the findings. The initial arrival ("first pass") of contrast agent causes an excessive broadening of color areas, known as "blooming" (12), which occurs within the 1st minutes after the local arrival of contrast agent. This phenomenon may well be common in carcinomas (a finding consistent with our own visual experience), thus contributing to the early peak described above. Furthermore, a shadowing phenomenon (ie, an initial decrease in the number of color signals owing to signal attenuation by highly concentrated contrast agent) may also play a role (13). Finally, other features, such as the presence of arteriovenous shunts, may also influence the findings (14).

Other authors have reported longer persistence of enhancement in malignant lesions, up to a mean of approximately 5 minutes. In this study, baseline CPD was almost reached after 3 minutes. In contrast to previous studies, however, in this study the decline in CPD (directly after the peak) began earlier in carcinomas than in benign lesions. Although these different observations may be due to the composition of the patient sample, the different means of assessment (image-based, computerized quantification versus subjective estimation) may play a role. It might be tempting to compare the shape of the CPD curve with familiar enhancement curves in dynamic magnetic resonance imaging (15–18). The fundamentally different distribution of the applied contrast agent, however, prohibits any consideration beyond the question of whether findings are basically compatible.

To summarize, the data presented support the subjective impression that benign and malignant tumors of the breast behave differently at US in both degree and dynamics of enhancement after the injection of a contrast agent. In light of the different age distributions among patients with benign and malignant lesions, one must consider that circulatory differences in different age populations might bear on the results. Since malignant lesions are more common in older women and benign lesions in younger female patients, part of this age variation might simply reflect the realities of clinical practice.

Considering the complex shape of some time-CPD curves, it becomes clear, however, that it will be difficult to predict in a given case whether the lesion is benign or malignant. Characteristic curves as shown in Figures 1 and 2 are easy to interpret, and even weaker enhancement may be indicative of malignancy if an unambiguous, early peak can be identified (Fig 3). The shape of the curve in Figure 4, however, shows that estimation of the time to peak may be extremely unreliable, even with objective methods like those used in this study. This finding considered, we believe that mere subjective judgment is entirely unsuitable for this purpose.

If quantitative analysis of enhancement over time is to make sense, mathematic smoothing procedures must be applied. Unfortunately, the image acquisition frequency available to date is still too low to allow sensible smoothing.

Therefore, future development will be directed at devising methods for online, real-time image storage and analysis.

References

1. Dixon JM, Walsh J, Paterson D, Chetty U. Colour Doppler ultrasonography studies of benign and malignant breast lesions. Br J Surg 1992; 79:259–260.
2. Cosgrove DO, Bamber JC, Davey JB, McKinna JA, Sinnet HD. Color Doppler signals from breast tumors. Radiology 1990; 176:175–180.
3. Cosgrove DO, Kedar RP, Bamber JC, et al. Breast diseases: color Doppler US in differential diagnosis. Radiology 1993; 189:99–104.
4. Madjar H, Prömpeler H, Sauerbrei W, Wolfarth R, Pfleiderer A. Color Doppler flow criteria of breast lesions. Ultrasound Med Biol 1994; 20:849–858.
5. Delorme S, Anton HW, Knopp MV, et al. Breast cancer: assessment of vascularity by color Doppler. Eur Radiol 1993; 3:253–257.
6. Sohn C, Stolz W, Grischke EM, Wallwiener D, Bastert G, von Fournier D. Die Dopplersonographische untersuchung von mammatumoren mit hilfe der farbdopplersonographie, der duplexsonographie und des CW-Dopplers. Zentralbl Gynäkol 1992; 114:249–253.
7. Kedar RP, Cosgrove D, McCready VR, Bamber JC, Carter ER. Microbubble contrast agent for color Doppler US: effect on breast masses—work in progress. Radiology 1996; 198:679–686.
8. Huber S, Delorme S, Knopp MV, et al. Breast tumors: computer-assisted quantitative assessment with color Doppler US. Radiology 1994; 192:797–801.
9. Delorme S, Weisser G, Zuna I, et al. Quantitative characterization of color Doppler images: reproducibility, accuracy and limitations. JCU 1995; 23:537–550.
10. Fein M, Delorme S, Weisser G, Zuna I, van Kaick G. Quantification of color Doppler for the evaluation of tissue vascularization. Ultrasound Med Biol 1995; 21:1013–1019.
11. Kedar RP, Cosgrove DO, Bamber JC, Bell DS. Automated quantification of color Doppler signals: a preliminary study in breast tumors. Radiology 1995; 197:39–43.
12. Forsberg F, Liu JB, Burns PN, Merton DA, Goldberg BB. Artifacts in ultrasonic contrast agent studies. J Ultrasound Med 1994; 13:357–365.
13. Bos LJ, Piek JJ, Spaan AE. Effects of shadowing on the time-intensity curves in contrast echocardiography: a phantom study. Ultrasound Med Biol 1996; 22:217–227.
14. Vaupel P. Durchblutung und mikrozirkulation in malignen tumoren (abstr). Zentralbl Radiol 1991; 143:707.
15. Boetes C, Barentsz JO, Mus RD, et al. MR characterization of suspicious breast lesions with a gadolinium-enhanced Turboflash subtraction technique. Radiology 1994; 193:777–781.
16. Barentsz JO, Jager GJ, van Vierzen PBJ, et al. Staging urinary bladder cancer after transurethral biopsy: value of fast dynamic contrast-enhanced MR imaging. Radiology 1996; 201:135–193.
17. Verstraete KL, De Deene Y, Roels H, Dierick A, Uyttendale D, Kunnen M. Benign and malignant musculoskeletal lesions: dynamic contrast-enhanced MR imaging—parametric "first-pass" images depict tissue vascularization and perfusion. Radiology 1994; 192:835–843.
18. Knopp MV, Hoffmann U, Brix G, Hawighorst H, Junkermann H, van Kaick G. Schnelle MR-kontrastmitteldynamik zur charakterisierung von tumoren. Radiologe 1995; 35:964–972.

Book Review

Radiographic Anatomy and Positioning: An Integrated Approach

Andrea Gauthier Cornuelle, MS, RT(R), and Diane H. Gronefeld, MEd, RT(R)

Stamford, Conn: Appleton & Lange, 1998. ISBN 0-8385-8238-9. Hardcover, $95.00; pp 508; 895 figures; tables.

Applications Manual for Radiographic Anatomy and Positioning

Diane H. Gronefeld, MEd, RT(R), and Mary L. Madigan, RT(R)(M)

Stamford, Conn: Appleton & Lange, 1998. ISBN 0-8385-8247-8. Softcover, $29.95; pp 312; 94 figures.

Competency Manual for Radiographic Anatomy and Positioning

Andrea Gauthier Cornuelle, MS, RT(R)

Stamford, Conn: Appleton & Lange, 1998. ISBN 0-8385-8239-7. Softcover, $29.95; pp 324; 139 figures; tables.

Pocket Manual for Radiographic Anatomy and Positioning

Andrea Gauthier Cornuelle, MS, RT(R), Diane H. Gronefeld, MEd, RT(R), and Mary L. Madigan, RT(R)(M)

Stamford, Conn: Appleton & Lange, 1998. ISBN 0-8385-8237-0. Softcover, $21.95; pp 300; 145 figures.

Radiographic Anatomy and Positioning: An Integrated Approach is a series of books designed to work together to provide radiography students with a survey of standard radiographic procedures, as well as procedures related to mammography and the cardiovascular system. These books can be used in radiographic procedures courses. All the authors are registered radiologic technologists and are in the educational field.

This book contains 18 chapters, one of which is an introduction to the entire radiographic process. Topics of other chapters include the skeletal and respiratory systems, contrast material–enhanced studies, mammography, and the cardiovascular system. Each chapter typically includes sections on anatomy, procedural considerations, and radiographic positioning. In addition, topics for critical thinking and application, as well as images for critique with questions, are included. Related terminology is defined in appropriate chapters.

The *Applications Manual* is a student workbook that provides positioning worksheets for coloring and labeling, fill-in-the-blank study questions, and case studies. The *Competency Manual* details each position in a step-by-step manner and provides a checklist for use by the instructor. The *Pocket Manual,* for clinical use, provides a brief description of each position along with a photograph that demonstrates correct positioning, centering, and collimation.

Radiographic Anatomy and Positioning: An Integrated Approach is well organized, is clearly written, and includes all of the radiographic procedures one would expect in basic procedures classes. The book is of very good quality and contains excellent photographs and duplicate side-by-side radiographs, with the salient anatomic information outlined in color on one side. The anatomic drawings—which are shaded and in which color is used to give the appearance of depth—though attractive, do not seem to provide as much detail as standard drawings. The related medical terminology is helpful, and the radiograph critique and critical thinking questions are well written and a good challenge for the student.

The *Applications Manual* and the *Competency Manual* seem to have a more limited value than *Radiographic Anatomy and Positioning: An Integrated Approach.* The *Applications Manual,* a student workbook, devotes almost two-thirds of the book to simple line drawings of radiographic anatomy to be colored and labeled by the student, and it provides a full page to rewrite the key information about performing the position. These pages may be helpful to the student learning the material, but the amount of time needed to color and label each full-page diagram and detail the examination seems prohibitive. Study questions use the fill-in-the-blank format, which provides a limited method of self-testing. The *Competency Manual* may be of use to the new instructor, as it provides a step-by-step task analysis of each position in a checklist format, but the experienced instructor may find it cumbersome; filling out three forms for one examination may be required. In addition, these forms do not include any references to patient approach and handling, an important aspect of procedures.

The *Pocket Manual* provides basic information, with accompanying photographs, on the most common positions included in *Radiographic Anatomy and Positioning: An Integrated Approach.* Space is provided for the student to write notes and sample technical factors. The photographs in this book are the same as those in *Radiographic Anatomy and Positioning: An Integrated Approach,* and they provide clear information about each position discussed. However, the written material is often cursory and will possibly require the student to fill in details. No radiographs are included in the *Pocket Manual.*

Radiographic Anatomy and Positioning: An Integrated Approach provides a solid alternative for use in radiographic procedures classes. In particular, it includes an attractive, appealing, clear-cut approach to the material, along with some extras such as the related terminology and the outlined radiographic anatomy. However, the supplementary books provide less than optimal support for *Radiographic Anatomy and Positioning: An Integrated Approach.* The series is reasonably priced, but it is more limited in the material presented. Instructors of basic radiographic procedures, especially if dissatisfied with their current textbooks, should take a look at this series for possible adoption.

Reviewed by Elizabeth L. Meixner, RT(R)(MR)

S. Nahum Goldberg, MD
Peter F. Hahn, MD, PhD
Francis J. McGovern, MD
Robert M. Fogle, BA
Peter R. Mueller, MD
G. Scott Gazelle, MD, MPH

Benign Prostatic Hyperplasia: US-guided Transrectal Urethral Enlargement with Radio Frequency—Initial Results in a Canine Model[1]

Index terms:
Prostate, hyperplasia, 841.316, 844.316
Prostate, therapeutic radiology, 841.12112, 841.1234, 841.1269, 841.12989, 844.12112, 844.1234, 844.1269, 844.12989
Prostate, US, 841.12989, 844.12985, 844.12989
Radiofrequency (RF) ablation, 841.1269, 844.1269

Radiology 1998; 208:491–498

Abbreviations:
BPH = benign prostatic hyperplasia
RF = radio frequency
RUG = retrograde urethrography
TURP = transurethral resection of the prostatic urethra

[1] From the Departments of Radiology (S.N.G., P.F.H., R.M.F., P.R.M., G.S.G.) and Urology (F.J.M.), Massachusetts General Hospital, Harvard Medical School, Fruit St, Boston, MA 02114. Received October 15, 1997; revision requested December 23; revision received January 30, 1998; accepted March 4. Supported in part by a grant from Radionics. S.N.G. was a 1997 Cesare Gianturco/RSNA Fellow supported by the Cook Group. **Address reprint requests to** S.N.G.

PURPOSE: To enlarge the prostatic urethra with thermal coagulation with transrectal radio-frequency (RF) application in dogs.

MATERIALS AND METHODS: Eight aged dogs underwent RF ablation of periurethral prostatic tissue for 6 minutes. Eighteen-gauge electrodes were placed into the periurethral tissues with a transrectal approach and ultrasound (US) guidance. Prostatic and rectal temperatures were measured during RF application. US, conventional and computed tomographic (CT) retrograde urethrography (RUG), and CT were performed immediately (n = 8) and at 3–96 days (n = 6) after ablation. Histopathologic analysis was performed at sacrifice immediately (n = 2), at 28 days (n = 2), or at 3 months (n = 4) after treatment.

RESULTS: All procedures were successful with no complications and were performed in less than 30 minutes. Rectal mucosal temperature did not exceed 38°C. Immediately after treatment, CT and US demonstrated 1.2-cm foci of altered periurethral tissue that corresponded to solid coagulated tissue at histopathologic analysis. By day 3, CT, RUG, and US demonstrated that these foci had begun to cavitate, resulting in enlargement of the urethra. Complete cavitation was demonstrated by day 28. Minimal reduction in the degree of urethral enlargement was noted by day 60, but narrowing, urethral strictures, or fistulas were not observed at 3 months. At histopathologic analysis, focal cavitary enlargement with at least doubling of the urethral diameter and with normal urothelium was noted in all dogs surviving at least 28 days.

CONCLUSION: Transrectal RF urethral enlargement is feasible and safe in animals and merits investigation for alleviating urethral obstruction due to benign prostatic hyperplasia.

Benign prostatic hyperplasia (BPH) is a common affliction of elderly men. If untreated, this condition can lead to urinary retention, renal failure, and urosepsis. The mainstay of therapy for BPH is surgical transurethral resection of the prostatic urethra (TURP), as removal of excess prostatic tissue improves voiding and bladder emptying (1). This operation is performed nearly 400,000 times annually in the United States, and associated expenses are approximately $5 billion per year (2). Medical therapies, including androgen-deprivation therapy, inhibition of 5α-reductase activity, and the use of α-adrenergic antagonistic drugs, relieve urinary retention in some cases, but medical therapy fails and surgical TURP is ultimately required in a substantial number of cases. Because of the limitations of medical therapy and the expense of TURP, newer, minimally invasive methods for prostatic tissue ablation have been developed, including transurethral laser (3,4), microwave (5,6), and radio-frequency (RF) (7–11) ablation.

RF tissue ablation has been shown to produce a limited and reliably controlled volume of tissue destruction in cadaveric, animal, and human prostatic tissue (7–14). RF ablation results in tissue destruction by producing cytotoxic temperatures in precisely controlled volumes of tissue (15). Several investigators (8–11,13) have treated patients with moderate

Author contributions:
Guarantors of integrity of entire study, S.N.G., G.S.G.; study concepts, S.N.G., P.F.H., F.J.M., G.S.G.; definition of intellectual content, S.N.G., F.J.M., G.S.G.; literature research, S.N.G.; experimental studies, S.N.G., P.F.H., R.M.F.; data acquisition, S.N.G., R.M.F.; data analysis, S.N.G., R.M.F., P.F.H., G.S.G.; manuscript preparation, S.N.G.; manuscript editing, S.N.G., P.F.H., F.J.M., G.S.G.; manuscript review, S.N.G., P.F.H., F.J.M., P.R.M., G.S.G.

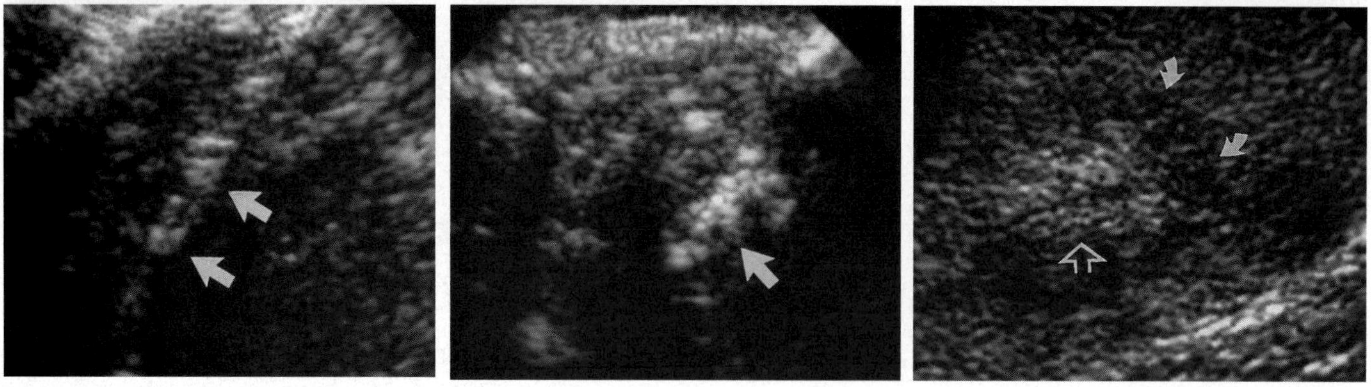

a. b. c.

Figure 1. US appearance during and immediately after transrectal RF ablation of the prostate. **(a)** US scan obtained after transrectal insertion of an 18-gauge electrode (arrows) into the prostate. **(b)** US scan shows that an irregularly shaped echogenic area (arrow) surrounds the electrode during RF application. **(c)** US scan obtained within 15 minutes of the procedure shows an 0.8-cm-diameter echogenic central region (open arrow) that surrounds the electrode track. A concentric, peripheral hypoechoic rim (solid arrows) also is seen. The overall diameter of the area with altered echogenicity measures 1.5 cm.

to severe prostatism by ablating prostatic tissue with placement of RF electrodes by using a transurethral approach. Improvement (50%–80% increase) in peak urinary flow and a 50%–80% decrease in prostatism symptom scores were documented in 60%–80% of patients 6 months after the procedure (9–11,13). In the remaining patients, failure of this technique to improve prostatism symptoms has often been attributed to "insufficient needle deployment" and to "undertreatment" (ablation of an insufficient amount of prostatic tissue) (9).

Imaging-guided percutaneous RF ablation has been used by interventional radiologists to treat osteoid osteomas (16), cerebral tumors (17), hepatic metastases (18–21), and hepatocellular carcinoma (18). In these studies, thin, insulated, metallic probes similar to biopsy needles are inserted percutaneously into the lesion by using computed tomographic (CT), magnetic resonance (MR) imaging, or ultrasonographic (US) guidance. These procedures are similar to US-guided transrectal prostate biopsy. We hypothesized that this type of real-time imaging guidance might aid in proper placement of RF electrodes in the periurethral prostatic tissue. The goal of this study was therefore to develop a method of enlarging the prostatic urethral channel by using transrectal RF application and to assess the feasibility, safety, and long-term sequelae of the procedure in a canine model.

MATERIALS AND METHODS

Studies were performed with the approval of the institutional subcommittee for research animal care. Eight aged, noncastrated, mongrel male dogs (7–12 years old) were used for this study. All procedures and follow-up diagnostic imaging were performed after the administration of a general anesthetic regimen (atropine sulfate [Phoenix Pharmaceuticals, St Joseph, Mo; 0.02–0.05 mg per kilogram of body weight administered intramuscularly] and propofol [Diprivan; Zeneca Pharmaceuticals, San Paolo, Italy; 6 mg/kg administered intravenously]). Halothane gas (Fluothane; Wyeth-Ayerst Laboratories, Philadelphia, Pa) was initially administered at 2% air flow by using a halothane vaporizer and a 2-L oxygen and room air carrier and was subsequently titrated to adequate anesthetic effect (1%–1.5% gas flow). To reduce the risk of infection, gentamicin sulfate (Fugisawa USA, Deerfield, Ill; 1–1.5 mg/kg) was administered intramuscularly before the procedure. The back of each animal was shaved, and a grounding pad was placed in contact with this area. Each animal had an 8-F catheter (Argyl tube; Sherwood Medical, St Louis, Mo) inserted through the urethra into the bladder.

RF Treatment

Experiments were performed by using a monopolar, 500-kHz RF generator (model 3-D; Radionics, Burlington, Mass). Monitoring capabilities for temperature, tissue impedance, and wattage are incorporated into the generator circuitry. Eighteen-gauge RF electrodes were constructed. The shafts of the electrodes were electrically insulated by coating the needle shaft with a thin layer of acrylic resin. The distal 0.5–1.0-cm part of the electrode was not coated, enabling focal RF deposition at the exposed metallic tip. Thermistors were embedded at the tip of the electrode and at 5, 10, and 15 mm from the tip. This enabled monitoring of temperatures not only at the site of ablation, but also within the periphery of the prostate and at the rectal mucosa.

Transrectal US of the prostate was performed by using B-mode scanning (model 128XP/10; Acuson, Mountain View, Calif) and an endocavitary, 7.5-MHz transducer (Acuson). After localization of the urethra, an RF electrode was inserted into the periurethral, intraprostatic tissue either unilaterally or bilaterally by using the transrectal approach (Fig 1). The urethra was easily identified by means of the anechoic urethral catheter. The RF electrode tip was then positioned 3–7 mm from the urethra by using the electronic biopsy-guide mode. Once proper electrode positioning was ascertained and before each RF application, the urethral catheter was withdrawn below the level of the prostate to prevent melting of the catheter during the ablation.

The electrode was connected to the RF generator. Five animals had an RF application in both the right and left periurethral tissues, and three animals had a single RF application, for a total of 13 RF applications. For each electrode placement, RF was applied for 6 minutes, with generator output adjusted to maintain a tip temperature of 90°C ± 2 (standard deviation; with ramping of the temperature to 90°C requiring no more than 60 seconds). Parameters were selected on the basis of previous use of these setting in other tissues to demonstrate maximal tissue coagulation without charring (22,23). During the procedure, the dogs were monitored for signs of distress or discomfort. Temperatures at the tip and along the shaft of the electrode, tissue impedance, and wattage were recorded at baseline and at 60-second intervals throughout the procedure. After the procedure, the RF electrode and urethral catheter were removed.

Postprocedural Animal Care

The first two dogs were selected as nonsurvival animals and were euthanized immediately after the postprocedural diagnostic imaging (described below) with an overdose (100 mg/kg) of pentobarbital sodium (Somlethal; Anpro Pharmaceutical, Arcadia, Calif) administered intravenously. The six surviving animals were allowed to recover. Animals were monitored clinically twice daily for the 1st postprocedural week and daily thereafter. Gentamicin sulfate (Fugisawa USA; total dose, 80 mg) was administered intramuscularly twice daily for 3 postprocedural days. All animals were given buprenex hydrochloride (Norwich Eaton, Norwich, NY; 0.1–0.3 mg/kg) every 12 hours for the first 24 hours after the procedure to minimize pain and duress. Two animals were euthanized at 28 days, and four were sacrificed at 90 days after the RF ablation.

Postprocedural Diagnostic Imaging Follow-up

To assess and characterize the imaging findings of in situ thermal coagulation in the prostate during the hyperacute, acute, subacute, and chronic phases of tissue response and repair, follow-up diagnostic imaging was performed. Immediately after the procedure, repeat transrectal US was performed in all eight animals to assess for changes in prostatic appearance. Additional postprocedural studies included CT of the pelvis without and with contrast material enhancement, conventional retrograde urethrography (RUG), and CT RUG. CT and conventional and CT RUG also were performed in all six surviving animals at 3, 10–14, and 21–28 days after the procedure and also in the four dogs surviving for longer periods at 42–63 days and 84–96 days. Follow-up US was performed at these time points only in the four dogs that had been selected for survival beyond 84 days.

Transrectal US was performed as described above. All CT and RUG examinations were performed by using a combined CT and fluoroscopy table (model TCT-900S/XII; Toshiba, Tokyo, Japan). Axial CT images were acquired with and without the intravenous administration of iohexol 350 (Omnipaque 350; Nycomed, Princeton, NJ; 2 mL/kg) by using a 5-mm section collimation, 120 kVp, 250 mA, and 2-second scanning time. Contrast material–enhanced images were obtained both 40 seconds and 5 minutes after the initiation of contrast material infusion. Images were analyzed by using soft-tissue (level, 50 HU; width, 350 HU) windows. Conventional RUG images were acquired by using a digital subtraction technique at 2.5 frames per second during manual injection of 10 mL of iohexol 150 (Omnipaque 150; Nycomed) through an 8-F catheter positioned in the infraprostatic urethra. Additional helical CT images of the prostate were then acquired (5-mm collimation, 120 kvp, 250 mA, 1:1 pitch) while 60 mL of iohexol 150 was injected at 3 mL/sec through the urethral catheter. These images were reconstructed at 1-mm intervals.

Postprocessing of the resultant data set was performed to create three-dimensional (volume-rendered) images by using CEMAX software (Cemax, Fremont, Calif) on a Sparc 10 workstation (Sun Microsystems, Sunnyvale, Calif). This program also was used to calculate the maximal change in cross-sectional area between the treated and untreated parts of the urethra for the day 21–28 scans.

Specimen Collection and Histopathologic Analysis

After euthanasia, the prostate was excised in toto to allow for histopathologic study and radiologic-pathologic correlation. Lesions were sectioned in the axial plane to correspond to the CT images. Specimens were then preserved in 10% formalin solution for microscopic analysis. A representative tissue sample was embedded in paraffin and sectioned by using a microtome. Hematoxylin-eosin staining was performed. Light microscopy was performed by using objective lenses of low (×4–×10) to high (×400) power. Histopathologic findings were correlated with diagnostic imaging findings.

RESULTS

Procedure

All procedures were technically successful and were performed in less than 30 minutes. Animals tolerated the RF ablation well; surviving animals awoke from anesthesia without undue delay. Generator output remained fairly constant throughout the procedure at 226 mA ± 62 (6.1 watts ± 3.0). Tissue impedance was stable throughout the procedure in all cases. While temperatures at the site of RF application measured 92°C ± 2, temperatures at 5 and 10 mm measured 46°C ± 3 and 40°C ± 2, respectively. In every case, the rectal mucosa was at least 15 mm from the tip of the electrode. Temperatures did not exceed 38°C (within 2°C of baseline) at 15 mm from the electrode tip during RF application.

Clinical Follow-up and Complications

Animals resumed their normal eating, sleeping, and voiding habits within 24 hours of the procedure. All animals were capable of voiding spontaneously from immediately after the procedure until scheduled euthanasia. One dog had hematuria for 2 days after the RF ablation, but this cleared without therapy. Postprocedural analgesia was not required beyond the initial 24 hours. No animal exhibited any signs of infection or fever. In addition, no animal developed incontinence or displayed signs of urinary retention.

Follow-up CT showed no evidence of abscess or urinoma formation. Conventional RUG demonstrated no evidence of periprostatic urinary leak, urethrorectal fistula, or urethral stricture in any animal.

Diagnostic Imaging

Ultrasonography.—During RF application, US demonstrated an echogenic irregular focus surrounding the electrode tip (Fig 1b). This region of echogenicity rapidly disappeared after the cessation of RF application. Within 10–15 minutes after the procedure, each individual RF treatment site showed an echogenic central region measuring 0.7–1.4 cm in diameter and surrounded by a peripheral hypoechoic rim (Fig 1c). The mean diameter of this treated area, including the hypoechoic zone, measured 1.1–1.7 cm (1.2 cm ± 0.4 [standard deviation]).

At 3 days after ablation, most of the treatment sites had changes in US appearance. An irregular, hypo- to anechoic region was present in the center of the treated zone. A well-defined communication with the urethra was demonstrated in two of four cases. Freely mobile echogenic debris partially filled the treatment site (Fig 2a). By day 14, this debris had cleared, and anechoic cavities communi-

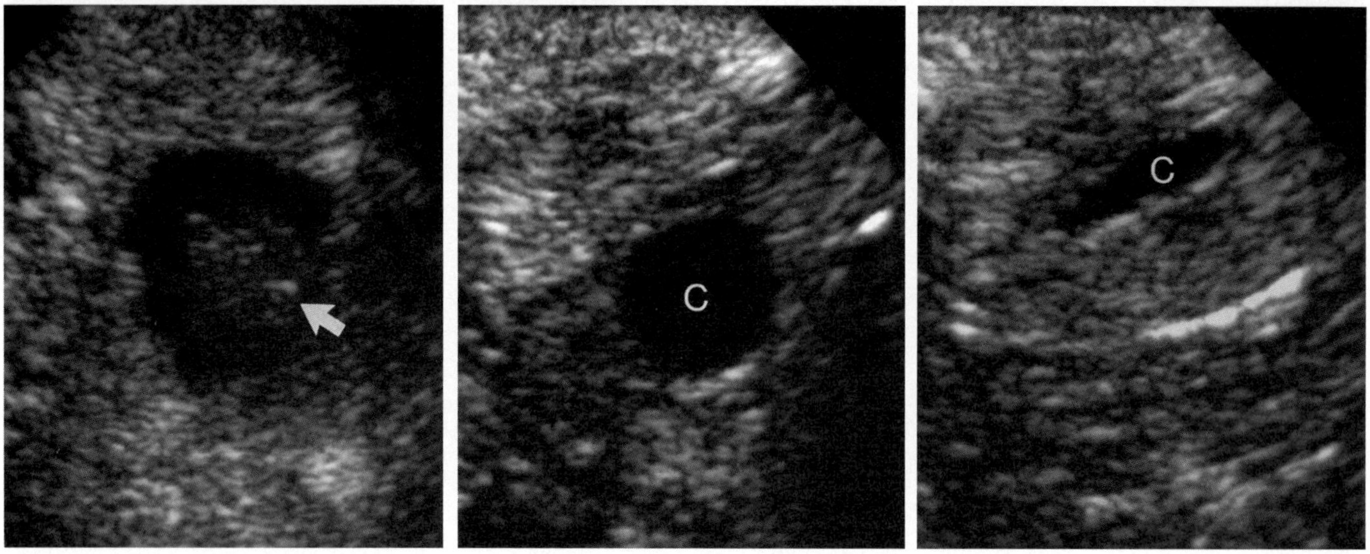

a. b. c.

Figure 2. US appearances during the subacute and chronic phases of tissue response after transrectal RF ablation of the prostate. **(a)** US scan obtained 3 days after ablation shows that the treated tissue has partially cavitated, with the development of an irregularly shaped, anechoic 1.1-cm-diameter center. Freely mobile echogenic debris (arrow) partially fills this cavity. **(b)** US scan obtained 21 days after ablation in the same animal demonstrates a smooth-walled anechoic cavity (*C*), which is free of debris. **(c)** US scan demonstrates that this cavity (*C*) is easily collapsible with ballottement by using the US transducer.

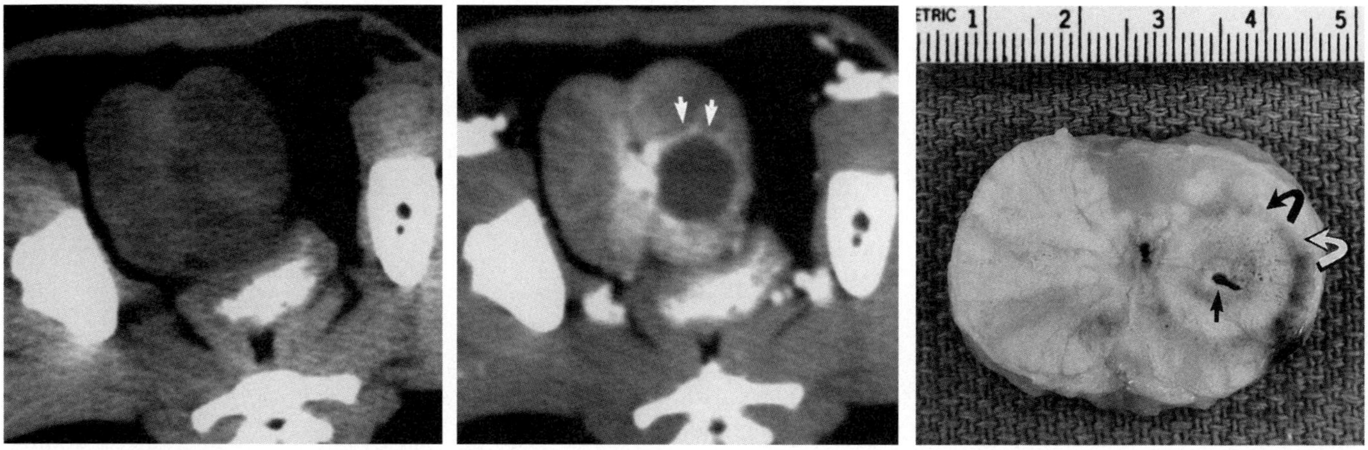

a. b. c.

Figure 3. CT appearance immediately after transrectal RF ablation. **(a)** Coagulation necrosis is not well visualized on this unenhanced CT image obtained within 1 hour after RF application. **(b)** Contrast-enhanced CT image shows a 1.4-cm focus of nonenhancing tissue. A 1-mm peripheral rim (arrows) of contrast material enhancement surrounds the region of nonenhancement. **(c)** Pathologic specimen shows a firm, 1.4-cm area (ruler is in centimeters) that corresponds to the treatment site. The electrode track (straight arrow) is seen in the center of the treatment focus. A 1-mm, dark, peripheral rim (curved arrows) demarcates the treatment area from the surrounding prostatic parenchyma. Histopathologic examination revealed necrotic cells in the center of the coagulated zone. Prostatic tissue peripheral to this rim was normal in histologic appearance.

cating with the urethra were present in all cases. Gas, instilled by prior RUG, collected in the antidependent portions of these cavities in several cases. By 21–28 days after the procedure, the anechoic cavities had smooth walls (Fig 2b). In addition, these cavities were collapsible with transducer ballottement and expandable with retrograde fluid instillation (Fig 2c). US findings changed little from the findings at 21–28 days at examinations performed beyond 28 days.

Computed tomography.—Areas of coagulation necrosis were not well visualized on the initial postprocedural unenhanced images (Fig 3a). By day 14, ill-defined regions of fluid attenuation that lacked discrete borders were identified in the treated regions of the prostate on the unenhanced images (Fig 4a). For each RF application, contrast-enhanced images showed foci of nonenhancement that measured 0.9–1.8 cm (1.3 cm ± 0.3) immediately after the procedure (Fig 3b). These foci did not change in size on images obtained during the first 28 postprocedural days. A faint peripheral rim of contrast material enhancement was seen on the earlier images in a majority of cases. The periurethral unenhanced re-

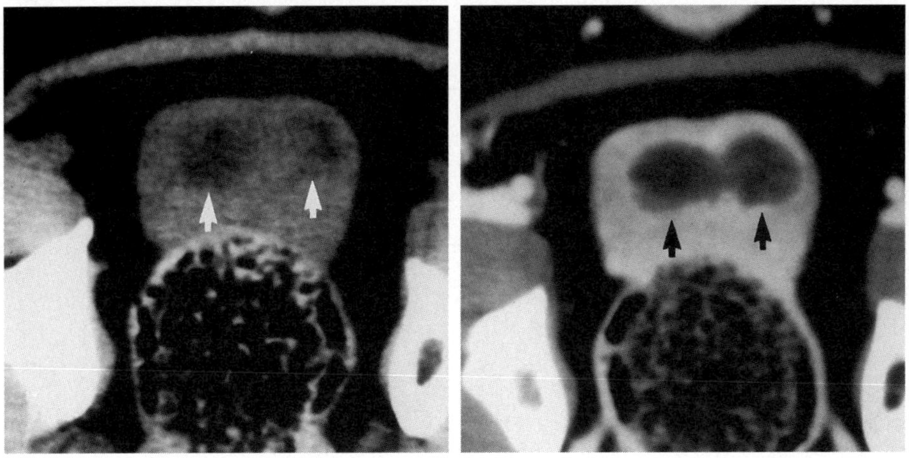

a. b.

Figure 4. CT appearance during the subacute phase of tissue response after transrectal RF ablation. **(a)** Two ill-defined regions of hypoattenuation (arrows) are identified in the periurethral portions of the prostatic parenchyma on this unenhanced CT image obtained 14 days after bilateral RF ablation. **(b)** CT image obtained after the administration of contrast material shows a bilobed unenhanced region that incorporates both hypoattenuating foci (arrows). This unenhanced region corresponded to cavitary enlargement at conventional RUG and histopathologic analysis.

gions were of fluid attenuation (≤10 HU) on all images obtained at least 3 days after the procedure (Fig 4). These abnormalities correlated within 2 mm to the regions of altered echotexture at US. Excreted intravenous contrast material flowed passively from the bladder and pooled in the enlarged urethral cavity in six of the 14 scans (43%) obtained at 28 postprocedural days or later.

Retrograde urethrography.—Immediately after the procedure, the urethra was of normal caliber and appearance in six of eight (75%) cases (Fig 5). In two cases, faint linear wisps of contrast material extended into the prostatic parenchyma. CT findings confirmed that this extravasation was limited to the region of treated prostatic tissue. By day 3, all animals had irregularly shaped cavities that communicated with the urethral lumen (Fig 5b). This cavity had a thin neck in three of the eight cases. By day 14, a bilobed region of urethral enlargement was seen in all four surviving dogs treated with bilateral RF application (Fig 5c). At 14 days after the procedure, residual irregularity in the contour of the RF-induced cavity was present. However, by day 28, a smooth, widened urethral channel was seen in all six cases. The maximal urethral widening was mildly decreased on images obtained 42–90 days after the procedure as compared to that on images obtained 28 days after the procedure, but neither further narrowing nor stricture formation was observed at 90 days.

CT RUG findings obtained during retrograde transurethral instillation of contrast material confirmed both the conventional axial CT and conventional urethrographic findings. Retrograde instillation of contrast material distended both treated and untreated portions of the urethra as compared with the urethra on CT images (Fig 5). Urethral enlargement, as measured by comparing the enlarged RF-treated urethral segment with an immediately adjacent untreated portion of the urethra, increased the cross-sectional area of the urethra from 36.6 mm^2 ± 18.7 to 173.7 mm^2 ± 64.3 (579.4% ± 35.5). As for conventional RUG, minimal reduction in the degree of urethral enlargement was noted by 60 days, but marked urethral widening over the baseline persisted at 90 days.

Pathologic analysis.—The prostate was excised in toto in all cases. No scars or adhesions were observed on the prostatic capsule. The rectal serosa was intact and without evidence of scarring or perforation.

Prostates in two animals were obtained at autopsy on the day of the procedure. One of these animals had undergone one and the other two separate RF applications. Three foci of altered tissue that measured 1.2–1.6 cm in diameter were identified in the areas treated with RF application (Fig 3c). These regions were of uniform beige color and of firmer consistency than were the untreated portions of the prostate. Surrounding this region was a 1–2-mm reddish-brown peripheral rim demarcating the treatment area from the surrounding prostatic parenchyma. Treated regions were limited to the prostatic parenchyma and did not extend to the prostatic capsule. In addition, the electrode track was readily identifiable only in the center of the treated region.

Specimens examined at 28 postprocedural days (n = 2) and at 3 months (n = 4) showed cavitary enlargement of the urethral cavity in the treated region (Fig 5f). No residual coagulated tissue was identified, as the remaining prostatic tissue was normal in appearance. In the four specimens examined at 3 months after ablation, the pearly white urethral cavities had a 1-mm-thick shiny lining. At 3 months, the urethral cavities were partially collapsed but easily distended with blunt instruments. The surrounding prostatic tissue was unremarkable.

Histologic analysis.—For the two specimens obtained immediately after the procedure, histologic findings matched the pathologic findings. The central portion of the treated region had necrotic cells with pyknotic or karyorrhectic nuclei and cytoplasmic hypereosinophilia. An acute inflammatory response of hemorrhage, congestion, and margination corresponded to the reddish brown rim surrounding the coagulated tissue. Prostatic tissue peripheral to this rim was normal in histologic appearance.

In the specimens obtained on day 28 and beyond, no coagulated tissue was identified. Continuous urothelium several cell layers in depth lined the enlarged urethral cavity. Peripheral prostatic tissue was normal in histologic appearance. In the four animals that survived 86–96 days, normal mature urothelium lined the cavitated areas of the urethra (Fig 5g).

Radiologic-pathologic correlation.—The mean difference between the extent of coagulated tissue in specimens harvested on the day of the procedure as determined with CT or US and histopathologic examination was 1–3 mm. No histopathologic correlate was demonstrated to account for the concentric echogenic pattern observed at US. Cavitary enlargement of the urethra on day 28 or at 3 months as visualized at CT, US, and RUG was also within 3 mm of the measurement at pathologic analysis.

DISCUSSION

RF ablation has been used to coagulate benign and malignant tissues in the liver, the central nervous system, and the mus-

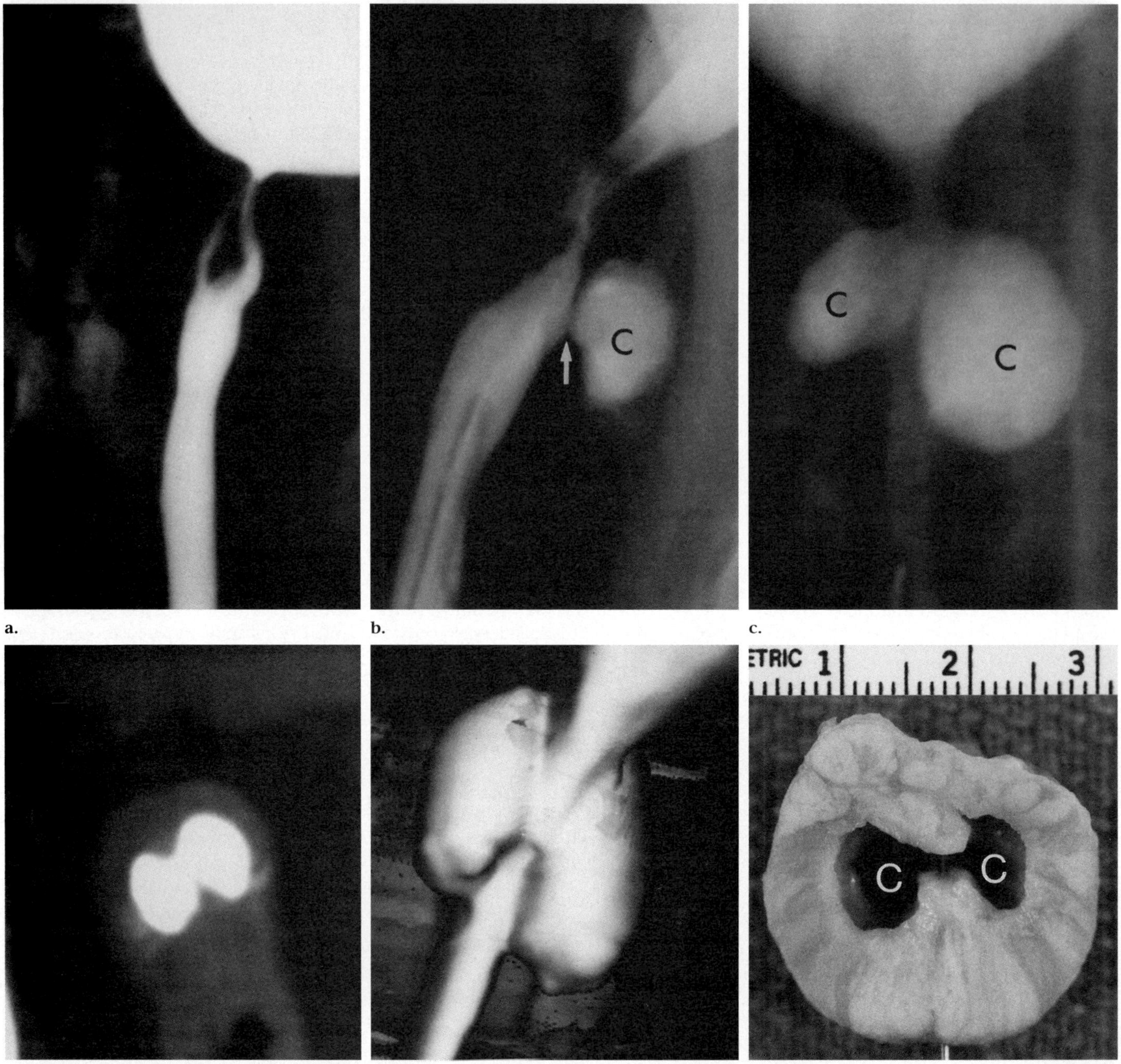

a. b. c.

d. e. f.

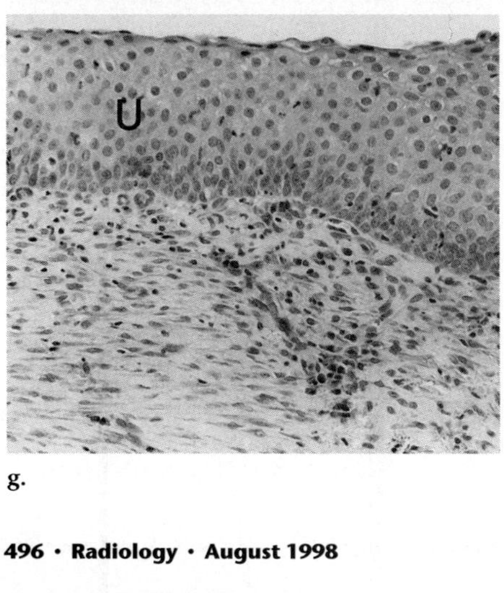

g.

Figure 5. RUG appearance of transrectal RF ablation. **(a)** Conventional anteroposterior RUG image obtained immediately after bilateral RF application shows that the urethra is of normal caliber and appearance. **(b)** Conventional RUG image obtained on day 3 shows a round cavity (*C*) that is in communication with the urethral lumen. This cavity communicates with the urethra by means of a thin neck (arrow), which is best seen in the left posterior oblique view with steep tube angulation. **(c)** Anteroposterior conventional RUG images obtained at 14 days after ablation demonstrate progressive urethral enlargement. Two regions of urethral enlargement (*C*) extend into the periurethral tissues. **(d)** Full extent of this bilobed urethral enlargement with a wide zone of communication to the native urethra is appreciated on a CT image obtained during transurethral instillation of contrast material. **(e)** Three-dimensional reconstruction of **d** demonstrates the extent of the cavitary enlargement. **(f)** Pathologic specimen of the prostate obtained 86 days after RF ablation confirms the patency of the enlarged urethra. Anatomic correlates of the two visualized lobes of focal urethral enlargement (*C*) are seen. Ruler is in centimeters. **(g)** Histopathologic specimen demonstrates mature urothelium (*U*) lining the new, enlarged urethral cavity. (Hematoxylin-eosin stain; original magnification, ×41.)

culoskeletal system (16–21). In addition, several investigators have demonstrated the feasibility of transurethral prostate ablation by using RF application in animals, and this technique recently has begun to be used to treat patients with benign prostatic hyperplasia (7–11,13). However, very little has been done to investigate the potential role of transrectal RF application, despite the fact that the transrectal approach is commonly used to perform US-guided biopsy.

McGahan et al (14), in an attempt to develop a technique for the treatment of prostate cancer, studied the acute effects of RF on the peripheral zone of the prostate in a nonsurvival study in six dogs. However, they did not investigate either the effects of RF on periurethral tissues or the potential to increase urethral patency. In the current study, we performed transrectal RF ablation of the prostate gland with the goal of increasing the caliber of the urethral lumen, and we have demonstrated that our results approximate the extent of urethral enlargement seen with TURP.

In our study of eight dogs, the use of real-time US guidance enabled rapid and accurate positioning of the electrodes. In all cases, we were able to complete the procedures within 30 minutes and demonstrate the safety of local heat deposition in the prostate. By measuring temperatures along the shaft of the RF electrodes, we also were able to demonstrate that the periphery of the prostate and rectal wall were never heated to a temperature greater than 40°C, well below the threshold for cytotoxicity (50°C for 6 minutes), for the duration of heating. No serious complications were observed in any animal during this study.

Histopathologic studies in two animals sacrificed immediately after ablation confirmed that small volumes of coagulation necrosis were induced acutely with the applications of RF. Histopathologic findings in the animals sacrificed during the acute phase of tissue response were similar to those of Goldwasser et al (7), who studied the histopathologic evolution of transurethral prostate ablation in 11 dogs, and to those of McGahan et al (14). Histopathologic findings from animals sacrificed 28 days or later in our study demonstrated cavitary enlargement of the urethra with relining of the cavity with urothelium by 28 days. Similar findings have been reported for transurethral ablation of the prostatic urothelium by using laser or microwave energy sources (3–6), as well as for transurethral RF ablation in some animals (7).

Cavitary enlargement of the urethra was observed more often in our study than in that of Goldwasser et al (7), who noted cavities within the prostatic parenchyma containing necrotic coagulum that did not communicate with the urethra in several animals after transurethral RF application. This difference is likely attributable to a technique often used with transurethral RF in which an insulating sheath prevents heating of the urethra. Similar cavities have been observed at histopathologic analysis in human prostates treated with the transurethral RF approach. In our study, no attempt was made to protect urethral tissue; thus, cavities created by necrosis of periurethral tissue communicated with and, as a result, enlarged the urethral lumen in all cases.

The use of multimodality imaging techniques in our study not only enabled description of imaging findings after the procedure, but also shed light on the pathophysiology of the treatment. US and conventional RUG demonstrated early cavitation by 3 postprocedural days, with subsequent ongoing remodeling of this region of cavity enlargement into smooth-walled cavities by 1 postprocedural month. Distention and compressibility of these cavities was also demonstrated at US, CT with retrograde urethral contrast material instillation, or both. CT after intravenous contrast material administration demonstrated passive flow of contrast material into the prostatic urethra in a substantial number of cases (six [43%] of 14). These findings are similar to the passive flow of contrast material into the prostatic urethra seen after TURP. Peripheral enhancement surrounding coagulated tissue on contrast-enhanced CT images, however, has not been reported after TURP but is similar to peripheral contrast material enhancement seen after RF ablation in the liver (19–21). Imaging also helped to confirm the absence of complications such as abscess, urinoma, or hematoma formation, or the development of urethrorectal fistulas or urethral strictures.

Transrectal RF ablation may offer several potential benefits over the transurethral method of RF ablation. One key element is the use of imaging guidance, which permits optimal positioning of the electrode near the bladder base, or at any site where the urethra appears focally compressed. Imaging also allows for the avoidance of placing the electrode near the nerves and urogenital diaphragm, which, if treated, could result in impotence, incontinence, or both. Transrectal US has been used to guide transurethral RF ablation (13), but this combined approach is cumbersome as it requires simultaneous cystoscopy and endocavitary transducer insertion.

Imaging of the prostate immediately before ablation may also allow tailoring of the volume of tissue to be treated. This is especially important, as failure of transurethral RF ablation to improve urinary symptom scores has been attributed to inadequate treatment of a given prostate volume. The linear extent of induced coagulation is determined by the length of exposed electrode, which can thus be selected after imaging. By inserting the RF electrode parallel to the urethra, which is readily accomplished by using transrectal US, cylindric enlargement of the prostatic urethra can be accomplished. Although the diameter of coagulation attainable with our electrodes is 1.6 cm, this extent will likely be adequate for most treatments, as this diameter represents a multifold increase over the normal urethral diameter. If larger diameters of coagulation are required, modified internally cooled electrodes, which can produce a coagulation diameter in excess of 4 cm, could be used (24). In comparison, the relatively small electrodes used for transurethral RF ablation can only be used to ablate tissues adjacent to a small portion of the urethral circumference.

In addition to the advantages of imaging guidance, our electrode system may help limit the potential complications of damaging the rectal wall or periprostatic tissues with overtreatment. The use of a monopolar electrode makes overtreatment unlikely, as the diameter of necrosis produced around the tip of the electrode reaches a maximum of 1.6 cm after 4–6 minutes of heating (22,23). In addition, multiple thermistors along the shaft of the electrode permit temperatures to be measured so that peripheral tissues, particularly the rectal wall, urogenital diaphragm, and neurovascular structures are not damaged. In comparison, monitoring of rectal mucosal temperatures during transurethral RF ablation has required transrectal thermistor application.

After transurethral RF application with urethral sparing, symptoms initially worsen for the 1st several weeks in 20%–42% of patients, presumably because of periurethral tissue swelling (7–11,13). Conversely, with transrectal RF application, cavitary communication permits necrotic tissue to be expelled into the urinary stream by 3–14 days. This rapid marsupialization of the treatment focus likely reduces pressure and prevents obstruction of the urethra. As a result, no animal experienced even transient urinary retention in our study, even though the urethral catheter was removed immediately after the procedure. Conversely, urethral catheters are generally left in place for 1–10 days after transurethral ablation procedures to prevent urinary retention (8–11).

The procedure we describe is similar in many respects to transrectal US-guided biopsy of the prostate. Transrectal US guidance for the placement of prostatic biopsy needles is standard practice, with accuracy of needle placement to within 2 mm. Complications of biopsy are low, with fewer than 1% of patients requiring hospitalization, transfusion for hemorrhage, or intravenous antibiotics for infection (25).

In this study, we enlarged the prostatic urethra in dogs at a distance from the bladder neck. This is in contradistinction to the common practice of surgical resection (TURP) in humans, where the urethra is widened at the bladder neck. Unfortunately, anatomic limitations of our model precluded treatment at this exact site. The prostate in the dog is intraperitoneal and situated at a slight distance from the bladder. Thus, treatment of the most superior aspect of the urethra could have led to perforation, with free spillage of urine into the peritoneum. To prevent this complication, we, like prior investigators (3,7), purposefully treated the intraprostatic urethra. We are unaware of another commonly available animal model of benign prostatic hyperplasia that possesses anatomy more comparable to humans.

This imaging-guided, minimally invasive therapy may have a role in the treatment of benign prostatic hyperplasia. On the basis of these initial, preliminary results, we believe that clinical trials in patients with moderate to severe prostatism, in whom medical therapy has failed and who are deemed poor surgical candidates are warranted. These trials will be necessary to overcome the limitations of our model, make relevant conclusions concerning clinical efficacy, and rule out the possibility of delayed complications such as stricture formation, infection, and impotence.

Practical applications: Transrectal US-guided RF tissue ablation can be used to create urethral enlargement in the canine model. Our method enables real-time imaging, ablation of prostatic tissue, and monitoring of peripheral, off-target heating by using a method analogous to trans- rectal prostatic biopsy. Transrectal RF application therefore offers the prospect of a minimally invasive, imaging-guided method for treating patients with benign prostatic hyperplasia.

Acknowledgments: The authors thank Marek Trocha, DVM, Diane Kierstead, BS, and Geoff Bessin, BS, for animal care, and Mary Theresa Shore, RTR, for diagnostic imaging assistance. We also thank Robert H. Young, MD, for assistance with histopathologic interpretation.

References

1. Oesterling JE. Benign prostatic hyperplasia: medical and minimally invasive treatment options. N Engl J Med 1995; 332:99–109.
2. Graversen PH, Gasser TC, Wasson JH, Hinman F Jr, Bruskewitz RC. Controversies about indications for transurethral resection of the prostate. J Urol 1989; 141:475–481.
3. Roth RA, Aretz HT. Transurethral ultrasound-guided laser-induced prostatectomy (TULIP procedure): a canine prostate feasibility study. J Urol 1991; 146:1128–1135.
4. McCullough DL, Roth RA, Babayan RK, et al. Transurethral ultrasound-guided laser-induced prostatectomy: national human cooperative study results. J Urol 1993; 150:1607–1611.
5. Harada T, Etori K, Kumazaki T, Nishizawa O, Noto H, Tsuchida S. Microwave surgical treatment of diseases of the prostate. Urology 1985; 26:572–576.
6. Ogden CW, Reddy P, Johnson H, Ramsay JW, Carter SS. Sham versus transurethral microwave thermotherapy in patients with symptoms of benign prostatic bladder outflow obstruction. Lancet 1993; 341: 14–17.
7. Goldwasser B, Ramon J, Engelberg S, et al. Transurethral needle ablation (TUNA) of the prostate using low-level radiofrequency energy: an animal experimental study. Eur Urol 1993; 24:400–405.
8. Viguier JL, Dessouki T, Castelo A, et al. Benign prostatic hypertrophy treatment by transurethral radiofrequency hyperthermia with Thermex II. Eur Urol 1993; 23:318–321.
9. Zlotta AR, Peny MO, Matos C, Schulman CC. Transurethral needle ablation of the prostate: clinical experience in patients in urinary acute retention. Br J Urol 1996; 77:391–397.
10. Issa MM. Transurethral needle ablation of the prostate: report of initial United States clinical trial. J Urol 1996; 156:413–419.
11. Mostafid AH, Harrison NW, Dawkins GP, Fletcher MS. Interstitial radiofrequency therapy of the prostate: results of a pilot study. J Urol 1996; 155:1946–1948.
12. Ramon J, Goldwasser B, Shenfeld O, Engelberg S, Rasor JS, Edwards SD. Needle ablation using radio frequency current as a treatment for benign prostatic hyperplasia: experimental results in ex vivo human prostate. Eur Urol 1993; 24:406–410.
13. Schulman CC, Zlotta AR, Rasor JS, Hourriez L, Noel JC, Edwards SD. Transurethral needle ablation: safety, feasibility, and tolerance of a new office procedure for treatment of benign prostatic hyperplasia. Eur Urol 1993; 24:415–423.
14. McGahan JP, Griffey SM, Budenz RW, Brock JM. Percutaneous ultrasound-guided radiofrequency electrocautery ablation of prostate tissue in dogs. Acad Radiol 1995; 2:61–66.
15. Cosman ER, Nashold BS, Ovelman-Levitt J. Theoretical aspects of radiofrequency lesions in the dorsal root entry zone. Neurosurgery 1984; 15:945–950.
16. Rosenthal DI, Springfield DS, Gebhart MC, Rosenberg AE, Mankin HJ. Osteoid osteoma: percutaneous radiofrequency ablation. Radiology 1995; 197:451–454.
17. Anzai Y, Lufkin R, DeSalles A, Hamilton DR, Farahani K, Black KL. Preliminary experience with MR-guided thermal ablation of brain tumors. AJNR 1995; 16: 39–48.
18. Rossi S, DiStasi M, Buscarini E, et al. Percutaneous RF interstitial thermal ablation in the treatment of hepatic cancer. AJR 1996; 167:759–768.
19. Solbiati L, Ierace T, Goldberg SN, et al. Percutaneous US-guided RF tissue ablation of liver metastases: long-term follow up. Radiology 1997; 202:195–203.
20. Livraghi T, Goldberg SN, Monti F, et al. Saline-enhanced radiofrequency tissue ablation in the treatment of liver metastases. Radiology 1997; 202:205–210.
21. Solbiati L, Goldberg SN, Ierace T, Livraghi T, Sironi S, Gazelle GS. Hepatic metastases: radiofrequency ablation with cooled-tip electrodes. Radiology 1997; 205:367–374.
22. McGahan JP, Brock JN, Tessluk H, Wei-Zhong G, Schneider P, Browning PD. Hepatic ablation with use of radiofrequency electrocautery in the animal model. JVIR 1992; 3:291–297.
23. Goldberg SN, Gazelle GS, Dawson SL, Rittman WJ, Mueller PR, Rosenthal DI. Tissue ablation with radiofrequency: effect of probe size, gauge, duration and temperature on lesion volume. Acad Radiol 1995; 2:399–404.
24. Goldberg SN, Gazelle GS, Solbiati L, Rittman WJ, Mueller PR. Radiofrequency tissue ablation: increased lesion diameter with a perfusion electrode. Acad Radiol 1996; 3:636–644.
25. Clements R, Aideyau OU, Griffiths GJ, Peeling WB. Side effects and patient acceptance of transrectal biopsy of the prostate. Clin Radiol 1993; 47:125–126.

Tatsuo Torizuka, MD
Susan J. Fisher, BA
Raya S. Brown, PhD
Richard L. Wahl, MD

Index terms:
Breast neoplasms, experimental, 00.329
Breast neoplasms, PET, 00.12163
Breast neoplasms, radionuclide studies, 00.12163
Diabetes mellitus
Fluorine
Glucose
Metabolism

Radiology 1998; 208:499–504

Abbreviation:
FDG = 2-[fluorine-18]-fluoro-2-deoxy-D-glucose

[1] From the Departments of Internal Medicine (T.T., S.J.F., R.S.B., R.L.W.) and Radiology (R.L.W.), Division of Nuclear Medicine, University of Michigan Medical Center, 1500 E Medical Center Dr, B1G412, Ann Arbor, MI 48109-0028. Received August 28, 1997; revision requested November 13; revision received February 27, 1998; accepted April 10. Supported by National Cancer Institute grants CA52880, CA53172, and CA56731. **Address reprint requests to** R.L.W.

Author contributions:
Guarantor of integrity of entire study, R.L.W.; study concepts, T.T., R.L.W.; study design, T.T., S.J.F., R.S.B., R.L.W.; definition of intellectual content, T.T., R.S.B., R.L.W.; literature research, T.T., R.S.B., R.L.W.; experimental studies, T.T., S.J.F., R.S.B., R.L.W.; data acquisition, T.T., S.J.F., R.S.B.; data analysis, T.T., S.J.F., R.S.B., R.L.W.; statistical analysis, T.T., S.J.F.; manuscript preparation, T.T.; manuscript editing, T.T., R.L.W.; manuscript review, T.T., S.J.F., R.S.B., R.L.W.

Effect of Insulin on Uptake of FDG by Experimental Mammary Carcinoma in Diabetic Rats[1]

PURPOSE: To determine whether insulin improves tumor uptake of 2-[fluorine-18]-fluoro-2-deoxy-D-glucose (FDG) in diabetic rats with mammary carcinoma.

MATERIALS AND METHODS: Rats were inoculated subcutaneously with mammary carcinoma cells. Four weeks later, diabetes was established with streptozocin while controls were given saline. Two weeks later, after overnight fasting, 12 diabetic and 11 control rats received saline and five diabetic rats received insulin 60 minutes before FDG injection (100 μCi [3.7 MBq]). Three diabetic rats received insulin 30 minutes before FDG injection. One hour after FDG injection (ie, at sacrifice), F-18 activity in tumor and normal tissues was measured.

RESULTS: Insulin significantly reduced blood glucose levels in diabetic rats at sacrifice. Tumor FDG uptake, which significantly declined with untreated diabetes ($P < .005$ vs controls), was not significantly different between insulin-treated and untreated diabetic rats. Insulin significantly improved tumor/lung and tumor/liver uptake ratios in diabetes ($P < .005$), although the tumor/muscle uptake ratio significantly decreased to 40% of the diabetic value with insulin ($P < .005$).

CONCLUSION: Diabetes markedly impairs tumor targeting with FDG. In diabetic patients, the judicious use of insulin may improve tumor/nontumor uptake ratios in specific organs such as the liver or lung, although insulin consistently reduces tumor/muscle uptake ratios.

Accelerated rates of glucose uptake and metabolism are frequent characteristics of malignant neoplasms (1,2). An analogue of glucose, 2-[fluorine-18]-fluoro-2-deoxy-D-glucose (FDG), has been widely used to detect a variety of malignant lesions with positron emission tomography (PET) (3–7). The high sensitivity of PET allows more accurate staging of cancers and quantitative assessment of metabolic responses to treatment (8–11). In the past several years, it has been realized that low blood glucose levels in the fasting state without insulin treatment are preferable to high glucose levels for tumor targeting with FDG PET. We have previously demonstrated that FDG accumulation in cancer cells is inversely related to media glucose levels in vitro and that acute hyperglycemia induced by glucose infusion markedly inhibits tumor FDG uptake in vivo, presumably owing to the direct competition between FDG and glucose for tumor uptake (12). In clinical PET studies, it has been reported that tumor FDG uptake is significantly decreased during the glucose-loaded state, as compared with the fasting state (13,14).

We recently reported, in an animal study of normal nondiabetic rats (15), that FDG uptake into experimental rat mammary carcinoma is significantly impaired with insulin-induced hypoglycemia, probably because hyperinsulinemia shifts FDG from the blood and tumor to the skeletal muscle and fat tissues, which have large numbers of highly insulin-sensitive Glut 4 glucose transporters. We also noted in this study that tumor/nontumor ratios of FDG uptake were significantly decreased with insulin in most normal organs.

When patients with cancer have poorly controlled diabetes, tumor imaging with FDG

PET is expected to be impaired because of hyperglycemia. To our knowledge, however, no report has compared tumor targeting with FDG between diabetic and nondiabetic patients in vivo. In the present study, with a streptozocin-induced diabetic rat model, we compared FDG uptake of tumor and normal organs between diabetic and nondiabetic rats. We also evaluated the effect of insulin treatment on the biodistribution of FDG in diabetic rats with cancer to determine if tumor targeting could be enhanced.

MATERIALS AND METHODS

Animals

Animal studies were conducted with the approval of the Unit of Laboratory Animal Medicine, a certified animal care organization, following the current National Institutes of Health guidelines for laboratory animal care. All studies were conducted in a manner to minimize both sample size and pain, including providing humane euthanasia.

Inbred Lewis rats (Charles River Breeding Laboratories, Kingston, NY) were injected with 1 million cells of transplantable rat mammary tumor cell line 1–9 (16) into the interscapular fat pads. Rat mammary tumor cells 1–9 were obtained from the carcinogen 7,12-dimethylbenz(a)anthracene–induced mammary carcinoma. The origin and in vivo growth characteristics of these cells have been described previously (16). FDG uptake by the mammary cancer cells is not acutely affected by insulin in vitro (12).

FDG Uptake Study

Four weeks after tumor inoculation, diabetes was established in the rats by means of intravenous injection of streptozocin (50 mg per kilogram of body weight), whereas control tumor-bearing rats received intravenous injection of saline (2 mL/kg) (Fig 1). Two weeks later, after overnight fasting, the control (n = 11) and diabetic (n = 12) rats received intraperitoneal injection of saline (1 mL/kg), whereas the insulin-treated diabetic rats (n = 8) received intraperitoneal injection of insulin (25 IU/kg). Sixty minutes after intraperitoneal injection of saline or insulin, the control and untreated diabetic rats and five of the eight insulin-treated diabetic rats were injected intravenously with approximately 100 μCi (3.7 MBq) of FDG, as previously described (12). To evaluate the time course of response to insulin treatment, the remaining three insulin-treated diabetic rats were intravenously injected with approximately 100 μCi (3.7 MBq) of FDG 30 minutes after intraperitoneal injection of insulin. All the rats were sacrificed 60 minutes after FDG injection. Tumor and normal tissues were excised and weighed, and F-18 activity in the tissues was determined with a gamma counter. The percentage of decay-corrected F-18 activity per gram of tissue was also obtained, normalized for animal weight (percentage of injected dose [per gram of tissue] per kilogram of animal weight), as previously reported (12,15).

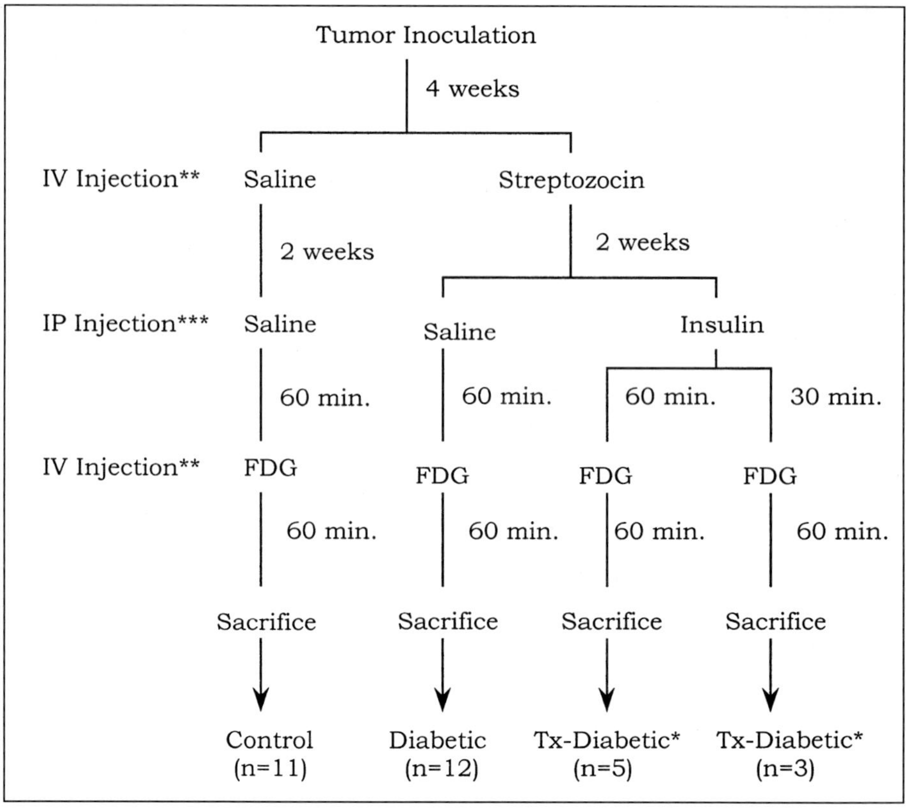

Figure 1. Flowchart of the animal experiment. *Tx-Diabetic** = insulin-treated diabetic rats, *IV injection*** = intravenous injection, *IP injection**** = intraperitoneal injection.

Blood samples were obtained at the time of each saline or insulin injection, at FDG injection, and at sacrifice. Blood glucose levels were measured (Accu-Chek IIm and Chemstrip bG; Boehringer Mannheim, Indianapolis, Ind). Plasma insulin levels in the same samples were determined with a double-antibody radioimmunoassay. Plasma insulin levels were not measured at the time of FDG injection to avoid excessive and nonphysiologic blood loss in the rats. Data were analyzed with paired or unpaired two-tailed t tests. A P value less than .02 was considered statistically significant (12,15).

Immunohistochemistry

To estimate the expression of Glut 1 glucose transporter, tumor samples from seven animals (two controls, two untreated diabetic rats, and three diabetic rats treated with insulin 60 minutes before FDG injection) were frozen in iso-pentane (2-methylbutane) cooled in liquid nitrogen and stored at −70°C. Formalin-fixed fresh frozen sections (6 μm thick) were used to study Glut 1 expression. The sections were incubated with anti–Glut 1 (Chemicon International, Temecula Calif), and the bound antibody was visualized by means of the avidin-biotin conjugate immunoperoxidase procedure (17) by using the Vectastain Elite kit (Vector, Burlingame, Calif), as previously described (18). Consecutive sections incubated with normal rabbit immunoglobulin G or with a mixture of the anti–Glut 1 with excess of the C-terminus peptide antigen (CGLFHPLGADSQV) were used as negative controls. Sections from paraffin-embedded kidney from normal fasted rat were used as positive controls.

TABLE 1
Blood Glucose Levels

Animal Group	Blood Glucose Level (mg/dL) At Saline or Insulin Injection	At FDG Injection (60 min)	At Sacrifice (120 min)
Rats injected with saline			
Control ($n = 11$)	101 ± 3	91 ± 2	113 ± 5
Diabetic ($n = 12$)	319 ± 12	307 ± 13	351 ± 14
Diabetic rats treated with insulin			
Time (min) insulin injected before FDG			
60 ($n = 5$)	290 ± 34	99 ± 8	78 ± 9
30 ($n = 3$)	338 ± 18	257 ± 41	126 ± 10

Note.—Data are the mean ± standard error of the mean. For conversion to SI units, 1 mg/dL = 0.05551 mmol/L.

TABLE 2
Biodistribution of FDG

Tissue	Rats Injected with Saline: Control ($n = 11$)	Diabetic ($n = 12$)	Diabetic Rats Treated with Insulin before FDG: At 60 min ($n = 5$)	At 30 min ($n = 3$)
Tumor	0.392 ± 0.028	0.126 ± 0.014*	0.177 ± 0.016	0.103 ± 0.016
Blood	0.028 ± 0.002	0.045 ± 0.004*	0.016 ± 0.004†	0.016 ± 0.002‡
Muscle	0.015 ± 0.001	0.014 ± 0.001	0.062 ± 0.016†	0.031 ± 0.003†
Fat	0.009 ± 0.002	0.032 ± 0.007§	0.043 ± 0.006	0.041 ± 0.006
Heart	0.145 ± 0.021	0.031 ± 0.004*	0.359 ± 0.032†	0.091 ± 0.047‖
Liver	0.041 ± 0.003	0.055 ± 0.006	0.021 ± 0.007†	0.017 ± 0.001‡
Spleen	0.185 ± 0.017	0.143 ± 0.019	0.129 ± 0.023	0.075 ± 0.007
Kidney	0.101 ± 0.009	0.121 ± 0.011	0.108 ± 0.026	0.049 ± 0.007‡
Lung	0.091 ± 0.008	0.087 ± 0.009	0.077 ± 0.016	0.039 ± 0.005
Small bowel	0.198 ± 0.015	0.104 ± 0.008*	0.149 ± 0.011‡	0.083 ± 0.011
Brain	0.339 ± 0.031	0.127 ± 0.018*	0.257 ± 0.055‡	0.085 ± 0.011

Note.—Data are the mean ± standard error of the mean (in percentage of injected dose [per gram] per kilogram of animal weight).
* $P < .005$ versus Control.
† $P < .005$ versus Diabetic (injected with saline).
‡ $P < .01$ versus Diabetic (injected with saline).
§ $P < .01$ versus Control.
‖ $P = .019$ versus Diabetic (injected with saline).

RESULTS

Blood Glucose Levels and Plasma Insulin Levels

Diabetes was successfully established in the animal model after the intravenous injection of streptozocin (Table 1). The mean blood glucose level in the diabetic rats (319 mg/dL ± 12 [17.7 mmol/L ± 0.67]) was significantly higher than the control value (101 mg/dL ± 3 [5.6 mmol/L ± 0.2]) at the time of saline injection ($P < .001$). With insulin treatment 60 minutes before FDG injection, mean blood glucose level in the insulin-treated diabetic rats was significantly reduced from 290 mg/dL ± 34 (16.1 mmol/L ± 1.9) to 99 mg/dL ± 8 (5.5 mmol/L ± 0.4) at FDG injection (60 minutes after insulin injection) and to 78 mg/dL ± 9 (4.3 mmol/L ± 0.5) at sacrifice (120 minutes after insulin injection) (each, $P < .005$). On the other hand, when insulin was administrated 30 minutes before FDG injection in the diabetic animals, mean glucose level at FDG injection (257 mg/dL ± 41 [14.3 mmol/L ± 2.3]) was not significantly lower than the baseline value (338 mg/dL ± 18 [18.8 mmol/L ± 0.9]), although mean glucose level at sacrifice (90 minutes after insulin injection) significantly decreased (126 mg/dL ± 10 [6.9 mmol/L ± 0.6], $P < .005$ vs the baseline value).

Plasma insulin levels were less than 6.0 μU/mL (43 pmol/L) in all the rats at the time of saline or insulin injection. At sacrifice, plasma insulin levels in the insulin-treated rats rose to more than 1,000.0 μU/mL (7,175 pmol/L), whereas those in the control and untreated diabetic rats remained less than 6.0 μU/mL (43 pmol/L), except in one control rat with a level of 11.7 μU/mL (84 pmol/L).

Biodistribution of FDG in Diabetic Rats

Table 2 summarizes the biodistribution of FDG, and Table 3 presents tumor/nontumor ratios of FDG uptake in each animal group. In the control rats, the tumor had the highest FDG uptake, which was 14.1 ± 0.6 times, 28.3 ± 1.9 times, and 51.8 ± 4.8 times greater than FDG uptake by the blood, muscle, and fat, respectively (Table 3). In the diabetic rats, however, mean tumor FDG uptake was significantly reduced to 32.1% of the control value, whereas F-18 levels in the blood and fat significantly increased as compared with the control values (Table 2). Thus, in the diabetic rats, tumor/blood and tumor/fat uptake ratios were significantly lower than the control values (Table 3). In addition, tumor/nontumor uptake ratios in the muscle, liver, spleen, kidney, lung, and small bowel significantly decreased in the diabetic rats as compared with the control values. On the other hand, FDG uptake by the heart, small bowel, and brain in the diabetic rats significantly declined to 21.4%, 52.5%, and 37.5% of the control values, respectively. Table 3 clearly demonstrates that streptozocin-induced diabetes reduced tumor/nontumor ratios of FDG uptake for most organs to 12%–91% of the control values, whereas only the tumor/heart uptake ratio increased with diabetes.

Biodistribution of FDG in Insulin-treated Diabetic Rats

When the diabetic rats were treated with insulin 60 minutes before FDG injection, tumor FDG uptake increased slightly (40.5%), although not significantly ($P = .051$), as compared with the diabetic value, whereas FDG uptake by the muscle and heart significantly increased to 4.4- and 11.6-fold of the diabetic values, respectively (Table 2). Thus, in the insulin-treated diabetic rats, tumor/muscle and tumor/heart ratios of FDG uptake were significantly lower than the diabetic values (Table 3). Tumor/fat uptake ratio in the insulin-treated diabetic rats was also reduced to 70.3% of the diabetic value, but the decrease was not significant. In contrast, FDG uptake by the blood and liver was significantly reduced with insulin, which resulted in significant increases in tumor/blood and tumor/liver uptake ratios (4.6- and 4.8-fold of the diabetic values, respectively). In addition, insulin treatment significantly increased tumor/spleen, tumor/kidney, and tumor/lung uptake ratios (Table 3).

When the diabetic rats were treated with insulin 30 minutes before FDG injection, tumor FDG uptake slightly, but not significantly, decreased as compared with the diabetic values (Table 2). In these insulin-treated diabetic rats, FDG uptake by the muscle and heart significantly increased to 2.2- and 2.9-fold of the diabetic values; thus, tumor/muscle and tumor/heart uptake ratios were significantly lower than the diabetic values (Table 3). In contrast, tumor/nontumor uptake ratios in the blood, liver, spleen, kidney, and lung in these insulin-treated diabetic rats were significantly higher than the diabetic values.

TABLE 3
Tumor/Nontumor Ratios of FDG Uptake

	Rats Injected with Saline		Diabetic Rats Treated with Insulin before FDG	
Tissue	Control (n = 11)	Diabetic (n = 12)	At 60 min (n = 5)	At 30 min (n = 3)
Blood	14.112 ± 0.616	2.919 ± 0.357*	13.321 ± 2.387†	6.475 ± 1.255†
Muscle	28.253 ± 1.898	9.119 ± 0.662*	3.815 ± 0.772†	3.422 ± 0.601†
Fat	51.808 ± 4.824	6.401 ± 1.465*	4.503 ± 0.332	2.578 ± 0.195
Heart	3.296 ± 0.478	4.271 ± 0.258	0.541 ± 0.074†	1.647 ± 0.566†
Liver	9.915 ± 0.319	2.371 ± 0.213*	11.436 ± 0.002†	6.361 ± 1.182†
Spleen	2.198 ± 0.111	0.956 ± 0.061*	1.647 ± 0.348‡	1.382 ± 0.167‡
Kidney	4.012 ± 0.199	1.071 ± 0.097*	2.191 ± 0.642‡	2.111 ± 0.283†
Lung	4.458 ± 0.225	1.505 ± 0.101*	2.861 ± 0.528†	2.639 ± 0.099†
Small bowel	2.006 ± 0.099	1.197 ± 0.072*	1.296 ± 0.179	1.231 ± 0.031
Brain	1.191 ± 0.079	1.084 ± 0.071	0.851 ± 0.159	1.222 ± 0.127

Note.—Data are the mean ± standard error of the mean.
* $P < .005$ versus Control.
† $P < .005$ versus Diabetic (injected with saline).
‡ $P < .02$ versus Diabetic (injected with saline).

Immunohistochemistry

All tumors were positive for Glut 1 glucose transporter (Fig 2). The staining appeared as cytoplasmic granules in all the positive cancer cells. In areas of densely packed cancer cells and around necrotic foci, strong membrane staining was seen. Qualitatively, more Glut 1–positive areas were found in tumors from the control rats than in tumors from the diabetic or the insulin-treated diabetic rats, but the differences in intensity were relatively subtle. Two of three insulin-treated diabetic rats had higher intensity Glut 1 tumor staining, whereas the remaining rat had lower intensity tumor staining, as compared with the diabetic rats. No staining was observed in sections incubated with a mixture of antibody and antigen. In the kidneys, staining was observed in the epithelium of renal tubules.

DISCUSSION

Findings in this animal study demonstrate that tumor FDG uptake is markedly impaired with streptozocin-induced diabetes. When diabetic rats were treated with insulin 60 minutes before FDG injection, tumor FDG uptake increased, although not significantly. In diabetic animals, insulin significantly improved tumor/nontumor ratios of FDG uptake for the blood, liver, spleen, kidney, and lung, but the tumor/muscle uptake ratio significantly declined with insulin. The latter is particularly important in clinical PET studies, in which images can be interpreted by means of tumor/muscle ratios of FDG uptake (4,19).

Findings in previous in vitro and in vivo studies (12) have demonstrated that FDG accumulation in cancer cells is markedly impaired with acute hyperglycemia, probably because of direct competition between FDG and D-glucose for uptake and incorporation by cancer cells. Findings in human PET studies (13,14) have also shown that tumor FDG uptake significantly decreases during the glucose-loaded state as compared with the fasting state in nondiabetic patients. Minn et al (20) have reported that tumor FDG uptake in two diabetic patients with hyperglycemia were much lower than those in 44 nondiabetic patients with normoglycemia, although the number of diabetic patients was small. These results emphasize the necessity for taking blood glucose levels into consideration when FDG uptake by cancer cells is estimated.

Because many patients are diabetic and some diabetic patients have cancers, we studied the effect of diabetes on FDG uptake by tumor and normal organs by means of a syngeneic rat mammary tumor model. Our data indicate that streptozocin-induced diabetes significantly reduced tumor FDG uptake, probably owing to the direct competition between glucose and FDG for tumor uptake during hyperglycemia. Diabetes also significantly reduced FDG uptake by the heart, small bowel, and brain while increasing FDG uptake by the blood and fat (Table 2). The heart uptake showed the most significant decline with diabetes, almost certainly owing to the lack of insulin-induced Glut 4 translocation to the membrane in the low-insulin diabetic state. Thus, as shown in Table 3, tumor/nontumor ratios of FDG uptake significantly decreased for most of the organs in the diabetic rats, except for the heart and brain, indicating that tumor targeting with FDG is impaired in diabetes, much as it is under conditions of acute hyperglycemia induced by glucose infusion.

We have recently demonstrated that insulin-induced hypoglycemia significantly reduced FDG uptake by the same experimental rat mammary tumor in normal rats to 35.4% of the control value (15). In contrast, FDG uptake by the muscle and fat was significantly increased after insulin injection to 5.2- and 5.8-fold of the control values, respectively. Thus, tumor/muscle and tumor/fat ratios of FDG uptake were markedly reduced with insulin-induced hypoglycemia. Because about 45% of the body weight of the rats is estimated to be from skeletal muscle and 15% from fat (21), insulin may shift FDG from tumor to these two tissues with a large mass, which have large numbers of highly insulin-sensitive Glut 4 transporters (22,23). Thus, it appears that insulin redirects FDG away from tumor to the skeletal muscle and fat tissues in nondiabetic animals.

It can be argued that pretreatment with insulin may increase tumor FDG uptake by decreasing blood glucose levels. However, the insulin effect may be divergent; use of insulin before FDG injection in diabetic rats may improve tumor FDG uptake, but it can also reduce tumor FDG uptake owing to re-targeting of FDG to muscle or fat. Indeed, our results indicate that, with insulin treatment 60 minutes

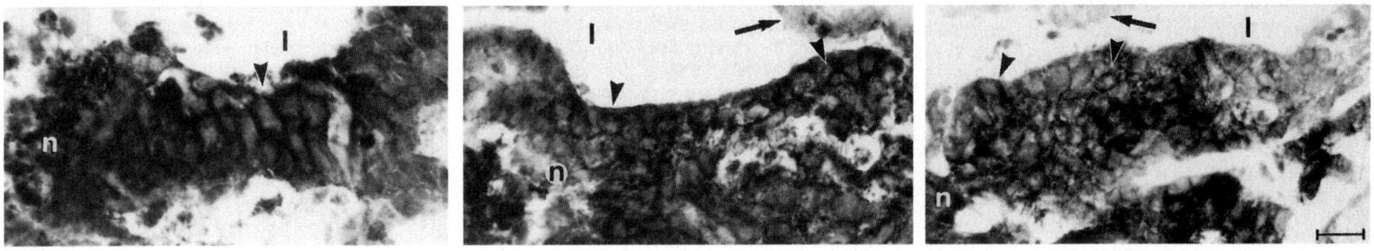

a. b. c.

Figure 2. Glut 1 expression in rat mammary tumors. As described in Materials and Methods, sections of tumors were obtained in **(a)** a control rat, **(b)** a diabetic rat, and **(c)** an insulin-treated diabetic rat. The sample in **a** shows higher intensity of tumor Glut 1 staining in the cell membrane (arrowheads) as compared with that in **b** and **c**, although the differences in intensity were subtle. Arrows indicate Glut 1–negative cancer cells, *l* = lumen, and *n* = necrotic area. Rule in **c** indicates 20 μm. (Original magnification, ×250.)

before FDG injection, tumor FDG uptake slightly, but not significantly in the sample size studied, increased in the diabetic rats, whereas muscle uptake increased to 4.4-fold and fat uptake increased to 1.3-fold of the diabetic values (Table 2). It should be noted that the insulin-induced increases in FDG uptake by the muscle and fat were smaller in the diabetic rats, as compared with those in the normal rats (4.4- vs 5.2-fold for the muscle and 1.3- vs 5.8-fold for the fat). These findings suggest that the insulin-induced shifts of FDG from tumor to these insulin-sensitive tissues may be attenuated in diabetic rats. In fact, Glut 4 transporter contents have been reported to decrease in the muscle and fat tissues of diabetic rats (24–26). Garvey et al (24) have demonstrated that the amount of Glut 4 transporter messenger RNA per unit cellular DNA was reduced by 30% in the skeletal muscle and 59% in the fat tissue in streptozocin-induced diabetic rats, as compared with control rats.

As shown in Table 2, insulin treatment 60 minutes before FDG injection significantly reduced F-18 levels in the blood and liver, probably partly because of decreases in the glucose levels in the blood pool and partly because of the shift of FDG to the insulin-sensitive tissues such as the muscle and fat. In the liver, glucose-6-phosphatase may be activated because of insulin-induced reduction of blood glucose levels. Insulin also reduced FDG uptake by the spleen, kidney, and lung, although not significantly. Thus, insulin improves tumor/nontumor ratios of FDG uptake for these organs in diabetes (Table 3).

It has been reported that chronic hyperglycemia downregulates the expression of Glut 1 transporter in several normal tissues of rats, possibly because high levels of glucose could be toxic to cells (27,28). FDG accumulation in the rat mammary cancer cells we used has been shown to be significantly correlated to their Glut 1 expression (18). Thus, one may speculate that decreased tumor FDG uptake in the diabetic rats may result partly from downregulation of Glut 1 expression in tumors and partly from direct competition between FDG and glucose for tumor uptake. In our study, the Glut 1 expression in cancer cell membranes of the untreated diabetic rats appeared lower as compared with that in the control rats. This finding may suggest that the regulation of glucose uptake by rat mammary cancer cells in diabetic rats may partly involve the reduction of membranous expression of Glut 1 transporter. However, it appears that the difference in tumor Glut 1 expression between the control and diabetic rats was not as remarkable as the difference of their tumor FDG uptake. Indeed, it is still not known to what extent FDG uptake depends on Glut 1 expression. For example, an increase of 150% of glucose uptake was associated with a 50% increase in membranous Glut 1 expression of the heart muscle to anoxia (29). Findings in our preliminary clinical studies indicate that in untreated primary breast cancer, the total extent of FDG uptake may be more directly related to the phosphorylation of FDG than to the membrane transport step (30,31). On the other hand, the intensity of Glut 1 tumor staining increased in two of three insulin-treated diabetic rats, as compared with that in untreated diabetic rats. This observation suggests that insulin may increase, at least in some cases, tumor Glut 1 expression in diabetes. However, the number of diabetic animals studied was too small to clarify the meaning of the findings, and further studies are necessary to evaluate and substantiate our hypothesis.

The time between insulin treatment and FDG injection likely affects the degree of change in FDG biodistribution. We found that when the diabetic rats were treated with insulin 30 minutes before FDG injection, the blood glucose levels were still high at the time of FDG injection (Table 1). In addition, such insulin treatment increased FDG uptake by the heart and muscle to only 2.9- and 2.2-fold of the diabetic values, respectively (Table 2). It is probable that FDG injection 30 minutes after insulin treatment was too early for insulin to exert sufficient biologic effect on biodistribution of FDG in diabetic rats.

In the control and untreated diabetic rats, mean blood glucose levels at sacrifice (120 minutes after saline injection) were significantly higher than those at FDG injection (60 minutes after saline injection) (Table 1). A similar phenomenon was observed in our previous study in normal, normoglycemic rats (15). During the experiment, the rats were exposed to stresses—such as multiple ether exposures, blood withdrawals, and intraperitoneal and intravenous injections—which may cause substantial hyperglycemic responses through activation of the adrenergic nervous system (32).

It has been demonstrated that long-term insulin treatment induces insulin resistance of glucose transport in adipose cells from obese or type II diabetes patients (33); therefore, further studies are needed to determine the effect of prolonged insulin treatment on FDG uptake by tumor and nontumor organs in diabetes. Additional studies are also necessary to evaluate FDG uptake by other tumors in diabetes, because some cancer cells are known to be somewhat insulin dependent for glucose uptake in vitro (34,35).

FDG uptake in experimental rat mammary cancer is significantly impaired in rats with streptozocin-induced diabetes. Tumor FDG uptake in these diabetic animals is not significantly changed by insulin treatment 60 minutes before FDG injection. In select instances, it may be possible to achieve improved tumor/nontumor uptake ratios in specific organs such as the liver or lung through the judicious use of insulin in diabetics. Although insulin treatment markedly reduced tumor/muscle ratio of FDG uptake in diabetes, it may improve relative targeting of lung cancer and metastatic liver cancer with FDG because of increased tumor/lung and tumor/liver uptake ratios. Further studies in diabetic patients with cancer are warranted to determine the clinical importance of these findings.

Practical application: In diabetic patients, tumor targeting with FDG will be markedly impaired. It is possible that the use of insulin before FDG injection can improve relative targeting of lung cancer and metastatic liver cancer with FDG because of increased tumor/lung and tumor/liver uptake ratios. Tumor/muscle uptake ratios of FDG are often used for quantitative evaluation of tumor FDG uptake in clinical settings. However, insulin should probably be used with considerable caution in FDG PET imaging of patients with cancer and diabetes, because (*a*) insulin treatment will significantly reduce tumor/background uptake ratios in the muscle tissue and (*b*) adequate insulin dose and time between insulin and FDG injections need to be determined for human studies.

References

1. Warburg O. The mechanism of tumors. New York, NY: Smith, 1931; 129–169.
2. Flier JS, Mueckler MM, Usher P, Lodish HF. Elevated levels of glucose transport and transporter messenger RNA are induced by *ras* or *src* oncogenes. Science 1987; 235:1492–1495.
3. Inokuma T, Tamaki N, Torizuka T, et al. Evaluation of pancreatic tumors with positron emission tomography and F-18 fluorodeoxyglucose: comparison with CT and US. Radiology 1995; 195:345–352.
4. Kubota K, Matsuzawa T, Fujiwara T, et al. Differential diagnosis of lung tumor with positron emission tomography: a prospective study. J Nucl Med 1990; 31:1927–1932.
5. Jabour BA, Choi Y, Hoh CK, et al. Extracranial head and neck: PET imaging with 2-[F-18]fluoro-2-deoxy-D-glucose and MR imaging correlation. Radiology 1993; 186: 27–35.
6. Vitola JV, Delbeke D, Sandler MP, et al. Positron emission tomography to stage suspected metastatic colorectal carcinoma to the liver. Am J Surg 1996; 171:21–26.
7. Wahl RL, Cody RL, Hutchins GD, Mudgett EE. Primary and metastatic breast carcinoma: initial clinical evaluation with PET with the radiolabeled glucose analogue 2-[F-18]-fluoro-2-deoxy-D-glucose. Radiology 1991; 179:765–770.
8. Steinert HC, Hauser M, Allemann F, et al. Non–small cell lung cancer: nodal staging with FDG PET versus CT with correlative lymph node mapping and sampling. Radiology 1997; 202:441–446.
9. Torizuka T, Tamaki N, Inokuma T, et al. Value of fluorine-18-FDG-PET to monitor hepatocellular carcinoma after interventional therapy. J Nucl Med 1994; 35:1965–1969.
10. Wahl RL, Zasadny K, Helvie M, Hutchins GD, Weber B, Cody R. Metabolic monitoring of breast cancer chemohormonotherapy using positron emission tomography: initial evaluation. J Clin Oncol 1993; 11:2101–2111.
11. Wahl RL, Quint LE, Greenough RL, Meyer CR, White RI, Orringer MB. Staging of mediastinal non–small cell lung cancer with FDG PET, CT, and fusion images: preliminary prospective evaluation. Radiology 1994; 191:371–377.
12. Wahl RL, Henry CA, Ethier SP. Serum glucose: effects on tumor and normal tissue accumulation of 2-[F-18]-fluoro-2-deoxy-D-glucose in rodents with mammary carcinoma. Radiology 1992; 183: 643–647.
13. Langen KJ, Braun U, Rota Kops E, et al. The influence of plasma glucose levels on fluorine-18-fluorodeoxyglucose uptake in bronchial carcinomas. J Nucl Med 1993; 34:355–359.
14. Lindholm P, Minn H, Leskinen-Kallio S, Bergman J, Ruotsalainen U, Joensuu H. Influence of the blood glucose concentration on FDG uptake in cancer: a PET study. J Nucl Med 1993; 34:1–6.
15. Torizuka T, Fisher SJ, Wahl RL. Insulin-induced hypoglycemia decreases uptake of 2-[F-18]fluoro-2-deoxy-D-glucose into experimental mammary carcinoma. Radiology 1997; 203:169–172.
16. Ethier SP, Cundiff KC. Importance of extended growth potential and growth factor independence on in vivo neoplastic potential of primary rat mammary carcinoma cells. Cancer Res 1987; 47:5316–5322.
17. Hsu SM, Raine L, Fanger H. Use of avidin-biotin-peroxidase complex (ABC) in immunoperoxidase techniques: a comparison between ABC and unlabeled antibody (PAP) procedures. J Histochem Cytochem 1981; 29:577–580.
18. Brown RS, Leung JY, Fisher SJ, Frey KA, Ethier SP, Wahl RL. Intratumoral distribution of tritiated-FDG in breast carcinoma: correlation between Glut-1 expression and FDG uptake. J Nucl Med 1996; 37:1042–1047.
19. Adler LP, Blair HF, Makley JT, et al. Noninvasive grading of musculoskeletal tumors using PET. J Nucl Med 1991; 32:1508–1512.
20. Minn H, Leskinen-Kallio S, Lindholm P, et al. [18F]Fluorodeoxyglucose uptake in tumors: kinetic vs steady-state methods with reference to plasma insulin. J Comput Assist Tomogr 1993; 17:115–123.
21. Goodman MN, Ruderman NB. Starvation in the rat. I. Effect of age and obesity on organ weights, RNA, DNA, and protein. Am J Physiol 1980; 239:E269–E276.
22. Gould GW, Holman GD. The glucose transporter family: structure, function and tissue-specific expression. Biochem J 1993; 295:329–341.
23. Ismail-Beigi F. Metabolic regulation of glucose transport. J Membr Biol 1993; 135:1–10.
24. Garvey WT, Huecksteadt TP, Birnbaum MJ. Pretranslational suppression of an insulin-responsive glucose transporter in rats with diabetes mellitus. Science 1989; 245:60–63.
25. Gerrits PM, Olson AL, Pessin JE. Regulation of the GLUT4/muscle-fat glucose transporter mRNA in adipose tissue of insulin-deficient diabetic rats. J Biol Chem 1993; 268:640–644.
26. Bourey RE, Koranyi L, James DE, Mueckler M, Permutt MA. Effects of altered glucose homeostasis on glucose transporter expression in skeletal muscle of the rat. J Clin Invest 1990; 86:542–547.
27. Gjedde A, Crone C. Blood-brain glucose transfer: repression in chronic hyperglycemia. Science 1981; 214:456–457.
28. Simmons RA, Flozak AS, Ogata ES. Glucose regulates Glut 1 function and expression in fetal rat lung and muscle in vitro. Endocrinology 1993; 132:2312–2318.
29. Wheeler TJ. Translocation of glucose transporters in response to anoxia in heart. J Biol Chem 1988; 263:19447–19454.
30. Brown RS, Leung JY, Zasadny KR, Flint A, Wahl RL. Relationship between SUV-lean and Glut-1 expression in untreated human lung and breast cancer (abstr). J Nucl Med 1996; 37(suppl):65P.
31. Torizuka T, Zasadny KR, Wahl RL. Comparison of FDG kinetic rate constants in patients with untreated lung cancer and untreated breast cancer (abstr). J Nucl Med 1997; 38(suppl):244P.
32. Garber AJ, Cryer PE, Santiago JV, Haymond MW, Pagliara AS, Kipnis DM. The role of adrenergic mechanisms in the substrate and hormonal response to insulin-induced hypoglycemia in man. J Clin Invest 1976; 58:7–15.
33. Sinha MK, Taylor LG, Pories WJ, et al. Long-term effect of insulin on glucose transport and insulin binding in cultured adipocytes from normal and obese humans with and without non–insulin-dependent diabetes. J Clin Invest 1987; 80:1073–1081.
34. Babia T, Denis-Pouxviel C, Murat JC, et al. Insulin controls key steps of carbohydrate metabolism in cultured HT29 colon cancer cells. Biochem J 1989; 261:175–179.
35. Delicado E, Torres M, Miras-Portugal MT. Effects of insulin on glucose transporters and metabolic patterns in Harding-Passey melanoma cells. Cancer Res 1986; 46: 3762–3767.

Leonard R. Goldfarb, MD
Naomi P. Alazraki, MD
Dennis Eshima, PhD
Lorie A. Eshima, MS
Stephen C. Herda, CNMT
Raghuveer K. Halkar, MD

Index terms:
Lymphatic system, radionuclide studies, 99.12974
Melanoma, 99.8332
Radionuclide imaging, technology, 99.12974
Radionuclide imaging, transit studies, 99.12974
Radionuclides, 99.12974

Radiology 1998; 208:505–509

[1] From the Department of Radiology, Division of Nuclear Medicine, Emory University, Atlanta, Ga (L.R.G., N.P.A., D.E., L.A.E., S.C.H., R.K.H.), and the Department of Nuclear Medicine, Veterans Affairs Medical Center, 1670 Clairmont Rd, Atlanta, GA 30033 (L.R.G., N.P.A., R.K.H.). From the 1997 RSNA scientific assembly. Received December 5, 1997; revision requested February 27, 1998; revision received March 30; accepted April 13. **Address reprint requests to** N.P.A.

Author contributions:
Guarantors of integrity of entire study, L.R.G., N.P.A.; study concepts, L.R.G., N.P.A., D.E.; study design, L.R.G., N.P.A.; definition of intellectual content, L.R.G., N.P.A., D.E.; literature research, L.R.G., N.P.A.; clinical studies, L.R.G., N.P.A., L.A.E., S.C.H.; data acquisition, L.R.G., N.P.A., L.A.E., S.C.H.; data analysis, L.R.G.; statistical analysis, L.R.G., R.K.H.; manuscript preparation, editing, and review, L.R.G., N.P.A.

Lymphoscintigraphic Identification of Sentinel Lymph Nodes: Clinical Evaluation of 0.22-μm Filtration of Tc-99m Sulfur Colloid[1]

PURPOSE: To evaluate the use of 0.22-μm filtration of technetium-99m sulfur colloid particles in the optimization of lymphoscintigraphy.

MATERIALS AND METHODS: Forty-one consecutive lymphoscintigraphic studies obtained with 0.22-μm filtration of Tc-99m sulfur colloid in 41 patients (26 men, 15 women; average age, 55.4 years) and 41 consecutive studies obtained with 5.0-μm filtration in 41 patients (20 men, 21 women; average age, 54.5 years) were retrospectively, randomly reviewed. Studies were evaluated for lymphatic channel depiction and sentinel lymph node depiction. Studies included immediate flow images (obtained at 10 seconds per frame) and multiview static images obtained up to 2 hours after intradermal Tc-99m sulfur colloid injection.

RESULTS: The number of drainage beds visualized was 52 with 5.0-μm filtration and 51 with 0.22-μm filtration ($P = .570$). The number of lymphatic channels visualized was 45 with 5.0-μm filtration and 75 with 0.22-μm filtration ($P = .006$). The number of lymph nodes visualized was 102 with 5.0-μm filtration and 123 with 0.22-μm filtration ($P = .123$). The number of studies judged as optimal (ie, depicted lymphatic channels leading to sentinel nodes) was 10 with 5.0-μm filtration and 19 with 0.22-μm filtration ($P = .038$). The number of studies with depicted lymph nodes but no depicted lymphatic channel was 15 with 5.0-μm filtration and six with 0.22-μm filtration ($P = .023$).

CONCLUSION: The use of 0.22-μm filtration in the preparation of Tc-99m sulfur colloid substantially improves study quality and increases the diagnostic certainty in the identification of sentinel lymph nodes.

Lymphoscintigraphy has recaptured the interest of physicians involved in the diagnosis and treatment of melanoma (1–5). The use of lymphoscintigraphy with the intraoperative gamma probe (C-Track Probe; Care Wise, Morgan Hill, Calif) substantially aids physicians in the surgical management and staging of melanoma (6–8). Linking the scintigraphic identification of the sentinel node to the intraoperative identification and excision of these nodes is not always a simple process. To be properly performed, lymphoscintigraphy requires the optimal selection and preparation of the radiopharmaceutical and the imaging protocol (9).

Linking the transit of radiolabeled particles from a primary melanoma site to a sentinel lymph node ideally is based on the visualization of lymphatic channels that lead to a sentinel node. Retention of radiolabeled particles within sentinel lymph nodes is required for the identification of these nodes at subsequent surgical exploration (usually 1–3 hours after imaging was completed) aided by the handheld gamma probe. Particle size is a major

1) 150 mCi (5.6 MBq) Tc-99m sodium pertechnetate and syringe A (hydrochloric acid) are added to vial
2) The vial is heated for 3 minutes in a rolling water bath
3) Cool for 2 minutes at room temperature
4) Add syringe B (sodium hydroxide and sodium biphosphate) to the vial
5) The patient dose of 1-2 mCi (37–74 MBq) is withdrawn through a 0.22-μm polycarbonite filter into a 3-mL tuberculin syringe
6) Dose is diluted to a volume of 1–2 mL (final concentration, 1mCi/mL [37 MBq/mL])

Figure 1. Steps of radiopharmaceutical preparation: modification of the TechneScan Sulfur Colloid Kit (Mallinckrodt Medical, St Louis, Mo).

1) The patient is positioned appropriately to maximize comfort and provide ease in performing the examination. The position should match that planned for subsequent surgery.
2) The area around the melanoma lesion is prepared in a sterile fashion.
3) 0.25–0.50 mCi (9.25–18.5 MBq) of Tc-99m sulfur colloid in a volume of 0.25–0.50 mL of normal saline solution is injected intradermally circumferentially in equal injections at four to six areas at the periphery of the lesion or excision scar. An injection that is too large or too distant from the lesion margin could result in the entering of colloid into lymphatic vessels that do not drain the lesion.
4) Dynamic images are obtained with a scintillation camera at 10-second intervals for 10 minutes.
5) Static images of 5 minutes each are obtained for 30 minutes with the patient in the optimal position for visualizing the nodal uptake. Note: Additional imaging may be needed if nodal uptake is delayed for 1 hour or longer.
6) The skin overlying the region of the nodal uptake is marked.
7) Transmission images obtained with a cobalt-57 source are recommended for optimal anatomic localization; a Tc-99m flood source or tank can also be used.

Figure 2. Steps of patient preparation and lymphoscintigraphy.

factor that affects the entrance of particles into the lymphatic system, their rate of transit, and their degree of retention by lymph nodes (10); therefore, optimization of imaging and identification of sentinel nodes intraoperatively is dependent on choice of suitable particle size of the radiocolloidal agent.

The purpose of the current investigation was to evaluate the effectiveness of using a 0.22-μm polycarbonite filter in the radiopharmaceutical preparation of technetium-99m sulfur colloid for lymphoscintigraphy, to be followed by surgical probe localization of sentinel lymph nodes on the basis of findings of the analysis of clinical studies.

MATERIALS AND METHODS

Lymphoscintigraphy at Emory University Hospital, Atlanta, Ga, was performed with a large-field-of-view, single-head camera (Starcam 400 AC or 500 AC; GE Medical Systems, Milwaukee, Wis) more than 250 times from April 1994 to January 1997. Studies were performed for the evaluation of lymphatic drainage and for the identification of sentinel nodes in patients with a diagnosed primary melanoma. A modified preparation of Tc-99m sulfur colloid (Technescan Sulfur Colloid Kit; Mallinckrodt Medical, St Louis, Mo) (11,12), in which the radiopharmaceutical was put through a 5.0-μm filter to eliminate very coarse clumped particles, initially was used. The use of fine 0.22-μm filtration in the preparation of Tc-99m sulfur colloid was initiated in April 1996 (Fig 1). A random selection of 41 consecutive studies obtained by using 0.22-μm filtration in 41 patients (26 men, 15 women; average age, 55.4 years) and 41 consecutive studies obtained by using 5.0-μm filtration in 41 patients (20 men, 21 women; average age, 54.5 years) were retrospectively reviewed in random order. The review included the immediate 10-second-per-frame flow images from a 10-minute dynamic acquisition and multiview static images obtained 10–60 minutes after the intradermal Tc-99m sulfur colloid injection at four to six points around the primary tumor site (Fig 2). The injections contained 100 μCi (3.7 MBq) per 0.1 mL; each intradermal administration was approximately 0.1 mL. All Tc-99m sulfur colloid was prepared by using a modified protocol of decreased heating time (3.0 minutes instead of 5.0 minutes) to minimize particle size (12).

Two nuclear medicine and radiology physicians (L.R.G., N.P.A.) retrospectively reviewed the studies. A study was judged to be optimal if lymphatic channels were well defined on both the dynamic flow images and the static delayed images. The numbers of lymphatic drainage basins, distinct channels visualized, and nodes demonstrating focal radiotracer uptake were recorded for each study. A sentinel node was identified with diagnostic certainty as a focus of retained activity that appeared as the first accumulation of radiotracer along a well-defined channel that could be traced from the lesion site to the node. A secondary node was identified as a more distal focus of retained radiotracer along a lymphatic channel that was in series with a sentinel node but that filled with radiopharmaceutical after the sentinel node. Any node that was not associated with a visualized channel was indeterminate. It was assumed for surgical purposes that an indeterminate node represented a sentinel node; therefore, excisional biopsy was performed on these nodes.

Results Summary: Frequency of Diagnostic Features

	Filtration 5.0 μm	Filtration 0.22 μm	*P* Value
Studies	41	41	NA
Drainage beds*	52	51	.570
Lymphatic channels visualized	45	75	.006
Lymph nodes visualized	102	123	.123
Studies judged to be optimal†	10	19	.038
Studies without visualized channel‡	15	6	.023

Note.—NA = not applicable.
* Axillary, inguinal, cervical, subclavian, and posterior auricular beds.
† Lymphatic channels leading to sentinel nodes were visualized.
‡ Lymph nodes visualized, but lymphatic channels not visualized.

For statistical analyses, the examinations were considered as two independent Bernoulli trials. Successful (optimal) studies were characterized as those depicting lymphatic channels that led to sentinel nodes on flow and static images. The diagnostic features were statistically evaluated (*z* test), with a *P* value of less than .05 considered to indicate a statistically significant difference (Table).

RESULTS

Figures 3–5 contain images from lymphoscintigraphic studies obtained with no

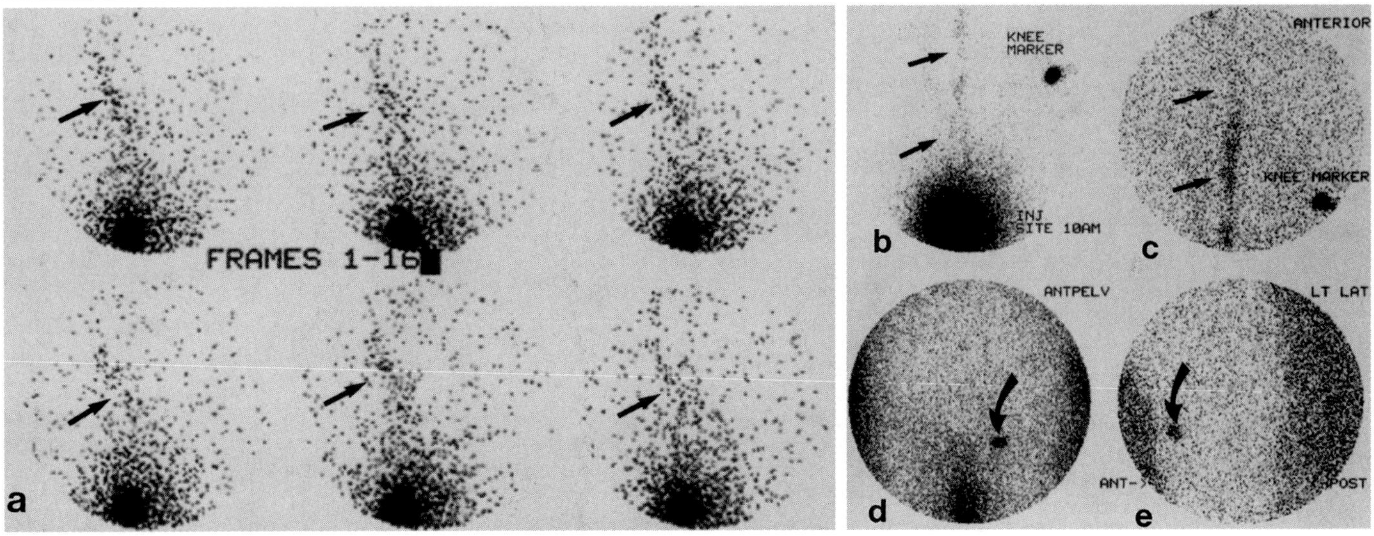

Figure 3. Lymphoscintigraphic images obtained after injection of 5.0-μm filtered Tc-99m sulfur colloid show a single node and poor channel definition in a 55-year-old woman with a primary melanoma site on the left lower extremity below the knee. *a,* Immediate 10-second per frame flow images show migration of the radiotracer (arrows) from the injection site ("hot spot" at lower end of image) along the medial aspect of the left lower extremity. Anterior static images at the, *b,* knee level and, *c,* thigh level show the pathway of flow (arrows in *b* and *c*) from the injection (*INJ*) site relative to a knee marker. Subsequent *d,* anterior pelvic (*ANTPELV*) and *e,* left lateral pelvic (*LT LAT*) views demonstrate retention of the radiotracer in a sentinel node in the left inguinal region (arrow in *d* and *e*). Radiotracer in a lymphatic channel that leads to the node is not depicted. *ANT* = anterior, *POST* = posterior.

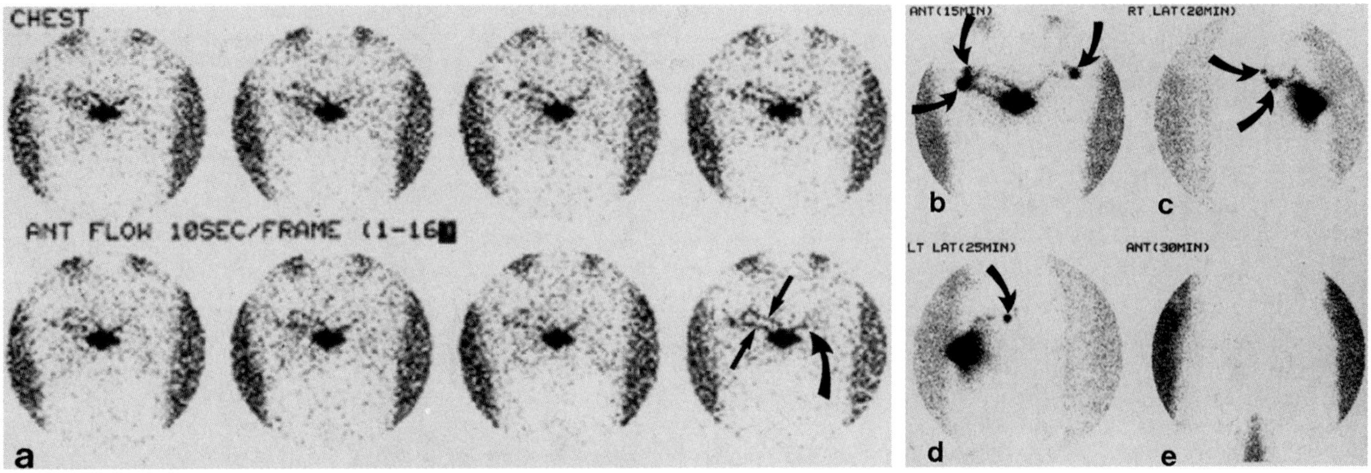

Figure 4. Lymphoscintigraphic images obtained after injection of 0.22-μm filtered Tc-99m sulfur colloid at the site of the primary melanoma excision (largest hot spot in *a–d*) on the middle part of the back in a 49-year-old man show multiple, well-defined channels and multiple sentinel nodes. *a,* anterior view flow (*ANT FLOW*) images show radiotracer in two well-defined lymphatic channels (straight arrows) extending to the right axilla and one well-defined channel (curved arrow) extending to the left axilla. Static images obtained in the *b,* anterior (*ANT*), *c,* right lateral (*RT LAT*), and *d,* left lateral (*LT LAT*) views distinctly depict three sentinel nodes (arrows). *e,* Anterior (*ANT*) view static image of the lower abdomen and pelvis silhouetted by a sheet source helps to exclude unsuspected pathways of lymphatic flow to other nodal basins.

microfiltration (5.0-μm filtration) (Fig 3) or with microfiltration (0.22-μm filtration) (Figs 4, 5). A consistently better definition of lymphatic channels that lead to a sentinel node is seen when microfiltration is used in preparation of the Tc-99m sulfur colloid radiopharmaceutical.

The total number of lymph nodes visualized in each imaging study was tabulated for those cases in which 0.22-μm filtration was used and for those in which 5.0-μm filtration was used (Table). Figure 6 graphically displays the distribution of the frequency of nodal visualization according to the filtration used. Similar numbers of lymph nodes were visualized whether 0.22-μm filtration was used or not. Figure 7 shows the distribution of the frequency of lymphatic channel depiction for the two groups. The distribution is significantly (P = .023) shifted toward nonvisualization (zero lymphatic channels seen) in the group of studies in which 0.22-μm filtration was not used. This is also indicated by the differences in the total numbers of channels depicted: 45 in the 5.0-μm filtration group compared to 75 in the 0.22-μm filtration group (P = .006).

DISCUSSION

The total number of lymph nodes and the total number of lymphatic drainage beds depicted were not significantly different ($P = .123$ and $P = .570$, respectively) for the two sizes of filters used. This suggests that there was no statistically significant difference in nodal retention for the different particle size profiles.

Studies in which no channel was seen on flow or static images were considered suboptimal for the purposes of definitive identification of sentinel lymph nodes, because a sentinel lymph node cannot be definitively identified as such without visualization of its afferent lymphatic channel coursing from the primary tumor site. Absence of lymphatic channel visualization was noted significantly more often ($P = .023$) when 0.22-μm filtration was not used. Studies in which all sentinel nodes are identified at the time of surgical exploration (even those with some secondary nodes mislabeled as sentinel nodes) are considered adequate. Reduction in the time and extent of the surgical exploration, however, is best achieved with an optimal lymphoscintigraphic mapping study so that only those nodes that are truly sentinel nodes are identified with the probe and excised. Studies were judged to be optimal with significantly greater frequency ($P = .038$) when 0.22-μm filtration was used (Fig 7): The total number of channels visualized was significantly greater ($P = .006$) when 0.22-μm filtration was used. The channels better define the "road map" of lymphatic drainage and improve the discrimination between sentinel and secondary lymph nodes.

The issues surrounding the optimal radiopharmaceutical selection for lymphoscintigraphy and intraoperative gamma-probe localization of sentinel nodes relate to radiopharmaceutical particle size and the timing of the imaging and surgical lymph node excisions. In the United States, Food and Drug Administration approval and therefore availability for clinical use is limited to Tc-99m sulfur colloid and Tc-99m human serum albumin. Tc-99m antimony sulfide colloid has a range and distribution of particle size (0.003–0.03-μm range) that has been reported to produce lymphatic maps of satisfactory quality (13). Tc-99m human serum albumin is not widely used for this procedure because, although it has the advantage of rapid uptake into the lymphatic system, it also has the likely disadvantage of poor retention in lymph nodes. Its molecular weight is about 65,000 Da, which has been translated into a particle size of about 0.004 μm.

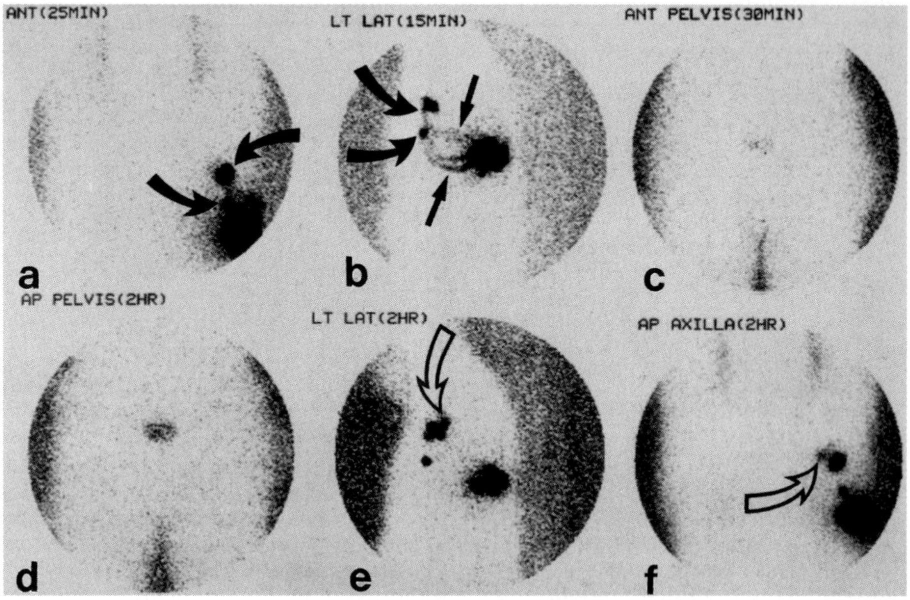

Figure 5. Lymphoscintigraphic images obtained after injection of 0.22-μm filtered Tc-99m sulfur colloid show multiple, well-defined channels and multiple sentinel nodes in a 37-year-old man with a primary melanoma site on the left lateral aspect of the chest. *a,* Anterior chest (*ANT*), *b,* left lateral chest (*LT LAT*), and *c,* anterior pelvic (*ANT PELVIS*) images were obtained within the 1st hour after injection. *d,* Anteroposterior pelvic (*AP PELVIS*), *e,* left lateral chest (*LT LAT*), and *f,* anteroposterior axillary (*AP AXILLA*) images were obtained after 2 hours. The largest hot spot corresponds to the injection site in *a, b, e,* and *f.* The early static images show four well-defined channels (straight arrows in *b*) and two clusters of sentinel nodes (solid curved arrows in *a* and *b*). The later static images show retention of radiotracer in sentinel nodes and an additional node (open curved arrow in *e* and *f*). *c* and *d* show a small amount of excreted activity in the urinary bladder, with no sentinel node uptake in this region.

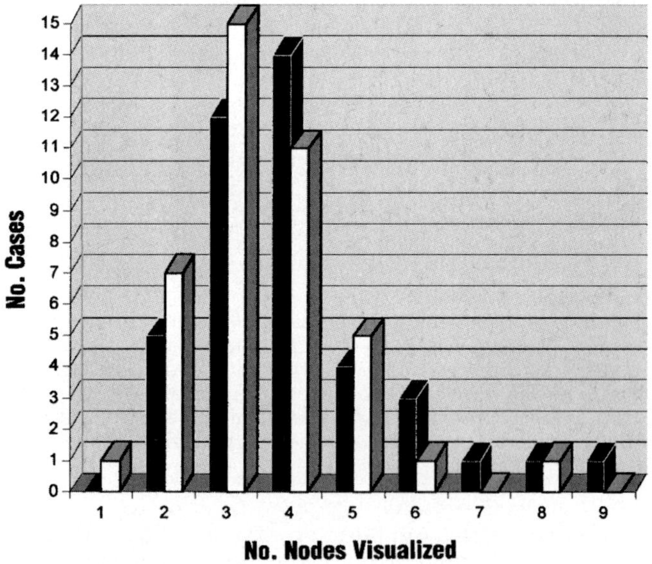

Figure 6. Distribution of the frequency of nodal visualization. ■ = 0.22-μm filtration, □ = 5.0-μm filtration.

Standard preparation of a Tc-99m sulfur colloid produces a large colloid particle, with the disadvantages of very slow lymphatic uptake and transit. Modifications in such factors as the age of Tc-99m eluate, the heating time of the sulfur colloid (11), and the use of microfiltration (14–16) yield a preparation that provides for better imaging and more desirable sentinel node retention characteristics (12). The true test of whether a particular radiolabeled particle prepara-

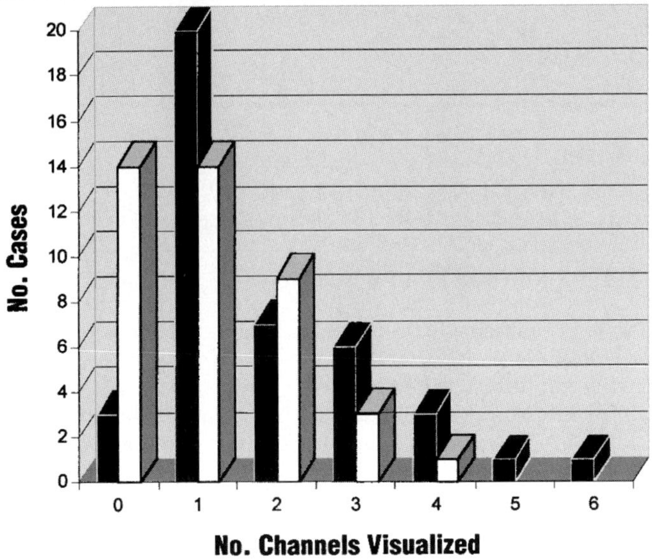

Figure 7. Distribution of the frequency of channel visualization. ■ = 0.22-μm filtration, □ = 5.0-μm filtration.

tion is optimal for lymphoscintigraphy tests not only its in vitro characteristics, but also, more important, whether it ultimately achieves a noticeable and substantial improvement in image quality. This should result in increased diagnostic certainty, which improves the identification of sentinel lymph nodes in clinical studies for surgical probe localization.

Discrimination between sentinel lymph nodes and secondary lymph nodes may not always be possible with diagnostic certainty if the lymphoscintigraphic examination is not optimal; that is, discreet lymphatic channels must be seen leading from the tumor site to the sentinel lymph nodes. Lymphoscintigraphic imaging studies obtained with a modified preparation of Tc-99m sulfur colloid demonstrate that 0.22-μm filtration results in substantially more definitive sentinel lymph node identification and optimal studies.

References

1. Morton DL, Wen DR, Wong JH, et al. Technical details of intraoperative lymphatic mapping for early stage melanoma. Arch Surg 1992; 127:392–399.
2. Morton DL, Wen DR, Foshag LJ, et al. Intraoperative lymphatic mapping and selective cervical lymphadenectomy for early-stage melanomas of the head and neck. J Clin Oncol 1993; 11:1751–1756.
3. Uren RF, Hofman-Giles RB, Shaw HM, et al. Lymphoscintigraphy in high risk melanoma of the trunk: predicting drainage node groups, defining lymphatic channels and locating the sentinel node. J Nucl Med 1993; 34:1435–1440.
4. Berman C, Norman J, Cruse CW, Reintgen DS, Clark RA. Lymphoscintigraphy in malignant melanoma. Ann Plast Surg 1992; 28:29–32.
5. Norman J, Cruse CW, Espinosa C, et al. Redefinition of cutaneous lymphatic drainage with the use of lymphoscintigraphy for malignant melanoma. Am J Surg 1991; 162:432–437.
6. Alex JC, Krag DN. Gamma probe guided localization of lymph nodes. Surg Oncol 1993; 2:137–143.
7. Alex JC, Weaver DL, Fairbank JT, Rankin BS, Krag DN. Gamma probe guided lymph node localization in malignant melanoma. Surg Oncol 1993; 2:303–308.
8. Krag DN, Meijer SJ, Weaver DL, et al. Minimal-access surgery of malignant melanoma. Arch Surg 1995; 130:654–658.
9. Taylor AT, Murray D, Herda SC, et al. Dynamic lymphoscintigraphy to identify sentinel and satellite nodes. Clin Nucl Med 1996; 21:755–758.
10. Bergqvist L, Strand SE, Persson BRR. Particle sizing and biokinetics of interstitial lymphoscintigraphic agents. Semin Nucl Med 1993; 12:9–19.
11. Eshima D, Eshima L, Gotti NM, et al. Technetium-99m-sulfur colloid for lymphoscintigraphy: effects of preparation parameters. J Nucl Med 1996; 37:1575–1578.
12. Alazraki NP, Eshima D, Eshima LA, et al. Lymphoscintigraphy, the sentinel node concept, and the intraoperative gamma probe in melanoma, breast cancer, and other potential cancers. Semin Nucl Med 1997; 27:55–67.
13. O'Brien CJ, Uren RF, Thompson JF, et al. Prediction of potential metastatic sites in cutaneous head and neck melanoma using lymphoscintigraphy. Am J Surg 1995; 170:461–466.
14. Larson SM, Nelp WB. Radiopharmacology of a simplified technetium-99m colloid preparation for photoscanning. J Nucl Med 1966; 7:817–826.
15. Dragotakes SC, Callahan RJ, LaPointe LC, et al. Particle size characterization of a filtered Tc-99m sulfur colloid preparation for lymphoscintigraphy (abstr). J Nucl Med 1995; 36:80P.
16. Hung JC, Wiseman GA, Wahner HW, et al. Filtered technetium-99m-sulfur colloid evaluated for lymphoscintigraphy. J Nucl Med 1995; 36:1895–1901.

Book Review

Handbook of Health Physics and Radiological Health. 3rd ed.

Edited by Bernard Shleien, PharmD, MSHyg, CHP, FAPHA, FHPS, Lester A. Slaback, Jr, CHP, and Brian Kent Birky, PhD
Baltimore, Md: Williams & Wilkins, 1998. ISBN 0-683-18334-6. Hardcover, $115.00; pp 946; 184 figures; tables.

Handbook of Health Physics and Radiological Health is a compendium of facts and data intended to serve as a ready reference book for those who regularly need radiologic health information in their day-to-day work. Its principal audience is the health physicist, although it may be of value to other professionals in the radiation field. The book covers the entire scope of radiation use and exposure, and it includes a number of useful sections on medical sources of radiation exposure.

The book is divided into 12 chapters. Much of the information presented is taken from sources such as the National Council on Radiation Protection and Measurements, International Commission on Radiological Protection, Nuclear Regulatory Commission, Food and Drug Administration, and Environmental Protection Agency, thus serving as a digest of much of the radiologic information provided by these organizations. The chapters on estimated radiation doses from various sources, patient doses, bioeffects and risk, and nonionizing radiation will be of interest to radiologists. Much of the handbook contains data on health physics and radiation safety, which will be of principal value to those who work in these areas.

This handbook is one of the most comprehensive compendiums on radiologic health data available. The material is presented in an organized and clear manner. There are many tables and graphs, and all of the information is referenced. The facts presented in the 1992 edition have been updated, and material has been added to this edition where appropriate.

Handbook of Health Physics and Radiological Health is meant mainly to be a reference for health physicists; not every radiologist needs a copy. However, it may be a valuable resource in a department library as a reference on radiologic health issues.

Reviewed by Dean W. Broga, PhD

Takuhito Tada, MD
Kazuo Minakuchi, MD
Mayuko Koda, MD
Noriyuki Masuda, MD
Kaoru Matsui, MD
Ichiro Kawase, MD
Toshifumi Nakajima, MD
Masayuki Nishioka, MD
Masahiro Fukuoka, MD
Takahiro Kozuka, MD

Index terms:
Lung neoplasms, 60.3213
Lung neoplasms, therapeutic radiology, 60.1299
Lung neoplasms, therapy, 60.1299

Radiology 1998; 208:511–515

[1] From the Department of Radiology (T.T., K. Minakuchi, M.K., T.K.) and the Second Department of Internal Medicine (N.M., K. Matsui, I.K.), Osaka Prefectural Habikino Hospital, 3-7-1 Habikino, Habikino-city, Osaka 583-0872, Japan; the Department of Radiology, Tenri Hospital, Japan (T.N.); the Department of Radiology, Osaka City University, Japan (M.N.); and the Fourth Department of Internal Medicine, Kinki University, Osakasayama, Japan (M.F.). Received September 3, 1997; revision requested November 19; final revision received and accepted March 3, 1998. **Address reprint requests to** T.T.

Author contributions:
Guarantor of integrity of entire study, T.T.; study concepts and design, T.T.; clinical studies, T.T., N.M., K. Matsui, I.K., M.N., M.F., T.K.; data acquisition, T.T., M.K.; data analysis, T.T., K. Minakuchi, T.N.; statistical analysis, T.T.; manuscript preparation, T.T.; manuscript review, K.M., T.N., N.M.

Limited-Stage Small Cell Lung Cancer: Local Failure after Chemotherapy and Radiation Therapy[1]

PURPOSE: To evaluate radiation therapy regimens for improvement in local control in patients with limited-stage small cell lung cancer.

MATERIALS AND METHODS: Radical radiation therapy results in 117 patients with limited-stage small cell lung cancer were retrospectively reviewed. The protocols in 90 patients were 40 Gy in 20 fractions ($n = 28$), 50 Gy in 25 fractions ($n = 32$), and 45 Gy in 30 fractions (accelerated hyperfractionation, $n = 30$). The other 27 patients received thoracic irradiation (dose range, 20–60 Gy; median dose, 54 Gy). All patients underwent systemic chemotherapy.

RESULTS: The 5-year Kaplan-Meier survival rates in the patients with N0, N1, N2, and N3 disease were 26%, 34%, 18%, and 0%, respectively; the rates of in-field relapse were 25%, 36%, 26%, and 25%, respectively; and the rates of marginal relapse were 0%, 9%, 15%, and 29%, respectively. In 56% of patients with marginal relapse, the relapse site was at the upper margin. The 4-year in-field control rates for the patients who underwent 40, 50, and 45 Gy were 51%, 70%, and 56%, respectively.

CONCLUSION: Patients with N3 limited-stage small cell lung cancer should undergo a separate protocol, and the upper margin should be extended in patients with N2 or N3 disease.

Approximately 30% of patients with small cell lung cancer have limited-stage cancer, which is defined as a tumor confined to one hemithorax and the regional lymph nodes, exclusive of the contralateral hilar lymph nodes. Even in patients with limited-stage small cell lung cancer, however, undetected metastatic disease is often present. Systemic chemotherapy is therefore considered to be the primary modality of treatment.

The results of several prospective studies (1–4) have indicated that thoracic radiation therapy improves the survival time of patients with limited-stage small cell lung cancer. As a consequence, further studies of ways to optimize thoracic radiation therapy have been performed. Takada et al (5) reported the preliminary results of their prospective study of concurrent versus sequential thoracic radiation therapy in combination with cisplatin and etoposide; they found that the median survival time in the patients who received concurrent therapy was 31.3 months. The complete-response rate of 38% was insufficient, however, and further improvement in survival time could be expected. We performed a retrospective study to investigate the patterns of local failure in patients with limited-stage small cell lung cancer.

MATERIALS AND METHODS

Patients

The study group consisted of consecutive patients with limited-stage small cell lung cancer who underwent radical radiation therapy at Osaka Prefectural Habikino Hospital (Japan) between 1986 and 1993. Three patients with two concurrent types of cancer and two patients who underwent surgical resection were excluded. The remaining 117 patients constituted the study group, and their characteristics are summarized in Table 1. Performance status was evaluated on the basis of the Eastern Cooperative Oncology Group criteria (6).

Staging of Disease

Diagnoses were established on the basis of histopathologic examination results in specimens obtained at bronchoscopic biopsy, sputum acquisition, or needle biopsy. Stage of disease was determined by means of chest radiography; computed tomography (CT) of the chest, upper abdomen, and brain; bone scintigraphy; and bone marrow biopsy. Physical examination, routine blood analysis (blood count and blood chemistry determination), and pulmonary function studies were also performed.

Treatment

Thoracic irradiation was performed with 10 MV of photons from a linear accelerator (model ML15-MIII; Mitsubishi, Tokyo, Japan). The dose distribution was calculated with a two-dimensional treatment planning system (MODULEX; Computerized Medical System, Maryland Heights, Mo). A CT simulator was not used.

Three dose-fraction schedules were used: 40 Gy in 20 fractions (in 28 patients treated between January 1986 and August 1988), 50 Gy in 25 fractions (in 32 patients treated between September 1988 and August 1990), and 45 Gy in 30 fractions (in 30 patients treated between September 1990 and December 1993 with accelerated hyperfractionation [1.5 Gy administered twice daily at an interval of 4–6 hours]). Twenty-seven patients in this study either could not receive the full dose or underwent treatment with protocols that had not been established. The radiation doses in these latter patients ranged from 20 to 60 Gy (median, 54 Gy). Four patients received doses of less than 40 Gy.

From September 1990 to December 1993, the radiation field was defined as the area that contained the primary tumor, a margin of 15 mm, the bilateral upper mediastinal lymph nodes, the subcarinal lymph nodes, and the regional enlarged lymph nodes (Fig 1). After initial irradiation with a dose of 30 Gy, off-cord (ie, the spinal cord was outside the field), oblique boost fields were used. In the patients who underwent treatment between January 1986 and August 1990, however, the field was not well defined, and off-cord oblique boost fields were not used. Between January 1986 and August 1988, radiation fields in 16 patients with N2 disease contained supraclavicular lymph nodes in five (31%) patients and upper mediastinal lymph nodes without supraclavicular lymph nodes in five (31%) patients. In the other six (38%) patients, the radiation field did not contain upper mediastinal lymph nodes. On the other hand, in three (60%) of five patients with N3 disease, the radiation field contained supraclavicular lymph nodes.

Between September 1988 and August 1990, in the patients who received a dose of 50 Gy, the last dose of 10 Gy was administered by using boost fields that contained only the primary tumor. Initial fields contained supraclavicular lymph nodes in one (6%) of 16 patients with N2 disease and upper mediastinal lymph nodes without supraclavicular lymph nodes in 13 (81%) patients. In the other two (12%) patients, the initial fields did not contain upper mediastinal lymph nodes. On the other hand, in six (55%) of 11 patients with N3 disease, the initial radiation field contained supraclavicular lymph nodes. In most patients, prechemotherapy volumes were treated. In at least three patients who received a dose of 40 Gy and in three patients who received a dose of 50 Gy, however, only postchemotherapy volumes were treated. These patients included three with N2 disease and three with N3 disease.

TABLE 1
Patient Characteristics

Characteristics	No. of Patients
Sex	
Male	93 (79)
Female	24 (21)
Performance status*	
0–1	101 (86)
2	13 (11)
3	3 (3)
Stage	
I	4 (3)
II	9 (8)
IIIA	54 (46)
IIIB	50 (43)
N factor	
0	9 (8)
1	11 (9)
2	67 (57)
3	30 (26)

Note.—Values in parentheses are percentages. Average age was 64 years (age range, 41–80 years).
* Evaluated on the basis of Eastern Cooperative Oncology Group criteria.

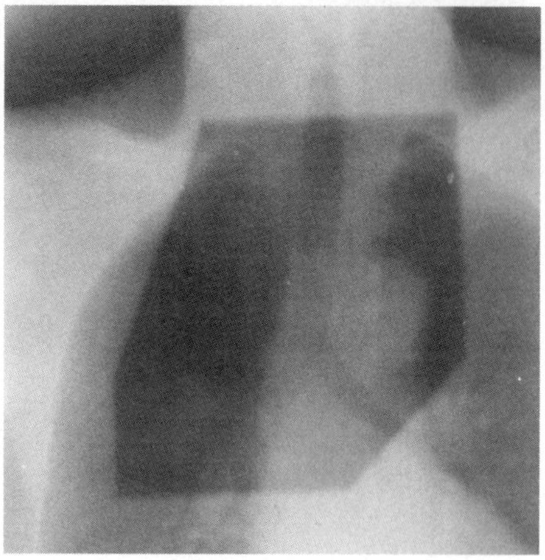

Figure 1. Portal localization radiograph shows a typical radiation field in a patient with N3 disease.

TABLE 2
Systemic Chemotherapy in Patients with Small Cell Lung Cancer

Regimen	No. of Patients
Cisplatin and etoposide	67 (58)
Cyclophosphamide, doxorubicin, and vincristine, with cisplatin and etoposide	19 (16)
Cisplatin with vincristine sulfate, doxorubicin, and etoposide	10 (9)
Carboplatin plus etoposide	9 (8)
Cyclophosphamide, doxorubicin, and vincristine	7 (6)
Other	4 (3)

Note.—Numbers in parentheses are percentages.

TABLE 3
Frequency of Pneumonitis

Dose	RTOG Grade* III	IV	V
40 Gy (n = 28)	4	0	1
45 Gy (n = 30)†	2	0	1
50 Gy (n = 32)	2	0	0
60 Gy (n = 12)	2	0	2
Other (n = 15)	2	0	1

* RTOG = Radiation Therapy Oncology Group.
† Accelerated hyperfraction.

All patients underwent systemic chemotherapy. The chemotherapy protocols are summarized in Table 2. Ninety-seven (83%) patients received a combination of cisplatin and etoposide. In many patients who underwent treatment between September 1988 and

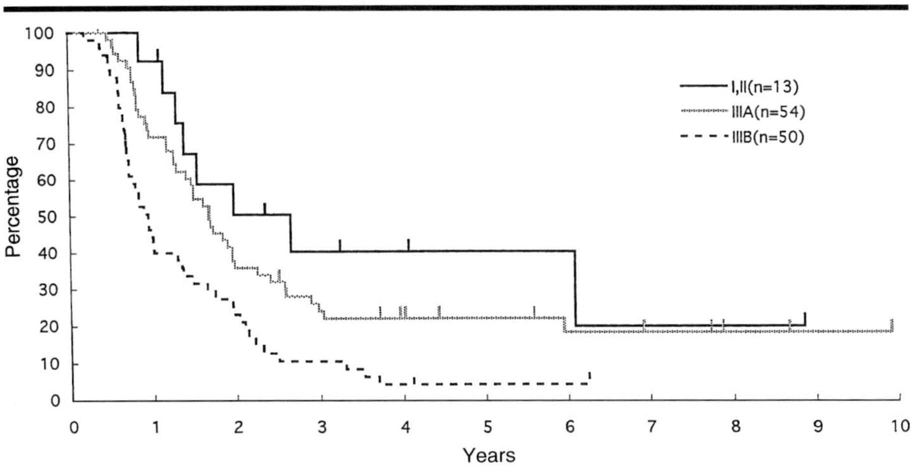

Figure 2. Kaplan-Meier survival curves for patients subgrouped according to cancer stage.

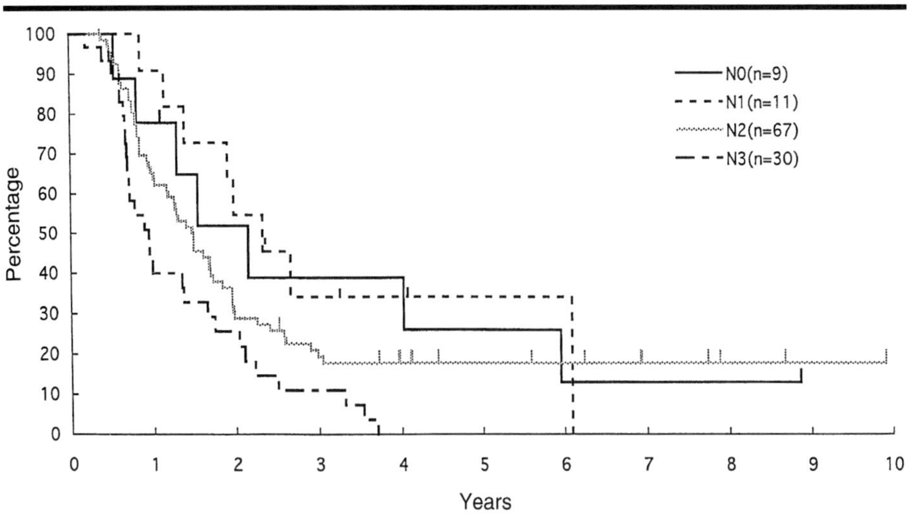

Figure 3. Kaplan-Meier survival curves for patients subgrouped according to N factor.

December 1993, chemotherapy and radiation therapy were performed concurrently. In the patients who received doses of 50 Gy and 45 Gy, respectively, 21 (66%) of 32 and 16 (53%) of 30 underwent chemotherapy and radiation therapy concurrently.

Toxicity

All patient records were analyzed with respect to treatment-induced pneumonitis. Criteria of the Radiation Therapy Oncology Group were used in the scoring of the patient data (Table 3).

Analysis

Survival rates were calculated with the Kaplan-Meier method. Statistical analysis was performed with the generalized Wilcoxon signed-rank test.

RESULTS

The overall complete-response rate was 44% (51 of 117 patients), and the partial-response rate was 48% (56 of 117 patients). Six patients died during the study period, and three were lost to follow-up.

The Kaplan-Meier survival curves of patients subgrouped with respect to stage and to N factor are shown in Figures 2 and 3, respectively. The median survival time associated with stage I–II, IIIA, and IIIB disease was 28, 20, and 11 months, respectively; the overall 2-year survival rate was 50%, 36%, and 23%, respectively; and the 5-year survival rate was 40%, 22%, and 4%, respectively. There was a significant difference between the survival rate of patients with stage IIIA disease and that of patients with stage IIIB disease ($P < .01$). The median survival time associated with N0, N1, N2, and N3 disease was 26, 28, 18, and 11 months, respectively; the overall 2-year survival rate was 52%, 55%, 29%, and 25%, respectively; and the 5-year survival rate was 26%, 34%, 18%, and 0%, respectively. There was a significant difference in survival rate between patients with N2 disease and those with N3 disease ($P < .05$).

Sites of relapse in the patients who had responses to treatment are summarized according to N factor in Table 4. Local relapse was subgrouped according to in-field relapse and marginal relapse, that is, relapse with respect to the radiation field. (Marginal relapse was defined as locoregional relapse and cervical lymph node metastases outside the initial radiation field or at the edge of the radiation field.) In two patients with N2 disease who received a dose of 50 Gy, relapse occurred at the edge of the local boost field. Relapse in these two patients was classified as in-field relapse, because it occurred within the initial field. Only sites of the first local failure were reported, whether the failure was an in-field relapse or a marginal relapse. Local relapse and distant metastases, however, partly overlapped. In nine patients with N2 disease and in eight patients with N3 disease, marginal relapse occurred. There was a small but notable difference in marginal relapse rates between patients with N2 disease and those with N3 disease ($P = .08$). Follow-up in the 19 relapse-free patients was 39–128 months (median, 75 months). Four patients died of complications related to the treatment, two died of other diseases, and three were lost to follow-up.

The site of marginal relapse in 10 patients was the upper margin, including the cervical lymph nodes in three patients, the supraclavicular lymph nodes in five, and the upper mediastinal lymph nodes in two. Marginal relapse occurred in the peripheral area of the lung in five patients, the contralateral mediastinal or hilar lymph nodes in three, and the lower mediastinal lymph nodes in one. (The data for marginal relapse partly overlap).

In 67 of the 117 patients, 95 sites of distant metastases were observed. The sites were the brain ($n = 40$), liver ($n = 17$), bone ($n = 9$), lung ($n = 8$), adrenal gland ($n = 7$), skin ($n = 5$), abdominal lymph nodes ($n = 5$), and other tissues ($n = 4$).

The distribution of patients according to N factor with respect to radiation dose is presented in Table 5. Because the distribution was too skewed for evaluation of the survival time, only the in-field local control rate was investigated (Fig 4). In this part of the study, only target volumes that received the full dose were evaluated. Therefore, relapse at the edge of the local boost fields in the 50-Gy group was classified as marginal relapse. The 4-year in-field Kaplan-Meier control rates were 51%, 56%, and 70%, respectively, for the patients treated with doses of 40, 45, and 50 Gy. There was no significant difference in local control rate between doses of 40 and 45 Gy, 40 and 50 Gy, or 45 and 50 Gy ($P > .05$).

In six patients, postchemotherapy volumes were treated. Marginal relapse, in-field relapse, and brain metastases occurred in three patients, two patients, and one patient, respectively.

Four patients died of pneumonitis related to the chemotherapy and radiation therapy. The radiation doses were 40, 45, and 54 Gy in one each of these patients and 60 Gy in two patients.

TABLE 4
Sites of Relapse

	Local Relapse		Distant Metastases				
N Factor	In-field	Marginal	Distant Metastases Only	Distant Metastases with Local Relapse	No Relapse	Other*	No. Responding/ Total
0	2	0	3	2	2	1	8/9
1	4	1	2	3	4	0	11/11
2	16	9	19	15	13	4	61/67
3	7	8	9	9	0	4	28/30
Total	29	18	33	29	19	9	108/117

* The category Other includes deaths related to treatment (n = 4), deaths due to other diseases (n = 2), and patients lost to follow-up (n = 3).

TABLE 5
Distribution of Patients by N Factor and Dose

	No. of Patients			
Dose	N0	N1	N2	N3
40 Gy (n = 28)	1 (4)	5 (18)	17 (60)	5 (18)
45 Gy (n = 30)*	1 (3)	4 (13)	19 (64)	6 (20)
50 Gy (n = 32)	3 (9)	0 (0)	17 (53)	12 (38)
Other (n = 27)	4 (15)	2 (7)	14 (52)	7 (26)

Note.—Numbers in parentheses are percentages.
* Accelerated hyperfraction.

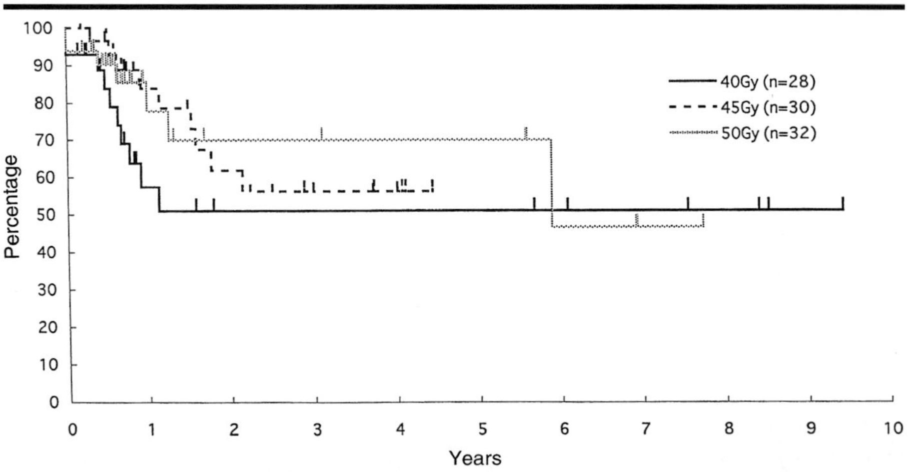

Figure 4. Kaplan-Meier curves of in-field control for patients subgrouped according to radiation dose.

DISCUSSION

To optimize thoracic radiation therapy in patients with limited-stage small cell lung cancer, the optimal timing in relation to chemotherapy, the optimal dose-fractionation schedule, and the extent of disease to be irradiated (whether pre- or postchemotherapy tumor volume) must be determined. The results of recent studies have improved our understanding of each of these factors.

With regard to the timing or radiation therapy, Komaki et al (7) compared the interdigitating method with the concurrent method, and Takada et al (5) compared the sequential method with the concurrent method. In both studies, the concurrent method produced superior results. The median survival time of 31.3 months for patients who underwent the concurrent method in the later study by Takada et al was excellent.

The optimal dose for radiation therapy may vary with the chemotherapy with which it is combined, the timing in relation to chemotherapy, and the fractionation (conventional or accelerated hyperfractionation). Arriagada et al (8) reported that an increase of the dose from 45 to 55 or 65 Gy resulted only in a lengthening of the term of local control, not in improvement of the long-term local control rate (ie, short-term control was improved, but long-term control was not). In the present study, the in-field control rate curve for the patients who underwent 40-Gy irradiation had a plateau level of approximately 50% (Fig 4). A dose escalation to 45 or 50 Gy shifted the curve to the right but did not improve the plateau level. These results are considered to support the data of Arriagada et al.

The extent of disease to be irradiated is a controversial issue. Healey and Abner (9) recommended that the radiation fields be limited to the postchemotherapy tumor volume. When chemotherapy and radiation therapy are performed concurrently, however, the prechemotherapy tumor volume is necessarily entirely contained in the radiation field. The present results suggest that the upper margin should be extended in patients with N2 or N3 disease, because marginal relapse seems to occur often at this site.

In the present study, long-term local control could not be achieved in patients with N3 disease. In general, for the prevention of radiation-induced myelopathy, an oblique photon beam is used during the later part of the radiation therapy schedule in patients with lung cancer. It is difficult to irradiate the tumor volume with a full dose in patients with N3 disease. This incomplete irradiation may cause poor local control. Therefore, it is considered to be worthwhile to irradiate without the oblique beam. In this application, the dose-fraction schedule of 44.4 Gy in 37 fractions over 3.7 weeks (hyperfractionation) is one of the options, because to our knowledge there is no report of the occurrence of radiation-induced myelopathy when 1.2-Gy fractions are administered twice daily, up to a total dose of approximately 45 Gy (10). The result that dose escalation did not improve long-term local control rates is considered to support the use of this method. On the other hand, two of our patients with T4 disease survived 4 years without recurrence. This result did not surprise us, because the tumor volume in patients with T4 disease can be irradiated with the full dose.

The frequency of brain metastases increases with the length of survival. The indication for prophylactic cranial irradiation, however, remains a controversial issue. The present results indicate that patients with N3 disease, even those with a complete response to concurrent chemotherapy and radiation therapy, are not good candidates for prophylactic cranial irradiation because, at present, a cure is not expected in them.

The optimization of thoracic irradiation in patients with limited-stage small cell lung cancer needs further examination. Our results suggest that patients with N3 disease should undergo a protocol separate from that used in other patients and that the upper margin of the radiation field should be extended in patients with N2 or N3 disease.

References

1. Arriagada R, Ihde DC, Johnson DH, Perry MC, Pignon JP, Souhami RL. Meta-analysis of randomized trials evaluating the role of thoracic radiotherapy in limited small cell lung carcinoma (SCLC) (abstr). Lung Cancer 1991; 7(suppl):98.
2. Warde P, Payne D. Does thoracic irradiation improve survival of local control in limited stage small cell carcinoma of the lung? a meta-analysis. J Clin Oncol 1992; 10:890–895.
3. Bunn PA, Lichter AS, Makuch RW, et al. Chemotherapy alone or chemotherapy with chest radiation therapy in limited stage small cell lung cancer: a prospective randomized trial. Ann Intern Med 1987; 106:655–662.
4. Kies MS, Mira JG, Crowley JJ, et al. Multimodal therapy for limited small-cell lung cancer: a randomized study of induction combination chemotherapy with or without thoracic radiation in complete responders; and with wide-field versus reduced-field radiation in partial responders—a Southwest Oncology Group study. J Clin Oncol 1987; 5:592–600.
5. Takada M, Fukuoka M, Furuse M, et al. Phase III study of concurrent versus sequential thoracic radiotherapy (TRT) in combination with cisplatin (C) and etoposide (E) for limited-stage (LS) small cell lung cancer (SCLC): preliminary results of the Japan Clinical Oncology Group (JCOG) (abstr). Proc Am Soc Clin Oncol 1996; 15:372.
6. Oken MM, Creech RH, Tormey DC, et al. Toxicity and response criteria of the Eastern Cooperative Oncology Group. Am J Clin Oncol 1982; 5:649–655.
7. Komaki R, Shin DM, Glisson BS, et al. Interdigitating versus concurrent chemotherapy and radiotherapy for limited small cell lung cancer. Int J Radiat Oncol Biol Phys 1995; 31:807–811.
8. Arriagada R, Pellae-Cosset B, Guevara JCL, et al. Alternating radiotherapy and chemotherapy schedules in limited small cell lung cancer: analysis of local chest recurrences. Radiother Oncol 1991; 20:91–98.
9. Healey EA, Abner A. Thoracic and cranial radiotherapy for limited-stage small cell lung cancer. Chest 1995; 107(suppl 6): 249S–254S.
10. Schultheiss TE, Kun LE, Ang KK, Stephens LC. Radiation response of the central nervous system. Int J Radiat Oncol Biol Phys 1995; 31:1093–1112.

Choroidal Neovascular Membranes: Treatment with Reirradiation[1]

Charles S. Cathcart, MD
Joshua N. Halpern, MD
Christopher M. Seery, MD
Ahmed Abdelsalam, MD
Marco A. Zarbin, MD

Index terms:
Eye, diseases, 2245.899
Eye, effects of irradiation on, 224.47
Eye, therapeutic radiology, 224.1269
Therapeutic radiology, experimental, 224.1269

Radiology 1998; 208:517–519

Abbreviation:
CNVM = choroidal neovascular membrane

[1] From the Departments of Radiology (C.S.C., J.N.H.) and Ophthalmology (C.M.S., A.A., M.A.Z.), University of Medicine and Dentistry of New Jersey–New Jersey Medical School, Newark. From the 1997 RSNA scientific assembly. Received December 1, 1997; revision requested December 24; revision received February 9, 1998; accepted March 5. **Address reprint requests to** C.S.C., Division of Radiation Oncology, University Hospital, Rm A1020, 195 S Orange Ave, Newark, NJ 07103.

PURPOSE: To evaluate re-treatment with an additional course of low-dose irradiation in patients with progressive or recurrent choroidal neovascular membranes (CNVMs).

MATERIALS AND METHODS: Ten patients who had received 14 Gy of external-beam radiation therapy in seven fractions for subfoveal CNVMs were found to have recurrent or persistent neovascularization at follow-up. They received an additional 15 Gy of radiation therapy administered in five daily fractions with a standard lens-sparing technique. Before reirradiation, visual acuity ranged from 20/80 to counting fingers. The median time between radiation courses was 6.5 months (range, 2–16 months). After re-treatment, the patients were followed up with angiography and visual field testing. The median follow-up was 18.5 months (range, 12–21 months).

RESULTS: Eight of 10 patients (80%) maintained their visual acuity at 1 year and three of seven (43%) at 18 months. Visual acuity was stabilized in five of the 10 patients at their last follow-up. No acute or late side effects of irradiation were noted.

CONCLUSION: Additional radiation therapy in selected patients with CNVMs who have failed to benefit from previous irradiation is well tolerated and appears to stabilize the disease process in a substantial proportion of these patients.

Recently, numerous studies have shown that therapeutic external-beam irradiation shows promise in the treatment of the wet form of age-related macular degeneration (1–8). In these studies, patients with macular degeneration who were not eligible for laser surgery received low-dose radiation therapy to the affected eye. Currently, randomized trials are being performed in Great Britain to evaluate the benefits of radiation therapy compared with no treatment in patients who are not eligible for laser treatment. Radiation therapy seems to be effective in both improving the patient's condition and stabilizing the disease. Chakravarthy et al (1) initially showed a stabilization rate for visual acuity of 63% at 9 months with radiation therapy. At 2-year follow-up, these patients had a stabilization rate for visual acuity of 65% (8). Other groups report a stabilization rate for visual acuity of 48%–79% at follow-up of 1 year or less (2–7).

The target tissues of the radiation are choroidal neovascular membranes (CNVMs). They are most often located in the subfoveal region of the retina and therefore cannot be treated safely with laser surgery. In the initial studies, several fractionation schedules were applied. In the most common regimens, 180–300 cGy was given daily for an overall dose of 1,000–1,500 cGy (1,3,5–8). Bergink et al (4) delivered higher daily doses; patients received either 800 cGy for one fraction, 600 cGy for two fractions, 600 cGy for three fractions, or 600 cGy for four fractions. The responses to these regimens were similar; however, a single dose of 800 cGy did not seem to control the disease as well as the more protracted schedules (2,4).

Twenty percent to 30% of patients who receive radiation therapy for macular degeneration have persistent or recurrent neovascularization. Persistent neovascularization can be defined as continued vessel growth and leakage within several weeks to months of the irradiation after no or partial response to radiation therapy. Recurrent disease is neovascularization that occurs after an initial long-term (>6-month) response to radiation therapy. Both persistent and recurrent vessel growth can be associated with a rapid decrease in vision, and there are virtually no treatment options for such neovascularization.

Author contributions:
Guarantor of integrity of entire study, C.S.C.; study concepts, C.S.C., J.N.H., C.M.S., M.A.Z.; study design, C.S.C., J.N.H.; definition of intellectual content, C.S.C.; literature research, C.S.C., A.A.; data acquisition, C.S.C., A.A.; data analysis, C.S.C.; statistical analysis, C.S.C.; manuscript preparation and editing, C.S.C.; manuscript review, C.S.C., J.N.H.

TABLE 1
Results of Initial and Repeat Irradiation in 10 Patients with CNVMs

Patient	VA before Initial Treatment	Month and Year of Initial Treatment	VA after Initial Treatment	Reason for Re-treatment of CNVMs	Month and Year of Repeat Treatment	VA at 12-month Follow-up	VA at 18-month Follow-up
1	20/150	September 1995	20/200	Persistence	March 1996	20/400	20/400
2	20/50	April 1995	20/80	Recurrence	March 1996	20/80	20/200
3	CF at 6 inches*	October 1995	CF at 8 inches	Persistence	February 1996	CF at 8 inches	CF at 8 inches
4	20/100	December 1995	20/100	Persistence	April 1996	20/150	No data
5	20/100	August 1995	20/200	Recurrence	April 1996	20/200	20/200
6	20/200	October 1995	20/200	Recurrence	October 1996	20/200	No data
7	20/100	November 1994	20/100	Recurrence	March 1996	20/100	20/200
8	20/400	January 1996	20/200	Persistence	March 1996	20/200	20/200
9	20/100	January 1996	20/100	Persistence	July 1996	20/100	No data
10	20/200	July 1995	20/200	Recurrence	April 1996	20/200	20/400

Note.—CF = counting fingers, VA = visual acuity.
*One inch = 2.5 cm.

At New Jersey Medical School, a cohort of 42 patients with CNVMs were treated between November 1994 and January 1996 with 1,400 cGy of radiation given in seven fractions. These patients were closely followed up, and 10 developed progressive or recurrent neovascularization with rapid clinical deterioration of vision in the affected eye. We believed that re-treatment could prevent further disease progression and eventual blindness in these patients. Therefore, we performed a pilot study to evaluate re-treatment with an additional course of low-dose irradiation in patients with progressive or recurrent choroidal neovascularization.

MATERIALS AND METHODS

Between February and October 1996, 10 patients who had been treated with radiation therapy for choroidal neovascularization were referred to the radiation oncology unit at our institution. Institutional review board approval and written informed consent had been obtained for the initial radiation therapy. All of these patients had received a total dose of 1,400 cGy, which was given in seven fractions over 1½ weeks to a 4 × 4-cm lens-sparing field with 8-MeV photons. All 10 had been regularly followed up in the ophthalmology department; five were found to have progressive neovascularization, and five were found to have recurrence. The median time to persistence of disease was 4.6 months (range, 3–6 months), and the median time to recurrence was 10.6 months (range, 6–12 months). Fluorescein angiography was performed in all patients for diagnosis and documentation. None of these patients were eligible for laser treatment, and all were actively losing visual acuity. The overall visual acuity before the second course of irradiation was poor and ranged from 20/80 to counting fingers. The median age of these patients was 81 years (range, 55–85 years).

Written informed consent was obtained, and simulation for radiation therapy was performed with computed tomographic treatment planning. All patients then received five fractions of 300 cGy for a total dose of 1,500 cGy. The patients were followed up regularly in the ophthalmology department with visual acuity testing and angiography when indicated. The median follow-up after reirradiation was 18.5 months (range, 12–21 months).

RESULTS

The results of re-treatment are shown in Table 1. At 1 year, eight of the 10 patients (80%) maintained their pretreatment visual acuity and showed disease stabilization. Three of the 10 patients have not been followed up to 18 months (one missed the scheduled appointment; two had not reached the 18-month posttreatment period at this writing). Of the seven patients who were followed up for 18 months or longer, three (43%) continued to have their visual acuity preserved. Overall, five of the 10 patients maintained their pretreatment visual acuity at the last follow-up. Although four patients stated that their eyesight was subjectively better 1 month after reirradiation, none of the patients showed an improvement in vision at direct testing.

Five patients were treated for persistent CNVMs and five for recurrent CNVMs. The results in these two groups are compared in Table 2. Of the five patients re-treated for persistent disease, three showed disease stabilization at 1 year; two of the three patients followed up for at least 18 months showed continued disease stabilization. Of the five patients re-treated for recurrent disease, all five had stable visual acuity at 1 year; however, only one of four had stable visual acuity at 18 months.

TABLE 2
Results by Type of Disease

Type of Disease	Stable VA at 12 Months	Stable VA at 18 Months
Persistent	3/5 (60)	2/3 (67)
Recurrent	5/5 (100)	1/4 (25)
All cases	8/10 (80)	3/7 (43)

Note.—Values are patients with stable visual acuity/total patients in group; values in parentheses are percentages. VA = visual acuity.

There were no short- or long-term side effects in these re-treated patients.

DISCUSSION

Radiation therapy has been used successfully in the recent past to treat the wet form of macular degeneration when no other treatment options are available. The failure rate for radiation therapy is 20%–50%. Unfortunately, for the majority of patients who fail to benefit from radiation therapy, no treatment options exist. There are two patterns of treatment failure for irradiation: persistence or recurrence. In both of these situations, the expected clinical outcome is blindness.

We used additional radiation therapy to treat 10 such patients who had been treated initially at our institution. Five of them had persistent disease. We hypothesized that altering the fractionation by escalating the daily increments to 300 cGy might be more effective in treating a benign proliferative process such as choroidal neovascularization. This regimen was also administered to the five patients who initially responded to their first course of radiation but had recurrent CNVMs. The increased daily dose was meant to act as a "second-line" form of radiation therapy. The overall dose given during primary irradiation and reirradiation was meant to be within the tolerance of the retina, optic chiasm, and brain parenchyma.

Our results show that additional radiation therapy may be beneficial in patients in whom initial irradiation for CNVMs has been a failure. One year after re-treatment, eight of the 10 patients maintained the same visual acuity as before reirradiation. These results are in the same range as those in patients after initial irradiation for CNVMs. By 18 months, the rate of disease stabilization dropped to 43%. However, it appears that cases of recurrent disease make up the bulk of treatment failures between 12 and 18 months.

Analysis of the data by comparing the two failure patterns, persistence and recurrence, may also suggest differences in benefits of reirradiation. Patients re-treated because of persistent disease had a response rate at 1 year of only 60%. In contrast, all patients in the recurrence group maintained visual acuity at 1 year. This result suggests that some patients with persistent disease do not respond well to radiation therapy given in short courses. Their disease persisted through treatment with 1,400 cGy in seven fractions and then through additional treatment 3–6 months later. Some patients in this group did respond to treatment; in these patients, the reirradiation might have been more useful as a boost to the primary irradiation if they had been noted to have no stabilization 1 month after the first course of radiation therapy. Such re-treatment would theoretically occur at a more radiobiologically advantageous time.

The five patients re-treated for recurrence seemed to respond well in the short term to reirradiation. However, as time passed, they developed new CNVMs. This was the same pattern as that which led these patients to require reirradiation after they had initially responded to primary radiation therapy with 1,400 cGy. This result suggests that these patients might best be served with multiple (two or more) courses of radiation therapy given 6–18 months apart, with the total dose kept within a safe range. Such a regimen could potentially protract the benefits of radiation therapy for years.

Most important, the treatment was well tolerated by all patients, with no short-term side effects occurring in any patient. Long-term side effects such as nervous tissue damage or second malignancy are of some concern when large total doses are given to large volumes. In the case of radiation therapy for a benign disease such as macular degeneration, the benefits must far outweigh the risks. Owing to the small volume irradiated and the advanced age of the patients, the benefits do appear to far outweigh the risks in this clinical situation.

In conclusion, additional radiation therapy in selected patients with choroidal neovascularization who have failed to benefit from previous irradiation is well tolerated and appears to stabilize the disease process in a substantial proportion of these patients.

References

1. Chakravarthy U, Houston RF, Archer DB. Treatment of age-related subfoveal neovascular membranes by teletherapy: a pilot study. Br J Ophthalmol 1993; 77:265–273.
2. Bergink GJ, Deutman AF, van den Broek JF, van Daal WA, van der Maazen RW. Radiation therapy for subfoveal choroidal neovascular membranes in age-related macular degeneration. Graefes Arch Clin Exp Ophthalmol 1994; 232:591–598.
3. Sasai K, Murata R, Mandai M, et al. Radiation therapy for ocular choroidal neovascularization (phase I/II study): preliminary report. Int J Radiat Oncol Biol Phys 1997; 39:173–178.
4. Bergink GJ, Deutman AF, van den Broek JF, van Daal WA, van der Maazen RW. Radiation therapy for age-related subfoveal choroidal neovascular membranes: a pilot study. Doc Ophthalmol 1995; 90:67–74.
5. Finger PT, Berson A, Sherr D, Riley R, Balkin RA, Bosworth JL. Radiation therapy for subretinal neovascularization. Ophthalmology 1996; 103:878–889.
6. Freire J, Longton WA, Miyamato CT, et al. External radiation therapy in macular degeneration: technique and preliminary subjective responses. Int J Radiat Oncol Biol Phys 1996; 36:857–860.
7. Berson AM, Finger PT, Sherr DL, et al. Radiotherapy for age-related macular degeneration: preliminary results of a potentially new treatment. Int J Radiat Oncol Biol Phys 1996; 36:861–865.
8. Hart PM, Chakravarthy U, MacKenzie G, Archer DB, Houston RF. Teletherapy for subfoveal choroidal neovascularization of age-related macular degeneration: results of follow up in a non-randomized study. Br J Ophthalmol 1996; 80:1046–1050.

Science to Practice
RSNA '98

Integrating Science Into Practice

Associated Sciences Program at RSNA 1998

Workshop: Saturday, Nov. 28, 1998, 10:15 am - 4:30 pm, McCormick Place Sou

Refresher Courses: Sunday, Nov. 29, 1998 through Friday, Dec. 4, 1998

Credits: $4\frac{1}{4}$ hours and an additional $1\frac{1}{2}$ hours credit for attendance at the Basic Physics Lecture

Welcome and Introduction
10:15 am
Samuel L. Hissong, MD, Chair, Associated Sciences Consortium and Committee
Eugene D. Frank, MA, RT(R), Coordinator, Associated Sciences Consortium

Keynote Presentation
10:30 - 11:50 am
Impact of Telematic Technologies on Image-Guided Medicine (AIA-AAH)
Heinz U. Lemke, PhD

Break
11:50 am - 12:10 pm

Special Luncheon Program
12:10 - 1:20 pm
Networking for the New Millennium - Important Factors to Consider (SMRT)
Bruce Johnson, BSEE

Break
1:20 - 1:30 pm

Panel Presentation
1:30 - 2:50 pm
The Reality of Computerization (AERS, AHRA, SROA)
Richard Carlton, MS, RT(R)
Robert Seely, MBA, RT(R)
Heinz U. Lemke, PhD

AAPM/RSNA Basic Physics Lecture for the Radiologic Technologist: Vascular Imaging Physics
Organized by Gerald A. White, Jr., MS
3:00 - 4:30 pm
$1\frac{1}{2}$ hours credit

Refresher Courses

(Each Refresher Course is approved for $1\frac{1}{2}$ hours credit)

Sunday RC 124
Organizational Culture and Health System Change
Cornelius J. Rater, MD (AERS)
Harry J. Granito, MS (RBMA)
Douglas R. Hanson (ASRT)

Monday RC 224
Liability Issues Arising from the Changing Health Care Environment
Ann Obergfell, JD, RT(R) (ASRT)
Perry Smith, JD, RDMS (SDMS)

Monday RC 324
Organizational Change In Radiology: Preparing Radiology for the Next Millennium
Monte G. Clinton (AHRA)
Donna L. Wright, EdD, RT(R) (AERS)
Loretta L. Hanwell, MPA (AHRA)

Tuesday RC 424
Competency, Continuity, and Compliance
Susan S. Weiss, CNMT (SNM-TS)
Kate Little, RN (ARNA)

Wednesday RC 524
Managing a Multisite Radiology Network
Larry Ranahan, MBA (RBMA) Moderator
Sherry Rader (RBMA)
Charles Deschamps, RT(R)(MR) (SMRT)
Rebecca Shanahan, JD (RBMA)

Thursday RC 624
Specialized Accreditations: A Cost of Doing Business
Luann J. Culbreth, MEd, RT(R)(MR) (SMRT) Moderator
John Kovelski, RT(R)(MR) (SMRT)
Karol Handrahan, RT(R) (SMRT)
Linda Zanin, MS, PhD (SDMS)
Ronald F. Bernardi, BA, RT(R)(N) (AHRA)

Thursday RC 724
Multidisciplinary Standards for the New Millennium
Susan S. Weiss, CNMT (SNM-TS), Moderator
William R. Poller, MD (SNM-TS)
Michael R. Bloyd, RT(R), BSN (ASRT)
Liz Anderson, MBA (AVIR)

Friday RC 824
Marketing Radiology: Getting the Message Out
Ronald F. Bernardi, BA, RT(R)(N), Moderator
Cherrill Farnsworth (AHRA)
Michael R. Favreau, FAHRA (AHRA)

Registration Information

Advance registration for the RSNA Scientific Assembly ends October 30. Onsite registration begins at 12:00 noon on Saturday, November 28, at McCormick Place. RSNA shuttle bus service to McCormick Place will be available beginning at 10:00 am on Saturday. Advance registration is not required for the Saturday workshop; however, to receive continuing education credit, you must register.

Advance registration information appears in the July issue of *Radiology*. Brochures are also available from your association or from the RSNA, 2021 Spring Road, Suite 600, Oak Brook, IL 60523-1860. Phone: 630/571-7862.

Registration for the RSNA Scientific Assembly includes registration for the Associated Sciences Workshop. A box lunch will be available for purchase to facilitate your attendance at the workshop. These lunches must be purchased with your advance registration for the RSNA Meeting. **If you wish to purchase a box lunch, please check the appropriate box on the RSNA Advance Registration form and enclose your $11.50 payment.**

If you would like a copy of the published Associated Sciences Proceedings, please call 630/571-7877.

Sponsoring Organizations

- American Healthcare Radiology Administrators (AHRA)
- American Institute of Architects — Academy on Architecture for Health (AIA-AAH)
- American Radiological Nurses Association (ARNA)
- American Society of Radiologic Technologists (ASRT)
- Association of Educators in Radiological Sciences (AERS)
- Association of Vascular and Interventional Radiographers (AVIR)
- Radiological Business Management Association (RBMA)
- Society for Radiation Oncology Administrators (SROA)
- Society of Diagnostic Medical Sonographers (SDMS)
- Society of Magnetic Resonance Technologists (SMRT)
- Society of Nuclear Medicine — Technologists Section (SNM-TS)

RSNA®
Radiological Society of North America
Founded in 1915
2021 Spring Road, Suite 600
Oak Brook, Illinois 60523-1860
630/571-2670 FAX: 630/571-7837
www.rsna.org

Associated Sciences

Appropriate Imaging in Children with Skull Fractures and Suspicion of Abuse[1]

Kirsten I. Mogbo, MD
Thomas L. Slovis, MD
Alexa I. Canady, MD
David J. Allasio, MSW, CSW
Cynthia L. Arfken, PhD

Index terms:
Children, injuries, 10.41
Computed tomography (CT), in infants and children, 10.1211
Infants, injuries, 10.41
Radiography, in infants and children, 10.11
Skull, fractures, 10.41

Radiology 1998; 208:521–524

[1] From the Departments of Pediatric Imaging (K.I.M., T.L.S.), Pediatric Neurosurgery (A.I.C.), and Social Work, Child Protection Team (D.J.A.), Children's Hospital of Michigan, 3901 Beaubien Blvd, Detroit, MI 48201-2196, and the Department of Psychiatry and Behavioral Neurosciences, Wayne State University, Detroit, Mich (C.L.A.). Received November 28, 1997; revision requested February 13, 1998; revision received April 3; accepted April 13. **Address reprint requests to** T.L.S.

Author contributions:
Guarantors of integrity of entire study, K.I.M., T.L.S.; study concepts, K.I.M, T.L.S.; study design, T.L.S.; definition of intellectual content, K.I.M., T.L.S., A.I.C., D.J.A., C.L.A.; literature research, K.I.M., T.L.S.; clinical studies, K.I.M., T.L.S.; data acquisition and analysis, K.I.M., T.L.S.; statistical analysis, C.L.A.; manuscript preparation, K.I.M., T.L.S., A.I.C., D.J.A., C.L.A.; manuscript editing and review, K.I.M., T.L.S.

PURPOSE: To define the role of computed tomography (CT) in children aged 2 years and younger with head trauma, suspected abuse, and normal neurologic findings.

MATERIALS AND METHODS: From 1992 through 1995, 87 consecutive children with skull fractures visible at plain radiography were referred to child protective services for evaluation of suspected abuse. Their cases were retrospectively reviewed.

RESULTS: Of 67 children with normal neurologic findings, 35 (52%) were not referred for CT. No patient in this group developed delayed findings requiring further evaluation. Of the 32 (48%) who underwent head CT, only six (19%) had evidence of acute intracranial injury, despite the presence of minimal depression and stellate, multiple, and diastatic fractures. Of 20 children with acute neurologic findings, 16 (80%) had positive CT scans, which led to neurosurgical intervention in nine (45%).

CONCLUSION: No child with normal neurologic findings had a clinically important abnormality depicted at CT. CT scans did not alter clinical management, clinical outcome, or legal outcome. Thus, routine CT of all patients with skull fractures in this population may be unnecessary.

Radiography of the skull is appropriately performed as a screening study in children with suspected abuse and a history of head trauma. When a skull fracture is demonstrated, both clinicians and radiologists, however, are reluctant to forego computed tomographic (CT) examination in neurologically normal children. The American College of Radiology specifically advises that for a child aged 2 years or younger with head trauma but no focal findings or neurologic abnormality, brain CT should be performed (1).

To our knowledge, data are lacking to support the recommendation for head CT in children aged 2 years or younger who present with head trauma and suspected abuse. Use of imaging algorithms alone, without clinically important data, often leads to excessive imaging. Therefore, we retrospectively studied the cases of children referred to child protective services for evaluation of suspected abuse who had plain radiographic evidence of skull fractures. The purpose of this study was to determine whether CT of the brain altered the outcome or clinical management in this patient population and to discern any clinical variables that would help in the decision regarding which children need to undergo CT.

MATERIALS AND METHODS

This study involved a retrospective review of the cases of 87 consecutive children aged 2 years and younger who were seen in the Children's Hospital of Michigan Emergency Department between 1992 and 1995. These children were referred to child protective services with skull fractures and suspected abuse. We reviewed their cases for (*a*) skull radiographic findings, (*b*) CT findings, (*c*) clinical status at presentation, (*d*) clinical outcome, and (*e*) legal outcome (final placement of the child). To limit the study population to children with proved head trauma, only those with skull fractures visible at plain radiography were included. Head CT scans obtained within 10 hours of the skull radiographs were evaluated for evidence of intraparenchymal traumatic injury as well as for extra-axial abnormalities. The medical charts were reviewed for other associated diseases

TABLE 1
Patients with Skull Fractures on Plain Radiographs

Neurologic Examination Findings	No. with Normal CT Scans	No. with Abnormal CT Scans*	No. with No CT	Total
Normal	26	6†	35	67
Abnormal	4	16‡	0	20
Total	30	22	35	87

* The difference in the number of patients with abnormal CT scans between the neurologically normal group and the neurologically abnormal group is statistically significant ($P = .00003$; Fisher exact test).

† Subdural hematomas, two patients; epidural hematoma, one patient; subarachnoid hemorrhage, two patients; surface contusion, one patient.

‡ Acute subdural hematomas, 13 patients; chronic subdural hematoma, five patients; subarachnoid hemorrhages, two patients; epidural hematoma, one patient; intraventricular hemorrhage, one patient.

TABLE 2
Clinical Variables and Outcomes

Clinical Variable	Normal Neurologic Findings (*n* = 67) CT (*n* = 32)	Normal Neurologic Findings (*n* = 67) No CT (*n* = 35)	Abnormal Neurologic Findings (*n* = 20) CT (*n* = 20)
Multiple skull fractures	10 (31)*	2 (6)*	7 (35)
Diastatic fractures	2 (6)	1 (3)	8 (40)
Depressed fractures	3 (9)	1 (3)	0 (0)
Other traumatic injury	5 (16)	1 (3)	11 (55)
Medical disease	5 (16)†	1 (3)‡	
Hospital admission	29 (91)§	10 (29)§	20 (100)
Average length of stay (d)			
With medical disease	10.6	5.0	
Trauma only	1.95	1.75	
Overall	3.6	2.1	
Court-ordered out-of-home placement at discharge	10 (31)	10 (29)	15 (75)
Substantiated abuse	15 (47)	17 (53)	13 (65)
Death	0 (0)	0 (0)	1 (0)

Note.—Data are the number of patients. Numbers in parentheses are percentages.

* Statistically significant difference between groups ($P = .01$).

† Failure to thrive, two patients; asthma, two patients; sepsis, one patient.

‡ Otitis media.

§ Statistically significant difference between groups ($P = .0001$).

and, specifically, for neurologic status at presentation, including level of consciousness, deep tendon reflexes, cranial nerve abnormalities, extremity paresis or paralysis, seizure activity, vomiting, or inconsolable irritability. The clinical course of the patient was also evaluated, including the need for neurosurgical intervention, hospital admission or nonadmission, and length of hospital stay. Legal outcomes were identified in terms of whether out-of-home placement was ordered by the court at discharge and, on the basis of further follow-up findings, whether abuse was substantiated.

The statistical significance of differences between groups was determined with the Fisher exact test. Differences with a P value less than .05 were considered significant.

RESULTS

Of the 87 children, 67 had normal neurologic examination results. Of these 67 children, 35 were not referred for CT examination, and 32 underwent head CT (Table 1). None of these 67 patients developed delayed findings requiring further evaluation or intervention at our institution. The patients who were referred for CT tended to have multiple or more complex skull fractures as well as additional injuries or illness (Table 2). Of the 32 neurologically normal patients who underwent head CT, six (19%) had evidence of acute intracranial injury, but these findings were limited to small, focal hemorrhages adjacent to the fracture (Figs 1, 2). Five of these patients had small amounts of extra-axial blood adjacent to the fracture, all without mass effect, and the sixth had a small hemorrhagic surface contusion. In no case did the CT findings require intervention or alter clinical management.

Of the 32 neurologically normal children who underwent CT, 29 were admitted to the hospital. Their average length of stay was 3.6 days. Excluding admissions for medical disease other than the head trauma, the average length of stay was 1.9 days. Ten of these patients had court-ordered out-of-home placements at discharge, and in 15 cases the abuse ultimately was deemed to be substantiated.

Of the 35 patients who did not undergo CT, 10 were admitted. Their average length of stay was 2.1 days; excluding medical admissions, the average length of stay was 1.75 days. Ten of these patients had court-ordered out-of-home placement at discharge, and in 17 cases the abuse ultimately was deemed to be substantiated.

Abnormal neurologic findings were associated with the acute head trauma in 20 children. These findings included altered levels of activity and responsiveness, ranging from inconsolable irritability and lethargy to unresponsiveness and the need for intubation. Other findings included new seizure activity, hypertonicity, vomiting, respiratory distress, apnea, optic neuropathy, a sixth-nerve palsy, and bulging fontanelle. Of these 20 patients, 16 (80%) had positive CT scans. Of these 16 findings, three were minor injuries and 13 were major. Major findings included acute and chronic subdural hemorrhages; subarachnoid hemorrhage; intraventricular, epidural, and parenchymal hemorrhages; pneumocephalus; encephalomalacia; and parenchymal edema. These findings led to neurosurgical intervention in nine patients (45%), one of whom died. Fifteen of these patients had court-ordered out-of-home placement at discharge, and in 13 cases the abuse ultimately was deemed to be substantiated.

DISCUSSION

As many as 650,000 cases of severe or life-threatening injuries and 2,000 deaths secondary to physical abuse are estimated to occur in the United States each year (2,3). Head trauma is the leading cause of morbidity and mortality in abused children, especially among those aged less than 2 years. It is estimated that 10% of neurologic developmental abnormalities can be traced to nonaccidental trauma (4). Billmire and Myers (5) found that 95% of clinically important intracranial injuries in a group of 64 infants resulted from abuse. Their findings were that acci-

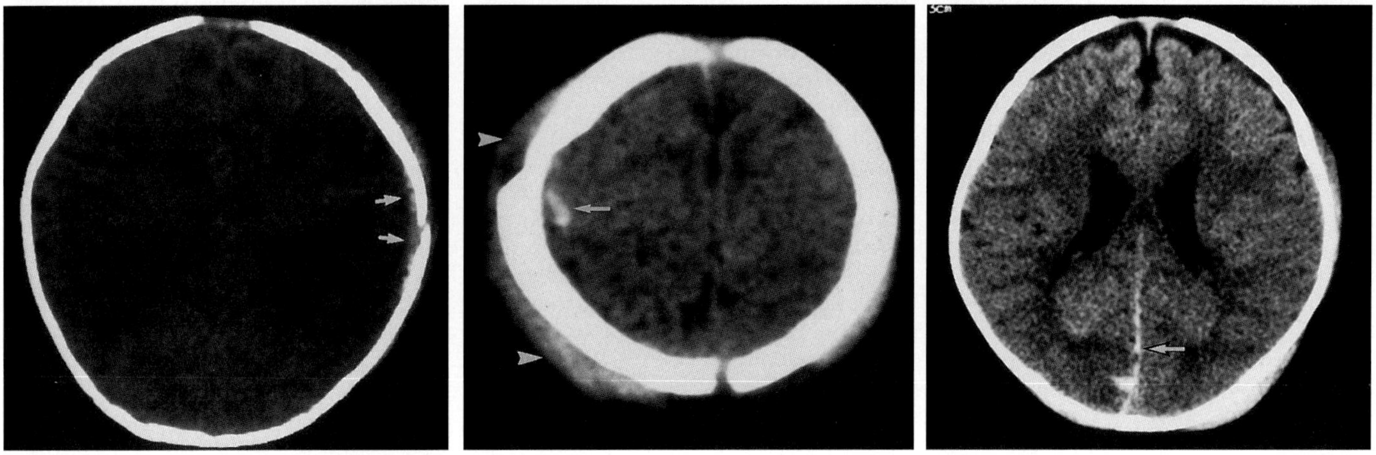

a. b. c.

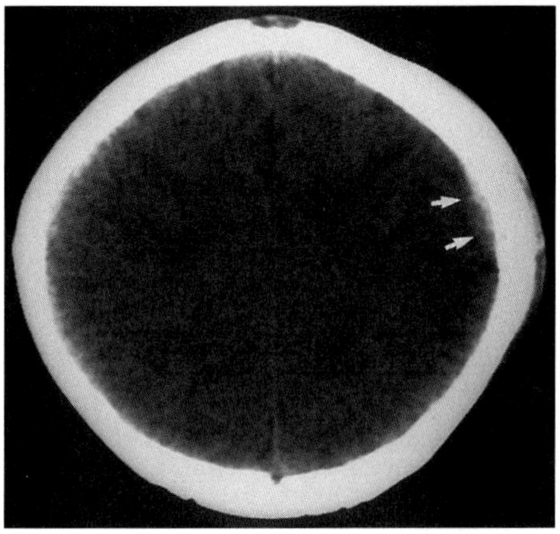

d.

Figure 1. Nonenhanced CT scans depict findings associated with skull fractures in neurologically normal patients. **(a)** Subdural blood (arrows) adjacent to a left parietal fracture is seen on scan obtained with subdural window settings at the centrum semiovale. **(b)** Superficial parenchymal contusion (arrow) associated with a depressed right skull fracture is depicted on the high-convexity image. (Scan obtained with bone window settings is not shown.) Note the scalp hematomas (arrowheads). **(c)** Image obtained at the level of the atria reveals subarachnoid blood along the posterior falx (arrow) associated with a left parietal fracture. (Scan obtained with bone window settings is not shown). **(d)** Epidural blood (arrows) without noticeable mass effect adjacent to a left parietal fracture is depicted on the high-convexity image.

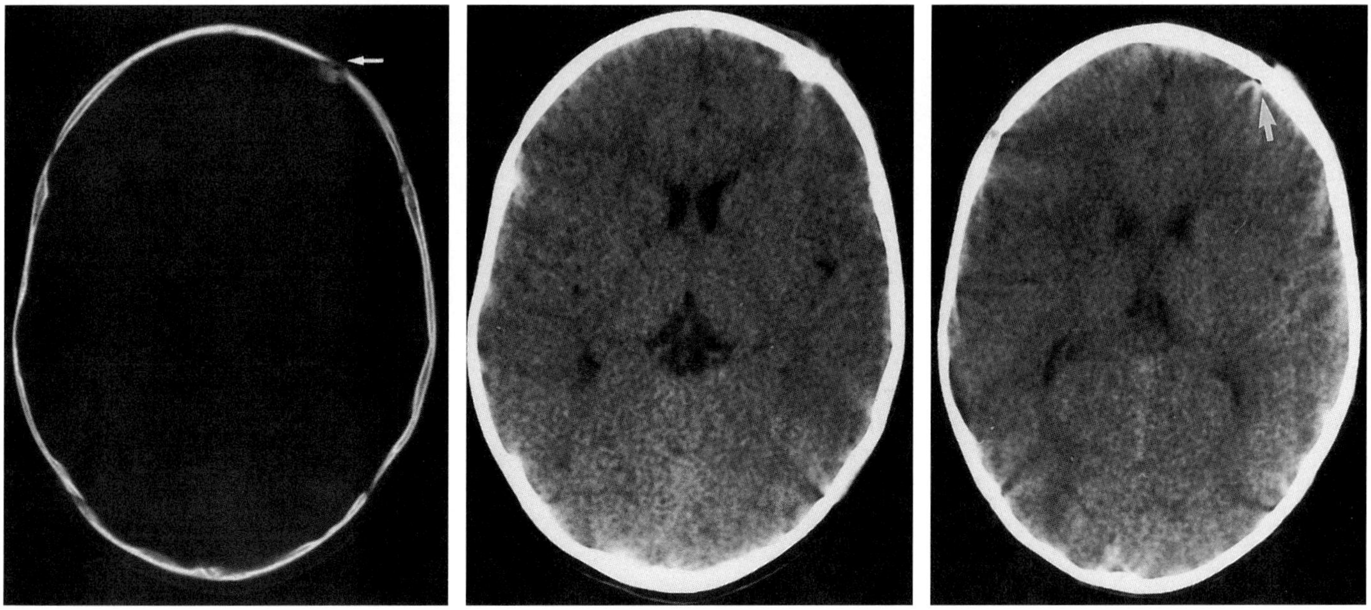

a. b. c.

Figure 2. Nonenhanced CT scans depict findings associated with skull fractures in neurologically normal patients. **(a)** Depressed left frontal fracture fragments (arrow) are depicted on scan obtained with bone window settings at the level of the frontal horns. **(b, c)** In another patient, minimal intracranial blood and air (arrow in **c**) on scans obtained with conventional brain window settings at the level of the frontal horns.

dental trauma in this age group rarely, if ever, causes intracranial injury.

The role of radiologic studies in the care of these children is twofold. First, acute injury must be identified and evaluated for appropriate treatment. Second, such studies document evidence of the nonaccidental nature of the injury for legal protection of the child. The question then becomes how this is most efficiently and effectively accomplished.

When searching for occult evidence of trauma in an infant or toddler whose symptoms at presentation raise the question of abuse, a skeletal survey and, if necessary, bone scanning should be performed to document injury (especially regarding multiplicity of sites or varying age of injuries) (1). Currently, without neurologic signs or skull fracture, few physicians would recommend referral for CT. In a child presenting with new neurologic signs or symptoms and with suspicion of abuse, CT of the head is appropriate regardless of whether a skull fracture is present. CT clearly is the most important imaging study in the evaluation of acute traumatic intracranial injury (1). The specific question addressed by our study was whether head CT is a value-added study for treatment or documentation in children with suspected abuse and known head trauma—as discovered on the basis of findings in the patient history, physical examination, or skeletal survey—but without a neurologic abnormality,

In terms of documentation, the fracture itself is much easier to detect on a plain radiograph than on a CT scan (6). There is no direct correlation between the presence of a skull fracture and the presence of an intracranial injury (2,7–12). Harwood-Nash (7) stated that, "In a child of any age, the presence of a linear skull fracture does not indicate any increased likelihood of significant intracranial injury; contrarily, its absence does not lessen the likelihood of intracranial damage." Merten et al (9) found that although 45% of abused children with clinically noticeable intracranial injury had skull fractures, 55% did not. In addition, only 56% of those with skull fractures had an intracranial injury. This lack of correlation has caused many to conclude that all children with suspicion for or history of head trauma should undergo CT to help detect occult intracranial injury. It appears, however, that the more appropriate criterion is not the presence or absence of head trauma or skull fracture but rather of neurologic abnormalities. The role of plain radiography of the skull is as part of a skeletal survey to document multiplicity of injuries, and the role of CT is in the evaluation of abnormal neurologic findings—not in the follow-up of the finding of a skull fracture.

In the studies by Zimmerman et al (8) and Merten et al (9), patients who were alert and responsive and had either no or minimal neurologic findings were excluded from CT examination. Our review suggests that when neurologically normal children undergo CT, regardless of the clinical findings, there is no difference in outcome, but there are substantial financial effects. Neurologically normal children with a minor CT finding were admitted more frequently and had longer hospital stays than children who did not undergo CT. The measurable outcome, however, was unchanged during a follow-up of 6 months to 4 years. We did not find any case for which, in the absence of neurologic signs or symptoms, head CT provided any information of clinical use or disclosed additional injuries for legal documentation.

The one potential setting in which cross-sectional imaging of the head may be warranted despite a normal neurologic examination is when there is high suspicion for abuse and findings in the skeletal survey and at bone scanning are normal. In this setting, with or without known head trauma, the need to document injury may demand further imaging. Magnetic resonance (MR) imaging would be the examination of choice, because CT may fail to depict deep parenchymal injuries or scar tissue and cannot help distinguish chronic subdural hematomas from prominent extra-axial fluid. Sato et al (13) cite the cases of three patients in whom MR imaging evidence of intracranial injury was the only objective finding of abuse; they also note there are instances in which the visual clarity of the MR image makes it much more convincing than a CT scan in a courtroom setting. Obviously these are cases that require individual management, and they do not fit a set of general screening criteria.

No child with a normal neurologic examination had a clinically important abnormality depicted at CT. Findings on CT scans did not alter clinical management, clinical outcome, or legal outcome. Thus, routine CT screening of all patients with skull fractures in this population may not be necessary.

References

1. American College of Radiology Task Force on Appropriateness Criteria. Imaging of the child with suspected physical abuse. In: ACR appropriateness criteria for imaging and treatment decisions. Reston, Va: American College of Radiology, 1995; chapter PD 5.
2. Ball WS. Nonaccidental craniocerebral trauma (child abuse): MR imaging. Radiology 1989; 173:609–610.
3. Sirotnak AP, Krugman RD. Child abuse diagnosis. Pediatr Rev 1994; 15:394–399.
4. Radkowski MA, Merten DR, Leonidas JC. The abused child: criteria for the radiologic diagnosis. RadioGraphics 1983; 3:262–297.
5. Billmire ME, Myers PA. Serious head injury in infants: accident or abuse? Pediatrics 1985; 75:340–342.
6. Saulsbury FT, Alford BA. Intracranial bleeding from child abuse: the value of skull radiographs. Pediatr Radiol 1982; 12:175–178.
7. Harwood-Nash DC. Abuse to the pediatric central nervous system. AJNR 1992; 13: 569–575.
8. Zimmerman RA, Bilaniuk LT, Gennarelli T, Bruce D, Dolinskas C, Uzzell B. Cranial computed tomography in diagnosis and management of acute head trauma. AJR 1978; 131:27–34.
9. Merten DF, Osborne DRS, Radkowski MA, Leonidas JC. Craniocerebral trauma in the child abuse syndrome: radiologic observations. Pediatr Radiol 1984; 14:272–277.
10. Harwood-Nash DC, Hendrick EB, Hudson AR. Significance of skull fractures in children: a study of 1,187 patients. Radiology 1971; 101:151–155.
11. Harwood-Nash DC. Craniocerebral trauma in children. Curr Probl Radiol 1973; 3:3–42.
12. Cohen RA, Kaufman RA, Myers PA, Towbin RB. Cranial computed tomography in the abused child with head injury. AJR 1986; 146:92–102.
13. Sato Y, Yuh WTC, Smith WL, Alexander RC, Kao SCS, Ellerbroeck CJ. Head injury in child abuse: evaluation with MR imaging. Radiology 1989; 173:653–657.

Tara C. Noone, MD
Richard C. Semelka, MD
Suvipapun Worawattanakul, MD
Hani B. Marcos, MD

Intraperitoneal Abscesses: Diagnostic Accuracy of and Appearances at MR Imaging[1]

Index terms:
Abdomen, abscess, 791.21
Abdomen, MR, 791.121411, 791.121415, 791.12143
Gadolinium
Pelvic organs, abscess, 80.211
Peritoneum, abscess, 791.21

Radiology 1998; 208:525–528

Abbreviations:
GRE = gradient-echo
RARE = rapid acquisition with relaxation enhancement

[1] From the Department of Radiology, CB 7510, University of North Carolina, 101 Manning Dr, Chapel Hill, NC 27599-7510. Received October 10, 1997; revision requested December 18; revision received February 17, 1998; accepted April 3. **Address reprint requests to** R.C.S.

PURPOSE: To prospectively investigate the diagnostic accuracy of and appearances at magnetic resonance (MR) imaging of patients clinically suspected to have intraperitoneal abscesses.

MATERIALS AND METHODS: Sixty-seven consecutive patients underwent MR imaging for suspected intraperitoneal abscesses. MR images were prospectively interpreted for intraperitoneal abscesses; the results were correlated with surgical, histopathologic, and laboratory findings.

RESULTS: MR imaging revealed 25 fluid collections consistent with intraperitoneal abscesses in 22 of 67 patients (33%). Of these collections, 22 were intraperitoneal abscesses; one, a giant sigmoid diverticulum; and two, sterile fluid collections. The latter two patients had been receiving antibiotic therapy. MR imaging allowed exclusion of intraperitoneal abscesses in 45 patients (67%). All collections demonstrated decreased signal intensity on T1-weighted images; on T2-weighted images, 13 collections demonstrated homogeneously increased signal intensity and 12 demonstrated heterogeneously increased signal intensity. The abscesses were best demonstrated on gadolinium-enhanced T1-weighted fat-suppressed images as well-defined fluid collections with peripheral rim enhancement. Sensitivity was 100%; specificity, 94% (95% confidence interval = 83%, 99%); positive predictive value, 88% (95% confidence interval = 69%, 97%); negative predictive value, 100%; and accuracy, 96% (95% confidence interval = 88%, 99%).

CONCLUSION: MR imaging has high diagnostic accuracy in evaluation of acute intraperitoneal abscesses.

Intraperitoneal abscesses occur primarily in patients with preexistent medical conditions and fever of unknown origin. This serious complication may occur in the setting of an immunocompromised state, inflammatory bowel disease, pelvic inflammatory disease, appendicitis, pancreatitis, diverticulitis, or prior abdominal or pelvic surgery (1–5). Intraperitoneal abscesses are associated with high morbidity and mortality; therefore, immediate recognition and prompt management with antimicrobial drugs, as well as interventional or surgical drainage, are imperative (2,5). Accurate, noninvasive diagnosis is necessary to appropriately direct drainage or to avoid unnecessary intervention in these patients.

Demonstration of intraperitoneal abscesses with magnetic resonance (MR) imaging has been reported in several studies, predominantly in the setting of Crohn disease. These reports described isolated abscesses discovered incidentally during the investigation of active Crohn disease (1,4,6). Demonstration of tubo-ovarian abscesses with MR imaging has also been described (3,7). MR imaging with a gadolinium-enhanced breath-hold fat-suppressed spoiled gradient-echo (GRE) technique has been shown to be effective at demonstrating peritoneal metastases secondary to the dramatic decrease in T1 achieved with gadolinium (8). It is reasonable to hypothesize that this technique would be sensitive for the detection of peritoneal inflammatory disease and abscesses as well.

To our knowledge, the accuracy of MR imaging in the evaluation of intraperitoneal abscesses has not been established. The purpose of this study, therefore, was to prospectively investigate the diagnostic accuracy of and appearances at MR imaging of intraperitoneal abscesses in patients with sepsis or fever of unknown origin.

Author contributions:
Guarantor of integrity of entire study, T.C.N.; study concepts, T.C.N., R.C.S.; study design, T.C.N.; definition of intellectual content, T.C.N., R.C.S.; literature research, T.C.N.; clinical studies, T.C.N., R.C.S.; data acquisition, T.C.N., S.W., H.B.M.; data analysis, T.C.N., R.C.S., S.W., H.B.M.; statistical analysis, T.C.N.; manuscript preparation, T.C.N.; manuscript editing and review, R.C.S.

MATERIALS AND METHODS

Patients

All patients at our institution who were known or suspected to have intraperitoneal abscesses and who underwent MR imaging between May 1995 and December 1997 were included in the study. A total of 67 consecutive patients (35 male, 32 female; age range, 7–89 years; mean age, 47 years) was accrued. Sixty-three patients did not have previously detected abscesses; four patients had abscesses detected with an earlier imaging study. Twelve patients had been included in a smaller study, which investigated the MR imaging appearances of bowel-related abscesses (9). All patients were referred for clinical investigation for either detection or confirmation of intraperitoneal abscesses. No specific selection or exclusion criteria were employed.

Fifty-eight patients presented with persistent fever of unknown origin, 41 with abdominal or pelvic pain, and 35 with both pain and fever. The greatest number of patients (21 of 67) lacked an underlying medical condition and had sepsis or fever of unknown origin. Among the remaining patients, 17 had an underlying malignancy, 12 had a generalized immunocompromised status, eight had recently undergone surgery, and nine had inflammatory bowel disease.

Twelve patients had undergone computed tomography (CT) within the previous 2 weeks. The reasons for subsequent referral for MR imaging were artifacts that hindered interpretation (n = 2), suboptimal examination secondary to lack of intravenously administered contrast material (n = 2), and CT findings that required further evaluation (n = 8). The artifacts that hindered interpretation consisted of retained, highly concentrated, intraluminal barium and excessive beam hardening due to surgical clips. Of the eight patients referred for further evaluation of CT findings, three required differentiation between poorly opacified bowel and abscess, two required differentiation between abscess and malignancy, two required determination of the total number of abscesses present, and one required further evaluation of the extent of adjacent muscle involvement.

Fifty-five of the 67 patients had not previously undergone CT. Thirty-four of these patients had an elevated serum creatinine level, which was considered to preclude evaluation with iodinated contrast material. The mean serum creatinine level in these patients was 2.3 mg/dL (203 μmol/L) (reference range = 0.6–1.0 mg/dL [53–88 μmol/L]). Six patients were evaluated with MR imaging because of underlying conditions that predisposed them to recurrent episodes of renal failure. Five patients underwent MR imaging due to the need to evaluate other, concomitant disease processes. Four patients had allergies to iodinated contrast media. Two gravid patients did not undergo CT due to radiation risks. Four patients underwent MR imaging due to a specific request by the patient or clinician. Fifty-four of these 55 patients underwent gadolinium-enhanced MR imaging as the initial imaging investigation for intraperitoneal abscess; one patient did not receive gadolinium contrast material due to his refusal to cooperate.

MR Imaging

MR imaging was performed with a 1.5-T unit (SP4000 or VISION; Siemens Medical Systems, Iselin, NJ). Pulse sequences included unenhanced T1-weighted breath-hold spoiled GRE imaging (repetition time msec/echo time msec = 130–143/4, 80° flip angle, 13–22 sections acquired in a 20-second breath hold) and T2-weighted fat-suppressed spin-echo or turbo (fast) spin-echo imaging (2,300–4,500/80–100). Spoiled GRE imaging was repeated immediately and 45 seconds after administration of 0.1 mmol/kg gadopentetate dimeglumine (Magnevist; Berlex Laboratories, Wayne, NJ). T1-weighted fat-suppressed spin-echo (500/14) or fat-suppressed spoiled GRE (130–140/2–4) images were acquired beginning 90 seconds after administration of contrast material. Spoiled GRE imaging was performed 5–10 minutes after contrast material administration in all patients.

Additional T1-weighted fat-suppressed spoiled GRE imaging in the sagittal plane and either half-Fourier rapid acquisition with relaxation enhancement (RARE) (single-shot technique, echo time = 90 msec) or T2-weighted turbo spin-echo (2,300–4,500/80–100) imaging in the coronal and sagittal planes were performed through the pelvis in 51 patients.

Image Interpretation

Prospective interpretation of all MR images was performed by one experienced radiologist (R.C.S.) as the official clinical interpretation. The clinical interpretation was used to evaluate the performance of MR imaging in the detection of abscesses. The interpreter was aware of the clinical suspicion of abscess but was blinded to biochemical findings. MR imaging studies were classified as positive or negative for the presence of a focal fluid collection consistent with an abscess. Additional retrospective review was performed by two board-certified radiologists (T.C.N., R.C.S.) to evaluate the specific features of the identified abscesses.

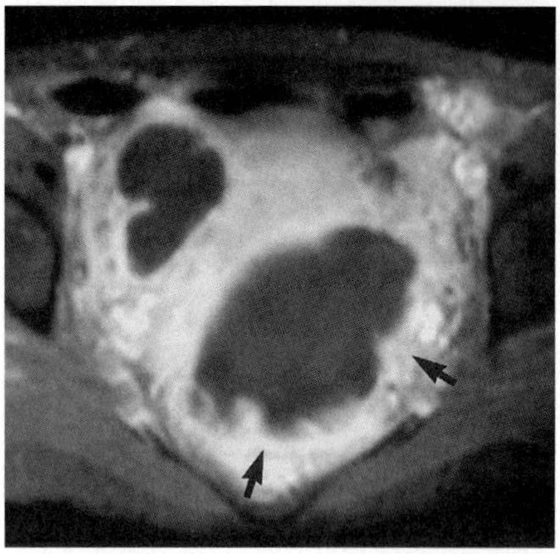

Figure 1. Abscess with peripheral rim and perilesion enhancement. Transverse gadolinium-enhanced fat-suppressed spoiled GRE image (130/2) shows a complex fluid collection in the pelvis with extensive rim and perilesion enhancement (arrows).

MR imaging features of focal fluid collections that were evaluated to determine whether they represented intraperitoneal abscesses included the following: (*a*) an enhancing, thickened rim on gadolinium-enhanced images; (*b*) perilesion enhancement on gadolinium-enhanced fat-suppressed images; (*c*) layering low-signal-intensity debris within the collection on T2-weighted images; (*d*) air within the collection; and (*e*) coexistent fistulous tracts. Several of these features were described in a recent study (9). The final MR imaging diagnosis was then correlated with surgical, laboratory, and histopathologic information obtained from patient charts 2 weeks to 30 months after MR imaging. The sensitivity, specificity, positive predictive value, negative predictive value, and accuracy for detecting intraperitoneal abscesses were also determined.

RESULTS

MR imaging revealed 25 fluid collections interpreted as intraperitoneal abscesses in 22 of the 67 patients (33%); surgical, laboratory, and histopathologic data confirmed the findings in 22 of the 25 collections (88%). MR imaging allowed exclu-

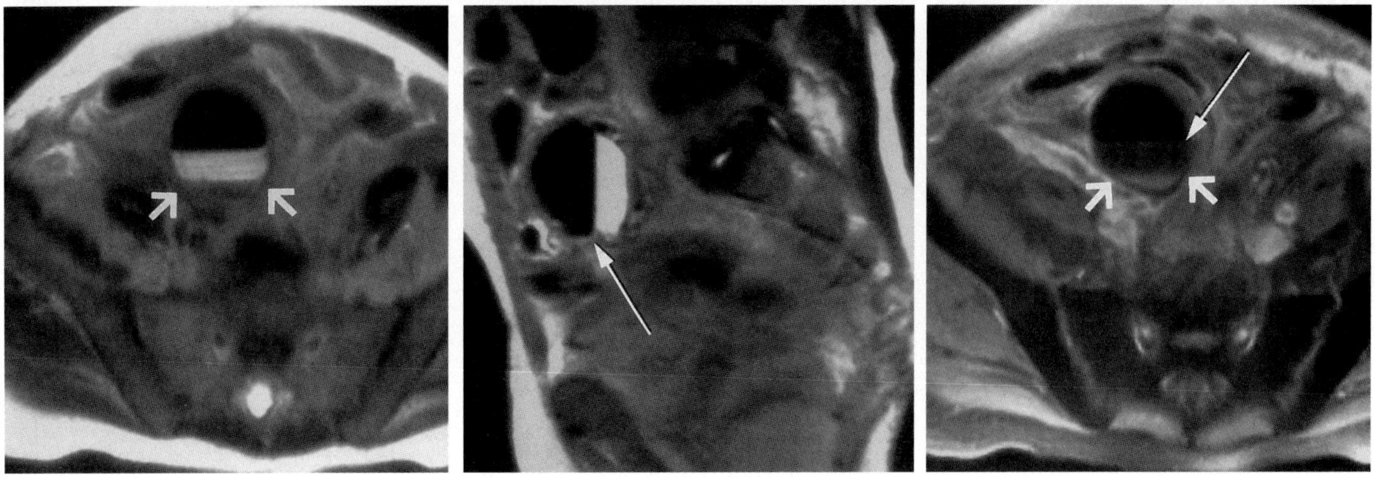

a. b. c.

Figure 2. Abscess containing layering debris and air. **(a)** Transverse and **(b)** sagittal half-Fourier RARE images (single shot/90) and **(c)** transverse gadolinium-enhanced fat-suppressed spoiled GRE image (140/4) show a rounded fluid collection in the right lower quadrant that contains air-fluid (arrow in **b**, long arrow in **c**) and fluid-debris (arrows in **a**, short arrows in **c**) levels. Also note the extensive perilesion enhancement on the gadolinium-enhanced image **(c)**.

sion of intraperitoneal abscesses in 45 of the 67 patients (67%). No patient had a subsequently diagnosed intraperitoneal abscess not revealed with MR imaging. Accurate MR imaging diagnosis was achieved in 64 of the 67 patients (96%) regardless of the predisposing medical condition.

Ten fluid collections were found in the midpelvis, six in the midabdomen, two in the right upper quadrant, five in the right lower quadrant, one in the left upper quadrant, and one in the left lower quadrant. The mean greatest dimension of the collections was 7.4 cm (range, 2.2–18.0 cm); the mean smallest dimension was 4.3 cm (range, 1.0–10.0 cm).

Two collections were treated with percutaneous aspiration, 17 with percutaneous drainage, and six with surgical drainage. Twenty-two of the 25 collections were subsequently proved to represent abscesses; one, a giant sigmoid diverticulum; and two, sterile fluid collections. Twenty-four of the collections were sampled and sent for laboratory analysis; the giant sigmoid diverticulum was resected. Four samples showed growth of gram-positive bacteria, two showed growth of gram-negative bacteria, and 16 showed growth of mixed flora, including gram-positive, gram-negative, and anaerobic species. Two samples contained polymorphonuclear white blood cells but did not show growth of bacteria; both patients had been receiving antibiotic therapy before sampling.

All 25 collections demonstrated decreased signal intensity on T1-weighted images; on T2-weighted images, 13 collections demonstrated homogeneously increased signal intensity and 12 demonstrated heterogeneously increased signal intensity. MR imaging findings in patients subsequently determined to have intraperitoneal abscesses included an enhancing, thickened rim in 21 of 24 collections (88%) imaged with gadolinium enhancement; perilesion enhancement in 18 of 24 collections (75%) imaged with gadolinium enhancement (Fig 1); air within the collection in 14 of 25 collections (56%) (Fig 2); layering debris within the collection on T2-weighted images in 12 of 25 collections (48%); and coexistent fistulous tracts in two of 25 collections (8%).

The detection of rim enhancement and perilesion enhancement was facilitated by the addition of fat suppression to the T1-weighted spin-echo or spoiled GRE images acquired 90 seconds after contrast material administration. Low-signal-intensity, dependently layering debris within the collection was detected on T2-weighted turbo spin-echo or half-Fourier RARE images. Intralesion gas was most perceptible on T2-weighted turbo spin-echo or half-Fourier RARE images. Pelvic abscesses were well shown with a combination of transverse and sagittal imaging.

One of the three patients with a false-positive MR imaging diagnosis of intraperitoneal abscess had a large pancreatic pseudocyst with inflammatory changes but no evidence of bacterial, fungal, or viral growth in repeated aspirates. Laboratory findings were confounded by prior antibiotic administration. Another patient had a complex fluid collection in the right lower quadrant; despite aspiration of complex fluid that contained extensive particulate matter, there was no growth at culturing. This patient had been receiving antibiotic therapy before percutaneous drainage of the collection. The third patient had a giant sigmoid diverticulum, which was misinterpreted as a diverticular abscess. Overall, sensitivity was 100%; specificity, 94% (95% confidence interval = 83%, 99%); positive predictive value, 88% (95% confidence interval = 69%, 97%); negative predictive value, 100%; and accuracy, 96% (95% confidence interval = 88%, 99%).

DISCUSSION

The results of our study suggest that MR imaging has high diagnostic accuracy in evaluation of suspected intraperitoneal abscesses. The addition of fat suppression to T1-weighted spin-echo or spoiled GRE imaging after administration of gadolinium contrast material increases the conspicuity of enhancement of both the abscess wall and adjacent soft-tissue inflammatory changes.

T2-weighted turbo spin-echo or half-Fourier RARE imaging was useful in the detection of layering intralesion debris. Intralesion gas was best appreciated on T2-weighted turbo spin-echo or half-Fourier RARE images due to the high contrast between signal void air and high-signal-intensity fluid. Application of fat suppression to T2-weighted turbo spin-echo or half-Fourier RARE sequences may aid differentiation of complex fluid and debris from surrounding increased-signal-intensity fat.

Our results for the detection of pelvic abscesses were comparable to the high detection rate (100%) of MR imaging in a previous study (3). The results of that study suggested that the combination of debris and gas within the collection is a helpful diagnostic feature, a conclusion supported by our results. Similar findings have also been reported in CT evaluation of patients suspected to have intraperitoneal abscesses (2,5).

The most frequently observed combination of specific MR imaging findings in patients with subsequently proved intraperitoneal abscesses was rim enhancement and perilesion enhancement (9). These enhancement features enabled differentiation of abscesses from other fluid collections with similar signal intensity characteristics on unenhanced T1- and T2-weighted images. Layering intralesion debris or air, although occurring less frequently, added to the specificity of interpretation.

A fluid collection with an enhancing rim may occasionally reflect chronic, aseptic inflammation (2). Culture results also may be adversely affected by prior antibiotic administration, as occurred in two of our three false-positive cases. Perilesion enhancement within the soft tissues may also reflect recent radiation therapy (10,11). Thus, caution should be exercised when evaluating patients who lack additional MR imaging and laboratory findings consistent with intraperitoneal abscesses, as inflammatory disease and neoplastic disease after radiation therapy may have similar appearances. The clinical history is therefore crucial in the evaluation of patients with complicated underlying disease processes.

Additional information provided by MR imaging, including assessment of tumor stage and recurrence, may prove particularly useful in the evaluation of patients with gynecologic malignancies and clinical suspicion of fistulas (1,3,6,10–12). The usefulness of MR imaging in the assessment of disease activity in inflammatory bowel disease makes these patients ideal candidates for MR imaging as well (1, 4,6,13,14).

Our study was limited by the lack of accurate laboratory data in two of the three false-positive cases. Percutaneous aspirates obtained after antibiotic administration precluded accurate assessment for bacterial overgrowth. This study also did not assess the cost-effectiveness of MR imaging in the setting of clinically suspected intraperitoneal abscesses. An important drawback of use of MR imaging for evaluation of possible intraperitoneal abscesses is the inability to perform concomitant abscess drainage. Such drainage can be performed with both CT and ultrasonographic guidance. Interventional MR imaging is currently being developed (15,16). However, it has not yet been determined whether interventional MR imaging will prove practical for routine percutaneous drainage.

Currently, because of ease of patient handling, uncooperative or critically ill patients are better imaged with CT, even when iodinated contrast material is contraindicated. An additional disadvantage of current MR imaging protocols is lack of intraluminal contrast material, potentially rendering distinction between abscesses and bowel or bowel diverticula difficult. However, demonstration of contrast material entering a structure does not exclude an abscess, nor does lack of contrast material entering a structure exclude a bowel diverticulum. In fact, the patient with the giant sigmoid diverticulum underwent a CT examination during which gastrointestinal contrast material failed to enter the diverticulum. This result was reflected in the final CT interpretation, in which the lesion was also considered an abscess. Ideally, a prospective study that compares CT and MR imaging in the detection of intraperitoneal abscesses in the same patient population should be performed. Finally, further investigation is needed to develop clinical appropriateness criteria.

In summary, this study demonstrates that MR imaging has high diagnostic accuracy in evaluation of suspected intraperitoneal abscesses. These observations have the potential to affect the treatment of patients with varied underlying disease processes. The potential benefits to patients with elevated serum creatinine levels, recently administered high-density barium, metallic implants, underlying malignancy, inflammatory bowel disease, and clinically suspected fistulas require further investigation.

Acknowledgment: The authors gratefully acknowledge Caroline Reinhold, MD, for her assistance with statistical analyses.

References

1. Madsen SM, Thomsen HS, Munkholm P, Schlichting P, Davidsen B. Magnetic resonance imaging of Crohn disease: early recognition of treatment response and relapse. Abdom Imaging 1997; 22:164–166.
2. Montgomery RS, Wilson SE. Intraabdominal abscesses: image-guided diagnosis and therapy. Clin Infect Dis 1996; 23:128–136.
3. Ha HK, Lim GY, Cha ES, et al. MR imaging of tubo-ovarian abscess. Acta Radiol 1995; 36:510–514.
4. Haggett PJ, Moore NR, Shearman JD, Travis SPL, Jewell DP, Mortensen NJ. Pelvic and perianal complications of Crohn's disease: assessment using magnetic resonance imaging. Gut 1995; 36:407–410.
5. Fukuya T, Hawes DR, Lu CC, Barloon TJ. CT of abdominal abscess with fistulous communication to the gastrointestinal tract. J Comput Assist Tomogr 1991; 15: 445–449.
6. Rafal RB, Nichols JN, Cennerazzo WJ, Kazam E, DeCosse JJ. MRI for evaluation of perianal inflammation. Abdom Imaging 1995; 20:248–252.
7. Zweemer RP, Scheele F, Verheijen RH, Hummel P, Schats R. Ovarian abscess during pregnancy mimicking a leiomyoma of the uterus: a complication of transvaginal ultrasound-guided oocyte aspiration. J Assist Reprod Genet 1996; 13:81–85.
8. Low RN, Barone RM, Lacey C, Sigeti JS, Alzate GD, Sebrechts CP. Peritoneal tumor: MR imaging with dilute oral barium and intravenous gadolinium-containing contrast agents compared with unenhanced MR imaging and CT. Radiology 1997; 204:513–520.
9. Semelka RC, John G, Kelekis NL, Burdeny DA, Worawattanakul S, Ascher SM. Bowel-related abscesses: MR demonstration—preliminary results. Magn Reson Imaging (in press).
10. Weber TM, Sostman HD, Spritzer CE, et al. Cervical carcinoma: determination of recurrent tumor extent versus radiation changes with MR imaging. Radiology 1995; 194:135–139.
11. Blomlie V, Rofstad EK, Tvera K, Lien HH. Noncritical soft tissues of the female pelvis: serial MR imaging before, during, and after radiation therapy. Radiology 1996; 199:461–468.
12. Semelka RC, Hricak H, Kim B, et al. Pelvic fistulas: appearances on MR images. Abdom Imaging 1997; 22:91–95.
13. Shoenut JP, Semelka RC, Silverman R, Yaffe CS, Micflikier AB. Magnetic resonance imaging in inflammatory bowel disease. J Clin Gastroenterol 1993; 17: 73–78.
14. Shoenut JP, Semelka RC, Magro CM, Silverman R, Yaffe CS, Micflikier AB. Comparison of magnetic resonance imaging and endoscopy in distinguishing the type and severity of inflammatory bowel disease. J Clin Gastroenterol 1994; 19:31–35.
15. Joensuu RP, Sepponen RE, Lamminen AE, Standertskjold-Nordenstam CG. Interventional MR imaging. Acta Radiol 1997; 38:43–46.
16. Steiner P, Erhart P, Heske N, Dumoulin CL, von Schulthess GK, Debatin JF. Active biplanar MR tracking for biopsies in humans. AJR 1997; 169:735–738.

Fecal Incontinence in Scleroderma: Assessment of the Anal Sphincter with Thin-Section Endoanal MR Imaging[1]

Nandita M. deSouza, MD, FRCR
Andreanna D. Williams, DCR
Helen J. Wilson, BA
David J. Gilderdale, PhD
Glyn A. Coutts, PhD
Carol M. Black, MD, FRCP

Index terms:
Anus, abnormalities, 757.613, 757.792
Anus, MR, 757.121411, 757.121417, 757.12143
Scleroderma, 757.613

Radiology 1998; 208:529–535

[1] From the Robert Steiner MR Unit, Imperial College School of Medicine, Hammersmith Hospital, Du Cane Rd, London W12 0HS, England (N.M.d.S., A.D.W., D.J.G., G.A.C.), and the Department of Rheumatology, Royal Free Hospital, London, England (H.J.W., C.M.B.). From the 1997 RSNA scientific assembly. Received November 12, 1997; revision requested January 23, 1998; revision received February 13; accepted March 9. D.J.G. supported in part by Picker International, Highland Heights, Ohio. **Address reprint requests to** N.M.d.S.

PURPOSE: To compare the magnetic resonance (MR) imaging appearance of the anal sphincter in patients with fecal incontinence and scleroderma with that in patients with fecal incontinence alone, scleroderma alone, or neither.

MATERIALS AND METHODS: The study population comprised 14 patients with fecal incontinence and scleroderma, four with scleroderma alone, 13 with incontinence alone, and six with neither. T1- and T2-weighted spin-echo, magnetization transfer contrast–weighted, and dynamic gadolinium-enhanced images were obtained and analyzed for the integrity, thickness, and length of sphincter components. Magnetization transfer contrast ratios and T2 were calculated to assess fibrosis of the internal sphincter. The percentage enhancement above baseline was calculated at 30-second intervals for the internal and the external sphincter.

RESULTS: Eleven patients with incontinence and scleroderma showed descent of rectal air and feces into the anterior anal canal, with forward deviation of the significantly ($P < .05$) atrophied internal sphincter, which showed a slower gadolinium-enhancement pattern compared with that in other groups. Patients with incontinence alone showed no evidence of internal sphincter deviation or altered vascularity but had a significant reduction ($P < .05$) in deep external sphincter bulk.

CONCLUSION: In patients with fecal incontinence and scleroderma, endoanal MR imaging helps delineate the anterior sphincter deformity and shows the slower gadolinium-enhancement pattern on dynamic studies of the internal sphincter.

Scleroderma (systemic sclerosis) is characterized by a chronic inflammatory process, fibrous connective tissue proliferation, and vasculitis that affects multiple organs (1). Gastrointestinal tract involvement is common, and the esophageal manifestations have been studied extensively because impaired peristalsis and acid reflux result in debilitating symptoms due to erosive esophagitis and stricture formation (2). Anorectal disease in these patients is often neglected not only because of a social stigma but also because it has not been possible to demonstrate the detailed anatomic appearances of the anal sphincter. Recently, endoanal magnetic resonance (MR) imaging has enabled the acquisition of thin-section images, with high spatial resolution, of the various muscle components of the anal sphincter complex (3–6). The purpose of this study was, therefore, to compare the MR imaging appearance of the anal sphincter in patients with scleroderma and fecal incontinence with that in patients with fecal incontinence but without scleroderma, in asymptomatic patients with scleroderma, and in control subjects. In addition, fibrosis of the internal sphincter in each group was quantified by using magnetization transfer contrast ratios, and the vascularity of the sphincter was compared among the groups by using dynamic contrast material–enhancement curves.

Author contributions:
Guarantor of integrity of entire study, N.M.d.S.; study concepts and design, N.M.d.S.; definition of intellectual content, N.M.d.S., C.M.B.; literature research, N.M.d.S., H.J.W.; clinical studies, H.J.W., C.M.B.; data acquisition, A.D.W., G.A.C., D.J.G.; data analysis, N.M.d.S., A.D.W.; statistical analysis, N.M.d.S.; manuscript preparation, N.M.d.S., A.D.W.; manuscript editing, N.M.d.S., C.M.B.; manuscript review, N.M.d.S.

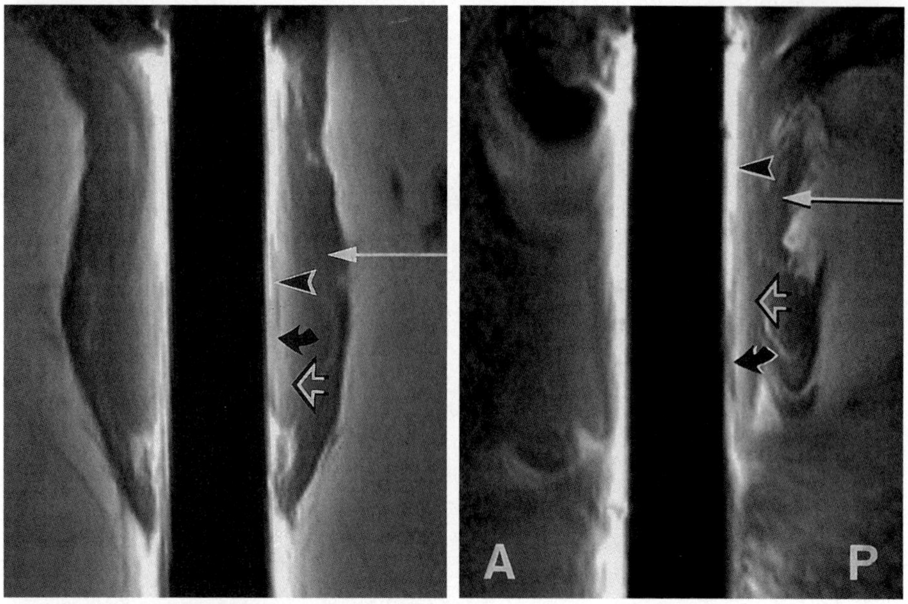

a.

b.

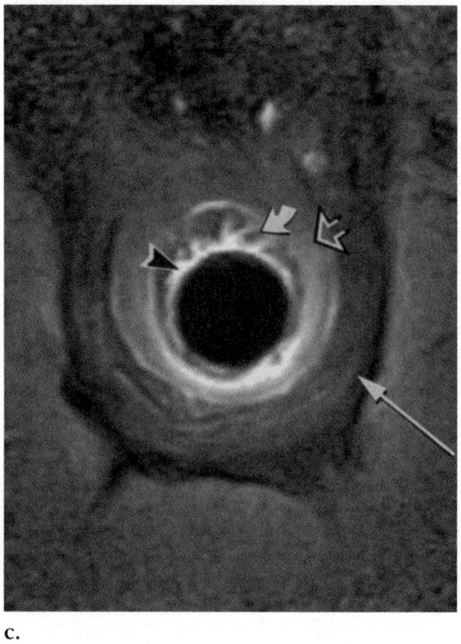

c.

Figure 1. **(a)** Coronal and **(b)** sagittal T1-weighted spin-echo images (720/20) and **(c)** transverse T2-weighted spin-echo image (2,500/80) obtained at the level of the middle of the sphincter show normal anatomy in a 57-year-old female control subject. The coil is seen as a central signal void. The mucosa (arrowhead) has very high signal intensity on all images. The submucosa (curved arrow) has low signal intensity on all images. The internal sphincter is seen as a homogeneous band (open arrow) and has particularly high signal intensity in **c**. The external sphincter (straight solid arrow) has relatively low signal intensity on all images. The sphincter is shorter anteriorly than posteriorly, and the deep component of the external sphincter does not form a complete ring anteriorly. This is best appreciated in **c**. In **b**, *A* = anterior, *P* = posterior.

MATERIALS AND METHODS

Patients

Thirty-seven patients were included in this study. The study was approved by our internal review board, and, after the procedure had been explained to the patients, written informed consent was obtained. Consecutive symptomatic patients were recruited during a 12-month period. During this period, asymptomatic, age-matched control subjects with or without scleroderma were recruited from those willing to participate. Exclusion criteria included the presence of a cardiac pacemaker and/or aneurysm clips and claustrophobia.

Fourteen patients (12 women, two men; age range, 26–78 years; mean, 57 years ± 12 [standard deviation]), had scleroderma and fecal incontinence. Two of the 14 patients had diffuse and 12 had limited cutaneous scleroderma. Of the women in this group, two were nulliparous and 10 were multiparous. Thirteen women (age range, 34–79 years; mean, 60 years ± 16) with fecal incontinence but without scleroderma were similarly examined: Twelve patients in this group were multiparous. Four other women (age range, 33–65 years; mean, 48 years ± 19) had scleroderma but no symptoms of fecal incontinence. Of these patients, one was nulliparous and three were multiparous. Finally, six asymptomatic control subjects (four women and two men without bowel problems; age range, 25–81 years; mean, 51 years ± 20) were included: Three of the four women were multiparous. The small numbers of patients and subjects without fecal incontinence reflect the difficulty in recruiting asymptomatic patients.

Fecal incontinence was graded according to the system of Miller et al (7), who considered the frequency of loss of solid, liquid, and gaseous material. Given a maximum possible score of 18, the mean score ± 1 standard deviation of the patients with fecal incontinence and scleroderma was 14 ± 4 (range, 5–18), whereas the mean score of the patients with fecal incontinence without scleroderma was 13 ± 4 (range, 7–18). In the other two groups, the scores were zero.

Anorectal manometry was performed as part of the routine clinical investigation at the referring hospital in nine of the 14 patients with fecal incontinence and scleroderma and in 12 of the 13 patients with fecal incontinence alone. Of the nine patients with fecal incontinence and scleroderma, six showed a reduction in resting pressure (median reduction, 25% below the norm for that laboratory) and five showed a reduction in squeeze pressure (ie, peak pressure at maximal voluntary contraction of the anal sphincter; median reduction, 50%). Of the 12 patients with fecal incontinence alone, 11 showed a reduction in resting pressure (median reduction, 47% below the norm for that laboratory); all 12 patients showed a reduction in squeeze pressure (median reduction, 43%).

Imaging Technique

The endoanal receiver coil was of a single-saddle design, 12 mm in diameter and 9 cm in length. The receiver coil was mounted on a Delrin former (Du Pont, Geneva, Switzerland) and was encased in a rigid outer cover with a rounded proximal end for ease of insertion. The coil incorporated integral tuning and matching and decoupling circuitry. Details of the endoanal coil have been described previously (3,4).

With the subject or patient in the lateral decubitus position, the receiver coil (covered in a rubber sheath) was positioned within the anal canal. The subject or patient was then turned supine, and the coil was immobilized with an external clamp, the base of which was under the thighs of the subject or patient. Initial examinations performed without the clamp produced considerable image degradation due to coil motion.

Imaging was performed with a 0.5-T unit (Asset; Picker International, Highland Heights, Ohio). Transverse T1-weighted spin-echo (repetition time msec/

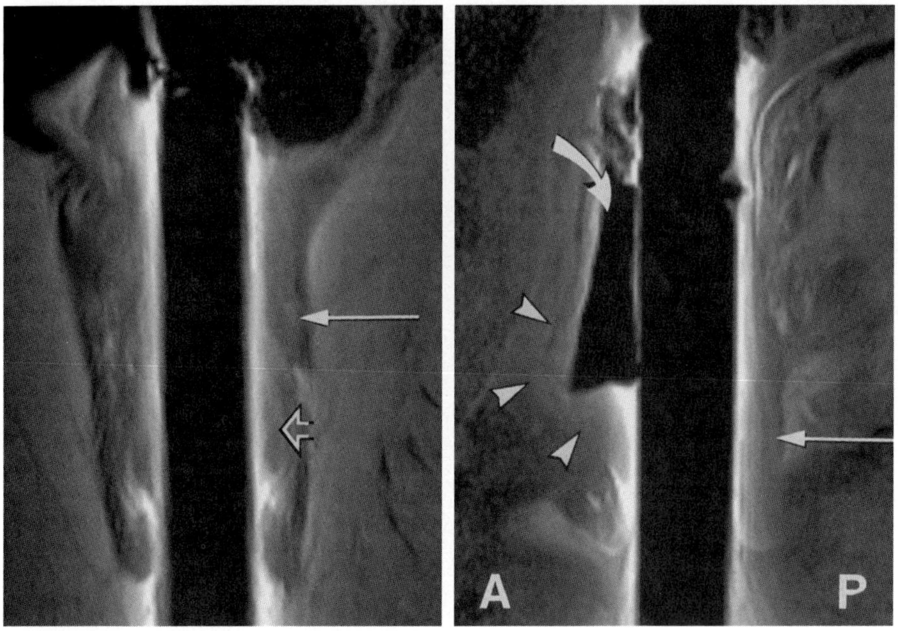

a. b.

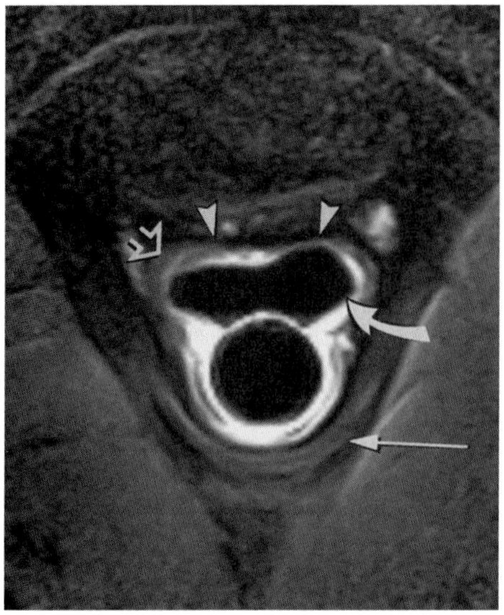

c.

Figure 2. (**a**) Coronal and (**b**) sagittal T1-weighted spin-echo images (720/20) and (**c**) transverse T2-weighted spin-echo image (2,500/80) obtained at the level of the middle of the sphincter show sphincter anatomy in a 78-year-old female patient with fecal incontinence and scleroderma. The coil is seen as a central signal void. The anterior part of the internal sphincter is buckled forward (arrowheads in **b** and **c**), with descent of rectal air (curved arrow in **b** and **c**) into the upper part of the sphincter. The atrophic internal sphincter (open arrow in **a** and **c**) is best appreciated in **c**. The external sphincter (straight solid arrow) is relatively normal. In **b**, *A* = anterior, *P* = posterior.

echo time msec, 720–820/20) images were obtained with and without a saturating radio-frequency pulse of 1,000 Hz off resonance to provide magnetization transfer contrast. Proton-density–weighted and T2-weighted spin-echo (2,500/20, 80) and short inversion time inversion-recovery (repetition time msec/echo time msec/inversion time msec, 2,500/30/107) images were also obtained in the transverse plane. In addition, coronal and sagittal T1-weighted (720–820/20) images were obtained. Contiguous 3-mm-thick sections were obtained with a 192 × 256 matrix, two to four signals acquired, and a 12-cm field of view. Dynamic images in three section positions (acquisition time, 10 seconds per section) were obtained through the thickest part of the internal sphincter during injection of a bolus of gadopentetate dimeglumine (Omniscan, Nycomed, Oslo, Norway; 0.1 mg gadolinium per kilogram of body weight) in all but two subjects, who were asymptomatic patients without scleroderma. Gadolinium–enhanced T1-weighted images were obtained in the transverse and coronal planes by using parameters that were identical to those used for unenhanced images.

Image Analysis

Images were assessed visually for the integrity of the internal sphincter and for each of the three components (subcutaneous, superficial, and deep) of the external anal sphincter. Deficiencies and any asymmetry of each muscle group were noted.

The maximum thickness of the internal sphincter was measured on T2-weighted transverse images. Measurements were made at the 3-o'clock and 9-o'clock positions, and an average was calculated. Likewise, the maximum thickness of each of the components of the external sphincter was measured at the 3-o'clock and 9-o'clock positions on T2-weighted transverse images, and an average was obtained. In cases where there was a substantial (>2 mm) discrepancy between right- and left-sided measurements due to hemiatrophy, only the values from the unaffected side were used.

The maximum length of the internal sphincter and of each of the three components of the external sphincter was measured on midline coronal T1-weighted images on the right and left sides, and an average was obtained.

Identical regions of interest were drawn in the internal sphincter and the components of the external sphincter on the T2-weighted, proton-density–weighted, and magnetization transfer contrast–weighted images. With these data, the T2 and the magnetization-transfer ratios were calculated for the internal sphincter and the external sphincter components.

Of the three sections obtained in the dynamic series, the third was used to draw regions of interest in the internal and external sphincters. The same regions of interest were used for subsequent acquisitions of that section after injection of the contrast material. The percentage increase above baseline in signal intensity over time was calculated and plotted, and the time to reach half the maximum enhancement was noted.

Statistical Analysis

Because of the skewness of the data, the nonparametric Mann-Whitney *U* test was used for the comparisons. For each of the four patient groups, the mean thickness and length (±1 standard deviation) of each sphincter component were calculated and compared.

The mean T2 and magnetization transfer contrast ratios (±1 standard deviation) for the internal sphincter were also calculated for each patient group and were compared, as was the percentage increase in enhancement of the internal and external sphincter relative to baseline at each time point.

RESULTS

Sphincter Anatomy

The normal anatomy of the internal sphincter and the three components of the external sphincter, along with their relationship to the pelvic floor, is shown in Figure 1. Of the 14 patients with scleroderma and fecal incontinence, 11 (nine women, two men) showed a striking abnormality of the musculature of the anterior sphincter. There was buckling of the anterior rectal wall forward, with descent of rectal air and feces below the levators into the upper half of the anal canal. This was best appreciated on the sagittal images (Fig 2). This appearance was also seen in one of the four patients with scleroderma but without fecal incontinence. It was not seen in any of the patients with fecal incontinence alone (Fig 3) or in the control subjects.

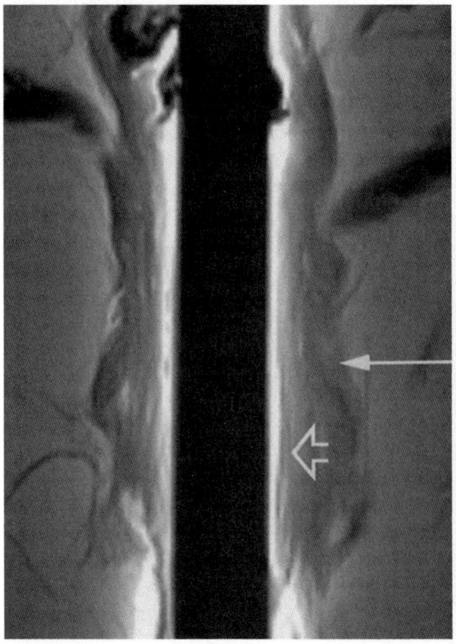

a.

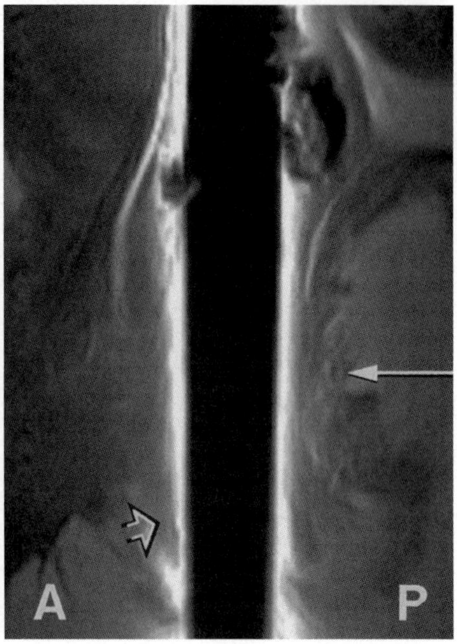

b.

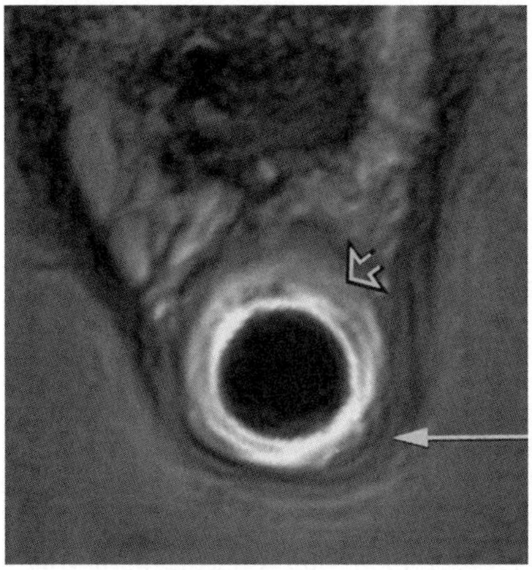

c.

Figure 3. **(a)** Coronal and **(b)** sagittal T1-weighted spin-echo images (720/20) and **(c)** transverse T2-weighted spin-echo image (2,500/80) obtained at the level of the middle of the sphincter show sphincter anatomy in a 75-year-old female patient with fecal incontinence without scleroderma. The coil is seen as a central signal void. In **a**, a normal-looking internal sphincter (open arrow) and atrophic external sphincter (solid arrow) are noted. There is no evidence of descent of rectal air below the pelvic floor in **b** or **c**. In **b**, *A* = anterior, *P* = posterior.

Sphincter Bulk

The Table lists the thickness and length measurements of each sphincter component for all patient groups. There was a significant reduction ($P < .05$) in the thickness of the internal sphincter in patients with scleroderma and fecal incontinence compared with that in all other groups. There was no significant difference, however, in internal sphincter thickness between patients with scleroderma but without fecal incontinence and control subjects. Likewise, patients with fecal incontinence alone did not have a significant reduction in internal sphincter bulk compared with control subjects.

There was a significant reduction ($P < .05$) in the thickness of the deep component of the external sphincter in patients with fecal incontinence alone compared with that in control subjects. Neither of the groups with scleroderma showed any significant change in external sphincter bulk compared with control subjects.

Length measurements for the internal sphincter and external sphincter components, when compared between groups, did not reach statistical significance in any instance.

T2 and Magnetization Transfer Contrast Ratio

The T2 and the magnetization transfer contrast ratio for the internal sphincter were 48 msec ± 10 and 75% ± 13, respectively, for patients with fecal incontinence and scleroderma; 58 msec ± 11 and 68% ± 4, respectively, for patients with fecal incontinence alone; 49 msec ± 8 and 71% ± 8, respectively, for patients with scleroderma alone; and 50 msec ± 5 and 65% ± 8, respectively, for control subjects. There were no significant differences for either of these parameters between any of the groups at the $P < .05$ level.

Gadolinium-Enhancement Patterns

The curves for gadolinium enhancement of the internal and the external sphincter for all groups are shown in Figure 4. The time to half the maximum enhancement of the internal sphincter was 90 seconds for patients with scleroderma and fecal incontinence, 75 seconds for patients with fecal incontinence alone, 60 seconds for patients with scleroderma alone, and 50 seconds for control subjects. There was a significant ($P < .05$) reduction in the percentage enhancement above baseline of the internal sphincter at 30, 60, and 90 seconds after contrast material administration between patients with fecal incontinence and scleroderma, patients with fecal incontinence without scleroderma, and control subjects. There was no statistically significant difference in percentage enhancement at any time points between patients with fecal incontinence and scleroderma and those with scleroderma without incontinence.

The enhancement of the external sphincter did not show statistically significant differences at any time points between any of the groups.

DISCUSSION

In this study, we defined the anatomic abnormality of the anterior part of the anal sphincter seen in patients with scleroderma who have developed fecal incontinence. In women, the anterior component of the sphincter complex is shorter

Thickness and Length of the Components of the Anal Sphincter Complex

Group	Thickness (cm)				Length (cm)			
	Internal Anal Sphincter	External Anal Sphincter			Internal Anal Sphincter	External Anal Sphincter		
		Subcutaneous	Superficial	Deep		Subcutaneous	Superficial	Deep
Patients with scleroderma and fecal incontinence (n = 14)	0.28 ± 0.10*	0.39 ± 0.09	0.28 ± 0.02	0.48 ± 0.10	3.7 ± 0.6	1.6 ± 0.3	1.6 ± 0.4	2.0 ± 0.5
Patients with fecal incontinence alone (n = 13)	0.36 ± 0.08	0.39 ± 0.15	0.29 ± 0.07	0.44 ± 0.13*	3.5 ± 0.6	1.4 ± 0.3	1.5 ± 0.4	1.9 ± 0.4
Patients with scleroderma without fecal incontinence (n = 4)	0.37 ± 0.10	0.48 ± 0.10	0.25 ± 0.04	0.54 ± 0.10	3.8 ± 0.7	1.5 ± 0.1	1.5 ± 0.2	1.9 ± 0.3
Control subjects (n = 6)	0.42 ± 0.13	0.40 ± 0.11	0.30 ± 0.06	0.59 ± 0.12	4.2 ± 0.3	1.6 ± 0.3	1.7 ± 0.3	2.1 ± 0.5

Note.—Data are the mean ± 1 standard deviation.
* Result was significantly different ($P < .05$) when compared with results in other groups.

than the posterior component and, thus, more easily compromised. This short anterior segment may prove to be a pitfall with current methods of assessment, particularly if it is buckled forward. Noncontact with the anterior sphincter by an ultrasound (US) probe or manometric balloon catheter may result in the false assumption of a sphincter defect. This was indeed the case in one of the patients in our study. In such cases, endoanal MR imaging provides detailed anatomic information about the presence, deformity, and integrity of the various sphincter components.

MR imaging with a body coil was initially used in anal sphincter imaging to assess anorectal atresias (8). Use of an endovaginal coil in adults provides some improvement over body coil techniques in terms of spatial resolution (9), but the angle between the vagina and rectum makes the anal sphincter difficult to visualize in its entirety. Endoanal MR imaging clearly demonstrates the configuration of the various muscle components of the sphincter and helps delineate the short anterior segment in women (3). Although this varies from findings obtained with the body coil (10), it is in keeping with models from anatomic dissections (11). In addition to the muscles of the sphincter, endoanal MR imaging also allows delineation of the mucosa and the submucosa (3,5,6). Endoanal MR imaging may, therefore, be used to define small tracks in perianal sepsis (12) and the extent of tumors of the lower rectum (13).

In patients with scleroderma, the forward deviation of the anterior part of the sphincter is a feature of the increased rigidity of the normally elastic internal sphincter and is in keeping with what is known about smooth muscle in other parts of the gastrointestinal tract (14). It is in contrast with the appearance in patients with fecal incontinence without scleroderma, in whom atrophy of the external sphincter is seen (15). Although anorectal function and motility have been studied in small cohorts of such patients in recent years (16,17), the detailed imaging appearances have until now been documented only with endoanal US in isolated cases (18). The deformity of the anterior part of the sphincter was not associated with mucosal prolapse on these static images in any of the patients in our study. MR imaging during straining can demonstrate rectal prolapse (19); hence, real-time imaging of the pelvic floor during squeeze and strain maneuvers with the use of a tracking technique (20) is the subject of an ongoing study.

Fecal continence depends not only on the integrity of the anal sphincter complex but also on its function (and thus its muscle bulk) (21). High pressure within the canal is generated by means of the internal sphincter at rest (22). The striated sphincter muscles—namely, the external sphincter and puborectalis muscles—display continuous tonic electromyographic activity (23). The combined effect is to maintain opposition of the walls of the anal canal, which, with appropriate sensory information, prevents fecal leakage in normal circumstances (24). In the future, a combination of structural information from thin-section MR images and functional data from physiologic studies will provide a more complete method for investigating and monitoring anorectal disease in these patients.

Gastrointestinal smooth muscle may be involved early in patients with scleroderma, before the onset of clinical symptoms and physiologic abnormalities (25). Examples of gastrointestinal smooth muscle involvement include reduced rectal compliance (25), low resting pressure but normal squeeze pressure, and absence of the rectoanal inhibitory reflex in up to 71% of patients (16,17). Despite this, fecal incontinence remains poorly recognized, and its prevalence is unknown. Our results showing anterior buckling of the rectal wall, even in asymptomatic patients with scleroderma, suggest that the underlying abnormality is present early. The true frequency of fecal incontinence in scleroderma may be masked by the social implications of the disease.

The internal anal sphincter shares several similarities with the lower esophageal sphincter. In histologic terms, both are smooth muscle. In functional terms, both contract constantly, and both are involved pathologically in scleroderma (26). The esophageal abnormalities in scleroderma (eg, lowered basal pressure, loss of competence and peristalsis) are believed to be secondary to early replacement of the smooth muscle with collagen (1) and the resultant fibrosis. Although fibrosis in muscles has shown correlation with a shorter T2 (27), the increased amount of collagen deposited in the internal sphincter in our study was not measurable as a shortening of T2 or a change in the magnetization transfer contrast ratio.

In the later stages of the disease, collagenous replacement of smooth muscle aggravates muscle dysfunction and leads to atrophy (14). In scleroderma–induced gastrointestinal involvement, however, it has also been postulated that the primary event is a neural lesion leading to smooth muscle atrophy (28). In our study, there was a statistically significant reduction in the thickness of the internal sphincter in patients with fecal incontinence and scleroderma but not in the asymptomatic patients with scleroderma; this further supports the evidence that incontinence is related to smooth muscle atrophy in these patients.

The pathogenesis of neuropathy may be caused by compression of nerve fibers by means of collagen, as postulated in the etiology of peripheral neuropathy (29); or an arteriolar change in the vasa nervorum may play a role (14). This relationship between neuropathy and vasculopathy is further supported by the finding of decreased esophageal blood flow in patients with Raynaud phenomenon (30), with neuropathy leading to visceral vasospasm. Vasculopathy of arterioles is common in scleroderma, and fibrous replacement of the internal sphincter may be partly ischemic in origin. This would account for the slower rates of gadolinium enhancement in the internal sphincter of the patients with fecal incontinence and scleroderma in our study. A more detailed gadolinium-enhancement profile involving more time points in the 1st minute may help to identify more clearly those patients in whom ischemia is present.

In this study, we established the anatomic changes in the anal sphincter complex in patients with fecal incontinence and scleroderma. The exquisite tissue contrast between the internal and external sphincter provided by using MR imaging enables the differentiation of patients in whom the internal sphincter is primarily affected from those in whom an external sphincter abnormality may be contributing to symptoms. Some patients have reportedly (10) experienced relief of their symptoms after repair of the external sphincter (posterior anal repair), and selection of these patients by means of the preoperative establishment of the thickness of the external sphincter would be an advantage. The ischemic nature of the perineal tissues in these patients indicates that surgical procedures to promote continence often fail due to poor healing of tissues. Delineation of the anatomic abnormalities aids decision making with regard to available treatment modalities. Patients with no anatomic breach of the sphincter may be better treated with nerve stimulators than with surgery, particularly if there is any associated atrophy of the external sphincter. Endoanal MR imaging is an easy method for monitoring the progression of anorectal disease in these patients and may also be of particular value for assessing the effect of various drug regimens.

In conclusion, thin-section endoanal MR imaging enables anatomic assessment of fecal incontinence by allowing evaluation of the bulk of the component muscles of the anal sphincter. In patients with fecal incontinence and scleroderma, endoanal MR imaging helps delineate the anterior sphincter deformity and shows the slower gadolinium-enhancement pattern on dynamic studies of the internal sphincter.

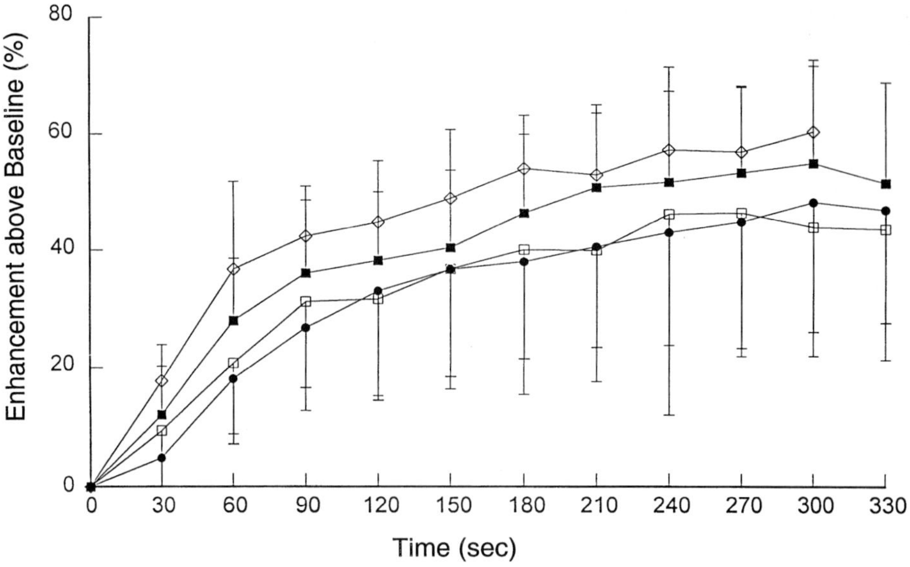

a.

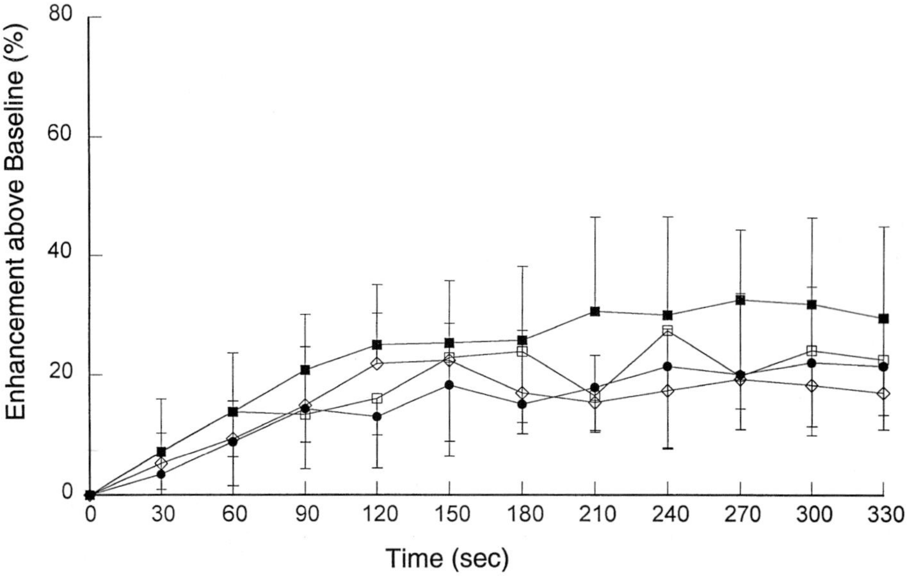

b.

Figure 4. Graphs show dynamic gadolinium-enhancement patterns for **(a)** the internal anal sphincter and **(b)** the external anal sphincter. In **a** and **b**, ● = patients with scleroderma and fecal incontinence, ■ = patients with fecal incontinence alone, □ = patients with scleroderma alone, ◇ = control subjects. **(a)** Patients with fecal incontinence and scleroderma show a small but statistically significant reduction in enhancement at 30, 60, and 90 seconds after injection of gadopentetate dimeglumine compared with that in control subjects. **(b)** There is no significant difference in enhancement rates between groups.

Acknowledgment: We are grateful to Mary C. Crisp for her secretarial assistance.

References

1. Scott JT, ed. Copeman's textbook of the rheumatic disease. 6th ed. New York, NY: Livingstone, 1986; 1364–1381.
2. Poirier TJ, Rankin GB. Gastrointestinal manifestations of progressive systemic sclerosis based on a review of 364 cases. Am J Gastroenterol 1972; 58:30–44.
3. deSouza NM, Puni R, Kmiot WA, Bartram CI, Hall AS, Bydder GM. MRI of the anal sphincter. J Comput Assist Tomogr 1995; 19:745–751.
4. deSouza NM, Puni R, Gilderdale DJ, Bydder GM. Magnetic resonance imaging of the anal sphincter using an internal coil. Magn Reson Med 1995; 11:45–46.
5. deSouza NM, Kmiot WA, Puni R, Hall AS, Bartram CI, Bydder GM. High resolution magnetic resonance imaging of the anal sphincter using an internal coil. Gut 1995; 51:284–287.
6. Hussain SM, Stoker J, Lameris JS. Anal sphincter complex: endoanal MR imaging of normal anatomy. Radiology 1995; 197: 671–677.
7. Miller R, Bartolo DC, Lock-Edmunds JC, Mortensen NJ. Prospective study of conservative and operative treatment for faecal incontinence. Br J Surg 1988; 75:101–105.
8. Peng HC, Chen HC, Wu JJ, Chong WT, Lee T. Evaluation of anorectal malformation using magnetic resonance imaging. Chung Hua I Hsueh Tsa Chih Taipei 1991; 48:190–196.
9. Muller-Schimpfle M, Franz H, Lobinger B, Claussen CD. High resolution magnetic resonance tomography of the anal sphincter using an intravaginal surface coil. ROFO 1995; 162:478–481. [German]
10. Aronson MP, Lee RA, Berquist TH. Anatomy of anal sphincters and related structures in continent women studied with magnetic resonance imaging. Obstet Gynecol 1990; 76:846–851.
11. Oh C, Kark AE. Anatomy of the external anal sphincter. Br J Surg 1972; 59:717–723.
12. Stoker J, Hussain SM, van Kempen D, Elevelt AJ, Laméris JS. Endoanal coil in MR imaging of anal fistulas. AJR 1996; 166:360–362.
13. deSouza NM, Hall AS, Puni R, Gilderdale DJ, Young IR, Kmiot WA. High resolution magnetic resonance imaging of the anal sphincter using a dedicated endoanal coil: comparison of magnetic resonance imaging with surgical findings. Dis Colon Rectum 1996; 39:926–934.
14. D'Angelo WA, Fries JF, Masi AT, Shulman LE. Pathologic observations in systemic sclerosis (scleroderma): a study of fifty-eight autopsy cases and fifty-eight matched controls. Am J Med 1969; 46:428–440.
15. deSouza NM, Puni R, Zbar A, Gilderdale DJ, Coutts GA, Krausz T. MR imaging of the anal sphincter in multiparous women using an endoanal canal: correlation with in vitro anatomy and appearances in fecal incontinence. AJR 1996; 167:1465–1471.
16. Chiou AWH, Lin JK, Wang FM. Anorectal abnormalities in progressive systemic sclerosis. Dis Colon Rectum 1989; 32:417–421.
17. Leighton JA, Valdovinos MA, Pemberton JH, Rath DM, Camilleri M. Anorectal dysfunction and rectal prolapse in progressive systemic sclerosis. Dis Colon Rectum 1993; 36:182–185.
18. Engel AF, Kamm MA, Talbot IC. Progressive systemic sclerosis of the internal anal sphincter leading to passive fecal incontinence. Gut 1994; 35:857–859.
19. Healy JC, Halligan S, Reznek RH, Watson S, Phillips RK, Armstrong P. Patterns of prolapse in women with symptoms of pelvic floor weakness: assessment with MR imaging. Radiology 1997; 203:77–81.
20. Coutts GA, Gilderdale DJ, Chui MK, Kasuboski L, deSouza NM. Integrated position tracking and imaging of interventional tools and devices. Magn Reson Med (in press).
21. Floyd WF, Walls EW. Electromyography of the sphincti ani externus in man. J Physiol 1953; 122:599–609.
22. Denny-Brown D, Robertson EG. An investigation of the nervous control of defecation. Brain 1935; 58:256–310.
23. Goligher JC, Hughes ESR. Sensibility of the rectum and colon: its role in the mechanism of anal incontinence. Lancet 1951; 1:543–548.
24. Duthie HL, Bennett RC. The relation of sensation in the anal canal to the functional anal sphincter: a possible factor in anal incontinence. Gut 1963; 4:179–182.
25. Whitehead WE, Taitelbaum G, Wigley FM, Schuster MM. Rectosigmoid motility and myoelectric activity in progressive systemic sclerosis. Gastroenterology 1989; 96:428–432.
26. Hamel-Roy J, Devroede G, Arhan P, et al. Comparative esophageal and anorectal motility in scleroderma. Gastroenterology 1985; 88:1–7.
27. Johnson RJ, Jenkins JP, Isherwood I, James RD, Schofield PF. Quantitative magnetic resonance imaging in rectal carcinoma. Br J Radiol 1987; 601:761–764.
28. Treacey WL, Baggenstoss AH, Slocoumb CH, et al. Scleroderma of the esophagus: a correlation of histologic and physiologic findings. Ann Intern Med 1963; 59:351–356.
29. Di Trapani G, Pocchiori M, Masullo C, Albanese A, Tulli A. Peripheral neuropathy in the course of progressive systemic sclerosis: light and ultrastructural study. Ital J Neurol Sci 1982; 3:341–348.
30. Belch JJF, Land D, Park RHR, et al. Decreased oesophageal blood flow in patients with Raynaud's phenomenon. Br J Rheum 1988; 27:426–430.

Pancreatic Arterial Anatomy: Depiction with Dual-Phase Helical CT[1]

Maria Chong, MD[2]
Patrick C. Freeny, MD
Udo P. Schmiedl, MD

Index terms:
Arteries, pancreatic, 95.92, 95.99
Computed tomography (CT), helical, 770.12115
Pancreas, CT, 770.12112, 770.12115

Radiology 1998; 208:537–542

[1] From the Department of Radiology, University of Washington School of Medicine, Box 357115, 1959 Pacific Ave, Seattle, WA 98195. From the 1997 RSNA scientific assembly. Received December 11, 1997; revision requested March 2, 1998; revision received March 24; accepted April 13. Supported in part by grants from Mallinckrodt Medical, St Louis, Mo, and GE Medical Systems, Milwaukee, Wis. **Address reprint requests to** P.C.F.

[2] Current address: Mallinckrodt Institute of Radiology, Washington University, St Louis, Mo.

PURPOSE: To determine the efficacy of arterial phase helical computed tomography (CT) for the depiction of small pancreatic arteries.

MATERIALS AND METHODS: Arterial phase helical CT (3-mm collimation, 1-mm reconstruction interval) was performed during power injection of 180 mL of ioversol at 5 mL/sec. Two radiologists reviewed 100 consecutive arterial phase helical CT scans of the pancreas in patients with normal glands and recorded the frequency of visualization of the major visceral (celiac, hepatic, splenic, gastroduodenal, superior mesenteric) and small pancreatic (dorsal pancreatic, right branch of the dorsal pancreatic, pancreaticomagna, caudal pancreatic, transverse pancreatic, anterior and posterior arcade, and inferior pancreaticoduodenal) arteries.

RESULTS: Scans in 87 patients were technically satisfactory and were included in the analysis. The major visceral arteries were seen in all patients. The following secondary pancreatic arteries were seen: dorsal pancreatic, 82 (94%) patients; pancreaticomagna, 45 (52%); caudal pancreatic, 34 (39%); transverse pancreatic, 36 (41%); right branch of the dorsal pancreatic, eight (9%); anterior arcade, 47 (54%); posterior arcade, 63 (72%); and inferior pancreaticoduodenal, 73 (84%).

CONCLUSION: Small pancreatic arteries can be delineated on arterial phase helical CT scans by using optimized techniques.

High-detail images obtained with dual-phase helical computed tomography (CT) during the arterial and venous phases of contrast material enhancement can potentially help improve the staging of pancreatic carcinoma. Several investigators (1–8) have described the value of dual-phase helical CT for the detection and staging of pancreatic carcinoma when thin-section collimation and ancillary computerized techniques are used to display the helical CT data sets for evaluation of the pancreatic arteries and veins.

It has been shown (9) that arterial phase helical CT can accurately display the major visceral arteries, the celiac axis and its branches, and the superior and inferior mesenteric arteries. At a review of cases at our institution in which helical CT angiograms were obtained, we noted that the small peripancreatic arteries—including the dorsal pancreatic, the right branch of the dorsal pancreatic, the pancreaticomagna, the caudal pancreatic, the transverse pancreatic, the inferior pancreaticoduodenal, and the anterior and posterior pancreaticoduodenal arcade arteries—often could be visualized. Angiographic depiction of tumor involvement of the visceral arteries and their major branches to the pancreas has been effective for the staging of pancreatic ductal adenocarcinoma (10–12). We postulated that if these small arteries could be depicted frequently at helical CT, they could potentially be used in concert with the evaluation of the adjacent small peripancreatic veins (7) to improve the accuracy of pancreatic carcinoma staging. The purpose of this study was to determine the efficacy of arterial phase helical CT scans for the depiction of the small peripancreatic arteries.

MATERIALS AND METHODS

Dual-phase helical CT is the standard examination at our institution for the evaluation of patients before anticipated liver resection or transplantation, for the initial detection and

Author contributions:
Guarantor of integrity of entire study, P.C.F.; study concepts and design, M.C., P.C.F., U.P.S.; definition of intellectual content, P.C.F.; literature research, M.C., P.C.F.; clinical studies, M.C., P.C.F., U.P.S.; data acquisition, M.C., P.C.F., U.P.S.; data analysis, M.C., P.C.F.; manuscript preparation, M.C., P.C.F.; manuscript editing, P.C.F.; manuscript review, M.C., P.C.F., U.P.S.

characterization of benign or malignant hypervascular liver tumors, and for the diagnosis and staging of pancreatic carcinoma. From the series of dual-phase helical CT studies performed in those patients evaluated for liver disease at our institution, 100 consecutive studies obtained during 3 years (June 7, 1994, to January 21, 1997) were reviewed retrospectively. None of the patients (age range, 36–75 years) had known or subsequently developed pancreatic disease during this study. Eighty-seven of the 100 patients underwent technically successful arterial phase helical CT of the pancreas, and the results in these patients form the basis of this report.

All dual-phase helical CT scans were obtained by using a HiSpeed Advantage scanner (GE Medical Systems; Milwaukee, Wis). The studies were optimized for imaging during the arterial phase by using a technique of bolus timing developed at our institution (9); a series of nonenhanced scans were obtained to determine the inferior level of the pancreas and the origin of the superior mesenteric artery. An initial test bolus of 20 mL of ioversol (Optiray 320; Mallinckrodt Medical, St Louis, Mo) was power injected via an antecubital vein at a rate of 5 mL/sec, and sequential low-dose CT scans were obtained at the level of the celiac artery (T12 vertebra). A cursor was placed on the aorta, and CT computer software was used to calculate the time of peak aortic enhancement. The arterial phase scanning delay was determined by subtracting 2 seconds from the time of peak aortic enhancement.

Dual-phase helical CT was then performed during power injection of 180 mL of ioversol at a rate of 5 mL/sec. Arterial phase scanning (120 kVp, 170–280 mA) began 2.5 cm below the origin of the superior mesenteric artery and/or pancreatic head and proceeded in a cranial direction to the dome of the liver; 3-mm collimation and a variable pitch of up to 1.9 were used to cover the entire pancreas and liver during a single breath hold. (The portal venous phase scanning sequence was initiated 60 seconds after the administration of ioversol, but these scans were not evaluated for this study.) All patients received 600–900 mL of water as an oral contrast agent 30 minutes before scanning and an additional 600–900 mL immediately before scanning, in accordance with our standard protocol for upper abdominal CT (13).

Arterial phase helical CT data were reconstructed with a standard soft algorithm at 1-mm increments and were saved on an optical disk or a digital-audio tape. The data were then transferred to a workstation (Advantage Windows; GE Medical Systems) and were displayed as a cine loop. At the workstation, three radiologists, one initially working independently (M.C.) and then two working simultaneously (M.C. and P.C.F. or M.C. and U.P.S.), assessed the data by viewing the cine loop and manually cine paging through the 1-mm-thick reconstructed axial images. The radiologists then recorded the frequency of visualization of the major visceral arteries (celiac, hepatic, splenic, gastroduodenal, and superior mesenteric arteries) and the small peripancreatic arteries (dorsal pancreatic, pancreaticomagna, caudal pancreatic, transverse pancreatic, right branch of the transverse pancreatic, inferior pancreaticoduodenal, and the anterior and posterior pancreaticoduodenal arcades).

The pancreatic arterial anatomy as described by Michels (14) was used as the reference for the evaluation of the arterial phase helical CT scans (Fig 1). Arteries were considered to be positively identified if the origin and anatomic course of the vessel could be traced by the readers and if the vessel anatomy agreed with the Michels description and classification. In the case of a discrepancy in identification between the two radiologists, a consensus was reached by reviewing the study together in the cine page mode.

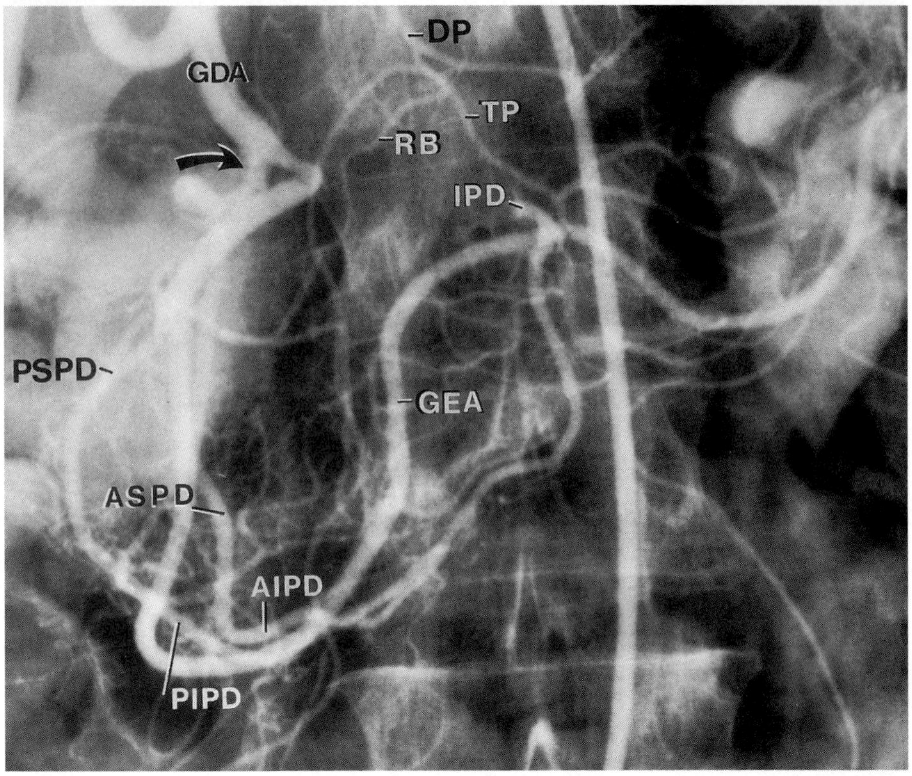

Figure 1. Pancreatic arteries. Selective gastroduodenal arteriogram shows the normal arterial anatomy of the pancreas as defined by Michels (14). Arrow = origin of the posterior superior pancreaticoduodenal artery, *AIPD* = anterior inferior pancreaticoduodenal artery, *ASPD* = anterior superior pancreaticoduodenal artery, *DP* = dorsal pancreatic artery, *GDA* = gastroduodenal artery, *GEA* = gastroepiploic artery, *IPD* = inferior pancreaticoduodenal artery, *PIPD* = posterior inferior pancreaticoduodenal artery, *PSPD* = posterior superior pancreaticoduodenal artery, *RB* = right branch of the dorsal pancreatic artery, *TP* = transverse pancreatic artery.

RESULTS

In 87 of the 100 patients, technically satisfactory arterial phase helical CT scans of the entire pancreas were obtained and formed the basis for this study. In the remaining 13 patients, the scans were technically unsatisfactory. These unsatisfactory images resulted from acquisition with 5-mm collimation in two patients and 7-mm collimation in three, patient-positioning errors that caused portions of the pancreatic head to be missed in six, and scanner malfunction during image acquisition that resulted in the loss of data in two.

The major visceral arteries were identified in all 87 patients. (The frequency of

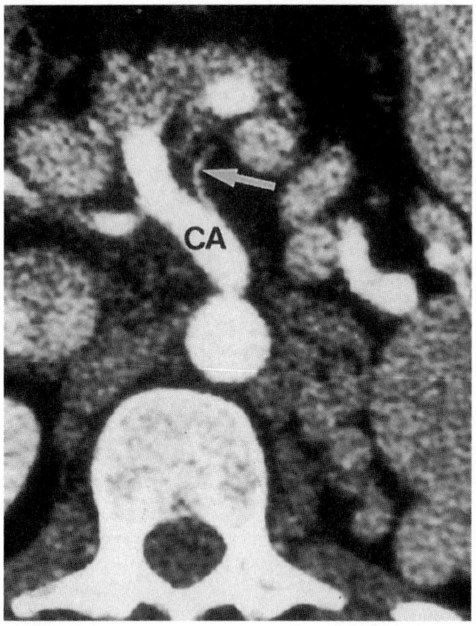

a.

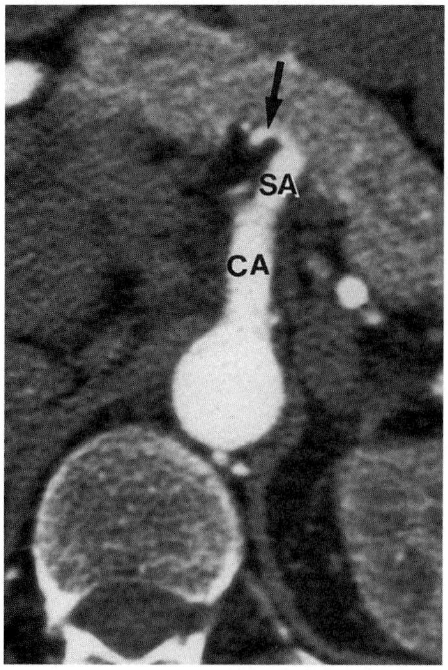

b.

Figure 2. Arterial phase helical CT scans show the origins of the dorsal pancreatic artery. **(a)** The dorsal pancreatic artery (arrow) is seen to arise from the celiac artery (*CA*) in a 46-year-old man. **(b)** In a 56-year-old man, the dorsal pancreatic artery (arrow) is seen to arise from the splenic artery (*SA*). *CA* = celiac artery.

visualization of the small pancreatic arteries is discussed later in this article.) The reader should be aware that vessel identification, branch origin, and anatomic course are easily assessed at dynamic viewing of the axial data set in the manual cine page mode. The images included in this report represent selected, individual axial CT scans, and, without knowledge of the cine mode, it may be difficult to ascertain the identity of a vessel on the basis of a single image, which cannot depict the anatomy of the entire vessel.

The dorsal pancreatic artery, which is the largest artery to the body of the pancreas, was visualized in 82 (94%) of the 87 patients (Figs 2, 3). It originated from the celiac axis in 14 (17%) of these 82 patients, the proximal part of the hepatic artery in 13 (16%) patients, the splenic artery in 34 (41%) patients, or the superior mesenteric artery in 21 (26%) patients. The dorsal pancreatic artery coursed ventrally from its origin along the posterior margin of the pancreas and divided into two branches.

The right branch of the dorsal pancreatic artery courses to the right, inferior to the neck of the gland, and quickly penetrates into the parenchyma. This artery was identified in only eight (9%) of the 87 patients (Fig 3b).

The transverse pancreatic artery, which is the major branch of the dorsal pancreatic artery, courses to the left along the posterior margin of the pancreatic body and tail and penetrates into the gland parenchyma. This artery was visualized in 36 (41%) of the 87 patients (Figs 3b, 4).

The splenic artery courses along the posterior margin of the pancreas and gives rise to two major arteries that supply the pancreatic body and tail. The pancreaticomagna artery, which is the largest artery supplying the tail of the gland, originated from the middle portion of the splenic artery and entered the pancreas at the posterior margin of the gland. It was visualized in 45 (52%) of the 87 patients (Fig 3b, 3c). The caudal pancreatic artery, a smaller branch supplying the pancreatic tail, originated from the distal portion of the splenic artery and gave off small branches to the gland. It was visualized in 34 (39%) patients (Fig 3d).

The nomenclature of the pancreaticoduodenal arcades is complex. For this study, we used the nomenclature defined by Michels (14); that is, we used Michels' type I (a single anterior and a single posterior arcade) to describe the pancreatic arcades (Fig 1). The anterior arcade is formed by the anterior superior pancreaticoduodenal artery, which arises as one of the two terminal branches of the gastroduodenal artery (the other branch being the right gastroepiploic artery). It anastomoses with the anterior inferior pancreaticoduodenal artery, which is one of the two branches of the inferior pancreaticoduodenal artery. The anterior arcade artery was seen to course inferiorly along the anterolateral surface of the pancreatic head in 47 (54%) patients (Fig 3d–3f).

The posterior arcade is formed by the posterior superior pancreaticoduodenal artery, which is the first branch of the gastroduodenal artery. This vessel is also called the retroduodenal artery. It courses along the posterior margin of the gland, anastomosing inferiorly with the posterior inferior pancreaticoduodenal artery. The posterior arcade artery was seen in 63 (72%) patients (Fig 3d–3f).

The inferior pancreaticoduodenal artery arises as the first branch of the superior mesenteric artery and divides into the anterior and posterior inferior pancreaticoduodenal arteries along the caudal margin of the pancreatic head. These vessels constitute the inferior portion of the anterior and posterior arcades and anastomose with the corresponding superior anterior and superior posterior arcade vessels (Fig 3e, 3f). The origin of the inferior pancreaticoduodenal artery was seen in 73 (84%) patients (Fig 3e). The anterior branch of the inferior pancreaticoduodenal artery could be traced along the anteroinferior margin of the pancreatic head, where it anastomosed with the anterior-superior branch (Fig 3e, 3f). Only short segments of the posterior branch usually were seen; they were identified in cross section along the posterior margin of the pancreatic head as they turned superiorly to parallel the intrapancreatic segment of the distal part of the common bile duct (Fig 3f).

The frequency of visualization of seven small pancreatic arteries in each of the 87 patients is as follows: only one vessel was identified in two (2%) patients, two vessels were identified in three (3%), three vessels were identified in 17 (20%), four vessels were identified in 21 (24%), five vessels were identified in 26 (30%), six vessels were identified in 11 (13%), and all seven vessels were identified in seven (8%).

DISCUSSION

These results show that small pancreatic arteries can often be identified on arterial phase helical CT scans (Table 1). Overall, three to six of the seven small arteries were seen in 75 (86%) of the 87 patients. These results differ from those of two previous reports (3,8), which indicated that depiction of these small vessels is infrequent on arterial phase helical CT scans. In the studies by Kaneko et al (3) and Sim et al (8), the dorsal pancreatic

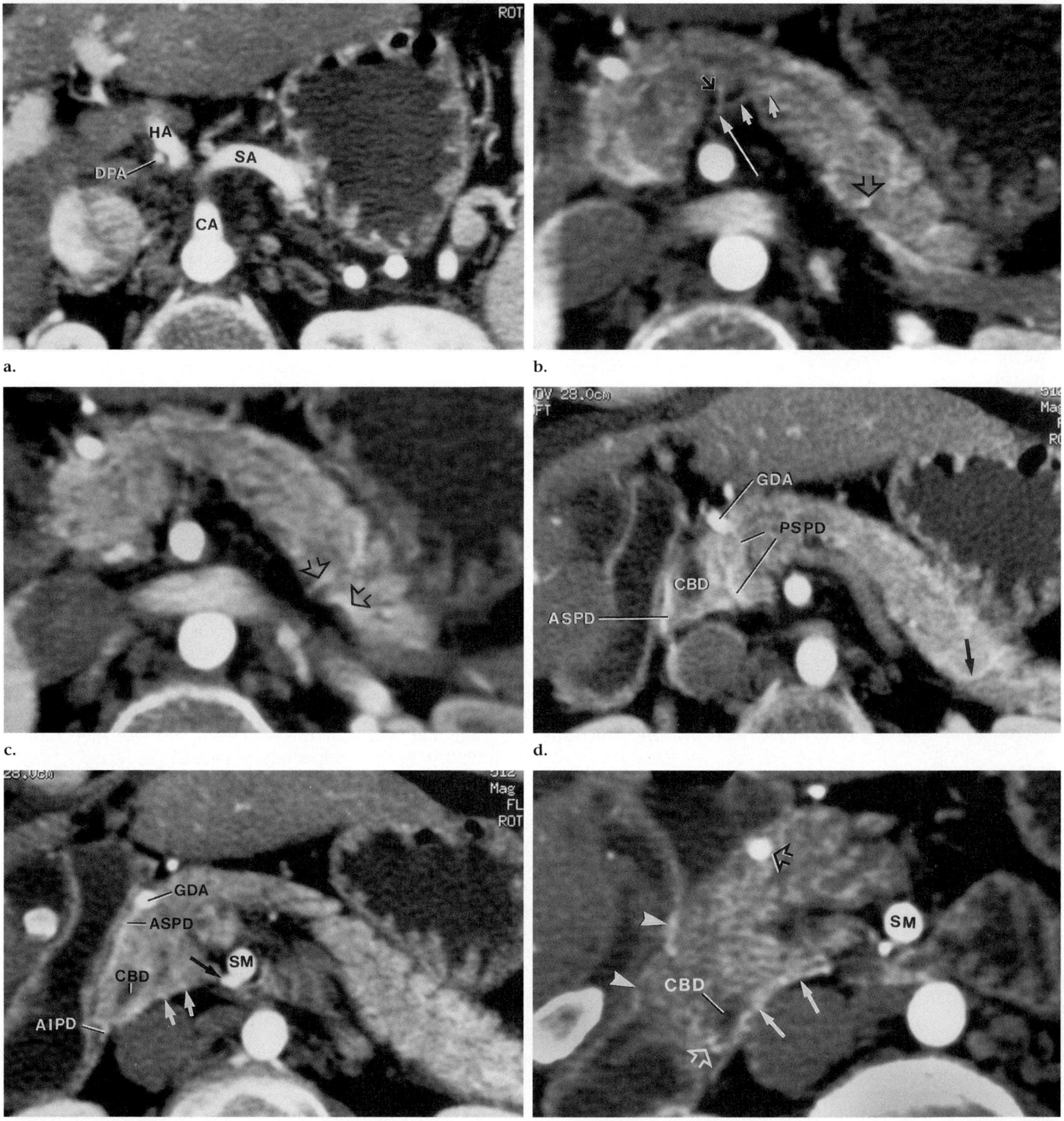

Figure 3. Arterial phase helical CT scans of the pancreatic arteries in a 30-year-old woman. **(a)** The dorsal pancreatic artery (*DPA*) is seen to arise from the hepatic artery (*HA*). *CA* = celiac artery, *SA* = splenic artery. **(b)** Scan obtained 21 mm below **a** shows the distal dorsal pancreatic artery (long white arrow) dividing into a small right branch (solid black arrow) and a left branch or transverse pancreatic artery (small white arrows). Open black arrow = pancreaticomagna artery. **(c)** Scan obtained 3 mm below **b** shows two branches of the pancreaticomagna artery (arrows) in the middle portion of the pancreatic tail. **(d)** Scan obtained 5 mm below **c** shows the posterior superior pancreaticoduodenal artery (*PSPD*) arising from the gastroduodenal artery (*GDA*) and coursing posteriorly within the pancreatic head. A segment of the anterior superior pancreaticoduodenal artery (*ASPD*) is seen, as is the caudal pancreatic artery (arrow) in the pancreatic tail. *CBD* = common bile duct. **(e)** Scan obtained 6 mm below **d** shows the anterior superior pancreaticoduodenal artery (*ASPD*) arising from the gastroduodenal artery (*GDA*), coursing along the anterolateral margin of the pancreatic head, and anastomosing inferiorly with the anterior inferior pancreaticoduodenal artery (*AIPD*). The inferior pancreaticoduodenal artery (black arrow) arises from superior mesenteric artery (*SM*), with posterior branches (white arrows) coursing along the posteroinferior margin of the pancreatic head. *CBD* = common bile duct. **(f)** Scan obtained 10 mm below **e** shows the anterior inferior pancreaticoduodenal artery (arrowheads) coursing along the inferior anterolateral margin of the pancreatic head. The posterior inferior pancreaticoduodenal artery (solid white arrows) is seen along the posteroinferior margin of the pancreatic head, with two small branches (open white arrow) ascending along the distal common bile duct (*CBD*). Open black arrow = gastroduodenal artery, *SM* = superior mesenteric artery.

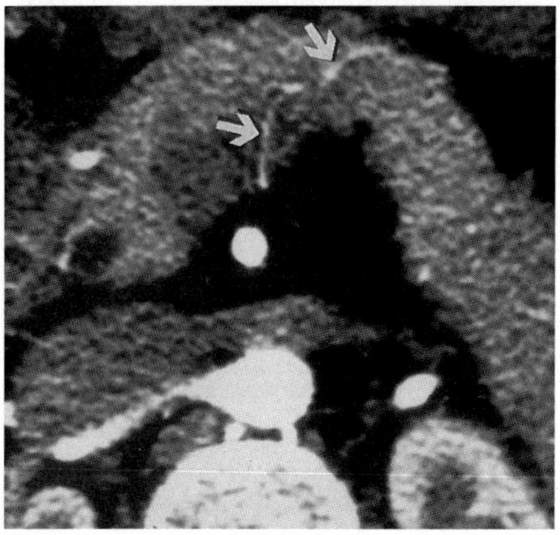

Figure 4. Arterial phase helical CT scan in a 52-year-old woman shows the intrapancreatic segment of the transverse pancreatic artery (arrows) coursing within the body of the pancreas.

TABLE 1
Visualization of Visceral and Pancreatic Arteries in 87 Patients

Artery	No. Visualized
Splenic	87 (100)
Superior mesenteric	87 (100)
Celiac	87 (100)
Hepatic	87 (100)
Gastroduodenal	87 (100)
Dorsal pancreatic	82 (94)
Transverse pancreatic	36 (41)
Right branch of dorsal pancreatic	8 (9)
Pancreaticomagna	45 (52)
Caudal pancreatic	34 (39)
Posterior arcade	63 (72)
Anterior arcade	47 (54)
Inferior pancreaticoduodenal	73 (84)

Note.—Numbers in parentheses are percentages.

TABLE 2
Origins of the Dorsal Pancreatic Artery

Origin	Present Study (*n* = 82)	Michels' Study (*n* = 200)*
Splenic artery	34 (41)	80 (40)
Hepatic artery	13 (16)	Not stated
Celiac artery	14 (17)	44 (22)
Superior mesenteric artery	21 (26)	28 (14)

Note.—Data are the number of arteries. Numbers in parentheses are percentages.
* Reference 14.

artery was seen in only 12% and 20% of cases, respectively; the transverse, caudal pancreatic, and pancreaticomagna arteries in no cases in either study; and the inferior pancreaticoduodenal artery in 4% and 20% of cases, respectively.

There are several technical differences between our study and those of Kaneko et al (3) and Sim et al (8) that potentially explain our improved results. These include differences in the reconstruction interval, the volume of intravenously administered contrast material, and the timing of the arterial phase helical acquisition.

In our study, arterial phase helical CT was performed by using 3-mm collimation and a 1-mm reconstruction interval. Kaneko et al (3) used 5-mm collimation with no retrospective reconstructions; Sim et al (8) used 3-mm collimation with a 3-mm reconstruction interval. Thin-section collimation and a 1-mm reconstruction interval are crucial for the visualization of small vessels (15). For example, the diameter of the dorsal pancreatic artery ranged from 1 to 4 mm (Figs 2, 3). We chose 1-mm reconstruction intervals on the basis of earlier work by Winter et al (9) and Brink et al (15).

A volume of 180 mL of contrast material was used in our study compared with a volume of 100 mL used by Kaneko et al (3) and Sim et al (8). In addition, the scanning delay used by Kaneko et al and Sim et al was 40 and 35 seconds, respectively, whereas the delay we used was calculated from the initial timing bolus (average scanning delay, 12 seconds). In both of the previous studies, the results indicated that small intrapancreatic vessels were difficult to visualize because they were obscured by pancreatic tissue. The larger volume of contrast material and the bolus timing of the arterial phase scanning sequence used in our study, as well as the 3-mm collimation and 1-mm reconstruction interval, likely combined to account for the improved conspicuity of small pancreatic vessels within the pancreatic parenchyma (Figs 3, 4).

A potential limitation of our study was that conventional catheter angiography was not performed as an anatomic reference standard. Because there was no clinical indication for catheter angiography in these patients, angiography was not considered to be justified. We believe, however, that the accuracy of vessel identification in our study was indirectly verified because our data essentially agreed with the anatomic data in Michels' (14) description of the origins and anatomic locations of the pancreatic vessels (Table 2).

Our results show that it is possible to delineate small pancreatic arteries on arterial phase helical CT scans by using the optimized techniques we have described. In the past, angiographic depictions of these small vessels were used extensively for the diagnosis and staging of pancreatic ductal adenocarcinoma. Tumor involvement of the major visceral vessels or of the origins of the small pancreatic arteries—particularly the gastroduodenal artery, the pancreatic arcades, the dorsal pancreatic artery, the caudal pancreatic artery, and the pancreaticomagna artery—was a reliable indicator of tumor extension beyond the margins of the gland and, hence, of surgical incurability (10–12,16). With the advent of CT, however, angiography essentially disappeared from the list of studies used for such diagnosis and staging (17). Thin-section helical CT has subsequently been shown to be superior to angiography for the depiction of vascular invasion from pancreatic carcinoma, and the CT analysis of small pancreatic veins has been shown (1–8,18) to improve the accuracy of staging of carcinoma of the head of the pancreas. We believe that the ability to assess the small pancreatic arteries may further improve the accuracy of helical CT in the staging of pancreatic carcinoma. This is the topic of current, ongoing research.

References

1. Choi BI, Chung MJ, Han JK, et al. Detection of pancreatic adenocarcinoma: relative value of arterial and late phases of spiral CT. Abdom Imaging 1997; 22:199–203.
2. Fuhrman GM, Charnsangavej C, Abbruzzese JL, et al. Thin-section contrast-enhanced computed tomography accurately predicts the resectability of malignant pancreatic neoplasms. Am J Surg 1994; 167: 104–113.
3. Kaneko K, Honda H, Hayashi T, et al. Helical CT evaluation of arterial invasion in pancreatic tumors: comparison with angiography. Abdom Imaging 1997; 22: 204–207.
4. Lu DSK, Reber HA, Krasny RM, et al. Local staging of pancreatic cancer: criteria for unresectability of major vessels as revealed by pancreatic-phase thin-section helical CT. AJR 1997; 168:1439–1443.
5. Mori H, Miyake H, Aikawa H, et al. Dilated posterior superior pancreaticoduodenal vein: recognition with CT and clinical significance in patients with pancreaticobiliary carcinomas. Radiology 1991; 181: 793–800.
6. Raptopoulos V, Steer ML, Sheiman RG, et al. The use of helical CT and CT angiography to predict vascular involvement from pancreatic cancer: correlation with findings at surgery. AJR 1997; 168:971–977.
7. Hommeyer SC, Freeny PC, Crabo LG. Carcinoma of the head of the pancreas: evaluation of the pancreaticoduodenal veins with dynamic CT—potential for improved accuracy in staging. Radiology 1995; 196:233–238.
8. Sim JS, Choi BI, Han JK, et al. Helical CT anatomy of the pancreatic arteries. Abdom Imaging 1996; 21:517–521.
9. Winter TC, Freeny PC, Nghiem HV, et al.

Hepatic arterial anatomy in transplantation candidates: evaluation with three-dimensional CT arteriography. Radiology 1995; 195:363–370.
10. Rösch J, Holman D. Superselective arteriography of the pancreas. In: Anacker H, ed. Efficiency and limits of radiologic examination of the pancreas. Acton, Mass: Publishing Sciences, 1975; 159–167.
11. Tylen U, Arnesjo B. Resectability and prognosis of carcinoma of the pancreas evaluated by angiography. Scand J Gastroenterol 1973; 8:691–697.
12. Freeny PC, Lawson TL. Radiology of the pancreas. New York, NY: Springer-Verlag, 1982.
13. Winter TC, Ager JA, Nghiem HV, et al. Upper gastrointestinal tract and abdomen: water as an orally administered contrast agent for CT. Radiology 1996; 201: 365–370.
14. Michels N. Blood supply and anatomy of the upper abdominal organs. Philadelphia, Pa: Lippincott, 1955.
15. Brink JA, Lim JT, Wang G, et al. Technical optimization of spiral CT for depiction of renal artery stenosis: in vitro analysis. Radiology 1995; 194:157–163.
16. Ariyama J. Radiology in disorders of the liver, biliary tract and pancreas. Tokyo, Japan: Igaku-Shoin, 1981.
17. Freeny PC, Marks WM, Ball TJ. Impact of high-resolution computed tomography of the pancreas on utilization of ERCP and angiography. Radiology 1982; 142:35–39.
18. Loyer EM, David CL, Dubrow RA, et al. Vascular involvement in pancreatic adenocarcinoma: reassessment by thin-section CT. Abdom Imaging 1996; 21:202–206.

Hyun-Jung Jang, MD
Byung Ihn Choi, MD
Tae Kyoung Kim, MD
Eun Joo Yun, MD
Kyoung Won Kim, MD
Joon Koo Han, MD
Man Chung Han, MD

Index terms:
Angioma, gastrointestinal tract, 761.3194
Computed tomography (CT), contrast enhancement, 761.12114
Computed tomography (CT), helical, 761.12115
Liver neoplasms, CT, 761.12114, 761.12115, 761.3194
Liver neoplasms, diagnosis, 761.3194

Radiology 1998; 208:543–548

Abbreviations:
FLASH = fast low-angle shot
HAP = hepatic arterial phase
PVP = portal venous phase

[1] From the Department of Radiology, Seoul National University College of Medicine, 28, Yongon-dong, Chongno-gu, Seoul 110-744, Korea. Received October 23, 1997; revision requested January 5, 1998; revision received February 17; accepted March 27. **Address reprint requests to** B.I.C.

Author contributions:
Guarantors of integrity of entire study, H.J.J., B.I.C.; study concepts, J.K.H.; study design, H.J.J., T.K.K.; definition of intellectual content, B.I.C.; literature research, H.J.J., E.J.Y.; clinical studies, J.K.H., B.I.C., T.K.K.; data acquisition, H.J.J., K.W.K., E.J.Y.; data analysis, B.I.C., J.K.H., T.K.K., E.J.Y.; manuscript preparation, H.J.J.; manuscript editing, H.J.J., T.K.K.; manuscript review, M.C.H., B.I.C.

Atypical Small Hemangiomas of the Liver: "Bright Dot" Sign at Two-Phase Spiral CT[1]

PURPOSE: To determine if a tiny enhancing dot is characteristic of small hemangiomas with low attenuation during the hepatic arterial phase (HAP) and portal venous phase (PVP) of two-phase spiral computed tomography (CT).

MATERIALS AND METHODS: Among 249 consecutive patients with 377 hemangiomas who underwent two-phase spiral CT (performed 30 and 65 seconds after the start of injection), 34 hemangiomas in 20 patients were less than 2 cm in diameter, had low attenuation during the HAP and PVP, and showed characteristic findings on dynamic contrast material–enhanced magnetic resonance (MR) images. The CT scans were retrospectively reviewed for tiny enhancing dots and correlated with the MR images.

RESULTS: Tiny enhancing dots were found in 26 of 34 hemangiomas (76%). The dots were seen during the HAP and PVP in 15 lesions (58%) and during the PVP alone in 11 lesions (42%). The lesions showed a tendency toward slow fill-in at MR imaging (only four lesions completely filled with contrast material within 5 minutes). The dots seen at CT corresponded to the initial enhancing area at MR imaging.

CONCLUSION: Small hemangiomas with persistent low attenuation at two-phase spiral CT can be diagnosed with the "bright dot" sign.

Hemangiomas are the most common benign tumors of the liver. The characteristic enhancement patterns of hepatic hemangiomas at conventional contrast material–enhanced computed tomography (CT) and dynamic incremental CT have been well documented (1–9). Two-phase spiral CT during maximal arterial enhancement (hepatic arterial phase [HAP]) and during maximal hepatic parenchymal enhancement (portal venous phase [PVP]) is now widely used, with many supporting reports of superior characterization (10,11) and superior detection of focal hepatic lesions, particularly small nodules (12). At our institution, two-phase spiral CT is routinely performed for evaluation of all focal hepatic lesions.

To our knowledge, there have been no reports that describe the appearances of hemangiomas at two-phase spiral CT during the HAP and PVP. In our earlier series (13), large hemangiomas (>2 cm in diameter), which show typical globular enhancement at dynamic incremental CT, seemed to show essentially the same feature at two-phase spiral CT; there is seldom doubt about the diagnosis of these tumors. Small hemangiomas (<2 cm in diameter) seem to be detected more frequently with two-phase spiral CT, whereas they are occasionally overlooked at conventional CT due to a tendency to be isoattenuating (2,14). Most small hemangiomas show a well-known characteristic finding—homogeneous high attenuation or peripheral globular enhancement—at two-phase spiral CT.

However, not infrequently, we encounter atypical small hemangiomas that show low attenuation during the HAP and PVP. Because this finding is considered nonspecific, the clinical situation rather than the imaging findings leads us to a tentative diagnosis among several possibilities (eg, metastases, nodules associated with chronic liver disease, inflammatory lesions, atypical hemangiomas). Recently, we have found a distinctive feature in atypical small hemangiomas: the "bright dot" sign. This feature has not been previously described, to our knowledge. To determine whether this sign is commonly applicable, we retrospectively studied all proved small hemangiomas that showed low attenuation at spiral CT performed with our current two-phase protocol.

MATERIALS AND METHODS

Selection of Cases

We obtained a list of all patients who underwent hepatic spiral CT performed with a two-phase (HAP and PVP) protocol at our institution between June 1994 and December 1996. After review of all radiologic reports and the clinical records in particular cases, 249 consecutive patients with 377 hemangiomas were included. The confirmatory diagnosis was made with dynamic contrast-enhanced magnetic resonance (MR) imaging (n = 80), surgery (n = 5), percutaneous biopsy (n = 2), or ultrasound (US) (n = 162). Criteria for US diagnosis were typical findings at initial US with no growth at follow-up US over 6 months or longer (range, 6–35 months; mean, 14 months).

Among these cases, 229 hemangiomas in 131 patients were less than 2 cm in diameter. Of these small lesions, 59 hemangiomas (26%) in 34 patients showed low attenuation during the HAP and PVP. Because the CT findings were considered atypical, we excluded 25 lesions diagnosed solely with follow-up US; they were excluded to avoid possible inclusion of other benign lesions with US appearances similar to that of hemangiomas and to correlate the CT findings with those of dynamic MR imaging.

The final inclusion criteria were (*a*) diameter less than 2 cm, (*b*) low attenuation during the HAP and PVP with no progressively enhancing areas or globular enhancing nodules, (*c*) characteristic MR imaging findings (high signal intensity relative to that of cerebrospinal fluid on T2-weighted images and globular enhancement that progressed centripetally on dynamic contrast-enhanced images), and (*d*) no change in size at follow-up US over 6 months. Ultimately, 20 patients (seven men and 13 women aged 25–67 years [mean, 49.7 years]) with 34 hemangiomas were included in the study. The mean diameter of the hemangiomas was 13.2 mm (range, 7–20 mm).

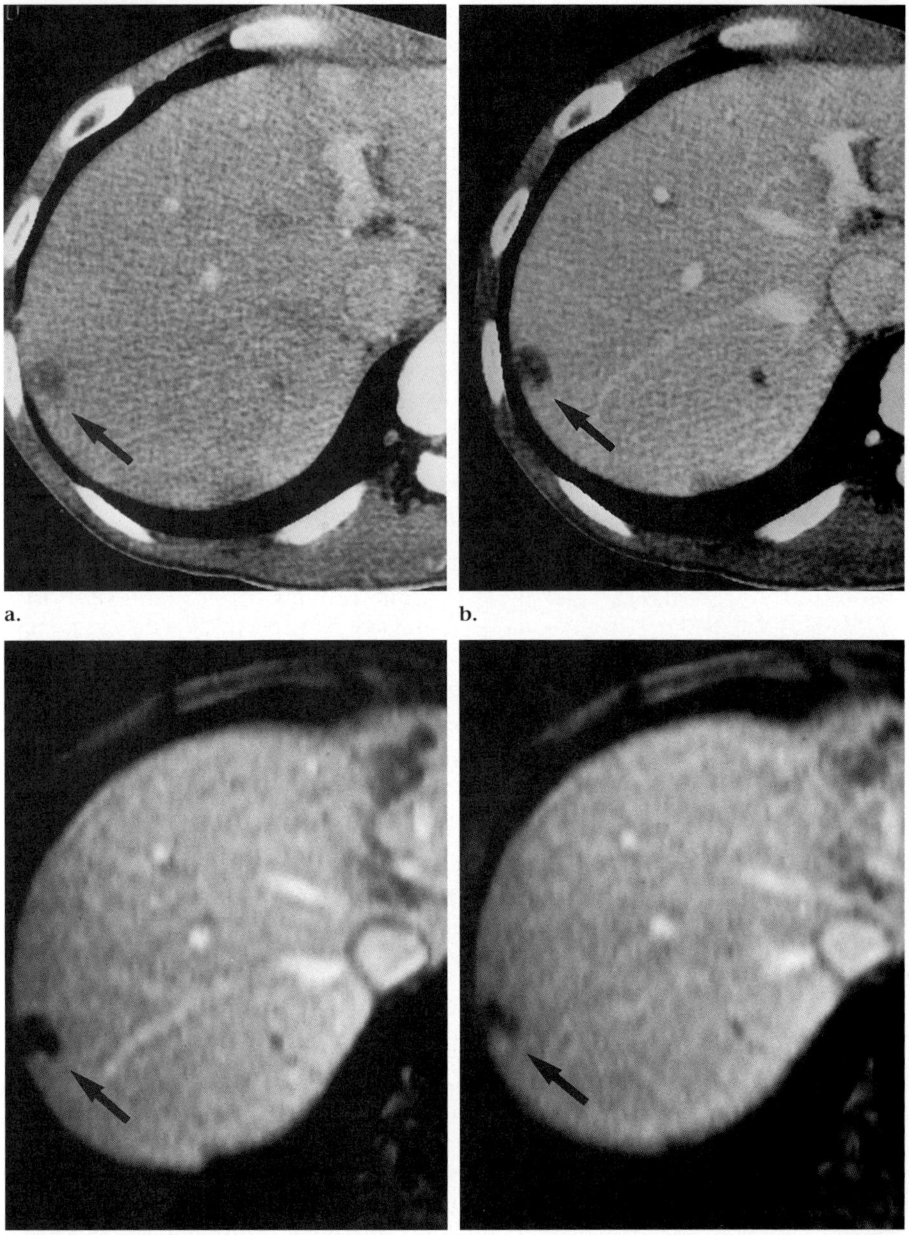

a. b. c. d.

Figure 1. Atypical small hemangioma with the bright dot sign during the HAP and PVP. **(a)** HAP and **(b)** PVP CT scans show a hypoattenuating mass (arrow) in the right hepatic lobe. A tiny enhancing dot is seen in the right posterior aspect of the tumor during both phases. Another tiny enhancing dot is suspected near the right lateral aspect of the lesion. Dynamic FLASH MR images (160/6.6) obtained **(c)** 1 minute and **(d)** 5 minutes after injection of contrast material show a hypointense mass (arrow) with an enhancing globule in the same location as the enhancing dots in **a** and **b**. The enhancing area is slightly enlarged in **d**; however, a large area of persistent hypointensity still remains.

Imaging Methods

CT was performed with a Somatom Plus S (Siemens, Erlangen, Germany) or HiSpeed Advantage (GE Medical Systems, Milwaukee, Wis) spiral scanner. Contrast material was injected into an antecubital vein with a power injector. In 21 lesions, 120 mL of Ultravist 300 (iopromide; Schering, Berlin, Germany) was injected at 3.0 mL/sec; in 13 lesions, 100 mL of Ultravist 370 (iopromide; Schering) was injected at 2.5 mL/sec. HAP imaging was begun 30 seconds after the start of injection, and PVP imaging was begun 65 seconds after the start of injection. A beam collimation of 10 mm and table speed of 10 mm/sec (pitch of 1:1) were used. Images were reconstructed at 7-mm intervals.

MR imaging was performed with a 1.0-T (Magnetom Expert; Siemens) or 1.5-T (Magnetom SP, Siemens, or Signa, GE Medical Systems) imager. All MR examinations included T2-weighted fast spin-echo imaging (repetition time msec/echo time msec = 3,000–5,000/90–117, echo train length of six to 15), as well as two-dimensional dynamic fast low-angle shot (FLASH) imaging (130–153/5–6, 70°

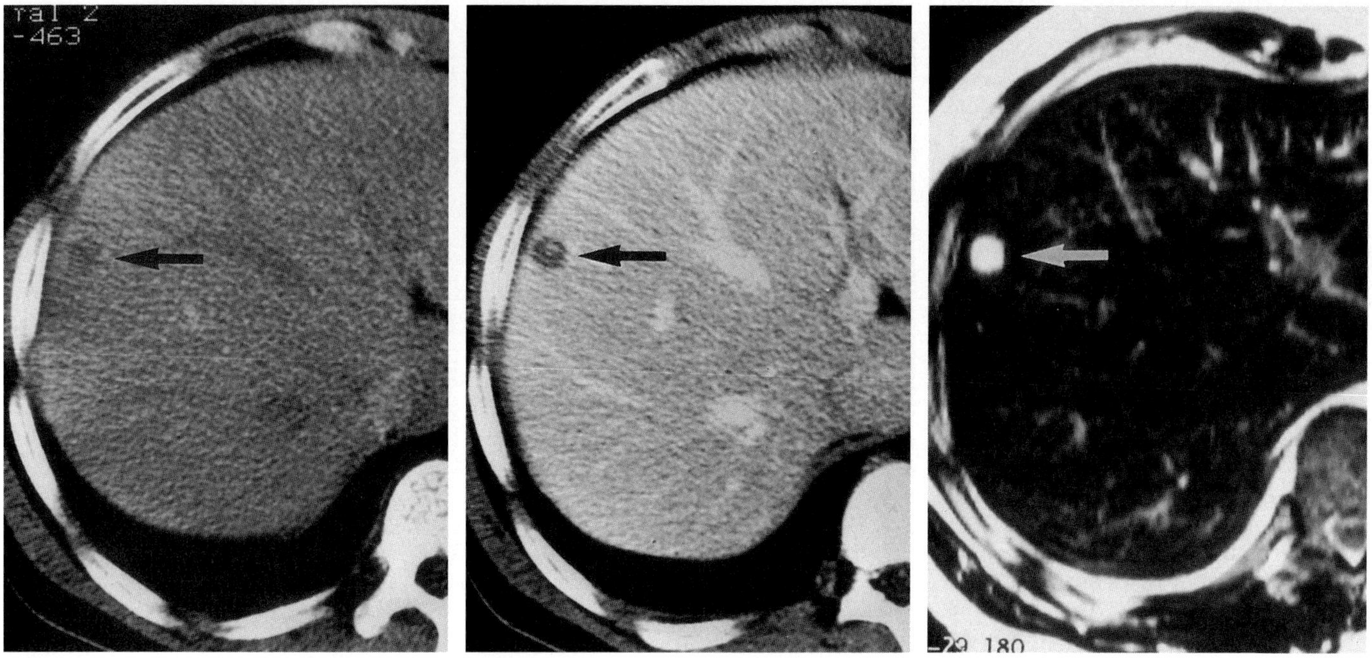

a. b. c.

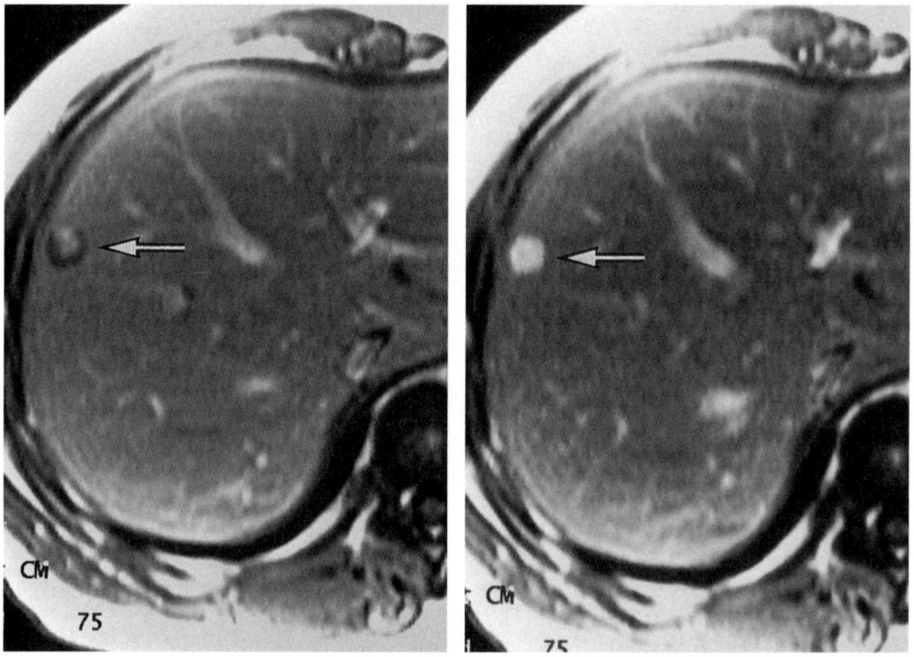

d. e.

Figure 2. Atypical small hemangioma with the bright dot sign during the PVP. **(a)** HAP CT scan shows a hypoattenuating mass (arrow) in the right lobe of the liver. **(b)** PVP CT scan shows a tiny enhancing dot in the anterior aspect of the mass (arrow). **(c)** T2-weighted fast spin-echo MR image (3,500/138) shows typical hyperintensity of the tumor (arrow). **(d)** Dynamic FLASH MR image (160/6.6) obtained 1 minute after injection of contrast material shows a hypointense mass (arrow) with globular enhancement in the same location as the enhancing dot in **b**. **(e)** Dynamic FLASH MR image (160/6.6) obtained 5 minutes after injection of contrast material shows uniform enhancement of the mass (arrow).

flip angle) performed before and immediately, 1 minute, 3 minutes, and 5 minutes after rapid bolus intravenous injection of 0.1 mmol/kg gadopentetate dimeglumine (Magnevist; Schering).

Image Analysis

The bright dot sign was defined as a tiny enhancing dot within hemangiomas that did not progress to the focus of globular enhancement described by Quinn and Benjamin (2). The possibility that the dot represented neighboring vascular structures was excluded by comparing the image with adjacent images. All CT images were retrospectively reviewed by four abdominal radiologists (B.I.C., T.K.K., E.J.Y., J.K.H.). Each evaluated the presence of such dots, the number and locations of any dots, and the brightness of the dots relative to the hepatic arteries during the HAP and relative to the portal veins during the PVP. Disagreement between the reviewers was resolved by means of consensus. Each HAP and PVP image was also compared with the gadolinium-enhanced dynamic MR images.

RESULTS

Although all 34 hemangiomas had been interpreted as hypoattenuating during the prospective reading, we found tiny enhancing dots in 26 hemangiomas (76%). This finding was seen during the HAP and PVP in 15 lesions (58%) (Fig 1) and during the PVP alone in 11 lesions (42%). Only one dot was seen in 17 lesions (65%) (Fig 2); two or more dots were seen in nine lesions (35%) (Fig 3). During the PVP, the attenuation of the dots was equal to that of the portal vein in 20 lesions (77%) and lower in six lesions (23%) at visual assessment. During the

HAP, the dots were as bright as the hepatic arteries in only seven lesions (47%) and less bright in eight lesions (53%). The dots were at the periphery of the lesion in 21 cases (81%) and in the center of the lesion in five cases (19%).

On dynamic contrast-enhanced MR images, all 34 lesions showed the globular centripetal enhancement characteristic of hemangiomas, although the CT findings in these lesions were considered atypical. The lesions all demonstrated a tendency toward slow fill-in for their small size; only four lesions (12%) completely filled with contrast material in 5 minutes. All of the dots in hemangiomas on CT scans corresponded to the initial enhancing area on MR images. Among the 26 hemangiomas with tiny enhancing dots at CT, the initial enhancing area on MR images appeared immediately after injection of contrast material in 17 lesions (65%), at 1 minute in six lesions (23%), and at 3 minutes in three lesions (12%). Among the eight hemangiomas without tiny enhancing dots (Fig 4), the initial enhancing area appeared immediately after injection of contrast material in two lesions (25%), at 1 minute in two lesions (25%), and at 3 minutes in four lesions (50%).

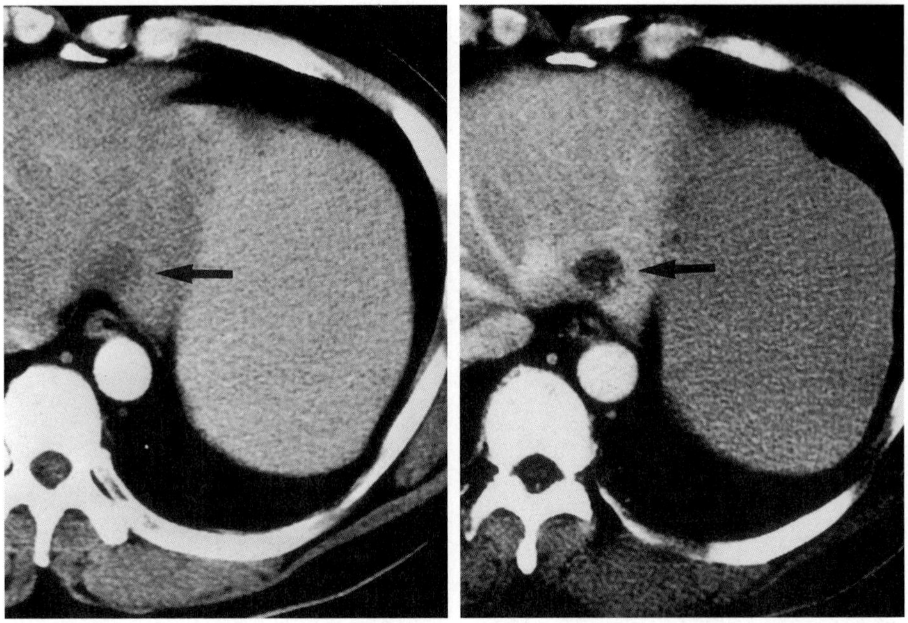

a. b.

Figure 3. Atypical small hemangioma with two bright dot signs. **(a)** HAP CT scan shows a hypoattenuating mass (arrow) in the left lobe of the liver. **(b)** PVP CT scan shows two tiny enhancing dots in the posterior aspect of the mass (arrow). MR images (not shown) demonstrated the typical features of hemangioma.

DISCUSSION

With the advent of spiral CT, more small hemangiomas can be detected and more atypical small hemangiomas are seen. A recent study (1) performed with two-phase dynamic incremental CT (30–71-second and 96–137-second delays) found a considerable proportion of atypical hemangiomas (11 of 51 [22%]), which changed from hyper- to isoattenuating (seven of 51 [14%]) or showed persistent low attenuation during both phases (four of 51 [8%]). On the basis of our previous report (13), we expect some differences from these initial results (1) with earlier scanning at each phase: (*a*) A larger proportion of hemangiomas will show persistent low attenuation during both phases, but this appearance will still be atypical, and (*b*) the hemangiomas that changed from hyper- to isoattenuating at dynamic incremental CT might be more likely to remain hyperattenuating during the PVP.

Because immediate and persistent homogeneous enhancement is the most frequent pattern in small hemangiomas, persistent hyperattenuation is fairly typical of these tumors, which usually contain small blood pools (1,14). In contrast, the differential diagnosis for a small nodule with persistent low attenuation can include various diseases. In the prospective reading of our images, the first-choice diagnosis was atypical hemangioma ($n = 16$), hypovascular hepatocellular carcinoma or dysplastic nodule ($n = 8$), focal fatty infiltration ($n = 2$), eosinophilic abscess ($n = 3$), and metastasis ($n = 5$).

In our experience, atypical small hemangiomas are not uncommon. In our series, 59 of 377 hemangiomas (16%) had persistent low attenuation and were less than 2 cm in diameter. (These 59 lesions, which included nodules that were sonographically confirmed, may have been more representative of the true prevalence. The prevalence of atypical hemangiomas among those confirmed with MR imaging is inexact because of a tendency to perform MR imaging in hemangiomas with more atypical appearances.) We focused on hemangiomas less than 2 cm in diameter because no larger lesions lacked recognizable typical enhancement in our series (13).

At two-phase spiral CT, a hypoattenuating small hemangioma seems to be the most common type to cause a diagnostic dilemma. It is therefore important to find a helpful diagnostic clue for such hemangiomas on the basis of two-phase spiral CT findings, thus reducing the rate of further invasive or expensive studies. In our study, all small hemangiomas that were atypical at two-phase spiral CT had a typical appearance at MR imaging and were confidently diagnosed without difficulty. Contrast enhancement appears to occur faster and be more conspicuous at dynamic MR imaging than at spiral CT: In our study, 23 of 26 hemangiomas with tiny enhancing dots at CT (88%) and four of eight without such dots (50%) showed a typical enhancing globule on MR images within 1 minute after contrast material injection (a delay similar to the PVP at CT). Possible reasons for the better demonstration of globular enhancement at MR imaging are (*a*) the inherently superior soft-tissue contrast and (*b*) the more compact retention of contrast material due to the relatively small amount injected with the bolus technique (15).

Although the MR images showed unequivocal appearances for confident diagnosis, the hemangiomas in this series had a tendency toward slow fill-in for their small size. In the large series of Semelka et al (14), most (89%) small hemangiomas (<1.5 cm in diameter) showed immediate uniform enhancement (43%) or peripheral nodular enhancement that progressed to uniform enhancement (46%), whereas peripheral nodular enhancement with persistent hypointensity (even at 10 minutes) occurred in only 11%. In contrast, 30 of 34 hemangiomas (88%) in our study showed the latter form of enhancement. Recently, Yamashita et al (16) correlated

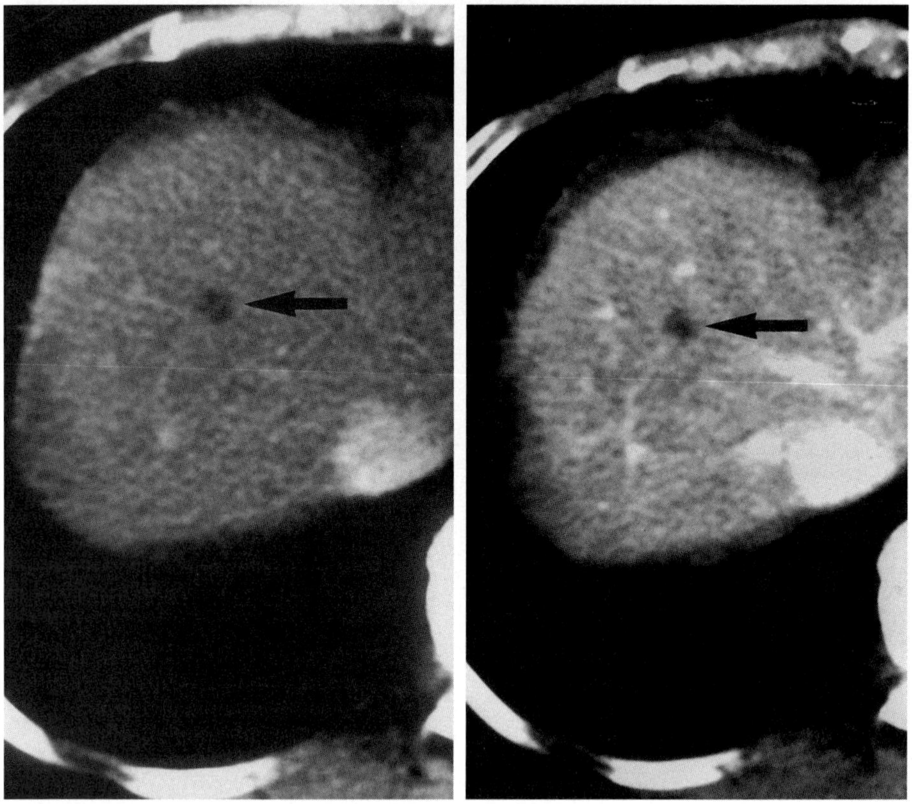

a. b.

Figure 4. Atypical small hemangioma without the bright dot sign. **(a)** HAP and **(b)** PVP CT scans show a hypoattenuating mass (arrow) in the dome of the liver. No enhancing area is discernible within the lesion. The typical features of hemangioma were seen on MR images (not shown).

the pathologic features of cavernous hemangiomas with the enhancement patterns at dynamic contrast-enhanced CT. They concluded that the various dynamic enhancement patterns correlated with the collective sizes of the constituent vascular spaces of the hemangiomas. Tumors with slow fill-in had relatively large vascular spaces, and tumors with rapid enhancement had small vascular spaces and a large interstitium. The results of another pathologic correlative study (17) suggest that there is no histologic difference in the sizes of the vascular spaces between hemangiomas less than 2 cm in diameter and larger hemangiomas. On the basis of these studies and the fairly frequent occurrence of atypical small hemangiomas at two-phase spiral CT, it makes more sense to regard persistently hypoattenuating small hemangiomas as tumors with large vascular spaces rather than as atypical.

Because the tiny enhancing dots at two-phase spiral CT corresponded well to the initial enhancing globule at dynamic MR imaging, the bright dot sign appears to represent substantially the same process that gives rise to an enhancing globule. The bright dot sign is thought to be a variant of globular enhancement that reflects the small size of the lesion and the earlier scanning in two-phase spiral CT, as well as the propensity for slow fill-in of this particular type of hemangioma.

In addition to the pattern of enhancement, the attenuation of enhancing globules is also reported to be characteristic of hemangioma (7,9,18). Because enhancing areas consist of vascular spaces directly supplied by arteries, the attenuation of such areas is theoretically identical to that of the aorta. Leslie et al (9) found that globular enhancement isointense to the aorta was 67% sensitive and 100% specific for hemangiomas. Conversely, Quinn and Benjamin (2) found that the qualitative attenuation of hemangioma nodules was similar to that of the adjacent hepatic and portal veins but lower than that of the aorta. In our study, the tiny enhancing dots were as bright as the portal vein during the PVP in 20 of 26 lesions (77%); during the HAP, however, the dots were less bright than the hepatic arteries in eight of 15 lesions (53%). A partial-volume-averaging effect due to the small size of the dots might have affected our results. However, most of the dots were relatively bright for their small size, a finding that is sufficient to indicate vascular spaces.

Our study had several limitations. First, the images were reviewed retrospectively; it is uncertain whether the sign would be recognized with the same frequency during a prospective reading. Second, the images were reviewed not independently but by four radiologists who worked together. Such analysis precludes assessment of interobserver variability, which could affect the results in evaluation of this subtle sign. Third, we used 10-mm collimation, which is relatively thick for evaluation of such small lesions. Partial volume averaging due to the imaging technique could have had an effect on the appearance of the lesions. Fourth, because the study did not include other lesions that may have low attenuation, it cannot be determined whether the sign is specific for hemangioma. Because the tiny enhancing dots are thought to be a form of the enhancing globules seen at correlative dynamic MR imaging, we suggest that the bright dot sign is as reliable as the globular enhancement seen in previous studies (2,7,9).

The bright dot sign is tiny and is difficult to recognize if one is unfamiliar with it. Therefore, despite the limitations of our study, we believe that knowledge of the bright dot sign could be helpful in diagnosing small hemangiomas with nonspecific hypoattenuation at two-phase spiral CT.

In summary, small hemangiomas with slow enhancement occasionally appear as low-attenuation nodules at two-phase spiral CT. Such hemangiomas are easily characterized with MR imaging. However, awareness of a tiny enhancing dot, which is likely to be overlooked, could lead to a correct diagnosis of atypical small hemangioma with two-phase spiral CT.

References

1. Hanafusa K, Ohashi I, Himeno Y, Suzuki S, Shibuya H. Hepatic hemangioma: findings with two-phase CT. Radiology 1995; 196:465–469.
2. Quinn SF, Benjamin GG. Hepatic cavernous hemangiomas: simple diagnostic sign with dynamic bolus CT. Radiology 1992; 182:545–548.
3. Freeny PC, Marks WM. Hepatic hemangioma: dynamic bolus CT. AJR 1986; 147: 711–719.
4. Itai Y, Furui S, Araki T, Yashiro N, Tasaka A. Computed tomography of cavernous hemangioma of the liver. Radiology 1980; 137:149–155.

5. Johnson CM, Sheedy PF, Stanson AW, Stephens DH, Hattery RR, Adson MA. Computed tomography and angiography of cavernous hemangiomas of the liver. Radiology 1981; 138:115–121.
6. Ashida C, Fishman EK, Zerhouni EA, Herlong FH, Siegelman SS. Computed tomography of hepatic hemangioma. J Comput Assist Tomogr 1987; 11:455–460.
7. Leslie DF, Johnson CD, MacCarty RL, Ward EM, Ilstrup DM, Harmsen WS. Single-pass CT of hepatic tumors: value of globular enhancement in distinguishing hemangiomas from hypervascular metastases. AJR 1995; 165:1403–1406.
8. Barnett PH, Zerhouni EA, White RI Jr, Siegelman SS. Computed tomography in the diagnosis of cavernous hemangioma of the liver. AJR 1980; 134:439–447.
9. Leslie DF, Johnson CD, Johnson CM, Ilstrup DM, Harmsen WS. Distinction between cavernous hemangiomas of the liver and hepatic metastases on CT: value of contrast enhancement patterns. AJR 1995; 164:625–629.
10. Choi BI, Han JK, Cho JM, et al. Characterization of focal hepatic tumors: value of two-phase scanning with spiral computed tomography. Cancer 1995; 76:2434–2442.
11. Kim TK, Choi BI, Han JK, Jang HJ, Cho SG, Han MC. Peripheral cholangiocarcinoma of the liver: two-phase spiral CT findings. Radiology 1997; 204:539–543.
12. Hollett MD, Jeffrey RB Jr, Nino-Murcia M, Jorgensen MJ, Harris DP. Dual-phase helical CT of the liver: value of arterial phase scans in the detection of small (<1.5 cm) malignant hepatic neoplasms. AJR 1995; 164:879–884.
13. Yun EJ, Jang HJ, Kim TK, Han JK, Choi BI. Hepatic hemangiomas: contrast enhancement patterns on two-phase spiral CT. J Korean Radiol Soc 1998; 38:93–98.
14. Semelka RC, Brown ED, Ascher SM, et al. Hepatic hemangiomas: a multi-institutional study of appearance on T2-weighted and serial gadolinium-enhanced gradient-echo MR images. Radiology 1994; 192: 401–406.
15. Yamashita Y, Mitsuzaki K, Yi T, et al. Small hepatocellular carcinoma in patients with chronic liver damage: prospective comparison of detection with dynamic MR imaging and helical CT of the whole liver. Radiology 1996; 200:79–84.
16. Yamashita Y, Ogata I, Urata J, Takahashi M. Cavernous hemangioma of the liver: pathologic correlation with dynamic CT findings. Radiology 1997; 203:121–125.
17. Tung GA, Vaccaro JP, Cronan JJ, Rogg JM. Cavernous hemangioma of the liver: pathologic correlation with high-field MR imaging. AJR 1994; 162:1113–1117.
18. Gaa J, Saini S, Ferrucci JT. Perfusion characteristics of hepatic cavernous hemangioma using intravenous CT angiography (IVCTA). Eur J Radiol 1991; 12:228–233.

Letters to the Editor

Intratumoral Blood Flow in Cavernous Hemangioma of the Liver: Radiologic-Pathologic Correlation.

From:
Jeong-Sik Yu, MD, Myeong-Jin Kim, MD, and Ki Whang Kim, MD

Department of Diagnostic Radiology, YongDong Severance Hospital, Yonsei University College of Medicine
146-92 Dokok-Dong, Kangnam-Ku, Seoul 135-270, South Korea

Editor:
In their article in the April 1997 issue of *Radiology,* Yamashita and colleagues (1) gave three classifications of hepatic hemangiomas that depended on the pattern of contrast material fill-in and the timing of enhancement during dynamic computed tomography (CT). They concluded that the dynamic enhancement patterns of cavernous hemangiomas are related to the collective size of their constituent vascular spaces. Furthermore, they assumed that small hemangiomas with slow fill-in have relatively large vascular spaces and that tumors with rapid enhancement have small vascular spaces and a large interstitium. We cannot agree with their conclusions, because they are different from our experience and findings of previous studies (2,3) and are not clear from their own data.

Among their cases, a majority of type 1 hemangiomas with typical globular fill-in were large enough (mean, 7.7 cm) for degenerative changes to manifest as a heterogeneous internal architecture, which is far from the classic appearance of hemangioma. The histologic findings and the timing of contrast material fill-in were not clearly stated for each case according to the size of each tumor. According to their description, the vascular space in the central area of a type 1 hemangioma was larger than the periphery of the tumor, even if the central area was intermingled with fibrotic scar tissue.

Actually, cavernous hemangioma is understood as a congenital hamartoma (4). The enlargement of hemangioma is known to originate from dilatation of intratumoral vascular channels rather than from true neoplastic growth. As a result of progressive dilation of cavernous spaces, the large hemangioma peripherally contains vascular channels that are partially compressed by surrounding liver parenchyma and that are narrower than those in the areas apart from the margin. Regardless of the size of individual vascular spaces, it is not strange to think that the cavernous hemangioma, as a large, spongelike, conglomerated vascular channel, would become enhanced gradually and centripetally. No or minimal enhancement of the central area may be also explained in terms of degenerative changes, including organizing thrombus, hemorrhage, or fibrotic scar, rather than in terms of wider vascular space.

In type 2 cavernous hemangiomas, diffuse enhancement throughout the tumor in the arterial dominant phase and at subsequent washout mimicked hypervascular neoplasm (1,2,5). The volume of type 2 hemangiomas was substantially smaller than that of type 1 hemangiomas in their cases, and the distance from the periphery to the center of the tumors was short. As a matter of course, there may be a high chance of fill-in to the central area within a short time in smaller tumors. Two hemangiomas classified as type 3 showed enhancement only in the periphery of the tumor; however, the sizes of their vascular spaces were considerably different from each other.

We experienced several small hemangiomas with rapid, diffuse enhancement in the arterial dominant phase that showed relatively wide vascular space with thin septa (Figure). A delayed or minimal contrast-enhanced area contained smaller vascular channels intermingled with abundant fibrotic interstitium in another small hemangioma. For these reasons, we believe that the net size of their vascular spaces is not enough to determine the pattern of contrast material fill-in in cavernous hemangiomas. Meanwhile, the total volume of the tumor, the degree of fibrosis of tumoral interstitium intermingled with the vascular channels, the arterial pressure and circulation time related to the individual cardiac output, and intratumoral degeneration must be taken into account in classifying on the basis of the enhancement pattern and speed of contrast material fill-in.

References

1. Yamashita Y, Ogata I, Urata J, Takahashi M. Cavernous hemangioma of the liver: pathologic correlation with dynamic CT findings. Radiology 1997; 203:121–125.
2. Takayasu K, Moriyama N, Shima Y, et al. Atypical radiographic findings in hepatic cavernous hemangioma: correlation with histologic features. AJR 1986; 146:1149–1153.
3. Chang JC, Han KS. Relation of internal echo patterns and hemodynamics by incremental dynamic CT in hepatic cavernous hemangioma. J Korean Radiol Soc 1993; 29:775–782. [Korean]
4. Kojimahara M. Ultrastructural study of hemangiomas. IV. Cavernous hemangioma of the liver. Acta Pathol Jpn 1986; 36:1477–1485.
5. Hanafusa K, Ohashi I, Himeno Y, Suzuki S, Shibuya H. Hepatic hemangioma: findings with two-phase CT. Radiology 1995; 196: 465–469.

Dr Yamashita responds:

We appreciated the comments made by Dr Yu and colleagues and their interest in our study (1). As everybody knows, cavernous hemangiomas show various radiologic features, but radiologic-pathologic correlation has been very rarely performed. Therefore, experiences among authors can be different.

In our cases, type 1 hemangiomas were large and symptomatic. Type 2 and type 3 tumors showed an atypical enhancement pattern. In that sense, there was a selection bias in our case materials. Although type 1 hemangiomas showed a typical enhancement pattern, the tumors were apparently larger than classical hemangiomas. At macroscopic and microscopic observation, the size of the vascular channel was statistically significantly larger than that of the periphery in those hemangiomas. It may be speculated that the fill-in of contrast material is more gradual in large vascular channels than it is in small vascular channels. This was evident in type 2 hemangiomas, which showed rapid fill-in.

As pointed out by Dr Yu, degenerative changes, including organizing thrombus, hemorrhage, and fibrotic scar, were almost always present in our cases. These degenerative changes

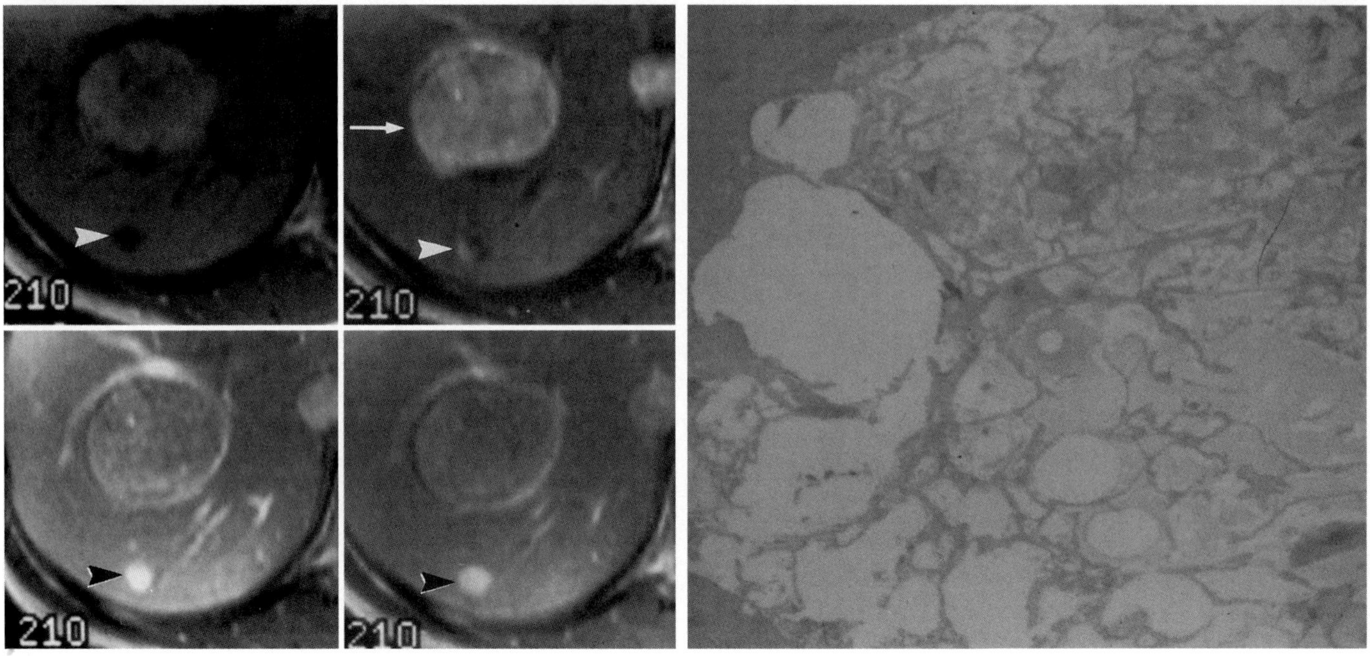

a. b.

Small cavernous hemangioma in the right lobe of the liver. **(a)** Dynamic fast multiplanar spoiled gradient-recalled-echo MR images (210/4.2 [repetition time msec/echo time msec]) obtained after the intravenous administration of contrast material show rapid fill-in of contrast material into the tumor (arrowheads). (Upper left image was obtained before contrast material administration, upper right image obtained 10 seconds after the start of contrast material injection, lower left image obtained at 45 seconds, lower right image obtained at 5 minutes.) Another larger tumor (arrow) above the hemangioma was an angiomyolipoma. **(b)** Photomicrograph shows relatively wide vascular channels with thin septa. (Hematoxylin-eosin stain; original magnification, ×20.)

usually do not show enhancement on the delayed CT image. Connective tissue was thicker in type 2 hemangiomas than in type 1 hemangiomas. As expected, more extensive sclerosis may result in minimal enhancement.

Dr Yu and colleagues discuss the size of the tumor. First, we emphasize that we obtained CT images in the good arterial phase. As pointed out, in tumors smaller than 2 cm, we often experience complete fill-in in the arterial phase. This can be due to either rapid fill-in, lower temporal resolution of the scan, or both. In their Figure, wide vascular space is seen even in a small hemangioma. In the early phase image (obtained at 10 seconds after contrast material injection), only peripheral enhancement is observed. If images are obtained at only 45 seconds, tumors may appear hypervascular. As can be seen in this case as well as in our experience, there is no question that scanning timing is an important factor for the radiologic appearance of hemangiomas. It should be noted, however, that some sclerosing hemangiomas show very rapid fill-in, which usually makes it difficult to distinguish them from hypervascular malignant tumors, our type 2 hemangiomas.

In conclusion, we agree that the net vascular size is not the only factor in the imaging pattern. The imaging technique and size of the tumor and arterial pressure may contribute. However, as we stated in the article, vascular size and degenerative changes are the most important factors for the speed of fill-in. The rapid imaging technique will further clarify the hemodynamics of hemangiomas.

Reference

1. Yamashita Y, Ogata I, Urata J, Takahashi M. Cavernous hemangioma of the liver: pathologic correlation with dynamic CT findings. Radiology 1997; 203:121–125.

Yasuyuki Yamashita, MD
Department of Radiology, Kumamoto University School of Medicine 1-1-1 Honjo, Kumamoto, 860 Japan

Three-dimensional MR Imaging of Neurovascular Compression in Trigeminal Neuralgia

From:

Karsten Papke, MD,* Georg Bongartz, MD,† Harald Masur, MD,‡ and Gerhard Schuierer, MD*
Institute for Clinical Radiology, University of Münster
Albert-Schweitzer-Strasse 33, D-48129 Münster, Germany*

Department of Medical Radiology, Kantonsspital Basel, University Clinics
Petersgraben 4 CH-4301 Basel, Switzerland†

Edith Stein Clinic for Neurology and Orthopedics
Am Wonneberg, D-76887 Bad Bergzabern, Germany‡

Editor:

We read with interest the article by Majoie and colleagues (1) in the August 1997 issue of *Radiology*. The authors compared the feasibility of two different magnetic resonance (MR) imaging techniques to demonstrate neurovascular contact in trigeminal neuralgia. They concluded that both fast imaging with steady-state precession (FISP) and magnetization-prepared rapid gradient-echo (MP-RAGE) MR imaging are useful in the detection of vascular contact at the nerve root entry zone.

In our own study (2) on this subject in 18 patients with typical unilateral trigeminal neuralgia, we used one of the techniques (three-dimensional FISP, 64 partitions, single-section thickness of 0.8 mm, in-plane resolution of 0.78×0.78 mm) used by Majoie and colleagues. We agree with Majoie and colleagues that this technique is suited to clearly depicting the relevant neural and vascular structures involved in the pathogenesis of trigeminal neuralgia.

It is a merit of the study by Majoie and colleagues that a large number of healthy control subjects were included, whereas in our study (2), the asymptomatic nerves of the patients served as the control nerves, with a potentially higher prevalence of asymptomatic neurovascular contact.

However, even in the study by Majoie and colleagues, neurovascular contact was seen in 7% of asymptomatic nerves; in the other studies cited by the authors, the prevalence of asymptomatic neurovascular contact was 8%–32%.

In our own study (2), a simple contact was observed in the asymptomatic sides of 10 of the 18 patients. Correlating clinical and radiologic findings, we therefore considered it important to take into account the intensity of the neurovascular contact and to make a distinction between simple neurovascular contact on the one hand and a dislocation or compression of the nerve at its root entry zone on the other hand. In our study, a dislocation or compression of the nerve was always associated with symptoms of trigeminal neuralgia and was observed in seven of 16 judgable nerves. We concluded that a simple neurovascular contact is not always sufficient to explain trigeminal neuralgia, with possible implications for the potential benefit of neurovascular decompression.

This view is supported by the clinical, intraoperative, and autopsy findings of a study by Hamlyn and King (3), which was based on the autopsy findings in 30 patients without a history of trigeminal neuralgia. They reported that the percentage of nerves with vessels adjacent or in simple contact increased from 16% to 40% after perfusion of the vessels with physiologic pressure (arteries, 50–100 mm Hg initially, followed by 200 mm Hg for 5 minutes; veins, 0–15 mm Hg initially, followed by 40 mm Hg for 5 minutes). A distortion or compression of the nerve, however, was never observed in the normal cadaveric material. In contrast, a vessel was intraoperatively found to distort and create a groove in the nerve in 37 of 41 patients who had undergone neurovascular decompression because of trigeminal neuralgia.

We therefore ask whether Majoie and colleagues have made similar observations when taking into account the intensity of the neurovascular contact (ie, simple contact vs dislocation or compression of the nerve). Comparing the intensities of the neurovascular contacts would be of particular interest in the six patients who underwent successful surgery and in the healthy control subjects.

For a better understanding of the pathologic meaning of neurovascular contact and the prognostic importance of MR tomographic findings, prospective studies will be necessary in which the MR tomographically defined intensity of neurovascular contact is compared with the intraoperative findings and the postoperative outcome.

References

1. Majoie CBLM, Hulsmans FJH, Verbeeten B, et al. Trigeminal neuralgia: comparison of two MR imaging techniques in the demonstration of neurovascular contact. Radiology 1997; 204:455–460.
2. Masur H, Papke K, Bongartz G, Vollbrecht K. The significance of three-dimensional MR-defined neurovascular compression for the pathogenesis of trigeminal neuralgia. J Neurol 1995; 242:93–98.
3. Hamlyn PI, King IT. Neurovascular compression in trigeminal neuralgia: a clinical and anatomical study. J Neurosurg 1992; 76:948–954.

Dr Majoie and colleagues respond:

We thank Dr Papke and colleagues for their interest in our article in the August 1997 issue of *Radiology* (1). We agree with Papke et al that three-dimensional FISP imaging (with an effective section thickness of 0.8–1 mm) is a good technique for depicting neurovascular contacts at the root entry zone of trigeminal nerves in patients with trigeminal neuralgia (1,2). We found neurovascular contacts in 77% of symptomatic and in 7% of asymptomatic control nerves ($P < .001$; χ^2 test) (1).

These results correspond to results of previous studies in which the same techniques were used. Meaney et al (3,4) found neurovascular contacts in 8%–9% of asymptomatic and in 70%–76% of symptomatic trigeminal nerves with three-dimensional FISP. The 32% of neurovascular contacts in asymptomatic nerves was found by authors (5) of an earlier study who used another technique, namely, coronal T1-weighted spin-echo imaging with a 3-mm section thickness. This relatively high percentage might be due to partial volume averaging caused by the small vessel size in relation to the section thickness (3). Microvascular decompression is recommended as the procedure of choice for the treatment of trigeminal neuralgia in patients who have undergone unsuccessful medical therapy (6). Without preoperative imaging, no cause of symptoms can be found at surgery in 10%–30% of patients. MR imaging can be used to determine which patients may benefit from microvascular decompression, that is, select those patients with trigeminal neuralgia that demonstrate neurovascular contacts at the root entry zone of the symptomatic trigeminal nerves.

Papke and colleagues (2) advocate evaluation of the intensity of the neurovascular contact. Whether the MR finding of deformity of the root entry zone will contribute in the selection of those patients who will ultimately benefit the most from this operation is a matter of debate. In our experience, and those experiences of previous authors (4,7), we think that the deformity of the nerve is not the criterion to use to select patients for microvascular decompression but that the finding of vessel contacts at the root entry zone of ipsilateral symptomatic nerves is sufficient. Previous study findings have shown that patients with trigeminal neuralgia that showed neurovascular contacts at the root entry zone of ipsilateral symptomatic nerves without grooving or deformity were symptom-free postoperatively (3,4,7).

We agree with Meaney et al (4) that, at present, given the absence of definitive criteria for determining the intensity of neurovascular contact, the finding of neurovascular contact in a patient with trigeminal neuralgia must be assumed to be clinically important even in the absence of nerve distortion or grooving. When definite criteria of the intensity of neurovascular compression and dislocation can be established, prospective studies comparing contact intensities as depicted at MR imaging with surgical outcome will be interesting.

References

1. Majoie CBLM, Hulsmans FJH, Verbeeten B, et al. Trigeminal neuralgia: comparison of two MR imaging techniques in the demonstration of neurovascular contact. Radiology 1997; 204:455–460.
2. Masur H, Papke K, Bongartz G, Vollbrecht K. The significance of three-dimensional MR-defined neurovascular compression for the pathogenesis of trigeminal neuralgia. J Neurol 1995; 242: 93–98.
3. Meaney JFM, Miles JB, Nixon TE, Whitehouse GH, Ballantyne ES, Eldridge PR. Vascular contact with the fifth cranial nerve at the pons in patients with trigeminal neuralgia: detection with 3D FISP imaging. AJR 1994; 163:1447–1452.
4. Meaney JFM, Eldridge PR, Dunn LT, Nixon TE, Whitehouse GH, Miles JB. Demonstration of neurovascular compression in trigeminal neuralgia with magnetic resonance imaging. J Neurosurg 1995; 83:799–805.
5. Tash RR, Sze G, Leslie DR. Trigeminal neuralgia: MR imaging features. Radiology 1989; 172:767–770.
6. Barker FG, Janetta PJ, Bissonette DJ, Larkins MV, Jho HD. The long-term outcome of microvascular decompression for trigeminal neuralgia. N Engl J Med 1996; 334:1077–1083.
7. Nagaseki Y, Horikoshi T, Omata T, et al. Oblique sagittal magnetic resonance imaging visualizing vascular compression of the trigeminal or facial nerve. J Neurosurg 1992; 77:379–386.

Charles B. L. M. Majoie, MD,* Frans-Jan H. Hulsmans, MD, PhD,* Jonas A. Castelijns, MD, PhD,† and Jacob Valk, MD, PhD†
Department of Radiology, Academic Medical Center
Meibergdreef 9, 1105 AZ, Amsterdam, The Netherlands*

Department of Radiology, Free University Hospital
P.O. Box 7057, 1007 MB, Amsterdam, The Netherlands†

Reducing Artifacts in MR Imaging of the Shoulder

From:
H. Peter Higer, MD
MR-Zentrum am Krankenhaus Nordwest
Haingrabenstr 72, D-60488 Frankfurt, Germany

Editor:
An article by Dr McGee et al (1) in the November 1997 issue of *Radiology* deals with motion artifacts during magnetic resonance (MR) imaging examination of the shoulder. Doubtless, this is a problem that needs to be solved, and we should use what we can to prevent motion artifacts and improve image quality. This method might be one way. I was, however, alarmed by the statement that "observable motion corruption was present in the majority of the 143 MR examinations in the shoulder. . . ." A look at Materials and Methods left a remarkable blank for the coil applied; however, the design of the coil and the immobilization of the patient and the coil during the examination are the most important cornerstones of the MR examination of the shoulder. In my experience, image quality improved remarkably when we changed from a wrap-around coil to a coil that is fixed on the table by the patient's weight and is designed like a cap, tightly fitted to the shoulder. I have observed quality-diminishing motion artifacts only in a small minority of MR examinations of the shoulder. Proper positioning and immobilization should be the first step; the application of artifact-reducing algorithms should be the second step.

Reference

1. McGee KP, Grimm RC, Felmlee JP, Rydberg JR, Riederer SJ, Ehman RL. The shoulder: adaptive motion correction of MR images. Radiology 1997; 205:541–545.

Dr McGee and colleagues respond:

Thank you for giving us an opportunity to respond to the letter submitted by Dr Higer with regard to our article (1).

We thank Dr Higer for his comments. In our study of motion effects in shoulder MR imaging, we used a dedicated shoulder coil that is the standard model supplied by the manufacturer of our 1.5-T imagers (GE Medical Systems, Milwaukee, Wis). Although we have not evaluated the shoulder MR imaging coil described in his letter, it seems plausible that a stability-enhancing design might reduce motion artifacts to some extent. Unfortunately, immobilization does not prevent transmitted respiratory motion, and it is simply not feasible to eliminate all voluntary motion in this region by means of fixation pressure alone.

Our experience indicates that subjective judgments about the prevalence of motion artifacts in clinical examinations can be unreliable. In our study, we addressed this issue by using a panel of four independent observers to assess motion artifacts and by quantitatively measuring motion amplitude with navigator echoes in a series of 143 consecutive shoulder examinations (1). It is difficult without conducting a comparable trial to assess the observation by Dr Higer that substantial motion artifact is present "only in a small minority of MR examinations."

Reference

1. McGee KP, Grimm RC, Felmlee JP, Rydberg JR, Riederer SJ, Ehman RL. The shoulder: adaptive motion correction of MR images. Radiology 1997; 205:541–545.

Kiaran P. McGee, MS, Roger C. Grimm, MS, Joel P. Felmlee, PhD, John R. Rydberg, MD, PhD, Stephen J. Riederer, PhD, Richard L. Ehman, MD.
Department of Diagnostic Radiology, Mayo Clinic
200 First Street SW, Rochester, MN 55905

Mammographic Artifact due to Film

From:
Laurie Margolies, MD
Connecticut Radiology Associates
300 Seymour Drive, Derby, CT 06418

Editor:
I avidly read the article by Hedrick et al (1) in the March 1998 issue of *Radiology*. They describe an artifact that I noticed after

one of our mammography sites had switched to MIN-R 2000 film (Kodak, Rochester, NY). Until reading this article, I was unable to obtain any guidance with regard to this artifact.

I hope that this article will prompt the film manufacturer to rectify the problem or at least to inform users that there is a problem that can be fixed by paying attention to which side of the film is placed down in the processor.

Reference

1. Hedrick WR, Poulton TB, Starchman DE, Tobias TE. Unusual artifact with mammography film. Radiology 1998; 206:835–837.

Beware the Pseudo Guinea Worm!

From:

Shella Farooki, MD, Leanne L. Seeger, MD, Richard H. Gold, MD

Department of Radiological Sciences, University of California at Los Angeles School of Medicine

200 UCLA Medical Plaza, Suite 165-59, Los Angeles, CA 90095-6952.

Editor:

A 65-year-old woman was referred for a radiographic examination because of a 1-year history of left hip and knee pain. Radiographs revealed extensive calcification-like, punctate opacities projected over the soft tissues of the left buttock and thigh (Fig 1). The opacities were distributed linearly, an appearance characteristic of the calcified guinea worm, *Dracunculus medinensis* (Fig 2). Because the patient had a history of extensive travel in Egypt, a diagnosis of dracunculiasis was considered.

Several weeks later, a radiograph of the abdomen of a 2-month-old male infant revealed similar opacities projected over the abdomen, as well as beyond the lateral abdominal wall. By questioning the technologist, we learned that iodinated contrast material (Hypaque-76 [diatrizoate meglumine and diatrizoate sodium injection], Nycomed, Princeton, NJ) had been spilled on the mat covering the radiographic table. A radiograph of the mat (Fig 3) revealed linear opacities identical to those in the radiographs obtained in both patients. Although attempts had been made to clean the mat, residual contrast material remained within clefts of the plastic surface.

Dracunculiasis, or guinea worm disease, is a potentially disabling infection caused by *D medinensis*. It is endemic to the Nile Valley, central and western Africa, India, Pakistan, Iran, and other parts of the Arabian peninsula. Infection occurs with the ingestion of water contaminated with larvae, which eventually migrate to the subcutaneous tissues. There, the female larvae become mature worms, mate, and expel their larvae through the skin. If a female worm dies before reaching the skin surface, it may calcify within the subcutaneous tissues. Calcification is the usual fate of the male worm

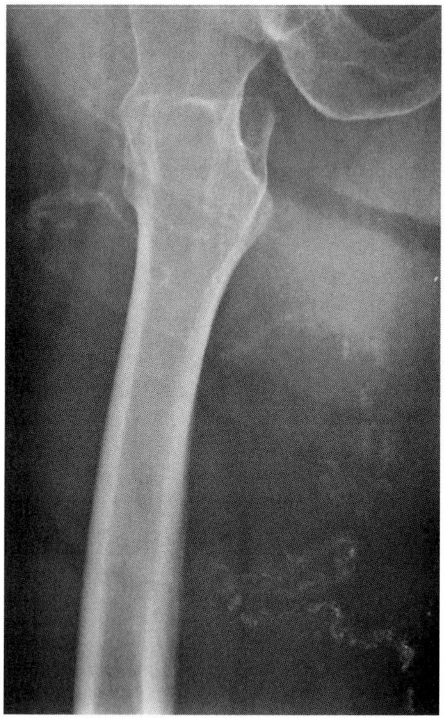

Figure 1. Lateral radiograph obtained in a 65-year-old woman shows extensive linear opacities projected over the soft tissues of the thigh.

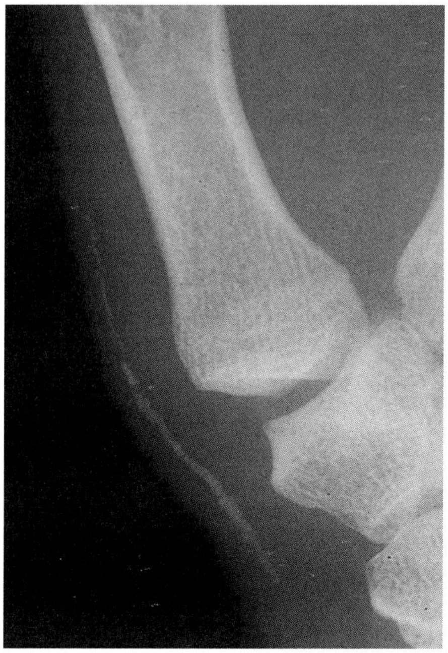

Figure 2. Collimated posteroanterior radiograph of the hand of a patient with documented dracunculiasis.

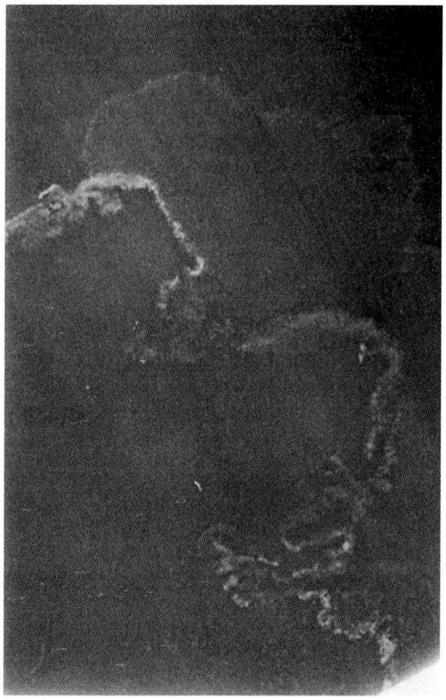

Figure 3. Radiograph of the mat covering the radiographic table demonstrates linear opacities that can be exactly superimposed on those in Figure 1.

(1,2). The radiologic finding of a calcified guinea worm is common in endemic areas, and there have been anecdotal reports of calcified guinea worms in radiographs obtained in patients in the eastern United States (2). It has been reported that 89% of patients who were found to have calcified guinea worms were asymptomatic (2).

Artifacts are commonly encountered in radiographic images, and their recognition is an essential part of radiologic diagnosis. Under most circumstances, their cause is readily apparent, and their unimportance is understood. As in our case, however, an artifact may closely simulate human disease and lead to an incorrect diagnosis. When rare or unusual soft-tissue "calcifications" are encountered, it is prudent to consider the possibility of contamination with radiopaque material on or in mats, positioning devices, or the equipment itself.

References

1. Markell EK, Voge M, John DT. Medical parasitology. 7th ed. Philadelphia, Pa: Saunders, 1992; 324–327.
2. Muller R. *Dracunculus* and dracunculiasis. In: Dawes B, ed. Advances in parasitology. New York, NY: Academic Press, 1971; 73–140.

Cost of PACS and Computed Radiography in the United States

From:
André J. Duerinckx, MD, PhD,* Edward G. Grant, MD†
Radiology Service, Mail Route W114, Magnetic Resonance Imaging Clinic, Building 507,
West Los Angeles Veterans Affairs Medical Center
11301 Wilshire Boulevard, Los Angeles, CA 90073*

Department of Radiology, University of California Los Angeles Medical Center, CA 90095†

Editor:
I read with interest, but great concern, the article by Pratt et al in the January 1998 issue of *Radiology* (1). I believe that the authors' conclusion that full picture archiving and communication system (PACS) and computed radiographic (CR) implementation would not provide cost savings for a large subspecialized department can be misleading to our radiology community. Both our group (Duerinckx et al [2]) and Pratt et al (3) presented a cost analysis of a full PACS-CR implementation during the 1997 Society of Photo-Optical Instrumentation Engineers–, or SPIE-, sponsored International Symposium on Medical Imaging in February 1997 in Newport Beach, Calif. We performed a cost analysis for a PACS-CR system with a teleradiology network connecting four major veterans affairs medical centers and several large clinics in a Veterans Integrated Service Network in Southern California. Our Veterans Integrated Service Network–wide cost analysis included an evaluation of incremental costs of department-wide implementation of a PACS and CR system in individual hospitals. Specifically, we performed a detailed cost analysis for the West Los Angeles Veterans Affairs Medical center, a tertiary Veterans Affairs referral center, with 500 medical-surgical beds and an additional 700 nursing home and psychiatric beds. About 120,000 radiologic studies are performed per year at our center. Pratt et al never stated the number of beds and procedures performed per year.

Our cost model was very similar to the one presented by Pratt et al in the January 1998 issue of Radiology. We also determined all capital and operational costs associated with PACS-CR implementation. The economic effects were identified, adjusted for time value, and used to calculate the net present value of a PACS-CR system for the whole department. The yearly net present value, which starts out as a negative value, indicates how much the PACS-CR system has cost the radiology department up to that year. It is hoped that after a number of years of semifilmless operation, the net present value of a PACS-CR system becomes $0 and then later becomes positive, indicating a net profit. Because we made different assumptions about the gradual implementation of our PACS-CR system and its base cost, our conclusions are different (4).

First, the total cost base of our PACS was only U.S. $2.8 million, unlike the $9.2 million assumed by Pratt et al. This is one of several substantial differences in the two models. It is important for the readers of *Radiology* to realize that one does not have to spend close to $10 million to have a workable PACS-CR system. The cost of individual CR units and digital chest units has substantially decreased to the point where $2.8 million will be adequate to cover most moderately sized hospitals.

Second, we assumed that we would achieve an 80% reduction in the use of film for chest radiography, bone imaging, and fluoroscopy within 4 years, as opposed to the 90% reduction within 8 years in the model by Pratt et al. We could take this difference one step further and for a moment assume that an 80% film-use reduction could be achieved within 1 year, which, although unrealistic, will help clarify our point. The change in net present value for both scenarios, a 4-year versus a 1-year transition to 80% filmless operation, is shown in the Figure. Our model assumes that half the radiographic studies are performed with CR units and half with direct digital chest units. The graphs are for a $2.8 million base cost, with 5-year amortization (with a 5% yearly discount rate but without interest payments, as it is a federal government facility).

If there is an 80% reduction in film use within the 1st year, then the net present value decreases during the first 5 years down to −$1.75 million before it starts to increase. This is because the yearly amortization cost ($756,000) is greater than the yearly projected savings ($529,560). After 5 years, the equipment has been paid for and the net present value increases to reach $0 after 3 years before it becomes positive (curve for 1 year in the Figure). This differs from the case in which the 80% film-use reduction is gradually achieved over 4 years (curve for 4 years in the Figure). When a PACS-CR system is in place and less than 80% film-use reduction is achieved, the net present value decreases much more during the first 5 years, down to −$2.49 million, before it starts to increase. It then takes the net present value slightly more than 4 years to become $0 (curve for 4 years in the Figure).

Although one could conservatively interpret this as meaning that it took 7–9 years for the PACS-CR system purchase to pay for itself, there is another way of looking at these data. If

80% filmless operation is achieved within 1 year, then the actual cost to the hospital of the purchase of the PACS-CR equipment never exceeds $1.75 million with a cost base of $2.8 million. After 8 years, the net present value is only −$170,000, a very small price tag (less than 10% of the base cost) for a $2.8 million PACS-CR system. Even if it takes 4 years to become 80% filmless, the net present value after 8 years is only −$900,000 (and $0 after 9 years), again a small fraction of the total base cost. Either way, this represents a substantial discount on the purchase of PACS-CR equipment. But it also points out substantial added savings when one tries to go filmless as quickly as possible (ie, within 1 year rather than over 4 years). And this does not even begin to take into account the nonfinancial benefits of PACS that have been publicized since the very beginning of scientific and commercial activity in the PACS arena in 1982 by Duerinckx et al (5).

Another important difference in our cost model and the one presented by Pratt et al is that we opted to amortize the purchase price over 5 years. Pratt et al instead assumed that all hardware investment cash flows occurred at time 0. If one opts for a scenario where all hardware investment cash flows occur at time 0, then the net present value decreases to −$3.26 million during the 2nd year and then increases to become $0 after 8 years (curve $2.8M-zero in the Figure). Although the time needed to pay for the PACS-CR system (ie, the time needed for the net present value to become $0) is 1 year less than it is with a 5-year amortization, the actual cost at any one time is very different, as the total incremental costs to the department during the 1st years will exceed the base cost of the PACS-CR system.

On the basis of these considerations, it is important that the radiology community realize that the purchase of large-scale PACS and CR systems can be cost-effective. Not only will the system pay for itself within 7–8 years in most moderately sized hospitals, but also, if the use of radiographic film can be reduced more rapidly, it may allow the purchase of PACS-CR equipment for less then half the cost base. Using a hardware investment cash flow that occurs at time 0 instead of a 5-year amortization will increase the incremental cost during the 1st years after the PACS-CR system purchase, but it will also reduce the overall time to reach a $0 net present value.

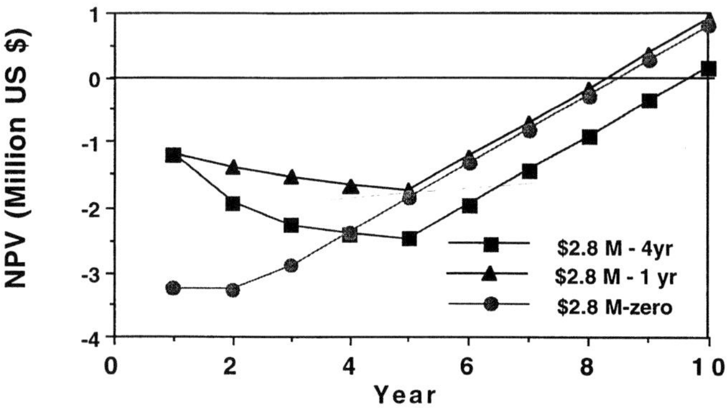

Changes in the net present value (*NPV*), as a function of years in service, associated with a new PACS-CR system installation in a moderately sized hospital. The results are for a PACS-CR system base cost of $2.8 million and three scenarios: (*a*) a gradual film-use reduction of 80% over 4 years with 5-year amortization (■); (*b*) a film-use reduction of 80% within 1 year with 5-year amortization (▲); and (*c*) a film-use reduction of 80% within 4 years, but with all investment cash flow occurring at time 0 (●). *M* = million, *yr* = year.

References

1. Pratt HM, Langlotz CP, Feingold ER, Schwartz JS, Kundel HL. Incremental cost of department-wide implementation of a picture archiving and communication system and computed radiography. Radiology 1998; 206:245–252.
2. Duerinckx AJ, Hayrapetian AS, Kenagy JJ, Grant KG. Teleradiology for Veterans Integrated Service Networks. In: Proceedings of the SPIE's International Symposium on Medical Imaging 1997: PACS design and evaluation—engineering and clinical issues. Vol 3035. Bellingham, Wash: SPIE, 1997; 124–131.
3. Pratt HM, Langlotz CP, Feingold ER, Schwartz IS, Kundel HL. Incremental cost of a department-wide PACS implementation. In: Proceedings of the SPIE's International Symposium on Medical Imaging 1997: PACS design and evaluation—engineering and clinical issues. Vol 3035. Bellingham, Wash: SPIE, 1997; 413–423.
4. Duerinckx AJ, Kenagy JJ, Grant KG. Planning and cost-analysis of picture archiving and communication systems (PACS) and computed radiography (CR) services for a Veterans Integrated Service Network in the USA. J Telemed Telecare (in press).
5. Duerinckx AJ. PACS status review: 1983. In: Proceeding of the second International Conference and Workshop on Picture Archiving & Communication Systems (PACS II) for Medical Applications. Vol 418. Bellingham, Wash: SPIE, 1983; 68–73.

Dr Langlotz and colleagues respond:

Drs Duerinckx and Grant raise several concerns with regard to our recent article (1) addressing the cost of PACS-CR systems. Their concerns relate to our estimated PACS purchase price, our assumptions with regard to the time to transition to filmless operation, and the "amortization period" chosen for our system purchase. We will address each in turn.

Drs Duerinckx and Grant assert that our PACS cost estimate is exorbitant because they estimate a PACS for their hospital would cost $2.8 million. There are many potential reasons for this difference, which cannot be ascertained without the benefit of their full report. Some of the differences may be due to the power of their governmental institution (a Veterans Affairs medical center) to demand a low price. Most of the difference is likely attributable to a lower examination volume at their institution, which is 40% lower than our own. Since an institution that performs fewer examinations will also have smaller savings from a filmless system, it is not clear that the difference in purchase price will result in different model conclusions, as Drs Duerinckx and Grant suggest.

Our system design was the result of an exhaustive analysis of digital imaging needs for each section of our department. For example, we carefully examined the number of reading areas, image alternators, and radiologist full-time equivalents to estimate workstation needs. We studied the average and peak imaging volumes hour-by-hour throughout the day to estimate the number of CR reader units needed. We calculated data capacities by using image file size and image volumes. We therefore stand by our estimate of PACS costs and believe it accurately reflects the needs of our department.

Drs Duerinckx and Grant also question our assumption that film use would decline gradually to 10% of its original value over 8 years. We made this conservative assumption for two reasons. First, studies performed before PACS implementation must be maintained on film for a time, both for clinical comparisons and for legal reasons. Second, because we are a tertiary referral center, a large fraction of our patients make an isolated visit to our hospital to see a specialist and to undergo specialized imaging examinations. These patients and their physicians often wish to bring a hard-copy record of their imaging examinations back to their community, where the images can be used to guide subsequent treatment. Since our original report, we have confirmed the results in the table 4 of our article: Substantially different assumptions with regard to film use cause economic changes much smaller than the $1.5 million that would be required to make PACS a break-even proposition for our institution.

The authors also suggest that the method we chose to finance the project is suboptimal. These comments may reflect a misunderstanding of the net present value method of economic analysis. A net present value calculation converts a series of cash flows (costs and cost savings) over time to an equivalent expenditure (or gain) in the present. The net present value method uses a discount rate that reflects the fact that a sum of money today is more valuable than the same amount of money in the future. For example, $100,000 in 8 years is calculated to be worth only $71,068 in present dollars by using a 5% interest rate. Likewise, a payment plan requiring $100,000 payment each year for 8 years has a net present value of −$678,637 (see the Table). Thus, the net present value method makes no assumptions about the amortization period or about how a project will be financed (eg, cash purchase, lease, or loan). Since net present value has meaning only in the present (which is when we must make the economic decision), we presume that the y axis in the Figure reflects not net present value, but cumulative cash flow. The Figure supports our point, since the cash purchase line (circles in the Figure) and the 5-year amortized purchase line (triangles in the Figure) are superimposed after the amortization period, reflecting no net economic effect of the financing method on cumulative cash flow.

Finally, we thank Drs Duerinckx and Grant for providing us an opportunity to correct a typographic error in our original report (1) that may have caused some confusion. The third column of table 3, which reflected the total examination volume of the department over the 8 years analyzed, was erroneously given the units "gigabytes" rather than "examinations" (1). Thus, our total estimated examination volume over 8 years is 1.57 million, corresponding to approximately 200,000 examinations annually.

So, while it at first may appear that Drs Duerinckx and Grant's soon-to-be-published economic analysis of PACS (3) is at odds with our own, further analysis suggests that their results may be quite consistent with ours, when considering the differences between our institutions and the assumptions of our models. Rapid technologic changes are occurring in PACS hardware and software—in fact, our department is in the midst of implementing a PACS different than the one we envisioned when we began this analysis 2 years ago. Nevertheless, as PACS and CR technologies and their costs change, our analysis can serve as a stable economic reference point for departments like our own (2).

Net Present Value Calculation for a 5% Interest Rate

Year	Cash Flow ($)	Net Present Value ($)
0	−100,000	−100,000
1	−100,000	−95,238
2	−100,000	−90,703
3	−100,000	−86,384
4	−100,000	−82,270
5	−100,000	−78,353
6	−100,000	−74,622
7	−100,000	−71,068
Total	−800,000	−678,637

Note.—A payment of $100,000 annually for 8 years has a net present value of $678,637. $100,000 in 7 years has a net present value of $71,068.

References

1. Pratt HM, Langlotz CP, Feingold ER, Schwartz JS, Kundel HL. Incremental cost of department-wide implementation of a picture archiving and communication system and computed radiography. Radiology 1998; 206:245–252.
2. Langlotz CP, Pratt HM, Feingold ER, Horii SC, Kundel HL. Factors determining the adoption of digital imaging systems. In: Proceedings of Medical Imaging: PACS design and evaluation—engineering and clinical issues. Bellingham, Wash: SPIE, 1998.
3. Duerinckx AJ, Kenagy JJ, Grant KG. Planning and cost-analysis of picture archiving and communication systems (PACS) and computed radiography (CR) services for a veterans integrated service network in the USA. J Telemed Telecare (in press).

Curtis P. Langlotz, MD, Steven C. Horii, MD, Hugh M. Pratt, MD, Harold L. Kundel, MD

Department of Radiology, University of Pennsylvania Medical Center

3600 Market Street, Suite 370, Philadelphia, PA 19104-2641

Erratum

"Hyperechoic Liver Nodules: Characterization with Proton Fat-Water Chemical Shift MR Imaging." Radiology 1998; 207:325–330.

On page 326, the first sentence of the first full paragraph in the middle column should read as follows: "In patients with a primary tumor, liver nodules were diagnosed as metastases when a slightly hyperintense nodule **on T2-weighted images** had a pattern of contrast enhancement with a persistent continuous peripheral hyperintense rim **on gradient-echo images.**

Abstracts of Current Literature

Genitourinary System

Three-dimensional Transrectal Ultrasound Guided Cryoablation for Localized Prostate Cancer in Nonsurgical Candidates: A Feasibility Study and Report of Early Results. Joseph L. Chin, Donal B. Downey, Michael Mulligan, et al. *J Urol* 1998; 159:910–914. (J.L.C., 800 Commissioners Rd E, London, Ontario, Canada N6A 4G5)

Purpose: A three-dimensional (3D) transrectal ultrasound (US) imaging system was incorporated into the cryoablation routine for prostate cancer to assess its feasibility and use. The objective was to improve visibility for probe placement and for intraoperative monitoring. *Materials and Methods:* A commercially available transrectal US unit was coupled with a custom-designed software system to construct 3D prostate images. Fifty-two patients with clinically localized prostate cancer in whom radiation therapy had failed (n = 45) or who were otherwise judged to be nonsurgical candidates (n = 7) were treated with cryoablation with 3D transrectal US used for intraoperative guidance. *Results:* In all cases, the intraoperative 3D transrectal US images provided a unique coronal view of the prostate, by revealing useful information and facilitating more precise probe placement and treatment monitoring. Early postoperative histologic and biochemical results and complication rates compared well with those of other contemporary series. *Conclusions:* Although the precise role of cryoablation in the management of prostate cancer remains unclear and long-term results are pending, incorporation of a 3D transrectal US imaging system into the cryoablation routine proved feasible, appeared a worthwhile effort to facilitate the procedure, and deserves further evaluation.
Authors' Abstract

Magnetic Resonance Imaging of Clinically Localized Prostatic Cancer. Saana Ikonen, Päivi Kärkkäinen, Leena Kivisaari, et al. *J Urol* 1998; 159:915–919. (From the Departments of Radiology and Urology, Helsinki University Central Hospital, Finland)

Purpose: The authors assess the accuracy of endorectal coil magnetic resonance (MR) imaging for detection of tumor localization, capsular penetration, and seminal vesicle invasion in clinically organ-confined prostate cancer. They also evaluate intraobserver and interobserver agreement in interpretation of MR imaging studies. *Materials and Methods:* MR imaging studies of 51 consecutive patients (mean age, 61 years) with biopsy-proved prostate cancer were retrospectively read twice by two radiologists in random order. Both radiologists marked tumor localization, capsular penetration, and seminal vesicle invasion on standard tumor maps. These findings were compared with the histopathologic results in radical prostatectomy specimens. *Results:* The overall accuracy for detection of cancer localization was 61%. The detection rate for cancer foci of less than 5 mm was only 5%, but for lesions greater than 10 mm it was 89%. There was 91% and 80% accuracy for detecting capsular penetration and seminal vesicle invasion, respectively. Sensitivity and specificity were 60% and 63%, 13% and 97%, and 59% and 84% for localization, capsular penetration, and seminal vesicle invasion, respectively. Intraobserver and interobserver agreement ranged from fair to good (κ coefficient, 0.240–0.647). *Conclusions:* Endorectal MR imaging seems to be better than previously reported for help in detection of seminal vesicle invasion and tumor foci in the anterior half of the prostate. Sensitivity for detection of minor capsular penetration of the tumor was low but can probably be improved by means of methodologic development. MR imaging may be useful for locating cancer foci in patients with high prostate-specific antigen values but repeatedly negative biopsy findings.
Authors' Abstract

Male Pelvic Anatomy Reconstructed from the Visible Human Data Set. James D. Brooks, Wen-Min Chao, John Kerr. *J Urol* 1998; 159:868–872. (J.D.B., Department of Urology, Rm S287, Stanford University Medical Center, Stanford, CA 94305-5118)

Purpose: To improve understanding of the male pelvic anatomy pertinent to urologic surgery, the authors performed computer-generated, three-dimensional reconstruction of the male pelvis from the Visible Human data set. *Materials and Methods:* A total of 18 discrete anatomic structures, including the prostate, bladder, urethra, rectum, and pelvic musculature, were segmented from the Visible Human cross-sectional data obtained from the National Library of Medicine. With use of high-speed computing and rendering software, three-dimensional models of each structure were generated and assembled into composite figures. *Results:* These reconstructions offer a revised view of pelvic anatomy as it has been traditionally depicted. The lateral surfaces of the levator ani muscle are oriented vertically in the pelvis and are directly applied to the entire lateral surface of the prostate. The bladder rests primarily anterior to the prostate rather than directly above it, as has been commonly depicted. In the cross-sectional data and reconstructions, the trigone and anterior fibromuscular stroma of the prostate appear as a single unit in continuity, which may have functional implications for understanding of the mechanisms of continence at the bladder neck. The striated urethral sphincter appears circular, with abundant tissue posteriorly. This sphincteric muscle has greater length anteriorly than posteriorly. *Conclusions:* These three-dimensional reconstructions provide unique insights into male pelvic anatomy. They are a useful teaching tool for investigation and virtual reality modeling of the male pelvis.
Authors' Abstract

Three-dimensional Computerized Tomography and Virtual Reality Endoscopy of the Reconstructed Lower Urinary Tract. Arnulf Stenzl, Renate Frank, Robert Eder, et al. *J Urol* 1998; 159:741–746. (From the Departments of Urology and Radiology II, University of Innsbruck Medical Center, Austria)

Purpose: The authors describe postoperative surgical anatomy after orthotopic reconstruction of the lower urinary tract by using three-dimensional (3D) computed tomography (CT) and virtual reality endoscopy. *Materials and Methods:* Electronic-beam CT was performed in 39 men and 15 women (mean age, 60 years) with an orthotopic ileal neobladder (n = 50) or ureteroileal rectosigmoidostomy (n = 4), followed by 3D reconstruction of the pelvic anatomic structures by using specialized computer hardware and software. The mean interval between surgery and CT was 15 months (range, 3–110 months), and the mean interval between two subsequent 3D CT studies in 22 patients was 6 months (range, 3–9 months). *Results:* CT time with the patient on the table was 45 minutes, and computerized 3D reconstruction time with the patient off the table was 4–5 hours. The pouch had a smooth ovoid shape in 66% and 82% of the patients on the first and second 3D CT studies, respectively. The mean length of the antireflux nipple was 4 cm (range, 2.5–8.0 cm), and the mean length of the afferent limb was 6 cm (range, 3–15 cm). There were no radiologically meaningful sex-specific differences in the shape or dimensions of the urinary reservoirs, except for a tendency toward more acute angles between the pouch and remnant urethra. No pathologic findings were visible on 3D CT images that were not also evident on conventional CT images. *Conclusions:* Three-dimensional CT may be clinically useful for surgical planning of a lower abdominal reoperation or unexplained findings and symptoms in patients with bladder substitutions. Cost and time expenditures for processing preclude its routine use in all cases. Virtual reality endoscopy may be a valuable tool for teaching and scientific purposes.
Authors' Abstract

Cardiovascular System

A Comparison of Recombinant Urokinase with Vascular Surgery as Initial Treatment for Acute Arterial Occlusion of the Legs. Kenneth Ouriel, Frank J. Veith, Arthur A. Sasahara, et al. *N Engl J Med* 1998; 338:1105–1111. (K.O., Department of Surgery, University of Rochester, 601 Elmwood Ave, Rochester, NY 14642)

Background: Recent controlled trials suggest that thrombolytic therapy may be an effective initial treatment for acute arterial occlusion of the legs. A major potential benefit of initial thrombolytic therapy is that limb ischemia can be managed with less invasive interventions. *Methods:* In this randomized, multicenter trial

conducted at 113 North American and European sites, the authors compared vascular surgery (eg, thrombectomy or bypass surgery) with thrombolysis by catheter-directed intraarterial recombinant urokinase; all patients (272 per group) had acute arterial obstruction of the legs for 14 days or less. Infusions were limited to a period of 48 hours (mean [±standard error], 24.4 hours ± 0.86), after which lesions were corrected by means of surgery or angioplasty if needed. The primary end point was the amputation-free survival rate at 6 months. *Results:* Final angiograms, which were available for 246 patients treated with urokinase, revealed recanalization in 196 (79.7%) and complete dissolution of thrombus in 167 (67.9%). Both treatment groups had similar significant improvements in the mean ankle–brachial blood pressure index. Amputation-free survival rates in the urokinase group were 71.8% at 6 months and 65.0% at 1 year, compared with 74.8% and 69.9% in the surgery group; the 95% confidence intervals for the differences were −10.5% to 4.5% at 6 months (P = .43) and −12.9% to 3.1% at 1 year (P = .23). At 6 months, the surgery group had undergone 551 open operative procedures (excluding amputations), as compared with 315 in the thrombolysis group. Major hemorrhage occurred in 32 patients in the urokinase group (12.5%) as compared with 14 patients in the surgery group (5.5%) (P = .005). There were four episodes of intracranial hemorrhage in the urokinase group (1.6%), one of which was fatal. By contrast, there were no episodes of intracranial hemorrhage in the surgery group. *Conclusions:* Despite its association with a higher frequency of hemorrhagic complications, intraarterial infusion of urokinase reduced the need for open surgical procedures, with no significantly increased risk of amputation or death.
Authors' Abstract

Vein Graft Surveillance: Is Graft Revision without Angiography Justified and What Criteria Should Be Used? Mirza M. Idu, Jacob Buth, Wim C. J. Hop, et al. *J Vasc Surg* 1998; 27:399–413. (J.B., Department of Surgery, Catharina Hospital, PO Box 1350, 5602 ZA Eindhoven, The Netherlands)

Purpose: The objective of this study was to assess the accuracy of color duplex flow surveillance parameters to detect infrainguinal vein graft stenoses and to investigate whether graft revision without angiography is justified. *Methods:* In a prospective study in which three centers participated, the data of graft surveillance in 300 patients were analyzed. For the evaluation of surveillance criteria, all patients underwent digital subtraction angiography if a graft stenosis was suspected. A consented digital subtraction angiography was also performed in patients with normal grafts to create a control group. From these data, the accuracy of seven duplex and three ankle blood pressure–derived variables was assessed. The relation between various surveillance criteria and continued graft patency was determined by means of life table analysis with the transient state method. *Results:* The mean follow-up period was 20 months (range, 1–40 months). At univariate and multivariate analysis, the peak systolic velocity (PSV) ratio provided the best correlation with angiographic stenoses of 70% or greater (PSV ratio cutoff, 3.0; sensitivity, 80%; specificity, 84%). This finding did not differ between the participating centers. With life table methods, it was demonstrated that the best combination of efficacy (limitation of the number of unnecessary revisions), safety (minimal number of correctable lesions missed), and reduction of angiograms was obtained by a two-parameter surveillance algorithm. This algorithm included a PSV ratio of less than 2.5 to delineate patients in whom a conservative approach without angiography or revision was appropriate, a PSV ratio of at least 4.0 to indicate patients in whom vein graft revision without angiography could be scheduled, and a group with PSV ratios between 2.5 and 4.0 in whom angiography was to be performed to determine clinical management on the basis of the stenosis severity. This algorithm had a positive predictive value of 93% and a negative predictive value of 89%. In addition, it reduced the number of angiograms by 49%, compared with a policy of performing angiography in all patients with a PSV ratio of at least 2.5. *Conclusions:* The best criterion to identify a failing graft is the PSV ratio. With a two-parameter algorithm for vein graft surveillance, the incidence of unnecessary revisions and of missed high-grade lesions was acceptably low, whereas the number of angiograms was reduced by one-half.
Authors' Abstract

The Value of Computed Tomography in the Assessment of Suspected Ruptured Abdominal Aortic Aneurysm. Donald J. Adam, Andrew W. Bradbury, Wesley P. Stuart, et al. *J Vasc Surg* 1998; 27:431–437. (D.J.A., Vascular Surgery Unit, University Department of Surgery, Royal Infirmary, Edinburgh EH3 9YW, Scotland)

Objective: The objective of this study was to determine the diagnostic value of computed tomography (CT) in patients with suspected ruptured abdominal aortic aneurysm. *Study Design:* The study was an interrogation of a prospectively gathered computerized database. *Setting:* The study was performed at a regional vascular surgery unit. *Subjects:* Six hundred fifty-two consecutive patients were admitted to this unit with suspected ruptured abdominal aortic aneurysm between January 1, 1989, and December 31, 1996. Seventy-four patients (11.3%) in whom the diagnosis was in doubt on clinical grounds alone underwent urgent CT. A total of 47 men and 27 women with a median age of 73 years (age range, 52–86 years) were evaluated. *Main Outcome Measures:* CT and operative findings were compared. *Results:* CT correctly demonstrated rupture in 22 of 28 patients who underwent operation and correctly excluded rupture in 30 of 39 patients who underwent operation. The sensitivity and specificity of CT when compared with operative findings were therefore 79% and 77%, respectively. *Conclusions:* These data indicate that CT has little additional diagnostic value. If an experienced vascular surgeon judges that rupture cannot be excluded on clinical grounds alone, and that the patient has no medical contraindications to abdominal aortic aneurysm repair, the patient should be taken directly to the operating department.
Authors' Abstract

Endoleak after Endovascular Graft Repair of Experimental Aortic Aneurysms: Does Coil Embolization with Angiographic "Seal" Lower Intraaneurysmal Pressure? Bettina Marty, Luis A. Sanchez, Takao Ohki, et al. *J Vasc Surg* 1998; 27:454–462. (L.A.S., Division of Vascular Surgery, Montefiore Medical Center, 111 E 210th St, New York, NY 10467)

Purpose: To investigate the relation between endoleaks (the presence of flow outside endovascular grafts) and intraaneurysmal pressure (IAP) and the effect of coil embolization in the management of endoleaks. *Methods:* The infrarenal aorta of a dog (n = 15) was replaced by a polytetrafluoroethylene aneurysm containing a pressure transducer. Group 1 (n = 4) had untreated aneurysms. Group 2 (n = 4) had endovascularly excluded aneurysms without an endoleak. Group 3 (n = 7) had aneurysms excluded by means of grafts with a defect that represented the source of an endoleak. After 4 weeks of follow-up study, the endoleaks in group 3 dogs were subjected to coil embolization. Systolic IAP was measured daily and expressed as a ratio of systolic blood pressure obtained from a forelimb cuff. Arteriography, duplex ultrasonography, and spiral contrast computed tomography (CT) were performed to evaluate endoleaks. *Results:* In group 1, the IAP remained close to systolic blood pressure (ratio, 0.96 ± 0.06), whereas in group 2 the IAP ratio showed a decline to 0.34 ± 0.16 (P = .0009, group 1 vs group 2). After an initial decrease, the IAP ratio in group 3 stabilized at 0.75 ± 0.18 (P = .003, group 2 vs group 3). Aneurysms with an endoleak remained pulsatile with a pulse pressure of 30 mm Hg ± 16, which was less than that of untreated aneurysms (62 mm Hg ± 15; P < .001, group 1 vs group 3). Arteriography and CT revealed "sealing" of endoleaks after coil embolization, but IAP ratio did not decrease (0.76 ± 0.14) after coil embolization. *Conclusions:* Incomplete endovascular aneurysm exclusion caused by an endoleak fails to reduce IAP ratio and may subject the aneurysm to a continued risk for rupture. Although coil embolization resulted in angiographic and CT sealing, it failed to reduce the IAP ratio.
Authors' Abstract

Ex Vivo Human Carotid Artery Bifurcation Stenting: Correlation of Lesion Characteristics with Embolic Potential. Takao Ohki, Michael L. Marin, Ross T. Lyon, et al. *J Vasc Surg* 1998; 27:463–471. (T.O., Division of Vascular Surgery, Montefiore Medical Center, 111 E 210th St, New York, NY 10467)

Purpose: To develop an ex vivo human carotid artery stenting model that can be used for the quantitative analysis of risk for emboliza-

tion associated with balloon angioplasty and stenting and to correlate this risk with lesion characteristics to define lesions suitable for balloon angioplasty and stenting. *Methods:* Specimens of carotid plaque (n = 24) were obtained circumferentially intact from patients undergoing standard carotid endarterectomy. Carotid lesions were prospectively characterized on the basis of angiographic and duplex findings before endarterectomy and clinical findings. Specimens were encased in a polytetrafluoroethylene wrap and mounted in a flow chamber that allowed access for endovascular procedures and observations. Balloon angioplasty and stenting were performed under fluoroscopic guidance with either a Palmaz stent or a Wallstent endoprosthesis. Ex vivo angiograms were obtained before and after intervention. Effluent from each specimen was filtered for released embolic particles, which were microscopically examined, counted, and correlated with various plaque characteristics by means of multivariate analysis. *Results:* Balloon angioplasty and stenting produced embolic particles that consisted of atherosclerotic debris, organized thrombus, and calcified material. The number of embolic particles detected after balloon angioplasty and stenting was not related to preoperative symptoms, sex, plaque ulceration or calcification, or artery size. However, echopenic plaques generated a higher number of particles compared with echogenic plaques ($P < .01$). In addition, increased lesion stenosis also significantly correlated with the total number of particles produced by balloon angioplasty and stenting ($r = .55$). Multivariate analysis revealed that these two characteristics were independent risk factors. *Conclusions:* Echopenic plaques and plaques with stenosis of at least 90% produced a higher number of embolic particles and therefore may be less suitable for balloon angioplasty and stenting. This ex vivo model can be used to identify high-risk lesions for balloon angioplasty and stenting and can aid in the evaluation of new devices being considered for carotid balloon angioplasty and stenting.
Authors' Abstract

Efficacy and Safety of a Hemostatic Puncture Closure Device with Early Ambulation after Coronary Angiography. Samuel R. Ward, Paul Casale, Russell Raymond, et al. *Am J Cardiol* 1998; 81:569–572. (Conrad Simpfendorfer, Department of Cardiology, Desk F-25, Cleveland Clinic Foundation, 9500 Euclid Ave, Cleveland, OH 44195)

Failure to achieve puncture site hemostasis after coronary angiography can result in prolonged hospital stay, patient discomfort, and vascular complications. Various attempted strategies to achieve hemostasis have included use of smaller sheath sizes, C clamps, or pneumatic compression devices, plus a variety of through-the-sheath arterial closure devices. A collagen hemostatic puncture closure device has been developed as an alternative to traditional manual pressure techniques for achieving effective femoral arterial hemostasis after coronary angiography. The purpose of this study was to determine whether patients receiving this device can ambulate safely at 1 hour compared with patients receiving traditional manual pressure and bed rest after sheath removal for diagnostic cardiac catheter placement. Patients (n = 304) were randomized to either the device group (n = 202) with ambulation at 1 hour after sheath removal or to the manual pressure control group (n = 102) with ambulation at 4–6 hours after sheath removal. The device group achieved earlier time to hemostasis (0.9 minutes ± 3 vs 17.0 minutes ± 8; P = .001) and faster time to outpatient discharge (5.0 hours ± 4 vs 7.7 hours ± 4; P = .001) compared with the control group. There was bleeding or vascular complications in 19 patients (9%) in the device group and in six patients (6%) in the manual pressure group, but this difference was not significant (P = .397). In patients undergoing diagnostic coronary angiography, this device, compared with traditional techniques for achieving hemostasis after sheath removal, allows effective hemostasis to be achieved more quickly, with resultant earlier discharge from the hospital.
Patricia A. Randall, MD
SUNY Health Science Center at Syracuse, NY

Comparison of Exercise Electron Beam Computed Tomography and Sestamibi in the Evaluation of Coronary Artery Disease. Matthew J. Budoff, Robert Gillespie, Demetrios Georgiou, et al. *Am J Cardiol* 1998; 81:682–687. (M.J.B., Saint John's Cardiovascular Research Center, 1124 W Carson St, RB-2, Torrance, CA 90502)

Exercise testing is a well-established, noninvasive method for detecting obstructive coronary artery disease. Many imaging studies have been performed during stress testing. This blinded, single-center study prospectively compared exercise electron-beam computed tomography (CT) with stress technetium-99m sestamibi single-photon emission CT (SPECT) in 33 patients undergoing coronary angiography for evaluation of chest pain. Patients undergoing routine cardiac catheter placement for the diagnosis of possible coronary artery disease as a cause of chest pain were imaged at rest with electron-beam CT. Patients exercised on a semisupine ergometer, and exercise electron-beam CT was immediately followed by injection of Tc-99m sestamibi for assessment of myocardial ischemia. At peak exercise, Tc-99m SPECT, followed immediately by nonionic contrast material, was injected intravenously to compare these two imaging techniques directly. Patients underwent repeat imaging with Tc-99m SPECT while at rest 24–48 hours after stress. Exercise electron-beam CT, the findings of which were analyzed by using a global ejection fraction method, had a sensitivity of 81% and a specificity of 76% compared with angiography. By using the development of a new regional wall motion abnormality as evidence of coronary artery disease, electron-beam CT yielded a specificity of 100% and a sensitivity of 88%. Reversible perfusion defects identified at SPECT, as evidence of obstructive coronary artery disease, revealed a sensitivity of 75% and a specificity of 71%. This specificity of regional wall motion analysis by electron-beam CT was significantly better ($P < .01$) than in this population. The results of this study demonstrate regional wall motion assessed by electron-beam CT to be as sensitive as and more specific than SPECT regional perfusion imaging in demonstrating obstructive coronary artery disease as defined by angiography.
Patricia A. Randall, MD
SUNY Health Science Center at Syracuse, NY

Coronary Angioplasty Outcomes in the Healthcare Cost and Utilization Project, 1993–1994. Charles Maynard, Michael K. Chapko, Nathan R. Every, et al. *Am J Cardiol* 1998; 81:848–852. (James L. Ritchie, Division of Cardiology, Box 356422, University of Washington, Seattle, WA 98195)

It is estimated that over 400,000 percutaneous transluminal coronary angioplasty (PTCA) procedures are performed in the United States annually. This article reports patient characteristics and outcomes for 163,527 PTCAs performed in 214 hospitals in 17 states from 1993 to 1994. These hospitals were a 20% random sample of hospitals in the Healthcare Cost and Utilization Project, which was designed to reflect hospitalization in the United States generally. PTCA was defined as International Classification of Disease, Ninth Revision, Clinical Modification procedure codes 36.01, 36.02, and 36.05, and all such cases were categorized as to whether acute myocardial infarction (AMI) was the principal discharge diagnosis. The average age of 44,270 (27%) patients with AMI diagnoses at discharge was 62 years ± 12, and that of 119,257 (73%) non-AMI patients was 64 years ± 11; one-third of both groups were female patients, 88% were white, and almost 90% had Medicare or private insurance as the primary payer. The states contributing the most cases were Florida (26%), California (12%), and Wisconsin (10%). The hospital mortality rate was 1.7% overall, 3.8% for AMI, and 0.8% for non-AMI cases. The incidence of bypass surgery performed during the same admission was 3.5% overall and was 4.5% and 3.0% for AMI and non-AMI cases, respectively. Multivariate analysis showed that advanced age, diabetes, female sex, and Medicaid payer status were associated with increased risk of mortality. National estimates from this 20% sample indicate that over 850,000 PTCAs were performed in the 2 years, with 452,319 cases estimated for 1994. In 1994, there were an estimated 2,789 deaths and 9,903 bypass surgeries in the non-AMI subset of 327,856 procedures. For the AMI group of 124,463 procedures, there were 4,486 deaths and 5,799 bypass surgeries in 1994. This study of PTCA outcomes contains the largest number of cases, as well as the most representative sample reported to date.
Patricia A. Randall, MD
SUNY Health Science Center at Syracuse, NY

Intravascular Ultrasound Evaluation of Plaque Distribution at Curved Coronary Segments. Hiroshi Tsutsui, Masakazu Yamagishi, Masaaki Uematsu, et al. *Am J Cardiol* 1998; 81:977–981. (M.Y., Cardiology Division of Medicine, National Cardiovascular Center, 5-7-1 Fujishiro-dai, Suita, Osaka 565, Japan)

The intravascular ultrasound (US) imaging technique has enabled recognition of the morphology and distribution of atherosclerotic plaque even in the absence of angiographically depicted stenosis. However, it is difficult to demonstrate exact plaque distribution in clinical settings because of technical difficulties. The determination of plaque distribution may be particularly important in deciding on the strategy of the interventional procedure. Although the distribution of atherosclerosis at the curved coronary segment has implications for atherogenesis and interventional procedures, few data exist regarding the plaque distribution in these sites. Therefore, the authors prospectively analyzed the intravascular US images of 55 coronary sites in 37 patients in whom intravascular US simultaneously demonstrated atherosclerotic plaque and pericardium. The pericardial images were defined as a high-intensity linear-echo image that moved outside the vessel wall during the cardiac cycle. By the line that was parallel to the pericardial image, the vessel area was divided into two semicircles with the same area, namely myocardial and pericardial sides. In each side, the maximal thickness, area, and percentage area of plaque were measured. The mean (±standard deviation) plaque thickness and area of the myocardial side were significantly greater (1.5 mm ± 0.5, 4.9 mm^2 ± 2.1 or 66%, respectively) than those of the pericardial side (1.1 mm ± 0.4, 3.5 mm^2 ± 2.1 or 45%, respectively; $P < .01$). The maximal plaque thickness was positioned at the point with a mean angle of 139° ± 37 from the point just facing the pericardial image, indicating that atherosclerosis was eccentrically located on the opposite side of the pericardium in these coronary segments and suggesting that the side of the pericardial image represents the outer curvature of the coronary artery. These results indicate that the pericardial images can be seen with intravascular US, facilitating the recognition of the disease distribution in situ. The eccentric plaque located on the inner wall at the curved coronary segments, probably due to uneven local shear stress, may have implications for the interventional procedures for these segments.

Patricia A. Randall, MD
SUNY Health Science Center at Syracuse, NY

Musculoskeletal System

Knee Osteoarthritis after Meniscectomy: Prevalence of Radiographic Changes after Twenty-One Years, Compared with Matched Controls. Harald Roos, Mårten Laurén, Torsten Adalberth, et al. *Arthritis Rheum* 1998; 41:687–693. (H.R., Department of Orthopedics, Lund University Hospital, S-221 85, Lund, Sweden)

Objective: To study the long-term outcome of surgical removal of a meniscus in the knee with regard to radiographic signs of osteoarthritis. *Methods:* Of the 123 patients who underwent an open meniscectomy due to an isolated meniscus tear in 1973 at Lund University Hospital, 107 were followed up 21 years later by means of clinical examination and review of knee radiographs obtained with weight bearing. Seventy-nine of the 107 patients were men, and the mean age of the total study group at examination was 55 years (age range, 35–77 years). Sixty-eight sex- and age-matched individuals with healthy knees served as control subjects. *Results:* Mild radiographic changes were found in 76 (71%) of the knees, while more advanced changes, comparable with a Kellgren-Lawrence grade of 2 or higher, were seen in 51 (48%). The corresponding prevalence values in the control group were 12 (18%) and 5 (7%), respectively. The relative risk for the presence of the more advanced radiographic changes representing definite radiographic tibiofemoral osteoarthritis was 14.0 (95% confidence interval, 3.5, 121.2), with age- and sex-matched pairs used for comparison. No correlation with sex, localization to compartment, type of meniscus tear, or workload was found. Knee symptoms were reported twice as often in the study group as in the control group. *Conclusion:* Surgical removal of a meniscus after knee injury represents a significant risk factor for radiographic tibiofemoral osteoarthritis, with a relative risk of 14.0 after 21 years.

Authors' Abstract

Classified Services

POLICY

As a service to its readers, *Radiology* accepts classified advertising, and every effort is made to ensure that the ads are relevant to the practice of radiology. Acceptable categories include positions available, positions sought, fellowships, announcements of postgraduate courses or symposia, practices for sale, medical facilities for rent or sale, used radiologic equipment and apparatus for sale, medical employment bureau advertising, academic posts to be filled, available posts for interns and residents, and malpractice insurance. We retain the right to refuse any advertisement considered not relevant, and respondents are advised to investigate each offer since we cannot assume responsibility for the offers or claims of advertisers.

RATES (per month, per insertion)

Line ads in *Radiology* (no agency commission)

50 words or less $90.00

51–100 words $135.00

Each word over 100—$1.00 per word.

Box Number—$30.00 additional per each insertion (this service is optional).

TERMS

Payment must accompany order.* Make checks payable to **Radiological Society of North America.** We accept American Express, VISA, Mastercard, and Diners Club for classified ads. Call for details. Send payment to:

RSNA, Radiology Classified Ad Department
Accounts Payable, 2021 Spring Road, Suite 600
Oak Brook, IL 60523-1860 USA.

*Purchase Order Numbers are accepted with prior approval.

Please mark each issue:

❒ Jan ❒ Feb ❒ Mar ❒ Apr ❒ May ❒ June
❒ July ❒ Aug ❒ Sept ❒ Oct ❒ Nov ❒ Dec

Send invoice and tearsheet to:

____
____
____
____

Advertisers who cancel ads will not receive refunds.

DEADLINE

Copy must be received by the **20th of the second month preceding issue.** Please submit copy typed and double-spaced. Initials or abbreviations equal one word. Telephone numbers with area code equal one word.

CLASSIFIED DISPLAY ADVERTISING

Black and white frequency rates are based on the total number of insertions used within a 12-month period from date of first insertion.

Ad Space	Size	1X	6X	12X
1 page	7" x 9-1/2"	$2250	2170	2090
2/3 pg vert	4-1/2" x 9-1/2"	$1900	1830	1760
1/2 pg horzt	7" x 4-1/2"	$1350	1300	1250
1/2 pg vert	3-3/8" x 9-1/2"	$1350	1300	1250
1/2 pg island	4-1/4" x 7-1/2"	$1350	1300	1250
1/3 pg vert	2-1/4" x 9-1/2"	$1085	1045	1005
1/3 pg square	4-1/2" x 4-1/2"	$1085	1045	1005
1/4 page	3-3/8" x 4-1/2"	$ 850	820	790
1/6 page	2-1/4" x 4-1/2"	$ 605	585	565
1/9 page	2-1/4" x 3"	$ 420	400	380

Preferred materials are composite negatives, right-reading, emulsion side down. (Conversion materials such as positive film, repro proofs, and camera-ready artworks are acceptable at additional charge.)

Customer supplied negative: cost as noted
Customer supplied mechanical: add 10%
Customer supplied copy to be set and ad prepared: add 20%

Call Production Department for additional information. Address for correspondence, insertion orders, copy, proofs, box number, and payment:

***Radiology* Advertising Production Office**
2021 Spring Road, Suite 600
Oak Brook, IL 60523-1860

To respond to a box number ad, send your CV and/or any other information to the above address; on the front of the envelope, please indicate the appropriate box number.

For further information:
Carissa Muccianti, *Advertising Coordinator*
630.571.7817
630.571.7837 (fax)

Positions Available

RADIOLOGIST-BREAST IMAGING—The Department of Diagnostic Radiology and Nuclear Medicine at Rush Medical College and Rush-Presbyterian-St. Luke's Medical Center is seeking a Board certified radiologist with fellowship training or equivalent subspecialty experience in breast imaging. The department has dedicated outpatient facilities for breast imaging including a stereotactic unit for needle biopsy. Rank and salary are commensurate with experience. Interested parties should contact Peter Jokich, MD, Director of the Section of Breast Imaging, Department of Diagnostic Radiology and Nuclear Medicine, Rush-Presbyterian-St. Luke's Medical Center, 1653 W Congress Parkway, Chicago, IL 60612. Rush is an equal opportunity/affirmative employer.

HARVARD MEDICAL SCHOOL COMMUNITY TEACHING HOSPITAL—Has an unexpected opening for a 1st-year (PGY-2) radiology resident for July, 1998. ACGME accredited program. Contact Michael Shortsleeve, MD, Program Director, Mount Auburn Hospital, 330 Mt. Auburn St, Cambridge, MA 02238; 617-499-5070, fax 617-499-5138.

LAKE MICHIGAN - LAKESHORE RESORT COMMUNITY—A 6-member progressive private practice seeks an additional Board certified radiologist to join our rapidly expanding practice. Strongly prefer an individual who is fellowship trained in angiography/interventional. New partner would join an established interventional practice but would also be required to interpret CT, MRI, mammography, ultrasound, Doppler, nuclear medicine and general radiographs, and cover teleradiology call on a rotating basis. Position is partnership track in a fee-for-service environment, with generous salary, benefit and vacation package. This community has four seasons, abundant recreational activities including fabulous boating on beautiful Lake Michigan. Reply to Box R-080.

ANGIOGRAPHER/INTERVENTIONAL RADIOLOGIST—There is an excellent opportunity to join a progressive group of 17 Board certified radiologists practicing at Lehigh Valley Hospital, a 600-bed university affiliated hospital. The applicant should be a fellowship trained interventionalist, capable of performing a wide range of examinations in a department that does over 4,000 angio/interventional procedures per year. The position also requires skills in diagnostic radiology including body imaging. There is a competitive salary and benefit package that leads to full partnership. The hospital is located 1-hour from Philadelphia and 1 ½ hours from NY. For further information, contact Robert Kricun, MD, Department of Radiology, Lehigh Valley Hospital, PO Box 689, Allentown, PA 18105-1556; telephone 610-402-8088, fax 610-402-1023.

CARDIOVASCULAR/INTERVENTIONAL RADIOLOGY - FULL-TIME ACADEMIC POSITION—The Department of Radiology, University Hospital at State University of New York College of Medicine, Syracuse is seeking a fellowship trained, full-time cardiovascular/interventional radiologist at the Assistant/Associate Professor level. ABR/CAQ certification eligibility in vascular/interventional radiology is required. This position will work at two centers, a 350-bed acute care university hospital and tertiary referral center and an adjacent 200-bed VA Hospital. Both centers have state-of-the-art digital equipment. In excess of 4,000 examinations a year are performed and include the full range of diagnostic and interventional vascular and non-vascular procedures. There is an ACGME accredited fellowship program with one and potentially two fellows each year. The duties of faculty members include teaching and research. The radiologists are organized as a limited liability partnership, offering very competitive salaries and excellent fringe benefits. For further information, contact Dr Paramjit S. Chopra, at 315-464-7439 or send resume to Department of Radiology, University Hospital, State University of New York Health Science Center, 750 E. Adams St, Syracuse, NY 13210 or fax to 315-464-7458. You may also send e-mail to *choprap@mailbox. hscsyr.edu.* State University of New York, Syracuse is an equal opportunity employer and encourages applications from women and members of minority groups.

ESTABLISHED PRACTICE IN SOUTHERN CALIFORNIA—Is seeking a Board certified, fellowship trained breast imaging radiologist and general diagnostic radiologist. Our practice is located in a beautiful coastal community with both hospital and free-standing imaging center business. Please mail your CV to Digital & Radiologic Imaging Associates, Inc, 26161 Marguerite Parkway, Suite D, Mission Viejo, CA 92691; attn: Kerry Jones.

DIAGNOSTIC RADIOLOGIST WITH BODY CT/ULTRASOUND FELLOWSHIP—Or special interest wanted for partnership track position. Will spend half of time in a small rural hospital and half in large metropolitan hospital in desert southwest. Excellent benefits provided. Send curriculum vitae to Box R-081.

WANTED: BOARD CERTIFIED RADIOLOGISTS IN NE PENNSYLVANIA—Radiological Consultants, Inc, has a demand for several radiologists secondary to both retiring members as well as an expanding service area. We are group of 17 radiologists in northeast Pennsylvania covering two hospitals in Scranton, one hospital in Wilkes Barre, one hospital in Nanticoke, as well as an MRI center which houses two 1.5 Tesla magnets as well as an open 0.3 Tesla magnet. We are currently targeting fellowship trained or an equivalent experienced radiologist. Competitive salary and benefits are being offered for this excellent opportunity. Reply to Radiological Consultants, Inc, c/o John J. Culliney, MD, 751 Keystone Industrial Park, Dunmore, PA 18512. Phone 717-346-8272 or fax CV to 717-346-4872.

RADIOLOGIST/PEDIATRIC—The Department of Radiology at the University of Minnesota has a full-time position available in the pediatric section at the rank of Assistant Professor (tenure-track or clinical track), Associate Professor (tenured or clinical-track), or Professor (tenured or clinical-track) beginning as soon as possible. At the Assistant Professor level, minimum requirements are Board certification in radiology, a minimum of 1-year post residency specialty training. Appointment at the rank of Associate Professor requires Board certification in radiology, a minimum of 4-years post residency specialty training or experience in pediatric radiology, a professional distinction in research and writing, and demonstrated effectiveness in teaching and advising. Appointment at the rank of Professor requires Board certification in radiology, a minimum of 6-years post residency specialty training or experience in pediatric radiology, a national reputation in research and writing, and evidence of leadership in candidate's professional field in addition to other qualifications listed for Assistant and Associate Professor status. Responsibilities will include all facets of pediatric radiology as well as graduate and undergraduate medical education. For tenure-track and tenured positions, research performance will be strongly encouraged and evaluated. Salary is negotiable and competitive, and is dependent upon past scholarly productivity and post MD experience. Applicants must be licensed or able to obtain a license to practice medicine in the state of Minnesota before appointment date. Applications will be accepted through September 15, 1998. Send letters to Dr Becky Carpenter, Associate Professor and Director of Pediatric Radiology, Departments of Radiology and Pediatrics, Box 292 Mayo Bldg, University of Minnesota, 420 Delaware St SE, Minneapolis, MN 55455. The University of Minnesota is an equal opportunity educator and employer.

WOMEN'S CENTER RADIOLOGIST—Suburban Atlanta, GA. Progressive 13-member subspecialized group seeking mammographer. State-of-the-art women's facility is on main hospital campus with large interventional mammography, obstetrical and neonatal services. Please send replies to Robert Eisenberg, MD, Promina Gwinnett Health System, 1000 Medical Center Blvd, Lawrenceville, GA 30045-7694; 770-995-4440.

NUCLEAR MEDICINE (FULL-TIME)—The Department of Radiology, University of Maryland Medical System in Baltimore is seeking a recent fellowship trained full-time nuclear radiologist at the Assistant Professor level who desires an academic career. ABR certification with special competence in nuclear radiology or ABNM certification is required. The medical center is a 800-bed acute care hospital and tertiary referral center. A new affiliated, all digital (PACS) VA Hospital with 324-beds is connected to the University. The full range of diagnostic, interventional and therapeutic procedures are performed. The division plans to move into all new space during the second half of 1998. Six SPECT capable cameras, four with multiple detectors, a PACS environment and a state-of-the-art multi-media work and conference facility. The division currently has two full-time ABNM trained radiologists, a full-time, on-site nuclear physicist, and a fellow. The duties of faculty members includes research, teaching, and clinical service. The radiologists are organized as a professional corporation offering excellent fringe benefits. For further information, contact Dr Philip A. Templeton at 410-328-3477 or send resume to Department of Radiology, University of Maryland Medical System, 22 S Greene St, Baltimore, MD 21201 or fax 410-328-0641. The University of Maryland at Baltimore is an AA/EOE/ADA employer and encourages applications from women and members of minority groups.

OPEN RANK—The University of Arizona Department of Radiology is seeking a Board certified/eligible academic radiologist for Section Chief of Body Imaging, Assistant Professor, Associate Professor or Professor, TT/NTE. Required, fellowship training in MRI, demonstrated knowledge of MRI and CT technology and application and eligibility for medical licensure in the state of Arizona. This position will open July 1, 1998. Review applications will commence September 1, 1998 and continue until the position is filled. The applicant must be able to obtain an Arizona license prior to the starting date. Letters of inquiry and CV should be sent to Theron W Ovitt, MD, Chair, Department of Radiology, AHSC, PO Box 245067, Tucson, AZ 85724-5067. For more information see web site *http://w3.arizona.edu/~ahschr/jobs.htm.* The University of Arizona is an EEO/AA employer. M/W/D/V.

THE UNIVERSITY OF MISSISSIPPI MEDICAL CENTER—Department of Radiology is seeking a general radiologist with interest in mammography. Some fellowship training preferred. The department currently has four mammographic units, stereotactic biopsy and breast ultrasound. Compensation will be based on qualifications and productivity. Interested parties should contact Dr Brent Harrison at 601-984-2515. EOE, M/F/D/V.

RADIOLOGIST—TTUHSC at El Paso, Department of Radiology seeks a Board eligible or certified radiologist with fellowship training in body imaging. This is an interesting and challenging position in a county hospital that is the trauma center for a community of 650,000 and the primary inpatient and outpatient care giver for a large indigent and undeserved population of 250,000. Our equipment is current with a new MRI, second CT scanner, and combined cardiovascular machine soon to be installed. Our mammography program is a center of excellence. Our ultrasound and mammography sections are ACR accredited. This is an ideal position for a recent trainee who desires to affiliate with a medical school and become a part of an active clinical service. Salary is commensurate with training and experience. Benefits including retirement are generous. El Paso is a delightful city of 650,000 with a year-round warm dry climate and the ease of southern living. Send correspondence to Dr Lloyd K. Mark, Professor and Regional Chairman, Department of Radiology, Texas Tech University HSC at El Paso, 4800 Alberta St, El Paso, TX 79905, fax 915-545-6607, e-mail *radelkm@ttuhsc.edu* or call me at 915-545-6845.

DEPARTMENT OF RADIOLOGY, MASSACHUSETTS GENERAL HOSPITAL, HARVARD MEDICAL SCHOOL—The neuroradiology division at the Massachusetts General Hospital invites applications from interested, qualified radiologists for a faculty position in interventional neuroradiology at the Instructor or Assistant Professor level. Candidates must be Board certified in radiology, have completed a 2-year fellowship in interventional neuroradiology, and have experience in clinical and laboratory research. The successful individual will be joining two fellowship trained interventional neuroradiologists in a busy clinical service spanning all aspects of interventional neuroradiology, and participating in a broad range of teaching and research opportunities. The MGH and Harvard Medical School strongly encourage applications from women and minority candidates. Please send CV and a list of three references to Christopher M. Putman, MD, Interventional Neuroradiology, GRB 289, Massachusetts General Hospital, 55 Fruit St, Boston, MA 02114; e-mail *putman.christopher@mgh.harvard.edu.*

RADIOLOGIST—VA Central Iowa Health Care System seeks full-time, BC radiologist for inpatient and outpatient services. This position offers state-of-the-art equipment and challenging work environment. In excess of 35,000 examinations a year are performed and include full range of diagnostic and interventional procedures. ACGME accredited internal medicine and general surgery residency programs offer some teaching opportunities. Ability to perform angiography an asset. Des Moines, IA is an outstanding community with excellent schools with numerous recreational and cultural activities. Position offers generous pay salary and excellent fringe benefit package. Applicants must be U.S. citizens and will be subject to federal hiring regulations and random drug screening procedures. For consideration, please send CV to Dr Bert Ammann, Radiology Service, VA Central Iowa Health Care System, 3600 30th St, Des Moines, IA 50310; e-mail address *ammann@vacihs.med.va.gov.* EOE.

BC RADIOLOGIST CERTIFIED OR ELIGIBLE FOR CAQ IN IR—Prefer fellowship training in IR to join five person group practice in Eugene-Springfield, OR. Must also have expertise in general radiography to include mammography, CT, US, MRI and nuclear medicine. Competitive salary, excellent benefits and partnership opportunity. Please send CV to Paul Longstreth, MD, McKenzie Medical Imaging, 960 N 16th St, Suite 103, Springfield, OR 97477.

DIAGNOSTIC RADIOLOGISTS - NORTHEAST FLORIDA—The University of Florida Health Science Center/Jacksonville is seeking two staff radiologists for full-time positions. Requirements: MD degree and BC/BE in diagnostic radiology. Special interest, expertise, or fellowship training in abdominal imaging (CT, MRI and ultrasound), musculoskeletal or pediatric radiology, neuroradiology or nuclear medicine is desirable. Fringe benefits are excellent; salary is negotiable. Academic appointments will be based on training, background and experience. Tenure track: Instructor, Assistant Professor, Associate Professor or Professor; non-tenure track: Clinical Instructor, Clinical Assistant Professor, Clinical Associate Professor or Clinical Professor. Application deadline is August 31, 1998 with anticipated start date October 15, 1998. Send CV and references to Chairman, Search Committee, Department of Radiology, 655 W 8th St, Jacksonville, FL 32209. Equal employment opportunity/affirmative action employer.

NATIONAL UNIVERSITY HOSPITAL, SINGAPORE—Excellence our mission, a commitment. The National University Hospital is a 900-bed multi-specialty teaching hospital. An opportunity exists to share in our mission of achieving excellence in patient care, medical education and research through the provision of quality patient care with state-of-the-art medical technology; consultant/senior registrar/registrar (diagnostic imaging). Applicants must hold a basic and postgraduate medical degree registrable with the Singapore Medical Council and any of the following postgraduate qualifications: FRCR, FRACR, FRCP Canada, American Board Certified. Commencing salary will be competitive depending on qualifications and experience. Please give full personal particulars, professional qualifications, career history and expected salary together with medical testimonials, certificate of registration, recent photograph and telephone number to Chairman, Medical Board, Medical Affairs Department, National University Hospital, 5 Lower Kent Ridge Rd, Singapore 119074. Telefax 65-775-6757; telephone 65-772-5920; web site *http://www.nuh.com.sg;* enquiries *leesm,@nuh.com.sg;* closing date, three weeks from date of publication.

BREAST IMAGING RADIOLOGIST/COASTAL CAROLINA AREA—Large, diversified and progressive radiology practice in the coastal Carolina area seeking a Board certified radiologist with fellowship training in breast imaging. General diagnostic skills are required. Associate salaried position with possible advancement. Excellent time-off. Social, cultural and recreational amenities abundant. Please send CV to Box R-082.

UT MEDICAL GROUP IN MEMPHIS—Is actively recruiting a pediatric radiologist whose primary site of practice would be LeBonheur Children's Medical Center. The successful applicant will receive an appointment with the University of Tennessee, Memphis. Applicant must be certified by or eligible for examination by the American Board of Radiology. He or she also should have completed a fellowship in pediatric radiology and either have or be eligible to sit for the certificate of added qualification in pediatric radiology. An interest in neuroradiology is particularly desirable. Minorities, women and individuals with disabilities are encouraged to apply. UT Medical Group is an equal employment opportunity/title IX/section 504/ADA affirmative action employer. Send curriculum vitae to Robert E. Gold, MD, Chair, Department of Radiology, The University of Tennessee, Memphis, 800 Madison Ave, Memphis, TN 38163.

ALLEGHENY UNIVERSITY OF THE HEALTH SCIENCES AT HAHNEMANN AND MCP—The Department of Radiology at AUHS seeks a Board certified, fellowship trained neuroradiologist. Faculty rank will be commensurate with experience. AUHS is an equal opportunity employer. Interested applicants send CV to Allegheny University of the Health Sciences/HU, F.Y. Tsai, MD, FACR, Department of Radiology/MS 206, Broad & Vine Sts, Philadelphia, PA 19102.

ALLEGHENY UNIVERSITY OF THE HEALTH SCIENCES AT HAHNEMANN AND MCP—The Department of Radiology at AUHS seeks a Board certified, fellowship trained interventional radiologist. Faculty rank will be commensurate with experience. AUHS is an equal opportunity employer. Interested applicants send CV to Allegheny University of the Health Sciences/HU, F.Y. Tsai, MD, FACR, Department of Radiology/MS 206, Broad & Vine Sts, Philadelphia, PA 19102.

ALLEGHENY UNIVERSITY OF THE HEALTH SCIENCES AT HAHNEMANN AND MCP—The Department of Radiology at AUHS seeks a Board certified, fellowship trained general diagnostic radiologist. Faculty rank will be commensurate with experience. AUHS is an equal opportunity employer. Interested applicants send CV to Allegheny University of the Health Sciences/HU, F.Y. Tsai, MD, FACR, Department of Radiology/MS 206, Broad & Vince Sts, Philadelphia, PA 19102.

ALLEGHENY UNIVERSITY OF THE HEALTH SCIENCES AT HAHNEMANN AND MCP—The Department of Radiology at AUHS seeks a Board certified, fellowship trained body imager, MRI, CT, US. Faculty rank to commensurate with experience. AUHS is an equal opportunity employer. Please send CV to Allegheny University of the Health Sciences, F.Y. Tsai, MD, FACR, Department of Radiology/MS 206, Board & Vine Sts, Philadelphia, PA 19102.

PEDIATRIC RADIOLOGIST—KK Women's and Children's Hospital (KKH) has an opening for a fellowship trained pediatric radiologist to join four full-time staff members. Requirements include Board certification/FRCR or equivalent, and at least 1-year's pediatric radiology fellowship experience (the latter can be arranged). Compensation and rank will be commensurate with experience and qualifications. KKH is the newest (1997) and largest women's and children's hospital in Singapore, performing 75,000 examinations/year. Please send current curriculum vitae and photograph to Manager, Human Resource Department, KK Women's and Children's Hospital, 100 Bukit Timah Rd, Singapore 229899. Enquiries Dr Anne Tan Kendrick, *annetan@kkh.com.sg* or fax 65-394-2254.

A LARGE PRIVATE RADIOLOGY GROUP—In the hill country of central Texas seeks an ABR certified radiologist. The practice includes nine hospitals and 13 clinics. Must have skills in general radiology, mammography, ultrasound, CT and nuclear medicine. Interested persons should send their CVs to Thomas Fletcher, MD, PO Box 4099, Austin, TX 78765 or fax 512-795-5122 or e-mail *ARAadmin@eden.com.*

THE DEPARTMENT OF RADIOLOGY OF SUNY SCHOOL OF MEDICINE AT STONY BROOK—Is seeking a fourth interventional radiologist for an increasing range and volume of procedures at University Hospital, a 540-bed tertiary care center on the highly desirable north shore of Long Island, 60 miles from New York City. Highly competitive salary. Send CV to John A. Ferretti, MD, Chief, Division of Interventional Radiology and Special Procedures, Department of Radiology School of Medicine, Health Sciences Center, Level 4, State University of New York at Stony Brook, Stony Brook, NY 11794-8460. SUNY, Stony Brook is an affirmative action/equal opportunity employer.

VASCULAR/INTERVENTIONAL FULL-TIME POSITION—Private practice, partnership position. Two tertiary care hospitals, 900-beds, 1,800+ procedures/year. There are 21 diagnostic radiologists and four radiation oncologist seeking fellowship trained interventionalist competent in vascular access and magnetic resonance angiography. Some general radiology required. Practice in Sioux Falls, SD, called by Money Magazine in 1992, "the best place to live in America." Forward curriculum vitae to Mr Gerald Larson, Medical X-Ray Center, PC, 1417 S Minnesota Ave, Sioux Falls, SD 57105.

SPECIALIZED MEDICAL CENTER, RIYADH, KINGDOM OF SAUDI ARABIA—A large multispecialty medical group practice which involves a state-of-the-art imaging service and day surgery center seeks experienced Board certified radiologists with North American training and qualifications. A competitive benefits plan awaits the physicians selected. Interested physicians should send CV, certificates and references to fax 966-1-419-1614 or e-mail address *smcltd @khaleej.net.bh* to the attention of Michael Wilson, FACHE, Chief Operating Officer, Specialized Medical Company Limited, PO Box 66548, Riyadh 11586, Kingdom of Saudi Arabia.

BODY IMAGING—Raleigh Radiology Associates in Raleigh, NC, seeks fellowship trained body imaging radiologist for partnership track position. A 10-person high volume hospital-based practice with outpatient imaging center. Must have recently completed body imaging fellowship with experience in abdominal/pelvic MRI, MRA, and interventional procedures utilizing CT and ultrasound guidance. Inquiries to Gregory C. Hinn, MD, 4020 WestChase Blvd, Suite 350, Raleigh, NC, 27607; e-mail *GCHINNRRA @AOL.COM.*

MAMMOGRAPHY/WOMEN'S IMAGING—A full-time position is available with a large private practice radiology group in Cincinnati, OH practicing at the Christ and Jewish Hospitals. Radiologist with formal training and extensive experience in mammography or women's imaging, fellowship training preferred. Experience to include stereotactic and ultrasound-guided breast biopsies. This position will be available starting in July, 1999 or earlier if available. Candidate must be Board certified. This is a partnership tract position with excellent salary and benefits. Please submit curriculum vitae and three letters of reference to Raymond C. Rost, Jr, MD, Co-CEO, Professional Radiology, Inc, 3481 Central Pkwy, Suite 200, Cincinnati, OH 45223-3300.

FACULTY POSITIONS-INTERVENTIONAL RADIOLOGY—The Department of Radiology of the University of Medicine and Dentistry of New Jersey - School of Osteopathic Medicine, seeks two BC/BE interventional radiologists to join our active department based at Kennedy Memorial Hospital-UMC, Stratford, NJ. Interventional radiology practice has expanded during the past 3-years and coverage is now provided for a second division. Two new interventional suites are under construction at our base in Stratford. Applicants must be willing to assist in other areas of the department. Benefit package and salary are competitive; faculty rank will be commensurate with experience. Please forward CV, letter outlining salary requirements and date of availability to Harvey A. Koolpe, MD, Section Chief-Interventional Radiology, Department of Radiology, UMDNJ-SOM, 40 E Laurel Rd, Suite 222, Stratford, NJ, 08083 or fax to 609-566-6256. UMDNJ is an affirmative action/equal opportunity employer.

SOUTHERN CALIFORNIA—Radiology group seeking a qualified radiologist with fellowship training in MRI, CT, body imaging, mammography, angio/interventional, musculoskeletal, and/or women's imaging. This growing practice is undergoing new and progressive upgrades, including new MRI center, ultrasound facilities, and comprehensive information systems. Clinical potential is superb. This service area of over 380,000 people has a strong patient referral base. Practice is affiliated with a 350-bed medical center. Outstanding compensation package, exceptional financial potential, and partnership option. Abundant cultural, educational, and recreational amenities. Contact Michael Kirschner, American Medical Consultants, Inc, 800-519-4868, fax 954-370-1341; e-mail *amcfl@bellsouth.net.*

SECTION HEAD- NEURORADIOLOGY - BOSTON UNIVERSITY—Boston University School of Medicine/Boston Medical Center seeks an individual to serve as Section Head of Neuroradiology. Boston Medical Center is a large integrated healthcare system performing approximately 250,000 exams per year with a full range of advanced imaging capability including three helical CT scanners, two advanced high field MRI systems, and networked PACS technology. The Department of Radiology has a strong commitment to clinical research. Candidates with a record of accomplishment in academics will be preferred. Administrative and teaching responsibilities are included with the position. Board certification in diagnostic radiology and full Massachusetts state license are required. Salary and academic rank negotiable. Please forward curriculum vitae to E. Kent Yucel, MD, Chair, Neuroradiology Search Committee, Department of Radiology, Boston Medical Center, 88 E Newton St, Boston, MA 02118.

THE DEPARTMENT OF RADIOLOGY OF THE UNIVERSITY OF MISSOURI-KANSAS CITY—Is seeking a staff radiologist with subspecialty training or interest in musculoskeletal radiology, GI/GU, mammography or ultrasound. Contact Dr Martin L. Goldman; 816-556-3926. EOE.

WISCONSIN (SE) - DIAGNOSTIC RADIOLOGIST OPPORTUNITY—A six-member radiology group seeking BE/BC radiologist. Practice includes general radiology, nuclear medicine, ultrasound, CT, MRI, mammography, and special procedures in hospital and clinic environments. Please contact William Brauer, MD, 2420 Pasadena Blvd, Wauwatosa, WI 53226, phone 414-334-8344 or fax 414-334-8293.

SEATTLE AREA, GENERAL RADIOLOGIST—Puget Sound based Radia Medical Imaging, a 34-member radiologist practice serving five hospitals, one large multi-specialty clinic and various outpatient radiology sites, is seeking a Board certified general radiologist with cross-sectional imaging expertise for "nighthawk" position. Candidates with fellowship training are preferred. Implementation of 24-hour emergency services coverage via a teleradiology network and elevated exam volumes have increased the need for radiologists. If you are interested in 1) working with a progressive practice, 2) living in an environment that allows access to a multitude of metropolitan and outdoor activities, please forward your curriculum vitae to Sanjiv Parikh, MD, c/o Cheryl West, Radia Medical Imaging, 728 134th St, SW #120, Everett, WA 98204; fax 425-297-6250.

EVENING/WEEKEND DIAGNOSTIC RADIOLOGISTS—Midwest group seeking Board certified (eligible) individuals to rotate coverage. General, CT, US, nuclear medicine skills needed. Basic angio helpful. Salaried position; 810-412-9944 ask for Judi.

DIAGNOSTIC RADIOLOGIST, SEATTLE—Group Health Permanente currently has two openings available. We are well-established, physician managed, multi-specialty group recently affiliated with the Kaiser Permanente system. Currently seeking radiologist with a fellowship in nuclear medicine. Candidate should have ultrasound, mammography, CT and body MRI experience. Also, seeking an interventional radiologist who has an interest in body imaging, CT, ultrasound and body MRI. For further information, call 800-543-9323 or fax CV and cover letter to 206-448-6191.

MRI RADIOLOGIST—Large physician outpatient multispecialty clinic seeking fellowship trained radiologist to head up beginning MRI services. Candidate should be fellowship trained in MRI, body imaging, or neuroradiology but realize position involves no angio/interventional work. Will join three general radiologists. Must be willing to participate in all imaging modalities (except mammography). No call at present and this is an equal partnership track position. Fax CV and cover letter in confidence to Robin Baltimore, Physician Recruitment; 704-344-2619.

CARDIOVASCULAR AND INTERVENTIONAL RADIOLOGIST—The State University of New York/Health Science Center at Brooklyn seeks a Board certified/eligible radiologist with fellowship training in interventional radiology for a faculty position. The institution is a 1,300 bed facility, including the Kings County, the State University, and the Brooklyn Veterans Hospitals. The medical center performs approximately 2,000 diagnostic and interventional procedures including angioplasty, TIPS, embolization, caval filters, covered stents, gastrointestinal, genitourinary, and pulmonary interventions. There are five new digital vascular rooms (three Philips, one Siemens, and one GE). Research time and facilities are available. Rank and salary are commensurate with qualifications. Curriculum vitae should be addressed to Joshua A. Becker, MD, SUNY Health Science Center at Brooklyn, Department of Radiology, 450 Clarkson Ave, Brooklyn, NY 11203; 718-270-1603. An EO/AA.

INTERVENTIONAL RADIOLOGIST—Well-established group in southern Oregon seeks fellowship trained, Board certified interventionalist to join busy practice of 13 members in a regional referral center. Expertise needed in both vascular and non-vascular studies, but proficiency expected in other modalities of radiology. Generous compensation package with 2-years to partnership. Outstanding lifestyle with numerous cultural and recreational activities available in a beautiful area. Send a current CV to Seth M. Hofstetter, MD, 842 E Main St, Medford, OR 97504.

MRI-ANGIOGRAPHY OPPORTUNITY—Department of Veterans Affairs, Central Texas Veterans Health Care System (CTVHCS), in Temple, TX in affiliation with Texas A&M Health Science Center has an immediate position for BE/BC radiologist with experience or recent training in MRI and angiography to work at Temple, TX. The position will include some general radiology and teaching of residents/medical students. Applicants should be qualified for academic appointment. Citizenship or permanent resident status required. Excellent benefits package. Competitive salary. Central Texas enjoys moderate climate, recreational and cultural activities. No state income tax and is ideally located between Dallas and Austin. Fax CV to Mary Doerfler, Physician Recruiter, CTVHCS, 1901 S First St, Temple, TX 76504; fax 254-899-4007, voice 254-899-4049. Applicants are subject to drug testing. Equal opportunity employer.

IF YOU WANT TO MAKE A DIFFERENCE AND SERVE IN A CARING COMMUNITY—Wallace Thomson Hospital has an immediate need for a staff radiologic technologist. Registered or registry eligible in SC, with 2+-years experience in the acute care setting. ACLS, NALS and PALS cert pref to serve a rural 143-bed hospital, near the big cities, in the beautiful foothills of SC. Hospital offers attractive, competitive salary generous package of fringe benefits plus sign on bonus, shift and weekend differentials. If interested in a pastoral environment without the traffic, fax your resume to Human Resource Director, Wallace Thomson Hospital, PO Box 789, Union, SC 29379; fax 864-429-2653. EOE\M\F\H\V.

LARGE STABLE MINNEAPOLIS BASED PRIVATE PRACTICE—Radiology group seeks skilled mammographer to assist with expanding full service breast centers. Radiologist must be certified by the American Board of Radiology. Fellowship training in mammography is desired. Duties would include approximately one-half time spent doing full service mammography including stereotactic and ultrasound guided core biopsies. The remainder of the time would be spent providing coverage as a general radiologist in other areas of the practice. Interested parties should send curriculum vitae to Steven J. Miller, MD, at the following address Consulting Radiologists, Ltd, Abbott Northwestern Hospital, Radiology Department, 800 E. 28th St, Minneapolis, MN 55407; phone 612-863-4261; fax 612-863-3587; website *http://www.medi-maging.com.*

THE DEPARTMENT OF RADIOLOGY, VIRGINIA COMMONWEALTH UNIVERSITY, MEDICAL COLLEGE OF VIRGINIA, RICHMOND, VA—Seeks candidates for several faculty positions in diagnostic radiology. These include positions in musculoskeletal/emergency radiology, angiography/interventional radiology, and abdominal imaging. ABR certification or eligibility required. Fellowship training and interest in teaching and research are preferred. MCV Hospital is a 1,058-bed facility and a level 1 trauma center. Individuals should have experience working in a culturally diverse environment. Academic rank and salary commensurate with experience. For position description, or to submit CV, write or phone B.J. Manaster, MD, PhD, Department of Radiology, PO Box 980470, Richmond, VA 23298-0470; 804-828-6600; fax 804-828-6129. VCU/MCV is an equal opportunity/affirmative action employer. Women, minorities, and persons with disabilities are encouraged to apply.

Nuclear Medicine

Marshfield Clinic, one of the nation's most respected and recognized integrated health care systems is seeking to replace a retiring nuclear medicine physician.

We desire a BC/BE radiologist, fellowship trained in nuclear medicine. The successful candidate will practice at the main campus in Marshfield and at the adjacent 524-bed hospital.

As a 540 physician multispecialty group, Marshfield Clinic is at the forefront of today's medical practice and offers physician specialists a stimulating opportunity for clinical practice, teaching and research. Family focus lifestyle, four-season recreational activities and an excellent compensation package further enhance this outstanding opportunity.

Interested candidates may send their curriculum vitae and three letters of reference to Timothy L. Swan, M.D., Chairman, Department of Radiology, Marshfield Clinic, 1000 North Oak Avenue, Marshfield, WI 54449. Telephone: 1-800-782-8581, extension 93474. Fax: (715) 387-5240.

MARSHFIELD CLINIC

SORRY, NOT A HEALTH PROFESSIONAL SHORTAGE AREA
An Equal Opportunity/Affirmative Action Employer m/f/h/v

Radiologist

Gundersen Lutheran is seeking a board certified/board eligible Radiologist who has completed a fellowship in Magnetic Resonance Imaging to add to our rapidly expanding department. A new Siemens 1.5 T Vision unit and open system have just recently been installed.

Gundersen Lutheran is a large multi-specialty group practice with over 320 physicians located in La Crosse, WI. It's main campus is attached to a 402 bed acute care hospital. The Gundersen Lutheran system includes 36 regional community clinics based throughout western Wisconsin, eastern Minnesota and northeastern Iowa. Gundersen Lutheran is a modern state-of-the-art facility that has a service area for a population base of over 530,000. Gundersen Lutheran is also the designated western campus of the University of Wisconsin Medical School.

La Crosse, Wisconsin, nestled between towering bluffs, is located where the Mississippi, La Crosse, and Black Rivers merge. The area was untouched by the glaciers, leaving many hills and valleys. The metropolitan area of La Crosse, with its 100,000 people, offers exceptional year round opportunities for recreational activities. The area also offers outstanding public and private schools, low crime rates, and cultural activities.

We offer competitive salaries and excellent fringe benefits. Interested candidates should send a letter of application and curriculum vitae to Frank Perez-Guerra, Director, Recruitment, Retention, and Resource Planning, Gundersen Lutheran, 1836 South Avenue, La Crosse, WI 54601; or call 800-362-9567, Ext. 6325.

Gundersen Lutheran

Equal Opportunity Employer

Classified Services

SOUTH DENVER SUB-SPECIALTY RADIOLOGY GROUP—Seeks Board certified, fellowship trained body imager with extensive experience in body MRI. Experience in MR/CT angiography or cardiovascular MRI is desirable. Multiple hospital and out-patient sites. Research interests encouraged. Send CV to Marti Heck, Administrative Assistant, RIA, 3333 S. Bannock St, Suite 740, Englewood, CA 80110, or fax 303-788-6546.

SOUTH DENVER SUB-SPECIALTY RADIOLOGY GROUP—Seeks Board certified radiologist with fellowship in emergency radiology. Interventional body imaging skills are desirable. Research interests encouraged. Send CV to Marti Heck, Administrative Assistant, RIA, 3333 S. Bannock St, Suite 740, Englewood, CO, 80110, or fax 303-788-6546.

ANGIO/INTERVENTIONAL RADIOLOGIST—Allegheny University - Graduate Hospital is seeking applications for a interventional radiologist. Candidates must be eligible for or certified by the American Board of Radiology and also be eligible for or have passed the CAQ examination. Candidate must possess strong clinical skills and communication abilities. The hospital is affiliated with Allegheny University of the Health Sciences. The department offers a private practice opportunity. The hospital has strong history of excellence in gastroenterology, oncology, orthopedics and cardiology. The department is outfitted with state-of-the-art equipment. In addition, there is a free standing imaging center. Philadelphia offers numerous cultural, historical and recreational activities. Please send letter of interest and current curriculum vitae to Arthur P. Staddon, MD, Radiology Search Committee, AUH-Graduate, 1840 S St, 2nd Fl, Philadelphia, PA 19146.

RADIOLOGY DEPARTMENT CHAIRMAN—Allegheny University - Graduate Hospital is seeking applications for the Chair of the Department of Radiology. Candidates must be certified by the American Board of Radiology and should possess strong clinical skills with excellent organizational and management abilities. The hospital is affiliated with Allegheny University of the Health Sciences. The department offers a private practice opportunity. The hospital has a strong history of excellence in gastroenterology, oncology, orthopedics and cardiology. The department is outfitted with state-of-the-art equipment. In addition, there is a free-standing outpatient imaging center. Philadelphia offers numerous cultural, historical and recreational activities. Please send letter of interest and current curriculum vitae to Arthur P. Staddon, MD, Radiology Search Committee, AUH-Graduate, 1840 S St, 2nd Fl, Philadelphia, PA 19146.

DIVISION DIRECTOR, ABDOMINAL RADIOLOGY—The Department of Radiology, Emory University School of Medicine, seeks a fellowship trained abdominal radiologist for Director of the Abdominal Division. Divisional activity includes CT, US, MR, fluoroscopy, urography and imaging guided interventional procedures. Appointment will be at the academic rank of Associate Professor or Professor. Candidate must be certified by the American Board of Radiology and have significant clinical, teaching and research experience in abdominal radiology. Curriculum vitae and letter describing interest, background and qualifications should be sent to William Casarella, MD, Chairman, Department of Radiology, Emory University Hospital, 1364 Clifton Rd, NE, Atlanta, GA 30322. Phone 404-712-4996; fax 404-712-7839. EOE/AA employer.

SE MICHIGAN—Progressive group seeks Board certified body imager with special expertise in vascular ultrasound to head up ultrasound department at new suburban hospital. Practice includes busy MR center as well as general radiology. A 440-bed hospital located between Detroit and Flint, with state-of-the-art equipment. Completely filmless digital department. Partnership track is available. Generous compensation and vacation package. Send or fax CV to Eugene Brown, MD, 10775 S Saginaw St, Suite D, Grand Blanc, MI 48439; fax 810-695-6615.

EVENING/WEEKEND DIAGNOSTIC RADIOLOGISTS—Midwest group seeking Board certified (eligible) individuals to rotate coverage. General, CT, US, nuclear medicine skills needed. Basic angio helpful. Salaried position; 810-412-9944 ask for Judi.

Radiology Positions - Mayo Health System

A Mayo Health System regional radiology practice, which has recently been established in Mankato, south central Minnesota, is looking for two radiologists to join two others. Candidates should be familiar with all diagnostic imaging modalities and have skills in inverventional radiology, nuclear medicine, ultrasound or other sub-speciality of radiology.

The practice is based at the Immanuel St. Joseph's-Mayo Health System facility, a regional acute care hospital licensed for 272 beds. ISJ-MHS's Radiology Department is equipped with helical CT, MRI, two cath labs, two linear accelerators, ultrasound, nuclear, and a wide range of other diagnostic equipment. The practice provides services to several nearby communities which, together with ISJ-MHS and the Mayo Clinic Rochester Department of Radiology, are interconnected with T1 teleradiology lines. In addition, appropriate teleradiology equipment will also be installed in the radiologists' homes.

Mankato, connected to Minneapolis/St. Paul 75 miles away via a four-lane highway, has been rated as one of the most livable micropolitan areas in the United States. This attests to the high quality of life here. The local population, some 60,000 within 5 miles, is large enough to ensure a wide variety of amenities yet small enough to avoid the magnitude of serious problems common to most urban and some suburban areas. We offer a very low crime rate; excellent schools, including two National Schools of Excellence; several colleges; outstanding four-season recreational activities; and many other fine quality-of-life characteristics. This part of Minnesota has a diverse business and industrial base and is economically stable.

Interested candidates should FAX or e-mail a CV and cover letter to: Frank Ellesmere, Director, Physician Placement. FAX: 507-625-1847. Toll-free Tel: 800-628-3707. E-mail: ellesmere.frank@mayo.edu. General DR positions available elsewhere. See: www.isj-mhs.net

LOUISIANA - GENERAL DIAGNOSTIC RADIOLOGY—No nights, no call, no weekends, no holidays, no pressure! Live in a wonderful community known for its horse farms and its sailing, 80 miles outside of New Orleans. Become part of a large, university trained radiology group who will be your back-up via teleradiology. Enjoy your day working with well-trained, friendly people as you build the volume, allowing you to make substantially more each year. Exceptional starting salary, pension, six weeks vacation and much more. Candidate must be service minded and Board certified. For consideration, please fax your CV and call Teresa Duggan, 733 Turnpike St, Suite 116, N Andover, MA 01845; Voice 888-950-5864, fax 978-682-9422, e-mail *tduggan@physicianjobs. com*, website *http://www.physicianjobs.com*.

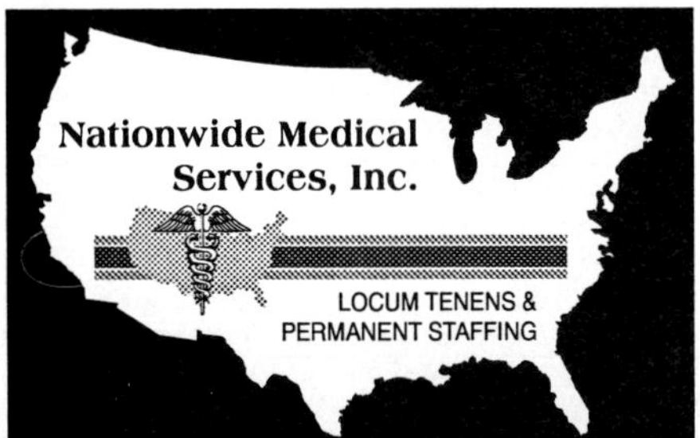

1-800-841-2291

If you're a Physician interested in Locum Tenens *or* Permanent opportunities through NATIONWIDE MEDICAL SERVICES, INC. Call Jennifer or Fax your CV to (919) 493-7763.

For information about how we can quickly and efficiently schedule your next Locum Tenens or Permanent vacancy, call Joan or Beth at 1-800-841-2291.

E-Mail Us Or Visit Our Web Page
Radiology@nationwide-med.com
www.nationwide-med.com

OREGON - GENERAL RADIOLOGIST—Wanted for job sharing position. Work 26 weeks per year. Flexible schedule. Low stress practice with up-to-date equipment in pleasant SW Oregon town. No mammography/angiography; very limited interventional; average two call-backs per month. Fax CV and references to L. Taylor 541-440-1368.

DIRECTOR, BREAST IMAGING—Emory University and the Emory Clinic, Atlanta, GA, is seeking an experienced breast imager to lead a large, academic breast division. The division covers two full service sites as well as satellite screening clinics. The primary sites house nine mammography units, two stereotactic biopsy tables with digital capability, and three dedicated breast ultrasound units. MRI, PET scanning and NM also available. Primary duties are responsible for the leadership and development of all aspects of breast imaging as well as development of women's imaging in our new cancer center. Candidate should be familiar with all aspects of breast imaging and intervention. Fellowship training in breast imaging preferred; equivalent experience will be considered. Salary and rank commensurate with experience. Board certification and GA licensure required. Send CV to William Casarella, MD, Chairman, Department of Radiology, Emory University Hospital, 1364 Clifton Rd, NE, Atlanta, GA 30322. Phone 404-712-4996; fax 404-712-7839. EOE/AA employer.

NORTH FLORIDA GULF COAST—An eight man group seeks Board certified candidate with fellowship training in MRI with interest in musculoskeletal imaging. Practice includes four MRI units. Partnership track and excellent benefits. Respond to Box R-084.

FLORIDA GULF COAST GROUP—Seeks Board certified fellowship trained neuroradiologist. Practice includes both hospital and outpatient centers. Partnership track and excellent benefits. Respond to Box R-085.

BREAST RADIOLOGIST—The Department of Radiology at Indiana University School of Medicine is pleased to announce the availability of a faculty position in the Division of Breast Imaging. Candidates must be Board certified in diagnostic radiology and have fellowship training or substantial equivalent experience in breast imaging. This is a tenure track position and the successful candidate will have clinical and academic responsibilities. We seek an individual

Radiology Opportunities in Virginia

Lexington, Virginia

Metro American Radiology, a Team Health affiliate, is seeking a radiologist to join our group in Lexington, Virginia. The position involves a commitment of approximately 35 weeks per year. Candidates must be board certified and well trained in all imaging modalities, including MRI.

Lexington is a 19th century college town located in the heart of the Shenandoah Valley of Virginia. The town is rich in history and is the home of Washington and Lee University and the Virginia Military Institute.

Richlands, Virginia

Metro American Radiology, a Team Health affiliate, is seeking a full-time radiologist for a two-physician practice in Richlands, Virginia. Candidates must be board certified and comfortable with all imaging modalities, including interventional procedures.

Richlands, rich in history, is located near the Tri-Cities area of Tennessee, which includes the cities of Bristol, Kingsport and Johnson City.

Full-time benefits include malpractice coverage, medical and life insurance, a 401k retirement plan and generous CME allowance. At Team Health, we offer practice opportunities designed to preserve physician incomes and maximize quality of life in today's rapidly changing healthcare environment.

For more information on these opportunities, please call Kathryn Watson at

(800) 662-6387

or fax your CV to David Forsberg, MD
(423) 693-4064
www.team-health.com

TEAM HEALTH
Right Team, Right Now

NATIONAL UNIVERSITY HOSPITAL
SINGAPORE

Excellence Our Mission, A Commitment

The National University Hospital is a 900-bed multi-specialty teaching hospital. An opportunity exists to share in our mission of achieving excellence in patient care, medical education and research through the provision of quality patient care with state-of-the-art medical technology.

CONSULTANT/SENIOR REGISTRAR/REGISTRAR
(DIAGNOSTIC IMAGING)

Applicants must hold a basic and postgraduate medical degree registrable with the Singapore Medical Council and any of the following postgraduate qualifications:

1. FRCR
2. FRCP Canada
3. FRACR
4. American Board Certified

Commencing salary will be competitive depending on qualifications and experience. Please give full personal particulars, professional qualifications, career history and expected salary together with medical testimonials, certificate of registration, recent photograph and telephone number to:

Chairman, Medical Board
Medical Affairs Department
National University Hospital
5 Lower Kent Ridge Road
Singapore 119074

Telefax: (65)7756757 • Tel. No.: (65)7725920
Website: *http://www.nuh.com.sg* • Enquires: *leesm@nuh.com.sg*

Closing date: September 1998

Classified Services

who has a demonstrated research interest and has clinical skills in the following areas; screening and diagnostic mammography, breast sonography, image-guided needle localization and core needle biopsy using ultrasound and stereotactic guidance. Our division consists of two experienced breast imagers and performs approximately 17,000 examinations per year. Salary and academic rank will be commensurate with experience and qualifications. Interested applicants should send their curriculum vitae to Handel E. Reynolds, MD, Department of Radiology, Indiana University Hospital, Room 0279, 550 N University Blvd, Indianapolis, IN 46202-5253. Indiana University is an equal opportunity/affirmative action employer.

RADIOLOGIST NEEDED IN IOWA—Join outstanding group of five radiologists within a MSG. Perform all aspects of general diagnostic radiology. Fellowship training desired in either nuclear medicine or body imaging. Radiologist with experience/interest in assisting the department develop the area of nuclear medicine, or ultrasound and non-neuro MR will be strongly considered. Safe, Midwestern community of 200,000. Excellent schools! The arts and universities available in the community. Call Germaine Lorbert, 800-765-3055, ID#5957RA, fax 314-726-3009, e-mail *glorbert@cejka.com.*

THE DIVISION OF DIAGNOSTIC IMAGING OF THE UNIVERSITY OF TEXAS MD ANDERSON CANCER CENTER—Is recruiting for a Board certified, fellowship trained breast imaging radiologist at the Assistant Professor level for appointment effective July, 1998. Applicants must be committed to patient care, teaching and research. Approximately 16,000 breast related radiological examinations are performed in the Section of Breast Imaging and 2,500 in the Section of Ultrasound. A new breast diagnostic Center opened in April, 1997 and is well-equipped with four mammography units, three US units, a stereotactic prone biopsy table and a pathology laboratory. A new mobile screening mammography van was acquired in October, 1996. The division is staffed by 30 radiologists, 10 of whom are involved in breast imaging. Letters of interest should be addressed to Carol B. Stelling, MD, The University of Texas MD Anderson Cancer Center, Division of Diagnostic Imaging, Box 57, 1515 Holcombe Blvd, Houston, TX 77030. UT MD Anderson Cancer Center is an equal/opportunity affirmative action employer. Women and minorities are encouraged to apply.

FAIRFAX RADIOLOGICAL CONSULTANTS, PC—Is a 30-member quality oriented and aggressive diagnostic radiology private practice group with six full service outpatient imaging centers and a tertiary 650-bed hospital in northern Virginia (Washington, DC metropolitan area). Fairfax Radiological Consultants, PC is actively seeking several fellowship trained general radiologists with a broad range of skills and experience in CT imaging, ultrasound, and mammography. Fellowship or junior academic staff experience in body imaging or women's imaging activities preferred. Openings are available immediately and are partnership tract positions

BODY IMAGER

The Department of Radiology of the Roswell Park Cancer Institute, Buffalo, New York, seeks a Board-Certified, fellowship-trained, Body Imager to fill an unexpected entry level (Assistant Professor) opening, commencing 8/1/98. Familiarity with all body imaging modalities — MR, CT, ultrasound, and fluoroscopy — is required, as well as a high comfort level with a wide variety of CT and ultrasound-guided percutaneous interventional procedures. Roswell Park is a SUNY Buffalo affiliate, with academic appointments for its staff, protected academic time, and a highly competitive salary/benefits package. The department includes state-of-the-art imagining technology in a new $240 million hospital/institute complex. Please fax cover letter and CV to **Zachary D. Grossman, M.D., Chairman, Department of Radiology, 716-845-8759**. RPCI and the University at Buffalo are M/F/H/V Affirmative Action Employers.

ROSWELL PARK CANCER INSTITUTE

100 YEARS

PATIENT CARE · RESEARCH · EDUCATION

DIAGNOSTIC RADIOLOGIST
GROWING MIDWEST CITY

16-physician radiology group, income potential in the top 5%, 13 weeks vacation/CME, partnership opportunity. Premier radiology group seeks a BC/BE radiologist to join a rapidly expanding practice. Position offers a full range of diagnostic radiology services with state-of-the-art equipment including both high field and open M.R.I. units, DEXA, and teleradiology. In this position you will join 16 board certified colleagues providing expertise in all areas of radiology. A fellowship in one of the following subspecialty areas is required: Musculoskeletal, MRI, Mammography, or Nuclear Medicine.

Contact:
Barb Kennington, 1-800-765-3055
ID#: 5865RA Fax: 314-726-3009
e-mail: bkennington@cejka.com

which offer a highly competitive salary and benefits package. Please submit your curriculum vitae with letters of recommendation to Fairfax Radiological Consultants, PC, 2722 Merrilee Dr, Suite 230, Fairfax, VA 22031 or fax to 703-698-2176.

NIGHT RADIOLOGISTS—Bay Imaging Consultants Medical Group, Inc, a large San Francisco Bay area private practice radiology group with multiple outpatient and hospital sites, is seeking night radiologists for the night rotation. The night rotation is comprised of 12-hour rotations from 7:00pm to 7:00am. Must be Board certified. Competitive salary. Start date as soon as possible. Please submit your CV, a cover letter and the names of three references to Human Resources, 175 Lennon Ln, Suite 100, Walnut Creek, CA 94598. EOE.

BOARD CERTIFIED RADIOLOGISTS—Rapidly growing group in northeastern Pennsylvania seeks two aggressive Board certified radiologists with fellowship trainining in nuclear medicine and body imaging/MRI. State-of-the-art equipment including: GE LCA digital angio suite, GE Spiral CT with SUN workstation, two digital fluoroscopy suites, ATL HDI 5000 and Ultramark 9, Siemans Dual Head E Cam, fixed GE MRI, stereotactic breast. Outstanding opportunity to practice general radiology and to build the practice in your area of expertise. Excellent financial package with early partnership. Address inquiries to David Fontaine, MD, Chairman, 717-621-4420. Fax CV to 717-621-4582.

RADIOLOGIST—Private progressive hospital based practice located in South central Kentucky is seeking Board certified. The practice has multiple hospital and outpatient locations, but is linked by teleradiography. The facilities offer state-of-the-art technology. The practice includes MRI, ultrasound, angiography, CT, mammography, nuclear medicine, and general radiology. The position offers an excellent compensation package. Please provide a curriculum vitae and names of references to Mona Wood, Physician Recruiter, 800 Park St, PO Box 9867, Bowling Green, KY 42102; fax 502-745-1518.

INTERVENTIONAL RADIOLOGIST—The Department of Diagnostic Radiology and Nuclear Medicine of Rush Medical College, Chicago, IL is seeking two vascular/interventional radiologists. The position will include teaching responsibilities at Rush-Presbyterian-St. Luke's Medical Center, a 600-bed acute and tertiary care facility. The section performs approximately 6,000 vascular and non-vascular interventions per year. In this private practice group in an academic teaching hospital, CAQ eligibility is required. Interested parties should contact Terence A.S. Matalon, MD, Rush Presbyterian-St. Luke's Medical Center, 1653 W Congress Pkwy, Chicago, IL 60612. Rush-Presbyterian-St. Luke's Medical Center is an equal opportunity/affirmative action employer. Women and minority candidates are encouraged to apply.

TWO RADIOLOGIST - CONNECTICUT Fellowship-trained radiologist with CAQ eligibility and fellowship trained body imaging specialist sought by growing, progressive, subspecialty-oriented group of 15 radiologists. Yale affiliated, community hospital-based private practice with residents and separate outpatient facilities. Position available now, but will wait for right person. Responsibilities divided between subspecialty area and general office and hospital radiology. Excellent opportunities with expectation for partnership. Send CV to Alan Kaye, MD, 777 Commerce Dr, Fairfield, CT 06432, or fax to 203-384-4363.

MRA AND FMRI ARE ESSENTIAL—Interest in research and teaching are important and opportunities exist to work with MS, alzeheimers disease, movement disorder, epilepsy, and stroke centers. Faculty rank dependent on publication and academic accomplishments. Send curriculum vitae to Michael S. Huckman, MD, Director of Neuroradiology, Rush-Presbyterian-St. Luke's Medical Center, 1653 W Congress Pkwy, Chicago, IL 60612. Phone 312-942-5781, fax 312-942-2114, e-mail *mhuckman@rush.edu*. RPSLMC is an AA/EOE employer.

LOVELACE HEALTH SYSTEMS - ALBUQUERQUE, NM—A 300-physician multi-specialty practice, 14-member radiology department seeks two BC/BE radiologists: one interventional radiologist, CAQ preferred, and one fellowship trained body imaging radiologist. Comprehensive benefits package and state-of-the-art equipment. Contact Cheryl DeVita, 222 S Central Ave, Suite 400, St. Louis, MO 63105. Phone 800-678-7858, ID#5869RA, fax 314-726-0026, e-mail *cdevita@cejka.com*.

INTERVENTIONALIST NEEDED—Looking for young superstar interventionalist to earn his/her way into full partnership in the premier radiology group in the mid-Hudson Valley. Maintain skills in all aspects of imaging with state-of-the-art equipment and expert colleagues while helping to lead the interventional department of a 300-bed tertiary care hospital. Many outpatient offices also including multiple MRI/CT sites. Send CV or call V. Gaines, MD, Department Imaging, Vassar Brothers Hospital, Reade Place, Poughkeepsie, NY 12601; 914-431-5644.

IMMEDIATE OPENING FOR TWO RADIOLOGISTS WITH CROSS-SECTIONAL IMAGING BACKGROUND, FELLOWSHIP PREFERRED BUT NOT A REQUIREMENT—Large progressive group near metropolitan Chicago in northwest Indiana. Covering four hospitals, several clinics and a free-standing imaging center, four MRIs, several CTs, state-of-the-art ultrasound and in-home PET scanner. Please send CV to Radiologic Associates of Northwest Indiana, Inc, 825 E. Lincolnway, Valparaiso, IN 46383 or call Dr James Forde at 219-464-4891.

NEURORADIOLOGIST—Georgetown University has a unique opportunity to join an academic radiology group in Washington, DC. The neuroradiology section includes four faculty and four fellows. Excellent collaborative research opportunities exist with the Georgetown Imaging Science and Information Systems group, the Georgetown Institute for Cognitive and Computational Sciences, and the neighboring National Institutes of Health in Bethesda, MD. The candidate should exhibit special interest and knowledge in neuro MRI. Experience with non-anatomic or functional MRI and background in research are desirable. Working skills in traditional invasive techniques (diagnostic angiography, myelography, etc), Board certification, and a certificate of added qualification in neuroradiology (or eligibility) are required. The Department of Radiology operates two 1.5T Siemens magnets (Vision), three advanced GE CT scanners (two helical) and a new Siemens Neurostar angio/interventional suite. The position is expected to be filled on or before July 1, 1999. Interested parties should contact Michael J. Pentecost, MD, Professor and Chairman, Department of Radiology, Georgetown University Medical Center, 3800 Reservoir Rd, NW, Washington, DC, e-mail *pentecom@gunet.georgetown.edu*, fax 202-687-1804.

DIAGNOSTIC RADIOLOGIST, ISLAND OF GUAM—Immediate opening available in a recently opened private imaging office. GE spiral CT, Accuson sonography and general radiography support a full cancer treatment center as well as outpatient referrals. Opportunity for cross coverage with an affiliated Maui, HI based diagnostic radiology group. Partnership track, apartment and auto provided. Please send CV and direct inquiries ro Mr Nick Gladdis, Administrative Director, 221 Mahalani St, Wailuku, HI 96793; phone 808-242-2054, fax 808-242-1940, e-mail *mrc@maui.net*.

MAUI, HI—Hospital based radiology group seeks Board certified radiologist for evening and night coverage position. This 200-bed facility includes diagnostic radiology, interventional/angiography, nuclear medicine, computerized tomography, ultrasound and magnetic resonance. Basic angiography/interventional skills are a plus. As part of the interview process candidates will be required to spend a minimum of one week in locum tenens position in the hospital environment. Please send CV and direct inquiries to Mr Nick Gladdis, Administrative Director, 221 Mahalani St, Wailuku, HI 96793; phone 808-242-2054, fax 808-242-1940, e-mail *mrc@maui.net*.

SOUTHERN LOUISIANA—Growing community of 104,000 population is seeking a particular type of radiologist. We need a women's health specialist. Focus is to work at the Women's hospital. No MRI work involved. Primarily, breast biopsy, mammography, and CT. Call coverage 1:2 with a salary of $180,000 plus full benefits; 1-year to partnership! Great practice and community! Area has large university and metro amenities. Easy access ro LSU and New Orleans! For details, call David at 800-677-7987 or fax CV to 800-440-2676; e-mail *dbgmsg@ swbell.net*, website *www.medopps-hka.com*.

PUGET SOUND BASED RADIA MEDICAL IMAGING—A 32-member radiologist practice serving five hospitals, one large multi-specialty clinic and various outpatient radiology sites, is seeking a Board certified general radiologist with cross-sectional imaging experience. Candidates with fellowship training are preferred. Implementation of 24-hour emergency services coverage via a teleradiology network and elevated exam volumes have increased the need for radiologists. If you are interested in working with a progressive practice, developing and promoting your area of subspecialization, sharing evenings and night work rotation, and living in an environment that allows access to a multitude of metropolitan and outdoor activities, please forward your curriculum vitae to Sanjiv Parikh, MD, Radia Medical Imaging, 3822 Colby Ave, Everett, WA 98201. Fax 425-339-8322.

FLORIDA - GENERAL RADIOLOGIST—Central Florida West Coast group seeks BE/BC radiologist. Interventional fellowship and/or body imaging fellowship desirable. Competitive compensation/benefits. CVs may be faxed to 813-898-4505.

RADIOLOGIST—We are seeking two Board certified radiologists to join a rapidly growing practice in Albert Lea, MN. The practice includes general radiology and all cross sectional imaging. The practice includes a busy outpatient practice and a 110-bed hospital. Albert Lea Medical Center is part of the Mayo Health System in southern Minnesota. For consideration, send a current CV to Jeffrey P. Lotts, MD, Medical Director, 1602 Fountain St, Albert Lea, MN, 56007 or fax 507-377-4826.

SOUTH FLORIDA, IMMEDIATE OPENINGS—Desirable private practice with two hospitals in need of fellowship trained MRI radiologist, fellowship trained interventional radiologist, and a fellowship trained pediatric radiologist. The successful candidates must be willing to do general radiology as well. Excellent positions for excellent individuals. Please send CVs to fax 561-488-8347.

STAFF RADIOLOGIST, CHEST SECTION—The Department of Radiology at the Brigham and Women's Hospital and Harvard Medical School is recruiting a full-time staff radiologist for a faculty position in its chest section. Radiology is a subspecialty oriented academic department with excellent programs in clinical service, research and teaching. Outstanding high technology equipment, including digital radiography, CT fluoroscopy and interventional MR is available. Candidates should be Board certified in diagnostic radiology, completed a fellowship in thoracic radiology and demonstrate competence in all clinical aspects of thoracic radiology. Faculty rank is expected to be Instructor or Assistant Professor level. Curriculum vitae and letter describing interest, background and qualifications should be sent to Steven E. Seltzer, MD, Chairman, Department of Radiology, Brigham and Women's Hospital, 75 Francis St, Boston, MA 02115. Brigham and Women's Hospital/Harvard Medical School is an affirmative action/equal opportunity educator and employer.

PUGET SOUND BASED RADIA MEDICAL IMAGING—A 32-member radiologist practice serving five hospitals, one large multispecialty clinic and various outpatient radiology sites, is seeking a Board certified general radiologist subspecializing in nuclear medicine with Board certification. Practice at a progressive 200-bed community hospital with state-of-the-art equipment. Practice involves developing and promoting nuclear medicine, working in other areas, sharing evening and night work rotation. Live in an environment that allows access to a multitude of metropolitan and outdoor activities, good schools and cultural diversity. Please forward your CV to Sanjiv Parikh, MD, c/o Cheryl West, Radia Medical Imaging, 3822 Colby Ave, Everett, WA 98201.

ALASKA - EXCITING OPPORTUNITY—Department of Veterans Affairs (VA) Medical and Regional Office Center is seeking Board certified radiologist for the position of Chief, Radiology Service. Excellent opportunity to work in state-of-the-art teleradiology hub. Anchorage is a cosmopolitan center within a pristine wilderness, which offers boundless cultural and recreational opportunities. No state income tax, plus tax-free COLA salary supplement, (COLA may be subject to change in the future). Travel and/or relocation expenses offered. U.S. citizenship is a condition of employment. Send

RADIOLOGISTS

Group Practice in the Hudson Valley Region is seeking Board Certified Radiologists for the following positions:

- **General Radiologist with mammography expertise**
- **Radiologist with MRI Body Imaging/MRI training or Neuroradiology**
- **Interventional Radiologist**

Competitive salary with incentives and partnership track.

Please forward CVs to

Barbara Enny
Practice Administrator
PO Box 199
Jefferson Valley, NY 10535
or FAX to 914-245-8962. EOE

CV with letter of interest to Christine Swink (11CP), VA Medical and Regional Office Center, 2925 Debarr Rd, Anchorage, AK 99508; 907-257-5485 or fax 907-257-3718. Position subject to drug testing. VA is an equal opportunity employer.

GENERAL DIAGNOSTIC RADIOLOGIST—Board certified or eligible, fellowship trained a plus. Partnership tract opportunity with a five person radiology group. Candidate will possess ability to provide quality radiology services including angiography, MRI, CT, US, nuclear, mammography and general radiology. Board certification required by 2nd-year. Group provides radiology services to a 300-bed Level 1 trauma center tertiary care hospital in Bismark, ND and several rural hospitals. Bismarck is a family-centered community with numerous outdoor recreational opportunities, located on the Missouri River. Excellent school system with both private and public schools. Generous benefit package, competitive starting salary and partnership opportunity. Please send CV to Douglas Peterson, MD, Central Dakota Radiologists, PC, 810 E Rosser Ave, Suite 201, Bismarck, ND 58501. Phone 701-224-7480; fax 701-224-8320; e-mail *Cendakrad@aol.com.*

RADIOLOGIST - OPENINGS IN NORTH GEORGIA, NORTH FLORIDA, SOUTH CAROLINA, NORTH CAROLINA, NEW MEXICO, AND TEXAS—Community based outpatient imaging company needs BC radiologist for new state-of-the-art imaging centers, MRI and CT, Monday through Friday, excellent compensation and benefits. Send CV to HR Manager, 3295 River Exchange Dr, Suite 275, Norcross, GA 30092, or call Mark Rooney at 800-849-3713 or fax CV to 770-734-9652.

LEXINGTON, KY—BC/BE diagnostic radiologist for salaried position in a six person radiology group. No weekend, on-call or holiday responsibilities. Expertise in general radiology, mammography, CT, nuclear medicine, and ultrasound required. Interest in women's imaging is a plus. MRI and angiography are a plus, but not required. Competitive salary and benefits. Please send CV to Scott Stevens, MD, Radiology, 1740 S Nicholasville Rd, Lexington, KY 40503.

ABR CERTIFIED RADIOLOGIST—Needed for nighthawk coverage in Raleigh, NC metropolitan area. Responsibilities include general, nuclear medicine, CT, ultrasound, and basic MR. Excellent salary, generous benefits and time off. Please send CV to William H. Johnson, Administrator at Wake Radiology, PO Box 19366, Raleigh, NC 27619.

A 14-MEMBER RADIOLOGY GROUP—Seeking two Board certified radiologists: one with fellowship training in musculoskeletal or MRI with strong general radiology skills; and one general radiologist. Please reply to B.L. Storm, MD, PO Box 12219, Tallahassee, FL 32317-2219. Office telephone 850-942-4497; fax 850-942-1610.

NEW ORLEANS, LA—Outstanding opportunity for Board certified radiologist with recent fellowship in interventional radiology. Practice includes state-of-the-art interventional suite, 1.5T MRI, CT/US, mammography, nuclear medicine and general diagnostic. Candidate will spend 50% of time in interventional and rest in imaging and diagnostic radiology. Progressive group in acute care hospital and one outpatient clinic with teleradiology call coverage. Generous salary and benefits with opportunity for full partnership. Generous salary and benefits with opportunity for full partnership. Please reply with CV to PO Box 1827, Harvey, LA 70058.

VASCULAR/INTERVENTIONAL RADIOLOGIST—The Department of Radiology at Saint Louis University Health Sciences Center is seeking an ABR eligible or certified, fellowship trained vascular/interventional radiologist for a full-time, faculty position open in July, 1998. The rapidly expanding practice has a case load including diagnostic angiography (including pulmonary angiography), angioplasty, central venous access, thrombolysis, embolization, IVC Filter placement, biliary and uroradiology, TIPS, percutaneous biopsy and percutaneous gastrostomy. A broad range of teaching and research opportunities is available. Appointment is anticipated at the Assistant Professor level. For information, contact Thomas Bocchini, MD, Chief, Section of Interventional Radiology, Department of Radiology, Saint Louis University Health Sciences Center, 3635 Vista at Grand Boulevard, St. Louis, MO 63110-0250. Phone 314-268-5784; fax 314-268-5116. Saint Louis University Health Sciences Center is an equal opportunity employer M/F/D/V.

THE RADIOLOGY GROUP—Affiliated with the Stratford General Hospital and environs is seeking a radiologist to join their group. The successful individual must have experience with numerous modalities including ultrasound, mammography, CT and interventional procedures. The interested candidate should send his/her CV to Dr. Yale A. Erenberg, Radiologist in Chief, c/o Department of Medical Imaging, Stratford General Hospital, 46 General Hospital Dr, Stratford, Ontario N5A 2Y6. Phone 519-272-8210 ext 2278, fax 519-272-8221.

ASHEVILLE, NC— A third board certified radiologist is needed for night, weekend day, and holiday call coverage of 21 person group practice in major referal center. Salaried position with excellent time off and benefits package in beautiful mountain vacation area. Send CV to Ms. Sue Spivey, P.O. Box 2959, Asheville, NC 28802

PENNSYLVANIA—Growing practice in community hospital is seeking a Board certified general radiologist with MRI skills. University town with excellent living and year round recreational activities. Send CV to T.J. Heromin, MD, PO Box 488, Bloomsburg, PA 17815.

DIAGNOSTIC RADIOLOGIST—Broadly trained general radiologist needed to join two others in hospital practice in Fremont, OH, 35 miles from Toledo. Practice performs approximately 33,000 studies per year, including MRI, CT, US, nuclear, and interventional/angio. Fellowship training is not required but is welcome. Additional coverage in an outpatient center in Toledo is also required. Generous vacation allowance and compensation package. Please send CV to Dr. Daniel Dessner, Toledo Radiological Associates, Inc, 4841 Monroe Street, Suite 103, Toledo, OH 43623, or fax to 419-479-6078.

HARTFORD, CT—Large, private radiology group in Hartford, CT is seeking well-trained individual for part or full-time position. The practice includes Hartford Hospital (a large community hospital with Level 1 Trauma Center with an independent radiology residency program) and three suburban offices. Please send CV to Steven K. Sussman, MD, Jefferson X-Ray Group, 85 Seymour St, Suite 200, Hartford, CT 06106.

Position Sought

EXPERIENCED ABR-CERTIFIED—Fellowship-trained (neuroradiology), ASNR senior member seeks full-time position. Neuroradiology, general radiology, or interventional or some combination. Administrative experience. Available 1/1/99. Prefer midwest, but other locations considered. Reply to Box R-083.

Fellowships

ACCREDITED FELLOWSHIPS IN PEDIATRIC RADIOLOGY—The Department of Radiology, Children's Hospital and Harvard Medical School, Boston, MA, offers a 2-year accredited (residency review committee for radiology of ACGME) fellowship in pediatric radiology beginning July 1, 2000. There are 1-year pediatric neuroradiology and pediatric vascular/interventional fellowship programs also available. Children's Hospital is a 350-bed institution and performs over 112,000 radiological examinations annually in one of the largest pediatric medical centers in North America. The department has 24 faculty pediatric radiologists, three PhD research faculty, one physicist, 10 pediatric radiology fellows, six neuroradiology fellows, and many resident trainees. Up to five pediatric radiology, one pediatric neuroradiology, and one pediatric vascular/interventional fellowship positions are available annually. Training includes all aspects of pediatric imaging including neonatal radiology, neuroimaging, musculoskeletal radiology, cardiovascular and thoracic imaging, abdominal imaging, oncologic imaging, ultrasonography, nuclear medicine, computed tomography, MRI, and vascular/interventional radiology. The department has an extremely active clinical service with state-of-the-art equipment as follows: two digital fluoroscopy rooms; five ultrasound units with Doppler and color-flow Doppler capabilities; planar and SPECT gamma cameras; two GE High-Speed Advantage Helical CT scanners, two 1.5T GE MRI systems with spectroscopy and MR angiography; and two vascular/interventional suites with digital imaging. The department provides extensive academic support; the Stem Memorial Radiology Library and a departmental librarian are valuable resources. The fellowship provides a broad clinical experience in pediatric radiology as well as numerous opportunities to participate in clinical, basic, and health services research. There are opportunities for collaborative research efforts at Children's Hospital, other Harvard teaching hospitals, Harvard Medical School, and the Harvard School of Public Health. Candidates must be Board certified or Board qualified in diagnostic radiology and must obtain a Massachusetts medical license. Salary and fringe benefits are competitive. Applications are due no later than November 1, 1998 with interviews scheduled during the fall of 1998. Many career opportunities are available in pediatric radiology. To receive more information about careers in pediatric radiology in general or the fellowships at Children's Hospital in particular, please contact Carlo Buonomo, MD, Director, Fellowship Program, Children's Hospital, Department of Radiology, 300 Longwood Ave, Boston, MA 02115; 617-355-6496. Children's Hospital and Harvard Medical School are affirmative action/ equal opportunity employers.

BREAST IMAGING FELLOWSHIP—University of Illinois College of Medicine at Peoria and the Susan G. Komen Breast Center an affiliate of OSF St. Francis Medical Center, an advanced care, teaching hospital, are offering a 1-year intensive fellowship in all aspects of breast imaging, beginning July 1, 1999. Please contact S. Horatio Slawson, MD, at 309-683-6626 or Karol Burton at 309-683-6623 or c/o The Susan G. Komen Breast Center, 4911 Executive Dr, Peoria, IL 61615 for information and an application packet.

ACCREDITED FELLOWSHIP IN PEDIATRIC RADIOLOGY—The Division of Pediatric Radiology, Rainbow Babies and Childrens Hospital of the University Hospitals of Cleveland/Case Western Reserve University, Cleveland, OH, is offering a 1-year fellowship in pediatric radiology. Rainbow Babies and Childrens Hospital is a 244-bed institution. Over 45,000 pediatric radiological examinations are performed yearly. The fellowship provides a broad clinical experience with training in all aspects of pediatric imaging including radiography, fluoroscopy, sonography, computed tomography, nuclear medicine, MRI and interventional radiology. The fellowship also provides opportunities to participate in research. A new, modern patient tower was just completed and pediatric radiology recently moved into fully renovated facilities. Salary and fringe benefits are highly competitive. We are currently interviewing for positions beginning of July, 1999 and July 2000. To receive more information, please contact Carlos J. Sivit, MD, Director, Pediatric Radiology, Rainbow Babies and Childrens Hospital of University Hospitals of Cleveland, 11100 Euclid Ave, Cleveland, OH 44106-5056. Telephone 216-844-1172; e-mail *sivit@uhrad.com*. EEO/AA.

FELLOWSHIP IN ABDOMINAL IMAGING AVAILABLE JULY, 1999—Department of Radiology, Louisiana State University Medical School at New Orleans. The Louisiana State University Department of Radiology has a 1-year position open for July, 1999. The division is staffed by eight radiologists with extensive specialization experience or fellowship training. Equipment includes two MRI scanners including a 1.5T GE Signa. Three Siemens Somatom Plus S CTs are in place with plans for at least two more CTs and upgrades in the near future. Nine ultrasound machines with color and power doppler capabilities are currently in use. One of the ultrasound departments is currently filmless and a hospital wide PACS is being implemented. All ultrasound and CT-guided procedures including chest procedures are performed by imaging fellows. Option for combination with musculoskeletal fellowship. Direct inquiries to Thomas R. Beidle, MD, RVT, LSU Radiology, Rm 308, 1542 Tulane Ave, New Orleans, LA 70112; e-mail *tbeidl@lsumc.edu*, phone 504-568-4968.

THE MAYO CLINIC DEPARTMENT OF RADIOLOGY—Rochester, MN, has an unanticipated opening for a fellowship beginning June 26, 1999. There is the potential for a fellowship position in the following areas: nuclear medicine, cross-sectional imaging (ultrasound, CT, MR), thoracic imaging and musculoskeletal imaging. Address correspondence to Thomas E. Hartman, MD, Department of Radiology, Mayo Clinic, 20 First St, SW, Rochester, MN, 55905.

FELLOWSHIP IN NEURORADIOLOGY AVAILABLE 1998—Department of Radiology, Louisiana State University Medical Center. LSU neuroradiology section has one unexpected fellowship opening for 1998. This ACGME accredited program is staffed by four full-time academic neuroradiologist and one full-time neuro-interventionalist and covers the 400-bed Charity Hospital of New Orleans as well as the adjacent 400-bed University Hospital. Candidate will get significant exposure to all aspects of neuroradiology, including low/high field MR, helical CT, myelography, diagnostic and interventional neuroangiography, and ENT radiology. Send CV to Albert Alexander, MD, LSU Medical School, Rm 212, 1542 Tulane Ave, New Orleans, LA 70112.

THORACIC RADIOLOGY FELLOWSHIP POSITION 1999—Department of Radiology, Louisiana State University Medical Center. The Louisiana State University School of Medicine program in New Orleans is offering a fellowship position beginning July of 1999. The fellow will rotate between two primary teaching hospitals; one being the major trauma center for the region. Both campuses are equipped with spiral CT, and one with digital radiography and PACS. A strong pulmonary medicine program and a large and varied case load contribute to the learning experience. Apply to Lisa Diethelm, MD, Department of Radiology, 1542 Tulane Ave, New Orleans, LA 70112.

UNEXPECTED CALIFORNIA INTERVENTIONAL FELLOWSHIP AVAILABLE 7/98—Interventional, MRI and cross-sectional imaging fellowship in tertiary care hospital, with 1.5T MRI, spiral CT and state-of-the-art digital angiography suite. Contact A.M. Levan, MD, at St. Mary Medical Center, 1050 Linden Ave, Long Beach, CA 90813 or call 562-491-9900.

NEURORADIOLOGY FELLOWSHIP—Unexpected opening has developed for a 2-year fellowship position starting July 1, 1999, with clinical, research and teaching duties. Also we have three openings for our 2-year fellowship program beginning July 1, 2000. Applicants must be Board certified and must have completed their residency in radiology by starting date. Interested candidates may contact Daniel K. Kido, MD, Neuroradiology Section, Mallinckrodt Institute of Radiology, Washington University School of Medicine, 510 S Kingshighway Blvd, St. Louis, MO 63110. Phone 314-362-5950; fax 314-362-4886.

THE UNIVERSITY OF MASSACHUSETTS MEDICAL CENTER—Offers fellowship positions in neuroradiology, vascular/interventional and body imaging/MRI. The University of Massachusetts includes a medical school and a 388-bed hospital and trauma center located 40 miles West of Boston. The radiology department performs approximately 170,000 exams per year. State-of-the-art equipment includes two vascular/interventional, two CT, and two 1.5 telsa MRI units. The positions include teaching of medical students and residents with opportunities for research and conference attendance. The neuroradiology and vascular/interventional fellowships are approved by ACGME. For information contact John Knorr, DO, for neuroradiogy. David Phillips, MD, for vascular/interventional. Ashley Davidoff, MD, for body imaging at University of Massachusetts Medical Center, Department of Radiology, 55 Lake Ave North, Worcester, MA 01655; 508-856-2215.

Practice for Sale

BOSTON—Medical imaging suite with radiography, mammography and ultrasound. Administrative offices. Located in Longwood medical area. Reply to Box R-079.

Used Equipment

COMPLETE MAMMOGRAPHY SYSTEM—A 1997 (only 6 months old) Advanced Kodak M35A-MX-OMAT film processor $11,500. A 1992 GE Stenographie 600TS mammography unit (1997 tube) $20,000. Original owners, under service plan, excellent condition, generous discount if purchased together! Call 314-432-2459 or e-mail *neal@writemail.com.*

RSNA®

RSNA Executive Offices • 2021 Spring Road, Suite 600
Oak Brook, IL 60523 • (630) 571-2670

Bulletin Board

August 1998

- ✓ RSNA President-elect Honored by Alma Mater
- ✓ RSNA '98: Registration Update
- ✓ Society's Headquarters Construction Moving Right Along
- ✓ New, Remodeled Hotels Open in Time for RSNA '98

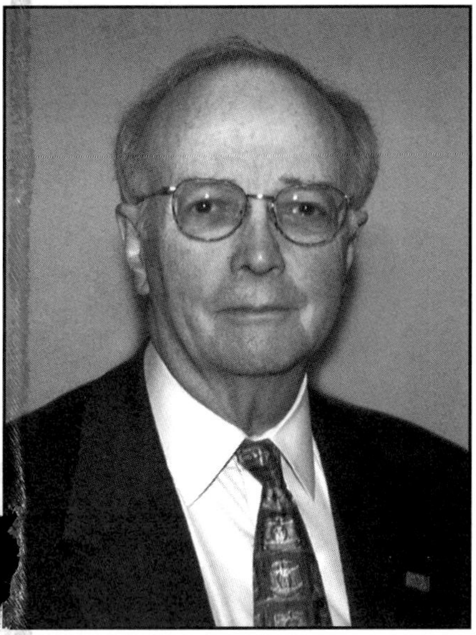

Seymour H. Levitt, MD

■ The University of Colorado School of Medicine Alumni Association presented Seymour H. Levitt, MD, RSNA president-elect, with its 1998 Silver and Gold Award at a ceremony held May 15, 1998, at the Denver Museum of Natural History. The highest recognition bestowed by the Alumni Association, the Silver and Gold Award recognizes alumni for their distinguished professional achievement and community service. Dr Levitt, who received his medical degree from the University of Colorado School of Medicine in 1954, expressed gratitude after accepting his award. "I am very honored to be recognized not only by my colleagues in clinical practice, but by peers at my alma mater," said Dr Levitt.

■ The Refresher Course Enrollment, Scientific Program, Advance Registration, and Housing registration booklet for the Society's 84th Scientific Assembly and Annual Meeting was sent to over 30,000 RSNA members in mid-June. The same booklet also was included with the July issue of *Radiology*. All are encouraged to fill out the registration materials included in the booklet and submit them by the appropriate deadline: October 30, 1998, for North American registrants, and October 2, 1998 for non-North American registrants. Non-North American registrants who wish to receive meeting materials prior to the 84th Scientific Assembly and Annual Meeting must send their registration forms so they are received by October 2, 1998. Registration forms received after that date will be processed, but materials will not be mailed. Instead, materials can be picked up at McCormick Place beginning Saturday, November 28.

■ Construction of the RSNA's new headquarters building is steadily progressing. The 101,000 square-foot structure, shown here in a photograph taken on June 12, 1998, is scheduled for completion in fall 1998. Watch for additional building updates in *RSNA News* and check out RSNA *Link* at *www.rsna.org,* where you'll find more photographs that chronicle the construction.

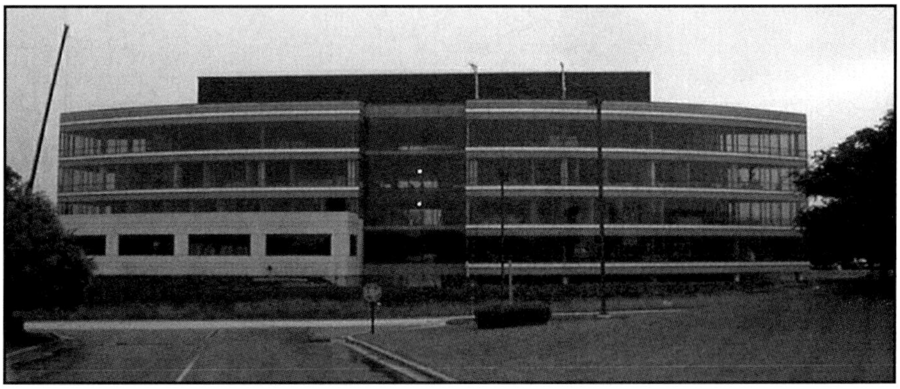

■ The RSNA is pleased to add the following hotels to the 1998 housing block: Crowne Plaza Silversmith, Hampton Inn and Suites, Hotel Allegro Chicago, Hyatt Regency McCormick Place, and Raphael Chicago. These additional hotels will provide more than 1,300 rooms, which will be available to attendees and exhibitors. Looking toward the future, several hotels are presently under construction and are expected to open in 1999.

■ The following is a list of applicants for RSNA membership, published as provided by the bylaws of the Society. Society members are asked to review these names. Should a member have a question concerning the eligibility of an applicant, within 30 days of the publication of this list, the member should request that the applicant's membership be withheld pending investigation and reconsideration by the Membership and Credentials Board. Please mark your signed letter of protest "Confidential" and address it to Secretary-Treasurer, RSNA, 2021 Spring Road, Suite 600, Oak Brook, IL 60523. Please note that listed here are only the locations in which the prospective members reside and the counselors for those areas.

ALABAMA
Counselor: Leon W. Bell III, MD
Michael S. Zinsmeister, MD, Birmingham

CALIFORNIA
Counselors: Deborah S. Ablin, MD
Gary R. Hansen, MD
Eric W. Olcott, MD
Zbigniew Petrovich, MD
Dolores H. Pretorius, MD
Morton Wexler, MD
Daniel M. Dorsey, MD, Yuba City
Torben B. Kristensen, MD, Sunnyvale
Barry R. Paull, MD, Santa Ana
Mauricio T. Schrader, MD, Chico
Daniel J. Valentino, PhD, Los Angeles
J. P. Wheelock, MD, Rolling Hills Estate

CONNECTICUT
Counselor: Marc Glickstein, MD
Barry Stein, MD, Hartford

FLORIDA
Counselor: John A. Arrington, MD
Richard N. Edelstein, MD, Delray Beach
Marilin F. Espino-Maya, MD, Tampa
Paul A. Phillips, DO, Tampa
Moises Roizental, MD, Miami
Holly B. Saunders, MD, Orlando

ILLINOIS
Counselors: Boyd E. Nelson, MD
Steven M. Pinsky, MD
Reni S. Butler, MD, Des Plaines
Janis P. O'Malley, MD, Bourbonnais

INDIANA
Counselor: Smari Thordarson, MD
Nina F. Johnson, MD, Granger
David M. Kurlander, MD, Indianapolis

LOUISIANA
Counselor: David R. Hunter, MD
Edwin Rivera, MD, Shreveport

MASSACHUSETTS
Counselor: Robert H. Cleveland, MD
Timothy J. Hough, MD, Beverly

MICHIGAN
Counselors: Judith M. Bender, MD
Walter W. Laidlaw, MD
Frederick J. Brodeur, Jr, MD, Bay City

MINNESOTA
Counselor: Deborah L. Day, MD
June D. Krivach, MD, Minneapolis

NEW HAMPSHIRE
Counselor: Ronald C. Oliver, MD
Mark D. Wellens, MD, Acworth

NEW JERSEY
Counselor: Karen L. Karlson, MD
Richard R. Jacobs, MD, Lakewood
Stefanie S. Jacobs, MD, Short Hills
Judith H. Murphy, MD, Princeton
Steven N. Sireci, MD, Princeton

NEW YORK
Counselors: Mario A. Grosso, MD
David M. Panicek, MD
Arthur J. Segal, MD
Christopher G. Filippi, MD, New York
Shuichi Higano, MD, PhD, Rochester
Elizabeth W. Lazzara, MD, Scarsdale

NORTH DAKOTA
Counselor: Robert J. Shook, MD
Leszek J. Jaszczak, MD, Williston

OHIO
Counselors: Michael A. Geisinger, MD
Jonathan S. Moulton, MD
Sina S. Hazneci, MD, Findlay
Hasel W. Slone, MD, Powell

PENNSYLVANIA
Counselors: Nilima Dash, MD
Kathryn A. Evers, MD
John E. Madewell, MD
Laurie A. Abrams, MD, Huntingdon Valley
Britton Chance, PhD, DSc, Philadelphia
Andrew W. Loftus, MD, Harrisburg
Laurence Parker, PhD, Philadelphia

TEXAS
Counselors: Karl A. Glastad, MD
Franz J. Hallermann, MD
Timothy W. Lillick, MD
Patrick W. Barr, MD, Dallas
Pamela Nurenberg, MD, Dallas
Vani Velamati, MD, Plano

VIRGINIA
Counselors: Deborah A. Kuban, MD
Arnold J. Kuta, MD
Pamela H. Burdett, MD, Norfolk

WEST VIRGINIA
Counselor: Gary D. Marano, MD
Harry A. Bishop, MD, Bridgeport

ARMY
Counselor: Michael P. Brazaitis, MD
Andrew M. Moran, MD, APO
Brice T. Smith, MD, APO

CANADA

ONTARIO
Counselor: Giles W. Stevenson, MD
Wopco M. Cnoop-Koopmans, MD, Oshawa
David J. Peck, MD, BSc, London
Markus P. Prieditis, MD, Toronto

CORRESPONDING
Mohammad T. Akhtar, MBBS, Pakistan
David M. Allan, MBChB, DMRD, United Kingdom
Takeshi Arita, MD, Japan
Charles Arteaga, MD, France
Sven G. Barkelius, MD, Sweden
Timothy J. Beale, MBBS, United Kingdom
Rene Bokobza, MD, France
Alison J. Bradley, MBChB, United Kingdom
Kieran M. Carroll, MBBCh, United Kingdom
Pablo E. Cikman, MD, Argentina
Adriana D. Coppola, MD, Argentina
Tejinder S. Dhillon, MBBS, MD, India
Duncan F. Ettles, MBChB, MD, United Kingdom
Jose Emmanuel G. Flandes, MD, Philippines
Marcello Greco, MD, Italy
Harald Grosse Hokamp, MD, Germany
Gertraud Heinz-Peer, MD, Austria
Carlos I. Hernandez Rojas, MD, Peru
Shuzo Kanasaki, MD, Japan
Susumu Kandatsu, MD, Japan
Sangam G. Kanekar, MBBS, DMRD, Bahrain
Tarek H. Khalil, MD, Egypt
Kimihiko Kichikawa, MD, Japan
Yoshihisa Kodama III, Japan
Peter Kullnig, MD, Austria
Andrea Laghi, MD, Italy
Torsten K. Larsson, MD, Sweden
Peter P. Leyman, MD, Belgium
Hans T. Lindgren, MD, Sweden
Jorge E. Lopera, MD, Colombia
Galvao A. Lopes, MD, Brazil
Babak Madani, MD, Austria
Asem H. Mansour, MD, Jordan
Hisayasu Matsuo, MD, Japan
Kunizo Mochizuki, MD, Japan
Teruhito Mochizuki, MD, Japan
Kiyoshi Mori, MD, Japan
Yukiko Ochiai, MD, Japan
Simon P. Padley, MBBS, United Kingdom
Dirk Perdieus, MD, Belgium
Virginia G. Rafaelli, MD, Argentina
Andrew P. Richards, MBChB, United Kingdom
Maria Zelia D. Silva, MD, Brazil
Osvanir Simonato, MD, Brazil
Roman B. Sokiranski, MD, Germany
Andrea S. Souza, MD, Brazil
Myrsini Stassinopoulou, MD, Greece
Christiane B. Strauss, MD, France
Simon Strauss, MBChB, Israel
Richard I. Thompson, MBBS, Australia
Alvan H. Troughton, MD, United Kingdom
Rajasekaran K. Vaheesan, MD, India
Mario C. Wilenmann, MD, Chile
Michio Yamasaki, MD, Japan
Kyu-Tong Yoh, MD, South Korea
Jorge M. Yokochi, MD, Brazil
Paul M. Yoong, MBBS, DMRD, Australia
Shigeyuki Yoshida, MD, Japan

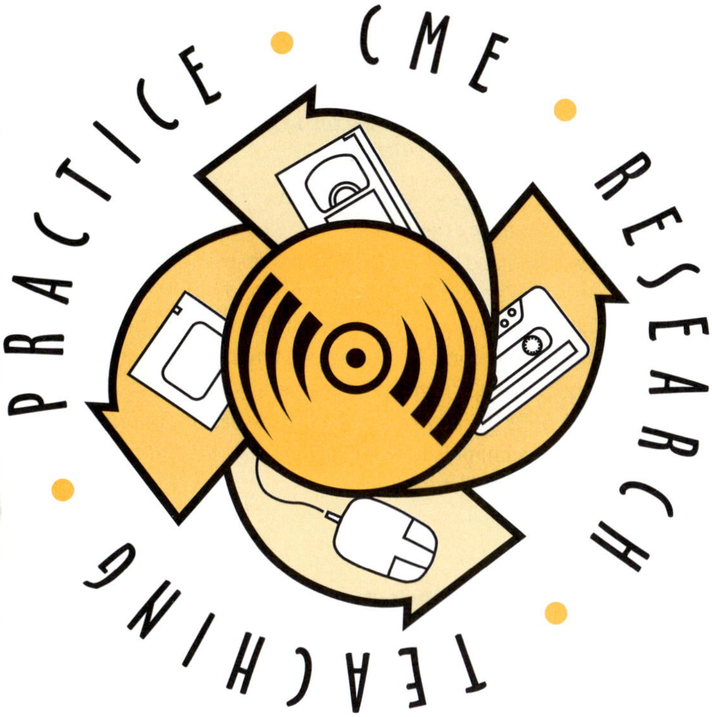

Radiation Oncology

Learning Center Resources

August 1998

Featured Topics

- Brachytherapy Delivery Systems
- Calculational Algorithms for Brachytherapy
- Brachytherapy: Quality Assurance and Human Factors
- Brachytherapy Physics: Calibration and Dose Measurement

New Service

The entire 1997–1998 Learning Center Resources Catalog is now available on the RSNA Link, the Web site of the Radiological Society of North America, on the Internet.

You can reach us through the World Wide Web (WWW) by entering the uniform resource locator: http://www.rsna.org

We invite you to browse through the catalog, search for specific courses of interest, then simply order via our fax or 800 phone number.

RSNA® | Radiological Society of North America Founded in 1915

Detach and store for your future use.

The following 10 Radiation Oncology titles are now available in the Learning Center Resources Library. All videotapes are available for purchase or rental (U.S., Canada, and Mexico). All video programs may be purchased in NTSC, PAL, and SECAM television standards. Slides and audiotapes are available for purchase only.

For more information, call or fax the RSNA Learning Center Resources at the numbers listed on the order form. To order by mail, use the form on the back.

New!

Brachytherapy: Templates and Their Applications *RSP 640*
Arthur J. Olch, PhD

This case-based review describes interstitial treatment of the prostate, rectum, vagina and parametria, breast, and brain with templates. *Learning objectives:* (1) To understand the potential benefits and pitfalls of using commercial templates for brachytherapy. (2) To become familiar with volumetric implants and the associated dosimetry. (3) To review cases in which templates were used. (4) To learn rules for source placement and differential loading.

59 slides/audiotape *M$140, N$160*
Not available on videotape

New!

Brachytherapy Delivery Systems *RSP 650*
Bruce R. Thomadsen, Ph
Geoffrey S. Ibbott, PhD

Brachytherapy Source Material
Bruce R. Thomadsen, PhD

Learning objectives: (1) To understand the "ideal" brachytherapy source. (2) To understand how encapsulation works with source material to achieve the goals of the application. (3) To learn the appropriate tests to perform on brachytherapy sources to ensure that they perform as desired.

Brachytherapy Delivery Systems
Geoffrey S. Ibbott, PhD

The designs of representative brachytherapy devices are reviewed and compared, and the advantages and disadvantages of each are discussed. *Learning objectives:* (1) To learn about the evolution of brachytherapy delivery systems. (2) To understand the development and benefits of afterloading. (3) To compare the designs and advantages of remote afterloading systems.

86 slides/2 audiotapes *M$205, N$225*
VHS *M$205, N$225*

New!

Brachytherapy Dose Calculations: Localization *RSP 651*
Jerome A. Meli, PhD

Several localization methods are reviewed. The advantages, disadvantages, and accuracy of each are compared, and ways to improve and verify localization accuracy are discussed. *Learning objectives:* (1) To become familiar with various localization methods and their limitations. (2) To understand ways to improve localization accuracy. (3) To recognize what to look for in a brachytherapy planning system.

VHS *M$140, N$160*
Not available in slide/audiotape

New!

Calculational Algorithms for Brachytherapy *RSP 652*
Keith A. Weaver, PhD

This presentation reviews the basic physical processes in brachytherapy dose deposition. Common algorithms are described and relationships between commonly used parameters are explained. *Learning objectives:* (1) To understand the fundamental concepts that underlie brachytherapy dose calculations. (2) To become familiar with common brachytherapy algorithms, especially the one promulgated by AAPM Task Group 43. (3) To understand when Monte Carlo techniques might be useful in brachytherapy

48 slides/audiotape *M$140, N$160*
VHS *M$140, N$160*

New!

Radiobiology—Biologic Aspects and Practical Application *RSP 653*
Colin G. Orton, PhD

Understanding the basic radiobiology of brachytherapy is essential if one is to maximize benefit and minimize risk, particularly when converting from traditional LDR regimens to HDR, MDR, or PDR. *Learning objectives:* (1) To identify important radiobiological principles in brachytherapy. (2) To understand the radiobiologic differences between LDR, MDR, HDR, PDR, and permanent implants. (3) To learn how to use the L-Q model to predict these radiobiologic differences and to convert from one modality to the other.

69 slides/2 audiotapes *M$205, N$225*
Not available on videotape

New!

Brachytherapy: Dose Specification, Prescription, and Implant Evaluation *RSP 654*
Mary K. Martel, PhD

Learning objectives: (1) To review the 3D treatment planning system tools used to evaluate brachytherapy implants. (2) To compare 3D dose specification with traditional calculation points and methods. (3) To review results of the use of 3D target and normal organ dose specification and clinical outcome.

68 slides/audiotape *M$140, N$160*
Not available on videotape

M/N = Member/Nonmember prices
To order call 800-272-2920 or FAX 708-409-9703

New!

Brachytherapy Object-oriented Treatment Planning Based on Three-dimensional Image Guidance *RSP 655*

Kenneth J. Weeks, PhD

This program covers various aspects of brachytherapy object-oriented treatment planning. Examples of low-dose-rate traditional brachytherapy, such as tandem and ovoids for carcinoma of the uterine cervix and customized needle templates for vaginal implants, are presented. *Learning objectives:* (1) To review how 3D visualization facilitates brachytherapy treatment planning. (2) To illustrate reconstruction of source-applicator orientation on serial images.

VHS *M$140, N$160*

Not available in slide/audiotape

New!

Optimization in Brachytherapy *RSP 656*

Gary A. Ezzell, PhD

Historical approaches to optimization are reviewed, with reference made to classic systems of brachytherapy. This presentation sets the context for optimization goals in brachytherapy, which can differ for various implant sites and methods. Modern optimization methods applied to brachytherapy are reviewed. *Learning objectives:* (1) To learn the concepts fundamental to different optimization techniques in order to better appreciate their advantages, disadvantages, and ranges of applicability. (2) To learn how to apply at least one quantitative method for evaluating optimized implants, such as the natural dose-volume histogram.

VHS *M$140, N$160*

Not available in slide/audiotape

New!

Brachytherapy: Quality Assurance and Human Factors *RSP 657*

Jeffrey F. Williamson, PhD

Bruce R. Thomadsen, PhD

Quality Assurance of Brachytherapy Treatment Delivery and Planning Devices

Jeffrey F. Williamson, PhD

This presentation emphasizes the detailed device quality assurance (QA) program recommended by the recently completed AAPM Task Group 56 Report, "Brachytherapy Physics Code of Practice." *Learning objectives:* (1) To acquire a working knowledge of the physical test and measurement procedures used to assess brachytherapy equipment performance with respect to accuracy and safety end points. (2) To appreciate the principles governing design of device QA protocols. (3) To acquire a working knowledge of the TG-56 model QA program for brachytherapy delivery and planning devices.

Quality Assurance and Human Factors

Bruce R. Thomadsen, PhD

Learning objectives: (1) To learn about techniques for analysis of human error. (2) To become familiar with the principles for establishing a QA program to intercept human errors. (3) To understand the application of the principles in exemplary situations.

78 slides/2 audiotapes *M$205, N$225*

Not available on videotape

New!

Brachytherapy Physics: Calibration and Dose Measurement *RSP 658*

Larry A. DeWerd, PhD

Cynthia L. Thomason, PhD

Source Strength

Larry A. DeWerd, PhD

This program covers the uncertainties of calibration. Medical physics metrology procedures are reviewed for low-dose-rate (LDR) sources and well chambers and for high-dose-rate (HDR) chambers. *Learning objectives:* (1) To review the need of calibration for LDR and HDR sources. (2) To summarize primary calibration techniques at NIST and the ADCLs. (3) To review methods of calibration transfer to the clinic. (4) To review methods for source calibration not having national standards. (L.A.D. owns stock in Standard Imaging.)

Calibration and Dose Measurement

Cynthia L. Thomason, PhD

This program discusses techniques used by select institutions for characterizing new computational techniques, applicators, or sources and those used for clinical quality assurance. *Learning objectives:* (1) To identity the problems in brachytherapy dose measurement. (2) To outline the desirable properties of a detector to be used for dose measurement. (3) To describe the radiation detectors and techniques used for dose measurement, including limitations, advantages, and disadvantages. (4) To suggest how to choose a technique based on isotope and treatment site and technique.

127 slides/2 audiotapes *M$205, N$225*

Not available on videotape

Place Stamp Here

TO: RSNA LEARNING CENTER RESOURCES
PO BOX 5316
OAK BROOK, IL 60522-5316
USA

FOLD HERE

Order Form

You may mail or fax this form. To fax your order, dial 708-409-9703. Please print.

☐ *RSNA Member* ☐ *Nonmember*

NAME

RSNA MEMBER # (REQUIRED FOR MEMBER PRICING)

ADDRESS

CITY

STATE/COUNTRY

ZIP

PHONE

FAX

Order Information (for purchase and rentals)

Course Number	*Showing Date (Rental Only)*	*Format (Purchase Only)*	*Price*

FOLD HERE

Check one:

☐ *Rental*

☐ *Purchase*

Subtotal

Shipping & Handling

Total

Shipping Information

United States

1 program = $7
2 – 3 programs = $10
4 – 6 programs = $20
7 programs and up = $30

Rental

No charge for shipping to renter. Renter is responsible for return shipping charges.

Outside United States

1 program = $10
Each additional program = $5

All orders from outside the U.S. must be prepaid, either by MasterCard, VISA, AMEX or Diner's Club or a check in U.S. dollars, drawn on a U.S. bank.

Payment Information

☐ Payment by check

☐ Payment by credit card: ☐ VISA ☐ MasterCard ☐ AMEX ☐ Diner's Club

CARD NUMBER

SIGNATURE

EXP. DATE

For faster service, phone 800-272-2920 or fax 708-409-9703.

TEAR HERE

Foto-Comm Corporation is the distributor of RSNA Learning Center Resources.

RAD 8.98

September 1998
Volume 208 • Number 3
RADLAX 208 (3) 561–840

1923-1998 75th ANNIVERSARY

Radiology

Subspecialty Society Messages	561
Editorial	571
Special Report	573
Review	577
Gastrointestinal Imaging	591
Diagnosis Please: Case 6	619
Case 2 Answer	621
Vascular and Interventional Radiology	625
Ultrasonography	649
Neuroradiology	663
Signs in Imaging	687
Head and Neck Imaging	689
Technical Developments	695
Breast Imaging	717
Genitourinary Imaging	729
Radiation Oncology	739
Thoracic Imaging	749
Pediatric Imaging	783
Obstetric Imaging	795
Experimental Studies	799
Cardiac Imaging	807
Musculoskeletal Imaging	815
Letters to the Editor	829
Publishers' Row	61A

THE RADIOLOGICAL SOCIETY OF NORTH AMERICA

RSNA® **84th Scientific Assembly and Annual Meeting**
Chicago, November 29–December 4, 1998

Radiology

September 1998
Volume 208
Number 3

RSNA®

A monthly journal devoted to clinical radiology and allied sciences, owned and published by THE RADIOLOGICAL SOCIETY OF NORTH AMERICA, INC.

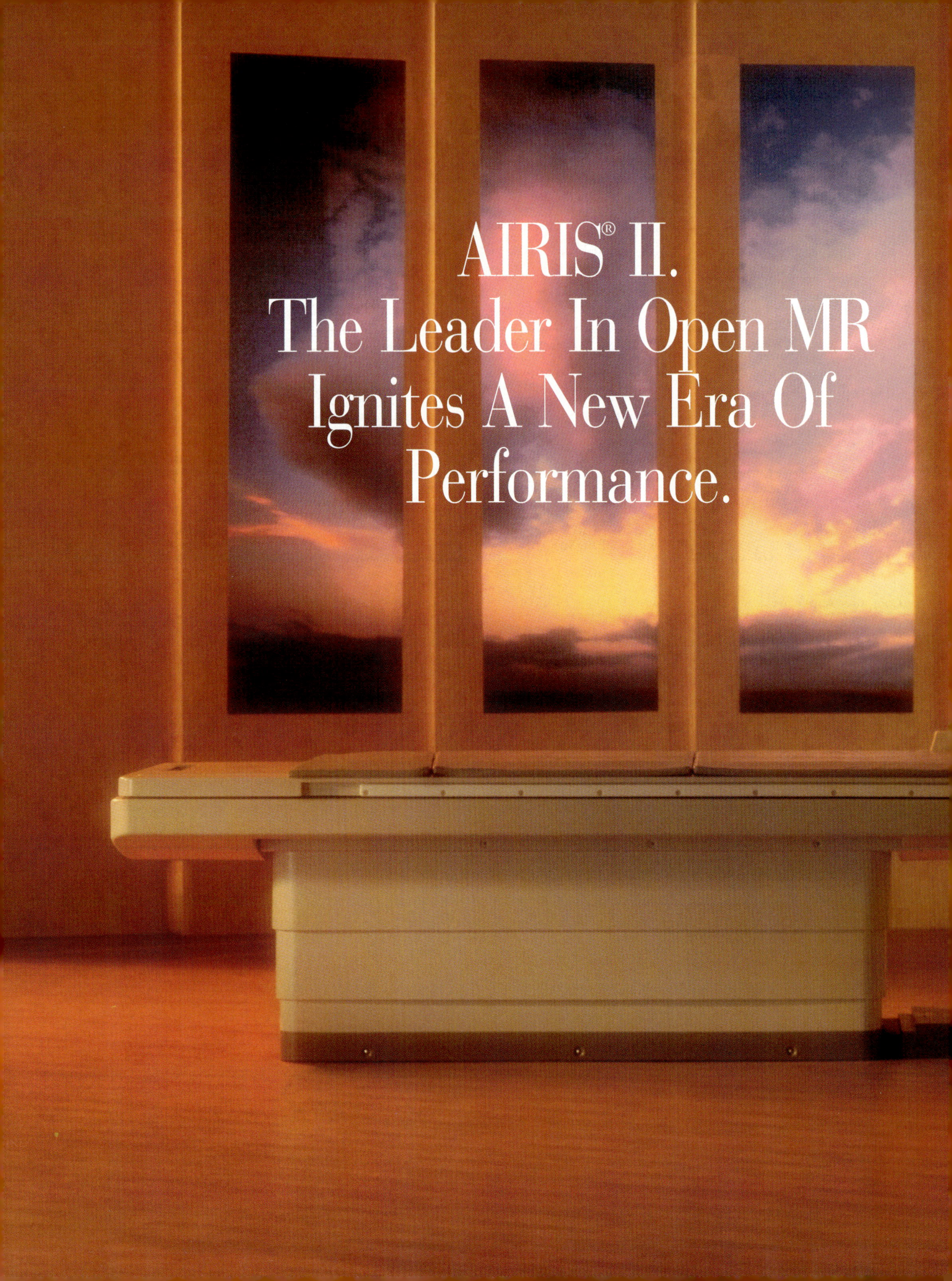
AIRIS® II.
The Leader In Open MR
Ignites A New Era Of
Performance.

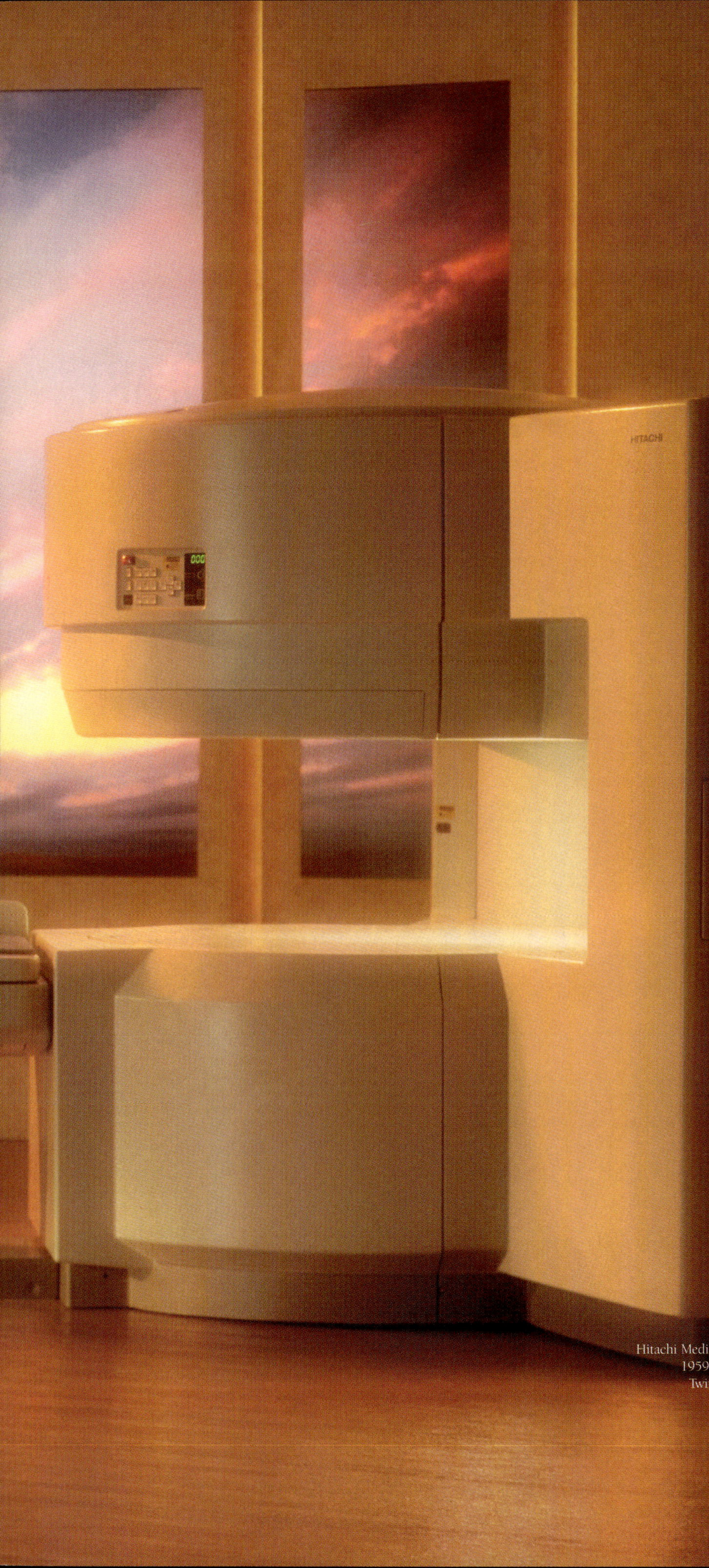

September 1998
Volume 208 • Number 3

Radiology

A monthly journal devoted to clinical radiology and allied sciences, owned and published by the Radiological Society of North America, Inc.

RSNA

Future Directions of Imaging Research: Subspecialty Society Messages

561 *The International Skeletal Society—*
Musculoskeletal Imaging
Holger Pettersson and Donald Resnick
No, we are not clairvoyant, but we believe that the subdiscipline of musculoskeletal imaging is in good health today and the outlook for future development and refinement is promising.

563 Commentary
The Right Stuff
Jeremy J. Kaye
Musculoskeletal radiologists can ensure a prominent role in the future of medicine by possessing a greater knowledge of diseases through education and continuing education, by accurately and completely reporting studies in a timely fashion, by being pioneers and ready participants in information and imaging transfer, and by performing scientific research, especially on diseases.

565 *The American Society of Emergency Radiology—*
Emergency Radiology Practice and Research beyond the Millennium
Frederick A. Mann, Michael I. Zucker, and William R. Mower
As members of a dynamic specialty, we radiologists must not only think about changes needed in this rapidly evolving medical environment but also begin to enhance our critical roles in emergent patient care.

568 Commentary
American Society of Emergency Radiology: Research Revisited
John H. Harris, Jr
As with emergency physicians who are clinical "generalists," emergency radiologists must also be "generalists" comfortable with the use of all imaging modalities in the evaluation of patients of all ages with unexpected or acute conditions affecting all organ systems.

Editorial

571 **Coronary Arterial Calcium Screening: Ready for Prime Time?**
Scott D. Flamm
Radiologists should be leading the way in refining and optimizing the techniques and completing large-scale studies that demonstrate the cost-effectiveness and predictive value of coronary arterial calcium screening before selling it to an anxious and often ill-informed health care–consuming public.

Special Report

573 **Cardiac MR Imaging: Report of a Working Group Sponsored by the National Heart, Lung, and Blood Institute**
Thomas F. Budinger, Alan Berson, Elliot R. McVeigh, Roderic I. Pettigrew, Gerald M. Pohost, John T. Watson, and Samuel A. Wickline
The Working Group recommends areas of research and development that could lead to more extensive clinical use of MR methods to improve the diagnosis and management of cardiovascular and cardiopulmonary disorders.

Review

577 **Diagnostic Pitfalls and Artifacts in Abdominal MR Imaging: A Review**
Scott A. Mirowitz
Many sources of potential diagnostic error are encountered on abdominal MR images; it is important to be aware of the manifestations and causes of these entities.

Gastrointestinal Imaging

591 **Gastric Stromal Sarcomas: Correlation of MR Imaging and Histopathologic Findings in Nine Patients**
Shinichi Hasegawa, Richard C. Semelka, Tara C. Noone, John T. Woosley, Hani B. Marcos, Phillip J. Kenney, and Evan S. Siegelman
Multiplanar MR imaging with breath-hold (eg, spoiled gradient-recalled-echo) and breathing-independent (eg, half-Fourier rapid acquisition with relaxation enhancement) techniques is helpful in evaluating the gastric origin and varied appearances of gastric stromal sarcomas.

597 **Nontumorous Arterioportal Shunt Mimicking Hypervascular Tumor in Cirrhotic Liver: Two-Phase Spiral CT Findings**
Tae Kyoung Kim, Byung Ihn Choi, Joon Koo Han, Jin Wook Chung, Jae Hyung Park, and Man Chung Han
Typical two-phase spiral CT findings can suggest the possibility of nontumorous arterioportal shunt in the cirrhotic liver, which is one of the causes of hypervascular pseudolesions.

605 **Mucin-producing Tumor of the Pancreas: Diagnostic Value of Diffusion-weighted Echo-planar MR Imaging**
Yasuyuki Yamashita, Tomohiro Namimoto, Katsuhiko Mitsuzaki, Joji Urata, Tadatoshi Tsuchigame, Mutsumasa Takahashi, and Michio Ogawa
Diffusion-weighted echo-planar MR imaging is a promising technique for characterizing cystic masses on the basis of differences in apparent diffusion coefficients, although its value awaits further evaluation in a larger number of cases.

611 **Right Colonic Diverticulitis: US and CT Findings—New Insights about Frequency and Natural History**
Louk F. I. J. Oudenhoven, Robert K. J. Koumans, and Julien B. C. M. Puylaert
Our results show that right-sided colonic diverticulitis occurs much more frequently than was previously assumed, and its natural history is benign, which allows primarily nonsurgical treatment.

Diagnosis Please

619 **Case 6**
Patrick M. Rao and Robert A. Novelline

621 **Case 2: Embryonal Rhabdomyosarcoma of the Biliary Tree**
Lane F. Donnelly, George S. Bisset III, and Donald P. Frush
The age, sex, clinical presentation, and bulky intraductal common bile duct masses shown in the case example are all consistent with the diagnosis of embryonal rhabdomyosarcoma of the biliary tree.

Vascular and Interventional Radiology

625 **Uterine Arterial Embolization for the Management of Leiomyomas: Quality of Life Assessment and Clinical Response**
Robert L. Worthington-Kirsch, George L. Popky, Francis L. Hutchins, Jr
Uterine arterial embolization shows great promise as a primary treatment of symptomatic leiomyomas, because the procedure is well tolerated and effective, with the potential for considerable advantages over traditional therapies.

631 **Deep Venous Thrombosis: Gradient-recalled-Echo MR Imaging Changes over Time—Experience in 10 Patients**
Charles E. Spritzer, Priscilla Trotter, and H. Dirk Sostman
The gradient-recalled-echo MR imaging findings we have reported should facilitate the distinction between acute and chronic deep venous thrombosis.

Continued—

Radiology is published monthly by the Radiological Society of North America, Inc, 2021 Spring Rd, Suite 600, Oak Brook, IL 60523 (ISSN 0033-8419). Printed in USA. Periodical class postage paid at Oak Brook, Ill, and additional mailing offices. The nonmember subscription rate for the USA is $215.00 per year; for all other countries, $260.00 (includes postage). Information about subscription rates for residents is available on request. (Air freight is available; rates are furnished on request.) Single copies are $25.00 ($36.00 to a non-U.S. address). Notice of missing issues or change of address (include old mailing label and new address) should be sent to RSNA Subscriptions Department, 2021 Spring Rd, Suite 600, Oak Brook, IL 60523. Inquiries via e-mail should be directed to *subscrib@rsna.org*. POSTMASTER: Send address correction "changes" to: *Radiology*, RSNA, 2021 Spring Rd, Suite 600, Oak Brook, IL 60523.

Claims for copies lost in the mail are allowed within 90 days of the date of issue. Claims are not allowed for issues lost as a result of insufficient notice of change of address.

Membership in the Radiological Society of North America is by formal application. Membership information should be secured from the Executive Director, the Radiological Society of North America, Inc, 2021 Spring Rd, Suite 600, Oak Brook, IL 60523. Dues are payable annually in January. In accordance with U.S. postal regulations, $107.50 of active membership dues is allocated to a subscription to *Radiology*.

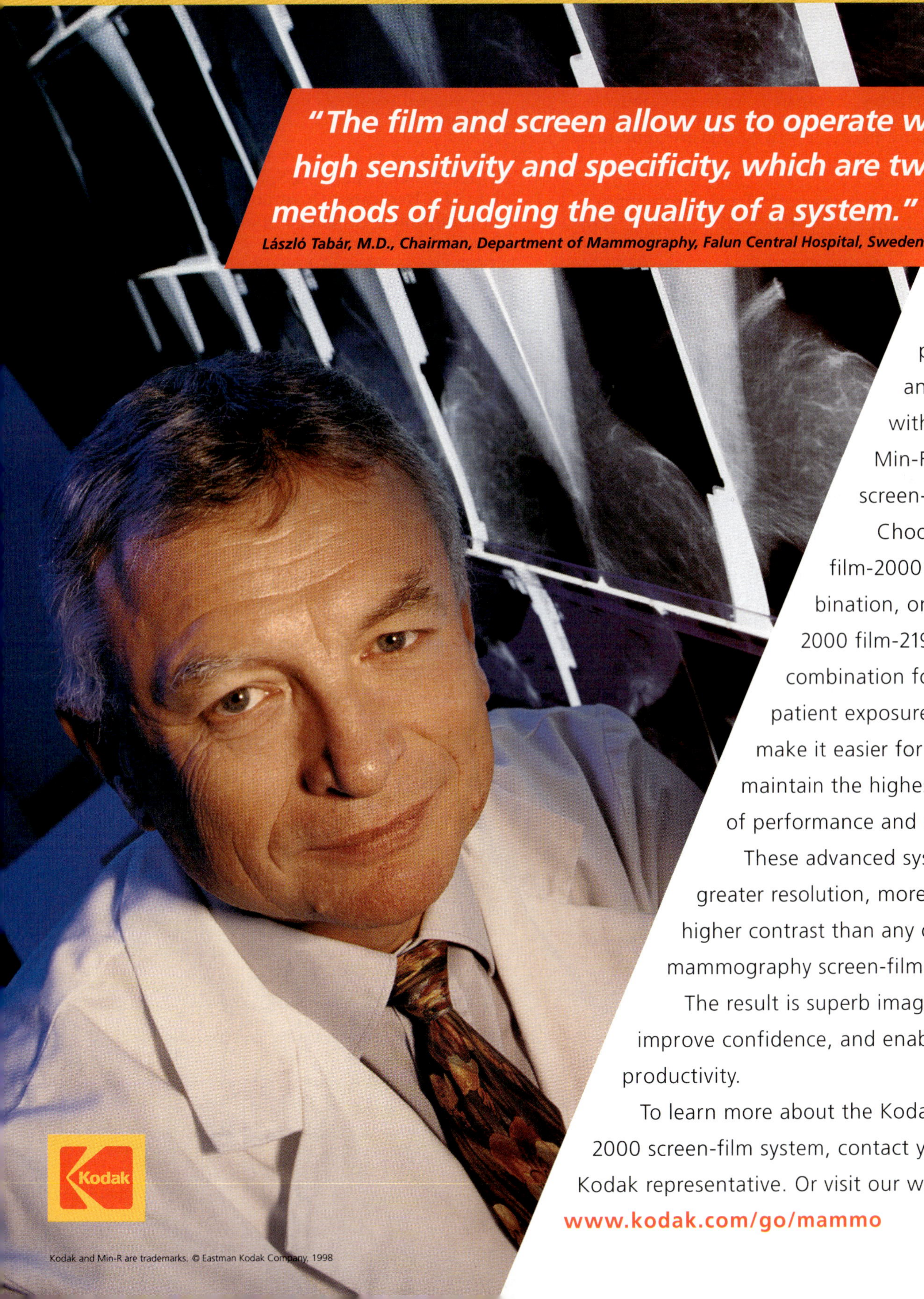

641 **Iliac Arterial Occlusive Disease: Cost-effectiveness Analysis of Stent Placement versus Percutaneous Transluminal Angioplasty**
Johanna L. Bosch, Eric Tetteroo, Willem P. T. M. Mali, and Maria G. M. Hunink, For the Dutch Iliac Stent Trial Study Group
Our results suggest that percutaneous transluminal angioplasty with selective stent placement is a cost-effective strategy, compared with percutaneous transluminal angioplasty alone, for the treatment of iliac arterial occlusive disease and that the gain in effectiveness justifies the additional costs.

Ultrasonography

649 **Hypoechoic Plaque at US of the Carotid Artery: An Independent Risk Factor for Incident Stroke in Adults Aged 65 Years or Older**
Joseph F. Polak, Lynn Shemanski, Daniel H. O'Leary, David Lefkowitz, Thomas R. Price, Peter J. Savage, William E. Brant, and Cheryl Reid, For the Cardiovascular Health Study
The authors performed this study to prospectively evaluate the association between incident ischemic stroke and the in vivo appearance of carotid plaque on US images obtained in a cohort of asymptomatic individuals aged at least 65 years with an average follow-up of 3.3 years.

655 **Hemodialysis Access Graft Stenosis: US Detection**
Michelle L. Robbin, Rachel F. Oser, Michael Allon, Michael W. Clements, Jeanne Dockery, Therese M. Weber, Kay M. Hamrick-Waller, J. Kevin Smith, Brian C. Jones, Desiree E. Morgan, and Souheil Saddekni
US of hemodialysis access grafts with use of peak systolic velocity criteria and color flow imaging is highly sensitive in the detection of graft and drainage vein stenoses.

Neuroradiology

663 **Cerebral Toxoplasmosis and Lymphoma in AIDS: Perfusion MR Imaging Experience in 13 Patients**
Thomas M. Ernst, Linda Chang, Mallory D. Witt, Howard A. Aronow, Marcia E. Cornford, Irvin Walot, and Mark A. Goldberg
The addition of perfusion MR imaging to existing MR imaging protocols in patients with acquired immuno deficiency syndrome who have focal brain lesions may help improve the clinical diagnosis and, possibly, the disease prognosis, if these patients receive the appropriate treatment earlier.

671 **Unselected Brain 0.5-T MR Imaging: Comparison of Lesion Detection and Characterization with Three T2-weighted Sequences**
Antoine J. Maubon, Agnès Pothin, Jean Michel Ferru, Vincent M. Berger, Jean Pierre Daurès, and Jean Pierre Rouanet
It is of value to associate a black cerebrospinal fluid T2-weighted sequence with the usual white cerebrospinal fluid T2-weighted sequences in routine unselected brain MR imaging.

679 **MR Imaging of the Inner Ear: Comparison of a Three-dimensional Fast Spin-Echo Sequence with Use of a Dedicated Quadrature-Surface Coil with a Gadolinium-enhanced Spoiled Gradient-recalled Sequence**
Shinji Naganawa, Tokiko Ito, Hiroshi Fukatsu, Takeo Ishigaki, Tsutomu Nakashima, Nobuyasu Ichinose, Yukimori Kassai,and Mitsue Miyazaki
MR imaging of the inner ear with a three-dimensional asymmetric fast spin-echo sequence with a quadrature-surface phased-array coil allows the reliable detection of vestibular schwannoma in the cerebellopontine angle and internal auditory canal without the need for gadolinium enhancement.

Signs in Imaging

687 **The Hyperdense Middle Cerebral Artery Sign**
Nicola Petitti
The hyperdense middle cerebral artery sign is an indirect sign of cerebral ischemia that corresponds to arterial occlusion of the middle cerebral artery.

Head and Neck Imaging

689 **Lacrimal System Obstruction Treated with Lacrimal Polyurethane Stents: Outcome of Removal of Occluded Stents**
Ho-Young Song, Deok Hee Lee, Hyosook Ahn, Jae-Ho Kim, Sung-Gwon Kang, Hyun-Ki Yoon, and Kyu-Bo Sung
Recurrence of epiphora after placement of lacrimal plastic stents was treated by removing the occluded stents and irrigating with saline solution through the lacrimal point in 33% of cases, with the result of a patent lacrimal system after stent removal.

Technical Developments

695 **Mandibular Sigmoid Notch: A Window for CT-guided Biopsies of Lesions in the Peripharyngeal and Skull Base Regions**
James J. Abrahams
This easy method allows biopsy of difficult-to-reach lesions of the peripharyngeal and skull base regions by means of traversal of the sigmoid notch of the mandible.

Continued—

700 **Cochlear Implants: In Vitro Investigation of Electromagnetic Interference at MR Imaging—Compatibility and Safety Aspects**
Christian Teissl, Christian Kremser, Erwin S. Hochmair, and Ingeborg J. Hochmair-Desoyer
It is an absolute necessity to consult the manufacturer of a cochlear implant to determine whether the particular MR imaging procedure intended to be performed in a patient with a cochlear implant is considered safe.

709 **Mammography of a Phantom and Breast Tissue with Synchrotron Radiation and a Linear-Array Silicon Detector**
Fulvia Arfelli, Valter Bonvicini, Alberto Bravin, Giovanni Cantatore, Edoardo Castelli, Ludovico Dalla Palma, Marco Di Michiel, Renata Longo, Alessandro Olivo, Silvia Pani, Diego Pontoni, Paolo Poropat, Michela Prest, Alexander Rashevsky, Giuliana Tromba, and Andrea Vacchi
Images obtained with a linear-array, silicon pixel detector capable of counting single photons show good contrast resolution.

Breast Imaging

717 **US-guided Core Breast Biopsy: Use and Cost-effectiveness**
Laura Liberman, Timothy L. Feng, D. David Dershaw, Elizabeth A. Morris, and Andrea F. Abramson
Percutaneous biopsy of a nonpalpable breast mass with either US guidance or stereotactic guidance is less expensive than surgery, but the cost savings are greater if the biopsy is performed with US guidance.

725 **Breast Cancer in Women Who Undergo Screening Mammography: Relationship of Hormone Replacement Therapy to Stage and Detection Method**
Marilyn A. Roubidoux, Todd E. Wilson, Richard J. Orange, J. Thomas Fitzgerald, Mark A. Helvie, and Sasha A. Packer
Our findings indicate that in women who participate in screening mammography, hormone replacement therapy does not impair the mammographic detection of breast cancer and is not associated with differences in stages of breast cancer.

Genitourinary Imaging

729 **Renal Blood Flow: Measurement in Vivo with Rapid Spiral MR Imaging**
Graham Sommer, Geraldine Corrigan, Jill Fredrickson, Anne Sawyer-Glover, Jan-Ray Liao, Bryan Myers, and Norbert Pelc
Sources of error in flow computation can be minimized with cine phase-contrast MR imaging techniques, and the accuracy of in vivo renal blood flow determination appears acceptable for clinical application.

735 **Small Cell and Anaplastic Prostate Cancer: Correlation between CT Findings and Prostate-specific Antigen Level**
Lawrence H. Schwartz, Linda R. LaTrenta, Ermelinda Bonaccio, William K. Kelly, Howard I. Scher, and David M. Panicek
Despite the rapid progression of disease, the prostate-specific antigen levels in most were not elevated—unlike in patients with typical advanced adenocarcinoma of the prostate.

Radiation Oncology

739 **Stage I Hodgkin Disease: Radiation Therapy and Chemotherapy at The University Of Texas M. D. Anderson Cancer Center, 1967–1997**
Maria T. Vlachaki, Chul S. Ha, Frederick B. Hagemeister, Lillian M. Fuller, Maria A. Rodriguez, Mark A. Hess, Susan L. Tucker, Fernando Cabanillas, and James D. Cox
Subtotal nodal irradiation is recommended for patients with favorable prognostic factors, with chemotherapy reserved for those with less favorable factors.

Thoracic Imaging

749 **Epstein-Barr-Virus–associated Lymphoproliferative Disease of the Lung: CT and Histologic Findings**
Jannette Collins, Nestor L. Müller, Ann N. Leung, Georgeann McGuinness, Patricia J. Mergo, Julia D. Flint, Thomas F. Warner, Charles Poirier, James Theodore, Dani Zander, and Herman T. Yee
In our series of patients, most of whom either had acquired immunodeficiency syndrome, or AIDS, or had undergone bone marrow or solid organ transplantation, the two most common diagnoses were polyclonal lymphoproliferative disease and malignant lymphoma; the most common CT findings for both diagnoses included multiple nodules, large and small, with a peribronchovascular and subpleural distribution, involving the middle and lower lung zones.

761 **Volume Rendering of the Tracheobronchial Tree: Clinical Evaluation of Bronchographic Images**
Martine Remy-Jardin, Jacques Remy, Dominique Artaud, Marc Fribourg, and Alain Duhamel
The volume-rendered images improved the recognition of mild cylindric bronchiectasis and stenosis and helped identification of congenital or acquired complex airway anatomy.

771 **Thoracic Spiral CT: Influence of Subsecond Gantry Rotation on Image Quality**
Geoffrey D. Rubin, Ann N. Leung, Valerie J. Robertson, and Paul Stark
On the basis of results in this study, an additional advantage of subsecond scanning is improved thoracic image quality as a result of diminished motion artifacts, particularly in regions closest to the heart.

Continued—

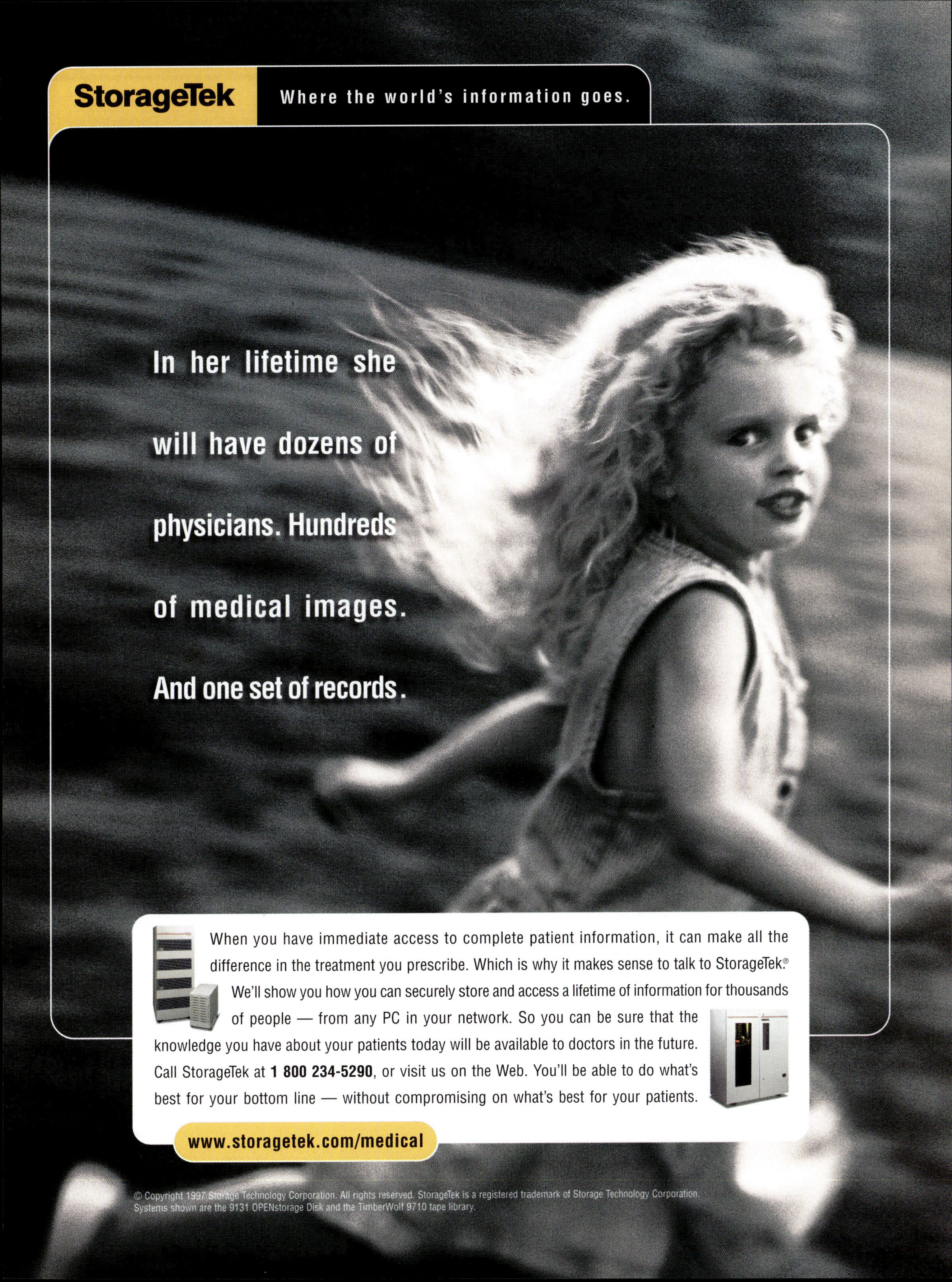
StorageTek
Where the world's information goes.
In her lifetime she will have dozens of physicians. Hundreds of medical images. And one set of records.
When you have immediate access to complete patient information, it can make all the difference in the treatment you prescribe. Which is why it makes sense to talk to StorageTek.® We'll show you how you can securely store and access a lifetime of information for thousands of people — from any PC in your network. So you can be sure that the knowledge you have about your patients today will be available to doctors in the future. Call StorageTek at 1 800 234-5290, or visit us on the Web. You'll be able to do what's best for your bottom line — without compromising on what's best for your patients.
www.storagetek.com/medical
© Copyright 1997 Storage Technology Corporation. All rights reserved. StorageTek is a registered trademark of Storage Technology Corporation.
Systems shown are the 9131 OPENstorage Disk and the TimberWolf 9710 tape library.

777 **Invasive Pulmonary Aspergillosis: Prediction at Thin-Section CT in Patients with Neutropenia—A Prospective Study**
Hyung Jin Won, Kyung Soo Lee, Jung-Eun Cheon, Jung Hwa Hwang, Tae Sung Kim, Hong Ghi Lee, and Joungho Han
Thin-section CT findings of invasive pulmonary aspergillosis are nonspecific, and similar findings can be seen in patients with neutropenia and mucormycosis, organizing pneumonia, or pulmonary hemorrhage.

Pediatric Imaging

783 **Bronchiolitis Obliterans Syndrome: Thin-Section CT Diagnosis of Obstructive Changes in Infants and Young Children after Lung Transplantation**
Debra M. Lau, Marilyn J. Siegel, Charles F. Hildebolt, and Alan H. Cohen
Although the sample size was small, the findings support the continued use of thin-section CT as an adjunctive study to confirm the diagnosis of bronchiolitis obliterans syndrome.

789 **Vascular Lesions in Children: Percutaneous MR Imaging–guided Interstitial Nd:YAG Laser Therapy—Preliminary Experience**
Frank K. Wacker, Dietmar Cholewa, Andre Roggan, Andreas Schilling, Jürgen Waldschmidt, and Karl-Jürgen Wolf
An open MR imager can be used to guide interstitial laser therapy of hemangiomas and vascular malformations in children.

Obstetric Imaging

795 **Enlarged Fetal Gallbladder: Prognostic Importance for Aneuploidy or Biliary Abnormality at Antenatal US**
Barbara S. Hertzberg, Mark A. Kliewer, James D. Bowie, and Patricia J. McNally
Fetal cholecystomegaly does not appear to be associated with a substantially increased risk for chromosomal aneuploidy or a particular anatomic malformation.

Experimental Studies

799 **Transjugular Intrahepatic Portosystemic Shunt: Effect of Bile Leak on Smooth Muscle Cell Proliferation**
Gao-Jun Teng, Michael A. Bettmann, P. Jack Hoopes, Robert J. Wagner, Byeong-Ho Park, Li Yang, and Brian R. Baxter
As early occlusion of a transjugular intrahepatic portosystemic shunt (TIPS) in humans is rare, bile leak in a TIPS is probably not a detrimental occurrence and may, on the basis of the findings here, actually aid patency.

Cardiac Imaging

807 **Coronary Artery Disease: Improved Reproducibility of Calcium Scoring with an Electron-Beam CT Volumetric Method**
Tracy Q. Callister, Bruce Cooil, Sai P. Raya, Nicholas J. Lippolis, Donald J. Russo, and Paolo Raggi
Our analysis allowed us to determine which level of change in the calcium volumetric score can be considered to be reliable evidence of the true progression of disease rather than mere replication error, thus providing important information for the practicing physician.

Musculoskeletal Imaging

815 **Submaximal Delayed-Onset Muscle Soreness: Correlations between MR Imaging Findings and Clinical Measures**
Gregory F. F. Evans, Ronald G. Haller, Philip S. Wyrick, Robert W. Parkey, and James L. Fleckenstein
Submaximal workloads are adequate to produce delayed-onset muscle soreness, and correlations between conventionally measured indexes of injury may be enhanced at more modest workloads.

821 **Musculoskeletal Tumors: Does Fast Dynamic Contrast-enhanced Subtraction MR Imaging Contribute to the Characterization?**
Henk-Jan van der Woude, Koenraad L. Verstraete, Pancras C. W. Hogendoorn, Anthonie H. M. Taminiau, Jo Hermans, and Johan L. Bloem
Fast, dynamic, contrast-enhanced subtraction MR imaging is a readily available technique that may be useful in the differentiation between benign and malignant soft-tissue masses.

Letters to the Editor

829 **The Meaning of Words**
John R. Wilcox, Jr

829 **Reply**
Richard M. Friedenberg

829 **Aunt Minnie**
Rita L. Teele and N. Thorne Griscom

830 **Reply**
Leonard Berlin

830 **CT Features of Cystic Dystrophy of the Duodenal Wall**
Lionel Arrivé and Jean-Pierre Saint-Maurice

831 **Reply**
Carlo Procacci, Rossella Graziani, Giuseppe Zamboni, Giorgio Cavallini, Paolo Pederzoli, Alessandro Guarise, Giuseppe Bogina, Carlo Biasiutti, Giovanni Carbognin, Ivo Andrea Bergamo-Andreis, and Gianfranco Pistolesi

Continued—

Evolution Continues on the New DynaView™ II

The Aloka SSD-1700 DynaView diagnostic ultrasound system has received worldwide acclaim since its introduction and is presently a best seller* thanks to its high performance and advanced functions. Now Aloka is proud to introduce the highly evolved DynaView II with field-proven reliability and enhanced performance that will ensure confident diagnosis and higher patient throughput.

*Over 2,000 systems have been ordered and the number is still growing.

DICOM-compatible DMS

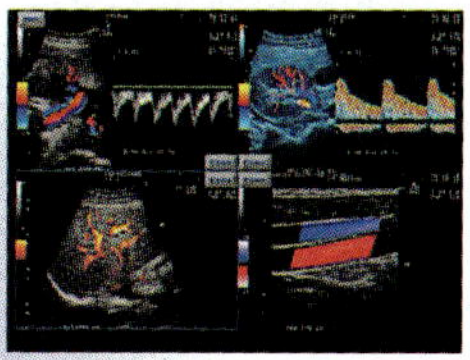

DynaView II
ALOKA
SSD-1700

The DMS (Data Management Subsystem) built-in digital interface option enables efficient digital data management. Fully digital output and lossless compression deliver original image quality with no degradation. Images can be transmitted directly to the DICOM file server and printer. Up to 4,000 grayscale images or 1,500 color images can be stored per 540MB MO disk. Loading of images into personal computers as bitmap files is also possible.

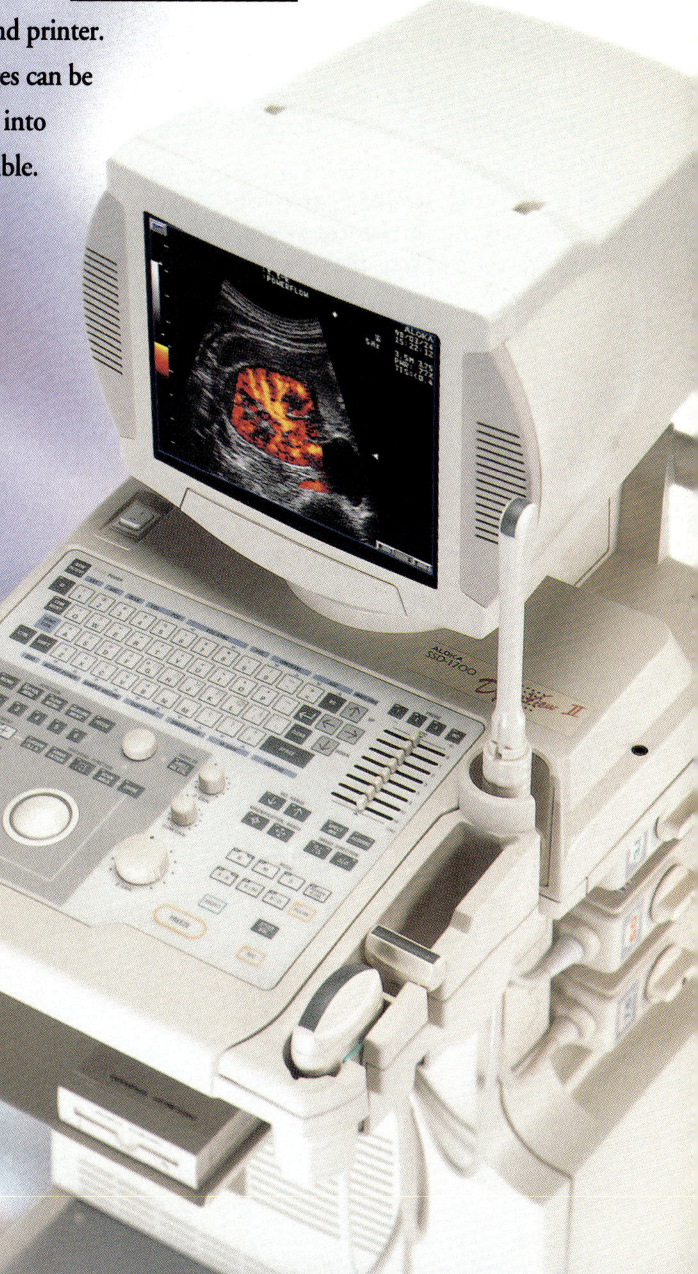

New Volume Mode

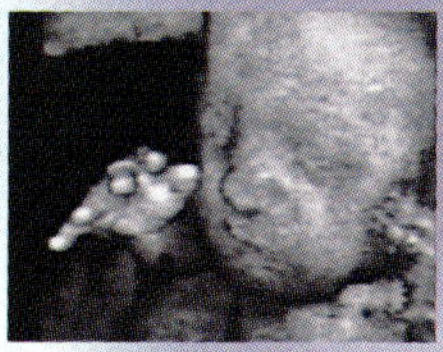

Courtesy of Chulalongkorn University, Thailand

Amazing photo realistic images can be quickly obtained using Aloka's proprietary Volume Mode technology. The Volume Mode image can then be rotated and zoomed.

QFI (QuintFrequency Imaging)

Frequent probe changing, to adjust sensitivity and resolution in accordance with the examination purpose, is unnecessary since up to five transmission frequencies for grayscale and four transmission frequencies for Doppler/Color flow imaging are independently selectable.

Dynamic PowerFlow and Precise Color Doppler

ALOKA
Science & Humanity

ALOKA CO., LTD. 6-22-1 Mure, Mitaka-shi, Tokyo 181-8622, Japan Tel: +81 422 45 6049 Fax: +81 422 45 4058 Telex: 02822-344 Cable Address: ALOKA MITAKA URL: http://www. aloka. co. jp
ALOKA CO., LTD, U.S. OFFICE 10 Fairfield Boulevard, Wallingford, CT 06492 Tel.: 800-872-5852 Fax.: 203-269-6075 mail@aloka.com

831 Comparing Test Bolus Injections with Full Bolus Injections during MR Angiography
George X. Zaleski and Brian Funaki

831 Reply
Jae K. Kim, Richard I. Farb, and Graham A. Wright

832 Normal Endometrial Signals at Color and Spectral Doppler US
Michael Applebaum

833 Reply
Stephanie R. Wilson and Peter M. Burns

833 Residual Metal Shavings and Fragments Associated with Large-Core Biopsy Needles: A Follow-up
Charles A. Finder, Richard W. Kisielewski, and Anita M. Kedas

Book Reviews

590 Imaging of Anorectal Disease
604 Practical Nuclear Medicine. 2nd ed.
624 Functional Imaging
640 Diagnostic Ultrasound: A Logical Approach
686 Imaging of the Temporal Bone. 3rd ed.
748 Basic Clinical Radiobiology. 2nd ed.

Interludes

570 A Different Kind of Radiologic Ghost
662 Photographs from South Africa
670 Photographs from Arizona and Utah

Departments

835 Abstracts of Current Literature
834 Errata
16A Advertisers' Index
15A RSNA Quick Reference
51A *Radiology* Business Information
21A Announcements and Books, Audiovisual Materials, and Software Received
27A Continuing Medical Education
55A Publication Information for Authors
59A *Radiology* Manuscript Categorization Terms
54A Copyright and Certifications Agreement
81A Classified Services
99A RSNA Bulletin Board
61A Publishers' Row
50A Associated Sciences Workshop 1998

RSNA® Radiological Society of North America Founded in 1915

2021 Spring Road, Suite 600
Oak Brook, Illinois 60523
630/571-2670
FAX: 630/571-7837

Quick Reference

RSNA PURPOSE

The purpose of the Radiological Society of North America is to promote and develop the highest standards of radiology and related sciences through education and research. The Society seeks to provide radiologists and allied health scientists with educational programs and materials of the highest quality, and to constantly improve the content and value of these educational activities. The Society seeks to foster closer fellowship among all radiologists and greater cooperation among radiologists and members of other branches of medicine and allied health care professionals.

RSNA OFFICERS FOR 1998

President, **David B. Fraser, MD,** Halifax, NS

President-Elect, **Seymour H. Levitt, MD,** Minneapolis, MN

First Vice-President, **Carol B. Stelling, MD,** Houston, TX

Second Vice-President, **Miguel E. Stoopen, MD,** Mexico City, Mexico

Third Vice-President, **Guy H. Simmons, Jr, PhD,** Lexington, KY

Historian, **William R. Eyler, MD,** Beverly Hills, MI

RSNA BOARD OF DIRECTORS FOR 1998

C. Douglas Maynard, MD, Chairman of the Board, Winston-Salem, NC

Jerry P. Petasnick, MD, Liaison for Education, Northbrook, IL

R. Nick Bryan, MD, PhD, Liaison for Publications, Baltimore, MD

Peggy J. Fritzsche, MD, Liaison for Annual Meeting Arrangements, Riverside, CA

Brian C. Lentle, MD, Liaison Designate for Education, Vancouver, BC

David B. Fraser, MD, President, Halifax, NS

Seymour H. Levitt, MD, President-Elect, Minneapolis, MN

Delmar J. Stauffer, Executive Director

RSNA IMPORTANT TELEPHONE NUMBERS

MAIN TELEPHONE	(630) 571-2670	MEMBERSHIP	(630) 571-7873
FAX	(630) 571-7837	RESEARCH DEVELOPMENT	(630) 368-3756
ACCOUNTING	(630) 571-7812	PROGRAM SERVICES	(630) 571-7874
EXECUTIVE	(630) 571-7866	RESEARCH & EDUCATION FUND	(630) 571-7816
LEARNING CENTER	(630) 368-3753	ADVERTISING	(630) 571-7817
MARKETING COMMUNICATIONS	(630) 571-7830	CLASSIFIED ADVERTISING	(630) 571-7817
MEETINGS	(630) 571-7850	RSNA LINK	http://www.rsna.org
PERMISSIONS	(630) 571-7829	SUBSCRIPTIONS	(630) 571-7873 e-mail: subscrib@rsna.org

RSNA MEETING DATES AND LOCATIONS

1998 November 29 to December 4
McCormick Place, Chicago

1999 November 28 to December 3
McCormick Place, Chicago

2000 November 26 to December 1
McCormick Place, Chicago

RSNA YEAR-AT-A-GLANCE

September 1–2, 1998
R&E Fund Trustee Meeting

September 9–10, 1998
RSNA Board of Directors Meeting

September 15, 1998
Third Seed Grant Deadline

October 30, 1998
Deadline for Advance Registration Forms for RSNA Scientific Assembly

November 29 to December 4, 1998
RSNA 84th Scientific Assembly and Annual Meeting

January 1, 1999
Call for Scientific Papers, Scientific Exhibits, and *info*RAD Exhibits

January 9, 1999
Deadline for receipt of all RSNA R&E Fund Grant Materials

January 15, 1999
First Seed Grant Deadline

February 19–21, 1999
RSNA Board of Directors Meeting

March 1, 1999
Roentgen Centennial Fellow "Preliminary Letter of Interest" Deadline

March 23-24, 1999
R&E Fund Trustee Meeting

April 15, 1999
Deadline for Submission of Scientific Paper, Scientific Exhibit, and *info*RAD Applications

May 15, 1999
Second Seed Grant Deadline

June 16–20, 1999
RSNA Board of Directors Meeting

Advertisers' Index

RSNA Advertising Policy

According to the advertising policy of the Radiological Society of North America, the information describing radiological equipment, products, and services offered by vendors in their advertisements should be ethical, educational, professional, of value in furthering the radiologic evaluation and treatment of patients and furthering the education of the radiologists and allied scientists. The guidelines below should be followed for advertising in RSNA journals.

- All advertising must be directed to radiologic diagnosis, therapy, research, communication and/or to the professional and managerial roles of radiologists and allied scientists. Advertising material should be consistent with the highest standards of professionalism.

- RSNA reserves the right to reject copy which, in its opinion, is not in good taste, is unprofessional, or is inappropriate for a radiology publication, or offers products or services not in the best interest of the patient or the Society. Advertisements that are constructed to resemble the journal's editorial pages will not be accepted in that form.

- Acceptance of advertising does not mean endorsement by RSNA of the products or services advertised, the advertisers, or the claims made.

For media kits and questions about advertising ONLY, contact:
Jim Drew, *Director of Advertising*
RSNA Publications
2021 Spring Road, Suite 600
Oak Brook, IL 60523
(630) 571-2670
FAX (630) 571-7837

For all other RSNA department telephone numbers, see "RSNA Quick Reference"; consult "Departments" in the Table of Contents for page.

Able Software Company 26A
Aloka 13A
M.D. Anderson Cancer Center 94A

Bioscan 28A
Bracco/SCA&I Fellowship Program 96A

CompHealth 89A
Cook Inc 37A–44A

Daniel & Yeager 83A
Dartmouth-Hitchcock Medical Center 93A
Diversified Diagnostic Products, Inc 22A, 35A, 49A

Eastman Kodak Company 7A
E-Z-EM, Inc 23A

C.B. Fleet 53A
Fuji Medical Systems IFC

GE Medical Systems OBC
Gundersen Lutheran 86A, 94A

Hitachi Medical Systems America, Inc 2A–3A

Imation 9A
InterAmerican Congress of Radiology 47A

Jackson & Coker 91A

Locum Medical Group 85A

Marshfield Clinic 86A
MetroHealth Medical Center 87A, 93A

National Institutes of Health 97A
Nationwide Medical Services, Inc 88A

RadioGraphics 80A
Radiology 806
Radiology Resources 85A
RADX 31A
Rhode Island Hospital 87A
RSNA Associated Sciences 50A, 724
RSNA *EJ* 36A, 596
RSNA Learning Center 610, 630, 101A–104A
RSNA Membership 30A
RSNA Online Journals 32A, 48A
RSNA ORD 45A, 760
RSNA Research & Education Fund 24A–25A, 34A
RSNA Resident Membership 19A–20A
RSNA Scientific Assembly and Annual Meeting 17A–18A, IBC

Society of Cardiovascular and Interventional Radiology 26A
Staff Relief, Inc 89A
StorageTek 11A

Charles C. Thomas, Publisher, Ltd 33A
Toshiba 4A
Trex Medical 716

U.S. Army Reserve 28A
USPHS Indian Health Service 88A

Village of Willowbrook 21A
Vista Staffing Solutions 83A

Announcement

3rd Residents' Review Course

The "3rd Residents' Review Course," sponsored by the Radiology Education Foundation, will take place on October 22–25, 1998, at the Tata Memorial Hospital Auditorium, Mumbai (Bombay), India. It is an intense, all-India review course for radiology residents, featuring didactic lectures and sessions on all specialties and modalities. Topics include radiology of the head and neck, gastrointestinal system, and the chest, as well as obstetrics and gynecology, neurology, and magnetic resonance imaging. Faculty: Bhaya, Chaubal, Desai, B. B. Jankharia, B. G. Jankharia, Joshi, Kohli, Merchant, Ramakantan, Ramamoorthy, Shetty, Shroff, Ursekar. Fee: Rs 500. For further information, contact Dr Bhavin Jankharia, "F," 1st Fl, Bhaveshwar Vihar 383, Sardar VP Rd, Mumbai 400 004, India; telephone 91 22 389-3551; fax 91 22 382-9595; e-mail *bhavinj@giasbm01.vsnl.net.in; http://www.jankharia.com/ref.html.*

Books, Audiovisual Materials, and Software Received

Radiology carries a complete listing of all books, CD-ROMs, and other material received by the Radiological Society of North America. If the material is later reviewed, the reviews of books will be printed in *Radiology* and the reviews of CD-ROMs and electronic material will appear in *RadioGraphics*.

Send publications for review to Richard A. Szucs, MD, Book Review Editor, *Radiology* Editorial Office, 1001 E Broad St, Suite 310, Richmond, VA 23219.

Functional Computed Tomography. Edited by Kenneth Miles, Peter Dawson, Martin Blomley. Hardcover, $150.00; 176 pp, 99 illustrations. ISBN: 1-899066-39-X. Oxford, England: Isis Medical Media, 1997.

Hepatobiliary and Pancreatic Radiology: Imaging and Intervention. Edited by G. Scott Gazelle, MD, MPH, Sanjay Saini, MD, Peter R. Mueller, MD. Hardcover, $182.00; 912 pp, 675 illustrations. ISBN: 3-13-109721-3. Stuttgart, Germany: Georg Thieme Verlag, 1998.

Imagerie Dynamique des Troubles Pelvi-Périneaux de la Femme [Dynamic medical imaging of pelvic floor disorder in women]. Albert Kujas, Alain Coussement, Richard Villet. Hardcover, $58.00; 144 pp, 131 illustrations. ISBN: 2-7114-1650-0. Paris, France: Éditions Vigot, 1998.

Introduction to Clinical Radiation Oncology. 3rd ed. Lawrence R. Coia, MD, David J. Moylan, MD. Softcover, $48.95; 618 pp, 11 illustrations. ISBN: 0-944838-70-7. Madison, Wis: Medical Physics Publishing, 1998.

New Developments in Cardiac Nuclear Imaging. Edited by Ami E. Iskandrian, MD, Mario S. Verani, MD. Hardcover, $85.00; 300 pp, 106 illustrations. ISBN: 0-87993-670-3. Armonk, NY: Futura, 1998.

Pediatric Radiology Case Base: The Baby Minnie of Pediatric Radiology. Joanna J. Seibert, MD, Charles A. James, MD. Softcover, DM 148; 656 pp, 701 illustrations. ISBN: 3-13-107891-X. Stuttgart, Germany: Georg Thieme Verlag, 1998.

RSNA®

Research & Education Fund

Now Available

Application/Nomination Information

The deadline for most 1999 Grant Programs is January 8, 1999. Most grants begin on July 1, 1999.

Seed Grant Program and Roentgen Centennial Fellow Program have additional deadlines and start dates. See the respective sections for details.

For additional information and application/ nomination materials, please contact the RSNA Research and Education Fund office at 630-368-7885.

Scholar

Purpose –To support young faculty members by freeing at least one–half of their time to gain experience in research early in their academic careers.

Amount –$60,000 annually for two years, payable to the institution, to be used exclusively as stipend.

Requirements –Nominee should:
- have advanced training completed, including residency, fellowship, doctorate, etc.;
- be Board Certified or eligible to sit for certifying exams;
- be a faculty member of a North American educational institution at time of award commencement;
- be within five years of initial faculty appointment;
- and have not served as principal investigator on a major ($50,000 or more) grant.

Only one nominee per department.

Medical Student/Scholar Assistant

Purpose –To provide promising medical students an opportunity to experience radiology research while assisting second year RSNA Scholars.

Amount –$5,000 per year payable to the institution.

Requirements –Candidates must be nominated by a current RSNA Scholar grant recipient and must be medical students at the time of nomination. Medical students who receive this award will devote 100% of their time to the research activity during an initial period of vacation or elective time, and will continue on a part–time basis throughout the academic year.

Notes: Parties from institutions that are hosts to current RSNA Research and Education Fund Scholars and Fellows interested in applying for these awards, should be aware that the Trustees have developed policies regarding the equitable distribution of awards. Please contact the Society office for details on these policies.

Awards, with the exception of the Seed grant award, are restricted to citizens of North American countries and to individuals in the process of becoming citizens of the same.

Medical Student Department Program

Purpose –To enable departments of diagnostic radiology/radiation oncology/nuclear medicine allied with medical schools to provide research opportunities to medical students.

Amount –$1,000 per month to be matched by department for a period of 3 or more months.

Requirements –Awards restricted to departments of diagnostic radiology/radiation oncology/nuclear medicine allied with fully accredited North American medical schools. Departments must describe the following: commitment to research, student project that will require 100% of student's time, and proposed benefit for both medical student and the designated scientific advisor/project manager. The method by which student will be selected must also be identified.

Note: Name of student must be advised prior to grant disbursement.

Research Fellow

Purpose –To provide educational opportunities for young investigators not yet professionally established in radiologic sciences to gain further insight into scientific investigation, or to develop competence in research and educational techniques and methods.

Amount –$35,000 Fellow stipend for one year, with opportunity to renew for a second year at $40,000. Upon request, $5,000 is given to the institution to be applied directly to expenses.

Requirements –Nominee should:
- hold a degree of MD, DO, DVM, DDS, DMD, or the equivalent as recognized by the American Medical Association, and
- be nearing the end of prescribed training and/or have completed the prerequisite training to sit for certifying exams.

It is expected that Fellows will devote, essentially, their full time to research under the guidance of a scientific advisor of their choice.

Research Resident

Purpose –To provide educational opportunities for radiology residents to gain further insight into scientific investigation, or to develop competence in research and educational techniques and methods.

Amount –$30,000 grant for one year, payable to the department, to be used as stipend.

Requirements –Nominee should:
- possess an academic degree acceptable for the radiology residency, and
- at time of nomination, be in a residency program.

It is expected that the Research Resident will devote 90% of his or her time to the program outlined.

Seed Grant

Purpose –To assist young investigators in testing hypotheses and defining objectives before they apply for major grants from corporations, foundations, or government agencies.

Amount –One-year grant of $25,000 or less, payable to the department in equal installments.

Requirements –Applicant should hold full–time faculty position,
- have completed all advanced training, and
- have not served as principal investigator in a major ($50,000 or more) grant.

Any area of radiology–related research is eligible, including basic, clinical, developmental, health care planning and delivery, efficacy studies, and education.

Note: Applicant need not be citizen/resident of a North American country.

The Seed Grant Program will be offered three times each year. Deadlines are:
January 15 for July 1 start date
May 15 for November 1 start date
September 15 for March 1 start date

Roentgen Centennial Fellow Program

Purpose –To permit experienced practitioners the opportunity to explore and apply innovative solutions to key issues facing the radiology community. Such activity may include, but is not limited to: research studies, or program delivery focusing on topics such as health care policy/economics; educational methodology; evaluation methodology/outcomes research; basic or clinical research; rural health care delivery; or technology assessment.

Amount –This $100,000 award is designed to support a one–year program of study and/or research.

Requirements –Nominee should be beyond initial radiologic training and have several years of experience.

The individual who receives this award will devote a majority of his or her time to the proposed activity for a period of one year.

Application details differ for this program. Detailed letter of interest outlining applicant's innovative idea should be received at the Fund's office by March 1 each year.

Outstanding Researcher Award

Purpose –To honor one senior physician or radiology researcher who has made a career of significant contributions to the field of radiology or radiologic sciences through research.

Amount –$25,000 award payable to the recipient.

Requirements –Nominee must demonstrate a long–term commitment to radiology research.

Nomination packets must include:
- letter of nomination that addresses individual's appropriateness for award;
- corroborating letter of support; and
- nominee's CV, which includes a summary of candidate's grant support and research activities.

Nominations must be made by June 15. Nominee need not be a member of the RSNA.

Roentgen Resident/Fellow Research Award

Purpose –To recognize and encourage outstanding residents and fellows in radiologic research.

Recognition Award –Each participating residency program will receive an award plaque. Plaque includes place for additional names. Each year the Fund will provide a memento for the department to present to the selected resident or fellow.

Requirements –The director of the residency program or the department chair will identify an individual based on the following criteria:
- presentations or scientific papers at regional or national meetings,
- publication of scientific papers in peer-reviewed journals,
- receipt of a research grant, or
- other research activities.

The R&E Fund does not make the selections. Each department simply submits the name and address of the resident/fellow selected with a description of the individual's research activities. Nomination is to be submitted no later than April 1.

Continuing Medical Education

NOTE: Notices of continuing medical education programs will be considered for publication in *Radiology* if the program is directly relevant to medical imaging and if the following information is included: (*a*) dates and location, (*b*) a brief description of the course, (*c*) a listing of local and visiting faculty, (*d*) fees, and (*e*) number of category 1 credits that are available. Such notices should be submitted *at least* 5 months before the meeting date. Announcements of CME programs we consider not pertinent will not be published. We assume no responsibility for the content of CME programs appearing here. **Address announcements to** Julie Pietryla, RSNA Publications, 2021 Spring Rd, Suite 600, Oak Brook, IL 60523.

Continuing medical education programs are listed according to diagnostic discipline; interdisciplinary programs are grouped under the predominant or first-listed specialty.

Diagnostic Imaging

Mini-Fellowship in Radiology

The Department of Radiology and Office of Continuing Medical Education, University of Texas–Houston Medical School, is offering its "Mini-Fellowship in Radiology: A Hands On Approach" on an ongoing basis at the University of Texas Medical School, Houston. Participants may register for this fellowship during any consecutive period of 4–8 weeks (6 weeks is suggested); a 1-week course is also offered. The course will provide radiologists an opportunity to increase their skill levels in subspecialty areas such as magnetic resonance imaging, computed tomography, and ultrasound. Upon completion of the course, participants should be able to (*a*) demonstrate and employ a wide variety of advanced subspecialty procedures, (*b*) evaluate and recognize the risks and benefits of procedures, (*c*) demonstrate their increased skill level in performing procedures, and (*d*) develop and produce enhanced practice patterns for patient care in their home hospital setting. Course directors: Cohen, Goldman. Fee: $2,000 for the first week, $1,000 for subsequent weeks; 40 hours of category 1 credit will be available per week. For further information, contact Mary Ann Henderson, Department of Radiology, University of Texas–Houston Medical School, 6431 Fannin, Ste 2.132 MSB, Houston, TX 77030-1503; telephone (713) 500-7632; fax (713) 500-7639; e-mail *maryannh@msrad3.med.uth.tmc.edu; http://msrad3.med.uth.tmc.edu/mfp.htm.*

Radiology Refresher Course

A "Radiology Refresher Course," sponsored by the Department of Radiology, University of Minnesota, will take place on September 16–19, 1998, at the Silverado Country Club and Resort, Napa Valley, Calif. This course is designed to provide an overview of up-to-date techniques used in everyday clinical practice. After attending the course, participants will be able to identify current applications of ultrasound, computed tomography, and magnetic resonance imaging in radiology and demonstrate effective imaging approaches to common clinical situations. Course directors: Engeler, Everson, Thompson, Trenkner. Faculty: Carpenter, Galle, Helms, Ikeda, Moss, Pugatch, Thompson, Truwit, Walsh. Fee: $695; 18 hours of category 1 credit will be available. For further information, contact the Office of Continuing Medical Education, University of Minnesota, 615 Washington Ave SE, Ste 107, Minneapolis, MN 55414; telephone (800) 776-8636 or (612) 626-7600; fax (612) 626-7766; *http://www.cee.umn.edu:80/cme/.*

Radiology/98: Thoracoabdominal Imaging and Mammography

The Department of Radiology, University of Minnesota, is sponsoring the "61st Annual Radiology/98: Thoracoabdominal Imaging and Mammography" course, to be held on October 8–10, 1998, at the Radisson Hotel Metrodome, Minneapolis, Minn. Participants in this course will learn about diverse imaging techniques, including ultrasound and magnetic resonance, used in the evaluation of thoracoabdominal disorders, as well as current procedures in mammography. Course directors: Engeler, Everson, Thompson, Trenkner. Guest faculty: Bird, Carlson, Cody, Collins, Day, Hattery, Johnson, McCarty, Pugatch, Semelka, Stephens. Fee: $395; 20 hours of category 1 credit will be available. For further information, contact the Office of Continuing Medical Education, University of Minnesota, 615 Washington Ave SE, Ste 107, Minneapolis, MN 55414; telephone (800) 776-8636 or (612) 626-7600; fax (612) 626-7766; *http://www.cee.umn.edu:80/cme/.*

23rd Annual San Diego Postgraduate Radiology Course

The 23rd Annual San Diego Postgraduate Radiology Course, sponsored by the University of California–San Diego School of Medicine, will be held on October 26 to November 1, 1998, at the Hotel del Coronado, San Diego, Calif. This course, intended for practicing radiologists, will be a comprehensive review of the recent advances and most difficult subject material within each subspecialty. Emphasis is placed on practical and useful clinical information and understanding clinical problems. Program directors: Bergin, Wong. Fee: $995 ($700 for residents, fellows, and technologists); 39 hours of category 1 credit will be available. For further information, contact Ryals & Associates, Inc, PO Box 1925, Roswell, GA 30077-1925; telephone (770) 641-9773; fax (770) 552-9859; e-mail *webmaster@ryalsmeet.com; http://www.ryalsmeet.com.*

Radiology in Sydney

"Radiology in Sydney," a course co-sponsored by the Cleveland Clinic Foundation, will take place on March 21–28, 1999, at the Sheraton on the Park Hotel, Sydney, Australia. This course is designed to be an overview of cutting-edge, practical radiology. Topics include helical computed tomography, mammography, Doppler ultrasound, neuroradiology, and magnetic resonance imaging of the bones, joints, abdomen, chest, and central nervous system. Course director: Crawford. Faculty: Brant, Earwaker, Federle, Helms, Masaryk, Read, Rickard, Sagel, Whyte, Young. Fee: $795 until September, $895 thereafter; 32 hours of category 1 credit will be available. For further information, contact Betsy Birchenough, director, Radiology International, Inc, 340 Cleverdale Rd, PO Box 95, Cleverdale, NY 12820; telephone (888) 656-3104 or (518) 656-3104; fax (518) 656-9815; e-mail *betsy@radiologyintl.com; http://www.radiologyintl.com.*

Computed Tomography

CT-MRI State of the Art

The Department of Medical Imaging, University of Toronto, is sponsoring a course entitled "CT-MRI State of the Art," to take place on October 15–18, 1998, at the Hamilton Princess Hotel, Hamilton, Bermuda. This 18-hour course will emphasize recent advances in helical computed tomography and magnetic resonance imaging in the diagnosis and treatment of diseases of the chest, abdomen, musculoskeletal system, and central nervous system. Program directors: Kucharczyk, Rappaport. Faculty: Asch, Fishman, Kucharczyk, Merchant, Montanera, Rappaport, Salonen. Fee: Can $650 (Can $460 for residents, fellows, and technologists); 18 hours of category 1 credit will be available. For further information, contact Ryals & Associates, Inc, PO Box 1925, Roswell, GA 30077-1925; telephone (770) 641-9773; fax (770) 552-9859; e-mail *webmaster@ryalsmeet.com; http://www.ryalsmeet.com.*

CT for Pulmonary Embolism: Getting Started

"CT for Pulmonary Embolism: Getting Started," a course sponsored by the Department of Radiology, Medical College of Wisconsin, will be held on October 17, 1998, at the Medical College of Wisconsin, Milwaukee. This course is designed to provide a practical approach to diagnosing pulmonary embolisms for those beginning to use computed tomography. Program objectives are to evaluate current approaches, present scanning protocols, review normal anatomy and variants, and present multiple cases for hands-on demonstrations. Course director: Goodman. Faculty:

Goodman, Lipchik, Karabulut, Malone, Mayo. Fee: $150 ($75 for residents and fellows); 4.5 hours of category 1 credit will be available. For further information, contact Sylvia Bartz, Department of Radiology, Froedtert Memorial Lutheran Hospital, 9200 W Wisconsin Ave, Rm 2803, Milwaukee, WI 53226-3596; telephone (414) 805-3120; fax (414) 476-7503; e-mail *sylbartz@mcw.edu.*

Neuroradiology

Computed Tomography and Magnetic Resonance Imaging of the Brain, Head, Neck and Spine

The 25th Annual Course on Computed Tomography and Magnetic Resonance Imaging of the Brain, Head, Neck and Spine, sponsored by the Department of Diagnostic Radiology, Rush-Presbyterian-St Luke's Medical Center, will be held on October 22–23, 1998, at the Westin River North Hotel, Chicago, Ill. Topics include brain tumor imaging and classification, imaging of "brain attack," clinical uses of diffusion-weighted imaging, and atypical manifestations of demyelinating disease. Guest faculty: Castillo, Hasso, Haughton, Kucharczyk, Murtagh, Naidich, Osborn, Ramsey, Russell, Som. Local faculty: Cambray, Geremia, Huckman. Fee: $525 ($395 for persons in training); 15 hours of category 1 credit will be available. For further information, contact Michael S. Huckman, MD, Department of Diagnostic Radiology, Rush-Presbyterian-St Luke's Medical Center, 1653 W Congress Pkwy, Chicago, IL 60612; telephone (312) 942-5781; fax (312) 942-2114; e-mail *mhuckman@rush.edu.*

Nuclear Medicine

Central Chapter, Society of Nuclear Medicine

The Central Chapter of the Society of Nuclear Medicine is holding its 1998 Fall Meeting on September 26–27, 1998, at the Hilton Hotel, Milwaukee, Wis. This year's course is entitled "Positrons and Other Oncological Topics." Emphasis is placed on the use of positron-emitting radiopharmaceuticals in the diagnosis and treatment of disease. Topics include detection of positrons with collimated and coincidence SPECT cameras, positron-emission tomography in clinical oncology, the clinical role of F-18 FDG in lymphoma and prostate carcinoma, and therapy with antibodies and receptor agents. Program chairmen: Priem, Weir. Fee: $100 for physician nonmembers, $75 for physician members ($70 for technologist nonmembers, $60 for technologist members); category 1 accreditation pending. For further information, contact Vincent J. Sodd, PhD, executive director, Central Chapter, SNM, Inc, 5987 Turpin Hills Dr, Cincinnati, OH 45244-3946; telephone (513) 231-5274.

Southeastern Chapter, Society of Nuclear Medicine

The Southeastern Chapter of the Society of Nuclear Medicine is holding its 39th Annual Meeting on October 16–18, 1998, at the Wynfrey Hotel, Birmingham, Ala. This year's course is entitled "Expanding the Clinical Application of Nuclear Medicine." Topics include oncology, cardiology, managed care, positron-emission tomography, and radiopharmaceutical development. Approximately 35 companies will exhibit their nuclear medicine–related instrumentation, radiopharmaceuticals, and supplies. Program chairman: Mountz. Fee: $25; category 1 accreditation pending. For further information, contact Vincent J. Sodd, PhD, executive director, Southeastern Chapter, SNM, Inc, 5987 Turpin Hills Dr, Cincinnati, OH 45244-3946; telephone (513) 231-6955.

Greater New York/New England Chapters, Society of Nuclear Medicine

The 12th Annual Northeast Regional Scientific Meeting, sponsored by the Greater New York/New England Chapters, Society of Nuclear Medicine, will be held on November 6–8, 1998, at the Newport Marriott Hotel, Newport, RI. This year's course is entitled "Clinical Applications: 1998." A broad range of lectures will address nuclear medicine as applied to cardiology, endocrinology, gastroenterology, neurology, oncology, orthopedics, and pediatrics. Joint presentations by specialists in nuclear medicine and other imaging modalities will emphasize the value of correlating functional and anatomic information. Interactive, case-oriented "Read with the Expert" sessions will enable participants to gain insight into clinical challenges from recognized leaders in the field. Course directors: Connolly, Tikofsky. Fee: $200 for physician nonmembers, $170 for physician members ($90 for technologist nonmembers, $50 for technologist members, $40 for residents and fellows); 15.75 hours of category 1 credit will be available. For further information, contact Mitchell Stromer, Northeast Regional Scientific Meeting, SNM, Inc, 360 Cedar Ln, East Meadow, NY 11554; telephone (718) 405-8468; fax (718) 824-1369.

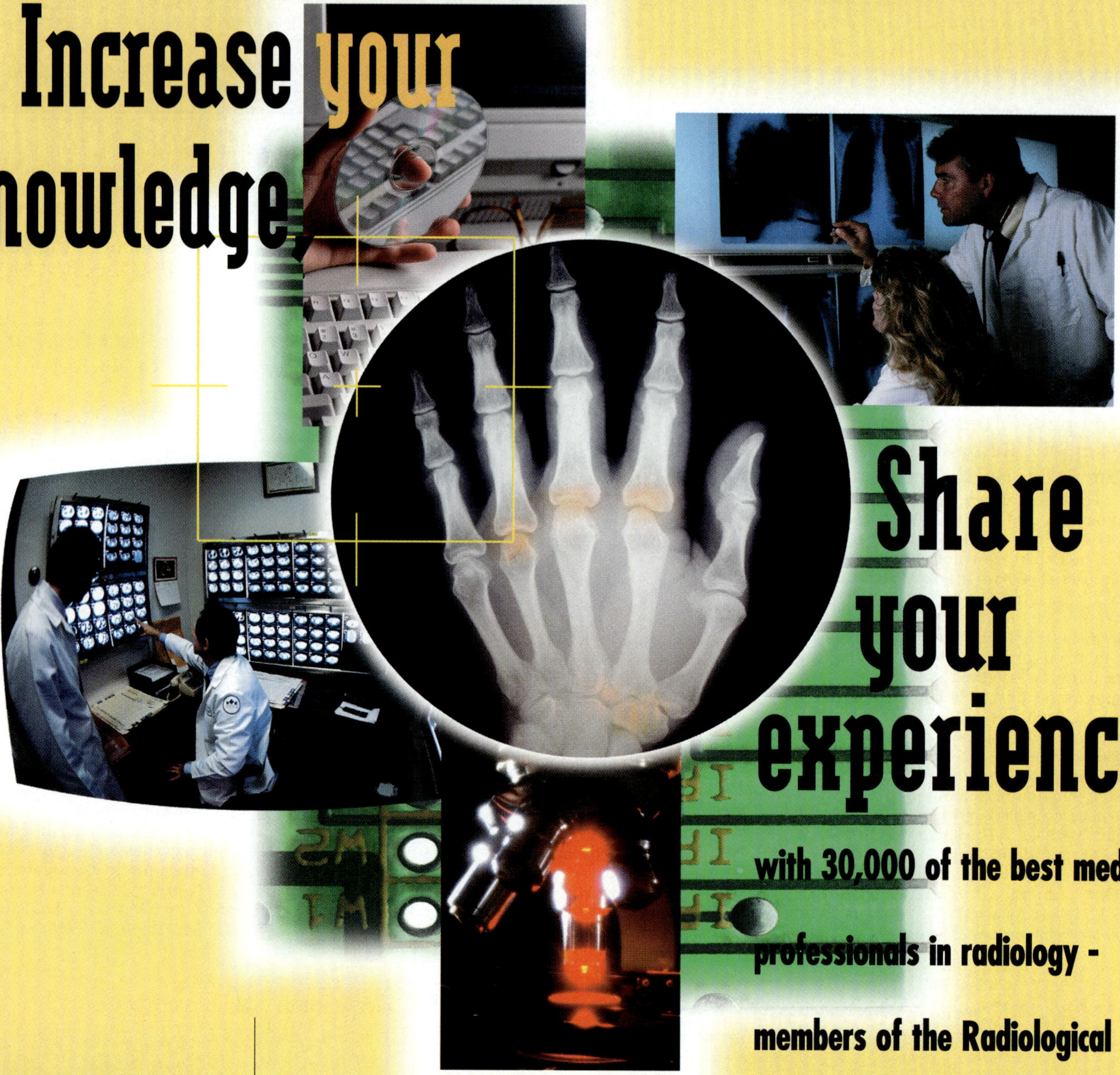

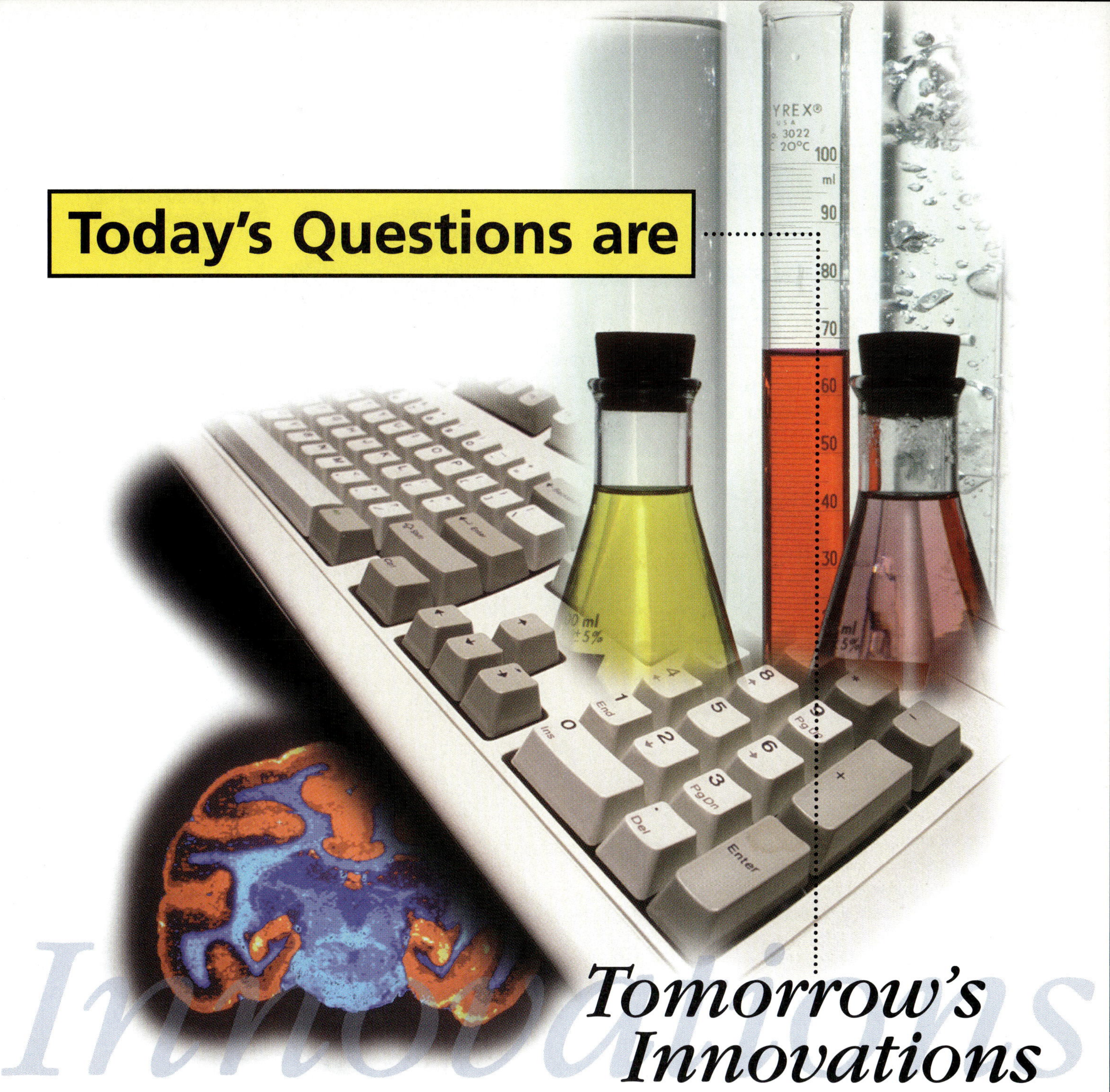
Today's Questions are
Tomorrow's
Innovations

Science to Practice
RSNA '98

Integrating Science Into Practice

Associated Sciences Program at RSNA 1998

Workshop: Saturday, Nov. 28, 1998, 10:15 am - 4:30 pm, McCormick Place South

Refresher Courses: Sunday, Nov. 29, 1998 through Friday, Dec. 4, 1998

Credits: $4\frac{1}{4}$ hours and an additional $1\frac{1}{2}$ hours credit for attendance at the Basic Physics Lecture

Welcome and Introduction
10:15 am
Samuel L. Hissong, MD, Chair, Associated Sciences Consortium and Committee
Eugene D. Frank, MA, RT(R), Coordinator, Associated Sciences Consortium

Keynote Presentation
10:30 - 11:50 am
Impact of Telematic Technologies on Image-Guided Medicine (AIA-AAH)
Heinz U. Lemke, PhD

Break
11:50 am - 12:10 pm

Special Luncheon Program
12:10 - 1:20 pm
Networking for the New Millennium - Important Factors to Consider (SMRT)
Bruce Johnson, BSEE

Break
1:20 - 1:30 pm

Panel Presentation
1:30 - 2:50 pm
The Reality of Computerization (AERS, AHRA, SROA)
Richard Carlton, MS, RT(R)
Robert Seely, MBA, RT(R)
Heinz U. Lemke, PhD

AAPM/RSNA Basic Physics Lecture for the Radiologic Technologist: Vascular Imaging Physics
Organized by Gerald A. White, Jr., MS
3:00 - 4:30 pm
$1\frac{1}{2}$ hours credit

Refresher Courses

(Each Refresher Course is approved for $1\frac{1}{2}$ hours credit)

Sunday RC 124
Organizational Culture and Health System Change
Cornelius J. Rater, MD (AERS)
Harry J. Granito, MS (RBMA)
Douglas R. Hanson (ASRT)

Monday RC 224
Liability Issues Arising from the Changing Health Care Environment
Ann Obergfell, JD, RT(R) (ASRT)
Perry Smith, JD, RDMS (SDMS)

Monday RC 324
Organizational Change In Radiology: Preparing Radiology for the Next Millennium
Monte G. Clinton (AHRA)
Donna L. Wright, EdD, RT(R) (AERS)
Loretta L. Hanwell, MPA (AHRA)

Tuesday RC 424
Competency, Continuity, and Compliance
Susan S. Weiss, CNMT (SNM-TS)
Kate Little, RN (ARNA)

Wednesday RC 524
Managing a Multisite Radiology Network
Larry Ranahan, MBA (RBMA) Moderator
Sherry Rader (RBMA)
Charles Deschamps, RT(R)(MR) (SMRT)
Rebecca Shanahan, JD (RBMA)

Thursday RC 624
Specialized Accreditations: A Cost of Doing Business
Luann J. Culbreth, MEd, RT(R)(MR) (SMRT) Moderator
John Kovelski, RT(R)(MR) (SMRT)
Karol Handrahan, RT(R) (SMRT)
Linda Zanin, MS, PhD (SDMS)
Ronald F. Bernardi, BA, RT(R)(N) (AHRA)

Thursday RC 724
Multidisciplinary Standards for the New Millennium
Susan S. Weiss, CNMT (SNM-TS), Moderator
William R. Poller, MD (SNM-TS)
Michael R. Bloyd, RT(R), BSN (ASRT)
Liz Anderson, MBA (AVIR)

Friday RC 824
Marketing Radiology: Getting the Message Out
Ronald F. Bernardi, BA, RT(R)(N), Moderator
Cherrill Farnsworth (AHRA)
Michael R. Favreau, FAHRA (AHRA)

Registration Information

Advance registration for the RSNA Scientific Assembly ends October 30. Onsite registration begins at 12:00 noon on Saturday, November 28, at McCormick Place. RSNA shuttle bus service to McCormick Place will be available beginning at 10:00 am on Saturday. Advance registration is not required for the Saturday workshop; however, to receive continuing education credit, you must register.

Advance registration information appears in the July issue of *Radiology*. Brochures are also available from your association or from the RSNA, 2021 Spring Road, Suite 600, Oak Brook, IL 60523-1860. Phone: 630/571-7862.

Registration for the RSNA Scientific Assembly includes registration for the Associated Sciences Workshop. A box lunch will be available for purchase to facilitate your attendance at the workshop. These lunches must be purchased with your advance registration for the RSNA Meeting. **If you wish to purchase a box lunch, please check the appropriate box on the RSNA Advance Registration form and enclose your $11.50 payment.**

If you would like a copy of the published Associated Sciences Proceedings, please call 630/571-7877.

Sponsoring Organizations

- American Healthcare Radiology Administrators (AHRA)
- American Institute of Architects — Academy on Architecture for Health (AIA-AAH)
- American Radiological Nurses Association (ARNA)
- American Society of Radiologic Technologists (ASRT)
- Association of Educators in Radiological Sciences (AERS)
- Association of Vascular and Interventional Radiographers (AVIR)
- Radiological Business Management Association (RBMA)
- Society for Radiation Oncology Administrators (SROA)
- Society of Diagnostic Medical Sonographers (SDMS)
- Society of Magnetic Resonance Technologists (SMRT)
- Society of Nuclear Medicine — Technologists Section (SNM-TS)

RSNA®
Radiological Society of North America
Founded in 1915

2021 Spring Road, Suite 600
Oak Brook, Illinois 60523-1860
630/571-2670 FAX: 630/571-7837
www.rsna.org

Associated Sciences

Radiology Business Information

Radiology, a monthly journal devoted to clinical radiology and allied sciences, is owned and published by

The Radiological Society of North America, Inc (RSNA)
2021 Spring Road, Suite 600
Oak Brook, IL 60523 USA
(630) 571-2670 • FAX (630) 571-7837
RSNA Link *http://www.rsna.org*

Delmar J. Stauffer, *Executive Director and Business Manager for Publications*

■ JOURNAL BUSINESS

Send new manuscripts to the address given in the Publication Information for Authors.

Correspondence concerning accepted or published material should be addressed to

Anthony V. Proto, MD–Editor, *Radiology*
Radiology Editorial Office • 1001 East Broad Street
Suite 310 • Richmond, VA 23219
(804) 644-5667 FAX (804) 644-5672
e-mail: *proto@rsna.org*

■ COPYRIGHT AND PERMISSIONS

■ PHOTOCOPYING

Authorization to photocopy items for internal or personal use, or the internal or personal use of specific clients and educators, is granted by RSNA, provided that the appropriate fee is paid directly to Copyright Clearance Center, Inc (CCC), 222 Rosewood Dr, Danvers, MA 01923 (phone 978-750-8400; FAX 978-750-4744).

Consent for photocopying does not extend to copying for general distribution, resale, or advertising and promotional purposes, or for creating new collective works. Permission for the latter categories may be sought by writing to the Permissions Coordinator, RSNA Publications, Oak Brook, IL (address above).

■ SUBSCRIPTION INFORMATION

The nonmember subscription rate for the USA is $215.00 per year; for outside USA, $260.00 (includes postage). (Air freight is available; rates are furnished on request.) Residents who are members of the RSNA may subscribe to **both** *Radiology* and *RadioGraphics* for a special rate of $80.00 (for North American addresses; residents from outside North America, add $60.00 for postage). Single copies are $25.00 (air freight, $11.00). Orders for subscriptions, remittances, and questions about subscriptions should be sent to

RSNA Subscriptions Department
2021 Spring Road, Suite 600
Oak Brook, IL 60523 USA
(630) 571-7873
FAX (630) 571-7837
e-mail: *subscrib@rsna.org*

The page containing advertising information (Advertisers' Index) may be located by consulting the Departments section in the Table of Contents.

■ CHANGE OF ADDRESS

The Post Office will not forward your journal to a new address. To avoid missing any issues, you must notify us of a change in address. At least 5 weeks before you move, please send (*a*) your **new address**, with zip code, and (*b*) your **current mailing label** with your old address to the address above.

■ MISSING ISSUES AND BACK COPIES

Claims for copies lost in the mail are allowed within 90 days of issue. Claims are not allowed for issues lost as a result of insufficient notice of change of address. To replace a missing issue or order a back copy contact RSNA Subscriptions Department at the address above. Back copies cost $25.00 (air freight, $11.00).

■ REPRINTS

The first footnote on the first page of each *Radiology* article contains the name and address of the author who answers requests for reprints. For reprint orders of 100 or more, contact

(continued)

RSNA DEPARTMENT TELEPHONE NUMBERS

Accounting	(630) 571-7812
Advertising	(630) 571-7817
Copyrights and Permissions	(630) 571-7829
Executive	(630) 571-7866
Learning Center	(630) 368-3753
Meetings	(630) 571-7850
Membership	(630) 571-7873
Office of Research	(630) 368-3756
Permissions	(630) 571-7829
Program	(630) 571-7874
Research and Education Fund	(630) 571-7816
Reprints	(610) 250-7244
Subscriptions	(630) 571-7873
Syllabus sales	(800) 272-2920
Main telephone	(630) 571-2670
FAX	(630) 571-7837

Radiology Reprints
1991 Northampton St
Easton, PA 18042-3189 USA
(610) 250-7244

For reprints of advertisements, contact the Advertising Production Manager (address under Advertising).

■ MICROFORM

Radiology is available in microfilm and microfiche from

University Microforms International
300 N Zeeb Road
Ann Arbor, MI 48106 USA
(800) 521-3044

■ INDEXES

Radiology is included in the *RSNA Index to Imaging Literature,* a 3-year cumulative subject and author index of *Radiology* and 41 radiologic journals, available for $35.00 per copy (air freight, $11.00). Subscribers to the Journal receive the index free of charge. *Radiology* is indexed in *Current Contents/Clinical Medicine,* available from the Institute for Scientific Information, and *Index Medicus,* available from the National Library of Medicine.

■ BOOK REVIEWERS AND BOOKS FOR REVIEW

Any person who would like to help in reviewing books for *Radiology* should contact

Richard A. Szucs, MD, Book Review Editor
Radiology Editorial Office
1001 E Broad St
Suite 310
Richmond, VA 23219

Publishers wishing to have books reviewed should send them to the same address.

■ PUBLISHERS' ROW

As a service to readers and colleagues in medical publishing, *Radiology* publishes a list of current imaging publications of interest to radiologists and allied scientists. Complete addresses and phone numbers of participating publishers are included. Publishers' Row is featured quarterly, in the March, June, September, and December issues. For information on publishing a list, contact Mary Ann Morrissey at RSNA Publications (address under Journal Business).

■ ADVERTISING

The advertising policy appears on the Advertisers' Index of each issue. Questions about advertising and billing, advertising contracts, and insertion orders and requests for media kits should be addressed to

James F. Drew, *Director of Advertising*
RSNA Publications
2021 Spring Road, Suite 600
Oak Brook, IL 60523 USA
(630) 571-7819
FAX (630) 571-7837

Questions about advertising production should be addressed to:

Pat Hollingsworth, *Advertising Production Manager*
RSNA Advertising Department
2021 Spring Rd, Suite 600
Oak Brook, IL 60523 USA
(630) 571-7818
FAX (630) 571-7837

■ CLASSIFIED ADVERTISING

As a service to readers, *Radiology* accepts classified advertising, and every effort is made to ensure that the ads are relevant to the practice of radiology. For more details on the classified advertising policy and procedures, see the Classified Advertising section in each issue (consult the Departments section in the Table of Contents for page number) or contact the Advertising Production Manager (address under Advertising).

CHANGE OF ADDRESS FORM

Please allow 90 days for change to take effect

Name: ______________________________

Previous Address

Address: ______________________________

____

____

City/State/Zip: ______________________________

New Address

Address: ______________________________

____

____

City/State/Zip: ______________________________

Mail to:
RSNA Subscriptions Department • 2021 Spring Road • Suite 600 • Oak Brook, IL 60523 USA **FAX:** (630) 571-7837

Transfer of Copyright and Certifications Agreement

Manuscript No. (for Editorial Office use only)____________________

Complete copyright to the article entitled:

____

____

is hereby transferred to the Radiological Society of North America (for **U.S. government employees:** to the extent transferable), effective if and when the article is accepted for publication in ***Radiology,*** printed or electronic format. In the case of authors who are officers or employees of the U.S. government, the Radiological Society of North America recognizes that works prepared by them as part of their official government duties are in the public domain.

Authors reserve the following rights:

A. Other than copyright, all proprietary rights including patent rights relating to the subject matter of the article.
B. The license for personal use in lectures, lecture notes, and exhibits.

Please return this form as soon as possible. The signed statement **must** be received by the Editor **before** the manuscript can be processed for publication.

A. All authors certify that this material or similar material has not been and will not be submitted by them or by colleagues in their institution to any other publication prior to its appearance in ***Radiology.***

B. All authors certify that they have read the Publication Information for Authors found in the most recently published issue of ***Radiology*** at the time the manuscript is submitted. They further certify their compliance with the various requirements found therein.

C. All authors certify that they have submitted all required permissions and that all required statements have been inserted in the text where appropriate.

D. All authors certify that all individuals who have participated sufficiently in the conception and design of this work, in the analysis of the data, and in the writing of the manuscript have been listed as authors. All authors further certify that they have read the final version of the manuscript and approve it for submission for publication.

E. All authors certify that the Editor may correspond with the designated *corresponding author* regarding acceptance, rejection, revision of the manuscript and that the corresponding author is responsible for informing all other authors of the same.

F. All authors certify that responses, revisions received by the Editor from the designated *corresponding author* will be treated as if from all authors and that the corresponding author is responsible for informing all other authors of the same.

G. All authors certify that: **(must check one)**

- ❐ they have no direct or indirect financial interest in the products under investigation or subject matter discussed in this manuscript, or
- ❐ one or more (please name) authors do have a direct or indirect financial interest in the products under investigation or subject matter discussed in this manuscript. A separate statement is attached that details this proprietary interest, and the authors hereby grant permission to publish this information or an appropriate summary thereof with the manuscript if the manuscript is published.

TO BE SIGNED BY ALL AUTHORS:

Name (print) (First) ____________________ Signature ____________________

Name (print) ____________________ Signature ____________________

Name (print) ____________________ Signature ____________________

Name (print) ____________________ Signature ____________________

Name (print) ____________________ Signature ____________________

Name (print) ____________________ Signature ____________________

Use additional page if necessary.

This signed form (a photocopy is acceptable) must be submitted with all proffered works.

Radiology Publication Information for Authors

Radiology is published under the supervision of the Board of Directors of the Radiological Society of North America, Inc, which appoints the Editor who selects all material submitted for publication, including advertisements. No responsibility is accepted by the Board of Directors or the appointed Editor for the opinions expressed by the contributors. Please note that the instructions below are in accord with the *Uniform Requirements for Manuscripts Submitted to Biomedical Journals* (*Annals of Internal Medicine* 1997; 126:36-47). Although *Radiology* will receive material prepared and submitted according to these instructions, the right is reserved to introduce any changes necessary to make the contributions conform to the individual editorial standards of this Journal.

Full manuscripts should be addressed to:
Anthony V. Proto, MD—Editor, *Radiology*
Radiology Manuscripts • RSNA Publications
2021 Spring Road, Suite 600 • Oak Brook, IL 60523 USA
FAX (630) 571-7837

All other submissions and correspondence concerning accepted or published material should be addressed to:
Anthony V. Proto, MD—Editor, *Radiology*
Radiology Editorial Office • 1001 East Broad Street
Suite 310 • Richmond, VA 23219
(804) 644-5667 FAX (804) 644-5672
e-mail: *proto@rsna.org*

Assistant to the Editor: Deborah L. Hogan
Office Coordinator: Donna L. Schulze, Beth A. Stephenson

Inquiries about manuscript status and preparation, as well as letters to the editor, can be directed to *radiolog@ rsna.org*

The page containing advertising information (Advertisers' Index) may be located by consulting the Departments section in the Table of Contents.

■ TRANSFER OF COPYRIGHT AND CERTIFICATIONS AGREEMENT

Please send the copyright and certifications agreement with the initial submission of all proffered works. This may be accomplished by using a copy of the form that appears in this issue. **All** authors of any single composition must sign this agreement. In the case of officers or employees of the U.S. government, the Society recognizes that works prepared as part of their official government duties are in the public domain, but they must still sign the copyright and certifications agreement.

■ FINANCIAL INTEREST

Authors must describe any direct or indirect financial interest they may have in the subject matter of a submitted manuscript, and they must authorize the Society to publish this financial disclosure with the article if deemed appropriate. The Society's Financial Disclosure policy is as follows:

"Each author shall describe (*a*) any direct financial interest that author has in the subject matter discussed in the submitted manuscript, and (*b*) any affiliation or financial involvement that author has with or in any organization having a direct financial interest in the subject matter discussed in the submitted manuscript. Such information will be held in the confidence of the journal Editor during the review process. If necessary, in the Editor's view, this information may be shared with reviewers after discussion between the Editor and author. The submission of a manuscript to *Radiology* grants permission for RSNA to publish the financial information described above, or an appropriate summary thereof, with the manuscript if the manuscript is accepted for publication."

■ MANUSCRIPT PREPARATION

Original writings will be accepted only with the understanding that they are contributed solely to *Radiology*. Manuscripts should be typewritten and **double-spaced (all pages)** on only one side of the paper with at least 3-cm margins. Each manuscript component should begin on a **new page** in this order: title pages, abstract, text, acknowledgments, references, tables (each on a separate page), and captions for illustrations. The title pages and abstract page should not be numbered. Sequential numbering should begin with the text. To ensure anonymity in the review process, authors' names should appear on only the full title page; names of authors or the institution should **not** be given in the text or on the illustrations. **Three copies** of the manuscript and three complete sets of mounted illustrations should be submitted. The author should retain a complete copy of the manuscript, since accepted manuscripts will not be returned and only the illustrations of rejected manuscripts will be returned. All manuscripts are acknowledged; please allow 2-3 weeks from the time you mailed the manuscript for receipt of an acknowledgment.

■ TITLE PAGES, AUTHOR CONTRIBUTIONS

Full Title Page: This page should include the title of the manuscript, the first and last names, middle initials, and degrees of all authors, the name and street address (not a postal box) of the institution from which the work originated, the telephone number, the FAX or Telex number, and the e-mail address (if available) of the **corresponding author**, and information concerning grants. The address for reprint requests should include

(continued)

the **complete** name, street address (not a postal box), and zip code. It is important to indicate on this title page whether your paper has been presented at an RSNA meeting (please give year) or has been accepted for presentation at a future meeting.

Abbreviated Title Page: This page should include only the title of the manuscript so as to allow for anonymity during the review process.

Author Contributions: Authors are required to identify their manuscript contributions, for which they are responsible. The author(s) responsible for the integrity of the entire study should also be identified. Please list the following phrases on a separate page, to follow the *"Abbreviated Title Page,"* and beside each indicate the name(s) of the author(s) to whom these phrases apply:

- guarantor of integrity of entire study
- study concepts
- study design
- definition of intellectual content
- literature research
- clinical studies
- experimental studies
- data acquisition
- data analysis
- statistical analysis
- manuscript preparation
- manuscript editing
- manuscript review

For those phrases that do not apply, please list them and so indicate.

■ ABSTRACT, KEY WORDS, CATEGORIZATION TERMS, AND SUMMARY STATEMENT

An abstract of 200 words or less must be submitted with each manuscript of a major paper. The abstract must be divided into four paragraphs with the following headings.

Purpose: State the hypothesis being tested or the procedure being evaluated.

Materials and Methods: Briefly state what was done and what materials were used, including number of subjects. Also include the methods used to assess the data and to control bias.

RESULTS: Provide the findings of the study, including indicators of statistical significance. Include actual numbers, as well as percentages.

CONCLUSION: Summarize in one or two sentences the conclusion made on the basis of the findings.

Below the abstract, please list three to six key words as derived from the terms used in the most recent 3-year *RSNA Index to Imaging Literature.* Also, on the Manuscript Categorization Terms form provided at the end of these instructions, please select as many terms as are appropriate for your manuscript. It is important that you comply with this request, since the terms you select are utilized to match your manuscript with the appropriate reviewers.

On the reverse side of the Manuscript Categorization Terms form, the *author should reproduce from the text the one statement that best conveys or summarizes the message of the study.*

An abstract of 60 words or less must be submitted for each case report or Technical Developments paper. The abstract must state (*a*) what was done, (*b*) what was found, and (*c*) what was concluded.

■ TEXT

The text of observational and experimental studies is arranged in sections with the headings Introduction, Materials and Methods, Results, and Discussion. Lengthy papers may need subheadings within some sections to clarify their content, especially within the Results and Discussion sections.

Introduction: Clearly state the hypothesis or purpose of the study. Give only strictly pertinent references, and do not review the literature extensively.

Materials and Methods: Describe clearly the number and selection of the subjects studied (patients or experimental animals, including controls). Identify the methods, instrumentation (manufacturer's name and address in parentheses), and procedures in sufficient detail to allow other workers to reproduce the results. To ensure anonymity in the review process, do **not** include the name of the institution where the work was performed, either within the text or at the top of each manuscript page. Give references to established methods, including statistical methods that have been published but are not well known; describe new or substantially modified methods and give reasons for using these techniques. Include numbers of observations and the statistical significance of the findings when appropriate. Detailed statistical analyses, mathematical derivations, and the like should be presented in one or more appendixes.

Results: Present the results in logical sequence in the text, along with tables, and illustrations. Do not repeat in the text all the data in the tables and/or illustrations; summarize only important observations.

Discussion: Emphasize the new and important aspects of the study and conclusions that follow from them. Do not repeat in detail the data given in the Results section. Include in the Discussion the implications of the findings and their limitations, in particular with reference to the use of modified methods, statistical or otherwise. Relate the observations to other relevant studies. Link the conclusions with the goals of the study, but avoid unqualified statements and conclusions not supported completely by the data. Avoid claiming priority and alluding to work that has not been completed. State new hypotheses when warranted, but clearly label them as such. Recommendations, when appropriate, may be included.

For experimental studies, please describe the potential importance of your conclusions as they relate to future practical applications. Please identify this paragraph with the title "Practical Application(s)."

■ ACKNOWLEDGMENTS

List here those who have contributed substantially to the work reported in the manuscript, such as editorial and writing assistance, but who are not authors of the study. Authors are expected to obtain written permission of those acknowledged, and to submit the same, as readers might interpret that those acknowledged agree with the data and conclusions of the study.

■ REFERENCES

Number references consecutively in the order in which they are first mentioned. The abbreviations used for periodicals cited in the references should follow the style of *Index Medicus.* For journal articles, list surnames and initials of all authors when six or less, such as:

1. Stuart MJ, Elrad H, Graeber JE, Hakanson DO, Sunderji SG, Barvinchak MK. Increased synthesis of prostaglandin endoperoxides and platelet hyperfunction in infants of mothers with diabetes mellitus. J Lab Clin Med 1979; 94:12–26.

When seven or more authors are listed, only the first three names need to be identified, followed by "et al," such as:

1. Hibbard CT, Campbell S, Sabbagha RE, et al. Demonstration of tissue interfaces within the body by ultrasonic echo sounding. Br J Radiol 1961; 34:539–549.

Abstracts, editorials, and letters to the Editor should be noted as such. In the case of books, the authors of a chapter, title of the chapter, editor(s), title of the book, edition, city, publisher, year, and specific pages must be provided.

1. Brown M, Gray L. Indications for hematology. In: Wintrobe MM, ed. Clinical hematology. 3rd ed. Philadelphia, Pa: Lea & Febiger, 1975; 1146–1167.

It is the responsibility of the author(s) to ensure that all references are listed accurately.

■ TABLES

Tables should be numbered in Arabic numerals and should have a title. All abbreviations used in the table should be explained in a footnote.

Tables should be presented in the style used in recent issues of the Journal. No vertical lines or shading should be included. Avoid excessive use of horizontal lines within the table.

■ CAPTIONS FOR ILLUSTRATIONS

A caption must be supplied for each illustration, including drawings and graphs. It should not duplicate text material and should follow the style used in recent issues of the Journal. All captions should appear collectively on one or more pages separate from the text, and each caption should also appear below the corresponding illustration. It is essential that the caption describes all labels placed on the print of an illustration.

■ ILLUSTRATIONS

Illustrations should be limited to those required to show the essential features described in the manuscript. Space constraints prevent us from publishing redundant or excessive illustrations. Unretouched glossy prints no larger than 12.7 × 17.8 cm (5 × 7 inches) are desirable. Prints to be combined into one array, such as posteroanterior and lateral views, should be the same height or the same width to facilitate reproduction. They should correspond in appearance to the tonal relations of the original radiograph (ie, showing the bones white on a dark background, with the patient's right to the observer's left; computed tomograms and MR images should employ the "view from below"). If an image has been enhanced electronically, explain the alterations that have been made and send an original image along with the enhanced one. Drawings and charts should be rendered professionally in India ink on white paper. In computer-generated artwork, shading should be done in continuous tones (ie, solid black, solid gray, solid white): **Do not use dotted shadings.**

Since the size of the illustration printed in the Journal is typically smaller than that submitted by the author(s), it is essential that each submitted illustration show only the area(s) of interest with enough surrounding area for orientation puposes (e.g., to illustrate a cavity at the right lung apex, show only that area with enough surrounding area for orientation, rather than the entire chest).

All illustrations must be numbered and the top indicated on the back. For protection against loss or damage, each illustration should then be neatly attached to paper (one illustration per page), and the number and top should be reindicated on this page. For attachment, **avoid using glue, staples, or corner mounts.** Because it holds the illustration securely to the page without damage, we recommend Scotch Removable Magic Tape (3M, St Paul, Minn). **Please** do not add letters or numbers to the **face** of the illustration to identify the figure (such as 1A or 1B).

Arrows and other labels should be placed only on the final print, should be of professional quality, and should be **removable**. Professional artist service for such items is available to authors without charge. The desired additions may simply be indicated on tissue or a transparent overlay attached securely to the print.

Illustrations of accepted manuscripts become the property of the RSNA and will be stored for 2 years after publication. Illustrations will be returned only upon receipt of a written request from the corresponding author. We suggest that authors make and keep a set of illustrations in addition to the three sets submitted to the Journal.

■ UNITS AND ABBREVIATIONS

Radiation measurements and laboratory values should be given in the *International System of Units (SI)* (resources: SI Units in Radiation Protection and Measurements, NCRP Report no. 82 [August 1985]; "Now Read This: The SI Units Are Here," *JAMA* 1986; 255:2329–2339). Abbreviations should be spelled out when first used in the text, such as "cerebrospinal fluid (CSF)." Laboratory slang, clinical jargon, and uncommon abbreviations should be avoided.

■ INFORMED CONSENT

Manuscripts reporting the results of experimental studies on human subjects must include a statement in Materials and Methods to the effect that informed consent was obtained after the nature of the procedure(s) had been fully explained. In addition, a statement affirming approval of the appropriate institutional review board is required. If a review board does not exist, then the Declaration of Helsinki principles should be followed and a statement affirming the same should be made (41st World Medical Assembly. Declaration of Helsinki: recommendations guiding physicians in biomedical research involving human subjects. Bull Pan Am Health Organ 1990; 24: 606-609).

The maintenance and care of experimental animals to provide humane treatment and to ensure reliable results are described in the National Institutes of Health guidelines for use of laboratory animals. Authors must affirm compliance with these guidelines or approval of the appropriate institutional review board in the Materials and Methods section.

■ RIGHTS AND PERMISSIONS

Written permission (we require a copy) must be granted by the publisher and author to reproduce any previously published figures, including permission to reproduce in both print and electronic formats; any such material must be clearly noted and its source given in the manuscript. A signed letter of permission must be included with your manuscript for any individual who might be identified due to written descriptions, photographs (masking the eyes in photographs is not sufficient protection of anonymity), or otherwise. Informed consent, which requires that the individual be shown the manuscript, should be affirmed in the Materials and Methods section.

If reference is made in the text to personal communication (oral or written) as a source of information, a signed statement of permission is required from each such source.

AUTHOR RESPONSIBILITY

Authors must be certain that no manuscript on the same or similar material has been or will be submitted to another journal by themselves or others at their institution before their work appears in *Radiology*. The submission by authors of similar material to advertising media must be indicated at the time *Radiology* receives the manuscript.

ELECTRONIC SUBMISSION OF ACCEPTED MANUSCRIPTS

Manuscripts that have been **accepted** for publication must be submitted on computer disk (required for text, desirable for illustrations). A hard copy should accompany the disk and should match the disk file exactly. The disk should be labeled with its assigned manuscript number, the first author's last name, the word processing program used, and the file name.

Text File: Submit text on high-density 3½-inch disk prepared with an IBM- or Macintosh-compatible computer. Manuscripts should be prepared in WordPerfect 6.1 or Microsoft Word for PC (7.0) or Mac (5.0 or higher). Files prepared in any other word-processing program should be saved in an unformatted, text-only ASCII file and the program used should be indicated.

The entire article should be submitted as a single text file, with the elements in the standard order: title pages, abstract, text, acknowledgments, references, tables, captions. Only the final version of the article should be on the submitted disk. Keep the text file as free from formatting codes as possible: Do not use boldface, italic, underlining, strange fonts, codes for centering, unnecessary line spacing, etc. Use the default settings of the word-processing program; especially do not use right-justified margins. Use tabs to indent at the beginnings of paragraphs, and insert only one space after end punctuation marks. Use hard returns only at the ends of paragraphs or between sections of the manuscript; do not insert them mid-paragraph. Do not insert tabs in references; use only one hard return at the end of each reference.

Illustrations File: Although not required, submission of illustrations on 3½" disk, ZIP disk, or Syquest cartridge will improve image quality. For black and white images, we require that they be submitted in PC Tiff or PC eps format with a dot range of 5%–95% and resolution of 500 dpi. Four-color images should also be PC Tiff or PC eps format with a maximum of 280% total tonal density and resolution of 300 dpi. Each image file should be named, and with the disk or cartridge the following should be provided: a hard-copy inventory with specific information on the image, two sets of proofs obtained at 800–1,800 dpi, and one set of proofs obtained with a laser printer to be used as a reference set.

BOOK REVIEWERS

Any person who would like to help in reviewing books for *Radiology* should contact

Richard A. Szucs, MD, Book Review Editor
Radiology Editorial Office
1001 E Broad St
Suite 310
Richmond, VA 23219

BOOKS FOR REVIEW

Publishers wishing to have books reviewed should send them to the address above.

✔ **Checklist of Requirements:**

❒ 1. Send 3 copies of manuscript and 3 copies of illustrations.
❒ 2. Mount each illustration on a separate page, 8½ × 11 inches. Indicate figure number and top.
❒ 3. Double space all parts of manuscript.
❒ 4. Send copyright and certifications agreement with signatures of all authors.
❒ 5. Send institutional affiliation for each author and corresponding author's name, address, phone number, FAX or Telex number, and e-mail address.
❒ 6. Send a **brief** abstract: 200 words or less for regular articles, 60 words or less for case reports and Technical Developments papers.
❒ 7. Give SI units for radiation measurements and laboratory values.
❒ 8. Send copy of letter of permission to reprint any figure that was published previously or for any other reasons as noted in the instructions found above.
❒ 9. Send a completed copy of the Manuscript Categorization Terms form. Please remember to reproduce from the text the one statement that best conveys or summarizes the message of your study.

Radiology Manuscript Categorization Terms

Please PRINT your name: ______________________________

Please print the title of your manuscript ______________________________

____

For each section, please categorize your manuscript by checking off **as many terms as are appropriate.**

Modalities/Techniques

- ___ Absorptiometry/ Bone Densitometry
- ___ Angiography
- ___ Arthrography
- ___ Conventional Radiography
- ___ CT
- ___ CT-Angiography
- ___ CT-Electron Beam
- ___ CT-High Resolution
- ___ CT-Spiral
- ___ Dacryocystography
- ___ Defecography
- ___ Digital Radiography
- ___ Echocardiography
- ___ Fluoroscopy
- ___ Hysterosalpingography
- ___ Image Manipulation/ Reconstruction
- ___ Lymphography
- ___ MR-Angiography
- ___ MR-Diffusion/Perfusion
- ___ MR-Functional Imaging
- ___ MR-Imaging
- ___ MR-Spectroscopy
- ___ Neural Networks
- ___ PACS
- ___ PET
- ___ Radionuclide Studies
- ___ Sialography
- ___ SPECT
- ___ Ultrasound
- ___ Ultrasound-Color Doppler
- ___ Ultrasound-Doppler
- ___ Ultrasound-Power Doppler
- ___ Ultrasound-Spectral Doppler

Procedures

- ___ Angioplasty
- ___ Angioscopy
- ___ Balloon Insertions
- ___ Biopsy/Drainage
- ___ Dilation
- ___ Embolization
- ___ Endoscopy
- ___ Filter Insertions
- ___ Interventional Other ______________
- ___ Intraoperative
- ___ Laser
- ___ Lithotripsy
- ___ Localization
- ___ Myelography
- ___ Percutaneous
- ___ Radiation Therapy/Oncology
- ___ Radionuclide Therapy
- ___ Shunts
- ___ Stents
- ___ Thrombolysis

Areas/Systems

- ___ Abdomen
- ___ Biliary
- ___ Breast
- ___ Cardiac
- ___ CNS
- ___ Ear/Nose/Throat
- ___ Genital/Reproductive
- ___ GI
- ___ Head/Neck
- ___ Hematologic
- ___ Lymphatic
- ___ Muscular
- ___ Nervous-Peripheral
- ___ Skeletal-Appendicular
- ___ Skeletal-Axial
- ___ Soft Tissues/Skin
- ___ Thorax
- ___ Urinary
- ___ Vascular

Structures

- ___ Adrenal
- ___ Ankle
- ___ Anus
- ___ Aorta
- ___ Appendix
- ___ Arteries
- ___ Bile Ducts
- ___ Bladder
- ___ Brain/Brain Stem
- ___ Breast
- ___ Cervix
- ___ Diaphragm
- ___ Duodenum
- ___ Ear
- ___ Elbow
- ___ Esophagus
- ___ Extremities
- ___ Eye
- ___ Face
- ___ Fallopian Tubes
- ___ Foot
- ___ Gallbladder
- ___ Hand
- ___ Heart
- ___ Hip
- ___ Jaw
- ___ Joints
- ___ Kidney
- ___ Knee
- ___ Lacrimal Glands
- ___ Large Bowel
- ___ Larynx
- ___ Ligaments
- ___ Liver
- ___ Long Bones
- ___ Lung
- ___ Marrow
- ___ Mediastinum
- ___ Meninges
- ___ Mesentery
- ___ Omentum
- ___ Orbit
- ___ Ovaries
- ___ Pancreas
- ___ Paranasal Sinuses
- ___ Parathyroid
- ___ Pelvis
- ___ Pelvocalyceal
- ___ Penis
- ___ Pericardium
- ___ Peritoneum
- ___ Pharynx
- ___ Pineal
- ___ Pituitary
- ___ Pleura
- ___ Prostate
- ___ Pylorus
- ___ Rectum
- ___ Retina
- ___ Retroperitoneum
- ___ Ribs
- ___ Salivary Glands
- ___ Scrotum
- ___ Shoulder
- ___ Skull
- ___ Small Bowel
- ___ Spinal Cord
- ___ Spine-Cervical
- ___ Spine-Lumbar

Continued

Structures, continued

___ Spine-Sacrum/Coccyx
___ Spine-Thoracic
___ Spleen
___ Stomach
___ Tendons
___ Testes
___ Thymus
___ Thyroid
___ Tongue
___ Tracheobronchial Tree
___ Ureters
___ Urethra
___ Uterus
___ Vagina
___ Valves
___ Veins
___ Vena Cava
___ Wrist

Topics

___ Abscess
___ Acceptance Testing
___ Acute
___ Adults
___ AIDS
___ Anatomy
___ Aneurysms
___ Animal Investigations
___ Arteriosclerosis
___ Arthritides
___ Artifacts
___ Atelectasis
___ Athletic Injuries
___ AVM
___ Axilla
___ Biological Effects
___ Biostatistics
___ Blood
___ Calcifications/Calculi
___ Cardiac Assist Devices
___ Catheters
___ Cavitation
___ Cerebral Palsy
___ Chemistry
___ Chronic Obstructive Airways Disease
___ Cirrhosis
___ Comparative Studies
___ Complications
___ Computer Applications-3D
___ Computer Applications-Teleradiology
___ Computer Applications-Virtual Imaging
___ Computer Applications-Other____________________
___ Congenital
___ Connective Tissue Disorders
___ Contrast Agents-Intravenous
___ Contrast Agents-Oral
___ Cost-effectiveness
___ CSF
___ Cysts
___ Dementia
___ Demineralization-Bone
___ Dilatation
___ Dissection
___ Diverticula
___ Dosimetry
___ Drugs/Reactions
___ Dysplasias
___ Eating Disorders
___ ECMO
___ Edema
___ Education
___ Efficacy Studies
___ Embolism
___ Endocrine Disorders
___ Equipment
___ Ethics
___ Experimental Investigations
___ Fetus
___ Fistula
___ Foreign Bodies
___ Forensics
___ Genetic Defects
___ Grafts
___ Health Policy and Practice
___ Hemangioma
___ Hematologic Diseases
___ Hemodynamics/Flow Dynamics
___ Hemorrhage
___ Hernia
___ History
___ Hyperplasia/Hypertrophy
___ Hypertension
___ Imaging Sequences
___ Infection
___ Inflammation
___ Instrumentation
___ Ischemia/Infarction
___ Laboratory Tests
___ Leukemia
___ Lymphoma
___ Medicolegal Issues
___ Metabolic Disorders
___ Metastases
___ Monoclonal Antibodies
___ Motility
___ Neoplasms-Primary
___ Normal Variants
___ Observer Performance
___ Obstetrics
___ Obstruction/Occlusion
___ Occupational/Environmental Hazards
___ Outcomes Analysis
___ Parasites
___ Pathology
___ Pediatric Population-Adolescents
___ Pediatric Population-Children
___ Pediatric Population-Infants
___ Pediatric Population-Neonates
___ Physics
___ Physiological Studies
___ Pregnancy
___ Prostheses
___ QA/QC
___ Radiation Effects
___ Radiation Safety
___ Radiobiology
___ Safety
___ Screening
___ Sedation
___ Seizure Disorders
___ Socioeconomic Issues
___ Speech Disorders
___ Staging
___ Statistics
___ Surgery
___ Technical Aspects
___ Technology Assessments
___ Tissue Characterization
___ Transplantation
___ Trauma
___ Treatment Effects
___ Tropical Diseases
___ Varices
___ Volvulus

Please reproduce here the **one sentence** from the text that best conveys or summarizes the message of your study.

____

____

Please provide author initials by appropriate author contribution category.

________ Guarantor of integrity of entire study
________ Study concepts
________ Study design
________ Definition of intellectual content
________ Literature research
________ Clinical studies
________ Experimental studies
________ Data acquisition
________ Data analysis
________ Statistical analysis
________ Manuscript preparation
________ Manuscript editing
________ Manuscript review

This form *must be* included with your manuscript submission.

Holger Pettersson, MD ▎ Donald Resnick, MD

The International Skeletal Society

Musculoskeletal Imaging[1]

In common with other subdisciplines in radiology, musculoskeletal imaging has been affected dramatically by the profound technologic developments that have taken place during the past 2 decades. As examples, although computed tomography (CT) and magnetic resonance (MR) imaging were initially applied to clinical problems other than those that affect the musculoskeletal system, both methods now are used by many on a daily basis to investigate disorders of bones, joints, and soft tissues. They provide information that, until now, was considered impossible to gather in a noninvasive fashion, and, further, they hold great promise for future endeavors related to clinical practice, as well as to research. The opportunities are endless and truly exciting, but with these opportunities has come a challenge. Compared with routine radiography, the images generated with MR imaging and to some extent CT scanning are far more numerous, the planes of section are highly variable, the displays are affected dramatically by the precise imaging parameters that are chosen, and the need to know regional anatomy has never been greater.

Historical Aspects

Routine radiography of the skeleton began shortly after the discovery of the x-ray more than 100 years ago. Worldwide, routine radiography of the skeleton remains one of the most commonly performed procedures and, indeed, in some countries that lack the necessary resources, routine radiography remains the only means by which most disorders of the skeleton are studied. Whereas conventional radiography is excellent as a method to investigate morphologic changes in bones, radionuclide techniques, which were introduced later, provided information regarding the metabolic function of the skeleton. Subsequently, with the introduction and refinement of ultrasonography (US), the morphology not only of the skeleton but also of the soft tissues was investigated. Indeed, US now enjoys great popularity in certain parts of the world (less so in the United States) as a method that can be used effectively to determine the presence and nature of an abnormality located in those parts of the musculoskeletal system that are accessible to a probe placed on the surface of the body. With the later development of CT scanning and MR imaging came the ability to study normal and abnormal tissues with improved contrast resolution and with sectional displays. An initial pessimistic view that MR imaging would not be valuable in the assessment of osseous abnormalities soon disappeared as the unique signal intensity characteristics of marrow were recognized, allowing early identification of a number of disorders that would replace, displace, or infiltrate this tissue. Subsequently, the unmatched diagnostic capabilities of MR imaging when used to study soft tissues and, especially, intra- and periarticular structures became apparent, such that this method now is regarded by many as an indispensable aid in determining the precise cause of dysfunction of virtually any human joint.

Current Status

Advances in recent years have been no less dramatic, based in large part on the further nurturing of the marriage of diagnostic imaging and computer technology, a union that currently is rock solid. Digital radiography enables accurate and direct assessment of precise trabecular architecture and, indirectly, allows evaluation of bone density and strength. Pseudo–three-dimensional displays on the basis of imaging data derived from CT scanning or MR imaging and true three-dimensional displays afforded by holography are increasingly vivid and allow clinical colleagues in orthopedics to view pathologic conditions in a way similar to that seen in the surgical suite. Computer-generated models of diseased areas and the ability to operate first by manipulation of data on the screen rather than by dissection of living tissues are not a future dream but rather a current reality. Further, the newest generations of equipment allow real-time CT and MR fluoroscopy, open-configuration MR units provide the access required by interventional radiologists, and low-field-strength dedicated MR units make possible a direct and inexpensive means to survey the extremities (1). The acquisition of three-dimensional, high-resolution images derived from standard MR imaging and CT or MR arthrography makes virtual arthroscopy a real possibility (2). Think of it. One can explore every recess of a joint without ever having to introduce a bulky arthroscope!

Also, in recent years, radiologists have assumed an ever-increasing role as interventionalists. In musculoskeletal imaging, this has translated into a clear demand for radiology participation in a number of procedures that previously had been performed by orthopedic surgeons, neurosurgeons, or anesthesiologists. Therapeutic injections of painful joints, percutaneous biopsy of tumors and tumorlike processes, and resection of localized neoplasms are among the invasive techniques that currently are performed by radiologists. The certain advantages of such participation in patient care include the ability to place a needle, trocar, or catheter precisely in a structure and to document correct placement by recording the site of injection, biopsy, or tissue removal through fluoroscopic, CT, or even MR imaging guidance. Percutaneous resection of tumors and tumorlike processes of the musculoskeletal system has been popular in cases of osteoid osteoma, eosinophilic granuloma, and simple bone cysts; instillation of methyl

Index terms:
Bones, 30.**2, 40.**
Joints, 30.**, 40.**
Muscles, 30.**, 40.**
Radiology and radiologists, research
Subspecialty society messages

Radiology 1998; 208:561–562

[1] From the Department of Radiology, University Hospital, Lund S-221 85, Sweden (H.P.), and the Department of Radiology, Veterans Administration Hospital, San Diego, Calif (D.R.).
Received January 6, 1998; accepted February 11. **Address reprint requests to** H.P.
[2]** Entire organ system or region.

See also the article by Kaye (pp 563–564) in this issue.

methacrylate cement and other substances provides stability in instances of skeletal metastasis; and ablation of vascular lesions of the musculoskeletal system through percutaneous embolization is possible. Because careful monitoring of the interventional procedure is ideal, the development of open magnets, rapid imaging sequences, and needles and instruments compatible with magnetic fields has received new attention.

The development of contrast agents compatible with MR imaging has also received recent attention. Although the value of intravenous administration of a gadolinium-containing agent has been well documented in cases of musculoskeletal tumor or infection, this same method appears to have important potential in the investigation of synovial inflammatory diseases and, when delivered as a bolus injection, of benign versus malignant tumors of bone and soft tissue. Direct MR arthrography employing such contrast agents has been used in the investigation of glenohumeral joint instability, recurrent symptoms after meniscal surgery, and osteochondritis dissecans, leading to, respectively, an increased understanding of capsulolabroligamentous variations and disorders of the shoulder, a means to differentiate changes associated with prior surgical invention and those indicative of a new meniscal lesion, and a method that allows detection of instability of an osteochondral fragment (3).

Future Directions

Few of us are clairvoyant enough to be able to predict with any certainty what the future may hold. We believe, however, that technologic, turf, and training issues will receive emphasis. With regard to technology, further advances in MR imaging clearly will occur. Very high tesla magnets will provide increasingly crisp and detailed images of musculoskeletal structures, allowing a degree of magnification similar to that seen through the microscope (4). Pathophysiologic data will be readily available regarding cartilage perfusion, bone and muscle metabolism, and tumor dynamics (5). With regard to muscle, for example, noninvasive imaging should allow the careful monitoring of gene therapy for inherited disorders, the response of inflammatory diseases to innovative therapeutic regimens, the recovery of tissue in patients with neuromuscular disorders, and the effectiveness of training methods in elite athletes, and skeletal muscle motion will be studied by using such recently described methods as phase-contrast velocity-encoded MR imaging and Doppler tissue US. By employing faster MR imaging sequences coupled with open magnet configurations, the normal and abnormal dynamics of countless joints will be explored. By combining three-dimensional imaging acquisition and new computer software programs, real-time and noninvasive exploration of the marrow ("osteoscopy") and spinal canal ("myeloscopy") should be possible. Real-time imaging displays of soft-tissue processes will simulate those seen surgically as tissue planes are peeled away, layer by layer.

The frequency and complexity of musculoskeletal interventional procedures also are likely to increase. Radiologists will compete with anesthesiologists to perform procedures designed to alleviate symptoms related to spinal and extraspinal diseases and, by necessity, will be required to possess an increased understanding of pharmacologic effects of a number of existing or new drugs. Substances will be developed that can be administered percutaneously to replace or reinforce disease processes of bone.

The issues of turf will become ever more complex (6). Even today, the necessity for review of routine musculoskeletal imaging studies by radiologists is being challenged by colleagues in other subspecialties (eg, emergency room physicians, orthopedic surgeons, and rheumatologists) who believe that they are equally (or more) qualified to interpret these studies. Small fluoroscopic units currently are available for use by clinicians in the emergency room or in offices to monitor reduction of displaced fractures and subsequent fracture healing. Further, the increased popularity of dedicated extremity-only MR units, which are being purchased by orthopedic surgeons for office use, leads to the sobering thought that resultant images will be interpreted independent of review by radiologists.

The turf of the radiologist of the future also will be defined by an ever increasingly constringent health care economy. As in other areas of diagnostic imaging, the musculoskeletal radiologist will become a manager of imaging assessment, as he or she will weigh the benefits of an examination or procedure and its cost. The answers to two basic questions will dominate his or her thinking. Will the results of the imaging examination (or examinations) influence the treatment of the patient and, if so, what is the most direct (ie, cost-effective) way to obtain these results? A shift of emphasis from diagnostic imager to imaging consultant will be necessary, as the musculoskeletal radiologist will be required to provide guidance in the choice of a specific protocol from a list that will become increasingly long and complex. Indeed, it will be this very diversity of available imaging methods and techniques that will lead even the highly specialized orthopedic surgeon and rheumatologist to more often seek the opinion of the radiologist.

As they are now, issues of training also will be dominant in the future. Clearly, musculoskeletal specialists in radiology will be required who know the language of the orthopedic surgeon and rheumatologist and who can use this language to communicate with them in a meaningful fashion. How many such specialists will be necessary and just how specialized they need to be (ie, amount of specialized training) are not clear. Accreditation of musculoskeletal imaging fellowships currently is offered in the United States, and certification of trainees in these fellowships may not be far behind. International and, more recently, European and American societies of musculoskeletal radiologists (and, in some instances, colleagues in related specialties as well) now exist whose agendas include, among other things, discussions of some of these issues of technology, turf, and training.

No, we are not clairvoyant, but we believe that the subdiscipline of musculoskeletal imaging is in good health today and the outlook for future development and refinement is promising. Obstacles surely will be encountered in the years ahead, but, as has occurred in the past, they will be negotiated successfully.

References

1. Erickson SJ. High-resolution imaging of the musculoskeletal system. Radiology 1997; 205:593–618.
2. Dupuy DE, Hanger DH, Zachazewski JE, et al. Kinematic CT of the patellofemoral joint. AJR 1997; 169:211–215.
3. Hodler J, Resnick D. Current status of imaging of articular cartilage. Skeletal Radiol 1996; 25:703–709.
4. Johnson GA, Benveniste H, Black RD, et al. Histology by magnetic resonance microscopy. Magn Reson Q 1993; 9:1–30.
5. Beckmann N, Bruttel K, Mir A, Rudin M. Noninvasive 3D MR microscopy as a tool in pharmacological research: application to a model of rheumatoid arthritis. Magn Reson Imaging 1995; 13:1013–1017.
6. Ferris EJ. Expanding the role of the diagnostic imaging specialist: new opportunities for today and tomorrow. Radiology 1997; 202:593–596.

Jeremy J. Kaye, MD

Commentary

The Right Stuff[1]

In this issue of *Radiology,* Pettersson and Resnick (1) have provided thoughts about the past, present, and future of musculoskeletal radiology. I have been asked to provide a commentary on their thoughts and to provide my additional reflections. Although there is clearly overlap in these areas, I would like to provide my commentary under several headings: historical aspects, technology, training, practice patterns, research, and the future.

Historical Perspective

Pettersson and Resnick (1) provide a brief history of the development of technical aspects of musculoskeletal imaging. The intellectual aspects of this discipline need to be re-emphasized. In patients with musculoskeletal disorders, radiologists (and other physicians) use imaging studies for a number of purposes: to detect disease, to establish the diagnosis, to determine the extent of disease, to assess disease activity and evaluate progression of disease, to evaluate the effectiveness of therapy, to help select surgical candidates and help choose the appropriate procedure, and to recognize the complications of disease and of therapy (2).

Index terms:
Bones, 30.**[2], 40.**
Joints, 30.**, 40.**
Muscles, 30.**, 40.**
Radiology and radiologists, research
Subspecialty society messages

Radiology 1998; 208:563–564

[1] From the Department of Radiology, Saint Vincents Hospital and Medical Center, 153 W 11th St, New York, NY 10011. Received January 26, 1998; accepted February 11. **Address reprint requests to** the author.
[2] . ** Entire organ system or region

See also the article by Pettersson and Resnick (pp 561–562) in this issue.

To do all of these tasks intelligently, it became apparent that additional knowledge was necessary. Thus, musculoskeletal radiology was developed as a subspecialty discipline, in response to *need* (3). Initially, musculoskeletal radiologists were found in orthopedic hospitals. As the advantages of their greater knowledge and expertise became apparent, especially for training of residents, academic institutions sought subspecialists, including musculoskeletal radiologists. As the demands have increased for better communication and relationships between radiologists and their referring physicians, especially orthopedic surgeons, rheumatologists, and emergency room physicians, practice opportunities in nonacademic hospitals and private practices have evolved. In short, musculoskeletal radiology developed out of the need for radiologists with *the right stuff.*

Technology

Pettersson and Resnick (1) discuss the evolution of technologic developments and current status of technology applicable to musculoskeletal imaging. They also predict some future technologic advancements. Additional imaging-guided procedures, including those that use ultrasonography, computed tomography (CT), and magnetic resonance imaging, will develop, perhaps bringing to everyday use the "operating room of the future" (4). Real-time CT fluoroscopy will be used for biopsies and other CT-guided procedures (5). Musculoskeletal radiologists are, however, not unique because of their understanding and ability to apply technology, but are distinguished by their knowledge. If they understand diseases and their natural histories, complications, and treatment, then they have *the right stuff.*

Training

The virtual explosion of technology in recent years has had a strong influence on residency training programs. Even with the extension of the length of residency training to 4 years beyond a clinical year, residents are confronted with a bewildering amount of physics, technology, and techniques as a part of their training. Recently, Heitzman (6) has wondered whether it is time for our residency training programs to include more time in certain organ-oriented subspecialties, including musculoskeletal radiology. This commentator is in agreement with this proposal; we seem to be losing perspective. As technology develops and evolves, it will be extremely important to emphasize the intellectual disciplines in radiology rather than the techniques and technologies. Let us not overly dilute the knowledge of diseases and organs with too much training time devoted to the tools of our trade, some of which eventually may become obsolete.

While a diagnostic radiology residency should produce knowledgeable and competent general radiologists, residency is not the time to develop the skills or the knowledge of a subspecialist. Fellowship training programs have become numerous for those with an interest in musculoskeletal radiology, as noted by Pettersson and Resnick (1). In this observer's opinion, these should be encouraged, for they will provide the musculoskeletal radiologists of the future and they will be the intellectual leaders guaranteeing the future of the subspecialty. If we are unable to provide the intellectual skills and leadership in the future, guaranteeing *the right stuff* will be available, radiology could lose battles in future turf wars.

Practice Patterns

Subspecialization has evolved in virtually all areas of medical practice, especially in internal medicine and surgery. Referring physicians wish to consult only those physicians who are knowledgeable about the diseases they are treating and the problems they might encounter. This provides further support for subspecialized knowledge in musculoskeletal radiology being *the right stuff* for us to relate properly to referring orthopedic surgeons, rheumatologists, and emergency room physicians.

What will be the role of the musculoskeletal radiologist in these days of managed care? Emphasizing quality and appropriate studies is an important part (7). It is important to recognize that quality includes the interpretation, based on knowledge of musculoskeletal disorders—*the right stuff.*

Will radiologists, including musculoskeletal radiologists, become "gatekeepers" of studies, a consultant to guide the referring physician (8)? Perhaps, but the effectiveness of this will be based on knowledge of diseases and their manifestations—*the right stuff.* As indicated by Ferris (8), this does not mean that we should all become general radiologists. Subspecialization continues to be a desirable goal.

Research

Radiologists need to initiate and be primary investigators of imaging manifestations of diseases affecting the musculoskeletal system. To do so effectively requires subspecialized knowledge of diseases in an organ system rather than the technology (9). Radiologists, especially musculoskeletal radiologists, should encourage, initiate, and participate in studies comparing accuracy and completeness of interpretation of imaging studies. These should be participated in, however, only if the "playing field" is level and strict and precise scientific methods are followed.

This commentator is opposed to the term frequently employed: "added value." Use of this term implies that there is inherent value to a nonradiologist's interpretation and that the interpretation is correct. Judgments of "value" or "added value" should be based on scientific research. Often they are not, leading radiologists and musculoskeletal radiologists into assuming a defensive posture. It is far easier to call on radiologists to establish "added value" than to participate in real comparative research studies.

Musculoskeletal radiologists should be in the best position to carry out research using imaging techniques. Nevertheless, even brief perusal of nonradiology journals reveals many publications devoted to imaging in which radiologists do not participate. Furthermore, radiologists may be added as authors only because they helped in data collection or in some aspect of the study. Musculoskeletal radiologists should take the lead in promoting imaging research and should control, in a scientific manner, the research methods. Then we will be able to establish that we have *the right stuff.*

The Future

Unfortunately, science-fiction writers seem to be better than scientists in predicting the future. It seems possible that the future will bring some new imaging method not heretofore considered. Certainly, there will be further developments, refinements, and applications of existing technology.

Alas, with the greater competition for funds in health care, it is easy to predict that the future will hold more disputes and "turf battles" for imaging, especially musculoskeletal imaging. These battle lines are forming even today.

There are a large number of factors to be considered concerning the supply of radiologists and musculoskeletal radiologists (10). In particular, the overall increase in age of the population should increase the need for musculoskeletal radiologists. As the population ages, the prevalence of arthritis increases, as does the frequency with which patients present to physicians with arthritic complaints (11). This should increase the need for musculoskeletal radiologists. The need for musculoskeletal radiologists in the nonacademic and private practices should also increase in the future; a lack of knowledge about diseases will place radiologists at a disadvantage in the future "turf battles."

Musculoskeletal radiologists can ensure a prominent role in the future of medicine by possessing a greater knowledge of diseases through education and continuing education, by accurately and completely reporting studies in a timely fashion, by being pioneers and ready participants in information and imaging transfer, and by performing scientific research, especially on diseases. These will ensure all that we have *the right stuff.*

References

1. Pettersson H, Resnick D. Musculoskeletal imaging. Radiology 1998; 208:561–562.
2. Kaye JJ. Arthritis: roles of radiography and other imaging techniques in evaluation. Radiology 1990; 177:601–608.
3. Taveras JM. Subspecialization in radiology: response to a need. AJR 1987; 148: 465–469.
4. Jolesz FA. Image-guided procedures and the operating room of the future. Radiology 1997; 204:601–612.
5. Katada K, Kato R, Anno H, et al. Guidance with real-time CT fluoroscopy: early clinical experience. Radiology 1996; 200:851–856.
6. Heitzman ER. Time will tell. Radiology 1998; 206:14–15.
7. Holman BL. Can radiology save managed care? preserving quality in the face of managed competition. AJR 1998; 170:3–7.
8. Ferris EJ. Expanding the role of the diagnostic imaging specialist: new opportunities for today and tomorrow. Radiology 1997; 202:593–596.
9. Taveras JM. Subspecialization in radiology: what approach should we take? Invest Radiol 1986; 21:91.
10. Friedenberg RM. Future physician requirements: radiologists. Radiology 1996; 200: 51A–54A.
11. Centers for Disease Control. Prevalence of arthritic conditions: United States, 1987. MMWR Morb Mortal Wkly Rep 1990; 39:99–102.

Frederick A. Mann, MD ■ Michael I. Zucker, MD ■ William R. Mower, MD

The American Society of Emergency Radiology

Emergency Radiology Practice and Research beyond the Millennium[1]

. . .the future has a disturbing tendency to go its own way . . . (1)

Emergency department physicians in the United States see nearly 100 million patients each year and attend to time-sensitive "emergency" conditions, whose sequelae are among the most common causes of disability and death for almost all age groups (2) (Table). Over the past decade, emergency radiology has evolved into a distinct discipline that specifically responds to the imaging needs of emergency department patients and physicians, including imaging-guided diagnosis and therapy for medical and surgical conditions that either are unexpected or demand immediate action.

Leading Causes of Death in the United States by Age Group

	Age Group (y)					
Cause	1–4	5–14	15–24	25–44	46–64	≥65
Unintentional trauma (vehicular, falls, industrial)	1st	1st	1st	1st	4th	
Homicide	4th	3rd	2nd	6th		
Suicide		5th	3rd	5th		
Cancer	3rd	2nd	4th	3rd	1st	2nd
Cardiovascular diseases	5th	6th	5th	4th	2nd	1st
Cerebrovascular diseases					3rd	3rd
Congenital anomalies	2nd	4th				
Diabetes mellitus						6th
Hepatobiliary diseases (cirrhosis), chronic					6th	
Human immunodeficiency virus			6th	2nd		
Pneumonia (bacterial or viral)	6th					5th
Pulmonary diseases, chronic					5th	4th

Source.—References 3 and 4.

Change is the only constant in these millenarian times. While the futures of radiology and emergency radiology promise to be as spectacular as they will be interesting, the haze of incomplete knowledge and habituation to practices (clinical and political) of dubious merit are likely to make the road both tortuous and bumpy. We believe there are four determinants of positive change: strong values, clear clinical goals, enabling technology, and the capacity to overcome constraints.

The American Society of Emergency Radiology (ASER) strongly values timely, accessible, safe, cost-effective, and clinically relevant imaging consultations; continuous education of medical practitioners, allied personnel, and the public about the optimal practice of emergency radiology; and new skills refined through collaborative, multidisciplinary research focused on the strategic patient-care needs of our clinical and administrative colleagues. We believe that these values and purposes will guide our future.

Important enabling technologies are evolving within biomedical, computer, pharmaceutical, and telecommunications industries. Four important trends should substantially affect medical practices for emergencies and trauma: miniaturization of components and processes; incremental and novel improvements in spatial, contrast, and temporal resolution; rapidly increasing telecommunications bandwidth and reach; and sophisticated decision-analysis methods and software tools to acquire and analyze very large real-time databases. A limited sampling of these four "techno-trends" would include application-specific integrated circuits and liquid crystal displays, user-definable World Wide Web search engines, and self-educating neural and evolutionary-logic networks. Improved resolution could be obtained with very high-frequency ultrasonography (US), magnetic resonance (MR) spectroscopy, and "functional" MR imaging. Telecommunications using global-coverage satellite networks with nondestructive data compression and multiinstitutional, multidisciplinary databases would be the basis on which efficiency, cost-effectiveness, and outcomes research could address now statistically intractable medical and policy issues.

Predicting how "enabling technologies" will affect the future of emergency radiology is an imprecise matter. However, the imaging research domains into which potential future advances will fall include (*a*) development and elaboration

Index terms:
Emergency medical service system
Radiology and radiologists, research
Subspecialty society messages

Radiology 1998; 208:565–567

[1] From the Department of Radiology, Harborview Medical Center, 325 Ninth Ave, Box 359728, Seattle, WA 98104-2499 (F.A.M.), and the Divisions of Emergency Radiology and Emergency Medicine, UCLA Medical Center, Los Angeles, Calif (M.I.Z., W.R.M.). Received January 9, 1998; accepted February 27. **Address reprint requests to** F.A.M.

See also the article by Harris (pp 568–569) in this issue.

of novel techniques for imaging (5,6), consulting, and real-time knowledge synthesis; (*b*) descriptive elucidation "of the anatomic, histologic, and functional effects of various disease processes" essential to the "the art and science of image interpretation" (7); and (*c*) explication of information and skills necessary to manage the intellectual, human, and physical resources for "optimal" patient outcomes (7). Examples of research in these domains might include (*a*) technical innovations such as a hand-held US unit, mobile CT and MR imaging, improved MR spectroscopy, electrical impedance tomography, magnetic source imaging; consulting with computer-assisted artificial intelligence and telemedicine; and data synthesis with online, linked World Wide Web–based databases with national and/or worldwide real-time entry of pharmaceutical, device, and procedural outcomes; (*b*) classic descriptive research with use of newly developed devices and techniques; and (*c*) medical "management" techniques specifying methods to tailor cost-effective practice guidelines to local disease prevalence and expertise, and organizational and management strategies to optimize throughput.

As part of our strategic planning for the ASER, we queried 100 "emergency" physicians (including specialists in anesthesiology, cardiology, critical care, emergency medicine, neurologic surgery, orthopedic surgery, pediatrics, pulmonary medicine, radiology, and trauma surgery) (8) as to how individual imaging goals and needs (Figure) might be positively affected by each of these enabling technology trends, and what imaging roles the innovations might play. We offer the following four examples to portray the potential that might result from favorable interactions of values, goals, and enabling technologies.

First, the decentralization of imaging can be expanded by component and process miniaturization, making sophisticated modalities more portable. In most major North American cities, emergency medical scene response times are less than 5 minutes. Provision of high-capability portable imaging equipment (eg, a hand-held US unit) and therapeutic equipment (eg, high-intensity focused ultrasound beam therapy) may make more of the "golden hour" available for intervention and, thus, allow detection and provisional treatment of ongoing hemorrhage from blunt torso injury (transcutaneous coagulative hemostasis of arterial bleeding induced by using a tightly focused, high-intensity ultrasound beam). In a similar fashion, evolution of mobile CT and MR imaging equipment will decentralize imaging and image-guided intervention from fixed-position sources to sites closer to patients (eg, the accident scene, the battlefield, or in operating theaters and intensive care units). Although this may increase imaging by nonradiologists, the demand for radiologists should increase as global screening expands the need for expert imaging consultants whose services will be largely delivered by means of telemedicine.

- Management: Increasing Value and Capacity
  - Accessibility and timeliness
  - Accurate clinical data and prior reports
  - Adequate reimbursement
  - Communications
    - Clarity
    - Alacrity
  - In-field diagnostic imaging
  - Knowledge
  - Methods for
    - Costing
    - Cost-efficiency
  - Research funding
  - Risk management
  - Safety
  - Special populations
    - Pediatric
    - Geriatric
    - Pregnant
  - Throughput, decreasing fixed costs per patient
- Nontrauma: Recognition and Intervention
  - Acute abdominal pain, not limited to
    - Surgical (appendicitis, infarction, obstruction)
    - Nonsurgical (infection, pancreatitis, obstruction)
  - Acute chest pain
    - Acute coronary syndromes
    - Thromboembolism
  - Brain attacks (stroke)
  - Chemical (drugs and alcohol) dependency
  - Infection
    - Tuberculosis
    - Human immunodeficiency virus
    - Other
  - Syncope
- Trauma: Decreasing Secondary Injury and Morbidity
  - Blunt torso
    - Chest and great vessels
    - Abdomen
      - Solid organs
      - Hollow organs
    - Pelvis
      - Bones
      - Genitourinary
  - Burns
  - Closed head
  - Firearms
  - Occupational
    - Soft tissues
    - Spinal cord

Abbreviated top 25 common goals and opportunities for emergency radiology research.

Second, improved spatial resolution should provide better grading of and treatment planning for thermal burns. Large-area US and MR imaging at very high spatial resolution (50–100 μm) can show exquisite detail of the dermal-epidermal junction (9) and may allow prediction of the need for and timing of skin grafting. Also, image-guided local instillation of transforming growth factor β may prevent formation of physically and socially disabling scar tissue (10).

Third, mapping extent and physiologic (ie, functional) severity of traumatic soft-tissue injuries may allow more cost-effective tailoring of patient therapy. Although a national disability database is not available and the literature is inconclusive, lower extremity injuries are probably the third leading cause of disability preventing men aged 18–35 years from returning to work. Total creatine level correlates with muscle exercise performance. MR spectroscopic quantification of total creatine (11) in leg muscle compartments may improve grading and prognosis of soft-tissue injuries and guide end points of rehabilitation. Regardless of the target organ (eg, brain, liver, muscle), such "functional" imaging requires sophisticated molecular biochemical knowledge, not common among today's emergency radiologists.

Fourth, wide-area networks with interrelated and intelligent databases can support the rapid acquisition of data sets through real-time, multiuser data entry. With use of mathematic evolutionary logic, data can be constantly searched to establish associations that are similar to those already known. Early recognition of associations that require large numbers of observed events, such as rare complications following medical device use, may promote shorter product development cycles and more profitable investment in "orphan" products (eg, vaccines), and support existing trends toward noninvasive and minimally invasive diagnostic tests and nonsurgical therapies. Certainly, resolving many of the existing medical and fiscal conundrums will require more efficient research designs and exploitation of all attainable data, so as to obtain necessary clinical and statistical power.

Emergency radiologists must champion the techniques of "evidence-based medicine"—the use of all kinds of evidence to treat patients, but particularly that gathered from the critical appraisal of the medical literature—to add scientific weight to our practices, and to broaden the "bandwidth" of imaging research to include health care delivery systems (12,13).

The fixed and operating costs (per hour or per patient) of the typical emergency department is exceeded only by those of operating rooms. Increasing unit (ie, patient) throughput is usually central to effective cost-minimization strategies and reduces fixed costs per patient. Few emergency departments, however, can interactively coordinate the numerous clinical services (eg, laboratory medicine, respiratory therapy, radiology, subspecialty consultants, transportation) necessary to deliver both excellent and expedient diagnosis and patient disposition. Although a few editorials hint at possible cost and time savings attendant to propitious use of "high-tech" imaging interventions, to our knowledge essentially no research addresses the practicalities of system cost-effectiveness. We, therefore, need to develop new research methods that are an addition to more traditional organ- and disease-specific morphologic and functional imaging research, with which to train a new generation of radiology-clinician researchers. The ASER vigorously advocates the cost and life-saving advantages of funding this type of research and supports close collaboration with academic practitioners of emergency medicine and trauma surgery.

There remain myriad clinical dilemmas for which knowledge is demonstrably incomplete and often seemingly contradictory. After a potential spine injury, for example, what role does CT play? Should it be used only to answer specific questions raised by the radiographic series or should it be part of the imaging protocol in addition to a complete or limited preliminary radiographic examination? Are any radiographs needed if CT is performed? Can some trauma patients safely forego all spine imaging if they fulfill certain clinical criteria? What is the role of MR imaging in the evaluation of a cervical spine injury? Should it remain solely the standard of reference for cord injuries or should it supplant flexion and extension views to evaluate ligament injury or be used as a primary screen for all bone, soft-tissue, and cord injuries?

And what of emergency department US? US may replace diagnostic peritoneal lavage, a surgically invasive procedure, in the search for intraperitoneal fluid in blunt trauma. It appears to have a role in the investigation of blunt and penetrating vascular injuries of the neck, symptomatic abdominal aortic aneurysm, acute biliary tract disease, and hemopericardium. It can and does provide clinicians with definitive real-time information necessary for many critical clinical decisions. As many researchers and practitioners of emergency department US are nonradiologists, some concern has been voiced regarding physician roles and practice credentialing.

Nonetheless, patients are best served when diagnostic and therapeutic interventions, including US, are performed by optimally trained and readily available persons. We believe that radiologists who provide timely service 24 hours per day relieve emergency department physicians from the burden of performing time-consuming imaging examinations and thus afford them more time to spend on direct patient care.

As far as the temporal horizon is visible, change will mandate change. As members of a dynamic specialty, we radiologists must not only think about changes needed in this rapidly evolving medical environment but also begin to enhance our critical roles in emergent patient care. Research is the vehicle to formulate the proactive changes needed for the next millennium, and the time to make the necessary adjustments is now. While we may not be able to predict the future, we can, in the words of Louis Pasteur, prepare for it: "Chance favors the prepared mind."

References

1. Berlin L. Perspectives: on the accuracy of prophecies. Radiology 1997; 204(2):32A–33A.
2. Runge JW. The cost of injury. Emerg Med Clin North Am 1993; 11:241–253.
3. National Center for Health Statistics, U.S. Department of Health and Human Services, Public Health Service: Monthly Vital Statistics Report, Advance Report of Final Mortality Statistics, 1992; 43:1–76.
4. Jacobs BB, Jacobs LM. Epidemiology of trauma. In: Feliciano DV, Moore EE, Mattox KL, eds. Trauma. 3rd ed. Stamford, Conn: Appleton & Lange, 1996.
5. Young IR. Review of modalities with a potential future in radiology. Radiology 1994; 192:307–317.
6. Katz DS, Lane MJ, Sommer FG. Unenhanced helical CT of ureteral stones: incidence of associated urinary tract findings. AJR 1996; 166:1319–1322.
7. Ehman RL. Limitations of tried-and-true imaging signs with new modalities. Radiology 1997; 205:39–40.
8. Hunter JC, Mann FA. The role of radiologists in emergency care: how we are viewed by our surgical and medical colleagues and how we see ourselves. Presented at the 17th Annual Oration of the Society of Skeletal Radiology, Phoenix, Ariz, February 23–26, 1994.
9. Erickson SJ. High-resolution imaging of the musculoskeletal system. Radiology 1997; 205:593–618.
10. Rivara FP. Pediatric injury control in 1997: Where do we go from here? Presented at the 1997 Annual Oration of the Society for Pediatric Research, Washington, DC, May 3, 1997.
11. Bottomley PA, Lee Y, Weiss RG. Total creatinine in muscle: Imaging and quantification with proton MR spectroscopy. Radiology 1997; 204:403–410.
12. Gyatt GH. Evidence-based emergency medicine. Ann Emerg Med 1977; 30:675–676.
13. Waecherle JF, Cordell WH, Wyer P, Osborn HH. Evidence-based emergency medicine: integrating research into practice. Ann Emerg Med 1997; 30:626–628.

John H. Harris, Jr, MD

Commentary

American Society of Emergency Radiology: Research Revisited[1]

The American Society of Emergency Radiology (ASER) is a relatively new society with approximately 325 members who have a primary interest in imaging acutely ill or injured patients seen in the emergency department. Its membership includes academic and nonacademic radiologists. As with emergency physicians who are clinical "generalists," emergency radiologists must also be "generalists" comfortable with the use of all imaging modalities in the evaluation of patients of all ages with unexpected or acute conditions affecting all organ systems.

"To promote research in Emergency Radiology by clinical and basic science investigators" (1) is one of the principles adopted by the founding members of the ASER. From that principle, Drs Mann, Zucker, and Mower (2) have masterfully identified the developing "enabling technologies" that offer the potential for effecting dramatic change in the way emergency radiology is taught and practiced.

It is very difficult, if not impossible, to predict the future of emergency radiology particularly with the dramatic explosion of imaging technology of the past decade serving as a prologue. A decade and a half ago, Yoram Ben-Menachem, MD, a world-renowned angiographer, predicted that the initial imaging procedure in evaluation of a multiply-injured patient would be whole-body computed tomography. With but minor variations of that theme, Dr Ben-Menachem's predication is today's reality in some major trauma centers.

At an international meeting to discuss the future of radiology convened by the American College of Radiology (ACR) in 1980, internationally recognized radiologic physicists stated, unequivocally, that nuclear magnetic resonance would never have clinical application. The inappropriatness of that predication is obvious today. To quote Dr Heitzman (3), "time will tell" whether, in the future, an emergency medical technician's instituting medical care under the direction of a remote physician who had been provided data obtained from a portable MR imaging unit operated by the same emergency medical technician at the scene will be a reality.

Research opportunities exist in other of the principles formulated to create ASER as follows:

1. "Establish Emergency Radiology as an area of special interest" (1)(a unique body of knowledge). ASER has achieved some of the objectives to meet this goal by being an invited participant at the past two annual meetings of the ACR Summit. For the first time, in 1997 ASER was represented by a seat on the Council of the ACR. While these are objective signs that emergency radiology is recognized as a radiologic subspecialty by the ACR, much research remains to have emergency radiology recognized as such in our imaging journals and as a sectional area by the American Board of Radiology.

2. "Improve methods of education in Emergency Radiology" (1). This goal is intended to establish, or expand, opportunity for medical student education in emergency radiology, to establish or expand emergency radiology as a required component of the radiology resident program curriculum, and to foster emergency radiology fellowships. Implementation of each of these objectives requires diligent research in the development of compelling reasons for presentation to medical school curriculum committees, radiology department chairs, and residency program directors. Expanding or introducing emergency radiology into already crowded medical school curricula will require very imaginative research. Alterations in radiology residency programs to accommodate appropriate training in emergency radiology should be somewhat easier because of the curriculum for emergency radiology developed by Mann and Wilson (4). Those academic radiology departments associated with hospitals with level I trauma centers should be encouraged to establish an emergency radiology fellowship program. The existing emergency radiology fellowship programs should seek accreditation through the American Council for Graduate Medical Education. Creation of emergency radiology fellowships are extremely important because of the increasing demand and short supply of radiologists with this special training.

3. "Provide a mechanism for presentation of scientific papers on various aspects of Emergency Radiology" (1). The 9th annual scientific session of the ASER was held in St Petersburg, Fla, on April 4–8, 1998. Approximately 350 registrants attended the 1997 annual meeting; this is a far cry from the 35 members who attended the 1st annual 1-day scientific session 9 years ago. *Emergency Radiology*, the journal of the ASER, is starting its 5th year of presenting refereed original scientific papers, review articles, case reports, challenge cases, pictorial essays, and reviews of articles pertinent to emergency radiology published in other journals. Even though ASER is a dynamic and

Index terms:
Emergency medical service system
Radiology and radiologists, research
Subspecialty society messages

Radiology 1998; 208:568–569

[1] From the Department of Radiology, University of Texas Houston Medical School, 6431 Fannin, Ste 2.100 MSB, Houston, TX 77030. Received February 24; accepted February 27. **Address reprint requests to** the author.

See also the article by Mann et al (pp 565–567) in this issue.

growing society, and the quality of articles selected for publication in *Emergency Radiology* is comparable to that of major radiology journals, the research appropriate to this goal involves the development of methods of attracting more of the radiologists who provide imaging services for the emergency department to take advantage of the educational opportunities available through the annual session and *Emergency Radiology*, the subtitle of which is *A Journal of Practical Imaging*. The focus of both the annual scientific session and *Emergency Radiology* is limited to the imaging aspects of patients seen in the emergency department.

With its "past as prologue," ASER anticipates an exciting and expanding role in the initial treatment of acutely ill and injured patients.

References

1. By-laws. Oak Brook, Ill: American Society of Emergency Radiology.
2. Mann FA, Zucker MI, Mower WR. Emergency radiology practice and research beyond the millennium. Radiology 1998; 208: 565–567.
3. Heitzman ER. Time will tell. Radiology 1998; 206:14–15.
4. Mann FA, Wilson AJ. A curriculum for emergency radiology. Emerg Radiol 1966; 70–81.

Interlude

A Different Kind of Radiologic Ghost

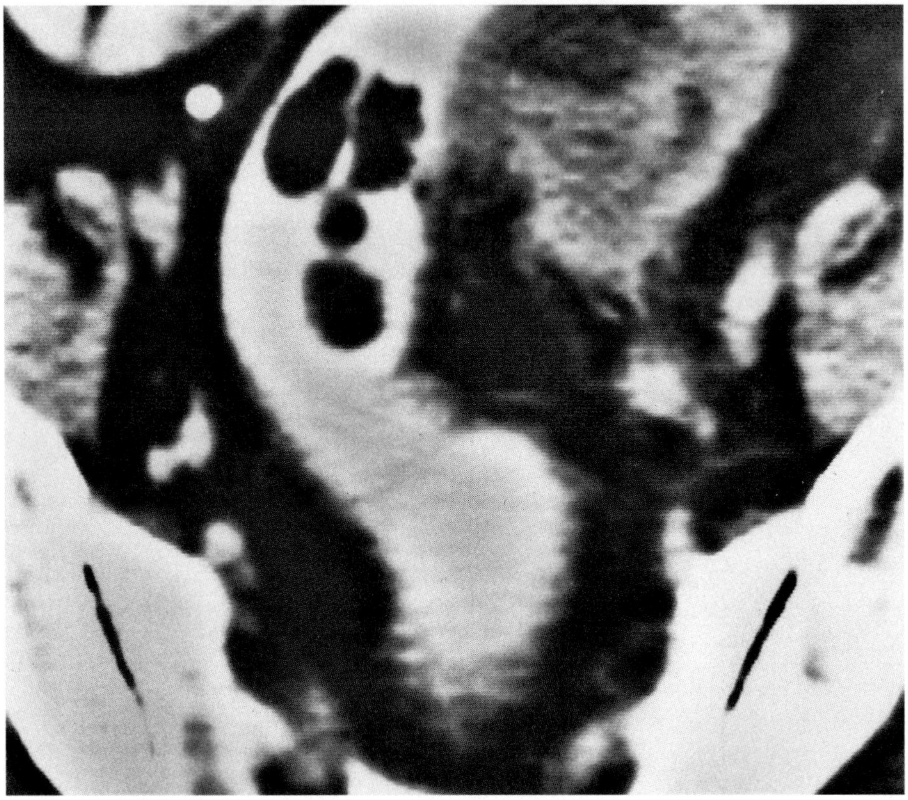

Courtesy of Herman I. Libshitz, MD, Houston, Tex

Editorial

Scott D. Flamm, MD

Coronary Arterial Calcium Screening: Ready for Prime Time?[1]

The relationship of severe coronary arterial calcification in patients with coronary arterial disease is well known from pathologic and epidemiologic studies (1). The noninvasive detection of coronary arterial calcification has been progressively improved by means of the introduction of methods from plain radiography to fluoroscopy, cine fluoroscopy, and standard axial computed tomography (CT). These techniques have allowed a qualitative assessment of coronary arterial calcification; however, quantitative measurements eluded us until the development of electrocardiographically (ECG) triggered electron-beam CT.

Current electron-beam CT protocols are used for measuring coronary arterial calcification by acquiring a stack of contiguous 3-mm-thick sections. Scanning is triggered to the diastole, but before atrial contraction, so that the heart is relatively immobile, with each section obtained in 100 msec. A complete set of images of the coronary arteries is usually obtained in two breath holds. The calcium score, as originally proposed by Agatston et al (2), is determined on the basis of the product of the total area of a calcified plaque and an arbitrary scoring system for those pixels with an attenuation greater than 130 HU. Theoretically, this multisection data set should give a clear representation of the amount of calcification in the major coronary arterial tree, yet high interscan variability has impaired the ability to measure coronary arterial calcification precisely and repeatedly (3–6).

Interscan variability also presents challenges in measuring changes in coronary arterial calcium in individuals over time. This variability has demanded large changes in an individual patient's calcium score before investigators can be confident of the progression of coronary arterial calcification (3,7,8). Multiple factors account for the wide range of variability, although interscan misregistration and the arbitrary attenuation scaling factor likely play the greatest roles.

Electron-beam CT measurement of coronary arterial calcification in large groups of individuals has provided important epidemiologic statistics regarding the relationship between coronary arterial calcification and coronary events such as myocardial infarction (9–11). However, two primary questions need to be addressed before electron-beam CT for coronary arterial calcium measurement is perceived as a useful and effective technique for planning patient care. The first question concerns whether we can measure coronary arterial calcification in *individuals* with reasonable certainty and precision, as well as repeatedly over meaningful time intervals. Without this ability, the effect of treatment regimens on the progression of coronary arterial calcium in individual patients cannot be determined. The second critical question concerns whether changes in coronary arterial calcification serve as a reliable marker for future coronary events in individual patients. We cannot begin to address the latter question until the former has been resolved.

More specifically, the calcified atherosclerotic plaques that are detected at electron-beam CT are believed to be relatively stable as opposed to the unstable, lipid-rich, noncalcified atherosclerotic plaques that cannot be identified at electron-beam CT (12,13). The latter group of plaques are also those that are more prone to rupture, which can result in acute coronary events (14). Further, the calcified plaques are often not the sites of hemodynamically significant stenoses; instead, hemodynamically significant lesions often are noncalcified and distant from the calcified plaques (15–17). These clearly are different kinds of atherosclerotic lesions with different implications regarding detection and treatment.

Multiple questions logically follow: (*a*) Can electron-beam CT help discern a correlation between these calcified and noncalcified lesions? (*b*) Can calcified plaques be used as a marker for the presence of noncalcified lesions? (*c*) Does an increase in coronary arterial calcium in an individual patient imply an increased likelihood of future coronary events, or is it simply the case that previously unstable lesions are stabilizing? (*d*) Does a decrease in coronary arterial calcification in an individual patient foretell a decreased likelihood of an acute coronary event?

In this issue of *Radiology,* Callister et al (18) describe a volumetric method for improving the reproducibility of scoring of coronary arterial calcification detected with electron-beam CT. They applied a postprocessing technique called isotropic interpolation (by using specialized software and a dedicated workstation) to electron-beam CT data in 52 patients who underwent two separate examina-

Index terms:
Arteriosclerosis, 54.76
Calcium
Computed tomography (CT), electron beam, 54.12119
Coronary vessels, calcification, 54.76
Coronary vessels, CT, 54.12111, 54.12119
Editorials

Radiology 1998; 208:571–572

[1] From the Division of Radiology/MRI-L10, Cleveland Clinic Foundation, 9500 Euclid Ave, Cleveland, OH 44195. Received June 3, 1998; accepted June 8. **Address reprint requests to** the author.

See also the article by Callister et al (pp 807–814) in this issue.

tions to determine reproducibility and interscan variability. Their method demonstrated a statistically significant improvement over the standard calcium scoring method when the latter was applied to the same data sets. Callister et al studied an additional 27 patients on two separate occasions (1 year apart) who had known cardiac risk factors; they found changes in coronary arterial calcium scores that were significantly greater than the determined interscan variability of the technique.

The volumetric score described by Callister et al substantially improves interscan reproducibility in the scoring of coronary arterial calcification. The technique refines the traditional calcium scoring method in two ways. First, it eliminates the attenuation scaling factor that arbitrarily gives greater weight to atherosclerotic plaques with greater attenuation (Hounsfield units). Second, by using isotropic interpolation techniques, the CT data set is reconstructed into a more precise volumetric map of coronary arterial calcium. The technique allows simpler and more precise measurement of the total coronary arterial calcification volume without the application and resultant distortion of scaling factors and, therefore, more reliable serial evaluations of the coronary arterial calcium burden. At present, the technique requires a separate computer workstation, which may result in greater expense and longer postprocessing time for data analysis to obtain the calcium score. However, continuing rapid advances in computer software and declining costs of computer hardware lessen these minor impediments.

This is not to suggest, however, that this method of calcium volume determination is the best we might hope to achieve. The section-misregistration problems encountered with electron-beam CT will likely persist, imposing a limit on the precision of the calcium score. Further improvements may come from coupling the postprocessing technique of isotropic interpolation with true volumetric imaging data. The advent of fast ECG-triggered helical CT may yet provide the best input data for the quantification of coronary arterial calcium volume.

The relationship of coronary arterial calcification to coronary arterial disease remains a contentious and problematic issue. Yet it is one that radiologists can neither ignore nor afford to plunge into carelessly. The deluge of radio and billboard advertisements for coronary arterial calcium screening in most major urban centers is a testament to how "hot" this topic is in the public eye. However, serious ethical considerations arise from the aggressive promotion of coronary arterial calcium screening when there currently is no consensus about the meaning of the results in those individuals being evaluated (19). Radiologists should be leading the way in refining and optimizing the techniques and completing large-scale studies that demonstrate the cost-effectiveness and predictive value of coronary arterial calcium screening before selling it to an anxious and often ill-informed health care–consuming public.

The volumetric method for quantifying coronary arterial calcification reported by Callister et al is a notable improvement and a step in the right direction in the process of optimizing the reproducibility of calcium scoring. The usefulness of the volumetric method must be confirmed in the hands of other investigators to document the method's robustness; also, when fast ECG-triggered helical CT is widely available, the method should be applied to true volumetric imaging data to learn if further improvements in precision and reproducibility can be attained. With these advances, we can begin to define the effects of treatment regimens on coronary arterial calcification and to determine whether changes in coronary arterial calcification in individual patients have predictive value for future coronary events.

References

1. Doherty TM, Detrano RC. Coronary arterial calcification as an active process: a new perspective on an old problem. Calcif Tissue Int 1994; 54:224–230.
2. Agatston AS, Janowitz WR, Hildner FJ, Zusmer NR, Viamonte M Jr, Detrano R. Quantification of coronary artery calcium using ultrafast computed tomography. J Am Coll Cardiol 1990; 15:827–832.
3. Devries S, Wolfkiel C, Shah V, Chomka E, Rich S. Reproducibility of the measurement of coronary calcium with ultrafast computed tomography. Am J Cardiol 1995; 75:973–975.
4. Shields JP, Mielke CH Jr, Rockwood TH, Short RA, Viren FK. Reliability of electron beam computed tomography to detect coronary artery calcification. Am J Card Imaging 1995; 9:62–66.
5. Bielak LF, Kaufmann RB, Moll PP, McCollough CH, Schwartz RS, Sheedy PF II. Small lesions in the heart identified at electron beam CT: calcification or noise? Radiology 1994; 192:631–636.
6. Hernigou A, Challande P, Boudeville JC, Sene V, Grataloup C, Plainfosse MC. Reproducibility of coronary calcification detection with electron-beam computed tomography. Eur Radiol 1996; 6:210–216.
7. Wang S, Detrano RC, Secci A, et al. Detection of coronary calcification with electron-beam computed tomography: evaluation of interexamination reproducibility and comparison of three image-acquisition protocols. Am Heart J 1996; 132:550–558.
8. Hoeg JM, Feuerstein IM, Tucker EE. Detection and quantitation of calcific atherosclerosis by ultrafast computed tomography in children and young adults with homozygous familial hypercholesterolemia. Arterioscler Thromb Vasc Biol 1994; 14:1066–1074.
9. Janowitz WR, Agatston AS, Viamonte M Jr. Comparison of serial quantitative evaluation of calcified coronary artery plaque by ultrafast computed tomography in persons with and without obstructive coronary artery disease. Am J Cardiol 1991; 68:1–6.
10. Janowitz WR, Agatston AS, Kaplan G, Viamonte M Jr. Differences in prevalence and extent of coronary artery calcium detected by ultrafast computed tomography in asymptomatic men and women. Am J Cardiol 1993; 72:247–254.
11. Detrano RC, Wong ND, Doherty TM, Shavelle R. Prognostic significance of coronary calcific deposits in asymptomatic high-risk subjects. Am J Med 1997; 102: 344–349.
12. Lee RT, Grodzinsky AJ, Frank EH, Kamm RD, Schoen FJ. Structure-dependent dynamic mechanical behavior of fibrous caps from human atherosclerotic plaques. Circulation 1991; 83:1764–1770.
13. Mintz GS, Popma JJ, Pichard AD, et al. Patterns of calcification in coronary artery disease: a statistical analysis of intravascular ultrasound and coronary angiography in 1155 lesions. Circulation 1995; 91:1959–1965.
14. Cheng GC, Loree HM, Kamm RD, Fishbein MC, Lee RT. Distribution of circumferential stress in ruptured and stable atherosclerotic lesions: a structural analysis with histopathological correlation. Circulation 1993; 87:1179–1187.
15. Mautner SL, Mautner GC, Froehlich J, et al. Coronary artery disease: prediction with in vitro electron beam CT. Radiology 1994; 192:625–630.
16. Budoff MJ, Georgiou D, Brody A, et al. Ultrafast computed tomography as a diagnostic modality in the detection of coronary artery disease: a multicenter study. Circulation 1996; 93:898–904.
17. Sangiorgi G, Rumberger JA, Severson A, et al. Arterial calcification and not lumen stenosis is highly correlated with atherosclerotic plaque burden in humans: a histologic study of 723 coronary artery segments using nondecalcifying methodology. J Am Coll Cardiol 1998; 31:126–133.
18. Callister TQ, Cooil B, Raya SP, Lippolis NJ, Russo DJ, Raggi P. Coronary artery disease: improved reproducibility of calcium scoring with an electron-beam CT volumetric method. Radiology 1998; 208:807–814.
19. Wexler L, Brundage B, Crouse J, et al. Coronary artery calcification: pathophysiology, epidemiology, imaging methods, and clinical implications—a statement for health professionals from the American Heart Association. Circulation 1996; 94: 1175–1192.

Thomas F. Budinger, MD, PhD
Alan Berson, PhD
Elliot R. McVeigh, PhD
Roderic I. Pettigrew, MD, PhD
Gerald M. Pohost, MD
John T. Watson, PhD
Samuel A. Wickline, MD

Index terms:
Heart, MR, 51.1214
Magnetic resonance (MR), vascular studies, 51.1214
Special reports

Radiology 1998; 208:573–576

[1] From the Center for Functional Imaging, Lawrence Berkeley National Laboratory, University of California, Berkeley (T.F.B.); the National Heart, Lung, and Blood Institute, National Institutes of Health, 9000 Rockville Pike, Bethesda, MD 20892 (A.B., J.T.W.); the Department of Biomedical Engineering, Johns Hopkins University School of Medicine, Baltimore, Md (E.R.M.); the Department of Radiology, Emory University Hospital, Atlanta, Ga (R.I.P.); the Division of Cardiovascular Disease, University of Alabama, Birmingham (G.M.P.); and the Department of Internal Medicine, Jewish Hospital, St Louis, Mo (S.A.W.). Received August 7, 1997; accepted May 8, 1998. **Address reprint requests to** A.B.

This article is also to be published in the *Journal of Cardiovascular Magnetic Resonance* (in press) in view of the importance of the material to the different audiences reached by *Radiology* and the *Journal of Cardiovascular Magnetic Resonance*, with agreement by both Editors.

Cardiac MR Imaging: Report of a Working Group Sponsored by the National Heart, Lung, and Blood Institute[1]

Dramatic progress has been made over the past several years in the research and development of magnetic resonance (MR) techniques for imaging biologic structure and function, and much of this work has been supported by the National Institutes of Health (NIH). MR imaging has capabilities that are unique, as compared with other imaging modalities, for measurement and monitoring of biologic processes in vivo. Despite these capabilities, the use of MR imaging by cardiovascular and cardiopulmonary clinicians remains limited; in many institutions, clinicians rarely refer patients for MR examinations. The principal reasons for this include long imaging times with associated patient discomfort, low postprocessing speeds, inadequate access to patients during imaging, and lack of understanding of MR processes and benefits by clinicians and their associates.

On October 28–29, 1996, the National Heart, Lung, and Blood Institute (NHLBI) sponsored a Working Group to explore the potential of MR for imaging the heart, lung, and vasculature. They recommend areas of research and development that could lead to more extensive clinical use of MR methods to improve the diagnosis and management of cardiovascular and cardiopulmonary disorders. Approximately 50 scientists, bioengineers, and clinicians from academia, industry, and government convened at the NIH Natcher Conference Center, Bethesda, Md.

OVERVIEW OF PRESENTATIONS

Several sessions were organized with the aim of having cardiologists present their views on needs in diagnosis and patient care.

There is a changing paradigm for cardiovascular medicine that focuses on the features of outpatient examinations that are noninvasive and patient-friendly, with the consideration of atherosclerosis and its sequelae as a chronic disease requiring a long-term approach. The MR imaging examination must consolidate many tests into one to produce an examination that requires 1 hour or less for complete diagnosis. It must be cost-effective relative to other standard examinations. The principal capabilities that influence diagnosis and patient care that can be currently accomplished with MR imaging of the heart are in anatomic and functional assessments, including volumetric and deformation evaluation, vascular lumina, and assessment of myocardial perfusion and viability.

Visualization of Coronary Arteries

Imaging of the coronary arteries at a resolution equivalent to that of conventional angiography remains a crucial goal that has not yet been achieved. MR angiography is continually progressing, but considerable additional research is required before it can replace conventional x-ray angiography for both clinical and epidemiologic applications. Clinical acceptance of cardiac MR imaging will not occur until diagnostic quality images are achieved in a cost-effective manner for most of the coronary tree. Development of suitable intravascular contrast agents may be essential for accomplishing this. Success in this area will allow medical management on the basis of noninvasive and low-cost measures of disease progression and regression.

Functional Assessment of the Ventricles

MR imaging of structure and function should provide optimal ability to assess (*a*) detection of ischemia through stress testing, (*b*) risk stratification in coronary artery disease, (*c*) remodeling, (*d*) right ventricular disease and the response of the right ventricle to pulmonary hypertension, (*e*) chemotherapy cardiotoxicity, (*f*) allograft rejection, and (*g*) risk stratification in valvular and congenital volume overload states.

Although ventricular evaluation with MR imaging has been predominantly aimed at the left ventricle, MR imaging also allows evaluation of the right ventricle. Assessment of its function in response to diseases such as chronic obstructive pulmonary disease, relevant congenital heart disease, and primary pulmonary hypertension is enabled by improved MR imaging strategies.

Myocardial Flow, Perfusion, and Viability

Ischemic heart disease leads to greater mortality than any other single cardiovascular disease. MR methods currently exist for blood flow measurements, but there is a clinical need for improvements in quantitation and volume coverage, especially for assessment of low flow. MR methods are potentially capable of assessing the distribution of myocardial perfusion with high resolution. Innovations in contrast agents are helping to achieve this potential. Several MR approaches have the potential to assess viability. One approach is the use of cine MR imaging before and during the infusion of a myocardial stimulant such as dobutamine in low doses. Another approach makes use of the ability of MR spectroscopy to assess high-energy phosphate metabolism. Viability studies with metabolite MR spectroscopy require improvements in hardware and collaborations between researchers and manufacturers. Basic research in chemistry, physics, and bioengineering are needed to accomplish this.

Vascular Disease and Tissue Characterization

Major clinical applications of MR imaging are in the evaluation of the carotid arteries and the iliofemoral vascular systems. Imaging of these structures with MR is now possible with high resolution, with use of intravascular contrast agents. Atherosclerotic plaque, particularly the unstable plaque, is now understood to greatly influence coronary events and/or stroke. The evaluation of plaque constituents and the characterization of tissue within and around the plaque with use of MR imaging and spectroscopic techniques may allow investigators to differentiate between stable and unstable plaque. This is an important research area that has high risks in terms of its clinical success, but also has potentially high clinical benefits.

Myocardial Dynamics and Fiber Architecture

Evaluation of myocardial function is fraught with uncertainties and errors that include the inability to track a specific tissue volume because of through-plane and in-plane motion, nonobjective measures of wall function, the transmural variation of motion, and limited views of the heart. Wall motion MR techniques of tagging and velocity tracking offer ways to solve these problems. This is a research area that holds great promise and is near the stage of validating its accuracy and efficacy. Well-characterized multicenter clinical studies should be undertaken to assess sensitivity and specificity compared with those of contemporary methods

The unique capabilities of MR imaging to enable visualization and quantification of myocardial muscle microstructure with diffusion imaging have been reported in preliminary studies. The ability to measure and monitor muscle microstructure over time is still under development but may open doors into basic physiology of muscle during phases of myocardial development and progression and regression of disease, particularly congestive heart failure.

A database of normal hearts can now be obtained for the construction of the "normal human heart model." Additionally, a cohort of patients with heart failure can be tracked in a longitudinal study from the preclinical condition to full heart failure. These data can be used to increase our understanding of this disease and manage dose levels of drugs with an objective measurement of response and disease progress.

Hardware and Software

The major limitations of current MR imaging systems are associated with efficiency, safety, patient comfort, and cost-effectiveness. MR systems should incorporate integrated continuous patient modular monitoring of functions such as Po_2, electrocardiograms, and blood pressure. Needed improvements that should make cardiac and vascular MR imaging more accurate and acceptable are in electrocardiographic- and respiratory-gating techniques and in the standardization of imaging protocols.

The inability to have data presentation during or immediately after imaging is a serious impediment to clinical acceptance. It is crucial that results be presented in near real time or within a few minutes of the patient study. This would include standard sets of views as a basis set and convenient provision of images for referring physicians to facilitate rapid decision making. Methods should be standardized and automated to the extent possible for clinical applications in both resting and stress conditions (eg, radiofrequency tagging; phase contrast to assess ventricular function, perfusion, and viability). Efficiency and patient friendliness will benefit from more comfortable and accessible magnet configurations, reduced imaging times, noise abatement, and faster postprocessing of data. Patient safety needs to be enhanced by being able to monitor patients in real time during the imaging procedure.

Substantial gains in signal-to-noise ratio can be achieved through advances in coil design. Phased arrays have been developed for cardiac imaging, but more efficient arrays are still needed for the improved spatial resolution and patient comfort demanded by clinical cardiologists. MR-compatible implants, stents, sutures, clips, and pacemakers are important so that the ever-increasing number of patients with these devices can be accepted for MR studies.

The following principal achievable technical specifications are essential for advancements in cardiac MR imaging:

1. The optimum range for magnets designed for cardiovascular MR imaging is 0.5–2.0-T field strength, homogeneity of at least 2.5 parts per million across a 45–50-cm diameter, with 0.65-m-diameter free access in the bore.

2. Gradients of 2–5 G/cm are acceptable for most imaging applications. Some velocity-encoding techniques may require higher than 2 G/cm; diffusion-encoding gradients should be as high as possible.

3. Switching rate of gradient fields must take into account physiologic limits minimizing the tissue-induced electric fields related to dB/dt (rate of change in magnetic field) in nonimaged regions of the patient.

4. The magnet configuration should take into account patient comfort for a 1-hour examination and allow easy access to the patient by the physician.

5. Audio noise should be minimized to allow communication with the patient and for patient comfort.

6. Image reconstruction should be performed at rates up to 30 frames per second.

ACCEPTANCE OF MR METHODS

In addition to the above research and technical areas, the Working Group considered two issues that need to be addressed as they importantly affect the acceptance of MR methods into clinical cardiology.

Cost-effectiveness

Appropriate clinical studies must be designed to demonstrate improvement in outcome and in physician acceptance for selected diagnostic problems. Questions of the value of MR methods to replace other methods in a cost-effective way must be resolved. Models of cost-effectiveness using preliminary data may begin this effort for specific disease entities, such as ischemic heart disease and heart failure. These modeling strategies can provide an initial estimate of the cost-effectiveness of MR methods.

The Working Group discussed a model for research wherein the NIH would take a leadership role for the strategy and development of research followed by the initiation of carefully designed clinical trials. The problem is that a protocol for MR cardiac studies could become obsolete during the course of the clinical trial. It is important that the trials not prematurely test applications that require more sophisticated capabilities than are widely available, that they include a mechanism for, as rapidly as possible, recognizing and incorporating technologic advances as they occur, and that by a concurrent analysis strategy they point to directions required to achieve or improve the desired results. This is different from the conventional clinical trial, and the strategy development should receive careful attention by the NIH and experienced scientific investigators. The trial design must take into account the fact that MR technology is rapidly improving.

Training

Training must be available for researchers and clinicians who specialize in cardiovascular MR studies. In contrast to many other imaging modalities, MR imaging has greater versatility but at the same time is more complex in the underlying physics and engineering. Trainees must be made aware of cardiovascular physiology, of the risks in cardiac patients, of other cardiovascular procedures, and of the contraindications for MR studies. Training must include basic physics, an understanding of the variety of MR imaging and spectroscopic methods, the cost-effectiveness of MR methods, and a firm grounding in the other noninvasive imaging modalities. The initiative for training programs is a shared responsibility of the NIH and the professional cardiology, radiology, and bioengineering societies.

WORKING GROUP RECOMMENDATIONS

The Working Group recommends that the scientific and engineering communities of academia and industry vigorously continue the following tasks of enhancing the value of MR imaging for clinical decision making:

1. Efficiency: Systems must be optimized for high-speed imaging so as to complete a cardiac examination of anatomy and function within 1 hour, including patient preparation time.

2. Monitoring and patient safety: Electrocardiographic- and respiratory-gating techniques that can be applied during the imaging procedure without the need for breath holding must be developed, including real-time monitoring during stress testing. The MR system should also be designed for integrated patient monitoring of such functions as Po_2 and blood pressure during imaging.

3. Display of results: Processing time of image data must be substantially reduced to provide images in near real time, and readily comprehended image displays must be available nearly as fast as the data are acquired. Fast and interactive imaging is critically necessary. Additionally, standardization of imaging protocols is needed to facilitate clinical testing and comparison among laboratories.

These following activities are recommended for immediate implementation:

1. Cost-effectiveness: Under the NIH, models for estimating the cost-effectiveness should be developed in anticipation of a method of clinical evaluation of a rapidly developing technology. Trials should begin to establish those applications that have the potential for cost-effectiveness.

2. Training: The NIH should initiate training opportunities for researchers and clinicians in MR imaging.

3. Magnet configuration: Diagnosis and patient care are hampered by the inability to have access to patients during imaging. Industry designers must concentrate on changing the magnet architecture to resolve this problem. At the same time, this will address the issue of physician and patient acceptance.

The following high-risk/high-benefit activities are recommended as foci for academic researchers and as special areas of emphasis for the NIH:

1. Coronary artery visualization and flow quantitation: Replacing conventional coronary angiography with MR angiography could lead to considerable cost savings with the ability to perform repeat examinations with no risk to patients. The potential has been realized for visualizing the proximal major coronary arteries with near diagnostic quality. Continued efforts are needed to improve spatial resolution and motion compensation so as to image most of the coronary tree with a resolution approaching that of conventional x-ray angiography. Fast imaging methods and effective intravascular contrast agents will be needed to accomplish this. Evaluation of the coronary arteries should ideally include the quantitation of coronary blood flow. The clinical importance of this is very high, and the potential for MR angiography to accomplish this with high accuracy should be a specific focus.

2. Plaque characterization: The potential for characterizing important compositional components of atherosclerotic plaque with MR methods should lead to vastly improved predictive capability in identifying unstable plaque. The results of several preliminary studies suggest MR imaging and/or spectroscopy could be successful including use of intraluminal coils. The goal should be to obtain compositional information of plaque in vivo that is comparable to measurements of excised tissue in the pathology laboratory. This is an ambitious goal with considerable risk for success, but the impact would be extremely high.

3. Cardiac wall strain: Myocardial dynamics may be an important marker of physiology associated with heart failure and ischemic heart disease. Quantitation of cardiac wall strain in vivo is a unique capability of MR imaging that has been demonstrated in preliminary studies. It is timely to conduct additional research, including human clinical studies, to validate the accuracy and clinical utility of these techniques.

4. Heart muscle function and orientation: Results of preliminary research in high-resolution MR imaging of heart muscle demonstrates that it may be possible to quantitate myocyte fiber architecture and that structural aberrations may be an early manifestation of ineffectual heart contractile activity. The in vivo assessment of fiber architecture is one of the several unique potential capabilities of MR imaging techniques to evaluate congestive heart failure.

5. Contrast imaging agents: Although a principal advantage of MR imaging is its relative noninvasiveness, substantial image improvement may be obtained with the use of appropriate intravenously administered intravascular blood pool agents. Such agents offer the promise for visualizing the entire vascular system, including coronary arteries, in a cost-effective way.

SUMMARY OF SCIENTIFIC PRIORITIES AND IMPLEMENTATION STRATEGIES

If MR imaging is to achieve greater credibility among cardiovascular and cardiopulmonary clinicians, academic and industry researchers must continue to address the issues of reduced imaging time, higher postprocedure processing speeds, more friendly and accessible magnet configurations, standardized protocols for image processing and display, real-time display, and improved gating and monitoring during imaging. Some of these activities are supported by the NIH through regular and small-business research grants, and this should continue. Industry efforts should be much more aggressive, responding to the priorities and needs of the practitioners responsible for cost-effective patient care.

Scientific priorities that require specific government support relate to the cost-effectiveness and accuracy of MR imaging methods and to the training of researchers involved in cardiovascular imaging. It is now timely to develop models to evaluate cost-effectiveness and to show the potential sensitivity, specificity, and outcomes of imaging structure and function in specific patient groups with those MR technologies, taking into account the continuing rapid advances.

Long-term research support by the NIH can ensure that several high-risk/high-benefit potentials of MR imaging be pursued to determine whether or not they can be clinically useful and cost-effective. Some areas worthy of special attention are coronary artery imaging, plaque characterization, cardiac wall strain, heart muscle microstructure, and intravascular contrast agents.

Five recommendations are offered by the Working Group that require actions by the NIH, academic researchers, and industry researchers and developers:

1. The NIH must initiate trials to establish the cost-effectiveness of dynamic functional MR imaging of the heart, imaging of the coronary artery tree and perfusion imaging, and evaluate the clinical utility for important disease entities such as ischemic heart disease and heart failure.

2. The NIH must initiate training opportunities in MR imaging for researchers and clinicians within the next 3 years.

3. The NIH must maintain its leadership in this field by continuing its support of research. There is a high likelihood that advances will occur in the near future in coronary artery imaging and in the development and use of contrast agents that will have great impact on clinical acceptance of MR functional and perfusion imaging. In coronary artery imaging, improved resolution is necessary to allow visualization of most of the coronary artery tree so that MR may replace conventional angiography in a cost-effective manner for many applications. Contrast agents for enhancing images may be necessary to achieve clinically acceptable structural and functional images. Research is expected to continue in quantitation of perfusion imaging of the entire myocardium.

4. As MR imaging offers a unique technique for discoveries through the measurement and monitoring of physical and biochemical data in vivo and noninvasively, several high-risk/high-benefit research areas should be considered for special NIH emphasis: imaging of cardiac wall strain, delineation and quantitation of muscle fiber orientation, characterization of atherosclerotic plaque, imaging of myocardial metabolites, and multinuclear selected-region spectroscopy. Each of these applications is critically important for advancing our knowledge of the physiology and pathophysiology of the heart and vascular system.

5. There is an urgent need for close industry and academic research cooperation and collaboration in developing solutions to several important problems that currently limit the usefulness of MR imaging. Industry in particular must respond aggressively to the needs for cost-effective patient care. These problems include system architecture to address patient comfort and accessibility; imaging protocols to allow complete cardiac examinations within 60 minutes; postprocessing of data to access images in near real time; monitoring of physiologic parameters such as P_{O_2}, electrocardiograms, and blood pressure during imaging; development of MR-compatible materials for improved safety; and ways to allow acceptance of patients with implants (eg, catheters, stent materials, pacemakers).

The Working Group participants shared the NIH's interest and optimism in the challenges and opportunities that exist in this exciting area of science and medicine. Implementing the recommendations will lead to important benefits for patients through improved and earlier diagnosis and improved patient care and cost-effective strategies and the advancement of scientific knowledge of heart and vascular physiology and pathophysiology.

Acknowledgments: The authors acknowledge the important input from many of the participants at the meeting and especially wish to thank the following individuals whose comments on early drafts were particularly valuable: Leon Axel, PhD, MD, University of Pennsylvania; S. Morry Blumenfeld, PhD, GE Medical Systems; Paul Bottomley, PhD, Johns Hopkins University School of Medicine; Michael Jerosch-Herold, PhD, University of Minnesota; Albert Macovski, PhD, Stanford University; and Norbert Wilke, MD, University of Minnesota.

Scott A. Mirowitz, MD

Index terms:
Abdomen, abnormalities, 761.93, 761.94, 770.93, 770.94, 775.93, 775.94, 81.93, 81.94, 86.93, 86.94
Abdomen, MR, 761.1214, 770.1214, 775.1214, 81.1214, 86.1214
Magnetic resonance (MR), technology, 761.1214, 770.1214, 775.1214, 81.1214, 86.1214

Radiology 1998; 208:577–589

Abbreviations:
SNR = signal-to-noise ratio
TE = echo time
TR = repetition time

[1] From the Mallinckrodt Institute of Radiology, Washington University School of Medicine, 216 S Kingshighway Blvd, St Louis, MO 63110. Received December 2, 1997; revision requested January 23, 1998; revision received March 4; accepted April 28. **Address reprint requests to** the author.

Diagnostic Pitfalls and Artifacts in Abdominal MR Imaging: A Review[1]

Magnetic resonance (MR) imaging has demonstrated considerable clinical usefulness in many abdominal applications. Experience with this modality has also revealed a number of entities that can result in misdiagnosis. Diagnostic pitfalls include the simulation of abnormalities that do not exist, the obscuration of abnormalities that do exist, and interference with the characterization of abnormalities. These pitfalls may be related to technical MR artifacts, visual or perceptive errors, or anatomic variation. This review will focus on the most clinically important and frequently encountered pitfalls in abdominal MR imaging. Additional information concerning other pitfalls in MR imaging is available elsewhere (1). It is the objective of this review to describe the manifestations of these pitfalls as well as the tools that are available to resolve the diagnostic issues they may create.

LIVER

Partial Volume Averaging

Partial volume averaging occurs when voxels encompass more than one adjacent tissue. As a result, the voxel's net signal intensity is determined by the relative proportion and signal intensity of each component. Partial volume averaging usually occurs along the section-selection direction of the image, which is the direction in which the voxel dimension is the greatest. Partial volume averaging can simulate or obscure lesions or interfere with their characterization.

Structures that commonly undergo partial volume averaging with the liver and thereby simulate hepatic lesions include the hepatic flexure of the colon, the gallbladder, the duodenum, and exophytic right adrenal or renal lesions. Those structures that contain fluid create high-signal-intensity pseudolesions on T2-weighted images; the colon has variable signal intensity, depending on its contents. High-signal-intensity blood in the left ventricular cavity can simulate a focal left hepatic lobe lesion on flow-compensated T2-weighted images. Left ventricular myocardium, which has T2 relaxation properties similar to those of the liver, appears to represent normal hepatic tissue surrounding the abnormality. Fat contained in the falciform ligament or hepatic fissures can also create high-signal-intensity pseudolesions on T1-weighted images or fast spin-echo T2-weighted images.

Careful inspection of contiguous images usually allows partial volume averaging to be distinguished from an actual pathologic entity. When doubt remains, partial volume averaging can be reduced by making the voxel size smaller. This is achieved by decreasing the field of view, increasing the number of matrix elements, and particularly by decreasing the section thickness. It may also be helpful to acquire images in alternate planes. For example, coronal images often clarify the nature of partial volume effects that are encountered on transaxial images.

Vascular Structures

The portal and hepatic veins have signal intensity characteristics that are similar to those of many lesions on both T1-weighted images and flow-compensated T2-weighted images (Fig 1). Consequently, these vessels can be confused with hepatic lesions. For example, when hyperintense hepatic foci are seen on a T2-weighted image, it can be difficult to distinguish those that represent vessels from those that could represent lesions. Close evaluation of contiguous images usually allows vessels to be recognized as tubular structures that ultimately join the main portal vein or inferior vena cava. In difficult cases, flow-compensated T1-weighted gradient-echo images are useful, as they display flowing blood as bright and most lesions as dark relative to the liver. Alternatively, T2-weighted images acquired by using spatial radio-frequency presaturation pulses and without flow compensation (ie, gradient moment nulling) display vessels as dark and most lesions as bright relative to the liver. These imaging techniques also allow bile ducts to be differentiated from vessels.

Flowing blood in abdominal vessels—particularly the aorta—creates phase errors that can simulate or obscure hepatic abnormalities (Fig 2). These artifacts traverse the phase-encoding direction of the image such that they intersect the lateral segment of the left hepatic lobe. Pulsation artifacts are recognized by their alignment with the aorta (or other vessel) along the phase-encoding direction and by their replication of the vessel's cross-sectional size and shape. However, the signal intensity of these artifacts usually differs from that of the actual vessel and alternates between foci that are bright and foci that are dark relative to the liver.

Vascular pulsation artifacts are made less prominent when radio-frequency presaturation bands cephalic to the acquired images are prescribed to decrease the signal intensity of inflowing blood. Gradient moment nulling helps to establish phase coherence among the population of moving protons at the time of echo formation, which also reduces these artifacts. Pulsation artifacts are generally more prominent on images acquired by using a prolonged echo time (TE) because of the reduced signal-to-noise ratio (SNR) and on gradient-echo images acquired by using relatively high excitation flip angles (2). Reorientation of the phase- and frequency-encoding gradients allows pulsation artifacts to be displaced so that they overlie the right hepatic lobe. This helps to confirm the artifactual nature of the observed signal intensity abnormality and allows the left hepatic lobe to be better

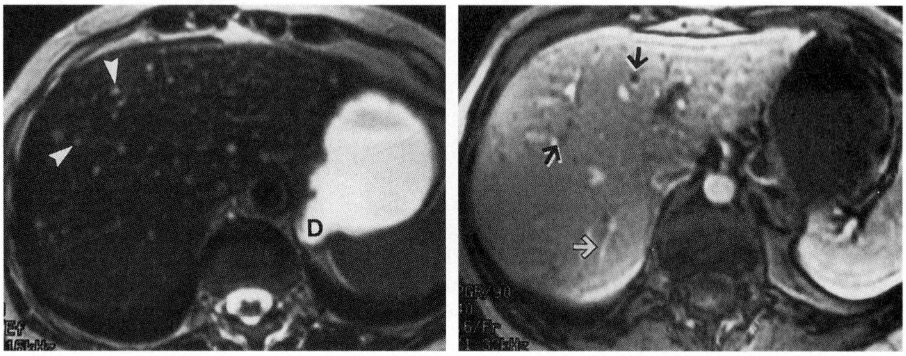

a. b.

Figure 1. **(a)** Multiple small, rounded hyperintense foci are distributed throughout the liver on this transaxial fast spin-echo T2-weighted MR image (3,300/128 [TR msec/TE msec]; echo train length, 16). It is difficult to distinguish which of these foci (arrowheads) represent lesions and which represent normal hepatic vessels on this image, which was acquired by using flow compensation (ie, gradient moment nulling) for artifact reduction. A posterior gastric diverticulum (*D*) is also present. **(b)** Gadolinium-enhanced, T1-weighted gradient-echo image (140/2.6, 90° flip angle) obtained in the same patient reveals an absence of enhancement in many of the foci in **a**. This absence of enhancement verifies that the foci (black arrows) represent simple hepatic cysts, whereas the larger hepatic vessels (white arrow) are enhanced.

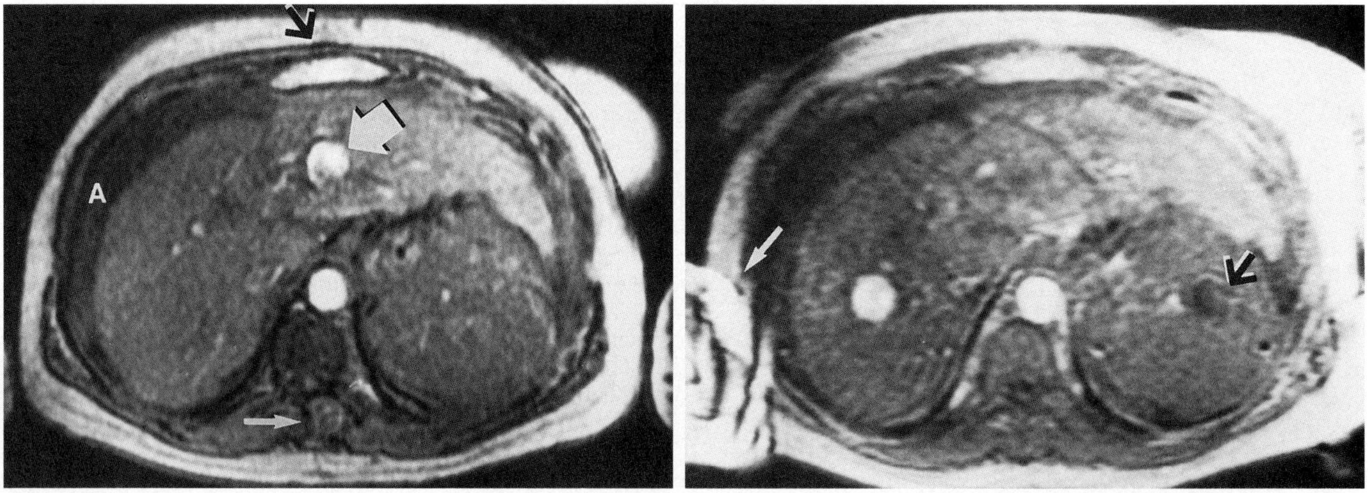

a. b.

Figure 2. **(a)** Axial T1-weighted gradient-echo MR image (120/3.1, 90° flip angle) shows a rounded focus of relatively increased signal intensity (large white arrow) in the left hepatic lobe. The cross-sectional shape and size of the apparent lesion resemble those of the aorta; however, the signal intensity of this lesion is lower than that of the aorta. Close inspection demonstrates a series of subtler artifacts with similar morphology but variable signal intensity oriented along the phase-encoding direction of the image (thin arrows). The patient is also noted to have ascites (*A*) and findings of hepatic cirrhosis, with decreased size of the right hepatic lobe, hypertrophy of the lateral segment of the left hepatic lobe, and a nodular hepatic surface. **(b)** Axial T1-weighted gradient-echo MR image (120/3.1, 90° flip angle) obtained after reorientation of the phase- and frequency-encoding gradients shows that the signal intensity abnormality overlies the right hepatic lobe and thus allows for confirmation of its artifactual nature (vascular pulsation artifact) and for better evaluation of the left lobe. A related focus of decreased signal intensity (black arrow) also projects over the left upper quadrant. With the phase-encoding gradient oriented along the horizontal axis of the body, aliasing (ie, wraparound) artifact occurs, with overlap of the signal that corresponds to the patient's arms (white arrow) along the lateral aspects of the image.

evaluated for lesions that could otherwise be obscured.

Motion Artifacts

Respiratory movement of the abdominal wall also interferes with lesion detection on MR images and can occasionally simulate abnormalities. As protons in the abdominal wall move with respiration, they have an inconsistent location and signal intensity during the acquisition of successive phase-encoding steps. This creates phase errors or ghost artifacts that appear as replications of the moving tissue displayed along the phase-encoding direction of the image. Respiratory motion also leads to blurring throughout the image because of the lack of phase coherence among the population of moving protons at echo formation (3,4).

Although abdominal wall fat is usually the major contributor to respiratory motion artifacts, other high-signal-intensity structures, such as the gallbladder, spleen, or hyperintense hepatic lesions that move with respiration, can also generate phase errors that simulate hepatic abnormalities.

There are many approaches to reducing respiratory motion artifacts. The amplitude of respiratory motion can be mechanically restricted with abdominal binders or by imaging the patient in the prone position. These maneuvers are of limited usefulness and can, paradoxically, accentuate motion artifacts by contributing to patient discomfort. Respiratory gating limits data collection to the end-expiratory portion of the respiratory cycle and thereby allows for consistent location of the protons on successive data acquisitions. With this method, data collection is inefficient and imaging time is prolonged considerably. Respiratory-ordered phase encoding involves monitoring the patient's respiratory cycle during imaging so that data can be subsequently reordered to simulate a prolonged slow respiration. Gradient moment nulling (ie, flow compensation) involves the use of gradient pulses to rephase moving protons at echo formation. Intrinsic rephasing occurs on even-numbered echoes of multiecho pulse sequences and thus also reduces motion artifacts (5). Respiratory-ordered phase encoding and gradient moment nulling do not prolong imaging time and can be used simultaneously.

Respiratory (and other) motion artifacts are accentuated on long-TE images because of the reduced SNR. Spatial radio-frequency presaturation pulses applied along the anterior abdominal wall reduce the signal intensity of abdominal wall tissue and that of any motion artifacts that result from the movement of the anterior abdominal wall. Caution must be exercised to avoid presaturation of the anterior part of the liver, because presaturation of the liver can obscure hepatic lesions. Radio-frequency saturation of the lipid peak suppresses fat signal intensity throughout the field of view but may be incomplete in the presence of magnetic field inhomogeneities.

Each of the above-mentioned imaging techniques can help to reduce respiratory motion artifacts, although the only means of eliminating these artifacts is to acquire images during suspended respiration. Various spin-echo, gradient-echo, and echo-planar sequences can enable imaging of the entire liver during a single breath hold and thus allow respiratory-phase errors and blurring to be avoided.

Pulsatile cardiac motion transmitted to the underlying left hepatic lobe can produce dephasing artifacts. These manifest as areas of decreased hepatic signal intensity that can obscure lesions or simulate them on T1-weighted images (Fig 3). Options for reducing these artifacts include coordinating the data collection with the cardiac cycle by using electrocardiographic triggering, fast imaging pulse sequences, or reduced TEs.

Contrast Material

Gadolinium chelate contrast material improves the detection and characterization of some hepatic lesions and is being used with increased frequency for this purpose. Like iodinated contrast materials, gadolinium chelates rapidly equilibrate between the intravascular and interstitial tissue compartments. Consequently, many hepatic lesions become relatively isointense with the surrounding liver on images acquired more than 2 minutes after the injection of gadolinium chelate contrast material. Thus, effective use of gadolinium chelates in hepatic lesion detection requires the administration of contrast material by using rapid injection rather than slow infusion, coupled with rapid image acquisition (6,7) (Fig 4).

Immediately after the bolus injection of gadolinium chelate contrast material, an oval region of relatively increased contrast material enhancement can be observed in the medial segment of the

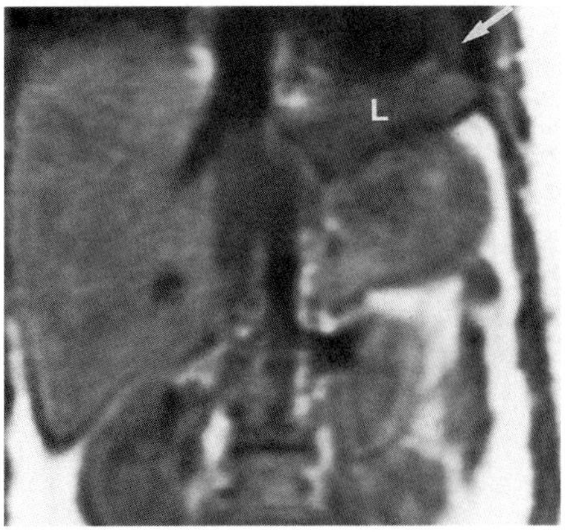

Figure 3. Because of dephasing caused by transmitted pulsations from the overlying left ventricle (arrow), the signal intensity is decreased throughout the left hepatic lobe (*L*) relative to the signal intensity in the remainder of the liver on this coronal T1-weighted MR image (670/12).

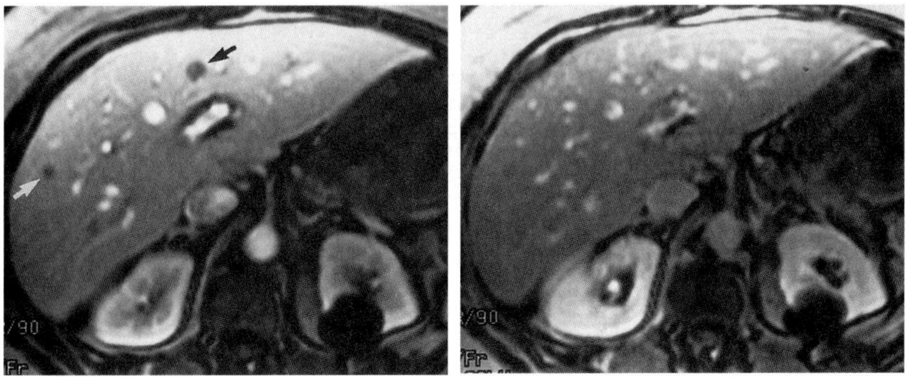

a. b.

Figure 4. **(a)** Liver metastases (arrows) secondary to appendiceal carcinoma are seen on a T1-weighted gradient-echo MR image (140/2.1, 90° flip angle) acquired immediately after bolus injection of gadolinium chelate contrast material. **(b)** These lesions are obscured on the T1-weighted MR image (610/12) acquired 5 minutes later.

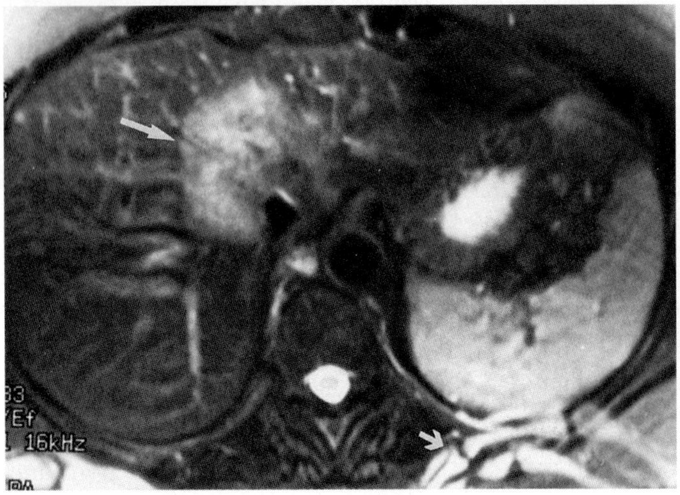

a.

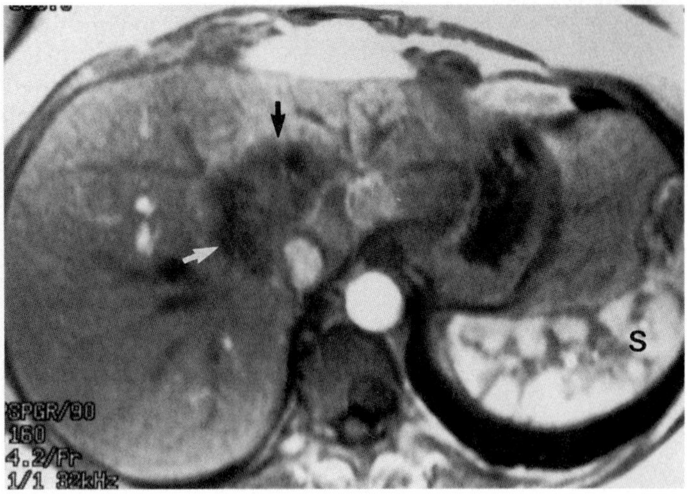

b.

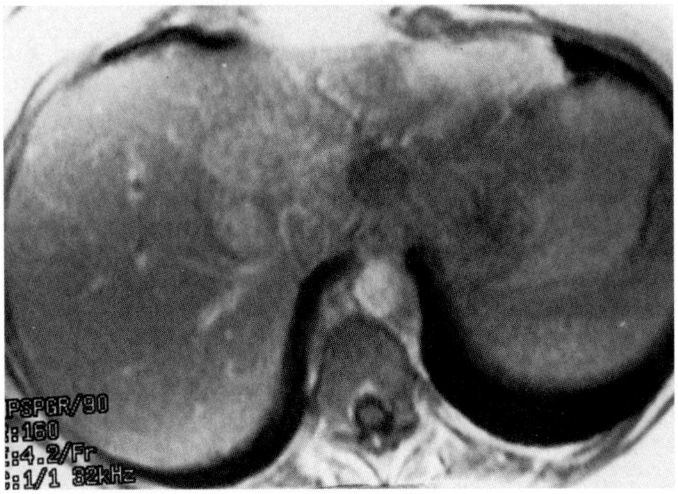

c.

Figure 5. **(a)** A large high-signal-intensity lesion (long arrow) is seen adjacent to the intrahepatic inferior vena cava on a transaxial fast spin-echo T2-weighted MR image (3,300/96; echo train length, 16). Aliasing (ie, wraparound) of the patient's fingers (short arrow) into the posterior aspect of the image is also demonstrated. **(b)** The lesion, representing cholangiocarcinoma, has decreased signal intensity relative to the signal intensity of the surrounding liver on the T1-weighted gradient-echo MR image (160/4.2, 90° flip angle) acquired during bolus intravenous injection of gadolinium chelate contrast material. Note the ring of peripheral enhancement (arrows). A markedly heterogeneous appearance of the spleen (*S*) is observed on this image, which was obtained during the arterial phase. **(c)** The lesion is enhanced homogeneously on a delayed image (160/4.2, 90° flip angle) acquired approximately 20 minutes after contrast material injection.

left hepatic lobe (8). This occurs during the arterial phase of contrast material enhancement and is believed to represent an area of increased hepatic arterial blood supply, an area of more rapid venous drainage, or both. Regional variations in hepatic perfusion are also hypothesized to cause transient segmental or subsegmental zones of relatively decreased hepatic enhancement on images acquired immediately after bolus injection of gadolinium chelate contrast material (9).

Gadolinium chelate contrast enhancement patterns are very useful in characterizing focal liver lesions, although some patterns are nonspecific and require differential diagnosis. Peripheral, ringlike enhancement, which is often associated with metastatic lesions, can also be seen with hepatocellular carcinoma and abscesses. Centripetal progression to complete enhancement is usually associated with cavernous hemangioma but can also be seen with metastases, hepatocellular carcinoma, and cholangiocarcinoma (Fig 5). Observation of a broken ring of nodular enhancement during the arterial phase of contrast material administration is key to the diagnosis of cavernous hemangioma. Diffuse nodular enhancement on arterial phase images can be seen with benign lesions, such as focal nodular hyperplasia or small hemangiomas, but it can also be seen with vascular primary or secondary hepatic malignancies (9–11).

In the liver, T2-shortening superparamagnetic iron oxide particles selectively accumulate in Kupffer cells and thereby render most hepatic lesions more conspicuous. However, lesions that contain Kupffer cells, such as focal nodular hyperplasia and some well-differentiated hepatocellular carcinomas, can also accumulate iron oxide; this accumulation can lead to isointensity with the surrounding liver tissue. Well-differentiated hepatocellular carcinomas can also become enhanced when manganese-based hepatocellular contrast material is administered, with similar results (12).

Pulse Sequences and Imaging Parameters

Appropriate selection of pulse sequences and imaging parameters is critically important in the detection of hepatic lesions. Conventional T1- and T2-weighted spin-echo sequences continue to be widely used in liver imaging. Focal hepatic abnormalities are most sensitively displayed when the repetition time (TR) and TE are optimized for tissue contrast (13–15). In T1-weighted imaging, a TR less than 500 msec and a TE less than 20 msec (preferably much less) are desirable, whereas in T2-weighted imaging, the TR and TE should be greater than 2,500 msec and 80 msec, respectively. In characterizing focal hepatic lesions, substantially greater T2 weighting is required, with TEs of 120 msec or greater. Both T1- and T2-weighted pulse sequences should always be used, since some lesions are

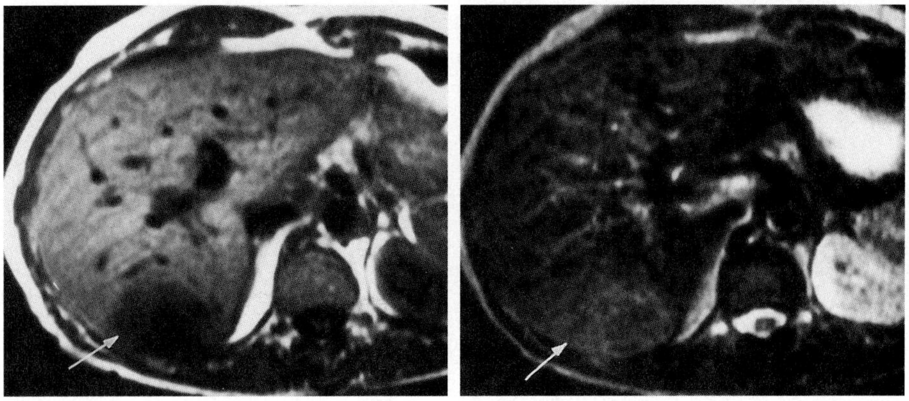

a. b.

Figure 6. **(a)** A large focus of abnormal signal intensity (arrow) that represents hepatic lymphoma is demonstrated on a T1-weighted MR image (500/11). **(b)** The focus (arrow) is much less conspicuous on the corresponding T2-weighted MR image (3,400/80).

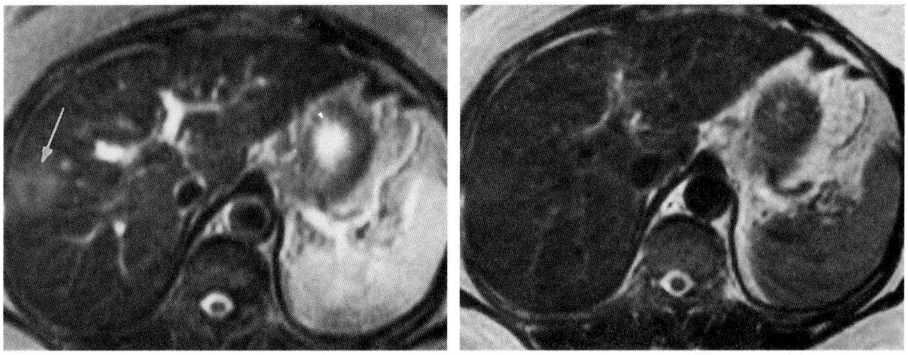

a. b.

Figure 7. T2-weighted MR images acquired by using **(a)** conventional (3,600/80) and **(b)** fast spin-echo (4,000/119; echo train length, 16) techniques. The colon carcinoma metastasis (arrow in **a**) in the anterior segment of the right hepatic lobe is much more visible on the conventional spin-echo image. Liver-spleen contrast is also increased in **a** as compared with that in **b**.

evident on images obtained with one sequence and not on images obtained with the other (Fig 6). T1-weighted images may be somewhat more sensitive in liver lesion detection at low magnetic field strength, and T2-weighted images may be more sensitive at high field strength, although this is of relatively limited relevance in individual patients (16).

Fast spin-echo pulse sequences are now widely used in hepatic imaging. These sequences substantially decrease imaging time while displaying features similar to those on conventional spin-echo images. However, subtle alterations in tissue contrast that can interfere with the detection of solid (but not cystic) hepatic lesions are seen on fast spin-echo T2-weighted images (17) (Fig 7). Reduced contrast on fast spin-echo images is attributed to two properties: (*a*) the increased off-resonance radio-frequency energy that is due to the multiple 180° pulses that are delivered and (*b*) the reduced dynamic range of tissue contrast display that is due to the relatively increased signal intensity of abdominal fat. Concordant with the latter explanation, tissue contrast on T2-weighted fast spin-echo images is markedly improved when fat saturation is used.

Fat suppression is also helpful in improving the conspicuousness of focal lesions in patients with diffuse hepatic fatty infiltration (18). Therefore, it is recommended that T2-weighted fast spin-echo images obtained with fat saturation be used for hepatic lesion detection and that fat saturation be omitted when attempting to characterize lesions. Blurring can interfere with lesion detection on fast spin-echo images, particularly when short TEs, long echo trains, or both have been prescribed (19).

Gradient-echo pulse sequences are also commonly used in liver imaging. Proton-density–weighted image contrast, which is unfavorable for liver lesion detection, results when inappropriate combinations of TR, TE, and flip angle are prescribed. For example, relatively long (eg, >100 msec) or very short (eg, 10 msec) TRs contribute to proton density weighting. On very short TR (ie, rapid, snapshot) gradient-echo images, T1- or T2-weighted contrast is improved when magnetization preparation pulses, such as a 180° inversion pulse or a 90°–80°–90°–pulse driven equilibrium module are used. Centric reordering of k space allows central data lines that encode image contrast and the SNR to be collected initially and thus improves these features (20). Of course, exogenous contrast materials, such as gadolinium chelates, are also frequently used in conjunction with gradient-echo imaging to promote lesion detection.

Fatty Hepatic Tissue

Fatty metamorphosis of the liver is often inapparent on conventional spin-echo MR images. However, prominent collections of fat can be seen as foci of relatively increased signal intensity on T1-weighted images. These findings can simulate other short T1 lesions, including hepatocellular carcinomas, metastatic melanomas, or hemorrhagic lesions (21) (Fig 8). Whereas hepatic fat is relatively inconspicuous on conventional spin-echo T2-weighted images, images obtained with fast spin-echo pulse sequences display fat as substantially more intense. Therefore, focal hepatic fat collections can have an appearance that is similar to that of metastases or other lesions on fast spin-echo T2-weighted images.

In patients with fatty liver tissue, focal lesions may also be obscured on T2-weighted fast spin-echo images acquired without fat suppression because of the increased signal intensity of fat. Similar results can occur on T1-weighted gradient-echo images that are acquired by using an opposed-phase TE; on these images, both the lesion and the background liver display reduced signal intensity (22) (Fig 9). Nondisplaced hepatic vessels coursing through a focus of abnormal signal intensity are often considered to be indicative of focal fat, although similar findings are observed in some neoplasms (23).

Patients with diffuse hepatic fatty infiltration may have focal sparing of a portion of the liver. In this situation, mildly increased signal intensity of hepatic fatty infiltration on T1-weighted images causes the spared portion to appear as a low-

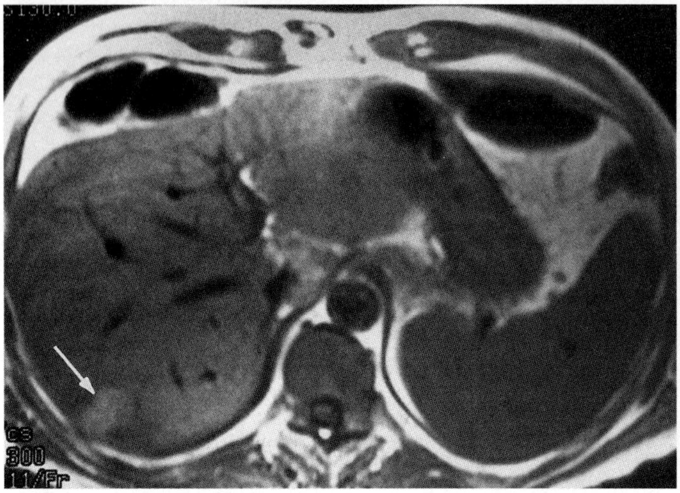

a.

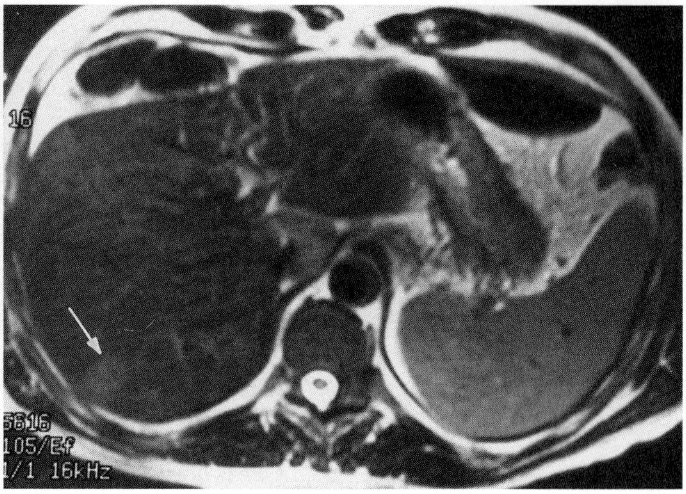

b.

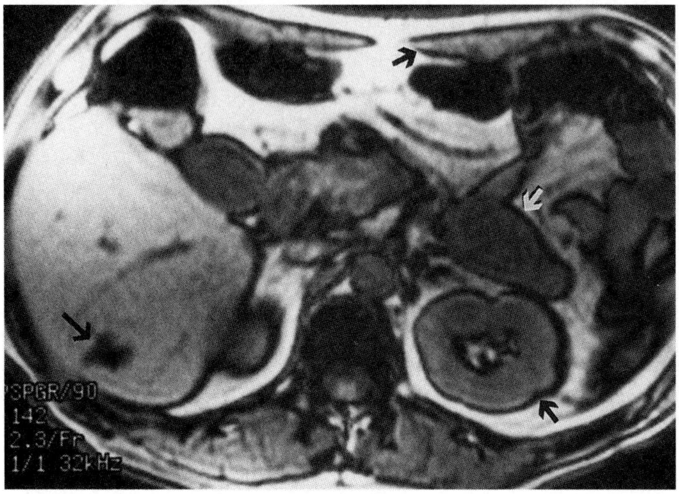

c.

Figure 8. **(a)** A rounded focus of relatively increased signal intensity (arrow) is observed in the posterior segment of the right hepatic lobe on a transaxial T1-weighted MR image (300/11). **(b)** The corresponding T2-weighted fast spin-echo MR image (5,600/105; echo train length, 16) demonstrates the abnormality (arrow) to have increased signal intensity compared with the remainder of the liver. This abnormality represents a focus of fatty infiltration, as verified on **(c)** the opposed-phase T1-weighted gradient-echo MR image (140/2.3, 90° flip angle), where the lesion (long black arrow) has markedly reduced signal intensity. Phase cancellation artifacts (short arrows) are also noted at fat-water interfaces throughout the abdomen.

signal-intensity lesion (Fig 10). Fat-specific imaging techniques, such as radio-frequency fat saturation and particularly opposed-phase chemical shift imaging, are useful for clarifying the above entities and distinguishing them from neoplastic involvement (24). Loss of signal intensity at the liver-fat interface may obscure small peripheral or capsular hepatic lesions on opposed-phase images. Chemical shift misregistration artifact can also produce similar results.

Cross Excitation

Radio-frequency section profile imperfections produce unintended excitation of the tissues adjacent to the section being imaged (25,26). As a result, these adjacent tissues can become saturated and display reduced contrast and SNR that contribute to poor lesion depiction. To avoid this situation, image acquisition can be interleaved such that alternating sections are initially acquired; subsequent acquisition of intervening sections allows for more complete relaxation of these tissues. Alternatively, an intersection gap of approximately 30%–50% of the nominal section thickness can be introduced to avoid cross excitation. Optimized (ie, square) radio-frequency pulses have also been used to reduce this artifact.

Lesion Characterization

Diffuse heterogeneous hepatic signal intensity can result from various benign liver conditions, including cirrhosis, hepatitis, cholestasis, and vascular thrombosis (24). These entities may be difficult to differentiate from diffuse metastatic involvement, which can have a similar appearance (Fig 11).

The signal intensity of lesions relative to the liver on T2-weighted images is often used to characterize hepatic lesions as benign (eg, cavernous hemangiomas or cysts) or malignant (eg, metastases or hepatocellular carcinomas). Because the liver is metabolically active, its signal intensity is subject to diffuse alteration, which may lead to lesion mischaracterization. For example, iron overload markedly reduces hepatic signal intensity. In this setting, metastases appear very bright and thus simulate benign abnormalities (27) (Fig 12). Conversely, inflammatory or other conditions that diffusely increase hepatic signal intensity cause focal abnormalities to appear less intense than they otherwise would. Thus, lesion signal intensity should be assessed relative to less metabolically active tissues, such as skeletal muscle or cerebrospinal fluid. Analysis of enhancement patterns after the administration of gadolinium chelate contrast material also is frequently helpful in lesion characterization.

Even in patients without diffuse liver disease, there is overlap in signal intensity characteristics between some malignant and benign lesions. Hypervascular or hemorrhagic metastases can display markedly increased signal intensity on T2-weighted images (28) (Fig 13). Conversely, low signal intensity can be observed in proteinaceous or hemorrhagic

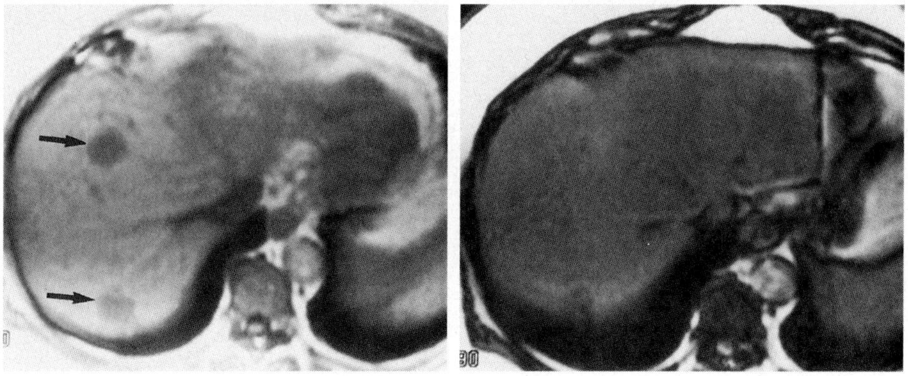

a. b.

Figure 9. Corresponding transaxial T1-weighted gradient-echo MR images acquired by using **(a)** in-phase (160/4.2, 90° flip angle) and **(b)** opposed-phase (140/2.3, 90° flip angle) TEs. The metastatic foci secondary to colon cancer (arrows in **a**) are considerably more conspicuous in **a** because of the mild, diffuse hepatic fatty infiltration that results in reduced signal intensity in the surrounding liver parenchyma in **b**.

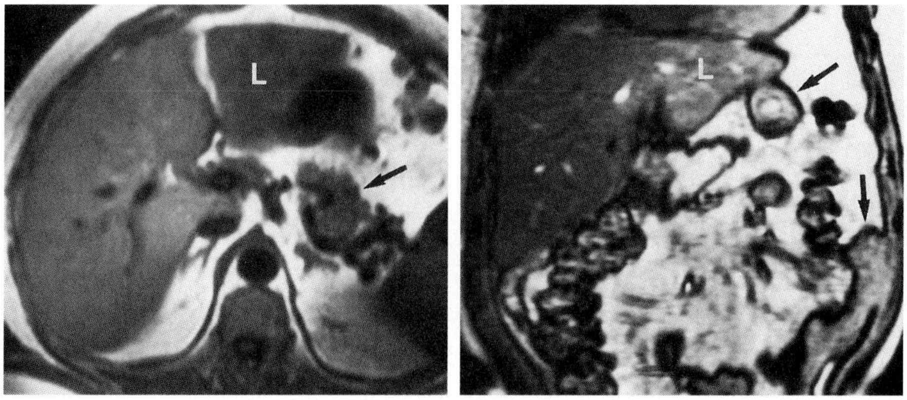

a. b.

Figure 10. **(a)** Relatively decreased signal intensity in the left hepatic lobe (*L*) is seen on this transaxial T1-weighted spin-echo MR image (500/12). This is due to focal sparing of diffuse hepatic fatty infiltration, as verified on **(b)** the coronal, opposed-phase T1-weighted gradient-echo MR image (113/2.6, 90° flip angle), which shows increased signal intensity in the left lobe (*L*) relative to the remainder of the liver. Phase-cancellation artifacts (arrows) are noted throughout **b** at fat-water interfaces, such as those surrounding the bowel loops and visceral organs. In **a**, lobular contour of the pancreas (arrow), a normal finding, is noted.

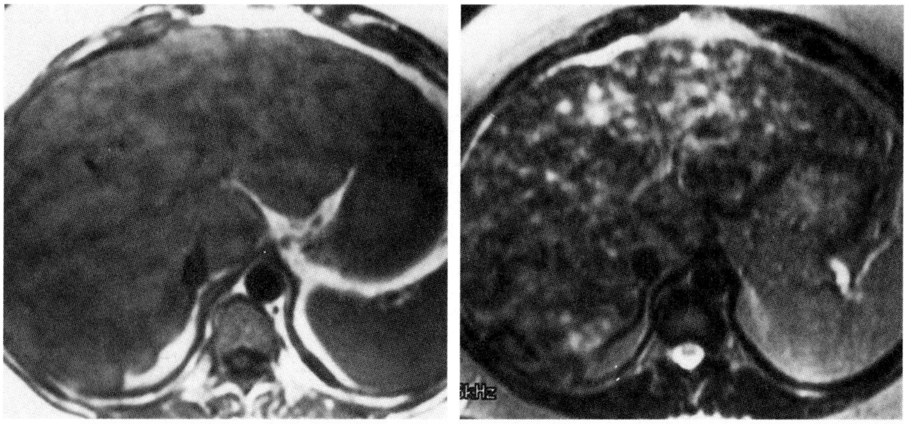

a. b.

Figure 11. **(a)** Transaxial T1-weighted (333/11) and **(b)** T2-weighted (3,800/80) MR images display markedly heterogeneous signal intensity throughout the liver in a patient with metastatic breast cancer. This pattern is similar to the appearance of other diffuse hepatic processes.

hepatic cysts and in fibrotic giant cavernous hemangiomas (29). Central scars, which are usually associated with focal nodular hyperplasia, can also occur with hepatic adenoma, fibrolamellar hepatocellular carcinoma, and cholangiocarcinoma (30).

SPLEEN

Partial volume averaging of the spleen with adjacent entities, such as tortuous splenic vessels, the gastric wall or gastric contents, ascitic fluid, or perisplenic fat, can simulate splenic lesions. Careful analysis of adjacent images, reduction of voxel dimensions (particularly section thickness), and use of alternate imaging planes are useful in problematic cases.

When the left hepatic lobe lies adjacent to the spleen, T1-weighted images may appear to depict a subcapsular splenic hematoma. This is due to the shorter T1 of hepatic tissue compared with that of the adjacent spleen. Lesions in this portion of the liver may appear to be of splenic origin.

Many splenic lesions are poorly depicted on both T1- and T2-weighted images, because these lesions have similar relaxation characteristics as normal splenic tissue (31,32). Therefore, exogenous contrast materials are important in the detection of focal and diffuse splenic abnormalities (32,33). As in the liver, in the spleen, gadolinium chelate contrast materials rapidly equilibrate between lesions and the surrounding splenic parenchyma. Standard T1-weighted spin-echo images acquired after gadolinium chelate contrast material administration or images acquired after slow infusion of contrast material are unlikely to be beneficial.

Images acquired immediately after gadolinium chelate contrast material injection show marked, heterogeneous contrast enhancement throughout the spleen before contrast material has equilibrated between the splenic sinusoids and pulp (Fig 14). Round, linear, or wedge-shaped foci of relatively decreased intensity are observed and should not be interpreted as lesions. Of course, such splenic heterogeneity can also interfere with the detection of focal lesions. This makes images acquired approximately 1 minute after contrast material injection critical, because, at this time, splenic enhancement is usually homogeneous, but focal lesions may not yet be obscured.

Superparamagnetic iron oxide is another contrast material that has shown

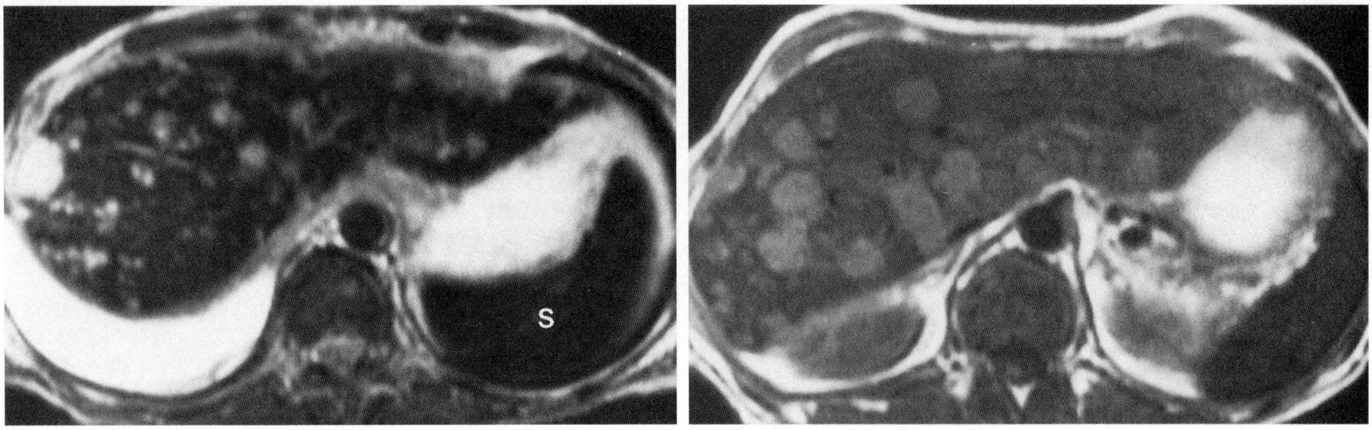

a. b.

Figure 12. (a) Multiple lesions that are of markedly increased signal intensity relative to the surrounding liver parenchyma are observed on a transaxial T2-weighted MR image (2,650/90). The spleen (*S*) has markedly reduced signal intensity, which is concordant with hemosiderosis. Although markedly increased signal intensity on T2-weighted images can suggest a benign lesion, such as a cavernous hemangioma or cyst, these breast cancer metastases appear as such because of the reduced background liver signal intensity from hepatic iron overload due to multiple blood transfusions. (b) The lesions are also of increased signal intensity relative to the surrounding liver on the corresponding T1-weighted MR image (500/12).

promise in the detection of focal and diffuse splenic abnormalities. After intravenous infusion, these particles accumulate in reticuloendothelial tissues and shorten T2. Thus, high-signal-intensity splenic lesions appear more conspicuous against a background of low-signal-intensity splenic tissue. Superparamagnetic iron oxide may be particularly helpful in distinguishing splenic enlargement due to benign granulomatous involvement from that due to lymphoma (34).

In some patients, the spleen appears to have markedly low signal intensity on T2-weighted images in the absence of exogenous contrast material. This is usually due to the accumulation of iron (ie, hemosiderosis), which is often related to repeated red blood cell transfusions. In other patients, including those who have not undergone previous transfusion, it is theorized that splenic signal intensity is reduced because of the iron accumulation that results from erythrocyte breakdown (31). Chemotherapeutic agents and perhaps other medications can also diffusely reduce splenic signal intensity.

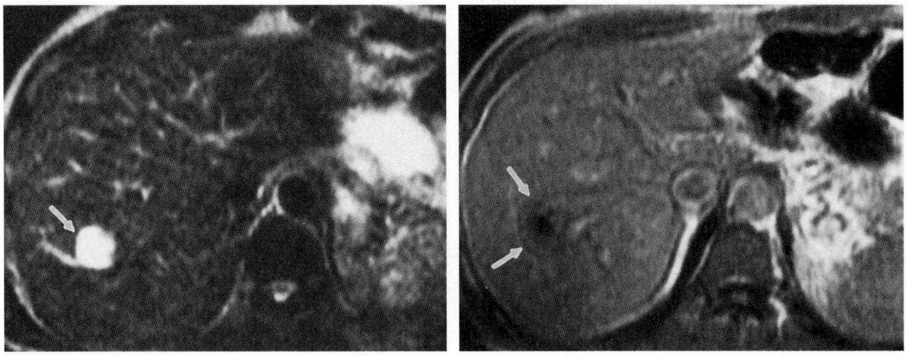

a. b.

Figure 13. (a) A lesion (arrow) in the right hepatic lobe demonstrates markedly increased signal intensity, which is suggestive of a hepatic cyst or cavernous hemangioma, on this transaxial T2-weighted MR image (3,300/120). Close inspection demonstrates a subtle irregularity in the medial wall of the lesion that raises suspicion of malignancy. (b) The T1-weighted gradient-echo MR image (160/4.2, 90° flip angle) obtained after the administration of gadolinium chelate contrast material reveals continuous peripheral enhancement of the lesion (arrows) that is compatible with metastatic disease. This is a necrotic metastasis in a patient with recurrent rectal carcinoma.

PANCREAS

Focal prominence of the pancreatic head or tail can appear to represent a mass; concordance of signal intensity with the remainder of the pancreas on images obtained with all pulse sequences allows for recognition of these normal variations (35) (Fig 15).

Partial volume averaging of tortuous splenic vessels with the pancreas can simulate pancreatic ductal enlargement (Fig 16). Vascular structures display a signal void on T2-weighted spin-echo images rather than the high signal intensity of ductal fluid. Flow-sensitive gradient-echo images can also be used to verify the presence of flowing blood. The fat plane that separates the pancreas from adjacent splenic vessels can simulate a prominent pancreatic duct (Fig 17). Fluid signal intensity characteristics are again absent on T2-weighted images, and fat-suppression techniques can be used if necessary. Blood flow within the superior mesenteric vein can also cause high signal intensity on entry sections and on flow-compensated T2-weighted images and thereby cause the vein to simulate a dilated common bile duct (Fig 18).

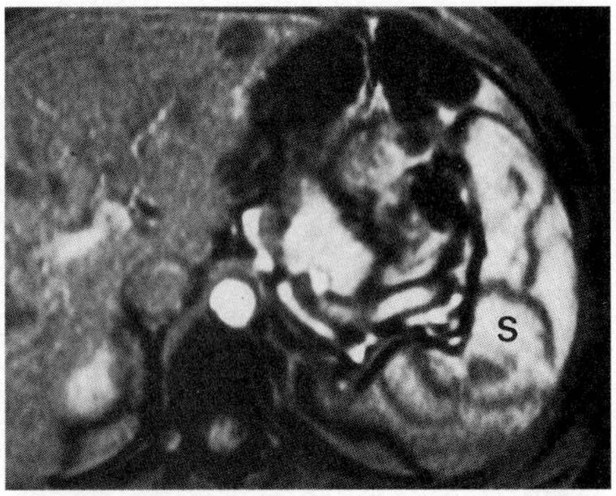

Figure 14. On this T1-weighted gradient-echo MR image (110/2.1, 90° flip angle) obtained during the arterial phase after bolus injection of gadolinium chelate contrast material, a heterogeneous pattern is present throughout the spleen (*S*).

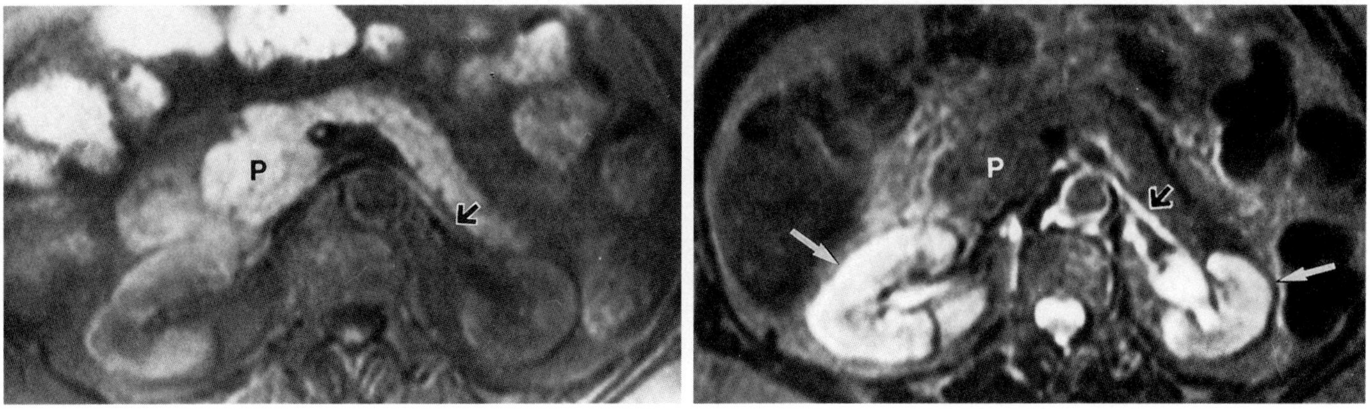

a. b.

Figure 15. Prominence of the pancreatic head (*P*) is demonstrated on **(a)** transaxial, fat-suppressed T1-weighted (430/11) and **(b)** T2-weighted (3,000/80) MR images. This is due to normal anatomic variation, as suggested by the concordance of the signal intensity of the pancreatic head with that of the remainder of the pancreas with both pulse sequences. In **b**, chemical shift misregistration artifact is observed surrounding the kidneys (white arrows). Relatively increased signal intensity in the proximal to middle left renal vein (black arrow) is also noted on both images.

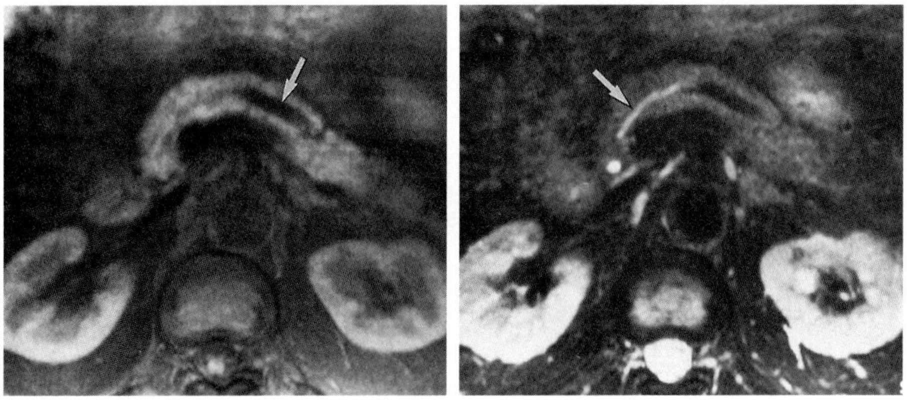

a. b.

Figure 16. **(a)** The pancreatic duct (arrow) appears enlarged on this transaxial, T1-weighted fat-suppressed fast spin-echo MR image (890/12; echo train length, three). This is due to volume averaging of the pancreas with the splenic vein, as confirmed on **(b)** the corresponding fat-suppressed T2-weighted fast spin-echo image (7,550/119; echo train length, 15), where the vessel displays a flow void rather than the high signal intensity of fluid. In **b**, a portion of a normal-caliber pancreatic duct (arrow) demonstrates high signal intensity.

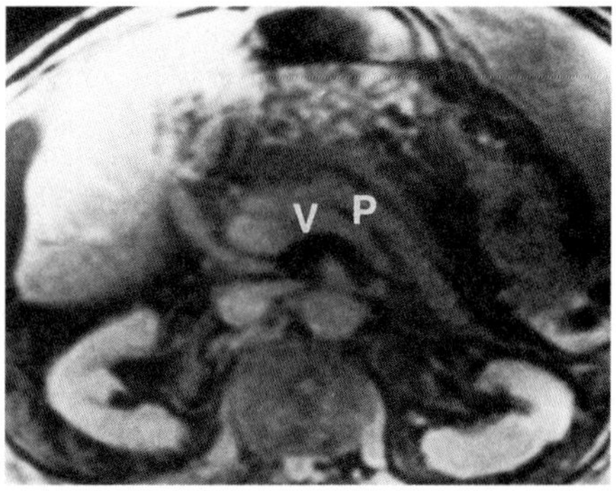

Figure 17. The fat plane that separates the posterior margin of the pancreas (*P*) from the anterior margin of the splenic vein (*V*) simulates a dilated pancreatic duct on this transaxial, fat-suppressed T1-weighted gradient-echo MR image (105/2.1, 30° flip angle) acquired after the administration of gadolinium chelate contrast material.

Fatty Pancreatic Tissue

The signal intensity of the pancreas on T1-weighted images increases with aging because of parenchymal fatty replacement. Focal collections of pancreatic fat can also be encountered. Pancreatitis is suggested when the pancreas appears less intense than the liver on T1-weighted images. This finding is most conspicuous on fat-suppressed images, where the normal pancreas appears to have relatively increased signal intensity.

Many pancreatic lesions are isointense with the surrounding pancreas on standard T1- and T2-weighted images (36). Fat saturation is again useful in improving the detection of these abnormalities because of the increased signal intensity of normal pancreatic tissue on fat-suppressed T1-weighted images (37). In addition, dynamic gadolinium-enhanced images (particularly those acquired by using fat suppression) can improve the sensitivity of pancreatic lesion detection and assist in the characterization of these lesions. The pancreas usually undergoes homogeneous contrast enhancement; a heterogeneous pattern can indicate chronic pancreatitis or other abnormalities.

Motion Artifacts

Respiratory motion artifacts can impair depiction of pancreatic abnormalities. Use of the methods previously discussed should be considered when performing pancreatic imaging. Peristaltic motion of the gastrointestinal tract is of particular concern in pancreatic imaging. Such motion results in image blurring, although structured phase artifacts can also be seen. Peristaltic motion is decreased when patients fast for several hours before imaging. Intramuscular glucagon or other antiperistaltic agents are also useful in improving the clarity of the pancreas. Because motion artifacts are proportional to the intensity of the moving tissue from which they originate, contrast materials that decrease the signal intensity of the gastrointestinal tract lumen are also helpful.

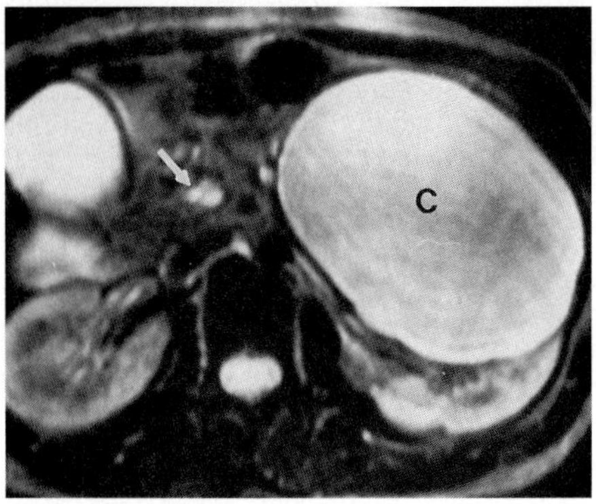

Figure 18. Transaxial T2-weighted MR image (3,100/80) depicts a structure that appears to represent a dilated distal common bile duct (arrow). This structure represents the superior mesenteric vein, which has increased intraluminal signal intensity owing to relatively slow blood flow and the use of flow compensation (ie, gradient moment nulling) for artifact reduction. A large left renal cyst (C) is also present.

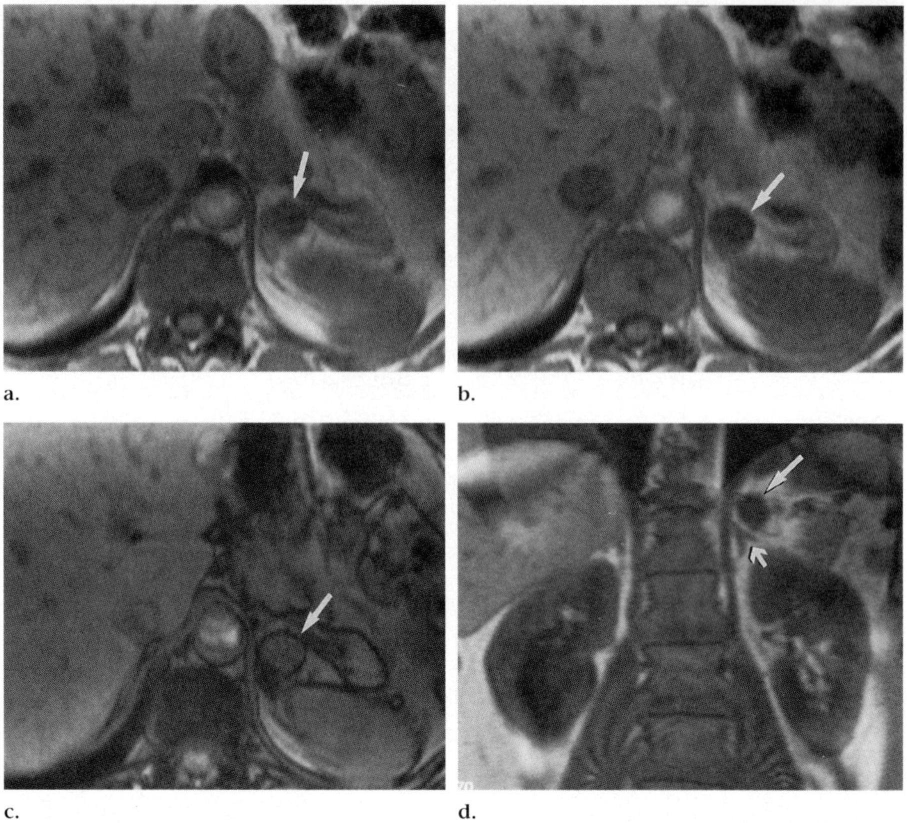

Figure 19. **(a, b)** Transaxial, T1-weighted gradient-echo MR images (250/4.0, 70° flip angle) obtained at adjacent levels and **(c)** the corresponding opposed-phase image (250/7.0, 70° flip angle) demonstrate a nodular left adrenal mass (arrow). **(d)** Coronal, in-phase T1-weighted gradient-echo MR image (156/4.0, 70° flip angle) demonstrates the mass (long arrow) to be separate from the adrenal gland (short arrow); additional images showed this mass to represent the gastric fundus.

Contrast Materials

Gastrointestinal contrast materials, including those that increase or decrease luminal signal intensity, are sometimes necessary to distinguish pancreatic masses from adjacent bowel loops. Among the many contrast materials that have been used to mark the gastrointestinal tract are oral preparations of dilute gadolinium chelate, iron oxides, nutritional support formula, perflubron, kaolin, and water.

Susceptibility Artifacts

Gastrointestinal air creates susceptibility artifacts that are particularly prominent on gradient-echo images. Although these artifacts can interfere with pancreatic evaluation, on occasion, they assist in recognizing bowel loops. Problematic susceptibility artifacts can be reduced when images are acquired by using shorter TEs, smaller voxel sizes, a lower magnetic field strength, and fast spin-echo pulse sequences.

ADRENAL GLANDS

Adjacent Structures

Various structures in the vicinity of the adrenal glands can simulate adrenal masses. Tortuous splenic vessels, gastric diverticula, or the pancreatic tail can simulate left adrenal masses (38) (Fig 19). The duodenum or hepatic flexure of the colon can have similar results on the right side, and the diaphragmatic crura or upper-pole renal masses can simulate masses on either side. These entities usually have signal intensity characteristics that are distinct from those of most adrenal masses.

Lesion Characterization

The major issue in characterizing adrenal lesions is distinguishing benign incidental adenomas from metastases. The relative signal intensity of adrenal masses on T2-weighted images has been used to make this distinction, with adenomas having lower signal intensity than malignancies. However, there is overlap in the T2 behavior of these lesions, as determined qualitatively or quantitatively (39). Characterization of adrenal masses by their rates of enhancement and washout at dynamic gadolinium-enhanced imaging has also been described (40) but is not widely used. Phase-contrast imaging is currently the most reliable method in distinguishing adrenal adenomas from malignancies. Gradient-echo images are obtained by using TEs with which fat and water protons are of a similar and an opposite phase (39,41).

The presence of microscopic lipid in adrenal adenomas causes them to undergo signal intensity loss on images in which fat and water protons are of an opposed phase. Phase-contrast imaging is generally more useful in identifying microscopic lipid in adrenal adenomas than is radio-frequency fat saturation. However, macroscopic fat, as may be present in adrenal myelolipoma, is not suppressed on opposed-phase images, although it is suppressed on radio-frequency fat-saturated images (Fig 20).

Although signal intensity decrease on opposed-phase images is usually specific for adrenal adenoma, some malignancies, including adrenal carcinoma and metastatic renal cell carcinoma, can contain lipid (41,42). Conversely, many benign adrenal lesions, including hemorrhages, cysts, inflammatory processes, and most pheochromocytomas, do not contain lipid. Therefore, attention to lesion size,

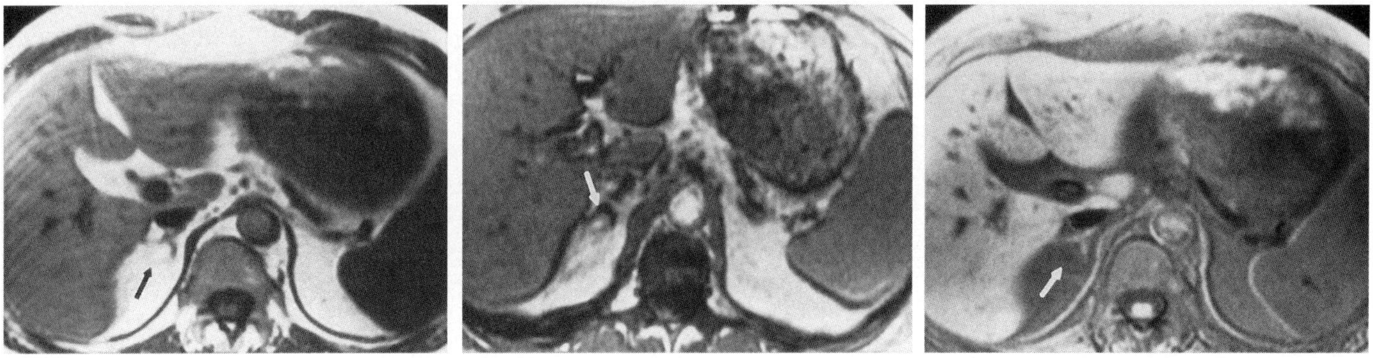

a. b. c.

Figure 20. (**a**) Transaxial T1-weighted MR image (610/11) depicts fat within a right adrenal mass (arrow), which indicates myelolipoma. (**b**) The fatty component fails to be suppressed on the T1-weighted opposed-phase gradient-echo MR image (150/6.3, 90° flip angle), because the component contains largely macroscopic fat. Phase-cancellation artifact (arrow) is observed at the interface between the fatty component and the adrenal crus. (**c**) Suppression of the fatty component is achieved, however, on a radio-frequency fat-saturated T1-weighted MR image (630/11) of the mass (arrow).

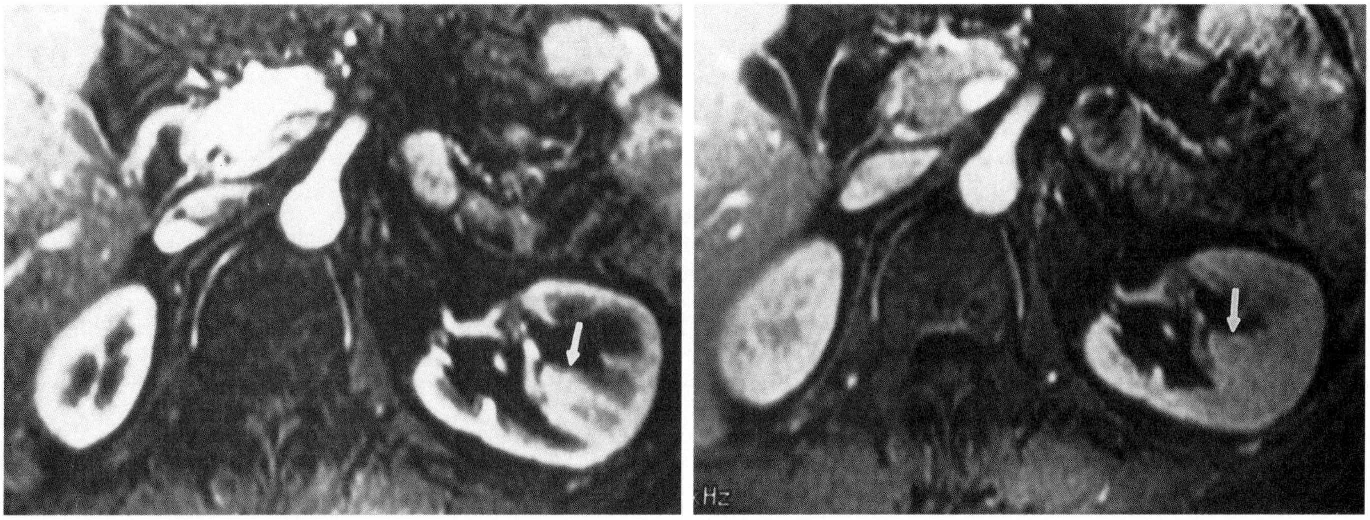

a. b.

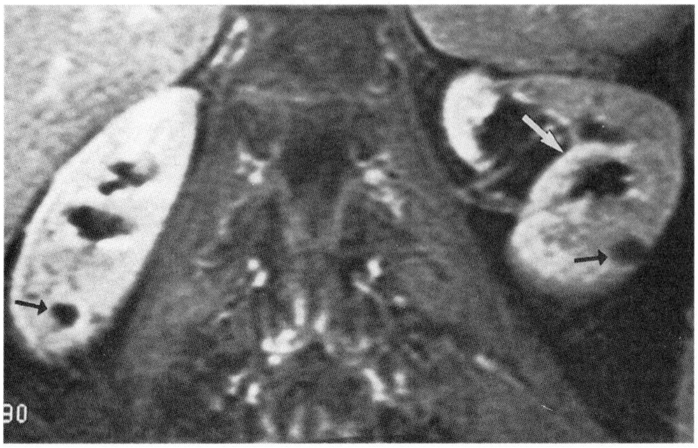

c.

Figure 21. (**a**) Transaxial, T1-weighted fat-suppressed gradient-echo MR image (130/1.6, 90° flip angle) acquired during bolus injection of gadolinium chelate contrast material demonstrates a column of Bertin (white arrow) that enhances concordantly with the renal cortex immediately and remains enhanced after several minutes on images acquired in the (**b**) transaxial and (**c**) coronal planes. Small cysts (black arrows in c) are present in the lower poles of both kidneys.

morphology, homogeneity, and clinical context remains important. Another potential pitfall occurs when small adrenal malignancies undergo partial volume averaging with adjacent fat (39). In this situation, although the lesion itself contains no lipid, signal intensity decrease occurs on opposed-phase images and leads to a false diagnosis of adenoma.

KIDNEYS

Anatomic Variations

The kidneys are subject to numerous anatomic variations that can simulate abnormalities. Among these are rotational abnormalities, crossed fused ectopia, renal lobulation, dromedary hump, splenic impression, column of Bertin (Fig

21), prominent hilar lip, horseshoe kidney, and cake kidney. Acquired renal contour alterations occur in patients who have previously undergone renal surgery or have had scarring from inflammatory disease, with compensatory hypertrophy of the spared renal parenchyma. MR imaging allows these pseudotumors to be distinguished from renal neoplasms when the apparent abnormality maintains the expected signal intensity of renal parenchyma, particularly on fat-suppressed T1-weighted images, and when it undergoes enhancement concordant with renal tissue at dynamic gadolinium-enhanced imaging. Coronal images are often useful in clarifying the nature of these variations.

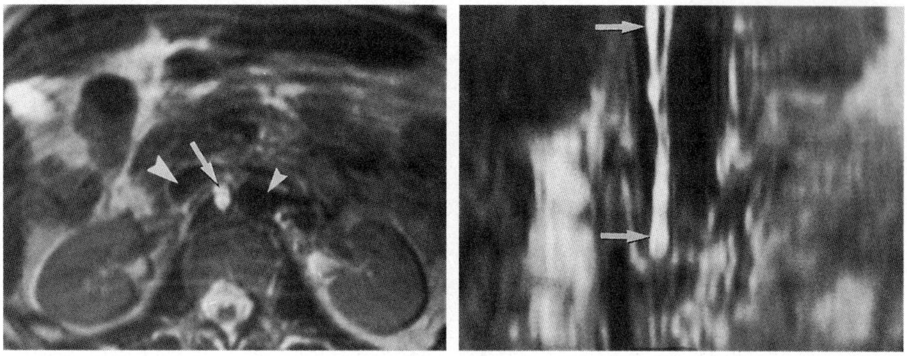

a. b.

Figure 22. **(a)** A rounded focus of increased signal intensity (arrow) that is suspicious for lymphadenopathy is observed between the abdominal aorta (small arrowhead) and the inferior vena cava (large arrowhead) on a transaxial T2-weighted fast spin-echo MR image (4,300/105; echo train length, 16). However, this focus represents slow blood flow in the azygos vein, as confirmed on **(b)** a coronal reformation of transaxial T2-weighted images that demonstrates continuity of that vascular structure (arrows) into the chest.

Chemical Shift Misregistration Artifact

Signal misregistration occurs at the interface between the kidney and adjacent fat, particularly on T2-weighted images (Fig 15). This misregistration can simulate perirenal fluid collections or can obscure small peripheral renal lesions. Chemical shift misregistration is usually observed along the frequency-encoding direction of the image but can occasionally occur along the section-selection direction (43). In the latter situation, displaced signal intensity can simulate lesions of the adrenal or upper renal pole. Misregistration is accentuated on images acquired with high magnetic field strength, reduced receiver bandwidth, and large voxel sizes and on T1-weighted images acquired after gadolinium chelate contrast material administration (44). Although some of these parameters can be altered to reduce misregistration, gradient reorientation, which allows the artifact to be displaced to another portion of the image, is often the simplest approach.

Lesion Characterization

Similar relaxation behavior in renal tissue and in most renal malignancies has led to poor depiction of renal carcinoma on conventional T1- and T2-weighted images (45,46). The use of gadolinium chelate contrast material—particularly in conjunction with fat-suppressed T1-weighted imaging—is helpful in lesion detection as well as in lesion characterization. The use of fat suppression accentuates subtle enhancement and thus allows for improved differentiation between neoplasms and cysts. Contrast enhancement may be particularly subtle in some hypovascular renal cell carcinomas, such as those of the papillary type.

Lack of enhancement is very helpful in characterizing complex cysts that have septa, nodularity, or hemorrhagic or proteinaceous contents. Heavily T2-weighted fast spin-echo sequences are also useful in identifying fluid within cystic lesions. Hemorrhagic or proteinaceous renal cysts often have high signal intensity on T1-weighted images. Distinction from angiomyolipoma can be made by using fat-suppression techniques, including fat saturation and phase-contrast imaging. Misdiagnosis of renal carcinoma as angiomyolipoma can result when carcinomas engulf perirenal fat or, rarely, when they contain visible fat owing to foci of ossification (47,48).

As with other cross-sectional imaging modalities, MR imaging has limited ability to enable differentiation of renal cell carcinoma from benign solid renal tumors, such as adenomas or oncocytomas (49). Although renal neoplasms are usually moderately intense on T2-weighted images, occasionally, carcinomas can appear to have low signal intensity, which raises the suspicion of renal fibroma (50). Partial volume averaging and respiratory motion artifacts can interfere with renal lesion detection and characterization as they do with liver lesions.

The staging of renal cell carcinoma by means of MR imaging includes regional evaluation of lesion extent, vascular involvement, and lymph node involvement. The left renal vein frequently demonstrates relatively increased signal intensity on transaxial T2-weighted images, which can simulate or obscure a tumor thrombus (Fig 15). This occurs because blood flow in the vein is in the plane of image acquisition and because of the rephasing effects of gradient moment nulling. Gradient-echo images, particularly in the sagittal plane, are useful in clarifying this issue. A number of entities can simulate enlarged retroperitoneal lymph nodes; these entities include nodularity of the diaphragmatic crura or psoas muscles, anterior vertebral osteophytes, a retroaortic or circumaortic left renal vein, a left-sided or duplicated inferior vena cava, a tortuous aorta or aortic aneurysm, and collateral retroperitoneal veins (Fig 22). Flow-sensitive pulse sequences and multiplanar imaging are useful in preventing misdiagnoses.

CONCLUSION

Many sources of potential diagnostic error are encountered on abdominal MR images; it is important to be aware of the manifestations and causes of these entities.

References

1. Mirowitz SA, ed. Pitfalls, variants, and artifacts in body MR imaging. St Louis, Mo: Mosby–Year Book, 1996.
2. Te Strake L, Freling NJM, Kamman RL, et al. Abdominal applications of fast MR imaging: a comparison of fast field echo (FFE) and spin echo (SE) pulse sequences. Magn Reson Imaging 1989; 7:297–303.
3. Wood ML, Runge VM, Henkelman RM. Overcoming motion in abdominal MR imaging. AJR 1988; 150:513–522.
4. Powers T, Lum A, Patton JA. Abdominal MRI artifacts. Semin Ultrasound CT MR 1989; 10:2–10.
5. Mitchell DG, Vinitski S, Burk DL Jr, et al. Multiple spin-echo MR imaging of the body image contrast and motion-induced artifact. Magn Reson Imaging 1988; 6:535–546.

6. Hamm B, Wolf KJ, Felix R. Conventional and rapid MR imaging of the liver with Gd-DTPA. Radiology 1987; 164:313–320.
7. Mirowitz SA, Lee JKT, Gutierrez E, et al. Dynamic gadolinium-enhanced rapid acquisition spin-echo MR imaging of the liver. Radiology 1991; 179:371–376.
8. Ito K, Choji T, Fujita T, et al. Early-enhancing pseudolesion in medial segment of left hepatic lobe detected with multisection dynamic MR. Radiology 1993; 187:695–699.
9. Schlund JF, Semelka RC, Kettritz U, Eisenberg LB, Lee JK. Transient increased segmental hepatic enhancement distal to portal vein obstruction on dynamic gadolinium-enhanced gradient echo MR images. JMRI 1995; 5:375–377.
10. Fan ZM, Yamashita Y, Harada M, et al. Intrahepatic cholangiocarcinoma: spin-echo and contrast-enhanced dynamic MR imaging. AJR 1993; 161:313–317.
11. Mahfouz AE, Hamm B, Taupitz M, et al. Hypervascular liver lesions: differentiation of focal nodular hyperplasia from malignant tumors with dynamic gadolinium-enhanced MR imaging. Radiology 1993; 186:133–138.
12. Rofsky NM, Weinreb JC, Bernardino MR, et al. Hepatocellular tumors: characterization with Mn-DPDP–enhanced MR imaging. Radiology 1993; 188:53–59.
13. Henkelman RM, Hardy P, Poon PY, et al. Optimal pulse sequence for imaging hepatic metastases. Radiology 1986; 161: 727–734.
14. Foley WD, Kneeland JB, Cates JD, et al. Contrast optimization for the detection of focal hepatic lesions by MR imaging at 1.5 T. AJR 1987; 149:1155–1160.
15. Paling MR, Abbitt PL, Mugler JP, et al. Liver metastases: optimization of MR imaging pulse sequences at 1.0 T. Radiology 1988; 167:695–699.
16. Steinberg HV, Alarcon JJ, Bernardino MR. Focal hepatic lesions: comparative MR imaging at 0.5 and 1.5 T. Radiology 1990; 174:153–156.
17. Catasca JV, Mirowitz SA. T2-weighted MR imaging of the abdomen: fast spin-echo vs conventional spin-echo sequences. AJR 1994; 162:61–67.
18. Schwartz LH, Seltzer SE, Tempany CMC, et al. Prospective comparison of T2-weighted fast spin-echo pulse sequences in the upper abdomen. Radiology 1993; 189:411–416.
19. Chien D, Mulkern RV. Fast spin-echo studies of contrast and small-lesion definition in a liver-metastasis phantom. JMRI 1992; 2:483–487.
20. Chien D, Atkinson DJ, Edelman RR. Strategies to improve contrast in turboFLASH imaging: reordered phase encoding and k-space segmentation. JMRI 1991; 1: 63–70.
21. Yates CK, Streight RA. Focal fatty infiltration of the liver simulating metastatic disease. Radiology 1986; 159:83–84.
22. Low RN, Francis IR, Herfkens RJ, et al. Fast multiplanar spoiled gradient-recalled imaging of the liver: pulse sequence optimization and comparison with spin-echo MR imaging. AJR 1993; 160:501–509.
23. Apicella P, Mirowitz SA, Weinreb JC. Extension of vascular structures through hepatic masses on MR and CT images. Radiology 1994; 191:135–136.
24. Mitchell DG. Focal manifestations of diffuse liver disease at MR imaging. Radiology 1992; 185:1–11.
25. Kucharczyk W, Crawley AP, Kelly WM, et al. Effect of multislice interference on image contrast in T2- and T1-weighted MR images. AJNR 1988; 9:443–451.
26. Schwaighofer BW, Yu KK, Mattrey RF. Diagnostic significance of interslice gap and imaging volume in body MR imaging. AJR 1989; 153:629–632.
27. Mirowitz SA, Heiken JP, Lee JKT. Potential MR pitfall in relying on lesion/liver intensity ratio in presence of hepatic hemochromatosis. J Comput Assist Tomogr 1988; 12:323–324.
28. Wittenberg J, Stark DD, Forman BH, et al. Differentiation of hepatic metastases from hepatic hemangiomas and cysts by using MR imaging. AJR 1988; 151:79–84.
29. Ros PR, Lubbers PR, Olmsted WW, et al. Hemangioma of the liver: heterogeneous appearance on T2-weighted images. AJR 1987; 149:1167–1170.
30. Rummeny E, Weissleder R, Sironi S, et al. Central scars in primary liver tumors: MR features, specificity, and pathologic correlation. Radiology 1989; 171:323–326.
31. Hahn PF, Weissleder R, Stark DD, Saini S, Elizondo G, Ferrucci JT. MR imaging of focal splenic tumors. AJR 1988; 150:823–827.
32. Mirowitz SA, Brown JJ, Lee JKT, et al. Dynamic gadolinium-enhanced MR imaging of the spleen: normal enhancement patterns and evaluation of splenic lesions. Radiology 1991; 179:681–686.
33. Semelka RC, Shoenut JP, Lawrence PH, et al. Spleen: dynamic enhancement patterns on gradient-echo MR images enhanced with gadopentetate dimeglumine. Radiology 1992; 185:479–482.
34. Weissleder R, Elizondo G, Stark DD, et al. The diagnosis of splenic lymphoma by MR imaging: value of superparamagnetic iron oxide. AJR 1989; 152:175–180.
35. Mitchell DG, Shapiro M, Schuricht A, et al. Pancreatic disease: findings on state-of-the-art MR images. AJR 1992; 159:533–538.
36. Semelka RC, Ascher SM. MR imaging of the pancreas. Radiology 1993; 188:593–602.
37. Mitchell DG, Vinitski S, Saponaro S, et al. Liver and pancreas: improved spin-echo T1 contrast by shorter echo time and fat suppression at 1.5 T. Radiology 1991; 178: 67–71.
38. Dunnick NR. Adrenal imaging: current status. AJR 1990; 154:927–936.
39. Mitchell DG, Crovello M, Matteucci T, et al. Benign adrenocortical masses: diagnosis with chemical-shift MR imaging. Radiology 1992; 185:345–351.
40. Krestin GP, Friedmann G, Fishbach R, Neufang KF, Allolio B. Evaluation of adrenal masses in oncologic patients: dynamic contrast-enhanced MR vs CT. J Comput Assist Tomogr 1991; 15:104–110.
41. Tsushima Y, Ishizaka H, Matsumoto M. Adrenal masses: differentiation with chemical shift, fast low-angle short MR imaging. Radiology 1993; 186:705–709.
42. Reinig JW. MR imaging differentiation of adrenal masses: has the time finally come? (editorial). Radiology 1992; 185:339–340.
43. Wachsberg RH, Mitchell DG, Rifkin MD, et al. Chemical shift artifact along the section-select axis. JMRI 1992; 2:589–591.
44. Apicella PL, Mirowitz SA, Borrello J. Chemical shift misregistration artifacts: increased conspicuity following intravenous administration of gadopentetate dimeglumine. Magn Reson Imaging 1994; 12:675–678.
45. Quint LE, Glazer GM, Chenevert TL, et al. In vivo and in vitro MR imaging of renal tumors: histopathologic correlation and pulse sequence optimization. Radiology 1988; 169:359–362.
46. Hricak H, Thoeni RF, Carroll PR, et al. Detection and staging of renal neoplasms: a reassessment of MR imaging. Radiology 1988; 166:643–649.
47. Helenon O, Chretien Y, Paraf F, et al. Renal cell carcinoma containing fat: demonstration with CT. Radiology 1993; 188: 429–430.
48. Davidson AJ, Davis CJ Jr. Fat in renal adenocarcinoma: never say never (editorial). Radiology 1993; 188:316.
49. Palmer WE, Chew FS. Renal oncocytoma (clinical conference). AJR 1991; 156:1144.
50. Sussman SK, Glickstein MF, Krzymowski GA. Hypointense renal cell carcinoma: MR imaging with pathologic correlation. Radiology 1990; 177:495–497.

Book Review

Imaging of Anorectal Disease

Shahid M. Hussain, MD

Oxford, England: Oxford Medical Publications, 1998. ISBN 1-900151-36-7.
Hardcover, £69.50; pp 164; 95 figures.

Imaging of Anorectal Disease is intended to help radiologists and surgeons understand and perform the new techniques available in the imaging of the anus and rectum. The author is well known as a leader in this area and has put together a short but fairly comprehensive book.

The book contains an initial discussion of normal anatomy and normal imaging findings with a separate chapter on ultrasonography (US) and magnetic resonance (MR) imaging. The remainder of the book covers specific diseases and topics including anal fistulas, perianal Crohn disease, fecal incontinence, functional abnormalities, and anorectal tumors.

The organization of the text is sound, and the author has made liberal use of illustrations, many of which have accompanying anatomic correlation. Particularly helpful is the use of side-by-side comparisons of MR and US images. A guide at the beginning of the book helps readers grasp the numerous color schematics, which are visually striking but difficult to use. The overall quality of all the illustrations is excellent.

Some radiologists may find the discussion of the physics of the imaging techniques superfluous, while surgeons, the other intended audience, may find it too complicated for practical use. The specific descriptions of normal anatomy are difficult to follow, but this may simply reflect the anatomic complexity of this region of the body. The brief but thorough description of the history of various investigators' studies of this region is a distinctive contribution. The section dealing with specific diseases and clinical problems provides excellent illustrations and many points of practical value.

Most interpreters of images of the anorectal area will find *Imaging of Anorectal Disease* an exceptional, solid reference textbook. The cost may deter some, particularly residents, from purchasing it.

Reviewed by James M. Messmer, MD

Shinichi Hasegawa, MD
Richard C. Semelka, MD
Tara C. Noone, MD
John T. Woosley, MD
Hani B. Marcos, MD
Phillip J. Kenney, MD
Evan S. Siegelman, MD

Index terms:
Sarcoma, 72.322
Stomach, MR, 72.121412, 72.12143
Stomach, neoplasm, 72.322

Radiology 1998; 208:591–595

Abbreviations:
GRE = gradient-recalled echo
RARE = rapid acquisition with relaxation enhancement

[1] From the Department of Radiology, Hamamatsu Medical Center, Japan (S.H.); the Departments of Radiology (R.C.S., T.C.N., H.B.M.) and Pathology (J.T.W.), University of North Carolina Hospitals, CB 7510, Old Clinic Bldg, Chapel Hill, NC 27599-7510; the Department of Radiology, University of Alabama–Birmingham (P.J.K.); and the Department of Radiology, University of Pennsylvania, Philadelphia (E.S.S.). Received December 22, 1997; revision requested March 19, 1998; revision received April 6; accepted April 13. **Address reprint requests to** R.C.S.

Author contributions:
Guarantors of integrity of entire study, S.H., T.C.N., R.C.S.; study concepts and design, S.H.; definition of intellectual content, S.H., R.C.S.; literature research, S.H.; clinical studies, R.C.S., P.J.K., E.S.S.; data acquisition, all authors; data analysis, S.H., T.C.N., J.T.W.; manuscript preparation, S.H., T.C.N., R.C.S.; manuscript editing, T.C.N., R.C.S.; manuscript review, J.T.W.

Gastric Stromal Sarcomas: Correlation of MR Imaging and Histopathologic Findings in Nine Patients[1]

PURPOSE: To define the appearance of gastric stromal sarcomas at magnetic resonance (MR) imaging.

MATERIALS AND METHODS: Nine patients with gastric stromal sarcoma underwent MR imaging with the following sequences: nonenhanced and gadolinium-enhanced breath-hold, T1-weighted, spoiled gradient-recalled echo (n = 9); fat-suppressed, T2-weighted, fast spin echo (n = 9); and breathing-independent, half-Fourier rapid acquisition with relaxation enhancement (n = 6). Lesion morphology, signal intensity features, and relationships to the gastric wall and surrounding organs were retrospectively evaluated. The diagnosis of gastric stromal sarcoma was histologically proved in all patients.

RESULTS: The nine tumors were solitary, multilobulated, shaped irregularly, predominantly exophytic, and large (diameter range, 7–28 cm [mean, 15.8 cm]). The epicenters of all lesions were extrinsic to the stomach, and all lesions arose from the gastric cardia or body. Regions of necrosis and hemorrhage were detected in all cases. Marginal definition on MR images corresponded to histologic grade: High-grade neoplasms possessed ill-defined margins, and low-grade neoplasms demonstrated more well-defined margins. Relationships to surrounding organs depicted at MR imaging corresponded well with histopathologic findings.

CONCLUSION: Gastric stromal sarcomas demonstrate characteristic MR imaging features, which correspond well with histopathologic findings. The direct multiplanar capability of MR imaging facilitates delineation of relationships of the tumors to the stomach and surrounding organs.

Gastrointestinal stromal tumors are relatively rare neoplasms that originate in the submucosal layer of hollow viscera in the gastrointestinal tract; they compose 1%–3% of malignant gastric tumors (1). A minority of these neoplasms fulfill modern pathologic criteria for subclassification into leiomyomas or leiomyosarcomas, leiomyoblastomas (epithelioid leiomyomas or leiomyosarcomas), schwannomas, glomus tumors, and neurofibromas or ganglioneuromas. As defined with current standards, the majority of stromal tumors of the gastrointestinal tract demonstrate either incomplete or no features of differentiation. As a result, the generic designation of "gastrointestinal stromal tumors," or "gastrointestinal stromal sarcomas," has been widely adopted (2,3).

In this study, we explored the appearance of gastric stromal sarcomas at magnetic resonance (MR) imaging. The computed tomographic (CT) and ultrasonographic (US) features of gastric leiomyosarcomas have been reported previously (1,4–8). To our knowledge, however, few articles included a description of the appearance of gastric leiomyosarcomas on MR images (9).

MR imaging with current techniques, including breath-hold sequences performed with and without gadolinium enhancement, has been shown to be useful in the characterization of pathologic conditions within the bowel (10,11). The purpose of this study was to describe the appearance of gastric stromal sarcoma at MR imaging with current techniques,

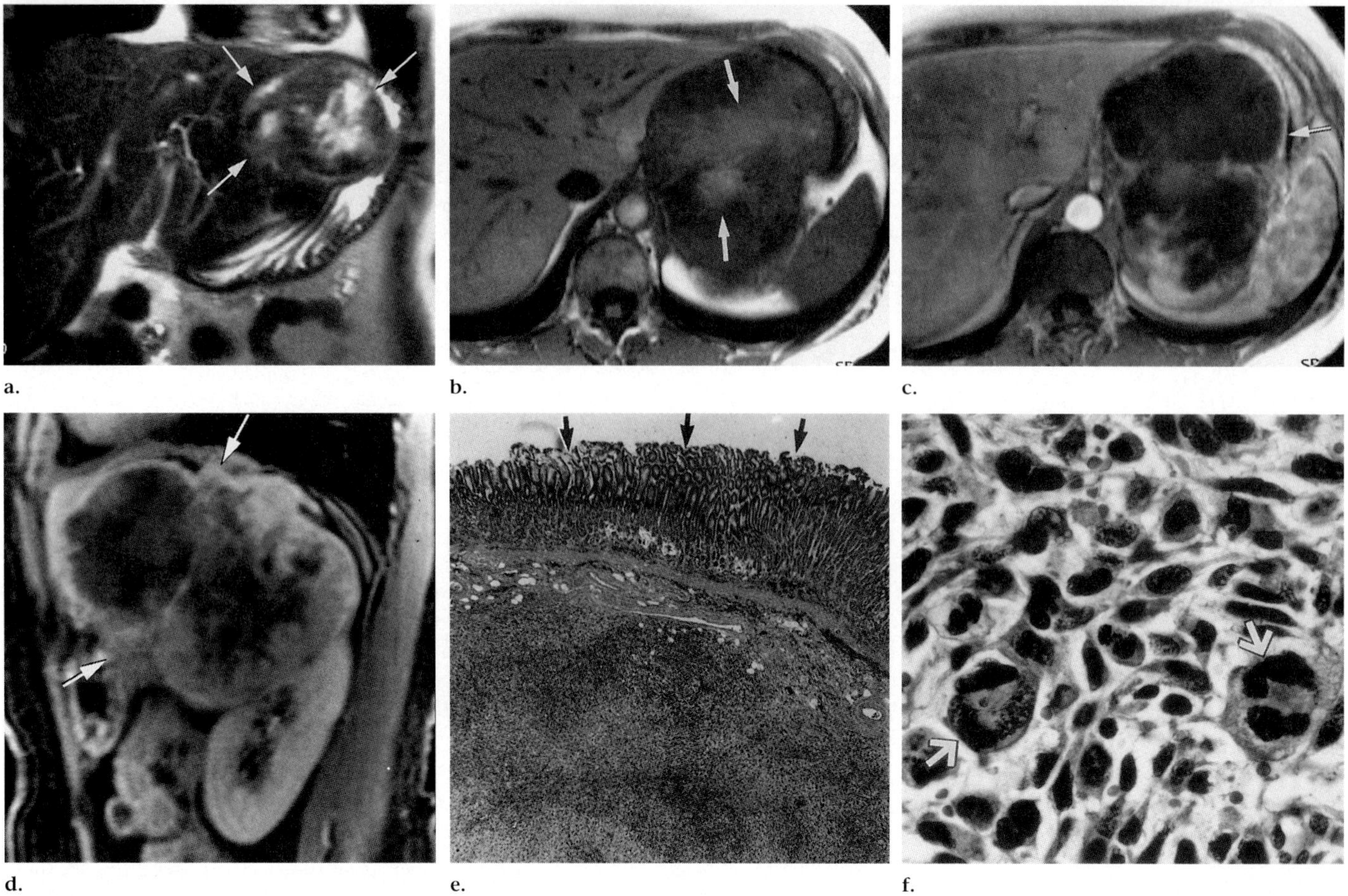

Figure 1. High-grade gastric stromal sarcoma in a 55-year-old woman. (a) Coronal half-Fourier RARE T2-weighted image; (b) transverse, nonenhanced spoiled GRE T1-weighted image; (c) transverse, gadolinium-enhanced spoiled GRE image obtained immediately after injection of contrast material; (d) sagittal, gadolinium-enhanced, fat-suppressed, spoiled GRE image obtained at 90 seconds after administration of contrast material; and (e, f) photomicrographs of histologic specimens (e, hematoxylin-eosin stain, original magnification, ×10; f, hematoxylin-eosin stain, original magnification, ×60). In **a**, a dumbbell-shaped tumor (arrows) arises from the gastric fundus and body. In **b**, the lesion is depicted with heterogeneous signal intensity secondary to focal areas of hemorrhage and necrosis (arrows). In **c**, high signal intensity of normal, overlying gastric mucosa (arrow) corresponds directly with histopathologic findings (arrows in **e**). In **d**, the solid portion of the tumor exhibits ill-defined margins (arrows) that correspond to high-grade cellular features seen at histopathologic examination (arrows in **f**). Persistent low-signal-intensity foci in **d** indicate tumor necrosis.

including dynamic imaging with gadolinium enhancement. MR imaging findings were correlated with histologic findings in all cases.

MATERIALS AND METHODS

Patients were included in this study on the basis of retrospective review of the pathologic records in the authors' institutions. All patients with histologically proved gastric stromal sarcoma who underwent MR imaging with current techniques, including dynamic gadolinium-enhanced examination, were included. Between March 1993 and December 1997, nine patients (five women and four men; age range, 28–71 years; mean age, 53 years) with gastric stromal sarcoma underwent MR imaging examination. In all patients, the diagnosis of gastric stromal sarcoma was proved histologically after resection of the mass.

MR imaging was performed with 1.5-T MR imaging systems (Vision, Siemens Medical Systems, Iselin, NJ [six patients]; SP4000, Siemens Medical Systems [one patient]; Signa, GE Medical Systems, Milwaukee, Wis [two patients]). Images were acquired with the following sequences: transverse, fat-suppressed, fast spin echo (repetition time msec/echo time msec = 5,000–5,600/20, 85–90; echo train length, five to eight) (all patients); breathing-independent, half-Fourier rapid acquisition with relaxation enhancement (RARE) (HASTE; Siemens Medical Systems) (∞/90 [effective]; echo train length, 150) (five patients); T1-weighted, breath-hold, spoiled gradient-recalled echo (GRE) (114–140/4.1; flip angle, 70°–80°; 20 sections in a 20- to 36-second breath hold) (seven patients); and T1-weighted spin echo (500–700/10–15) (two patients). T1-weighted spoiled GRE imaging was performed immediately after administration of a bolus of gadopentetate dimeglumine (Magnevist; Berlex Laboratories, Wayne, NJ) in a dose of 0.1 mmol per kilogram of body weight (nine patients) and later at 45 and 90 seconds and 5 minutes after administration (seven patients). Fat suppression was applied in the 90-second gadolinium-enhanced spoiled GRE sequence.

MR images were retrospectively reviewed by two investigators (S.H., T.C.N). Gastric stromal sarcomas were evaluated for size, location, morphology (including

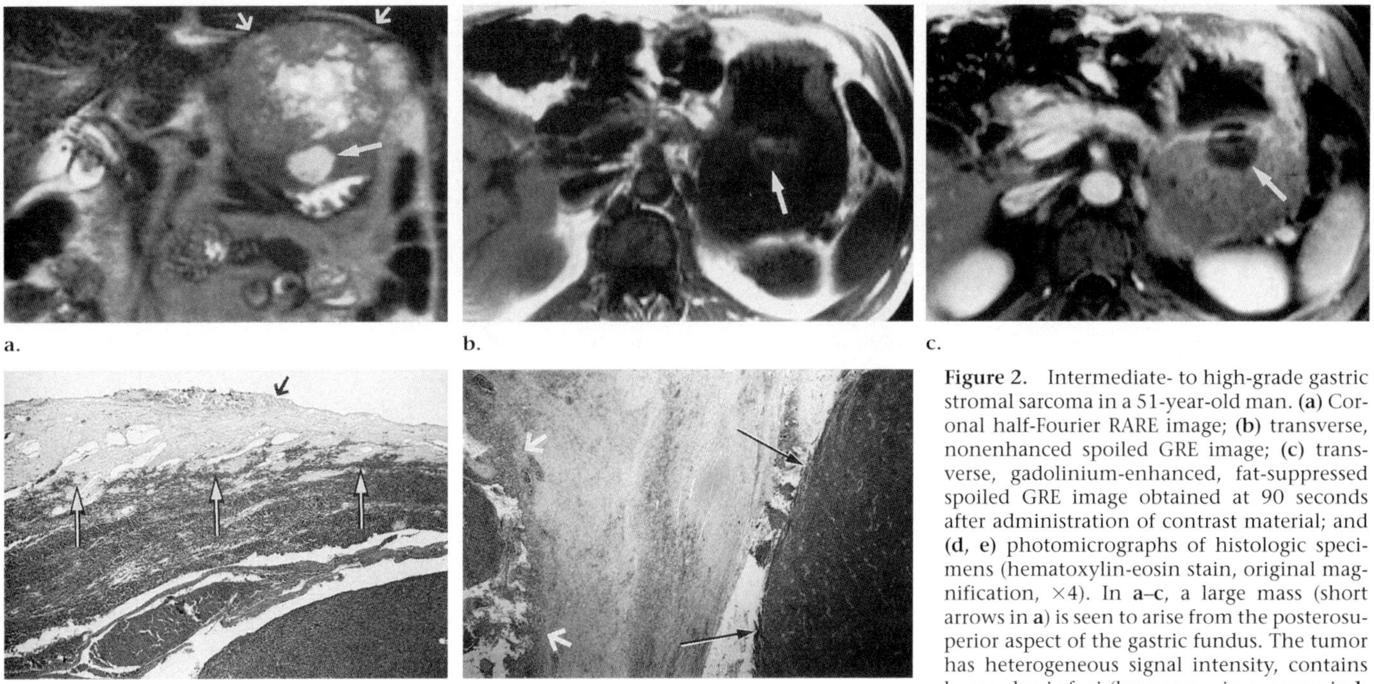

Figure 2. Intermediate- to high-grade gastric stromal sarcoma in a 51-year-old man. **(a)** Coronal half-Fourier RARE image; **(b)** transverse, nonenhanced spoiled GRE image; **(c)** transverse, gadolinium-enhanced, fat-suppressed spoiled GRE image obtained at 90 seconds after administration of contrast material; and **(d, e)** photomicrographs of histologic specimens (hematoxylin-eosin stain, original magnification, ×4). In **a–c**, a large mass (short arrows in **a**) is seen to arise from the posterosuperior aspect of the gastric fundus. The tumor has heterogeneous signal intensity, contains hemorrhagic foci (long arrow in **a**, arrow in **b** and **c**), and demonstrates moderate signal intensity. The mass has a long interface with the left hemidiaphragm and surrounding organs, but there is no evidence of deep invasion. These findings were confirmed at histologic evaluation. In **d**, the proximity of the tumor (white arrows) to the left hemidiaphragm is apparent, but there is no invasion of the muscular layer (black arrow). In **e**, the tumor (white arrows) is contiguous with the spleen (black arrows), but there is no direct invasion.

margination and internal architecture), signal intensity patterns on nonenhanced and gadolinium-enhanced MR images, intratumoral hemorrhagic necrosis or cystic components, enhancement of overlying mucosa, direct invasion of surrounding organs, peritoneal dissemination, liver metastases, and lymphadenopathy.

RESULTS

Three gastric stromal sarcomas were histologically diagnosed as high grade (Fig 1), one as intermediate to high grade (Fig 2), and four as low grade (Fig 3). Another gastric stromal sarcoma demonstrated biphasic histologic findings with low-grade features superficially and high-grade features deep within the tumor. All nine lesions arose from the gastric cardia or body (five masses from the posterior wall and four from the anterior wall).

All tumors were solitary, multilobulated, shaped irregularly, predominantly exophytic, and large (diameter range, 7–28 cm; mean, 15.8 cm). The four low-grade sarcomas and the histologically biphasic sarcoma were well defined and demonstrated no direct invasion of surrounding organs (Fig 3). The solid portions of the intermediate- to high-grade sarcoma and two of the high-grade sarcomas were ill defined and had contiguous borders with surrounding organs, including the spleen, pancreas, lateral segment of the left hepatic lobe, left adrenal gland, and left kidney. There was, however, no distinct evidence of deep invasion into these organs (Fig 2). The solid portions of the third high-grade sarcoma were ill defined and directly invaded the pancreatic tail, spleen, and left hemidiaphragm. All findings of surrounding organ invasion were histopathologically confirmed.

Review of the original MR image interpretations revealed that the gastric origins of the gastric stromal sarcomas were reported with confidence in five cases and were not established with confidence in three. The uncertainty of gastric origin reflected the large exophytic nature of the tumors, their relatively small gastric pedicles (Fig 3), and lack of mucosal invasion.

All gastric stromal sarcomas demonstrated markedly heterogeneous internal signal intensity on T1- and T2-weighted images. This finding corresponded to the histopathologic findings that all lesions contained intratumoral hemorrhage or liquefactive necrosis, which accounted for 40%–90% of tumor bulk. In our study, however, there was no direct correlation between the percentage of hemorrhagic or necrotic components and tumor grade. Signal intensity of these portions varied from low to high on both T1- and T2-weighted images, depending on the age of the hemorrhage. Foci of high signal intensity on T1- and T2-weighted images helped confirm the presence of subacute hemorrhage in six tumors (Figs 1, 2). Owing to their lack of contrast enhancement, necrotic areas were most easily discerned on gadolinium-enhanced images (Figs 1, 3).

On the immediate gadolinium-enhanced, spoiled GRE images, five tumors demonstrated intense enhancement, which corresponded to the hypervascular nature of gastric stromal sarcomas. One low-grade tumor demonstrated moderate signal intensity on the immediate postcontrast images. Solid components of the tumors demonstrated persistent enhancement from the capillary phase to the interstitial phase.

One tumor was associated with a small mucosal ulceration; histopathologic examination did not reveal whether it was intrinsic to the tumor or was the result of prior biopsy. Gastric wall thickening adjacent to the tumor was not present on either MR images or histopathologic specimens. Hyperintensity of the overlying gastric mucosa was depicted on interstitial phase (at 90 seconds) gadolinium-

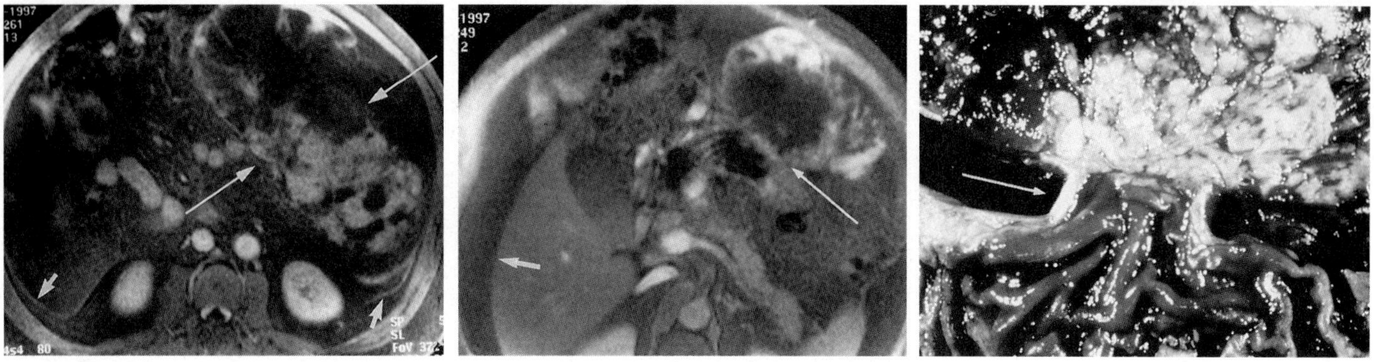

a. b. c.

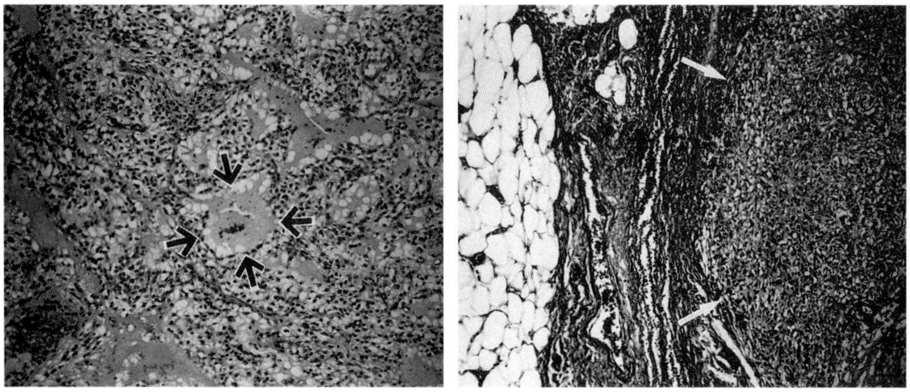

d. e.

Figure 3. Low-grade gastric stromal sarcoma in a 71-year-old man. **(a, b)** Transverse, gadolinium-enhanced, fat-suppressed spoiled GRE images obtained at 90 seconds after administration of contrast material; **(c)** photograph of gross pathologic specimen; and **(d, e)** photomicrographs of histologic specimens (hematoxylin-eosin stain, original magnification, ×20). In **a** and **b**, heterogeneous enhancement is depicted in a large, well-defined mass (long arrows in **a**) with a narrow attachment to the gastric wall (long arrow in **b**) that corresponds to gross pathologic findings (arrow in **c**). Increased peritoneal signal intensity (short arrows in **a**) and a large volume of ascites (short arrow in **b**) are also depicted. In **d**, the solid portions of the tumor contain large and small cystic components (arrows) that correspond to protein- or blood-filled spaces. In **e**, a tiny distant metastatic nodule (arrows) was found in the mesenteric fat, although this tumor was cytologically a low-grade gastric stromal sarcoma.

enhanced MR images obtained in two patients (Fig 1).

The gadolinium-enhanced, fat-suppressed images obtained at 90 seconds revealed thin, linear peritoneal high signal intensity associated with ascites in one patient (Fig 3). At surgery, the tumor extended into the omentum; however, surgical biopsy specimens did not reveal peritoneal metastases. Calcifications were detected in only one lesion in histopathologic specimens, but they were not detected on MR images.

Hepatic metastases were demonstrated in one patient, who had a low-grade sarcoma. The signal intensity characteristics of the metastatic lesions, which demonstrated moderate signal intensity after administration of contrast material, were similar to those of the primary gastric stromal sarcoma. In two cases, small lymph nodes were detected both on MR images and at surgery, but histopathologic findings of all sampled nodes were consistent with reactive hyperplasia.

DISCUSSION

Patients with gastric stromal sarcomas may have a wide age distribution, but they are predominantly middle aged or elderly (2,12). Men are affected more often than women (12). These tumors usually grow exophytically from the stomach and, thus, often remain clinically silent until remarkable size is achieved.

Tumor grade is determined on the basis of the degree of increased cellularity, high nuclear-to-cytoplasmic ratios, and mitotic activity (2). Areas of hemorrhage and necrosis are commonly observed in high-grade tumors (2). The finding of heterogeneous enhancement of the tumors in our study agrees with findings in previous studies involving CT (1,4,8). MR imaging findings can help confirm the presence of blood products at various stages owing to differences in the signal intensity of blood products of different ages (13,14).

In our study, solid components of the high-grade gastric stromal sarcomas possessed ill-defined borders, whereas those of the low-grade gastric stromal sarcomas were well defined. These ill-defined borders correlated directly with serosal invasion in histopathologic specimens. The external margins of large intratumoral hemorrhagic or liquefactive necrotic regions in the high-grade gastric stromal sarcomas were smooth and corresponded histologically to the lining of internal cystic areas, most likely formed as a result of adjacent reactive inflammation.

The results of our study suggest that careful scrutiny of solid tumor components is necessary to detect the locally aggressive features of high-grade gastric stromal sarcoma. Although we observed a correlation between margination of solid tumor components and histologic grade in our study, results of grading did not appear to correlate directly with distant spread of disease. In our study, only one tumor, which was a low-grade gastric stromal sarcoma, was associated with multiple hepatic metastases and another was associated with a small, distant mesenteric metastasis (Fig 3).

Gastric stromal sarcomas that arise from the posterior gastric wall may be misdiagnosed as retroperitoneal tumors. In these cases, the direct multiplanar capability of MR imaging can help delineate the relationship of gastric stromal sarcomas to the gastric wall. In difficult cases, selective angiography may be required to trace the origin of the lesion by determining the predominant blood supply (1).

Several features may help differentiate between gastric stromal sarcomas and exophytic adenocarcinomas. Exophytic growth is rarely demonstrated by gastric adenocarcinomas, but occasionally these tumors may be confused with gastric stromal sarcomas. Lee et al (15) reported that thickening of the gastric wall adjacent to the mass appeared to be a finding specific to exophytic adenocarcinomas. In our study, no gastric stromal sarcomas were associated with thickening of the adjacent gastric wall. In addition, gastric stromal sarcomas commonly arise from the proximal portion of the stomach, whereas gastric adenocarcinomas tend to arise from the distal portion. Although large gastric adenocarcinomas are often accompanied by perigastric lymphadenopathy, gastric stromal sarcomas usually are not. In our study, two tumors were associated with enhancing overlying mucosa on gadolinium-enhanced, breath-hold, T1-weighted spoiled GRE images (Fig 1). If this finding is present, exophytic adenocarcinoma may be excluded.

Relatively recent innovations in MR imaging employed in this study include breathing-independent half-Fourier RARE, breath-hold spoiled GRE, and fat suppression. These techniques reduce artifacts caused by breathing and peristalsis. Thus, image quality and, therefore, evaluation of gastrointestinal disease processes are improved (16). Direct multiplanar capabilities and the high soft-tissue contrast resolution of MR imaging help determine relationships between the mass and gastric wall or surrounding organs and help detect intratumoral hemorrhage or necrosis, or both. Although calcifications are better detected with CT, these lesions rarely contain calcifications (1,4,8), and only one tumor in histopathologic specimens in our series contained calcifications.

The use of oral contrast agents may facilitate delineation of the wall of the stomach in relation to the tumor (17–19). Use of these agents in combination with a high-quality surface coil and breathing-independent or breath-hold sequences could provide even greater anatomic detail.

Findings in our study are limited by the relatively small number of patients, which reflects the rarity of this tumor. This limitation was addressed by including multi-institutional data. In this study, we also did not evaluate the ability of MR imaging to help prospective diagnosis or staging of gastric stromal sarcoma; this limitation also reflects tumor rarity. In fact, one unusual feature of these tumors is that, owing to their exophytic nature, their organ of origin may be difficult to determine prospectively. Thus, the classic rule regarding determination of the organ of origin from the location of the epicenter of a tumor does not apply in these cases. Prospective interpretations in three of the nine cases in this study failed to clearly define the gastric origins of the tumors. Therefore, the findings of large cystic or solid masses with internal hemorrhage that have even a small region of contact with the stomach should prompt consideration of gastric stromal sarcomas.

In conclusion, findings in this study demonstrate the MR imaging findings in nine patients with proved gastric stromal sarcomas. These tumors are large and hypervascular and contain extensive necrotic components. Gastric stromal sarcomas are exophytic and may have a small gastric mural attachment. Multiplanar MR imaging with breath-hold (eg, spoiled GRE) and breathing-independent (eg, half-Fourier RARE) techniques is helpful in evaluating the gastric origin and varied appearances of gastric stromal sarcomas.

References

1. Megibow AJ, Balthazar EJ, Hulnick DH, et al. CT evaluation of gastrointestinal leiomyomas and leiomyosarcomas. AJR 1985; 144:727–731.
2. Suster S. Gastrointestinal stromal tumors. Semin Diagn Pathol 1996; 13:297–313.
3. Mazure MT, Clark HB. Gastric stromal tumors: reappraisal of histogenesis. Am J Surg Pathol 1983; 7:507–519.
4. McLeod AJ, Zornoza J, Shirkhoda A. Leiomyosarcoma: computed tomographic findings. Radiology 1984; 152:133–136.
5. Balfe D, Koehler R, Karstaedt N, et al. Computed tomography of gastric neoplasms. Radiology 1981; 140:431–436.
6. Nauert TC, Zornoza J, Ordonez N. Gastric leiomyosarcomas. AJR 1982; 139:291–297.
7. Lerner M, Farman J, Cho K, et al. Leiomyoblastoma: varied CT appearance. Clin Imaging 1992; 16:194–197.
8. Scatarige JC, Fishman EK, Jones B, et al. Gastric leiomyosarcoma: CT observations. J Comput Assist Tomogr 1985; 9:320–327.
9. Marcy PY, Francois E, Bruneton JN, et al. Gastric leiomyosarcoma: ultrasonographic endoscopy and MRI. J Radiol 1993; 74:583–588.
10. Semelka RC, John G, Kelekis NL, et al. Small bowel neoplastic disease: demonstration by MRI. JMRI 1996; 6:855–860.
11. Semelka RC, Shoenut JP, Silverman R, et al. Bowel disease: prospective comparison of CT and 1.5-T pre- and postcontrast MR imaging with T1-weighted fat-suppressed and breath-hold FLASH sequences. JMRI 1991; 1:625–632.
12. Appelman H, Helwig E. Gastric epithelioid leiomyoma and leiomyosarcoma (leiomyoblastoma). Cancer 1976; 38:708–728.
13. Hahn PF, Saini S, Stark DD, et al. Intraabdominal hematoma: the concentric-ring sign in MR imaging. AJR 1987; 148:115–119.
14. Rubin JI, Gomori JM, Grossman RI, et al. High-field MR imaging of extracranial hematomas. AJR 1987; 148:813–817.
15. Lee DH, Choi BI, Lee MG, et al. Exophytic adenocarcinoma of the stomach: CT findings. AJR 1994; 163:77–80.
16. Semelka RC, John G, Kelekis NL, Burdeny DA, Ascher SM. Small bowel neoplastic disease: demonstration by MRI. JMRI 1996; 6:855–860.
17. Hirohashi S, Hirohashi R, Uchida H, et al. MR imaging oral contrast agent mixed with milk for the small intestine. Nippon Igaku Hoshasen Gakkai Zasshi 1994; 54:784–788.
18. Burton SS, Liebig T, Frazier SD, Ros PR. High-density oral barium sulfate in abdominal MRI: efficacy and tolerance in a clinical setting. Magn Reson Imaging 1997; 15:147–153.
19. Pels Rijcken TH, Davis MA, Ros RR. Intraluminal contrast agents for MR imaging of the abdomen and pelvis. JMRI 1994; 4:291–300.

Tae Kyoung Kim, MD
Byung Ihn Choi, MD
Joon Koo Han, MD
Jin Wook Chung, MD
Jae Hyung Park, MD
Man Chung Han, MD

Index terms:
Liver, angiography, 761.1242, 952.1242
Liver, cirrhosis, 761.794, 958.79
Liver neoplasms, CT, 761.12113, 761.12114, 761.12115
Shunts, arterioportal, 761.49

Radiology 1998; 208:597–603

Abbreviations:
HAP = hepatic arterial phase
PVP = portal venous phase
TACE = transcatheter arterial chemoembolization

[1] From the Department of Radiology and the Institute of Radiation Medicine, Seoul National University College of Medicine, 28 Yongon-dong, Chongno-gu, Seoul 110-744, South Korea. From the 1997 RSNA scientific assembly. Received December 1, 1997; revision requested February 23, 1998; revision received March 24; accepted April 28. **Address reprint requests to** B.I.C.

Author contributions:
Guarantors of integrity of entire study, B.I.C., M.C.H.; study concepts, T.K.K., J.H.P., J.W.C.; study design, T.K.K., J.H.P.; definition of intellectual content, B.I.C., J.K.H.; literature research, T.K.K.; clinical studies, T.K.K., J.H.P., J.W.C.; data acquisition, T.K.K., J.K.H.; data analysis, T.K.K., B.I.C., J.K.H., J.H.P.; manuscript preparation, T.K.K.; manuscript editing, B.I.C., J.K.H., J.W.C.; manuscript review, J.H.P., M.C.H.

Nontumorous Arterioportal Shunt Mimicking Hypervascular Tumor in Cirrhotic Liver: Two-Phase Spiral CT Findings[1]

PURPOSE: To determine the two-phase (hepatic arterial phase [HAP] and portal venous phase [PVP]) spiral computed tomographic (CT) findings of a nontumorous arterioportal shunt in the cirrhotic liver that can mimic a hypervascular tumor.

MATERIALS AND METHODS: For 14 months, 803 patients with known or suspected hepatocellular carcinoma were referred for initial or repeated transcatheter arterial chemoembolization (TACE). Twenty-nine hyperattenuating lesions on HAP CT images obtained in 25 patients (23 men, two women; age range, 39–70 years) were regarded as nontumorous arterioportal shunts and were included in this study. The diagnosis of nontumorous arterioportal shunt was established by four radiologists who reviewed the two-phase spiral CT images and hepatic angiograms.

RESULTS: The longest dimension of the lesion was 1.0–7.9 cm (mean dimension, 2.9 cm). The morphology at HAP CT was wedge-shaped in 25 (86%), geographic (ie, focal area with irregular outline) in two (7%), and nodular in two (7%) lesions. All lesions were homogeneous in attenuation. Hyperattenuating linear branching structures that represented early opacification of portal veins were demonstrated during the HAP in nine (31%) lesions. PVP CT images showed these lesions as isoattenuating (n = 20 [69%]) or slightly hyperattenuating (n = 9 [31%]). Iodized oil CT images showed faint or no accumulation of iodized oil in all lesions.

CONCLUSION: In cirrhotic liver, nontumorous arterioportal shunts can be a cause of pseudolesions that mimic hypervascular tumors at two-phase spiral CT. Lesions that have the typical wedge-shaped and homogeneous appearance with or without internal linear branching structures during the HAP and that are isoattenuating or slightly hyperattenuating during the PVP can suggest this unusual condition.

The recently widespread use of two-phase spiral computed tomography (CT) during the hepatic arterial phase (HAP) and the portal venous phase (PVP) has led to an improvement in the detection of hypervascular tumors and hemodynamic alterations (1–3). In our experience, however, nontumorous hyperenhancing foci on HAP CT images are occasionally seen, especially in the cirrhotic liver. We found that most of these lesions were located in the subcapsular portion at the periphery of the liver and showed a wedge-shaped appearance. Similar experiences were also reported in prior reports (1–3). Although organic or functional arterioportal shunts, with or without obstruction of portal or hepatic venous flow, have been suggested as one of the causes of these pseudolesions (1), to our knowledge, small nontumorous arterioportal shunts that result in focal hyperenhancing areas on HAP CT images have not been proved as causes yet.

Structural distortion in the cirrhotic liver can produce various hemodynamic changes. Potential communications between the hepatic artery and the portal vein in the cirrhotic liver that are not associated with hepatocellular carcinoma have been proved with many clinical and experimental studies (4–9). Recently, Yu et al (4) documented radiologic findings of small nontumorous arterioportal shunts in the cirrhotic liver. They reported that angiographic findings of a tumorfree area accompanied by early filling (ie, contrast material enhancement) of the small branches of the portal vein and subsequent contrast enhancement of focal hepatic parenchyma are strongly suggestive of a nontumorous arterioportal shunt.

We thought that similar pseudolesions in the corresponding area of the nontumorous arterioportal shunt on hepatic angiograms could be expected to be depicted on CT images obtained during the HAP. Thus, we carried out a study of the two-phase spiral CT findings of nontumorous arterioportal shunts that were confirmed at hepatic angiography. A large population of patients who are known or suspected to have hepatocellular carcinoma associated with liver cirrhosis are referred to our department for transcatheter arterial chemoembolization (TACE). With a careful analysis of two-phase spiral CT and angiographic images obtained in these patients, we could collect cases of focal hyperattenuating lesions seen on HAP CT images that corresponded to the lesions that demonstrated typical angiographic findings of nontumorous arterioportal shunts.

Therefore, the purpose of this study was to determine the two-phase spiral CT findings of a nontumorous arterioportal shunt in cirrhotic liver that can mimic a hypervascular tumor.

MATERIALS AND METHODS

For 14 months, 803 patients who were known or suspected to have hepatocellular carcinoma were referred for initial or repeated TACE. With review of the medical records and radiologic findings in these patients, 29 hyperattenuating lesions at spiral CT during the HAP in 25 patients (23 men, two women; age range, 39–70 years; mean age, 55 years) were regarded as nontumorous arterioportal shunts and were included in this study. All 25 patients gave their full written informed consent, and institutional review board approval was obtained.

The diagnosis of nontumorous arterioportal shunts was established by four radiologists (T.K.K., B.I.C., J.K.H., J.H.P.) who reviewed the two-phase spiral CT images and hepatic angiograms. The diagnostic criteria of nontumorous arterioportal shunts were (*a*) a focal contrast-enhanced lesion on HAP CT images and on hepatic angiograms that demonstrated no increase in size for at least 4 months, (*b*) early opacification of small portal veins and subsequent focal parenchymal contrast enhancement on hepatic angiograms in the corresponding area of the lesion seen on HAP CT images, and (*c*) no evidence of compact nodular uptake of iodized oil by the lesion in patients who underwent iodized oil CT within 1 month after TACE.

We excluded lesions adjacent to other hypervascular tumors because of the possible presence of transtumoral arterioportal shunts instead of nontumorous lesions. We also excluded lesions in the area where percutaneous needle biopsy or percutaneous ethanol injection therapy had been performed, because an iatrogenic arterioportal fistula could manifest as a similar hyperattenuating lesion on HAP CT images (10).

On the basis of the clinical course and radiologic findings, liver cirrhosis associated with viral hepatitis was diagnosed in all 25 patients. Twenty patients had one (n = 9) or more (n = 11) additional hypervascular lesions in the liver at HAP CT; these lesions were diagnosed as hepatocellular carcinomas. The diagnosis of hepatocellular carcinoma in these patients was based on the results of percutaneous needle biopsy (n = 2) or on the results of typical clinical or laboratory testing (including elevated α-fetoprotein levels) in combination with the typical angiographic appearance and progression of disease on follow-up images (n = 18). Ten of the 29 lesions in this study developed after 1–14 TACE sessions (mean, 3.9 sessions). The remaining 19 lesions were found at the first TACE session.

CT examinations were performed with a HiSpeed Advantage spiral scanner (GE Medical Systems, Milwaukee, Wis) or a Somatom Plus-S scanner (Siemens Medical Systems, Erlangen, Germany). Each patient received 120 mL of ionic (Rayvist 300 [ioglycate]; Schering, Berlin, Germany) or nonionic (Ultravist 370 [iopromide]; Schering) contrast material through an 18-gauge, angiographic catheter inserted into a forearm vein by using an MK-IV dedicated CT injector (Medrad, Pittsburgh, Pa) at a rate of 3 mL/sec. Spiral CT was performed with the following parameters: 20-second acquisition time, 10-mm collimation, and 1:1 table pitch.

Spiral CT images were obtained during the HAP and the PVP 30 and 65 seconds, respectively, after the initiation of injection of contrast material. Each spiral acquisition through the liver was accomplished during the patient's breath hold. Contiguous axial reconstructions were obtained every 7 mm. In cases of a slightly hyperattenuating lesion on images obtained with soft-tissue windows, images with narrow window width were also obtained to identify the HAP CT findings.

TACE was performed with a mixture of iodized oil (Lipiodol; André Guerbet, Aulnay-sous-Bois, France), which is a radiopaque chemoembolization material, and doxorubicin hydrochloride (Adriamycin; Kyowa Hakko Kogyo, Tokyo, Japan) dissolution in all 25 patients (29 lesions). Follow-up CT without the administration of ionic or nonionic contrast material was performed 9–25 days (mean, 13 days) after TACE in 17 patients (21 lesions).

Follow-up hepatic angiography for additional TACE after the development of nontumorous arterioportal shunts was performed in 18 patients (22 lesions). There were 1–6 follow-up hepatic angiography sessions (mean, 2.1 sessions) during 4–33 months (mean, 13 months). Thirteen patients (16 lesions) were followed up with two-phase spiral CT 5–44 months (mean, 15 months) after the development of nontumorous arterioportal shunts. All 25 patients were followed up with angiography, two-phase spiral CT, or both at least 4 months after the detection of the lesion, which demonstrated no increase in size.

The radiologic studies were evaluated by four radiologists (T.K.K., B.I.C., J.K.H., J.H.P.) in one session and interpreted by consensus.

RESULTS

The longest dimension of the lesion on HAP CT images was 1.0–7.9 cm (mean dimension, 2.9 cm). All lesions were located in the subcapsular portion at the periphery of the liver. The mean size of the 10 lesions that developed after previous TACE was 4.7 cm, whereas that of the 19 lesions found at the initial TACE was 2.0 cm. All of the lesions that developed after previous TACE were identified in the area of the liver that was chemoembolized.

All lesions showed homogeneous hyperattenuation on the CT images obtained during the HAP. On several consecutive images, the three-dimensional morphology of the lesions was mostly wedge-shaped (25 [86%] lesions) (Figs 1, 2). Two (7%) lesions had a focal area with an irregular outline (Fig 3), and two (7%) lesions had a nodular shape (Fig 4). Small, tubular, contrast-enhanced structures within the lesion, representing early opacification of small portal venous branches, were demonstrated in nine (31%) lesions on HAP CT images (Figs 2,3). During the PVP, the lesions were seen as slightly hyperattenuating (nine [31%] lesions) or as isoattenuating (20 [69%] lesions) relative to the attenuation

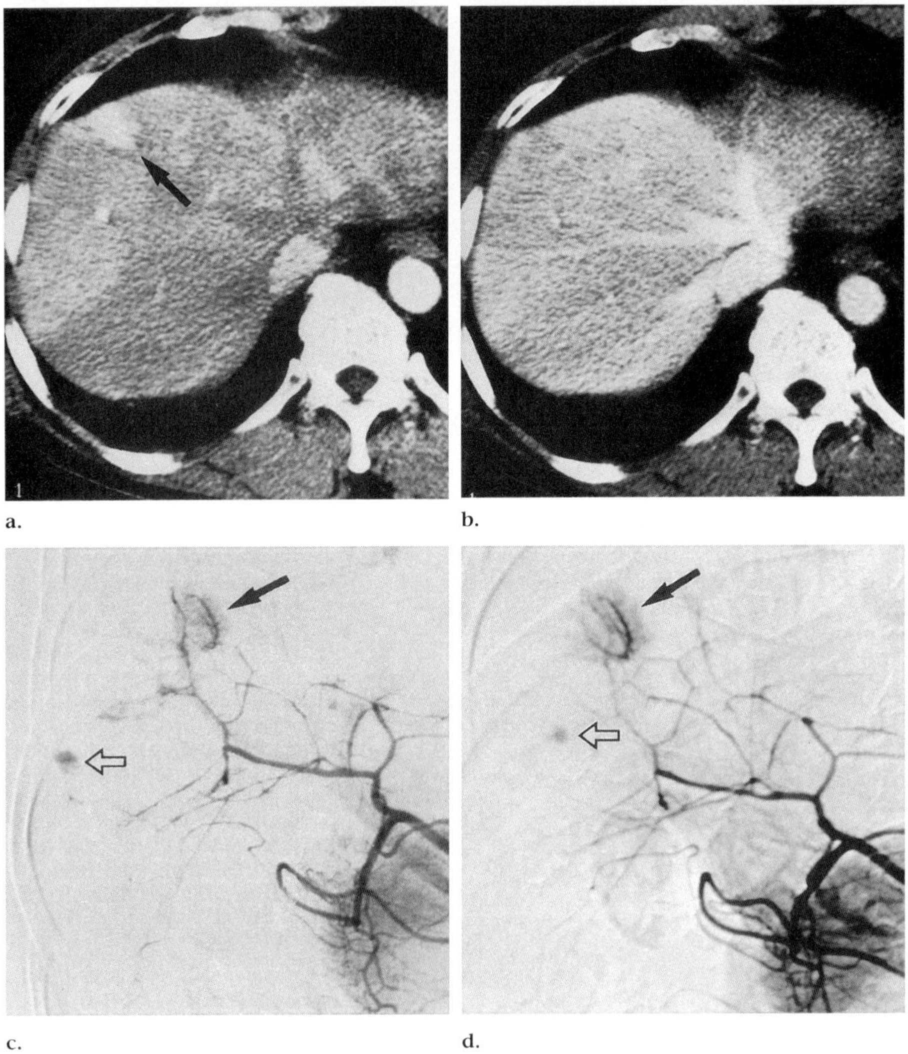

Figure 1. Nontumorous arterioportal shunt with a wedge-shaped appearance in a 68-year-old man. **(a)** CT image obtained during the HAP shows a small, wedge-shaped, hyperattenuating lesion (arrow) in the subcapsular portion of the right lobe of the liver. **(b)** The lesion in **a** is not seen on the CT image obtained during the PVP. **(c)** Hepatic angiogram shows small branching structures (solid arrow) that represent early filling of the small portal venous branches and focal contrast enhancement of the hepatic parenchyma in the corresponding area of the hyperattenuating lesion on the HAP CT image. Another small nodular contrast-enhanced lesion (open arrow) that suggests hepatocellular carcinoma is noted in the right lobe of the liver. **(d)** Nine-month follow-up hepatic angiogram demonstrates no change of the small arterioportal shunt (solid arrow). A tiny contrast-enhanced nodule (open arrow) that suggests a recurring hepatocellular carcinoma is seen in the right lobe of the liver.

of the liver (Figs 1–4). Of nine lesions that showed early opacification of portal venous branches on HAP CT images, six (67%) were seen as slightly hyperattenuating on images obtained during the PVP. No lesion was seen as hypoattenuating on PVP CT images. On follow-up two-phase spiral CT images, which were obtained in 13 patients (16 lesions), eight (50%) lesions demonstrated no change in size (Fig 2), and the remaining eight lesions (50%) disappeared without any evidence of the uptake of iodized oil.

Of the 21 lesions in which follow-up iodized oil CT was performed, five (24%) showed no uptake of iodized oil (Fig 4), and the remaining 16 (76%) demonstrated faint, irregular uptake without any area of compact nodular uptake.

DISCUSSION

CT images obtained during the HAP can demonstrate various hemodynamic changes in the liver that are usually undetected during the PVP (10,11). Before spiral CT was introduced, dynamic contrast-enhanced CT imaging at the same level was used in the evaluation of hepatic hemodynamics (12–15). Small, unexpected hemodynamic changes could not be evaluated, however, because only a single section could be imaged. With the advent of spiral CT, imaging of the entire liver during the HAP has become possible, and subtle attenuation changes caused by hemodynamic changes during the HAP can be detected.

Because the results of prior studies (16,17) have shown that HAP CT images are better for depicting hepatocellular carcinoma than are PVP and delayed-phase CT images, HAP images should be obtained to enable detection of hepatocellular carcinoma in patients with liver cirrhosis. A hyperattenuating focal hepatic lesion at HAP CT in the cirrhotic liver usually represents a hepatocellular carcinoma (18). In our experience, however, focal hyperattenuating lesions that seem to be nontumorous rather than malignant are occasionally seen on HAP CT images in the cirrhotic liver. At our hospital, a large proportion of patients with such lesions underwent hepatic angiography for TACE; thus, we could investigate the hemodynamic changes associated with these lesions.

Circulatory changes play an important role in the structural changes in liver cirrhosis and vice versa. Although extensive studies (4–9) have been concerned with the clarification of microcirculatory changes in cirrhosis, several problems, such as changes in arterioportal anastomoses, are still unresolved or are being debated. Occlusion of small hepatic venules and retrograde filling of portal flow by way of arterioportal anastomoses has been suggested as a cause of arterioportal communication in cirrhosis (5). Occlusion of the hepatic vein results in increased sinusoidal pressure and reverses the pressure gradient between the sinusoidal and portal veins. Therefore, the affected area is supplied with arterial blood only, and the portal veins become the draining veins in the occluded area. This phenomenon was proved in clinical studies (19,20) in which CT was performed after temporary occlusion of the hepatic vein with a balloon catheter. Portal venous obstruction can also result in increased hepatic arterial flow within the affected liver parenchyma and a functional arterioportal shunt (21).

There are several arterioportal communication systems, including transsinusoidal, transvasal, and transplexal routes (5,11,22). The results of a recent scanning

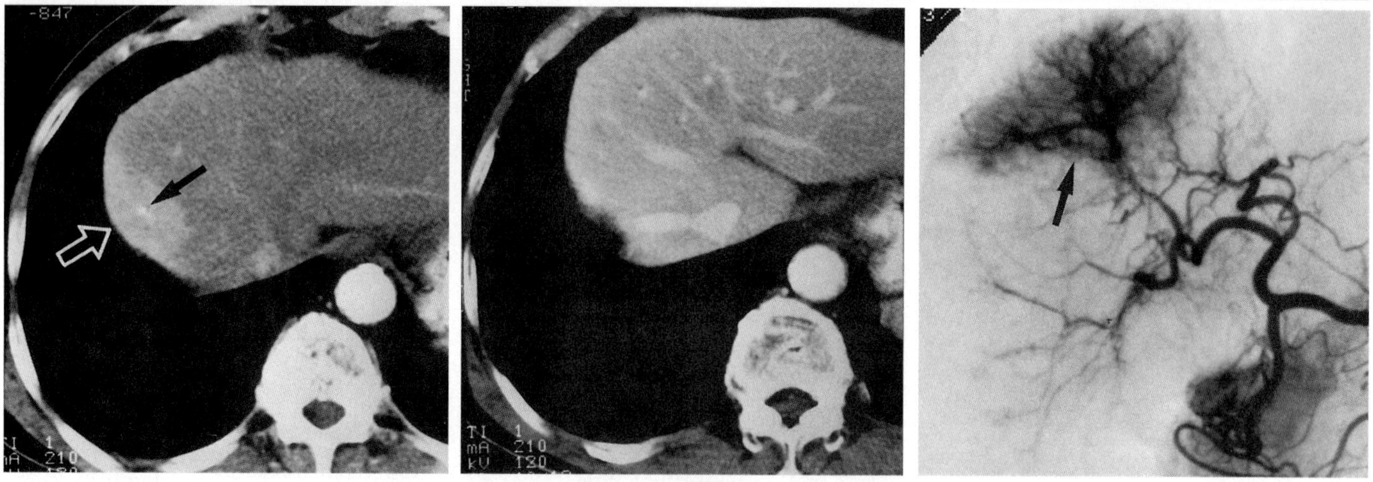

a. b. c.

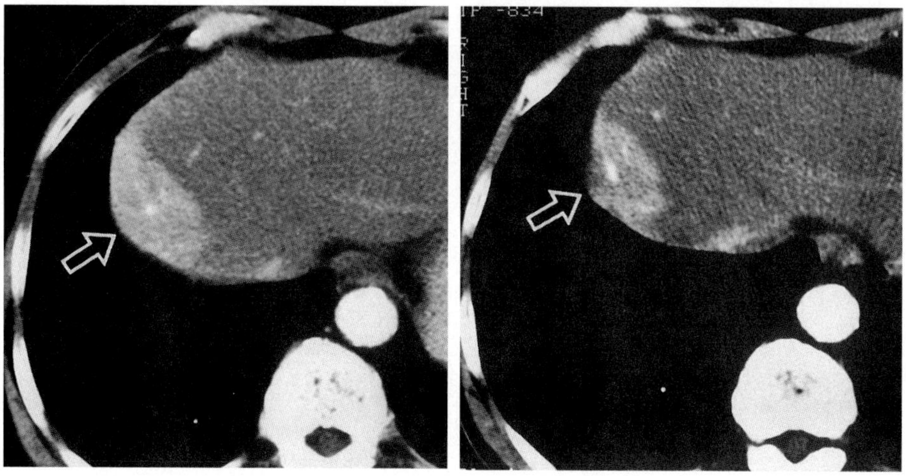

d. e.

Figure 2. Nontumorous arterioportal shunt with a wedge-shaped appearance in a 70-year-old man. **(a)** CT image obtained during the HAP shows a wedge-shaped, hyperattenuating lesion (open arrow) in the subcapsular portion of the right lobe of the liver. A tiny contrast-enhanced dot (solid arrow) that represents early opacification of a portal venous branch is seen within the lesion. **(b)** The lesion in **a** is not seen on the CT image obtained during the PVP. **(c)** Hepatic angiogram shows early filling of the branches of the portal vein and wedge-shaped parenchymal contrast enhancement (arrow) in the corresponding area of the hyperattenuating lesion on the HAP CT image. **(d, e)** Follow-up HAP CT images obtained after **(d)** 8 months and **(e)** 33 months show no change in the lesion (arrow in **d** and **e**).

electron microscopic study (6) demonstrated that hypertrophy of the peribiliary plexus and direct anastomosis in the peripheral area of the liver were major routes of arterioportal communication in experimental studies of rat cirrhosis. In addition, the formation of capillaries and the abnormal permeability of hepatic sinusoids were proved to be present with in vitro studies (7,8) in isolated human liver with cirrhosis; therefore, the formation of capillaries and the permeability changes of sinusoids might also be related to arterioportal communications of the cirrhotic liver.

Recently, Yu et al (4) reported that a small arterioportal shunt could be a cause of a pseudolesion at hepatic imaging. They described angiographic findings of a tubular vascular structure that represented a peripheral branch of the portal vein during the HAP and subsequent focal parenchymal contrast enhancement around the vascular structure that were suggestive of a nontumorous arterioportal shunt. CT images obtained during arterial portography showed these lesions as perfusion defects. No focal, nodular iodized oil uptake was identified on iodized oil CT images. Neither magnetic resonance imaging nor intraoperative ultrasonography demonstrated the lesions. Among four patients who underwent dynamic contrast-enhanced CT in that study, three had a contrast-enhanced lesion that corresponded to the arterioportal shunt at angiography. From these results, one can speculate that these lesions may be a cause of hyperattenuating pseudolesions at spiral CT during the HAP.

Hyperattenuating pseudolesions at HAP CT have also been documented by several authors. Hollett et al (2) noted two cases of false-positive detection of hypervascular lesions at HAP CT. In both cases, the HAP image showed a homogeneous and wedge-shaped lesion in the subcapsular portion of the liver that was invisible on the PVP image. Bonaldi et al (3) observed focal areas with irregular outlines or wedge-shaped focal areas of contrast enhancement on HAP CT images in 32 of 103 patients with various focal hepatic lesions. The flow abnormalities were attributed to evident portal venous obstruction in eight of these 32 patients but were unexplained in the remaining 24 patients.

Oliver and Baron (1) described their experiences with small, peripheral transient hyperenhancing foci at HAP CT. Similar experiences at dynamic incremental CT (12) and dynamic magnetic resonance imaging (23) also have been documented. Idiopathic obstruction of portal venous flow peripherally or arterioportal shunts were suggested causes of these pseudolesions (1); however, this hypothesis should be confirmed.

The results of our study showed that a nontumorous arterioportal shunt could be a cause of the wedge-shaped pseudolesions seen on HAP CT images. All lesions were homogeneous, and their attenuation during the PVP never decreased

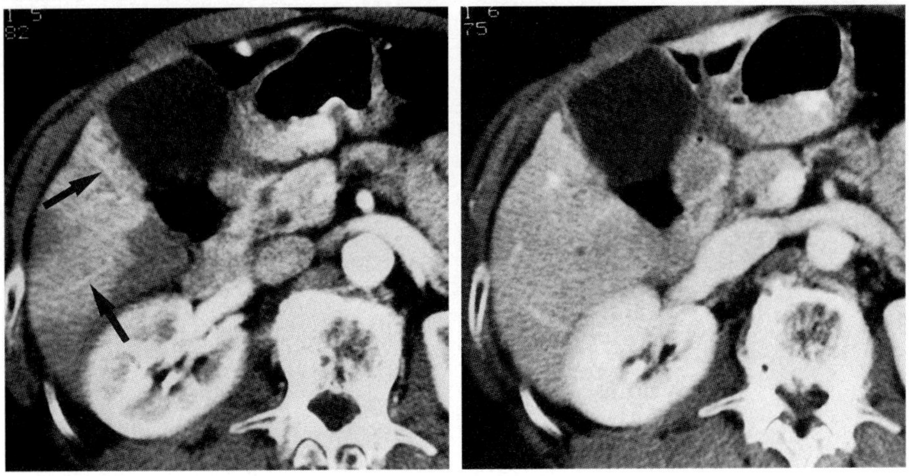

a. b.

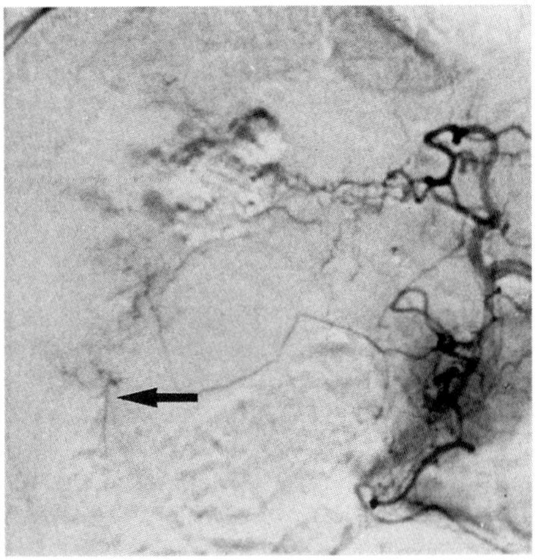

c.

Figure 3. Nontumorous arterioportal shunt with a focal area with an irregular outline in a 61-year-old man. **(a)** CT image obtained during the HAP shows a homogeneously hyperattenuating lesion with an irregular outline in the right lobe of the liver. Linear contrast-enhanced structures (arrows) that represent early opacification of the portal veins are seen within the lesion. **(b)** The lesion in **a** is not seen on the CT image obtained during the PVP. **(c)** Hepatic angiogram shows severe damage of the right hepatic artery due to previous, repeated TACE and early filling of the small branches of the portal vein (arrow) in the inferior portion of the right lobe.

below that of the surrounding liver parenchyma. A wedge shape and straight-line margin were seen in most cases. These features can help differentiate these lesions from hypervascular tumors, which are usually heterogeneous and seen as isoattenuating or hypoattenuating during the PVP.

In contrast to hepatic angiography, spiral CT during the HAP demonstrated early opacification of portal venous branches within the lesion in only 31% (nine lesions) of cases. This may be due to the limited resolution of CT in demonstrating small portal branches in the liver. Therefore, although the early opacification of the portal branches within the lesion at HAP CT can be suggestive of an arterioportal shunt, the frequency of this finding seems to be relatively low. However, the limited demonstration of portal venous branches within the lesions at HAP CT in our study might have been related in part to our use of 10-mm collimation. It is possible that with 5- or 7-mm collimation, early opacification of portal venous branches might have been demonstrated in a higher percentage of lesions.

Although most nontumorous arterioportal shunts are obviously wedge-shaped or have focal areas with irregular outlines, round or nodular lesions can develop because of the three-dimensional structure of the lesions and the plane of the CT scanning. In relatively large lesions, it is not difficult to differentiate the wedge-shaped appearance with careful observation of several contiguous CT images (11). However, it could be impossible to note the typical wedge-shaped appearance of small lesions. In our series, two (7%) lesions had a nodular appearance at HAP CT (Fig 3).

Nontumorous arterioportal shunts are closely related to nontumorous subcapsular wedge-shaped defects that are occasionally seen in the cirrhotic liver on CT images obtained during arterial portography (24–28), because a focal increase in portal venous pressure caused by small arterioportal shunts can produce wedge-shaped defects at CT during arterial portography. Also, these lesions are one of the causes of nontumorous subsegmental contrast enhancement at CT during hepatic arteriography (29,30).

In this study, we excluded small, wedge-shaped hyperattenuating lesions, which did not demonstrate early opacification of a branch of the portal vein at angiography, even if these lesions were regarded as nontumorous lesions at follow-up imaging. However, it is still possible that tiny arterioportal shunts, which could not be detected at angiography because of limited resolution and overlapping liver parenchyma or bowel, were present.

Possible benign causes of wedge-shaped hyperattenuating lesions at HAP CT other than arterioportal shunts include (*a*) aberrant venous drainage into the peripheral portal vein (eg, drainage of the gastric or cystic vein into the peripheral portal vein) (31), (*b*) transient increased attenuation in the gallbladder bed in patients with gallbladder disease (32), and (*c*) areas of high attenuation such as focal calcifications or siderotic regenerating nodules (1). The early contrast enhancement on images obtained in patients with aberrant venous drainage can be explained by the early inflow of contrast material into the focal area as a result of aberrant venous drainage compared with the inflow of contrast material into the surrounding liver parenchyma, which receives contrast material mainly from the splenic and superior mesenteric veins (31). The transient contrast enhancement near the gallbladder on images obtained in patients with gallbladder disease can also be attributed to the increased blood flow from the dilated aberrant cystic vein of the diseased hypervascular gallbladder (32). Although the reported hyperattenuating pseudolesions with these causes were in a characteristic location such as at the dorsomedial edge of the medial segment or in the area adjacent to the gallbladder, theoretically, it may be possible for similar pseudolesions to develop in the subcapsular portion as a result of aberrant portal venous supply.

Our results also suggest that TACE may be a cause of nontumorous arterioportal shunts. Ten of the 29 lesions in this study developed after one or more sessions of TACE. Because angiograms obtained before the development of the lesions did not show evidence of the arterioportal shunts, and all nontumorous arterioportal shunts that developed after TACE were in the area of the liver that was chemoem-

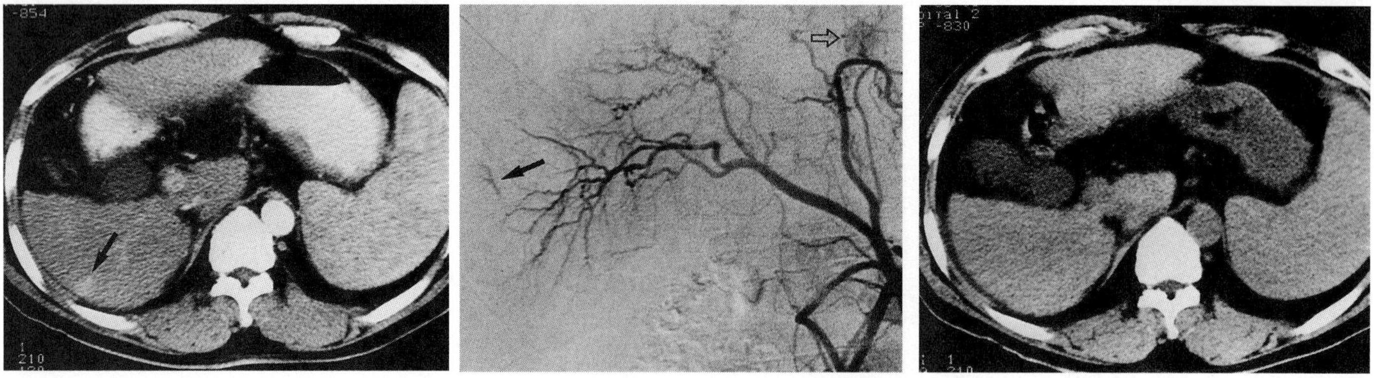

a. c. e.

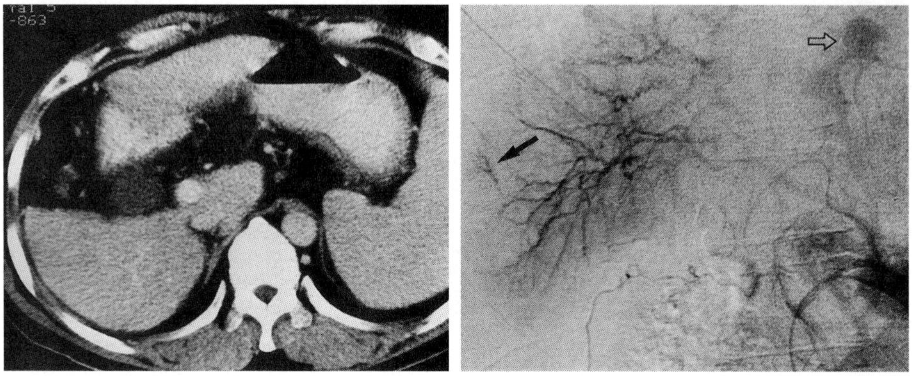

b. d.

Figure 4. Nontumorous arterioportal shunt with a nodular appearance in a 53-year-old man. **(a)** CT image obtained during the HAP shows a small, nodular, hyperattenuating lesion (arrow) in the subcapsular portion of the right lobe of the liver. **(b)** The lesion in **a** is not seen on the CT image obtained during the PVP. **(c, d)** Hepatic angiograms show small branching structures that represent **(c)** early filling of the small branches of the portal vein (solid arrow) and **(d)** subsequent focal parenchymal contrast enhancement (solid arrow) in the area that corresponds to the area of the hyperattenuating lesion on the HAP CT image. A nodular contrast-enhanced lesion (open arrows in **c** and **d**) that suggests a nodular hepatocellular carcinoma is seen in the left lobe. **(e)** Iodized oil CT image obtained 9 days after TACE demonstrates no uptake of iodized oil in the arterioportal shunt in the right lobe.

bolized, a relationship between the development of arterioportal shunts and prior TACE could be hypothesized. We found the lesions that developed after TACE tended to be larger than those that developed without TACE. The etiology of arterioportal shunts that develop after TACE is not known. We believe that vascular injury that results from the use of chemoembolic agents or a superselective microcatheter and a guide wire might be a cause of this phenomenon.

If all the typical CT findings of a nontumorous arterioportal shunt are present in a certain lesion at two-phase spiral CT, the invasive procedure (ie, TACE and iodized oil CT) may not be needed to exclude the presence of tiny tumors. However, according to our anecdotal experiences, follow-up two-phase spiral CT must be performed to exclude a tumor with a wedge-shaped transtumoral shunt, because a tiny tumor with a transtumoral arterioportal shunt can show the same findings as a nontumorous arterioportal shunt on HAP CT images. In these cases, iodized oil CT performed after TACE can demonstrate a tiny nodular uptake of iodized oil in a small portion of the wedge-shaped lesion, and the lesion usually has progressed at follow-up imaging. In this study, we ruled out the possibility of coexistent tumors by demonstrating no compact iodized oil uptake at iodized oil CT and no increase in size at follow-up CT or angiography.

The limitation of this study was that the subjects were patients who had been referred for TACE. Therefore, the results of this study preclude any reliable estimation of the frequency of nontumorous arterioportal shunts in the cirrhotic liver.

In conclusion, typical two-phase spiral CT findings can suggest the possibility of nontumorous arterioportal shunt in the cirrhotic liver, which is one of the causes of hypervascular pseudolesions. Lesions with the typical wedge-shaped appearance, homogeneous attenuation, early visualized portal branches during the HAP, and areas of isoattenuation or slight hyperattenuation during the PVP can be suggestive of nontumorous arterioportal shunts on two-phase spiral CT images. However, follow-up radiologic studies must be performed to exclude the possibility of coexistent tumors.

References

1. Oliver III JH, Baron RL. Helical biphasic contrast-enhanced CT of the liver: techniques, indications, interpretation, pitfalls. Radiology 1996; 201:1–14.
2. Hollett MD, Jeffrey RB Jr, Nino-Murcia M, Jorgensen MJ, Harris DP. Dual-phase helical CT of the liver: value of arterial phase scans in the detection of small (≤1.5 cm) malignant hepatic neoplasms. AJR 1995; 164:879–884.
3. Bonaldi VM, Bret PM, Reinhold C, Atri M. Helical CT of the liver: value of an early arterial phase. Radiology 1995; 197:357–363.
4. Yu JS, Kim KW, Sung KB, Lee JT, Yoo HS. Small arterial–portal venous shunts: cause of pseudolesions at hepatic imaging. Radiology 1997; 203:737–742.
5. Bookstein JJ, Cho KJ, Davis GB, Dail D. Arterioportal communications: observations and hypotheses concerning transsinusoidal and transvasal types. Radiology 1982; 142:581–590.
6. Haratake J, Hisaoka M, Yamamoto O, Horie A. Morphological changes of hepatic microcirculation in experimental rat cirrhosis: a scanning electron microscopic study. Hepatology 1991; 13:952–956.
7. Villeneuve JP, Dagenais M, Huet PM, Roy A, Lapointe R, Marleau D. The hepatic microcirculation in the isolated perfused human liver. Hepatology 1996; 23:24–31.
8. Hirooka N, Iwasaki I, Horie H, Ide G. Hepatic microcirculation of liver cirrhosis studied by corrosion cast/scanning electron microscope examination. Acta Pathol Jpn 1986; 36:375–387.
9. Demachi H, Matsui O, Kawamori Y, Ueda K, Takashima T. The protective effect of

portoarterial shunts after experimental hepatic artery embolization in rats with liver cirrhosis. Cardiovasc Intervent Radiol 1995; 18:97–101.
10. Lee SJ, Lim JH, Lee WJ, Lim HK, Choo SW, Choo IW. Transient subsegmental hepatic parenchymal enhancement on dynamic CT: a sign of postbiopsy arterioportal shunt. J Comput Assist Tomogr 1997; 21:355–360.
11. Itai Y, Matsui O. Blood flow and liver imaging. Radiology 1997; 202:306–314.
12. Itai Y, Hachiya J, Makita K, Ohtomo K, Kokubo T, Yamauchi T. Transient hepatic attenuation differences on dynamic computed tomography. J Comput Assist Tomogr 1987; 11:461–465.
13. Nakayama T, Hiyama Y, Ohnishi K, et al. Arterioportal shunts on dynamic computed tomography. AJR 1983; 140:953–957.
14. Itai Y, Moss AA, Goldberg HI. Transient hepatic attenuation difference of lobar or segmental distribution detected by dynamic computed tomography. Radiology 1982; 144:835–839.
15. Itai Y, Furui S, Ohtomo K, et al. Dynamic CT features of arterioportal shunts in hepatocellular carcinoma. AJR 1986; 146:723–727.
16. Choi BI, Lee HJ, Han JK, Choi DS, Seo JB, Han MC. Detection of hypervascular nodular hepatocellular carcinomas: value of triphasic helical CT compared with iodized-oil CT. AJR 1997; 168:219–224.
17. Hwang GJ, Kim MJ, Yoo HS, Lee JT. Nodular hepatocellular carcinomas: detection with arterial-, portal-, and delayed-phase images at spiral CT. Radiology 1997; 202: 383–388.
18. Lee HM, Lu DSK, Krasny RM, Busuttil R, Kadell B, Lucas J. Hepatic lesion characterization in cirrhosis: significance of arterial hypervascularity on dual-phase helical CT. AJR 1997; 169:125–130.
19. Murata S, Itai Y, Asato M, et al. Effect of temporary occlusion of hepatic vein on dual blood supply in the liver: evaluation with spiral CT. Radiology 1995; 197:351–356.
20. Murata S, Itai Y, Satake M, et al. Changes in contrast enhancement of hepatocellular carcinoma and liver: effect of temporary occlusion of a hepatic vein evaluated with spiral CT. Radiology 1997; 202:715–720.
21. Matsui O, Takashima T, Kitagawa K, et al. Segmental staining on hepatic arteriography as a sign of intrahepatic portal vein obstruction. Radiology 1984; 152:601–606.
22. Itai Y, Murata S, Kurosaki Y. Straight border sign of the liver: spectrum of CT appearances and causes. RadioGraphics 1995; 15:1089–1102.
23. Schlund JF, Semelka RC, Kettritz U, Weeks SM, Kahlenberg M, Cance WG. Correlation of perfusion abnormalities on CTAP and immediate postintravenous gadolinium-enhanced gradient echo MRI. Abdom Imaging 1996; 21:49–52.
24. Soyer P, Lacheheb D, Levesque M. False-positive CT portography: correlation with pathologic findings. AJR 1993; 160:285–289.
25. Peterson MS, Baron RL, Dodd GD III, et al. Hepatic parenchymal perfusion defects detected with CTAP: imaging-pathologic correlation. Radiology 1992; 185:149–155.
26. Nelson RC, Thompson GH, Chezmar JL, Harned RK II, Fernandez M. CT during arterial portography: diagnostic pitfalls. RadioGraphics 1992; 12:705–718.
27. Soyer P, Bluemke DA, Fishman EK. CT during arterial portography for the preoperative evaluation of hepatic tumors: how, when, and why? AJR 1994; 163:1325–1331.
28. Bluemke DA, Soyer P, Fishman EK. Nontumorous low-attenuation defects in the liver on helical CT during arterial portography: frequency, location, and appearance. AJR 1995; 164:1141–1145.
29. Freeny PC, Marks WM. Hepatic perfusion abnormalities during CT angiography: detection and interpretation. Radiology 1986; 159:685–691.
30. Kanematsu M, Hoshi H, Imaeda T, et al. Nonpathological focal enhancements on spiral CT hepatic angiography. Abdom Imaging 1997; 22:55–59.
31. Matsui O, Kadoya M, Yoshikawa J, et al. Aberrant gastric venous drainage in cirrhotic livers: imaging findings in focal areas of liver parenchyma. Radiology 1995; 197:345–349.
32. Ito K, Awaya H, Mitchell DG, et al. Gallbladder disease: appearance of associated transient increased attenuation in the liver at biphasic, contrast-enhanced dynamic CT. Radiology 1997; 204:723–728.

Book Review

Practical Nuclear Medicine. 2nd ed.

Edited by Peter F. Sharp, Howard G. Gemmell, and Francis W. Smith
New York, NY: Oxford University Press, 1998. ISBN 0-19-262841-0.
Softcover, $59.50; pp 364; 258 figures; tables.

This second edition of *Practical Nuclear Medicine* is an attractive, well-organized book that consists of 19 chapters, each of which is written by one or more distinguished medical scientists. The stated purpose of the first edition of this book was to provide the basic facts of nuclear medicine in a concise, practical, manual format, and I believe the authors have achieved this goal in this edition. The chapters are well written and are presented from a very practical and clinical viewpoint, making them easily readable for the busy clinician. Because of the lack of in-depth technical discussions, it is not an adequate textbook for radiologists, nuclear medicine physicians, or imaging residents.

The first seven chapters deal with some of the more basic principles of radionuclide imaging. For example, chapter 3 is new and deals specifically with the nonimaging techniques performed in nuclear medicine laboratories, chapter 5 addresses quality assurance issues in a comprehensive manner, chapter 6 features a short discussion of the principles of radiopharmacy, and chapter 7 presents an excellent discussion of the basic concepts of radiation biology used to form the present guidelines for radiation protection. Chapters 8–17 cover commonly used nuclear medicine procedures and are organized by the major organ systems in the body, and chapter 18 includes an interesting presentation on the various applications of technetium pertechnetate. These chapters contain discussions of standard imaging protocols of conventional nuclear medicine techniques in each organ system, along with sections on the clinical value of each technique. Chapter 19, the final chapter, is also new and deals with the basic principles of positron emission tomography. It serves as an excellent introduction to this imaging modality for the beginner.

Although this book presents a very basic, practical look at the entire field of nuclear medicine, the images used to illustrate various studies and scintigraphic findings do not appear to be state of the art. However, the summary tables are excellent and the references are adequate. As an introductory nuclear medicine textbook for medical students, residents in nonimaging specialties, and referring physicians, it serves its purpose well, and the price is reasonable. Practicing radiologists and nuclear medicine physicians would be better served by a more comprehensive treatment of the field as mentioned above.

Reviewed by Michael J. Blend, PhD, DO

Mucin-producing Tumor of the Pancreas: Diagnostic Value of Diffusion-weighted Echo-planar MR Imaging[1]

Yasuyuki Yamashita, MD
Tomohiro Namimoto, MD
Katsuhiko Mitsuzaki, MD
Joji Urata, MD
Tadatoshi Tsuchigame, MD
Mutsumasa Takahashi, MD
Michio Ogawa, MD

Index terms:
Pancreas, cysts, 770.312, 770.32
Pancreas, MR, 770.121411, 770.121415, 72.121416, 770.12149
Pancreas, neoplasms, 770.312, 770.32

Radiology 1998; 208:605–609

Abbreviations:
ADC = apparent diffusion coefficient
MPT = mucin-producing tumor

[1] From the Departments of Radiology (Y.Y., T.N., K.M., J.U., T.T., M.T.) and Second Surgery (M.O.), Kumamoto University School of Medicine, 1-1-1 Honjo, Kumamoto 860, Japan. Received October 30, 1997; revision requested January 20, 1998; revision received March 16; accepted April 17. **Address reprint requests to** Y.Y.

Author contributions:
Guarantor of integrity of entire study, Y.Y.; study concepts and design, Y.Y., J.U.; definition of intellectual content, T.T.; literature research, K.M.; clinical studies, Y.Y., T.N.; data acquisition, T.N.; data analysis, Y.Y.; statistical analysis, T.N.; manuscript preparation, Y.Y.; manuscript editing, M.T.; manuscript review, M.T., M.O.

PURPOSE: To determine whether diffusion-weighted echo-planar magnetic resonance (MR) imaging can help differentiate mucin-producing tumors of the pancreas from other cystic lesions.

MATERIALS AND METHODS: Diffusion-weighted echo-planar 1.5-T MR imaging was performed in patients with mucin-producing tumor (n = 15), pseudocyst (n = 15), or serous microcystic tumor (n = 2). Images were obtained with diffusion-sensitizing gradients of 30 and 300 sec/mm^2. The apparent diffusion coefficient (ADC) was calculated.

RESULTS: At 30 sec/mm^2, all cystic lesions had very high signal intensity. The dilated main pancreatic duct was depicted in eight patients with mucin-producing tumor and in six with pseudocyst. The mean (± standard deviation) ADCs of mucin-producing tumors (2.7×10^{-3} mm^2/sec $\pm 0.9 \times 10^{-3}$) and pseudocysts (3.2×10^{-3} mm^2/sec $\pm 1.0 \times 10^{-3}$) were significantly lower ($P < .01$) than those of serous cysts or cerebrospinal fluid (5.8×10^{-3} mm^2/sec $\pm 2.0 \times 10^{-3}$). At 300 sec/mm^2, cysts and the main pancreatic ducts had high signal intensity in cases of mucin-producing tumor, indicative of the presence of mucinous products in both the cystic cavity and the main pancreatic duct. The signal intensity of cystic fluid in pseudocysts was high on diffusion-weighted images, but that of the pancreatic duct was decreased (ADC = 5.1×10^{-3} mm^2/sec $\pm 1.7 \times 10^{-3}$).

CONCLUSION: Diffusion-weighted MR imaging can help characterize cystic lesions of the pancreas. Findings suggestive of viscous fluid in mucin-producing tumors are present on such images.

Cystic lesions of the pancreas include pseudocysts, serous tumors, and mucinous tumors, some of which are malignant. Duct ectatic mucinous cystic tumor, or mucin-producing tumor (MPT) of the pancreas, is considered to be a specific type of mucinous tumor. This tumor is characterized by the presence of a mass that represents cystic dilatation of the side branch of the main pancreatic duct, which contains thick mucoid secretions.

Endoscopic retrograde pancreatography enables the diagnosis of this disease by demonstrating cystic lesions that communicate with the pancreatic duct (1). The cystic ducts are lined by the mucin-secreting epithelium, and there is a known risk of malignant transformation of the epithelium. Mucin plugging of the papilla of Vater is often found at endoscopic observation (2–4).

The analysis of cystic fluid for cytologic findings, the presence of a tumor marker, and viscosity has been proposed as an aid for the differential diagnosis of pancreatic cystic lesions (5). Diffusion-weighted magnetic resonance (MR) imaging is sensitive to molecular diffusion, which is the random thermal motion of molecules (known as Brownian motion), because random motion in the field gradients produces incoherent phase shifts that result in signal attenuation (6). In cystic fluid, proton diffusion is strongly correlated with the viscosity of the fluid. MR imaging is the only method that can demonstrate the molecular diffusion process in vivo. Because diffusion directly reflects molecular mobility, measurement of diffusion with MR imaging has been shown (7,8) to have substantial promise in

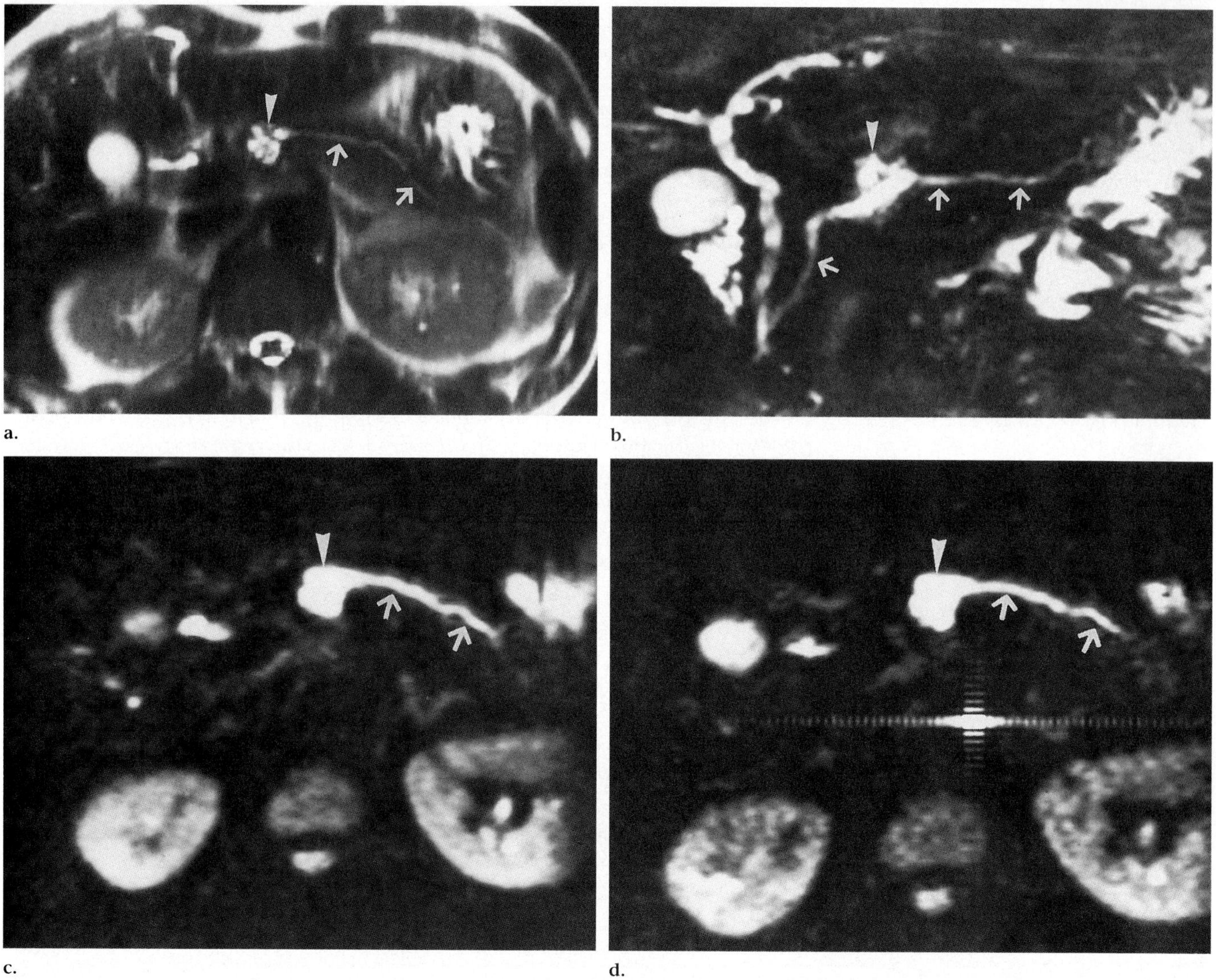

Figure 1. MPT of the pancreas in a 58-year-old man. **(a)** Axial and **(b)** oblique coronal half-Fourier single-shot turbo spin-echo MR cholangiographic maximum intensity projection images (∞/87) show a multiloculated cystic mass (arrowhead) and a slightly dilated main pancreatic duct (arrows). The cyst appears to have a connection with the main pancreatic duct. **(c)** Axial diffusion-weighted echo-planar MR image (∞/123) obtained with a *b* value of 30 sec/mm² shows high signal intensity in both the cyst (arrowhead) and the main pancreatic duct (arrows). **(d)** Diffusion-weighted echo-planar MR image (∞/123) with a *b* value of 300 sec/mm² shows that the decrease in the signal intensity of the cyst (arrowhead) and the main pancreatic duct (arrows) is small. The ADCs of the cyst and pancreatic juice are 3.3×10^{-3} and 3.4×10^{-3} mm²/sec, respectively.

clinical applications. At present, the most important clinical application of this imaging technique is the detection and characterization of cerebral ischemia (9,10). The use of echo-planar MR imaging with a preparation pulse that is sensitive to diffusion (diffusion-weighted echo-planar MR imaging) allows diffusion-weighted images to be obtained in the abdomen with a single breath hold (11).

We postulated that serial echo-planar MR imaging with different diffusion-sensitizing gradients might be used to help detect viscous fluid within MPTs. In the present study, we attempted to detect mucinous fluid in the MPT on the basis of the apparent diffusion coefficient (ADC) calculated from serial echo-planar MR images obtained with different diffusion-sensitizing gradients. Our purpose was to determine whether diffusion-weighted echo-planar MR imaging can help differentiate mucin-producing tumors of the pancreas from other cystic lesions.

MATERIALS AND METHODS

After oral informed consent had been obtained, diffusion-weighted echo-planar MR imaging was performed with a 1.5-T whole-body imager (Vision; Siemens, Erlangen, Germany) equipped with a phased-array body coil. The study population comprised 32 patients (20 men, 12 women; age range, 43–78 years; mean age, 64 years) with a cystic pancreatic lesion (15 patients with an MPT, 15 with a pseudocyst, and two with a microcystic serous tumor). Presence of MPTs and microcystic tumors were proved with surgical results. The diagnosis of a pseudocyst was rendered on the basis of clinical history and typical radiologic findings from ultrasonography (US), computed tomography (CT), and endoscopic retrograde cholangiopancreatography. The diameter of the MPTs was 15–50 mm (mean,

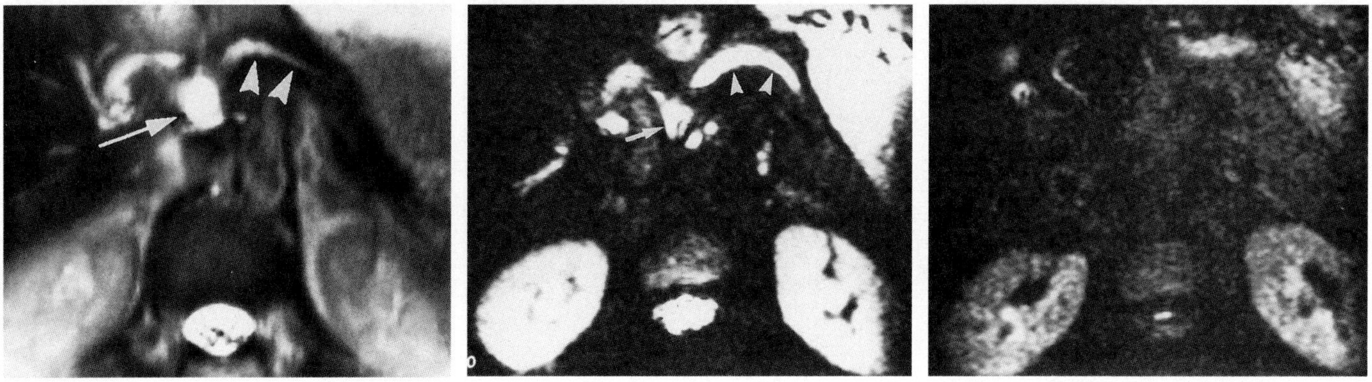

a. b. c.

Figure 2. Pseudocyst of the pancreas associated with chronic pancreatitis in a 64-year-old man with a long history of pancreatitis. The size of the cyst had decreased spontaneously at follow-up. **(a)** Axial half-Fourier single-shot turbo spin-echo MR image (∞/87) shows a unilocular cystic mass (arrow) and the dilated main pancreatic duct (arrowheads). **(b)** Axial diffusion-weighted echo-planar MR image (∞/123) with a *b* value of 30 sec/mm^2 shows high signal intensity in both the cyst (arrow) and the main pancreatic duct (arrowheads). Another small cyst is also visible. The image is slightly distorted because of a susceptibility artifact caused by gas in the stomach. The ADCs of the cyst and pancreatic juice are 3.5×10^{-3} and 7.2×10^{-3} mm^2/sec, respectively. **(c)** On a diffusion-weighted echo-planar MR image (∞/123) obtained with a *b* value of 300 sec/mm^2, both the cyst and the main pancreatic duct are no longer visible.

22 mm), and that of the pseudocysts was 20–85 mm (mean, 42 mm). The diameters of the two microcystic tumors were 28 and 35 mm.

Before echo-planar MR imaging was performed, all patients underwent MR imaging with a half-Fourier single-shot turbo spin-echo sequence (repetition time msec/echo time msec, ∞/87) performed in the axial plane. The matrix was 128 × 256, with one signal acquired, a 26–34-mm field of view, an 8-mm section thickness, and a 0.8-mm (10%) intersection gap. Axial images were obtained without fat suppression, and oblique coronal images were obtained with fat suppression; these images were postprocessed with a maximum intensity projection algorithm. These MR examinations were followed by multisection T2-weighted respiratory-triggered turbo spin-echo imaging with a repetition time that varied from 3,180 to 8,638 msec (mean, 4,657 msec), according to the period of the respiratory cycle; an effective echo time of 90 msec; an echo train length of seven; and one signal acquired. The field of view varied according to patient size and was 26–34 cm. The section thickness was 8 mm, and the intersection gap was 1.6 mm (20%).

For diffusion-weighted MR imaging, we used a spin-echo type of echo-planar sequence that combined diffusion gradients with an echo-planar imaging readout to perform diffusion-weighted imaging of the abdomen. Sequential sampling of k space was used, with an echo time of 123 msec, a bandwidth of 1,250 Hz/pixel, and 128 lines of data acquired in 0.3 second. The other parameters were a 340-mm field of view, a 128 × 128 matrix, an 8-mm section thickness, and one signal acquired. The sequence was modified by adding large diffusion gradients on both sides of the 180° pulse in the section-select direction. A short 2- or 3-msec diffusion gradient pulse, with gradient strengths of up to 25 mT/m, was applied. Images were obtained with breath holding to avoid respiratory motion.

First, the decrease in the signal intensity of masses was visually analyzed in comparison with that of the cerebrospinal fluid. Second, the ADC for the serial diffusion-weighted echo-planar sequences was calculated with two different *b* values (30 and 300 sec/mm^2) during each of the breath holds (see the Appendix for details). The analysis was performed in regions of interest placed over different organs or areas of pathologic tissue. The difference in ADCs among the cysts, the pancreatic duct, and cerebrospinal fluid in the spinal canal was analyzed by using the Student *t* test.

RESULTS

With the half-Fourier single-shot turbo spin-echo sequence, the details of the wall of the cyst and septa and the relationship with the pancreatic duct were clearly visualized (Figs 1, 2). On diffusion-weighted echo-planar images, a slight degree of image distortion due to susceptibility artifacts was seen in six patients, and a chemical shift artifact in the abdominal wall was observed in all patients. However, these artifacts did not preclude the evaluation of the cystic lesions, and calculation of the ADCs was possible for all cystic fluids. Dilatation of the main pancreatic duct was seen in eight patients with MPT (Fig 1), in six patients with a pseudocyst (Figs 2, 3), and in none with a microcystic serous tumor; calculation of the ADCs for pancreatic juice in the main pancreatic duct was possible in these patients.

On diffusion-weighted MR images with a *b* value of 30 sec/mm^2, all cystic lesions and the dilated main pancreatic duct had very high signal intensity (Figs 1c, 2b, 3b). On diffusion-weighted images with a *b* value of 300 sec/mm^2, all MPTs and six of 10 pseudocysts had high signal intensity (Figs 1d, 3c), whereas all serous cysts and four pseudocysts were not visible (Fig 2c). The ADCs of each tissue are shown in the Table. The average ADCs of MPTs (2.7×10^{-3} mm^2/sec $\pm$ 0.9×10^{-3} [standard deviation]) and pseudocysts (3.2×10^{-3} mm^2/sec $\pm$ 1.3×10^{-3}) were significantly lower ($P < .01$ in each case) than those of serous cysts or cerebrospinal fluid (5.8×10^{-3} mm^2/sec $\pm$ 2.0×10^{-3}). There was no significant difference between the ADCs of MPTs and those of pseudocysts. Both ADCs were significantly ($P < .01$) lower than those of CSF or microcystic serous tumors. In MPTs, the cysts and main pancreatic ducts (average ADC for pancreatic juice, 2.1×10^{-3} mm^2/sec $\pm$ 0.8×10^{-3}) had a similar signal intensity on diffusion-weighted MR images obtained with two diffusion gradients (Fig 1), which indicated the presence of mucinous products in both the cystic

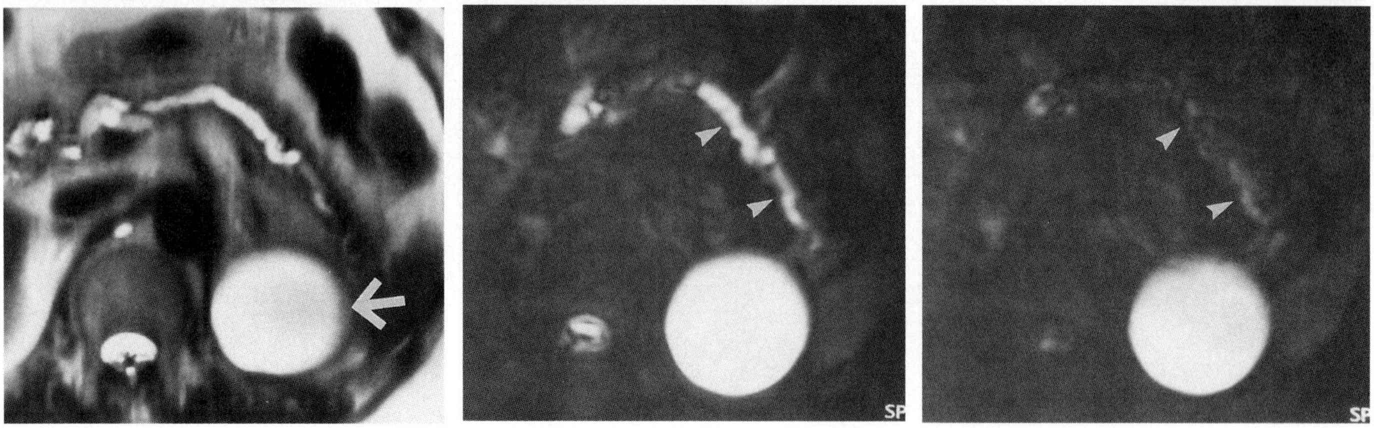

a. b. c.

Figure 3. Pseudocyst caused by acute pancreatitis in a 41-year-old man. **(a)** Axial half-Fourier single-shot turbo spin-echo MR image (∞/87) shows a unilocular cystic mass (arrow) in the hilum of the spleen. **(b)** Diffusion-weighted echo-planar MR image (∞/123) obtained with a *b* value of 30 sec/mm^2 shows high signal intensity in the lesion and the main pancreatic duct (arrowheads). **(c)** On a diffusion-weighted echo-planar MR image (∞/123) obtained with a *b* value of 300 sec/mm^2, the signal intensities of both the main pancreatic duct (arrowheads) and the cyst are markedly decreased relative to those in **b**, but both entities are still visible. The ADCs of the cyst and pancreatic juice are 4.1×10^{-3} and 6.0×10^{-3} mm^2/sec, respectively.

cavity and the main pancreatic duct. Although the signal intensity of cystic fluids in pseudocysts was high (average ADC, 3.1×10^{-3} mm^2/sec $\pm$ 0.8×10^{-3}) on diffusion-weighted images, that of the pancreatic duct was decreased (Fig 3).

DISCUSSION

Efforts have been directed to characterize various cystic lesions of the pancreas (12–16). It has been reported (12) that the total number of cysts and the size of most of the cysts within the mass are the two important criteria for the differentiation of the microcystic serous form from the mucinous subtype. However, clinical and radiologic criteria may not permit preoperative differentiation of the different types of pancreatic cystic lesions (3).

In histologic terms, MPT has been described (4,13,17) as an entity identical to a mucinous cystic neoplasm. An MPT is characterized by the presence of a mass that manifests as cystic dilatation of the side branch of the main pancreatic duct, which contains thick mucoid secretions. The mass consists of a conglomeration of communicating cysts covered by a rim of normal pancreatic parenchyma and a thin fibrous capsule. The cysts represent a dilated duct that is lined with papillary hyperplastic, atypical, or overtly malignant epithelium. Both the cystic cavity and the pancreatic duct are filled with mucinous secretions, and the papilla of Vater is occasionally dilated with mucous plugs.

In cases of MPT, US, CT, and MR imaging (especially MR cholangiopancreatography) demonstrate small lobulated or slightly irregularly marginated cystic masses; however, a definite diagnosis of MPT has been established on the basis of endoscopic retrograde cholangiopancreatographic findings, which include plugging of the papilla of Vater, mucin extrusion from the papillary orifice after intraductal injection of contrast medium, filling defects in the main pancreatic duct, and dilated main and branch pancreatic ducts in the absence of an obstructive ductal stricture (2). Localized cystic dilatation of a side branch duct, with grape-like clusters of contrast material pools, is often found. However, these multiloculated, conjugated cystic lesions have been confused with serous microcystic tumors or pseudocysts secondary to pancreatitis.

Cystic fluid analysis for cytologic findings, presence of tumor markers and enzymes, and viscosity has been proposed as an aid in the differential diagnosis of pancreatic cystic lesions (5). Cystic fluid may be obtained at CT-guided or US-guided needle aspiration. The viscosity of the cystic fluid has proved (18) to be useful for distinguishing mucinous tumors from other cystic lesions, with 89% sensitivity and 100% specificity. It has been reported (5) that a viscosity value greater than that of normal serum is virtually diagnostic for a mucinous tumor, whereas a value less than that of normal serum is seen in pseudocysts, serous tumors, and occasionally in mucinous tumors with a low mucin content.

ADC of Tissues at Diffusion-weighted MR Imaging

Lesion and Tissue	ADC (mm^2/sec)
Mucinous tumor	
Cystic fluid (n = 11)	$2.9 \times 10^{-3} \pm 0.9 \times 10^{-3}$*
Main pancreatic duct (n = 6)	$2.1 \times 10^{-3} \pm 0.8 \times 10^{-3}$*
Pseudocyst	
Cystic fluid (n = 10)	$3.2 \times 10^{-3} \pm 1.0 \times 10^{-3}$*
Main pancreatic duct (n = 7)	$5.1 \times 10^{-3} \pm 1.7 \times 10^{-3}$
Microcystic tumor (n = 2)	4.1×10^{-3}, 3.9×10^{-3}†
Cerebrospinal fluid (n = 13)	$5.9 \times 10^{-3} \pm 2.0 \times 10^{-3}$

Note.—Data are the mean ± standard deviation, unless otherwise noted.

* ADC was significantly different from that of cerebrospinal fluid ($P < .01$).

† Standard deviation not calculated because there were only two patients. Numbers are data for each patient.

Diffusion is a measure of motion freedom and is a sensitive parameter with which to characterize tissue at the microscopic level (19,20). Diffusion-weighted MR imaging may prove to be helpful in the characterization of pathologic conditions in abdominal organs, although in vivo abdominal diffusion-weighted MR imaging studies have had limitations, primarily as a result of motion artifacts (21). With the evolution of echo-planar MR imaging, high-speed imaging has become possible by obtaining all spatial-encoding information after a single radio-frequency excitation, thus reducing the motion artifacts during image acquisition. It is now possible to perform echo-planar–based diffusion studies with commercially available imagers owing to the evolution of enhanced gradient systems.

Because diffusion is closely related to the viscosity of the fluid, the characterization of cystic fluid may be possible with diffusion-weighted echo-planar MR imaging. Both MPTs and pseudocysts had a lower ADC than cerebrospinal fluid. This is to be expected, because these lesions are composed of viscous fluid collections or necrotic tissue, and water mobility is relatively limited. In a population of randomly moving molecules (Brownian motion), motion along the direction of the gradient is different for each molecule, which results in a distribution of different phase shifts and a loss of signal. However, the difference in ADCs between MPTs and pseudocysts was not statistically significant. Presumably, the contents of a pseudocyst may vary, depending on the stage of pancreatitis. Instead, the ADC of the main pancreatic duct in patients with MPT was less than that in patients with a pseudocyst. This is probably because mucinous fluid often occupies the main pancreatic duct in patients with MPT, whereas serous pancreatic juice is found in patients with a pseudocyst.

We obtained ADCs of the fluid at the two gradients (*b* values). However, all fluids with a high ADC had high signal intensity on diffusion-weighted images obtained with a large *b* value. In clinical practice, therefore, we can assume the fluid to be viscous when diffusion-weighted images obtained with a large diffusion gradient show high signal intensity, which would obviate the need for calculating ADCs.

Our approach to the characterization of cystic tumors of the pancreas on the basis of diffusion-weighted echo-planar MR imaging findings may have several limitations. First, with this echo-planar imaging technique, there was severe image distortion due to susceptibility effects and chemical shift artifacts along the phase-encoding axis. Therefore, the ADCs of small lesions may be somewhat unreliable. Second, we needed to perform several acquisitions with different ADCs. There can be some section misregistration in the acquisition of ADCs. Third, some MPTs may show low viscosity and may not communicate with the main pancreatic duct. In such cases, a diagnosis of MPT may be difficult.

In conclusion, molecular diffusion appears to be a unique parameter for help in characterizing the fluid in pancreatic cystic lesions. The demonstration of viscous fluid in both the cystic cavity and the main pancreatic duct is suggestive of MPT. Diffusion-weighted echo-planar MR imaging is a promising technique for characterizing cystic masses on the basis of differences in ADCs, although its value awaits further evaluation in a larger number of cases.

APPENDIX

Diffusion through a magnetic field gradient causes intravoxel dephasing and a loss of signal intensity and is expressed as $S/S_0 = \exp(-bD)$, where S/S_0 is the signal intensity ratio between two images acquired with and without diffusion-sensitizing gradients, and D is the diffusion coefficient, which characterizes the ratio of diffusion motion. In biologic systems, perfusion, water transport, or bulk motion may contribute to signal loss; therefore the term "apparent diffusion coefficient" is used instead of D. In diffusion-weighted echo-planar MR imaging, a pair of diffusion-sensitizing gradients of equal area are applied around the 180° pulse to dephase and cause signal loss from moving protons but not from stationary protons. The b value is the factor that depends on the strength, duration, and separation of the diffusion-sensitizing gradients (22). The ADC for serial diffusion-weighted echo-planar MR sequences can be calculated as ADC $= (1/b)\ln(S/S_0)'$, where S and S_0 are the signal intensity in the regions of interest obtained with two b values.

References

1. Itai Y, Ohhashi K, Nagai H, et al. "Duct ectatic" mucinous cystadenoma and cystadenocarcinoma of the pancreas. Radiology 1986; 161:697–700.
2. Tenner S, Carr-Locke DL, Banks PA, et al. Intraductal mucin-hypersecreting neoplasm "mucinous ductal ectasia": endoscopic recognition and management. Am J Gastroenterol 1996; 91:2548–2554.
3. Warshaw A, Compton C, Lewandrowski K, et al. Cystic tumors of the pancreas: new clinical, radiologic, and pathologic observations in 67 patients. Ann Surg 1990; 212:432–445.
4. Furukawa T, Takahashi T, Kobari M, Matsuno S. The mucin-hypersecreting tumor of the pancreas: development and extension visualized by three-dimensional computerized mapping. Cancer 1992; 70: 1505–1513.
5. Lewandrowski K, Lee J, Southern J, Centeno B, Warshaw A. Cyst fluid analysis in the differential diagnosis of pancreatic cysts: a new approach to the preoperative assessment of pancreatic cystic lesions. AJR 1995; 164:815–819.
6. Le Bihan D, Breton E, Lallemand D, Aubin ML, Vignaud J, Laval-Jeantet M. Separation of diffusion and perfusion in intravoxel incoherent motion MR imaging. Radiology 1988; 168:497–505.
7. Le Bihan D. Molecular diffusion nuclear magnetic resonance imaging. Magn Reson Q 1991; 7:1–30.
8. Le Bihan D, Turner R, Douek PP. Diffusion MR imaging: clinical applications. AJR 1992; 159:591–599.
9. Moseley ME, Kucharczyk J, Mintorovitch J, et al. Diffusion-weighted MR imaging of acute stroke: correlation with T2-weighted and magnetic susceptibility–enhanced MR imaging in cats. AJNR 1990; 11:423–429.
10. Warach S, Chien D, Li W, Ronthal M, Edelman RR. Fast magnetic resonance diffusion-weighted imaging of acute human stroke. Neurology 1992; 42:1717–1723.
11. Turner R, Le Bihan D, Maier J, et al. Echo-planar imaging of intravoxel incoherent motion. Radiology 1990; 177:407–414.
12. Johnson CD, Stephens DH, Charbouneau JW, Carpenter HA, Welch TJ. Cystic pancreatic tumors: CT and sonographic assessment. AJR 1988; 151:1133–1138.
13. Itai Y, Moss AA, Ohtomo K. Computed tomography of cystadenoma and cystadenocarcinoma. Radiology 1982; 145:419–425.
14. Friedman AC, Lichtenstein JE, Dachman AH. Cystic neoplasms of the pancreas: radiologic-pathologic correlation. Radiology 1983; 149:45–50.
15. Ros PR, Hamrick-Turner JE, Chiechi MV, Ros LH, Gallego P, Burton SS. Cystic masses of the pancreas. RadioGraphics 1992; 12: 673–686.
16. Wolfman NT, Ramquist NA, Karstaedt N, Hopkins MB. Cystic neoplasms of the pancreas: CT and sonography. AJR 1982; 138:37–41.
17. Agostini S, Choux R, Payan MJ, et al. Mucinous pancreatic duct ectasia in the body of the pancreas. Radiology 1989; 170:815–816.
18. Lewandrowski K, Southern J, Pins MR, Compton CC, Warshaw A. Cyst fluid analysis in the differential diagnosis of pancreatic cysts: a comparison of pseudocysts, serous cystadenomas, mucinous cystic neoplasms, and mucinous cystadenocarcinoma. Ann Surg 1993; 217:41–47.
19. Carr HY, Purcell EM. Effects of diffusion on free precession in nuclear magnetic resonance experiments. Phys Rev 1954; 94:630–635.
20. Steijskal EO, Tanner JE. Spin diffusion measurements: spin echoes in the presence of a time-dependent field gradient. J Chem Phys 1965; 42:288–292.
21. Müller MF, Prasad P, Siewert B, Nissenbaum MA, Raptopoulos V, Edelman RR. Abdominal diffusion mapping with use of a whole-body echo-planar system. Radiology 1994; 190:475–478.
22. Edelman RR, Wielopolski P, Schmitt F. Echo-planar MR imaging. Radiology 1994; 192:600–612.

Louk F. I. J. Oudenhoven, MD
Robert K. J. Koumans, MD, PhD
Julien B. C. M. Puylaert, MD, PhD

Right Colonic Diverticulitis: US and CT Findings—New Insights about Frequency and Natural History[1]

Index terms:
Colon, CT, 75.12112
Colon, diverticula, 75.273
Colon, US, 75.12981

Radiology 1998; 208:611–618

[1] From the Departments of Diagnostic Radiology (L.F.I.J.O., J.B.C.M.P.) and Surgery (R.K.J.K.), Westeinde Hospital, Lijnbaan 32, 2512 VA The Hague, The Netherlands. Received June 23, 1997; revision requested September 4; final revision received March 20, 1998; accepted April 23. **Address reprint requests to** J.B.C.M.P.

PURPOSE: To evaluate how the use of ultrasonography (US) and computed tomography (CT) has changed insights on the frequency and natural history of right colonic diverticulitis.

MATERIALS AND METHODS: Clinical findings, US and CT images, and clinical and surgical records in 44 patients with a final diagnosis of right colonic diverticulitis seen over 11 years were retrospectively studied.

RESULTS: Of the 44 patients, three underwent diverticulectomy, and 41 were successfully treated conservatively. Follow-up US demonstrated a consistent change in the pattern of the findings of diverticulitis over time, with eventual spontaneous evacuation of the contents of the inflamed diverticulum into the colonic lumen. Five patients had recurrent symptoms; two of them underwent elective surgery. The frequency of right colonic diverticulitis was one in 34 appendectomies, which is nine times higher than that reported to date.

CONCLUSION: Right colonic diverticulitis is more common than has been previously reported. US and CT findings are characteristic and show a consistent pattern of changes over time. The natural history is benign, and surgical intervention can be avoided in the vast majority of patients.

Right-sided colonic diverticulitis is considered to be a rare condition in Western countries. Most often, it is an unexpected finding at surgery for presumed appendicitis (1–3). The reported frequency is about one in 300 appendectomies (4–10).

In contrast to sigmoid diverticula, which are acquired and are usually multiple, right-sided colonic diverticula are mostly congenital and solitary. Whereas sigmoid diverticula are false diverticula (ie, herniations of the mucosa through the muscularis), right-sided colonic diverticula are usually true diverticula, that is, outpouchings of the colonic wall consisting of all layers of the wall. Not surprisingly, in view of its congenital character, right-sided colonic diverticulitis can occur at any age. The peak prevalence is in patients aged 35–45 years (2,3).

The patient's history, when compared with the history in patients with appendicitis, generally is more protracted. Nausea and vomiting are less frequent, the pain is milder, and the point of maximum tenderness is more variable in location (usually higher up). This explains why the clinical diagnosis of cholecystitis is occasionally considered. In about one-third of cases, a palpable mass is present, which can be misinterpreted as an appendiceal mass or a cecal tumor (2).

The stage of the disease determines the surgical management of right-sided colonic diverticulitis. In the early stage, the inflamed diverticulum is resected, as is the appendix, to prevent possible confusion in the future. Resection is not attempted if an extensive inflammatory peridiverticular mass is found and is correctly recognized as diverticulitis. Preferential treatment in such cases is conservative, which has been successful in all reported cases (11,12). The diagnosis of right-sided colonic diverticulitis is, however, far from clear at surgery: In over 40% of cases, a right hemicolectomy is performed because of presumed malignancy (2,12–16).

Author contributions:
Guarantor of integrity of entire study, J.B.C.M.P.; study concepts and design, J.B.C.M.P.; definition of intellectual content, R.K.J.K., J.B.C.M.P.; literature research, L.F.I.J.O.; clinical studies, R.K.J.K., J.B.C.M.P., L.F.I.J.O.; data acquisition, L.F.I.J.O.; data analysis, R.K.J.K., L.F.I.J.O.; statistical analysis, R.K.J.K.; manuscript preparation, L.F.I.J.O.; manuscript editing, J.B.C.M.P.; manuscript review, L.F.I.J.O., R.K.J.K., J.B.C.M.P.

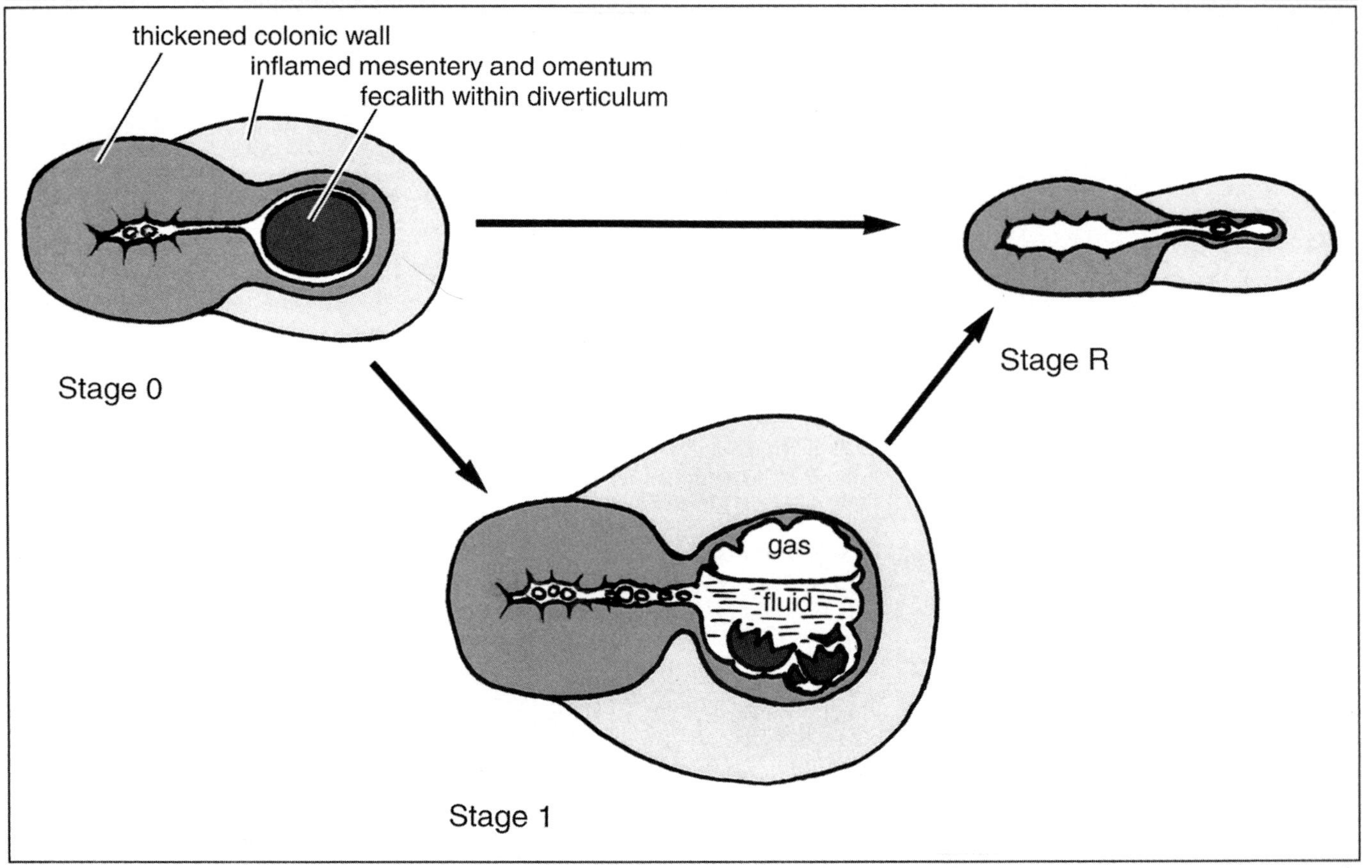

Figure 1. Schematic reconstruction of the natural history of right-sided colonic diverticulitis. The starting point is stage 0 inflammation of the diverticulum, which contains a fecalith and is surrounded by inflamed fat that represents mesentery and omentum. There is local, circumferential thickening of the colonic wall. Evacuation of the contents of the diverticulum takes place either directly (stage 0 evolving to stage R) or by means of the intermediate development of a small pericolonic abscess (stage 0 evolving to stage 1 evolving to stage R). The common end point after spontaneous evacuation is stage R, which is characterized by gradual resolution of the inflammatory abnormalities.

The authors of several reports have emphasized the role of ultrasonography (US) (17–21) and computed tomography (CT) (20,22,23) in the diagnosis of right-sided colonic diverticulitis and have reported (17,19) successful conservative management. The purpose of this study was to evaluate how the use of US and CT has changed insights about the frequency and natural history of right-sided colonic diverticulitis.

MATERIALS AND METHODS

From May 1985 to June 1996, a discharge diagnosis of right-sided colonic diverticulitis was established in 44 patients (19 male and 25 female patients; mean and median age, 37 years; age range 14–70 years) at our 600-bed community hospital; these patients constituted the study group. One patient was Asian, all others were white.

US was performed in all 44 patients according to the routine policy at our hospital with regard to patients with acute abdominal pain. CT was performed subsequently in 29 patients, with and without the use of a contrast agent. A number of US and CT units and various CT contrast agents were used during the course of this study. Follow-up US was performed in 29 patients, and follow-up clinical examination results were available in all 44. All US and CT images, reports, and clinical charts were studied retrospectively by two radiologists (L.F.I.J.O, J.B.C.M.P.). The original report made at the time of the initial US and CT examinations was the only basis for the assessment of the sensitivity of US and CT for the diagnosis of right-sided colonic diverticulitis. The images were correlated with clinical symptoms and laboratory data and were reviewed for changes in patterns over time.

The US criteria for the diagnosis of right-sided colonic diverticulitis that we used were (*a*) direct visualization of the diverticulum manifesting as a hyperechoic or hypoechoic outpouching of the right colonic wall and (*b*) localized circumferential wall thickening of the colon at the level of the diverticulum. The presence of a fecalith within the diverticulum and inflamed fat around the diverticulum provided additional support for the US diagnosis (17–21). The US criterion for a fecalith was the presence of a round or ovoid hyperechoic structure with a "clean" acoustic shadow (ie, with sharp boundaries). The US criterion for an abscess was the presence of irregular collections of gas, with or without fluid, in the diverticulum or in a cavity in the hyperechoic tissue adjacent to the colon. The US criterion for inflamed fat was the presence of hyperechoic, noncompressible tissue surrounding the diverticulum. In addition, the appendix should either have been not visible or have had a diameter of less than 6 mm.

The CT criterion for the diagnosis of right-sided colonic diverticulitis that we used was direct visualization of the diver-

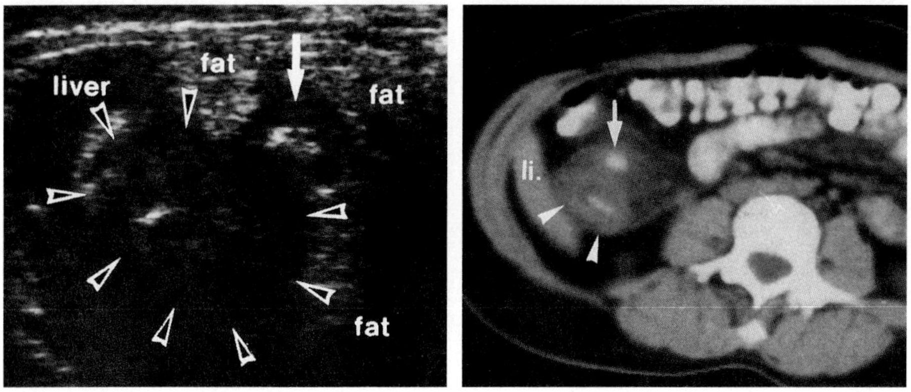

a. b.

Figure 2. Stage 0 right-sided colonic diverticulitis. **(a)** Axial US image through the ascending colon shows marked wall thickening (arrowheads) with the adjacent inflamed diverticulum (arrow), which contains a fecalith and is surrounded by inflamed fat. **(b)** Corresponding axial CT image shows the colon (arrowheads), with a small amount of contrast material in the collapsed lumen, and the diverticulum (arrow), which contains hyperattenuating material. In view of the US findings, this is probably a calcified fecalith. *li.* = liver.

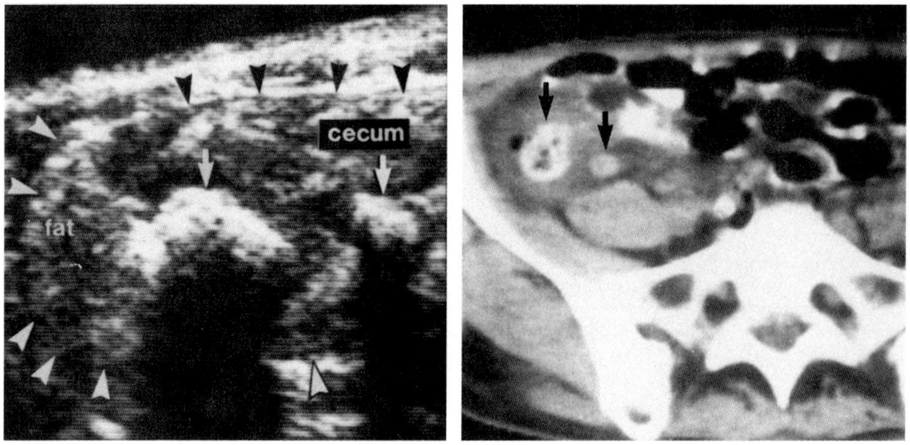

a. b.

Figure 3. Stage 0 cecal diverticulitis. **(a)** US image shows mural thickening of the cecum (black arrowheads) and two adjacent fecaliths (arrows). The larger fecalith is surrounded by a large mass of inflamed fat (white arrowheads). **(b)** CT image confirms the presence of the two calcified fecaliths (arrows). The small gas collection adjacent to the large fecalith and the surrounding inflammatory changes confirm the presence of inflammation.

ticulum as an outpouching of the right-sided hemicolon at the level of maximum circumferential wall thickening. The diverticulum was expected to contain gas, fluid, or calcified material with hyperattenuating strands in the surrounding fatty tissue adjacent to the diverticulum. There should be no evidence of appendicitis (20,22,23)

Disease in the patients was staged according to the method of Neff and vanSonnenberg (24) for the staging of sigmoid diverticulitis. Stage 0 represents the earliest stage of diverticulitis, with only phlegmonous changes around the diverticulum containing a fecalith (Figs 1–3). Stage 1 implies the presence of a small pericolonic abscess. We introduce here stage R diverticulitis, a residual stage of the disease after spontaneous evacuation: The diverticulum is empty, and the bowel wall thickening and the amount of surrounding inflamed fat have decreased (Fig 1).

The initial clinical diagnosis, the time from the onset of symptoms until hospital admission, and the total duration of symptoms were recorded. Body temperature at admission was measured, as were the maximum white blood cell count and erythrocyte sedimentation rate over the course of the disease. The pathology and surgical notes for seven patients who underwent surgery were reviewed. During the same 11 years, a total of 1,485 appendectomies were performed at our hospital.

RESULTS

Clinical Findings

Clinical and laboratory findings were comparable with those reported in the literature (1–3). The average duration of symptoms before hospital admission was 3.2 days (range, 1–12 days). The average total duration of symptoms was 5.9 days (range, 2–14 days). The average maximum erythrocyte sedimentation rate during the clinical course was 34 mm/h (range, 1–87 mm/h). The maximum white blood cell count during the course of the disease was 12.2×10^9 cells per liter (range, $4.8–20.3 \times 10^9$/L). The mean body temperature at the time of admission was 37.6°C (range, 36.0°C–38.8°C). The presumptive clinical diagnosis was acute appendicitis in 26 patients, an appendiceal mass in 10 patients, cholecystitis in four patients, right-sided colonic diverticulitis in three patients who had undergone appendectomy, and salpingitis in one patient.

US and CT Findings

The initial US examination was requested by the family practitioner in 10 patients, by the attending emergency room physician in 26, and by staff at the outpatient clinic in eight.

US enabled a confident diagnosis of right-sided colonic diverticulitis in 40 patients, which was reported as such at the time of the initial US examination. In the other four patients, US findings were suggestive of the diagnosis as one possibility but were not helpful in the differentiation of diverticulitis from appendicitis.

CT was performed in 29 patients. The diagnosis of right-sided colonic diverticulitis was confirmed in 27, but in the other two it was not possible to differentiate diverticulitis reliably from appendicitis. These two were part of the group of four patients in whom US findings were also equivocal.

The US features in the 44 patients corresponded to those described in the literature (17–19,25). Marked segmental circumferential wall thickening with preservation of the layer structure of the right-sided colonic wall was noted in 37 patients. Wall thickening was maximal at the level of the inflamed diverticulum, whereas the lumen of the colon at this location appeared collapsed. In seven patients, wall thickening was not circumferential but was limited to the side of the diverticulum. The diverticulum was identified with confidence in 40 patients; in four patients, it was impossible to differentiate it from a partially visualized appendix. In 26 patients, the diverticulum contained a fecalith with a clean acoustic shadow; in six patients, there were irregular gas collections with (n = 2) or without (n = 4) fluid, which were consistent with a pericolonic abscess; and in 12 patients, the diverticulum was small and hypoechoic, suggestive of a collapsed, empty diverticulum. In nine of these latter 12 patients, the diverticulum contained a very small gas collection. In all 44 patients, the diverticulum was surrounded by hyperechoic, noncompressible, fatty tissue, which represented mesentery and omentum. At graded compression US, the complex of the thickened colon, the diverticulum, and the surrounding inflamed fatty mesentery and omentum manifested as a single, firm, noncompressible mass.

The CT findings corresponded to the US features and were in agreement with those of previous reports (20,22,23). Of the 29 patients who underwent CT, 27 had findings of circumferential wall thickening. In the remaining two patients, there was only localized wall thickening at the side of the diverticulum. The diverticulum was identified in 27 patients; in two patients, it was impossible to differentiate it from an inflamed appendix. The surrounding fat had higher attenuation than normal in all patients. A calcified fecalith was identified in 17 patients; in 13 of these 17, there were areas of gas attenuation within the fecalith. An irregularly shaped gas collection without fluid was found in three patients, and an irregular gas collection with fluid was found in one patient. Seven patients had material with water attenuation and a very small gas collection within the diverticulum, and one patient had only water-attenuation material.

By using the combined US and CT data and the staging method for sigmoid diverticulitis proposed by Neff and vanSonnenberg (24), we categorized the 44 patients according to the stage of their diverticulitis at the time of admission. Twenty-six patients had stage 0 diverticulitis at admission. The mean diameter of the fecalith in these patients was 12 mm (range, 7–25 mm). In 20 of these 26 patients, a follow-up US study was available. The first US follow-up was performed 1–5 days (mean, 1.8 days) after admission to the hospital. A second US follow-up was performed in 15 patients 1–9 days (mean, 3.2 days) after the first follow-up, and a third US follow-up was performed in eight patients 1–15 days (mean, 4.5 days) after the second follow-up. The fecalith eventually resolved and was no longer visible in 18 patients in whom US depicted an empty diverticulum that manifested as a hypoechoic structure with, in 15 patients, a small gas collection (stage R; Figs 4, 5). These residual features slowly resolved in 1–2 weeks but markedly lagged behind the clinical improvement, which occurred quite abruptly and coincided with the disappearance of the fecalith (stage 0 evolving to stage R). Two of the 20 patients in whom US follow-up was performed developed, in due course, a small pericolonic abscess (stage 1) at the side of the diverticulum; in both patients, the contents of these abscesses evacuated into the colonic lumen (stage 0 evolving to stage 1 evolving to stage R; Fig 6).

Six of 44 patients had stage 1 diverticulitis at admission. The pericolonic abscess

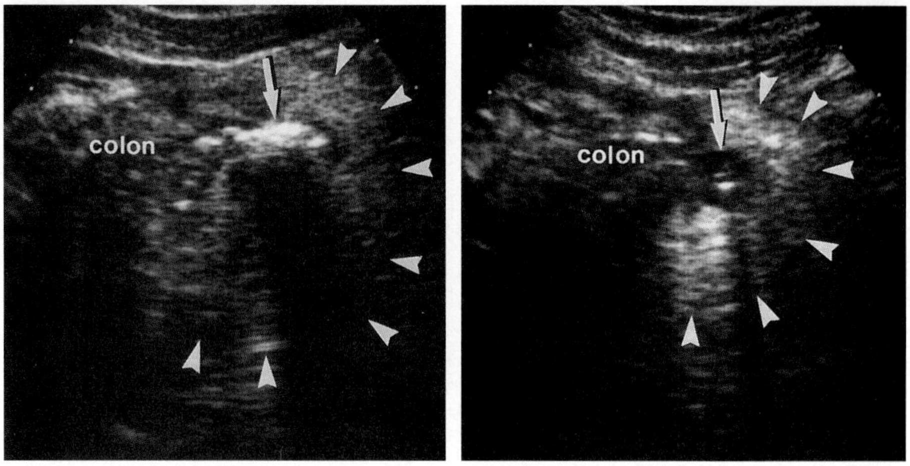

a. b.

Figure 4. Stage 0 evolving to stage R right-sided colonic diverticulitis. **(a)** US image shows a large fecalith (arrow) within the colonic diverticulum. The surrounding inflamed fat (arrowheads) was noncompressible. **(b)** US image obtained 1 day after **a** shows that the fecalith has been evacuated to the colonic lumen, and the diverticulum (arrow) is empty. There is still a considerable mass of inflamed fat (arrowheads) around the diverticulum, but the patient was symptom free.

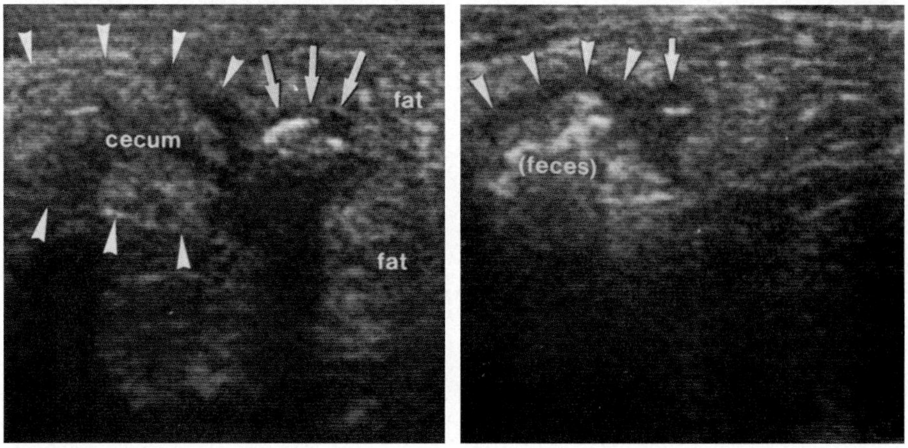

a. b.

Figure 5. Stage 0 evolving to stage R cecal diverticulitis. **(a)** US image shows the contracted, thickened cecum (arrowheads) and a diverticulum (arrows) containing a large fecalith. The diverticulum is surrounded by inflamed, noncompressible fat. **(b)** US image obtained 4 days after **a** shows that the fecalith has been evacuated to the cecal lumen, and the diverticulum (arrow) contains only a residual gas collection. The cecal wall (arrowheads) is thinner, and the lumen contains feces again, which is evidence of regained bowel function. The patient recalled the passage of a "grayish stone" in the stool 1 day before this image was obtained.

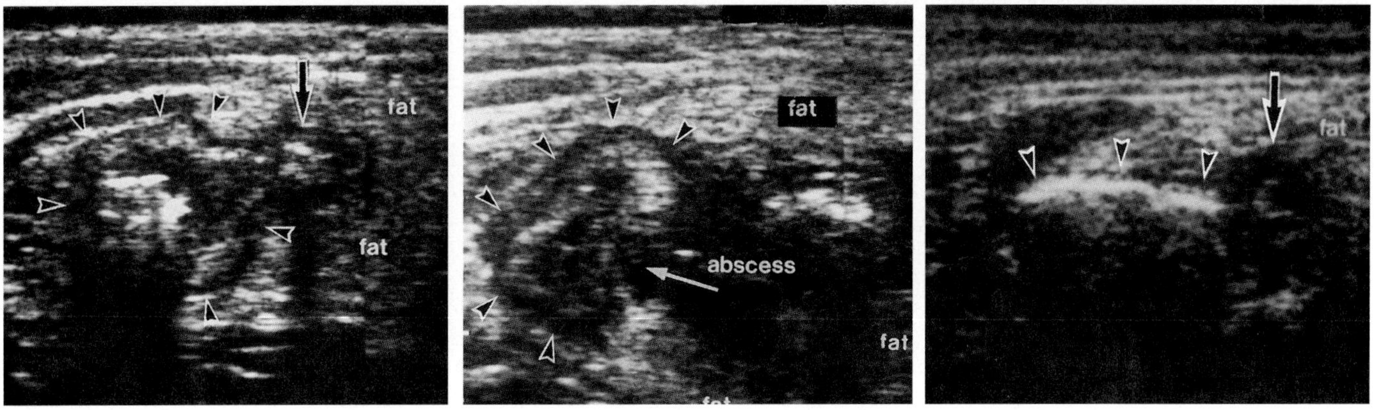

a. b. c.

Figure 6. The three stages of right-sided colonic diverticulitis in one patient. **(a)** Stage 0. Transverse US image shows the ascending colon (arrowheads) and the diverticulum, which contains a fecalith (arrow). Note the large mass of surrounding, inflamed fat. **(b)** Stage 1. US image obtained 4 days after **a** shows that the inflamed diverticulum has changed into a 3-cm-diameter pericolonic abscess (arrow) and is still surrounded by hyperechoic, noncompressible tissue. This represents the fatty mesentery and omentum, which is in the process of sealing off the abscess. Note the bulging of the abscess into the lumen of the colon (arrowheads), which may be a sign of impending evacuation. **(c)** Stage R. US image obtained 9 days after **b** shows that the abscess has completely evacuated to the colonic lumen, and the inflammatory mass surrounding the empty diverticulum (arrow) has largely resolved. The colon (arrowheads) now has a normal, thin wall and contains feces, indicating the return of normal function.

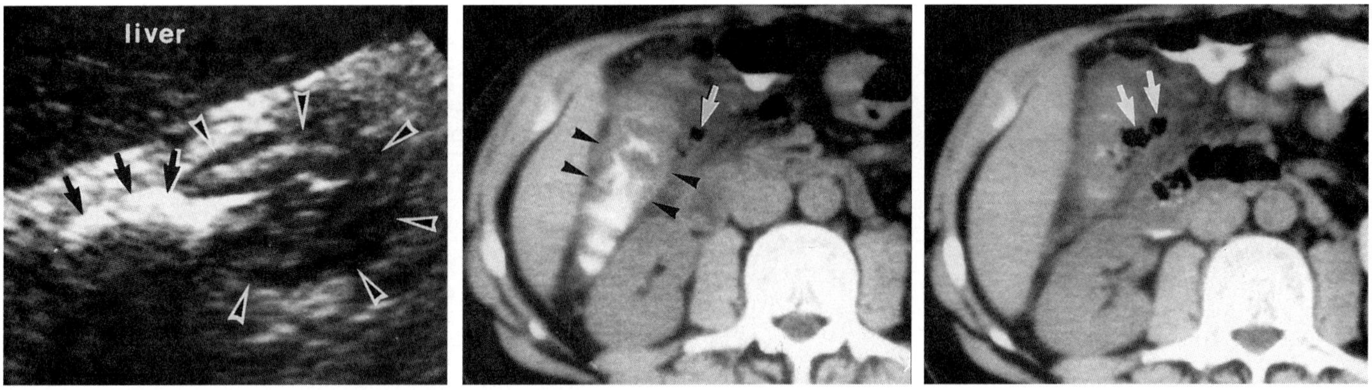

a. b. c.

Figure 7. Stage 1 right-sided colonic diverticulitis of the hepatic flexure of the colon. **(a)** US image obtained medial to the right lobe of the liver reveals marked colonic wall thickening (arrowheads). Adjacent to the colon is an abscess (arrows), with hyperechoic contents, in continuity with the lumen. This gas-filled tract indicates impending evacuation. **(b, c)** Contiguous axial CT sections confirm colonic wall thickening (arrowheads in **b**) and a 2-cm-diameter pericolonic abscess (arrow in **b**, arrows in **c**) surrounded by inflamed fat. The patient experienced an uneventful recovery after conservative treatment.

contained gas or both gas and fluid and had a mean diameter of 16 mm (range, 10–28 mm; Figs 7, 8). In four, a gas-filled tract between the diverticulum and the colonic lumen was visible (Figs 7, 8). In the three patients in whom follow-up US was performed, this situation evolved to stage R, with eventual complete resolution of all abnormalities (stage 1 evolving to stage R; Fig 9).

The remaining 12 patients had stage R diverticulitis at admission, and all 12 were already showing clinical improvement at that time.

The exact location of the inflamed diverticulum was established in all 29 patients who underwent CT (Fig 10).

Clinical Treatment

Of the 26 patients with a clinical diagnosis of acute appendicitis, seven underwent appendectomy. In three of these seven patients, the inflamed diverticulum was resected; in the other four, the diverticulum was not resected. Further conservative management was successful. The remaining 19 patients were treated conservatively. In seven of these 19 patients, a scheduled appendectomy was canceled on account of the US and CT findings.

In the 10 patients with a clinically suspected appendiceal mass, who were scheduled to undergo a postponed appendectomy, the operation was eventually canceled on the strength of the US and CT findings. In one patient with clinically suspected salpingitis, an intended laparoscopy was not performed because of the US and CT findings.

Altogether, 41 patients were treated conservatively, including the four who underwent appendectomy but did not undergo resection of the inflamed diverticulum. Three patients received antibiotics, and two received parenteral nutrition. All 41 patients recovered without further surgical intervention. Thirty-six remained symptom free (follow-up range, 4–139 months; mean, 60 months). Five patients had recurrent diverticulitis that was again successfully treated conservatively; two of these five had a history of recurrent attacks of diverticulitis; one eventually underwent an elective diverticulectomy, and the other, a right hemicolectomy. At no time did we observe large abscesses, free perforation to the peritoneal cavity, or other complications.

DISCUSSION

Frequency

Before the advent of US and CT, the diagnosis of right-sided colonic diverticulitis was almost exclusively made at laparotomy, which was performed in most cases for presumed appendicitis. The frequency of right-sided colonic diverticulitis in Western countries, calculated on the basis of accumulated reports (4–9) is one case in 300 appendectomies. On the basis of the 44 patients in 11 years and the 1,485 appendectomies performed during that same period, the frequency at our hospital is one case per 34 appendectomies, which is approximately nine times higher than the reported frequency.

A ready explanation for the high frequency of right-sided colonic diverticulitis in our study is our liberal use of US in patients with abdominal pain. Over the past decade, essentially all patients with acute or subacute abdominal pain have undergone US in an early stage of their diagnostic work-up (26,27). As a result, the correct diagnosis of right-sided colonic diverticulitis, which would otherwise have been overlooked, was established. Overlooking the correct diagnosis could have occurred in patients with relatively mild symptoms, in whom immediate surgery is not considered, and in patients with a clinical diagnosis of an appendiceal mass, in whom the usual treatment is conservative. Because the latter group of patients would undergo a postponed appendectomy—if they undergo an appendectomy at all—inflammatory signs will have disappeared by then, and with those signs, the chance to make the correct diagnosis.

Some cases of right-sided colonic diverticulitis may remain undetected even at laparotomy. In two of seven patients in our study who underwent an immediate appendectomy, the inflamed diverticulum was situated too far cranially and could not be reached via the gridiron incision. Only after extension of the incision and surgical mobilization of the right side of the colon, as suggested by the US findings, was the diverticulum detected.

In a considerable number of patients,

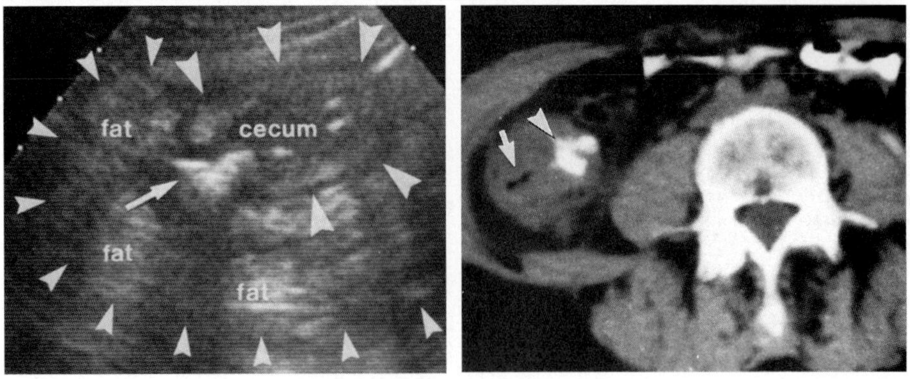

a. b.

Figure 8. Stage 1 cecal diverticulitis. **(a)** US image shows hyperechoic material in the diverticulum (arrow) and a gas-filled tract from the diverticulum to the cecal lumen. The cecal wall (large arrowheads) is thickened, and the diverticulum is surrounded by a large quantity of inflamed fat (small arrowheads). **(b)** Corresponding CT image confirms the presence of gas collections in a small pericolonic abscess (arrow) and a little contrast material in the collapsed cecal lumen (arrowhead).

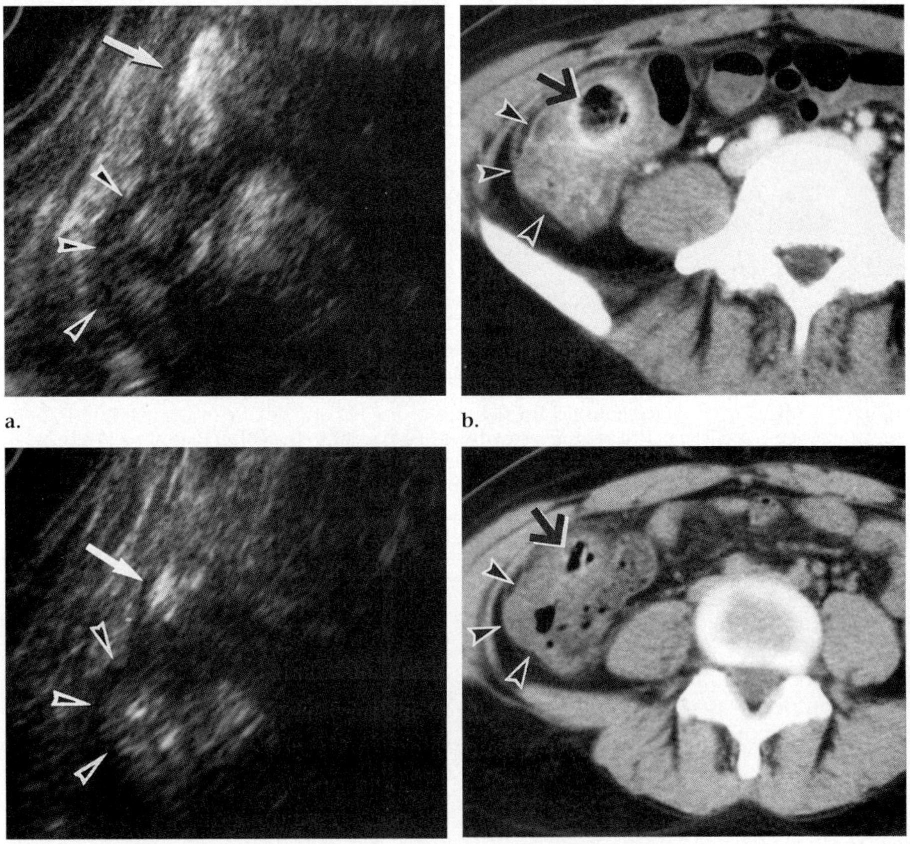

a. b. c. d.

Figure 9. Stage 1 evolving to stage R right-sided colonic diverticulitis. **(a)** US image reveals a pericolonic abscess (arrow) next to the contracted colon (arrowheads). **(b)** CT image confirms the presence of a 2-cm-diameter abscess (arrow) with a contrast-enhanced wall next to the colon (arrowheads), which has a markedly thickened wall and a collapsed lumen. **(c)** US image obtained 3 days after **b** shows that the abscess (arrow) is now much smaller, and the colonic wall (arrowheads) is thinner. The patient reported feeling better. **(d)** CT image confirms the marked decrease in both the size of the abscess (arrow) and the thickness of the colonic wall (arrowheads).

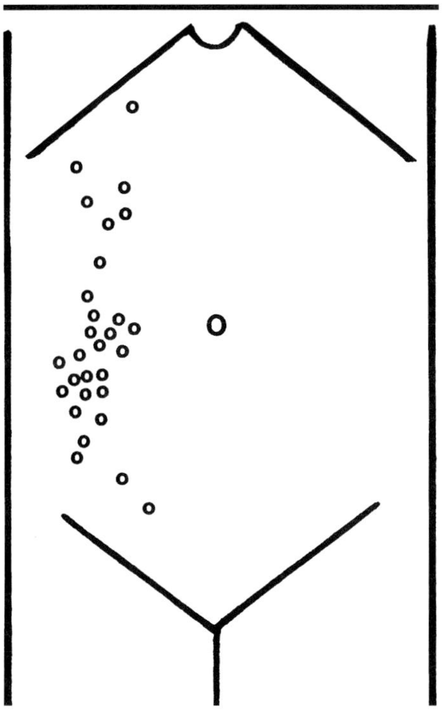

Figure 10. Schematic shows the variation in location of the inflamed diverticulum (○). These locations were determined on the basis of the CT findings in 29 patients.

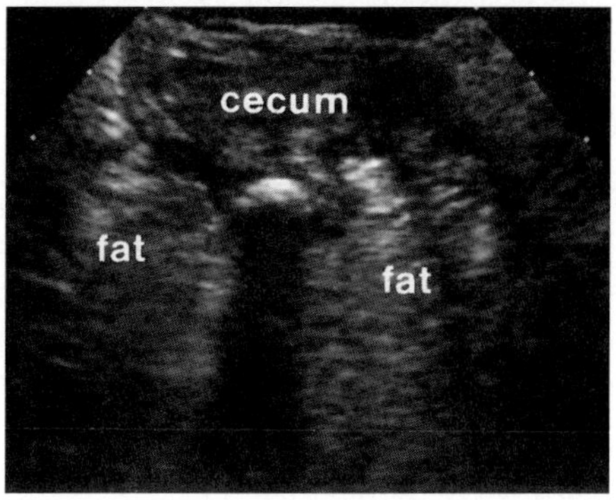

Figure 11. Pitfall in the US diagnosis of right-sided colonic diverticulitis. US image depicts cecal wall thickening and a fecalith within an outpouching of the cecum, which is surrounded by inflamed fat. The appendix is not visible. The US diagnosis was cecal diverticulitis. At surgery, appendicitis was found, with a fecalith in the base of the appendix.

therefore, the correct diagnosis will never be established without the use of imaging findings. The frequency of one case in 34 appendectomies found in this study, as well as the incidence of four cases per year at our 600-bed hospital, suggests that right-sided colonic diverticulitis is more common than has been previously assumed.

Diagnosis

The contents of the inflamed diverticulum have been variously described as hyperechoic or hypoechoic on US images (18,19,28) and as hyperattenuating or hypoattenuating areas on CT images (22,23). Our findings readily explain the variety among these observations by showing a pattern of change over time on the US and CT images. By reconstructing the corresponding morphologic-pathologic events, right-sided colonic diverticulitis appears to begin as stage 0, with the involved diverticulum containing a fecalith. This fecalith is relatively large, with a mean diameter of 12 mm (range, 7–25 mm; Fig 3). After a variable period of inflammation, the fecalith evacuates into the colonic lumen, either directly or by means of the intermediate development of a small pericolonic abscess (stage 1; Fig 6). The final stage—stage R—is the same for both the stage 0 and the stage 0 evolving to stage 1 pathways. A schematic reconstruction of the course of these events is illustrated in Figure 1. Bear in mind that it is not always possible to distinguish at US between stage 0 and stage 1, especially when the abscess is very small. It is also impossible at US or CT to differentiate a pus collection confined to the boundaries of the diverticulum from a pus collection in the surrounding tissue adjacent to the colon and outside the boundaries of the diverticulum. We have used the term pericolonic abscess to describe both situations.

In six of eight patients with a pericolonic abscess, US showed an obvious gas-filled tract between the diverticulum and the colonic lumen, which presumably indicated the onset of evacuation. A gas-filled tract was also seen in six patients with stage R diverticulitis. Once the diverticulitis had reached stage R, the clinical symptoms resolved (Figs 4–6, 9), with erythrocyte sedimentation rates slowly returning to normal. Resolution of the US abnormalities markedly lagged behind the clinical improvement.

When patients with right-sided colonic diverticulitis undergo surgery during an advanced stage of the disease, a large mass can be palpated in the colon. The sonographic substrate of this mass can be visualized during graded compression US when the complex of the thickened colonic wall, diverticulum, and surrounding inflamed fatty mesentery and omentum responds to compression as a single, firm mass.

US facilitated a confident diagnosis of right-sided colonic diverticulitis in 40 of 44 patients. Subsequent CT was performed in 29 of 44 patients. CT was performed in four patients because the US results were equivocal. In the other 25 patients, CT was performed because the surgeon wanted the highest level of confidence possible in view of the considerable consequence of the correct diagnosis on clinical decision making with regard to surgical versus nonsurgical treatment. The difficulty in convincing the surgeons is illustrated by the fact that, in the early years of our study, three patients underwent appendectomy despite a confident US diagnosis of right-sided colonic diverticulitis.

US and CT findings of right-sided colonic diverticulitis are, in most cases, quite characteristic. At US, however, confusion with appendicitis remains possible. In four of the patients in our study, we were unable to differentiate appendicitis from cecal diverticulitis on the basis of US results, and in two of these four we were also unable to render a confident diagnosis on the basis of CT findings. As a result, these four patients were selected to undergo surgery; all four had cecal diverticulitis. In three other patients who were evaluated early in the study, US facilitated a definite diagnosis of right-sided colonic diverticulitis, but the surgeons still decided to operate because the clinical findings strongly suggested appendicitis.

All in all, we had surgical proof in only seven of 44 patients. This low rate of surgical confirmation is the direct consequence of our first aim, namely, to prevent unnecessary surgery in patients. One might argue that one or more of the 37 patients without surgical proof in fact had a self-limiting condition other than right-sided colonic diverticulitis. One possibility is an appendiceal mass that, like right-sided colonic diverticulitis, may successfully respond to conservative treatment and may have identical clinical findings. If the secondary colonic wall thickening, the fecalith, and the inflamed fat associated with the appendiceal mass are visualized on US and CT images but the inflamed appendix is overlooked, an incorrect diagnosis of right-sided colonic diverticulitis might be made. In our opinion, however, it is unlikely that this happened in many patients.

Other possible pitfalls are epiploic appendagitis or right-sided segmental infarction of the omentum (29–32), which also have a benign, self-limiting course and clinical and laboratory findings similar to those of right-sided colonic diverticulitis. In cases of epiploic appendagitis and omental infarction, however, there is no fecalith or abscess present. Colonic wall thickening may be present in epiploic appendagitis but is usually subtle and not circumferential. Confusion of epiploic appendagitis or omental infarction with right-sided colonic diverticulitis on US and CT images is therefore unlikely. Confusion of right-sided colonic diverticulitis on US and CT images with ileocecal Crohn disease or cecal carcinoma is possible, but these diagnoses would eventually have been established during follow-up.

With only seven surgically proved cases and 37 cases with a final diagnosis based on a combination of clinical course and follow-up findings, any calculation of the sensitivity of US and CT is of limited value. In this retrospective study that included only patients with a final diagnosis of right-sided colonic diverticulitis, the sensitivity of US and CT for the diagnosis of right-sided colonic diverticulitis can be calculated to be 91% and 93%, respectively. Our data do not permit an estimate of the specificity, because there were no reliable records to establish the number of patients in whom a US or CT diagnosis of right-sided colonic diverticulitis was rendered but who in fact had appendicitis. To the best of our knowledge, in the 11 years of our study we have rendered a false-positive diagnosis in only two patients, which in one case led to a 12-hour delay before surgery. In both patients appendicitis was found, with a fecalith in the appendiceal base (Fig 11). Another potential pitfall, which we did not encounter, is confusion with a cecal carcinoma (20).

Natural History and Therapy

To date, more than 900 patients with right-sided colonic diverticulitis have been described in the literature (2,12,15,23,33). To our knowledge, formation of a large abscess has been reported in only two cases (2), and free perforation to the peritoneal cavity has never been described. This underlines the benign and self-limiting character of right-sided colonic diverticulitis. Our finding that all 41 patients treated conservatively recovered without problems supports the notion that the natural history of right-sided colonic diverticulitis is essentially benign, and that treatment can be primarily nonsurgical.

The use of antibiotics in the treatment of diverticulitis is controversial: At our hospital, as at most institutes in The Netherlands, antibiotics are not administered routinely in patients with diverticulitis. Therefore, only three patients in our study received antibiotics, because of persistent fever (>39°C) that lasted longer than 2 days.

Five patients in our study had recurrent symptoms after pain-free intervals of 6, 13, 19, 37, and 58 months. In three of these five patients, an elective barium enema study showed multiple diverticula confined to the right hemicolon. One of the five patients continued to complain of nagging pain and eventually underwent an elective diverticulectomy. Another patient with multiple diverticula underwent a right hemicolectomy after experiencing four bouts of right-sided colonic diverticulitis. The other three patients were successfully treated conservatively for the second time and thereafter remained symptom free.

Conclusion

Our results show that right-sided colonic diverticulitis occurs much more frequently than was previously assumed and its natural history is benign, which allows primarily nonsurgical treatment. US—complemented with CT, if necessary—permits a rapid and reliable diagnosis, thus preventing an unnecessary appendectomy or other more extensive surgical procedures such as a right hemicolectomy. Follow-up US can be used to monitor the natural evolution of the disease, which shows a consistent and recognizable pattern.

Acknowledgment: The authors are indebted to Arie M. Rijke, MD, of the University of Virginia, Charlottesville for his assistance in the preparation of the manuscript.

References

1. Scully RE, Mark EJ, McNeely WF, McNeely BU. A 46-year-old man with right-lower-quadrant pain and thickening of the wall of the cecum. Massachusetts General Hospital Case Records, case 33-1987. N Engl J Med 1987; 317:432–434.
2. Wagner DE, Zollinger RW. Diverticulitis of the cecum and ascending colon. Arch Surg 1961; 83:124–131.
3. Beranbaum SL, Zausner J, Lane B. Diverticular disease of the right colon. AJR 1972; 115:334–348.
4. Silberman VA. Appendectomy in a large metropolitan hospital: retrospective analysis of 1013 cases. Am J Med 1981; 142:615–618.
5. Pieper R, Kager L, Nasman P. Acute appendicitis: a clinical study of 1082 cases of emergency appendectomy. Acta Chir Scand 1982; 148:51–62.
6. Lewis FR, Holcroft JW, Boey J, Dunphy JE. Appendicitis: a critical review of diagnosis and treatment in 1000 cases. Arch Surg 1975; 110:677–684.
7. Gilmore OJA, Brownett JP, Griffin PH, et al. Appendicitis and mimicking conditions. Lancet 1975; 2:421–424.
8. Jess P, Bjerregaard B, Brynitz S, Holst-Christensen J, Kalaja E, Lund-Kristensen J. Acute appendicitis: prospective trial concerning diagnostic accuracy and complications. Am J Surg 1981; 141:232–234.
9. Fischer MG, Farkas AM. Diverticulitis of the cecum and ascending colon. Dis Colon Rectum 1984; 7:454–458.
10. Chang FC, Hogle HH, Welling DR. The fate of the negative appendix. Am J Surg 1973; 126:752–754.
11. Ngoi SS, Chia J, Goh MY, Sim E, Rauff A. Surgical management of the right colon diverticulitis. Dis Colon Rectum 1992; 35:799–802.
12. Crist DW, Fishman EK, Scatarige JC, Cameron JL. Acute diverticulitis of the cecum and ascending colon diagnosed by computed tomography. Surg Gynecol Obstet 1988; 166:99–102.
13. Markham NI, Li AKC. Diverticulitis of the right colon: experience from Hong Kong. Gut 1992; 33:547–549.
14. Mealy K. Solitary caecal diverticula presenting with right iliac fossa pain. Br J Hosp Med 1989; 41:284–285.
15. McFee AS, Sutton PG, Ramos R. Diverticulitis of the right colon. Dis Colon Rectum 1982; 25:254–256.
16. Kaufman Z, Shpits B, Reina A, Dinbar A. Cecal diverticulitis presented as a cecal tumor. Am Surg 1990; 56:675–677.
17. Puylaert JBCM. Caecal diverticulitis. In: Ultrasound of appendicitis and its differential diagnosis. Berlin, Germany: Springer-Verlag, 1990; 81–84.
18. Townsend RR, Jeffrey RB, Laing FC. Cecal diverticulitis differentiated from appendicitis using graded compression sonography. AJR 1989; 152:1229–1230.
19. Wada M, Kikuchi Y, Doy M. Uncomplicated acute diverticulitis of the cecum and ascending colon: sonographic findings in 18 patients. AJR 1990; 155:283–287.
20. Jeffrey RB. The gastrointestinal tract. In: Jeffrey RB, ed. CT and sonography of the acute abdomen. New York, NY: Raven, 1989; 201–259.
21. Wilson SR. Gastrointestinal tract sonography. Abdom Imaging 1996; 21:1–8.
22. Balthazar EJ, Megibow AJ, Gordon RB, Hulnick D. Cecal diverticulitis: evaluation with CT. Radiology 1987; 162:79–81.
23. Scatarige JC, Fishman EK, Crist DW, Cameron JL, Siegelman SS. Diverticulitis of the right colon: CT observations. AJR 1987; 148:737–739.
24. Neff CC, vanSonnenberg E. CT of diverticulitis: diagnosis and treatment. Radiol Clin North Am 1989; 27:743–752.
25. Wilson SR, Toi A. The value of sonography in the diagnosis of acute diverticulitis of the colon. AJR 1990; 154:1199–1202.
26. Puylaert JBCM, Rutgers PH, Lalisang RI, et al. A prospective study of ultrasonography in the diagnosis of appendicitis. N Engl J Med 1987; 317:666–669.
27. Puylaert JBCM. When in doubt, sound it out (editorial). Radiology 1994; 191:320–321.
28. Yacoe ME, Jeffrey RB. Sonography of appendicitis and diverticulitis. Radiol Clin North Am 1994; 32:899–912.
29. Rioux M, Langis P. Primary epiploic appendagitis: clinical, US, and CT findings in 14 cases. Radiology 1994; 191:523–526.
30. Rao PM, Wittenberg J, Lawrason JN. Primary epiploic appendagitis: evolutionary changes in CT appearance. Radiology 1997; 204:713–717.
31. Puylaert JBCM. Right-sided segmental infarction of the omentum: clinical, US, and CT findings. Radiology 1992; 185:169–172.
32. Karak PK, Millmond SH, Neumann D, Yamase HT, Ramsby G. Omental infarction: report of three cases and review of the literature. Abdom Imaging 1998; 23:96–98.
33. Anderson L, Minn R. Acute diverticulitis of the cecum. Surgery 1947; 22:479–488.

Diagnosis Please

Patrick M. Rao, MD
Robert A. Novelline, MD

Case 6[1]

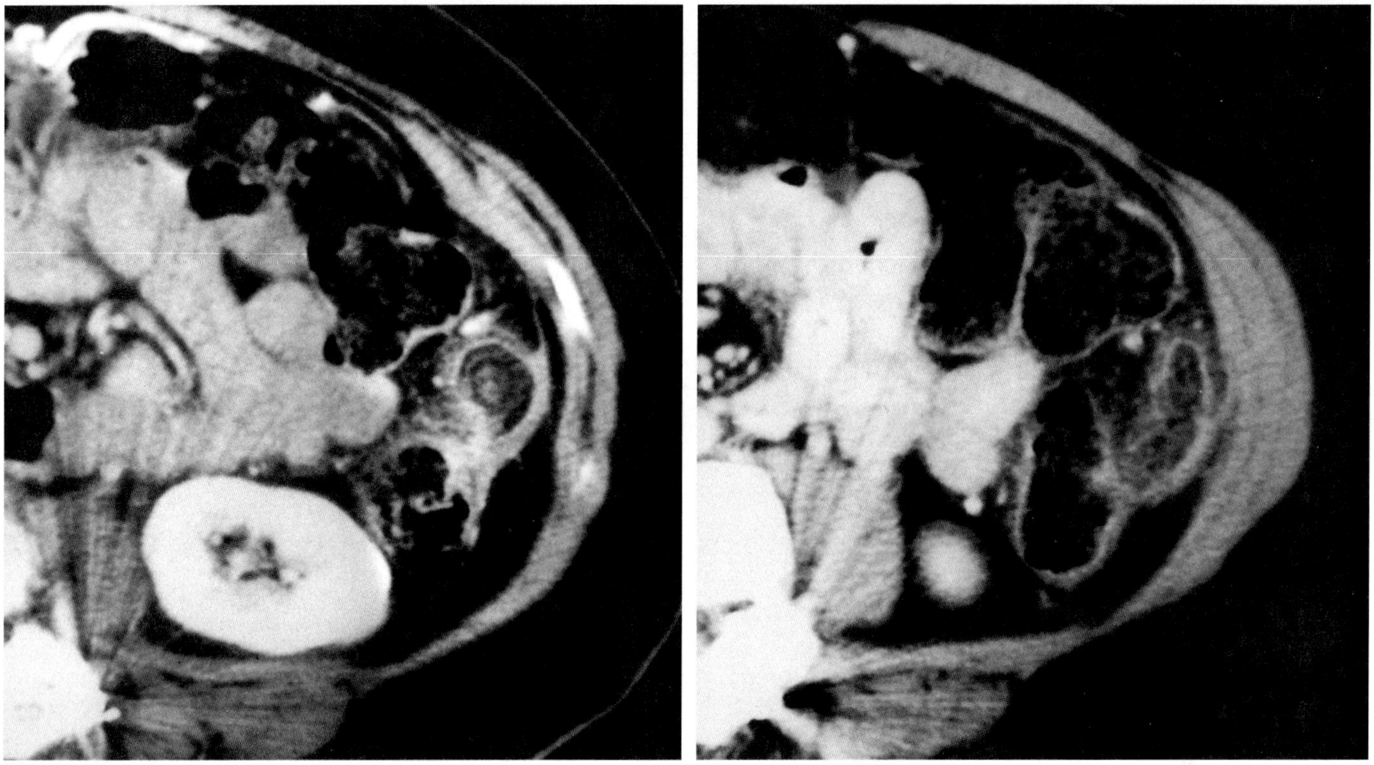

a. b.

Figure 1. Initial abdominopelvic CT scan obtained after oral and intravenous administration of contrast material (a) at the level of the left renal hilum and (b) at the level of the inferior pole of the left kidney.

HISTORY

A 46-year-old woman presented to our emergency department with left lower abdominal quadrant pain of 3 days duration.
(continued)

Index term:
Diagnosis please

Radiology 1998; 208:619–620

[1] From the Department of Radiology, Massachusetts General Hospital, 32 Fruit St, Boston, MA 02114. Received January 15, 1998; revision requested March 10; revision received March 23; accepted April 28. **Address reprint requests to** P.M.R.

Submit the most likely diagnosis to *dxplease@rsna.org* (use ***only*** for submission of diagnosis). Include case number, your name (as you would want it to appear in the journal), address, phone and fax numbers. Multiple diagnoses, multiple submissions, submissions without a case number will not be considered. ***Deadline:*** November 13, 1998. Answer will appear in the January 1999 issue. See also the editorial by Proto (p 1) in the April 1998 issue.

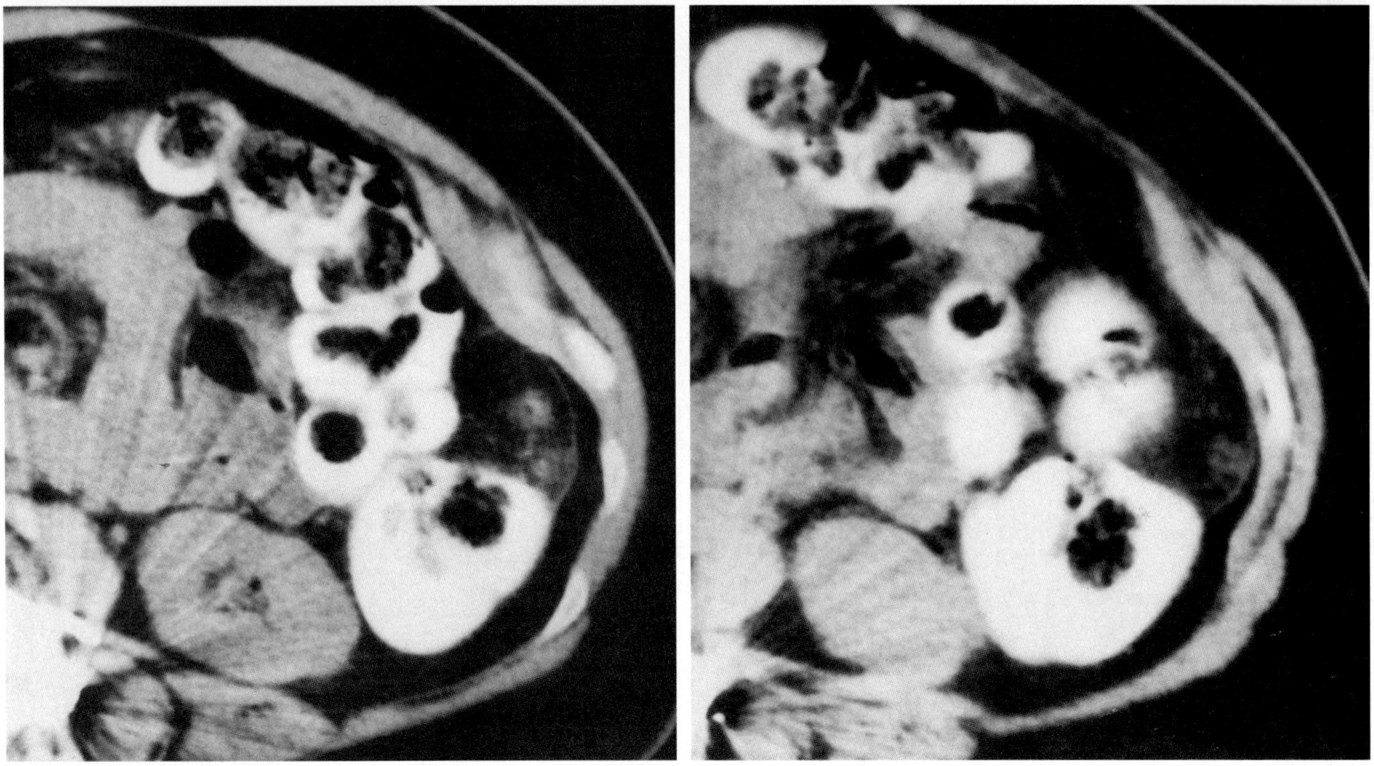

a. b.

Figure 2. Five-week follow-up abdominopelvic CT scan obtained, after the administration of colon contrast material, **(a)** at the level of the left renal hilum and **(b)** at the level of the lower pole of the left kidney.

The pain was sudden in onset, sharp in nature, and relatively constant. It worsened with cough, deep breathing, and abdominal stretching. She denied associated nausea, vomiting, anorexia, diarrhea, constipation, or fever.

On physical examination, the patient's tenderness was localized to the left lower abdominal quadrant, and there was associated rebound tenderness and guarding. No other physical findings were evident. Laboratory values were unremarkable, including a normal white blood cell count of 7,300/mm^3 (7.3×10^9/L) .

The patient underwent an abdominopelvic computed tomographic (CT) examination (Fig 1). A diagnosis was made, and the patient was discharged from the emergency department. Seven days after onset of symptoms, her pain subsided and did not recur. Five weeks after the initial CT examination, she underwent follow-up CT (Fig 2).

Lane F. Donnelly, MD
George S. Bisset III, MD
Donald P. Frush, MD

Case 2: Embryonal Rhabdomyosarcoma of the Biliary Tree[1]

CLINICAL HISTORY

A 2-year-old, previously healthy boy presents with a 2-month history of malaise, fever, and jaundice.

IMAGING FINDINGS

Computed tomography (CT) of the abdomen shows marked intrahepatic and extrahepatic bile duct dilatation (Fig 1). There is a soft-tissue mass within the porta hepatis, in the expected location of the lower common bile duct (Fig 1b). The mass is indistinguishable from the pancreatic head and second portion of the duodenum. There is retroperitoneal and mesenteric lymphadenopathy (Fig 1c).

Intraoperative cholangiogram shows a large, lobulated, intraluminal mass distending and obstructing the common bile duct (Fig 2). There is marked bile duct dilatation proximal to the mass. The greatest degree of bile duct dilatation, however, is at the level of the mass within the common bile duct, rather than in the ducts proximal to the obstruction. There is a second intraluminal mass within the biliary tree at the confluence of the right and left hepatic ducts (Fig 2).

DISCUSSION

Embryonal rhabdomyosarcoma of the biliary tree is a rare tumor that most commonly arises from the common bile duct (1–9). In a 1985 article, the Intergroup Rhabdomyosarcoma Group reported on 10 cases (1). Other descriptions have been limited to case reports and review articles (2–9). It is histologically the same as sarcoma botryoides, which is more commonly a sarcoma arising from the bladder or vagina of children. Most patients present with malaise, fever, and jaundice (1), symptoms often mistaken for the more common viral hepatitis (1–6). It is a disease of young children, with the median age at manifestation of the tumor being 3 years (most tumors manifest before the child is aged 5 years)(1–3). There is a slight male predominance (2,3).

At pathologic examination, the tumor arises as an intraluminal biliary mass or cluster of grapelike masses, similar to rhabdomyosarcomas that occur in the urinary bladder or vagina. The tumor distends and obstructs the bile duct and often grows through the bile ducts into the liver (1–5). The masses are usually large (8–20 cm), most commonly arise from the common bile duct, and often adhere to the adjacent duodenum, stomach, and pancreas (4). Metastatic disease is present at diagnosis in up to 30% of patients (1). CT most commonly shows a heterogeneous mass within the porta hepatis with bile duct dilatation (3–5). Cholangiography typically shows a large, bulky intraluminal mass or grapelike cluster of intraluminal masses that is completely or nearly completely obstructing (6). The ducts proximal to the obstructing mass are usually dilated to a lesser degree than is the portion of duct that contains the tumor (6).

The age, sex, clinical presentation, and bulky intraductal common bile duct masses shown in the case example are all consistent with the diagnosis of embryonal rhabdomyosarcoma of the biliary tree. The presence of retroperitoneal and mesenteric lymphadenopathy is consistent with metastatic disease. This patient also had multiple lung metastases identified at chest CT (not shown).

Jaundice is related to elevation of serum bilirubin levels. Laboratory evaluation of which type of bilirubin predominates—conjugated (direct) or unconjugated (indirect)—can help limit the differential diagnosis. Elevation of conjugated bilirubin is associated with conditions that obstruct the biliary system, cause hepatic injury, or are associated with inborn errors in hepatic metabolism. Elevated unconjugated bilirubin is seen with hemolysis, hematoma, swallowed blood, increased enterohepatic circulation, or Gilbert disease. This patient had a predominance of conjugated bilirubin.

The differential diagnosis for jaundice, fever, and malaise in a child of this age would include medical causes such as hepatitis, drug-induced jaundice, benign recurrent cholestasis, and cholangitis, as well as obstructive causes such as choledocholithiasis, choledochal cyst, parasitic disease, and neoplastic masses

Index terms:
Bile ducts, neoplasms, 76.322
Diagnosis please
Myosarcoma, 76.322

Radiology 1998; 208:621–623

[1] From the Department of Radiology, Division of Pediatric Radiology, Duke University Medical Center, Box 3808, Durham, NC 27710. Received November 11, 1997; revision requested December 12; revision received December 17; accepted January 9, 1998. **Address reprint requests to** L.F.D.

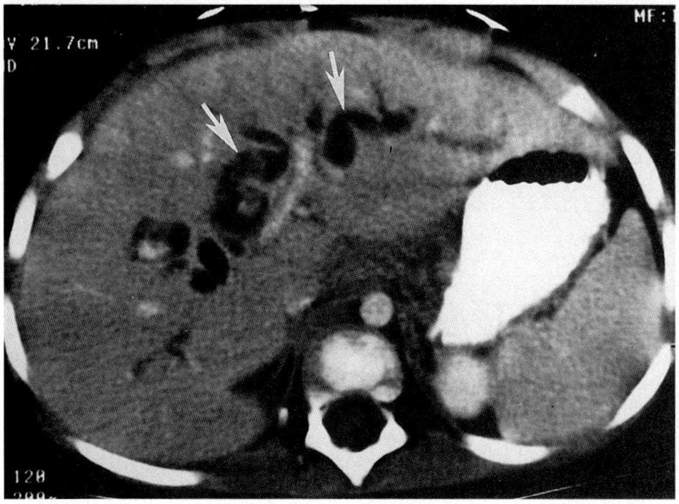

a.

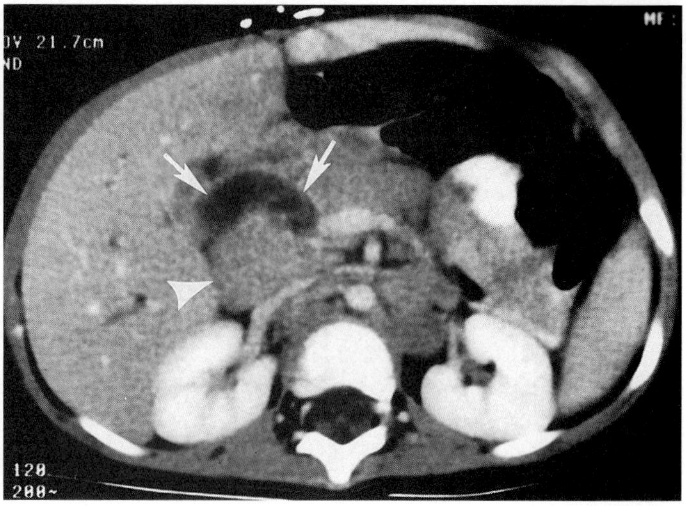

b.

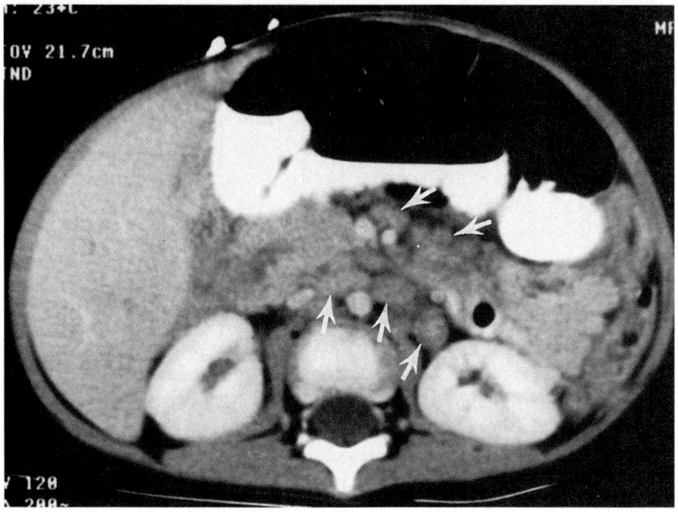

c.

Figure 1. Contrast material–enhanced CT scans show **(a)** dilatation of the intrahepatic bile ducts (arrows); **(b)** a soft-tissue mass (arrowhead) in the region of the porta hepatis, distending the dilated common bile duct (arrows); and **(c)** retroperitoneal (lower arrows) and mesenteric (upper arrows) lymphadenopathy.

(1,7). The presence of dilatation of the bile ducts seen on the CT scan is consistent with an obstructive cause. Medical causes can therefore be excluded. The presence of a soft-tissue mass in the porta hepatis excludes choledocholithiasis and choledochal cyst as potential causes.

There are multiple neoplasms that may manifest with a porta hepatis mass and bile duct dilatation in children. These would include liver masses, such as hepatoblastoma or undifferentiated embryonal sarcoma and hepatocellular carcinoma, or pancreatic neoplasms, such as pancreaticoblastoma and papillary cystic tumor of the pancreas (1,4,7). Hepatic masses can lead to bile duct obstruction by extrinsically compressing or invading the bile ducts. However, the appearance of a purely intraductal biliary mass, as seen in the test case, is consistent with a neoplastic process within the biliary system and would not be typical of any of these diagnoses. Systemic processes such as lymphoma, metastatic disease, or granulomatous infections can cause retroperitoneal lymphadenopathy, lung nodules, and liver masses. In addition, the liver masses that result from these systemic processes can occasionally cause bile duct obstruction. But, again, the presence of an intraductal mass in the case example makes these diagnoses unlikely. Concerning diseases primary to the biliary tree in children, there are really

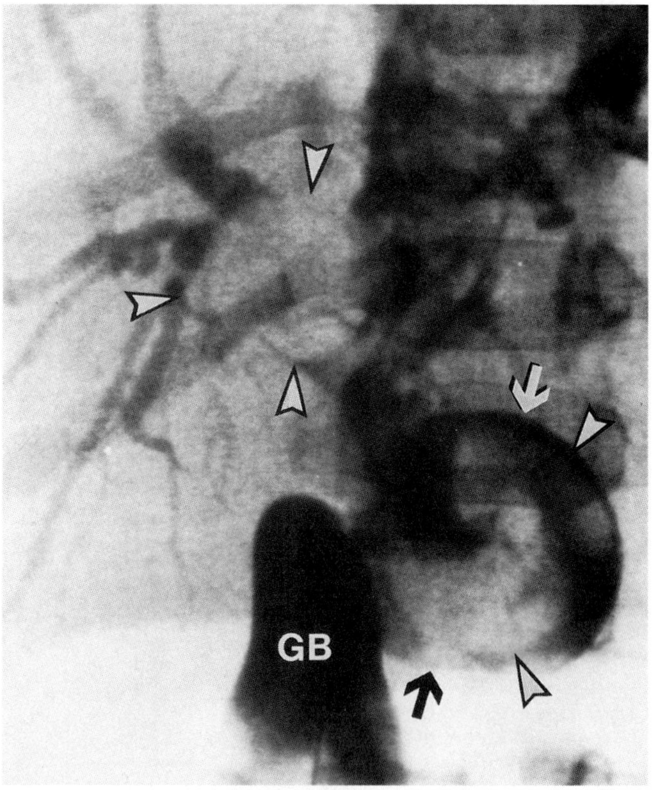

Figure 2. Intraoperative cholangiogram obtained after injection of the gallbladder (*GB*) shows multiple lobulated intrabiliary masses (arrowheads), the largest of which is in the markedly distended common bile duct (arrows). There is also dilatation of the intrahepatic bile ducts.

no neoplasms other than embryonal rhabdomyosarcoma of the biliary tree that arise from the bile ducts. Cholangiocarcinoma is primarily a disease of adults.

Embryonal rhabdomyosarcoma of the biliary tree is the diagnosis, which was confirmed with surgical biopsy.

References

1. Ruymann FB, Raney RB, Crist WM, Lawrence W, Lindberg RD, Soule EH. Rhabdomyoscarcoma of the biliary tree in childhood. Cancer 1985; 56:575–581.
2. Davis GL, Kissane JM, Ishak KG. Embryonal rhabdomyosarcoma of the biliary tree. Cancer 1969; 24:333–341.
3. Geoffray A, Couranet D, Montagne JP, Leclere J, Flamant F. Ultrasonography and computed tomography for diagnosis and follow-up of biliary duct rhabdomyosarcomas in children. Pediatr Radiol 1987; 17:127–131.
4. Davey MS, Cohen MD. Imaging of gastrointestinal malignancy in childhood. Radiol Clin North Am 1996; 34:717–742.
5. Friedburg H, Kauffmann GW, Bohm N, Fieldler L, Jobke A. Sonographic and computed tomographic features of embryonal rhabdomyosarcoma of the biliary tract. Pediatr Radiol 1984; 14:436–438.
6. Janes JO, Laughlin CL, Goldberger LE, Berk RN. Differential features of some unusual biliary tumors. Gastrointest Radiol 1982; 7:341–348.
7. Donnelly LF, Bisset GS III. Pediatric liver imaging. Radiol Clin North Am 1998; 36:413–427.
8. Sanz N, de Mingo L, Florez F, Rollan V. Rhabdomyosarcoma of the biliary tree. Pediatr Surg Int 1997; 12:200–201.
9. Caty MG, Oldham KT, Prochownik EV. Embryonal rhabdomyosarcoma of the ampulla of Vater with long-term survival following pancreaticoduodenectomy. J Pediatr Surg 1990; 25:1256–1258.

Our congratulations to the 24 individuals who submitted the most likely diagnosis (embryonal rhabdomyosarcoma of the biliary tree) for Diagnosis Please, Case 2. Their names are as follows:

Lionel Arrivé, MD, *Paris, France*
Edward L. Baker, MD, *San Francisco, Calif*
Jack Diel, MD, *Mineola, NY*
Edward P. Feutz, MD, *Clayton, MO*
Arnold C. Friedman, MD, *New York, NY*
Burton M. Gold, MD, *Mineola, NY*
Carlos Holguera Blßzquez, MD, *Madrid, Spain*
Lowrey H. Holthaus, MD, *Richmond, VA*
Douglas S. Katz, MD, *Mineola, NY*
António José Madureira, MD, *Matosinhos, Portugal*
Julio Mata, MD, *Camden, NJ*
Steven L. Meshkov, MD, *Yardley, PA*
Mehran Midia, MD, *Ringfield, Ill*
Hidetoshi Miyake, MD, *Oita, Japan*
Sergio J. Moguillansky, MD, *Rio Negro, Argentina*
David M. Panicek, MD, *New York, NY*
Narendrakumar Patel, MD, *Newburgh, NY*
Roberto E. Perez Gautrin, MD, *Sonora, Mexico*
Shawn P. Quillin, MD, *Charlotte, NC*
Enrique Remartinez Escobar, MD, *Melilla, Spain*
Derek J. Roebuck, FRACR, *Hong Kong, China*
Stuart A. Roya, MS, MD, *Birmingham, Ala*
Joanne B. Speigle, MD, *Richmond, Va*
J. Keith Thompson, MD, *Richmond, Va*

Book Review

Functional Imaging

Edited by Gustav K. van Schulthess, MD, PhD, and Juergen Hennig, PhD
Philadelphia, Pa: Lippincott-Raven, 1998. ISBN 0-397-51606-1.
Hardcover, $150.00; pp 485; 306 figures; tables.

The editors of this book have undertaken the ambitious goal of providing a broad framework that encompasses the common elements of functional organ imaging in medicine. To a large degree, they have succeeded by recruiting various experts in a wide variety of traditional and not-so-traditional imaging disciplines to write a well-annotated volume on this subject. Topics of chapters vary from standard radiologic modalities such as magnetic resonance imaging, nuclear medicine, x-ray imaging, and ultrasonography to unusual methods such as optical techniques, electroencephalography, and magnetoencephalography. Discussion focuses on the conceptual and physical basis of imaging by using clinical applications to illustrate methods. Chapters on contrast agents, physiologic modeling, and digital image processing round out the topics covered. Plentiful black-and-white and color illustrations are provided, and $150 is certainly a reasonable cost for a textbook of this length and quality.

The authors strive to develop commonality between various imaging modalities, and to a certain degree this devolves into mathematical descriptions of the imaging methods and physiologic processes studied. The editors have endeavored to employ a "two-leveled approach" that constrains formal mathematical notation to boxes interspersed within a less technical narrative. It is therefore difficult to appreciate this volume fully without a superior understanding of mathematics, although a more cursory reading of the text will still convey considerable information.

Functional Imaging would be an excellent choice for an engineering or applied physics textbook and can also serve as a valuable reference for technically oriented individuals. To a remarkable degree, the editors have achieved their stated goal of providing specialists versed in specific imaging techniques with complementary information regarding other imaging modalities.

Reviewed by Lionel S. Zuckier, MD

Robert L. Worthington-Kirsch, MD
George L. Popky, MD
Francis L. Hutchins, Jr, MD

Uterine Arterial Embolization for the Management of Leiomyomas: Quality-of-Life Assessment and Clinical Response[1]

Index terms:
Alcohol, 856.1264
Angiography, 854.1247
Arteries, chemotherapeutic embolization, 986.1264
Arteries, uterine, 986.1264
Uterine neoplasms, therapy, 854.1264
Uterine neoplasms, US, 854.1298, 854.315

Radiology 1998; 208:625–629

Abbreviation:
PVA = polyvinyl alcohol

[1] From the Department of Radiology, Philadelphia College of Osteopathic Medicine, Philadelphia, Pa (R.L.W.K., G.L.P.); the Section of Interventional Radiology, Delaware Valley Imaging, 301 City Ave, Suite G1, Bala Cynwyd, PA 19004 (R.L.W.K.); the Department of Obstetrics and Gynecology, Allegheny University Medical School, Philadelphia, Pa (F.L.H.); and the Department of Obstetrics and Gynecology, Thomas Jefferson University Medical School, Philadelphia, Pa (F.L.H.). Received November 14, 1997; revision requested February 16, 1998; revision received April 2; accepted May 8. **Address reprint requests to** R.L.W.K.

PURPOSE: To determine the effectiveness of uterine arterial embolization as a primary therapy in the management of symptomatic leiomyomas.

MATERIALS AND METHODS: Uterine arterial embolization was performed in 53 patients (age range, 33–58 years) with menorrhagia, bulk-related symptoms (frequency of urination, sensation of pressure, sensation of mass), or both, due to leiomyomas. The effectiveness of this therapy in the control of symptoms and the patients' acceptance of the treatment were measured by means of the information from patient interviews 3 months after the procedure.

RESULTS: Fifty-two (98%) of the 53 patients had technically successful procedures and were interviewed 3 months after embolization. Forty-six (88%) of these patients reported marked improvement in their abnormal bleeding. Twenty-nine (94%) of the 31 patients with bulk-related symptoms reported marked improvement in these symptoms. Follow-up ultrasonographic examinations showed a mean 46% reduction in uterine volume. Forty-one patients interviewed (79%) would choose this procedure again, eight (15%) would consider choosing this procedure again, and only three (6%) would choose another treatment option.

CONCLUSION: Uterine arterial embolization is an effective therapy in the management of symptomatic leiomyomas and may prove to be a valuable alternative to myomectomy, hysterectomy, or other surgical procedures. Further investigation is warranted.

Uterine myomas are the most frequent cause of nonacute abnormal uterine bleeding (1). They can also cause symptoms related to their bulk, such as frequency of urination, sensation of pressure, or sensation of mass. Unfortunately, all of the primary treatments of symptomatic leiomyomas—hysterectomy, myomectomy, myolysis, cryoablation, and hormonal therapy—have substantial disadvantages (1–4). Hysterectomy carries all of the risks associated with a major surgical procedure and eliminates fertility. Myomectomy has similar associated risks, and approximately 20%–25% of women undergoing myomectomy will have a recurrence of symptoms, requiring further intervention (2). Myolysis and cryoablation both also require laparotomy or laparoscopy and general anesthesia, and reported results have been mixed (3). Hormonal therapy is effective for short-term control but requires continued medication and has associated side effects, such as hot flashes, mood swings, insomnia, and dyspareunia (1).

Uterine arterial embolization, a recognized treatment of acute pelvic hemorrhage (4–8), has recently been applied to the management of nonacute uterine hemorrhage due to leiomyomas (9–12). The purpose of this study was to evaluate the effectiveness of uterine arterial embolization in relieving menorrhagia and bulk-related symptoms in patients with leiomyomas.

Author contributions:
Guarantor of integrity of entire study, R.L.W.K.; study concepts, R.L.W.K., F.L.H., G.L.P.; study design, R.L.W.K.; definition of intellectual content, R.L.W.K., G.L.P.; literature research, R.L.W.K.; clinical studies, R.L.W.K., F.L.H.; data acquisition, R.L.W.K., F.L.H.; data analysis, R.L.W.K.; manuscript preparation, R.L.W.K., F.L.H.; manuscript editing, G.L.P., R.L.W.K.; manuscript review, G.L.P.

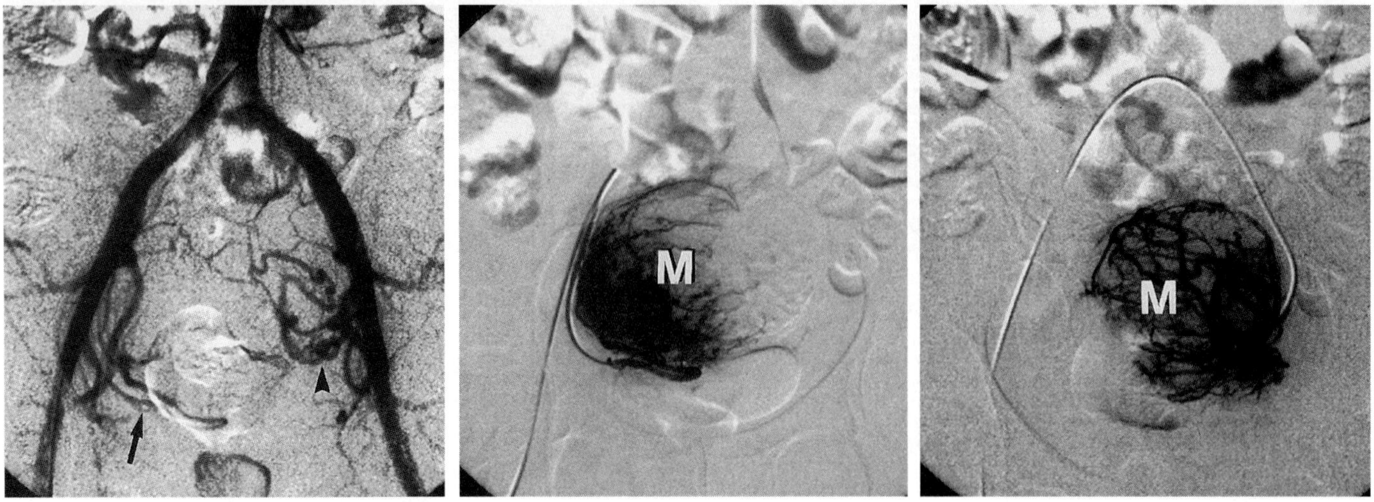

a. b. c.

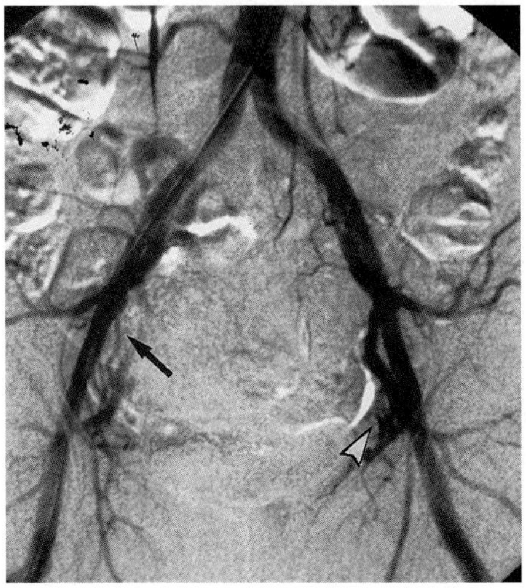

d.

(**a**) Mapping arteriographic image obtained after aortic injection of contrast material shows bilaterally enlarged and tortuous right (arrow) and left (arrowhead) uterine arteries. (**b**) Arteriographic image obtained after selective injection of contrast material into the right uterine artery shows marked hypervascularity of the myomatous uterus. The hypervascular mass (*M*) in the center is the leiomyoma. (**c**) Ateriographic image obtained after selective injection of contrast material into the left uterine artery shows marked hypervascularity of the myomatous uterus. The hypervascular mass (*M*) in the center is the leiomyoma. (**d**) Postprocedural arteriographic image obtained after aortic injection of contrast material shows no visible flow into either uterine artery. The origins of the right (arrow) and left (arrowhead) uterine arteries are marked.

MATERIALS AND METHODS

Patient Selection

Fifty-three adult women (age range, 33–58 years; mean age, 43 years) constituted the study population. All had complaints of severe menorrhagia and had a previous diagnosis of uterine myomas. Thirty-one women (58%) also complained of bulk-related symptoms. All women underwent pelvic ultrasonographic (US) studies that demonstrated leiomyomas, and all were premenopausal. Twenty-one were anemic because of chronic menorrhagia. Of the 21 women who were anemic (hemoglobin level < 120 g/L), the range of hemoglobin levels was 5.8–11.5 g/dL (58–115 g/L; mean, 9.6 g/dL [96 g/L]). All 53 patients had a strong desire to avoid surgery. Five patients were Jehovah's Witnesses and thus had a strong desire to avoid any surgery because of a religious prohibition against receiving blood products.

None of the women had additional gynecologic problems. Two women had insulin-dependent diabetes mellitus. One woman had a chronic seizure disorder, one had asthma and required daily nebulizer treatments, and one had sarcoidosis. The remainder of the women had no major current medical problems. All 53 were examined by an experienced gynecologist (F.L.H.), who determined that the patients' leiomyomas were the sole or major cause of their symptoms and that their symptoms were sufficiently severe to warrant intervention. Four patients had previously been treated with hormonal therapy alone, with good response, but had to abandon hormonal therapy because of intolerable side effects. Four had undergone myomectomy (one patient had undergone two myomectomies), and two had undergone both hormonal therapy and myomectomy. All patients who had undergone myomectomy experienced recurrence of symptoms within 2 years of surgery. All patients complained of menometrorrhagia. Thirty-one (58%) of the 53 patients also complained of bulk-related symptoms. Written informed consent was obtained from all patients.

Patient Preparation

Immediately before arteriography, all women were treated with one dose of prophylactic antibiotics (cefazolin sodium, 1 g administered intravenously; clindamycin phosphate, 300 mg administered intravenously in patients with a history of penicillin allergy) and underwent a pelvic US examination (model 128; Acuson, Mountain View, Calif).

Embolization Procedure

Pelvic arteriography (Angiography Suite; Shimadzu America, Columbia, Md) was performed by means of the right femoral approach. A 5-F diagnostic catheter (Imager Cobra 1, Medi-tech/Boston Scientific, Watertown, Mass; H1, Cook, Bloomington, Ind; or Levin-1, Cook) was used. Two patients required bilateral punctures because their anatomy precluded catheterization of the ipsilateral uterine artery. In three patients, a coaxial microcatheter (Tracker 325; Target Therapeutics, Fremont, Calif) was used.

After a mapping arteriographic image was obtained after injection of iohexol 300 (Omnipaque 300; Nycomed, Princeton, NJ; dose, 75–175 mL [initial dose, 10 mL]), with the catheter tip just above the aortic bifurcation (Figure, part a), the uterine arteries were selectively catheterized. The catheter tip was positioned at or beyond the junction of the descending and horizontal portions of each uterine artery, and embolization was performed with 500–700-μm polyvinyl alcohol (PVA) particles (Biodyne; Cook). PVA particles

TABLE 1
Complications of Uterine Arterial Embolization

Patient No.	Complication	Outcome
1	Postembolization syndrome	Hysterectomy on postembolization day 12
22	Upper gastrointestinal bleeding, second-degree nausea and vomiting	Self-limited, no therapy required
23	Postembolization syndrome	Readmitted to hospital on postembolization day 4 for 24 h

were injected into each uterine artery until there was complete cessation of flow or reflux of contrast material into the anterior division of the internal iliac artery. In the first 25 patients, embolization coils (Gianturco Coils, Cook; or Tornado Coils, Target Therapeutics) were inserted after PVA embolization. However, after we reviewed the protocols used in other radiology departments (12), coils were placed only if there was a question of the completeness of PVA embolization. A mean 350 mg (range, 100–700 mg) of PVA was used for the complete procedure. The average procedure time was approximately 60 minutes (range, 40–120 minutes).

All of the patients had a hypervascular uterus (Figure, parts b and c). At the completion of embolization, no flow was demonstrated in the uterine arteries (Figure, part d).

Sedation and Analgesia

Conscious sedation with a combination of narcotics (morphine sulfate, fentanyl citrate, or both) and benzodiazepines (midazolam hydrochloride) was used in all patients. All patients also received 60 mg of ketorolac tromethamine intravenously at catheterization of the first uterine artery. After the procedure, all patients were observed for at least 6 hours. Fifty-one patients stayed in the hospital overnight. All patients had pain and cramping similar to those seen both in cases of spontaneous infarction of uterine myomas and after embolization in other solid organs. Most patients were treated with oral nonsteroidal antiinflammatory drugs, or NSAIDs (typically ibuprofen, 800-mg oral loading dose followed by 600 mg orally every 4 hours). All patients had morphine sulfate available as a patient-controlled analgesic for the first 12–18 hours. The mean morphine sulfate dose used was 24 mg (range, 0–68 mg).

Forty-nine patients were discharged from the hospital on the 1st postprocedural day and were provided with prescriptions for oral pain medications (ibuprofen and oxycodone hydrochloride). Four patients required hospital stays longer than 24 hours for pain control (two patients were discharged on the 2nd postprocedural day, one on the 3rd postprocedural day, and one on the 4th postprocedural day).

Clinical Follow-up

All patients were contacted by telephone within 2 weeks of the procedure for initial follow-up and were contacted again 3 months after the procedure and interviewed either in person or by telephone. During the second interview, the patients were asked the following questions: (*a*) "How many days did it take to feel back to normal after the embolization?" (*b*) "How has the abnormal component of your bleeding changed?" Response options were as follows: stopped completely, greatly improved, moderately improved, slightly improved, unchanged, and worse. (*c*) "How have your bulk-related symptoms changed?" Response options were as follows: not applicable (those patients without bulk-related complaints), stopped completely, greatly improved, moderately improved, slightly improved, unchanged, and worse. (*d*) "If you had to do it over again, would you have an embolization procedure?" Response options were as follows: yes, maybe, and no.

In addition to the above questions, any complications of the procedure or hospitalization were discussed with the patient. Those patients whose charts indicated a desire for fertility were asked whether they were seeking to become pregnant or had conceived.

Follow-up US

All patients were requested to undergo follow-up US examinations at approximately 3 months after embolization. The percentage of reduction in uterine volume was calculated on the basis of measurements of the uterine longitudinal, transverse, and anteroposterior axes.

RESULTS

Technical Results

Bilateral embolization of the uterine arteries was accomplished in 52 (98%) of the 53 patients. The single technical failure was in a patient with a very small right uterine artery. Embolization of the left uterine artery was successful. The attempt to catheterize the right uterine artery caused dissection of its orifice, with thrombosis of the proximal portion of the vessel. However, because embolization was not performed in the peripheral vascular bed, the vessel was reconstituted by using collateral vessels. This patient had no clinical benefit from the procedure.

Complications

There were three patients with complications, as summarized in Table 1. Two patients were readmitted to the hospital for pain control of postembolization syndrome, which consisted of diffuse abdominal pain, mild fever, and mild leukocytosis. One of these patients had such severe abdominal pain that a hysterectomy was performed on postembolization day 12. The uterus weighed more than 7 kg and was almost completely replaced by a single leiomyoma. The leiomyoma was globally infarcted, while the residual normal myometrium was unremarkable. All culture findings were negative.

One patient developed severe nausea and vomiting several hours after the procedure and had a self-limited episode of hematemesis. This resolved without treatment and was thought to represent a small Mallory-Weiss tear caused by morphine-induced vomiting.

In many of the first 20 patients, postprocedural pain control with narcotics alone was very difficult. Nonsteroidal antiinflammatory drugs (usually ibuprofen) were added to the pain control regimen after the first 20 patients, with excellent results (as seen in the treatment of abdominal pain due to spontaneous infarction of a leiomyoma.) The postprocedural pain control regimen evolved to a point where pain control was excellent in most patients.

Follow-up US

Follow-up US was performed in 32 patients (60%). The mean reduction in uterine volume was 46% (range, 0%–84%) (Table 2). This agrees with findings in previously published articles (8,10,11).

Clinical Follow-up

Abnormal bleeding.—Forty-six (88%) of the 52 patients interviewed reported marked improvement in their abnormal bleeding starting with their first menses after embolization, 19 (37%) reported complete cessation of abnormal bleeding, 20 (38%) reported great improvement, and seven (13%) reported moderate improvement. Four patients (8%) reported only slight improvement, and two patients (4%) reported no change. No patients reported worsening of abnormal bleeding (Table 3).

Bulk-related symptoms.—Relief of bulk-related symptoms was also good, although not as dramatic as the change in abnormal bleeding. Twenty-nine (94%) of the 31 patients who had experienced marked bulk-related symptoms reported substantial improvement in these symptoms, with six (19%) reporting complete cessation of symptoms, 12 (39%) reporting great improvement, and 11 (35%) reporting moderate improvement. Two patients (6%) reported no change. No patients reported slight change in or worsening of these symptoms (Table 4).

Patient satisfaction.—If untreated, patients can experience marked pain after embolization. Institution of a simple oral analgesic regimen has permitted a high level of patient acceptance of the procedure. Forty-seven patients (90%) were able to return to normal activity within 10 days of embolization. The mean time for resolution of all postprocedural symptoms was 13 days. Forty patients (77%) reported complete resolution of symptoms in 14 days or less. The remainder reported recovery times of up to 60 days. No patients reported complications related to contrast material administration or puncture site. No patients reported any symptoms suggestive of nontarget embolization (such as urinary frequency, chronic pain, or sensory loss).

Forty-one (79%) of the patients interviewed would choose this procedure again; eight (15%) would consider choosing the procedure again. Only three (6%) would choose another treatment option. These three are those who had the least clinical benefit from the procedure.

TABLE 2
Change in Uterine Size at US

Patient No.	Uterine Volume (cm^2)	3 Months after Embolization	Percent Change
2	1,281	465	64
3	875	143	84
4	1,286	809	37
5	783	421	46
6	1,258	463	63
7	303	109	64
8	1,451	785	46
10	1,060	695	34
11	583	440	25
15	1,323	674	49
16	622	185	70
21	1,336	1,007	25
22	1,420	1,007	29
23	863	657	24
25	1,625	316	81
32	326	72	78
35	322	259	20
36	309	175	43
37	347	273	21
38	136	69	49
39	442	190	57
40	702	315	55
43	1,948	1,008	48
44	1,296	426	67
45	896	633	29
46	1,159	741	36
47	292	117	60
48	177	133	25
49*	286	286	0*
51	491	223	55
52	1,024	819	20
53	19,640	4,524	77

Note.—The mean volume reduction was 46%.
* Even though US showed no change in uterine volume, the patient reported that bleeding was greatly improved. She reported "not applicable" when asked about bulk-related symptoms at 3 months.

TABLE 3
Effect of Uterine Arterial Embolization on Menorrhagia

Menorrhagia	No. of Patients (*n* = 52)
Stopped completely	19 (37)
Greatly improved	20 (38)
Moderately improved	7 (13)
Slightly improved	4 (8)
No change	2 (4)
Worse	0 (0)

Note.—Number in parentheses is the percentage.

TABLE 4
Effect of Uterine Arterial Embolization on Bulk-related Symptoms

Symptoms	No. of Patients (*n* = 31)
Stopped completely	6 (19)
Greatly improved	12 (39)
Moderately improved	11 (35)
Slight improved	0 (0)
No change	2 (6)
Worse	0 (0)

Note.—Number in parentheses is the percentage.

DISCUSSION

Uterine arterial embolization is an established, safe, and effective treatment of the uterine hemorrhage that accompanies a number of conditions (4–8). Recently, it has also been described as useful in managing symptoms attributable to uterine myomas (9–12). It is a straightforward procedure in the myomatous uterus, because the vascular anatomy remains relatively normal. The uterine arteries are usually enlarged and tortuous (13). The enlargement of the uterine arteries due to the hypervascular leiomyomas actually makes the catheterization easier, although the increased tortuosity of the vessels can diminish this advantage.

It is impractical for a variety of reasons to selectively catheterize individual vessels supplying only leiomyomas. The major reason is that there are far too many branches for catheterization and embolization to be performed in an efficient and timely manner. Also, it is difficult to tell whether any one vessel supplies leiomyomas rather than normal myometrium. In many women, the myomatous involvement of the uterus is diffuse, and embolization of the entire uterine arterial distribution affords a global treatment for every myoma in the uterus.

Previously published reports (9–12) of uterine arterial embolization for the management of leiomyomas have involved smaller series of patients. Other investigators have used protocols slightly different from that in this study in the choice of PVA particle size (11,12) or the system used for catheterization of the uterine arteries (9). However, to our knowledge, all published articles to date have reported similar outcomes, which are confirmed by the findings in this larger series.

Uterine arterial embolization has the advantages of allowing preservation of uterine function (ie, normal menses and pregnancy) and prevention of a surgical procedure, such as myomectomy. Uterine arterial embolization does not appear to interfere with fertility (14), but whether it can restore fertility in situations of myoma-induced infertility has not been established. The procedure is well tolerated by patients and has a shorter recovery time than do surgical procedures in most patients.

A final clinical advantage is that, should uterine arterial embolization fail, the full range of other options for treatment of leiomyomas is still available. Indeed, surgery, if necessary, will be easier and safer because of the preoperative embolization (11).

There is a potential for substantial cost

savings with the use of uterine arterial embolization instead of traditional surgeries. However, an exact cost comparison has not yet been performed.

Uterine arterial embolization shows great promise as a primary treatment of symptomatic leiomyomas, because the procedure is well tolerated and effective, with the potential for considerable advantages over traditional therapies.

References

1. Wallach EE. Myomectomy. In: Thompson JD, Rock JA, eds. Te Linde's operative gynecology. 7th ed. Philadelphia, Pa: Lippincott, 1992; 647–662.
2. Hutchins FL. Abdominal myomectomy as a treatment for symptomatic uterine fibroids. Obstet Gynecol Clin North Am 1995; 22:781–789.
3. Phillips DR, Milim SJ, Nathanson HG, Haselkorn JS. Experience with laparoscopic leiomyoma coagulation and concomitant operative hysteroscopy. J Am Assoc Gynecol Laparosc 1997; 4:425–433.
4. Pais SO, Glickman M, Schwartz PE, Pingoud E, Berkowitz R. Embolization of pelvic arteries for control of postpartum hemorrhage. Obstet Gynecol 1980; 55:741–758.
5. Rosenthal DM, Colapinto R. Angiographic arterial embolization in the management of postoperative vaginal hemorrhage. Am J Obstet Gynecol 1985; 151:227–231.
6. Yamashita Y, Harada M, Yamamoto H, et al. Transcatheter arterial embolization of obstetric and gynecologic bleeding: efficacy and clinical outcome. Br J Radiol 1994; 67:530–534.
7. Gilbert WM, Moore TR, Resnik R, Doemeny J, Chin H, Bookstein JJ. Angiographic embolization in the management of hemorrhagic complications of pregnancy. Am J Obstet Gynecol 1992; 166: 493–497.
8. Greenwood CH, Glickman MG, Schwartz PE, Morse SS, Denny DF. Obstetric and nonmalignant gynecologic bleeding: treatment with angiographic embolization. Radiology 1987; 164:155–159.
9. Goodwin SC, Vedantham S, McLucas B, Forno AE, Perella R. Uterine artery embolization for uterine fibroids: results of a pilot study. JVIR 1997; 8:517–526.
10. McLucas B, Goodwin SC, Vedantham S. Embolic therapy for myomata. Minim Invasive Ther Allied Technol 1996; 5:336–338.
11. Ravina JH, Bouret JM, Fried D, et al. Value of preoperative embolization of uterine fibroma: report of a multicenter series of 31 cases. Contracept Fertil Sex 1995; 23: 45–49. [French]
12. Ravina JH, Herbreteau D, Ciraru-Vigneron N, et al. Arterial embolisation to treat uterine myomata. Lancet 1995; 346: 671–672.
13. Sampson JA. The blood supply of uterine myomata. Surg Gynecol Obstet 1912; 14: 215–234.
14. Stancato-Pasik A, Mitty HA, Richard HM III, Eshkar NS. Obstetric embolotherapy: effect on menses and pregnancy (abstr). Radiology 1996; 201(P):179.

Deep Venous Thrombosis: Gradient-recalled-Echo MR Imaging Changes over Time—Experience in 10 Patients[1]

Charles E. Spritzer, MD
Priscilla Trotter, RT
H. Dirk Sostman, MD[2]

Index terms:
Thrombosis, MR, 93.129412
Veins, MR, 93.129412
Veins, thrombosis, 93.411, 93.751

Radiology 1998; 208:631–639

Abbreviations:
DVT = deep venous thrombosis
GRE = gradient-recalled echo

[1] From the Department of Radiology, Duke University Medical Center, Box 3808, Erwin Rd, Durham, NC 27710. Received September 29, 1997; revision requested November 26; final revision received March 13, 1998; accepted April 10. **Address reprint requests to** C.E.S.

[2] Current address: Department of Radiology, New York Hospital-Cornell Medical Center, New York.

PURPOSE: To determine the gradient-recalled-echo (GRE) magnetic resonance (MR) imaging changes caused by intraluminal thrombus of the lower extremities over time and to establish GRE MR imaging criteria to help distinguish acute from previous deep venous thrombosis.

MATERIALS AND METHODS: Four women and six men, aged 38–76 years, underwent GRE MR imaging two to four times after the original diagnosis of deep venous thrombosis; eight also underwent confirmatory ultrasonography at that time. Follow-up was 3 months to 1½ years. All patients were treated with anticoagulants. Evidence of thrombus, signal intensity characteristics, and MR imaging appearance were evaluated.

RESULTS: Acute thrombosis was identified as an occlusion or prominent filling defect within the vessel. The luminal diameter of thrombosed veins was equal to or larger than that of a corresponding, unaffected vessel in each case. Acute thrombus signal intensity tended to be decreased initially and increased over time. Residual changes due to thrombosis included the web formation ($n = 3$), luminal narrowing ($n = 4$), and wall thickening and/or slow flow ($n = 5$). Vessels in three patients reverted to normal.

CONCLUSION: GRE MR imaging demonstrated progressive changes of venous thrombus over time. These criteria may help distinguish acute deep venous thrombosis from the residual changes of previous thrombosis.

Pulmonary emboli are a major source of morbidity and mortality in the United States. It has been estimated that 10,000–30,000 deaths per year are attributable to pulmonary embolism. Deep venous thrombosis (DVT) is a source of up to 90% of all pulmonary emboli. Between 100,000 and 300,000 hospitalizations each year are caused or complicated by acute DVT (1–4).

Although anticoagulation therapy is effective in preventing the propagation of acute DVT, it does entail some risk to the patient; the risk of intracranial hemorrhage is the most serious consequence. As such, accurate diagnosis is required to avoid unnecessary anticoagulation.

Because the clinical diagnosis of both pulmonary embolus and DVT is notoriously difficult and unreliable, imaging studies are needed to help in the accurate diagnosis of acute DVT. Venography and ultrasonography (US) have been shown to be reliable modalities for the demonstration of acute DVT (2–5).

More recently, magnetic resonance (MR) imaging performed with gradient-recalled-echo (GRE) sequences has been shown to be an accurate method for the assessment of acute DVT. When compared with venographic results or clinical outcome, reported (6–8) accuracies for thrombus in the thigh or pelvis have exceeded 95%. Much less has been written, however, about the attempt to distinguish acute DVT from more chronic thrombus. This is an important distinction because approximately 15% of patients have

Author contributions:
Guarantor of integrity of entire study, C.E.S.; study concepts and design, H.D.S., C.E.S.; definition of intellectual content, C.E.S.; literature research, C.E.S.; clinical studies, P.T.; data acquisition, P.T., C.E.S.; data analysis, C.E.S.; manuscript preparation, C.E.S.; manuscript editing and review, H.D.S., C.E.S.

TABLE 1
Findings Associated with DVT at Initial MR Imaging

Patient No.	Luminal Abnormality	Luminal Diameter*	Wall Thickness	Perivascular Edema	Cellulitis	Collateral Veins
1	Occlusion	Larger	Not distinct from adjacent thrombus	Absent	Present	Absent
2	Occlusion	Equal	Not distinct from adjacent thrombus	Absent	Absent	Present
3	Occlusion	Equal	Not distinct from adjacent thrombus	Absent	Present	Absent
4	Filling defect	Equal	Equal to unaffected vessel	Absent	Present	Absent
5	Filling defect	Larger	Equal to unaffected vessel	Absent	Absent	Absent
6	Occlusion	Larger	Not distinct from adjacent thrombus	Absent	Absent	Absent
7	Occlusion	Larger	Not distinct from adjacent thrombus	Absent	Absent	Present
8	Occlusion	Equal	Not distinct from adjacent thrombus	Equivocal	Absent	Present
9	Occlusion	Larger	Not distinct from adjacent thrombus	Present	Present	Absent
10	Filling defect	Larger	Equal to unaffected vessel	Absent	Absent	Absent

*Indicates luminal diameter of the thrombosed vessel relative to that of the contralateral, unaffected vessel.

repetitive episodes of DVT, and these episodes may be confused with postphlebitic syndrome (9). Although the clinical symptoms may be similar, acute DVT necessitates treatment with anticoagulation therapy, whereas changes due to more chronic thrombus (ie, venous stasis) are treated with conservative therapy, including leg elevation and applied heat.

The purpose of this study was to characterize the intraluminal thrombus and the vessel that contained the thrombus over time to determine the GRE MR imaging criteria for distinguishing acute DVT from residual changes caused by previous DVT. To our knowledge, such a study has not been previously reported.

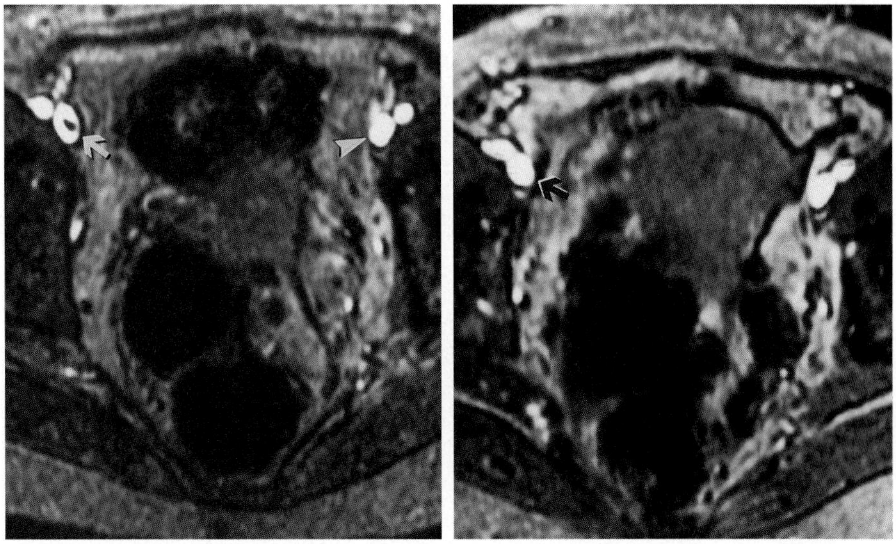

a. b.

Figure 1. GRE MR images (33/13, 60° flip angle) in a 61-year-old woman suspected of having a pulmonary embolus. **(a)** Transaxial image shows acute thrombus (arrow) partially filling the right external iliac vein. Note the unaffected left external iliac vein (arrowhead) for comparison. **(b)** Image obtained 3 months later shows complete resolution of the thrombus (arrow). Follow-up images obtained at 11 months (not shown) also appeared normal.

MATERIALS AND METHODS

Ten patients (four women, six men; age range, 38–76 years; mean age, 55 years) were examined two to four times after the initial diagnosis of acute DVT. All studies were performed with institutional review board approval, and written informed consent was obtained from the patients. Follow-up varied from 3 months to 1½ years. All patients received anticoagulant medications after the initial diagnosis of acute DVT. These medications consisted of intravenously administered heparin during the hospital stay, with conversion to warfarin sodium.

Eight of the 10 patients underwent confirmatory US at the time of the original diagnosis. One of these eight patients underwent US 48 hours before MR imaging, and the remaining seven patients underwent MR imaging and US within 24 hours of each other. In the ninth patient, US findings were negative, but the superficial femoral vein (the site of thrombus on MR images) was poorly seen, and a high-probability ventilation-perfusion study was obtained in this patient. Repeat US 1 week later confirmed thrombus in the area depicted on MR images. The 10th patient underwent no confirmatory studies at the time of diagnosis.

Three patients underwent follow-up US, one patient at 1 month and two patients at 3 months after the initial diagnosis. Two patients had previous DVT according to their clinical history, the exact location of which was unknown. In the remaining eight patients, the clinical history was negative for previous thromboembolic disease. The average duration of symptoms before initial diagnosis was 4 days (range, 1–33 days). This included two patients who complained of chest symptoms for 18 and 33 days before the detection of DVT.

MR imaging was performed at 1.5 T (Signa; GE Medical Systems, Milwaukee, Wis). GRE images were obtained in all patients. In the abdomen and thigh, typical imaging parameters were 33/13 (repetition time msec/echo time msec) with a 60° flip angle. In the calves, the parameters were 100/13 with a 60° flip angle. The field of view was 24–36 cm, and the matrix was 256 × 128 in the abdomen and thigh and 256 × 256 in the calf. Four signals were acquired in the pelvis, two were acquired in the thigh, and one to two were acquired in the calves. Section thickness was 5 mm, with a 5-mm inter-

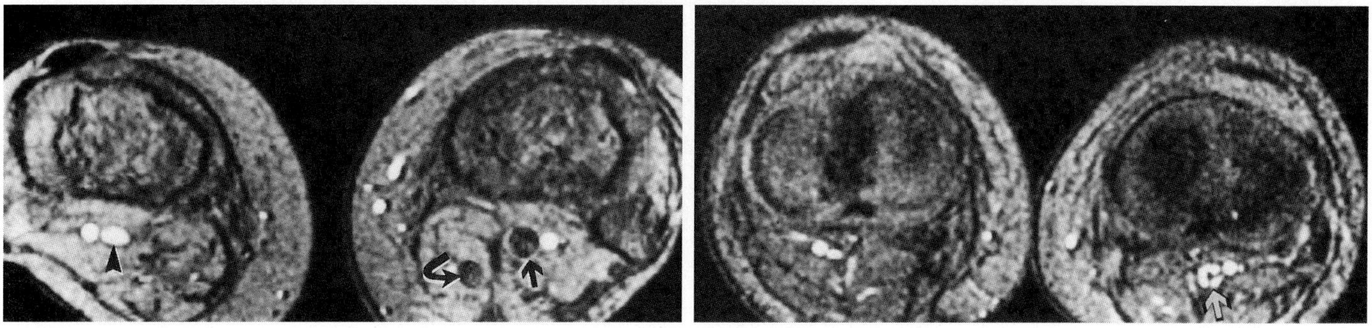

a. b.

Figure 2. GRE MR images (100/13, 60° flip angle) in a 66-year-old woman who presented with left lower extremity swelling. **(a)** Image obtained at the time of presentation shows thrombus (straight arrow) occluding the popliteal vein. Another thrombus (curved arrow) is also noted in an unnamed deep branch. The normal contralateral popliteal vein (arrowhead) is shown for comparison. **(b)** Image obtained 7 months later shows a residual web (arrow) in the popliteal vein.

TABLE 2
Follow-up Findings and Residual Changes in Patients with DVT at Final Follow-up MR Imaging

Patient No.	Luminal Abnormality	Luminal Diameter*	Wall Thickness†	Perivascular Edema	Cellulitis	Collateral Veins	Overall Appearance
1	Web	Equal	Thicker	Absent	Absent	Equivocal‡	Residual changes
2	Filling defect	Smaller	Thicker	Absent	Absent	Present	Residual changes
3	Web	Equal	Equal	Absent	Absent	Present	Residual changes
4	Patent	Equal	Equal	Absent	Absent	Absent	Normal
5	Patent	Equal	Equal	Absent	Absent	Absent	Normal
6	Occlusion	Smaller	Thicker	Absent	Absent	Absent	Residual changes
7	Patent	Smaller	Equal	Absent	Absent	Absent	Residual changes
8	Web	Equal	Thicker	Absent	Present§	Present	Residual changes
9	Occlusion	Smaller	Thicker	Absent	Absent	Present	Residual changes
10	Patent	Equal	Equal	Absent	Absent	Absent	Normal

* Indicates luminal diameter of the thrombosed vessel relative to that of the contralateral, unaffected vessel.
† Indicates wall thickness of thrombosed vessel relative to that of the contralateral, unaffected vessel. Findings include thickness and/or slow flow.
‡ Indicates a new episode of DVT.
§ Patient 8 had congestive heart failure.

section spacing. The frequency-encoding direction was right to left in each instance. A standard gradient set was used with a gradient strength of no greater than 1 G/cm (1 mT/m). The bandwidth was ±16 kHz in each instance.

Studies were retrospectively evaluated in a serial fashion by the senior author (C.E.S.). The location of the thrombus was noted as principally in the inferior vena cava, the common iliac veins, the external iliac veins, the superficial femoral veins, the popliteal vein, or the calf vessels. The length and diameter of the thrombus were assessed. Total or partial obstruction of the vessel was noted. Thrombus signal intensity was compared with that of cortical bone, muscle, and fat. Homogeneity at the center of the thrombus was noted. The presence of intraluminal webs, apparent wall thickening, and luminal diameter were recorded. Slow flow (as evidenced by means of decreased intraluminal signal intensity) was noted. In each instance, comparisons were made with the corresponding asymptomatic vessel. A change in diameter of 2 mm or more was noted. For the inferior vena cava, comparison was made with the patent vessel proximal to the thrombus.

Region-of-interest measurements of signal intensity were obtained on one to three images (depending on the extent of thrombus at the time of imaging) of the vessel that contained the thrombus. Region-of-interest measurements were also obtained from the corresponding, asymptomatic vessel on the same images. A region of interest that encompassed the entire width of the image posteriorly was obtained to measure background noise. The ratio of the signal intensity of the thrombosed vessel to that of the background region of interest divided by the ratio of the signal intensity of the normal vessel to that of the background region of interest was obtained and plotted. Measurements were obtained for each study performed in the patient. This included patients with complete resolution of the thrombus, with persistent webs, or with occlusion of the vessel.

Ancillary findings were also evaluated. Cellulitis was identified when an increase in the diameter of the extremity, a thickening and stranding of the subcutaneous tissues, and/or an accumulation of subcutaneous fluid were noted. If similar findings were noted in proximity to the vessels, perivascular edema was recorded. Collateral veins were also noted.

RESULTS

At the time of the initial diagnosis, thrombus was seen to extend through multiple vessels in five patients. Two had thrombus that extended from the superficial femoral vein to the inferior vena cava. In each of the remaining three patients, the

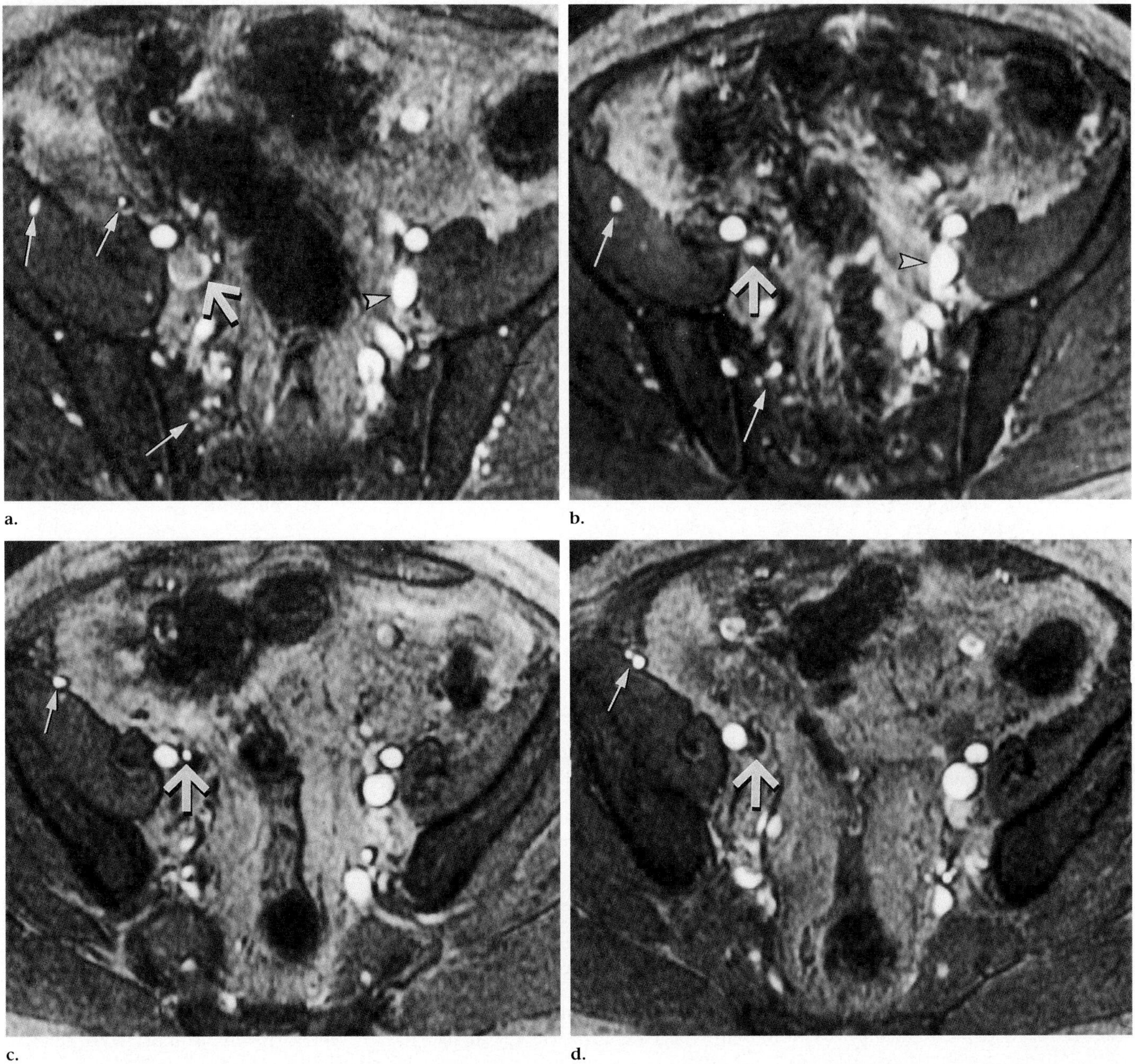

Figure 3. GRE MR images (33/13, 60° flip angle) in a 58-year-old man with right lower extremity swelling. **(a)** Initial image obtained at the time of diagnosis shows acute thrombus that extends from the inferior vena cava caudally into the superficial femoral vein. The thrombosed external iliac vein (large arrow) is markedly distended compared with the contralateral vein (arrowhead). Collateral venous return (small arrows) is present. **(b)** Image obtained 1 month after **a** shows wall thickening and/or slow flow (large arrow) in the involved vessel. The lumen of the vessel appears slightly smaller than that of the contralateral vein (arrowhead). Collateral venous return (small arrows) is present. **(c)** Image obtained 3 months after **a** shows the thick wall and diminutive lumen of the right external iliac vein (large arrow), with only mild residual flow. Collateral venous return (small arrow) is present. **(d)** Image obtained 6 months after **a** shows occlusion of the right external iliac vein (large arrow). Collateral venous return (small arrow) is present.

thrombus was located in (*a*) the external iliac vein and extending into the common iliac vein, (*b*) the popliteal vein and extending into the external iliac vein, and (*c*) a calf vessel and extending into the common femoral vein. In the remaining five patients, thrombus was localized to one segment. Two had isolated thrombus localized to the common iliac vein, two had thrombus isolated in the superficial femoral vein, and one had thrombus isolated in the calf (posterior tibial vein).

In the patient with thrombus initially isolated in the calf, propagation of thrombus into the popliteal vein and the distal superficial femoral vein was seen on follow-up MR studies. This patient had received subtherapeutic doses of warfarin sodium. For the purposes of the study, only the thrombus in the calf was evaluated. No other instances of thrombus propagation or recurrent DVT were documented in the remaining nine patients during the course of this study.

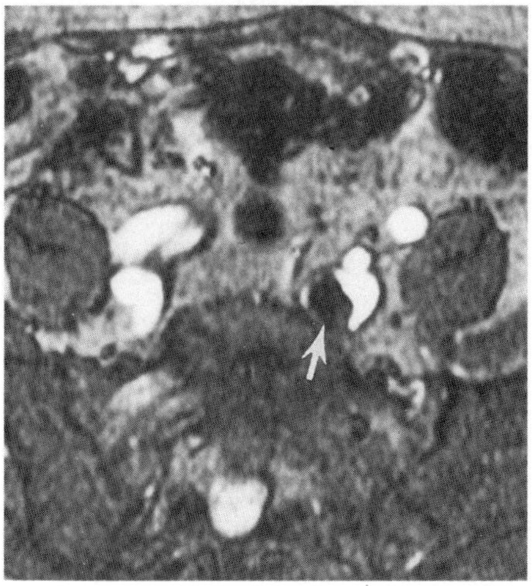

a.

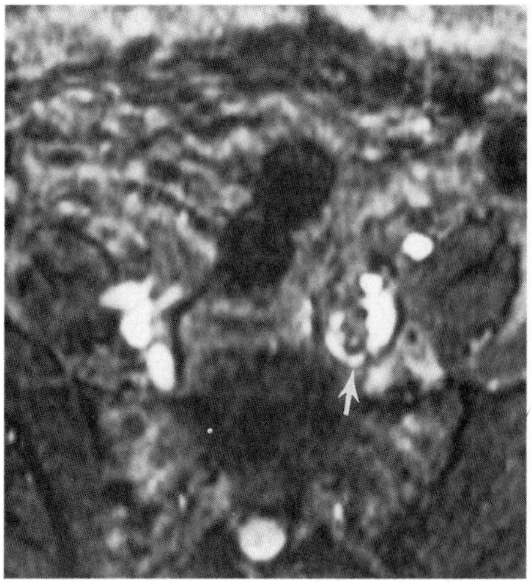

b.

Figure 4. GRE MR images (33/13, 60° flip angle) in a 76-year-old man with thrombus in the left common iliac vein. (a) At the time of diagnosis, the thrombus (arrow) has uniformly decreased signal intensity, which matches that of cortical bone. (b) Image obtained 1 week after a shows persistent thrombus (arrow) with slightly increased signal intensity and more heterogeneity.

Acute DVT Findings

Findings of acute DVT are summarized in Table 1. At the time of the diagnosis of acute DVT, the thrombus in seven patients occluded the vessel; in the remaining three patients, the thrombus manifested as a filling defect with flow evident around the thrombus (Figs 1a, 2a). In terms of signal intensity, the thrombus was essentially isointense compared with cortical bone in five patients, hyperintense compared with cortical bone but hypointense compared with muscle in three patients, and isointense compared with muscle in two patients (Figs 1a, 2a, 3a, 4a). The thrombus had a homogeneous appearance in eight of 10 patients and a mildly heterogeneous appearance in the remaining two patients. When compared with the corresponding unaffected vessel, the luminal diameter was increased in six patients and equal in four patients. The average increase in diameter was 0.55 cm (range, 0.2–1.6 cm). In no instance was the involved vessel smaller than the unaffected corresponding vein.

Ancillary findings of cellulitis, perivascular edema, or collateral veins were present in seven patients. In five patients, findings consistent with cellulitis were noted. In three patients, prominent collateral veins were identified. Findings of perivascular edema were present in one patient and equivocal in a second patient.

TABLE 3
Luminal Diameter at Initial and Last Follow-up MR Imaging Study

Patient No.	Thrombosed Vessel Diameter (cm): Initial Study	Thrombosed Vessel Diameter (cm): Follow-up Study	Contralateral Vessel Diameter (cm): Initial Study	Contralateral Vessel Diameter (cm): Follow-up Study
1	1.8	1.1	1.2	1.1
2	1.1	0.4	1.0	0.9
3	1.2	1.1	1.2	1.1
4	1.0	0.9	1.0	1.0
5	3.1	1.5	1.5	1.5
6	1.0	0.3	0.7	0.7
7	2.0	1.0	1.8	1.8
8	0.8	0.8	0.8	0.8
9	1.4	0.3	1.0	0.8
10	1.2	1.1	1.0	1.1

Follow-up Findings

Tables 2 and 3 summarize the follow-up MR imaging findings. At the time of the last MR examination in each patient, the veins in three patients had essentially reverted to normal (Fig 1b). The remaining seven patients showed residual changes.

Two patients showed occlusion of the vessel, and in both instances the luminal diameter was smaller than that on the initial study (Fig 3b–d). In a third patient, focal wall thickening or adherent thrombus was identified. An intraluminal web was identified in three additional patients (Fig 2b). In the remaining four patients, no intraluminal thrombus was identified.

In six patients, the diameter of the involved lumen was equal to that of the contralateral vein. In four patients, the luminal diameter was less than that of the contralateral vein. The average decrease in diameter in these patients was 0.4 cm (range, 0.2–0.5 cm). When compared with the corresponding initial study, luminal diameter decreased in six patients and remained unchanged in four patients. In five patients, there was increased wall thickness and/or slow flow. In five patients, wall thickness was equal to that on the unaffected, contralateral side, without evidence of slow flow.

In four patients, findings of prominent collateral veins were present; in a fifth patient, findings of collateral vessels were equivocal. In three of these patients, collaterals were visible on the initial MR images. In two patients, there were findings consistent with cellulitis. No perivascular edema was identified in any patient.

Thrombus Signal Intensity Changes over Time

Table 4 summarizes the changes in signal intensity of the thrombus over time. The signal intensity of the thrombus was assessed when a thrombotic mass could be clearly visualized. In three patients, there was no thrombus at the time of the first follow-up MR examination (obtained at 2, 3, or 6 months). In all but one of the seven remaining patients, the signal intensity of the thrombus increased between the initial and first follow-up examinations. The thrombus in five patients became heterogeneous between the initial and first follow-up studies (Fig 4a, 4b). In the other five patients, the thrombus remained homogeneous, albeit with a higher signal intensity. In the patient with a left calf thrombus that propagated into the popliteal vein after the initial study, the new popliteal thrombus appeared darker and homogeneous (nearly isointense to cortical bone).

A more quantitative analysis showed similar patterns at the time of the initial diagnosis. The signal intensity ratio of the thrombosed vessel to the unaffected vessel was 0.10–0.34. In all but two patients, the signal intensity increased between the first and second measurements. In the first patient with an interval decrease, the ratio decreased from 0.26 to 0.20. In the second patient, the ratio decreased from 0.33 to 0.14; in this patient, however, surgical clips and an air-filled bowel were near the imaged region, which may have affected the quantitative readings. In the remaining eight patients, the ratio increased by 0.1 to more than 1.0 (Fig 5).

TABLE 4
Changes in Signal Intensity over Time in Patients with DVT

Patient No.	Initial Study Findings	First Follow-up		Second Follow-up		Third Follow-up		Fourth Follow-up	
		Time	Findings	Time	Findings	Time	Findings	Time	Findings
1	Hypointense to muscle, homogeneous	1 mo	Hypointense to muscle, homogeneous	2 mo	Isointense to muscle, homogeneous	4 mo	No thrombus	NA	NA
2	Hypointense to muscle, homogeneous	1 wk	Isointense to muscle, heterogeneous	4 mo	No thrombus	NA	NA	NA	NA
3	Isointense to cortical bone, homogeneous	1 mo	Hypointense to muscle, heterogeneous	7 mo	No thrombus	NA	NA	NA	NA
4	Hypointense to muscle, heterogeneous	2 mo	No thrombus	NA	NA	NA	NA	NA	NA
5	Isointense to cortical bone, homogeneous	1 wk	Isointense to muscle, homogeneous	2 mo	Isointense to muscle, homogeneous	6 mo	No thrombus	NA	NA
6	Isointense to cortical bone, homogeneous	1 wk	Hyperintense to muscle, hypointense to fat, heterogeneous	1 mo	Hyperintense to muscle, hypointense to fat, heterogeneous	3 mo	Hyperintense to muscle, hypointense to fat, heterogeneous	6 mo	Occlusion
7	Isointense to cortical bone, homogeneous	3 mo	No thrombus	NA	NA	NA	NA	NA	NA
8	Isointense to cortical bone, homogeneous	2 mo	Hypointense to muscle, heterogeneous	5 mo	No thrombus	NA	NA	NA	NA
9	Hyperintense to muscle, hypointense to fat, heterogeneous	1 mo	Hyperintense to muscle, hypointense to fat, heterogeneous	3 mo	Hyperintense to muscle, hypointense to fat, heterogeneous	6 mo	Occlusion	NA	NA
10	Isointense to muscle, homogeneous	6 mo	No thrombus	NA	NA	NA	NA	NA	NA

Note.—NA = not applicable.

DISCUSSION

MR imaging has been shown (6–8,10–12) to be capable of demonstrating acute venous thrombosis in the lower extremities with an accuracy of more than 95% when compared with conventional venography. The diagnosis of acute DVT by using GRE MR images has relied on the identification of (*a*) a filling defect of low to almost absent signal intensity, with surrounding flow, or (*b*) an absence of flow within a vessel that appears distended with a low-signal-intensity thrombus. Perivascular inflammation, although infrequently identified on GRE MR images, has been considered a useful ancillary sign for acute DVT.

Little has been written, however, about the distinction of acute from chronic DVT in vivo by using GRE images (13). This is an important limitation of the technique because it has been estimated that 10%–15% of patients develop recurrent DVT (1,9). In addition, postphlebitic syndrome also occurs in a substantial percentage of patients after an episode of acute DVT (14). Unfortunately, the clinical distinction between these two entities is poor. As such, an ideal imaging study should be capable of helping distinguish between these two entities.

In histologic terms, an acute thrombus is composed of red blood cells, platelets, fibrin, and an occasional white blood cell. After the 1st week, clefts form between the thrombus and the wall of the vein (15–18). This is followed by penetration of capillaries from the venous wall and eventual recanalization. It has been shown (19) that clot composition changes most rapidly in the first 2 to 3 weeks after formation.

Much has been written about the MR imaging appearance of blood and blood products and how the appearance of blood changes with time. Factors known to affect the signal intensity of the thrombus include the oxygenation state and form of hemoglobin, the amount of fibrin, the presence of granulation tissue, the number of platelets, the number and integrity of red blood cells, the presence of recanalization, and the strength of the magnetic field (20–28).

Braun et al (21) described a patient with jugular venous thrombosis examined with a 0.5-T MR imager over 3 days. With age, the thrombus had higher signal intensity on both T1- and T2-weighted images, which was attributed to T1 shortening and T2 lengthening. Similar changes in T1 and T2 as demonstrated on spin-echo MR images have been reported by others (15,20,29).

Relatively little has been written about thrombus characterization on GRE MR images. Wu et al (23) used a fast GRE acquisition (repetition time, 8–18 msec) and commented that the faster GRE acquisitions tended to result in lower signal intensity in cases of acute thrombus. However, their clinical experience entailed only seven patients, and none of these patients were followed up serially.

Francis et al (13) used GRE sequences with a 1.5-T magnet to follow the acute changes of thrombus in two patients 3 days after the initiation of treatment (intravenous heparin in one, thrombolysis in the other). The patient treated with thrombolysis showed near complete resolution of the thrombus, with a minor vessel wall irregularity. The patient treated with heparin showed propagation of the thrombus, with areas of slightly higher signal intensity in the center of the thrombus.

Francis and Totterman (30) evaluated the signal intensity characteristics of thrombus on GRE images obtained in nine patients before and after fibrinolytic therapy but did not specifically comment on the changes in signal intensity characteristics after treatment. They noted, however, that in all of the cases in their series considered to be acute, the thrombi with the lowest signal intensity were typically present in patients with a symptom duration of less than 4 days. The authors also commented that in no instance at the time of the initial examination was there low-signal-intensity thrombus surrounded by higher signal intensity thrombus. More typically, the low-signal-intensity throm-

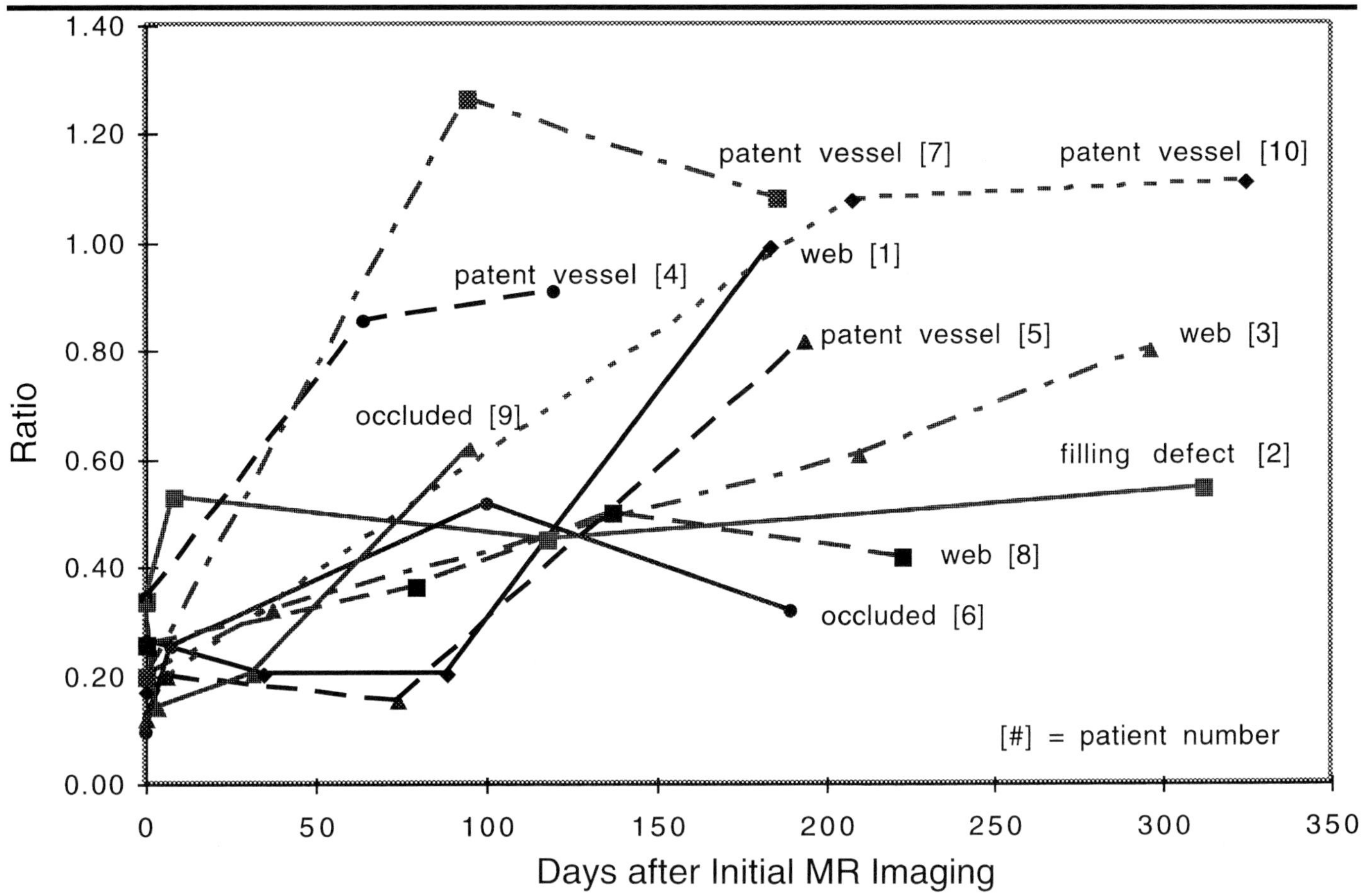

Figure 5. Graph shows signal intensity changes over time in the 10 patients. The signal intensity ratio of thrombus to noise divided by the signal intensity ratio of control vessel to noise is plotted. The number in brackets is the patient number.

bus was at the proximal and distal ends of the clotted segment. Having remarked that thrombolysis is more successful with less mature thrombi, Francis and Totterman found that a thrombus with a signal intensity less than that of muscle was more readily lysed with fibrinolytics than was a thrombus with a higher signal intensity. On the basis of these observations, they concluded that the most acute thrombus had the more uniform decrease in signal intensity.

In histologic terms, with recanalization of the vein there is concomitant loss of heme products. This loss of heme, as well as the reestablishment of flowing blood, contributes to the increased signal intensity seen as the thrombus ages.

In our series, bulky thrombus was present initially in all 10 patients and occluded the vein in six of the patients. In addition, the thrombus was homogeneous in nine patients and mildly heterogeneous in the remaining patient. With time and treatment, the signal intensity of the thrombus increased in each of the seven patients who did not have immediate resolution of the thrombus. In addition, the thrombus in only two of these patients remained homogeneous over time.

Even in the two instances where the affected vessel eventually became occluded, the signal intensity of the occluded vein increased between the initial and follow-up studies. As might be expected, the overall signal intensity of the thrombosed vein remained low relative to that of the control vessel, due to the presence of fibrin and the lack of flow. The fact that the signal intensity of the vessel increased at all over time suggests that the GRE sequence we used is especially sensitive to the presence of heme products and their gradual removal from the thrombus over time.

As we have already suggested, the variability in the ratios between the thrombosed and unaffected sides may in part be explained in terms of the differing ages of the thrombus at the time of the initial MR examination.

At the time of their last MR examination, only three patients had reversion to a completely normal-appearing vein. Abnormalities in vessel wall thickness and vessel diameter were the most striking residual changes. When compared with the initial study, luminal diameter decreased in six patients and remained unchanged in four. In five patients, there was an apparent increase in wall thickness and/or slow flow. Because phase-sensitive imaging, spin-echo imaging, and corroborative studies were not available, we did not attempt to distinguish between these two possibilities. In histologic terms, however, both wall thickening and abnormal flow are thought to occur (15,16).

At the time of the final examination, collateral vessels were identified with certainty in four patients and were questionable in a fifth patient. Three of these patients had collateral vessels identified on the initial study. In no instance did initially identified collateral vessels disappear on subsequent studies.

Persistent abnormalities after acute DVT have been reported (16,31,32) in both sequential venographic studies and US studies. Venographically demonstrated long-term abnormalities have been reported to occur in approximately 50% of people with DVT (33). In similar fashion, US demonstrates persistent abnormalities in up to 50% of patients months after the initial, acute episode of DVT (1,15,16,31). Included in these abnormalities are a narrowed vessel lumen, increased wall thickness, and abnormal compressibility. The difficulty arises in the attempt to determine whether these changes are due to postphlebitic syndrome or to recurrent DVT (16,31,32,34). Because both populations have abnormal vessels, compression (considered to be the most sensitive and specific means of diagnosing acute DVT at US) is rendered less effective.

By using the echogenecity of the thrombus and color flow imaging, US has been reported (1,15,16,35) to be helpful in the differentiation of acute from more chronic thrombus. Acute thrombus tends to be hypoechoic, whereas more chronic thrombus is hyperechoic. Despite the promise of these findings, others (16,36,37) have reported difficulty in using US to distinguish between recurrent or acute thrombus and more chronic thrombus.

US has other limitations, as well. When compared with MR imaging, the assessment of a thrombus above the inguinal ligament is difficult due to overlying bowel gas and the walls of the pelvic bones, even with color Doppler flow US (1); MR imaging has no such limitation (11,38–40). Evans et al (8) reported that in six of 61 patients, MR imaging demonstrated pelvic thrombi that were not seen at venography. Follow-up MR imaging and direct venous puncture studies confirmed thrombus in five of six cases. Dupas et al (41) reported, in a study with 25 patients (17 of whom underwent color Doppler US), that US did not demonstrate thrombi in the internal iliac vein in eight patients, whereas MR imaging did.

Our study has several limitations. First, we assumed that the initial evaluation was performed in patients with acute DVT. Eight of 10 patients in this series had no history of DVT. Nonetheless, it has been suggested (5,42) that as many as two-thirds of venous thrombi are silent. Thus, the possibility of previous DVT in these patients cannot be entirely excluded. Second, the time between the onset of symptoms and the establishment of the diagnosis of acute DVT was variable. This may account for some of the signal intensity differences of thrombi seen at the time of the initial diagnosis in our series. Third, our results lack corroboration. At the time of the initial diagnosis, positive US findings had been obtained in eight patients, and a high-probability ventilation-perfusion study had been obtained in one. More important, however, corroborative studies were not routinely available at the time of follow-up MR imaging. Fourth, all of the patients in our series underwent anticoagulation therapy because of presumed acute DVT. Therefore, an untreated thrombus was not assessed in vivo, and it is conceivable that an untreated thrombus may not behave similarly to a treated thrombus. Fifth, although to our knowledge ours is the largest such study to date, the number of patients is still relatively small. Finally, the studies were reviewed retrospectively in a nonblinded fashion so that identical areas of thrombus could be assessed over time. As such, observer bias was possible.

In conclusion, GRE MR images show that acute DVT tends to fill and/or distend the vessel. The thrombus generally has low signal intensity and is relatively homogeneous. With treatment and time, the thrombus shows increases in signal intensity and is less bulky, and the luminal diameter correspondingly decreases and is accompanied by slow flow and apparent wall thickening. Finally, in this small series, the majority of patients had residual changes from previous DVT. The GRE MR imaging findings we have reported should facilitate the distinction between acute and chronic DVT.

References

1. Dorfman GS, Cronan JJ. Venous ultrasonography. Radiol Clin North Am 1992; 30:879–893.
2. Cronan JJ. Venous thromboembolic disease: the role of US. Radiology 1993; 186: 619–630.
3. Stephen JM, Feied CF. Venous thrombosis: lifting the clouds of misunderstanding. Postgrad Med 1995; 97:36–42.
4. Wakefield TW, Greenfield LJ. Diagnostic approaches and surgical treatment of deep venous thrombosis and pulmonary embolism. Hematol Oncol Clin North Am 1993; 7:1251–1267.
5. Salzman EW. Venous thrombosis made easy. N Engl J Med 1986; 14:847–848.
6. Spritzer CE, Sostman HD, Wilkes DC, Coleman RE. Deep venous thrombosis: experience with gradient-echo MR imaging in 66 patients. Radiology 1990; 177:235–241.
7. Spritzer CE, Norconk JJ, Sostman HD, Coleman RE. Detection of deep venous thrombosis by MR imaging. Chest 1993; 104:54–60.
8. Evans AJ, Sostman HD, Knelson M. Detection of deep venous thrombosis: prospective comparison of MR imaging with contrast venography. AJR 1993; 161:131–135.
9. Dorfman GS, Cronan JJ. Asymptomatic pulmonary embolism in deep venous thrombosis: long-term follow-up (abstr). Radiology 1987; 165(P):205.
10. Erdman WA, Jayson HT, Redman HC. Deep venous thrombosis of extremities: role of MR imaging in the diagnosis. Radiology 1990; 174:425–431.
11. Carpenter JP, Holland GA, Baum RA, Owen RS, Carpenter JT, Cope C. Magnetic resonance venography for the detection of deep venous thrombosis: comparison with contrast venography and duplex Doppler ultrasonography. J Vasc Surg 1993; 18:734–741.
12. Sostman HD, Debatin JF, Spritzer CE, Grist TM, MacFall JR. MR imaging in venous thromboembolic disease. Eur Radiol 1993; 3:53–61.
13. Francis CW, Foster TH, Totterman S, Brenner B, Marder VJ, Bryant RG. Monitoring of therapy for deep vein thrombosis using magnetic resonance imaging. Acta Radiol 1989; 30:445–446.
14. Mudge M, Hughes LE. The long-term sequelae of deep vein thrombosis. Br J Surg 1978; 65:692–694.
15. Murphy TP, Cronan JJ. Evolution of deep venous thrombosis: a prospective evaluation with US. Radiology 1990; 177:543–548.
16. Cronan JJ, Leen V. Recurrent deep venous thrombosis: limitations of US. Radiology 1989; 170:739–742.
17. Flanc AC. An experimental study of the recanalization of arterial and venous thrombi. Br J Surg 1968; 55:519–524.
18. Thomas ML, McAllister V. The radiological progression of deep vein thrombus. Radiology 1971; 99:37–40.
19. Cox JT. The maturation and canalization of thrombi. Surg Gynecol Obstet 1963; 116:593–599.
20. Bass JC, Hedlund LW, Sostman HD. MR imaging of experimental and clinical thrombi at 1.5T. Magn Reson Imaging 1990; 8:631–635.
21. Braun IR, Hoffman JC Jr, Malko JA, Pettigrew RI, Dannels W, Davis PC. Jugular venous thrombosis: MR imaging. Radiology 1985; 157:357–360.
22. Erdman WA, Weinreb JC, Cohen JM, Buja LM, Chaney C, Peshock RM. Venous thrombosis: clinical and experimental MR imaging. Radiology 1986; 161:233–238.
23. Wu JJ, MacFall JR, Sostman HD, Hedlund LW. Clot-blood contrast in fast gradient echo MRI. Invest Radiol 1993; 28:586–593.
24. Stuhlmuller JE, Olson JD, Burns TL, Skorton DJ. Effect of varying fibrinogen and hematocrit concentrations on magnetic resonance relaxation times of thrombus. Invest Radiol 1992; 27:341–345.
25. Rapoport S, Sostman HD, Pope C, Camputaro CM, Holcomb W, Gore JC. Venous clots: evaluation with MR imaging. Radiology 1987; 162:527–530.
26. Cohen MD, McGuire W, Cory DA, Smith JA. MR appearance of blood and blood products: an in vitro study. AJR 1986; 146:1293–1297.
27. Macchi PJ, Grossman RI, Gomori JM, Goldberg HI, Zimmerman RA, Bilaniuk LT. High field MR imaging of cerebral venous thrombosis. J Comput Assist Tomogr 1986; 10:10–15.
28. Gomori JM, Grossman RI. Head and neck hemorrhage. Magn Reson Annu 1987; 71–112.
29. Blinc A, Keber D, Lahajnar G, Zupancic I, Zorec-Karlovsk M, Demsar F. Magnetic resonance imaging of retracted and nonretracted blood clots during fibrinolysis in vitro. Haemostasis 1992; 22:195–201.

30. Francis CW, Totterman S. MRI of deep vein thrombi correlates with response to thrombolytic therapy. Thromb Haemost 1995; 73:386–391.
31. Mantoni M. Deep venous thrombosis: longitudinal study with duplex US. Radiology 1991; 179:271–273.
32. Foley WD, Middleton WD, Lawson TL. Color Doppler ultrasound imaging of lower extremity venous disease. AJR 1989; 152:371–376.
33. Lipchik EO, DeWeese JA, Rogoff SM. Serial long-term phelobography after documented lower leg thrombosis. Radiology 1976; 120:563–566.
34. Krupski WC, Bass A, Dilley RB, Bernstein EF, Otis SM. Propagation of deep venous thrombosis identified by duplex ultrasonography. J Vasc Surg 1990; 12:467–475.
35. Belcaro G. Evaluation of recurrent deep venous thrombosis using colour duplex scanning: comparison with venography. Vasa 1992; 21:22–26.
36. Kolecki RV, Sigel B, Justin J, et al. Determining the acuteness and stability of deep venous thrombosis by ultrasonic tissue characterization. J Vasc Surg 1995; 21:976–984.
37. Baxter GM, Duffy P, MacKechnie S. Colour Doppler ultrasound of the postphlebitic limb: sounding a cautionary note. Clin Radiol 1991; 43:301–304.
38. Evans AJ, Sostman D, Witty L, et al. Detection of deep venous thrombosis: prospective comparison of MR imaging and sonography. JMRI 1996; 6:44–51.
39. Spritzer CE, Evans AC, Kay HH. Magnetic resonance imaging of deep venous thrombosis in pregnant women with lower extremity edema. Obstet Gynecol 1995; 85: 603–607.
40. Montgomery KD, Potter HG, Helfet DL. Magnetic resonance venography to evaluate the deep venous system of the pelvis in patients who have an acetabular fracture. J Bone Joint Surg [Am] 1995; 77: 1639–1649.
41. Dupas B, ElKouri D, Curtet C, et al. Angiomagnetic resonance imaging of iliofemorocaval venous thrombosis. Lancet 1995; 346:17–19.
42. Greenfield LJ. Venous thromboembolic disease. In: Moore WS, ed. Vascular surgery: a comprehensive review. Philadelphia, Pa: Saunders, 1991; 669–679.

Book Review

Diagnostic Ultrasound: A Logical Approach

Edited by John P. McGahan, MD, and Barry B. Goldberg, MD
Philadelphia, Pa: Lippincott-Raven, 1997. ISBN 0-397-51614-2.
Hardcover, $195.00; pp 1,309; 1,474 figures; tables.

This new diagnostic ultrasonography (US) textbook provides a complete overview of current practice excluding echocardiography. It covers the gamut of most US practices, including obstetric, abdominal, pelvic, small parts, and interventional US, and introduces innovative approaches that readers may not have seen previously.

The book begins with an excellent overview chapter on US physics and an outstanding chapter on artifacts. They are followed by chapters on interventional US, percutaneous procedures in radiology and obstetrics and gynecology, and intraoperative US procedures. Chapters 6–18 deal with obstetric US, while chapters 19–29 discuss US of the abdomen and pelvis. Separate chapters on US of the pelvis in pre- and postmenopausal women are an unusual feature. Gastrointestinal US is addressed in a distinct chapter and in a separate chapter on endoscopic US at the end of the book. Rectal US is not addressed. The chapters on vascular US of the extremities, carotid US, and transcranial Doppler are well organized and include good tables and diagrams. In particular, these chapters make liberal use of color images, which is appropriate for their respective topics. The chapter on the breast is very short; it does not discuss US-guided aspiration or biopsy of breast lesions or preoperative localization. With the exception of an extensive chapter on the pediatric head, there are no separate chapters dealing with pediatrics; pediatric diseases are discussed by using an organ systems approach. Short chapters on US contrast material, three-dimensional US, and US-guided therapy introduce readers to these new topics. The book concludes with a chapter on endoscopic US written by a gastroenterologist, which focuses on gastric, pancreatic, and biliary diseases.

Overall, the organization of this book is clear, and there is little redundancy. The writing is clear, and most chapters have good reference lists. Some of the obstetric US images have been reprinted from prior monographs. The figures are from 1995 or later and are of reasonably good quality. The overall printing quality is good. Figures and illustrations are liberally used but appropriately infused throughout the text. In some areas, this book lacks the detail and breadth of examples from recent two-volume US textbooks; however, it is a single volume and priced below these two-volume sets. Its particular strengths are its focus on interventional US and its up-to-date vascular US chapters.

Diagnostic Ultrasound: A Logical Approach would be appropriate for any general US laboratory. It is intended as a teaching and reference book and serves this purpose admirably. The tables and graphs, in addition to well-annotated gray-scale and color figures, make this work accessible for a wide readership from medical and US students to practicing sonographers and radiologists.

Reviewed by Deborah J. Rubens, MD

Johanna L. Bosch, PhD
Eric Tetteroo, MD, PhD
Willem P. T. M. Mali, MD, PhD
Maria G. M. Hunink, MD, PhD
For the Dutch Iliac Stent Trial Study Group

Index terms:
Arteries, grafts and prostheses, 98.1268, 98.128
Arteries, iliac
Arteries, stenoses or obstruction, 98.721
Arteries, transluminal angioplasty, 98.1268, 98.128
Cost-effectiveness
Economics, medical

Radiology 1998; 208:641–648

Abbreviations:
CI = confidence interval
DIST = Dutch Iliac Stent Trial
PTA = percutaneous transluminal angioplasty
QALY = quality-adjusted life year

[1] From the Dept of Health Sciences, University of Groningen, The Netherlands (J.L.B., M.G.M.H.); the Depts of Epidemiology and Biostatistics (J.L.B., M.G.M.H.) and Radiology (M.G.M.H.), Erasmus University Medical School, Rm EE21-40a, P.O. Box 1738, 3000 DR Rotterdam, The Netherlands; the Dept of Health Policy and Management, Keio University, Tokyo, Japan (J.L.B.); the Dept of Radiology, University Hospital of Utrecht, The Netherlands (E.T., W.P.T.M.M.); and the Dept of Health Policy and Management, Harvard School of Public Health, Boston, Mass (M.G.M.H.). Received Nov 10, 1997; revision requested Jan 27, 1998; revision received Mar 9; accepted Apr 17. Supported by a PIONIER award from the Netherlands Organization for Scientific Research and grant OG-93/001 from the Commission of Investigative Medicine of the Dutch National Health Insurance Council. **Address reprint requests to** M.G.M.H.

Author contributions:
Guarantors of integrity of entire study, J.L.B., E.T., W.P.T.M.M., M.G.M.H.; study concepts and design, J.L.B., M.G.M.H.; definition of intellectual content, J.L.B., W.P.T.M.M., M.G.M.H.; literature research, J.L.B., M.G.M.H.; clinical studies, J.L.B., E.T., W.P.T.M.M., M.G.M.H.; data acquisition, J.L.B., E.T., W.P.T.M.M., M.G.M.H., the Group; data analysis, J.L.B., M.G.M.H.; statistical analysis, J.L.B., M.G.M.H.; manuscript preparation, J.L.B.; manuscript editing, M.G.M.H.; manuscript review, E.T., W.P.T.M.M., the Group.

Iliac Arterial Occlusive Disease: Cost-effectiveness Analysis of Stent Placement versus Percutaneous Transluminal Angioplasty[1]

PURPOSE: To evaluate the relative benefits and cost-effectiveness of treating iliac arterial occlusive disease with various interventions.

MATERIALS AND METHODS: Cost-effectiveness was analyzed in a hypothetical cohort of patients with intermittent claudication caused by an iliac arterial stenosis. Primary stent placement, percutaneous transluminal angioplasty (PTA), and PTA with selective stent placement were analyzed. Reduction in the risk of failure after primary stent placement versus that after PTA with selective stent placement, quality of life, and cost data were derived from results of a randomized, controlled trial. Complication rates, patency results, and the reduction in risk of failure were derived from a published meta-analysis.

RESULTS: PTA with selective stent placement yielded equivalent complication rates, patency results, and quality-of-life outcomes compared with those of primary stent placement, and the latter cost $957 less (95% confidence interval = $726, $1,188). PTA with selective stent placement was more expensive than PTA alone but yielded higher patency results (relative risk of long-term failure, 0.61; 95% confidence interval = 0.49, 0.75) and quality-adjusted life expectancy (0.2 quality-adjusted life year [QALY] gained) and had an incremental cost-effectiveness ratio of less than $20,000 per QALY gained.

CONCLUSION: PTA with selective stent placement is a cost-effective treatment strategy compared with primary stent placement or PTA alone in the treatment of intermittent claudication caused by an iliac arterial stenosis.

During the past decade, stent placement has been introduced as an adjunct to percutaneous transluminal angioplasty (PTA) in the treatment of iliac arterial occlusive disease (1–9). Nonrandomized cohort studies have shown promising patency results after stent placement, and a meta-analysis of these studies demonstrated a reduction in the risk of long-term failure after stent placement compared with the risk after PTA (10).

Although stents are now commonly placed selectively when angioplasty results are suboptimal and are sometimes even used for primary treatment, to our knowledge the cost-effectiveness of either approach has not been demonstrated. Given current budgetary constraints, the cost of various strategies for the percutaneous treatment of iliac arterial lesions is an important consideration. Furthermore, in addition to the demonstrated improvement in patency results, one would like to have evidence that stent placement actually improves patients' quality of life. Finally, the most important question is whether the gain in the quality of life justifies the additional cost of stent placement, regardless of whether such placement is primary or selective.

The purpose of this study was to evaluate the relative benefits and cost-effectiveness of treating lifestyle-limiting claudication due to an iliac arterial stenosis with primary stent placement, PTA, or PTA with selective stent placement. A cost-effectiveness analysis was performed along with a randomized, controlled trial to compare primary stent placement and PTA with selective stent placement. PTA with selective stent placement comprised PTA followed immediately by stent placement for lesions with a residual mean pressure gradient of more than 10 mm Hg across the lesion with vasodilatation (11,12). By using a decision model and the results of a published meta-analysis (10), the cost-effectiveness analysis was extended to include a comparison with PTA alone, PTA followed by repeated PTA in cases of long-term failure, and PTA followed by selective stent placement in cases of long-term failure.

MATERIALS AND METHODS

The Model

A decision and cost-effectiveness analysis was performed by using a multistate transition (Markov process) model in which a hypothetical cohort of patients was followed up over time (13,14). The baseline analysis considered patients with lifestyle-limiting claudication due to stenoses in the iliac arteries for whom a percutaneous intervention was indicated; we did not examine alternative treatments such as drug therapy, exercise, or surgery. Six treatment strategies were evaluated, each consisting of an initial intervention followed by a secondary treatment for long-term failures during follow-up.

The initial interventions analyzed were primary (direct) stent placement, PTA with selective stent placement for immediate PTA failures, or PTA alone. The secondary treatment performed in the event of a long-term failure during follow-up was chosen to reflect commonly used strategies and was dependent on the invasiveness of the initial intervention. The secondary treatment strategies were PTA with selective stent placement (selective stent placement after primary stent placement, repeated selective stent placement, and selective stent placement after PTA), repeated PTA if PTA alone was initially performed, or conservative management after selective stent placement or PTA, with no further revascularization procedure.

The analysis was performed from a societal perspective (15). Costs and benefits (expressed as quality-adjusted life years [QALYs]) of the initial procedures and the events during follow-up were estimated. Future costs and benefits were discounted at a nominal rate of 3% per year (15). A strategy was considered to be "inferior by dominance" if another strategy yielded higher or equivalent effectiveness at a lower cost. Incremental cost-effectiveness ratios—that is, additional costs divided by the effectiveness gained in comparison with the next best strategy—were calculated when a more effective strategy was also more expensive. A strategy was considered to be "inferior by extended dominance" if another strategy yielded greater effectiveness and had a lower incremental cost-effectiveness ratio. After the strategies that were inferior by dominance or extended dominance were eliminated from further consideration, all incremental cost-effectiveness ratios were recalculated. Threshold incremental cost-effectiveness ratios of $20,000 and $50,000 per QALY gained were considered. The decision model was programmed in the C programming language (Borland, Scotts Valley, Calif).

Data and Assumptions

The model combined data from the randomized, controlled Dutch Iliac Stent Trial (DIST) (11,12) and from a published meta-analysis (10). The variables, their baseline values, and the ranges that were explored with the sensitivity analysis are listed in Table 1.

DIST data.—In the DIST, primary stent placement (n = 143) and PTA with selective stent placement (n = 136) were compared for the treatment of intermittent claudication or critical ischemia due to stenosis or occlusion of an iliac artery (11,12). Interviews, which included questions about costs and quality of life, were conducted with 131 patients (92%) in the primary stent placement group and with 123 patients (90%) in the PTA with selective stent placement group. Nonparticipation in the interviews was due to logistic reasons (ie, the time between enrollment in the study and the procedure was too short to perform the interview or patients could not be reached by telephone). The baseline characteristics of the included patients were not significantly different between the two groups (11,12).

Meta-analysis data.—In the meta-analysis of cohort studies, the short- and long-term results of PTA and stent placement (primary or after failed PTA) for the treatment of iliac arterial occlusive disease were estimated and compared. The meta-analysis included six PTA studies (1,300 patients) and eight stent studies (816 patients) that were published in 1990 or later. Each study's definition of success, which generally was the maintenance of symptomatic and hemodynamic improvement after revascularization, was used in the meta-analysis. Proportions were combined by using a random-effects model, and patency data were pooled, with adjustment for differences in the case mix (10). Pooled patency results after PTA and stent placement were calculated for subgroups, depending on lesion type (stenosis vs occlusion) and disease severity (disabling claudication vs critical ischemia).

Effectiveness

QALYs were estimated for each treatment strategy on the basis of the morbidity and mortality data, patency results, and quality-of-life data (Table 1).

Morbidity and mortality rates.—The results of both the meta-analysis and the DIST demonstrated that the procedural morbidity and mortality rates were low and not significantly different for PTA or stent placement. In the decision model, we included the procedural morbidity and mortality rates derived from the meta-analysis because these reflected a broader experience and the rates were comparable to those from the DIST. Postprocedural long-term survival was not affected by the percutaneous revascularization procedure performed. Nevertheless, we adjusted the long-term life expectancy on the basis of age- and sex-specific mortality rates from standard life tables of the general population and the excess mortality for peripheral arterial occlusive disease (16,17). For the sensitivity analysis, we used a relative risk ratio of 3.1 for the risk of dying among patients with peripheral arterial occlusive disease compared with the risk among individuals in the general population without the disease (17,18).

Patency.—The results of the DIST demonstrated that primary stent placement and PTA with selective stent placement yielded equivalent patency rates during a 2-year follow-up (12). Because failure rates are highest during the first 2 years after the procedure, we assumed that primary stent placement and PTA with selective stent placement would yield equivalent patency results for the entire life expectancy of the patient. The proportion of patients requiring stent placement due to an inadequate PTA result in the selective stent placement strategy was based on the DIST (43%), and a wide range (10%–90%) was explored in the sensitivity analysis.

To enable the comparison with PTA and to model the patency rates beyond 2 years, the primary patency results from the meta-analysis were included in the model (Table 1). We used the specific annual failure rate for the first 4 years

TABLE 1
Decision Model Variables, Baseline Values, and Estimates Used for the Sensitivity Analysis

Variable	Baseline Value	Range or Alternative Estimate*	Reference No. or Source†
Annual excess mortality rate due to peripheral arterial occlusive disease			
Ankle-brachial pressure index > 0.30	0.02	NA	16,17
Ankle-brachial pressure index ≤ 0.30	0.12	NA	16,17
Relative risk of mortality due to peripheral arterial occlusive disease	NA	3.1	16,18
Procedural mortality rate‡	0.01	0.00–0.03	10,12
Complication rate‡	0.05	0.02–0.07	10§
Proportion needing stent placement in selective placement strategy	0.43	0.10–0.90	12
Initial technical success rate			
Stent placement for stenoses	1.00	NA	10,12‖
Stent placement for occlusions	0.80	NA	10
PTA for stenoses	0.96	NA	10
PTA for occlusions	0.80	NA	10
Long-term patency after PTA for claudication and a stenosis, including technical failures			
Immediate	0.91	NA	10
1 y	0.74	NA	10
2 y	0.66	NA	10
3 y	0.61	NA	10
4 y	0.58	NA	10
Relative risk for long-term failure of patency			
Primary versus selective stent placement	1.00	NA	12
Stent versus PTA	0.61	0.49–0.75	10
Critical ischemia versus claudication	1.54	1.12–2.11	10
Quality-of-life score#			
Successful treatment	0.82	0.69–0.90	Present study
After failure	0.70	0.43–0.88	Present study
Procedural costs (1995 $)			
Primary stent placement	3,990	3,162–4,873	Present study
Selective stent placement	3,033	2,333–3,819	Present study
PTA	2,343	1,707–3,024	Present study
Cost of one stent	1,166	250–1,500	Present study
Bypass surgery	2,861	NA	Present study
Annual cost of follow-up (1995 $)			
1st year	457	NA	Present study
Subsequent years	229	NA	Present study
Discount rate (%)	3	0–7	15

* NA = not available.
† Reference 10 is a meta-analysis, reference 12 is a report of the DIST, reference 15 is a volume by Gold et al, reference 16 is a report by Fowkes, reference 17 is a report by Howell et al, and reference 18 is a report by Criqui et al.
‡ Includes only complications that necessitated treatment.
§ In the meta-analysis (10), the mortality and complication rates after stent placement or PTA were similar; in the DIST, these rates were similar for primary stent placement and PTA with selective stent placement.
‖ In the DIST, no significant differences were found for initial technical success rates between primary stent placement and PTA with selective stent placement.
\# Quality of life was similar after primary stent placement, PTA with selective stent placement, and PTA alone and was not affected by complications.

after revascularization and assumed a constant annual failure rate thereafter. The relative risk ratio of failure of 0.61 after stent placement relative to PTA was based on the results of the meta-analysis, and we explored the 95% confidence interval (CI) (95% CI = 0.49, 0.75) for the sensitivity analysis (Table 1). We assumed that the patency results after repeated procedures were equivalent to the patency results after the same procedure performed as an initial treatment (14). Furthermore, we assumed that repeated interventions were usually percutaneous interventions and that any surgical procedure performed owing to a long-term failure would yield patency results similar to those of a percutaneous procedure (10,12,19). Patients with an untreated failure were assumed to develop symptoms similar to their symptoms before treatment.

Quality of life.—Quality-of-life adjustments for untreated symptoms and for successful treatment were determined during interviews as part of the DIST (20). The interview consisted of a generic health status questionnaire (the RAND-36, which is equivalent to the Medical Outcomes Study Short Form-36 [21]) and several valuational measures. To assess quality-of-life values from the societal perspective, the McMaster Health-Utilities Index and the EuroQol-5D were used (22–25). Both measures include a descriptive classification system and a mathematic formula for calculating health state values. To assess quality-of-life values from the patient's perspective, the standard gamble, the time trade-off, and a rating scale were used. With these valuational measures, patients assigned numeric values or utilities to their present state of health averaged over the past 4 weeks on a scale from 0.0 (death) to 1.0 (full health comparable to that of healthy contemporaries) (10). The mean Health-Utilities Index values were used in the baseline analysis (to reflect the societal perspective), and the range found with the other valuational measures was explored for the sensitivity analysis.

Quality-of-life values after successful treatment and without long-term failure were shown to remain constant over time. Furthermore, the quality of life before intervention was not associated with age. Thus, within each health state we assumed that the quality adjustment was constant over time. Quality-of-life values after a procedure with complications were shown to be similar to those after a procedure with no complications. The observed complications were mostly inconsequential local complications such as hematomas (12). Therefore, no adjustments were made for quality of life after complications.

Cost Analysis

A cost analysis of primary stent placement and PTA with selective stent placement was performed among the corresponding patient groups of the DIST. The costs of PTA alone were estimated among the subgroup of patients in the selective stent group that did not have a residual intraarterial pressure gradient after treatment with PTA. Cost estimates included direct health care and non–health care costs incurred by the interventional radiology department, the hospital, and the patient and included the cost of treating complications (15). Costs of events during follow-up, including those of follow-up examinations and procedures performed for recurrent symptoms, were included in the decision model. Productivity losses associated with morbidity were considered to be reflected in the QALY estimate (15). The additional "friction" costs of lost productivity were considered, but because the majority of patients were retired and the mean convalescence time was less than a week, these costs were negligible (15,26). Furthermore, the costs of general medical care during follow-up were considered, but because the mean life expectancy was equivalent across strategies, these costs would cancel out in the incremental cost-effectiveness ratio calculation and were therefore omitted. All costs were converted to 1995 Dutch guilders by using the consumer price index and were subsequently converted to 1995 U.S. dollars by using the mean exchange rate for the year 1995 (ie, $1 = 1.61 guilders [27]).

The costs incurred by the interventional radiology department included the costs of personnel, materials, equipment and maintenance, and housing of the angiography room. Diagnostic angiography was considered to be an essential part of the interventional procedure. A time-and-motion study and cost accounting were performed for 16 procedures at the University Hospital of Utrecht, The Netherlands. The distribution of lesions and the number of stents needed to treat a lesion (mean, 1.4 stents) were calculated on the basis of data from the DIST. Because the cost of the stent prosthesis was an important component of the procedural cost of stent placement and because this cost varies across countries and the type of stent used, we explored the effect of varying this cost component for the sensitivity analysis (Table 1). Furthermore, a range of procedural cost estimates of PTA and stent placement was obtained by means of a survey among eight hospitals in The Netherlands. The range was explored for the sensitivity analysis (range for PTA, $1,707–$2,969; range for stent placement, $3,162–$4,873).

Hospital costs included those incurred by the interventional radiology department, room and board, and other hospital costs. The total costs for room and board and other hospital costs were calculated by multiplying the mean length of a hospital stay (determined in 254 patients with completed interviews in the DIST) by the price of a hospitalization day. The price of a hospitalization day was obtained from the University Hospital of Utrecht administration and included room and board and other costs such as those of medication, laboratory services, blood products, and nursing care. The mean cost per procedure due to complications was estimated by multiplying the probability of a complication by the reimbursements for the necessary treatment.

Follow-up costs consisted of the actual costs of two outpatient visits in the 1st year and one visit in following years and included medication, patient's travel expenses, time costs, and noninvasive diagnostic tests (treadmill testing, ankle pressure measurements, and duplex ultrasonography of the treated segment). The costs of the noninvasive tests were estimated on the basis of the duration of the test, the personnel involved, and the equipment, materials, and housing. The cost of an intervention during follow-up was estimated on the basis of the average cost of such an intervention in the DIST. Most interventions during follow-up (13 [81%] of 16) in the DIST were repeated percutaneous interventions, for which we had determined the costs as described; a few (three [19%] of 16) were surgical revascularizations, for which we used reimbursement data. Patient cost data were obtained among all patients who participated in the telephone interviews and included time costs, travel expenses, and out-of-pocket expenses (eg, purchase of walking equipment or hiring of housekeeping help). The time costs were estimated by multiplying the time expended for the intervention by the average wage for a 60-year-old man (15,27).

TABLE 2
Quality of Life and Clinical Outcome before and after Treatment

	Before Treatment		After Treatment	
Variable	Primary Stent Placement	PTA with Selective Stent Placement	Primary Stent Placement	PTA with Selective Stent Placement
Quality-of-life score				
Physical functioning*	40 ± 19	43 ± 20	74 ± 26	75 ± 26
Bodily pain*	50 ± 22	50 ± 25	78 ± 25	74 ± 26
Physical role functioning*	27 ± 36	32 ± 40	67 ± 43	64 ± 43
Time trade-off	0.82 ± 0.18	0.79 ± 0.21	0.87 ± 0.18	0.89 ± 0.15
Standard gamble	0.88 ± 0.17	0.89 ± 0.14	0.91 ± 0.15	0.92 ± 0.12
Rating scale	0.71 ± 0.17	0.72 ± 0.18	0.80 ± 0.17	0.79 ± 0.15
Health-Utilities Index mark II	0.68 ± 0.20	0.73 ± 0.21	0.81 ± 0.20	0.80 ± 0.19
EuroQol-5D	0.43 ± 0.13	0.43 ± 0.17	0.71 ± 0.28	0.69 ± 0.26
Clinical outcome				
Ankle-brachial index at rest	0.78 ± 0.20	0.77 ± 0.20	0.94 ± 0.19	0.93 ± 0.23
Ankle-brachial index after exercise	0.65 ± 0.30	0.63 ± 0.33	0.79 ± 0.27	0.83 ± 0.30
Walking distance (m)†	211 ± 94	226 ± 88	245 ± 80	257 ± 64

Note.—Data are the mean ± 1 standard deviation.
* The most limited health dimensions of the RAND-36 are reported.
† The maximum walking distance measured was 300 m.

RESULTS

Baseline Analysis

Findings from the randomized clinical trial demonstrated that primary stent placement and PTA with selective stent placement yielded equivalent complication rates (six [4%] of 143 for primary stent placement and 10 [7%] of 136 for selective stent placement [95% CI = −2%, 9%]), patency results (2-year cumulative patency rate of 71% for primary stent placement and 70% for selective stent placement; $P = .09$), and quality-of-life and clinical outcomes ($P > .05$; Table 2). Primary stent placement was more expensive than PTA with selective stent placement (incremental cost, $957; 95% CI = $726, $1,188; Table 3). Thus, primary stent placement was inferior by dominance to PTA with selective stent placement in the treatment of iliac arterial occlusive disease (Table 4).

For the baseline case in the decision model, we considered a 60-year-old man with intermittent claudication and an iliac arterial stenosis (Table 4). The comparison of PTA and selective stent placement with PTA alone yielded a higher patency rate (relative risk of long-term failure, 0.61; 95% CI = 0.49, 0.75) (10), higher quality-adjusted life expectancy (Table 4), and higher costs (Tables 3, 4). The incremental cost-effectiveness ratio, however, was well below $20,000 per QALY gained (Table 4). These findings were applicable irrespective of whether a repeated intervention was considered (in Table 4: PTA with selective stent placement followed by no revascularization [row 3] compared with PTA alone [row 2]; initial and repeated PTA with selective stent placement [row 6] compared with initial and repeated PTA [row 4] or PTA followed by PTA with selective stent placement [row 5]).

TABLE 3
Direct Procedural Costs in the Treatment of Iliac Arterial Occlusive Disease

Component	Primary Stent Placement (1995 $)	PTA with Selective Stent Placement (1995 $)	PTA (1995 $)
Radiology Department			
Personnel	324 ± 31	284 ± 30	257 ± 36
Materials	2,259 ± 136	1,352 ± 98	706 ± 35
Equipment	223 ± 27	214 ± 32	199 ± 56
Room	36 ± 4	35 ± 5	33 ± 7
Subtotal	2,842 ± 142	1,885 ± 108	1,195 ± 76
Additional Hospital Costs			
Room and board and other costs	807 ± 807	807 ± 807	807 ± 807
Complications	137	137	137
Subtotal	944 ± 807	944 ± 807	944 ± 807
Patient Costs			
Travel expenses	10 ± 12	10 ± 12	10 ± 12
Time expenses	194 ± 194	194 ± 194	194 ± 194
Out-of-pocket expenses	0	0	0
Subtotal	204 ± 194	204 ± 194	204 ± 194
Total	3,990 ± 842	3,033 ± 837	2,343 ± 834

Note.—Data are based on DIST results. Numbers are the mean ± 1 standard deviation.

TABLE 4
Quality-adjusted Life Expectancy, Costs, and Cost-Effectiveness Ratio for a 60-year-old Man with Claudication due to an Iliac Arterial Stenosis

Treatment Strategy	Quality-adjusted Life Expectancy (QALYs)*	Cost (1995 $)*	Incremental Cost-effectiveness Ratio†
No revascularization	10.30	3,368	Reference strategy
PTA followed by no revascularization	11.03	5,868	Inferior by extended dominance
PTA with selective stent placement followed by no revascularization	11.29	6,573	4,073
PTA and repeated PTA	11.36	7,145	Inferior by extended dominance
PTA followed by PTA with selective stent placement	11.47	7,504	Inferior by extended dominance
Initial and repeated PTA with selective stent placement	11.61	7,806	4,519
Primary stent placement followed by PTA with selective stent placement	11.61	8,763	Inferior by dominance

* Data are reported without discounting.
† Ratios are reported with 3%-per-year discounting of both costs and effectiveness.

Sensitivity Analysis

Similar results were found in a sensitivity analysis where we varied the relative risk of long-term failure after stent placement compared with the relative risk associated with PTA, the proportion of patients requiring stent placement after PTA (Fig 1), and the cost of a stent (Fig 2). The preferred treatment strategy was initial PTA with selective stent placement followed by repeated PTA with selective stent placement for long-term failures over a wide range of values for these variables; the incremental cost-effectiveness ratio was less than $20,000 per QALY gained. When we varied the relative risk of long-term failure after stent placement across the 95% CI (for risk reduction, 25%, 51%; for relative risk, 0.49, 0.75) the decision did not change regardless of the proportion requiring a stent (from 10% to 90%; Fig 1) and the cost of a stent (from $250 to $1,500; Fig 2). By using the baseline values for the proportion requiring a stent (59 [43%] of 136) and the cost of a stent ($1,166), the preferred strategy was PTA with selective stent placement (initial and for long-term failures), with an incremental cost-effectiveness ratio of less than $20,000 per QALY gained for a 15% or greater reduction in the risk of failure (relative risk ≤ 0.85).

In the event that the reduction in the risk of failure with stent placement was less than 25% (ie, relative risk greater than the upper limit of the 95% CI [0.75]), the preferred treatment strategy depended on the proportion requiring stent placement and the societal willingness to pay for such care (Fig 1). In similar fashion, if the reduction in the risk of failure with stent placement was less than 13% (relative risk > 0.87), the preferred treatment strategy was dependent on the cost of a stent and the societal willingness to pay for such care (Fig 2). PTA would be favored if the reduction in the risk of failures was much lower than expected (relative risk greater than the upper limit of the 95% CI), the proportion requiring stent placement in the selective stent strategy was high, the cost of a stent was high, and the societal willingness to pay was low. As expected, if stent placement and PTA yielded similar patency results (reduction in failure, 0%–1%; relative risk, 0.99–1.00), the optimal strategy was PTA followed by PTA for long-term failures, which cost less irrespective of the proportion requiring a stent and the cost of a stent.

The sensitivity analysis for patients treated because of an occlusion or critical ischemia in the iliac arteries yielded results similar to those of the baseline analysis. Variations in the quality-of-life values after successful treatment and after failure demonstrated that if the difference in utility between successful treatment and failure was 0.05 or greater, the optimal treatment strategy was PTA with selective stent placement (initial and for long-term failures), with a cost-effectiveness ratio of less than $20,000 per QALY gained. Finally, the decision for selective stent placement or PTA was insensitive to the explored variation (Table 1) in the procedural complication and mortality rates, excess mortality or relative increase in mortality rate due to the disease, discount rate, age group, sex, and costs for PTA and stent placement.

DISCUSSION

This study addressed the costs, benefits, and cost-effectiveness of various percutaneous treatment strategies for iliac arterial occlusive disease. Our results suggest that the optimal percutaneous treatment strategy is PTA followed by immediate stent placement to treat suboptimal results. Primary stent placement was equally effective compared with PTA with selective stent placement, but the former was more expensive. PTA with selective stent placement was more expensive than PTA alone, but the gain in effectiveness justified the additional cost. These results support the increasingly common practice of selective stent placement for the treatment of intermittent claudication due to stenosis in an iliac artery (1–7,9).

In this cost-effectiveness analysis, we included data from a randomized, controlled clinical trial (11,12) and from a meta-analysis (10). The hypothesis of the clinical trial was that primary stent placement may provide better initial angiographic and hemodynamic results compared with PTA with selective stent placement, with less chance of elastic recoil and improved sealing of intimal flaps. The results, however, demonstrated no difference between the two treatment strategies in terms of patency rates or quality of life (12).

It should be noted that the clinical trial started in November 1993, and the available follow-up period was thus limited to a mean of 9.3 months. It is still unclear what the effectiveness of a stent may be in the long term. Intimal proliferation may cause narrowing of the luminal diameter, and there may be risks associated with the presence of a foreign body. However, previous studies (28,29) demonstrated that the failure rate is highest in the 1st year after treatment; thus, a difference in failure rates beyond 1 year is unlikely.

The morbidity, mortality, and patency data included in our decision model were based on data from a meta-analysis (10) of six PTA studies and eight stent placement studies (primary placement or placement after PTA). The results of stent placement yielded similar complication rates compared with the results of PTA, a higher technical success rate in the treatment of stenoses, and a reduction in the long-term failure rate. A comparison was made with contemporary control subjects, and the patency data were adjusted for differences in case mix and reporting methods. Nevertheless, the results should be interpreted with caution because the patients were not randomly assigned to stent placement versus PTA, and success was not uniformly defined across the studies.

As with every simulation model, various assumptions were necessary to improve the tractability of the problem and the internal consistency of the model. First, we considered only percutaneous treatment and not alternatives such as exercise or medical therapy. Thus, our results apply only to those patients in whom noninvasive treatment has yielded inadequate results. Second, we assumed that stent placement and PTA had the same mortality and complication rates. Because no differences in these rates were found between the different treatment strategies in either the meta-analysis or the DIST, this assumption seemed justified. Third, we assumed that long-term failures would, in the majority of cases, be treated percutaneously. The cost estimates for interventions during follow-up were adjusted to include a small proportion of surgical interventions, but the patency rates after these few surgical interventions were assumed to be equivalent to those of a percutaneous intervention. Fourth, we assumed the same quality of life in patients who did and in those who did not have complications. In the DIST, patients with complications did not have differences in quality-of-life values compared with patients without complications. Finally, patients with complications did not have a longer hospital stay. Therefore, the effects of complications were only included as a cost incurred by the required treatment.

A limitation of our study was that we did not perform a formal cost analysis for the treatment of complications and for surgical interventions performed because of long-term failures; instead, we estimated these costs by using the reimbursements for the necessary treatment. Because the probability of complications was demonstrated to be equivalent irrespective of the initial treatment performed, this cost estimate will cancel out in the incremental cost-effectiveness ratio with respect to the initial treatment. Although they may be relevant in terms of a difference in subsequent repeated interventions, the probabilities of complications and surgical interventions during follow-up both were low. Thus, a small bias in the cost estimates for complica-

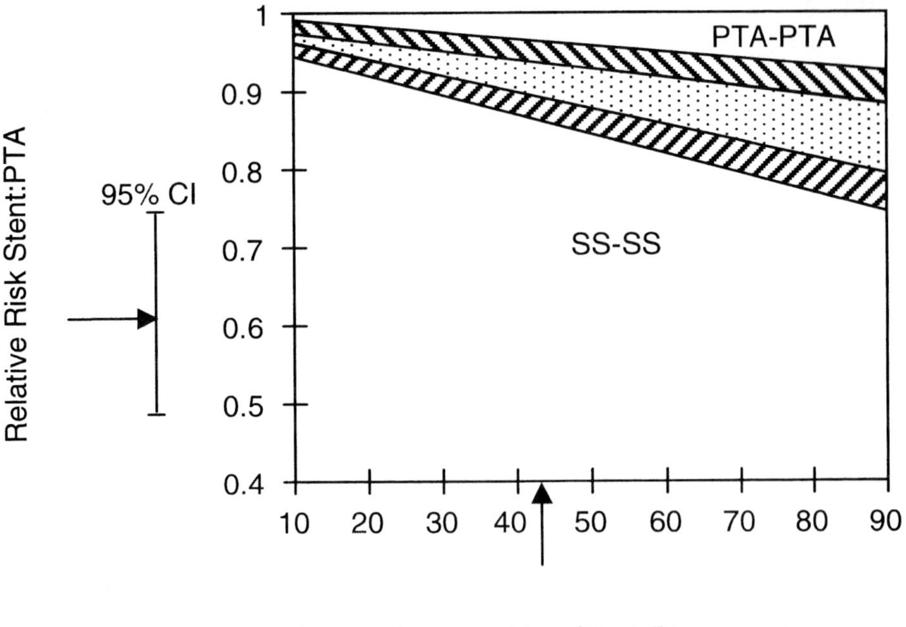

Figure 1. Graph shows the optimal treatment strategy in a two-way sensitivity analysis with varying relative risk of failure after stent placement compared with that for PTA and the proportion of patients requiring stent placement after PTA for threshold cost-effectiveness ratios of $20,000 per QALY and $50,000 per QALY. Indicated are the values used in the baseline analysis (arrows) and the 95% CI of the relative risk of failure after stent placement compared with that of failure after PTA. The optimal treatment strategy (ie, initial and repeated PTA [*PTA-PTA*], initial PTA and subsequent PTA with selective stent placement, or initial and repeated PTA with selective stent placement [*SS-SS*]) comprises an initial treatment (PTA alone or PTA with selective stent placement) followed by a secondary treatment performed in the event of a long-term failure. Top striped area = threshold ratio of $20,000 for initial and repeated PTA and of $50,000 for initial PTA and subsequent PTA with selective stent placement, dotted area = threshold ratio of $20,000 for initial and repeated PTA and of $50,000 for initial and repeated PTA with selective stent placement, bottom striped area = threshold ratio of $20,000 for initial PTA and subsequent PTA with selective stent placement and of $50,000 for initial and repeated PTA with selective stent placement.

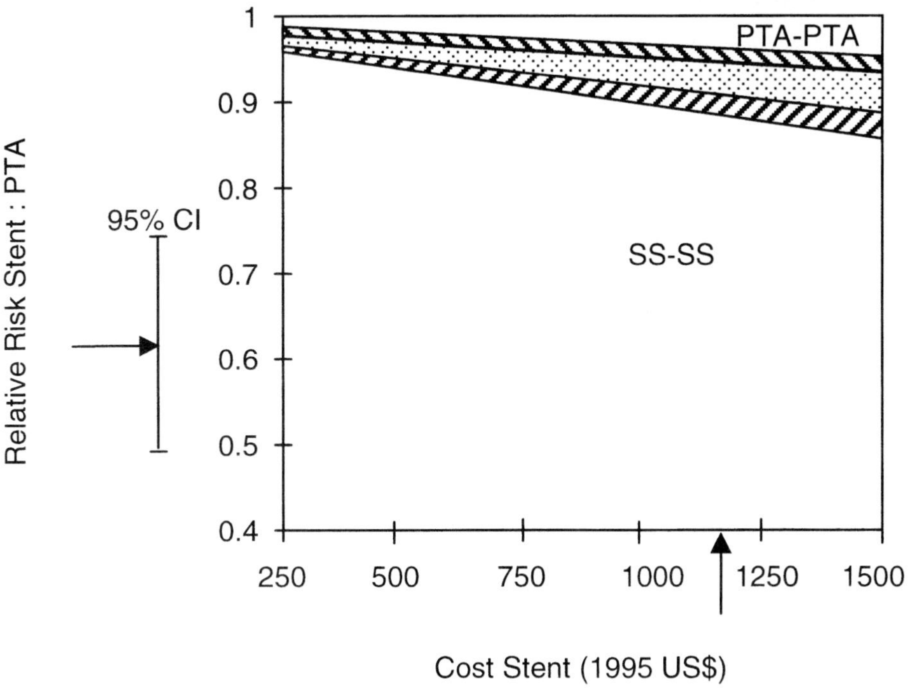

Figure 2. Graph shows the optimal treatment strategy in a two-way sensitivity analysis with varying relative risk of failure after stent placement compared with that for PTA and the cost of one stent prosthesis for threshold cost-effectiveness ratios of $20,000 per QALY and $50,000 per QALY. Indicated are the values used in the baseline analysis (arrows) and the 95% CI of the relative risk of failure after stent placement compared with that of failure after PTA. The optimal treatment strategy (ie, initial and repeated PTA [*PTA-PTA*], initial PTA and subsequent PTA with selective stent placement, or initial and repeated PTA with selective stent placement [*SS-SS*]) comprises an initial treatment (PTA alone or PTA with selective stent placement) followed by a secondary treatment performed in the event of a long-term failure. Top striped area = threshold ratio of $20,000 for initial and repeated PTA and of $50,000 for initial PTA and subsequent PTA with selective stent placement, dotted area = threshold ratio of $20,000 for initial and repeated PTA and of $50,000 for initial and repeated PTA with selective stent placement, bottom striped area = threshold ratio of $20,000 for initial PTA and subsequent PTA with selective stent placement and of $50,000 for initial and repeated PTA with selective stent placement.

tions and surgical interventions is unlikely to have had a major effect on our conclusions.

The estimated cost of PTA may have been underestimated, because this cost was determined among a specific subgroup in the selective stent strategy of the DIST, that is, those who were treated successfully with PTA alone and did not require stent placement. In practice PTA may be more expensive, because one would attempt to salvage the intervention by using a larger balloon or some other adjunct. Thus, our cost estimates of the initial PTA strategies (PTA with selective stent placement, PTA and repeated PTA, PTA followed by no revascularization) are probably underestimates. However, this implies that the cost difference between PTA with selective stent placement and PTA alone was possibly overestimated and that the corresponding incremental cost-effectiveness ratio was also overestimated. Because this ratio is well under the acceptable threshold and an extensive sensitivity analysis with changes in the cost of PTA showed similar results, the possible bias supports our argument that PTA with selective stent placement is cost-effective compared with PTA alone.

For the baseline case, we considered a 60-year-old man with a stenosis in the iliac artery who was undergoing treatment for intermittent claudication. The results were robust in a sensitivity analysis where each variable was varied over a plausible range: in particular, the relative risk of long-term failure after stent placement compared with the relative risk after PTA, the cost of a stent, the proportion of patients requiring stent placement after PTA, and quality-of-life outcomes. In fact, when the relative risk of long-term failure after stent placement was varied across the full 95% CI, the decision did not change.

The sensitivity analysis results in which the cost-effectiveness analysis was extended to patients with an occlusion in the iliac artery and to those treated for critical ischemia suggested that the preferred treatment strategy was PTA with selective stent placement. These results must be interpreted with caution, because the subgroup with occlusions or critical ischemia was underrepresented. In the meta-analysis (10), only 122 (15%) of 816 patients had critical ischemia at the time of presentation, and 254 (28%) of 906 lesions were occlusions. In the randomized clinical trial, only 18 (6%) of 279 patients were treated for critical ischemia, and 29 (8%) of 356 lesions were occlusions. It is likely that a selective stent placement strategy in patients with an occlusion would result in a high proportion of stent placements. In fact, of the 12 occlusions reported in the DIST (12) that were treated with an initial PTA, 10 (83%) required stent placement. This implies that the cost difference between primary stent placement and PTA with selective stent placement in this subgroup was only $285 and that patients with an occlusion may thus be more appropriately treated with primary stent placement. Furthermore, initial PTA for an occlusion followed by selective stent placement may increase the cost relative to primary stent placement if initial PTA is complicated because of thrombosis or extension of the site of the lesion. Although we did not find evidence for such an increase in costs, the number of patients with an occlusion was too small to demonstrate a clinically relevant difference.

Finally, the results of the randomized, controlled trial in which primary stent placement was compared with PTA with selective stent placement suggested that primary stent placement yields no additional long-term benefit and is more expensive. With an extensive cost analysis, including subsequent costs, we demonstrated that the main difference in the costs of these two strategies was the initial additional cost of the stents. In the population we studied, no cost savings were achieved with primary stent placement by means of a decrease in the use of other materials or a shorter duration of the procedure. Although we could not demonstrate a cost advantage with primary stent placement, this may be different in other settings where, for instance, a shorter procedural time can be attained, which may translate into large cost savings. In the United States, for example, a shorter procedural time would be associated with a large cost saving because of personnel costs that are high compared with those in The Netherlands. Furthermore, if multiple balloons are used in an attempt to optimize PTA results before stent placement, this would add procedural time and costs to the treatment strategy of PTA with selective stent placement. In addition, the price of a stent is lower in the United States than in The Netherlands. This implies that if the additional cost of a stent for a primary stent placement can be justified because of cost savings due to a shorter procedural time and the use of fewer other materials, primary stent placement would be cost-effective compared with PTA with selective stent placement.

In conclusion, our results suggest that PTA with selective stent placement is a cost-effective strategy, compared with PTA alone, for the treatment of iliac arterial occlusive disease and that the gain in effectiveness justifies the additional costs. In the treatment of patients with claudication and a stenosis, primary stent placement yielded no additional benefit and was more expensive compared with PTA followed by selective stent placement. In the treatment of patients with critical ischemia or an occlusion, the role of primary stent placement in comparison with selective stent placement remains to be elucidated.

Acknowledgments: The following centers in The Netherlands participated in the DIST Study Group (with investigators and numbers of patients included): St Antonius Hospital Nieuwegein (83 patients): T. T. C. Overtoom, MD, J. C. de Valois, MD, PhD, F. L. Moll, MD, PhD, and H. D. W. M. van de Pavoordt, MD, PhD; Slingeland Hospital Doetinchem (67 patients): J. H. Spithoven, MD, J. G. J. M. van Iersel, MD, and J. Seegers, MD; University Hospital Utrecht (50 patients): B. C. Eikelboom, MD, PhD, J. P. J. van Schaik, MD, PhD, F. J. A. Beek, MD, PhD, C. Haaring, BA, A. D. van Engelen, MD, and Y. van der Graaf, MD, PhD; University Hospital Rotterdam (35 patients): H. Pieterman, MD, and H. van Urk, MD, PhD; Twenteborg Hospital Almelo (33 patients): J. J. Kouwenberg, MD, F. H. B. Tuynman, MD, J. W. van den Heuvel, MD, and J. G. van Baal, MD, PhD; Catharina Hospital Eindhoven (11 patients): G. H. M. Landman, MD, PhD, A. V. Tielbeek, MD, PhD, and J. Buth, MD, PhD; University of Groningen: E. E. E. van Wijck, MSc.

References

1. Vorwerk D, Günther RW, Schurman K, Wendt G. Aortic and iliac stenoses: follow-up results of stent placement after insufficient balloon angioplasty in 118 cases. Radiology 1996; 198:45–48.
2. Long AL, Sapoval MR, Beyssen BM, et al. Strecker stent implantation in iliac arteries: patency and predictive factors for long-term success. Radiology 1995; 194:739–744.
3. Wolf YG, Schatz RA, Knowles HJ, Saeed M, Bernstein EF, Dilley RB. Initial experience with the Palmaz stent for aortoiliac stenoses. Ann Vasc Surg 1993; 7:254–261.
4. Strecker EPK, Hagen B, Liermann D, Schneider B, Wolf HRD, Wambsganss J. Iliac and femoropopliteal vascular occlusive disease treated with flexible tantalum stents. Cardiovasc Intervent Radiol 1993; 16:158–164.
5. Henry M, Amor M, Ethevenot G, et al. Palmaz stent placement in iliac and femoropopliteal arteries: primary and secondary patency in 310 patients with 2–4-year follow-up. Radiology 1995; 197:167–174.
6. Martin EC, Katzen BT, Benenati JF, et al. Multicenter trial of the Wallstent in the iliac and femoral arteries. JVIR 1995; 6:843–849.
7. Palmaz JC, Laborde JC, Rivera FJ, Encarnacion CE, Lutz JD, Moss JG. Stenting of the iliac arteries with the Palmaz stent: experience from a multicenter trial. Cardiovasc Intervent Radiol 1992; 15:291–297.
8. Laborde JC, Palmaz JC, Rivera FJ, Encarnacion CE, Picot MC, Dougherty SP. Influence of anatomic distribution of atherosclerosis on the outcome of revascularization with iliac stent placement. JVIR 1995; 6:513–521.
9. Zeitler E, Beyer-Enke S, Rompel O. Indications and results after Strecker-stent-application in iliac and SFA. Int Angiol 1993; 12:152–161.
10. Bosch JL, Hunink MGM. Meta-analysis of the results of percutaneous transluminal angioplasty and stent placement for aortoiliac occlusive disease. Radiology 1997; 204:87–96.
11. Tetteroo E, Haaring C, van der Graaf Y, et al. Intraarterial pressure gradients after randomized angioplasty or stenting of iliac artery lesions. Cardiovasc Intervent Radiol 1996; 19:411–417.
12. Tetteroo E, van der Graaf Y, Bosch JL, et al. Randomised comparison of primary stent placement versus primary angioplasty followed by selective stent placement in patients with iliac artery occlusive disease. Lancet 1998; 351:1153–1159.
13. Sonnenberg FA, Beck JR. Markov models in medical decision making: a practical guide. Med Decis Making 1993; 13:322–338.
14. Hunink MGM, Wong JB, Donaldson MC, Meyerovitz MF, De Vries JA, Harrington DP. Revascularization for femoropopliteal disease: a decision and cost-effectiveness analysis. JAMA 1995; 274:165–171.
15. Gold MR, Siegel JE, Russel LB, Weinstein MC. Cost-effectiveness in health and medicine. New York, NY: Oxford University Press, 1996.
16. Fowkes FGR. Epidemiology of atherosclerotic arterial disease in the lower limbs. Eur J Vasc Surg 1988; 2:283–291.
17. Howell MA, Colgan MP, Seeger RW, Ramsey DE, Sumner DS. Relationship of severity of lower limb peripheral vascular disease to mortality and morbidity: a six-year follow-up study. J Vasc Surg 1989; 9:691–697.
18. Criqui MH, Langer RD, Fronek A, et al. Mortality over a period of 10 years in patients with peripheral arterial disease. N Engl J Med 1992; 326:381–386.
19. De Vries SO, Hunink MGM. Long-term patency of bifurcation grafts for aortoiliac occlusive disease: a meta-analysis. J Vasc Surg 1997; 26:558–569.
20. Bosch JL, Hunink MGM. The relationship between descriptive and valuational quality-of-life measures in patients with intermittent claudication. Med Decis Making 1996; 16:217–225.
21. Hays RD, Sherbourne CD, Mazel RM. The RAND 36-item health survey 1.0. Health Econ 1993; 2:217–227.
22. Feeny D, Furlong W, Boyle M, Torrance GW. Multi-attribute health status classification systems: Health Utilities Index. Pharmacoeconomics 1995; 7:490–502.
23. Torrance GW, Furlong W, Feeny D, Boyle M. Multiattribute preference functions: Health Utilities Index. Pharmacoeconomics 1995; 7:503–520.
24. Essink-Bot ML, Stouthard MEA, Bonsel GJ. Generalizability of valuations on health states collected with the EuroQol-questionnaire. Health Econ 1993; 2:237–246.
25. van Hout B, McDonnell J. Estimating a parametric relation between health description and health valuation using the EuroQol instrument: EuroQol conference proceedings, Lund, Sweden, October 1991—IHE working paper. Swed Inst Health Econ 1992; 2:45–59.
26. Koopmanschap MA, Rutten FFH, van Ineveld BM, van Roijen L. The friction cost method for estimating the indirect costs of disease. J Health Econ 1995; 14:171–189.
27. Statistisch jaarboek centraal bureau voor de statistiek. The Hague, The Netherlands: Central Bureau for Statistics, 1997; 282.
28. Johnston KW. Iliac arteries: reanalysis of results of balloon angioplasty. Radiology 1993; 186:207–212.
29. Gallino A, Mahler F, Probst P, Nachbur B. Percutaneous transluminal angioplasty of the arteries of the lower limbs: a 5-year follow-up. Circulation 1985; 70:619–623.

Joseph F. Polak, MD, MPH
Lynn Shemanski, PhD
Daniel H. O'Leary, MD
David Lefkowitz, MD
Thomas R. Price, MD
Peter J. Savage, MD
William E. Brant, MD
Cheryl Reid, PhD
For the Cardiovascular Health Study

Index terms:
Carotid arteries, 1723.721
Carotid arteries, diseases, 1723.721
Carotid arteries, stenosis or obstruction, 1723.721
Carotid arteries, US, 1723.12983

Radiology 1998; 208:649–654

Abbreviations:
HDL = high-density lipoprotein
LDL = low-density lipoprotein
RR = relative risk

[1] From the Dept of Radiology, Brigham and Women's Hospital, 75 Francis St, Boston, MA 02115 (J.F.P.); CHS Coordinating Center, Univ of Washington, Seattle (L.S.); Dept of Radiology, Tufts–New England Medical Center, Boston (D.H.O.); Dept of Neurology, Bowman Gray School of Medicine, Winston-Salem, NC (D.L.); Dept of Neurology, Univ of Maryland Baltimore (T.R.P.); Epidemiology and Biometry Program, Div of Epidemiology and Clinical Applications, National Heart, Lung, and Blood Institute, Bethesda (P.J.S.); Dept of Radiology, Univ of California, Davis Medical Center (W.E.B.); and Div of Cardiology, Univ of California, Irvine (C.R.). Received Nov 28, 1997; revision requested Dec 30; revision received Mar 26, 1998; accepted May 8. Supported in part by NHLBI contracts N01-HC-5079 to N01-HC-85086. **Address reprint requests to** J.F.P.

Author contributions:
Guarantors of integrity of entire study, J.F.P., CHS Publication Committee; study concepts, all authors; study design, J.F.P., L.S.; definition of intellectual content, all authors; literature research, J.F.P., L.S., D.H.O.; clinical studies, J.F.P., D.H.O., D.L., T.R.P., P.J.S., W.E.B., C.R.; data acquisition, J.F.P., L.S., D.H.O., T.R.P.; data analysis, J.F.P., L.S.; statistical analysis, L.S.; manuscript preparation and editing, all authors; manuscript review, CHS Publication Committee

Hypoechoic Plaque at US of the Carotid Artery: An Independent Risk Factor for Incident Stroke in Adults Aged 65 Years or Older[1]

PURPOSE: To investigate the association between incident (first) stroke and the echogenicity of internal carotid arterial plaque at ultrasonography (US).

MATERIALS AND METHODS: A cohort of 4,886 individuals who, at baseline, were 65 years of age or older and without symptoms of cerebrovascular disease was followed up for an average of 3.3 years. Baseline clinical findings were from color Doppler and duplex US studies of the carotid arteries and a record of traditional risk factors: age, sex, presence of diabetes mellitus, pack-years of cigarette smoking, presence of hypertension, elevated systolic and diastolic blood pressures, elevated low-density lipoprotein cholesterol level.

RESULTS: Incident strokes, excluding hemorrhagic strokes and strokes of cardiac origin, were seen in 104 individuals (2.1%) at risk. Age- and sex-adjusted odds ratios for incident stroke were significant for hypoechoic plaque (odds ratio, 2.53; 95% CI, 1.42, 4.53). After controlling for risk factors in a Cox proportional hazards model, the relative risk (RR) of incident stroke was 1.72 (P = .015) for hypoechoic plaque and 2.32 (P = .004) for internal carotid arterial narrowing of at least 50%. In addition, hypoechoic plaque (RR, 2.78; CI, 1.36, 5.69) and 50%–100% stenosis (RR, 3.08; CI, 1.28, 7.41) were associated with ipsilateral, nonfatal stroke.

CONCLUSION: In asymptomatic adults aged 65 years or older, the risk of incident stroke was associated with two US features: hypoechoic internal carotid arterial plaque and an estimated internal carotid arterial stenosis of 50%–100%.

Incident (first) stroke has been related to the severity of internal carotid arterial stenosis in symptomatic (1–3) and asymptomatic (4) individuals. The internal structure of atherosclerotic plaque has also been associated with the risk of stroke, as carotid endarterectomy specimens from symptomatic patients have shown evidence of intraplaque hemorrhage (5). While it has not been possible to evaluate the internal structure of atherosclerotic plaque with arteriography, this has been achieved in vivo with carotid ultrasonography (US): Areas of intraplaque hemorrhage at histopathologic analysis have corresponded to hypoechoic zones on US images obtained before surgery (6,7). Hypoechoic areas on US images may also represent areas of increased fat deposition (8) and may be markers of plaques vulnerable to future rupture and cardiovascular events.

The results of cross-sectional cohort studies (9–13) have suggested that the US appearance of carotid plaque might be related to neurologic symptoms. While results from longitudinal studies have supported this possibility in patient populations with a high prevalence of carotid disease (11,14), the associations between incident stroke, severity of internal carotid arterial stenosis, and the US appearance of carotid plaque have not been studied in a cohort of free living individuals.

We performed this study to prospectively evaluate the association between incident ischemic stroke and the in vivo appearance of carotid plaque on US images obtained in a cohort of asymptomatic individuals aged 65 years or older with an average follow-up of 3.3 years.

MATERIALS AND METHODS

Population

Between June 1989 and May 1990, the Cardiovascular Health Study enrolled 5,201 men and women aged 65 years or older. The Cardiovascular Health Study cohort was recruited from a random sampling of the Health Care Financing Administration Medicare eligibility lists in four communities: Forsyth County, NC; Sacramento County, Calif; Washington County, Md; and Pittsburgh, Pa (15,16).

Participants were selected with a two-stage random sampling method (16). The basic sampling frame was a subsample of the Medicare eligibility lists provided by the Health Care Financing Administration; this yielded a sample of 5,000 individuals from the geographic area served by each field center. The Health Care Financing Administration estimated that the eligibility file was 98%–99% complete. The Cardiovascular Health Study coordinating center also performed further random sampling stratified by age and sex. A letter on Health Care Financing Administration stationery that defined the goals of the study and that requested participation was sent to potential enrollees.

The following were excluded: (*a*) institutionalized individuals; (*b*) those who were homebound; (*c*) persons receiving hospice treatment, radiation therapy, or chemotherapy for cancer (not including skin cancer); (*d*) those unable to give informed consent; (*e*) those requiring a proxy respondent during baseline studies; (*f*) those unable to communicate with the study interviewer; and (*g*) those planning to move out of the area during the subsequent 3 years. Local institutional review board approval was obtained at each field center, and all participants gave written informed consent.

Of the 5,201 participants, there were 2,239 men (43%) with an average age of 73.3 years ± 5.8 and 2,962 women (57%) with an average age of 72.4 years ± 5.4. Participants with definite stroke (n = 160), history of carotid endarterectomy (n = 66), or both (n = 24) were excluded, as were 65 individuals with a history of transient ischemic attack at baseline visit. Follow-up data were available for a mean of 3.3 years (range, 7–1,480 days) in the remaining 4,886 participants, who were asymptomatic at the time of the carotid US examination.

Clinical Variables

Initial data included demographic parameters such as age and sex. A carotid bruit was defined as a bruit heard in the middle of the neck. A transient ischemic attack was a documented episode of transient neurologic deficit with a duration of 24 hours or less that was reported at the baseline examination. Brachial blood pressure was determined from the average of two measurements. Hypertension was defined as present according to medical history and use of antihypertensive medications. Diabetes was defined as present according to a reported history of diabetes and use of insulin or oral hypoglycemic agents. Laboratory measurements, all processed at a central laboratory (17), included fasting total low-density lipoprotein (LDL) and high-density lipoprotein (HDL) cholesterol levels and serum glucose level.

Ultrasonography

Carotid US was performed at the four centers by using identically equipped devices: linear-array imaging probes (6.7 MHz, −3 dB cut point) with a pulsed Doppler US scanner (model SSA-270A; Toshiba America Medical Systems, Tustin, Calif). The internal carotid artery was defined to include the carotid artery bulb and the initial 10 mm of the part of the internal carotid artery distal to the bulb. Three sagittal images were obtained in each internal carotid artery: one anterior, one lateral, and one posterior. The sonographer was instructed to concentrate on any identifiable lesions and to optimize depiction of the interfaces between the lumen and the artery wall. All sonographers had been trained in the imaging protocol at a central US reading center. All had been certified after completing 20 imaging studies during a prepilot phase of the project (18).

Carotid arterial images were recorded on super-VHS videotape. An angle-corrected pulsed Doppler spectrum was recorded at the point of maximum peak systolic velocity in the internal carotid artery. In addition, images were digitized on site with a video frame grabber interfaced with a MacIntosh II microcomputer (Apple, Cupertino, Calif) and stored on an optical disk of 650-Mbyte capacity. Each week, the four field centers forwarded a super-VHS tape, a handwritten log, and one optical disk to a central reading center in Boston, Mass.

Images of the carotid arteries were reviewed at a central reading center (18). All measurements were done by readers who were blinded to all clinical variables. These readers had been trained in the reading protocol and certified to perform their evaluations after performing 20 readings in the prepilot study (18). Although the peak systolic blood flow velocities were recorded, the functional definition of a 50%–100% stenosis was selected for a cut point of 1.5 m/sec. This was selected instead of a lower cut point of 1.25 m/sec (19) to decrease the number of potential false-positive findings of a stenosis of 50%–100% of the luminal diameter (20). The maximum stenosis was defined as the maximum narrowing observed in the right or left internal carotid artery.

The echogenicity of each carotid arterial lesion, defined as a focal wall thickness of at least 1.5 mm, was categorized as follows (21): hypoechoic, isoechoic, or hyperechoic. The texture of the plaque was compared with the overall texture of hyperechoic structures seen in the soft tissues surrounding the carotid arteries: (*a*) hypoechoic lesions had an echogenicity the same as or less than that of the vessel lumen; (*b*) isoechoic lesions had an echogenicity the same as that of the surrounding soft tissues; and (*c*) hyperechoic lesions had a higher echogenicity than that of the surrounding soft tissues.

To maintain consistency in the subjective interpretations, the readers reviewed cases of interest biweekly with one of the co-investigators (J.F.P.). However, the original data that had been entered into the database for these selected cases were not modified. Rather, the review process was directed to establish a common reference for future interpretations. This strategy had a goal of minimizing reader variations during the year of the study. The dominant plaque in each carotid artery was classified as hypoechoic, isoechoic, or hyperechoic on the basis of the echogenicity of at least 50% of the visualized plaque volume. The plaque was classified as calcified when the ultrasound beam caused extensive shadowing and the internal structure of the plaque could not be visualized.

Outcome Variables

Incident strokes that could be ascribed to carotid arterial disease were considered as outcome variables in the analyses. Participants with possible subarachnoid and intracerebral hemorrhage, determined on the basis of stroke classifications made by an adjudication committee (22), were classified as not having incident stroke. Possible cardioembolic events, determined

TABLE 1
Relationships of Continuous Variables with Incident Stroke

Variable	Patients without Stroke	Patients with Stroke	*P* Value
Age (y)	72.6 ± 5.6 (*n* = 4,782)	75.2 ± 6.5 (*n* = 104)	<.001
LDL cholesterol (mg/dL)	133.1 ± 35.4 (*n* = 4,693)*	139.2 ± 35.3 (*n* = 104)†	.080
HDL cholesterol (mg/dL)	54.2 ± 15.7 (*n* = 4,752)‡	51.0 ± 16.9 (*n* = 103)§	.040
Systolic blood pressure (mm Hg)	135.3 ± 21.3 (*n* = 4,772)	145.5 ± 24.5 (*n* = 104)	<.001
Diastolic blood pressure (mm Hg)	70.1 ± 11.5 (*n* = 4,766)	73.4 ± 13.0 (*n* = 104)	.012
Pack-years smoked (all participants)	18.3 ± 26.3 (*n* = 4,709)	18.3 ± 30.4 (*n* = 104)	.990, NS
Pack-years smoked (among smokers)	34.3 ± 27.4 (*n* = 2,512)	40.4 ± 34.0 (*n* = 47)	.220, NS

Note.—NS = not significant.
* 3.44 mmol/L ± 0.92.
† 3.60 mmol/L ± 0.91.
‡ 1.40 mmol/L ± 0.41.
§ 1.32 mmol/L ± 0.44.

TABLE 2
Relationship of Dichotomous Variables with Incident Stroke

Variable	Patients without Stroke	Patients with Stroke	*P* Value
Male sex	1,998/4,782 (41.8)	49/104 (47.1)	.280
Diabetes mellitus present	331/4,782 (6.92)	19/104 (18.3)	<.001
Hypertension present	1,567/4,742 (33.0)	46/103 (44.7)	.013
Carotid bruit present	171/4,706 (3.63)	3/104 (2.88)	.710
Internal carotid arterial stenosis ≥50% present	255/4,706 (5.42)	15/102 (14.71)	<.001

Note.—Data are the number of patients. Number in parentheses is the percentage.

by means of an adjudication process (22), were also excluded and not considered as outcome variables. Additional analyses for strokes ipsilateral to carotid arterial lesions were performed only for nonfatal strokes. During follow-up, participants undergoing carotid endarterectomy or who were suspected to have had hemorrhagic or cardioembolic strokes were considered censored on the day after the event.

Statistical Methods

Participants with incident stroke were compared with participants without incident stroke by using the Student *t* test for continuous variables and the χ^2 test for categorical variables. The Fisher exact test was used for categorical variables when the assumptions of the χ^2 test were violated. Odds ratios adjusted for age and sex were calculated by using logistic regression models. Logistic regression and Cox proportional hazards models (SAS user's guide: basics version 6. SAS Institute, Cary, NC, 1990) were used to model incident stroke as a function of both clinically recognized risk factors for stroke and indicator variables for internal carotid arterial stenosis and lesion characteristics. In each participant, the stenosis severity and plaque echogenicity used in the analyses were the more extreme of those seen on either the right or the left side. Calcified lesions were not included in multivariate analyses, because the internal appearance of the plaque could not be evaluated. Proportional hazards models were generated, with cardiovascular risk factors and plaque characteristics included as covariates. Cox proportional hazards models were also generated, with presumed cardioembolic events included as outcomes. The reason for doing so was to determine whether any statistical association between atheroembolic events and carotid lesions would be attenuated by diluting the outcome events with cardioembolic strokes.

The association between carotid lesions and ipsilateral incident stroke was analyzed by considering each artery independently. Logistic regression analyses and a stepwise Cox proportional hazards model were then performed with incident nonfatal stroke as the outcome variable and ipsilateral carotid lesion characteristics (stenosis severity and lesion echogenicity) as predictor variables. Statistical test results were considered significant with a *P* value of .05; 95% CIs were calculated.

RESULTS

The incidence of a first stroke was 3.6% (175 of 4,886 individuals). With the exclusion of hemorrhagic and probable cardioembolic strokes, the prevalence of a first stroke was 2.1% (104 of 4,886 individuals). Eighteen primary hemorrhagic strokes (nine fatal, nine nonfatal) and 53 probable cardioembolic strokes (eight fatal, 45 nonfatal) were censored on the day after the event and were not treated as outcomes. In summary, 71 participants were excluded: Two of these participants had morbid followed by hemorrhagic strokes and two participants had nonfatal followed by fatal cardioembolic strokes. Thirty-two carotid endarterectomies were also censored on the day of surgery and were not treated as outcomes.

Variables positively associated with stroke (Tables 1, 2) were age, elevated systolic and diastolic blood pressures, diabetes mellitus, hypertension, and internal carotid arterial stenosis. An inverse association was seen between stroke and an elevated HDL cholesterol level. No significant association was seen between stroke and sex, elevated LDL cholesterol level, or pack-years of cigarette use. The rate of incident stroke was 1.9% (87 of 4,538 individuals) when internal carotid arterial narrowing was less than 50% and 5.6% (15 of 270 individuals) when narrowing was 50% of the diameter or more. After adjustment for age and sex, plaque echogenicity was positively associated with stroke (Table 3): Stroke was more likely with plaque that was hypoechoic (odds ratio, 2.53) or hyperechoic (odds ratio, 1.72).

The following variables were entered into a Cox proportional hazards model: age, sex, pack-years of cigarette use, 50%–100% stenosis, LDL and HDL cholesterol levels, diabetes, hypertension, and systolic and diastolic blood pressures. Hypoechoic plaque is the only index of plaque echogenicity that remained a statistically

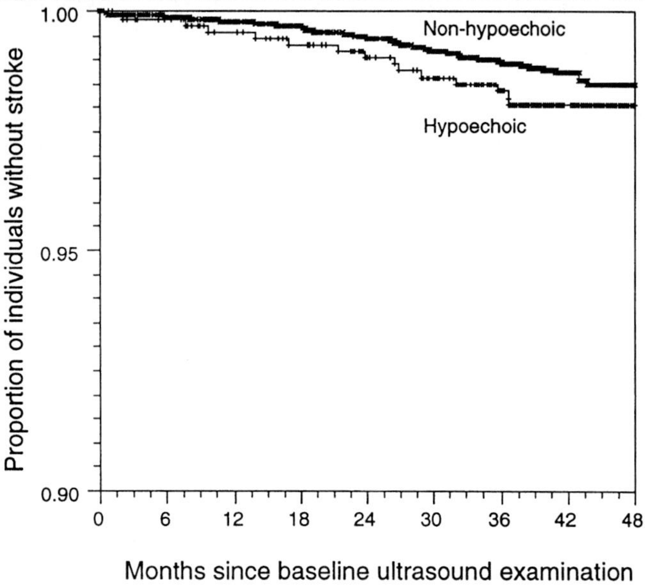

Figure 1. Graph of stroke-free survival curves for internal carotid arterial stenosis of less than 50%.

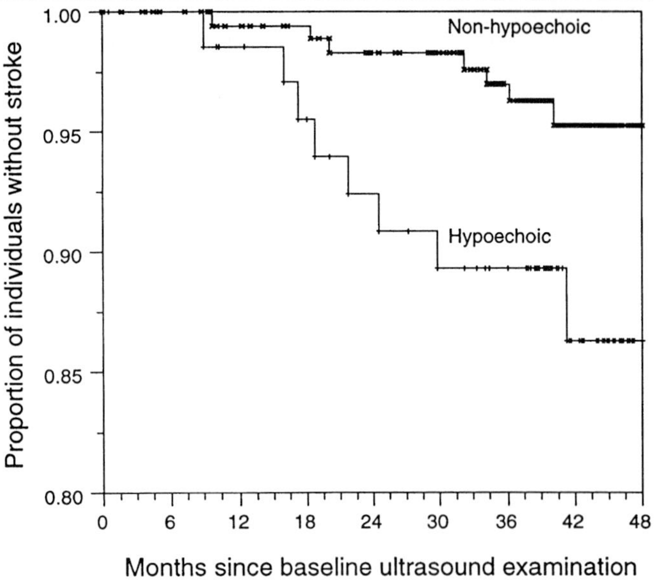

Figure 2. Graph of stroke-free survival curves for internal carotid arterial stenosis of 50% or more.

TABLE 3
Age- and Sex-adjusted Odds Ratios of Plaque Characteristics for Incident Stroke

Variable	Odds Ratio*	Incident Stroke Rate†
No plaque	1.0	20/1,587 (1.26)
Isoechoic plaque	1.39 (0.78, 2.46)	31/1,587 (1.95)
Hyperechoic plaque	1.72 (0.92, 3.24)	21/786 (2.67)
Hypoechoic plaque	2.53 (1.42, 4.53)	30/856 (3.50)
Calcified plaque	6.93 (0.8, 60.2)	1/9 (11)

* Parentheses contain the 95% CI.
† Parentheses contain the percentage.

TABLE 4
Variables Related to Incident Stroke in a Cox Proportional Hazards Model

Variable	RR	*P* Value
Diabetes mellitus	3.22	<.001
Stenosis ≥50%	2.32	.004
Hypoechoic plaque	1.72	.015
Age (for 10-y increase)	2.20	<.001
LDL cholesterol (for 10 mg/dL increase)*	1.06	.040
Systolic blood pressure (for a 10 mm Hg increase)	1.12	.040

Note.—Variables that are not significant but are forced into the model include sex, smoking history, pack-years of smoking, LDL cholesterol level, and diastolic blood pressure.
*For 0.26-mmol/L increase.

significant predictor when included in this statistical model.

Continuous variables associated with an increased relative risk (RR) of incident stroke (Table 4) were increased age (increased risk of 120% per decade), elevated LDL cholesterol levels (increased risk of 6% for every 10-mg/dL [0.26-mmol/L] increase), and elevated systolic blood pressure (increased risk of 12% for a 10-mm Hg blood pressure increase). Ordinal and nominal variables associated with an increased RR of stroke (Table 4) were diabetes (RR, 3.22), history of hypertension, and the presence of hypoechoic plaque (RR, 1.72). The association between stroke and 50%–100% internal carotid arterial stenosis was also significant (increased risk of 132%).

Kaplan-Meier curves for the incidence of stroke for hypoechoic and nonhypoechoic lesions showed a significantly increased risk of stroke for hypoechoic internal carotid arterial stenoses of less than 50% (Fig 1) and of 50%–100% (Fig 2).

The side of the neurologic event was clearly documented in 60 nonfatal incident strokes. The odds ratios for incident stroke were elevated for 50%–100% stenoses (odds ratio, 3.37; 95% CI, 1.44, 7.90) and for hyperechoic (odds ratio, 2.01; CI, 1.03, 3.91) or hypoechoic (odds ratio, 3.01; CI, 1.48, 6.11) plaques but not for isoechoic plaques (odds ratio, 1.2; CI, 0.58, 2.47) (Table 5). In a Cox proportional hazards model with lesion severity and echogenicity controlled for, 50%–100% stenosis (RR, 3.08; CI, 1.28, 7.41) and hypoechoic plaque (RR, 2.78; CI, 1.36, 5.69) were significantly associated with incident ipsilateral strokes, whereas isoechoic (P = .64) and hyperechoic (P = .15) plaques were not (Table 6).

The addition of adjudicated cardioembolic events to the outcome variables increased the number of events from 104 to 149. Two Cox proportional hazards models were generated: Both included all the risk factors used previously in addition to variables that described plaque echogenicity. One model used the original outcome variable, while the other used an outcome variable that included cases of presumed cardioembolic events. With the addition of cardioembolic events, the level of importance of internal carotid arterial stenosis decreased from a RR of 2.19 (P = .008) to 1.84 (P = .015), and the RR for stroke with hypoechoic plaque decreased from 1.98 (P = .024) to 1.67 (P = .045).

We further studied whether a change in the Doppler velocity cut point to 125

TABLE 5
Odds Ratios of Incident Ipsilateral Stroke in the Area of the Ipsilateral Carotid Artery

Variable	Odds Ratio	95% CI
No plaque	1.00	. . .
Echogenicity		
Isoechoic	1.20	0.58, 2.47
Hyperechoic	2.01	1.03, 3.91
Hypoechoic	3.01	1.48, 6.11
Stenosis		
<50%	1.00	. . .
≥50%	3.37	1.44, 7.90

TABLE 6
Predictors of Ipsilateral Incident Stroke

Variable	RR*	95% CI*
Stenosis ≥50%	3.08	1.28, 7.41
Hypoechoic plaque	2.78	1.36, 5.69

Note.—Hyperechoic and isoechoic plaque were kept in the model. Hyperechoic (P = .15) and isoechoic (P = .64) characteristics were not statistically significant predictors.
* Cox proportional hazards model.

cm/sec would have affected our findings: The curves derived from the Cox proportional hazards model were qualitatively similar to those shown in Figures 1 and 2. The prevalence of hypoechoic plaques varied by study center but had no effect in the full Cox proportional hazards models.

DISCUSSION

We report that the likelihood of a first incident stroke in asymptomatic adults aged 65 years or older is associated with hypoechoic plaques on US images of the internal carotid arteries. The positive association between hypoechoic plaque and incident stroke persists after controlling for risk factors such as diabetes mellitus, hypertension, elevated LDL cholesterol level, age, and the severity of internal carotid arterial stenosis. This positive association is stronger for ipsilateral incident strokes, even after controlling for the severity of ipsilateral carotid arterial narrowing.

We excluded, as an outcome variable, strokes thought to be of cardioembolic origin. Establishing the cause of strokes has been shown to be difficult and subject to marked interobserver variability (23). This problem has also been encountered in studies that look at the outcome of unilateral carotid endarterectomy (1,4). In these studies, strokes not associated with atheroembolism from carotid arterial plaques were as likely to be counted as positive outcomes for the study artery as they were for the contralateral artery.

For example, the European Carotid Study Trial, or ECST, study findings have shown that in patients with symptomatic, 70%–100% stenoses, 40% (n = 6) of 15 incident strokes were contralateral to the study artery in surgically treated participants and 17% (n = 9) of 53 incident strokes were contralateral to the study artery in nonsurgically treated participants (2). Some of these events may have originated from a cardiac source or from the aorta or may have been intracranial. In an analysis of all incident strokes in the Cardiovascular Health Study cohort, Manolio et al (24) reported a strong association between stroke and cardiac factors such as left ventricular dysfunction and atrial fibrillation.

Our analyses excluded strokes likely due to cardioembolism. While we have sacrificed some statistical power by excluding these events, in doing so, we should have made our analyses more relevant to atheroembolic events in the carotid arteries. Nevertheless, we did seek to determine whether the association between hypoechoic plaque and incident stroke would be weakened when the outcomes were diluted by the introduction of cases thought to represent cardioembolism. The Cox proportional hazards model with all events included showed a statistically significant, but attenuated, positive association between hypoechoic plaque and stroke. The results of these analyses support the existence of a positive association between hypoechoic plaque and the risk of a first stroke.

The association between incident stroke and plaque characteristics has almost certainly been confounded by increased systolic blood pressures, a known risk factor for stroke (24–26). The presence of elevated blood pressures has been shown to act as a risk factor for the development of atherosclerotic plaque (27). Distinguishing one association from the other was not possible given the limited longitudinal follow-up of our study.

The lack of significant sex or smoking status associations with stroke was surprising. This may have been due to a selection bias in favor of the survival of individuals in our cohort. Individuals who had died of diseases linked to the combined effects of age and cigarette smoking were likely to not have survived and possibly did not enter our cohort. Alternatively, these risk factors might have lost their importance as risk factors in individuals aged 65 years or older. A similar attenuation of the effect of cardiovascular risk factors with age has been reported: Kronmal et al (28) have reported a loss of the expected association between cholesterol levels and the risk of subsequent cardiovascular events in older adults.

The positive association that we observed between carotid arterial stenosis and incident stroke was not surprising. A similar finding has been shown in individuals with carotid bruits and carotid stenoses of 50%–100% at Doppler US (75%–100% stenosis of luminal area) (29). In the study by Chambers and Norris (29), the 5.5% incidence of stroke in individuals with 50%–100% diameter stenosis at Doppler US (at 22 months average follow-up) was greater than the 5.6% (at 3.3 years average follow-up) we now report. Because less than 4% of our subjects had carotid bruits (Table 2), whereas all individuals in the study by Chambers and Norris (29) had carotid bruits, it seems likely that the Chambers and Norris study was biased toward individuals who had more prevalent cardiovascular disease than had members of our cohort.

An association between stenosis severity and stroke has also been shown in trials such as the North American Symptomatic Carotid Endarterectomy Trial, or NASCET, and ECST in symptomatic patients. The incidences of stroke in the NASCET and ECST studies were higher than ours, which is likely a reflection of a difference in the composition of the cohorts. In NASCET and ECST, all individuals had neurologic symptoms, whereas no members of our cohort had recognized neurologic symptoms at the time of US.

In our study, we observed a low prevalence of carotid arterial disease. This prevalence is similar to that in the Framingham Study (27), where 8% of subjects had internal carotid arterial narrowing of 50% or more. We believe that this low prevalence contributes to the overall low incidence of stroke in our cohort.

At the outset, both hyperechoic and hypoechoic plaques showed a positive association with incident stroke. However, only hypoechoic plaque continued to be associated with stroke after controlling for the traditional risk factors linked to stroke. The loss of the association between hyperechoic plaque and stroke when these risk factors are controlled for is likely due to the inclusion of plaque size (stenosis severity) and subject age in the statistical model (9,21). This suggests that, once account is taken for the presence and size of atherosclerotic plaque, hypoechoic characteristics are predictive of future cardiovascular events. Although we cannot prove that the characteristics are linked to possible rupture of the carotid plaque and a subsequent event, this possibility is supported by our findings.

We have examined interreader reproducibility with a blinded rereading of carotid US images in 90 subjects (180 carotid arteries). The κ statistics were moderate for classifying plaque echogenicity ($\kappa = 0.56$) (30). This moderate κ value suggests that the process used to subjectively grade plaque characteristics might be improved on. A stronger κ value, and therefore reduced variability, might have increased the overall strengths of the association between hypoechoic plaque and stroke. This possibility suggests that quantitative methods of grading plaque characteristics (31) might increase the strength of the association between hypoechoic plaques and incident stroke (32). Subjective performance of plaque grading at US has been the subject of a recent international consensus panel, where Baud et al (33) reported lower κ values than ours, 0.31 and 0.41, when expert readers evaluated 53 carotid plaques.

Because the positive association between stroke and hypoechoic plaques persists after adjustment for other risk factors, hypoechoic plaque acts as an independent risk factor for incident stroke. The hypoechoic appearance should not necessarily be interpreted as representing intraplaque hemorrhage or rupture (34). Although intraplaque hemorrhage is hypoechoic on a real-time US image, smooth muscle cells or lipid accumulation appear the same (35). A direct histopathologic link between a hypoechoic plaque and a zone of recent plaque hemorrhage is unlikely to be the sole explanation for our findings: The incidence of stroke is much lower than the 18% prevalence (856 of 4,825) of hypoechoic plaques. It is likely that many of these plaques represented lipid-rich plaques at risk of future rupture (8). The US appearance may therefore relate to the biomechanical behavior of carotid plaque and therefore be linked to the future risk of intraplaque hemorrhage (36) and embolization. Again, longitudinal studies with quantitative methods of measuring plaque echogenicity might confirm our hypothesis.

We conclude that hypoechoic carotid plaques, as seen on US images of the carotid arteries in asymptomatic adults aged 65 years or older, are associated with increased risk of first stroke.

References

1. North American Symptomatic Carotid Endarterectomy Trial Collaborators. Beneficial effect of carotid endarterectomy in symptomatic patients with high-grade stenosis. N Engl J Med 1991; 325:445–453.
2. European Carotid Surgery Trialists' Collaborative Group. MRC European Carotid Surgery Trial: interim results for symptomatic patients with severe (70%–99%) or with mild (0%–29%) carotid stenosis. Lancet 1991; 337:1235–1243.
3. European Carotid Surgery Trialists' Collaborative Group. Endarterectomy for moderate symptomatic carotid stenosis: interim results for symptomatic patients from the MRC European carotid surgery trial. Lancet 1996; 347:1591–1593.
4. Executive Committee for the Asymptomatic Carotid Atherosclerosis Study. Endarterectomy for asymptomatic carotid artery stenosis. JAMA 1995; 273:1421–1428.
5. Lusby RJ, Ferrell LD, Ehrenfeld WK, Stoney RJ, Wylie EJ. Carotid plaque hemorrhage: its role in production of cerebral ischemia. Arch Surg 1982; 117:1479–1488.
6. O'Donnell TF, Erdoes L, Mackey WC, et al. Correlation of B-mode ultrasound imaging and arteriography with pathologic findings at carotid endarterectomy. Arch Surg 1985; 120:443–449.
7. Bluth EI, Kay D, Merritt CR, et al. Sonographic characterization of carotid plaque: detection of hemorrhage. AJR 1986; 146: 1061–1065.
8. Gronholdt MLM, Nordestgaard BG, Nielsen TG, Sillesen H. Echolucent carotid artery plaques are associated with elevated levels of fasting and postprandial triglyceride-rich lipoproteins. Stroke 1996; 27:2166–2172.
9. Leahy AL, McCollum PT, Feeley TM, et al. Duplex ultrasonography and selection of patient for carotid endarterectomy: plaque morphology or luminal narrowing. J Vasc Surg 1988; 8:558–562.
10. Steinke W, Hennerici M, Rautenberg W, Mohr JP. Symptomatic and asymptomatic high-grade carotid stenoses in Doppler color-flow imaging. Neurology 1992; 42: 131–138.
11. Belcaro G, Laurora G, Cesarone MR, et al. Ultrasonographic classification of carotid plaques causing less than 60% stenosis according to ultrasound morphology and events. J Cardiovasc Surg 1993; 34:287–294.
12. Hougaku H, Matsumoto M, Handa N, et al. Asymptomatic carotid lesions and silent cerebral infarction. Stroke 1994; 25: 566–570.
13. Holdsworth RJ, McCollum PT, Bryce JS, Harrison DK. Symptoms, stenosis and carotid plaque morphology: is plaque morphology relevant? Eur J Endovasc Surg 1995; 9:80–85.
14. Langsfeld M, Gray-Weale AC, Lusby RJ. The role of plaque morphology and diameter reduction in the development of new symptoms in asymptomatic carotid arteries. J Vasc Surg 1989; 9:548–557.
15. Fried LP, Borhani NO, Enright P, et al. The Cardiovascular Health Study: design and rationale. Ann Epidemiol 1991; 1:263–276.
16. Tell GS, Fried LP, Hermanson B, et al. Recruitment of adults 65 years and older as participants in the cardiovascular health study. Ann Epidemiol 1993; 3:358–366.
17. Ettinger W, Wahl P, Kuller L, et al. Lipoprotein lipids in older people: results from the cardiovascular health study. Circulation 1992; 86:858–869.
18. O'Leary DH, Polak JF, Wolfson SKJ, et al. The use of sonography to evaluate carotid atherosclerosis in the elderly: the cardiovascular health study. Stroke 1991; 22: 1155–1163.
19. Polak JF, Dobkin GR, O'Leary DH, Wang AM, Cutler AS. Internal carotid artery stenosis: accuracy and reproducibility of color-Doppler-assisted duplex imaging. Radiology 1989; 173:793–798.
20. Polak JF. Role of duplex US as a screening test for carotid atherosclerotic disease: benefit without cost? (editorial). Radiology 1995; 197:581–582.
21. Polak JF, O'Leary DH, Kronmal RA, et al. Sonographic evaluation of carotid artery atherosclerosis in the elderly: relationship of disease severity to stroke and transient ischemic attack. Radiology 1993; 188:363–370.
22. Price TR, Psaty B, O'Leary D, et al. Assessment of cerebrovascular disease in the cardiovascular health study. Ann Epidemiol 1993; 3:504–507.
23. Mohr JP, Caplan LR, Melski JW, et al. The Harvard cooperative stroke registry: a prospective registry. Neurology 1978; 28:754–762.
24. Manolio TA, Kronmal RA, Burke GL, et al. Short-term predictors of incident stroke in older adults: the cardiovascular health study. Stroke 1996; 27:1479–1486.
25. SHEP Cooperative Research Group. Prevention of stroke by antihypertensive drug treatment in older persons with isolated systolic hypertension. JAMA 1991; 265: 3255–3264.
26. Bikkina M, Levy D, Evans JC, et al. Left ventricular mass and risk of stroke in an elderly cohort: the Framingham Heart Study. JAMA 1994; 272:33–36.
27. Fine-Edelstein JS, Wolf PA, O'Leary DH, et al. Precursors of extracranial carotid atherosclerosis in the Framingham study. Neurology 1994; 44:1046–1050.
28. Kronmal RA, Cain KC, Ye Z, Omenn GS. Total serum cholesterol levels and mortality risk as a function of age: a report based on the Framingham data. Arch Intern Med 1993; 153:1065–1073.
29. Chambers BR, Norris JW. Outcome in patients with asymptomatic neck bruits. N Engl J Med 1986; 315:860–865.
30. Landis R, Koch G. The measurement of observer agreement for categorical data. Biometrics 1977; 33:159–174.
31. el-Barghouty N, Geroulakos G, Nicolaides A, Androulakis A, Bahal V. Computer-assisted carotid plaque characterization. Eur J Vasc Endovasc Surg 1995; 9:389–393.
32. el-Barghouty N, Nicolaides A, Bahal V, Geroulakos G, Androulakis A. The identification of the high risk carotid plaque. Eur J Vasc Endovasc Surg 1996; 11:470–478.
33. Baud JM, de Bray JM, Delanoy P, Coordinateurs de l'Étude AFFCA. Reproducibilité ultrasonore dans la charactérization des plaques carotides. In: deBray JM, Baud JM, Dauzat M, Gorge P, Tranquart F, eds. Plaques carotides: diagnostic, evaluation, prognostic. Montpellier, France: Sauramps Medical, 1997; 289–292.
34. Svindland A, Torvik A. Atherosclerotic carotid disease in asymptomatic individuals: a histological study of 53 cases. Acta Neurol Scand 1988; 78:506–517.
35. Widder B, Paulat K, Hackspacher J, et al. Morphological characterization of carotid artery stenoses by ultrasound duplex scanning. Ultrasound Med Biol 1990; 16:349–354.
36. Bassiouny HS, Davis H, Massawa N, et al. Critical carotid stenoses: morphologic and chemical similarity between symptomatic and asymptomatic plaques. J Vasc Surg 1989; 9:202–212.

Michelle L. Robbin, MD
Rachel F. Oser, MD
Michael Allon, MD
Michael W. Clements, RDMS, BS, RVT
Jeanne Dockery, RN
Therese M. Weber, MD
Kay M. Hamrick-Waller, MD
J. Kevin Smith, MD, PhD
Brian C. Jones, MD
Desiree E. Morgan, MD
Souheil Saddekni, MD

Index terms:
Arteries, extremities, 91.7229
Arteries, stenosis or obstruction, 91.7229
Dialysis, shunts, 91.7229, 91.79
Ultrasound (US), Doppler studies, 91.12983
Veins, extremities, 91.79
Veins, stenosis or obstruction, 91.79

Radiology 1998; 208:655–661

Abbreviations:
EDV = end diastolic velocity
PSV = peak systolic velocity
RI = resistive index

[1] From the Depts of Radiology (M.L.R., R.F.O., M.W.C., T.M.W., K.M.H.W., J.K.S., B.C.J., D.E.M., S.S.) and Nephrology (M.A.) and the Bone Marrow Transplant Service (J.D.), University of Alabama, 619 S 19th St, New Hillman Bldg 623, Birmingham, AL 35233. Received Sep 22, 1997; revision requested Nov 12; revision received Jan 30, 1998; accepted Apr 3. **Address reprint requests to** M.L.R.

Author contributions:
Guarantor of integrity of entire study, M.L.R.; study concepts and design, M.L.R., R.F.O., M.A.; definition of intellectual content, M.L.R., R.F.O., M.A.; literature research, M.L.R.; clinical studies, M.L.R., R.F.O., M.A., M.W.C., J.D., T.M.W., K.M.H.W., J.K.S., B.C.J., D.E.M., S.S.; data acquisition, all authors; data analysis, M.L.R., R.F.O., M.A.; statistical analysis, M.L.R., R.F.O.; manuscript preparation, M.L.R., R.F.O., M.A., B.C.J., D.E.M., J.K.S.; manuscript editing, M.L.R., R.F.O.; manuscript review, all authors.

Hemodialysis Access Graft Stenosis: US Detection[1]

PURPOSE: To prospectively evaluate the sensitivity of ultrasonography (US) in diagnosing stenosis of hemodialysis access grafts and their drainage veins in patients clinically suspected of having graft dysfunction.

MATERIALS AND METHODS: Thirty-eight patients in whom dysfunction of their hemodialysis access grafts was suspected underwent both Doppler US and angiography. Gray-scale and color US were combined with spectral analysis of the graft, anastomoses, and venous outflow. Flow velocity at anastomoses and suspected stenotic areas was measured. The volume of flow in the graft was also measured. The prospective US criterion for diagnosis of stenosis was a focal twofold or higher elevation of peak systolic velocity (PSV) compared with the PSV immediately upstream. A blinded angiographic evaluation of the graft and drainage veins followed US. Angiographic diagnosis of stenosis required at least 50% narrowing in luminal diameter. US and angiographic results were then compared.

RESULTS: Angiography allowed diagnosis of 43 stenoses in 34 patients. US depicted 92% (37 of 40) of these stenoses, with a 94% positive predictive value for any individual patient. Focal 2- to 2.9-times PSV elevation was associated with 50%–74% stenosis, while a threefold or greater increase was associated with 75% or greater stenosis. Graft flow volume and resistive index change did not correlate with stenosis.

CONCLUSION: US reliably depicts stenoses of hemodialysis access grafts and drainage veins in a clinically selected population when PSV criteria are used.

End-stage renal disease for which long-term hemodialysis is required affects about 200,000 Americans, with an annual cost of vascular access morbidity approaching $1 billion (1). Eighty percent of these patients rely on synthetic hemodialysis access grafts (2,3). The average 2-year patency rate of grafts has been reported to be 45%–80%, with the predominant range at 45%–60% (3–5). Graft failure in the 1st month after placement usually stems from surgical complications. After 1 month, however, more than 80% of graft failures result from progressive flow-limiting stenosis due to neointimal hyperplasia (6), with eventual graft thrombosis (7–10).

Detection of graft stenosis before thrombosis, with subsequent radiologic or surgical correction, increases graft longevity (11,12). This increase in graft longevity decreases the number of access sites needed in a patient's lifetime, thereby reducing the morbidity associated with graft failure.

Angiography is the traditional radiologic study for the evaluation of hemodialysis access grafts. Recently, however, ultrasonography (US) has emerged as an alternative method in the detection of graft stenosis (10,13–17). Unlike angiography, US is noninvasive and carries none of the risks associated with iodinated contrast material. Doppler US is also portable and requires less capital equipment cost than traditional angiography. These advantages are appealing to patients, referring physicians, and dialysis centers.

Our early experience with the US evaluation of dialysis access grafts suggested an association between focal elevations in peak systolic velocity (PSV) and stenosis of a graft or drainage vein. On the basis of this experience, as well as others' work involving the internal carotid artery (18,19) and synthetic lower-extremity arterial grafts (20,21), we formulated Doppler US criteria for the diagnosis of hemodialysis access graft and drainage vein stenoses. Using these criteria, we then performed a prospective study to evaluate the sensitivity of Doppler US in the detection of hemodialysis access graft and drainage vein stenosis in patients in whom stenosis is clinically suspected.

MATERIALS AND METHODS

Patients undergoing hemodialysis with synthetic grafts in whom stenosis of the graft or drainage veins was clinically suspected were recruited into this study, which was approved by the institutional review board of our institution. Informed consent was obtained after the procedures were fully explained. Each patient was scheduled to undergo US and angiographic evaluation of his or her graft and drainage veins. During the 6 months between August 1996 and January 1997, a total of 41 patients were enrolled. Three patients were excluded from analysis because they refused to undergo angiography. Angiography was performed on the same day as US in 31 patients. In the remaining seven patients, angiography was performed 2–17 days (mean, 7.7 days) after US. Delays in the performance of angiography were due to patient noncompliance.

Patients who met one or more of the following clinical criteria were recruited into the study: (*a*) dynamic blood pressure exceeding 100 mm Hg at a blood flow of 150 mL/min at three consecutive dialysis sessions, (*b*) abnormal graft auscultation (high-pitched or discontinuous bruit), (*c*) arm edema peripheral to the graft, (*d*) prolonged bleeding (>30 minutes) from the puncture site, and (*e*) delivered Kt/V (a dimensionless measure of the removal of urea during dialysis, where K is a constant, t is time, and V is the volume of urea distribution) more than 0.2 unit lower than the prescribed Kt/V.

Fifteen men and 23 women aged 31–76 years (mean, 55 years) were enrolled in the study. Seventeen (45%) of the 38 patients had diabetes mellitus, reflecting the dialysis patient population at our center. The graft anatomy consisted of 15 straight and 23 loop grafts, 23 located in the forearm and 15 in the upper arm. Each patient's graft status was followed for a minimum of 6 months or until August 1, 1997.

Technique for US Examination of the Graft and Drainage Veins

The patient's arm was positioned at approximately 45° from the body, in a comfortable position. Initial scanning of the entire upper extremity provided an overview of graft location and arterial and venous connections (16). All locations were described with the classic nomenclature of "proximal" and "distal" with respect to the heart. All vessels were examined in both transverse and longitudinal planes. Representative gray-scale and color images of all vessels and anastomoses were then obtained. Power Doppler US was used in cases of slow flow. Any other abnormalities, such as pseudoaneurysms or perigraft fluid collections, were also measured and recorded.

Spectral Doppler US waveforms were obtained at multiple locations in the upper extremity (Fig 1), with the angle of the transducer beam maintained at less than or equal to 60° to the vessel wall. Spectral Doppler US waveforms were obtained proximal to, at, and distal to any stenoses seen. Spectral waveform measurements included PSV, end diastolic velocity (EDV), and resistive index (RI). A PSV ratio was calculated (as in Fig 2) at sites of visible stenosis, areas with an increase in PSV, and anastomoses.

Duplex US clues in the graft and drainage veins that prompted closer examination of a focal area for stenosis were (*a*) tissue turbulence, (*b*) color aliasing, and (*c*) PSV elevations in the vessel. Although intragraft stenoses were usually visually apparent during US of the graft, the graft lumen was occasionally so irregular, with multiple small dilatations, that detection of stenosis was difficult. In such cases, comparison of luminal measurements with the known original graft diameter was useful. Flow direction in the feeding artery was documented distal to its anastomosis with the graft to assess for arterial steal.

Findings suggestive of stenosis, clot, or occlusion in the subclavian and proximal brachiocephalic vein were (*a*) small-diameter vein, (*b*) multiple small venous vessels in the area (probably collateral vessels), (*c*) a tortuous vessel, and (*d*) a vein not in direct proximity to the subclavian artery.

An attempt was made to directly visualize the brachiocephalic veins and superior vena cava for stenosis, thrombus, or occlusion. Transmitted cardiac pulsatility, respiratory variation, and deep inspiration and findings of the sniff and Valsalva maneuvers were assessed for indirect signs of central venous abnormality (22–26).

The technique for measurement of volume flow in the graft required selection of a nonstenotic midgraft location with parallel vessel walls. In the case of loop grafts, two locations were chosen, one from the central portion of each limb. At each site of volume measurement, measurement of the diameter of the graft (on a long-axis image) allowed the machine to automatically calculate average flow volume over three to five cardiac cycles. For loop grafts, the lowest of either the midarterial or midvenous measurement was used.

At completion of the examination, a staff sonographer recorded pertinent US information on a data work sheet designed for this study, under the supervision of a staff radiologist. All images (including waveforms and measurements) were archived to 5¼-inch magneto-optical disks. At a later date, a single sonologist (M.L.R.) reviewed all images to verify work sheet data and provided the final US interpretation.

All US was performed with an XP/128 ART or Sequoia unit (Acuson, Mountain View, Calif) in a laboratory accredited by the Intersocietal Commission for the Accreditation of Vascular Laboratory and the American College of Radiology.

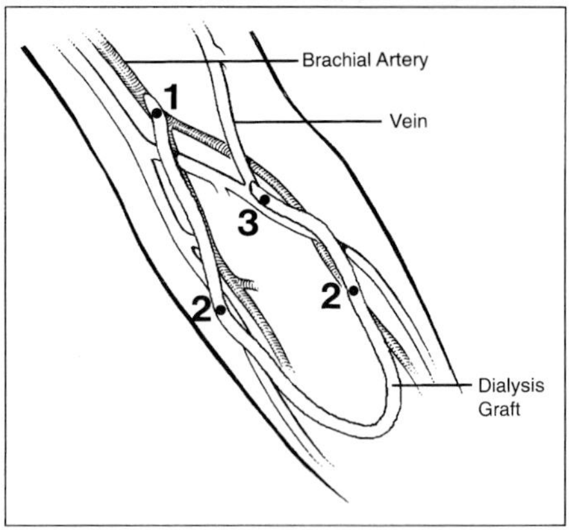

Figure 1. Drawing shows location of US measurements in the graft and drainage vein. Spectral waveform measurements were performed proximally, at, and distal to the following three locations: *1,* arterial anastomosis; *2,* middle of the graft (both arterial and venous limbs in a loop graft); and *3,* venous anastomosis. Representative waveforms were obtained in the drainage veins.

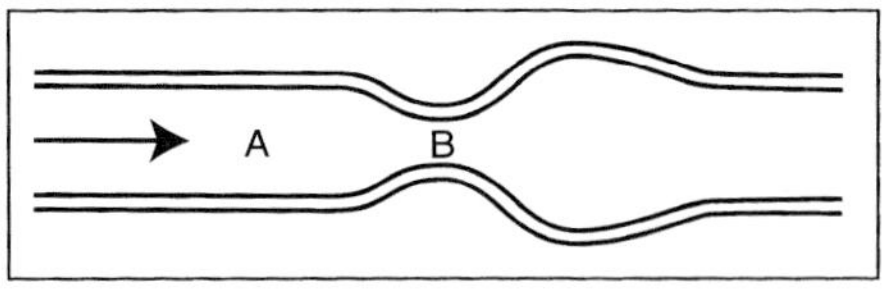

Figure 2. Drawing shows method for calculating the PSV ratio at a stenosis or anastomosis. PSV ratio = (PSV at *B*)/(PSV at *A*). The arrow indicates the direction of blood flow.

TABLE 1
Summary of US Findings versus Angiographic Findings

Location	No. of Stenoses at Angiography	Average Percentage of Stenosis at Angiography	Mean PSV	Mean EDV	Mean Volume Flow	Mean PSV Ratio
Graft	3	52.5	3.79	1.61	1,076.5	2.90
Venous anastomosis	27	65.5	4.21	2.58	919.5	3.40
Venous outflow	9	74.4	3.85	2.46	971.7	2.78
Central*	1	100.0	. . .	. . .	. . .	. . .

Note.—No US measurements were performed in false-negative cases.
* Central = brachiocephalic vein.

TABLE 2
Comparison of US Categorization with Angiographically Determined Percentage of Stenosis

Percentage of Stenosis at Angiography	Percentage of Stenosis at US: ≥50–74	≥75–100
≥50–74	13	4
≥75–100	5	15

Note.—κ coefficient = 0.512, indicative of a positive association between the US and angiographic results. Data are the number of cases.

US Criteria for Graft Stenosis

We used the following criteria to predict stenosis of the graft or its drainage veins: (*a*) PSV ratio across the stenosis of 2.0 or greater, (*b*) visual diameter reduction of at least 50% (usually used when multiple stenoses were present), and (*c*) borderline PSV ratios (≥1.9) at the venous anastomosis, with a PSV of at least 4 m/sec. We further predicted the degree of stenosis with PSV ratios: A PSV ratio of 2.0–2.99 was classified as 50%–74% stenosis and a PSV ratio of at least 3.0 as 75%–100% stenosis. Reduction in stenosis diameter was calculated with the following equation: diameter stenosis reduction = [1 − (minimal luminal diameter/nontapering adjacent normal luminal diameter)] × 100%.

If any of the above criteria were identified, the site was called stenotic. Focal stenoses that involved the drainage vein or graft within 1 cm of the venous anastomosis were called venous anastomotic stenoses.

Angiographic Evaluation of Synthetic Hemodialysis Access Grafts

Angiography was used as the standard for this study (3,27). The angiographers (R.F.O., K.M.H.W., S.S.) were blinded to the results of US. After sterile preparation of the arm, the graft was accessed with an 18-gauge needle or 4-F straight catheter. We routinely used a larger needle to access the graft, thus avoiding a second puncture, as the majority of our patients needed intervention at the time of imaging. Visualization of the arterial limb and arterial anastomosis was accomplished by means of compression of the graft or venous outflow during the injection of contrast material. If the arterial anastomosis was not adequately seen after several attempts and blood inflow appeared adequate at clinical examination, the procedure was terminated. Multiple views of each graft segment were obtained only when it was necessary to better define the graft anatomy. Luminal stenosis was considered significant with a luminal diameter reduction of at least 50% and was treated with angioplasty when necessary. At a later date, a single angiographer (R.F.O.) reviewed all angiograms on film and provided the final angiographic interpretation.

Statistical Analysis

Descriptive statistics for all quantitative variables were calculated from stenosis position. To measure the agreement between US diagnostic criteria and angiographic diagnosis, the κ coefficient was calculated. The relationship between velocity measurements and percentage of stenosis was analyzed by means of construction of scatterplots between the variables. The linear relationship between velocity measurements and percentage of stenosis was quantified by calculating correlation coefficients.

RESULTS

Forty-three stenoses were detected at initial angiography in 34 patients. Four patients had no angiographic evidence of stenosis. In two patients, lack of reflux of contrast material throughout the entire graft prevented initial visualization of three stenoses diagnosed at US, so we omitted these stenoses from our analysis. Subsequent thrombectomy procedures, however, helped confirm the presence of these stenoses.

Among patients with abnormal angiograms, the number of stenoses per patient averaged 1.3. Sixty-three percent of the stenoses (27 of 43) were located at or within 1 cm of the venous anastomosis. Another 21% (nine of 43) were located in the outflow veins, one of the nine in the subclavian vein. Only one of 43 stenoses was located in a central vein (ie, the brachiocephalic vein). Three intragraft and three periarterial anastomotic stenoses were identified. The average length of the stenoses was 2.4 cm. The average venous anastomotic stenosis was 2.2 cm long, and the average drainage vein stenosis was 1.7 cm long.

At US, 29 venous anastomotic stenoses were noted. Seven intragraft stenoses, seven stenoses and one occlusion in the outflow veins, and one brachiocephalic venous stenosis or occlusion were also seen.

No US criteria had been previously developed for arterial stenoses because of the rarity of arterial anastomotic problems. The arterial anastomosis is difficult to analyze with velocity ratios for two reasons: (*a*) Grafts are designed with a taper at the arterial side to more closely approximate the smaller feeding-artery caliber. (*b*) Despite the taper, there is often a change in diameter between the artery and the arterial end of the graft. Because previous experience demonstrated that the previously described criteria were not useful at the arterial anastomoses, the criteria were not applied. Thus, the three periarterial anastomotic stenoses seen at angiography were excluded from the following analysis, which left 40 stenoses in the graft and drainage veins that were detected at initial angiography.

The mean PSV, EDV, PSV ratio, and graft flow volume at each stenosis diagnosed at US and the percentage of angiographic stenosis are summarized in Table 1. At the venous anastomosis, the most common site of stenosis, the mean PSV, EDV, and PSV ratios were 4.21 m/sec ± 1.51 (standard deviation), 2.58 m/sec ± 0.96), and 3.40 m/sec ± 1.76, respectively. By using the criteria detailed above, the agreement between US criteria and positive angiographic findings of stenoses is shown in Table 2. A strong correlation between US and angiography was noted, with a κ coefficient of 0.512.

The sensitivity of US in the detection of

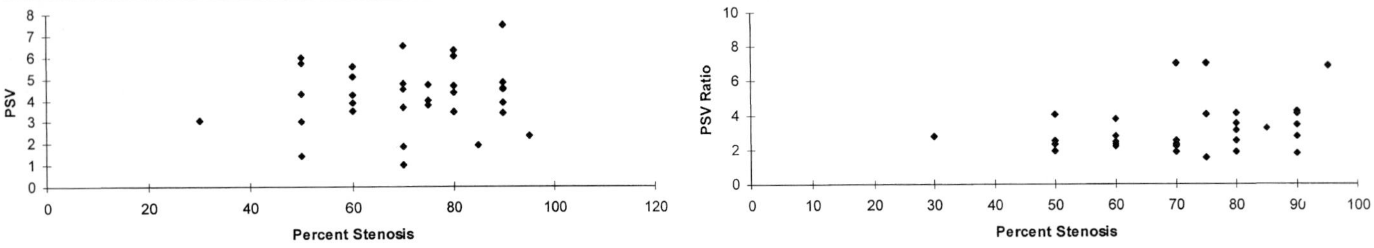

a. b.

Figure 3. Graphs show that both the (a) PSV and the (b) PSV ratio are not strongly linearly related to the percentage of stenosis at angiography. Thus, finer increments than 25% for the prediction of the percentage of stenosis by means of US are not possible with these data.

stenoses of at least 50% was 92% (37 of 40). The positive predictive value for stenosis detection in an individual patient was 94% (31 of 33). Specificity could not be reliably assessed with sufficient precision, as only four of 38 patients had completely negative findings for stenosis at angiography.

The development of a more detailed set of US velocity criteria with use of smaller intervals than 25% stenosis was not possible, as plots of PSV versus percentage of stenosis at angiography and of PSV ratios versus percentage of stenosis at angiography showed weak correlation (Fig 3). Likewise, weak correlation of the percentage of stenosis at angiography was shown with the RI at the stenosis, the change in the RI (RI distal to the stenosis minus RI proximal to the stenosis, according to Baird et al [28]), EDV, and volume flow. Thus, a multivariate analysis was not productive.

Eight patients had abnormal respiratory phasicity (respiratory flow patterns) and transmitted cardiac pulsatility in the subclavian or jugular veins; four of these patients had forearm grafts, and four had upper arm grafts. None of these patients had evidence of a central venous abnormality at angiography. The only patient with a central lesion (brachiocephalic occlusion) had proximal jugular venous occlusion and a large collateral vessel filling the jugular vein, causing flow reversal in the jugular vein. This patient had normal respiratory phasicity in both the jugular and subclavian veins but diminished transmitted cardiac pulsatility.

Twenty-four percent (eight of 34) of patients had reversal of flow in the artery distal to the graft takeoff (arterial steal) (29), and 12% (four of 34) had biphasic distal arterial flow. No patient had symptoms of arterial steal; thus, this US finding was not clinically important.

DISCUSSION

Several previous articles have described methods for the US detection of hemodialysis access graft stenoses. Tordoir et al (13) emphasized PSV measurements, while several authors (14–16) used combinations of visual stenosis measurement and color flow imaging. Others have advocated the use of flow volume measurements (10,17). PSV ratios have been used in vessels such as the internal carotid artery (18,19) and synthetic arterial grafts in the lower extremity (20,21); such ratios, however, have not been used widely in the detection of hemodialysis access graft problems. Our data suggest that a combination of PSV measurements, PSV ratios, and color flow imaging is highly sensitive in the detection of stenoses of hemodialysis access grafts and their drainage veins.

Venous Anastomotic Stenoses

The most frequent site of stenosis in this group of patients was found at the venous anastomosis, as in other studies (15). All venous anastomotic stenoses in the grafts were detected at US. A typical venous anastomotic stenosis is shown in Figure 4. All but three of the stenoses had a PSV ratio of at least 2.0. Two had a borderline PSV ratio (≥ 1.9) and a PSV of at least 4.0 m/sec, and the other was visually stenotic, with a hemodynamically significant drainage vein stenosis.

There were only two false-positive US diagnoses of venous anastomotic stenoses. The low morbidity associated with hemodialysis access graft angiography, along with the potential of substantially adverse consequences of missing these stenoses, probably justifies angiography in cases with borderline US findings.

Drainage Vein Stenoses

Drainage vein stenoses were more difficult to detect at US. In our patients, seven of nine drainage vein stenoses were detected with US. Most of these stenoses were within several centimeters of the venous anastomosis. They can be short (<0.5 cm in length), necessitating great care in US technique.

The cephalic vein frequently tapers at its insertion into the subclavian vein. This area may appear stenotic at US because of this normal narrowing, and PSVs may be elevated in this region. This area is the source of one of the false-positive US findings.

Because subclavian and proximal brachiocephalic veins are inaccessible to US transducer compression, it is more difficult to exclude clot or stenosis in these veins with confidence. Subclavian and central venous stenoses, however, occur in only about 6% of patients with grafts (9,30). The prevalence of subclavian venous stenoses has decreased in this institution and others, in large part because of recognition that placement of subclavian venous catheters is associated with a high prevalence of subclavian venous stenoses (3,31–33). Our only case of subclavian venous stenosis was not diagnosed prospectively with US, despite the recognition of multiple collateral vessels in the patient's arm. The presumed stenosis that caused the collateral vessels should have prompted a careful re-examination of the venous outflow.

Assessment of Central Stenosis

Transmitted cardiac pulsatility, respiratory phasicity, deep inspiration, and the sniff and Valsalva maneuvers can be useful in the assessment for a central stenosis, in both the lower and the upper extremities (22,34,35). In the presence of a hemodialysis access graft, however, these maneuvers are less meaningful (23). Normal accommodation of the outflow of a graft may overwhelm the low-amplitude velocity variations in the subclavian vein associated with transmitted cardiac pulsatility and respiration.

An abnormal flow pattern in the jugular vein, however, may still be a useful

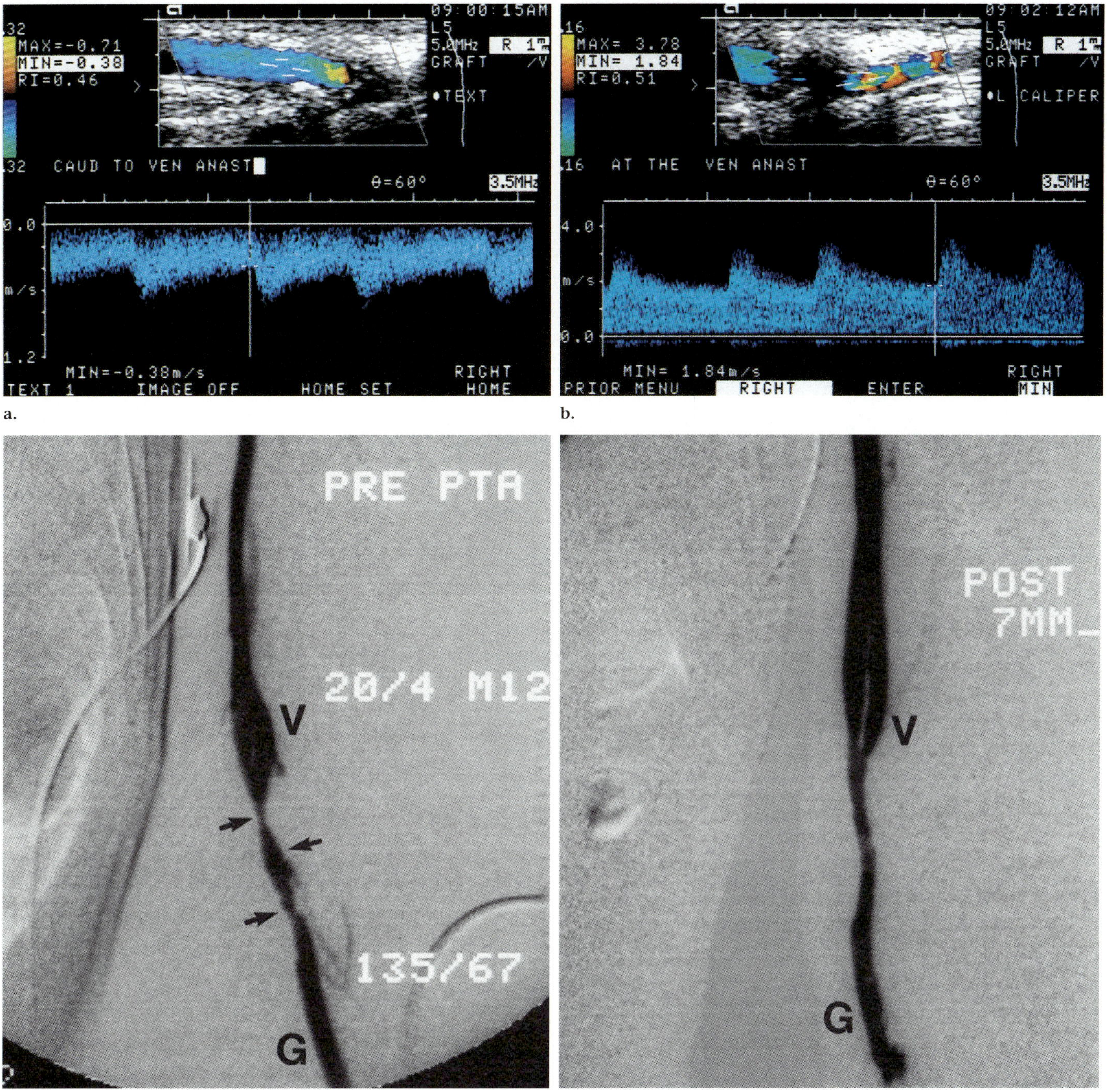

Figure 4. **(a)** Venous anastomotic stenosis in a 73-year-old man. Longitudinal duplex US image of graft distal to venous anastomotic stenosis. PSV measurement distal to the venous anastomosis is 0.71 m/sec. **(b)** Longitudinal duplex US image of graft at the venous anastomotic stenosis. Maximal PSV measurement at the venous anastomosis is 3.78 m/sec. The PSV ratio is 5.3, which is consistent with a stenosis of at least 75%. **(c)** Digital subtraction angiogram demonstrates a 90% 2-cm-long stenosis of the venous anastomosis and adjacent graft (arrows). (*PRE PTA, 20/4 M12,* and *135/67* are not relevant to this discussion.) **(d)** Digital subtraction angiogram obtained after percutaneous transluminal angioplasty shows improvement in the venous anastomotic stenosis. (*POST 7MM* is not relevant to this discussion.) In **c** and **d**, *G* = graft, *V* = vein.

sign of central venous stenosis or occlusion. We correctly identified the only patient with a brachiocephalic venous occlusion because of flow reversal in the cephalic portions of the internal jugular vein (Fig 5). Although the cardiac pulsatility was diminished, this patient's respiratory phasicity in the subclavian and jugular veins appeared to be within normal limits. This finding is probably secondary to extensive communication of collateral veins with the thoracic cavity.

Flow Volumes

Flow volume was an early US criterion used for detection of graft stenosis. Simplification of the complex graft fluid dynamics that vary with cardiac cycle and dis-

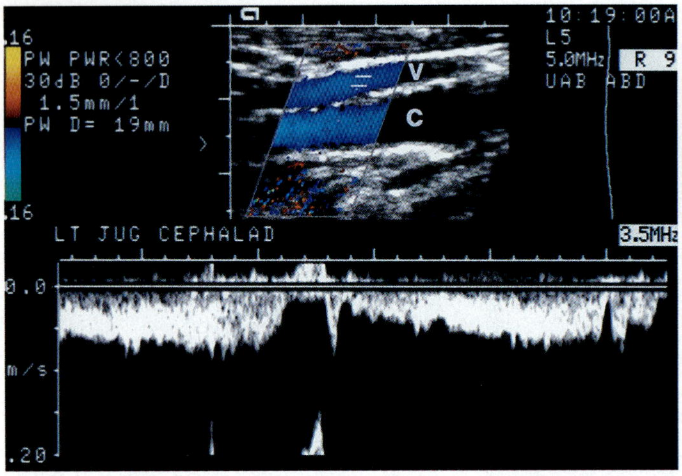

a.

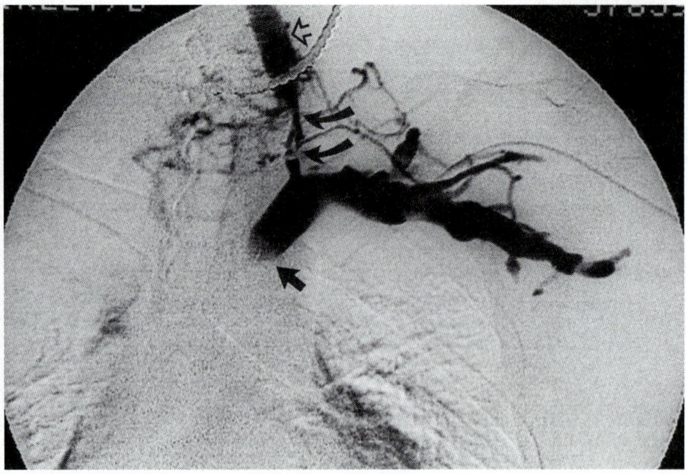

b.

Figure 5. **(a)** Longitudinal US scan of the jugular vein *(V)* in a 46-year-old man demonstrates reversed flow, consistent with a severe stenosis or occlusion of the ipsilateral brachiocephalic vein. Flow direction in the jugular vein is the same as that in the adjacent carotid artery *(C)*. Respiratory phasicity appears normal, although transmitted cardiac pulsatility is diminished. **(b)** Digital subtraction angiogram demonstrates brachiocephalic venous occlusion (straight solid arrow). The proximal jugular vein is occluded, and there is a large collateral vessel from the jugular vein to the subclavian vein (curved solid arrows). The open arrow indicates the patent jugular vein distally.

tance from the graft wall leads to flow volume, derived from an average velocity per unit of time multiplied by the volume of the region (36,37). Shackleton et al (38), in a series of 18 forearm loop grafts, found that a flow volume of less than 450 mL/min yielded a sensitivity of 83% and a specificity of 75% for episodes of thrombosis within the following 6 weeks.

Flow volumes, however, can vary by five- to 10-fold in normally functioning grafts (17,39). Within this large range of flow volumes, poor reproducibility of flow volumes in the same patient over time was found, with no apparent change in graft function (36,40).

Despite meticulous technique, we also found wide ranges of measured flow volumes with no association with the degree of stenosis. We postulate that the significant stenoses that affected nearly all our patients produced turbulent flow within the graft that rendered the flow volume measurements meaningless.

Recommendations

The multiple, careful PSV measurements that our technique requires can result in a relatively time-consuming examination (approximately 20–40 minutes per patient). Our experience suggests that 10–20 graft studies may be necessary to gain competence with the method, to avoid confusion and common errors from inexperience.

Limited US examinations may be sufficient in some patients. Because the venous anastomosis is the most common area of stenosis, this should be the first area examined after a brief initial survey to determine graft and vessel location. If there is a venous anastomotic stenosis and a patent drainage vein, the graft is probably amenable to percutaneous transluminal angioplasty. US can be concluded without a complete US evaluation of the remainder of the graft or drainage veins, as these will be assessed at angiography.

Screening versus Symptomatic Patients

In all patients in our study, there was a high degree of clinical suspicion of stenosis. US demonstrated a high (94%) positive predictive value in this population, with a high prevalence of disease. During the 6 months of the study, our institution had a 33% decrease in the number of hemodialysis access graft thromboses (4.8 per month) with respect to the previous 4 months (7.2 per month) (41). We believe this dramatic change was caused by intensive clinical surveillance for this study, resulting in increased stenosis detection and subsequently successful percutaneous treatment.

In our population, patients with a high clinical suspicion of stenosis have a high prevalence of stenosis. In those patients with a high clinical suspicion of stenosis, angiography should be performed primarily, as percutaneous transluminal angioplasty can be performed immediately after diagnostic angiography.

Our data suggest, however, that US may have an important role in patients with an intermediate level of suspicion of stenosis and in patients reluctant to undergo angiography. US also may be used to guide the correct placement of a needle into the graft for angiography when necessary.

In a population of patients who lack clinical signs of graft dysfunction, the prevalence of graft and drainage vein stenoses will be substantially decreased. To our knowledge, to date, no large prospective series has been studied to determine the sensitivity and specificity of US in a screening setting. Before we can recommend US screening of patients without signs of graft problems, further prospective studies are needed to determine the accuracy and cost-effectiveness of US.

US of hemodialysis access grafts with use of PSV criteria and color flow imaging is highly sensitive in the detection of graft and drainage vein stenoses. Abnormal results of US, with use of developed criteria, correlate strongly with results of angiography. Intensive clinical surveillance and aggressive percutaneous therapy can substantially decrease rates of graft thrombosis. Before the clinical use of US as a screening tool becomes routine, however, its accuracy and cost-effectiveness must be evaluated in a prospective, randomized trial.

Acknowledgments: We thank David Redden, PhD, Jill Barker, MS, and Jeannette Lee, PhD, for their statistical assistance. Angie French, Deonne Willis, and Beth Caminiti provided excellent secretarial assistance.

References

1. Feldman HI, Held PJ, Hutchinson JT, Stoiber E, Hartigan MF, Berlin JA. Hemodialysis vascular access morbidity in the United States. Kidney Int 1993; 43:1091–1096.
2. Windus D. Permanent vascular access: a nephrologist's view. Am J Kidney Dis 1993; 21:457–471.
3. Kumpe DA, Durham JD, Mann DJ. Thrombolysis and percutaneous transluminal angioplasty. In: Wilson SE, ed. Vascular access: principles and practice. St Louis, Mo: Mosby, 1996; 239–261.
4. Zibari GB, Rohr MS, Landreneau MD, et al. Complications from permanent hemodialysis vascular access. Surgery 1988; 104: 681–686.
5. Windus DW, Jendrisak MD, Delmez JA. Prosthetic fistula survival and complications in hemodialysis patients: effects of diabetes and age. Am J Kidney Dis 1992; 19:448–452.
6. Swedberg SH. Intimal fibromuscular hyperplasia at the venous anastomosis of PTFE grafts in hemodialysis patients. Circulation 1989; 80:1726–1736.
7. Kumpe DA, Cohen M. Angioplasty/thrombolytic treatment of failing and failed hemodialysis access sites: comparison with surgical treatment. Prog Cardiovasc Dis 1992; 34:263–278.
8. Sullivan KL, Besarab A, Bonn J, Shapiro M, Gardiner GA, Moritz MJ. Hemodynamics of failing dialysis grafts. Radiology 1993; 186:867–872.
9. Beathard GA. Percutaneous transvenous angioplasty in the treatment of vascular access stenosis. Kidney Int 1992; 42:1390–1397.
10. Sands J, Yound S, Miranda C. The effect of Doppler flow screening studies and elective revisions on dialysis access failure. ASAIO J 1992; 38:M524–M527.
11. Besarab A, Sullivan KL, Ross RP, Moritz MJ. Utility of intra-access pressure monitoring in detecting and correcting venous outlet stenoses prior to thrombosis. Kidney Int 1995; 47:1364–1373.
12. Schwab SJ, Raymond JR, Saeed M, Newman GE, Dennis PA, Bollinger RR. Prevention of hemodialysis fistula thrombosis: early detection of venous stenoses. Kidney Int 1989; 36:707–711.
13. Tordoir JHM, de Bruin HG, Hoeneveld H, Eikelboom BC, Kislaar JEHM. Duplex ultrasound scanning in the assessment of arteriovenous fistulas created for hemodialysis access: comparison with digital subtraction angiography. J Vasc Surg 1989; 10:122–128.
14. Dousset V, Grenier N, Douws C, et al. Hemodialysis grafts: color Doppler flow imaging correlated with digital subtraction angiography and functional status. Radiology 1991; 181:89–94.
15. Middleton WD, Picus DD, Marx MV, Melson GL. Color Doppler sonography of hemodialysis vascular access: comparison with angiography. AJR 1989; 152:633–639.
16. Finlay DE, Longley DG, Foshager MC, Letourneau JG. Duplex and color Doppler sonography of hemodialysis arteriovenous fistulas and grafts. RadioGraphics 1993; 13:983–999.
17. Strauch BS, O'Connell RS, Geoly K, Grundlehner M, Yakub YN, Tietjen DP. Forecasting thrombosis of vascular access with Doppler color flow imaging. Am J Kidney Dis 1992; 19:554–557.
18. Moneta GL, Edwards JM, Papanicolaou G, et al. Screening for asymptomatic internal carotid artery stenosis: duplex criteria for discriminating 60% to 99% stenosis. J Vasc Surg 1995; 21:989–994.
19. Carpenter JP, Lexa FJ, Davis JT. Determination of sixty percent or greater carotid artery stenosis by duplex Doppler ultrasonography. J Vasc Surg 1995; 22:697–705.
20. Beidle TR, Brom-Ferral R, Letourneau JG. Surveillance of infrainguinal vein grafts with duplex sonography. AJR 1994; 162: 443–448.
21. Polak JF. Arterial sonography: efficacy for the diagnosis of arterial disease of the lower extremity. AJR 1993; 161:235–243.
22. Gooding G, Hightower D, Moore E, Dillon W, Lipton M. Obstruction of the superior vena cava or subclavian veins: sonographic diagnosis. Radiology 1986; 159:663–665.
23. Nazarian GK, Foshager MC. Color Doppler sonography of the thoracic inlet veins. RadioGraphics 1995; 15:1357–1371.
24. Nack TL, Needleman L. Comparison of duplex ultrasound and contrast venography for evaluation of upper extremity venous disease. J Vasc Technol 1992; 16: 69–73.
25. Koksoy C, Kuzu A, Erden I, Turkcapra AG, Duzgun I, Anadol E. Predictive value of colour Doppler ultrasonography in detecting failure of vascular access grafts. Br J Surg 1995; 82:50–52.
26. Pucheu A, Evans J, Thomas D, Scheuble C, Pucheu M. Doppler ultrasonography of normal neck veins. J Clin Ultrasound 1994; 22:367–373.
27. England REM, Jackson A. Imaging of dialysis access: a review of 67 failing fistulas investigated by intravenous digital subtraction angiography. Br J Radiol 1993; 66:32–36.
28. Baird DE, Omdal DG, Yuill SC, et al. Doppler analysis of hemodialysis grafts: resistive index as a predictor of stenosis. J Ultrasound Med 1994; 13:791–796.
29. Valji K, Hye RJ, Roberts AC, Oglevie S, Ziegler T, Bookstein JJ. Hand ischemia in patients with hemodialysis access grafts: angiographic diagnosis and treatment. Radiology 1995; 196:697–701.
30. Kanterman RY, Vesely TM, Pilgram TK, Guy BW, Windus DW, Picus D. Dialysis access grafts: anatomic location of venous stenosis and results of angioplasty. Radiology 1995; 195:135–139.
31. Schillinger F, Schillinger D, Montagnac R, Milcent T. Post catheterization venous stenosis in haemodialysis: comparative angiographic study of 50 subclavian and 50 internal jugular accesses. Nephrol Dial Transplant 1991; 6:722–724.
32. Cimochowski GE, Worley E, Rutherford WE, Sartain J, Blondin J, Harter H. Superiority of the internal jugular over the subclavian access for temporary dialysis. Nephron 1990; 54:154–161.
33. Beenen L, van Leusen R, Deenik B, Bosch FH. The incidence of subclavian vein stenosis using silicone catheters for hemodialysis. Artif Organs 1994; 18:289–292.
34. Grassi CJ, Polak JF. Axillary and subclavian venous thrombosis: follow-up evaluation with color Doppler flow US and venography. Radiology 1990; 175:651–654.
35. Falk RL, Smith DF. Thrombosis of upper extremity thoracic inlet veins: diagnosis with duplex Doppler sonography. AJR 1987; 149:677–682.
36. Pagan-Marin H. Hemodialysis access imaging and intervention. In: Taveras JM, ed. Cardiac and vascular radiology. Philadelphia, Pa: Lippincott, 1996; 1–17.
37. Walter JP, McGahan JP, Lantz BMT. Absolute flow measurements using pulsed Doppler US. Radiology 1986; 159:545–548.
38. Shackleton CR, Taylor DC, Buckley AR, Rowley VA, Cooperberg PL, Fry PD. Predicting failure in polytetrafluoroethylene vascular access grafts for hemodialysis: a pilot study. Can J Surg 1987; 30:442–444.
39. Rittgers SE, Garcia-Valdez C, McCormick JT, Posner MP. Noninvasive blood flow measurement in expanded polytetrafluoroethylene grafts for hemodialysis access. J Vasc Surg 1986; 3:635–642.
40. Kirschbaum B, Compton A. Study of vascular access blood flow by angiodynography. Am J Kidney Dis 1995; 25:22–25.
41. Allon M, Bailey R, Deierhoi MH, et al. A multidisciplinary approach to hemodialysis access. Kidney Int 1998; 53:473–479.

Interlude

Photographs from South Africa

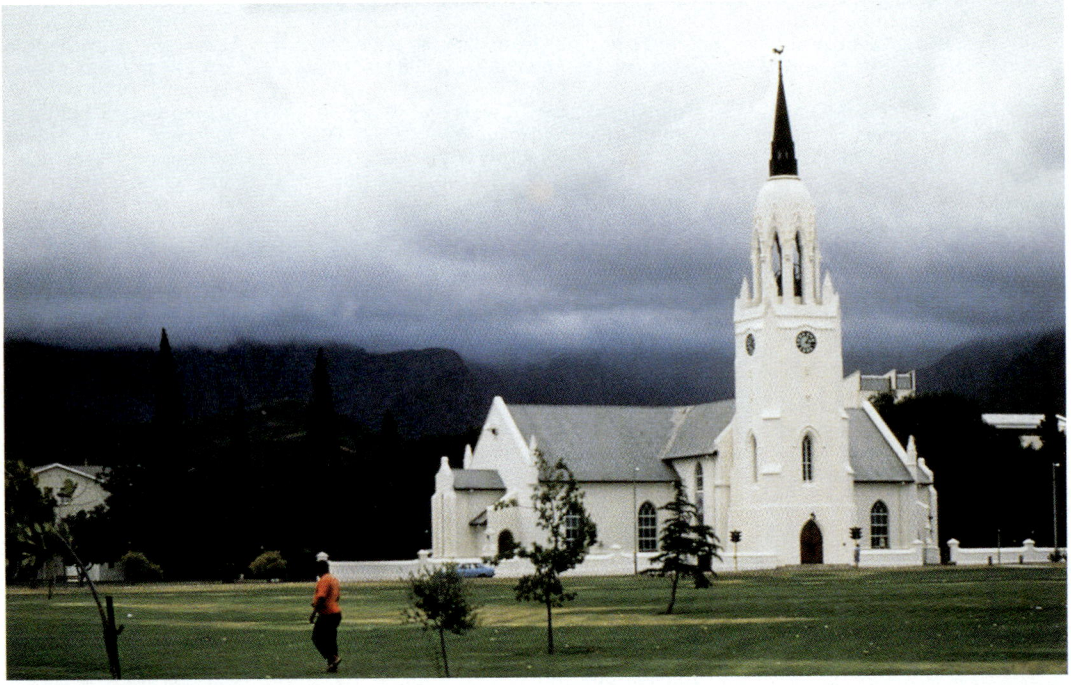

Church in Worcester, Cape Province

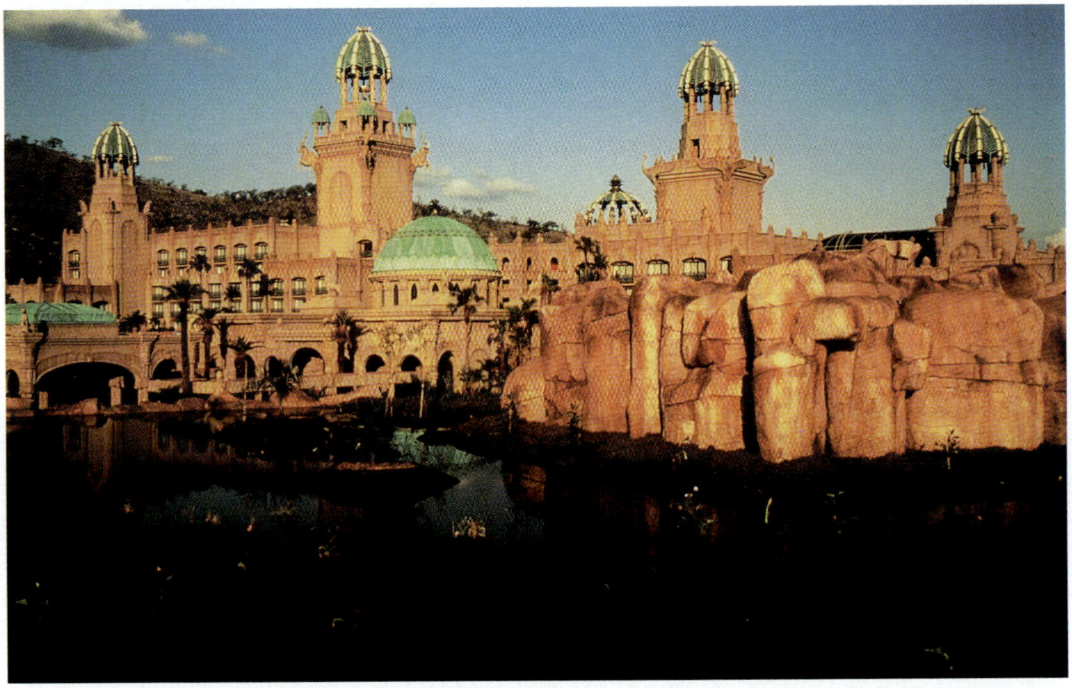

The Lost City

Photographs by Cyril Mazansky, MD, Boston, Mass

Thomas M. Ernst, PhD
Linda Chang, MD
Mallory D. Witt, MD
Howard A. Aronow, MD
Marcia E. Cornford, MD, PhD
Irvin Walot, MD
Mark A. Goldberg, MD, PhD

Index terms:
Acquired immunodeficiency syndrome (AIDS), 10.2068
Brain, MR, 10.121411, 10.121413, 10.121416
Brain neoplasms, diagnosis, 10.34
Lymphoma, 10.29, 10.34
Lymphomatoid granulomatosis, 10.3439, 10.629
Magnetic resonance (MR), perfusion study, 10.12144
Toxoplasmosis, 10.20746, 10.29

Radiology 1998; 208:663–669

Abbreviations:
AIDS = acquired immunodeficiency syndrome
HIV = human immunodeficiency virus
Ig = immunoglobulin
rCBV = regional cerebral blood volume

[1] From the Depts of Radiology (T.M.E., I.W.), Neurology (T.M.E., L.C., M.A.G.), Medicine (M.D.W.), and Pathology (M.E.C.), Harbor UCLA Medical Center, 1124 W Carson St, N-11, Torrance, CA 90502, and the Dept of Neurology and Medicine, University of Southern California Medical School, Los Angeles (H.A.A.). Received Dec 9, 1997; revision requested Feb 27, 1998; revision received Mar 23; accepted May 8. Supported in part by the NIH and State of California Universitywide AIDS Research program grant CC97 LA 175. L.C. supported in part by an NIH Scientist Development Award for Clinicians DA 00280. **Address reprint requests to** T.M.E.

Author contributions:
Guarantor of integrity of entire study, T.M.E.; study concepts and design, T.M.E., L.C.; definition of intellectual content, T.M.E., L.C.; literature research, T.M.E., L.C.; clinical studies, M.D.W., H.A.A., M.A.G.; data acquisition, T.M.E., L.C., M.D.W., H.A.A., M.E.C., I.W., M.A.G.; data analysis, T.M.E., L.C., I.W.; statistical analysis, T.M.E.; manuscript preparation, T.M.E.; manuscript editing, T.M.E., L.C.; manuscript review, T.M.E., M.D.W., H.A.A., M.E.C., I.W., M.A.G.

Cerebral Toxoplasmosis and Lymphoma in AIDS: Perfusion MR Imaging Experience in 13 Patients[1]

PURPOSE: To evaluate the perfusion magnetic resonance (MR) imaging characteristics of cerebral toxoplasmosis and lymphoma in patients with acquired immunodeficiency syndrome (AIDS).

MATERIALS AND METHODS: Perfusion MR imaging was performed prospectively in 13 patients with AIDS who had contrast material–enhancing focal brain lesions (six with active lymphoma, five with toxoplasmosis, one with treated lymphoma in remission, and one with toxoplasmosis plus lymphomatoid granulomatosis). Regional cerebral blood volume (rCBV) was determined by using dynamic echo-planar MR imaging during bolus injection of a gadolinium chelate.

RESULTS: The rCBV was decreased (44% ± 24 [standard deviation] of rCBV in the contralateral regions) throughout the toxoplasmosis lesions and in the surrounding edema of both lesion types, whereas all active lymphomas displayed areas of increased rCBV (258% ± 99). These differences were significant *(P* < .005).

CONCLUSION: Reduced rCBV in toxoplasmosis lesions is probably due to a lack of vasculature within the abscess; increased rCBV in lymphomas is probably due to hypervascularity in foci of active tumor growth; and decreased rCBV in the edema is probably due to vasoconstriction associated with increased interstitial pressure. Perfusion MR imaging is a rapid, noninvasive tool that may allow differentiation between cerebral lymphoma and toxoplasmosis in patients with AIDS.

Cerebral toxoplasmosis and primary brain lymphoma are two of the most common focal brain lesions in patients with acquired immunodeficiency syndrome (AIDS). These diseases typically occur when patients are severely immunocompromised. In radiologic terms, cerebral toxoplasmosis and lymphoma in patients with AIDS often present a diagnostic dilemma, because both lesions may appear as single or multiple lesions that show ring-shaped contrast material enhancement on computed tomographic (CT) or magnetic resonance (MR) images. Clinical variables and laboratory tests, including serologic tests and polymerase chain reaction analysis for toxoplasmosis or Epstein-Barr virus in the cerebrospinal fluid, are insensitive, nonspecific, or too slow to be useful for the establishment of the initial diagnosis (1,2). Because of substantial differences in the treatment for and prognosis of these diseases, there is a need for improved—and ideally noninvasive—techniques for the diagnosis of toxoplasmosis and lymphoma in patients with AIDS.

The aim of this study was to determine whether perfusion MR imaging can help differentiate cerebral toxoplasmosis and lymphoma in AIDS. The results of studies with nuclear medicine techniques such as single-photon emission CT (SPECT) and positron emission tomography (PET) suggest that lymphoma lesions are characterized by hypermetabolic foci, whereas toxoplasmosis lesions demonstrate decreased metabolism throughout the lesions (3–6). Because metabolism and perfusion are generally correlated and neoplastic lesions are often hypervascular, we predicted that cerebral lymphoma will have increased perfusion in the active tumor, whereas toxoplasmosis lesions will show uniform hypoperfusion.

MATERIALS AND METHODS

Thirteen patients with AIDS in whom a clinical diagnosis of either toxoplasmosis or lymphoma was established were recruited consecutively and evaluated prospectively. A summary of the patients' demographic characteristics, clinical signs, and MR imaging findings and the method used for diagnosis are shown in the Table. Six patients (age range, 23–50 years; mean age, 35 years; CD4 cell count, 0–49 cells per microliter [0–49 × 10^6/L]) had a diagnosis of active lymphoma. The presence of a lymphoma lesion was confirmed with biopsy or cytologic analysis results from cerebrospinal fluid in three patients; in addition, in two of these three patients, polymerase chain reaction results were positive for Epstein-Barr virus in the cerebrospinal fluid. In the remaining three patients, the diagnosis of lymphoma was based on their response to treatment. In addition, all six patients with active lymphoma had a negative *Toxoplasma* IgG titer, and none of these patients showed improvement while undergoing empiric anti-*Toxoplasma* therapy. One further patient (patient 4) was examined 2½ years after initial radiation therapy for lymphoma. This patient had a lymphoma lesion, proved at biopsy, that had resolved at the time of the perfusion MR imaging examination.

In five other patients (age range, 32–63 years; mean age, 40 years; CD4 cell count, 8–101 cells per microliter [8–101 × 10^6/L]), a diagnosis of toxoplasmosis was established: This was confirmed with the results of brain biopsy in two patients and with positive *Toxoplasma* IgG titer and response to anti-*Toxoplasma* therapy in all five patients. All five patients with toxoplasmosis also showed resolution of the lesion(s) on follow-up MR images obtained after treatment. Brain biopsy specimens in one further patient (patient 12), who had an HIV-2 infection, showed lymphomatoid granulomatosis (a prelymphomatous condition), with predominantly angiocentric, atypical B cells along with *Toxoplasma* organisms. This patient responded to both anti-*Toxoplasma* medications and dexamethasone treatment.

Verbal and written informed consent were obtained from all patients prior to MR imaging. The protocol was approved by our institutional review board.

MR Imaging Protocol

MR imaging was performed with a 1.5-T imager (Signa; GE Medical Systems, Milwaukee, Wis) equipped with model SR120 echo-planar imaging hardware. Conventional MR imaging consisted of the acquisition of sagittal T1-weighted images (repetition time msec/echo time msec, 500/11; section thickness, 5 mm; intersection gap, 2 mm; field of view, 24 cm), axial fast double spin-echo images (4,000/17, 102 [effective echo times]; section thickness, 5 mm; contiguous sections; field of view, 24 cm), and axial fluid-attenuated inversion recovery images (repetition time msec/echo time msec/inversion time msec, 11,000/142/2,600; section thickness, 5 mm; contiguous sections; field of view, 24 cm).

Perfusion MR imaging was performed with a single-shot gradient-echo echo-planar sequence (2,500/30; 12 6-mm-thick sections; intersection gap, 2 mm; field of view, 20 cm; matrix, 64 × 64). The entire brain was successively imaged 39 times (time resolution, 2.5 seconds). Thirty seconds into the image acquisition, a 20-mL bolus of gadoteridol (Prohance; Bracco Diagnostics, Princeton, NJ) was intravenously injected. Finally, axial gadolinium-enhanced T1-weighted images (500/11; section thickness, 5 mm; contiguous sections; field of view, 24 cm) were obtained.

Image Processing

Image analysis was performed on a workstation (DEC Alpha; Digital Equipment, Nashua, NH) by means of customized programs written in IDL (Research Systems, Boulder, Colo) specifically for the analysis of perfusion MR imaging data sets. Regional cerebral blood volume (rCBV) maps were reconstructed by using the inverse exponential relationship between the MR signal intensity and the concentration of the contrast material. The rCBV was calculated by means of numeric integration over the concentration-time curve (7).

The rCBV maps were aligned (ie, shifted and scaled) with the anatomic images for the drawing of regions of interest. Regions of interest were drawn manually on the gadolinium-enhanced T1-weighted images to include the central necrotic area, as well as the enhancing areas. Because the lesions were usually heterogeneous, the average and maximum rCBVs were calculated for each lesion. All values in the lesions were expressed as a percentage of the average value in the corresponding contralateral regions.

Statistical analyses were performed by using StatView software (Abacus, Berkeley, Calif). The Student t test was used to determine the statistical significance of differences between rCBVs in the six active lymphoma and the five toxoplasmosis lesions. Patient 4 (with lymphoma in remission) and patient 12 (with toxoplasmosis plus lymphomatoid granulomatosis) were excluded from the statistical analysis because they do not belong clearly in one of the two groups. A P value of less than .05 was considered to indicate statistical significance. All values are reported as means plus or minus 1 standard deviation.

RESULTS

All six patients in whom the diagnosis of active lymphoma was established consistently showed an elevated rCBV in the active tumor compared with that in the contralateral, normal-appearing brain region. Figure 1a shows a typical example (in patient 6) of a ring-shaped, enhancing (hereafter, ring-enhancing) lymphoma with a markedly increased rCBV in the lesion (182% of that in the contralateral region). Although it is commonly stated that lymphoma usually manifests as a single lesion, all of the patients in our study had two or three lesions each. All lymphoma lesions showed a mild to moderate degree of edema with mass effect. The pattern of gadolinium enhancement was homogeneous in lesions adjacent to the ventricles (n = 2) or ring-enhancing in lesions in the parenchyma (n = 4). The average rCBV of the lymphoma lesions was only mildly increased compared with that of normal tissue (135% ± 48 of that in the contralateral region). This result was due to low rCBV values in the necrotic areas of some lymphomas. The largest increases in the rCBV were observed in the enhancing regions, which showed an average maximum rCBV value of 258% ± 99 of that in the contralateral regions.

In contrast to lymphoma lesions, all five toxoplasmosis lesions showed a consistently decreased rCBV throughout, specifically, in central areas, in the enhancing rim, and in the surrounding edema. This is reflected by the greatly reduced average rCBV (44% ± 24 of that in the contralateral region); even the maximum rCBV values were below normal (92% ± 8 of that in the contralateral regions). All toxoplasmosis lesions were ring-enhancing. A typical example (in patient 8, who had a biopsy-proved toxoplasmosis lesion) is displayed in Figure 1b. At the time of presentation, this patient had a single right frontal lesion that showed ring enhancement and surrounding edema. It

Demographic, Clinical, Diagnostic, and MR Imaging Data in 13 Patients with AIDS

Patient No.	Age (y)/Sex	Diagnosis	Interval since Diagnosis (mo)	Symptoms	CD4 Count (cells/μL)*	Lesion Location	Confirmatory Diagnostic Test Results or Treatments†
1	38/M	Lymphoma	72	Headaches, nausea and vomiting, left homonymous hemianopsia; right arm weakness, dysphagia for 3 d	17	Three lesions in right basal ganglia and adjacent to anterior horn of lateral ventricle	Negative serum *Toxoplasma* IgG and IgM levels, deterioration with *Toxoplasma* therapy, improvement after dexamethasone
2	23/M	Lymphoma	48	Right-sided hemianopsia; right arm weakness and numbness for 2 mo	4	Two lesions in left basal ganglia and adjacent to anterior horn of lateral ventricle	Lymphoma confirmed at biopsy, negative serum *Toxoplasma* IgG and IgM levels, PCR positive for EBV and negative for *Toxoplasma* DNA in CSF, improvement after dexamethasone
3	23/F	Lymphoma	34	New onset of seizures for 3 wk	4	Three lesions in left periventricular area, left anterior temporal lobe, and right frontal lobe	Lymphoma confirmed at biopsy, negative serum *Toxoplasma* IgG and IgM levels, improvement after dexamethasone
4	33/M	Lymphoma, treated and in remission	103	Seizures at onset 30 months previously	300‡	Two lesions in left basal ganglia and adjacent to anterior horn of lateral ventricle	Lymphoma confirmed at biopsy, positive serum *Toxoplasma* IgG level, negative *Toxoplasma* IgM level, resolution with dexamethasone and radiation therapy
5	29/M	Lymphoma	72	Altered mental status; right hemiparesis for 1 mo	0	Two lesions in left caudate and adjacent to anterior horn of lateral ventricle	Negative serum *Toxoplasma* IgG and IgM levels, deterioration with *Toxoplasma* therapy, improvement with dexamethasone
6	50/M	Lymphoma	0	40-lb (88-kg) weight loss over 4 mo, dysphagia and forgetfulness for 3 wk	12	Two lesions in left basal ganglia and adjacent to left lateral ventricle	Cytologic analysis positive for B cells in CSF, PCR positive for EBV DNA in CSF, negative serum *Toxoplasma* IgG and IgM levels, improvement after dexamethasone
7	45/M	Lymphoma	2	Gait imbalance and aphasia for 2 wk	49	Two lesions in left temporal lobe and adjacent to posterior horn of lateral ventricle	Negative serum *Toxoplasma* IgG and IgM levels, deterioration after *Toxoplasma* therapy, improvement after dexamethasone
8	63/M	Toxoplasmosis	0.5	Left-sided weakness, right facial droop; right ptosis for 1.5 mo	63	One lesion in right frontal lobe white matter	Toxoplasmosis proved at biopsy, positive serum *Toxoplasma* IgG level, negative serum *Toxoplasma* IgM level
9	35/F	Toxoplasmosis	1.5	Headaches for 1 mo	101	One lesion in left frontal lobe white matter	Toxoplasmosis proved at biopsy, positive serum *Toxoplasma* IgG level
10	38/M	Toxoplasmosis	0.5	New onset of seizures and headaches for 2 wk	18	Three lesions in right and left thalami and left parietal lobe white matter	Response to *Toxoplasma* therapy, positive serum *Toxoplasma* IgG level, negative serum *Toxoplasma* IgM level
11	33/M	Toxoplasmosis	0	Acute left hemiplegia for 2 d	20	Two lesions in right dorsal frontal lobe and left subfrontal region	Response to *Toxoplasma* therapy, positive serum *Toxoplasma* IgG level, negative serum *Toxoplasma* IgM level
12§	47/M	Toxoplasmosis and lymphomatoid granulomatosis	0	New onset of headaches; nausea and vomiting, ataxia for 1 wk	19	One lesion in left medial cerebellum	Toxoplasmosis and lymphomatoid granulomatosis proved at biopsy, positive serum *Toxoplasma* IgG level, negative *Toxoplasma* serum IgM level
13	32/M	Toxoplasmosis	6	Headaches for 2 wk	8	One lesion in left subfrontal and caudate	Positive serum *Toxoplasma* IgG level, response to *Toxoplasma* therapy

* To convert to SI units (cells/L), multiply by 10^6.
† CSF = cerebrospinal fluid, EBV = Epstein-Barr virus, Ig = immunoglobulin, PCR = polymerase chain reaction.
‡ The CD4 count at the time of the initial diagnosis of lymphoma was fewer than 10 cells/μL (10^6 cells/L).
§ The patient was negative for human immunodeficiency virus (HIV)–1 antibodies and positive for HIV-2 antibodies.

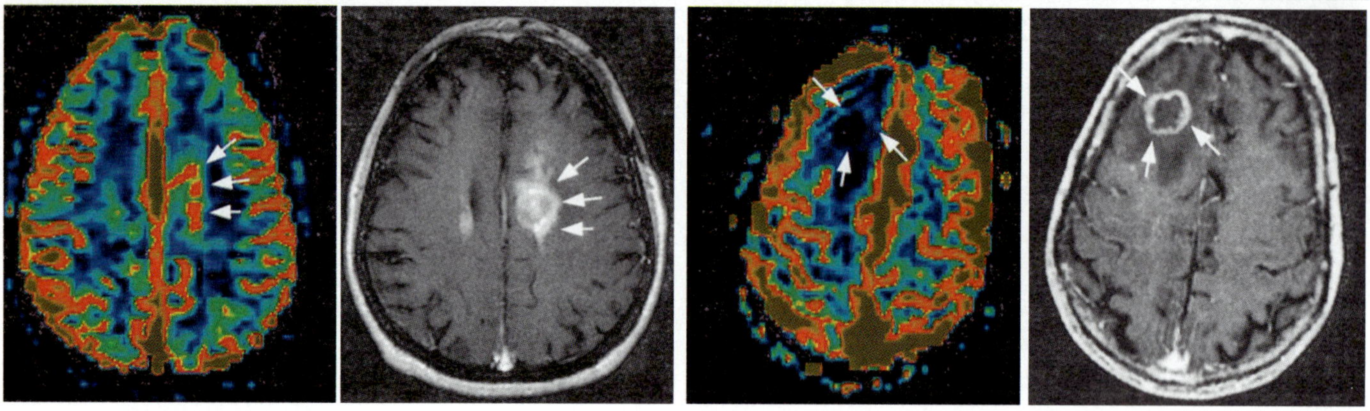

a.

b.

Figure 1. **(a) Patient 6.** Primary brain lymphoma lesion (arrows) in a 50-year-old man with AIDS. Left: rCBV map from perfusion MR imaging (2,500/30). Right: Gadolinium-enhanced T1-weighted image (500/11). The lymphoma lesion shows areas of greatly increased rCBV (arrows, left image); in this case, the maximum rCBV was 270% of that of the contralateral brain region. **(b) Patient 8.** Toxoplasmosis lesion (arrows) in a 63-year-old man with AIDS. Left: rCBV map from perfusion MR imaging (2,500/30). Right: Gadolinium-enhanced T1-weighted MR image (500/11). In contrast to **a**, the rCBV is consistently reduced in the central regions and in the enhancing rim of the toxoplasmosis lesion (arrows, left and right images), as well as in the surrounding edema; in this case, the maximum rCBV was 94% of that in the contralateral region.

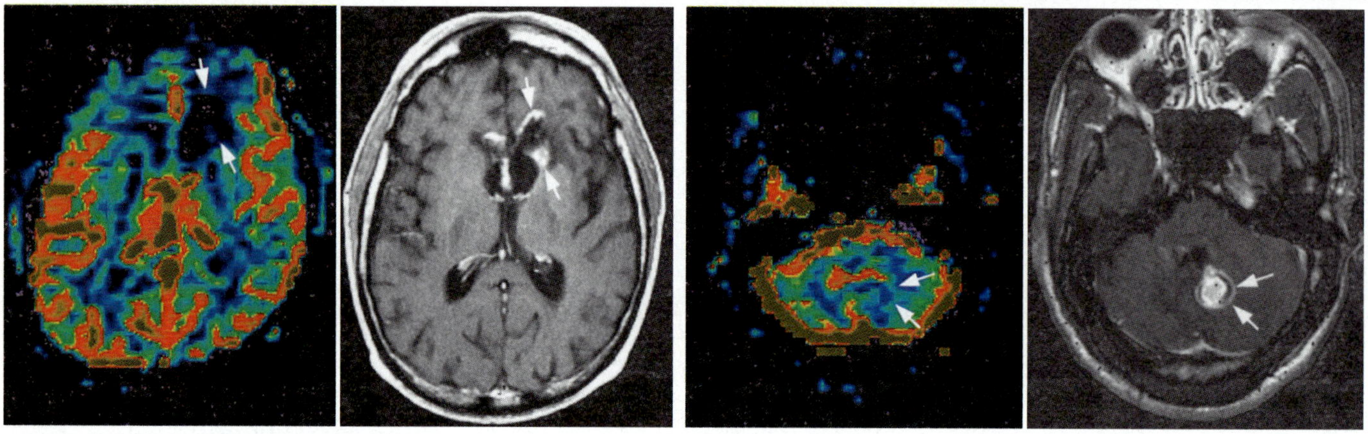

a.

b.

Figure 2. **(a) Patient 4.** Residual lymphoma lesion (arrows) in a 33-year-old man with AIDS. This patient was examined 2½ years after initial radiation therapy for lymphoma, which was in remission at the time of the perfusion MR examination. Left: rCBV map from perfusion MR imaging (2,500/30). Right: Gadolinium-enhanced T1-weighted MR image (500/11). The MR imaging study shows an enhancing residual lesion (arrows, right image), which is consistent with either residual tumor or radiation-induced necrosis. The perfusion MR image shows reduced or absent blood volume in the enhancing regions (arrows, left image), including the nodular region, which suggests radiation-induced necrosis (in agreement with the clinical course). **(b) Patient 12.** Toxoplasmosis and lymphomatoid granulomatosis in a 47-year-old man with AIDS. Left: The rCBV map from perfusion MR imaging (2,500/30) shows reduced rCBV (56% of that in the contralateral region) in the central part of the lesion (arrows) and the surrounding edema (56% of that in the contralateral region). The rCBV in the lateral rim of the lesion was similar to that in the contralateral region but higher than that in the central part and the edema (maximum rCBV, 101% of that in the contralateral region). Right: Gadolinium enhanced T1-weighted MR image (500/11) shows an enhancing lesion (arrows) surrounded by edema in the left cerebellum. Histopathologic results demonstrated a mixed lesion consisting of toxoplasmosis and lymphomatoid granulomatosis.

was not possible to differentiate between toxoplasmosis and lymphoma on conventional MR images. Perfusion MR images showed a virtually absent rCBV in the central part of the lesion, including the enhancing rim (14% of that in the contralateral region), as well as in the surrounding edema (43% of that in the contralateral region). In particular, there was no area of increased rCBV in the enhancing rim of the lesion (Fig 1b).

Two patients had unusual findings. Patient 4, with biopsy-proved lymphoma, was examined 2½ years after initial radiation therapy for lymphoma. The patient originally had a large, enhancing lesion along the left anterior horn of the lateral ventricle that extended into the basal ganglia. After radiation therapy, the patient showed clinical improvement, and the lesion was markedly decreased in size on MR images. The MR images obtained for the present study showed an enhancing residual lesion, which is consistent with either residual tumor or necrosis after irradiation. Gadolinium-enhanced T1-weighted images showed enhancement of a small nodule that protruded into the cerebrospinal fluid and some enhancement along the left anterior horn of the lateral ventricle (Fig 2a). Perfusion MR images showed a reduced or absent rCBV in the enhancing regions, includ-

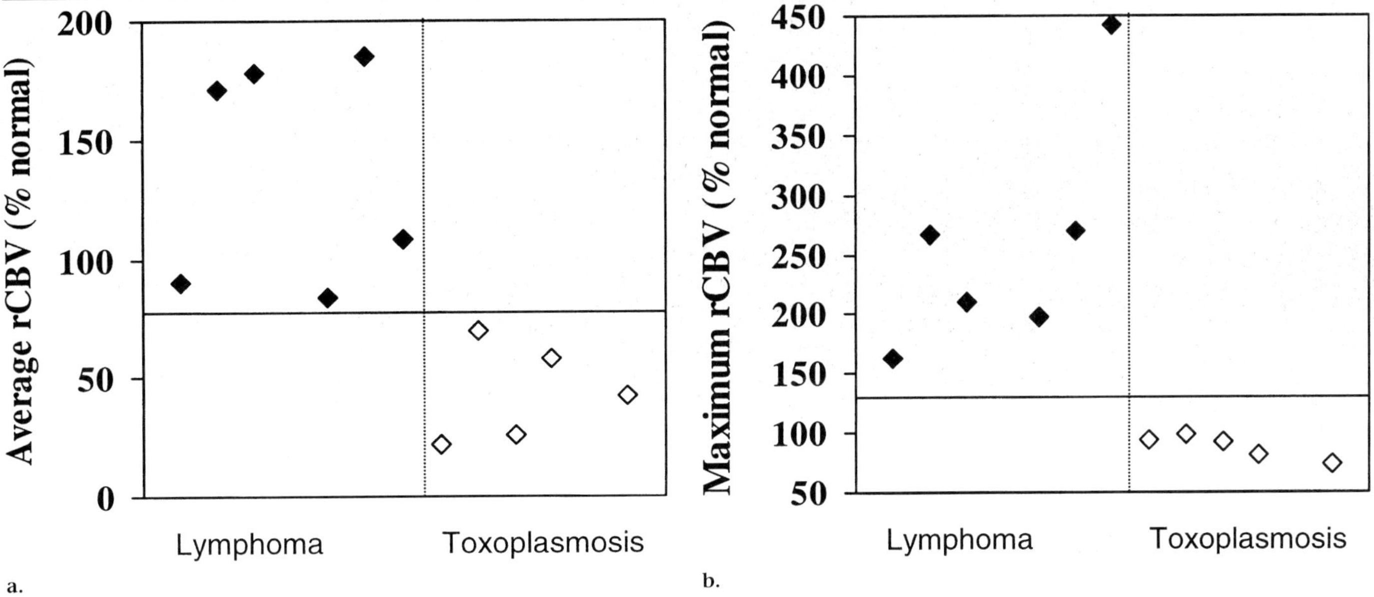

Figure 3. Plots show the **(a)** average and **(b)** maximum rCBV values for active toxoplasmosis (◇) and lymphoma (◆) lesions relative to the average rCBV values of the corresponding, normal-appearing contralateral regions. The individual data points are presented in order from left to right according to patient number. Data from patient 12, who had a mixed lesion, and patient 4, whose lymphoma was in remission after treatment, are not included in the plots. The difference between the toxoplasmosis and lymphoma lesions was statistically significant for both variables ($P < .005$). The maximum rCBV shows greater separation between toxoplasmosis and lymphoma.

ing the nodular region, which suggested the absence of hypervascularity (Fig 2a). Therefore, the clinical course and perfusion MR imaging findings were consistent with clinical remission of the lymphoma.

The second patient with an unusual MR imaging finding (patient 12) had an enhancing lesion, surrounded by edema, in the left cerebellum (Fig 2b). Perfusion MR images showed a reduced rCBV in the central part of the lesion (56% of that in the contralateral region) and the surrounding edema (56% of that in the contralateral region). The rCBV in the lateral rim of the lesion was similar to that of the contralateral side (101%) but was higher than that in the central part and the edema (Fig 2b). Histopathologic examination of brain tissue obtained at needle biopsy showed a mixed lesion that consisted of toxoplasmosis and lymphomatoid granulomatosis.

To determine whether perfusion MR imaging can help discriminate between active lymphoma and toxoplasmosis, we plotted the average and maximum rCBV values of the lesions in both groups (Fig 3; six active lymphoma and five toxoplasmosis lesions). The difference between the two groups was statistically significant for both variables ($P < .005$ for both variables; patients 4 and 12 were excluded from the analysis). However, the maximum rCBV (Fig 3b) showed greater separation between toxoplasmosis and lymphoma lesions than the average rCBV (Fig 3a) and therefore appears to be a promising variable for help in discriminating between the two types of lesions.

DISCUSSION

Our results suggest that perfusion MR imaging could help resolve some of the problems associated with the diagnosis of cerebral toxoplasmosis and lymphoma in patients with AIDS. Toxoplasmosis lesions were characterized by a consistently reduced rCBV with respect to both the average and the maximum rCBV within the lesions. The surrounding edema also showed a decreased rCBV. This consistent hypoperfusion is most likely caused by a lack of vasculature within the lesion and by vasoconstriction due to increased interstitial pressure in the surrounding edema. For the same reasons, large areas of decreased blood volume are also present in necrotic regions and in the surrounding edema of lymphomas. However, in contrast to toxoplasmosis lesions, all active lymphomas in our study exhibited an area of increased blood volume, which was most likely due to hypervascularity associated with the active neoplastic processes. As a result, the maximum perfusion values in lymphoma lesions were significantly higher than those in toxoplasmosis lesions.

Two patients had atypical lesions. In patient 12, who had combined toxoplasmosis and lymphomatoid granulomatosis, the rCBV map showed relatively normal blood volume in the lateral rim of the lesion. Thus, the lesion was not completely consistent with a pure toxoplasmosis lesion (which would have a decreased rCBV throughout) or a pure lymphoma (which would have an increased rCBV in the cellular regions and a decreased rCBV in the necrotic regions). Patient 4, who had a biopsy-proved lymphoma that was treated successfully and was in remission, showed no increased rCBV in the residual regions. This finding suggests that perfusion MR imaging might be useful for the differentiation of a recurrent neoplasm from radiation-induced necrosis, both of which may show contrast material enhancement (8).

The perfusion patterns seen with perfusion MR imaging appear to be similar to those observed with nuclear medicine techniques (3–6). PET scans show increased uptake of 2-[fluorine-18]fluoro-2-deoxy-D-glucose in lymphomas but not in toxoplasmosis lesions (3). Thallium-201 SPECT images also allow good differentiation between lymphoma and toxoplasmosis lesions in patients with AIDS (6). Another alternative diagnostic test for focal brain lesions in AIDS is proton, or hydrogen-1, MR spectroscopy (9–13). With H-1 MR spectroscopy, toxoplasmosis lesions show markedly elevated lactate and lipid levels and depleted levels of other normal brain metabolites; this characteristic chemical pattern is consistent with the anaerobic, acellular environment within a centrally necrotic abscess and the inflammatory response surrounding the abscess (9,10,14). In contrast, MR spectroscopy of central nervous system lymphoma in AIDS shows moderately increased lactate and lipid levels, a markedly elevated choline level, and decreased levels of the other normal metabolites. This pattern is probably due to increased cellularity caused by the small neoplastic lymphocytes, with ischemia and necrosis in the central portions of the lesion.

Perfusion MR imaging has several advantages over nuclear medicine techniques and MR spectroscopy: (*a*) Perfusion MR imaging has higher spatial resolution; (*b*) perfusion MR imaging may use the same contrast material (a gadolinium chelate) that is already given to patients with AIDS and brain lesions; (*c*) compared with localized spectroscopy, which is used to evaluate one lesion at a time, perfusion MR imaging can be used to evaluate the entire brain, including all the lesions; and (*d*) perfusion MR imaging adds less than 2 minutes to the acquisition time of an MR examination. Therefore, perfusion MR imaging can easily be added to the initial MR imaging session. Also, perfusion MR imaging is quite robust compared with H-1 MR spectroscopy. For example, we were able to obtain a high-quality rCBV map in patient 3 even though she was in severe pain and was agitated during the MR examination.

One potential problem with perfusion MR imaging is its sensitivity to blood in large vessels. This may make it difficult to determine whether hyperperfused areas are due to a neoplastic process or simply to the presence of a larger blood vessel, particularly when the lesion is close to the cortex. Most of the lesions in our study were located in subcortical regions, however, in which no large vessels are observed in healthy subjects. In addition, the influence of large vessels may be diminished by the use of spin-echo or asymmetric spin-echo techniques (15–18) or by means of image postprocessing (19).

An improved differential diagnosis between toxoplasmosis and lymphoma is important because the two lesions may be difficult to distinguish both clinically and by using standard radiologic techniques, despite marked differences in the histopathologic characteristics of the two conditions. Toxoplasmosis is caused by an opportunistic infection with the obligate intracellular protozoan *Toxoplasma gondii*. Serologic results for *Toxoplasma* are frequently positive, but the specificity for active brain infection is low (1). Recent studies (2) with polymerase chain reaction analysis for *T gondii* DNA in the cerebrospinal fluid demonstrated a sensitivity of only 50%. MR imaging of toxoplasmosis in patients with AIDS demonstrates single or multiple discrete foci with high signal intensity and surrounding edema on T2-weighted images; these lesions are mostly heterogeneous, with well-circumscribed margins that enhance after the administration of a gadolinium chelate (20–22). Perfusion MR imaging, however, shows a uniformly decreased rCBV throughout the lesion and the surrounding edema.

In contrast to toxoplasmosis, primary central nervous system lymphoma is a neoplastic process, nearly always of a high-grade B-cell type in AIDS. Because most cells contain the Epstein-Barr virus (23,24), it has been hypothesized that central nervous system lymphoma in AIDS may arise from Epstein-Barr virus–infected B cells (25).

At neuroimaging with CT and MR imaging, many lymphomas are indistinguishable from toxoplasmosis lesions. Like toxoplasmosis lesions, primary brain lymphomas may manifest as solitary or multicentric lesions (22,26) that are hypointense on T1-weighted images, are iso- to hyperintense on T2-weighted images, and have surrounding edema. Primary brain lymphoma in patients with AIDS rapidly becomes multicentric; multifocal lesions have been demonstrated in 80%–100% of patients with AIDS who were found at autopsy to have had lymphoma (27). Moreover, the lesions can more than double in size within weeks (28–30). This accelerated outward growth of the tumor may divert the vascular supply to the growing edge of the tumor, leading to central areas of necrosis and ring-enhancement after administration of a gadolinium chelate (22,29). This feature of lymphoma in AIDS blurs the conventional radiologic distinction from actually necrotic toxoplasmosis lesions. Perfusion MR imaging appears to be helpful for differentiating an active tumor from a toxoplasmosis abscess by demonstrating an elevated rCBV in the active tumor.

Before the advent of prophylactic therapy for toxoplasmosis, *Toxoplasma*-induced lesions occurred more frequently than lymphoma (31,32); therefore, most patients with AIDS and ring-enhancing brain lesions were empirically treated for toxoplasmosis for 2 weeks (2). Because tissue confirmation is necessary for the treatment of lymphoma with radiation therapy at many institutions (31), including ours, brain biopsy is generally performed if empiric treatment for toxoplasmosis is unsuccessful. With prophylactic therapy for toxoplasmosis in patients with AIDS as a new standard of care, however, we observed fewer patients with toxoplasmosis than with lymphoma. As a result, relatively more patients may be subjected to inappropriate empiric therapy for toxoplasmosis (with its potential side effects), while brain biopsy and the correct diagnosis are delayed. This is illustrated in the case of patient 3, who had cerebral lymphoma but was empirically treated for toxoplasmosis with sulfadiazene and pyrimethamine for 1 month. As the result of a severe allergic reaction to sulfadiazene, the patient developed Stevens-Johnson syndrome, which is characterized by extensive mucosal and skin dermatolytic lesions and fever. An improved diagnosis with noninvasive techniques would have prevented this complication. Therefore, safer and more efficient methods are needed for the early diagnosis in patients with AIDS who have enhancing brain lesions.

In summary, perfusion MR imaging shows an elevated rCBV in active lymphoma lesions and a decreased rCBV in toxoplasmosis lesions. These findings suggest that perfusion MR imaging may be a valuable tool for the rapid, noninvasive confirmation of suspected central nervous system lymphoma in patients with AIDS. Our preliminary observations, if further confirmed with a larger sample size, may help prevent empiric treatment with anti-*Toxoplasma* medication and the delay in radiation and steroid therapy in patients with AIDS. Ultimately, a combination of clinical variables, polymerase chain reaction analysis for Epstein-Barr virus in the cerebrospinal fluid, and perfusion MR imaging may have sufficient specificity to replace biopsy, especially when a biopsy is associated with a high risk or is contraindicated. The addition of perfusion MR imaging to existing MR imaging protocols in patients with AIDS who have focal brain lesions may help improve the clinical diagnosis and, possibly, the disease prognosis, if these patients receive the appropriate treatment earlier.

References

1. Derouin F, Thulliez P, Garin YJF. *Toxoplasma* serology in HIV-infected patients: value and limitations. Pathol Biol 1991; 39:255–259.
2. Antinori A, Ammassari A, De Luca A, et al. Diagnosis of AIDS-related focal brain le-

sions: a decision-making analysis based on clinical and neuroradiologic characteristics combined with polymerase chain reaction assays in CSF. Neurology 1997; 48:687–694.

3. Hoffman JM, Waskin HA, Schiffer T. FDG-PET in differentiating lymphoma from nonmalignant central nervous system lesions in patients with AIDS. J Nucl Med 1993; 34:567–575.
4. Ruiz A, Ganz WI, Post MJ, et al. Use of thallium-201 brain SPECT to differentiate cerebral lymphoma from *Toxoplasma* encephalitis in AIDS patients. AJNR 1994; 15:1885–1894.
5. Lorberboym M, Estok L, Machac J, et al. Rapid differential diagnosis of cerebral toxoplasmosis and primary central nervous system lymphoma by thallium-201 SPECT. J Nucl Med 1996; 37:1150–1154.
6. Ruiz A, Post MJ, Bundschu C, Ganz WI, Georgiou M. Primary central nervous system lymphoma in patients with AIDS. Neuroimaging Clin N Am 1997; 7:281–296.
7. Axel L. Cerebral blood flow determination by rapid-sequence computed tomography. Radiology 1980; 137:679–686.
8. Caramia F, Aronen HJ, Sorenson AG, Belliveau JW, Gonzalez RG, Rosen BR. Perfusion MR imaging with exogenous contrast agents. In: Le Bihan D, ed. Diffusion and perfusion magnetic resonance imaging. New York, NY: Raven, 1995; 255–267.
9. Yamagata NT, Miller BL, McBride D, et al. In vivo proton spectroscopy of intracranial infections and neoplasms. J Neuroimaging 1994; 4:23–28.
10. Chang L, Miller B, McBride D, et al. Brain lesions in patients with AIDS: H-1 MR spectroscopy. Radiology 1995; 197:527–531.
11. Chang L, Cornford ME, Chiang FL, Ernst TM, Sun NCJ, Miller BL. Radiologic-pathologic correlation: cerebral toxoplasmosis and lymphoma in AIDS. AJNR 1995; 16:1653–1663.
12. Walot I, Miller BL, Chang L, Mehringer CM. Neuroimaging findings in patients with AIDS. Clin Infect Dis 1996; 22:906–919.
13. Chang L, Ernst T, Tornatore C, et al. Metabolite abnormalities in progressive multifocal leukoencephalopathy by proton magnetic resonance spectroscopy. Neurology 1997; 48:836–845.
14. Confort-Gouny S, Vion-Dury J, Nicoli F, et al. A multiparametric data analysis showing the potential of localized proton MR spectroscopy of the brain in the metabolic characterization of neurological diseases. J Neurol Sci 1993; 118:123–133.
15. Kwong K, Chesler D, Zuo C, et al. Spin echo (T2, T1) studies for functional MRI (abstr). In: Proceedings of the 12th Annual Meeting of the Society of Magnetic Resonance in Medicine. Berkeley, Calif: Society of Magnetic Resonance in Medicine, 1993; 172.
16. Boxerman J, Hamberg L, Rosen B, Weisskoff R. MR contrast due to intravascular magnetic susceptibility perturbations. Magn Reson Med 1995; 34:555–566.
17. Bandettini PA, Wong EC, Jesmanowicz A, Hinks RS, Hyde JS. Spin-echo and gradient-echo EPI of human brain activation using BOLD contrast: a comparative study at 1.5T. NMR Biomed 1994; 7:12–20.
18. Chang SY, Talagala SL, Noll DC, Thulborn KR. Comparison of spin echo, asymmetric spin echo, and gradient echo echo-planar fMRI at 3.0 Tesla (abstr). In: Proceedings of the Fifth Annual Meeting of the International Society for Magnetic Resonance in Medicine. Berkeley, Calif: International Society for Magnetic Resonance in Medicine, 1997; 378.
19. Ernst T, Chang L, Itti L, Hsieh K. Elimination of large vessels improves reproducibility of perfusion MRI (abstr). In: Proceedings of the Fifth Annual Meeting of the International Society for Magnetic Resonance in Medicine. Berkeley, Calif: International Society for Magnetic Resonance in Medicine, 1997; 1791.
20. Kaissar G, Edwards M, Smith R. Neuroimaging of AIDS. Indiana Med 1991; 84:470–474.
21. Trenkwalder P, Trenkwalder C, Feiden W, Vogl T, Einhaupl KM, Lydtin H. Toxoplasmosis with early intracerebral hemorrhage in a patient with the acquired immunodeficiency syndrome. Neurology 1992; 42:436–438.
22. Dina T. Primary central nervous system lymphoma versus toxoplasmosis in AIDS. Radiology 1991; 179:823–828.
23. Rosenberg N, Hochberg F, Miller G, Kleinschimdt-DeMasters B. Primary central nervous system lymphoma related to Epstein-Barr virus in a patient with acquired immune deficiency syndrome. Ann Neurol 1986; 20:98–102.
24. Levine A. Acquired immunodeficiency syndrome–related lymphoma. Blood 1992; 80:8–20.
25. Bashir R, Luka J, Cheloha K, Chamberlain M, Hochberg F. Expression of Epstein-Barr virus proteins in primary CNS lymphoma in AIDS patients. Neurology 1993; 43: 2358–2362.
26. Ciricillo S, Rosenblum M. Use of CT and MR imaging to distinguish intracranial lesions and to define the need for biopsy in AIDS patients. J Neurosurg 1990; 73: 720–724.
27. Morgello S, Petito CK, Mouradian JA. Central nervous system lymphoma in the acquired immunodeficiency syndrome. Clin Neuropathol 1990; 9:205–215.
28. So Y, Beckstead J, Davis R. Primary central nervous system lymphoma in acquired immune deficiency syndrome: clinical and pathologic study. Ann Neurol 1986; 20:566–572.
29. Cordoliani Y, Derosier C, Pharaboz C, Jeanbourquin D, Schill H, Cosnard G. Primary cerebral lymphoma in patients with AIDS: MR findings in 17 cases. AJR 1992; 159:841–847.
30. Chiang F, Miller B, Chang L, McBride D, Cornford M, Mehringer CM. Fulminant cerebral lymphoma in AIDS. AJNR 1996; 17:157–160.
31. Levy RM, Mills CM, Posin JP, Moore SG, Rosenblum ML, Bredesen DE. The efficacy and clinical impact of brain imaging in neurologically symptomatic AIDS patients: a prospective CT/MRI study. J Acquir Immune Defic Syndr Hum Retrovirol 1990; 3:461–471.
32. Cornford M, Holden J, Boyd M, Berry K, Vinters H. Neuropathology of the acquired immune deficiency syndrome (AIDS): report of 39 autopsies from Vancouver, British Columbia. Can J Neurol Sci 1992; 19:442–452.

Photographs from Arizona and Utah

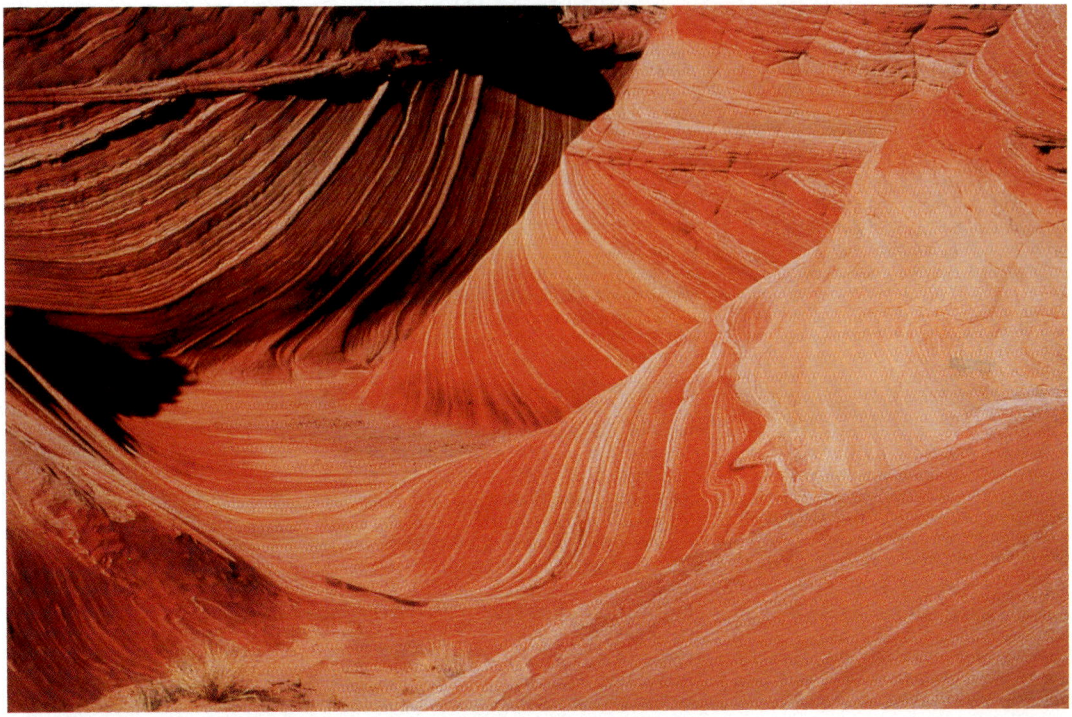

Sandstone Valley, Coyote Buttes area of northern Arizona

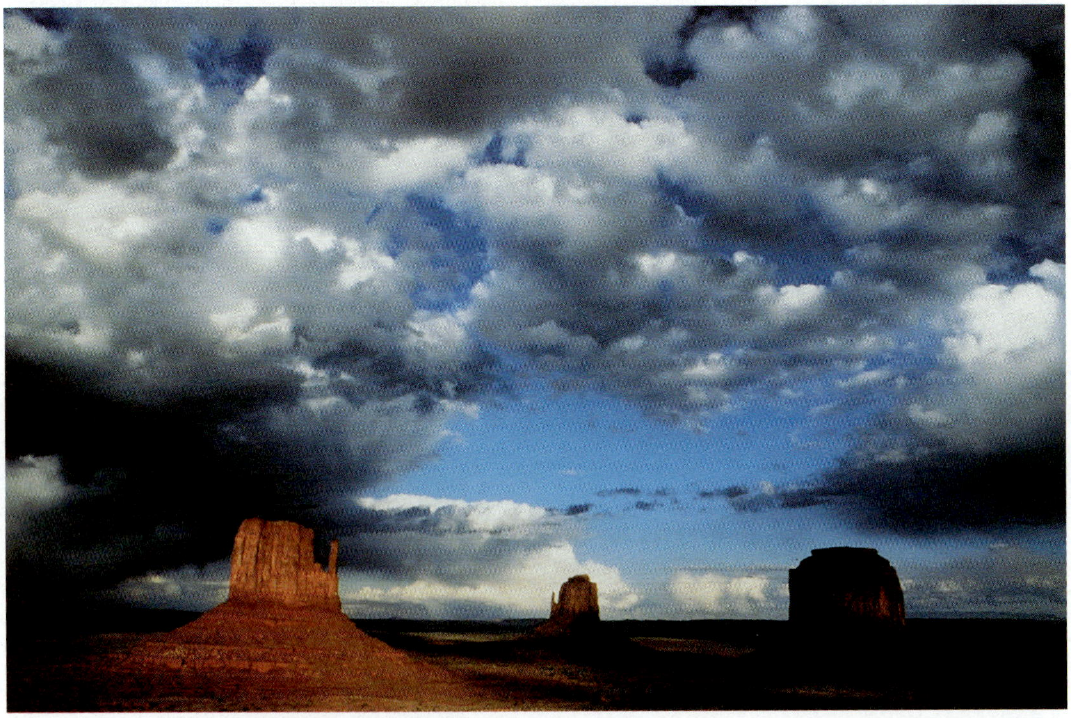

The Three Buttes, Monument Valley, Utah

Photographs by Cyril Mazansky, MD, Boston, Mass

Unselected Brain 0.5-T MR Imaging: Comparison of Lesion Detection and Characterization with Three T2-weighted Sequences[1]

Antoine J. Maubon, MD, PhD
Agnès Pothin, MD
Jean Michel Ferru, MD
Vincent M. Berger, MD
Jean Pierre Daurès, MD
Jean Pierre Rouanet, MD

Index terms:
Brain, abnormalities, 10.30, 10.43, 10.75, 10.78, 10.83, 10.871
Brain, MR, 10.12141
Magnetic resonance (MR), comparative studies, 10.121411, 10.121412, 10.121413, 10.121416
Magnetic resonance (MR), pulse sequences, 10.121411, 10.121412, 10.121413, 10.121416

Radiology 1998; 208:671–678

Abbreviations:
CNR = contrast-to-noise ratio
CSF = cerebrospinal fluid
EPI = echo-planar imaging
FLAIR = fluid-attenuated inversion recovery
GRASE = gradient and spin echo
ROI = region of interest
SE = spin echo

[1] From the Department of Medical Imaging, Centre Medico Chirurgical Beausoleil, 119 Ave de Lodeve, Montpellier, France (A.J.M., A.P., J.M.F., V.M.B., J.P.R.), and the Department of Medical Information, Centre Hospitaliea Universitaire, Montpellier, France (J.P.D.). Received September 30, 1997; revision requested December 15; revision received March 30, 1998; accepted April 28. **Address reprint requests to** A.J.M.

Author contributions:
Guarantor of integrity of entire study, A.J.M.; study concepts, A.J.M., A.P., V.M.B.; study design, A.J.M., A.P., J.M.F., J.P.D.; definition of intellectual content, A.J.M., J.P.R.; literature research, A.P., A.J.M.; clinical studies, A.J.M., A.P., J.M.F.; data acquisition, A.P.; data analysis, A.J.M., A.P., J.P.D.; statistical analysis, A.J.M., A.P., J.P.D.; manuscript preparation, A.J.M.; manuscript editing, A.J.M., A.P.; manuscript review, A.J.M., J.M.F., V.M.B.

PURPOSE: To compare the diagnostic values of three T2-weighted sequences in unselected brain 0.5-T magnetic resonance (MR) imaging examinations.

MATERIALS AND METHODS: MR imaging was performed in 102 patients because of neurologic symptoms or to follow up "previously known disease." The protocol comprised three T2-weighted sequences: turbo spin-echo (SE), turbo fluid-attenuated inversion-recovery (FLAIR), and gradient and SE (GRASE) sequences. In a prospective, blinded analysis, sequences were compared quantitatively and qualitatively by three independent readers for lesion detection and characterization.

RESULTS: Twenty-four patients had normal findings, and 78 had abnormal findings, with 121 final diagnoses. Quantitatively, the "white" cerebrospinal fluid (CSF) sequences, turbo SE and GRASE, had higher contrast-to-noise ratios (CNRs) than the "black" CSF sequence, FLAIR, with respect to the signal intensity of white matter, but lower CNRs than FLAIR with respect to the signal intensity of CSF. Qualitatively, for lesion detection, sensitivity and accuracy were significantly higher for FLAIR than for turbo SE or GRASE ($P < .05$); there was no statistically significant difference between turbo SE and GRASE. For lesion characterization, FLAIR was significantly superior to GRASE and turbo SE for white matter disease ($P < .05$), superior to only turbo SE ($P < .05$) for vascular disease, and not superior to GRASE or turbo SE for tumors.

CONCLUSION: The black CSF T2-weighted turbo FLAIR sequence is a useful adjunct to the usual white CSF T2-weighted sequences in unselected brain 0.5-T MR imaging.

T2-weighted sequences are very sensitive for lesion detection in brain magnetic resonance (MR) imaging (1); they are established as indispensable in brain MR imaging at most centers. Turbo spin-echo (SE) sequences have been shown to be as accurate as traditional SE sequences in a variety of diseases (2,3), with a substantial reduction in imaging times.

Since its introduction, the fluid-attenuated inversion-recovery (FLAIR) sequence, a T2-weighted sequence with a long echo time and a long repetition time but with cerebrospinal fluid (CSF) nulling, has shown promising results in brain and spinal disease (4,5), essentially through its high contrast resolution and decrease in the number of artifacts close to CSF. Nonetheless, it has been marred by long examination times, which are in excess of 15 minutes, according to an early report (6). Turbo FLAIR allows short imaging times, which are compatible with an active routine daily practice on a busy schedule, with preservation of high-contrast-resolution images. This sequence has now been tested in a variety of brain diseases and abnormalities—epilepsy (7), multiple sclerosis (8), cerebrovascular disease (9), and head injury (10)—at 1.5 T, but to our knowledge few articles on FLAIR at 0.5 T have been published (11,12).

Gradient and SE (GRASE) is a combination of turbo SE and echo-planar imaging (EPI); it is a fast imaging technique that allows heavily T2-weighted sequences (13). It has recently been tested in the brain (14), the liver (15), and the pelvis (16) but has not yet been fully evaluated in brain examinations at 0.5 T. Its rapid imaging time allows the use of a large matrix within clinically acceptable imaging times (17).

Our goal was to compare, in routine unselected brain MR imaging examinations, the diagnostic values of two recently available T2-weighted fast imaging sequences, FLAIR with black CSF and GRASE with white CSF, that are not yet fully validated, especially at 0.5 T, with the diagnostic value of the established T2-weighted turbo SE sequence. To our knowledge, a prospective comparison between these three sequences has not been published before.

TABLE 1
Difference in Signal Intensity between Lesions and White Matter or CSF and CNRs for White Matter and CSF

Parameter	Turbo SE	FLAIR	GRASE
Lesion contrast to white matter	1.32 ± 0.68	0.84 ± 0.80	1.98 ± 1.04
Lesion contrast to CSF	−0.15 ± 0.20	9.49 ± 6.20	−0.25 ± 0.20
CNR with respect to white matter	16.16 ± 8.30	8.45 ± 7.30	13.18 ± 6.80
CNR with respect to CSF	−5.68 ± 5.50	16.39 ± 8.69	−6.82 ± 6.20

Note.—Values are the mean ± standard error. $P < .001$ (Friedman test) for all comparisons.

TABLE 2
Lesion Detection by Three Reviewers

Statistic	Turbo SE	FLAIR	GRASE
Sensitivity (%)	88 (68 of 77)	92 (71 of 77)	86 (66 of 77)
Specificity (%)	100 (24 of 24)	100 (24 of 24)	100 (24 of 24)
Accuracy (%)	91 (92 of 101)	94 (95 of 101)	89 (90 of 101)

MATERIALS AND METHODS

Patients

Within 3 months (March to May 1996), 102 consecutive patients (61 male, 41 female; average age, 54.6 years ± 18.8; age range, 14–90 years) were examined.

Patients were outpatients referred by general practitioners or inpatients referred from the internal medicine, neurology, or surgery departments.

Indications for imaging were neurologic symptoms (transient ischemic attack [n = 3], ischemic stroke [n = 28], epilepsy [n = 12], headache [n = 6], miscellaneous neurologic symptoms [n = 32, including visual disorders, myoclonia, dizziness, walking disorders, and pyramidal or extrapyramidal syndrome], or confusion [n = 6]) or follow-up of previously known disease (brain tumor [n = 7], multiple sclerosis [n = 3], or arteriovenous malformation [n = 5]).

MR Imaging Examinations

All patients underwent a brain MR imaging examination performed with a commercially available standard 0.5-T superconducting magnet with a fast imaging pack (Gyroscan T5 NT; Philips, Best, The Netherlands) and a dedicated head coil.

In all cases, examination comprised one initial sagittal T1-weighted turbo SE sequence (433/15 [repetition time msec/echo time msec], 16 sections, 6-mm thickness with a 1-mm intersection gap, 256 × 180 matrix, 230-mm field of view, two signals acquired, 2 minute 36 second imaging time) and three T2-weighted axial sequences in the neuro-ocular plane.

The first sequence was a turbo SE sequence (3,000/120, 20 sections, 6-mm thickness with 0.6-mm intersection gap, 256 × 256 matrix, 240-mm field of view, three signals acquired, turbo factor of 19, 3 minute 18 second imaging time).

The second sequence was a turbo FLAIR sequence (8,000/130/2,000 [repetition time msec/echo time msec/inversion time msec], 20 sections, 6-mm thickness with 1.2-mm intersection gap, 256 × 230 matrix, 230-mm field of view, four signals acquired, turbo factor of 20, 5 minute 4 second imaging time). The high turbo factor (echo train length) reduces the acquisition time, thus allowing the use of a long repetition time for strong T2 weighting while retaining a sequence duration close to 5 minutes. Acquisition is interleaved, meaning that all the sections are excited once within a repetition time. The intersection gap, however, must be set at 20% of the section thickness to avoid signal intensity variations from section to section.

The third sequence was a GRASE sequence (5,263/130, 20 sections, 6-mm thickness with 0.6-mm intersection gap, 256 × 512 matrix, 240-mm field of view, five signals acquired, turbo factor of 19, EPI factor of three, 4 minute 7 second imaging time). After a single excitation, the number of profiles acquired is the turbo factor multiplied by the EPI factor, where the turbo factor is the number of 180° refocusing pulses and the EPI factor is the number of gradient alternations between refocusing pulses. Within the constraints of a 130-msec echo time and 4-minute imaging time, this sequence allows acquisition with a large (512 × 256) matrix.

When it was thought to be necessary for diagnosis, additional sequences were performed according to presentation: T1-weighted imaging, T2-weighted imaging, or both, in other imaging planes; gadolinium-enhanced T1-weighted imaging; and MR angiography. After the examination, a report was sent to the referring physician. This study received approval by our institutional review board, and patients gave written informed consent with regard to sequences performed in addition to our routine examination.

Image Analysis

Quantitative analysis.—On each image, automated measurements were made with an electronic cursor on a remote console (Easyvision, release 4.3; Philips).

Regions of interest (ROIs) of at least 50 pixels were chosen within lesions bigger than 0.5 cm (patients with smaller lesions were not included in this quantitative analysis). Measurements were made within normal white matter, within CSF, and laterally to the skull along the phase-encoding direction (right to left). ROIs in the same patient were of the same size in each structure.

We recorded the mean signal intensity of the ROIs within zones that were as homogeneous as possible, with an SD of signal intensity not higher than 60.

To be measured, lesions had to be seen in the same location with all three sequences. If a patient had more than one lesion, only the signal intensity of the biggest one was measured.

Owing to the low signal intensity of CSF at FLAIR (unlike the CSF signal intensity at the two other sequences), we measured contrast with respect to white matter and to CSF. (*a*) The lesion contrast–to–white matter ratio was as follows: $(S_L - S_W)/S_W$, where S_L is the signal inten-

TABLE 3
Percentages of Each Confidence Level When Reviewers Recognized a Normal Study

Pulse Sequence	Confidence Level 1	2	3
Turbo SE	12 (3 of 24)	58 (14 of 24)	29 (7 of 24)
FLAIR	0 (0 of 24)	12 (3 of 24)	88 (21 of 24)*
GRASE	8 (2 of 24)	46 (11 of 24)	46 (11 of 24)

* Statistically significant.

TABLE 4
Percentages of Each Confidence Level When Reviewers Recognized an Abnormality

Pulse Sequence	Confidence Level 1	2	3
Turbo SE	27 (21 of 77)	54 (41 of 77)	19 (15 of 77)
FLAIR	15 (12 of 77)	46 (35 of 77)	39 (30 of 77)
GRASE	19 (15 of 77)	56 (43 of 77)	25 (19 of 77)

Note.—None was statistically significant.

sity of the lesion and S_W is the signal intensity of the normal white matter. (*b*) The lesion contrast-to-CSF ratio was as follows: $(S_L - S_{CSF})/S_{CSF}$, where S_{CSF} is the signal intensity of the CSF. (*c*) The contrast-to-noise ratio (CNR) with respect to white matter was as follows: $(S_L - S_W)/S_N$, where S_N is the signal intensity of the noise. (*d*) The CNR with respect to the CSF was as follows: $(S_L - S_{CSF})/S_N$.

Qualitative analysis.—Six months after completion of the last examination, all images were reviewed. One examination was excluded owing to extreme patient motion, which made images obtained with all sequences nondiagnostic. The remaining 101 sets of images obtained with each of the three T2-weighted sequences were separated from all other sequences and then randomized.

Analysis was performed by three independent blinded readers (A.J.M., A.P., J.M.F.) unaware of the patient's status or of any clinical or biologic background information. Owing to obvious differences in the characteristic features of the sequences, readers were not blinded to the sequence used to obtain the image they were interpreting; the patient's birth date was also available. Sets of images obtained with each sequence were evaluated independently in random order, one at a time.

After preliminary study findings showed the absence of a statistically significant interobserver difference between the three readers, it was decided that each reader would study one sequence for each patient, so that each patient would have three readers (one for each sequence) and that each reader would read an equivalent number of images obtained with each sequence. After randomization, reader A studied 35 turbo SE sets, 32 FLAIR sets, and 34 GRASE sets of images; reader B, 31 turbo SE sets, 37 FLAIR sets, and 33 GRASE sets of images; and reader C, 35 turbo SE sets, 32 FLAIR sets, and 34 GRASE sets of images.

Lesion Detection

Because our patients were not selected for each sequence, the reader first had to classify the image as normal (absence of an intracerebral lesion) or abnormal (presence of at least one intracerebral lesion) with a three-point scale of confidence with regard to lesion detection: 1, not confident; 2, fairly confident; 3, very confident.

Lesion Characterization

If the examination findings were considered abnormal, the examination had to be classified as one of four predefined categories that corresponded to the most common abnormalities in our practice: vascular disease, tumoral disease, white matter disease, or atrophy. More than one diagnosis was possible in the same patient.

When possible, within these categories, the reader had to specify the size, number, location, and signal intensity of the lesions and the vascular abnormality (eg, hemorrhage, ischemia) and estimate the date of the vascular accident.

In addition, each patient's MR images were reevaluated by the three readers by means of consensus, with all the sequences and all relevant information available (MR imaging report at the time of examination, clinical examination findings and findings of subsequent consultations, biologic data, surgical results, histopathologic report (if any), telephone follow-up findings) to establish the MR imaging diagnosis to which the individual blinded interpretations would be compared.

Also, during this session, after establishing the MR imaging diagnosis, the readers rated the three sequences in rank order with regard to the ease of attaining the diagnosis retrospectively (1, the worst; 3, the best).

Statistical Analysis

Our goal was to compare the FLAIR and GRASE sequences with the turbo SE sequence, which was considered the standard. The null hypothesis was that the three sequences would be equivalent, with an α risk of 5%.

Quantitative analysis.—Differences in lesion contrast and CNR were compared by means of the Friedman test.

Qualitative analysis.—Characteristics of the readings were assessed with a κ correlation test to compare blinded and consensus readings. For lesion detection, we calculated the specificity, sensitivity, and accuracy of each sequence and compared them by means of the McNemar paired test. Differences in confidence levels were assessed by means of a χ^2 test. For lesion characterization, we compared (*a*) the mean confidence level of the various abnormal and normal findings for each of the three sequences by means of the nonparametric Kruskal-Wallis test and (*b*) the mean confidence level of each sequence for the same abnormality by means of the nonparametric Friedman test. When a difference was significant, we tried to determine the origin of this difference by pairing the results for each abnormality or each sequence. Image ranking data were compared by means of the nonparametric Friedman test.

RESULTS

Patient Studies

Of the 101 examinations included in the study, 24 had normal findings and 77 had abnormal findings, with 121 final diagnoses: 24 normal findings, 11 tumors (five benign tumors [all were meningiomas], six malignant tumors [four gliomas, one papilloma of the choroid plexus, one metastasis from mediastinal thymoma]), 37 vascular abnormalities (nine small vessel ischemia or infarction cases, 11 recent infarction cases, six late infarction cases, three hemorrhages, one subarachnoid hemorrhage, six vascular malformations, one chronic subdural hematoma), and 43 white matter disease cases (10 multiple sclerosis cases, 24 cases of leukopathy of vascular origin, two hydrocephaly cases, one metachromatic leukodystrophy case, six miscellaneous cases), six atrophy cases (three corticosubcortical cases, one hemiatrophy case, two postoperative cases).

TABLE 5
Number of Patients with Each Confidence Level in the Diagnosis of Vascular Disease, White Matter Disease, and Tumor

Pulse Sequence	Vascular Disease (n = 37) 1	2	3	White Matter Disease (n = 43) 1	2	3	Tumor (n = 11) 1	2	3
Turbo SE	17	19	1	25	17	1	5	5	1
FLAIR	11	4	22	0	3	40	4	3	4
GRASE	14	15	8	11	31	1	4	5	2

Note.—n = 91.

TABLE 6
Mean Confidence Level for Each Pulse Sequence and Each Diagnosis

Pulse Sequence	Vascular Disease	White Matter Disease	Tumor	Normal	P Value*
Turbo SE	1.568	1.442	1.638	1.917	.062
FLAIR	2.297	2.930	2.000	2.417	<.001
GRASE	1.838	1.767	1.818	2.292	.026
P value†	.016	<.001	.695	.067	. . .

* Kruskal-Wallis test.
† Friedman test.

Quantitative Analysis

The lesion contrast to white matter, lesion contrast to CSF, CNR with respect to white matter, and CNR with respect to CSF for each sequence are shown in Table 1.

Relative to the white matter signal intensity on the turbo SE images, the signal intensity of the lesions increased by an average of 150% on GRASE images and decreased by an average of 64% on FLAIR images. This difference in mean signal intensity was statistically significant between GRASE and FLAIR ($P < .05$), between GRASE and turbo SE ($P < .05$), and between turbo SE and FLAIR ($P < .05$, Friedman paired test). The CNR decreased by an average of 19% in GRASE and 48% in FLAIR. Differences in CNR were significant ($P < .05$, Friedman paired test) between turbo SE and FLAIR and between GRASE and FLAIR but not between turbo SE and GRASE.

Relative to the CSF signal intensity on the turbo SE images, the signal intensity of the lesions increased more than 10-fold on FLAIR images and decreased by an average of 60% on GRASE images. The difference was statistically significant ($P < .05$, Friedman paired test) between FLAIR and turbo SE, FLAIR and GRASE, and turbo SE and GRASE. The CNR increased by an average 280% in FLAIR and decreased by an average of 17% in GRASE. Differences in CNR were significant ($P < .05$, Friedman paired test) between FLAIR and turbo SE and between FLAIR and GRASE but not between turbo SE and GRASE.

Qualitative Analysis

To assess characteristics of the readings, we performed a κ correlation test between individual readings and the final diagnoses. A κ value higher than 0.4 indicates good agreement, and a value higher than 0.75 indicates very good agreement. The κ values were 0.761 ± 0.14, 0.847 ± 0.12, and 0.736 ± 0.14 for turbo SE, FLAIR, and GRASE, respectively. This indicates a very high correlation between the readings, no matter which sequence is considered, without significant differences in κ values between the three sequences ($P > .05$, χ^2 test).

TABLE 7
Results of Rank Order Analysis of Lesion Detection

Pulse Sequence	Lesion Detection Score: Median	Mean ± SD
Turbo SE	2	1.595 ± 0.59
FLAIR	3	2.553 ± 0.72
GRASE	2	1.909 ± 0.64

Note.—1 = worst, 2 = medium, 3 = best. N = 101. $P < .001$ for all scores (Friedman paired test).

Sequence Comparison for Lesion Detection

Sensitivities, specificities, and accuracies for lesion detection are given in Table 2. Differences in sensitivity and accuracy were statistically significant between FLAIR and turbo SE ($P < .05$, McNemar paired test) and between FLAIR and GRASE ($P < .05$) but not between GRASE and turbo SE.

Specificity was 100% for all three sequences: When examination findings were normal (absence of disease), they were in all cases confirmed by means of consensus reevaluation. Moreover, when findings of an examination were normal, confidence levels were significantly higher with the FLAIR sequence (Table 3) ($P < .001$ in favor of FLAIR versus turbo SE and GRASE, $P > .05$ in GRASE versus turbo SE, χ^2 test). When an abnormal diagnosis was made, there was also a tendency toward higher confidence levels with the FLAIR sequence, but without a significant difference ($P > .05$, χ^2 test) between sequences (Table 4).

Sequence Comparison for Lesion Characterization

We considered only the diagnoses of vascular abnormality (n = 37), white matter disease (n = 43), and tumor (n = 11), because the population of the subgroup *atrophy* was too small for analysis (n = 6).

The numbers of patients with each confidence level in lesion characterization for each of the three sequences are

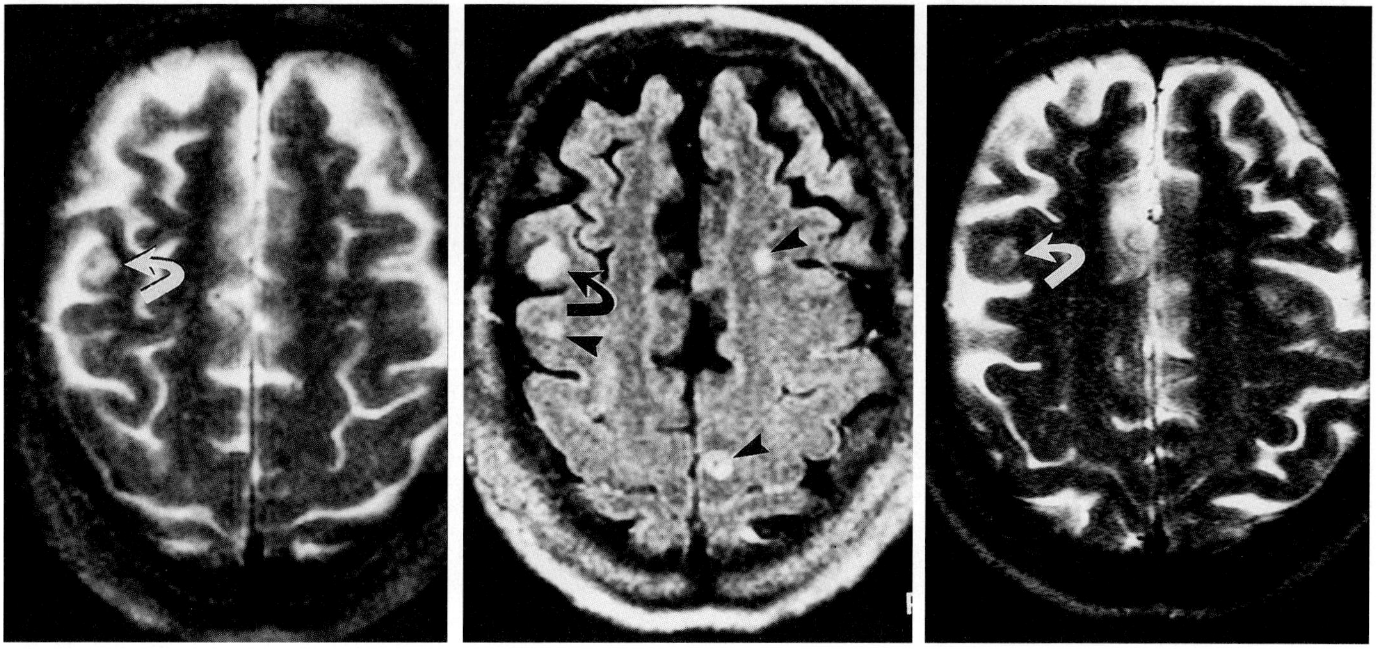

a. b. c.

Figure 1. Brain metastases of mediastinal thymoma in a 59-year-old woman. **(a)** Turbo SE image (3,000/120) shows a right frontal lesion (arrow). **(b)** FLAIR image (8,000/130/2,000) shows the right frontal lobe lesion (arrow) and three additional lesions (arrowheads). **(c)** GRASE image (5,263/130) shows only the right frontal lobe lesion (arrow). The three additional lesions were missed at the interpretation of turbo SE and GRASE images.

given in Table 5. For very confident diagnosis of vascular and white matter disease, we found significantly higher confidence levels in favor of the FLAIR sequence versus the other two sequences ($P < .025$ for vascular disease, $P < .014$ for white matter disease, χ^2 test). No significant difference was found between the three sequences for tumoral characterization.

Table 6 shows the mean confidence level for each of the three sequences and each diagnosis. A comparison of mean confidence levels with the turbo SE sequence for the various diagnoses showed no significant difference between abnormalities. The difference was significant in FLAIR ($P < .05$) between the confidence levels for white matter disease and all the other diagnoses and in GRASE between the confidence levels for white matter disease and normal findings only ($P < .05$).

When we compared mean confidence levels for one abnormality, the difference was statistically significant between FLAIR and the two other sequences ($P < .05$) for white matter disease, with no difference between GRASE and turbo SE. For vascular disease, the only difference was between FLAIR and turbo SE ($P < .05$), with no difference between FLAIR and GRASE or between GRASE and turbo SE. For findings of tumor and for normal findings, we found no statistically significant difference between sequences, but there was a tendency for FLAIR to be superior to GRASE and for GRASE to be superior to turbo SE.

So, globally, the FLAIR sequence had higher confidence levels for all diagnoses, with a significant difference over the other sequences for the diagnosis of white matter disease and vascular disease.

This was confirmed by means of the rank test established after the consensus reading (Table 7). For the 121 diagnoses, the readers preferred the FLAIR sequence for 84 diagnoses (69%), the GRASE sequence for 19 diagnoses (16%), and the turbo SE sequence for seven diagnoses (6%); confidence levels were even for 11 diagnoses (9%). Differences in rank means are significant between FLAIR and GRASE, between FLAIR and turbo SE, and between GRASE and turbo SE ($P < .05$, Friedman paired test).

DISCUSSION

Brain MR imaging is probably the most commonly performed MR imaging examination (18); thus, the question of the best possible sequence is of great importance. T2-weighted sequences are indispensable in brain MR imaging; they are very informative owing to their high contrast resolution (19). With the advent of every new fast imaging technique or sequence, the question is always to assess its value against that of established techniques. So far, turbo SE is the established T2-weighted sequence in brain MR imaging against which most comparative studies are performed (20,21). We wanted to compare the more established T2-weighted turbo SE sequence with two newly implemented T2-weighted fast imaging sequences. Specifically, one with "white" CSF, as in turbo SE and GRASE, and one with "black" CSF, as in FLAIR.

GRASE allows a thorough decrease in imaging times or, and this was our choice, a bigger matrix to be used with a comparable imaging time (17) to increase spatial resolution (voxel size was 5.23 mm^3 for turbo SE, 5.48 mm^3 for FLAIR, and 2.86 mm^3 for GRASE). The contrast in T2-weighted GRASE is similar to that in turbo SE, although the fat signal intensity is lower owing to the longer radio-frequency pulse interval. Another advantage is that the longer times between the radio-frequency pulses lead to a reduction in radio-frequency power in the patient relative to the power in turbo SE. Furthermore, blood flowing through intracranial arterial vessels has consistently uniform low signal intensity, allowing an approach of "black blood" MR angiography. Possible disadvantages of GRASE are

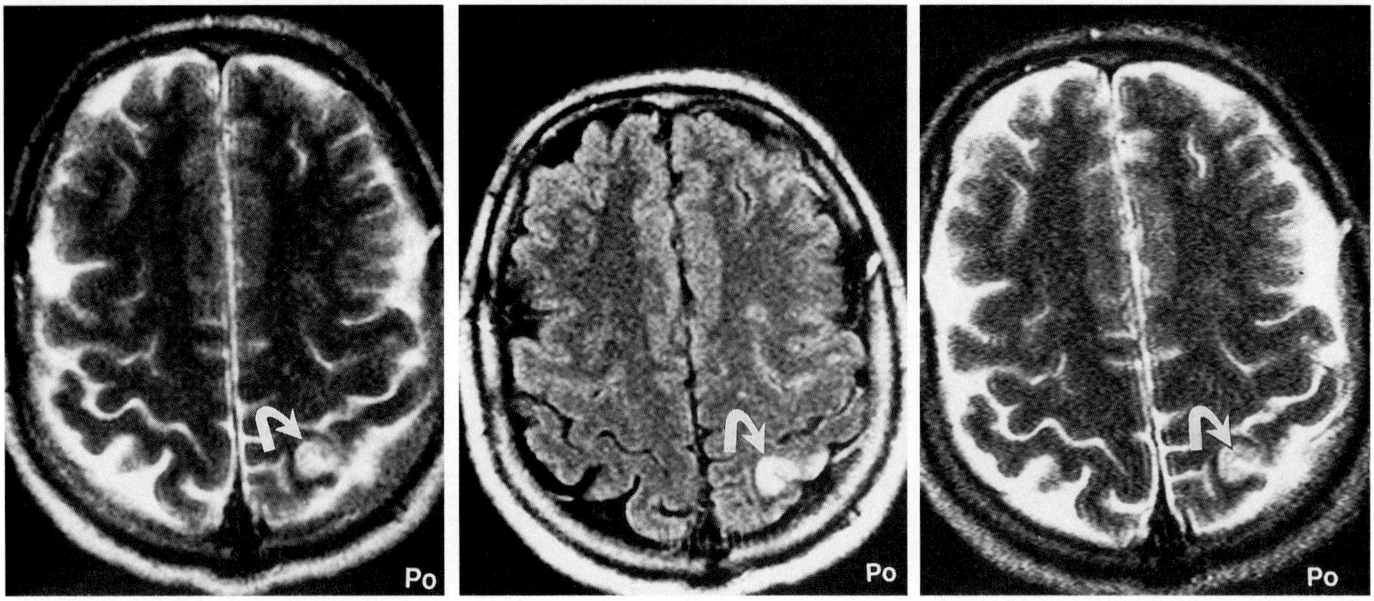

a. b. c.

Figure 2. MR images obtained in a 57-year old man with a partial, right-sided, hypoesthesia show a cortical infarction in the left parietal lobe. **(a)** Turbo SE (3,000/120), **(b)** FLAIR (8,000/130/2,000), and **(c)** GRASE (5,263/130) images. At interpretation, the vascular lesion (arrow) was missed in **a**, confidently described in **b** (confidence level 3), and described with less confidence in **c** (confidence level 1).

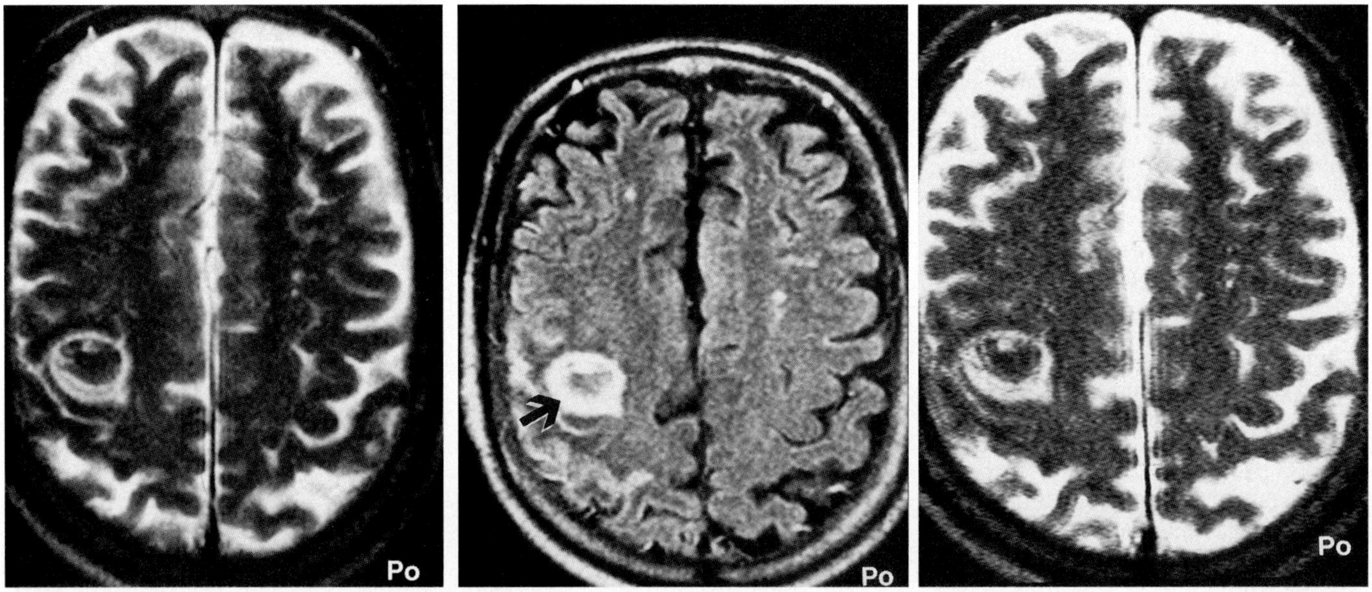

a. b. c.

Figure 3. MR images obtained 24 hours after the onset of clinical symptoms of an acute hematoma in the right frontal lobe in a 74-year-old man. **(a)** Turbo SE (3,000/120), **(b)** FLAIR (8,000/130/2,000), and **(c)** GRASE (5,263/130) images. Images obtained with all three sequences show the hematoma equally well, but only **b** shows high signal intensity (arrow) in the adjacent central fissure, indicating subarachnoid hemorrhage.

its greater sensitivity to susceptibility artifacts, which appear as blurring in the mildest cases, and a greater water-fat shift, which can be reduced by means of the spectral saturation of fat. These effects are, however, less pronounced than those in EPI (15).

Originally, FLAIR sequences were more than 10 minutes long (22) and were not compatible with a busy daily schedule. Interleaved turbo FLAIR allows a consistent shortening of imaging times but requires a 20% intersection gap; this is a potential pitfall. Nonetheless, it can be overcome by increasing the number of packages at the price of an increase in the imaging time (with our unit, it doubles the imaging time for this sequence, as only half the profiles would be acquired during one repetition time). Technically, recent study findings (23) demonstrated the superiority of the fast SE technique we have used over the multishot echo-planar technique for FLAIR imaging.

Unlike in previous studies (9,24–26), we did not perform a disease-oriented study but instead opted to study consecutive, unselected patients; thus, our patients are not homogeneous but have a variety of diseases. Our goal was simply to try to find which of these sequences was, or were, the most useful for a daily practice in which, in most cases, the MR imaging specialist does not a priori know what his or her patient has. So, the readers first had to assess the value of the sequences for gross lesion detection (ie, normal or abnormal findings) and then had to try to characterize which category of disease the case fit in. Difficulty was great for the readers who did not know which disease they were dealing with, if any. They also had only one sequence to use to come to a diagnosis, which is a major difference from everyday practice, in which reports are dictated with findings from all sequences of the examination. Nonetheless, although somehow artificial, interpretation of images obtained with one sequence at a time and not of a set of sequences was needed to stress the differences between sequences more.

Moreover, the consensus reevaluation and the rank test were performed for all sequences, including the T1-weighted sequence, and the high κ values show a very good correlation between the individual and consensus readings. This indicates that the fact that each reader interpreted images obtained with only one sequence in any given patient had no statistically significant effect on the final result. That could have been a strong bias.

We studied fast SE sequences only; they have a higher noise level than do conventional SE sequences (3,27), which is due to the echo train length (19 for turbo SE and GRASE, 20 for FLAIR), but the average noise was not significantly different for our three fast imaging sequences.

Quantitatively, the FLAIR sequence had lower lesion contrast and lower CNR relative to white matter than did the white CSF sequences but a much higher contrast and CNR relative to CSF. Moreover, the signal intensity of CSF was, on average, higher than that of the lesions (whatever their nature) in turbo SE and GRASE—it can be one of the explanations for the lesser conspicuity of lesions with these sequences compared with the conspicuity with FLAIR in this study. This result was expected owing to CSF nulling. These differences in contrast are especially beneficial for lesions close to CSF that appear bright next to the dark CSF and can be missed on bright CSF sequences (Figs 1, 2). The lower signal-to-noise ratio in the GRASE sequence can be explained, in part, by the smaller voxel size due to the higher matrix.

The nulling of the fluid signal in the FLAIR sequence brings about an advantage in addition to the higher conspicuity of white matter lesions, especially those close to the ventricles. The nulling of the highest signal (fluids) improves the apparent contrast between white matter, gray matter, and lesions because of a better use of the dynamics (highest signal intensity minus lowest signal intensity) during the acquisition.

Globally, sensitivity and accuracy were higher in FLAIR than in both white CSF T2-weighted sequences, with significantly higher confidence levels. These good results were obtained mainly in the white matter and vascular (Fig 3) disease categories. Conspicuity was greater in FLAIR for subcortical tumoral lesions, but the difference was not statistically significant among the three sequences in the tumoral category, a point that had already been noted (28), but in a relatively small number of patients.

The retrospective rank test confirmed the statistical superiority of FLAIR over GRASE and turbo SE and of GRASE over turbo SE, although the latter was less pronounced (29).

In our opinion, given the results of this study, it is of value to associate a black CSF T2-weighted sequence with the usual white CSF T2-weighted sequences in routine unselected brain MR imaging. It adds less than 5 minutes to the examination and improves diagnostic value and the confidence levels of the readers. When available on machines, a fast FLAIR sequence could be added to the usual T2-weighted sequences used in each center. The value of the fast FLAIR sequence as the only T2-weighted sequence in an examination will require further evaluation.

As a white CSF T2-weighted sequence, GRASE appeared slightly superior to turbo SE, probably owing to higher spatial resolution.

References

1. Brandt-Zawadzki M. MR imaging of the brain. Radiology 1988; 166:1–10.
2. Norbash AM, Glover GH, Enzmann DR. Intracerebral lesion contrast with spin-echo and fast spin-echo pulse sequences. Radiology 1992; 185:661–665.
3. Prenger EC, Beckett WW, Kollias SS, Ball WS. Comparison of T2-weighted spin-echo and fast spin-echo technique in the evaluation of myelination. JMRI 1994; 4:179–184.
4. Hajnal JV, De Coene B, Lewis PD, et al. High signal regions in white matter shown by heavily T2-weighted CSF nulled IR sequences. J Comput Assist Tomogr 1992; 16:506–513.
5. Rydberg JN, Hammond CA, Grimm RC, et al. Initial clinical experience in MR imaging with a fast fluid-attenuated inversion recovery pulse sequence. Radiology 1994; 193:173–180.
6. Noguchi K, Ogawa T, Inugami A, et al. MR of acute subarachnoid hemorrhage: a preliminary report of fluid-attenuated inversion recovery pulse sequence. AJNR 1994; 15:1940–1943.
7. Bergin PS, Fish DR, Shorvon SD, et al. Magnetic resonance imaging in partial epilepsy: additional abnormalities shown with the fluid attenuated inversion recovery (FLAIR) pulse sequence. J Neurol Neurosurg Psychiatr 1995; 58:439–443.
8. Hashemi RH, Bradley WG, Chen DY, et al. Suspected multiple sclerosis: MR imaging with a thin-section fast FLAIR pulse sequence. Radiology 1995; 196:505–510.
9. Alexander JA, Sheppard S, Davis PC, Salverda P. Adult cerebrovascular disease: role of modified rapid fluid-attenuated inversion-recovery sequences. AJNR 1996; 17:1507–1513.
10. Ashikaga R, Araki Y, Ishida O. MRI of head injury using FLAIR. Neuroradiology 1997; 39:239–242.
11. Von Keller E, Gieseke J, Kossack D, et al. Wertigkeit der Turbo-FLAIR-Sequenz in der diagnostik zerebraler bei 0.5 Tesla. ROFO 1995; 163:497–504.
12. Noguchi K, Ogawa T, Seto HS, et al. Subacute and chronic subarachnoid hemorrhage: diagnosis with fluid-attenuated inversion recovery MR imaging. Radiology 1997; 203:257–262.
13. Oshio K, Feinberg DA. GRASE (gradient- and spin-echo) imaging: a novel fast MRI technique. Magn Reson Med 1991; 20: 344–349.
14. Fellner F, Schmitt R, Trenkler J, Fellner C, Bohm-Jurkovic H. Turbo gradient-spin-echo (GRASE): first clinical experiences with a fast T2-weighted sequence in MRI of the brain. Eur J Radiol 1995; 19:171–176.
15. Jung G, Krahe T, Kugel H, et al. Prospective comparison of fast SE and GRASE sequences and echo planar imaging with conventional SE sequences in the detection of focal liver lesions at 1.0T. J Comput Assist Tomogr 1997; 21:341–347.
16. Fellner F, Held P, Fellner C, Schmitt R, Obletter N. Fast spin-echo (FSE) and gradient- and spin-echo (GRASE) in fast MRI of the pelvis. Magn Reson Imaging 1997; 15:517–524.
17. Feinberg DA, Kiefer B, Litt AW. High resolution GRASE MRI of the brain and spine: 512 and 1024 matrix imaging. J Comput Assist Tomogr 1995; 19:1–7.
18. Hisashige A. MR imaging in Japan and the United States: analysis of utilization and economics. AJR 1994; 162:507–510.
19. Brandt-Zawadzki M, Norman D, Newton TH, et al. Magnetic resonance of the brain: the optimal screening technique. Radiology 1984; 152:71–77.
20. Stevenson VL, Gawne-Cain ML, Barker GJ, Thompson AJ, Miller DH. Imaging of the spinal cord and brain in multiple sclerosis: a comparative study between fast FLAIR and fast spin echo. J Neurol 1997; 244:119–124.
21. Wieshmann UC, Free SL, Everitt AD, et al. Magnetic resonance imaging in epilepsy with a fast FLAIR sequence. J Neurol Neurosurg Psychiatr 1996; 61:357–361.

22. De Coene B, Hajnal JV, Gatehouse P, et al. MR of the brain using fluid-attenuated inversion recovery (FLAIR) pulse sequences. AJNR 1992; 13:1555–1564.
23. Sargent MA, Poskitt KJ. Fast fluid-attenuated inversion recovery (FLAIR) magnetic resonance imaging of the brain: a comparison of multi-shot echo-planar and fast spin-echo techniques. Pediatr Radiol 1997; 27:545–549.
24. Noguchi K, Ogawa T, Inugami A, et al. Acute subarachnoid hemorrhage: MR imaging with fluid-attenuated inversion recovery pulse sequences. Radiology 1995; 196:773–777.
25. Jack CR, Rydberg CH, Krecke KN, et al. Mesial temporal sclerosis: diagnosis with fluid-attenuated inversion recovery versus spin-echo imaging. Radiology 1996; 199:367–373.
26. Taoka T, Iwasaki S, Nakagawa H, et al. Fast fluid-attenuated inversion recovery (FAST-FLAIR) of ischemic lesions in the brain: comparison with T2-weighted turbo SE. Radiat Med 1996; 14:127-131.
27. Jones KM, Mulkern RV, Schwartz RB, et al. Fast spin-echo MR imaging of the brain and spine: current concepts. AJR 1992; 158:1313–1320.
28. Zheng J, Mayr NA, Yuh WT, Maeda M, Quets JP, Erhardt JC. Efficacy of FLAIR and STIR-FLAIR in the evaluation of brain glioma (abstr). Radiology 1996; 201(P):279.
29. Patel MR, Klufas RA, Shapiro AW. MR imaging of diseases of the brain: comparison of GRASE and conventional spin-echo T2-weighted pulse sequences. AJR 1995; 165:963–966.

Shinji Naganawa, MD
Tokiko Ito, MD
Hiroshi Fukatsu, MD
Takeo Ishigaki, MD
Tsutomu Nakashima, MD
Nobuyasu Ichinose, MS
Yukimori Kassai MS
Mitsue Miyazaki, PhD

Index terms:
Ear, abnormalities, 125.1419
Ear, anatomy, 125.92
Ear, MR, 125.121412
Nerves, abnormalities, 125.1419, 125.3641
Schwannoma, 125.3641

Radiology 1998; 208:679–685

Abbreviations:
SE = spin echo
SPGR = spoiled gradient-recalled
3D = three-dimensional

[1] From the Departments of Radiology (S.N., T. Ito, H.F., T. Ishigaki) and Otolaryngology (T.N.), Nagoya University School of Medicine, 65 Tsurumai, Shouwa-ku, Nagoya 466, Japan, and Toshiba, Tokyo, Japan (N.I., Y.K., M.M.). From the 1997 RSNA scientific assembly. Received November 28, 1997; revision requested February 17, 1998; revision received March 9; accepted April 17. **Address reprint requests to** S.N.

MR Imaging of the Inner Ear: Comparison of a Three-dimensional Fast Spin-Echo Sequence with Use of a Dedicated Quadrature-Surface Coil with a Gadolinium-enhanced Spoiled Gradient-recalled Sequence[1]

PURPOSE: To prospectively evaluate the sensitivity and specificity of magnetic resonance (MR) imaging in the inner ear with a long echo train, three-dimensional (3D), asymmetric Fourier-transform, fast spin-echo (SE) sequence with use of a dedicated quadrature-surface phased-array coil to detect vestibular schwannoma in the cerebellopontine angle and the internal auditory canal.

MATERIALS AND METHODS: In 205 patients (410 ears) with ear symptoms, 1.5-T MR imaging was performed with unenhanced 3D asymmetric fast SE and gadolinium-enhanced 3D spoiled gradient-recalled (SPGR) sequences with use of a quadrature-surface phased-array coil. The 3D asymmetric fast SE images were reviewed by two radiologists, with the gadolinium-enhanced 3D SPGR images used as the standard of reference.

RESULTS: Nineteen lesions were detected in the 410 ears (diameter range, 2–30 mm; mean, 10.5 mm ± 6.4 [standard deviation]; five lesions were smaller than 5 mm). With 3D asymmetric fast SE, sensitivity, specificity, and accuracy, respectively, were 100%, 99.5%, and 99.5% for observer 1 and 100%, 99.7%, and 99.8% for observer 2.

CONCLUSION: The unenhanced 3D asymmetric fast SE sequence with a quadrature-surface phased-array coil allows the reliable detection of vestibular schwannoma in the cerebellopontine angle and internal auditory canal.

Author contributions:
Guarantor of integrity of entire study, S.N.; study concepts and design, S.N.; definition of intellectual content, S.N.; literature research, S.N.; clinical studies, S.N., T. Ito, H.F., T. Ishigaki, T.N.; experimental studies, S.N., T. Ito, H.F., N.I., Y.K., M.M.; data acquisition, S.N., T. Ito, H.F.; data analysis, S.N., T. Ito; statistical analysis, S.N., T. Ito; manuscript preparation, S.N.; manuscript editing, S.N., M.M.; manuscript review, S.N., T. Ishigaki

The clinical usefulness of T2-weighted magnetic resonance (MR) imaging of the inner ear with a three-dimensional (3D) fast spin-echo (SE) sequence has recently been reported (1–7). To obtain images with higher resolution, high-speed pulse sequences and dedicated surface coils should be developed. With regard to pulse sequences, 3D fast SE with a long echo train and 3D asymmetric Fourier-transform fast SE have been developed, optimized, and clinically evaluated (4). In this study, with regard to coils, a dedicated quadrature-surface phased-array coil for examining the inner ear was developed for use with the 3D asymmetric fast SE sequence and evaluated in patients. Sensitivity values of 89%–94% were reported for MR imaging of vestibular schwannoma with a 3D constructive interference in steady state sequence with use of a head coil (8), and a sensitivity value of 98% was reported for two-dimensional fast SE imaging with a 3-inch (8-cm)-diameter phased-array receiver (9). However, the relatively high frequency of false-negative cases has hindered the widespread acceptance of unenhanced MR imaging as a screening study for vestibular

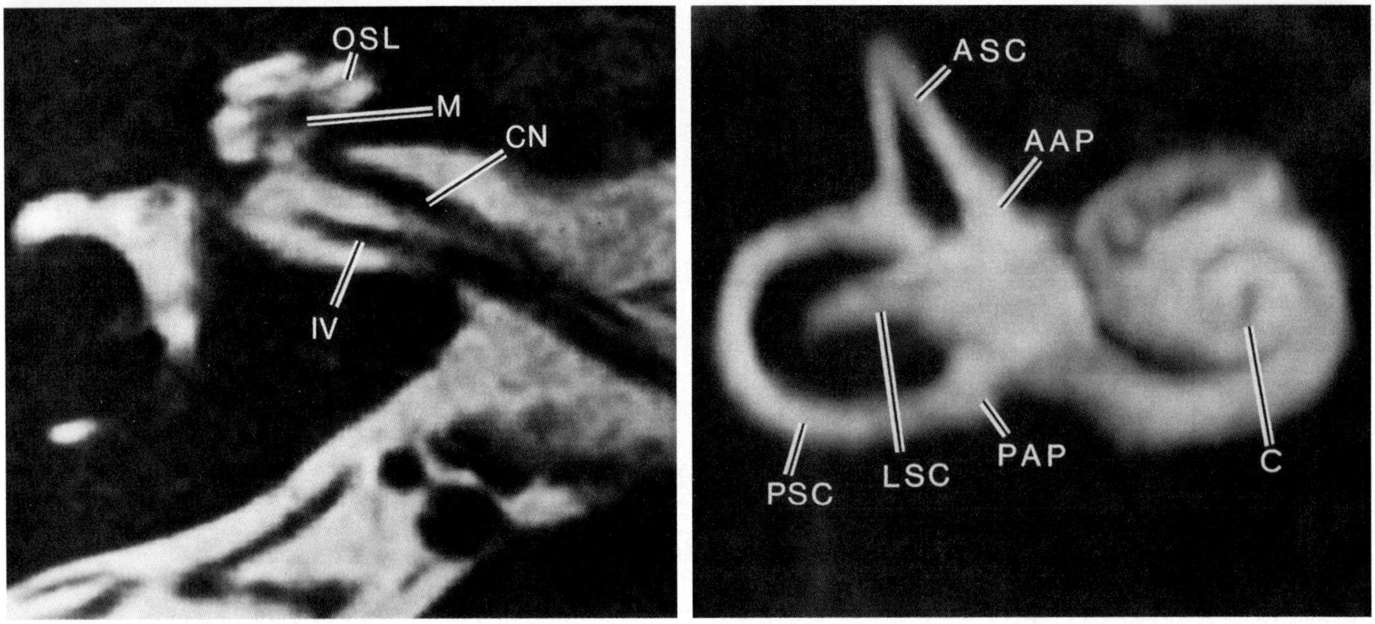

a. b.

Figure 1. Anatomic details of the labyrinth and internal auditory canal are clearly visualized in a normal ear. **(a)** A 3D asymmetric fast SE image at the level of the modiolus (*M*). *CN* = cochlear nerve, *IV* = inferior vestibular nerve, *OSL* = osseous spiral lamina. **(b)** Maximum intensity projection image of the labyrinth from the data for **a**. *AAP* = anterior ampulla, *ASC* = anterior semicircular canal, *C* = cochlea, *LSC* = lateral semicircular canal, *PAP* = posterior ampulla, *PSC* = posterior semicircular canal.

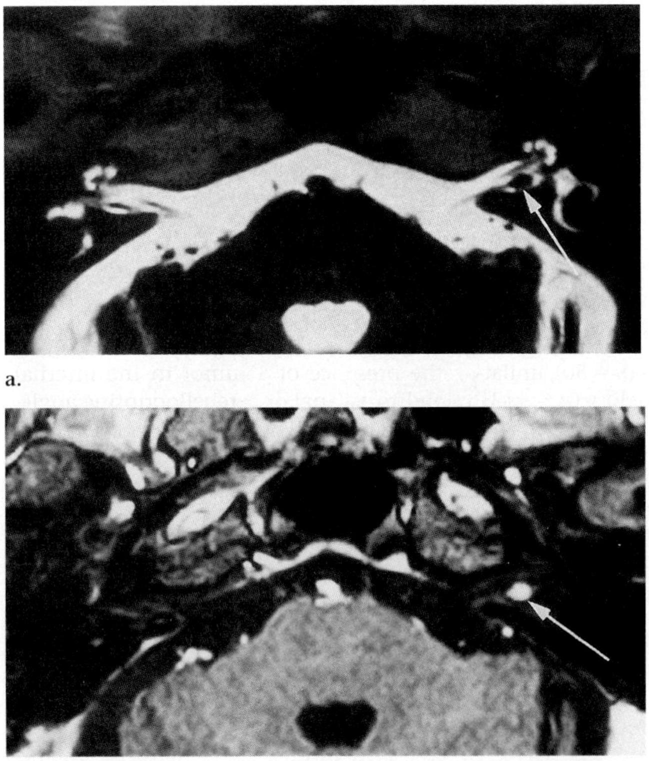

a.

b.

Figure 2. Inferior vestibular nerve schwannoma is depicted on **(a)** 3D asymmetric fast SE and **(b)** 3D SPGR images. The mass (arrow) is 2 mm in diameter.

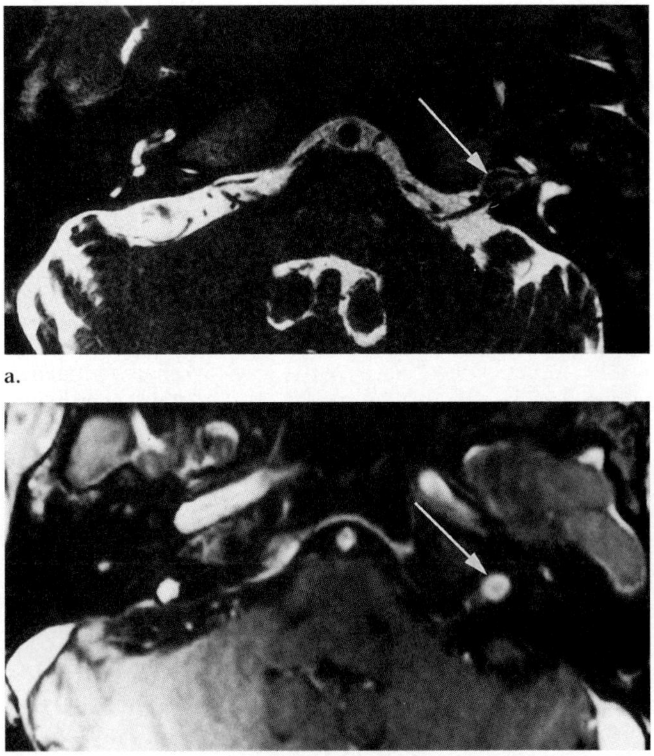

a.

b.

Figure 3. Another case of intracanalicular acoustic schwannoma (arrow) is depicted on **(a)** 3D asymmetric fast SE and **(b)** 3D SPGR images.

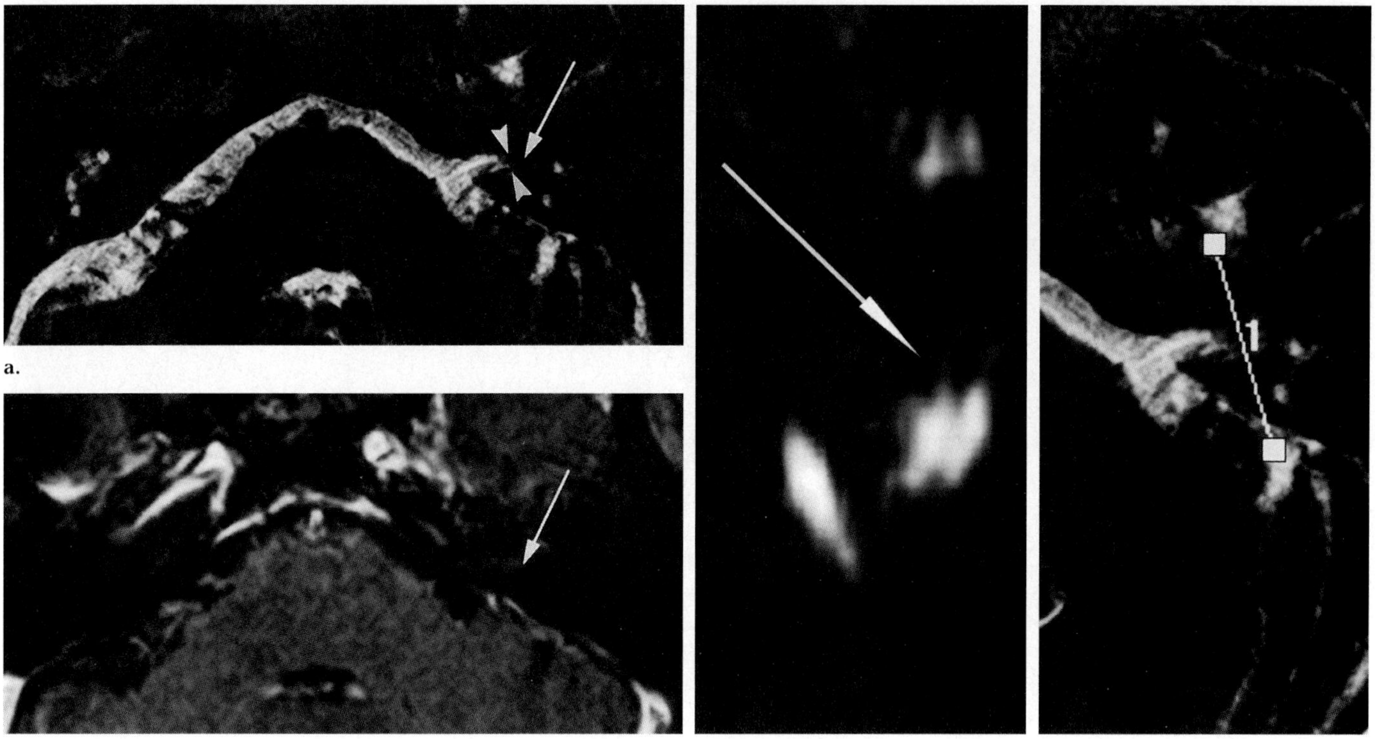

a. b. c. d.

Figure 4. False-positive case. **(a)** A filling defect (arrow) is noted on a 3D asymmetric fast SE image. **(b)** No enhancement is seen on a 3D SPGR image at the corresponding part of the internal auditory canal (arrow). **(c)** Oblique sagittal reformatted image of the data for **a** shows that the filling defect is a part of the wall of the narrow internal auditory canal (arrow). In retrospect, the facial and superior vestibular nerves (arrowheads in **a**) are depicted normally at the site of the filling defect. **(d)** The reference image for **c**. Line *1* indicates the plane orientation.

schwannoma (10). The purpose of this study was to prospectively evaluate visualization of pathologic conditions around the cerebellopontine angle and internal auditory canal with an unenhanced 3D asymmetric fast SE sequence with use of a dedicated quadrature-surface phased-array coil. Findings with a gadolinium-enhanced 3D spoiled gradient-recalled (SPGR) sequence were used as the standard of reference.

MATERIALS AND METHODS

All imaging was performed on a 1.5-T MR system (Visart; Toshiba, Tokyo, Japan) with use of a quadrature-surface phased-array coil. The quadrature-surface coil consists of figure-8-shaped and square elements. This coil has a curved configuration to fit the subject's temporal region. A pair of these quadrature-surface coils is used as a phased array and placed on both sides of the ear. Initially, the signal-to-noise ratios for a quadrature head coil, a 10-cm circular surface coil, and a quadrature-surface phased-array coil were measured with a phantom by means of the subtraction method (11).

Between April 1996 and May 1997, 205 consecutive patients (109 male and 96 female patients; age range, 12–79 years; mean age, 48.4 years ± 16.4 [standard deviation]) underwent MR imaging at the Nagoya University School of Medicine to evaluate ear symptoms. The distribution of 240 symptoms in the 205 patients (with 410 ears) is as follows: bilateral sensorineural hearing loss ($n = 50$), unilateral sensorineural hearing loss ($n = 113$), vertigo ($n = 47$), tinnitus ($n = 21$), and facial palsy ($n = 9$). All patients gave their written informed consent to be included in the investigation, which was approved by the institutional medical ethics committee.

MR imaging was performed with the following pulse sequences: (*a*) heavily T2-weighted 3D asymmetric fast SE (repetition time msec/echo time msec = 4,000/240; echo train length, 79; field of view, 16 cm; section thickness, 0.8 mm; matrix, 512 × 512 × 40; voxel size, 0.3 × 0.3 × 0.8 mm; one signal acquired; imaging time, 11 minutes 48 seconds); (*b*) gadolinium-enhanced (Magnevist; Berlex Laboratories, Wayne, NJ) T1-weighted 3D SPGR (23–40/7–10; flip angle, 30°; field of view, 16 cm; section thickness, 0.8 mm; matrix, 256 × 208 or 224 × 40; one signal acquired; imaging time, 6 minutes 25 seconds to 7 minutes 8 seconds).

Two radiologists (S.N., T. Ito), who were blinded to the patients' history and the results of gadolinium-enhanced 3D SPGR imaging, reviewed all 3D asymmetric fast SE images independently with regard to the presence of a tumor in the internal auditory canal or cerebellopontine angle. The findings on gadolinium-enhanced 3D SPGR images were used as the standard of reference. Sensitivity and specificity values were obtained for detection of vestibular schwannoma in the cerebellopontine angle and the internal auditory canal. Filling defects in the labyrinth and other abnormal labyrinthine findings such as labyrinthitis and inner ear malformation were also noted, but they were counted separately, because gadolinium-enhanced 3D SPGR imaging cannot be considered the standard of reference for these pathologic conditions. For example, labyrinthitis ossificans is depicted as a filling defect on 3D asymmetric fast SE images, but it is not always depicted with increased enhancement on gadolinium-enhanced 3D SPGR images.

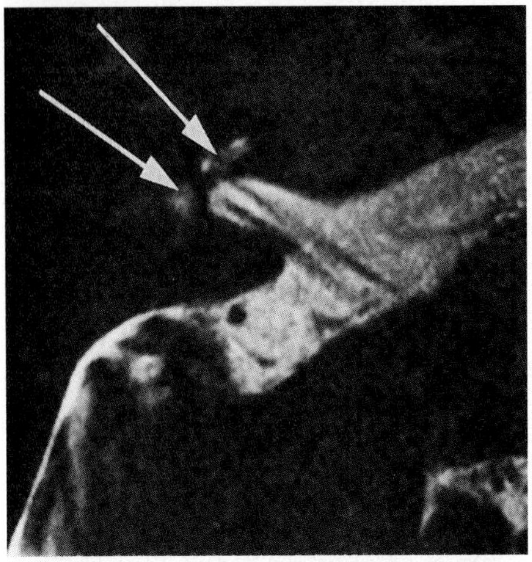

a.

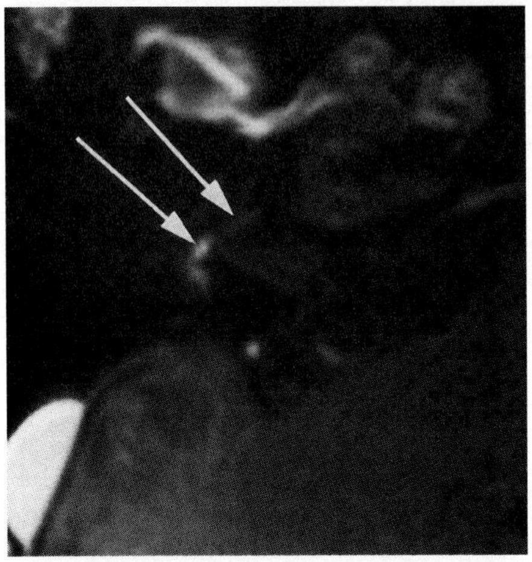

b.

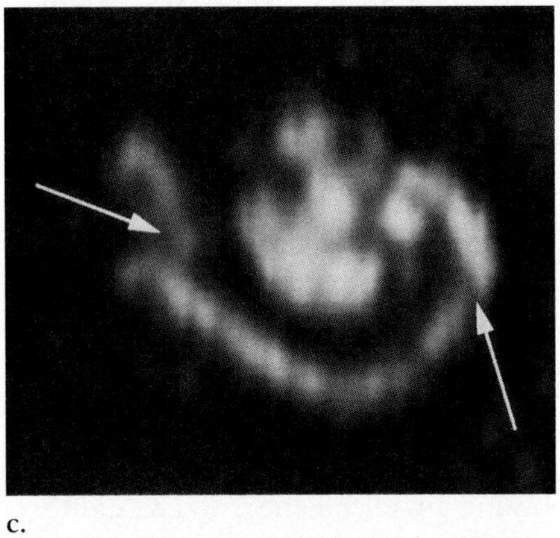

c.

Figure 5. Case of clinically diagnosed labyrinthitis in a patient with a typical history of hearing loss after meningitis. Filling defects (arrows) are seen in the cochlea and vestibule on **(a)** a 3D asymmetric fast SE image, but only minimal enhancement is seen on **(b)** a 3D SPGR image. **(c)** On a maximum intensity projection image from the data for **a**, the morphology of the filling defects (arrows) is more easily understood. Note that the margins of the enhancement are unclear compared with those of the intralabyrinthine schwannoma in Figure 7.

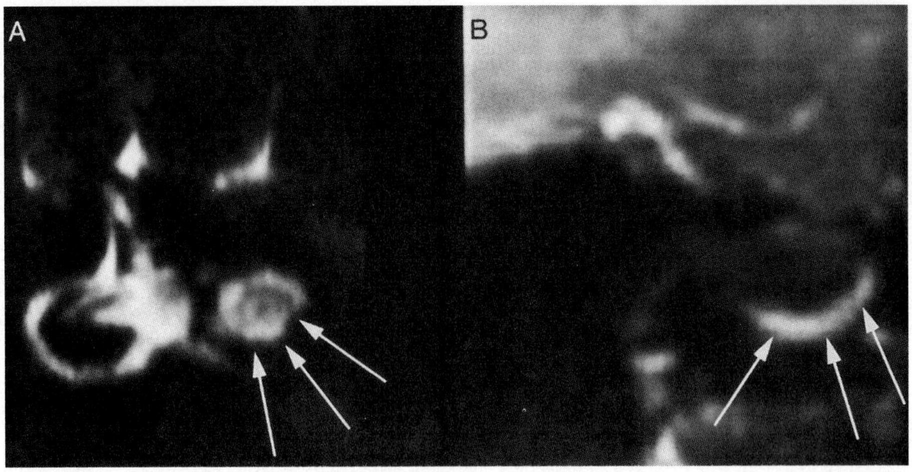

Figure 6. A case of presumed intracochlear schwannoma (clinically diagnosed but not surgically proved). *A*, A filling defect (arrows) is seen in the basal turn of the cochlea on the maximum intensity projection image from 3D asymmetric fast SE data. *B*, Marked enhancement (arrows) is seen on the maximum intensity projection image from 3D SPGR data.

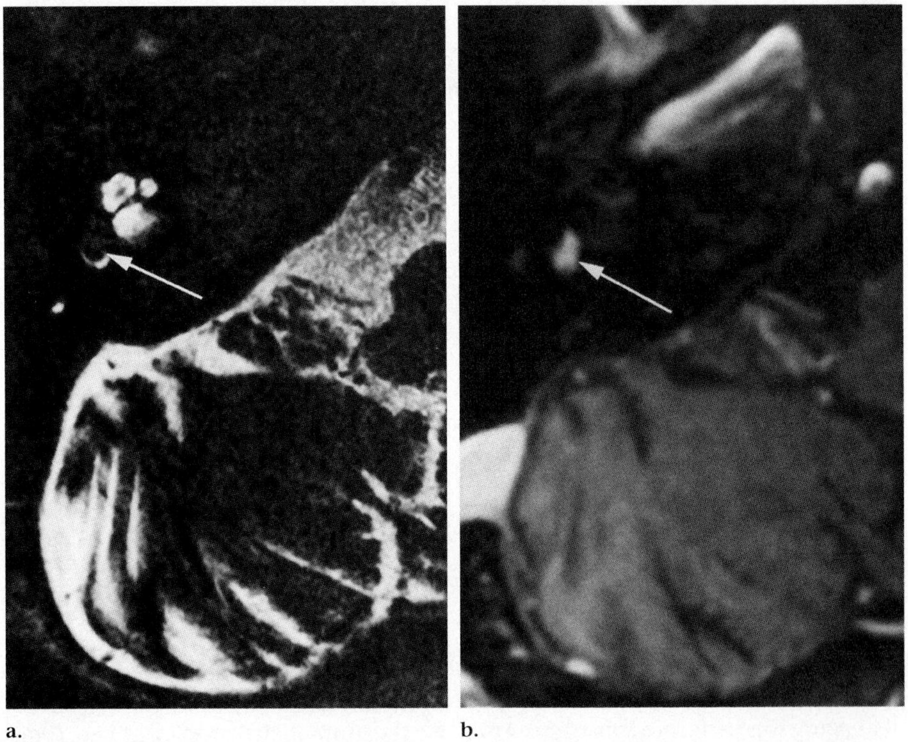

a. b.

Figure 7. A case of presumed intravestibular schwannoma (clinically diagnosed but not surgically proved). **(a)** A filling defect (arrow) is seen in the vestibule on a 3D asymmetric fast SE image. **(b)** Marked enhancement (arrow) is seen at the corresponding region on a 3D SPGR image.

RESULTS

Relative signal-to-noise ratios were measured at a depth of 5 cm from the surface: quadrature head coil, 1.0; 10-cm circular coil, 1.1; quadrature-surface phased-array coil, 1.6.

Anatomic details of the labyrinth and internal auditory canal were clearly visualized on 3D asymmetric fast SE images of the normal ear (Fig 1).

Results of evaluation in 410 ears for lesions in the cerebellopontine angle and internal auditory canal demonstrated 19 lesions (in 19 patients) (diameter range, 2–30 mm; mean diameter, 10.5 mm ±

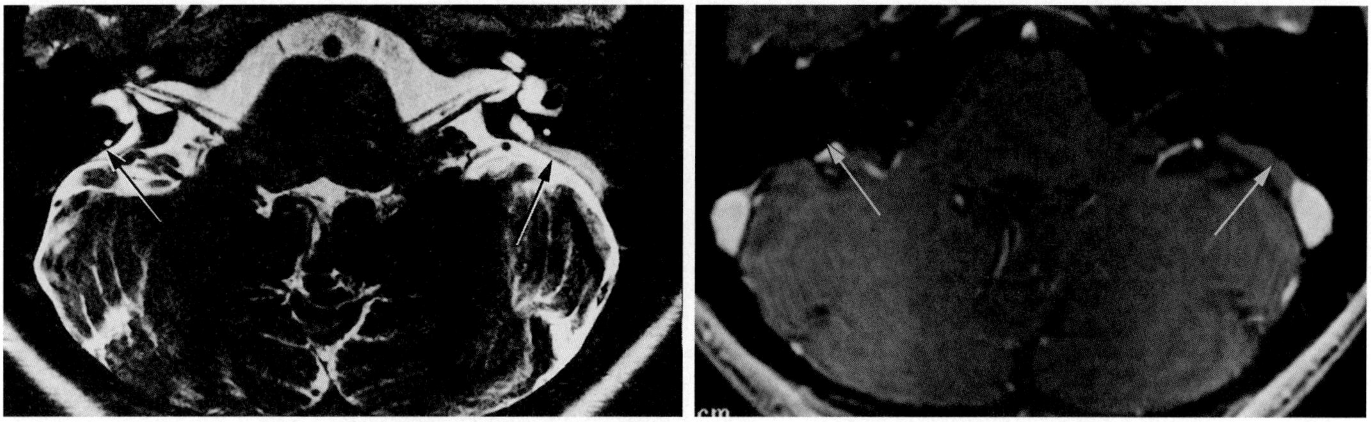

a. b.

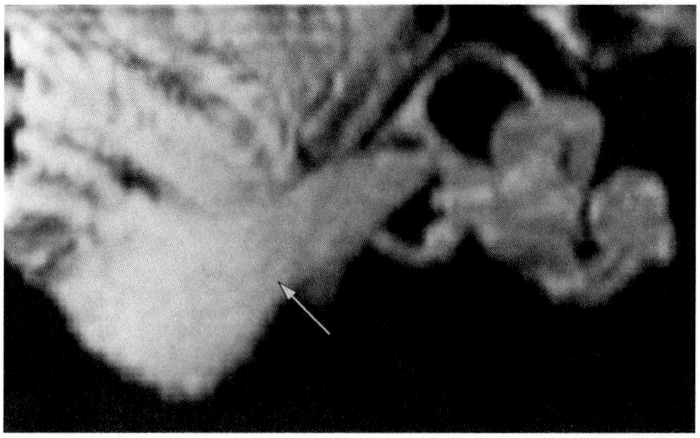

c.

Figure 8. Case of large vestibular aqueduct syndrome. The dilated endolymphatic duct and sac (arrows in **a** and **b**) are depicted on **(a)** 3D asymmetric fast SE and **(b)** 3D SPGR images. **(c)** On the maximum intensity projection image of the data for **a**, the relationship between the vestibule and the dilated endolymphatic duct (arrow) is clearly visualized. Note that the signal intensity of the left endolymphatic sac is slightly lower on **a** and higher on **b** than that on the right side. This is probably due to hemorrhage or protein containment.

6.4; five lesions were smaller than 5 mm). The maximum diameter of the masses was 2.0 mm or less ($n = 1$), 2.1–5.0 mm ($n = 4$), 5.1–10.0 mm ($n = 6$), 10.1–20.0 mm ($n = 7$), or greater than 20.1 mm ($n = 1$).

No false-negative findings (Figs 2, 3) and one or two false-positive findings (Fig 4) were noted on 3D asymmetric fast SE images. Interobserver variability was small with regard to lesions in the cerebellopontine angle and internal auditory canal. There was disagreement between the two observers in only one case, which was judged to be normal by one observer and to be positive by the other. There was no abnormal contrast enhancement on gadolinium-enhanced 3D SPGR images. For 3D asymmetric fast SE imaging, sensitivity, specificity, positive predictive value, negative predictive value, and accuracy, respectively, were 100%, 99.5%, 90.9%, 100%, and 99.5% for observer 1 and 100%, 99.7%, 95.2%, 100%, and 99.8% for observer 2.

In 13 ears (in eight patients), filling defects in the labyrinth were detected on 3D asymmetric fast SE images. Eleven ears (six patients) had a previous history of severe otitis media or meningitis. No or only minimal enhancement was seen in the labyrinth. Disease in these ears was clinically diagnosed as labyrinthitis (Fig 5). Two ears (two patients) had no history of otitis media or meningitis. Marked enhancement was seen in the labyrinth. Disease in these ears was clinically diagnosed as intralabyrinthine schwannoma (Figs 6, 7).

Other pathologic conditions found in the 410 ears included inner ear malformation and inflammatory disease. Inner ear malformations included large vestibular aqueduct syndrome (Fig 8) (five ears, three patients), Mondini malformation (Fig 9) (one ear, one patient), and hypogenesis of the lateral semicircular canal (one ear, one patient). These pathologic conditions were detected on 3D SPGR images in only two ears (one patient) with large vestibular aqueduct syndrome. Inflammatory disease (Ramsay Hunt syndrome, Fig 10) was found in one ear (one patient). This pathologic condition could not be detected on 3D asymmetric fast SE images.

DISCUSSION

In heavily T2-weighted MR imaging of the inner ear with a 3D asymmetric fast SE sequence, pathologic conditions can be recognized only when the morphologic details of a tissue surrounded by water have been visibly affected. Thus, inflammatory processes such as Bell palsy and Ramsay Hunt syndrome are difficult to diagnose. These diseases are not treated on the basis of MR imaging findings, however, so this does not appear to be a major problem for the 3D asymmetric fast SE sequence.

For the characterization of a small lesion at the edge of a narrow internal auditory canal, multiplanar reconstruction and gadolinium enhancement may be necessary. A 3D acquisition allows postprocessing such as maximum intensity projection or multiplanar reconstruction. High spatial resolution is necessary to detect slight morphologic changes. Imaging with a 3D asymmetric fast SE sequence with the use of a dedicated quadrature-surface phased-array coil is one solution.

Recent advances in MR imaging have enabled the preoperative visualization of intralabyrinthine pathologic conditions (12–18). The 3D structure of the labyrinth is very complicated (19–21). Even on reference images, it may sometimes be difficult to obtain a precise understanding of intralabyrinthine pathologic conditions, in which case, review of maximum intensity

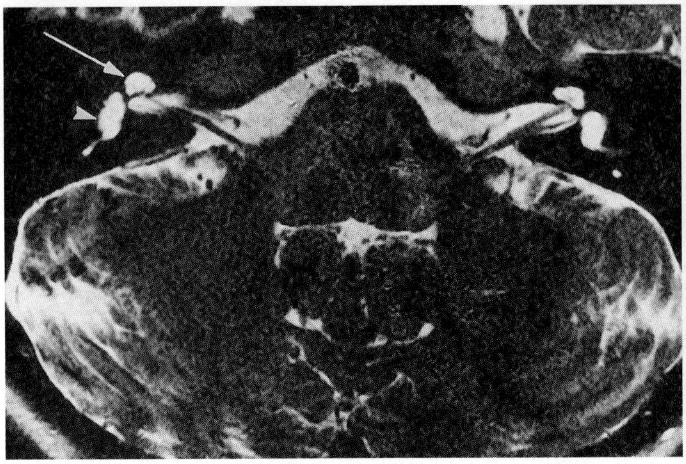

a.

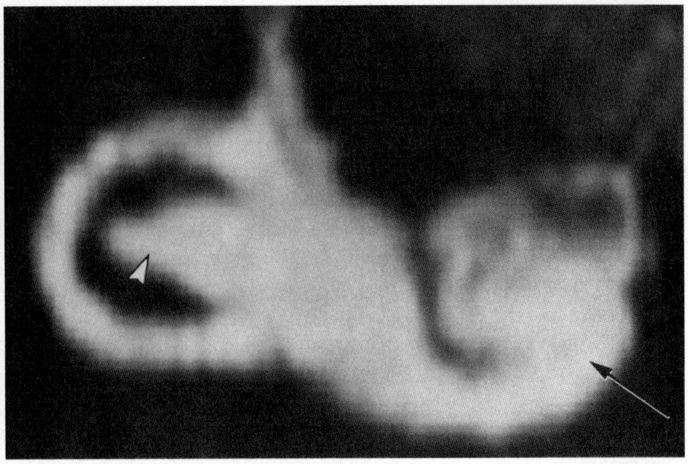

b.

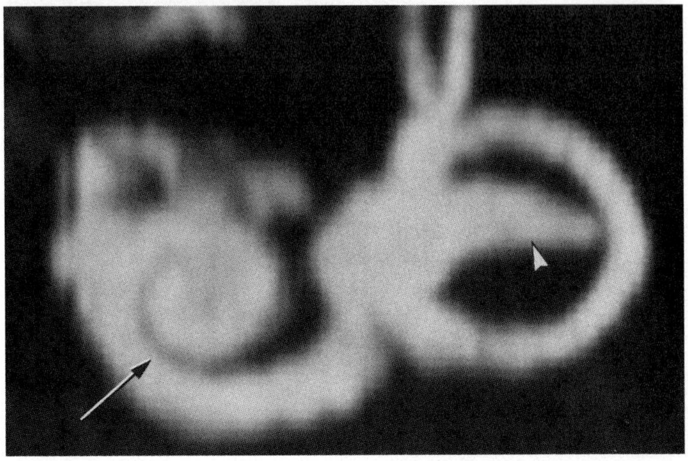

c.

Figure 9. Case of Mondini malformation. **(a)** Axial 3D asymmetric fast SE image and **(b, c)** maximum intensity projection images of the right (in **b**) and left (in **c**) inner ear. The cochlear turn (arrow) and lateral semicircular canal (arrowhead) are hypoplastic on the right side.

projection and multiplanar reconstruction images is helpful. Heavily T2-weighted images are highly sensitive for the detection of vestibular schwannoma without the need for gadolinium enhancement, (9,22–24), because the internal auditory canal mass is depicted with low signal intensity (23) and the images have high resolution (25–29). Sensitivity values of 89%–94% and specificity values of 94%–97% were reported for vestibular schwannoma with a 3D constructive interference in steady state sequence with use of a head coil (8), and a sensitivity value of 98% was reported for two-dimensional fast SE imaging with a 3-inch (8-cm)-diameter phased-array receiver (9). However, the relatively high frequency of false-negative cases has hindered the widespread acceptance of unenhanced MR imaging as a screening study for vestibular schwannoma (10). In our study, a sensitivity of 100% and a specificity of 99.5%–99.7% were obtained. These high values, which are superior to those reported previously, are attributable to the pulse sequence and the dedicated quadrature-surface coil employed in this study. False-positive findings are not a serious concern because these can be promptly resolved by performing gadolinium-enhanced MR studies (10). We now monitor all MR examinations for the screening of vestibular schwannoma, and if there is a positive finding on 3D asymmetric fast SE images, gadolinium-enhanced 3D SPGR imaging is performed to confirm whether this is a true- or false-positive finding. Although no false-negative finding occurred in this study, more patients should be studied to obviate the gadolinium-enhanced study. For this purpose, a multi-institutional study should be conducted in the future.

In conclusion, MR imaging of the inner ear with a 3D asymmetric fast SE sequence with a quadrature-surface phased-array coil permits the reliable detection of vestibular schwannoma in the cerebellopontine angle and internal auditory canal without the need for gadolinium enhancement.

References

1. Naganawa S, Yamakawa K, Fukatsu H, et al. High-resolution T2-weighted MR imaging of the inner ear using a long echo-train-length 3D fast spin-echo sequence. Eur Radiol 1996; 6:369–374.
2. Takehara Y, Ichijyo K, Tooyama N, et al. Three-dimensional projection images of the labyrinth acquired with multislab 3DFT fast spin-echo sequence and dual-array surface coil. AJR 1995; 165:645–646.
3. Naganawa S, Yamakawa K, Fukatsu H, et al. Visualization of the internal anatomy for the inner ear using a long echo train length 3D fast spin echo sequence (abstr). In: Proceedings of the Third Meeting of the International Society for Magnetic Resonance in Medicine. Berkeley, Calif: International Society for Magnetic Resonance in Medicine, 1995; 230.
4. Naganawa S, Fukatsu H, Ishigaki T, et al. High speed and high resolution MR imaging of the inner ear using ultra-long echo train length 3D fast spin echo and half Fourier imaging (abstr). In: Proceedings of the Fourth Meeting of the International Society for Magnetic Resonance in Medicine. Berkeley, Calif: International Society for Magnetic Resonance in Medicine, 1996; 631.
5. Naganawa S, Senda K, Ishigaki T, et al. High resolution MR imaging of the inner ear apparatus using 3D-fast spin echo sequence. Nippon Acta Radiol 1995; 55: 81–82.
6. Naganawa S, Ito T, Fukatsu H, et al. MR cisternography of the cerebellopontine angle using 3D fast SE (abstr). Radiology 1996; 201(P):450.
7. Kollias S, Samara C, Wichimann W, et al. High resolution anatomy and pathology of the inner ear using a long echo-train-length (ETL), 3D, fast spin echo sequence

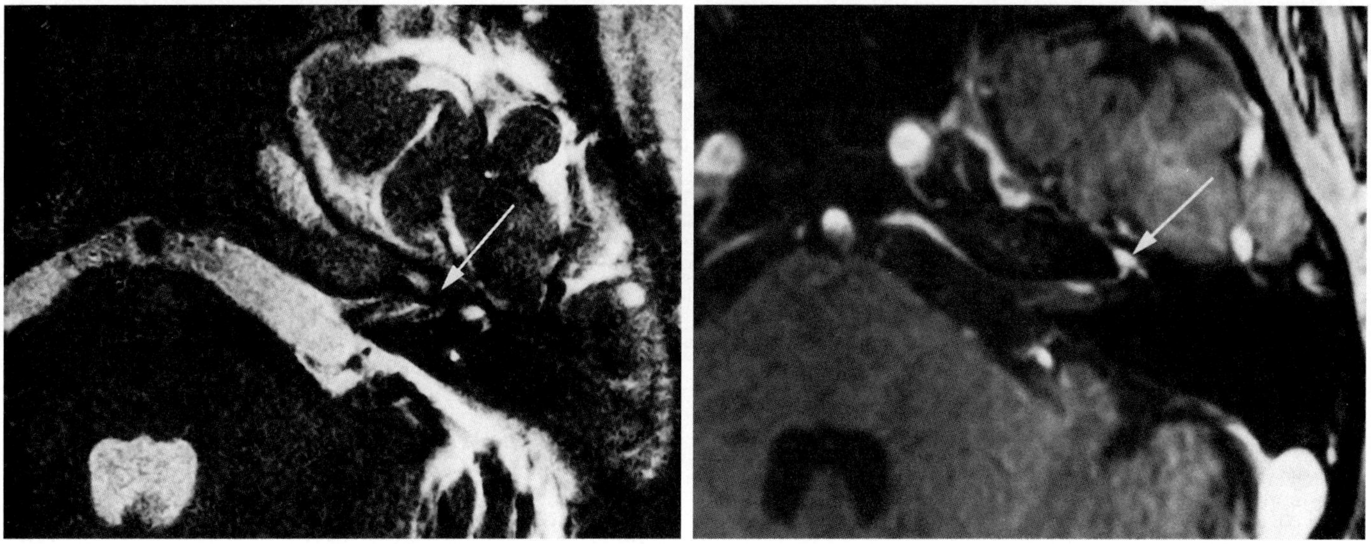

a. b.

Figure 10. Case of Ramsay Hunt syndrome. **(a)** On a 3D asymmetric fast SE image, no abnormality of the geniculate ganglion (arrow) is depicted. **(b)** On a 3D SPGR image, abnormally intense enhancement and swelling of the geniculate ganglion (arrow) is depicted. Enhancement of the geniculate ganglion is a common finding, but the intense enhancement and swelling depicted here should be interpreted as pathologic.

(abstr). In: Proceedings of the Fourth Meeting of the International Society for Magnetic Resonance in Medicine. Berkeley, Calif: International Society for Magnetic Resonance in Medicine, 1996; 635.

8. Hermans R, Goten AV, De Foer B, Baert AL. MRI screening for acoustic neuroma without gadolinium: value of 3DFT-CISS sequence. Neuroradiology 1997; 39:593–598.
9. Allen RW, Harnsberger HR, Shelton C, et al. Low-cost high-resolution fast spin-echo MR of acoustic schwannoma: an alternative to enhanced conventional spin-echo MR? AJNR 1996; 17:1205–1210.
10. Jackler RK. Cost-effective screening for acoustic neuroma with unenhanced MR: a clinician's perspective. AJNR 1997; 17: 1226–1228.
11. Price RR, Axel L, Morgan T, et al. Quality assurance methods and phantoms for magnetic resonance imaging: report of AAPM Nuclear Magnetic Resonance Task Group No. 1. Med Phys 1990; 17:287–295.
12. Mafee MF, Lachenauer CS, Kumar A, et al. CT and MR imaging of intralabyrinthine schwannoma: report of two cases and review of the literature. Radiology 1990; 174:395–400.
13. Seltzer S, Mark AS. Contrast enhancement of the labyrinth on MR scans in patients with sudden hearing loss and vertigo: evidence of labyrinthine disease. AJNR 1991; 12:13–16.
14. Brogan M, Chakeres DW. Gd-DTPA–enhanced MR imaging of cochlear schwannoma. AJNR 1990; 11:407–408.
15. Doyle KJ, Brackmann DE. Intralabyrinthine schwannomas. Otolaryngol Head Neck Surg 1994; 110:517–525.
16. Weed DT, Teague MW, Stewart R, Schwaber MK. Intralabyrinthine schwannoma: a case report. Otolaryngol Head Neck Surg 1994; 111:134–142.
17. Swarz JD. Sensorineural hearing deficit: a systematic approach based on imaging findings. RadioGraphics 1996; 16:561–574.
18. Wilson DF, Talbot JM, Hodgson RS. Magnetic resonance imaging: enhancing lesions of the labyrinth and facial nerve. Otolaryngol Head Neck Surg 1994; 120: 560–564.
19. Swartz JD, Daniels DL, Harnsberger HR, et al. Balance and equilibrium. II. The retrovestibular neural pathway. AJNR 1996; 17:1187–1190.
20. Daniels DL, Swartz JD, Harnsberger HR, et al. Hearing. I. The cochlea. AJNR 1996; 17:1237–1241.
21. Daniels DL, Swartz JD, Harnsberger HR, et al. Hearing. II. The retrocochlear auditory pathway. AJNR 1996; 17:1479–1481.
22. Stuckey SL, Harris AJ, Mannolini SM. Detection of acoustic schwannoma: use of constructive interference in the steady state three-dimensional MR. AJNR 1996; 17:1219–1225.
23. Fukui MB, Weissman JL, Curtin HD, Kanal E. T2-weighted MR characteristics of internal auditory canal masses. AJNR 1996; 17:1211–1218.
24. Weissman JL. Hearing loss. Radiology 1996; 199:593–611.
25. Takehara Y, Ichijo K, Tohyama N, et al. MR cisternography using "long echo train length fast spin echo sequence" for demonstrating the inner ear. Nippon Acta Radiol 1993; 53:859–861.
26. Phalps PD. Fast spin echo in otology. J Laryngol Otol 1994; 108:383–394.
27. Casselman JW, Kuhweide R, Deimling M, et al. Constructive interference in steady-state 3DFT MR imaging of the inner ear and cerebellopontine angle. AJNR 1993; 14:47–57.
28. Tien RD, Feisberg GJ, MacFall J. Fast spin-echo high-resolution MR imaging of the inner ear. AJR 1992; 159:395–398.
29. Casselman JW, Kuhweide R, Ampe W, Devlies F. Magnetic resonance examination of the inner ear and cerebellopontine angle in patients with vertigo and/or abnormal findings at vestibular testing. Acta Otolaryngol (Stockholm) 1994; 513(suppl):15–27.

Book Review

Imaging of the Temporal Bone. 3rd ed.

Edited by Joel D. Swartz, MD, and H. Ric Harnsberger, MD

Stuttgart, Germany: Georg Thieme Verlag, 1998. ISBN 3-13-688403-5.
Hardcover, $129.00; pp 510; 507 figures; tables.

Head and neck radiology has evolved from an overlooked, arcane field relegated to a minor role in neuroradiology and a subordinate role in body imaging to a vigorous and fertile area in which radiologists can actively participate in partnership with otolaryngologists to diagnose diseases and treat patients. However, despite the advances in technology, the topic of otologic imaging is still considered somewhat cryptic by residents and general radiologists because there is a large amount of anatomy packed into a small area of the body. Because computed tomography and magnetic resonance imaging provide such elegant anatomic detail, clinicians are requesting temporal bone imaging studies to evaluate such common symptoms as tinnitus, hearing loss, and dizziness, as well as for pre- and postoperative evaluation in cases of inflammatory disease, neoplasia, and Meniere disease. Therefore, a good reference book on imaging of the auditory apparatus is welcome. Such a book is *Imaging of the Temporal Bone*. This work has undergone two revisions since 1968, and both fundamental and contemporary knowledge is taught and demonstrated with each new edition.

Originally conceived as a monograph to give radiologists a solid background so they could assist otologic surgeons, the second edition expanded coverage to disseminate information on magnetic resonance imaging of the temporal bone. This third edition is a multiauthored reference work that has been expanded by more than 100 pages. Still, it retains the comforting feel of a monograph and did not become a formidable and daunting exhaustive treatise.

The book is organized into eight chapters and an appendix, and each chapter has been improved in one or more ways. Some sections have newer protocols and indications, while others have more illustrations. The enlarged appendix is now 16 pages, and three-letter mnemonic abbreviations replace numbers and arrows on the figure legends. There are exquisite color images of cochlear and labyrinth anatomy. The book has retained its familiar logical organization with an introductory chapter followed by sections on the external canal, the middle ear and mastoid, vascular diseases, the otic capsule, trauma, the facial nerve, and the vestibulocochlear nerve.

As in previous editions, the writing is lucid, the illustrations are superb and detailed, and the line drawings are excellent.

The legends are helpful yet unobtrusive. The use of mnemonics rather than numbers averts reader frustration by preventing the reader from bouncing back and forth between image and legend. The paper has changed from a high-gloss finish (used in the second edition) to a flat matte finish that is easier on the eyes. I have only a few minor suggestions for improvement. One would be to make a special effort in design to have each illustration on the same page as the text that refers to it. The value of the work would also be enhanced by a section illustrating embryology of the ear, particularly as it relates to malformations. Inclusion of gross images of pathologic specimens and histopathologic slides would also be appreciated. The chapter on vascular abnormalities of the ear was particularly strong and included very helpful imaging algorithms. However, there is essentially no discussion of vascular intervention for tumors or vascular malformations of the ear.

Currently, I know of only two books dedicated to imaging of the ear. *Imaging of the Temporal Bone* is the more recent and larger of the two. Although some works on head and neck imaging contain chapters on the temporal bone, by necessity the chapters cannot be as detailed as this monograph.

The editors have met their stated goals. This book is well worth the price. This book is a necessity for those who have a substantial head and neck imaging practice. For others who perform temporal bone imaging occasionally, this would be a good reference textbook.

Reviewed by David S. Martin, MD

Nicola Petitti, MD, PhD

The Hyperdense Middle Cerebral Artery Sign[1]

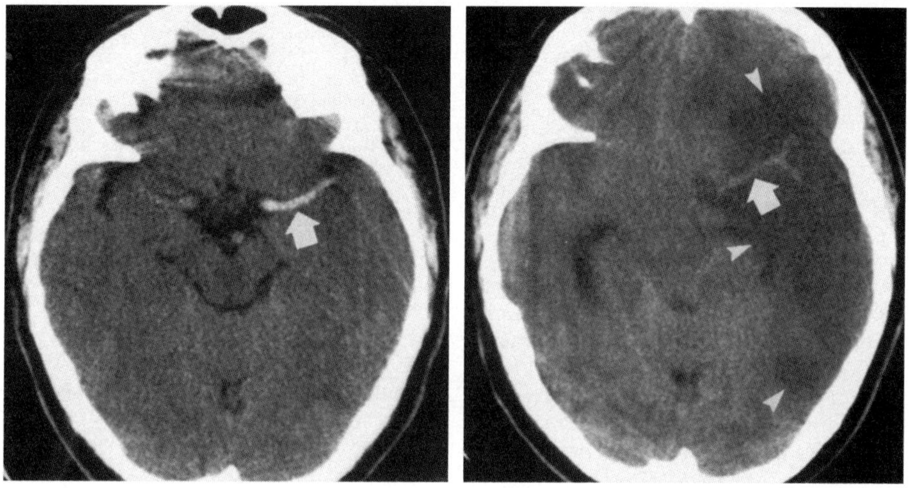

a. b.

The HMCA sign. **(a)** Unenhanced CT scan obtained after acute onset of right hemiplegia in a 48-year-old man demonstrates increased attenuation of the proximal left middle cerebral artery (arrow). **(b)** Unenhanced CT scan obtained in the same patient 24 hours later reveals a sharply defined area of hypoattenuation (arrowheads) that encompasses the entire left middle cerebral artery territory. The left middle cerebral artery (arrow) is still seen.

APPEARANCE

The hyperdense middle cerebral artery (HMCA) sign is sometimes seen on non–contrast material-enhanced computed tomographic (CT) scans (Figure) of the brain. It is recognized as an area of increased attenuation when compared to the contralateral side of the brain, along the course of the first or second segment of the middle cerebral artery.

Index terms:
Arteries, CT, 174.12111
Arteries, embolism, 174.771, 174.781
Brain, CT, 174.12111
Cerebral blood vessels, thrombosis, 174.7691, 174.781

Radiology 1998; 208:687–688

Abbreviation:
HMCA = hyperdense middle cerebral artery

[1] From the Department of Radiology, Wake Forrest University School of Medicine, Medical Center Blvd, Winston-Salem, NC 27157-1088. Received December 15, 1997; revision requested January 15, 1998; revision received February 11; accepted May 11. **Address reprint requests to** the author.

EXPLANATION

The HMCA sign is an indirect sign of cerebral ischemia that corresponds to occlusion of the middle cerebral artery. The hyperattenuating component of this sign represents occlusion of the middle cerebral artery by an intraluminal clot from a thrombus or an embolus (1–3). The attenuation of flowing blood, which is approximately 40 HU, is linearly related to the hemoglobin concentration. In a thrombus, there is an extrusion of serum, and the attenuation of a thrombus at CT is about 80 HU (4).

DISCUSSION

CT is often the first diagnostic test performed in patients with acute neurologic deficit. However, CT images of the brain often appear normal within the first few hours after a stroke. When brain imaging changes that are consistent with early ischemic infarction are present, they are often subtle at first and become more pronounced over time. Familiarity with some of the radiographic signs of acute infarction is helpful in identifying the cause of the acute neurologic deficit.

Early signs of middle cerebral artery infarction include the HMCA sign, loss of the insular ribbon, and hemispheric sulcal effacement. These signs may become evident on CT images of the brain within the first 6 hours after a stroke. The HMCA sign can theoretically be seen on CT images of the brain at the time of vascular occlusion, before other changes of acute stroke are manifested on the images. In addition, the HMCA sign is a transient phenomenon, as suggested in serial CT studies (3). The CT images obtained in most patients with acute stroke symptoms who have the HMCA sign do not show an HMCA sign after 1 week, which confirms the mobile nature of the clot (3).

In some studies (2,3) in patients who have stroke-related symptoms in the middle cerebral artery distribution, a substantial percentage of patients, perhaps as high as 35%–50%, have the HMCA sign. Angiographic follow-up findings, resolution of the increased attenuation at subsequent CT examinations, and attenuation measurements in the course of the affected middle cerebral artery suggest that the most likely cause of the HMCA sign is thromboembolism (1–3).

Caution is advised when the HMCA sign is seen, since it may not represent vascular occlusion (5). A false sign of occlusion can be produced by a high hematocrit level, which may increase the attenuation of the blood, or by calcification in the vessel walls, which is often associated with both diabetes mellitus (insulin-dependent and non–insulin-dependent) and hypertension. Strict adherence to the criteria used to define the HMCA sign is essential in diagnosing middle cerebral artery occlusion. The attenuation of the unilateral side of the middle cerebral artery must be greater than that of the contralateral middle cerebral artery and must not be caused by calcification or by an elevated hematocrit level (6).

Although its role is somewhat controversial, the HMCA sign may have a prognostic value in patients who have had strokes, as patients with this sign have been shown to have a substantially worse prognosis than other patients with acute ischemic infarction (7,8). The HMCA sign may be a stronger prognostic factor when it is associated with other early CT signs of brain infarction (6). However, unlike other signs of acute stroke, the presence of the HMCA sign does not exclude the use of thrombolytic therapy with tissue plasminogen activator (9). It is therefore crucial that CT scans of the brain are assessed by physicians with expertise in reading these imaging studies (9).

In conclusion, identification of increased attenuation along the course of the middle cerebral artery may be extremely valuable in the early CT diagnosis of infarction and in instituting an appropriate therapeutic regimen.

References

1. Pressman BD, Tourje EJ, Thompson JR. An early CT sign of ischemic infarction: increased density in a cerebral artery. AJR 1987; 149:583–586.
2. Schuknecht B, Ratzka M, Hofmann E. The "dense artery sign": major cerebral artery thromboembolism demonstrated by computed tomography. Neuroradiology 1990; 32:98–103.
3. Bastianello S, Pierallini A, Colonnese C, et al. Hyperdense middle cerebral artery CT sign: comparison with angiography in the acute phase of ischemic supratentorial infarction. Neuroradiology 1991; 33:207–211.
4. New PFJ, Aronow S. Attenuation measurements of whole blood and fractions in computed tomography. Radiology 1976; 121:635–640.
5. Rauch RA, Bazan C III, Larsson EM, Jinkins JR. Hyperdense middle cerebral arteries identified on CT as a false sign of vascular occlusion. AJNR 1993; 14:669–673.
6. Moulin T, Cattin F, Crepin-Leblond T, et al. Early CT signs in acute middle cerebral artery infarction: predictive value for subsequent infarct locations and outcome. Neurology 1996; 47:366–375.
7. Gacs G, Fox AJ, Barnett HJM, Vinuela F. CT visualization of intracranial arterial thromboembolism. Stroke 1983; 14:756–762.
8. Zorzon M, Mase G, Pozzi-Mucelli F, et al. Increased density in the middle cerebral artery by nonenhanced computed tomography: prognostic value in acute cerebral infarction. Eur Neurol 1993; 33:256–259.
9. Adams HP, Brott TG, Furlan AJ, et al. Guidelines for thrombolytic therapy for acute stroke: a supplement to the guidelines for the management of patients with acute ischemic stroke. Circulation 1996; 94:1167–1174.

Ho-Young Song, MD
Deok Hee Lee, MD
Hyosook Ahn, MD
Jae-Ho Kim, MD
Sung-Gwon Kang, MD
Hyun-Ki Yoon, MD
Kyu-Bo Sung, MD

Index terms:
Lacrimal gland and duct, 223.458
Lacrimal gland and duct, interventional procedure, 223.1299
Stents and prostheses, 223.1299

Radiology 1998; 208:689–694

[1] From the Departments of Diagnostic Radiology (H.Y.S., D.H.L., H.K.Y., K.B.S.), Ophthalmology (H.A.), and Otorhinolaryngology (J.H.K.), Asan Medical Center, University of Ulsan College of Medicine, 388-1, Poongnap-Dong, Songpa-Ku, Seoul, 138-040, Korea, and the Department of Diagnostic Radiology, Inha University Hospital, University of Inha College of Medicine, Inchon, Korea (S.G.K.). From the 1997 RSNA scientific assembly. Received November 6, 1997; revision requested January 27, 1998; revision received March 17; accepted April 23. Supported in part by a G7 Research Fund from the Korean Health and Welfare Ministry. **Address reprint requests to** H.Y.S.

Author contributions:
Guarantor of integrity of entire study, H.Y.S.; study concepts, H.Y.S., H.A., J.H.K.; study design, H.Y.S., K.B.S.; definition of intellectual content, D.H.L., H.K.Y.; literature research, S.G.K.; clinical studies, H.Y.S., H.A., J.H.K.; data acquisition and analysis, S.G.K., D.H.L.; statistical analysis, D.H.L.; manuscript preparation, H.Y.S., S.G.K.; manuscript editing, S.G.K.; manuscript review, H.K.Y., K.B.S.

Lacrimal System Obstruction Treated with Lacrimal Polyurethane Stents: Outcome of Removal of Occluded Stents[1]

PURPOSE: To describe the short- and long-term outcomes of the removal of occluded stents.

MATERIALS AND METHODS: With fluoroscopic guidance, 571 lacrimal polyurethane stents were placed in 502 patients with epiphora due to obstruction of the lacrimal system. Of the 571 stents, 142 were removed 2 weeks to 42 months (mean, 7 months) after placement because of recurrent epiphora, and the lacrimal system was irrigated with saline solution through the lacrimal point.

RESULTS: Stent removal was well tolerated. Mild epistaxis occurred in one patient and was controlled with a nasal pack. Recurrent epiphora was due to obstruction of the stent with mucoid material in 49 (35%) of 142 systems and granulation tissue in 93 (65%) systems. After stent removal, 73 (51%) of the 142 lacrimal systems showed improvement of epiphora, with a patent lacrimal system at 7-day follow-up dacryocystography. During the follow-up of 2 weeks to 49 months (mean, 22 months) after stent removal, patency was maintained in 24 (33%) of the 73 lacrimal systems.

CONCLUSION: Removal of an occluded lacrimal plastic stent was easy and safe. Recurrent epiphora after placement of lacrimal plastic stents can be treated with removal of the occluded stents and irrigation with saline solution through the lacrimal point, which resulted in a patent lacrimal system in 33% of cases in this study.

Fluoroscopic nonsurgical placement of an expandable metallic or plastic stent has yielded encouraging results in the treatment of epiphora due to obstruction of the lacrimal system (1–8). This procedure offers the following advantages over invasive surgical procedures: (*a*) General anesthesia is not needed; (*b*) the procedure is simple, safe, and cost-effective; (*c*) no facial scar is produced; (*d*) there is less bleeding; (*e*) there is no substantial anatomic alteration; and (*f*) the procedure is more easily tolerated by patients. Overall success rates of 95%–100% have been reported in studies (1–8) that have included more than four and fewer than 236 patients.

As lacrimal stents, however, metallic stents have limitations because, when the stents become blocked after placement, they cannot be removed without surgery (1,2). In addition, recurrent epiphora due to blockage of the stent by means of granulation tissue is common (2,9). Even in cases of plastic stent placement, the overall recurrence rate was 31% (81 of 262 lacrimal systems) (5).

It has been reported (5,6) that a lacrimal system with recurrent epiphora after stent placement could be recanalized by removing the occluded stent. These reports, however, have referred to only small numbers of lacrimal systems, with limited follow-up. Our purpose was to determine the short- and long-term outcomes of the removal of occluded plastic stents in 142 lacrimal systems in 125 patients.

MATERIALS AND METHODS

Patient Population

Beginning in April 1993, 6-F polyurethane nasolacrimal or canalicular stents (Song Naso-Lacrimal Duct Stent; Cook, Eight Mile Plains, Queensland, Australia) were success-

Results after Removal of Occluded Lacrimal Stents

Site of Obstruction	Total No. of Removed Stents	Contents in Removed Stents		Outcome of the Lacrimal System after Stent Removal				Obstruction of the Patent System during Follow-up			
				Mucus		Granulation		Mucus		Granulation	
		Mucus	Granulation	Patent	Occluded	Patent	Occluded	Yes	No	Yes	No
Canaliculus lacrimalis	16	1	15	1	0	9	6	0	1	6	3
Lacrimal sac	33	6	27	3	3	14	13	3	0	12	2
Junction	81	38	43	30	8	30	13	25	5	21	9
Nasolacrimal duct	12	4	8	3	1	6	2	1	2	4	2
Total	142	49	93	37	12	59	34	29	8	43	16

fully placed with fluoroscopic guidance in 571 lacrimal systems of 502 patients with epiphora, recurrent dacryocystitis, or both, due to complete obstruction of the lacrimal system. In 142 lacrimal systems of 125 patients, the stents were removed via the nose 2 weeks to 42 months (mean, 7 months) after placement, because of obstruction of the stent. The lacrimal system was then irrigated with saline solution through the lacrimal point (punctum lacrimale). Of the 125 patients, 103 were women and 22 were men; the patients were aged 32–80 years (mean, 56 years).

The sites of obstruction before stent placement were the junction between the lacrimal sac and the nasolacrimal duct in 81 systems, the lacrimal sac in 33, the canaliculus lacrimalis in 16, and the nasolacrimal duct in 12 (Table). We classified the 142 systems into two groups on the basis of the duration of stent placement. Fifty-one systems were classified as the short-duration group, with stents that were removed within 6 months after placement; 91 systems were classified as the long-duration group, with stents that were removed more than 6 months after placement.

Technique of Stent Removal

The stent was removed through the nose by using a hemostat with nasal endoscopic guidance or by using a stent retrieval hook that we made. Immediately after removal of the stent, dacryocystography through the inferior lacrimal point was performed with a 24-gauge needle (Cook) to verify the patency of the lacrimal system. Water-soluble contrast medium (meglumine ioxitalamate, Telebrix 30; Guerbet, Aulnay-sous-Bois, France) was used. The lacrimal system was then irrigated with saline solution through the inferior lacrimal point to wash out possible blood clots or mucoid material. In the last 12 lacrimal systems in our series that showed no patency despite irrigation with saline solution after removal of the stent, the superior lacrimal point was closed off by inserting a punctal dilator (Storz Instrument, St Louis, Mo) to avoid reflux of contrast medium or saline solution through the superior lacrimal point. Dacryocystography and irrigation with saline solution were then performed through a 24-gauge needle placed in the inferior canaliculus lacrimalis or lacrimal sac, with care taken not to cause extravasation. In patients with obstruction of the inferior lacrimal point, dacryocystography and saline irrigation of the lacrimal system were performed through the superior lacrimal point.

Clinical examinations and follow-up dacryocystography were performed 7 days after removal of the stent, to assess the patency of the lacrimal system. Additional clinical examinations and dacryocystography were performed only in patients with a patent lacrimal system 6 months and 1 year after removal of the stent. Thereafter, patients were advised to visit an outpatient clinic if they had a recurrence of symptoms, and all patients were contacted by telephone every 6 months to obtain information about epiphora.

Interpretation of Results

The overall initial patency rate and the maintained patency rate were analyzed in the 142 lacrimal systems (125 patients). Initial patency of the lacrimal system was defined as the flow of contrast medium through the lacrimal system into the inferior meatus of the nasal cavity as seen on dacryocystograms obtained immediately after stent removal. Maintained patency of the lacrimal system was defined as improvement in epiphora and patency of the lacrimal system on follow-up dacryocystograms. Therefore, for the evaluation of the maintained patency rate, we excluded lacrimal systems that showed no improvement in epiphora after removal of the stent or showed occlusion of the lacrimal system 7 days after removal of the stent.

We evaluated the results to determine whether the sites of obstruction before stent placement, the material that occluded the stent (granulation tissue or mucoid material), and the duration of stent placement (short- or long-duration group) made a difference in patency rate. The differences in initial patency rate between each group were evaluated with the χ^2 test. The long-term results were evaluated by using the Kaplan-Meier method to calculate the cumulative patency rates. The maintained patency rates in each group were compared with the Mantel-Haenszel χ^2 test.

RESULTS

Technical Results

Removal of the stent was well tolerated in all patients. No major complications occurred. The majority of patients had slightly bloodstained nasal discharge for 1 to 48 hours after the procedure, but this discharge stopped spontaneously. Mild epistaxis occurred in one patient and was controlled by means of a nasal pack. There was mucoid material in 49 removed stents and granulation tissue in the remaining 93 stents.

Initial Patency

Immediately after removal of the stents, 96 (68%) of the 142 lacrimal systems became patent (Fig 1), and the remaining 46 (32%) systems showed no patency (Fig 2). The causes of nonpatency after stent removal were obstruction of the common canaliculus lacrimalis in eight systems, stent placement through a false tract created owing to technical error in 16 systems, and material in the dilated lacrimal

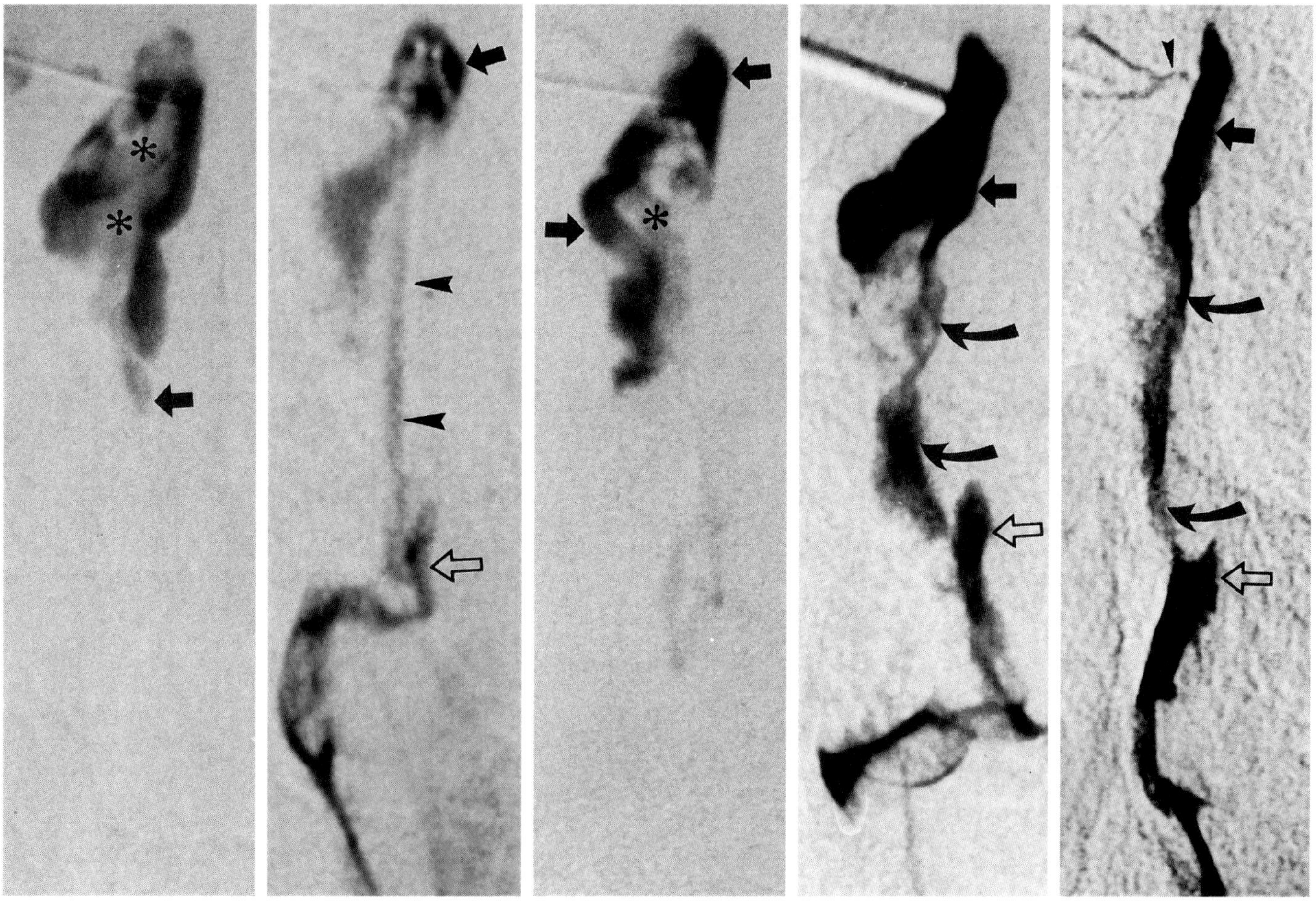

Figure 1. Subtraction dacryocystograms of a patent right lacrimal system after stent removal. **(a)** Complete obstruction at the junction (arrow) between the lacrimal sac and nasolacrimal duct and an irregular filling defect (*) due to mucoid material in the dilated lacrimal sac are seen. **(b)** Two months after stent placement, good passage of contrast medium through the stent (arrowheads) is seen from the upper portion of the lacrimal sac (solid arrow) to the inferior meatus of the nasal cavity (open arrow). **(c)** Eight months after stent placement, occlusion of the stent is seen, with an irregular filling defect (*) in the dilated lacrimal sac (arrows). **(d)** Immediately after stent removal, a patent lacrimal system is seen. The lacrimal sac (solid straight arrow), nasolacrimal duct (curved arrows), and inferior meatus of the nasal cavity (open arrow) are shown. **(e)** Two years after stent removal, a normal right lacrimal system is seen. Arrowhead = common canaliculus lacrimalis, open arrow = inferior meatus of the nasal cavity, solid straight arrow = lacrimal sac, curved arrows = nasolacrimal duct.

sac in the remaining 22 systems. Of the 12 lacrimal systems in which the superior lacrimal point was closed off by inserting a punctal dilator to avoid reflux of contrast medium or saline solution, five became patent.

The initial patency rates were 76% (37 of 49 systems) in the lacrimal systems in which the stent was occluded with mucoid material and 63% (59 of 93 systems) in those in which the stent was occluded with granulation tissue. Although the patency rate in the mucoid material group was slightly higher than that in the granulation tissue group, there was no significant difference between the two (P = .928).

As for the sites of obstruction before stent placement, the initial patency rates were 62% (10 of 16 systems) in the canaliculus lacrimalis, 52% (17 of 33 systems) in the lacrimal sac, 74% (60 of 81 systems) in the junction between the lacrimal sac and the nasolacrimal duct, and 75% (nine of 12 systems) in the nasolacrimal duct. There was no significant difference among the sites of obstruction (P = .116).

Maintained Patency

Twenty-three of 96 systems with initial patency showed no improvement in epiphora after removal of the stent and repeated occlusion of the lacrimal system at 7-day follow-up dacryocystography. In the remaining 73 systems, initial patency of the lacrimal system was maintained at 7-day follow-up dacryocystography, with improvement in epiphora. Among the 73 systems with maintained patency, reobstruction occurred in 48 systems during the first 6 months. Reobstruction occurred in one more lacrimal system during the second 6 months, which resulted in a 1-year patency rate of 33% (24 of 73 systems). This rate was unchanged at the 3-year follow-up. The cumulative patency rate appeared to plateau at 33% 28 weeks after removal of the stent (Fig 3).

The mean patency period of the long-duration group (70.1 weeks) was longer than that of the short-duration group (37.8 weeks), but this difference was not significant (P = .19) (Fig 4). There was also no significant difference (P = .31) in patency rates between the granulation tissue group and mucoid material group. The mean patency period was 49.4 weeks in the granulation tissue group and 54.5 weeks in the mucoid material group (Fig 5). Although the patency rates for the canaliculus lacrimalis group and the nasolacrimal duct group were higher than those for the lacrimal sac–nasolacrimal duct junction group and the lacrimal sac group, there also was no significant difference between them (P = .20) (Fig 6).

Treatment after Stent Removal

During a mean follow-up of 22 months (range, 2 weeks to 49 months) after removal of the stent, 24 of 142 systems needed no further treatment because obstruction of the lacrimal system and epiphora did not recur. In the remaining 118 systems with obstruction immediately after stent removal or during follow-up, a second stent was placed in 102, dacryocystorhinostomy was performed in six, and no further treatment was performed in the remaining 10 (which were in patients with low-grade epiphora with severe mucopurulent discharge before stent placement) because the resultant low-grade epiphora with improved mucopurulent discharge was not troublesome to the patients.

DISCUSSION

Fluoroscopically guided balloon dacryocystoplasty has been reported (10–15) to be a safe, easy nonsurgical treatment, with no major complications for complete or partial obstruction of the lacrimal system. Six-month patency rates of 20%–56% after this procedure, however, have not been encouraging in cases of complete obstruction of the lacrimal system (12–15). Lee et al (13) performed balloon dacryocystoplasty in 57 completely obstructed lacrimal systems. After the procedure, 54 (95%) of the 57 systems were seen to be patent on dacryocystograms obtained immediately afterward. Patency was maintained, with improvement of epiphora in 29 (54%) of these 54 patent systems at 7-day follow-up dacryocystography and in 11 (20%) systems at 6-month follow-up dacryocystography.

Of the 589 lacrimal systems in 513 patients treated at our institution because of complete obstruction of the lacrimal system, 571 (97%) systems showed a patent lacrimal system with improvement of epiphora at 7-day follow-up dacryocystography. Of these, 400 (70%) had maintenance of patency of the lacrimal system and improvement of epiphora during the mean follow-up of 28 months. These rates are higher than those associated with balloon dacryocystoplasty. Even in 24 (25%) of 96 systems that were patent after removal of the occluded stent, the epiphora could be treated by irrigating with saline solution; this result is comparable to the 2-year patency rate of balloon dacryocystoplasty reported by Lee et al (13).

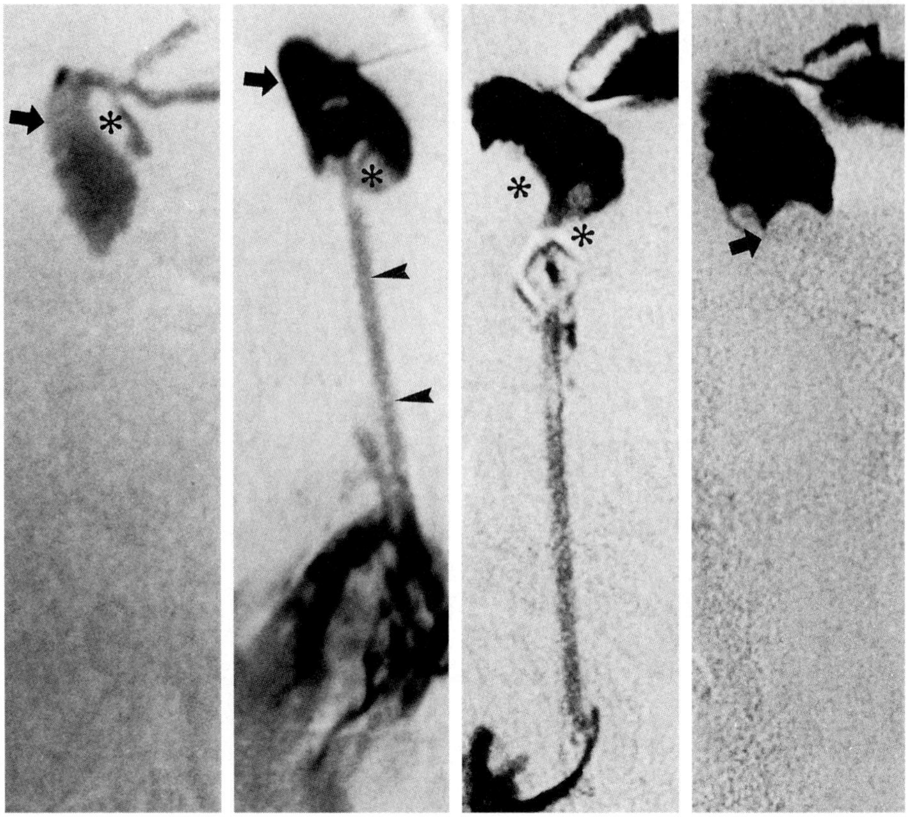

a. b. c. d.

Figure 2. Subtraction dacryocystograms of an obstructed left lacrimal system after stent removal. **(a)** Complete obstruction of the lacrimal system at the left lacrimal sac (arrow) and an irregular filling defect (*) in the dilated lacrimal sac are seen. The nature of the filling defect was not confirmed. **(b)** Immediately after stent placement, good flow of contrast medium through the stent (arrowheads) is seen, with a filling defect (*) at the bottom of the dilated lacrimal sac (arrow). **(c)** One year after stent placement, partial obstruction of the stent is seen, with an enlarged filling defect (*). **(d)** Immediately after stent removal, obstruction (arrow) of the left lacrimal system is seen.

The obstructive material identified on dacryocystograms obtained before and after stent removal could be blood clots, stones, impacted mucus, or a combination of these. Five of the 12 lacrimal systems in which dacryocystography showed no patency immediately after removal of the occluded stents became patent after saline solution irrigation through the inferior lacrimal point while the superior lacrimal point was closed off with a punctal dilator. We believe that some mucous debris or blood clots that were impacted in the lacrimal systems were flushed from the lacrimal system during saline solution irrigation. In patients with an obstructed lacrimal system after stent removal, it is now our policy to irrigate the lacrimal system vigorously with water-soluble contrast medium and then with saline solution through the inferior lacrimal point while the superior lacrimal point is occluded with a punctal dilator.

Dacryolithiasis has been considered an important cause of lacrimal obstruction and may cause recurrent dacryocystitis and mucopurulent discharge (16). Some investigators have reported that dacryolithiasis is associated with chronic dacryocystitis in 10%–30% of cases (17–19) and that the dacryoliths are likely to be fragmented (19,20). In our series, dacryoliths were detected in only three patients (<1%). The dacryoliths were radiopaque in one case and radiolucent in the other two cases. The radiopaque dacryoliths

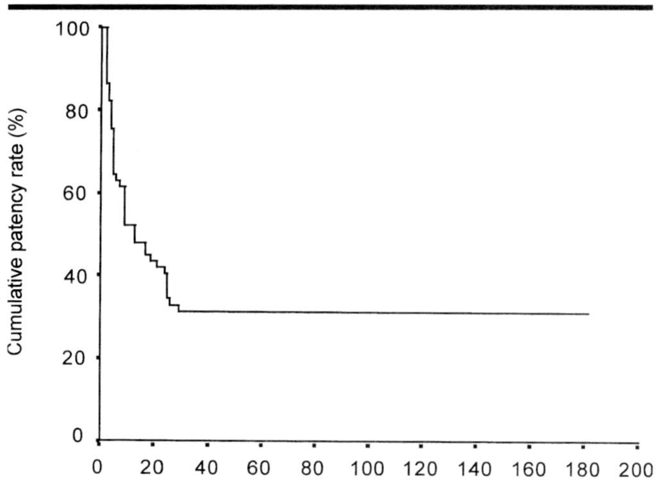

Figure 3. Curve shows the cumulative patency rate in 73 lacrimal systems during follow-up. The curve appears to plateau at 28 weeks after the removal of the occluded stents.

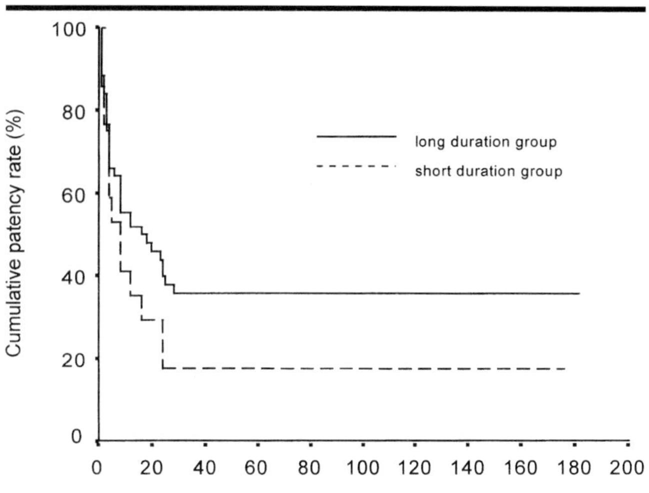

Figure 4. Curves show the difference in cumulative patency rates between the short-duration group and long-duration group.

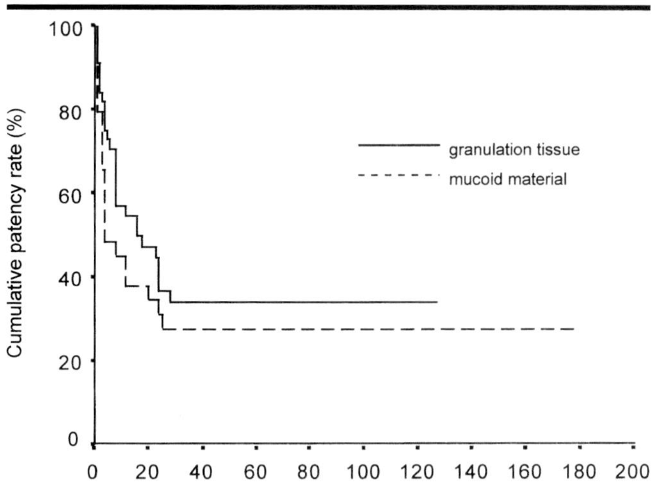

Figure 5. Curves show the difference in cumulative patency rates between the granulation tissue group and mucoid material group.

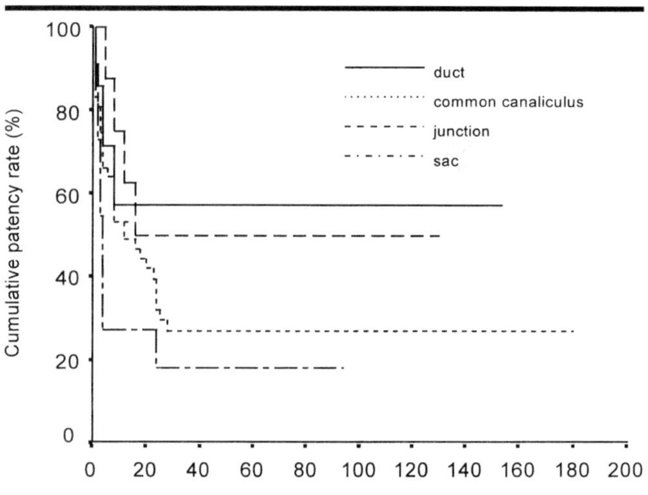

Figure 6. Curves show the cumulative patency rates according to the sites of obstruction.

were slowly broken into fragments from the moment that the guide wire was inserted until the sheath was withdrawn (7). The fragmented dacryoliths were passed through the stent into the pharynx, and the lacrimal system was irrigated with saline solution after the procedure. In the two cases of radiolucent dacryoliths, the dacryoliths were found during dacryocystorhinostomy, which was performed to treat recurrent epiphora after stent placement. We surmise that most dacryoliths are radiolucent and that there must have been more dacryoliths in our series that were removed partially or completely during stent placement without our being aware of their removal. Dacryocystorhinostomy, however, could be a better option than stent placement in patients with dacryoliths.

The proximal end ("mushroom" portion) of the stent used in this study has an outer diameter of 5 mm, and the body portion has an outer diameter of 2 mm (6-F) and an inner diameter of 1.5 mm. We believe that a 1.5-mm inner diameter is sufficient for the drainage of tears but not for the drainage of impacted mucus, dacryoliths, or blood clots. After removal of the stent, the diameter of the lacrimal system might be dilated to 2 mm, which is not sufficient for drainage of the materials. This problem seems to be solved by using a stent with a larger inner diameter. We are testing new stent designs with an inner diameter of 2–4 mm.

Among the 571 systems with successful placement, we retrospectively found that the stent was placed in a false tract created through the submucosa or periosteum of the lacrimal system in 16 systems. Seven of the 16 systems showed no resolution of epiphora after stent placement, and the remaining nine showed complete or partial resolution. All nine systems with improvement showed recurrence of epiphora due to obstruction of the stent less than 6 months after stent placement. After removal of the stent, all nine showed no patency of the lacrimal system. Therefore, it is important not to create a false tract while negotiating a guide wire through the obstructed lumen of the lacrimal system.

Ilgit et al (15) used a 20-gauge, soft, plastic, arterial sheath to negotiate a 0.016-inch guide wire through an obstruction of the lacrimal system during balloon dacryocystoplasty. They failed to cross the obstruction in 15 of 61 cases, but they did not experience any cases of a false tract. We agree that a false tract could be prevented by using a 0.016-inch guide wire and a 20-gauge, soft, plastic, arterial sheath.

In conclusion, the removal of an occluded lacrimal plastic stent is easy and safe. Recurrence of epiphora after placement of lacrimal plastic stents was treated by removing the occluded stents and irrigating with saline solution through the lacrimal point in 33% of cases, with the result of a patent lacrimal system after stent removal.

References

1. Song HY, Ahn HS, Park CK, Kwon SH, Kim CS, Choi KC. Complete obstruction of the nasolacrimal system. II. Treatment with expandable metallic stents. Radiology 1993; 186:372–376.
2. Ilgit ET, Yuksel D, Unal M, Akpek S, Isik S. Treatment of recurrent nasolacrimal duct obstructions with balloon-expandable metallic stents: results of early experience. AJNR 1996; 17:657–663.
3. Song HY, Jin YH, Kim JH, Sung KB, Han YM, Cho NC. Nasolacrimal duct obstruction treated nonsurgically with use of plastic stents. Radiology 1994; 190:535–539.
4. Song HY, Jin YH, Kim JH, et al. Nonsurgical placement of a nasolacrimal polyurethane stent. Radiology 1995; 194:233–237.
5. Song HY, Lee CO, Park S, et al. Nonsurgical placement of a nasolacrimal polyurethane stent: long-term effectiveness. Radiology 1996; 200:759–763.
6. Song HY, Lee CO, Park S, et al. Lacrimal canaliculus obstruction: nonsurgical treatment with a newly designed polyurethane stent. Radiology 1996; 199:280–282.
7. Song HY, Jin YH, Lee HK, Sung KB. Nonoperative management of dacryolithiasis. JVIR 1995; 6:647–650.
8. Pulido-Duque JM, Reyes R, Pinana C, et al. Epiphora: treatment with polyurethane stents (abstr). Cardiovasc Intervent Radiol 1997; 20(suppl 1):99.
9. Song HY. Interventional techniques in the lacrimal system. In: Castaneda-Zuniga WR, ed. Interventional radiology. 3rd ed. Baltimore, Md: Williams & Wilkins, 1997; 1679–1690.
10. Becker BB, Berry FD. Balloon catheter dilatation in lacrimal surgery. Ophthalmic Surg 1989; 20:193–198.
11. Munk PL, Lin DTC, Morris DC. Epiphora: treatment by means of dacryocystoplasty with balloon dilation of the nasolacrimal drainage apparatus. Radiology 1990; 177: 687–690.
12. Song HY, Ahn HS, Park CK, Kwon SH, Kim CS, Choi KC. Complete obstruction of the nasolacrimal system. I. Treatment with balloon dilatation. Radiology 1993; 186: 367–371.
13. Lee JM, Song HY, Han YM, et al. Balloon dacryocystoplasty: results in the treatment of complete and partial obstructions of the nasolacrimal system. Radiology 1994; 192:503–508.
14. Song HY, Lee CO, Park S, et al. Lacrimal canalicular obstructions: safety and effectiveness of balloon dilation. JVIR 1996; 7:929–934.
15. Ilgit ET, Yuksel D, Unal M, Akpek S, Isik S, Hasanreisoglu B. Transluminal balloon dilatation of the lacrimal drainage system for the treatment of epiphora. AJR 1995; 165:1517–1524.
16. Baratz KH, Bartley GB, Campbell RJ, Garrity JA. An eyelash nidus for dacryoliths of the lacrimal excretory and secretory systems. Am J Ophthalmol 1991; 111:624–627.
17. Berlin AJ, Rath R, Rich L. Lacrimal system dacryoliths. Ophthalmic Surg 1980; 11: 435–436.
18. Maltzman BA, Favetta JR. Dacryolithiasis. Ann Ophthalmol 1979; 11:473–475.
19. Wilkins RB, Pressly JP. Diagnosis and incidence of lacrimal calculi. Ophthalmic Surg 1980; 11:787–789.
20. Jones LT. Tear-sac foreign bodies. Am J Ophthalmol 1965; 60:111–113.

James J. Abrahams, MD

Index terms:
Computed tomography (CT), guidance, 279.1261
Neck, biopsy, 20.1261
Pharynx, biopsy, 279.1261
Pharynx, CT, 279.1211
Pharynx, neoplasms, 279.3

Radiology 1998; 208:695–699

[1] From the Department of Diagnostic Radiology, Yale University School of Medicine, 333 Cedar St, New Haven, CT 06520-8042. Received October 24, 1997; revision requested January 5, 1998; final revision received March 17; accepted April 28. **Address reprint requests to** the author.

Author contribution:
Guarantor of integrity of entire study, J.J.A.

Mandibular Sigmoid Notch: A Window for CT-guided Biopsies of Lesions in the Peripharyngeal and Skull Base Regions[1]

Biopsy of lesions in the peripharyngeal and skull base regions frequently is difficult with standard computed tomography–guided retromandibular and retromaxillary approaches. An alternative approach via the mandibular sigmoid notch (concave superior margin of the mandibular ramus) was used in 13 patients. It provided easy access to deep lesions and to areas such as the skull base and clivus, which are unapproachable with other methods.

Biopsy of parapharyngeal, masticator, retropharyngeal, carotid space, and skull base abnormalities is frequently challenging with fine-needle-aspiration or core-biopsy techniques because of the deep, central location of these lesions and the intervening osseous structures that surround them: the maxilla, mandible, and vertebral body.

To improve access to this region for computed tomographic (CT)-guided needle biopsy, I developed a technique in which a needle is inserted through the sigmoid notch of the mandible. The sigmoid notch is the concave, semicircular, superior border of the mandibular ramus that is bordered anteriorly by the coronoid process and posteriorly by the condyle (1) (Fig 1). The zygomatic arch runs in an anteroposterior direction just superior to the sigmoid notch and thus forms a window through which a needle can be inserted to gain access to the deeper, more medial regions. The borders of this window, therefore, are the zygomatic arch superiorly, coronoid process anteriorly, condyle posteriorly, and sigmoid notch inferiorly. The window is easily identified at CT as the space between the coronoid process and the condyle of the mandible (Fig 2b). This technique is potentially advantageous because it is simple, allows all regions to be approached from one entry point (rather than from different approaches for different regions), and may permit access to areas that were previously unapproachable (Fig 2).

Materials and Methods

CT scans obtained before biopsy in 13 patients (five women and eight men; age range, 54–84 years; mean age, 67 years) were reviewed to determine the various routes by which biopsy could be performed. Lesions in three patients (two clival lesions and one skull base lesion) were considered unapproachable by means of any route except through the sigmoid notch. In the remaining 10 patients, although lesions were approachable by means of standard routes, the sigmoid notch provided a window through which access was more direct and complete.

Written informed consent was obtained from the 13 patients before CT-guided needle biopsy. The patients were draped, and local anesthesia was provided with 1% lidocaine hydrochloride. Eleven patients were supine, and two were in the lateral decubitus position because they were unable to lie flat. In all patients, tape was used to hold their heads in position and prevent motion. A radiopaque marking grid (Fast-find Grid; E-Z-Em, Westbury, NY) was placed on the ipsilateral side of the face to overlie the sigmoid notch. Axial helical CT was performed (HiSpeed Advantage; GE Medical Systems, Milwaukee, Wis) to identify the

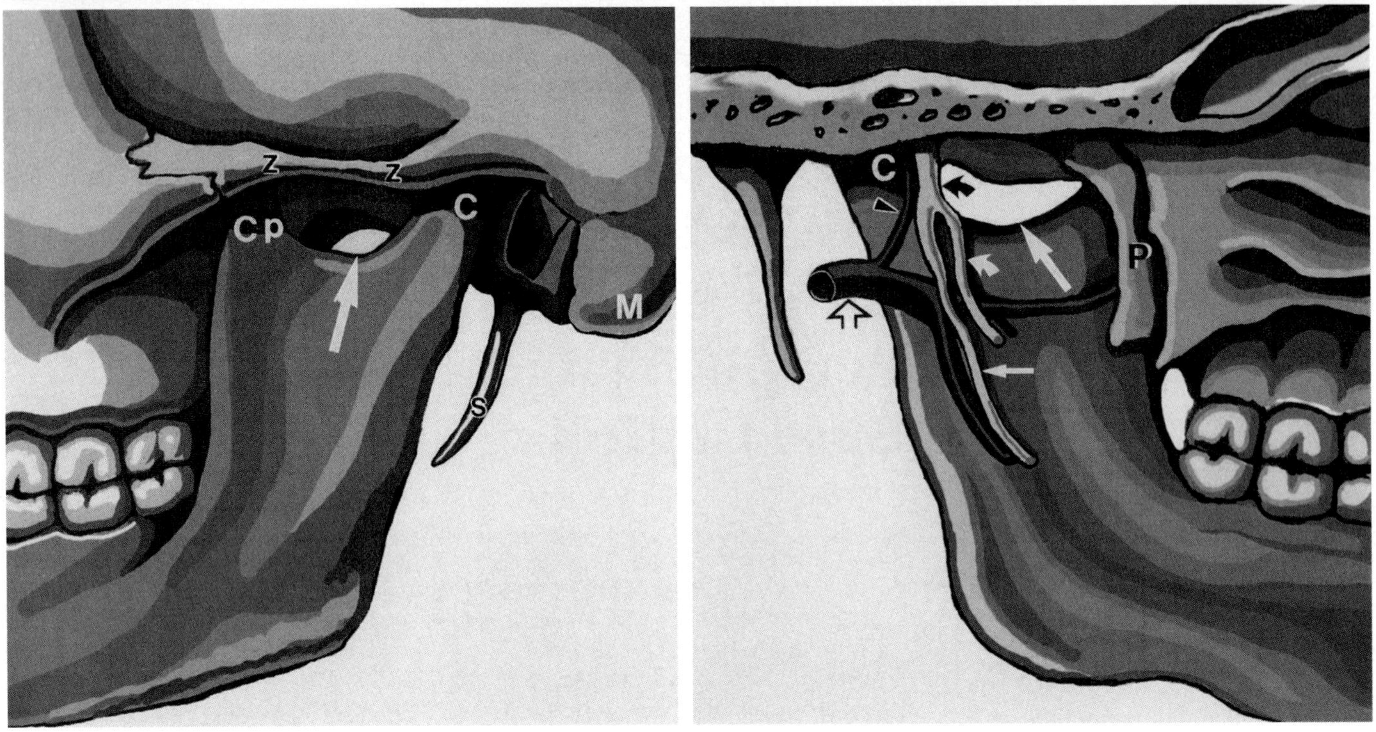

a. b.

Figure 1. Illustrations demonstrate the sigmoid notch and surrounding anatomic features. **(a)** Lateral surface of the mandibular ramus shows the sigmoid notch (arrow) bordered by the coronoid process (*Cp*) anteriorly, condyle (*C*) posteriorly, and zygomatic arch (*Z*) superiorly. *M* = mastoid process, *S* = styloid process. **(b)** Medial surface of the mandibular ramus shows the mandibular branch of the trigeminal nerve (curved black arrow), inferior alveolar nerve (short straight white arrow), lingual nerve (curved white arrow), maxillary artery (open arrow), and middle meningeal artery (arrowhead). The long straight white arrow indicates the sigmoid notch. *C* = condyle, *P* = pterygoid plate.

sigmoid notch and lesion. Five-millimeter-thick sections were imaged through the area of the lesion, and 3-mm-thick sections were imaged in the actual biopsy site. The marks on the grid were used to determine the site of entry, trajectory, and depth for the biopsy.

The sigmoid notch was identified on the axial images, and the grid marks were used to place a mark on the skin that overlay the notch. If the lesion was not in the same plane as the site of entry (sigmoid notch), then after the needle passed through the sigmoid notch, it was angled and advanced toward the lesion by means of axial CT guidance with 3-mm-thick sections over the needle tip. As an alternative, the gantry was placed at an angle and the needle was angled accordingly.

The biopsy needle was pushed through the sigmoid notch, and the needle angle was then corrected to the predetermined trajectory. The needle was advanced into the lesion and its position confirmed with CT. Contrast enhancement frequently was used at initial CT to help localize the carotid artery. Tissue samples were examined by means of cytopathologic, surgical pathologic, or bacteriologic examination, or a combination of the three, and the condition of the patients was followed up (1–3 hours) for possible complications.

The following biopsy needles were used: 18-, 20-, and 22-gauge Franseen needles (Manan Medical Products, Northbrook, Ill); a 20-gauge Green needle (Manan Medical Products); and a 20-gauge Temno coaxial biopsy system (Bauer Medical, Clearwater, Fla). The personal preference of the radiologist who performed the procedure (J.J.A.) determined which needle was used.

Results

The biopsy needle easily traversed the sigmoid notch and was confirmed, by means of CT, to be within the desired lesion in all 13 patients. Lesions involved the skull base in three patients, clivus in three, parapharyngeal region in two, masticatory region in two, retropharyngeal region in one, carotid and parapharyngeal regions in one, and hypoglossal canal and parapharyngeal region in one. Representative examples are shown in Figures 2 and 3.

Lesions included squamous cell carcinoma ($n = 6$), schwannoma ($n = 1$), esthesioneuroblastoma ($n = 1$), mesenchymal neoplasm ($n = 1$), granulation tissue ($n = 1$), malignant mixed salivary tumor ($n = 1$), and inflammation ($n = 2$). Among the 13 patients, results were positive in nine, the diagnosis was incorrect in three, and the amount of tissue obtained was insufficient in one. Although findings in some biopsy specimens did not allow correct diagnosis, the biopsy needle was confirmed by means of CT to be within the lesion and, therefore, access was successful in all 13 patients.

The procedure was tolerated well by all patients, and no immediate complications or unusual patient discomfort occurred. Thus, postprocedure CT was not performed. In one patient, a pseudoaneurysm of the buccal branch of the internal maxillary artery developed 3 months after the procedure. Whether this finding was caused by the biopsy needle or the patient's underlying cancer and irradiation, or a combination of the two, was undetermined. No patient had evidence of manipulation or injury of the mandibular nerve.

Discussion

Three techniques for access to these lesions have been described previously.

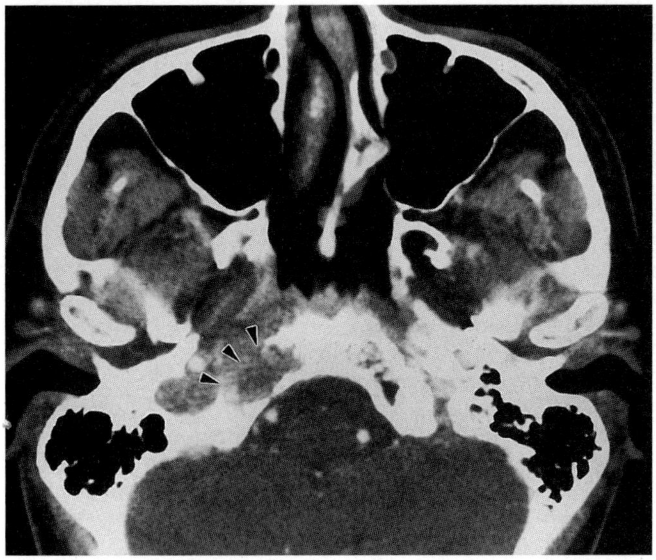

a.

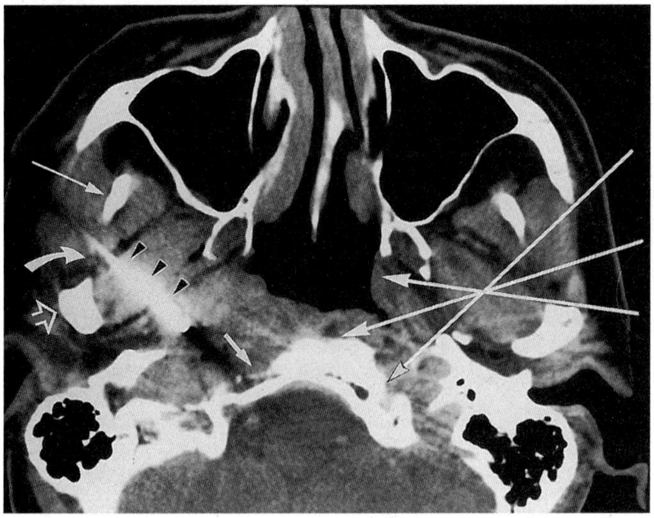

b.

Figure 2. CT-guided biopsy was performed with the sigmoid notch technique in a patient with undifferentiated squamous cell carcinoma that involved the clivus and parapharyngeal space. **(a)** Axial helical CT scan (level, 46 HU; width, 402 HU) demonstrates destruction of the clivus (arrowheads). **(b)** Axial helical CT scan obtained with the same window settings and slightly caudad to **a** demonstrates the biopsy needle (arrowheads) as it traverses the sigmoid notch (curved arrow) and enters the lesion (shortest straight white arrow). This lesion cannot be reached with a retromandibular or retromaxillary approach. The coronoid process (medium straight white arrow) and condyle (open arrow) are seen. On the patient's left, the longest straight white arrows indicate the anterior or posterior angulation of the needle that permits access to multiple areas. Superior and inferior angulation permit farther caudal and cephalic regions to be reached.

They include the peroral transmucosal approach (2); the percutaneous, CT-guided, retromandibular transparotid approach (3) (Fig 4); and the percutaneous, CT-guided, oblique retromaxillary approach (3) (Fig 4). Each of these techniques has its limitations. With the peroral approach, a needle is inserted, without CT guidance, through the pharyngeal mucosa via an open mouth. This approach is blind and is associated with the inherent risks that the lesion would be missed and that unintended structures would be hit and injured. It is also less accurate than the percutaneous CT-guided techniques (2,4–7).

When the retromandibular transparotid approach is used, the parapharyngeal region can be reached by inserting a needle percutaneously between the posterior aspect of the mandible and the mastoid process and then by traversing the parotid gland (Fig 4). Although relatively safe, traversal of the parotid gland may preclude the use of needles with larger bores and is associated with increased risk of injury to the gland, facial nerve, or adjacent vascular structures. This technique, however, is limited by the surrounding anatomic features. Because of the position of the carotid sheath behind the styloid process and the bony mastoid and mandible, it is necessary to angle the needle anteriorly; therefore, the more posterior prevertebral and cephalic skull base regions cannot be reached with this technique.

Last, the retromaxillary approach is also limited by the adjacent anatomic features. It is necessary to angle the needle, which is inserted posteriorly to the maxilla and anteriorly to the mandible, in a posterior trajectory because of the shape of the maxilla (Fig 4). This angulation limits the areas that can be reached with this technique.

To alleviate these problems, this easy method allows biopsy of difficult-to-reach lesions of the peripharyngeal and skull base regions by means of traversal of the sigmoid notch of the mandible. With this technique, a single access point (sigmoid notch) can be used to reach multiple areas, whereas with other methods, different approaches are required for different regions. This access to multiple areas through a single access point is possible because the sigmoid notch window is relatively superficial and allows the needle, once it passes through the window, to be angled easily in an anterior, posterior, cranial, or caudal direction. This ease provides flexibility regarding the areas that can be reached. Use of one approach also allows the development of greater expertise than does the use of several different approaches. With the retromaxillary or retromandibular methods, the needle cannot be angled because of bone constraints.

I found the Temno coaxial biopsy system to be most useful. The coaxial needle was 19 gauge, which provided some rigidity that made angulation of the needle easy after traversal of the sigmoid notch. The biopsy needle itself was 20 gauge, which provided a core of tissue for surgical pathologic study. When this needle was removed, it could be replaced through the 19-gauge coaxial needle with a 20-gauge aspiration needle to provide material for cytopathologic study. Biopsy needles compatible with magnetic resonance (MR) imaging may make this technique possible with MR guidance. Visualization of the bone landmarks, which is important for accurate and safe needle placement, however, is best with CT.

Locating the sigmoid notch is easy. If the index finger is placed just anterior to the external auditory canal, the mandibular condyle can be felt to translocate under the finger as the mouth is opened and closed. By sliding the finger anteriorly along the inferior margin of the zygomatic arch while the jaw is continually opened and closed, the radiologist can soon feel the coronoid process of the mandible slide under the finger. If the finger is then pressed between the condyle and coronoid process, at the inferior margin of the zygomatic arch, a vague depression the size of the index fingertip can be felt. That depression is the sigmoid

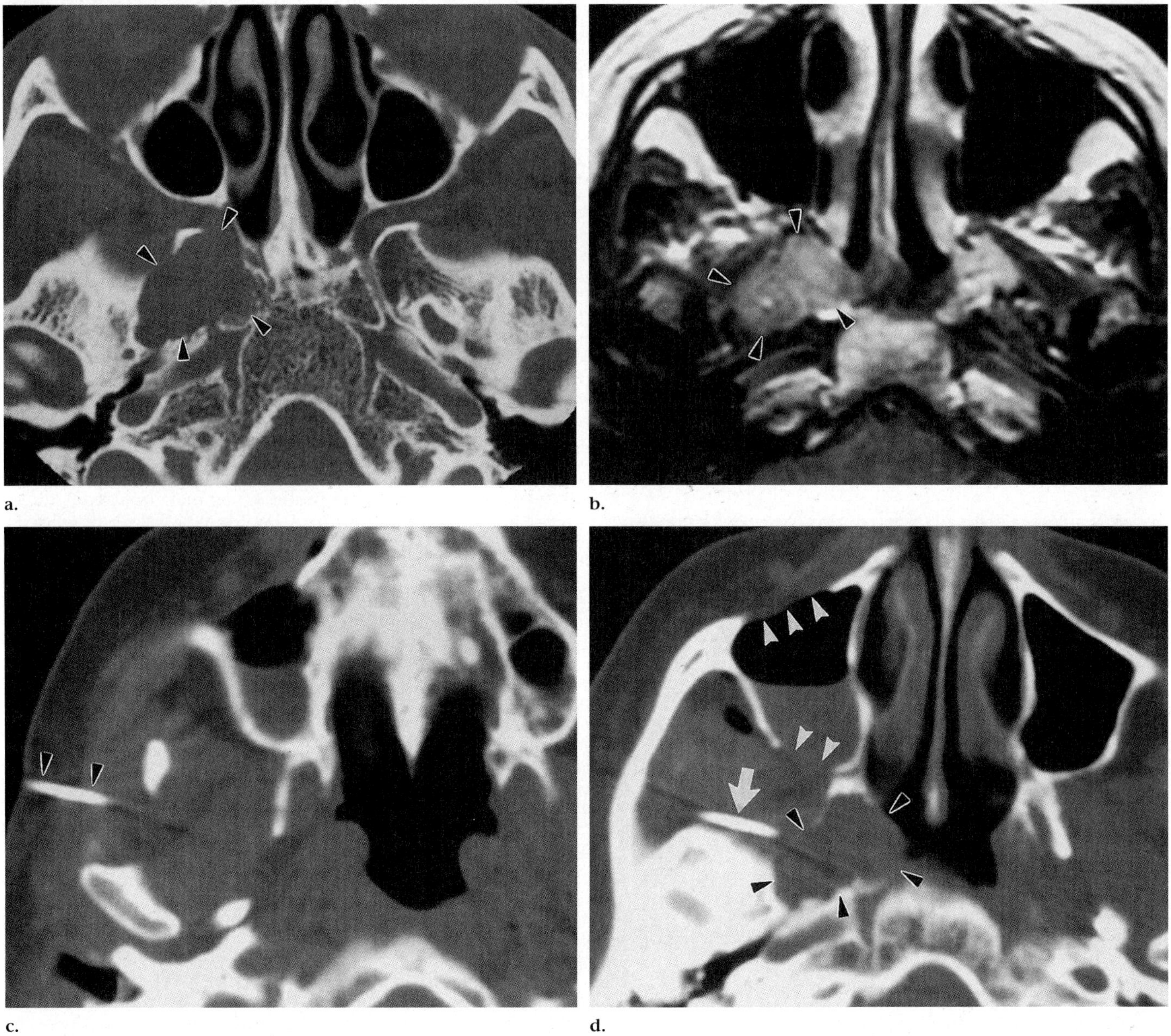

Figure 3. CT-guided needle biopsy of a mesenchymal neoplasm at the skull base was performed with the sigmoid notch technique. **(a)** Axial helical CT scan obtained with bone window settings (level, 87 HU; width, 3,746 HU) demonstrates a destructive lesion (arrowheads) in the skull base. **(b)** Gadolinium-enhanced T1-weighted axial MR image (repetition time, 550 msec; echo time, 25 msec; three signals acquired; 3 × 1-mm section thickness) demonstrates enhancement of the lesion (arrowheads). **(c)** Axial helical CT scan obtained with level of 195 HU and width of 1,316 HU shows a biopsy needle (arrowheads) as it enters the sigmoid notch. **(d)** Axial helical CT scan obtained with the same window settings and cephalad to c shows a biopsy needle (arrow) as it enters the lesion (black arrowheads). A defect in the anterior and posterior walls of the right maxillary sinus (white arrowheads) was caused by an unsuccessful attempt at surgical biopsy. This lesion is unapproachable with other CT-guided techniques.

notch. At axial CT, it is seen at the top of the ramus between the coronoid process and condyle (Fig 2b). If passage of the needle through the sigmoid notch is difficult, the mouth should be opened to widen the window. I found, however, that this maneuver was not necessary.

The major anatomic structures that could be affected with this approach are the mandibular branch of the trigeminal nerve and the carotid artery. The mandibular nerve exits the oval foramen of the sphenoid bone and travels inferior and deep to the posterior aspect of the sigmoid notch to enter the inner surface of the mandibular ramus (Fig 1b). Posterior to this, the middle meningeal artery travels superiorly near the condyle to enter the spinous foramen. Although the mandibular nerve could not be seen, no patient had any symptom related to manipulation or injury of the nerve during or after the procedure; thus, the nerve did not appear to present a problem. Injury to the nerve would be expected to produce sensory alterations in the chin. The carotid artery was easily identified after injection of radiographic contrast material and was thus avoided.

CT-guided biopsies of the peripharyngeal and skull base regions via the man dibular sigmoid notch seem to be advantageous. I found the technique to be easy

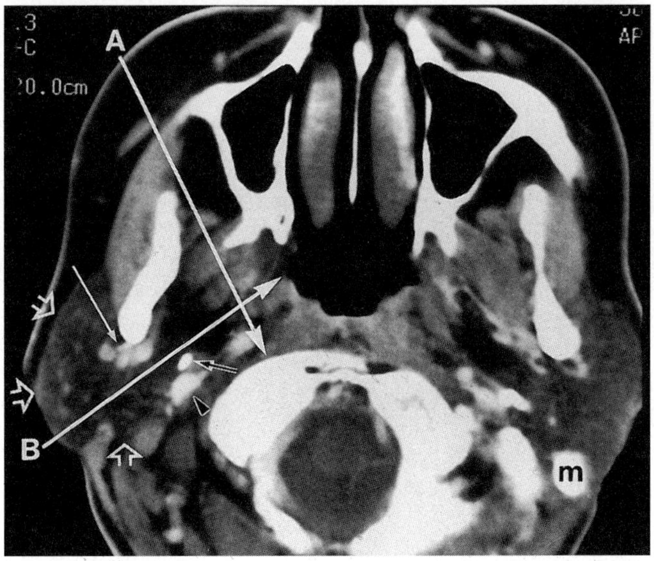

Figure 4. Axial helical CT scan (level, 25/400 HU; width, xxx HU) obtained in a patient without a lesion illustrates retromandibular transparotid and retromaxillary CT-guided biopsy techniques. Arrow *A* represents the needle trajectory for the retromaxillary approach, and arrow *B* represents the trajectory for the retromandibular approach. The following anatomic structures are seen: parotid gland (open arrows), retromandibular vein and facial nerve (white arrow), styloid process (black arrow), carotid artery and jugular vein (arrowhead), and mastoid process (*m*).

and safe and to provide great flexibility because it allowed biopsy of multiple regions through a single entry point. Of greatest importance, however, is that this technique permits access to areas such as the skull base that could not be reached previously.

References

1. Netter FH. Atlas of human anatomy. Summit, NJ: CIBA-Geigy, 1989; 9–11.
2. Mondal A, Raychoudhuri BK. Peroral fine needle aspiration cytology of parapharyngeal lesions. Acta Cytol 1993; 37:694–698.
3. Yousem DM, Sack MJ, Scanlan KA. Biopsy of parapharyngeal space lesions. Radiology 1994; 193:619–622.
4. Das DK, Gulati A, Bhatt NC, et al. Fine needle aspiration cytology of oral and pharyngeal lesions: a study of 45 cases. Acta Cytol 1993; 37:333–342.
5. Castelli M, Gattuso P, Reyes C, Solans EP. Fine needle aspiration biopsy of intraoral and pharyngeal lesions. Acta Cytol 1993; 37:448–450.
6. Meyers DS, Templer J, Davis WE, Balch JA. Aspiration cytology for diagnosis of head and neck masses. Otolaryngology 1978; 86:650–655.
7. Young JEM, Archibald SD, Shier KJ. Needle aspiration cytologic biopsy in head and neck masses. Am J Surg 1981; 142:484–489.

Christian Teissl, MS
Christian Kremser, PhD
Erwin S. Hochmair, PhD
Ingeborg J. Hochmair-Desoyer, PhD

Index terms:
Ear, prostheses, 2133.456
Magnetic resonance (MR), safety

Radiology 1998; 208:700–708

Abbreviations:
FLASH = fast low-angle shot
RARE = rapid acquisition with relaxation enhancement
RF = radio frequency
SE = spin echo

[1] From the Departments of Applied Physics (C.T., E.S.H., I.J.H.D.) and MR Imaging (C.K.), Institut für Angewandte Physik, Universität Innsbruck, Technikerstrasse 25, A-6020 Innsbruck, Austria. From the 1997 RSNA scientific assembly. Received December 2, 1997; revision requested February 23, 1998; revision received March 23; accepted April 28. Supported by Austrian Science Foundation grant P11755-TEC. **Address reprint requests to** C.T.

Author contributions:
Guarantors of integrity of entire study, C.T., C.K., E.S.H., I.J.H.D.; study concepts and design, C.T.; definition of intellectual content, C.T.; literature research, C.T.; experimental studies, C.T.; data acquisition and analysis, C.T.; statistical analysis, C.T.; manuscript preparation, C.T.; manuscript editing and review, C.T., C.K., E.S.H., I.J.H.D.

Cochlear Implants: In Vitro Investigation of Electromagnetic Interference at MR Imaging—Compatibility and Safety Aspects[1]

In vitro experiments were performed to determine the compatibility of a cochlear implant at 0.2- and 1.5-T magnetic resonance (MR) imaging. Except for the torque at 1.5 T, all electromagnetic interferences remained within acceptable limits. MR imaging should be performed only if there is a strong medical indication, by following appropriate safety procedures. MR imaging at 0.2 T should be safe; at 1.5 T, however, the relative risks will have to be assessed.

Cochlear implant systems are an accepted means for the treatment of profound bilateral deafness with direct electrical stimulation of the auditory nerve. The majority of these systems consist of an external sound processing device and the actual implant situated in a milled-out section in the side of the temporal bone (Fig 1a). The implant includes a receiver for reception of stimulation data via a transcutaneous inductive link and circuitry for stimulation via electrodes inserted into the inner ear (Fig 1b).

Currently, approximately 18,000 implants of various designs are used by adults and children worldwide. At some point in their lives, these cochlear implant wearers will most likely become candidates for magnetic resonance (MR) imaging examination, a diagnostic tool with a rapidly increasing range of applications. This makes the investigation of the compatibility of cochlear implants at MR imaging a timely research topic.

The electromagnetic fields appearing during an MR imaging session (static magnetic field, static gradients, switched gradients, radio-frequency [RF] pulses) interfere with the implant. Eddy currents in the conductive elements of the cochlear implant can result in heating accompanied by the hazard of burning of the surrounding tissue. Induced voltages in conductive loops (implant-receiver circuit, stimulation electrodes) due to RF fields can damage the implant. Force and torque on ferromagnetic parts of the implant due to magnetic field gradients and the homogeneous magnetic field can produce pain or impede the functionality of the implant.

Small internal magnets (rare-earth permanent magnets of cylindrical shape, magnetized along the main axis of symmetry, which is normal for the skin) are used to guarantee sufficient transmission quality between the external transmitter and the internal receiver by holding the external transmitter in place (1). The comparatively strong fields of the magnet can result in strong force and torque components and cause artifacts on the MR image (2). Furthermore, the magnet can be demagnetized, resulting in reduced implant functionality.

A series of different studies deal with the electromagnetic interferences between the fields generated in the MR imager and biomedical implants (2–10). Owing to the variety of interferences and existing MR equipment and implant types, these studies concentrate on certain specific topics such as displacement, deflection force, torque, or induced voltage.

The aim of this study was to determine the whole range of electromagnetic interferences of a multichannel cochlear implant system within a wide range of clinical MR imaging applications. Therefore, in vitro experiments were performed on 0.2- and 1.5-T MR imagers. RF sequences, RF absorption rates, and geometric positions were varied to determine the worst-case scenarios for the implant.

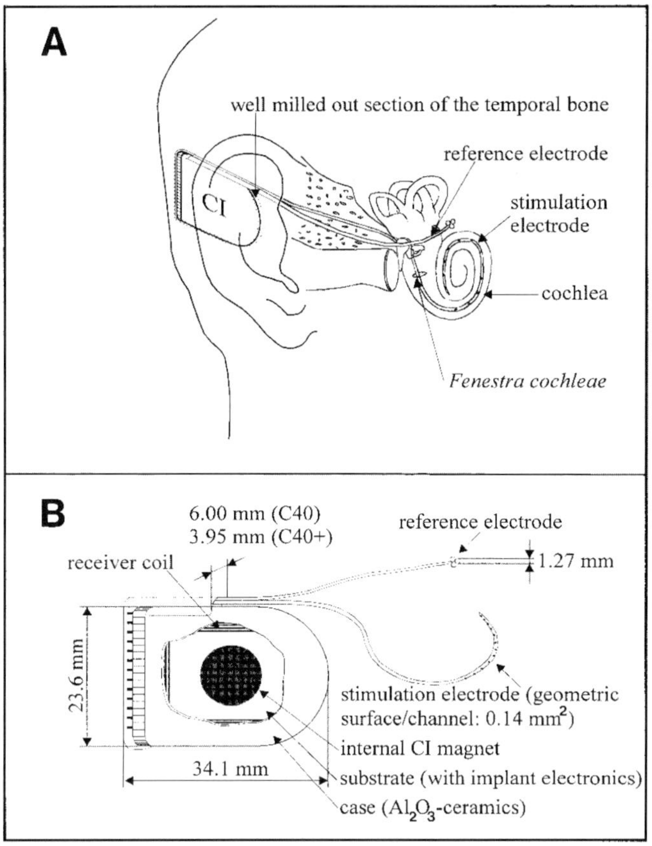

Figure 1. *A*, Schematic drawing of the clinical situation of an implanted cochlear implant (*CI*). The implant is placed in a milled-out well in the side of the temporal bone. The stimulation electrode is inserted into the cochlea, and the reference electrode is placed within the temporal muscle. The implant is fixed (eg, with some sutures), then the soft flap is sutured over the implant. *B*, Schematic drawing of the multichannel cochlear implant (*CI*) systems (*C40, C40+*) used in this study.

Materials and Methods

The MR imagers used in this study were a 0.2-T imager (Magnetom Open Viva; Siemens Medical Systems, Erlangen, Germany) and a 1.5-T imager (Magnetom Vision [active shielded magnet]; Siemens Medical Systems).

The cochlear implant tested was the Combi 40/40+ multichannel system (MedEl, Innsbruck, Austria) (11). In this type of cochlear implant, an amplitude-keyed, digital signal is received by a coil (center frequency tuned to 12 MHz; C40 receiver coil, seven concentrated windings, active total area, 2,100 mm^2; C40+ receiver coil, nine distributed windings, active total area, 2,130 mm^2). The plane of the coil is approximately parallel to the skin. Both stimulation information (selection of channel, stimulation pulse length and level) and supply voltage are derived from the received signal. The demodulated signal is processed by a microprocessor and triggers the current source for stimulation. Excitable tissue in the inner ear is stimulated by current pulses generated by the implant electronics. The stimulating current flows back to the implant via the implanted electrode contacts, the tissue, and the reference electrode.

For the present study, the electromagnetic interference between the cochlear implant and the MR imager was determined. The removable external transmitter and the external speech processor are removed from the patient. Therefore, the patient is unable to hear during the MR imaging examination. This inconvenience is outweighed, however, by the benefit of removing additional electromagnetic interference between the device and the MR unit (eg, the electromagnetic interference with the microphone and the external processor can influence the processed signal, which may lead to overstimulation). The electromagnetic radiation of the external speech processor can interfere with the weak nuclear MR signal and affect the detected signal from the MR receiver.

The following experiments were performed: (*a*) evaluation of artifact (0.2 and 1.5 T); (*b*) evaluation of demagnetization (1.5 T); (*c*) evaluation of movement, force, and torque (0.2 and 1.5 T); (*d*) temperature measurement (1.5 T); (*e*) induced voltages due to switched gradients (1.5 T) or RF (0.2 and 1.5 T); (*f*) performance test (0.2 and 1.5 T).

Evaluation of Artifacts at 0.2 and 1.5 T

Several micro–test plates (96 microtubes per plate) were filled with contrast medium solution (0.0001 mmol/mL gadodiamide, Omniscan; Nycomed, Oslo, Norway) and stacked on top of each other. They were then placed in the load phantom and positioned in the center of the head coil. Multisection two-dimensional spin-echo (SE) sequences (repetition time msec/echo time msec = 700/15; coronal orientation; section thickness, 4 mm; intersection gap, 12.6 mm; field of view, 150 × 150 mm; matrix, 256 × 256) were used for image acquisition. Vectors $\mathbf{V}_1$ and $\mathbf{V}_2$ were assigned with the help of the coronal MR images to each microtube before ($\mathbf{V}_1$) or after ($\mathbf{V}_2$) adding the internal magnet of the cochlear implant (the magnetic moment *m* of the internal magnet of the cochlear implant was orientated as in a clinical situation). The difference vectors, $\Delta\mathbf{V} = \mathbf{V}_2 - \mathbf{V}_1$, a measure for the distortion due to the field inhomogeneity, were calculated.

A specific region was called a "void" if it showed a pronounced reduction in contrast compared with that in undisturbed areas of the image.

Evaluation of Demagnetization at 1.5 T

Internal magnets, fastened on a plastic mounting in the center line of the main magnetic field, were moved several times into and out of the main magnetic field (magnetic moment in the x direction, usual head position; in the y direction, head turned 90° to the side; parallel and antiparallel [worst case] to the z direction). The magnetic field strength of the internal magnets before and after exposure to the main magnetic field was detected by means of Hall measurements.

Movement, Force, and Torque

Movement.—All individual elements of the cochlear implant were tested for deflection force during movement into the magnetic field and within the field of the imager. A method similar to that described in reference 4 was performed. Each element was placed in a transparent plastic box containing a ruler for position measurement. The box was smoothly moved into the magnetic field of the imager on the transport platform. Any displacement of the cochlear implant parts was recorded.

Force and torque.—The magnetic moment (m) of the internal magnet was determined with $m = T/B$, where T is the torque on the internal magnet determined by means of a balance condition (T in balance with a known mechanical torque) and B is the known magnetic field strength of a test field. Then, the distribution of the magnetic field B of the 1.5-T imager was measured with a magnetic field probe (F.W. Bell, Orlando, Fla). From these data, the spatial derivative of the field B was calculated.

The force (F) on the internal magnet was calculated with $F = \Delta(mB)$. The magnitude of the torque (T_1) on the internal magnet is given with $T_1 = mB \sin\phi$, where ϕ is the angle between m and B.

Temperature Measurement at 1.5 T

A thin layer of phosphorus material was placed on the reference electrode. The fluorescence signal of this phosphorus material has a variable decay time dependent on the ambient temperature. This signal was transmitted outside the RF cabin via an optical fiber to a calibrated thermometer (Fluoroptic, model 710; Luxtron, Mountain View, Calif) (12).

The measurement was carried out with a functioning implant, fixed on a head phantom. The reference electrode and the stimulation electrode were embedded in a piece of fresh meat (beef; dimensions, 100 × 100 × 20 mm) to simulate tissue impedance. The orientation of the loop formed by the cochlear implant, stimulation electrode, tissue, and reference electrode was sagittal (worst-case orientation). The surface temperature of the sample was measured during repeated turbo SE and half-Fourier rapid acquisition with relaxation enhancement (RARE) (HASTE; Siemens Medical Systems) sequences. Repetition time, echo spacing, and number of sections were selected to achieve a high specific absorption rate corresponding to that of the first level operating mode (13).

Induced Voltage Measurement

The induced voltage was converted into an optical signal at the test points by means of a specially designed, electro-optical transducer. The transducer was shielded with an aluminum box. The optical signal was transmitted via an optical fiber to an optical detector located outside the RF cabin, where it was converted to an electrical signal and amplified. The output signal of the optical detector was displayed by means of a digital storage oscilloscope. The setup was calibrated outside the RF cabin with RF pulses of known amplitude, which enabled absolute voltage measurements owing to the relation between the output signal and the RF voltage at the input of the electro-optical transducer. A schematic drawing of the induced voltage measurement setup is shown in Figure 2. The detection limit was 20 mV peak to peak; the time resolution was 5 μsec. The following voltage measurements were performed.

RF-induced voltage in the receiver circuit of the cochlear implant at 0.2 and 1.5 T.—The induced voltage was measured at the parallel resonant circuit of the implant receiver. The parallel resonant circuit was fixed on a head or body phantom; the orientation of the receiver coil of the cochlear implant was as in a real patient situation during MR imaging (sagittal). This was the worst-case orientation, because the magnetic field vector of the RF is perpendicular to the surface of the cochlear implant coil giving the largest induced voltage. With the 0.2-T imager, the head coil was used for RF transmission. To detect the maximum induced peak voltage, sequences were used that contained pulses with high RF peak amplitudes as 180° pulses in SE sequences and pulse trains of very short 180° pulses in turbo SE sequences. With the 1.5-T imager, both the head and body resonators were used for RF transmission. In addition to the SE and turbo SE sequences, sequences containing saturation pulses and adiabatic inversion pulses were used.

RF-induced voltage in the electrode loop at 1.5 T.—The induced voltage was detected between the stimulation electrode and the ground electrode. The implant, the electrode array, and the reference electrode were fastened within a plastic box; the electrodes were immersed in NaCl solution. This arrangement was fixed to a head phantom. The plane orientation of

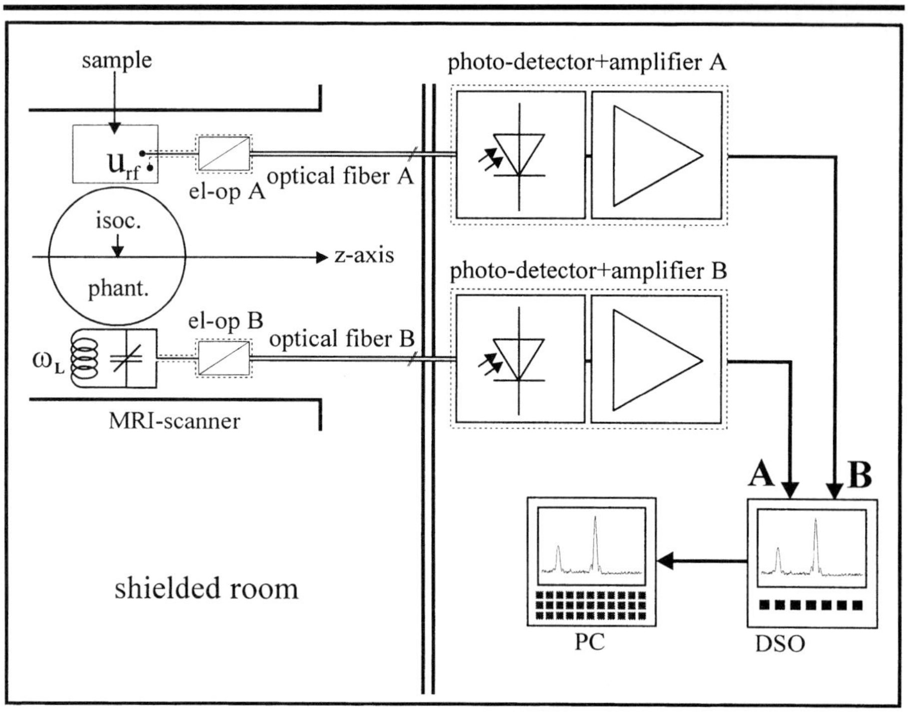

Figure 2. Arrangement for the measurement of the induced voltage. The induced voltage, u_{rf}, was converted into an optical signal by means of a shielded electro-optical (*el-op*) transducer (*el-op A*). The optical signal was transmitted via an optical fiber to a photo detector located outside of the shielded room. The detected signal was amplified and displayed by means of a storage oscilloscope (digital storage oscilloscope [*DSO*]). The measured signal was mapped with a calibration curve to the corresponding RF signal by using a personal computer (*PC*). As a trigger source, the induced voltage in a parallel resonant circuit (tuned to the Larmor frequency, ω_L) was used. *isoc.* = isocenter, *phant.* = phantom.

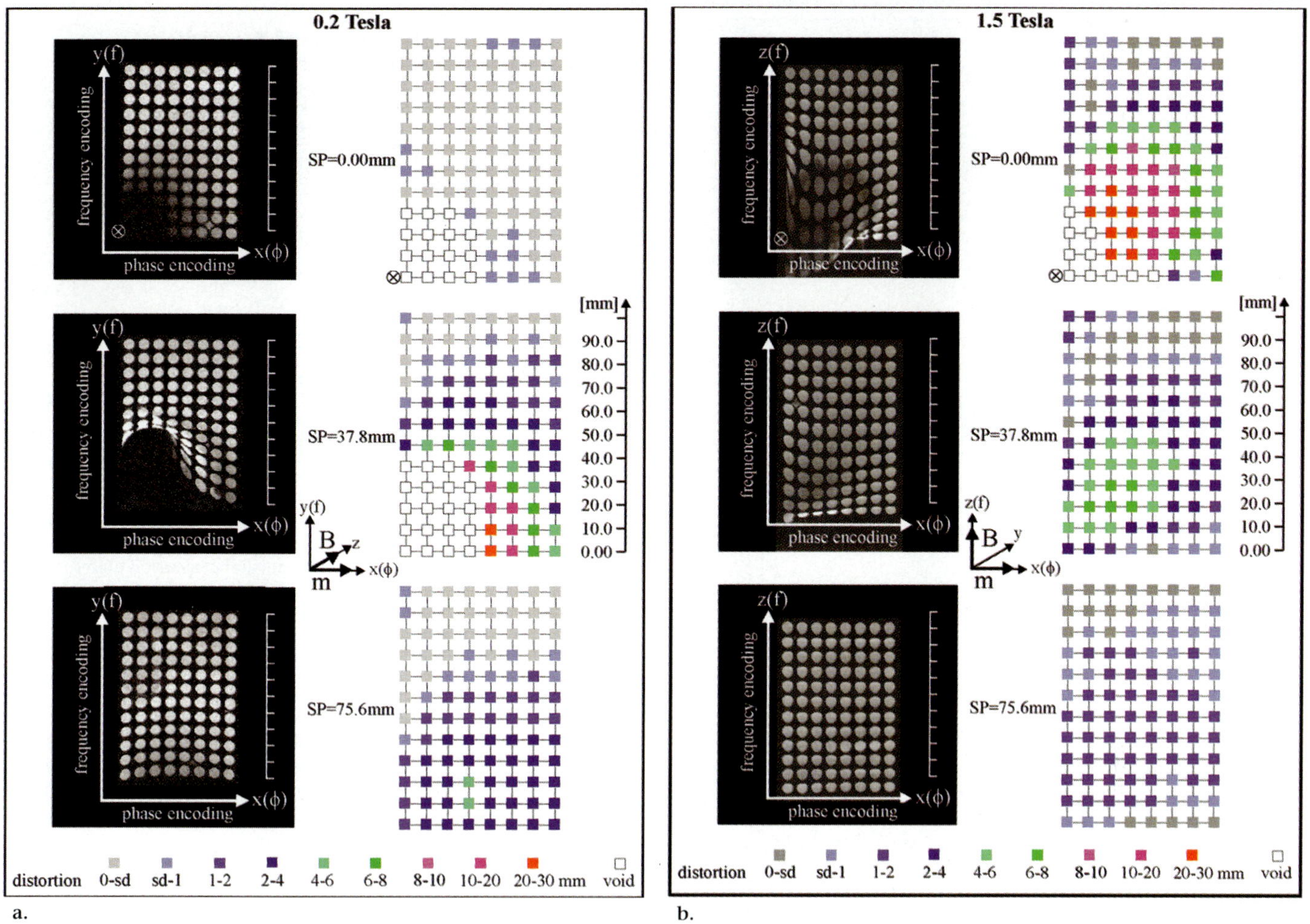

Figure 3. **(a)** Coronal images of a periodic structure (several micro–test plates stacked on top of each other) were obtained with SE sequences and a 0.2-T MR imager. A color-coded graphic representation of the distortions can be found to the right of each MR image. The respective colored square gives the value of the distortion vector generated at this distance from the internal magnet of the cochlear implant. The orientation of the main magnetic field (*B*) of the imager and the orientation of the magnetic moment (*m*) of the internal magnet of the cochlear implant are indicated. **(b)** Coronal images of a periodic structure were obtained with SE sequences and a 1.5-T MR imager. *sd* = standard deviation, *SP* = section position, ⊗ = position of the internal magnet of the cochlear implant.

the loop formed by the cochlear implant, electrode array, NaCl solution impedance, and reference electrode was sagittal (worst-case orientation). The head coil was used for RF transmission (SE sequences).

Induced voltage due to the switched gradients in the receiver coil of the cochlear implant at 1.5 T.—The induced voltage due to switched gradients in the receiver coil of the cochlear implant was performed by using the body resonator of the 1.5-T imager. The cochlear implant coil was fastened to a wooden mounting at a distance of 250 mm from the isocenter. The orientation of the cochlear implant coil was transverse; the x and y coordinates were selected to correspond to those in a real patient situation during MR imaging. With SE and echo-planar imaging sequences, field of view, section thickness, and section-selection direction were selected to produce high induced voltages.

Performance Test

The implant was fixed on a plastic mounting and placed in a plastic box filled with 1,000 mL of NaCl solution. The plane of the receiver coil and the plane formed by the electrodes was sagittal (worst-case orientation); the area between the electrode array and the reference electrode was comparable to that in a clinical situation. This arrangement was put in the head coil of the 0.2- and 1.5-T imagers. The implant was tested for functionality before and after exposure to worst-case sequences by means of a telemetering test (11) and a stimulation pulse test. The sequences used and parameters selected for the performance test are shown in Table 1.

Results

Evaluation of Artifacts at 0.2 and 1.5 T

Artifacts due to the internal magnet of the cochlear implant on different coronal images are shown in Figure 3. The scale of distortion of each grid point is given by means of a color-coded graphic representation. Since there was no distortion in the phase-encoding direction, the colored squares represent the distortion in the frequency-encoded direction.

Evaluation of Demagnetization at 1.5 T

Demagnetization of the internal magnet results in a mean decrease in mag-

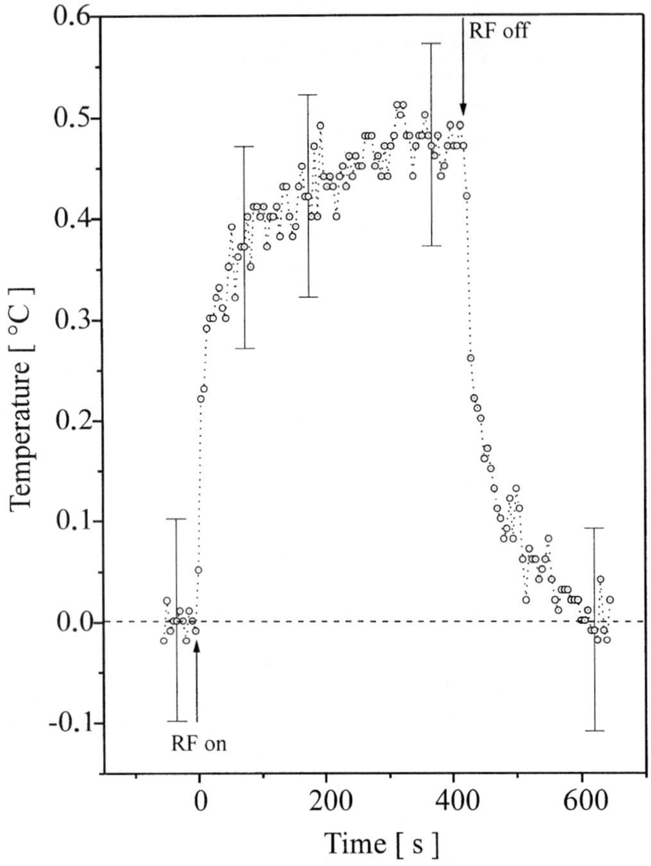

Figure 4. Temperature increase detected with the temperature measurement system at the reference electrode during a continuously repeated half-Fourier RARE sequence (repetition time, 8.2 msec; echo spacing, 66 msec; number of sections, 21 [selected parameters correspond to those of the first level operating mode]). Error bars indicate plus or minus 1 standard deviation.

TABLE 1
Performance Test Protocol

Magnet and Pulse Sequence	Repetition Time (msec)	Echo Time (msec)	Imaging Time (sec)
0.2 T			
Scout	40	10	19
SE	300	15	1,200
Turbo SE	2,800	1,100	1,506
1.5 T			
Scout	. . .	. . .	10
SE	300	15	944
Turbo SE*	800	76	120
Half-Fourier RARE*	11.9	95	260
Half-Fourier RARE*	11.9	95	60
Echo-planar, two-dimensional*	1.2	42.1	60
Turbo FLASH*†	2.7	1.2	15.2

* Specific absorption rate level corresponds to that in the first level operating mode.
† Contains adiabatic inversion pulses.

netic field strength of 38.3% ± 0.7% (standard deviation) in the worst-case orientation (magnetic moment antiparallel to the longitudinal main magnetic field). No demagnetization was detected in the usual head orientation.

Movement, Force, and Torque Measurement

Only the internal magnet of the cochlear implant experienced motion due to the main magnetic field of the MR imagers. The measured magnetic moment was a mean 0.117 Nm/T ± 0.006. The maximum longitudinal spatial derivative of the main field was $B_z = -2.517$ T/m at 941 mm from the isocenter. This results in a maximum force component $F_z = 0.29$ N on the internal magnet of the cochlear implant, the magnetic moment parallel to B_z. The main magnetic field strengths of the 0.2- and 1.5-T imagers within the isocenter result in a mean maximum torque (T_1) on the internal magnet of the cochlear implant (magnetic moment perpendicular to the main magnetic field) of $T_1 = 0.0234$ Nm ± 0.0012 (0.2 T) and $T_1 = 0.176$ Nm ± 0.009 (1.5 T), respectively.

Temperature Measurement at 1.5 T

Figure 4 shows the temperature increase at the reference electrode as a function of the imaging time. The mean maximum temperature increase was 0.48°C ± 0.1, with use of continuous, repeated half-Fourier RARE sequences (selected parameters corresponding to the first level operating mode [repetition time, 8.2 msec; echo spacing, 66 msec; number of sections, 21]).

Induced Voltage Measurement

RF-induced voltage in the receiver circuit of the cochlear implant at 0.2 and 1.5 T.—Figure 5 shows the output signal of the optical detector, u_{out}, during different sequences containing RF pulses with high RF peak amplitudes, measured at the parallel resonant receiver circuit of the cochlear implant, with use of a head coil for RF transmission. The corresponding maximum values for the induced RF voltage are summarized in Table 2.

Figure 6 shows the maximum induced voltage during SE sequences, as a function of the distance to the isocenter, with use of the body resonator for RF transmission.

The calibration curve, shown in Figure 5a, was used to determine the induced voltage, u_{RF}, from the recorded signal, u_{out}. The residual signals were taken into account.

RF-induced voltage in the electrode loop.—The induced voltage in the loop formed by the cochlear implant, reference electrode, tissue (NaCl solution), and stimulation electrode is shown in Figure 7 as a function of the area between the reference and stimulation electrodes.

Induced voltage due to the switched gradients in the receiver coil of the cochlear implant.—The maximum induced voltage due to the switched gradients measured during SE sequences (300/15; field of view, 35; section thickness, 2 mm) was a mean 156 mV peak (standard deviation, 6.9 mV). The maximum induced voltage due to the switched gradients measured during echo-planar, two-dimensional imaging (1.2/54; field of view, 220; section thickness, 3 mm) was a mean 83 mV peak (standard deviation, 6.9 mV).

Performance Test

Results of the performance tests did not show any influence on the functionality of

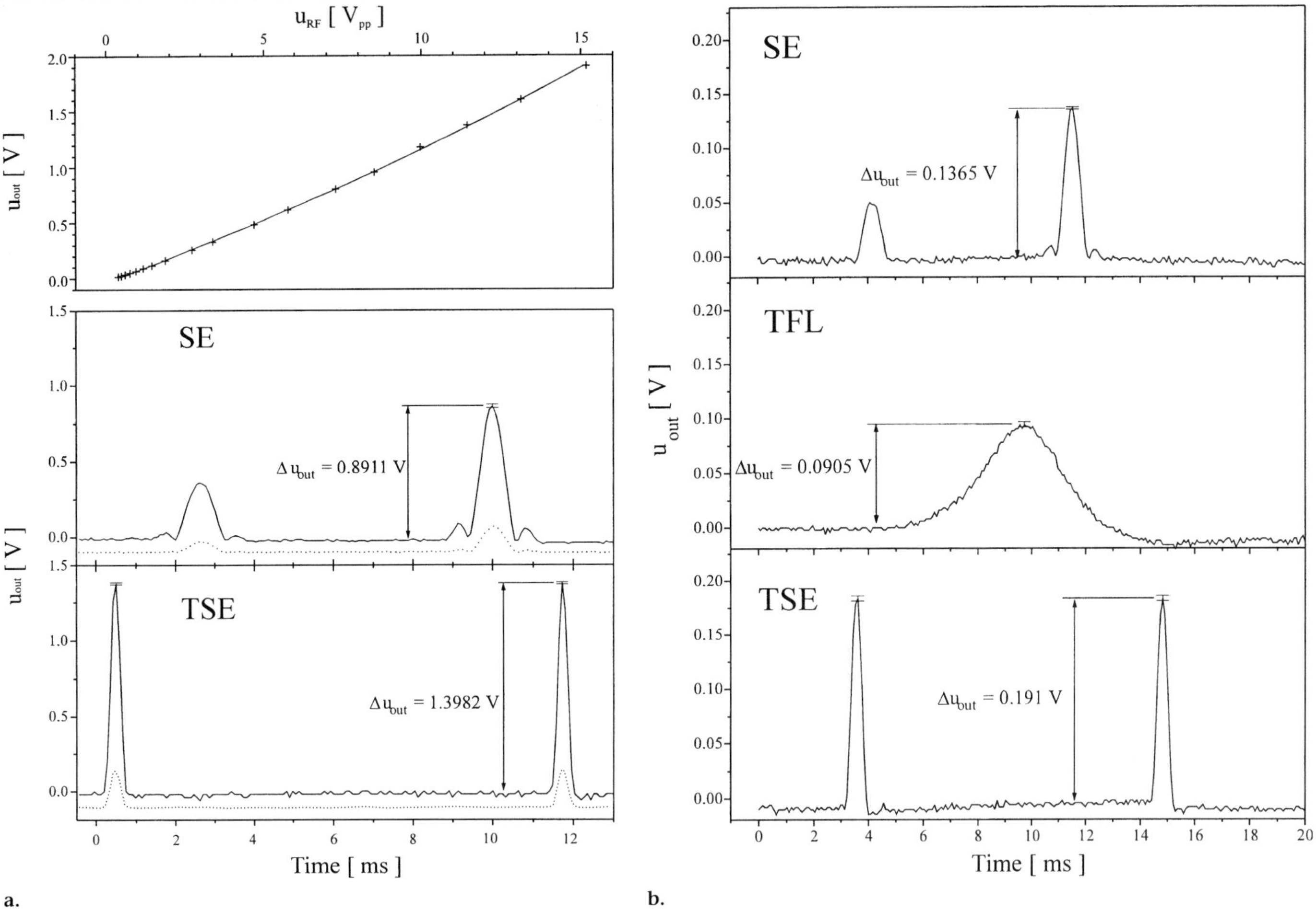

Figure 5. The output signal of the optical detector, u_{out}, during different sequences containing RF pulses with high RF peak amplitudes with **(a)** a 0.2-T imager and **(b)** a 1.5-T imager. The induced voltage, u_{RF}, was measured at the parallel resonant circuit of the receiver of the cochlear implant, by using a head coil for RF transmission. In **a** and **b**, the peak values of these signals are mapped by means of the calibration curve (top graph in **a**) to obtain the corresponding maximum values for the induced RF voltages, $u_{RF}[V_{pp}]$, summarized in Table 2. The residual signals (dotted lines in middle and bottom graphs in **a**) were considered. In **a** and **b**, *TSE* = turbo SE. In **b**, *TFL* = turbo FLASH.

TABLE 2
Maximum Induced RF Voltage at the Parallel Resonant Circuit of the Receiver Circuit of the Cochlear Implant

Pulse Sequence	Repetition Time (msec)	Echo Time (msec)	Mean Induced RF Voltage* At 0.2 T	Mean Induced RF Voltage* At 1.5 T
SE	300	15	3.03	0.834
Turbo SE	2,800	1,100	4.50	1.112
Turbo FLASH†	2.7	1.2	. . .	0.586

Note.—Data were acquired with a head coil for RF transmission.
* One standard deviation = 0.038.
† Contains adiabatic inversion pulses.

the cochlear implant after exposure to worst-case sequences in the 0.2- and 1.5-T imagers.

Discussion

Evaluation of Artifacts

Although coronal images obtained in a patient's head will be locally distorted, acceptable images may be obtained at regions a certain distance from the internal magnet of a cochlear implant. The influenced area increased with sequences more sensitive to magnetic field inhomogeneity (eg, echo planar or fast low-angle shot [FLASH]).

The distortion in frequency-encoding direction due to the field of the internal magnet of the cochlear implant can be reduced by increasing the receiver bandwidth. Since there was no distortion in the phase-encoding direction, the selection of the phase-encoding direction offers a possibility to reduce the influence of the artifact on the specific region of interest.

Evaluation of Demagnetization

Owing to the comparable high coercive electric field strengths (eg, 850–1,000 kA/m) of the internal permanent magnets of the cochlear implant, only partial demagnetization occurred in worst-case orientation within the static magnetic field of the 1.5-T MR unit. For the same reason, there will be no demagnetization at 0.2 T. Since there is no demagnetization in the usual head position, partial demagnetization at 1.5 T could be avoided

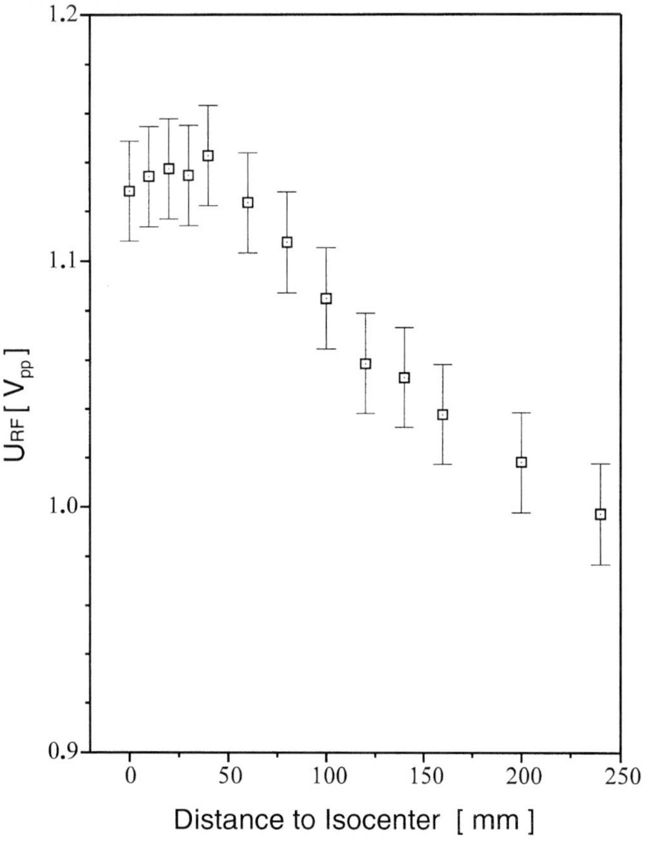

Figure 6. At 1.5 T, maximum induced peak voltage, $U_{RF}[V_{pp}]$, as a function of the distance to the isocenter with use of the body resonator and SE sequences. Induced signal was detected at the parallel resonant circuit of the receiver of the cochlear implant. Error bars indicate plus or minus 1 standard deviation.

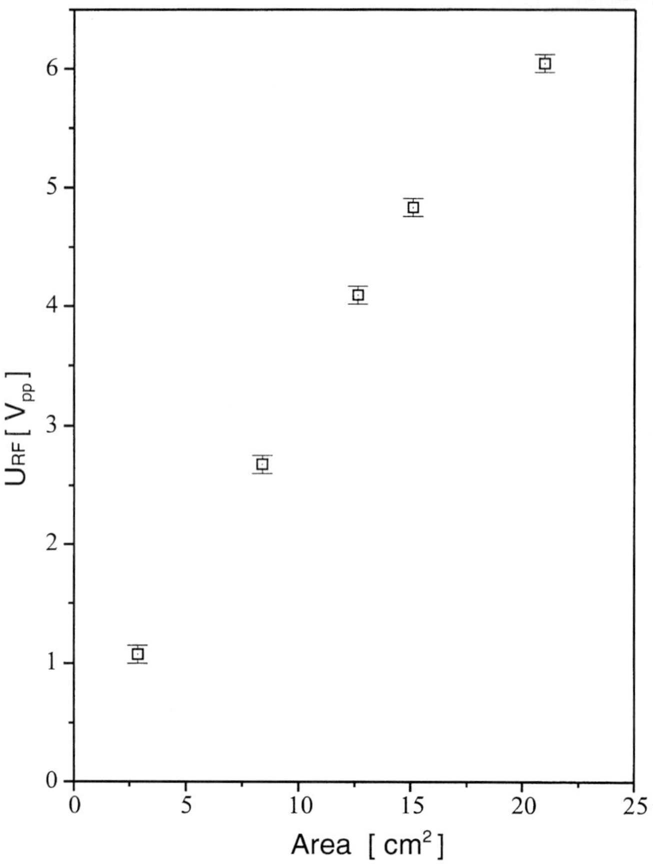

Figure 7. At 1.5 T, maximum induced peak voltage, $U_{RF}[V_{pp}]$, in the loop formed by the cochlear implant, reference electrode, tissue (NaCl solution), and stimulation electrode as a function of the area between the reference and stimulation electrodes. The head coil was used for the transmission; SE sequences were used to produce high induced voltages. Error bars indicate plus or minus 1 standard deviation.

by using a head orientation parallel to the magnetic field of the imager.

Temperature Measurement

The majority of the cochlear implant parts were of limited consequence concerning temperature increase, because the implant housing is made of ceramic and the reference electrodes as well as the stimulation electrode are isolated with a silicone coating. Since the surface-current density at the lamella of the reference electrode was comparable to that at the lamella of a single stimulation electrode, the temperature was determined at only the reference electrode. The maximum detected temperature rise was below the limit of the U.S. Food and Drug Administration for maximum allowable temperature increase of 1.0°C in the head region during MR imaging (14). The temperature increase due to RF-induced heating will be smaller at 0.2 T, since eddy currents will decrease with decreasing magnetic field strength.

Induced Voltage Measurement

The maximum levels of the induced voltages were given by the manufacturer. For the parallel resonant circuit of the receiver of the cochlear implant and the loop formed by the stimulation electrode, tissue, reference electrode, and the cochlear implant, the maximum allowed voltages were 6 V peak. All the induced voltages in these two tested loops were below the maximum allowed input voltage, even during RF-pulse trains of short 180° pulses in turbo SE sequences.

Although the transmitted RF power decreases with the square of the main field strength, the induced voltages in the receiver circuit of the cochlear implant at 0.2 T were higher than those at 1.5 T. This is due to the fact that the Larmor frequency of the 0.2-T imager (8.25 MHz) is closer to that of the 1.5-T imager to the carrier frequency of the cochlear implant (12 MHz).

The induced peak voltage in the receiver circuit of the cochlear implant due to the RF of the MR imager depends on the peak intensity of the transmitted MR RF signal, the bandwidth of the receiver circuit of the cochlear implant, and the difference between the carrier frequency of the cochlear implant and the MR transmission frequency. The bandwidths and carrier frequencies of receiver circuits of cochlear implants from various manufacturers are different, and details are available from each manufacturer. In general, as far as the induced voltage is concerned, use of the greatest possible separation between the MR transmission frequency and the carrier frequency of a cochlear implant, as well as a narrow bandwidth of the receiver of the cochlear implant, is helpful. From this, it is apparent that systems with low field strength and a correspondingly low Larmor frequency may not always be the best choice.

The induced voltages in the receiver coil of the cochlear implant due to switched gradients during SE and echo-planar imaging sequences were far below the maximum allowed input voltage. Since the total area of the receiver coil and the area of the electrode loop are of comparable sizes, the values of the induced voltages will be on the same order and, therefore, will be below the allowed input voltage.

With SE sequences at 1.5 T, the induced voltage in the electrode loop due to the RF was below the maximum allowed voltage. The induced voltage due to 180° RF pulses depends on the duration of the 180° pulse. For turbo SE sequences, short 180° pulses are usually used, which lead to high induced voltages. To guarantee a safety margin in the maximum allowed voltage, use of 180° RF pulses shorter than those shown in Figure 5b should be avoided. Since the RF power decreases with the square of the main magnetic field strength, the induced voltage in the electrode loop at 0.2 T will be negligible.

Data transmission from the external transmitter to the implanted receiver of the implant used in this study is performed in a digital format with error detection (11). Reliability tests of this error detection software were performed during development of the implant. Therefore, no accidental undesired stimulation during RF transmission is likely to occur.

Performance Test

The maximum currents delivered by the cochlear implant are limited by the implant circuitry to avoid physiologic damage. However, an uncomfortable sensation of loudness is possible due to destruction of the implant circuitry. This possible scenario can be excluded even for worst-case sequences, because results of all performance tests showed no influence on the functionality of the studied cochlear implants.

Movement, Force, and Torque Measurement

For the patient's comfort and safety, force and torque on the cochlear implant should be as low as possible, because of the risks associated with movement or dislodgment (3,15). Since force and torque on the fixation of the cochlear implant exist under normal conditions found in the everyday life of a patient with a cochlear implant (removal of the external transmitter, stress during chewing or biting), a reasonable value for the stress on the fixation of the implant housing may be set on the basis of the typical force produced by the external transmitter during its removal. This typical force is between 0.3 and 1.0 N, depending on the distance between the transmitter and receiver (typically, 8—4 mm, respectively). The magnetic coupling that occurs between a subcutaneous internal magnet within the implant and a magnet in the external transmitter coil is an accepted means to guarantee sufficient transmission quality (1).

The calculated values for the force on the cochlear implant produced by the spatial derivative of the 1.5-T main magnetic field were within these limits. Since the main static homogeneous magnetic field of the 0.2-T imager is lower by a factor of 7.5, it is unlikely that the spatial derivative of the 0.2-T imager will exceed that of the 1.5-T imager. Therefore, the resulting force on the cochlear implant will also remain within the reasonably acceptable force previously discussed. The switched gradients for spatial encoding are up to B = 25 mT/m, which is 100 times smaller than the static gradient on the entry of the bore. This produces a negligible force on the internal magnet (F = 0.0027 N) due to the switched gradients.

The stress on the fixation of the cochlear implant housing due to the torque can be calculated with the given implant geometry. The torque on the cochlear implant translates into a force of, depending on the implant orientation, between 0.78 and 1.05 N (80–107 g) at 0.2 T and between 5.9 and 7.8 N (600–800 g) at 1.5 T trying to pull the edge of the implant out from its proper position. The stress on fixation due to the torque at 0.2 T is within the discussed acceptable limits. For 1.5 T, this limit is exceeded by a factor of 7.8.

In general, the cochlear implant is fixed inside a milled out section of the temporal bone, and the stimulation electrode is placed into the cochlea. The electrodes are made of nonferromagnetic material. The associated risk for the patient arises from the possibility that the implant will turn and exert pressure on the brain. This risk is especially high with small children shortly after operation, in whom the bone underneath the implant is very thin or has been removed. The thickness of the bone underneath the implant can be determined at computed tomography (CT). In the great majority of cases, the bone will be sufficiently strong to eliminate this particular failure mode, and use of a compression bandage could provide additional stabilization.

Still, the implant, if not fixed sufficiently within its milled-out well in the side of the temporal bone, may turn a few degrees from its proper position and possibly damage the electrode leads as a result of shear forces, which would cause a partial or total loss of implant functionality.

A cautious approach is important, since a wide variety of surgical techniques are being used for implant fixation—such as use of dissolvable or undissolvable sutures, fixation with glass-ionomere cement, stimulation of new bone formation—that differ in strength. In addition, the influence of time elapsed since implantation has to be considered. Until now, no reliable indicators have been available to evaluate the strength with which the implant is anchored to the bone.

On the other hand, there is circumstantial evidence from several cases that the implants used in this study were sufficiently well fastened to withstand the torque induced.

Therefore, an MR imaging examination should not be denied under specific circumstances (ie, if the bone in the vicinity of the implant is sufficiently thick, as determined at CT; if evidence is available that fixation of the implant was adequate; and, as an additional safety measure, if pressure bandages are being used to restrict possible movement of the implant).

MR imaging examinations with a 0.2-T imager should be safe in patients with cochlear implants under these circumstances. Use of open MR systems offers an additional alternative for stabilization. The patient with a cochlear implant may be turned to the side, so that the magnetic moment of the internal magnet of the cochlear implant is parallel to the main magnetic field of the imager, and the implant plane is perpendicular to the main magnetic field B_z (magnetic moment antiparallel to B_z would represent an unstable alignment of the cochlear implant). The proper orientation can be determined by holding the external transmitter of the cochlear implant in the isocenter of the MR unit. The corresponding transmitter orientation must also be in the state of equilibrium (ie, no torque). Furthermore, in this orientation, the plane of the receiver coil of the cochlear implant is parallel to the polarization plane of the transmitted RF magnetic field of the MR unit; therefore the induced voltage equals zero.

At 1.5 T, some assessment of the relative risks involved (ie, possible electrode lead damage versus the risk of not providing the diagnostic capabilities of MR imaging) will have to be made.

It should be emphasized that the hazard remains of dislodging the implant as a result of the strong torque. Therefore, indispensable MR imaging examinations should, at present, be allowed under only very restricted conditions.

As a consequence of the great variety of equipment and procedures existing, it has not been possible to perform exhaustive tests on all available MR systems. Different nuclear MR imagers may generate shorter RF pulses that produce higher amplitudes and may lead to destruction of the implant. The induced voltage in the receiver circuit of the implant may increase in MR imagers with static magnetic field strengths different from those we tested, depending on RF power and center-to-center spacing of the affiliated MR imaging frequency and the transmission carrier frequency of the cochlear implant.

Further studies with different MR imagers and investigation of methods to determine the strength of a particular surgical technique for implant fixation will be the topics of further research.

It has to be noted that cochlear implant systems are offered by a limited number of manufacturers. At present, the most widely available multichannel cochlear implant systems are the Clarion 1.2 system (Advanced Bionics, Sylmar, Calif), the Nucleus 22 and 24 systems (Cochlear, Sydney, Australia [for a study on the MR imaging compatibility of the Nucleus 22 system, see reference 9]), and the Combi 40/40+ system (MedEl) used in this study.

Existing analog cochlear implant systems differ from these digital systems in the specific characteristics of their transcutaneous signal transmission and in the signal processing in the implant. In contrast to digital systems, the induced signal in the receiver circuit of the cochlear implant due to the RF field of the MR imager can reach the electrodes and could cause unintended stimulation signals.

The various models of cochlear implant systems are quite different (eg, transmission frequency, bandwidth, error detection, voltage endurance); therefore, no general conclusion can be drawn, and each device needs to be investigated carefully.

In any case, at present, it is an absolute necessity to consult the manufacturer of a cochlear implant to determine whether the particular MR imaging procedure intended to be performed in a patient with a cochlear implant is considered safe.

Acknowledgments: Access to the 0.2-T open MR imager was granted by Siemens Medical Systems, Erlangen, Germany. Access to the 1.5-T imager was granted by the Department for Magnetic Resonance Tomography at our institution.

References

1. Dormer K, Richard G, Hough J, Nordquist R. The use of rare-earth magnet couplers in cochlear implants. Laryngoscope 1981; 91:1812–1820.
2. Portnoy W, Matucci K. Cochlear implants as a contraindication to magnetic resonance imaging. Ann Otol Rhinol Otolaryngol 1991; 100:195–197.
3. Shellock F, Curtis J. MR imaging and biomedical implants, materials, and devices: an updated review. Radiology 1991; 180:541–550.
4. Applebaum E, Valvassori G. Further studies on the effects of magnetic resonance fields on middle ear implants. Ann Otol Rhinol Laryngol 1990; 99:801–804.
5. Kagetsu N, Litt A. Important considerations in measurement of attractive force on metallic implants in MR imagers. Radiology 1991; 179:505–508.
6. Shellock F, Crues J. High-field-strength MR imaging and metallic biomedical implants: an ex vivo evaluation of deflection forces. AJR 1988; 151:389–392.
7. Soulen R, Budinger T, Higgins C. Magnetic resonance imaging of prosthetic heart valves. Radiology 1985; 154:705–707.
8. Pavlicek W, Geisinger M, Castle L, et al. The effects of nuclear magnetic resonance on patients with cardiac pacemakers. Radiology 1983; 147:149–153.
9. Heller J, Brackmann D, Tucci D, Nyenhuis J, Chou C. Evaluation of MRI compatibility of the modified nucleus multichannel auditory brainstem and cochlear implants. Am J Otol 1996; 17:724–729.
10. Portillo F, McCreery D, Waluch V, Mobley J, Nelson R. Effects of magnetic resonance imaging on auditory brainstem implant. In: Hochmair-Desoyer IJ, Hochmair E, eds. Advances in cochlear implants: proceedings of the 3rd International Cochlear Implant Conference 1993. Vienna, Austria: Manz, 1993; 178–185.
11. Zierhofer C, Hochmair-Desoyer I, Hochmair E. Electronic design of a cochlear implant for multichannel high-rate pulsatile stimulation strategies. IEEE Trans Rehabil Eng 1995; 3:112–116.
12. Wickersheim K, Sun M. Fluoroptic thermometry. Med Electron 1987; February: 84–91.
13. International standard: medical electrical equipment. II. Particular requirements for the safety of magnetic resonance equipment for medical diagnosis. Geneva, Switzerland: International Electrotechnical Commission, 1995; 48–49.
14. U.S. Food and Drug Administration. Guidance for content and review of a magnetic resonance diagnostic device 510(k) application. Silver Springs, Md: U.S. Food and Drug Administration, 1988.
15. Shellock F. Biological effects and safety aspects of magnetic resonance imaging. Magn Reson Q 1989; 5:243–261.

Fulvia Arfelli, PhD
Valter Bonvicini, PhD
Alberto Bravin, PhD
Giovanni Cantatore, PhD
Edoardo Castelli, PhD
Ludovico Dalla Palma, MD
Marco Di Michiel, PhD
Renata Longo, PhD
Alessandro Olivo, MS
Silvia Pani, MS
Diego Pontoni, MS
Paolo Poropat, PhD
Michela Prest, PhD
Alexander Rashevsky, PhD
Giuliana Tromba, PhD
Andrea Vacchi, PhD

Mammography of a Phantom and Breast Tissue with Synchrotron Radiation and a Linear-Array Silicon Detector[1]

Index terms:
Breast neoplasms, radiography, 00.119, 00.128, 00.129
Breast radiography, technology, 00.119, 00.128, 00.129
Dosimetry
Phantoms
Synchrotron, 00.128

Radiology 1998; 208:709–715

Abbreviation:
SNR = signal-to-noise ratio

[1] From Istituto Nazionale di Fisica Nucleare, Sezione di Trieste, Italy (F.A., V.B., A.B., G.C., E.C., M.D.M., R.L., A.O., S.P., D.P., P.P., M.P., A.R., G.T., A.V.); Società Sincrotrone Basovizza, Trieste (F.A., G.T.); Department of Physics, Università di Trieste, via Valerio 2, 34100 Trieste, Italy (A.B., G.C., E.C., M.D.M., R.L., A.O., P.P., M.P.); and Istituto di Radiologia dell'Università di Trieste, Ospedale di Cattinara, Trieste (L.D.P.). From the 1996 RSNA scientific assembly. Received August 14, 1997; revision requested October 23; final revision received March 11, 1998; accepted April 17. **Address reprint requests to** R.L.

Author contributions:
Guarantors of integrity of entire study, E.C., L.D.P., R.L.; study concepts and design, all authors; definition of intellectual content, all authors; literature research, R.L.; experimental studies, F.A., A.B., G.C., M.D.M., R.L., A.O., S.P., G.T.; data acquisition, V.B., D.P., P.P., M.P., A.R., A.V.; data analysis, R.L., S.P., L.D.P.; manuscript preparation and editing, R.L.; manuscript review, G.C., F.A., L.D.P., R.L.

A linear-array, silicon pixel detector, capable of counting single photons, was applied to mammography by using a synchrotron radiation beam. Images were obtained of both a mammographic phantom and a breast-tissue sample. The phantom image was acquired with a mean glandular dose of 0.32 mGy. This detector combined with a synchrotron radiation beam allows acquisition of high-contrast, low-dose images of soft tissues.

Screen-film x-ray mammography has its limitations, particularly when radiographically dense breasts are being imaged (1). In fact, masses and microcalcifications, which are important indicators of cancer, are hardly visualized in very dense breasts, which occur in approximately 25% of women (2). To improve cancer diagnosis in dense breasts, it is possible to improve the performance of detectors (3,4) and to apply different x-ray spectra optimized for breast composition and thickness (5).

Findings in recent in vitro studies performed at facilities for synchrotron radiation demonstrate the high quality of mammographic images obtained with monochromatic beams. The doses delivered with a screen-film system (6) or a photostimulable storage phosphor plate (7) are comparable to or smaller than the doses delivered with clinical mammographic units.

In conventional mammography, the narrow dynamic range of radiographic film, which must be balanced against the need for wide latitude (8), determines the contrast and noise on images. To allow better detection of low contrast without changing the x-ray spectrum, it is necessary to apply different screen-film systems with different characteristic curves (ie, higher gamma, or γ; lower sensitivity) that increase the contrast or signal-to-noise ratio (SNR). In digital radiology, in which acquisition and display are separate processes, the detectability of low-contrast details is limited only by the SNR, which increases with exposure. Hence, display contrast can be enhanced after acquisition by performing simple manipulations of digital images. The development of digital detectors for mammography must conform to severe constraints in spatial and contrast resolution and dynamic range (9).

The development of and clinical trials with a linear-array digital detector for mammography, used in combination with a laminar beam, show that it is possible to apply a harder spectrum and reduce the delivered doses, even with the polychromatic spectrum emitted by an x-ray tube (10,11). Moreover, the slit technique is an efficient method for scatter reduction, which results in an increase in contrast.

Our group is working on x-ray imaging of soft tissues by employing both an innovative digital detector and an unconventional x-ray source. We use a tunable, monochromatic synchrotron radiation beam and a high-efficiency, linear-array digital detector. A synchrotron radiation beam is intrinsically laminar and polarized. Moreover, a monochromatic beam can be easily obtained within a continuous energy range. In this article, we present digital images of a mammographic test object and a breast tissue sample obtained at the Elettra Synchrotron Radiation Facility, Trieste, Italy, with use of a linear-array, silicon pixel detector capable of counting single photons (12). These are preliminary results of a feasibility study carried out at a beam line devoted to medical physics and with use of a small engineering prototypic detector based on the technology developed for high-energy physics experiments (13).

Materials and Methods

Synchrotron Radiation Beam Line

The source of radiation in our beam line is one of the 24 bending magnets of the ring. Figure 1 shows a schematic layout of the beam line. The radiation emitted from bending magnets is polychromatic; therefore, the beam line is equipped with a channel-cut silicon crystal monochromator that produces a beam with a bandwidth of about 20 eV in the energy range of 8–35 keV. The beam dimensions are defined by means of a slit system in front of the monochromator. At the experimental area, the maximal cross section of the beam is 120 × 4 mm. During acquisition of the images presented in this article, the beam dimensions were 50 × 0.2 mm, to match the detector area.

Each image was acquired by moving the object through the beam with use of a stepping motor controlled with a computer. Between the monochromator crystal and the holder of the test object, an ionization chamber was placed across the beam and used to determine the dose delivered to the sample. This large-area ionization chamber was built in our laboratory. We verified experimentally that the chamber response was close to the theoretic limit. The uniformity in spatial response of the sensitive area of the ionization chamber was also verified. The uncertainties associated with flux measurements were less than 5%.

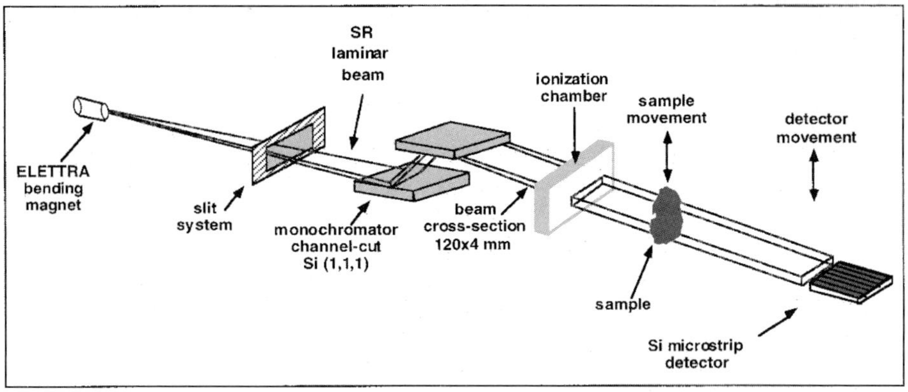

Figure 1. Schematic layout of the beam line. *ELETTRA* = Elettra Synchrotron Radiation Facility, Trieste, Italy; *Si* = silicon; *SR* = synchrotron radiation.

The Detector

A 5-cm-long linear-array detector with a pixel size of 200 × 300 μm was developed in our laboratory and manufactured by Canberra Semiconductors (Olen, Belgium). The detector consists of a silicon microstrip device used in a configuration in which radiation impinges on the side rather than on the surface of the chip. Pixel size is defined on the basis of strip pitch and detector thickness. The radiation strikes a 1-cm-deep silicon pixel. If the incident radiation energy is less than 30 keV, more than 95% of the photons are absorbed. A small, dead region on top of the pixel (average undepleted thickness, ~150 μm), due to the necessary separation between the implanted strips and the edge of the detector itself (14), limits detection efficiency; the photons absorbed in the dead region are not counted. As a consequence, the efficiency increases with energy. In the energy range of 18–30 keV, detection efficiency increases from 70% to 90%. More details about detector design and acceptance tests can be found in the articles by Arfelli et al (15) and Comes et al (16).

Figure 1 illustrates the detector geometry. The strips are parallel to the incoming radiation, and the active area of the detector is matched to the cross section of the beam. The readout electronics allow almost noiseless counting of single photons above a minimal threshold of 12 keV. These electronics consist of a series of 32-channel, analog-to-digital, very large scale of integration (or VLSI) chips, including a 16-bit counter, developed and produced in collaboration with the Laboratoire pour l'Ectronique e la Physique des Sistemes Instrumentaux (Strasbourg, France) (16). The maximal counting rate, with use of a periodic signal, is 100 kHz, but because of the Poisson distribution of the photons, the counting rate was kept at about 10 kHz per pixel to limit partial saturation of the readout chain, which decreases the efficiency of the detector. Under our experimental conditions, the efficiency of the readout electronics was greater than 90%. The exposure time was selected to count about 10,000 photons per pixel in the image background, which means an acquisition time of 1 second per step. To form images of objects larger than 5 cm in width, it was necessary to acquire two or more strips. Before visualization, pixel counts were normalized to correct for gain differences in the electronic channels; these corrections were less than 8%.

Spatial resolution of the images is related to the detector pixel size (300 μm in the scanning direction) and to the scanning step. In this study, we used a 100-μm step; hence, each image detail contributes to three consecutive acquisitions. The visibility of small details is greater than that with a 300-μm scanning step. During each acquisition step, the test object was kept stationary in front of the detector and was subsequently moved to the next position for a successive acquisition.

Test Object and Breast Tissue

The test object used in this study was an Ackermann mammographic phantom (RMI 160; Gammex, Middleton, Wis). It consists of a box (9 × 11 cm) containing various details (Mammochip; Gammex) and two uniform slabs of Lucite (polymerized methyl methacrylate) 1 cm and 3 cm thick. The box contains both small details and simulated tissue samples embedded in a homogeneous background (17).

Human breast tissue was unfixed and imaged within 12 hours after postmortem excision. The sample was 2.5 cm thick, and its dimensions in the image plane were 3 × 3 cm; during imaging, it was contained in a Plexiglas holder.

Conventional mammographic images of both the test object and breast tissue were acquired to compare delivered doses, as well as spatial and contrast resolution. The clinical mammographic unit (Senographe; GE Medical Systems, Milwaukee, Wis) has a molybdenum anode with 30-μm molybdenum filtration. A Trimax T2M screen cassette (3M; Ferrania, Italy) was used.

Dose Calculation

The mean glandular dose was calculated for the synchrotron radiation images by measuring the incident flux with an ionization chamber. We assumed the sample was composed of 50% glandular and 50% adipose tissue as in the breast model previously specified (18). This model includes a 0.5-cm-thick outer adipose layer.

The glandular dose (D_g) at depth x, in centimeters, is

$$D_g(x) = \phi E(\mu_{en/g} \div \rho_g) \times \exp[-(\mu_a 0.5)] \times \exp[-\mu_m(x - 0.5)],$$

where E is the photon energy, ϕ is the photon fluence incident on the breast surface, μ_a is the adipose tissue attenuation coefficient, μ_m is the glandular-adipose mixture attenuation coefficient, $\mu_{en/g}$ is the glandular absorption coefficient, and ρ_g is the glandular density.

The mean glandular dose (MGD) is evaluated from

$$\text{MGD} = [1/(t - 1)] \int_{0.5}^{(t-0.5)} D_g(x)\, dx,$$

where t is the breast thickness in centimeters and 0.5 cm is the thickness of the outer adipose layer. In the present dose calculation, the attenuation and absorption coefficients were taken from the article by Biggs (19).

Owing to dead time for movement of the object between two consecutive positions, the delivered dose was larger than the dose actually needed for image acquisition. In the dose evaluation, only the effective exposure time was considered, since we are developing a fast shutter to stop radiation during dead time. The errors in dose evaluation were not larger than 10% and included both the uncertainties in flux measurements and those in absorption and attenuation coefficients.

The mean glandular dose for the conventional mammographic images was evaluated according to the article by Dance (20).

Optimization of Beam Energy

To select the appropriate energy for mammographic images, the figures of merit for a ductal carcinoma and for a microcalcification were calculated for the standard breast composition (50% glandular, 50% adipose tissue) and different breast thicknesses. The outer layer of 0.5 cm of adipose tissue was taken into account. The figure of merit (FOM) is defined as

$$\text{FOM} = \text{SNR}/\text{MGD}^{1/2},$$

where MGD is mean glandular dose. The SNR of the lesion is defined according to Dance (21) as

$$\text{SNR} = (N_1 - N_2)/(N_1 + N_2)^{1/2},$$

where N_1 is the total number of photons detected on surface S_1, in the shadow of the lesion, and N_2 is the total number of photons detected on surface S_2, outside the shadow of the lesion. S_1 and S_2 contain the same number of pixels. The standard deviation of the signal is $(N_1 + N_2)^{½}$, according to the Poisson distribution of the photons.

For a certain lesion with a given SNR, a higher figure of merit means a lower mean glandular dose. On the basis of analysis of the figure of merit, it is possible to select the best energy for an examination, since the SNR allows determination of detail visibility in digital images.

In figure-of-merit calculations, the ductal carcinoma was modeled as a 1-mm-thick, 5-mm-diameter cylinder. The linear attenuation coefficients were taken from the study by Johns and Yaffe (22), and the absorption coefficients for glandular and fat tissue were taken from the study by Biggs (19). The figure of merit for microcalcifications was calculated with a calcium detail size of 300 × 300 × 300 μm. The dependence of detector efficiency on photon energy was taken into account.

Contrast Evaluation

The contrast (C_c) of a detail on a conventional mammogram is defined as

$$C_c = (I_2 - I_1)/I_2,$$

where I_1 and I_2 are the signal intensities evaluated in the detail region and in a surrounding uniform region, respectively. In the present study, the film optical densities were evaluated by using a densitometer (model 331; X-Rite, Grandville, Mich).

One of the advantages of using a digital imaging system is the possibility of contrast enhancement by means of display window settings. The contrast may be calculated both with the raw data and on the manipulated image. The image contrast (C_d) on a digital image is defined as

$$C_d = (C_2 - C_1)/C_2,$$

where C_1 and C_2 are the average signal intensity of the pixels in the detail region and in the surrounding uniform region, respectively. In our experimental condition, C_1 and C_2 are the average numbers of photons counted per pixel.

The enhanced contrast (C_e) is, on the other hand, defined as

$$C_e = (G_2 - G_1)/G_2,$$

where G_1 and G_2 are the average gray levels of the pixels that correspond to the detail and surrounding regions, respectively.

Results

Figure 2 shows the calculated figures of merit for a ductal carcinoma and for calcifications in a 50%-fat, 50%-glandular breast. The optimal energy increases as breast thickness increases. For a 5-cm-thick breast, the optimal monochromatic energy lies between 20 and 27 keV.

Images of the Ackermann phantom were acquired both at the clinical mammographic department, with a screen-film system, and at the synchrotron radiation facility, with the digital detector. With the conventional unit, the best result was obtained with 28 kVp (Fig 3). With the synchrotron radiation beam, after the figure-of-merit calculations, the test object was imaged at 22 keV. Figure 4 shows images of the entire Ackermann phantom obtained with two different gray scales for contrast enhancement of different regions of interest. On the first image (Fig 4a), the contrast of the simulated tissues is optimized; on the second image (Fig 4b), small details of different dimensions and contrasts are visible. In Figure 4a, a steel needle and a 50-μm-diameter copper wire are visible within the structure that represents a lymph node. In Figure 4b, the small, calibrated details are more clearly visible than they are on the conventional image. See Table 1 for a comparison of detail visibility between the digital monochromatic image and the mammogram obtained with the clinical unit. Moreover, the structures of the low-contrast simulated tissues are more clearly visible on the digital image (Fig 4b) than on the conventional image (Fig 3).

The contrast of the thickest (700-μm) polycarbonate disk was calculated as 6% on the mammogram, whereas image contrast and enhanced contrast on the monochromatic digital image were 4% and 19% (Fig 4b), respectively. Since the digital image was acquired in 5-cm-wide strips, which were then pasted together, some artifacts are visible.

The mean glandular dose delivered for acquisition of the digital image was 0.32 mGy, whereas that delivered with the clinical unit for the best image obtained (28 kVp) was 1.8 mGy. The detector exposure was 7.5 mR (1.935×10^{-3} mC/kg),

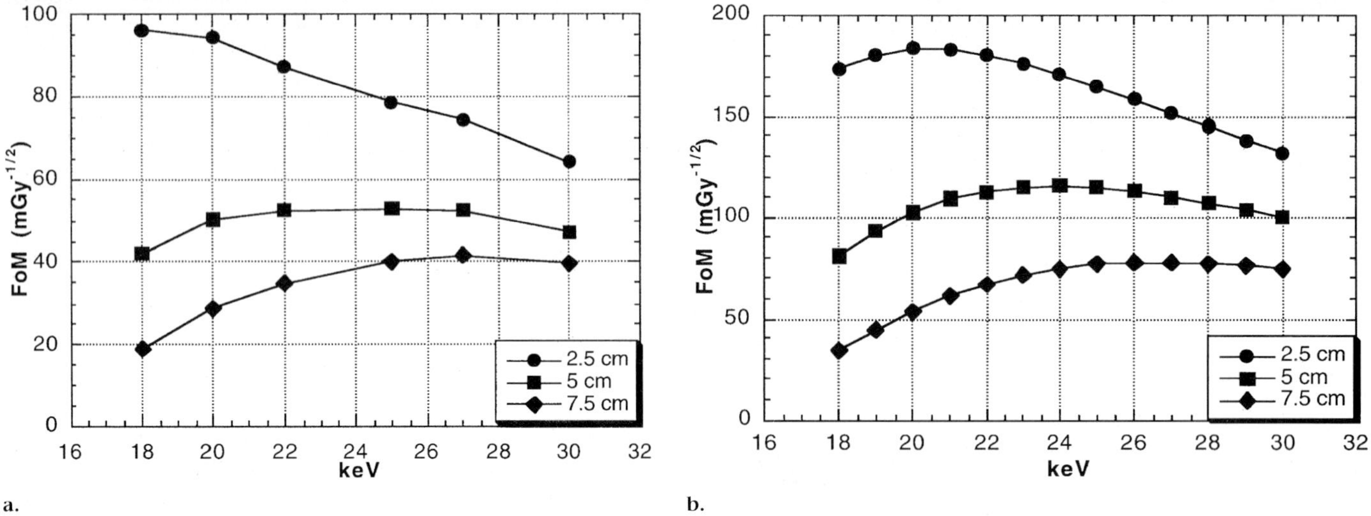

Figure 2. Graphs show figures of merit (*FoM*) for **(a)** ductal carcinoma and **(b)** microcalcifications in a 50%-fat, 50%-glandular breast. Figures of merit were calculated for different breast thicknesses, from published data (see Materials and Methods).

whereas our screen-film system needs 12 mR (3.096×10^{-3} mC/kg) for the correct exposure.

Figure 5 shows a digital image of a breast-tissue sample acquired with a 20-keV synchrotron radiation beam, and Figure 6 shows an image of the same sample obtained with the mammographic unit. The delivered mean glandular dose for the digital synchrotron radiation image was 0.17 mGy, whereas the mean glandular dose delivered with the clinical unit was 0.39 mGy. The detector exposure was 10 mR (2.58×10^{-3} mC/kg).

Eight digital images of the tissue sample were also acquired with the photon energy tuned within a range of 16–30 keV. Contrast on each image was evaluated for the region highlighted in Figure 5. Table 2 shows the image contrast, SNR, mean glandular dose, and figure of merit for details at the reported photon energy. The average number of counted photons per pixel was about 10,000 on all images. The SNR was calculated according to the Poisson distribution of photons. The decrease in delivered dose was greater than the decrease in contrast between 16 and 20 keV, when the number of counted photons was kept constant. At 20 keV, the mean glandular dose was 41% of that delivered at 16 keV, whereas the image contrast at 20 keV was 82% of the contrast at 16 keV. The experimental figure of merit obtained for the detail indicated in Figure 5 had its maximum in approximately the same region of the figure of merit calculated for a 2.5-cm-thick breast model (Fig 2).

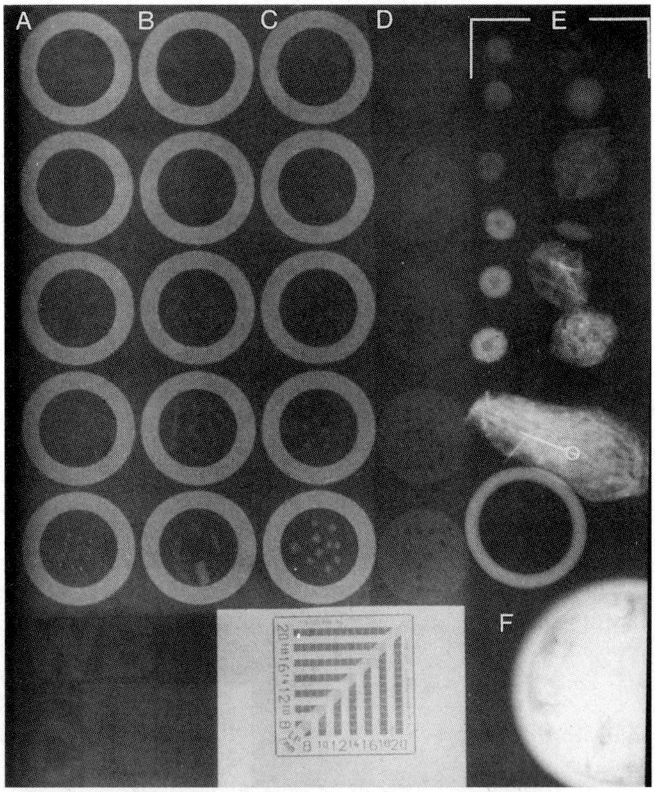

Figure 3. Image of the test object acquired with the clinical mammographic unit (28 kVp). *A,* Al_2O_3 specks from 250 μm (bottom) to 83 μm (top) in diameter mimic microcalcifications. *B,* Polyamide wires from 0.8 mm (bottom) to 0.3 mm (top) in diameter mimic fibrous structures. *C,* Carbohydrate spheres from 1.2 mm (bottom) to 0.35 mm (top) in diameter. *D,* Polycarbonate disks containing 0.6-mm-diameter holes are arranged to form single digits that indicate the depth of the hole in tenths of a millimeter. *E,* Simulated breast tissues of very low (top), low (middle), and normal (bottom) absorption. A steel needle and a copper wire are embedded in the structure (wire diameter, 50-μm) that represents a lymph node. *F,* Sample represents a dense breast.

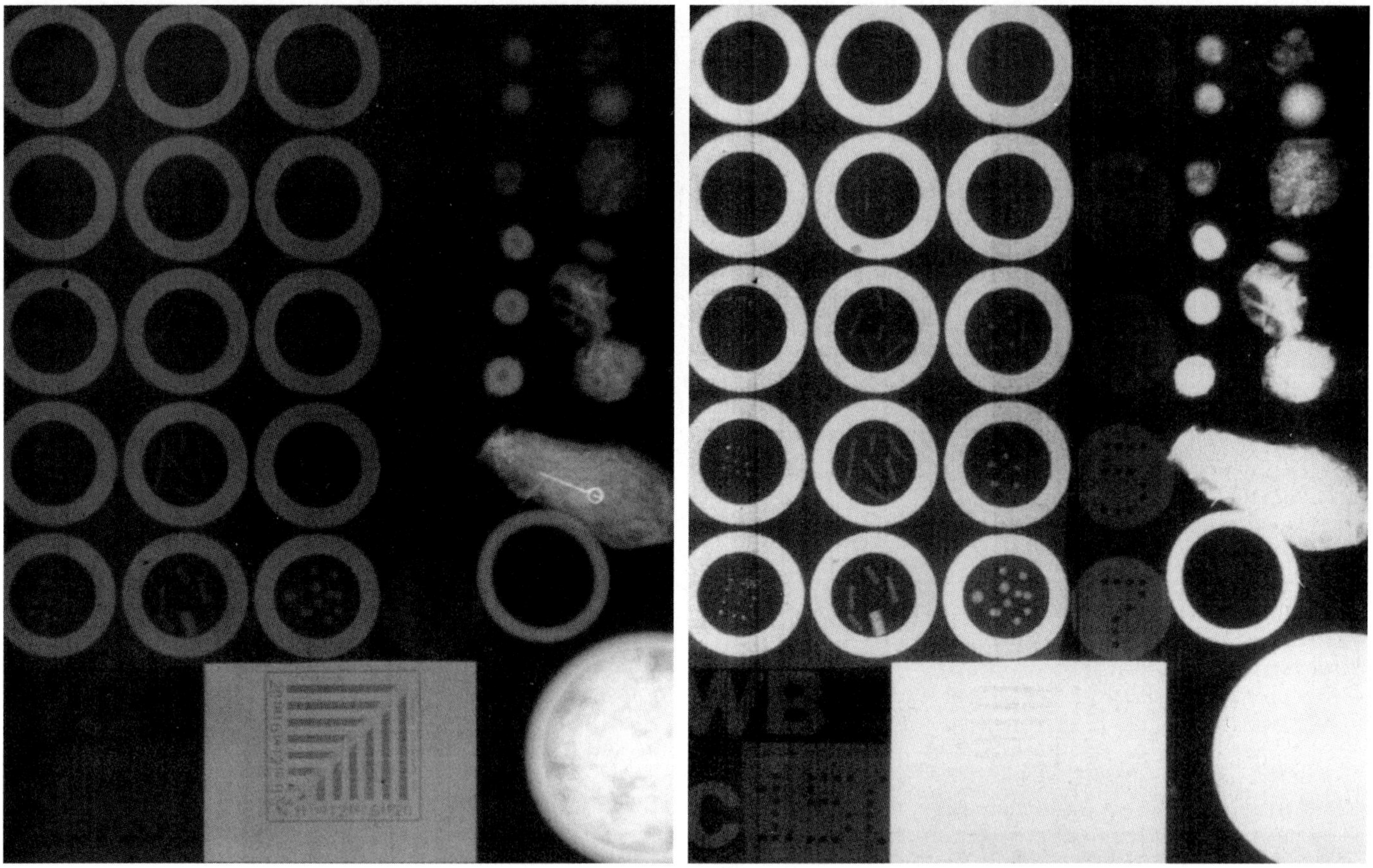

a. b.

Figure 4. Digital images of the Ackermann phantom, with the gray scale optimized for contrast enhancement of different regions. (**a**) Contrast of the simulated tissues is optimized. (**b**) Small details depicted in *A–D* in Figure 3 are visible. Beam energy is 22 keV, and mean glandular dose is 0.32 mGy.

TABLE 1
Visibility of Mammographic Phantom Details: Comparison between Digital and Conventional Images

Detail	Synchrotron Radiation and Digital Detector	Standard Mammographic Unit
Diameter (μm) Al_2O_3 specks (microcalcifications)	180	180
Carbohydrate spheres (nodules)	355–425	500–600, 355–425*
Polyammide fibers	300	400, 300*
Polycarbonate disks	200	200
Mean glandular dose (mGy)	0.32	1.8

*Radiologist interpretation, "doubtful visibility."

Discussion

Other authors have used conventional screen-film systems and photostimulable storage phosphor plates to evaluate mammographic applications of monochromatic synchrotron radiation beams (6,7). They obtained images with good contrast without a substantial reduction in the delivered dose compared with that of a conventional mammographic unit. In the present study, the x-ray source is still a synchrotron radiation beam but the detector is a new digital linear-array pixel detector.

One of the advantages of a digital imaging system is the possibility of contrast enhancement by means of display window settings. Our digital images have greater contrast than the conventional images, as shown with the contrast calculations regarding the polycarbonate disks within the test object. Even if the higher beam energy used at digital imaging results in image contrast less than that at conventional mammography, the enhanced contrast is three times greater than that on mammograms. Moreover, the large dynamic range of our digital detector allows acquisition of useful information in both high- and low-density regions with a single exposure (Fig 4). On our digital images, it is possible to detect low-contrast details not easily detectable on conventional images while delivering 20% of the mean glandular dose delivered with conventional mammographic equipment. This result is due to the good SNR obtained when a digital detector capable of counting single photons is used (12). A detector that counts single photons does not add noise to the acquired signal, and detail visibility is determined with Poisson statistics of only the photons. It is obvious that the spatial resolution of the present prototype does not allow recognition of the shape of very small calcifications, which is important information for the diagnosis of breast cancer.

Our results show a substantial decrease in mean glandular dose when a monochromatic x-ray beam is employed in combination with a linear-array, silicon pixel detector compared to that with a conventional mammographic unit. The reduction in dose is greater for medium or thick breasts, since full absorption of the softer components of polychromatic beams is more evident in thicker breasts. In such breasts, the softer components of the beam contribute greatly to the absorbed dose and do not increase image contrast (21). With a synchrotron radiation beam, which has continuous tunability, the energy is selected according to the figure of merit to obtain the best compromise between SNR and mean glandular dose, and the dose is not increased by lower energy components, which are absent.

Our results, which indicate 20–27 keV as the optimal energy range for x-ray imaging of standard 5-cm-thick breast tissue, stem from the combination of a monochromatic beam with a high-efficiency digital detector. The optimal energy changes with breast thickness. A 2.5-cm-thick breast requires 18–20 keV of photon energy, and a 7.5-cm-thick breast presents the best compromise between contrast and dose at about 27 keV. The optimal energy for our system is therefore higher than that determined in previous studies at synchrotron radiation facilities in which screen-film systems and imaging plates are used as detectors. In fact, the efficiency of our detector increases with energy up to 30 keV, whereas conventional detectors (screen-film systems or photostimulable storage phosphor plates) have lower efficiency at higher energy. The decrease in image contrast at higher energies may be balanced by the increase in SNR at constant mean glandular dose.

It is well known that the shape and edges of microcalcifications are important in the classification of benign or malignant behavior. With use of our detector to increase spatial resolution, it is possible to acquire an image with a small scanning step and then to apply filtered deconvolution to the data (23), which increases the delivered dose. Moreover, with a second-generation silicon pixel detector, the pixel size in the direction of the array could be decreased by a factor of 10, if necessary, and the detector thickness could be reduced by a factor of 2. In principle, images with a nominal pixel size of 50 × 50 μm could be obtained by using a 50 × 200-μm pixel size detector, an acquisition step of 50 μm, and filtered deconvolution. This postprocessing slightly decreases the SNR with respect to an image acquired under similar conditions with a detector of the same efficiency but a pixel size of 50 × 50 μm. More investigations must be carried out to establish the pixel dimensions and scanning step necessary for mammographic diagnosis with our detector. We will evaluate different acquisition schemes, with different step sizes and continuous movement of the test object, to obtain the best compromise among spatial resolution, SNR, and delivered dose.

To find a reasonable compromise between scatter suppression and acquisition time, we will assemble a multiline detector by stacking single elements, forming a "brick wall," to obtain an active surface of 125 × 4 mm, which will match the beam cross section. Our silicon detectors have been developed to allow easy and efficient assembly of a multilayer detector (14,15). Preliminary tests with a two-layer detector have been performed in our laboratory; the distance between layers was 50 μm (24). With the present prototype, the acquisition time is several minutes, which is too long for clinical practice. With use of a multilayer detector (ie, 10 layers to match the maximal beam cross section) and a faster photon counting chip (ie, photon counting rate, 200 kHz [25]), it will be possible to acquire a full breast image in a few seconds.

The detector in this study was developed to perform digital radiology with synchrotron radiation; a small prototype, however, was previously tested with use of a conventional x-ray source (12). To develop a linear-array, silicon pixel detector for use with a conventional x-ray source, the best results will probably be obtained by using trapezoidal strips to achieve convergence on the source (typically 60–70 cm from the surface) (26). It is obvious that a slit system must be applied and the tube must support a high flux and long acquisition time. If a filter is applied to obtain a broad but peaked radiation spectrum in the middle of the optimal energy range for the investigated sample, estimated with the figure of merit, it may be possible to obtain a substantial dose reduction by using a silicon strip detector and a conventional x-ray tube.

In conclusion, images obtained with a linear-array, silicon pixel detector capable of counting single photons show good contrast resolution. The present spatial resolution is sufficient to see microcalcifications as small as 180 μm in diameter. In this study, the image of the mammographic phantom at 22 keV was acquired with a mean glandular dose of 0.32 mGy, which is less than 20% of that delivered with a conventional mammographic unit.

The next step in our project is the development of a new prototypic multi-

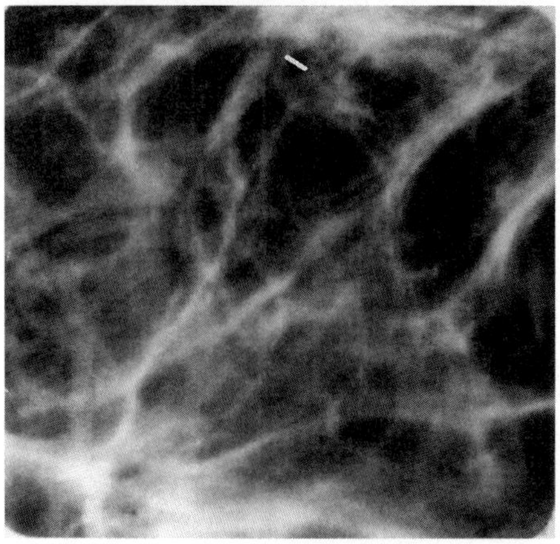

Figure 5. Digital image, acquired at the synchrotron radiation facility (beam energy, 22 keV), of a breast tissue sample (3 × 3 cm). White bar indicates the region used in the contrast calculations reported in Table 2.

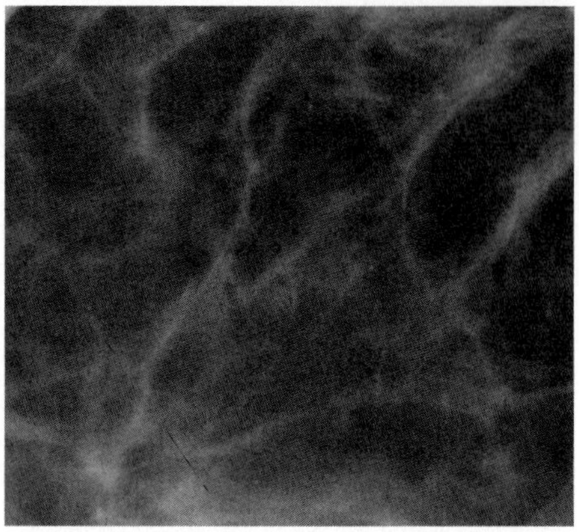

Figure 6. Image acquired with the clinical mammographic unit (20 kVp) of the same breast tissue sample depicted in Figure 5.

TABLE 2
Energy Dependence of Contrast, Dose, and Figure of Merit: Experimental Measurements

Energy (keV)	Image Contrast (%)	SNR	Mean Glandular Dose (mGy)	Figure of Merit $(mGy)^{-1/2}$
16	10.1	7.1	0.41	11
18	9.5	6.7	0.25	13
20	8.3	5.9	0.17	14
22	6.1	4.3	0.13	12
24	4.4	3.1	0.11	9
26	4.3	3.0	0.11	9
28	2.6	1.8	0.10	6
30	2.5	1.8	0.09	6

line detector of larger overall dimensions that will allow shorter acquisition times. With such a device, it will be possible to understand whether a linear-array, silicon pixel detector capable of counting single photons combined with a monochromatic x-ray beam can make a substantial contribution to the mammographic evaluation of dense breasts.

Acknowledgments: The authors acknowledge the support of Fabrizio Zanconati, MD, in preparation of tissue samples and Cristina Cressa, MD, for assistance with the acquisition of conventional images.

References

1. Jackson VP, Hendrick RE, Feig SA, Kopans DB. Imaging of the radiographically dense breast. Radiology 1993; 188:297–301.
2. Tabar L, Dean PB. Mammographic parenchymal patterns: risk indicator for breast cancer. JAMA 1982; 247:185–189.
3. Williams MB, Fajardo LL. Digital mammography: performance considerations and current detectors designs. Acad Radiol 1996; 3:429–437.
4. Sabel M, Aichinger H. Recent development in breast imaging. Phys Med Biol 1996; 41:315–368.
5. Jennings RJ, Quinn PW, Gagne RM, Fewell TR. Evaluation of x-ray source for mammography. SPIE 1993; 1896:259–268.
6. Burattini E, Cossu E, Di Maggio C, et al. Mammography with synchrotron radiation. Radiology 1995; 195:239–244.
7. Johnston RE, Washburn D, Pisano E, et al. Mammographic phantom studies with synchrotron radiation. Radiology 1996; 200:659–663.
8. Yaffe MJ. Digital mammography. In: Haus AG, Yaffe MJ, eds. Syllabus: a categorical course in physics—technical aspects of breast imaging. Oak Brook, Ill: Radiological Society of North America, 1992; 69–84.
9. Maidment AD, Fahrig R, Yaffe MJ. Dynamic range requirements in digital mammography. Med Phys 1993; 20:1621–1633.
10. Yaffe MJ. Direct digital mammography using a scanned-slot CCD imaging system. Med Prog Technol 1993; 19:13–21.
11. Fahrig R, Yaffe MJ. Optimization of spectral shape in digital mammography: dependence on anode material, breast thickness, and lesion type. Med Phys 1994; 21:1473–1481.
12. Arfelli F, Bonvicini V, Bravin A, et al. Linear array silicon pixel detector: images of a mammographic test object and evaluation of delivered doses. Phys Med Biol 1997; 42:1565–1573.
13. Damerell CJS. Developments in solid state vertex detectors. In: McDonough P, ed. The sixth quark. In: Proceedings of the Stanford Linear Acelerator Center. Stanford, Calif: Stanford Linear Acelerator Center, 1985; 43–117.
14. Arfelli F, Bonvicini V, Bravin A, et al. Design and evaluation of AC-coupled, FOXFET-biased, "edge-on" silicon strip detectors for x-ray imaging. Nucl Instrum Methods Phys Res 1997; 385(A):511–520.
15. Arfelli F, Barbiellini G, Bonvicini V, et al. An "edge-on" silicon strip detector for x-ray imaging. IEEE Trans Nucl Sci 1997; 44:874–880.
16. Comes G, Loddo F, Hu Y, et al. CASTOR: a VLSI CMOS mixed analog-digital circuit for low noise multichannel counting applications. Nucl Instrum Methods Phys Res 1996; 377(A):440–445.
17. Law J. A new phantom for mammography. Br J Radiol 1991; 64:116–120.
18. National Council on Radiation Protection and Measurements. Mammography: a user's guide. NCRP report no. 85. Washington, DC: Government Printing Office, 1986.
19. Biggs F. Analytical approximations for x-ray cross sections. Sandia report no. 7. Albuquerque, NM: Sandia National Laboratory, 1987.
20. Dance DR. Monte Carlo calculation of conversion factors for the estimation of mean glandular breast dose. Phys Med Biol 1990; 35:1211–1219.
21. Dance DR. Diagnostic radiology with x-ray. In: Webb S, ed. The physics of medical imaging. Bristol, England: Institute of Physics Publishing, 1988.
22. Johns PC, Yaffe MJ. X-ray characterization of normal and neoplastic breast tissue. Phys Med Biol 1987; 32:675–695.
23. Arfelli F, Barbiellini G, Cantatore G, et al. Silicon detectors for synchrotron radiation digital radiology. Nucl Instrum Methods Phys Res 1994; 353(A):366–370.
24. Arfelli F, Barbiellini G, Bonvicini V, et al. At the frontiers of digital mammography: SYRMEP. Nucl Instrum Methods Phys Res 1998; 909(A):529–533.
25. Beuville E, Cederström B, Danielsson M, et al. An application specific integrated circuit and data acquisition system for digital x-ray imaging. Nucl Instrum Methods Phys Res 1998; 906(A):337–392.
26. Beuville E, Cahn R, Cederstrorm B, et al. High resolution x-ray imaging using a silicon strip detector. In: Nalcioglu O, ed. Conference Record of the 1997 IEEE Nuclear Science Symposium [book on CD-ROM]. New York, NY: Institute of Electrical and Electronics Engineers, 1997.

Laura Liberman, MD
Timothy L. Feng, MD
D. David Dershaw, MD
Elizabeth A. Morris, MD
Andrea F. Abramson, MD

US-guided Core Breast Biopsy: Use and Cost-effectiveness[1]

PURPOSE: To determine the frequency with which ultrasonographically (US) guided core biopsy obviated diagnostic surgical biopsy of nonpalpable breast masses, to calculate the cost savings of diagnosis attributable to US-guided core biopsy, and to compare the costs of US-guided versus stereotactically guided core biopsy.

MATERIALS AND METHODS: US-guided core biopsy was performed in 151 consecutive solitary, nonpalpable breast masses in 151 women (age range, 23–80 years) by using a 14-gauge automated gun and needle. Clinical follow-up data were obtained. Cost savings were assessed by using national Medicare reimbursement costs of $385 for US-guided core biopsy, $610 for stereotactic core biopsy, and $1,332 for needle localization and surgical biopsy.

RESULTS: US-guided core biopsy obviated a surgical procedure in 128 (85%) of 151 women. The mean adjusted direct cost saving per US-guided core biopsy was $744 per case. Use of US-guided biopsy decreased the cost of diagnosis by 56% ($744/$1,332) over the cost of surgical biopsy. If biopsy had been performed with stereotactic rather than with US guidance, the mean adjusted direct cost saving would have been $519 per case, a 39% ($519/$1,332) decrease in the cost of diagnosis compared with the cost of surgical biopsy.

CONCLUSION: Percutaneous biopsy of a nonpalpable breast mass with either US or stereotactic guidance is less expensive than surgery, but cost savings are greater with US-guided biopsy.

Index terms:
Biopsies, technology, 00.1261, 00.1267, 00.12985
Breast, biopsy, 00.1261, 00.1267, 00.12985
Breast neoplasms, diagnosis, 00.31, 00.32
Stereotaxis, 00.1267
Ultrasound (US), guidance, 00.12985

Radiology 1998; 208:717–723

Abbreviations:
CPT = *Current Procedural Terminology*
DCIS = ductal carcinoma in situ

[1]From the Breast Imaging Section, Memorial Sloan-Kettering Cancer Center, 1275 York Ave, New York, NY 10021. Received December 24, 1997; revision requested February 10, 1998; revision received March 13; accepted April 23. **Address reprint requests to** L.L.

Percutaneous imaging-guided core biopsy is being used increasingly as an alternative to surgical biopsy for the diagnosis of breast lesions that are suspicious for or highly suggestive of malignancy (1–18). While stereotactic guidance is preferable for percutaneous biopsy of lesions that are evident as calcifications, most masses are amenable to percutaneous biopsy with either stereotactic guidance or ultrasonographic (US) guidance (4,8,9,13). US-guided percutaneous breast biopsy offers several advantages. There is no ionizing radiation; the procedure can be performed quickly; all areas of the breast and axilla are accessible; the breast is not compressed during the procedure, which may make biopsy more comfortable for the woman; and the needle position can be observed in real time (4,8,9).

US-guided, 14-gauge core breast biopsy was first described in 1993 by Parker et al (4) in a study of 181 lesions. In that study, there was a 100% correlation between the results of US-guided core biopsy and those of surgery in the 49 lesions, including 34 cancers, that were subsequently surgically excised. In the remaining 132 lesions, for which core biopsy results indicated benignity, no cancers were found at follow-up (range, 12–36 months). The procedure time averaged 20 minutes, and no complications occurred. Since the initial description of US-guided core biopsy, to our knowledge, few studies (7,8) have evaluated its usefulness, and none have assessed its cost-effectiveness. This study was undertaken to determine the frequency with which US-guided core biopsy obviated a surgical procedure in women with nonpalpable breast masses, to calculate the cost savings attributable to US-guided core breast biopsy in our patients, and to compare the costs of core biopsy with US versus stereotactic guidance.

Author contributions:
Guarantor of integrity of entire study, L.L.; study concepts and design, L.L.; definition of intellectual content, L.L., T.L.F., D.D.D., E.A.M., A.F.A.; literature research, L.L., T.L.F.; clinical studies, L.L., D.D.D., E.A.M., A.F.A.; data acquisition, L.L., T.L.F.; data analysis, L.L.; manuscript preparation, editing, and review, L.L., T.L.F., D.D.D., E.A.M., A.F.A.

MATERIALS AND METHODS

Clinical Protocol

US-guided core biopsy was performed in 179 nonpalpable breast masses from May 18, 1993, to June 30, 1997. Twenty-eight lesions in women who underwent biopsy of multiple lesions were excluded. The remaining 151 consecutive solitary, nonpalpable breast masses in 151 women (age range, 23–80 years; median age, 50 years) who underwent US-guided core biopsy formulate the basis of this study. The lesions were 0.6–5.5 cm (median, 1.4 cm). Written informed consent to perform all US-guided core biopsy procedures was obtained from all patients.

At our institution, US-guided automated core biopsy was offered as an alternative to surgical biopsy of nonpalpable breast lesions that were suspicious for or highly suggestive of malignancy unless (*a*) the thickness of the breast parenchyma was inadequate to accommodate the excursion of the needle, (*b*) the patient had a hemorrhagic diathesis, (*c*) the patient was unable to cooperate for the procedure, or (*d*) the lesion measured less than 5 mm. The 5-mm-diameter limit for automated core biopsy was observed to avoid removing the entire mammographic lesion, which could render subsequent needle localization more difficult.

For masses that were evident with mammography, percutaneous biopsy with stereotactic guidance was an additional alternative. The choice between stereotactic and US-guided percutaneous biopsy depended on several factors, including lesion visibility and accessibility, equipment availability, and patient and radiologist preference. During the study, stereotactic biopsy was performed in 678 nonpalpable lesions at our institution, and needle localization and surgical excision were performed in 2,252 lesions.

US-guided core biopsy was performed with the patients in the supine or supine oblique position by using high-resolution (7.5-MHz linear-array transducer) US equipment (128-XP, Acuson, Mountain View, Calif; or Ultramark 4 Plus, Advanced Technology Laboratories, Bothell, Wash). All biopsies were performed by using a 14-gauge cutting needle (Automatic Cutting Needle, Manan Medical Products, Northbrook, Ill; Biopty-Cut Needle, Bard Urological, Covington, Ga; or Ultra-Core Biopsy Needle, Medical Device Technologies, Gainesville, Fla) and a long-excursion, spring-loaded automated gun (Pro-Mag 2.2; Manan Medical Products or Biopty; Bard Urological). A median of four core biopsy specimens per lesion (range, 2–7 specimens per lesion) were obtained (19); three or more specimens were obtained in 139 (92%) of 151 lesions.

The histopathologic findings at US-guided core biopsy were correlated with the imaging findings, and specific follow-up recommendations were made to the patient and referring clinician. Follow-up recommendations were based on the following protocol: Repeat biopsy (either percutaneous or surgical) was suggested if inadequate tissue was obtained or if there was discordance between the histopathologic findings and the imaging characteristics. Women in whom US-guided core biopsy results revealed atypical ductal hyperplasia were referred for diagnostic surgical biopsy (6,10). Diagnostic surgical biopsy was also recommended if the histopathologic findings at US-guided core biopsy suggested the presence of a lesion that could be managed best with surgical excision, such as a phyllodes tumor (20). Phyllodes tumors may be histologically heterogeneous, with both benign and malignant areas; furthermore, even benign phyllodes tumors may be locally aggressive and warrant excision (20). Although it has been recommended that benign papillary lesions found at core biopsy be surgically excised (8), to our knowledge, there have been no reported cases of carcinoma in such lesions found at surgery. The recommendations for repeat biopsy were based on the pathologist's review of core biopsy findings and on the experiences in the core biopsy literature (Table 1).

If the US-guided core biopsy results revealed carcinoma, the patient was referred for definitive surgery. If the US-guided core biopsy results revealed benign findings concordant with the imaging characteristics, the patient was advised to return for follow-up imaging in 1 year.

TABLE 1
Published Experience with Benign or Atypical Lesions at 14-Gauge Automated Core Biopsy for Which Surgical Excision Was Suggested

Study	No. of Lesions Excised	Surgical Histopathologic Finding
Atypical ductal hyperplasia		
Jackman et al (6)	16	9 (56%) carcinomas
Liberman et al (9)	21	11 (52%) carcinomas
Burbank (21)	18	8 (44%) carcinomas
"Discordant" mammographic and histopathologic findings		
Dershaw et al (11)	11	7 (64%) carcinomas
Lee et al (16)	9	9 (100%) benign lesions
Fibroepithelial tumor (fibroadenoma or phyllodes tumor)		
Dershaw et al (11)	7	3 (43%) benign phyllodes tumors, 4 (57%) fibroadenomas
Radial scar		
Jackman et al (22)	6	2 (33%) carcinomas
Lee et al (16)	4	1 (25%) carcinoma
Papilloma		
Rubin et al (8)	7	7 (100%) benign papillomas

End Point Variables

The patient was considered to have been spared a surgical procedure if the US-guided core biopsy resulted in a diagnosis of a benign finding for which surgery was neither recommended nor performed. The patient was also considered to have been spared a surgical procedure in all cases of carcinoma in which the first operation after core biopsy was a therapeutic procedure that consisted of either lumpectomy with axillary lymph node dissection or mastectomy. Patients with carcinomas 1 cm or larger who were treated with lumpectomy as a one-stage procedure and patients with core biopsy–proved carcinomas who did not undergo subsequent surgery were also considered to have been spared a surgical procedure (10).

US-guided core biopsy was considered not to have spared the patient a surgical procedure in the following situations: (*a*) Repeat biopsy was recommended, performed, or both; (*b*) a small (<1-cm) core biopsy-proved carcinoma was excised without axillary lymph node dissection; or (*c*) a lesion yielded ductal carcinoma in situ (DCIS) at core biopsy and invasive carcinoma at surgery, and the patient returned for axillary lymph node dissection as a separate procedure.

Economic Modeling and Data Analysis

The *Current Procedural Terminology* (CPT) codes used in the economic analysis are shown in Tables 2–5. For automated core

TABLE 2
CPT Codes for Cost Analysis

CPT Code	Description	Cost per Service ($)*
00400	Anesthesia	96
19125	Excision of breast lesion identified by radiological marker	374
19125 SG	Excision of breast lesion identified by radiological marker, facility cost	466
19290	Preoperative placement of needle localization wire	72
19290 SG	Preoperative placement of needle localization wire, facility cost	165
76096	Preoperative placement of needle localization wire, radiological supervision and interpretation	74
76098	Radiological examination of the surgical specimen	23
88305	Surgical pathology, gross and microscopic	62
19100	Biopsy of breast, needle core	76
19101	Biopsy of breast, incisional	238
19120	Biopsy of breast, excisional	335
19120 SG	Biopsy of breast, excisional, facility cost	463
76942	US localization	85
76095	Stereotactic localization	310

* 1996 National Medicare average allowed cost per service for selected CPT-coded procedures and modifiers (William J. Sobaski, Health Care Financing Administration, written communication, June 1997).

TABLE 3
Direct Costs of US-guided Core Breast Biopsy of Nonpalpable Breast Masses

Procedure	Cost ($)
US localization	85
Biopsy of breast, incisional	238
Histopathologic analysis	62
Total	385

TABLE 4
Direct Costs of Stereotactic Core Breast Biopsy of Nonpalpable Breast Masses

Procedure	Cost ($)
Stereotactic localization	310
Biopsy of breast, incisional	238
Histopathologic analysis	62
Total	610

TABLE 5
Direct Costs of Needle Localization and Surgical Biopsy of Nonpalpable Masses

Procedure	Cost ($)
Needle localization	311*
Surgery	840†
Radiologic examination of the specimen (for all lesions)	23
Anesthesia	96
Histopathologic analysis	62
Total	1,332

* Amount is the sum of $72 for placement of the localizing wire (CPT code 19290), $74 for radiologic supervision and interpretation (76096), and the $165 facility cost (19290 SG).

† Amount is the sum of $374 for excision of the breast lesion identified by the radiologic marker (CPT code 19125) and the $466 facility cost (19125 SG).

biopsy, the CPT code 19101 (for "biopsy of breast, incisional") was used, per the recommendations published in the October 1997 Bulletin of the American College of Radiology (23).

The direct savings in cost attributable to the use of US-guided core biopsy were calculated by subtracting the cost of US-guided core biopsy from the cost that would have been generated if surgical biopsy had been performed. The adjusted direct savings in cost were calculated by taking into account the percentage of cases in which US-guided core biopsy was performed in addition to rather than in lieu of diagnostic surgical biopsy. For women who underwent surgical biopsy after core biopsy, the cost of diagnosis was the additive cost of the two procedures. In addition, a theoretic calculation was made of what the direct cost savings would have been if all biopsies had been performed with stereotactic guidance rather than with US guidance.

The data were entered into a computerized spreadsheet (EXCEL; Microsoft, Redmond, Wash) for analysis. Statistical calculations were performed by using EPI-INFO (version 5.0; Centers for Disease Control and Prevention, Atlanta, Ga).

RESULTS

US-guided core biopsy was performed on the same day as the initial diagnostic evaluation at our facility in 126 (83%) of 151 women. The histopathologic findings at US-guided core biopsy are shown in Table 6.

Surgery was not performed in five of 56 women with malignancy for the following reasons: two had stage IV breast cancer, two had other medical problems that precluded surgery, and one had lymphoma treated with chemotherapy. Three women chose to undergo diagnostic surgical biopsy rather than therapeutic surgery after a core biopsy–based diagnosis of carcinoma. The remaining 48 women with carcinoma at core biopsy underwent a therapeutic surgical procedure as the first operation after core biopsy; this procedure was mastectomy in eight women and breast-conserving surgery in 40 women. One of these women had a subcentimeter carcinoma that was excised without axillary lymph node dissection. Because the excisional biopsy may have been therapeutic, she was not considered to have been spared a surgical procedure by undergoing US-guided core biopsy.

In all women with infiltrating carcinoma at core biopsy, the presence of infiltrating carcinoma was confirmed at surgery. Of four women with DCIS at core biopsy, two (50%) had infiltrating carcinoma at surgery. In one of these two women, core biopsy yielded papillary carcinoma that was suspicious for invasion; surgery yielded a 1.8-cm papillary carcinoma with microscopic foci of invasion that was treated with excision alone. In the other woman, core biopsy yielded papillary DCIS; surgical excision revealed a papillary carcinoma with foci of invasion that measured up to 0.2 cm. She returned for axillary lymph node dissection at a later date and therefore was not spared a surgical procedure by undergoing US-guided core biopsy.

Prompt repeat biopsy was recommended in 15 (10%) women who underwent US-guided core biopsy. In five of these women, core biopsy yielded a fibroepithelial tumor that was thought to represent either a cellular fibroadenoma or a phyllodes tumor. Surgical excision was performed in three of these women and yielded fibroadenoma in two and a low-grade malignant phyllodes tumor in one. Repeat biopsy was also suggested in one woman with a radial scar and in one woman with a benign papilloma at core biopsy; surgical excision findings confirmed the core biopsy findings in both cases. In one woman, core biopsy yielded a fibroadenoma and focal atypical ductal hyperplasia. Surgical excision yielded a benign fibroadenoma.

In five women, repeat biopsy was recommended because of discordant imaging and histopathologic findings. Repeat biopsy, which was performed in four of these women, yielded benign findings in three and carcinoma in one. In the latter woman, US-guided core biopsy of an irregularly shaped mass with spiculated borders yielded fibrosis; prompt surgical excision revealed infiltrating ductal carcinoma.

In two women, US-guided core biopsy yielded inadequate tissue. In these women, the inner needle advanced, but the outer cannula did not advance over it, so no tissue sample was retrieved. Repeat biopsy yielded benign findings in both women.

Clinical follow-up data were available in 72 (90%) of 80 women in whom US-guided core biopsy findings were benign without atypia (median follow-up, 13 months; range, 5–48 months). No carcinomas have been detected in these women. Two of these women chose to undergo diagnostic surgical biopsy in spite of the diagnosis of a benign lesion at US-guided core biopsy. The surgical findings were benign and concordant with the core biopsy findings in these women. Follow-up mammography, follow-up US, or both were performed in 50 of the 80 women with benign core biopsy findings at a median of 20 months (range, 6–48 months) after core biopsy. No change was seen in 49 (98%) of these women. In one woman, the 6-month follow-up mammogram obtained after the core biopsy–based diagnosis of ductal hyperplasia and pseudoangiomatous stromal hyperplasia showed interval growth; surgical biopsy revealed pseudoangiomatous stromal hyperplasia.

In our series, use of US-guided core biopsy spared 128 (85%) of 151 women a surgical procedure. The histopathologic findings in the 23 women in whom US-guided core biopsy did not obviate a surgical procedure are shown in Table 7. The mean adjusted direct cost savings with US-guided core biopsy were calculated by using Medicare data and taking into account the percentage of patients who were not spared a surgical procedure by undergoing US-guided core biopsy (Table 8). The mean adjusted direct cost saving was $744 per case. The use of US-guided core biopsy resulted in a 56% ($744/$1,332) decrease in biopsy costs.

We used our clinical data to make a theoretic estimate of what the cost savings would have been if percutaneous biopsy had been performed with stereotactic guidance in our patient population (Table 8). If these 151 women had undergone biopsy with stereotactic guidance, and 128 (85%) of them had been spared a surgical procedure, the cost saving from using stereotactic biopsy rather than surgery would have been $519 per case, a 39% ($519/$1,332) decrease in the cost of diagnosis compared with the cost of diagnosis with surgical biopsy.

TABLE 6
Core Biopsy Histopathologic Findings in 151 Lesions

Histopathologic Finding	No. of Lesions*
Benign lesion	94 (62)
Imaging follow-up suggested†	80 (53)
Unusual histopathologic finding, excision suggested‡	7 (5)
Discordant imaging and histopathologic findings	5 (3)
Inadequate specimen	2 (1)
Atypical ductal hyperplasia	1 (<1)
Malignant lesion§	56 (37)

* Numbers in parentheses are percentages.
† Includes 38 cases of fibroadenoma; nine, fibroadenomatoid hyperplasia; nine, fibrosis; six, ductal hyperplasia; four, apocrine metaplasia; four, chronic inflammation; two, lymph node; two, pseudoangiomatous stromal hyperplasia; two, sclerosing adenosis; two, benign breast tissue; one, adenosis; and one, ductal stasis.
‡ Includes five fibroepithelial lesions, one radial scar, and one papilloma.
§ Core biopsy histopathologic findings were infiltrating carcinoma in 51 lesions, DCIS in four lesions, and lymphoma in one lesion.

TABLE 7
Histopathologic Findings in 23 Women Who Were Not Spared a Surgical Procedure with US-guided Core Breast Biopsy

Histopathologic Finding	No. of Women*
Benign histopathologic finding requiring further investigation	7 (30)
Fibroepithelial tumor	5 (22)
Papilloma	1 (4)
Radial scar	1 (4)
Discordant imaging and histopathologic findings	5 (22)
Inadequate tissue	2 (9)
Atypical ductal hyperplasia	1 (4)
Benign lesion†	3 (13)
Malignant lesion‡	5 (22)

* Numbers in parentheses are percentages of all women who were not spared a surgical procedure.
† Includes two women who chose to undergo surgical biopsy after benign core biopsy and one woman who underwent surgical biopsy because of an interval growth at 6-month follow-up mammography.
‡ Includes three women who chose to undergo diagnostic surgical biopsy after a core biopsy diagnosis of carcinoma, one with a subcentimeter carcinoma treated with excision without axillary dissection, and one with DCIS at core biopsy and invasive carcinoma at surgery who returned for axillary dissection at a later date.

DISCUSSION

Previous studies (10,15–17,24–26) of the cost-effectiveness of imaging-guided biopsy have involved analysis of stereotactic biopsy only. Lindfors and Rosenquist (15) reported that the marginal cost per year of life saved with screening was reduced by 23% with the use of stereotactic core biopsy rather than surgical biopsy. Liberman et al (10) found that stereotactic core biopsy decreased the cost of diagnosis by more than 50%; if these results were generalized to the national level, annual savings in the United States would approach $200 million. Liberman et al (10) and Lee et al (16) found that the cost savings with stereotactic biopsy are higher in masses than in calcifications, probably because failure to sample the lesion, "underestimates" of atypical ductal hyperplasia and DCIS, and DCIS lesions in which excision may be both diagnostic and therapeutic are more common when biopsy of calcifications is performed (18).

The cost savings with US-guided core biopsy should exceed those with stereotactic biopsy for two reasons. First, US equipment is less expensive. A stereotactic table with digital imaging capability costs more than $220,000 and is dedicated for one purpose only: interventional breast procedures. In contrast, US equipment is readily available and can be used for other purposes. This difference in cost is reflected in the Medicare reimbursements of $310 for stereotactic localization (CPT code 76095) versus $85 for US localization (CPT code 76942) (Tables 2–4).

Second, US guidance allows the needle position to be observed in real time. In one study (18), inaccurate needle placement was the most common cause of cancers missed at stereotactic core biopsy. These "misses" did not cause a substantial delay in diagnosis but did result in a recommendation for repeat biopsy owing

TABLE 8
Adjusted Direct Costs and Savings due to Percutaneous Core Biopsy with US or Stereotactic Guidance

Guidance Method	Surgery (A) ($)	Core Biopsy (B*) ($)	B/A Ratio (%)	Savings per Case (A − B) ($)
US	1,332	588	44	744
Stereotaxis†	1,332	813	61	519

* Mean adjusted direct cost of imaging-guided core biopsy, assuming that (*a*) unadjusted direct costs are $385 for US-guided core biopsy and $610 for stereotactic biopsy and (*b*) core biopsy is performed instead of a surgical procedure in 85% of cases and in addition to a surgical procedure in 15% of cases.
† The calculations for stereotactic biopsy are theoretical—that is, based on the clinical data from our patient population.

TABLE 9
Frequency of Spared Surgical Procedure due to Percutaneous Core Breast Biopsy

Study	Mammographic Finding*		
	Mass	Calcification	All
Liberman et al (10)†	91/108 (84)	49/74 (66)	140/182 (77)
Lee et al (16)†	220/254 (87)	108/151 (72)	328/405 (81)
Present study‡	128/151 (85)	. . .	128/151 (85)

* Numbers in parentheses are percentages.
† Biopsy with stereotactic guidance.
‡ Biopsy with US guidance.

to discordant imaging and histopathologic findings, with a resultant increase in cost (18). Real-time depiction of the needle with US should assist in accurate needle placement and diminish misses and thereby increase efficacy and diagnostic yield.

In this study, US-guided core biopsy obviated a surgical procedure in 128 (85%) of 151 women with nonpalpable breast masses, with a resultant 56% decrease in the cost of diagnosis. The frequency of obviating a surgical procedure with US-guided core biopsy in this study was comparable to the frequency of obviating a surgical procedure after stereotactic core biopsy of nonpalpable breast masses in previous studies (Table 9). Since US-guided core biopsy is less expensive than stereotactic biopsy and equally likely to spare a woman surgery, the cost savings are greater with core biopsy performed with US rather than stereotactic guidance. When it is possible to perform US-guided core biopsy on the same day as the initial diagnostic evaluation, as was the case in 126 (83%) of our patients, there are additional savings due to the decreased time lost from work, diminished patient anxiety, and lowered likelihood of attrition due to nonadherence to biopsy recommendations.

The 10% (15 of 151 women) frequency of recommending repeat biopsy after US-guided core biopsy in this study is lower than the 18% rate of repeat biopsy after stereotactic biopsy reported by Dershaw et al (11). The indications for repeat biopsy in that study also differed from those in our study. The most common reasons for recommending a repeat biopsy after US-guided core biopsy in our study were (*a*) benign histopathologic findings in which excision was suggested, such as a fibroepithelial tumor (ie, fibroadenoma vs phyllodes tumor) and (*b*) discordance between histopathologic findings and imaging study findings. The finding of atypical ductal hyperplasia, which accounted for more than half of the recommendations for repeat biopsy after stereotactic biopsy, was uncommon in our series of US-guided core biopsy, probably because atypical ductal hyperplasia is seen more often in biopsy of calcifications than in biopsy of masses (18).

Inadequate specimens are uncommon after automated large-core biopsy, but they led to a recommendation for repeat biopsy in two cases in this study. Failure of the outer cannula to advance over the needle most often occurs in patients with hard lesions, dense breast parenchyma, or both, and is audibly recognized as a dull "thud" rather than the usual sharp "click" of the automated needle (18). If this problem is encountered, it may be helpful to cock the needle in the breast and then remove it from the breast. One may then attempt to obtain a specimen from a different part of the lesion by using a new needle. If this problem is encountered repeatedly, it may be necessary to replace the gun's spring.

It is possible that obtaining a larger volume of tissue will improve the diagnostic yield in US-guided core breast biopsy. In a previous study by Liberman et al (19) of 14-gauge automated core biopsy of nonpalpable breast lesions with stereotactic guidance, the first specimen yielded diagnostic material in 84% of the masses; obtaining two, three, four, or five specimens per lesion resulted in a diagnosis in 91%, 98%, 98%, and 99% of the masses, respectively. Because US allows real-time depiction of the needle, one would expect the number of specimens required for US-guided core biopsy to be no greater than that required for stereotactic biopsy. It is our current practice to obtain a minimum of three 14-gauge automated core biopsy specimens per lesion in most cases. Additional specimens may be obtained on the basis of real-time assessment of the images and visual inspection of the tissue samples.

In this study, if US-guided biopsy yielded a specific diagnosis of benignity concordant with the imaging characteristics, the patient was referred for follow-up imaging in 1 year. Some other investigators (7,14,16,22,27) perform the first follow-up imaging examination 6 months after percutaneous biopsy reveals a benign finding. The follow-up interval influences the cost savings with percutaneous biopsy. Regardless of the time of the first imaging study, it is critical that follow-up be continued for a longer period (28–30). The cost of a delayed diagnosis of breast cancer is high, and without long-term follow-up data, the frequency of missed cancers cannot be determined. Lack of long-term follow-up data was a limitation of our study.

Technologies, including the directional, vacuum-assisted biopsy instrument (Mammotome; Biopsys/Ethicon Endo-surgery, Cincinnati, Ohio) (27,31–39) and the Advanced Breast Biopsy Instrumentation device (US Surgical, Norwalk, Conn) (40–42), are available for performing percutaneous biopsy of the breast. These instruments allow acquisition of larger volumes of tissue than are possible with 14-gauge automated large-core biopsy devices but are substantially more expensive (Table 10). Several studies (21,31–34) indicate that the directional, vacuum-assisted bi-

TABLE 10
Disposable Costs of Different Tissue Acquisition Devices for Percutaneous Breast Biopsy

Instrument	Cost ($)
14-gauge automated biopsy needle	
Manan Medical Products	14
Medical Device Technologies	14
Bard Urological	24
Directional vacuum-assisted biopsy instrumentation	
14-gauge probe*	146
11-gauge probe without clip†	226
11-gauge probe with clip†	301
Advanced breast biopsy instrumentation	
All cannulas	513

Note.—Data reflect listed prices as of December 1997.
* Costs are $135 for the 14-gauge probe, $6 for the disposable probe guide, and $5 for the vacuum cannister.
† Costs are $215 for the 11-gauge probe, $6 for the disposable probe guide, and $5 for the vacuum cannister; the localizing clip (MicroMark; Biopsys/Ethicon Endo-surgery), placed to facilitate subsequent localization if the lesion is removed, costs an additional $75.

opsy instrument has advantages over the automated needle in the assessment of calcifications. It remains to be determined whether these new technologies provide an increment in the diagnostic yield of percutaneous biopsy of nonpalpable breast masses and whether that yield increment justifies the additional costs.

Our data can be used to estimate what the national cost savings would be if US-guided core biopsy were used instead of surgical biopsy for histopathologic assessment of nonpalpable breast masses. If we assume that (*a*) approximately 1 million breast biopsies will be performed in the United States in 1998 (43), (*b*) at least 30% (n = 300,000) of the lesions on which biopsy is performed will be nonpalpable (44), and (*c*) at least one-third (n = 100,000) of the 300,000 nonpalpable lesions will be evident as masses (45), then if US-guided core biopsy is used rather than needle localization and surgical biopsy in 80% (n = 80,000) of these nonpalpable masses, the annual national savings in the cost of diagnosis would be $59,520,000. Percutaneous biopsy of a nonpalpable breast mass with either US or stereotactic guidance is less expensive than surgery, but the cost savings are greater if the biopsy is performed with US guidance.

Acknowledgments: The authors thank William J. Sobaski, MBA, of the Health Care Financing Administration for expert interpretation of Medicare information and David C. Perlman, MD, for invaluable assistance.

References

1. Parker SH, Lovin JD, Jobe WE, et al. Stereotactic breast biopsy with a biopsy gun. Radiology 1990; 176:741–747.
2. Parker SH, Lovin JD, Jobe WE, Burke BJ, Hopper KD, Yakes WF. Nonpalpable breast lesions: stereotactic automated large-core biopsies. Radiology 1991; 180:403–407.
3. Dowlatshahi K, Yaremko ML, Kluskens LF, Jokich PM. Nonpalpable breast lesions: findings of stereotaxic needle-core biopsy and fine-needle aspiration cytology. Radiology 1991; 181:745–750.
4. Parker SH, Jobe WE, Dennis MA, et al. US-guided automated large-core biopsy. Radiology 1993; 187:507–511.
5. Elvecrog EL, Lechner MC, Nelson MT. Nonpalpable breast lesions: correlation of stereotaxic large-core needle biopsy and surgical biopsy results. Radiology 1993; 188:453–455.
6. Jackman RJ, Nowel KW, Shepard MJ, Finkelstein SI, Marzoni FA. Stereotaxic large-core needle biopsy of 450 nonpalpable breast lesions with surgical correlation in lesions with cancer or atypical hyperplasia. Radiology 1994; 193:91–95.
7. Parker SH, Burbank F, Jackman RJ, et al. Percutaneous large-core breast biopsy: a multi-institutional study. Radiology 1994; 193:359–364.
8. Rubin E, Dempsey PJ, Pile NS, et al. Needle-localization biopsy of the breast: impact of a selective core needle biopsy program on yield. Radiology 1995; 195:627–631.
9. Liberman L, Cohen MA, Dershaw DD, Abramson AF, Hann LE, Rosen PP. Atypical ductal hyperplasia diagnosed at stereotaxic core biopsy of breast lesions: an indication for surgical biopsy. AJR 1995; 164:1111–1113.
10. Liberman L, Fahs MC, Dershaw DD, et al. Impact of stereotaxic core breast biopsy on cost of diagnosis. Radiology 1995; 195:633–637.
11. Dershaw DD, Morris EA, Liberman L, Abramson AF. Nondiagnostic stereotaxic core breast biopsy: results of rebiopsy. Radiology 1996; 198:323–325.
12. Brenner RJ, Fajardo L, Fisher PR, et al. Percutaneous core biopsy of the breast: effect of operator experience and number of samples on diagnostic accuracy. AJR 1996; 166:341–346.
13. Liberman L, LaTrenta LR, Dershaw DD, et al. Impact of core biopsy on the surgical management of impalpable breast cancer. AJR 1997; 168:495–499.
14. Kaye MD, Vicinanza-Adami CA, Sullivan ML. Mammographic findings after stereotaxic biopsy of the breast performed with large-core needles. Radiology 1994; 192:149–151.
15. Lindfors KK, Rosenquist CJ. Needle core biopsy guided with mammography: a study of cost effectiveness. Radiology 1994; 190:217–222.
16. Lee CH, Egglin TK, Philpotts L, Mainiero MB, Tocino I. Cost-effectiveness of stereotactic core needle biopsy: analysis by means of mammographic findings. Radiology 1997; 202:849–854.
17. Fajardo LL. Cost-effectiveness of stereotaxic breast core needle biopsy. Acad Radiol 1996; 3:521–523.
18. Liberman L, Dershaw DD, Glassman JR, et al. Analysis of cancers not diagnosed at stereotactic core breast biopsy. Radiology 1997; 203:151–157.
19. Liberman L, Dershaw DD, Rosen PP, et al. Stereotaxic 14-gauge breast biopsy: how many core biopsy specimens are needed? Radiology 1994; 192:793–795.
20. Liberman L, Bonaccio E, Hamele-Bena D, Abramson AF, Cohen MA, Dershaw DD. Benign and malignant phyllodes tumors: mammographic and sonographic findings. Radiology 1996; 198:121–124.
21. Burbank F. Stereotactic breast biopsy of atypical ductal hyperplasia and ductal carcinoma in situ lesions: improved accuracy with a directional, vacuum-assisted biopsy instrument. Radiology 1997; 202:843–847.
22. Jackman RJ, Finkelstein SI, Marzoni FA. Stereotaxic large-core needle biopsy of histologically benign nonpalpable breast lesions: false-negative results and failed follow-up (abstr). Radiology 1995; 197(P):203.
23. The American College of Radiology. 19101 approved for stereotactic breast biopsy, effective immediately. In: ACR Bulletin (newsletter). Reston, Va: American College of Radiology, October 1997; 53:5.
24. Hillner BE, Bear HD, Fajardo LL. Estimating the cost-effectiveness of stereotaxic biopsy for nonpalpable breast abnormalities: a decision analysis model. Acad Radiol 1996; 3:351–360.
25. Fajardo LL. Cost-effectiveness of stereotaxic core needle biopsy. Acad Radiol 1996; 3:S21–S23.
26. Nields MW. Cost-effectiveness of image-guided core needle biopsy versus surgery in diagnosing breast cancer. Acad Radiol 1996; (suppl 1) 3:138–140.
27. Burbank F. Mammographic findings after 14-gauge automated needle and 14-gauge directional, vacuum-assisted stereotactic breast biopsies. Radiology 1997; 204:153–156.
28. Kopans DB. Caution on core (devil's advocate). Radiology 1994; 193:325–328.
29. Goodman KA, Birdwell RL, Ikeda DM. Compliance with recommended follow-up after percutaneous breast core biopsy. AJR 1998; 170:89–92.
30. Berlin L. Tracking for breast cancer. AJR 1998; 170:93–95.
31. Burbank F, Parker SH, Fogarty TJ. Stereotactic breast biopsy: improved tissue harvesting with the Mammotome. Am Surg 1996; 62:738–744.
32. Liberman L, Hann LE, Dershaw DD, Morris EA, Abramson AF, Rosen PP. Mammographic findings after stereotactic 14-gauge vacuum biopsy. Radiology 1997; 203:343–347.
33. Jackman RJ, Burbank F, Parker SH, et al. Atypical ductal hyperplasia diagnosed at stereotactic breast biopsy: improved reliability with 14-gauge, directional, vacuum-assisted biopsy. Radiology 1997; 204:485–488.
34. Meyer JE, Smith DN, Dipiro PJ, et al. Stereotactic breast biopsy of clustered microcalcifications with a directional, vacuum-assisted device. Radiology 1997; 204:575–576.
35. Berg WA, Krebs TL, Campassi C, Magder LS, Sun CCJ. Evaluation of 14- and 11-gauge directional, vacuum-assisted biopsy probes and 14-gauge biopsy guns in a breast parenchymal model. Radiology 1997; 205:203–208.

36. Burbank F. Mammotomy: post-biopsy mammogram findings and CPT coding. Adm Radiol 1997; 16:14–19.
37. Burbank F. Stereotactic breast biopsy: comparison of 14- and 11-gauge Mammotome probe performance and complication rates. Am Surg 1997; 11:988–995.
38. Burbank F, Forcier N. Tissue marking clip for stereotactic breast biopsy: initial placement accuracy, long-term stability, and usefulness as a guide for wire localization. Radiology 1997; 205:407–415.
39. Liberman L, Dershaw DD, Morris EA, et al. Clip placement after stereotactic vacuum-assisted breast biopsy. Radiology 1997; 205:417–422.
40. Bird RE. A prospective and retrospective evaluation of the potential usefulness of the 2 cm core ABBI technology in breast biopsy. Presented at the Third Postgraduate Course of the Society of Breast Imaging, San Diego, Calif, April 16-19, 1997.
41. Ferzli GS, Hurwitz JB, Puza T, Vorst-Bilotti SV. Advanced breast biopsy instrumentation: a critique. J Am Coll Surg 1997; 185:145–151.
42. D'Angelo PC, Galliano DE, Rosemurgy AS. Stereotactic excisional breast biopsies utilizing the advanced breast biopsy instrumentation system. Am J Surg 1997; 174:297–302.
43. Mandis SH, Murray T, Bolden S, Wingo PA. Cancer statistics, 1998. CA Cancer J Clin 1998; 48:6–29.
44. Osteen RT, Cady B, Chmiel JS, et al. 1991 National Survey of Carcinoma of the Breast by the Commission on Cancer. J Am Coll Surg 1994; 178:213–219.
45. Jackman RJ, Marzoni FA. Needle-localized breast biopsy: why do we fail? Radiology 1997; 204:677–684.

Science to Practice
RSNA '98

Integrating Science Into Practice

Associated Sciences Program at RSNA 1998

Workshop: Saturday, Nov. 28, 1998, 10:15 am - 4:30 pm, McCormick Place Sou

Refresher Courses: Sunday, Nov. 29, 1998 through Friday, Dec. 4, 1998

Credits: 4¼ hours and an additional 1½ hours credit for attendance at the Basic Physics Lecture

Welcome and Introduction
10:15 am
Samuel L. Hissong, MD, Chair, Associated Sciences Consortium and Committee
Eugene D. Frank, MA, RT(R), Coordinator, Associated Sciences Consortium

Keynote Presentation
10:30 - 11:50 am
Impact of Telematic Technologies on Image-Guided Medicine (AIA-AAH)
Heinz U. Lemke, PhD

Break
11:50 am - 12:10 pm

Special Luncheon Program
12:10 - 1:20 pm
Networking for the New Millennium - Important Factors to Consider (SMRT)
Bruce Johnson, BSEE

Break
1:20 - 1:30 pm

Panel Presentation
1:30 - 2:50 pm
The Reality of Computerization (AERS, AHRA, SROA)
Richard Carlton, MS, RT(R)
Robert Seely, MBA, RT(R)
Heinz U. Lemke, PhD

AAPM/RSNA Basic Physics Lecture for the Radiologic Technologist: Vascular Imaging Physics
Organized by Gerald A. White, Jr., MS
3:00 - 4:30 pm
1½ hours credit

Refresher Courses

(Each Refresher Course is approved for 1½ hours credit)

Sunday RC 124
Organizational Culture and Health System Change
Cornelius J. Rater, MD (AERS)
Harry J. Granito, MS (RBMA)
Douglas R. Hanson (ASRT)

Monday RC 224
Liability Issues Arising from the Changing Health Care Environment
Ann Obergfell, JD, RT(R) (ASRT)
Perry Smith, JD, RDMS (SDMS)

Monday RC 324
Organizational Change In Radiology: Preparing Radiology for the Next Millennium
Monte G. Clinton (AHRA)
Donna L. Wright, EdD, RT(R) (AERS)
Loretta L. Hanwell, MPA (AHRA)

Tuesday RC 424
Competency, Continuity, and Compliance
Susan S. Weiss, CNMT (SNM-TS)
Kate Little, RN (ARNA)

Wednesday RC 524
Managing a Multisite Radiology Network
Larry Ranahan, MBA (RBMA) Moderator
Sherry Rader (RBMA)
Charles Deschamps, RT(R)(MR) (SMRT)
Rebecca Shanahan, JD (RBMA)

Thursday RC 624
Specialized Accreditations: A Cost of Doing Business
Luann J. Culbreth, MEd, RT(R)(MR) (SMRT) Moderator
John Kovelski, RT(R)(MR) (SMRT)
Karol Handrahan, RT(R) (SMRT)
Linda Zanin, MS, PhD (SDMS)
Ronald F. Bernardi, BA, RT(R)(N) (AHRA)

Thursday RC 724
Multidisciplinary Standards for the New Millennium
Susan S. Weiss, CNMT (SNM-TS), Moderator
William R. Poller, MD (SNM-TS)
Michael R. Bloyd, RT(R), BSN (ASRT)
Liz Anderson, MBA (AVIR)

Friday RC 824
Marketing Radiology: Getting the Message Out
Ronald F. Bernardi, BA, RT(R)(N), Moderator
Cherrill Farnsworth (AHRA)
Michael R. Favreau, FAHRA (AHRA)

Registration Information

Advance registration for the RSNA Scientific Assembly ends October 30. Onsite registration begins at 12:00 noon on Saturday, November 28, at McCormick Place. RSNA shuttle bus service to McCormick Place will be available beginning at 10:00 am on Saturday. Advance registration is not required for the Saturday workshop; however, to receive continuing education credit, you must register.

Advance registration information appears in the July issue of *Radiology.* Brochures are also available from your association or from the RSNA, 2021 Spring Road, Suite 600, Oak Brook, IL 60523-1860. Phone: 630/571-7862.

Registration for the RSNA Scientific Assembly includes registration for the Associated Sciences Workshop. A box lunch will be available for purchase to facilitate your attendance at the workshop. These lunches must be purchased with your advance registration for the RSNA Meeting. **If you wish to purchase a box lunch, please check the appropriate box on the RSNA Advance Registration form and enclose your $11.50 payment.**

If you would like a copy of the published Associated Sciences Proceedings, please call 630/571-7877.

Sponsoring Organizations

- American Healthcare Radiology Administrators (AHRA)
- American Institute of Architects — Academy on Architecture for Health (AIA-AAH)
- American Radiological Nurses Association (ARNA)
- American Society of Radiologic Technologists (ASRT)
- Association of Educators in Radiological Sciences (AERS)
- Association of Vascular and Interventional Radiographers (AVIR)
- Radiological Business Management Association (RBMA)
- Society for Radiation Oncology Administrators (SROA)
- Society of Diagnostic Medical Sonographers (SDMS)
- Society of Magnetic Resonance Technologists (SMRT)
- Society of Nuclear Medicine — Technologists Section (SNM-TS)

Marilyn A. Roubidoux, MD
Todd E. Wilson, MD
Richard J. Orange, MD
J. Thomas Fitzgerald, PhD
Mark A. Helvie, MD
Sasha A. Packer, BS

Index terms:
Breast neoplasms, 00.32
Breast radiography, 00.11
Cancer screening, 00.11
Hormones, 00.52

Radiology 1998; 208:725–728

Abbreviation:
HRT = hormone replacement therapy

[1]From the Department of Radiology, University of Michigan Hospitals/TC2910, 1500 E Medical Center Dr, Ann Arbor, MI 48109-0326 (M.A.R., T.E.W., M.A.H.); the Department of Medical Education, Towsley Center G1211, Ann Arbor, Mich (J.T.F.); the Department of Health Education, University of Utah, Salt Lake City (S.A.P.); and the Department of Radiology, Emory University, Atlanta, Ga (R.J.O.). Received October 14, 1997; revision requested January 12, 1998; revision received February 12; accepted April 3. **Address reprint requests to** M.A.R.

Author contributions:
Guarantor of integrity of entire study, M.A.R.; study concepts, M.A.R., T.E.W., S.A.P.; study design, M.A.R., T.E.W.; definition of intellectual content, M.A.R.; literature research, S.A.P., M.A.R.; clinical studies, M.A.H.; data acquisition, M.A.R., T.E.W., R.J.O.; data analysis, M.A.R., T.E.W.; statistical analysis, J.T.F.; manuscript preparation, M.A.R.; manuscript editing, M.A.R., M.A.H.; manuscript review, M.A.R., T.E.W., M.A.H.

Breast Cancer in Women Who Undergo Screening Mammography: Relationship of Hormone Replacement Therapy to Stage and Detection Method[1]

PURPOSE: To compare the breast cancer stages and detection methods in screened women who receive hormone replacement therapy (HRT) with those in screened women who do not receive HRT to determine whether HRT affects the stage or mammographic detection of malignancy.

MATERIALS AND METHODS: One hundred fifteen cases of breast cancer in women (age range, 55–65 years) in whom at least one screening mammogram had been obtained at least 24 months before diagnosis and in whom the history regarding HRT could be determined were reviewed retrospectively. Statistical analysis was performed with χ^2 analysis and the Fisher exact test.

RESULTS: The cancer stages in the 58 women who received HRT were stage 0 in 15 (26%), stage I in 28 (48%), stage II in 13 (22%), and stage III in two (3%) women. The stages in the 57 women who did not receive HRT were stage 0 in 19 (33%), stage I in 24 (42%), stage II in 11 (19%), stage III in two (4%), and stage IV in one (2%) woman. Cancers in 38 (67%) of the women who did not receive HRT and in 38 (66%) of those who did receive HRT were detected with mammography alone; false-negative mammograms were obtained in five (9%) women in the non–HRT group and in four (7%) women in the HRT group (P = .89).

CONCLUSION: Among screened women who developed breast cancer, there were no significant differences in cancer stages or in the number of mammographically detected cancers or false-negative mammograms between the HRT group and the non-HRT group.

Hormone replacement therapy (HRT) is an important component of preventive health care for postmenopausal women (1). The risk-benefit ratio of this popular therapy is complex, because HRT has been reported to not only increase the risk of breast cancer but also to decrease the sensitivity of screening mammography (2,3). Screening mammography is the most sensitive method in the detection of breast cancer, and if the accuracy of mammography is negatively affected by HRT, higher breast cancer stages and increased rates of palpable cancer and false-negative mammograms would be expected in these women (4). The purpose of this study was to evaluate cancers found in women who have undergone screening mammography and compare women who use HRT with those who do not use HRT.

MATERIALS AND METHODS

Through a retrospective search of the computerized tumor registry and breast imaging database, we reviewed the findings in 178 postmenopausal women aged 55-65 years with breast cancer found between January 1987 and May 1997 who underwent staging and final treatment at our institution and in whom the history regarding prior estrogen use and the dates of previously performed mammography could be determined. During the time of the study, a total of 856 patients had breast cancer diagnosed by using clinically directed or wire-localized biopsy performed at our institution. Of these 856 patients, 193 were aged 55–65 years. In 178 of these 193 patients, information regarding the dates of prior mammography, HRT, and the stage of disease was available. Excluded from the study were 15 patients in whom this information was not available. All patients with invasive breast cancer underwent surgical axillary dissection or the stage of their cancer was determined clinically.

Of the 178 women, 115 had at least one routine screening mammogram obtained within 24 months before diagnosis. Screening mammography was defined as that performed in women without clinical abnormalities. These 115 women were our study group, and 92 (80%) of them had their breast tumor malignancy detected solely at our institution. The remaining 23 (20%) patients had come to our institution for evaluation, biopsy, or both of a clinical or mammographic finding identified at another institution. The clinical, mammographic, and histologic records of these women were reviewed to determine the cancer stages, clinical findings, and dates of estrogen use and previous screening mammography.

Data regarding estrogen use were obtained from a computerized search of our pharmacy database and from the responses to questionnaires regarding mammography recorded by either the patients or the technologists. HRT was defined as oral or transdermal use of estrogen, with or without progesterone. Women who had received HRT were categorized in the HRT group if their duration of HRT was more than 6 months before the breast cancer diagnosis. Women who had not received HRT within 1 year of diagnosis were categorized in the non-HRT group. The intervals, in months, from the last previous screening mammogram were determined.

The study group of 115 women included women with all breast cancers regardless of the method of detection. The methods of detection were palpation alone, mammography alone, or mammography and palpation. All cancers were classified into one of these three categories.

The women in the study group were aged 55–65 years because estrogen use was most common in women in this age range at our institution and because the menopause status was more clearly distinguished in women in this age range.

Comparisons between the HRT group and the non–HRT group were made by using the χ^2 analysis for stages and detection methods. The combined early cancer stages (0 and I) and the combined late cancer stages (III and IV) in these women were evaluated by using the Fisher exact test. The Fisher exact test was also used to determine the differences between the two groups in positive findings for lymph nodes and in screening intervals.

RESULTS

The average age of the 115 women at the time of breast cancer diagnosis was 60 years. Fifty-seven women (mean age, 60 years) had not received HRT, and 58 women (mean age, 60 years) had received HRT. The duration of HRT was 6–170 months (mean duration, 68 months). The intervals, in months, from the last previous screening mammogram to the detection of cancer were compared between the non–HRT group (range, 4–24 months; mean, 12.8 months) and the HRT group (range, 5–24 months; mean, 12.4 months) (P = .99). In the 67 women who were screened at least 12 months before the detection of breast cancer, four of 34 cancers in women in the HRT group and five of 33 cancers in women in the non-HRT group manifested as "interval cancer," defined as a clinically detected malignancy that occurred before the next annual screening mammogram date.

The cancer stages and axillary metastases found in the HRT and non-HRT groups are summarized in Table 1. Cancers were diagnosed at an early stage (stage 0 or I) in 43 (74%) women who had received HRT and in 43 (75%) women who had not received HRT. No differences in the five stages of cancer (P = .75), positive findings for axillary lymph nodes (P = .65), or combined early (0 and I) or combined late (III and IV) stages (P = .99) were indicated between the two groups.

The cancer detection methods are summarized in Table 2. Cancers in 38 (67%) women who did not receive HRT and in 38 (66%) women who did receive HRT were detected with mammography alone; false-negative mammograms (cancers were detected with palpation alone) were obtained in five (9%) women in the non-HRT group and in four (7%) women in the HRT group (P = .89).

TABLE 1
Cancer Stages in Women Who Received HRT versus Those in Women Who Did Not Receive HRT

Cancer Stage*	HRT Group (n = 58)	Non-HRT Group (n = 57)
0	15 (26)	19 (33)
I	28 (48)	24 (42)
T1a	4 (7)	2 (4)
T1b	7 (12)	8 (14)
T1c	17 (29)	14 (25)
II	13 (22)	11 (19)
III	2 (3)	2 (4)
IV	0 (0)	1 (2)
Nodal metastases	11 (19)	13 (23)

Note.—Numbers in parentheses are percentages.
* P = .75 for differences between the HRT group and the non-HRT group in the number of women with stage I, II, III, or IV cancer. P = .65 for differences between the HRT group and the non-HRT group in the number of women with nodal metastasis.

TABLE 2
Cancer Detection Methods in Women Who Received HRT versus Those in Women Who Did Not Receive HRT

Cancer Detection Method	HRT Group	Non-HRT Group
Mammography alone	38 (66)	38 (67)
Palpation alone	4 (7)	5 (9)
Mammography and palpation	16 (28)	14 (25)
Total	58 (100)	57 (100)

Note.—P = .89 for differences in cancer detection methods between the HRT group and the non-HRT group.

Of the 86 women with early-stage (0 and 1) cancers, 35 of 43 (81%) women in the HRT group and 36 of 43 (84%) women in the non-HRT group had cancers that were detected by using mammography alone.

DISCUSSION

The survival and quality-of-life benefits of HRT for postmenopausal women, including relief of menopausal symptoms and prevention of cardiovascular disease and osteoporosis (1,5–7), are well established. However, endogenous gonadal hormones are known to have an important role in causing breast cancer, and exogenous HRT is reported to increase the risk of breast cancer 1.5–2.0-fold (3).

The results of a recent study (8) indicated that the risk of death caused by breast cancer increases 43% after 10 years of HRT; this increased risk could offset the expected survival advantages. Furthermore, estrogens may increase the growth of some breast cancer cells and thus accelerate the development of breast cancer (9).

It has also been reported (2) that the sensitivity and specificity of screening mammography are lower in women who receive HRT. In a subsequent report (10), a marginal decrease in only specificity was found; however, staging information was not provided. If the increased breast density seen on mammograms in women who receive HRT decreases the sensitivity of mammography in the detection of early breast cancer, then higher stages or greater proportions of palpable cancers may be expected in these women (2).

Despite concern regarding mammographic sensitivity in women who receive HRT, in several studies (11,12) it was found paradoxically that survival rates improved 10%–50% in women who received HRT and developed breast cancer. In previous studies (11–14) in which breast cancers in women who received HRT were compared with those in women who did not receive HRT, variable differences in lymph node status were found, and no differences were found in the other tumor indices of size, differentiation, or receptor status. The duration of HRT has not been reported to affect these parameters or lymph node status (12,14). The most important difference in tumor indices between the two groups was that smaller proportions of stage III and stage IV cancers were found in women who received HRT. Therefore, the improved survival rates were considered to be due to favorable cancer stages at diagnosis and not related to the cardiovascular benefits of estrogen. However, it was unclear whether the better stage at diagnosis was due to an intrinsic beneficial effect of estrogen on the tumor or to improved diagnostic detection because of wider use of screening in women who received HRT (14,15).

Various limitations in previous studies (10–14) of HRT and breast cancer have been the exclusion of patients with ductal carcinoma in situ, differences between the mean age of women who received HRT and that of women who did not receive HRT, select population groups, and the lack of staging information or detailed screening mammographic data. Since cancer stage at detection varies with use of screening mammography, comparisons of breast cancer stages must identify whether differences exist in rates of screening mammography between groups (4).

In contrast to the previous study (14) in which fewer stage III and stage IV cancers were found, we did not find differences in cancer stages. This suggests that previously reported differences may have been due to different screening rates between groups. Our study groups were homogeneous with regard to age and screening mammography history; the HRT and non-HRT groups had no differences in proportions of cancer stages, positive lymph node statuses, interval cancers, mammographically detected cancers, or false-negative mammograms. Despite previous evidence (16) that HRT increases breast density, our findings indicate that HRT does not impair the early detection of breast cancer in women who have undergone screening mammography; the findings do not indicate that women who receive HRT have improved survival because hormones predispose women to low-risk breast tumors (12,15–17).

Our study group included women with all breast cancers regardless of the method of detection. This way, the outcome is measured in terms of breast cancer stages determined within 2 years after screening mammography. The results were not limited to only those in women with cancers that were detected exclusively by means of screening mammography, a subgroup known to have favorable prognostic parameters (18). In our study groups, the proportions of positive axillary nodes and rates of interval cancers found before the next 12-month screening date were similar to those described in a previous study (14) of cancers found after a first screening round.

A limitation of this study was that women who had not been screened, including those who had received HRT and those who had not, were not included. Thus, it is unknown whether differences in stage or detection methods would be found between women in HRT and non-HRT groups who did not have the benefit of undergoing screening mammography within the previous 24 months. Another limitation was the lack of data on the role of clinical breast examination or self breast examination in cancer detection in women who receive HRT compared with those in women who do not receive HRT. Another limitation of this study was that data were not available regarding the type of preparation, administration, and dosage of estrogen. Therefore, it is unknown whether differences in any of these pharmacologic factors could affect the stage of cancer. Another limitation was that mammographic density, a factor that is reported to be altered with HRT, was not compared between the HRT and non-HRT groups. Therefore, it is unknown whether differences in mammographic density in these women might affect the cancer stage at detection.

Annual screening mammography has been advocated for women older than 40 years. There are conflicting findings in the literature (19) with regard to most factors that are thought to affect compliance with screening mammography guidelines, such as economic status, insurance, marital status, education, income, employment, and breast cancer risk factors. However, physician endorsement through referral and discussion with the patient is consistently found to be the most powerful motivation for patient participation in screening mammography (19,20).

Each woman and her physician must compare her personal health risks with the statistical risks and benefits of HRT. Our findings indicate that in women who participate in screening mammography, HRT does not impair the mammographic detection of breast cancer and is not associated with differences in stages of breast cancer.

Acknowledgments: The authors appreciate the manuscript preparation by Debra Harris and wish to thank Dottie M. Packer, who originally proposed the questions that initiated research into this topic.

References

1. Speroff L. Menopause and hormone replacement therapy. Clin Geriatr Med 1993; 9:33–55.
2. Laya MB, Larson EB, Taplin SH, White E. Effect of estrogen replacement therapy on the specificity and sensitivity of screening mammography. J Natl Cancer Inst 1996; 88:643–649.
3. Colditz GA, Hankinson SE, Hunter DJ, et al. The use of estrogens and progestins and the risk of breast cancer in postmenopausal women. N Engl J Med 1995; 332: 1589–1593.
4. Thurfjell EL, Lindgren JAA. Population-based mammography screening in Swedish clinical practice: prevalence and incidence screening in Uppsala County. Radiology 1994; 193:351–357.
5. Henderson BE, Paganini-Hill A, Ross RK. Decreased mortality in users of estrogen replacement therapy. Arch Intern Med 1996; 151:75–78.
6. Psaty BM, Heckbert SR, Atkins D, et al. A review of the association of estrogens and progestrins with cardiovascular disease in postmenopausal women. Arch Intern Med 1993; 153:1421–1427.
7. Riggs BL, Melton LJ. The prevention and treatment of osteoporosis. N Engl J Med 1992; 327:620–627.
8. Grodstein F, Stampfer MJ, Colditz GA, et al. Postmenopausal hormone therapy and mortality. N Engl J Med 1997; 336:1769–1775.

9. Khoo KS, Chick P. Sex steroid hormones and breast cancer: is there a link with oral contraceptives and hormone replacement therapy. Med J Aust 1992; 156:124–132.
10. Thurfjell EL, Holmberg LH, Persson IR. Screening mammography: sensitivity and specificity in relation to hormone replacement therapy. Radiology 1997; 203: 339–341.
11. Strickland DM, Gambrell RD Jr, Butzin CA, Strickland K. The relationship between breast cancer survival and prior postmenopausal estrogen use. Obstet Gynecol 1992; 80:400–404.
12. Bergkvist L, Persson I, Bergstrom R, Krusemo UB. Prognosis after breast cancer diagnosis in women exposed to estrogen and estrogen-progestogen replacement therapy. Am J Epidemiol 1989; 130:221–228.
13. Grodstein F, Stampfer MJ, Colditz GA, et al. Postmenopausal hormone therapy and mortality. N Engl J Med 1997; 336:1769–1775.
14. Jones C, Ingram D, Mattes E, Hahnel R. The effect of hormone replacement therapy on prognostic indices in women with breast cancer. Med J Aust 1994; 161:106–110.
15. Brinton LA, Schairer C. Postmenopausal hormone-replacement therapy: time for a reappraisal? N Engl J Med 1997; 336:1821–1822.
16. Cyrlak D, Wong CH. Mammographic changes in postmenopausal women undergoing hormonal replacement therapy. AJR 1993; 161:1177–1183.
17. Laya MB, Gallagher JC, Schreiman JS, Larson EB, Watson P, Weinstein L. Effect of postmenopausal hormonal replacement therapy on mammographic density and parenchymal pattern. Radiology 1995; 196:433–437.
18. Sickles EA. Quality assurance: how to audit your own mammography practice. Radiol Clin North Am 1992; 30:265–275.
19. Schapira DV, Levine RB. Breast cancer screening and compliance and evaluation of lesions. Cancer 1996; 80:15–25.
20. Fox SA, Siu AL, Stein JA. The importance of physician communication on breast cancer screening of older women. Arch Intern Med 1994; 154:2058–2068.

Renal Blood Flow: Measurement in Vivo with Rapid Spiral MR Imaging[1]

Graham Sommer, MD
Geraldine Corrigan, MD
Jill Fredrickson, PhD
Anne Sawyer-Glover, RT
Jan-Ray Liao, PhD
Bryan Myers, MD
Norbert Pelc, ScD

Index terms:
Blood, flow dynamics, 961.91, 966.91
Magnetic resonance (MR), phase imaging
Magnetic resonance (MR), technology
Renal arteries, flow dynamics, 961.91
Renal arteries, MR, 961.12949, 966.12949

Radiology 1998; 208:729–734

Abbreviations:
PAH = *p*-aminohippuric acid
RBF = renal blood flow

[1] From the Department of Radiology (G.S., J.F., A.S.G., J.R.L., N.P.) and the Division of Nephrology (G.C., B.M.), Stanford University Medical Center, 300 Pasteur Dr, Rm H-1307, Stanford, CA 94305-5105. Received December 22, 1997; revision requested March 17, 1998; revision received April 21; accepted May 8. Supported in part by grant RO1-DK48051 from the National Institutes of Health. **Address reprint requests to** G.S.

Author contributions:
Guarantor of integrity of entire study, G.S.; study concepts, G.S., N.P.; study design, G.S., N.P., B.M.; definition of intellectual content, G.S., N.P., B.M.; literature research, G.S., N.P.; clinical studies, G.S.; experimental studies, G.S., N.P., J.R.L., J.F.; data acquisition, G.S., A.S.G.; data analysis, G.S., G.C.; statistical analysis, G.S., G.C.; manuscript preparation, G.S.; manuscript editing, G.S.; manuscript review, G.S.

PURPOSE: To assess the ability of three cine phase-contrast magnetic resonance (MR) imaging techniques to measure normal human renal blood flow (RBF) in vivo.

MATERIALS AND METHODS: Eighteen healthy volunteers were studied with three cine phase-contrast MR imaging techniques: breath-hold, segmented k-space, two-dimensional, Fourier transform technique (ie, time-resolved imaging with automatic data segmentation, or TRIADS); a breath-hold rapid spiral acquisition; and a non–breath-hold rapid spiral acquisition that allowed resolution of both cardiac and respiratory cycles. In each case, total arterial RBF and blood flow per unit of renal volume were calculated. For each subject, RBF was measured with a standard technique of *p*-aminohippuric acid (PAH)-clearance hematocrit on the same day as the MR imaging examination was performed.

RESULTS: The range of agreement (2 standard deviations, or 95% confidence interval) between RBF measurements obtained with the PAH-clearance hematocrit technique and the various cine phase-contrast techniques varied from ±17.6% to ±26.5%. The best agreement was obtained with non–breath-hold rapid spiral data, by using data from the end-expiratory phase of respiration.

CONCLUSION: Findings with cine phase-contrast MR imaging employing rapid spiral acquisition are in good agreement with measurements made with PAH-clearance hematocrit and give the promise of clinical measurement of RBF.

Current methods for quantifying human renal blood flow (RBF) in vivo are either indirect, and subject to a variety of assumptions that may be incorrect, or unacceptably invasive. Cine phase-contrast magnetic resonance (MR) imaging techniques (1–8), on the other hand, offer the possibility of direct and accurate measurement of in vivo RBF noninvasively. Such determination of RBF could be of considerable value in better understanding renal physiology, since the renal circulation is known to play a critical role in glomerular filtration, tubular reabsorption, and renal hormone production. Additionally, the diagnosis of reduced RBF due to renal arterial stenosis would likely be facilitated by means of such a noninvasive measurement. Such compromise in RBF is an important clinical problem in the United States and has long been recognized as an important cause of both systemic hypertension and chronic renal failure (9,10).

Findings in prior studies have indicated that cine phase-contrast techniques are capable of accurate measurement of blood flow in phantoms, animal models, and in vivo human studies (2,11–16). In the measurement of human arterial RBF in vivo, one problem that has been noted is physiologic motion of the renal vessels with respiration, which can lead to substantial measurement inaccuracy. Prior studies of measurement of human arterial RBF employing cine phase-contrast MR imaging techniques with breath holding and a segmented k-space acquisition have indicated a potential for more accurate measurements (2). In the present study, results with cine phase-contrast techniques employing rapid spiral acquisitions were evaluated for the measurement of human RBF in vivo and compared to those obtained with the previous segmented k-space method and a standard technique of *p*-aminohippuric acid (PAH)-clearance hematocrit. Cine phase-contrast techniques employing spiral imaging of k space were thought to be promising for this application, since such techniques are suitable for very rapid acquisitions with either standard or enhanced magnetic field gradient hardware (15,16). Importantly, the spiral acquisition strategy has excellent behavior in the presence of flow and is therefore inherently well suited for flow determination, since each spiral data acquisition begins at the origin of k space, and gradient moments are periodically nulled due to the oscillatory nature of the gradients.

MATERIALS AND METHODS

Eighteen healthy volunteers (seven men, 11 women; age range, 23–45 years; mean age, 28 years) who had no history of renal disease and were not taking medications known to interfere with secretion of PAH were evaluated prospectively after giving written informed consent, according to a protocol approved by our human subjects review committee. In each subject, RBF was determined by means of both cine phase-contrast MR imaging and PAH-clearance hematocrit on the same day. RBF was measured with each technique by two different investigators, who were blinded to the results of the other study.

Subjects were admitted to the clinical research center at our institution to determine PAH-clearance hematocrit according to a standard procedure (17). They voided urine spontaneously. Diuresis was then established by means of oral water loading (10 mL per kilogram of body weight) and sustained thereafter by having the subject ingest water in a volume equal to that of the urine voided. A priming dose of PAH (16 mg/kg) was administered followed by a sustaining intravenous infusion to maintain plasma levels constant at around 1.5 mg/dL. One hour was allowed for equilibration, and then arterial blood pressure was determined and a blood sample was obtained from a peripheral vein. Subsequently, four timed urine collections were made, with a blood sample obtained before and after each collection. Plasma and urinary concentrations of PAH were assayed by using techniques described previously (17). Renal plasma flow (RPF) was calculated from the clearance rate of PAH divided by PAH extraction rate, assumed to be 0.9. RBF was calculated as RPF/(1 − Hct), where Hct is the hematocrit of venous blood.

After the clearance study was completed, each subject was transferred to the MR imaging facility. All patients underwent imaging in a 1.5-T MR imaging system with enhanced magnetic field gradients (Signa Echospeed 5.5; GE Medical Systems, Milwaukee, Wis). A posterior 5-inch (13-cm)-diameter surface coil was employed for all studies. Respiration was recorded by a means of a chest bellows, and gating of the cardiac cycle was performed by means of digital plethysmography.

Initial gradient-recalled-echo images were obtained to visualize the renal arteries in coronal and axial planes. Contiguous 5-mm-thick sections were obtained with repetition time msec/echo time msec of 19/12, a flip angle of 30°, field of view of 32 cm, and data acquisition matrix of 256 × 128 pixels. A dual-oblique approach was employed to allow acquisition of flow data in a plane as orthogonal as possible to the renal arteries, as shown in Figure 1. After the initial coronal gradient-recalled image was acquired (Fig 1a), oblique axial gradient-recalled images were obtained along planes parallel to each renal artery, as depicted on the initial images. Prior to quantitative imaging, magnetic field homogeneity over the volume to be imaged was optimized by using the automated shimming feature provided by the manufacturer. This was done once per subject (ie, the same shim setting was used for all vessels and all sequences). The acquisition plane for the various cine phase-contrast sequences was 4 mm thick and was positioned 1–2 cm from the origin of the renal artery on the basis of the resultant oblique axial image, with the acquisition plane perpendicular to the renal artery (Fig 1b).

Three cine phase-contrast techniques were then employed to acquire data in each renal artery. The techniques were (*a*) a segmented k-space, two-dimensional, Fourier transform technique (time-resolved imaging with automatic data segmentation, or TRIADS [12]) (hereafter, "segmented k space"); (*b*) a breath-hold technique employing rapid spiral acquisition (16) (hereafter, "breath-hold rapid spiral"); and (*c*) a recently described technique employing rapid spiral acquisitions that simultaneously resolves both cardiac and respiratory motion and does not require breath holding (18) (hereafter, "non–breath-hold rapid spiral"). Details of the three techniques are summarized in Table 1. As noted in this table, the non–breath-hold rapid spiral technique resolves the respiratory cycle into eight phases, and the imaging time is therefore about eight times longer than that for the breath-hold rapid spiral technique.

All pulse sequences were optimized for the available gradient amplitude (22 mT/m) and slew rate (120 mT/m/msec). For the segmented k-space technique, only six cardiac frames were acquired to limit imaging time to a breath-hold interval. The segmented k-space data were acquired with 19/7.9, a flip angle of 45°, a 20-cm field of view, and a data acquisition matrix of 256 × 128 pixels. For both the non–breath-hold and breath-hold rapid spiral techniques, sections were acquired with 55/6.3, a flip angle of 45°, a 20-cm field of view, 20 spiral interleaves, and a data acquisition matrix of 188 × 188 pixels. With the breath-hold and non–breath-hold rapid spiral techniques, spectral-spatial excitation pulses were used to reduce off-resonance effects, and piecewise linear spiral trajectories (19) were employed to reduce gradient slewing duty cycles. No problems or limitations were observed due to the use of piecewise linear trajectories.

In all cases, the maximum velocity chosen for flow encoding was 100 cm/sec. In cases of accessory renal arteries, separate dual-oblique localization of each

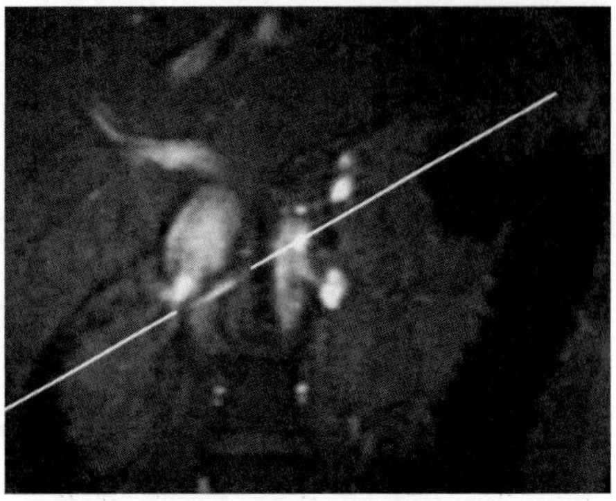

a.

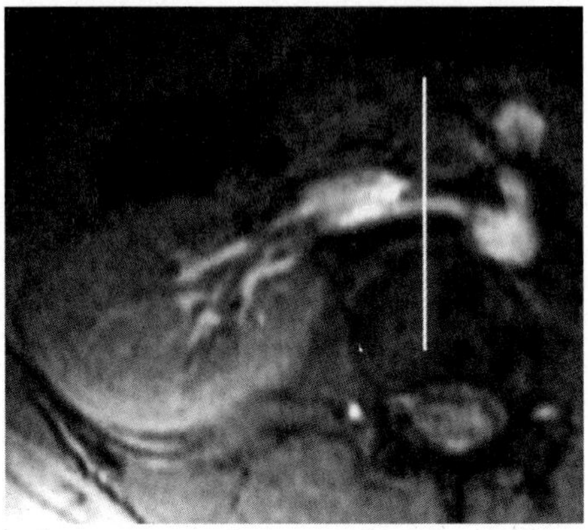

b.

Figure 1. Method for prescription of double-oblique acquisition. **(a)** On this coronal gradient-recalled image, the oblique axial plane (line) is prescribed parallel to the right renal artery. **(b)** On this oblique axial gradient-recalled image, the acquisition plane (line) for cine phase-contrast sequence is prescribed orthogonal to the right renal artery.

TABLE 1				
Characteristics of Three Phase-Contrast MR Imaging Techniques				

Phase-Contrast Technique	Type of Acquisition	Approximate Acquisition Time	No. of Cardiac Phases	No. of Respiratory Phases*
Segmented k space	Two-dimensional, Fourier transform	28 sec	6	NA
Rapid spiral				
Breath hold	Spiral	16 sec	16	NA
Non–breath hold	Spiral	2 min 30 sec	16	8

* NA = not applicable.

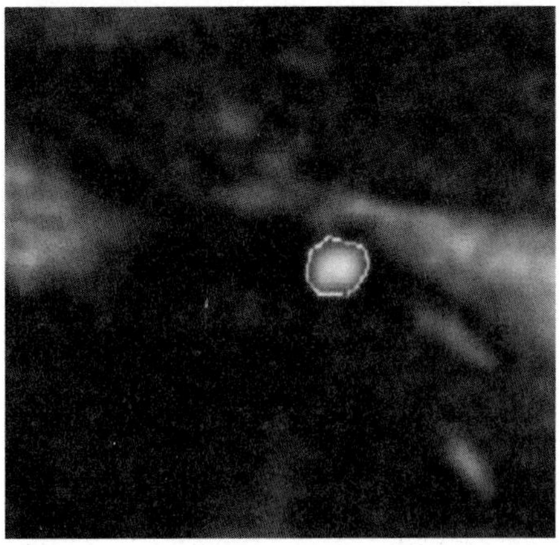

a.

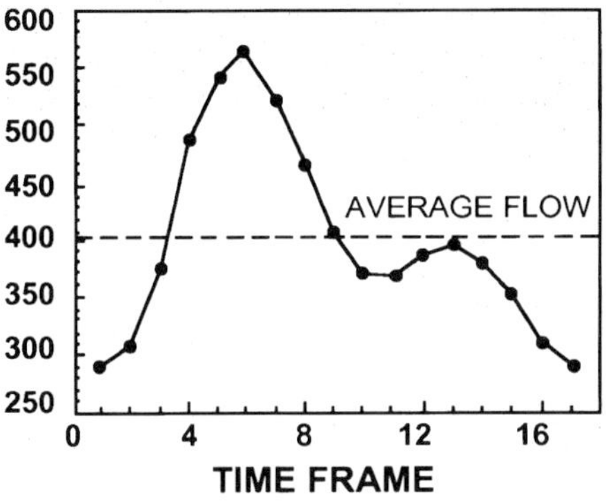

b.

Figure 2. Computation of flow in a right renal artery. **(a)** Breath-hold rapid spiral image is one of 16 frames of the cardiac cycle and depicts the automatically computed region of interest around the right renal artery. **(b)** Graph depicts the average flow profile over 16 cardiac frames computed for the right renal artery. The y axis indicates right arterial RBF (in milliliters per minute).

renal artery was performed, unless these arteries ran along essentially parallel courses, in which case single localization was performed. Whenever possible, dual-oblique localization of right and left renal veins was also performed in a manner similar to that outlined for the arterial acquisitions. The maximum velocity for flow encoding employed for venous acquisitions was 50 cm/sec. After cine phase-contrast acquisitions for flow measurement, breath-hold axial T1-weighted images were obtained throughout the kidneys with a fast multiplanar spoiled gradient-recalled, or FMPSPGR, technique with section thickness of 1 cm. These images were obtained to allow later measurement of bilateral renal volumes by summing the areas of the renal outlines on each axial image. Effects of partial volume averaging at the edges of the kidneys were minimized by tracing renal outlines at the center of the region of signal intensity gradation between the renal margin and the adjacent perinephric fat.

The breath-hold and non–breath-hold rapid spiral images were reconstructed off-line. The algorithm included a correction for constant and linearly varying field offsets as part of the grid application step (20). A single field map was used for all cine time frames. The reconstruction time for a 16-frame breath-hold rapid spiral image—including line interpolation, grid application, Fourier transformation, and phase difference processing—was about 2 minutes on a Sparc-10 workstation (Sun Microsystems, Palo Alto, Calif). The reconstruction time for a non–breath-hold rapid spiral image with eight respiratory frames was eight times longer.

Flow calculations were performed by using flow analysis software developed at our institution. For the non–breath-hold rapid spiral technique, data from both end expiration and end inspiration were analyzed separately to provide two corresponding values of RBF. Initially, a first-order background correction for phase shifts caused by factors other than blood flow (primarily, eddy currents) was performed with the aid of data from regions of interest outlined on static tissues. Flow for each renal artery was computed by using separate regions of interest for each phase of the cardiac cycle. The margins of each renal arterial region of interest were determined automatically by the software as the boundary at which the image signal intensity was 30% of the maximal signal intensity determined within the vessel. The 30% boundary criterion was based on the results of our earlier studies in arterial flow in phantoms and patients (2). Flow was then computed for all individual phases of the cardiac cycle, as illustrated in Figure 2, which shows arterial flow in a spiral acquisition. Venous RBF was computed in the same manner but with a boundary criterion of 40% of maximum, which we found empirically to give the best agreement between arterial and ipsilateral venous RBF values. Computation time for flow analysis is short, and processing time is limited by operator input.

Correlations were calculated by means of linear regression analysis.

RESULTS

For each of the three techniques in each subject, total arterial RBF measured with cine phase-contrast MR imaging as a function of the corresponding measurement with PAH-clearance hematocrit is shown in Figure 3. Results obtained at both end inspiration and end expiration are shown for the non–breath-hold rapid spiral technique. For the various techniques, technical problems with reconstruction of some images prevented computation of arterial RBF for several patients.

A visual impression of agreement between corresponding measurements was obtained by referring to the line of identity that was drawn. However, as noted by Bland and Altman (21), a better way to analyze the relationship between two methods designed to measure the same physiologic parameter, when neither is unequivocally correct, is to assess the degree of agreement. This was done by first plotting the individual differences between the arterial RBF as measured with MR imaging and PAH-clearance hematocrit against the corresponding mean values of the two measurements, as shown in Figure 4. The range of agreement for 2 standard deviations (95% confidence intervals) for the different cine phase-contrast techniques can be computed, as also shown in Figure 4. The 95% confidence intervals for the limits of agreement and the percentage bias in arterial RBF measurements with the four cine phase-contrast MR imaging techniques and PAH-clearance hematocrit are summarized in Table 2.

Native left renal vein blood flow measurement was not performed in two cases owing to the presence of venous anomalies and was successful in 14 (88%) of the 16 subjects without venous anomalies. The right renal vein was adequately visualized in only five (28%) of the 18 subjects. The short, oblique course of the right renal vein and the frequent presence of multiple right renal veins made acquisition of satisfactory data for these vessels difficult. Figure 5 shows the correlation between RBF measured in the left renal artery and the corresponding left renal vein of each subject at the end-expiratory phase of the non–breath-hold rapid spiral acquisition.

RBF per unit renal volume for the individual subjects was computed by dividing the value of arterial RBF for each subject as determined with PAH-clearance hematocrit by their total renal volume as calculated by summing the areas of each kidney on MR images, as described previously. The mean RBF value was 3.47 mL/min per cubic centimeter of renal parenchyma (standard deviation, 0.56; range, 2.57–4.30 mL/min/cm³).

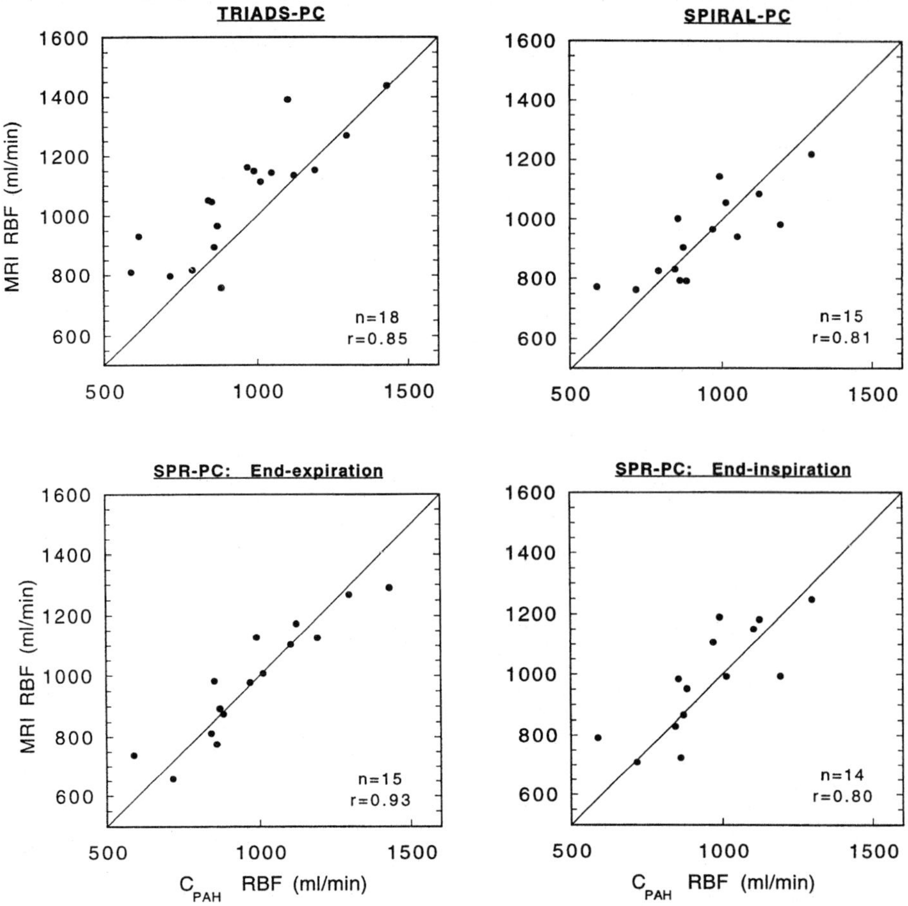

Figure 3. Plots of total arterial RBF measured with the four cine phase-contrast (*PC*) MR imaging (*MRI*) techniques as a function of measurements with PAH-clearance hematocrit (C_{PAH}). The best agreement was obtained with the non–breath-hold rapid spiral (*SPR*) technique in end expiration. *SPIRAL* = breath-hold rapid spiral, *TRIADS* = segmented k space. The number of subjects studied with the different techniques differs because some of the data acquired with rapid spiral acquisition could not be analyzed for technical reasons.

DISCUSSION

The best agreement between the measurements of arterial RBF with cine phase-contrast MR imaging and PAH-clearance hematocrit (Table 2) was with the non–breath-hold rapid spiral technique in end expiration. Measurements of arterial RBF with breath-hold rapid spiral technique and non–breath-hold rapid spiral technique at end expiration agreed less well with PAH-clearance hematocrit measurements, but there was little bias noted between the two former measurements. Agreement between measurements of arterial RBF with segmented k-space technique and PAH-clearance hematocrit was somewhat poorer, and there was a small positive bias. We do not fully understand this poorer agreement at this time, but it could be due in part to the poorer temporal resolution with this method. The lower temporal resolution can be expected to cause an underestimation of peak flow rate and an overestimation of average flow due to magnitude variations secondary to flow-related enhancement (22). It is also possible that the slightly lower and asymmetric spatial resolution of the segmented k-space method had an effect. It is not surprising that non–breath-hold rapid spiral data provided better agreement at end expiration than at end inspiration, since we observed the end-expiratory phase of respiration is generally longer. It is likely, therefore, that a degree of arterial motion during acquisition of data at end inspiration decreased the accuracy of measurement. Arterial RBF determined at end expiration resulted in somewhat better agreement with PAH-clearance hematocrit measurements than did the breath-hold rapid spiral data; this difference may be related to lack of complete breath holding throughout the entire acquisition in at least some subjects. Non–breath-hold rapid spiral technique may provide more accurate measurements of arterial RBF than did breath-hold rapid spiral technique owing to the altered hemodynamics during breath holding. In general, agreement was good between arterial RBF measurements with PAH-clearance hematocrit and those with both breath-hold and non–breath-hold rapid spiral techniques, particularly since comparisons between the latter techniques are likely associated with comparable degrees of measurement error. Our results give promise that these techniques may prove useful in the clinical determination of arterial RBF. The non–breath-hold rapid spiral technique at end expiration may be particularly practical to employ clinically, since it apparently provides accurate results without the need for breath holding, which might be impossible in young or very ill patients.

Venous RBF was measured, with calculations as discussed in Materials and Methods, to determine the degree of agreement that might be expected in healthy subjects between ipsilateral arterial and venous RBF measurements. These venous measurements were generally straightforward in the long left renal vein but were often not possible in the short, oblique right renal vein. Agreement between arterial and venous RBF measurements was quite good, as seen in Figure 5, indicating

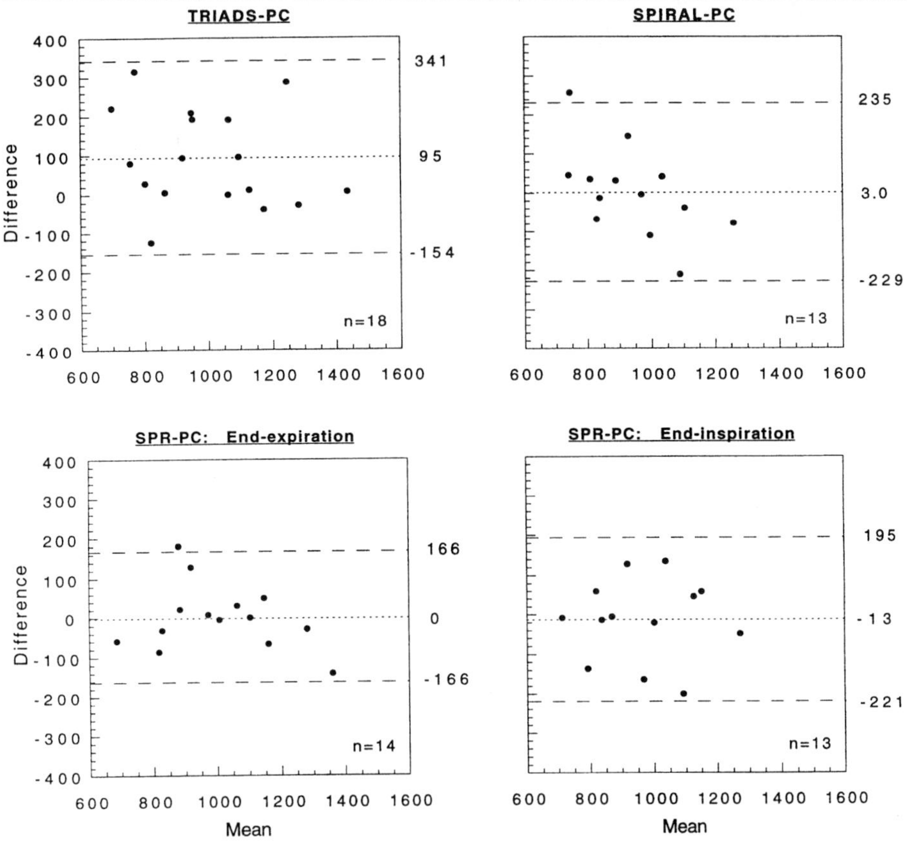

Figure 4. Plots of the differences in arterial RBF measured with the four cine phase-contrast (*PC*) MR imaging techniques and PAH-clearance hematocrit as a function of mean RBF measured with the two techniques. Dotted lines indicate the 95% confidence intervals for agreement, which are largest for the segmented k-space (*TRIADS*) technique and smallest for the non–breath-hold rapid spiral (*SPR*) technique in end expiration. The x and y axes indicate milliliters per minute. *SPIRAL* = breath-hold rapid spiral.

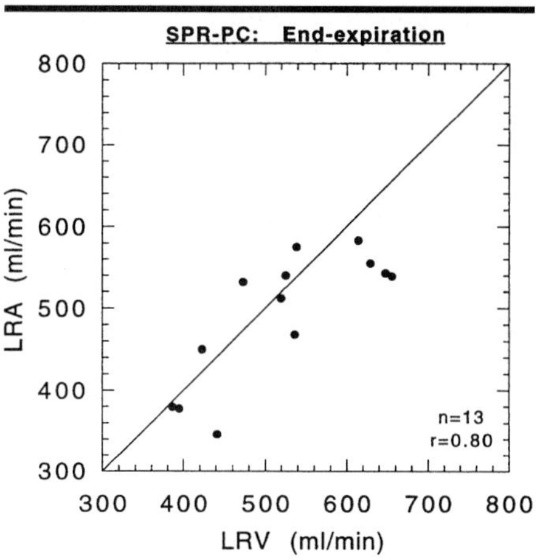

Figure 5. Plot of flow in the left renal vein (*LRV*) as a function of flow in the ipsilateral left renal artery (*LRA*) as computed with the non–breath-hold rapid spiral phase-contrast (*SPR-PC*) technique in end expiration. The reasonably good agreement indicates that venous flow measurement may be useful as a check of or alternative to arterial flow measurement.

TABLE 2
RBF Measurements with Cine Phase-Contrast versus PAH-Clearance Hematocrit Techniques

Phase-Contrast Technique	Bias (%)	95% Confidence Interval (%)
Segmented k space	+10.0	±25.0
Rapid spiral		
Breath hold	+0.3	±26.5
Non–breath hold		
End expiration	0.0	±17.6
End inspiration	−1.3	±23.0

that venous RBF might be determined for a particular kidney as either a check of or an alternative to the arterial measurement. One instance in which a venous measurement might prove useful would be as a check of an arterial RBF measurement obtained distal to a renal arterial stenosis, where turbulence could produce an erroneous flow measurement. Furthermore, direct arterial RBF measurement might be difficult or impossible after placement of a renal arterial stent, which would create a susceptibility void, whereas ipsilateral measurement of venous RBF might be possible.

RBF per unit volume of renal parenchyma was found to be 3.47 ± 0.56 mL/min/cm^3, and this value is in good agreement with that in the literature (23). This value has been of interest to us, because it may be a useful parameter in the diagnosis of renal ischemia. Since the literature suggests this parameter does not vary greatly among healthy individuals, RBF per unit volume might prove useful in assessment of the degree of ischemia in kidneys affected with ischemic atrophy (24).

Sources of error should be considered in measurement of either arterial or venous RBF with cine phase-contrast MR imaging. In order of diminishing importance, these sources include renal vascular motion during acquisition, effects on flow calculation of partial volume averaging at vessel margins and in the section direction, variation in size and shape of renal vessels throughout the cardiac cycle, and effects of phase shifts due to factors other than flowing blood. In our earlier work (7) with non-breath-hold techniques, we noted a poor correlation with PAH-clearance hematocrit values between arterial measurements of RBF in healthy subjects, apparently mainly due to vessel motion during acquisition. In the same study, a better correlation was obtained between venous measurements, probably because the renal veins move less during respiration as a percentage of their cross-sectional width. In subsequent work (2), substantial measurement error was introduced with phantoms as a result of motion of vessels during data acquisition, and breath-hold segmented k-space studies in humans in vivo gave arterial RBF measurements in good agreement with those determined with PAH-clearance hematocrit. Recently, rapid echo-planar techniques have been recommended for use in acquisition of breath-hold phase-contrast data in vivo (11), in addition to the rapid spiral techniques employed in the present study (14,16,18).

Effects of partial volume averaging at vessel margins are a substantial source of potential error in measurement of RBF with cine phase-contrast MR imaging techniques. This phenomenon, which has been discussed previously (7,15), is caused by the fact that the total signal recorded from voxels at the margin of vessels is the vector sum of the signal from both static and moving spins within that voxel, but the apparent phase shift is dominated by the moving spins due to flow-related enhancement. This phenomenon can result in marked overestimations of blood flow, particularly when the imaging plane is not perpendicular to the vessel or when there is relatively low spatial resolution on the MR images. The double-oblique acquisition in this study was performed to minimize these effects and to make possible a consistent strategy for determination of vessel edge.

Another source of error in RBF measurement is variation in the apparent size and shape of the vessel over the cardiac cycle, a factor considerably more important for renal arteries than for renal veins, which generally demonstrate continuous flow. Such variability is an important potential source of error, but, in our study, the vessel edge of both arteries and veins was determined on a per frame basis in each cardiac phase, or frame (segmented k space, six frames; breath-hold and non-breath-hold rapid spiral, 16 frames). This form of analysis likely minimized the effect of this variable on measurement inaccuracy.

Another source of error, which is probably relatively minor, is the need to account for phase shifts caused by factors other than flowing blood, primarily those due to eddy currents within the imager itself. In our computations, the first-order background correction performed in each case produced only relatively small corrections, on the order of 10–20 mL/min, to the flow to each kidney. Larger effects may be present with other systems.

Sources of error in flow computation can be minimized with cine phase-contrast MR imaging techniques, and the accuracy of in vivo RBF determination appears acceptable for clinical application. Phase-contrast techniques, particularly those with rapid spiral acquisitions, show promise for providing useful physiologic information about quantitative RBF. This information is complementary to that provided by means of anatomic visualization of conditions such as renal artery stenosis with contemporary MR angiographic techniques.

References

1. Cortsen M, Petersen LJ, Stahlberg F, et al. MR velocity mapping measurement of renal artery blood flow in patients with impaired kidney function. Acta Radiol 1996; 37:79–84.
2. Debatin JF, Ting RH, Wegmuller H, et al. Renal artery blood flow: quantitation with phase-contrast MR imaging with and without breath holding. Radiology 1994; 190: 371–378.
3. Lundin B, Cooper TG, Meyer RA, Potchen EJ. Measurement of total and unilateral renal blood flow by oblique-angle velocity-encoded 2D-cine magnetic resonance angiography. Magn Reson Imaging 1993; 11:51–59.
4. Maier SE, Scheidegger MB, Liu K, Schneider E, Bollinger A, Boesiger P. Renal artery velocity mapping with MR imaging. JMRI 1995; 5:669–676.
5. Myers BD, Sommer FG, Li K, et al. Determination of blood flow to the transplanted kidney: a novel application of phase-contrast, cine magnetic resonance imaging. Transplantation 1994; 57:1445–1450.
6. Schoenberg SO, Knopp MV, Bock M, et al. Renal artery stenosis: grading of hemodynamic changes with cine phase-contrast MR blood flow measurements. Radiology 1997; 203:45–53.
7. Sommer F, Noorbehesht B, Pelc N, et al. Normal renal blood flow measurement using phase-contrast cine magnetic resonance imaging. Invest Radiol 1992; 27: 465–470.
8. Wolf RL, King BF, Torres VE, Wilson DM, Ehman RL. Measurement of normal renal artery blood flow: cine phase-contrast MR imaging vs clearance of *p*-aminohippurate. AJR 1993; 161:995–1002.
9. Vaughan DE Jr. Renovascular hypertension. Kidney Int 1985; 27:811–827.
10. Jacobson HR. Ischemic renal disease: an overlooked clinical entity? Kidney Int 1988; 34:729–743.
11. Debatin JF, Leung DA, Wildermuth S, Botnar R, Felblinger J, McKinnon GC. Flow quantitation with echo-planar phase-contrast velocity mapping: in vitro and in vivo evaluation. JMRI 1995; 5:656–662.
12. Fredrickson JO, Pelc NJ. Time-resolved MR imaging by automatic data segmentation. JMRI 1994; 4:189–196.
13. Pelc LR, Pelc NJ, Rayhill SC, et al. Arterial and venous blood flow: noninvasive quantitation with MR imaging. Radiology 1992; 185:809–812.
14. Pike GB, Meyer CH, Brosnan TJ, Pelc NJ. Magnetic resonance velocity imaging using a fast spiral phase contrast sequence. Magn Reson Med 1994; 32:476–483.
15. Pelc NJ, Sommer FG, Li KC, Brosnan TJ, Herfkens RJ, Enzmann DR. Quantitative magnetic resonance flow imaging. Magn Reson Q 1994; 10:125–147.
16. Liao JR, Sommer FG, Herfkens RJ, Pelc NJ. Cine spiral imaging. Magn Reson Med 1995; 34:490–493.
17. Myers BD, Peterson C, Molina C, et al. Role of cardiac atria in the human renal response to changing plasma volume. Am J Physiol 1988; 254:F562–F573.
18. Fredrickson JO, Drangova M, Liao JR, Pelc NJ. Simultaneous resolution of cardiac and respiratory motion with a rapid spiral acquisition (abstr). In: Proceedings of the Fourth Meeting of the International Society for Magnetic Resonance in Medicine. Berkeley, Calif: International Society for Magnetic Resonance in Medicine, 1996; 393.
19. Liao JR, Pauly JM, Pelc NJ. MRI using piecewise-linear spiral trajectories. Magn Reson Med 1997; 38:246–252.
20. Irarrazabal P, Meyer CH, Nishimura DG, Macovski A. Inhomogeneity correction using an estimated linear field map. Magn Reson Med 1996; 35:278–282.
21. Bland JM, Altman DG. Statistical methods for assessing agreements between two methods of clinical measurement. Lancet 1986; 1:307–311.
22. Hangiandreou NJ, Rossman PJ, Riederer SJ. Analysis of MR phase-contrast measurements of pulsatile velocity waveforms. JMRI 1993; 3:387–394.
23. Lerman LO, Flickinger AL, Sheedy PF, Turner ST. Reproducibility of human kidney perfusion and volume determinations with electron beam computed tomography. Invest Radiol 1996; 31:204–210.
24. Zimmerman GG, Leung DA, Pelkonen P, Botnar R, Hany T, Debatin J. Detection of significant renal artery stenoses based on PC flow and renal volume measurements (abstr). In: Proceedings of the Fifth Meeting of the International Society for Magnetic Resonance in Medicine. Berkeley, Calif: International Society for Magnetic Resonance in Medicine, 1997; 811.

Lawrence H. Schwartz, MD
Linda R. LaTrenta, MD
Ermelinda Bonaccio, MD[2]
William K. Kelly, DO
Howard I. Scher, MD
David M. Panicek, MD

Index terms:
Genitourinary system, neoplasms, 844.30
Neoplasms, staging, 844.12112
Prostate, CT, 844.12112
Prostate, neoplasms, 844.30

Radiology 1998; 208:735–738

Abbreviation:
PSA = prostate-specific antigen

[1] From the Departments of Radiology (L.H.S., L.R.L., E.B., D.M.P.) and Medicine (W.K.K., H.I.S.), Memorial Sloan-Kettering Cancer Center, 1275 York Ave, New York, NY 10021. From the 1997 RSNA scientific assembly. Received December 24, 1997; revision requested January 26, 1998; final revision received April 20; accepted May 8. **Address reprint requests to** L.H.S.

[2] Current address: Elizabeth Wende Breast Clinic, Rochester, NY.

Author contributions:
Guarantors of integrity of entire study, L.H.S., L.R.L.; study concepts, L.H.S., H.I.S.; study design, L.H.S., E.B., D.M.P.; definition of intellectual content, H.I.S., L.H.S., W.K.K., D.M.P.; literature research, L.R.L., L.H.S.; clinical studies, H.I.S., W.K.K.; data acquisition, E.B., L.H.S.; data analysis, L.R.L., L.H.S.; statistical analysis, L.H.S., L.R.L.; manuscript preparation, L.H.S., L.R.L.; manuscript editing and review, L.H.S., L.R.L., E.B., W.K.K., H.I.S., D.M.P.

Small Cell and Anaplastic Prostate Cancer: Correlation between CT Findings and Prostate-specific Antigen Level[1]

PURPOSE: To evaluate the computed tomographic (CT) findings in patients with the anaplastic clinical variant of prostate cancer and to correlate these with prostate-specific antigen (PSA) levels.

MATERIALS AND METHODS: Twenty-seven men with the anaplastic clinical variant of prostate cancer, including 12 patients with small cell cancer of the prostate, underwent CT before platinum-based chemotherapy. CT findings were retrospectively reviewed for the extent of disease in the abdominal and pelvic lymph nodes, liver, bone, and prostate. CT findings were correlated with baseline PSA levels.

RESULTS: The overall mean PSA level was 59.9 ng/mL ± 23.3 (range, 0–583 ng/mL; median, 4 ng/mL), with a mean PSA level in the small cell cancer subgroup of 12.3 ng/mL ± 9.0 (range, 0–110 ng/mL; median, 1.7 ng/mL). Twenty-six patients (96%) had metastatic disease evident at CT, but only nine (33%) had PSA levels greater than 10 ng/mL. The mean PSA level in patients with pelvic lymphadenopathy was 12.8 ng/mL ± 7.9 (median, 1.6 ng/mL); that in the small cell cancer subgroup was only 2.8 ng/mL ± 1.4 (median, 1.6 ng/mL). Whereas 19 (70%) of all patients had osseous metastases and an average PSA level of 73 ng/mL ± 32 (median, 9.1 ng/mL), the seven (58%) with small cell cancer and bone metastases had an average PSA level of 18 ng/mL ± 13 (median, 4 ng/mL).

CONCLUSION: Unlike patients with advanced typical adenocarcinoma of the prostate, patients with the anaplastic clinical variant of prostate cancer often have extensive metastatic disease at CT despite relatively low PSA levels.

A small percentage of patients with adenocarcinoma of the prostate are considered to have an anaplastic clinical variant. This variant is defined clinically by one or more of the following: (*a*) rapid progression of clinical symptoms, (*b*) presence of visceral metastases, (*c*) poor response to androgen ablation therapy, and (*d*) relatively low serum prostate-specific antigen (PSA) levels. This clinical definition has implications for treatment, as these patients are relatively resistant to standard therapy and may benefit from platinum-based chemotherapy (1).

Although the most common histologic type of prostate cancer is adenocarcinoma, it has become increasingly recognized that prostatic tumors may also have neuroendocrine differentiation. This ranges from focal in the majority of cases to multifocal in 10% of tumors (2–4). Tumors with purely neuroendocrine histologic findings are less commonly reported on than those with coexistent adenocarcinoma (5). In mixed tumors, the neuroendocrine component does not secrete PSA and, therefore, does not contribute to an elevated PSA level (5). Although most patients with the anaplastic clinical variant have pure adenocarcinoma, histologic analysis either at the time of initial biopsy or at the time of repeat biopsy after treatment failure in some patients demonstrates a substantial component of neuroendocrine differentiation.

Small cell cancer of the prostate is a histologic subtype of neuroendocrine tumor, with only approximately 130 cases reported in the world literature (6). This histologic type has an aggressive clinical course characterized by widespread metastatic disease, lack of response to hormone therapy, and, rarely, paraneoplastic syndromes (7–10). An estimated 74% of patients with small cell cancer have metastatic disease at initial diagnosis, with a mean survival time of 9.8 months (range, 0–90 months) and a 5-year survival rate of 0.9% (6). Patients often present with symptoms related to metastatic disease, such as bone pain, or with rapid onset of symptoms related to bladder outlet obstruction. Effective therapy for small cell cancer has yet to be determined, but most cases are treated with a combination of radiation therapy and *cis*-platinum–based chemotherapy similar to that for small cell lung cancer (6).

This study was undertaken to evaluate the relevant soft-tissue and osseous findings at computed tomography (CT) in a group of patients with the anaplastic clinical variant, including a subgroup of patients shown to have a substantial histologic component of small cell cancer, and to correlate these findings with PSA levels.

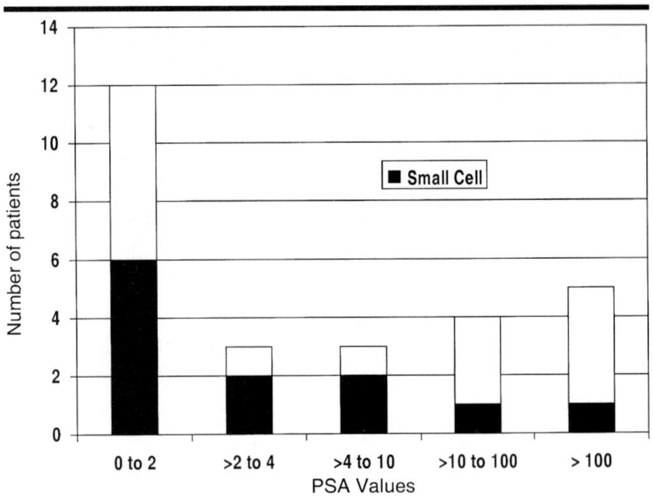

Figure 1. Bar graph shows the distribution of PSA levels in patients with the anaplastic clinical variant of prostate cancer. PSA levels are in nanograms per milliliter.

CT Findings in Patients with Small Cell and Anaplastic Prostate Cancer

	No. of Patients		Mean PSA Level (ng/mL)	
CT Findings	All Patients with Anaplastic Cancer (*N* = 27)	Small Cell Cancer Subgroup (*n* = 12)	All Patients with Anaplastic Cancer (*N* = 27)*	Small Cell Cancer Subgroup (*n* = 12)*
Prostatic mass	11 (41)	7 (58)	16.2 ± 9.6	4.9 ± 1.8
Liver metastases	16 (59)	5 (42)	83.4 ± 37.7	25.0 ± 21.3
Pelvic adenopathy	13 (48)	6 (50)	12.8 ± 7.9	2.8 ± 1.4
Retroperitoneal adenopathy	8 (30)	4 (33)	36.6 ± 19.4	5.1 ± 2.0
Osseous metastases	19 (70)	7 (58)	72.9 ± 32.2	18.0 ± 13.2

Note.—Number in parentheses is the percentage. Total of percentages exceeds 100 because some patients had more than one finding.
* Data are the mean ± standard error.

MATERIALS AND METHODS

Thirty men (age range, 45–79 years; mean age, 64 years) examined by two medical oncologists (W.K.K., H.I.S.) at our institution between February 1991 and February 1995 were retrospectively identified as having the anaplastic clinical variant of prostate cancer on the basis of new onset of symptoms or evidence of clinically aggressive disease at physical examination. Imaging studies in three patients were not available for review. Therefore, our study population consisted of 27 patients with the anaplastic clinical variant of prostate cancer, including 12 patients (44%) with a substantial histologic component of small cell cancer either at initial biopsy or at repeat biopsy after treatment failure.

Before the initiation of platinum-based chemotherapy, 26 patients underwent CT of the abdomen and pelvis; one other patient underwent abdominal CT and pelvic magnetic resonance (MR) imaging. All but one patient received oral contrast material for CT, and 21 (78%) of the 27 patients received intravenous contrast material for CT. Soft-tissue, lung, bone, and liver windows were available in 17 patients; only soft-tissue windows in four patients; and soft-tissue, lung, and liver windows in six patients. All scans were contiguous axial sections obtained with collimation of 10 mm or less.

CT findings were retrospectively reviewed by two radiologists (L.H.S., E.B.) in consensus for the extent of disease (including the presence and size of a prostatic mass), retroperitoneal or pelvic adenopathy, osseous metastasis, and focal or diffuse liver metastases. "Adenopathy" was defined as the presence of lymph nodes 1 cm or larger in the short axis. CT findings were correlated with baseline PSA levels (Tandem-E; Hybritech, San Diego, Calif).

RESULTS

Biochemical PSA levels

The overall mean PSA level at presentation was 59.9 ng/mL ± 23.3 (range, 0–583 ng/mL; median, 4 ng/mL). Nine patients (33%) had PSA levels greater than 10 ng/mL (Fig 1), and eight patients (30%) had PSA levels greater than 20 ng/mL (Fig 1). The average PSA level in the 12 patients with small cell cancer was 12.3 ng/mL ± 9.0 (range, 0–110 ng/mL; median, 1.7 ng/mL). In this subgroup, two patients (17%) had PSA levels greater than 10 ng/mL, and one patient (8%) had a PSA level greater than 20 ng/mL. The mean PSA levels, stratified by imaging findings, are presented in the Table.

Imaging Findings

Overall, 26 (96%) of the 27 patients had metastases in the abdomen or pelvis, and 19 (70%) had osseous metastases. Of the 26 patients with metastatic disease, 17 (65%) had PSA levels less than 10 ng/mL. Among those 26 patients with abdominal or pelvic metastases, the mean PSA level was 60 ng/mL ± 27. Among

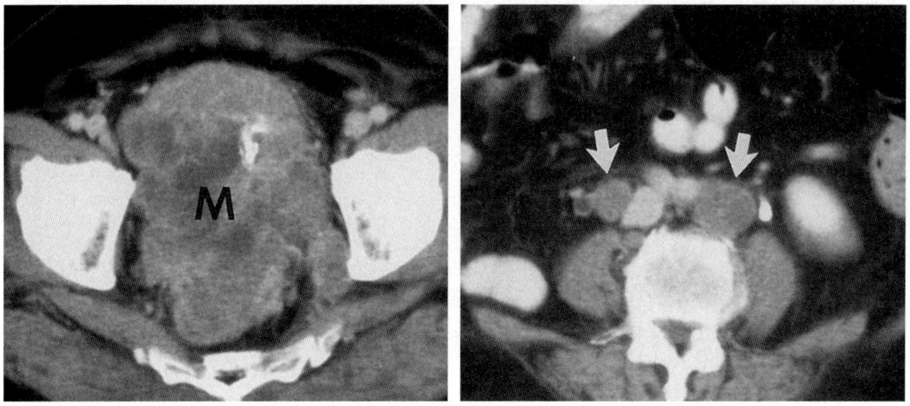

a. b.

Figure 2. CT images obtained in a 66-year-old man with small cell cancer of the prostate and a PSA level of 8 ng/mL at the time of imaging demonstrate **(a)** a large prostatic mass (*M*) and **(b)** retroperitoneal adenopathy (arrows).

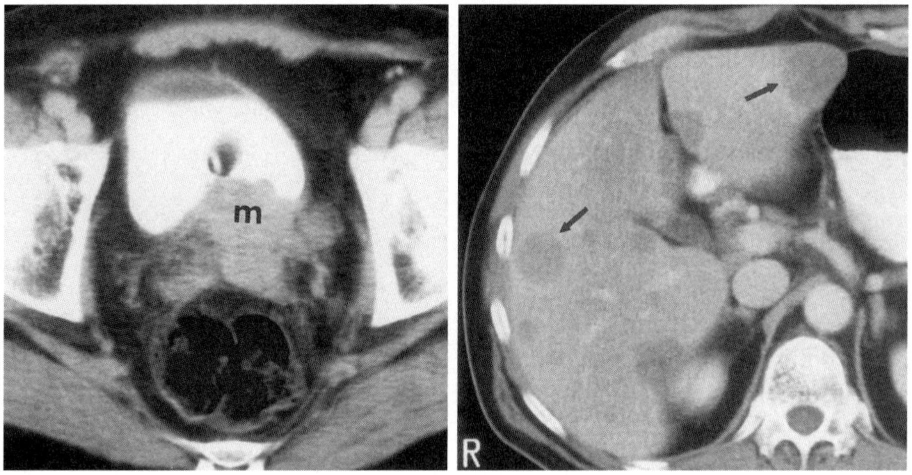

a. b.

Figure 3. CT images obtained in a 70-year-old man with anaplastic prostate cancer and a PSA level of 0.9 ng/mL at the time of imaging demonstrate **(a)** a prostatic mass (*M*) and **(b)** multiple liver metastases (arrows).

those 19 patients (70%) with osseous metastases, the mean PSA level was 72.9 ng/mL ± 32.2. Among those 18 patients (67%) with lymphadenopathy (either abdominal or pelvic), the mean PSA level was 19 ng/mL ± 9. In all 13 patients with pelvic adenopathy, the mean nodal size was 3.6 cm, with a mean of 3.0 cm in the six patients with pelvic adenopathy and small cell cancer. In all eight patients with retroperitoneal adenopathy, the mean nodal size was 1.9 cm, with a mean of 1.8 cm in the four patients with small cell cancer. Of the 19 patients with bone metastases evident at CT, 12 (63%) had blastic, three (16%) had lytic, and four (21%) had mixed lytic and blastic findings.

Of note, patients with small cell cancer and prostatic masses or abdominal or pelvic adenopathy (regardless of other sites of metastatic disease) had a mean PSA level of less than 10 ng/mL (Fig 2). Those seven patients with osseous metastases (regardless of other sites of metastatic disease) and small cell cancer had a mean PSA level of less than 20 ng/mL. Sixteen (59%) of all 27 patients had liver metastases (Fig 3).

DISCUSSION

The 27 patients in this study were a cohort of patients with the anaplastic clinical variant of prostate cancer, which was identified because of the rapid clinical progression of disease before the initiation of platinum-based chemotherapy. Despite the rapid progression of disease, the PSA levels in most were not elevated—unlike in patients with typical advanced adenocarcinoma of the prostate. For instance, 96% of patients in this group had metastatic disease, but 65% had PSA levels less than 10 ng/mL. Nine (47%) of the 19 patients with bone metastases had a PSA level in the normal range (0–4 ng/mL). Eleven (85%) of the 13 patients with pelvic adenopathy and nine (56%) of the 16 patients with liver metastases had a PSA level less than 20 ng/mL, with the majority of these levels within the normal range (0–4 ng/mL).

Although adenocarcinoma is the most common histologic type of prostate cancer, it is increasingly recognized that many prostatic tumors contain a neuroendocrine component, such as small cell cancer or a carcinoidlike histologic type. The neuroendocrine cells initially were thought to be part of an amine precursor and uptake decarboxylation system that had undergone malignant transformation. Currently, the neuroendocrine tumor cells are thought to arise from a common stem cell or multipotent cell, which can differentiate into multiple tissues (6). This latter theory would explain the heterogeneous cell population present in many prostate cancers, as well as the observation that the diagnosis of small cell cancer is often preceded by the diagnosis of adenocarcinoma of the prostate (1). Although uncommon, small cell cancer of the lung can metastasize to the prostate. However, primary small cell cancer of the prostate almost always coexists with adenocarcinoma of the prostate, whereas metastatic small cell cancer of the lung does not—an observation that can be used to distinguish between primary small cell cancer of the prostate and small cell cancer of the lung metastatic to the prostate.

Identification of a neuroendocrine component of prostate cancer is important, because its coexistence with adenocarcinoma is an independent variable that indicates a poor prognosis (11). The presence of a neuroendocrine component can also affect the clinical management, because the neuroendocrine components do not secrete PSA, which limits the usefulness of the PSA level for management. After biopsy to determine the histologic findings and pathologic grade of a prostatic tumor, determination of the serum PSA level is a critical part of the initial examination of patients with prostate cancer. PSA level is generally directly proportional to advancing clinical stage and can be used to select appropriate imaging for the staging of typical adenocarcinoma of the prostate (12,13). Oesterling et al (14) found that only 0.5% of 852 patients with a new diagnosis and PSA levels less than 10 ng/mL had positive bone scans and that no asymptomatic patients had a positive bone scan. Although abdominopelvic CT or MR imaging is often used to stage prostate cancer, Huncharek and Muscat (15) found that less than 1% of patients with PSA levels less than 20 ng/mL have positive findings from these tests. Therefore, in asymptomatic patients with newly diagnosed typical adenocarcinoma and a PSA level of less than 10 ng/mL, a staging bone scan is considered unnecessary by many clinicians. Furthermore, some believe that abdominopelvic CT or MR imaging is not needed if the PSA level is less than 20 ng/mL.

Because the PSA level generally reflects tumor burden, it is used to follow disease activity in patients who have undergone therapy (ie, radiation therapy, hormone therapy, or surgery). For example, PSA levels are used to detect residual tumor after radiation therapy; moreover, PSA levels correlate with patient outcome (16). Stamey et al (17) found that the PSA level measured 6 months after the initiation of antiandrogen therapy indicated whether the patient would achieve a favorable, prolonged response. Furthermore, in one study (18), all patients with a PSA level greater than 0.4 ng/mL after radical prostatectomy developed recurrent disease if they did not receive adjuvant therapy, indicating the presence of residual disease after surgery. Therefore, regardless of the treatment modality used, PSA levels can be used to detect residual or recurrent disease and determine the need for repeat imaging in patients with typical adenocarcinoma of the prostate.

A limitation of this study is that one might predict that these patients would have low PSA levels, given that one possible (but not required) feature of the anaplastic clinical variant of prostate cancer is a disproportionately low PSA level. However, as shown by the wide range of PSA levels (0–583 ng/mL) and the elevated mean PSA level (59.9 ng/mL ± 23.3) in this cohort, the absolute PSA level would be irrelevant in establishing the diagnosis of an anaplastic clinical variant if the tumor had aggressive clinical behavior. Because small cell cancer of the prostate does not secrete PSA, selection bias in favor of patients with small cell cancer accounts for the large number of patients in the cohort with this histologic type. Depending on the relative proportions of typical adenocarcinoma and small cell cancer present in a given tumor, variable amounts of PSA will be produced. This histologic ratio is not always determinable in a given patient because most patients with advanced disease will not undergo prostatectomy. In these patients, the results of a diagnostic needle biopsy would not yield a valid histologic ratio owing to sampling error.

PSA level alone should not be used to determine the threshold to restage disease in patients with an anaplastic clinical variant or small cell cancer of the prostate, because these patients have a high likelihood of extraprostatic disease spread, despite the relatively low PSA levels. Furthermore, because imaging studies in these patents may show extensive visceral metastases despite a low PSA level, the existence of a second primary tumor need not be postulated. Nor should it be implied that all patients with prostate cancer and a low serum PSA level need to undergo CT. Anaplastic prostate cancer is rare and should be considered only in the proper clinical setting. Once diagnosed, anaplastic prostate cancer is best followed up with CT, because PSA values alone are misleading in evaluating the extent of disease.

Our findings reemphasize the need for development of new serum tumor markers that accurately reflect the clinical activity of the anaplastic clinical variant and small cell cancer of the prostate. Such promising markers include serum tissue-specific polypeptide antigen, or TPS, and neuron-specific enolase (19). However, until such markers become clinically available, the limitations of using the absolute PSA level for assessing disease status in this subset of patients with prostate cancer needs to be recognized.

References

1. Frank SJ, Amsterdam A, Kelly WK, Liebertz C, Reuter V, Scher HI. Platinum-based chemotherapy for patients with poorly differentiated hormone-refractory prostate cancers (HRPC): response and pathologic correlation (abstr). Proc Am Soc Oncol 1995; 14:232.
2. di Sant'Agnese P. Neuroendocrine differentiation in carcinoma of the prostate: diagnostic, prognostic, and therapeutic implications. Cancer 1992; 70:254–268.
3. di Sant'Agnese P. Neuroendocrine differentiation in prostatic carcinoma: recent findings and new concepts. Cancer 1995; 75: 1850–1859.
4. di Sant'Agnese P. Neuroendocrine differentiation in prostatic malignancy. Cancer 1996; 78:357–361.
5. Turbat-Herrera EA, Herrera GA, Gore I, Lott RL, Grizzle WE, Bonnin JM. Neuroendocrine differentiation in prostatic carcinomas: a retrospective autopsy study. Arch Pathol Lab Med 1988; 112:1100–1105.
6. Abbas F, Civantos F, Benedetto P, Soloway MS. Small cell carcinoma of the bladder and prostate. Urology 1995; 46:617–630.
7. Oesterling JE, Hauzeur CG, Farrow GM. Small cell anaplastic carcinoma of the prostate: a clinical, pathological, and immunohistological study of 27 patients. J Urol 1992; 147:804–807.
8. Tetu B, Ro JY, Ayala AG, Johnson DE, Logothetis CJ, Orodonez NG. Small cell carcinoma of the prostate. I. A clinicopathologic study of 20 cases. Cancer 1987; 59:1803–1809.
9. Efros MD, Fischer J, Mallouh C, Choudhury M, Goergsson S. Unusual primary prostatic malignancies. Urology 1992; 39: 407–410.
10. Bolton DM, Chiu ST, Clarke S, Angus D. Primary small cell carcinoma of the prostate: unusual modes of presentation. Aust N Z J Surg 1994; 64:91–94.
11. Cohen RJ, Glezerson G, Haffejee Z. Neuroendocrine cells: a new prognostic parameter in prostate cancer. Br J Urol 1991; 68:258–262.
12. Oesterling JE. Prostate specific antigen: a critical assessment of the most useful tumor marker for adenocarcinoma of the prostate. J Urol 1991; 145:907–923.
13. Stamey TA, Kabalin JN. Prostate specific antigen in the diagnosis and treatment of adenocarcinoma of the prostate. I. Untreated patients. J Urol 1989; 141:1070–1075.
14. Oesterling JE, Martin SK, Bergstalh EJ, Lowe FC. The use of prostate specific antigen in staging patients with newly diagnosed prostate cancer. JAMA 1993; 269:57–60.
15. Huncharek M, Muscat J. Serum prostate-specific antigen as a predictor of radiographic staging studies in newly diagnosed prostate cancer. Cancer Invest 1995; 13:31–35.
16. Kabalin JN, Hodge KK, McNeal JE, Freiha FS, Stamey TA. Identification of residual cancer in the prostate following radiation therapy: role of transrectal ultrasound guided biopsy and PSA. J Urol 1989; 142: 326–331.
17. Stamey TA, Kabalin JN, Ferrari M, Yang N. Prostate specific antigen in the diagnosis and treatment of adenocarcinoma of the prostate. IV. Anti-androgen treated patients. J Urol 1989; 141:1088–1090.
18. Lange PH, Ercole CJ, Lightner DJ, Fraley EE, Vesella R. The value of serum prostate specific antigen determinations before and after radical prostatectomy. J Urol 1989; 141:873–879.
19. Tarle M, Frkovic-Grazio S, Kraljic I, Kovacic K. A more objective staging of advanced prostate cancer: routine recognition of malignant endocrine structures: the assessment of serum TPS, PSA and NSE values. Prostate 1994; 24:143–148.

Stage I Hodgkin Disease: Radiation Therapy and Chemotherapy at The University Of Texas M. D. Anderson Cancer Center, 1967–1997[1]

Maria T. Vlachaki, MD
Chul S. Ha, MD
Frederick B. Hagemeister, MD
Lillian M. Fuller, MD
Maria A. Rodriguez, MD
Mark A. Hess, BBA
Susan L. Tucker, PhD
Fernando Cabanillas, MD
James D. Cox, MD

Index terms:
Hodgkin disease, **.342[2], 67.342
Hodgkin disease, therapeutic radiology, **.342[2], 67.342
Hodgkin disease, therapy, **.342[2], 67.342
Lymphoma, **.342[2], 67.342
Lymphoma, therapeutic radiology, **.342[2]
Lymphoma, therapy, **.342[2]

Radiology 1998; 208:739–747

Abbreviations:
ABDIC = doxorubicin, bleomycin, dacarbazine, lomustine
CVPP = cyclophosphamide, vinblastine sulfate, procarbazine hydrochloride, and prednisone
EORTC = European Organization for Research and Treatment of Cancer
MOPP = nitrogen mustard, vincristine sulfate, procarbazine hydrochloride, and prednisone
NOVP = mitoxantrone hydrochloride, vincristine sulfate, vinblastine sulfate, and prednisone
OS = overall survival

[1] From the Div of Radiation Oncology (M.T.V., C.S.H., L.M.F., M.A.H., J.D.C.) and Depts of Hematology (F.B.H., M.A.R., F.C.) and Biomathematics (S.L.T.), University of Texas M. D. Anderson Cancer Center, 1515 Holcombe Blvd, Box 97, Houston, TX 77030. Received Sep 11, 1997; revision requested Nov 20; revision received Feb 9, 1998; accepted Apr 4. **Address reprint requests to** C.S.H.

[2] **. Multiple body systems

Author contributions:
Guarantors of integrity of entire study, M.T.V., C.S.H., J.D.C.; study concepts and design, C.S.H., J.D.C.; definition of intellectual content, C.S.H., J.D.C.; literature research, M.T.V.; clinical studies, M.T.V., C.S.H., F.B.H., L.M.F., M.A.R., F.C., J.D.C.; data acquisition, M.T.V.; data analysis, M.T.V., C.S.H., J.D.C., S.L.T., M.A.H.; statistical analysis, S.L.T., M.A.H.; manuscript preparation, M.T.V., C.S.H., J.D.C.; manuscript editing and review, M.T.V., C.S.H., F.B.H., L.M.F., M.A.R., M.A.H., S.L.T., F.C., J.D.C.

PURPOSE: To summarize 30 years of experience in treatment of and prognosis for stage I Hodgkin disease.

MATERIALS AND METHODS: The authors reviewed retrospectively the cases of 196 patients seen and followed up at one institution from 1967 to 1997. All patients were treated with radiation therapy, and 46 also received combination chemotherapy as part of their initial treatment. Radiation therapy techniques included involved- or regional-field irradiation in 83 patients, extended-field irradiation (mantle or inverted Y) in 74, and subtotal nodal irradiation in 39 (median radiation doses for subclinical and clinical disease were 30 and 40 Gy, respectively, at 1.5–2.0 Gy per fraction). Of 46 patients treated with combination chemotherapy and radiation therapy, 26 received subtotal nodal irradiation; in the remaining 20, chemotherapy was combined with more limited-field radiation therapy. Follow-up ranged from 3 to 356 months (median, 144 months).

RESULTS: The actuarial overall survival, disease-specific survival, and freedom from progression at 10 and 20 years were 82% and 66%, 94% and 91%, and 77% and 70%, respectively. In multivariate analysis, age adversely influenced overall survival, and female sex favorably affected freedom from progression. Mixed cellularity histology and mantle field technique adversely influenced disease-specific survival. Laparotomy significantly influenced disease-specific survival but not overall survival.

CONCLUSION: Radiation therapy results in an excellent outcome in patients with favorable stage I Hodgkin disease. Pathologic staging is no longer necessary.

Optimal treatment of patients with early-stage Hodgkin disease is still controversial. Different therapeutic approaches, including radiation therapy and chemotherapy, have resulted in an excellent outcome, particularly in patients with stage I Hodgkin disease. Because most patients are young at the time of diagnosis, concerns regarding late recurrence and treatment-related toxicity gain increasing importance. Current clinical trials focus on the identification of patient risk groups in which selective intensification or reduction of treatment will maintain the high rate of freedom from recurrence while limiting the frequency of late complications (1,2).

A retrospective review was conducted of the cases of patients with stage I Hodgkin disease treated and followed up at The University of Texas M. D. Anderson Cancer Center from 1967 to 1997. The purposes of this study were (*a*) to report the long-term outcome, (*b*) to identify prognostic factors for overall survival (OS) and freedom from progression of disease, (*c*) to describe the patterns of treatment failure and long-term treatment sequelae, and (*d*) to develop treatment recommendations for this group of patients.

MATERIALS AND METHODS

From 1967 to 1994, 196 patients (127 [64.8%] men and 69 [35.2%] women [ratio, 1.8:1]; age range, 16–76 years; median age, 30.5 years) with previously untreated stage I Hodgkin disease were treated at our institution. They were followed up from 1967 through 1997. Of the 196 patients, 132 were aged less than 40 years, and eight (4.1%) presented with B symptoms (unexplained fever, night sweats, weight loss greater than 10% of body weight in the past 6 months).

Their evaluation included a complete history and careful physical examination, hematologic and biochemical surveys, chest radiography, bipedal lymphangiography, and bone marrow aspiration and biopsy. Of the 196 patients, 109 (55.6%) underwent staging laparotomy. Laparotomy was usually not performed in patients with small suprahyoid or inguinal adenopathy, those receiving chemotherapy (after 1988), and those with medical contraindications (3). Computed tomography was performed of the chest, abdomen, and pelvis in 74 (37.8%) patients. The histologic diagnosis was reviewed and confirmed for each patient at the time of diagnosis. In all patients, Hodgkin disease was classified according to the Ann Arbor staging system (4).

The type of initial therapy varied according to the time when the patient was first seen. It included radiation therapy alone or a combination of radiation therapy and chemotherapy.

Radiation Therapy

All patients received radiation therapy. The extent of radiation therapy was categorized as follows: (*a*) involved field, treatment of one lymph node–bearing region (25 patients); (*b*) regional field, treatment of the involved field as well as the next level of lymph nodes (58 patients); (c) extended field, treatment of all lymph node–bearing regions on one side of the diaphragm (eg, mantle or abdominopelvic irradiation) (74 patients); (*d*) subtotal nodal irradiation, treatment of the mantle and upper abdomen (para-aortic and splenic pedicle and/or spleen in 14 patients and whole upper abdominal irradiation in 25 patients). The rationale for the treatment techniques is published elsewhere (3). All patients were treated with megavoltage photons (cobalt gamma rays or 6-MV x rays) Total doses ranged from 30 to 60 Gy at 1.5–4.0 Gy per fraction. Median total dose was 40 Gy, and median dose per fraction was 2 Gy. In the majority of patients, mediastinal radiation was administered via anteroposterior and posteroanterior portals weighted 2:1 or 3:2 in favor of the anteroposterior field. The anteroposterior field was treated daily at 2.0 Gy per fraction at maximum dose, or the Dmax, whereas the posteroanterior treatment was administered every other day at 2 Gy per fraction. The maximum radiation dose to the myocardium was calculated at the axial plane 2 cm above the lower edge of the irradiation field and 4 cm from the anterior surface of the thorax. In three patients, whole-lung radiation to 15 Gy was administered in addition to the mediastinal radiation. When whole-abdominal radiation was used, the dose to the liver and kidneys was limited to 25 Gy and 18 Gy, respectively.

Chemotherapy

Forty-six patients received chemotherapy. The indications for chemotherapy evolved over the years and were based on either clinical studies in effect at the time or on prognostic factors (mediastinal disease, bulky adenopathy, mixed cellularity histology) (3). The chemotherapeutic regimens included the following: (*a*) mitoxantrone hydrochloride, vincristine sulfate, vinblastine sulfate, and prednisone (NOVP) for three cycles in 26 patients (since 1988); (*b*) nitrogen mustard, vincristine sulfate, procarbazine hydrochloride, and prednisone (MOPP) for two, three, or six cycles in 15 patients; (c) doxorubicin, bleomycin, vinblastine sulfate, and dacarbazine, or ABVD, for two, three or six cycles in three patients; and cyclophosphamide, vinblastine sulfate, procarbazine hydrochloride, and prednisone (CVPP) with doxorubicin, bleomycin, dacarbazine, and lomustine (ABDIC) for eight cycles in one patient. Salvage treatment in one additional patient who experienced progression of disease while receiving multiple chemotherapeutic regimens (including NOVP, MOPP, and CVPP-ABDIC) was successful with high-dose chemotherapy and autologous bone marrow transplantation.

Recurrence and Late Complications

Recurrence was described as in field or marginal when disease recurred in a previously irradiated region; as adjacent, discontinuous, or transdiaphragmatic when disease recurred in nonirradiated nodal groups; and as visceral when disease recurred in bone marrow or liver. Transdiaphragmatic recurrence was seen in the initially uninvolved side of the diaphragm. Adjacent and discontinuous recurrence was seen on the same side of the diaphragm as the original disease. Adjacent recurrence was seen in the next level of lymph nodes, and discontinuous recurrence was seen in any group of lymph nodes except those adjacent to the original disease.

Late toxic effects of treatment were scored according to the Late Radiation Morbidity Scoring Scheme of the Radiation Therapy Oncology Group and the European Organization for Research and Treatment of Cancer (EORTC) (5).

Follow-up

Follow-up of surviving patients ranged from 3 to 356 months (median, 144 months). Follow-up included regular office visits and telephone communication with the patients or the physicians caring for them.

Statistical Methods

The Kaplan-Meier product limit method was used to calculate OS, disease-specific survival, and freedom from progression of disease, as well as the actuarial rate of cardiac-related death and second malignancies (6). The statistical significance of the difference between the life table curves was assessed by means of the log-rank method (7). The statistical test used in multivariate analysis was the Cox proportional hazards model (8).

RESULTS

Of the 196 patients, 178 (90.8%) had supradiaphragmatic disease, 17 had infradiaphragmatic disease, and one had primary Hodgkin disease in the brain. On the basis of histologic findings, lymphocyte predominance was seen in 36 (18.4%) patients, mixed cellularity in 81 (41.3%), and nodular sclerosis in 77 (39.3%). On the basis of the site of disease, the histologic findings and the extent of irradiation fields are presented in Table 1. The bulk of adenopathy was 5 cm or less in 143 (72.9%) patients and greater than 5 cm in 53 (27.0%). The bulk of mediastinal adenopathy was accounted for separately (<7.5 cm in 10 patients, ≥7.5 cm in 13 patients). The bulk of mediastinal adenopathy versus chemotherapy is presented in Table 1. Thirty-two of 87 pa-

TABLE 1
Number of Patients With Primary Findings

A: Site and Histologic Findings*

Site	Lymphocyte Predominance	Mixed Cellularity	Nodular Sclerosis	Total
Neck	18	66	47	131
Axilla	9	10	5	24
Mediastinum	0	2	21	23
Lower torso	9	3	4	16
Total	36 (18.6%)	81 (41.8%)	77 (39.7%)	194

B: Site and Extent of Irradiation Fields†

Site	Involved	Regional	Extended	Subtotal Nodal Irradiation	Total
Neck	20 (11)	34 (20)	50 (35)	27 (11)	131 (77)
Axilla	4 (3)	8 (5)	8 (5)	4 (0)	24 (13)
Mediastinum	0 (0)	3 (0)	12 (11)	8 (1)	23 (12)
Lower torso	0 (0)	13 (6)	4 (1)	0 (0)	17 (7)
Total	24 (14)	58 (31)	74 (52)	39 (12)	195‡ (109)

C: Bulk of Mediastinal Adenopathy and Chemotherapy†

Mediastinal Mass Size (cm)	Chemotherapy	No Chemotherapy	Total
≥7.5	6 (3)	7 (4)	13 (7)
<7.5	5 (0)	5 (5)	10 (5)
Total	11 (3)	12 (9)	23 (12)

* One additional patient had unclassified splenic Hodgkin disease, and another additional patient had primary brain Hodgkin disease.
† Numbers in parentheses are numbers of patients with pathologically staged disease.
‡ One additional patient had primary brain Hodgkin disease.

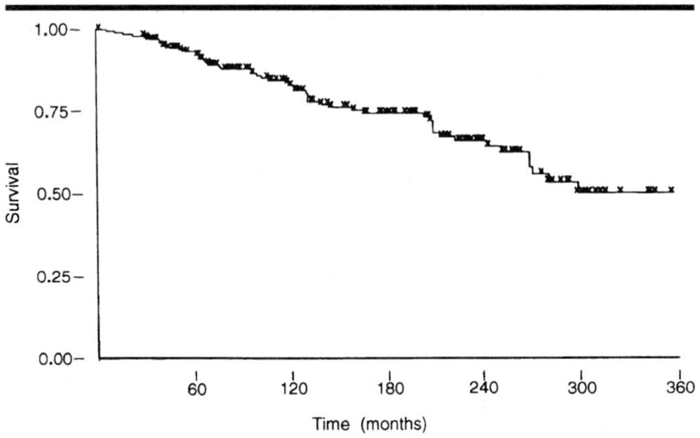

Figure 1. Overall survival in 196 patients with stage I Hodgkin disease.

tients with clinically staged disease and 14 of 109 patients with pathologically staged disease received chemotherapy.

Survival for the entire group is shown in Figure 1. Of the 196 patients, 143 were alive and only 13 had died of Hodgkin disease; the majority of the deaths occurred because of intercurrent disease (40 patients). The actuarial 10- and 20-year OS and disease-specific survival rates were 82% and 66% and 94% and 91%, respectively. The actuarial 10- and 20-year freedom-from-progression rates were 77% and 70%, respectively (Fig 2). Forty-seven of the 196 patients experienced recurrent disease.

Factors analyzed for statistical significance in terms of OS, freedom from progression, and disease-specific survival included the following: patient age and sex, histologic findings, site and bulk of primary adenopathy, laparotomy, B symptoms, extent of irradiation fields, and use of chemotherapy.

In univariate analysis, the statistically significant adverse risk factors for OS were age over 40 years ($P < .0001$), clinical versus pathologic staging ($P = .0003$), and irradiation fields other than subtotal nodal ($P = .0314$). For disease-specific survival, the only adverse risk factor was the presence of mixed cellularity histology ($P = .042$). For freedom from progression, the only significant adverse risk factor was sex ($P = .019$), with men faring worse than women (irradiation technique was marginally significant, $P = .057$). By irradiation technique, the 20-year actuarial OS and freedom from progression were the following: involved field, 57% and 46%; regional, 66% and 74%; extended, 66% and 74%; and subtotal nodal, 82% and 83%, respectively. For treatment with combined modality versus radiation therapy alone, the 20-year OS and freedom from progression, respectively, were 72% and 65% versus 79% and 70%.

In multivariate analysis, the statistically significant ($P = .05$) adverse risk factors for OS were older age (as a continuous variable) and mantle irradiation. Relative risk for mantle irradiation was 2.6 (95% confidence interval, 1.4, 4.7). Three factors significantly affected disease-specific survival: clinical versus pathologic staging (relative risk, 3.4; 95% confidence interval, 1.1, 10.5), mixed cellularity histology (relative risk, 4.7; 95% confidence interval, 1.4, 15.6), and mantle-field technique (relative risk, 3.6; 95% confidence interval, 1.2, 11.1). With a P value cutoff of .06, involved-field technique was an additional adverse prognostic factor (relative risk, 5.2). For freedom from progression, significant ($P = .05$) risk factors included male sex (relative risk, 2.3; 95% confidence interval, 1.1, 2.8) and involved-field technique (relative risk, 2.5; 95% confidence interval, 1.3, 5.0). Significant correlations were found between (*a*) mantle-field technique and pathologic staging ($P < .001$), (*b*) bulky disease (>5 cm) and the presence of mediastinal adenopathy ($P < .001$), (*c*) bulky disease (>5 cm) and treatment with chemotherapy ($P < .001$), (*d*) nonbulky disease and involved-field technique ($P < .001$), and (*e*) treatment with chemotherapy and mixed cellularity histology ($P = .026$).

Of the 196 patients, 47 (23.9%) experienced recurrent disease (13 died of Hodgkin disease after the first or subsequent recurrence). Median time to recurrence was 26 months. Actuarial recurrence rates at 10 and 20 years were 23%

and 30%, respectively. The site of recurrence according to the site of primary adenopathy and histologic findings is shown in Table 2. Seven patients experienced recurrent disease 10 years after the diagnosis and treatment of Hodgkin disease. Histologic types of disease at presentation were lymphocyte predominance in two patients, nodular sclerosis in two, and mixed cellularity in three.

Five recurrences were in field and five were marginal. The actuarial local failure rate was 5.5% at both 10 and 20 years. Two of the cases of marginal recurrence manifested as submental adenopathy after unilateral irradiation to the involved side of the neck. Of the remaining three cases of marginal recurrence, one occurred in the infraclavicular area after mantle treatment, one in the right hilum after mantle treatment for bulky mediastinal Hodgkin disease, and one in the left internal mammary lymph nodes after subtotal nodal irradiation (Table 3).

Recurrent disease in 26 (55.3%) of the 47 patients was in previously nonirradiated nodal regions, which accounted for the majority of recurrences. Actuarial recurrence rates in previously nonirradiated lymph nodes at 10 and 20 years were 13% and 15%, respectively. Five recurrences were adjacent, four discontinuous, and 17 (36.2%) transdiaphragmatic. Among the latter, 10 had been treated with involved- and regional-field technique and seven with extended-field irradiation. Twelve of 101 patients with pathologically staged disease and five of 44 patients with clinically staged disease developed transdiaphragmatic recurrent disease. In seven of the 47 patients, the pelvis was one of the sites of recurrence, and in six of the seven patients it was accompanied by para-aortic disease (Table 4).

Ten patients (21.3 %) experienced recurrent visceral disease with an actuarial rate of 4% and 8% at 10 and 20 years, respectively. One additional patient who had mixed-cellularity Hodgkin disease of the left supraclavicular area treated with mantle irradiation experienced recurrent disease 8 months after his initial diagnosis. Information about the site of recurrence and treatment of this patient was not available for review.

One of the eight patients with B symptoms and right cervical adenopathy with mixed cellularity histology at diagnosis experienced recurrent hepatic, splenic, and para-aortic disease after receiving combination chemotherapy and mantle irradiation. He died of Hodgkin disease despite intensive combination chemotherapy treatment (CVPP-ABDIC for seven cycles). The remaining seven patients have not experienced recurrent disease.

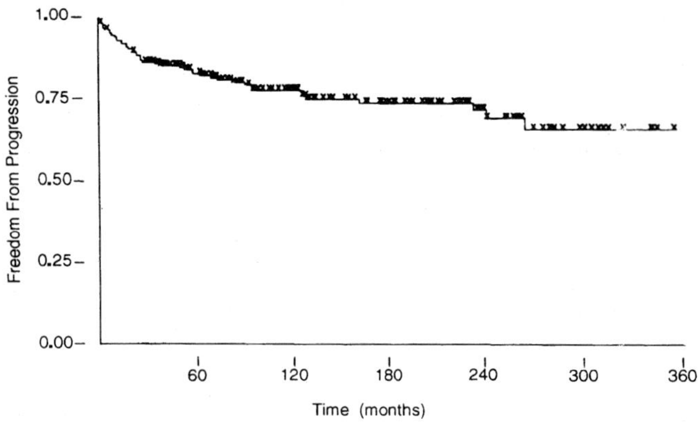

Figure 2. Freedom from progression of disease in 196 patients with stage I Hodgkin disease.

TABLE 2
Number of Patients with Recurrent Disease

A: Site of Primary and Recurrent Disease

Site of Recurrence	Primary Disease Site: Cervical	Axilla	Mediastinum	Lower Torso	Total
In field or marginal	8	0	2	0	10
Adjacent	4	1	0	0	5
Discontinuous	3	1	0	0	4
Transdiaphragmatic	12	4	0	1	17
Visceral	9	1	0	0	10
Total	36	7	2	1	46

B: Histologic Findings in Recurrent Disease

Site of Recurrence	Lymphocyte Predominance	Nodular Sclerosis	Mixed Cellularity	Total
In field or marginal	0	5	5	10
Adjacent	0	3	2	5
Discontinuous	2	0	2	4
Transdiaphragmatic	4	5	8	17
Visceral	1	5	4	10
Total	7	18	21	46

Note.—One additional patient experienced recurrent disease, but the records were not available for review.

Salvage treatment was effective in 34 of the 47 patients with recurrent disease. Actuarial OS rates at 5 and 10 years were 69.3% and 60%, respectively. Actuarial rates of freedom from second recurrence at 5 and 10 years were 63% and 55%, respectively. Records of salvage treatment were available for review for 44 of the 47 patients. Salvage treatment included radiation therapy in eight patients, combination chemotherapy plus radiation therapy in 19, and chemotherapy alone in 17. Irradiation fields were involved or regional in 13 patients, extended in nine, and subtotal nodal in four. Chemotherapy with MOPP was used in 15 patients and with CVPP-ABDIC in 17, and two underwent autologous bone marrow transplantation.

Sixty-two (31.6%) of the 196 patients developed late effects that could represent toxicity from the treatment. Two years after the completion of treatment with three cycles of NOVP and subtotal nodal irradiation, one patient developed pericardial tamponade (grade 4 cardiotoxicity) that necessitated placement of a pericardial window. Twenty-four (12.2%) patients developed ischemic heart dis-

TABLE 3
Findings for In-Field and Marginal Recurrent Disease

Type of Recurrence	Site of Primary Disease	Primary Histologic Finding	Site of Recurrent Disease	Irradiation Technique	Freedom from Progression of Disease (mo)
In field	Cervical	Mixed cellularity	Cervical	Regional	71
In field	Cervical	Mixed cellularity	Cervical	Mantle	37
In field	Cervical	Nodular sclerosis	Mediastinum	Mantle	64
In field	Axilla	Mixed cellularity	Mediastinum	Subtotal nodal*	26
In field	Mediastinum	Nodular sclerosis	Mediastinum	Subtotal nodal*	26
Marginal	Cervical	Mixed cellularity	Submental	Involved	6
Marginal	Cervical	Nodular sclerosis	Submental	Involved	4
Marginal	Mediastinum	Nodular sclerosis	Infraclavicular	Mantle	9
Marginal	Mediastinum	Mixed cellularity	Right hilum	Mantle	8
Marginal	Mediastinum	Nodular sclerosis	Mediastinum	Subtotal nodal*	19

* NOVP for three cycles.

TABLE 4
Recurrent Disease in Nonirradiated Areas

Type of Recurrence	Site of Recurrence	Site of Primary Disease	Histologic Finding	Irradiation Technique	Freedom from Progression of Disease (mo)
Adjacent	Right hilum and lung	Cervical	Nodular sclerosis	Regional	22
Adjacent	Bilateral axillae	Cervical	Nodular sclerosis	Involved	4
Adjacent	Right cervical, left axilla	Left cervical	Nodular sclerosis	Progressive disease*	1
Adjacent	Left cervical, right axilla	Left axilla	Mixed cellularity	Involved	2
Adjacent	Mediastinum	Cervical	Mixed cellularity	Involved	265
Discontinuous	Left axilla	Right axilla	Lymphocyte predominance	Regional	39
Discontinuous	Right cervical	Left cervical	Mixed cellularity	Involved	15
Discontinuous	Left axilla	Right cervical	Lymphocyte predominance	Regional	162
Discontinuous	Right inguinal	Cervical	Mixed cellularity	Subtotal nodal†	27
Transdiaphragmatic	Para-aortic	Cervical	Nodular sclerosis	Extended	8
Transdiaphragmatic	Para-aortic, pelvis	Cervical	Mixed cellularity	Extended	12
Transdiaphragmatic	Para-aortic, pelvis	Cervical	Lymphocyte predominance	Regional	96
Transdiaphragmatic	Para-aortic, spleen, right axilla	Cervical	Mixed cellularity	Regional	52
Transdiaphragmatic	Mediastinum, para-aortic	Cervical	Mixed cellularity	Regional	11
Transdiaphragmatic	Cervical, pelvis	Axilla	Lymphocyte predominance	Regional‡	84
Transdiaphragmatic	Left hilum, para-aortic	Cervical	Mixed cellularity	Involved	30
Transdiaphragmatic	Para-aortic	Axilla	Lymphocyte predominance	Involved	26
Transdiaphragmatic	Mediastinum	Lower torso	Mixed cellularity	Regional	22
Transdiaphragmatic	Para-aortic, pelvis	Cervical	Mixed cellularity	Regional	24
Transdiaphragmatic	Para-aortic, pelvis	Cervical	Nodular sclerosis	Extended	58
Transdiaphragmatic	Para-aortic	Axilla	Lymphocyte predominance	Regional	126
Transdiaphragmatic	Para-aortic	Axilla	Nodular sclerosis	Extended	94
Transdiaphragmatic	Para-aortic	Cervical	Nodular sclerosis	Extended	90
Transdiaphragmatic	Para-aortic, pelvis	Cervical	Nodular sclerosis	Extended	7
Transdiaphragmatic	Para-aortic, pelvis, inguinal	Cervical	Mixed cellularity	Extended	18
Transdiaphragmatic	Para-aortic	Cervical	Mixed cellularity	Involved	241

* NOVP for one cycle.
† NOVP for three cycles.
‡ MOPP for six cycles.

ease, only 14 of whom had received mediastinal irradiation. Eight deaths were cardiac related. The actuarial rates of mortality from coronary artery disease at 10 and 20 years were 2.1% and 7.4%, respectively. The median interval to the development of coronary artery disease was 9.9 years (range, 4–280 months). Among the irradiated patients, 13 were treated with cobalt gamma rays and one was treated with 6-MV photons, and the dose at the myocardium ranged from 33 Gy in 15 fractions to 50 Gy in 23 fractions. Five of the 15 patients who received mediastinal irradiation developed grade 5 cardiotoxicity and died of myocardial infarction, five survived after myocardial infarction (grade 4 cardiotoxicity), and four experienced grade 3 cardiotoxicity that resulted in triple-vessel bypass in two (Table 5). Differences were not statistically significant in the frequency of coronary artery disease in patients who received mediastinal irradiation compared with those who did not (14 of 112 vs 10 of 84 patients, $P = .9$). One of the 24 patients who developed coronary artery disease had also received chemotherapy as part of the initial treatment.

In two patients, Hodgkin disease was diagnosed simultaneously with other malignancies. One had a squamous cell carcinoma of the right true vocal cord, and the other had an adenoid cystic carcinoma of the hard palate. Twenty-four (12.2%) of the 196 patients developed second malignancies (median time, 9.7 years; range, 6–275 months). The actuarial rates of second malignancies at 10 and 20 years were 8.1% and 16.7%, respectively. Twenty-two (11.2%) patients developed secondary malignant solid tumors, 11 (5.6%) within the irradiated field. Two patients, one of whom received chemotherapy as part of the initial treatment, died of acute myelogenous leukemia. Time to development of acute leukemia was 4.5 years for the patient who had received chemotherapy and 9.5 years for the one who was treated with radiation therapy only. Non-Hodgkin lymphoma and lung and skin cancer were the most common secondary malignancies (Table 6). Differences were not statistically significant for the frequency of second malignant tumors between patients treated with adjuvant chemotherapy and those treated with radiation therapy alone (four of 46 vs 20 of 150 patients, respectively; $P = .401$).

Two patients developed severe grade 3 radiation fibrosis of the lung, which resulted in collapse of the right lower lobe in one patient and in phrenic nerve paralysis with diaphragmatic elevation in the other. The first patient received treatment to the mediastinum for recurrent disease to 30 Gy with a right hilar boost of 10 Gy. The second patient received a total dose of 50 Gy to the upper mediastinum and 55 Gy to the trachea at 5-cm depth with subsequent severe pulmonary fibrosis as well as laryngeal stenosis that necessitated placement of a permanent tracheostomy. Clinical hypothyroidism was documented in 23 (11.7%) of the 196 patients. One additional patient developed hyperparathyroidism. Sterility was documented in four patients, three of whom had received chemotherapy with MOPP, one as primary treatment and two for recurrent disease.

TABLE 5
Late Cardiotoxicity in 15 Patients Who Received Mediastinal Irradiation

		Radiation Therapy			
Patient Age (y)*	Late Toxic Effects†	Technique	Dose (Gy)	No. of Fractions	Outcome
27	Pericardial tamponade (G4)	Subtotal nodal	40	18	Alive
50	Triple bypass (G3)	Subtotal nodal	38	18	Alive
40	Triple bypass (G3)	Subtotal nodal	34	20	Alive
42	Severe coronary artery disease (G3)	Extended	48	20	Died of large cell lymphoma
46	Severe coronary artery disease (G3)	Extended	50	23	Alive
79	Myocardial infarction (G5)	Extended	36	15	Died of myocardial infarction
39	Myocardial infarction (G5)	Extended	40	20	Died of myocardial infarction
62	Myocardial infarction (G5)	Extended	34	15	Died of myocardial infarction
34	Myocardial infarction (G5)	Extended	33	15	Died of myocardial infarction
40	Myocardial infarction (G4)	Extended	39	20	Alive
29	Myocardial infarction (G4)	Extended	40	20	Alive
30	Myocardial infarction (G4)	Subtotal nodal	39	17	Alive
55	Myocardial infarction (G4)	Subtotal nodal	47	19	Died of lung cancer
39	Myocardial infarction (G4)	Subtotal nodal	40	18	Alive
29	Myocardial infarction (G5)	Subtotal nodal	40	17	Died of myocardial infarction

Note.—Ten additional patients who experienced cardiac events did not receive mediastinal irradiation and are not included in this table.
* Age at the time of manifestation of coronary artery disease.
† On the basis of the Radiation Therapy Oncology Group and EORTC Late Radiation Morbidity Scoring Scheme.

DISCUSSION

Patients with stage I Hodgkin disease have an excellent outcome. In this study, with a median and maximum follow-up of 12 and 29.6 years, respectively, the 10- and 20-year OS rates were 82% and 66%, and the 10- and 20-year freedom-from-progression rates were 77% and 70%, respectively. Our results are in accordance with published reports from other referral centers (9–12), even though only a few have reported the outcome of stage I disease separately (13,14). In the EORTC trials (15), the 12-year rates for stage I and II disease were 77% to 80% for OS and 68% to 85% for freedom from progression of disease. In a retrospective review of patients with stage I Hodgkin disease, the 15-year actuarial rates for OS and freedom from progression were 78% (13).

Several host-, disease-, and treatment-related factors have been found to influence outcome in patients with early-stage Hodgkin disease. In this retrospective review, the evolution of diagnostic and therapeutic strategies over 30 years, as well as the excellent outcome of patients with stage I Hodgkin disease, makes it difficult to single out specific factors as beneficial or deleterious in any treatment regimen. In multivariate analysis, older age was selected as an adverse prognostic factor for OS. In fact, the majority of deaths (40 of 53) resulted from intercurrent disease. In several studies of patients with either clinical or pathologic stage I and II Hodgkin disease, older age has been associated with both poorer disease-free survival and OS (16,17) and defines a high-risk patient group in which intensification of treatment with combination chemotherapy and radiation therapy may be warranted. Sex also influenced freedom from progression in multivariate analysis. In studies of patients with both clinically and pathologically staged disease, female sex often emerges as an independent favorable prognostic factor (2).

The histologic subtype of mixed cellularity was selected as an unfavorable factor for disease-specific survival in multivariate analysis (relative risk, 4.7). Mixed cellularity histology is known to be predictive of positive findings at laparotomy and, thus, of more extensive tumor burden in patients with clinically staged disease (16). In patients with pathologically staged disease, the role of histologic subtype is less well defined, and histologic data are not used by some investigators to determine major treatment decisions (10,18).

The presence of systemic symptoms, although rare in stage I Hodgkin disease,

TABLE 6
Second Malignancies Diagnosed in 22 Patients

Second Malignancy	No. in Nonirradiated Field	No. in Irradiated Field
Non-Hodgkin disease	1	2
Lung cancer	1	2
Skin cancer	4	1
Urethral cancer	0	1
Endometrial cancer	0	1
Colorectal cancer	2	0
Rectal melanoma	0	1
Squamous cell cancer of parotid gland	0	1
Adenocarcinoma of unknown primary site	1	0
Prostate cancer	1	0
Penile cancer	1	0
Breast cancer	0	2

Note.—Two additional patients, one of whom received chemotherapy as part of the initial treatment for Hodgkin disease, developed acute myelogenous leukemia.

has been associated with occult or extranodal disease dissemination. In this study, B symptoms did not influence outcome. However, most investigators have observed more frequent recurrences in patients with systemic symptoms, specifically fever and weight loss, and they recommend a more intensive therapeutic approach with chemotherapy and radiation therapy (16,17,19).

The site and bulk of primary adenopathy including mediastinal manifestations did not influence outcome in either univariate or multivariate analysis. In this study, two patients with large mediastinal adenopathy treated with radiation therapy alone experienced marginal recurrences. The presence of bulky mediastinal disease has been shown to be an independent adverse prognostic factor for disease-free survival and OS (10,20). In addition to combination chemotherapy, appropriate management of this disease requires careful design of the radiation therapy portals to adequately cover the volume of the disease. The role of whole-lung irradiation was established in the prechemotherapy era; it successfully treats microscopic tumor deposits in the pulmonary parenchyma and results in prolonged disease-free survival (21,22). However, concerns about cardiopulmonary toxicity and second malignant tumors in the irradiated field have limited its use to patients who are not candidates for chemotherapy. Some investigators believe that the presence of bulky adenopathy in sites other than the mediastinum is also prognostically important (18).

Laparotomy was selected as a favorable prognostic factor for disease-specific survival, but it did not influence OS in multivariate analysis. These results are in accordance with reports from other institutions (23,24). It seems that patients whose disease is staged pathologically experience a slightly prolonged disease-free interval than those whose disease is staged clinically (76% vs 68%, respectively, at 12 years), but the former are also subject to increased risk of death due to intercurrent disease. In addition, identification of factors that are predictive of recurrence or death in patients with clinically staged disease has limited the use of laparotomy (9,25).

In multivariate analysis, involved- and mantle-field irradiation emerged as unfavorable treatment-related factors for disease-specific survival; the mantle-field technique also adversely influenced OS. In addition, the long-term freedom-from-progression rates for involved-, regional-, and extended-field techniques were inferior to those for subtotal nodal irradiation (46%, 74%, 74%, and 83% at 20 years, respectively). These results are in agreement with previous observations from our institution (14). It is well known that mantle irradiation alone is not sufficient treatment for patients with clinically staged disease or for those with pathologically staged disease older than 40 years presenting with unfavorable histologic findings and/or systemic symptoms (16). Involved-field irradiation is also inadequate, even though some investigators may consider it appropriate in selected patients with suprahyoid cervical adenopathy and lymphocyte predominance histology (12). In the recent EORTC trials (H7 and the ongoing H8 trials), a selected favorable group of patients consisting of women aged 40 years or less with clinical stage IA disease, with lymphocyte predominance or nodular sclerosis histology, and without bulky mediastinal adenopathy are treated with mantle irradiation alone (2). Until the results of these trials mature, subtotal nodal irradiation remains the standard treatment for patients with clinically staged disease with favorable prognostic factors (14).

Chemotherapy did not emerge as a prognostic factor in this study. However, it was administered selectively to patients with mediastinal disease, bulky adenopathy, and mixed cellularity histology. In clinical stage I Hodgkin disease, chemotherapy is used to eradicate occult tumor, indicated by the presence of systemic symptoms or bulky mediastinal adenopathy, and it has been shown to result in prolonged recurrence-free survival (10,16,19,26). Currently, the optimal delivery of chemotherapy and radiation therapy is still debated and is being addressed in some ongoing clinical trials. At our institution, encouraging results have been reported with use of two cycles of MOPP or three cycles of NOVP and subtotal nodal irradiation (27,28). In addition, the most recent trial (H8) of the EORTC group—which compares four versus six cycles of the hybrid of MOPP and doxorubicin, bleomycin, vinblastine sulfate, or ABV, and involved-field irradiation—was performed to confirm the preliminary data from other nonrandomized studies.

The majority of relapses occurred in unirradiated lymph node regions (55.3%) and specifically in the upper abdomen (36.2%). These results are in accordance with the failure patterns reported by others (9,29) and verify the importance of subtotal nodal irradiation as the treatment of choice in patients with favorable prognostic factors. Limited experience with encouraging preliminary results has been reported with the use of mantle irradiation only in a selected group of patients aged 40 years or less with pathologic stage IA and IIA disease, lymphocyte predominance or nodular sclerosis histology, and without bulky mediastinal and/or hilar disease (9-year disease-free survival and OS rates of 69% and 94%, respectively) (1,9). In this study, we were unable to identify a subset of patients that would benefit from mantle irradiation alone.

Salvage treatment of patients with recurrent disease has been reported to be related to the primary treatment. The probability of successful salvage treatment is significantly lower for patients in whom chemotherapy with MOPP fails than for those in whom radiation therapy alone fails (15% vs 85%, respectively) (30,31). In this study, the salvage rates after initial treatment with radiation therapy versus combination chemotherapy plus radiation therapy were comparable (74% vs 75%, respectively) and may be attributed to the small number of events and the short follow-up period in patients treated with NOVP. Chemotherapy is recommended in patients with unfavorable manifestations or in those participating in clinical trials.

A substantial number of patients experienced recurrent disease long after they completed primary treatment. Late recurrence associated with stage I Hodgkin disease has been reported elsewhere (32,33) and indicates the need for prolonged surveillance to ensure prompt diagnosis and treatment.

The effect of late treatment-related sequelae was appreciated in patients with long-term follow-up. Cardiovascular toxicity has been associated with mediastinal irradiation and is reported to contribute significantly to the morbidity and death due to intercurrent disease in long-term survivors of Hodgkin disease (34–36). The risk is increased in younger patients and in those who have received mediastinal doses of more than 30 Gy (36). In our study, 58.3% of the patients who developed ischemic heart disease had been treated with mediastinal irradiation, and the actuarial rate of cardiovascular deaths in this group at 20 years was 7.4%. In a number of patients, cardiovascular events occurred at an unusually young age (≤40 years). Irradiation techniques such as the use of a cobalt beam, preferential weighting of the anterior field, and large daily fractions have been implicated in the development of late cardiac toxic effects. The same factors may have contributed to the development of severe pulmonary fibrosis in two patients (37).

In long-term survivors of Hodgkin disease, the frequency of secondary neoplasms exceeds the expected frequency of primary tumors in the general population (38,39). Data compiled from several medical centers indicate that second malignancies occur more frequently in younger patients treated with combined modality therapy and/or subtotal or total nodal irradiation (40). In addition, the frequency of acute myelogenous leukemia is most pronounced in cases of splenectomy or prior treatment with alkylating agents (41). In this review, the actuarial rate of secondary tumors was 16.7% at 20 years. Because of the few patients who developed second neoplasms, we were unable to identify a subgroup of patients at high risk for secondary malignancies.

In conclusion, stage I Hodgkin disease has an excellent outcome. Subtotal nodal irradiation is recommended for patients with favorable prognostic factors, with chemotherapy reserved for those with less favorable features. Staging laparotomy is no longer necessary. Treatment should be tailored according to prognostic factors. In our institution, it is the current practice to recommend subtotal nodal irradiation for patients with favorable prognostic factors and to reserve chemotherapy for patients older than 50 years or who present with B symptoms and/or bulky mediastinal disease. Prolonged surveillance is recommended for the early identification and management of late recurrences and/or toxic effects. Current investigations are focusing on the efficacy of subtotal nodal irradiation with three courses of different chemotherapeutic regimens for patients with unfavorable manifestations.

References

1. Mauch PM, Canellos GP, Shulman LN, et al. Mantle irradiation alone for selected patients with laparotomy staged IA to IIA Hodgkin's disease: preliminary results of a prospective trial. J Clin Oncol 1995; 13:947–952.
2. Noordijk EM, Carde P, Mandard AM, et al. Preliminary results of the EORTC-GPMC controlled clinical trial H7 in early stage Hodgkin's disease. Ann Oncol 1994; 5(suppl):S107–S112.
3. Fuller LM, Hagemeister FB, Sullivan MP, Velasquez WS. Hodgkin's disease in adults: stages I and II Hodgkin's disease and non-Hodgkin's lymphomas in adults and children. New York, NY: Raben, 1988; 208–222.
4. Carbone PP, Kaplan HS, Musshoff K, Smithers DW, Tubiana M. Report of the Committee on Hodgkin's Disease Staging Classification. Cancer Res 1971; 31:1860–1861.
5. Cox JD, Stetz J, Pajak TF. Toxicity criteria of the Radiation Therapy Oncology Group (RTOG) and the European Organization for Research and Treatment of Cancer (EORTC). Int J Radiat Oncol Biol Phys 1995; 31:1341–1346.
6. Kaplan EL, Meier P. Nonparametric estimation from incomplete observations. J Am Stat Assoc 1958; 53:457–481.
7. Mantel N. Evaluation of survival data and two new rank order statistics arising in its consideration. Cancer Chemother Rep 1966; 50:163–170.
8. Cox DR. Regression models and life tables (with discussion). J R Stat Soc Br 1972; 34:187–220.
9. Cosset JM, Henry-Amar M, Meerwaldt JH, et al. The EORTC trials for limited stage Hodgkin's disease. Eur J Cancer 1992; 28A:1847–1850.
10. Leslie NT, Mauch PM, Hellman S. Stage IA to IIB supradiaphragmatic Hodgkin's disease, long-term survival and relapse frequency. Cancer 1985; 55:2072–2078.
11. Hoppe RT, Horning SJ, Rosenberg SA. The concept, evolution and preliminary results of the current Stanford clinical trials for Hodgkin's disease. Cancer Surv 1985; 4:459–475.
12. Gospodarowicz MK, Sutcliffe SB, Clark RM, et al. Analysis of supradiaphragmatic clinical stage I and II Hodgkin's disease treated with radiation alone. Int J Radiat Oncol Biol Phys 1992; 22:859–865.
13. Ganesan TS, Wrigley PFM, Murray PA, et al. Radiotherapy for stage I Hodgkin's disease: 20 years experience at St. Bartholomew's Hospital. Br J Cancer 1990; 62:314–318.
14. Vlachaki MT, Hagemeister FB, Fuller LM, et al. Long term outcome of treatment for Ann Arbor stage I Hodgkin's disease: prognostic factors for survival and freedom from progression. Int J Radiat Oncol Biol Phys 1997; 38:593–599.
15. Tubiana M, Henry-Amar M, Hayat M, et al. The EORTC treatment of early stages of Hodgkin's disease: the role of radiotherapy. Int J Radiat Oncol Biol Phys 1984; 10:197–210.
16. Tubiana M, Henry-Amar M, Carde P, et al. Toward comprehensive management tailored to prognostic factors of patients with clinical stages I and II in Hodgkin's disease: the EORTC Lymphoma Group controlled clinical trials 1964–1987. Blood 1989; 73:47–56.
17. Gospodarowicz MK, Sutcliffe SB, Bergsagel DE. Radiation therapy in clinical stage I and II Hodgkin's disease. Eur J Cancer 1992; 28A:1841–1846.
18. Mendenhall NP, Cantor AB, Barré DM, Lynch JW Jr, Million RR. The role of prognostic factors in treatment selection for early-stage Hodgkin's disease. Am J Clin Oncol 1994; 17:189–195.
19. Crnkovich MJ, Leopold K, Hoppe RT, Mauch P. Stage I to IIB Hodgkin's disease: the combined experience at Stanford University and the Joint Center for Radiation Therapy. J Clin Oncol 1987; 5:1041–1049.
20. Johnson DW, Hoppe RT, Cox RS, Rosenberg SA, Kaplan HS. Hodgkin's disease limited to intrathoracic sites. Cancer 1983; 52:8–13.
21. Levitt SH, Lee CKK, Aeppli DM. Radical treatment of Hodgkin's disease with radiation therapy: results of a 15-year clinical trial (the 1985 Erskine Lecture). Radiology 1987; 162:623–630.
22. Levitt SH, Lee CKK, Aeppli D, Lindgren B, Peterson BA. The role of radiation therapy in Hodgkin disease: experience and controversy. Cancer 1992; 70:693–703.
23. Leibenhaut MH, Hoppe RT, Efron B. Prognostic indicators at laparotomy: findings in clinical stage I–II supradiaphragmatic Hodgkin's disease. J Clin Oncol 1989; 7:81–91.
24. Mauch P, Larson D, Osteen R. Prognostive factors for positive surgical staging in patients with Hodgkin's disease. J Clin Oncol 1990; 8:257–265.
25. Cox JD, Stoffel TJ. Clinical versus pathologic stage I and II Hodgkin's disease. Oncology 1980; 37:325–328.
26. Hughes-Davies L, Tarbell NJ, Coleman CN, et al. Stage IA–IIB Hodgkin's disease: management and outcome of extensive thoracic involvement. Int J Radiat Oncol Biol Phys 1997; 39:361–369.
27. Fuller LM, Hagemeister FB, North LB. The adjuvant role of two cycles of MOPP and low dose lung irradiation in stage IA through IIB Hodgkin's disease: preliminary results. Int J Radiat Oncol Biol Phys 1988; 14:683–692.
28. Hagemeister FB, Fuller LM, Laughlin M. NOVP and radiotherapy for early staged Hodgkin's disease: an interim analysis. Ann Oncol 1992; 3:587–590.
29. Hellman S, Mauch P. Role of radiation therapy in the treatment of Hodgkin's disease. Cancer Treat Rep 1982; 66:915–923.
30. Biti GP, Cimino G, Cartoni C, et al. Extended-field radiotherapy is superior to MOPP chemotherapy for the treatment of pathologic stage I–IIA Hodgkin's disease: eight year update of an Italian prospective

randomized study. J Clin Oncol 1992; 10:1367–1369.
31. Cimino G, Biti GP, Cartoni C, Magrini SM. Chemotherapy versus radiotherapy in early-stage Hodgkin's disease: evidence of a more difficult rescue for patients relapsed after chemotherapy. Eur J Cancer 1992; 28A:1853–1855.
32. Herman TS, Hoppe RT, Donaldson SS, Cox RS, Rosenberg SA, Kaplan HS. Late relapses among patients treated for Hodgkin's disease. Ann Intern Med 1985; 102:292–297.
33. Vlachaki MT, Hagemeister FB, Fuller LM, et al. Long term outcome of treatment for Ann Arbor stage I Hodgkin's disease: patterns of failure, late toxicity and second malignancies. Int J Radiat Oncol Biol Phys 1997; 39:609–616.
34. Boivin JF, Hutchinson GB, Lubin JH, Mauch P. Coronary artery disease mortality in patients treated for Hodgkin's disease. Cancer 1992; 69:1241–1247.
35. Cosset JM, Henry-Amar M, Pellae-Cosset B. Pericarditis and myocardial infarctions after Hodgkin's disease therapy. Int J Radiat Oncol Biol Phys 1991; 21:447–449.
36. Hancock SL, Tucker MA, Hoppe RT. Factors affecting late mortality from heart disease after treatment of Hodgkin's disease. JAMA 1993; 270:1949–1955.
37. Dubray B, Henry-Amar M, Meerwaldt JH, et al. Radiation induced lung damage after thoracic irradiation for Hodgkin's disease: the role of fractionation. Radiother Oncol 1995; 36:211–217.
38. Tucker MA, Coleman CN, Cox RS. Risk of second cancers after treatment for Hodgkin's disease. New Engl J Med 1988; 318:76–81.
39. Henry-Amar M, Hayat M, Meerwaldt JH, et al. Causes of death after therapy for early stage Hodgkin's disease entered on EORTC protocols. Int J Radiat Oncol Biol Phys 1990; 19:1155–1157.
40. Biti G, Cellai E, Magrini SM, Papi MG, Ponticelli P, Boddi V. Second solid tumors and leukemia after treatment for Hodgkin's disease: an analysis of 1121 patients from a single institution. Int J Radiat Oncol Biol Phys 1994; 29:25–31.
41. Rodriguez MA, Fuller LM, Zimmerman SO, et al. Hodgkin's disease: study of treatment of intensities and incidents of second malignancies. Ann Oncol 1993; 4:125–131.

Book Review

Basic Clinical Radiobiology. 2nd ed.

Edited by G. Gordon Steel, DSc

London, England: Edward Arnold, 1997. ISBN 0-340-70020-3.
Hardcover, $45.00; pp 254; 181 figures; tables.

This slender volume presents the basic radiobiologic principles that underlie the modern clinical practice of radiation oncology. Intended primarily for medical students and radiation therapy residents, this is the second edition of a book that first appeared in 1993 and was developed from a teaching course directed since 1990 by Professor Steel for the European Society for Therapeutic Radiology and Oncology. The 11 authors are internationally known contributors to the literature in the areas of experimental radiation biology and clinical radiation oncology.

The subject matter is organized into 25 chapters. The initial chapters introduce the concepts of how the cellular organization and proliferative characteristics of tumors and normal tissues form the basis of their response to radiation. Several chapters follow in which the concepts of DNA and cell damage and repair are presented. A variety of experimental assay systems used in quantitating these effects are described, and a chapter is devoted to mathematical models of radiation cell killing. The material then becomes more clinically oriented, starting with time-dose-fractionation relationships, the role of hypoxia in tumor response, and dose rate effects. Later chapters are devoted to discussions of particle beams, the use of radiation in combination with hyperthermia and chemotherapy, and the special problems of targeted radiation therapy with internal emitters. The final chapter deals with the current state of development of predictive assays intended to aid in tailoring treatment to individual patients.

The writing is clear and concise with a good balance and integration of scientific and clinical subject matter. The large number of figures and tables in the first edition, which are integral to the understanding of the text, have been preserved in this edition. The figures are uniform in appearance, are well labeled, and include extensive legends where necessary. I believe that the second edition benefits from the rearrangement and combination of several of the original chapters, which provide an improved flow to the presentation of the material. Much of the information in the first edition has been updated and expanded. New chapters have been added in three clinical areas: dose-response relationships, retreatment tolerance, and applications of combined radiation therapy and chemotherapy. The book is well edited, is virtually error free, and has a uniformity of style and context throughout. It contains a complete index, a useful glossary of radiation biology terms, and a listing of key points at the end of each chapter. As before, an excellent bibliography and recommendations for further reading are provided at the end of each chapter.

In my judgment, this book is as complete and up to date in terms of coverage of subject matter as any of the similarly intended volumes I have seen. It will serve as a useful primer for board examinations, as well as an excellent textbook around which to organize a radiation biology course for radiation oncology residents. At the budget-friendly cost of $45.00, I recommend that it be on every resident's bedside table.

Reviewed by John D. Wilson, PhD

Epstein-Barr-Virus–associated Lymphoproliferative Disease of the Lung: CT and Histologic Findings[1]

Jannette Collins, MD, MEd
Nestor L. Müller, MD, PhD
Ann N. Leung, MD
Georgeann McGuinness, MD
Patricia J. Mergo, MD
Julia D. Flint, MD
Thomas F. Warner, MD
Charles Poirier, MD
James Theodore, MD
Dani Zander, MD
Herman T. Yee, MD

Index terms:
Acquired immunodeficiency syndrome (AIDS), 60.2069, 60.2518
Epstein-Barr virus, 60.2069
Lung, transplantation, 60.459
Lung neoplasms, CT, 60.1211
Lymphoma, AIDS-related, 60.3439
Lymphoma, CT, 60.1211
Viruses, 60.2069

Radiology 1998; 208:749–759

Abbreviations:
AIDS = acquired immunodeficiency syndrome
EBV = Epstein-Barr virus
FK506 = tacrolimus
LPD = lymphoproliferative disease
OKT = Ortho Kung T cell

[1] From the Departs of Radiology (J.C.) and Pathology (T.F.W.), University of Wisconsin Hospital and Clinics, 600 Highland Ave, E3/311 Clinical Science Center, Madison, WI 53792-3252; Departs of Radiology (N.L.M.) and Pathology (J.D.F.), University of British Columbia, Vancouver; Departs of Radiology (A.N.L.) and Pulmonary and Critical Care Medicine (C.P., J.T.), Stanford University Medical Center, Calif; Departs of Radiology (G.M.) and Pathology (H.T.Y.), New York University Medical Center, NY; and Departs of Radiology (P.J.M.) and Pathology (D.Z.), University of Florida College of Medicine, Gainesville. From the 1997 RSNA scientific assembly. Received Nov 13, 1997; revision requested Jan 27, 1998; revision received Feb 18; accepted Apr 3. **Address reprint requests to** J.C.

Author contributions:
Guarantor of integrity of entire study, J.C.; study concepts, J.C., N.L.M.; study design, J.C., N.L.M.; definition of intellectual content, J.C., N.L.M.; literature research, J.C.; data acquisition, J.C., N.L.M., A.N.L., G.M., P.J.M.; data analysis, J.C., N.L.M., J.D.F., T.F.W., C.P., J.T., D.Z., H.T.Y.; manuscript preparation, J.C.; manuscript editing, J.C., N.L.M., A.N.L., G.M.; manuscript review, all authors.

PURPOSE: To assess the computed tomographic (CT) and histologic findings of intrathoracic lymphoproliferative disease (LPD) associated with the Epstein-Barr virus (EBV).

MATERIALS AND METHODS: The authors retrospectively reviewed the CT scans of the chest and the pathologic specimens obtained in 24 patients with histologically proved intrathoracic LPD and with positive serologic findings or immunohistochemical staining for EBV. Five patients had acquired immunodeficiency syndrome (AIDS); one had common variable immune deficiency; and 18 were receiving immunosuppressive therapy for heart, lung, or heart-lung (n = 15) or bone marrow (n = 2) transplantation and vasculitis (n = 1).

RESULTS: Final diagnoses included malignant lymphoma (n = 15), polyclonal LPD (n = 8), and hyperplasia of bronchus-associated lymphoid tissue (n = 1). CT findings included multiple nodules (n = 21), lymphadenopathy (n = 9), areas of ground-glass opacification (n = 8), septal thickening (n = 7), consolidation (n = 5), pleural effusion (n = 4), and solitary endobronchial lesion (n = 2). The nodules were 2–4 cm in diameter, involved mainly the middle and lower lung zones, and frequently had a predominantly peribronchovascular (n = 15) or subpleural (n = 14) distribution.

CONCLUSION: EBV-associated LPD may range from benign lymphoid hyperplasia to high-grade lymphoma. The most common CT manifestation consists of multiple nodules, frequently in a predominantly peribronchovascular or subpleural distribution.

Epstein-Barr virus (EBV) is a gamma-group herpes virus. It has been implicated in the pathogenesis of the African form of Burkitt lymphoma (1), nasopharyngeal carcinoma (2), B-cell lymphomas in immunosuppressed individuals (3), some T-cell lymphomas (4), and some cases of Hodgkin disease (5). EBV is usually associated with lymphoproliferative disease (LPD) in patients who have congenital or acquired immunodeficiencies and occasionally in patients with no apparent immunodeficiency (3). In adults, EBV-associated LPD is seen most commonly in organ transplant recipients who are treated with immunosuppressive therapy and in patients with acquired immunodeficiency syndrome (AIDS). The imaging manifestations of LPD in organ transplant recipients (6–10), in patients with AIDS (11–15), or in other immunocompromised patients (16,17) have been previously described. However, none of these previous studies assessed specifically EBV-associated LPD seen in a variety of different types of immunocompromised patients.

The purpose of this study was to review the computed tomographic (CT) and histologic findings of intrathoracic LPD in immunocompromised patients with documented EBV infection proved by means of positive serologic results or immunohistochemical staining.

MATERIALS AND METHODS

The authors retrospectively reviewed CT scans of the chest and pathologic specimens obtained in 24 immunocompromised patients from five major medical centers. All patients

TABLE 1
Clinical, CT, and Pathologic Findings in Patients with AIDS

Patient No./ Sex/Age (y)	Diagnosis	CT Findings	Pathologic Examination and Findings	Treatment and Follow-up
1/M/42	Lymphoma	Multiple nodules, anterior mediastinal adenopathy, bilateral septal thickening	Transbronchial biopsy: malignant lymphoma, not further classified	No treatment, patient died
2/M/34	Lymphoma	Multiple nodules, multiple areas of consolidation, multiple areas of ground-glass attenuation, subcarinal and bilateral hilar adenopathy	Transbronchial biopsy: non-Hodgkin malignant lymphoma, large cell type	Chemotherapy, no response, patient died
3/M/35	Lymphoma	Multiple nodules, multiple sites of ground-glass attenuation	Open lung biopsy: malignant lymphoma, large cell type; dense lymphoid infiltrate composed of small lymphoid cells (T cells) and focal areas with large atypical lymphoid cells (B cells); involvement of several blood vessels and bronchial walls by lymphoid infiltrate	No treatment
4/F/56	Lymphoma	Multiple nodules	Open lung biopsy: moderate to high-grade malignant lymphoma with B-cell immunoblastic pattern	Chemotherapy
5/M/41	Lymphoma	Solitary subpleural nodule, pleural effusion (<2 cm thick), 2-cm low-attenuation right lower lobe endobronchial mass with collapse of the right lower lobe	Transbronchial biopsy: B-cell lymphoma, large lymphoid cells, occasional smaller lymphocytes and scattered eosinophils	Chemotherapy with response

had histologically proved intrathoracic LPD associated with EBV diagnosed between July 1990 and August 1996. Immunosuppression was a result of AIDS (n = 5); heart, lung, or heart-lung transplantation (n = 15); bone marrow transplantation (n = 2); common variable immune deficiency (n = 1); and immunosuppressive therapy for vasculitis (n = 1). The time between transplantation and development of posttransplantation LPD ranged from 38 days to 10 months (median, 3 months). Final diagnoses included malignant lymphoma (n = 15), polyclonal LPD (n = 8), and hyperplasia of bronchus-associated lymphoid tissue (n = 1).

The time between CT examination and histologic diagnosis ranged from 0 to 69 days (median, 3 days). The study included a total of 24 patients (15 female and nine male patients) ranging in age from 14 to 65 years (mean, 32.2 years). The diagnosis of intrathoracic disease was proved by means of open lung biopsy (n = 6), transbronchial biopsy (n = 13), needle aspiration biopsy (n = 3), or autopsy (n = 2). The diagnosis of EBV infection was based on positive serologic results (n = 14) or positive histochemical staining in tissue (n = 10).

A variety of CT protocols were used at the five contributing institutions, and the scans were obtained on a variety of commercially available scanners. The CT scans were obtained with 10-mm-thick sections (n = 6), 7 mm (n = 3), 6 mm (n = 1), 5 mm (n = 1), 1.5 mm (n = 1), 1 mm (n = 5), 10 and 5 mm (n = 2), 10 and 3 mm (n = 2), 10 and 1 mm (n = 2), or 5 and 1.5 mm (n = 1). Scans with 1.0- and 1.5-mm-thick sections were reconstructed with a high-spatial-frequency algorithm. In four patients, the scans were obtained after intravenous administration of contrast material, and in one patient scans were obtained both before and after intravenous administration of contrast material. The images were obtained at window settings appropriate for assessment of the mediastinum (level, 30–40 HU; width, 400–450 HU) and lung parenchyma (level, −700 HU; width, 1,000–1,500 HU).

The CT scans were reviewed by two chest radiologists (J.C., N.L.M.) from different institutions who were not aware of the underlying diagnoses and causes of the immunocompromised state at the time of interpretation. The scans were initially interpreted independently by the observers, and final decisions were reached by consensus.

The observers assessed the presence, appearance, and distribution of parenchymal, mediastinal, and pleural disease, and they recorded information on a flow sheet. Ground-glass opacification was defined as a hazy increase in attenuation without obscuration of vascular markings and was considered to be present only when it could be seen on thin-section (1.0–1.5-mm section thickness) CT scans. Areas of consolidation were defined as areas of increased attenuation that caused obscuration of the underlying lung markings. Presence of interlobular lines and thickening of the interlobular septa was noted. Nodules were assessed according to diameter (<1 cm or ≥1 cm); distribution (peribronchovascular, subpleural, centrilobular, or random); location (upper, middle, or lower lung zone); whether solitary or multiple; margin characteristics (smooth or irregular); and whether the nodule was of low attenuation relative to other soft-tissue structures, had evidence of cavitation, or was associated with a halo of ground-glass opacification. Mediastinal or axillary lymphadenopathy was considered to be present when the short-axis diameter of the nodes was equal to or greater than 10 mm and hilar lymphadenopathy when the diameter was greater than 5 mm. The presence of pleural or pericardial effusions or thickening was noted.

The pathologic specimens were reviewed by the pathologist at each of the five participating institutions (J.D.F., T.F.W., D.Z., H.T.Y.). Definitions and classifications of LPD of the lung were based on the criteria of Craig and colleagues (18). Posttransplantation LPD was categorized into polymorphic and monomorphic categories, on the basis of the morphology of the lymphoid infiltrate. Polymorphic lesions were made up of a mixture of cell types including small mature lymphocytes, small and large follicular center cells, plasmacytoid cells, plasma cells, and immunoblasts. Mono-

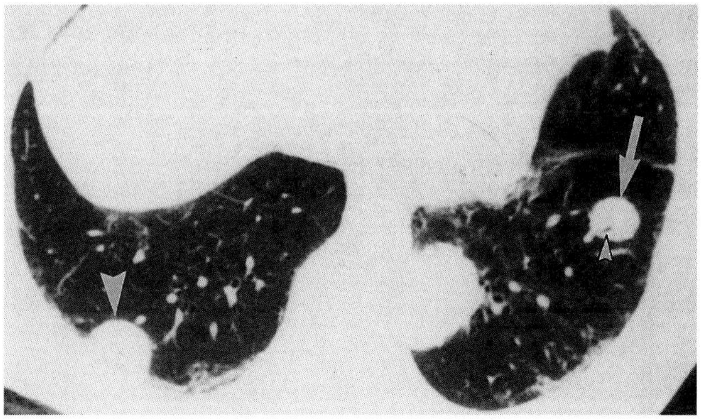

Figure 1. Malignant B-cell lymphoma in a 5-year-old boy with AIDS. Thin-section CT scan (1.0-mm section thickness) shows multiple nodules, greater than 1 cm in diameter, in a peribronchovascular (arrow) and subpleural (large arrowhead) distribution. The nodule margins are smooth and irregular. Note the air bronchogram (small arrowhead) in the left lower lobe nodule.

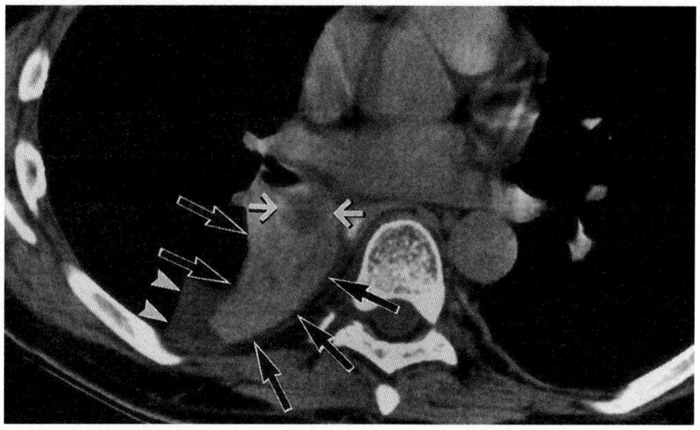

Figure 2. Malignant B-cell lymphoma in a 41-year-old man with AIDS. CT scan obtained with intravenous contrast material (3-mm section thickness) shows a 2-cm-diameter, low-attenuation endobronchial mass (white arrows) in the right lower lobe that is causing the lobe to collapse (black arrows). There is an associated right pleural effusion (arrowheads).

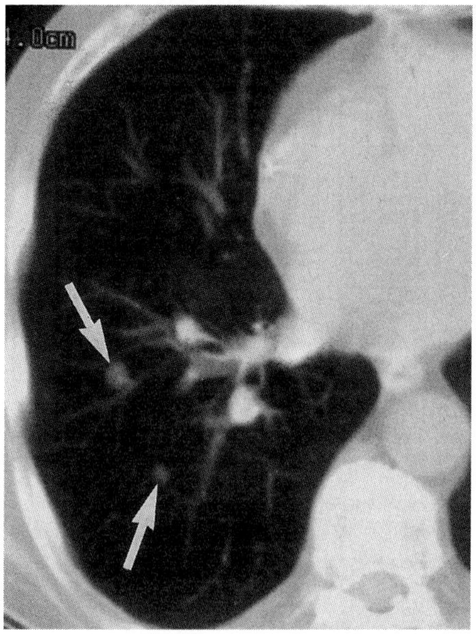

Figure 3. Polyclonal posttransplantation LPD in a 61-year-old male heart transplant recipient. CT scan (10-mm section thickness) shows small, well-circumscribed nodules (arrows) in the right lower lobe.

morphic lesions were histologically indistinguishable from immunoblastic lymphomas occurring in immunocompetent patients.

Medical records were reviewed to document the following: (*a*) type of immunosuppressive therapy the patient was receiving prior to development of LPD, (*b*) CD4 count in patients with AIDS, (*c*) time between transplantation and development of posttransplantation LPD, (*d*) presence of extrathoracic involvement of LPD, (*e*) therapy received for LPD, and (*f*) patient response to therapy. Eighteen patients were receiving immunosuppressive therapy for heart, lung, or heart-lung (n = 15) or bone marrow (n = 2) transplantation and vasculitis (n = 1). Immunosuppressive therapy in these patients included cyclosporine (n = 14), prednisone (n = 11), Ortho Kung T cell 3 (OKT3) monoclonal antibody (n = 6), azathioprine (n = 6), and tacrolimus (FK506) (n = 2). The CD4 count was available in three of the five patients with AIDS and ranged from 4–18 cells per cubic millimeter (normal range, 550–1,190 cells/ mm^3). Extrathoracic involvement was present in five patients, including central nervous system involvement (n = 1); liver and spleen (n = 1); lower extremity, larynx, and mesentery (n = 1); abdominal lymph nodes (n = 1); and disseminated lymphadenopathy (n = 1). After diagnosis of LPD, 15 patients were treated with a decrease in immunosuppressive therapy, six with chemotherapy, two with surgery, and four with treatment for EBV (two with acyclovir, one with ganciclovir, and one with hyperimmune globulin). Four patients received no treatment. The chemotherapy regimen consisted of cyclophosphamide, doxorubicin, vincristine, and prednisone, or CHOP. Disease responded to treatment in 11 patients, progressed with treatment in seven, and had little or no response in one; no follow-up was available for five patients.

RESULTS

The CT and histologic findings are presented according to the underlying cause for the immunodeficiency and are categorized as follows: patients with AIDS, patients who had undergone transplantation, and patients with other causes for immunodeficiency.

Patients with AIDS

All five patients with AIDS had EBV-associated malignant B-cell lymphoma (Table 1). At CT, four of the patients had multiple nodules with diameter greater than or equal to 1 cm (n = 1) or both less than and greater than or equal to 1 cm (n = 3) (Fig 1), and one had an endobronchial lesion (Fig 2). The nodules involved all lung zones and were located in a predominantly peribronchovascular and subpleural distribution. Three patients had mediastinal (n = 2) or hilar (n = 1) adenopathy. Open lung biopsy performed in one patient demonstrated angioinvasion and bronchial wall invasion by the lymphoid infiltrate, which accounted for the peribronchovascular distribution of nodules seen at CT.

Three of the patients had extrathoracic involvement of the central nervous system (n = 1); liver and spleen (n = 1); and lower extremity, larynx, and mesentery (n = 1). The CD4 counts were equal to or less than 18 cells/mm^3 (normal range, 550–1,190 cells/mm^3) for the three patients in whom this information was available. Disease in only one patient improved with chemotherapy (Table 1).

Posttransplantation LPD

Nine of the 17 patients who had undergone transplantation had malignant lym-

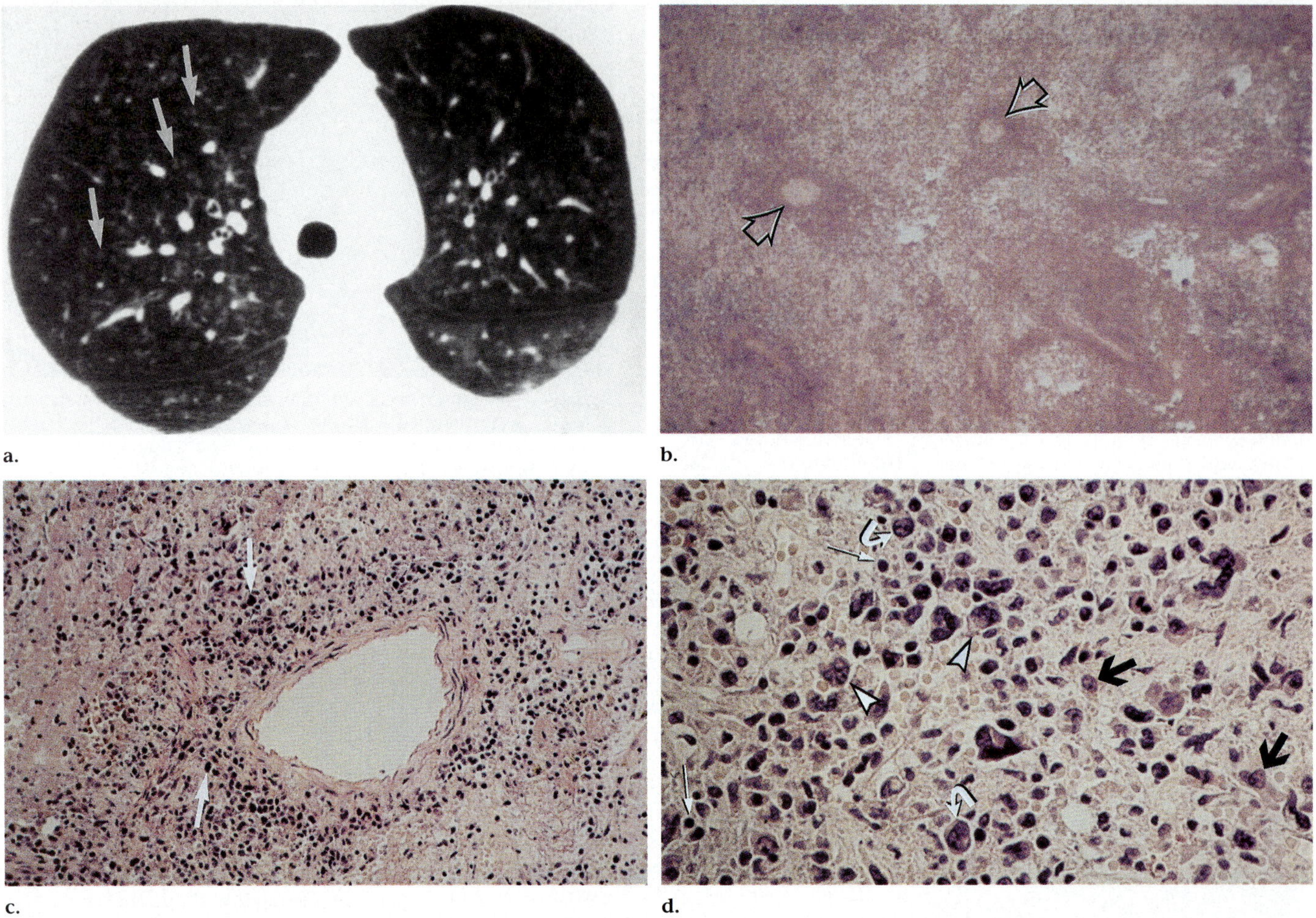

Figure 4. Malignant B-cell lymphoma in a 30-year-old man after bone marrow transplantation for acute lymphocytic leukemia. Diagnosis was made at autopsy. **(a)** Thin-section CT scan (1.0-mm section thickness) shows numerous small, ill-defined nodules (arrows) in a centrilobular distribution. **(b)** Photomicrograph of a lung nodule shows extensive necrosis and focal perivascular viable lymphoid infiltrates (arrows). (Hematoxylin-eosin stain; original magnification, ×40.) **(c)** Photomicrograph of a necrotic nodule shows remaining islands of viable perivascular atypical large lymphoid cells (arrows). (Hematoxylin-eosin stain; original magnification, ×100.) **(d)** Photomicrograph shows a heterogeneous population of cells including small lymphocytes (white straight arrows), plasma cells (black arrows), immunoblasts (curved arrows), and transformed lymphocytes (arrowheads). (Hematoxylin-eosin stain; original magnification, ×200.)

phoma and eight had polyclonal LPD (Table 2). Both types of LPD were seen among recipients of lung, heart, heart-lung, and bone marrow transplants. The most common CT finding was multiple pulmonary nodules; this findings was present in 15 (88%) of 17 patients. The nodules occurred in a peribronchovascular (n = 2), subpleural (n = 4), peribronchovascular and subpleural (n = 7), or random (n = 2) distribution, and they involved the middle and lower (n = 7), all (n = 5), lower (n = 2), or middle (n = 1) lung zones (Table 2). Nodule diameter in each patient was less than 1 cm (n = 2), greater than or equal to 1 cm (n = 3), or both (n = 10). Nodule margins were smooth (n = 2, Fig 3), irregular (n = 6), or both (n = 7). In two patients, the peribronchovascular nodules had a centrilobular distribution (Fig 4) at CT. Areas of ground-glass opacification were seen in five patients, four of whom also had nodules with halos of ground-glass opacification (Fig 5). Areas of consolidation were seen in four patients. Septal thickening, seen in six patients, was associated with surgically related pleural thickening. Five patients had mediastinal (n = 3) or hilar (n = 4) lymphadenopathy (Figs 6, 7).

Histologic examination showed evidence of peribronchovascular involvement in five patients who also had multiple nodules in a peribronchovascular distribution at CT (Table 2). In one patient who underwent open lung biopsy, pleural involvement was seen at histologic examination, which correlated with a subpleural distribution of multiple nodules seen at CT. In one patient with low-attenuation hilar lymphadenopathy at CT, aggregates of predominantly necrotic lymphoid tissue were seen at histologic examination of the transbronchial biopsy specimen.

Two patients had extrathoracic involvement including abdominal adenopathy (n = 1) and disseminated lymphadenopathy (n = 1). All but one of the patients were treated: Fifteen were treated by decreasing their dose of immunosuppression; two received chemotherapy; two underwent surgery; and four received treatment for EBV, including three with acyclovir, one with ganciclovir, and one with hyperimmune globulin. Disease in 11 patients responded to treatment and progressed in one, and four patients died. The untreated patient also died.

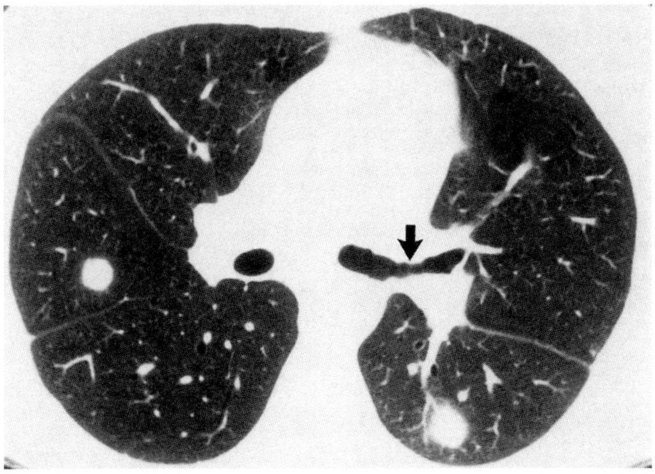

Figure 5. Polyclonal posttransplantation LPD in a 23-year-old female bilateral lung transplant recipient. Thin-section CT scan (1.0-mm section thickness) shows middle lung zone nodules greater than 1 cm in diameter, in a predominantly peribronchovascular distribution. The nodules have fairly smooth margins. There is mild narrowing of the left bronchial anastomosis (arrow).

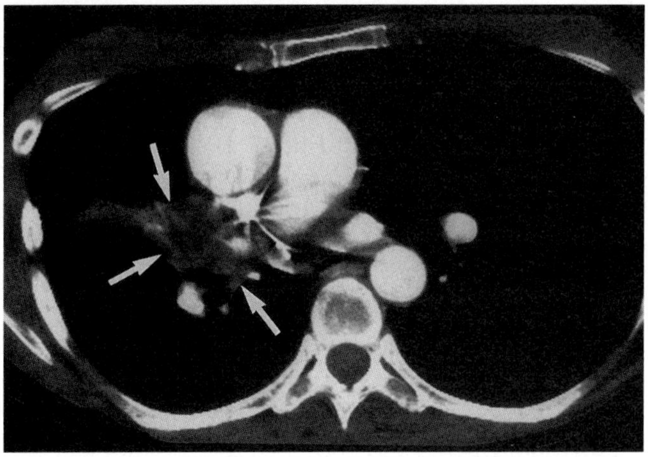

Figure 6. Polyclonal posttransplantation LPD in a 52-year-old woman after right lung transplantation for α_1-antitrypsin deficiency. CT scan (7.0-mm section thickness) obtained with intravenous contrast material shows an approximately 3 × 3-cm area of low-attenuation right hilar adenopathy (arrows).

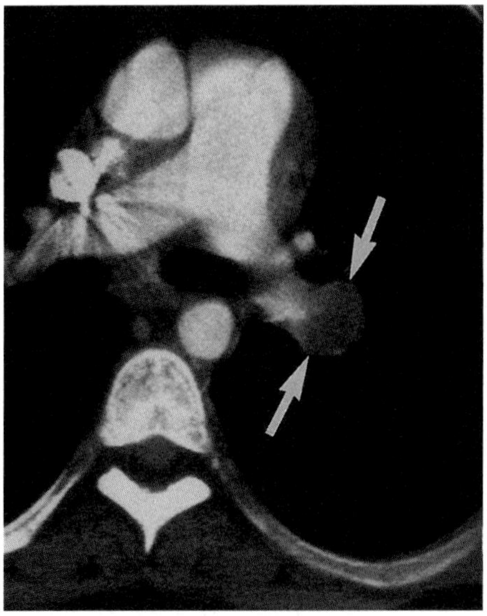

Figure 7. Malignant B-cell lymphoma in a 15-year-old girl after heart-lung transplantation for complex congenital heart disease. CT scan (7.0-mm section thickness) obtained with intravenous contrast material shows a 17 × 24-mm area of low-attenuation left hilar adenopathy (arrows).

Patients with Common Variable Immunodeficiency or Vasculitis

Both patients had multiple nodules less than 1 cm in diameter with irregular margins at CT (Table 3). In the patient with common variable immunodeficiency, the nodules were in a peribronchovascular distribution and were found at histologic examination to be due to hyperplastic bronchus-associated lymphoid tissue (Table 3). The nodules in the patient with vasculitis who was receiving azathioprine were in a centrilobular distribution and were found histologically to be due to large lymphomatous cells with a peribronchovascular distribution.

Neither patient presented with symptoms of extrathoracic LPD. The patient with vasculitis was treated with chemotherapy; the lymphoma rapidly progressed, resulting in extensive parenchymal consolidation, mediastinal adenopathy, and pleural effusions.

DISCUSSION

Posttransplantation LPD affects approximately 2% of all allograft recipients (19). Posttransplantation LPD associated with immunosuppressive drug therapy is unique for several reasons: a predilection for extranodal sites, varied morphologic appearance, a strong and probably causal association with EBV infection, a frequent absence of immunophenotypic or genotypic evidence of monoclonality, and a poor response to cytolytic chemotherapeutic or irradiation regimens (18). Posttransplantation LPD affects approximately 0.6% of patients after bone marrow transplantation (20), 1%–5% after renal graft transplantation (21), 1.8%–20.0% after cardiac transplantation (3,22–25), and 2% after liver transplantation (26). The incidence of posttransplantation LPD after lung transplantation ranges from 6.2% to 9.4% and is twofold higher than that seen after transplantation of other organs (27). Among heart and lung transplant recipients, the risk of developing posttransplantation LPD remains 5%–6% per year, and it is the third leading cause of mortality outside the perioperative period, accounting for 7% of the deaths in both groups (28). After lung or heart-lung transplantation, the death rate for posttransplantation LPD is approximately 40% but can be as high as 70% in cases of late-onset posttransplantation LPD (28). Compared with transplant recipients who die, survivors have fewer monoclonal lesions (26% of survivors vs 57% of patients who died) (3).

A three-step process leading to the development of posttransplantation LPD has been described (Fig 8): (*a*) infection of B lymphocytes with EBV, which causes increased proliferation of B cells (polyclonal B-cell expansion); (*b*) loss of immune control by T cells, which allows uncontrolled proliferation of EBV-infected B lymphocytes (oligoclonal); and (*c*) genetic mutation, which transforms some B-cell clones into malignant cells (18). The latter, with subsequent monoclonal proliferation of malignant cells, leads to development of aggressive malignant lymphomas that often cannot be treated successfully (3,29–31). Although the most common type of posttransplantation LPD involves B cells, 14% of posttransplantation LPD is of T-cell rather than B-cell origin (19,32).

EBV has been identified in the majority of cases of posttransplantation LPD by means of molecular techniques (18). The rate of primary or reactivated EBV infec-

TABLE 2
Clinical, CT, and Pathologic Findings in Patients after Transplantation

Patient No./ Sex/Age (y)	Type of Transplant and Immunosuppression Therapy	Diagnosis	CT Findings	Pathologic Examination and Findings	Treatment and Follow-up
1/F/23	Bilateral lung transplant, cyclosporine and OKT3	Polyclonal LPD	Multiple nodules	Open lung biopsy: B-cell polyclonal LPD, sheetlike growth with some areas of necrosis and vasoinvasion, pleural involvement obvious, tracking at the edge of the lesion along bronchovascular bundles, mixture of large immature lymphoid elements, some mature lymphocytes and scattered plasma cells	Decrease in immunosuppression, nodules resolved
2/F/21	Bilateral lung transplant, cyclosporine and OKT3	Lymphoma	Multiple nodules, multiple randomly distributed areas of ground-glass opacification	Transbronchial biopsy: B-cell malignant high-grade lymphoma, massive central necrosis with marked tendency toward vasoinfiltration	Decrease in immunosuppression, patient died
3/M/16	Heart-lung transplant, cyclosporine and OKT3	Lymphoma	Multiple nodules, multiple areas of ground-glass attenuation, right pleural thickening and effusion (<2 cm), mediastinal (paratracheal and subcarinal) and right hilar adenopathy	Transbronchial biopsy: B-cell malignant lymphoma	Decrease in immunosuppression, treatment with ganciclovir and hyperimmune globulin, disease progressed
4/M/30	Bone marrow transplant, cyclosporine and OKT3	Lymphoma	Multiple nodules, solitary area of consolidation, multiple randomly distributed areas of ground-glass opacification	Autopsy: B-cell malignant lymphoma with disseminated lymphadenopathy	No treatment, patient died
5/F/52	Bone marrow transplant	Polyclonal LPD	Multiple nodules	Autopsy: polyclonal LPD	Chemotherapy, surgery, patient died
6/F/45	Left lung transplant; FK506, prednisone, and azathioprine	Polyclonal LPD	Multiple low-attenuation nodules, solitary subpleural area of consolidation, multiple areas of randomly distributed ground-glass opacification, left pleural and pericardial thickening, bilateral septal thickening	Transbronchial biopsy: polyclonal LPD composed of large cells in a fine fibrous stroma	Decrease in immunosuppression, disease resolved
7/M/65	Heart transplant; cyclosporine, prednisone, and azathioprine	Lymphoma	Multiple nodules	Open lung biopsy: large cell malignant lymphoma, large lymphoid cells, 3-cm tumor mass involving the interatrial septum at autopsy	Decrease in immunosuppression, surgery, patient died
8/M/61	Heart transplant, FK506 and prednisone	Polyclonal LPD	Multiple nodules	Open lung biopsy: polyclonal LPD, diffuse infiltrate consisting of large and medium lymphoid cells, rare large vesicular cells with a large nucleolus that are multilobated	Decrease in immunosuppression, partial response
9/F/63	Left lung transplant; cyclosporine, prednisone, azathioprine, and OKT3	Lymphoma	Multiple nodules, left pleural and pericardial thickening, left septal thickening	Needle aspiration: malignant B-cell lymphoma	Decrease in immunosuppression, treatment with acyclovir, complete response
10/F/45	Left lung transplant; cyclosporine, prednisone, azathioprine, and OKT3	Lymphoma	Multiple nodules, bilateral septal thickening, left hilar adenopathy (4 cm)	Transbronchial biopsy: malignant large B-cell lymphoma	Decrease in immunosuppression, patient died

(Table 2 continues)

TABLE 2 (*continued*)
Clinical, CT, and Pathologic Findings in Patients after Transplantation

Patient No./ Sex/Age (y)	Type of Transplant and Immunosuppression Therapy	Diagnosis	CT Findings	Pathologic Examination and Findings	Treatment and Follow-up
11/F/39	Heart-lung transplant; cyclosporine, prednisone, and azathioprine	Polyclonal LPD	Multiple nodules, multiple areas of randomly distributed consolidation, right pleural thickening, bilateral septal thickening	Transbronchial biopsy: polyclonal LPD, perivascular lymphocytic infiltrate that extends into the adjacent interstitium of alveolar walls, atypical large lymphoid cells	Decrease in immunosuppression, partial response
12/F/14	Bilateral lung transplant, cyclosporine and prednisone	Polyclonal LPD	Multiple nodules, multiple areas of consolidation, mediastinal (paratracheal) and right hilar adenopathy (2 cm, low attenuation), bilateral septal thickening	Needle aspiration: polyclonal LPD; mixed population of cells including large and small lymphocytes; many atypical large lymphoid cells with scant cytoplasm; monocytoid cells, neutrophils, small groups of benign mesothelial cells and pulmonary macrophages; scattered mitotic figures	Decrease in immunosuppression, partial response
13/F/52	Right lung transplant, cyclosporine and prednisone	Lymphoma	Multiple nodules, right hilar adenopathy (3 cm)	Transbronchial biopsy: malignant B-cell lymphoma, atypical lymphoid infiltrate within airway wall, monotonous lymphoid cells resembling large cell lymphoma	Decrease in immunosuppression, partial response
14/F/19	Heart-lung transplant, cyclosporine and prednisone	Polyclonal LPD	Multiple nodules, left pleural thickening, left septal thickening	Needle aspiration: polyclonal LPD, numerous abnormal lymphoid cells appearing singly and in loosely arranged aggregates, occasional larger cells showing multiple irregular nuclei with macronucleoli and abundant cytoplasm, other cells with plasmacytoid features	Decrease in immunosuppression, treatment with acyclovir, partial response
15/F/15	Heart-lung transplant, cyclosporine and prednisone	Lymphoma	Low-attenuation left hilar adenopathy (2.4 cm)	Transbronchial biopsy: malignant B-cell lymphoma, aggregates of predominantly necrotic lymphoid tissue, monotonous population of atypical large cells, abundant necrosis, scattered mitotic figures	Decrease in immunosuppression, treatment with chemotherapy, partial response
16/F/44	Heart-lung transplant, cyclosporine and prednisone	Lymphoma	Left lower lobe endobronchial lesion, left pleural effusion (<2 cm)	Transbronchial biopsy: malignant B-cell lymphoma, monomorphic proliferation of atypical lymphoid cells with medium to large cleaved and noncleaved nuclear forms	Decrease in immunosuppression, treatment with acyclovir, partial response
17/F/52	Bilateral lung transplant, cyclosporine	Polyclonal LPD	Multiple nodules, multiple randomly distributed areas of ground-glass opacification, subcarinal adenopathy, left pleural effusion (<2 cm)	Open lung biopsy: polyclonal LPD; nodule with central zone of necrosis, rimming of vessels, and thin zone of lymphoid elements; some tracking down the adjacent bronchovascular bundles; more than one clone proliferating	Decrease in immunosuppression, partial response

TABLE 3
Clinical, CT, and Pathologic Findings in Patients with Common Variable Immunodeficiency and Vasculitis

Patient No./ Sex/Age (y)	Diagnosis	CT Findings	Pathologic Examination and Findings	Treatment and Follow-up
1/F/20	Lymphoma, azathioprine therapy for vasculitis	Multiple nodules, multiple randomly distributed areas of ground-glass opacification, bilateral septal thickening	Transbronchial biopsy: T-cell malignant lymphoma of high cytologic grade, large cells with prominent nucleoli with brisk mitotic activity, foci of necrosis, definite vasocentricity to the process with some peribronchial involvement, diffuse edema (representing areas of ground-glass attenuation)	Chemotherapy, disease progressed
2/M/32	Hyperplasia of bronchus-associated lymphoid tissue, underlying diagnosis of combined variable immunodeficiency	Multiple nodules, bilateral axillary adenopathy	Transbronchial biopsy: hyperplastic nodules of lymphoid tissue in the walls of bronchioles, lymphoid cells of normal size with an enlarged germinal center in one nodule	No treatment

tion has been found to be higher in patients with EBV-associated LPD (93%) than in the general transplantation population (30%) (33). Patients who are seronegative for EBV before transplantation are much more likely to develop posttransplantation LPD than those who are seropositive (27). However, some patients with posttransplantation LPD show no evidence of EBV at either lesion biopsy or serologic analysis. In addition, 60% of all transplant recipients may have evidence of EBV infection, but posttransplantation LPD develops in only 2%–3% of cases (34).

Symptoms of posttransplantation LPD can occur at variable intervals after transplantation, including up to several years. Symptoms of posttransplantation LPD occur at a mean 2–5 months after bone marrow, lung, or heart-lung transplantation and at a mean 23–32 months after kidney, heart, or liver transplantation (3). In our study group of 17 patients with posttransplantation LPD, 15 of whom were heart, lung, or heart-lung transplant recipients, the mean time to development of disease after transplantation was 2½ months. In one study of heart transplant recipients who developed posttransplantation LPD, no correlation was found between clinically aggressive disease (disseminated disease vs single site of lesion involvement) and the time to diagnosis of posttransplantation LPD (35). In patients treated with cyclosporine, posttransplantation LPD can occur within 1 month of transplantation (36). Cyclosporine prevents allograft rejection by blocking the activation of alloreactive cytotoxic T lymphocytes by means of a reduction in interleukin-2 production and interleukin-2 receptor expression. Cyclosporine also inhibits the activation of EBV-specific cytotoxic T lymphocytes, which hinders the patient's defense against EBV-induced B-cell proliferation. Cyclosporine also induces resistance of EBV-transformed B lymphocytes to immune cytolysis by blocking cell destruction as a result of apoptosis (18,37). Posttransplantation LPD can be considered a defect in the balance between cellular destruction and cellular proliferation; uncontrolled proliferation of B lymphocytes increases the likelihood of mutational oncogenesis (38). Treatment with OKT3 monoclonal antibody is also associated with a high incidence and early onset of posttransplantation LPD (39).

In previous studies, the most common intrathoracic manifestations of posttransplantation LPD have been found to consist of well-circumscribed pulmonary nodules, patchy air space consolidation, and mediastinal and hilar adenopathy (6,8–10,16). Our review of EBV-associated posttransplantation LPD showed the same findings. In three of our patients, two of whom were being treated with cyclosporine immunosuppressive therapy, the pulmonary nodule or nodal mass had a low-attenuation center (Fig 9); this finding has also been reported in patients who were not treated with cyclosporine (7). As in other studies, we had no cases of cavitary nodules. Pleural thickening and effusion have been noted with posttransplantation LPD (6); all of our cases with these findings were believed to be related to the transplantation surgery and not to posttransplantation LPD. In one of our patients with multiple areas of randomly distributed ground-glass opacification at CT, correlative histologic examination showed diffuse edema. Carignan et al (16) reported that posttransplantation LPD nodules were the result of dense infiltration with lymphocytes and the halo of ground-glass opacification resulted from

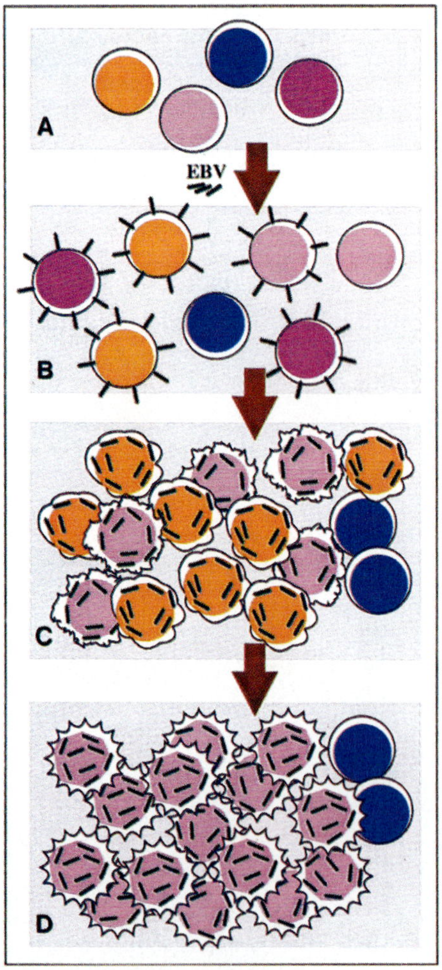

Figure 8. Schematic diagram of B-lymphocyte transformation by EBV. Each color refers to a different clone of B cells. *A*, Infection with EBV causes increased proliferation of B cells. *B*, Polyclonal B-cell expansion. *C*, Immunosuppression leads to loss of immune control by T cells, which allows uncontrolled proliferation of EBV-infected B lymphocytes (oligoclonal). *D*, Genetic mutation transforms some B-cell clones into malignant cells. (Adapted and reprinted, with permission, from reference 18.)

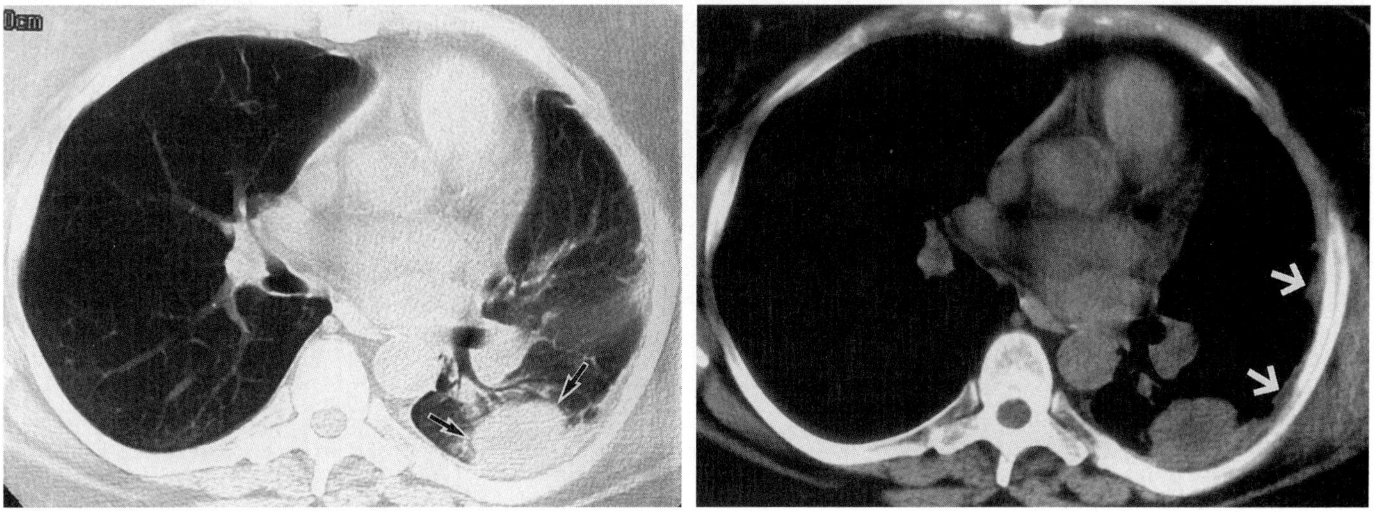

a. b.

Figure 9. Polyclonal posttransplantation LPD in a 45-year-old woman after left lung transplantation for α_1-antitrypsin deficiency. **(a)** Unenhanced helical CT scan (5-mm section thickness) shows a 3.5-cm-diameter subpleural mass (arrows) in the left lower lobe. Opacification in the left lung is secondary to increased perfusion to the lung transplant and the diminished volume of that lung, with mediastinal shift to the left due to the emphysematous native right lung. **(b)** Unenhanced helical CT scan (5.0-mm section thickness) obtained with mediastinal window settings shows the mass with a low-attenuation center. Pleural thickening (arrows) on the left is related to the transplantation surgery.

infiltration of the surrounding interstitium by less densely arranged cells, which was seen in one patient in our study.

With a reported incidence of approximately 2%, lymphoma occurs 40–100 times more frequently in patients with AIDS than in the general population (40). AIDS-related lymphomas are almost always of a non-Hodgkin type (41), are highly aggressive, and are associated with a poor prognosis (12). Immunologically, AIDS-related lymphomas are almost always intermediate- or high-grade B-cell lymphomas (42,43). Extranodal disease is common (90% of patients with AIDS-related lymphoma) and involves the central nervous system, lungs, liver, bowel, and bone marrow (40,44,45). In patients with AIDS-related lymphoma, primary pulmonary involvement was seen in 8%–15% (40,44–46) and intrathoracic involvement was seen in 40% (46).

The radiographic features of AIDS-related lymphoma have been described and include pleural effusions (most common radiographic abnormality, observed in approximately 50% of cases); hilar or mediastinal adenopathy (observed in approximately 25% of cases); and diffuse, bilateral, reticulonodular heterogeneous opacities (41). The nodules can demonstrate extremely rapid growth, with a doubling time of 4 to 6 weeks.

In one study of 38 patients with AIDS-related lymphoma involving the lungs or pleura, chest CT showed pulmonary nodules (50%), lobar infiltrates (27%), and lung masses (19%) as the most common parenchymal abnormalities (14). Pleural effusion and thoracic lymphadenopathy were also common findings, although the importance of lymphadenopathy was unclear, as many of the patients had concurrent diseases that could involve adenopathy. Furthermore, there were no correlations between CT and histologic findings and no blinded readings of the CT scans. Pleural effusion has been reported as the sole manifestation of the thoracic component of AIDS-related lymphoma in one patient (12). CT findings of pleural or pericardial effusions and ascites, in the absence of solid tumor masses or parenchymal abnormalities, have been described recently in patients with AIDS. This peculiar type of non-Hodgkin lymphoma, termed "body cavity–based lymphoma," is associated with infection by human herpesvirus 8 and in some cases by EBV (47). Endobronchial lesions have been reported in 19% of patients with AIDS-related lymphoma (14), compared with 20% in our AIDS patients. Mean CD4 count in patients with AIDS-related lymphoma have ranged from 67 cells/mm^3 ± 65 (standard deviation) to 189 cells/mm^3 (14,48); in our patients, the mean CD4 count of 11.6 cells/mm^3 was much lower than that reported by others.

Chemotherapeutic agents have been used less successfully in the treatment of AIDS-related lymphomas than in the treatment of lymphomas not related to human immunodeficiency virus, or HIV; complete responses are infrequent and tend to be short (42). Of our five patients with AIDS, the one with disseminated malignant lymphoma had a marked response to chemotherapy depicted at follow-up CT.

One of our patients, a 32-year-old man with congenitally acquired immunodeficiency (common variable immunodeficiency), developed benign reactive proliferations of bronchus-associated lymphoid tissue. CT findings in this patient consisted of multiple small nodules in a peribronchovascular distribution, which correlated with the anatomic distribution of bronchus-associated lymphoid tissue and the pathologic distribution of hyperplastic nodules of lymphoid tissue in the walls of bronchioles. Hyperplasia of bronchus-associated lymphoid tissue has also been described in children with AIDS and in solid organ transplant recipients (11). It has been theorized that chronic antigenic stimulation due to rejection, in conjunction with latent EBV genome in the bronchus-associated lymphoid tissue of the graft, results in development of posttransplantation LPD. Our patient with hyperplasia of bronchus-associated lymphoid tissue as a manifestation of LPD was not a transplant recipient.

Our study has several limitations. It is retrospective and includes a limited number of cases. In many cases, thin-section CT (1.0- or 1.5-mm section thickness) was not performed, which limits assessment for areas of ground-glass opacification. Because only five of the 24 CT examinations were performed with intravenous contrast material, we may have underestimated the frequency of mediastinal and hilar lymphadenopathy. With all types of biopsy, sampling error or artifact can be a problem and can limit CT-pathologic correlation. Transbronchial biopsy was the most common method of obtaining a tissue sample in our study, and the accuracy of this biopsy method in establishing the diagnosis of EBV-associated LPD in all patient populations has not been determined.

In conclusion, a spectrum of pulmonary LPD is associated with EBV, and in a heterogeneous population of patients with congenital and acquired immunodeficiencies, the CT findings are similar. In our series of patients, most of whom either had AIDS or had undergone bone marrow or solid-organ transplantation, the two most common diagnoses were polyclonal LPD and malignant lymphoma; the most common CT findings for both diagnoses included multiple nodules, large and small, with a peribronchovascular and subpleural distribution, involving the middle and lower lung zones. In patients with AIDS and those who undergo transplantation, these CT findings should prompt biopsy to determine the diagnosis of LPD. An early diagnosis, especially in the case of posttransplantation LPD, is critical to provide early treatment for a favorable clinical response. In patients with AIDS, the differential diagnoses include other malignancies (especially Kaposi sarcoma) and infection (especially fungus and mycobacteria). In patients after transplantation, the differential diagnoses include infection (eg, fungus or cytomegalovirus) or rejection.

Acknowledgment: We thank Betsy True, a gifted artist, for her illustration in Figure 8.

References

1. deThe G, Geser A, Day NE, et al. Epidemiological evidence for causal relationship between Epstein-Barr virus and Burkitt's lymphoma from Ugandan prospective study. Nature 1978; 274:756–761.
2. deThe G, Zeng Y. Population screening for EBV markers: toward improvement of nasopharyngeal carcinoma control. In: Epstein MA, Achong BG, eds. The Epstein-Barr virus: recent advances. New York, NY: Wiley, 1986; 237–249.
3. Cohen JI. Epstein-Barr virus lymphoproliferative disease associated with acquired immunodeficiency. Medicine 1991; 70:137–160.
4. Jones JF, Shurin S, Abramowsky C, et al. T-cell lymphomas containing Epstein-Barr viral DNA in patients with chronic Epstein-Barr virus infections. N Engl J Med 1988; 318:733–741.
5. Weiss LM, Movahed LA, Warnke RA, Sklar J. Detection of Epstein-Barr viral genomes in Reed-Sternberg cells of Hodgkin's disease. N Engl J Med 1989; 320:502–506.
6. Dodd GD, Ledesma-Medina J, Baron RL, Fuhrman CR. Posttransplant lymphoproliferative disorder: intrathoracic manifestations. Radiology 1992; 184:65–69.
7. Honda H, Barloon TJ, Franken EA Jr, Garneau RA, Smith JL. Clinical and radiologic features of malignant neoplasms in organ transplant recipients: cyclosporine-treated vs untreated patients. AJR 1990; 154:271–274.
8. Harris KM, Schwartz ML, Slasky BS, Nalesnik M, Makowka L. Posttransplantation cyclosporine-induced lymphoproliferative disorders: clinical and radiologic manifestations. Radiology 1987; 162:697–700.
9. Tubman DE, Frick MP, Hanto DW. Lymphoma after organ transplantation: radiologic manifestations in the central nervous system, thorax, and abdomen. Radiology 1983; 149:625–631.
10. Haramati LB, Schulman LL, Austin JHM. Lung nodules and masses after cardiac transplantation. Radiology 1993; 188:491–497.
11. Heitzman ER. Pulmonary neoplastic and lymphoproliferative disease in AIDS: a review. Radiology 1990; 177:347–351.
12. Sider L, Weiss AJ, Smith MD, VonRoenn JH, Glassroth J. Varied appearance of AIDS-related lymphoma in the chest. Radiology 1989; 171:629–632.
13. McGuinness G, Scholes JV, Jagirdar JS, et al. Unusual lymphoproliferative disorders in nine adults with HIV or AIDS: CT and pathologic findings. Radiology 1995; 197:59–65.
14. Eisner MD, Kaplan LD, Herndier B, Stulbarg MS. The pulmonary manifestations of AIDS-related non-Hodgkin's lymphoma. Chest 1996; 110:729–736.
15. Oldham SAA, Castillo M, Jacobson FL, Mones JM, Saldana MJ. HIV-associated lymphocytic interstitial pneumonia: radiologic manifestations and pathologic correlation. Radiology 1989; 170:83–87.
16. Carignan S, Staples CA, Müller NL. Intrathoracic lymphoproliferative disorders in the immunocompromised patient: CT findings. Radiology 1995; 197:53–58.
17. Bragg DG, Chor PJ, Murray KA, Kjeldsberg CR. Lymphoproliferative disorders of the lung: histopathology, clinical manifestations, and imaging features. AJR 1994; 163:273–281.
18. Craig FE, Gulley ML, Banks PM. Posttransplantation lymphoproliferative disorders. Am J Clin Pathol 1993; 99:265–276.
19. Nalesnik MA, Makowka L, Starzl TE. The diagnosis and treatment of posttransplant lymphoproliferative disorders. Curr Probl Surg 1988; 25:367–372.
20. Zutter MM, Martin PJ, Sale GE, et al. Epstein-Barr virus lymphoproliferation after bone marrow transplantation. Blood 1988; 72:520–529.
21. McCune JM. Epstein-Barr virus associated lymphoproliferative disease in mice and men. Lab Invest 1991; 65:377–380.
22. Cleary ML, Warnke R, Sklar J. Monoclonality of lymphoproliferative lesions in cardiac-transplant recipients: clonal analysis based on immunoglobulin-gene rearrangements. N Engl J Med 1984; 310:477–482.
23. Cleary ML, Sklar J. Lymphoproliferative disorders in cardiac transplant recipients are multiclonal lymphomas. Lancet 1984; 2:489–493.
24. Brusamolino E, Pagnucco G, Bernasconi C. Secondary lymphomas: a review on lymphoproliferative diseases arising in immunocompromised hosts—prevalence, clinical features and pathogenetic mechanisms. Haematologica 1989; 74:605–622.
25. Linder J, Purtilo DT. Current concepts of immunodeficiency disorders. Mod Pathol 1990; 3:524–544.
26. Starzl TE, Nalesnik MA, Porter KA, et al. Reversibility of lymphomas and lymphoproliferative lesions developing under cyclosporine-steroid therapy. Lancet 1984; 1:583–587.
27. Aris RM, Maia DM, Neuringer IP, et al. Post-transplantation lymphoproliferative disorder in the Epstein-Barr virus-naive lung transplant recipient. Am J Respir Crit Care Med 1996; 154:1712–1717.
28. Armitage JM, Kormos RL, Stuart S, et al. Posttransplant lymphoproliferative disease in thoracic organ transplant patients: ten years of cyclosporine-based immunosuppression. J Heart Lung Transplant 1991; 10:877–887.
29. Hanto DW, Frizzera G, Gajl-Peczalska KJ, Simmons RL. Epstein-Barr virus, immunodeficiency, and B cell lymphoproliferation. Transplantation 1985; 39:461–472.
30. Bird AG, Britton S. The relationship between Epstein-Barr virus and lymphoma. Semin Hematol 1982; 19:285–300.
31. Randhawa PS, Yousem SA, Paradis IL, et al. The clinical spectrum, pathology, and clonal analysis of Epstein-Barr virus–associated lymphoproliferative disorders in heart-lung transplant recipients. Am J Clin Pathol 1989; 92:177–185.
32. Nalesnik MA, Jaffe R, Starzl TE, et al. The pathology of post-transplant lymphoproliferative disorders occurring in the setting of cyclosporine A–prednisone immunosuppression. Am J Pathol 1988; 133:173–192.
33. Ho M, Miller G, Atchison RW, et al. Epstein-Barr virus infections and DNA hybridization studies in posttransplantation lymphoma and lymphoproliferative lesions: the role of primary infection. J Infect Dis 1985; 152:876–886.
34. Penn I, ed. Roundtable report: immunosuppression and lymphoproliferative disorders. Cincinnati, Ohio: University of Cincinnati, 1991; 10, 14.
35. Chen JM, Barr ML, Chadburn A, et al. Management of lymphoproliferative disorders after cardiac transplantation. Ann Thorac Surg 1993; 56:527–538.
36. Penn I. Cancers following cyclosporine therapy. III. Transplantation Proc 1987; 19:2211–2213.
37. Hudnall SD. Cyclosporine A renders target cells resistant to immunocytolysis. Eur J Immunol 1991; 21:221–226.
38. List AF, Greco FA, Vogler LB. Lymphoproliferative diseases in immunocompromised hosts: the role of Epstein-Barr virus. J Clin Oncol 1987; 5:1673–1689.
39. Swinnen LJ, Costanzo-Nordin MR, Fisher SG, et al. Increased incidence of lymphoproliferative disorder after immunosuppression with the monoclonal antibody OKT3 in cardiac-transplant recipients. N Engl J Med 1990; 323:1723–1728.
40. Polish LB, Cohn DL, Ryder JW, Myers AM, O'Brien RF. Pulmonary non-Hodgkin's

lymphoma in AIDS. Chest 1986; 96:1321–1326.
41. Goodman PC. Non-Hodgkin's lymphoma in the acquired immunodeficiency syndrome. J Thorac Imaging 1991; 6:49–52.
42. Kaplan LD. AIDS-associated lymphomas. Infect Dis Clin North Am 1988; 2:525–532.
43. DiCarlo EF, Amberson JB, Metroka CE, et al. Malignant lymphomas in the acquired immunodeficiency syndrome. Arch Pathol Lab Med 1986; 110:1012–1016.
44. Ioachim HL, Dorsett B, Cronin W, et al. Acquired immunodeficiency syndrome–associated lymphomas: clinical, pathologic, immunologic, and viral characteristics of 111 cases. Hum Pathol 1991; 22:659–673.
45. Dodd GD III, Greenler DP, Confer SR. Thoracic and abdominal manifestations of lymphoma occurring in the immunocompromised patient. Radiol Clin North Am 1992; 30:597–610.
46. Haskel ZJ, Lindan CE, Goodman PC. Lymphoma in the immunocompromised patient. Radiol Clin North Am 1990; 28:885–899.
47. Morassut S, Vaccher E, Balestreri L, et al. HIV-associated human herpesvirus 8–positive primary lymphomatous effusions: radiologic findings in six patients. Radiology 1997; 205:459–463.
48. Levine AM, Sullivan-Halley J, Pike MC, et al. Human immunodeficiency virus–related lymphoma. Cancer 1991; 68:2466–2472.

Volume Rendering of the Tracheobronchial Tree: Clinical Evaluation of Bronchographic Images[1]

Martine Remy-Jardin, MD, PhD
Jacques Remy, MD
Dominique Artaud, MD
Marc Fribourg, MD
Alain Duhamel, PhD

Index terms:
Bronchi, CT, 671.12117
Computed tomography (CT), technology, 671.12117
Computed tomography (CT), three-dimensional, 671.12117
Computed tomography (CT), volume rendering, 671.12117

Radiology 1998; 208:761–770

Abbreviation:
3D = three-dimensional

[1] From the Department of Radiology, Hôpital Calmette, Blvd Jules Leclerc, 59037 Lille, France. Received November 5, 1997; revision requested January 26, 1998; revision received February 23; accepted March 27. **Address reprint requests to** M.R.J.

PURPOSE: To evaluate the application of the volume-rendering technique to airway disease.

MATERIALS AND METHODS: Seventy-four spiral computed tomographic (CT) examinations (1- to 5-mm section thickness; pitch, 1.7–2.0) were performed for known or suspected abnormality of the airways, including (*a*) benign tracheobronchial stenosis (group 1, $n = 47$), (*b*) complex airway lesions (group 2, $n = 15$), and (*c*) bronchiectasis (group 3, $n = 12$). Two radiologists independently compared overlapping transverse CT scans and volume-rendered bronchographic images for detection of airway abnormalities and identification of lesion morphology and extent, with bronchoscopic correlation.

RESULTS: Bronchographic image quality was graded as excellent (73%) or good (24%), whereas motion-related artifacts led to poor image quality in 3% of cases (trapezoid parameters included window width of −700 to −350 HU, triangular trapezoid shape, parenchymal opacification of 70%, unshaded algorithm). Compared with transverse CT scans, volume-rendered images (*a*) provided supplemental diagnostic and/or morphologic information in 23 cases (31%) (group 1, 16 cases; group 3, seven), (*b*) improved confidence in the interpretation of congenital airway abnormalities in six cases (8%) (all from group 2), and (*c*) corrected interpretive errors in four cases (5%) (group 1, two cases; group 2, two).

CONCLUSION: Volume-rendered images improved the recognition of mild changes in airway caliber and the understanding of complex tracheobronchial anomalies.

With the emergence of spiral computed tomography (CT), there has been a renewed interest in three-dimensional (3D) medical imaging. Although these images contain no more information than do the corresponding series of transverse scans, there is a consensus that the viewer can better appreciate spatial relationships in a 3D display than in a series of sections (1). Among the numerous potential applications, these new imaging modalities have been widely applied to musculoskeletal and vascular imaging, but their role in the evaluation of airways has been little explored. The initial experience with 3D imaging of the bronchial tree was based on autopsy specimen studies that provided rudimentary images of central and peripheral airways (2,3). Since then, accurate representations of the tracheobronchial tree have been created from in vivo clinical studies to evaluate potential applications of 3D imaging of central airways as a complement to transverse imaging (4–9).

Among the postprocessing techniques available, most attention has been focused on shaded surface displays (4–9) and, to a lesser degree, minimum intensity projection images, with specific attention to their respective advantages and limitations (9). Volume rendering is a third method of generating a two-dimensional image that can convey 3D spatial information inherent in a 3D volume data set. As recently emphasized by Johnson et al (10) for vascular applications, the reconstruction algorithm and display technology used in volume rendering yield a number of advantages over minimum intensity projection images and shaded surface displays. Details of the technical aspects of volume-rendered 3D images of the bronchial tree have been recently reported, suggesting the possibility of

Author contributions:
Guarantors of integrity of entire study, M.R.J., J.R.; study concepts, J.R.; study design, M.R.J., J.R.; definition of intellectual content, M.R.J., J.R.; literature research, J.R.; clinical studies, M.R.J., J.R., D.A., M.F.; data acquisition, M.R.J., J.R., A.D., M.F.; data analysis, M.R.J., J.R., A.D.; statistical analysis, A.D.; manuscript preparation, editing, and review, M.R.J., J.R.

creating images similar to conventional bronchograms applicable in clinical practice (11). The purpose of this study was to determine whether such images could assist radiologists in better analyzing airway lesions.

MATERIALS AND METHODS

Population

Seventy-four spiral CT examinations of the tracheobronchial tree were performed in 71 consecutive patients referred to our department of radiology for a CT evaluation of suspected or known airway lesions. Examinations were repeated in two transplant recipients to determine whether there was any change in the appearance of the anastomosis over time. One patient who did not undergo transplantation underwent repeat CT because of worsening symptoms. The population comprised 65 adults (35 men and 30 women) and six children, ranging in age from 3 months to 71 years (mean, 47 years). In three of the six children (aged 3 months, 2 years, and 3 years), the spiral CT examinations were obtained under general anesthesia. Spiral CT studies were obtained to evaluate known or suspected abnormality or abnormalities of central airways, including (*a*) benign tracheobronchial stenosis (group 1, n = 47), (*b*) congenital or acquired complex airway lesion (group 2, n = 15), and (*c*) bronchiectasis (group 3, n = 12).

Clinical indications in group 1 included (*a*) known or suspected tracheal stenosis (n = 19) (secondary to previous intubation or tracheotomy [n = 14], extrinsic compression from a thyroid goiter [n = 3], osteochondroplastic tracheobronchopathy [n = 1], airway reconstruction after tumor resection [n = 1]), (*b*) follow-up of bronchial anastomoses after lung transplantation (n = 12), and (*c*) pretherapeutic evaluation of bronchial stenosis (n = 16) at the level of the main-stem (n = 5), lobar (n = 5), and segmental (n = 6) bronchi (secondary to benign endobronchial tumor [n = 3], broncholithiasis [n = 2], posttransplantation ischemic lesion [n = 1]).

In group 2, spiral CT examinations were performed to evaluate congenital or acquired complex airway anatomy: (*a*) suspicion of abnormal bronchial branching patterns (n = 10) and (*b*) evaluation of fistulous tracts of tumoral (n = 3) or infectious (n = 2) origin.

Spiral CT examinations in group 3 were indicated for (*a*) suspicion of bronchiectasis on conventional thin-section CT scans (n = 6) and (*b*) presurgical evaluation of focal varicose bronchiectasis (n = 6).

CT findings were correlated with findings at fiberoptic bronchoscopy in all cases.

CT Examination

Data acquisition.—All scans were obtained with a Somatom Plus 4A scanner (Siemens Medical Systems, Erlangen, Germany). Spiral CT examinations consisted of a focal acquisition through the region of clinical interest, which was selected on the conventional CT study of the entire thorax obtained at the same session.

The spiral CT protocol was performed at 171 mA and 140 kV (scanning time, 0.75 second per revolution). The scanning volume was selected to place the airway of interest within the center of the imaged volume. Section thickness and duration of breath holding varied according to the region of clinical interest: (*a*) 3-mm section thickness and pitch of 1.7 for evaluation of the trachea, (*b*) 2-mm section thickness and pitch of 2 for evaluation of the main-stem and lobar bronchi, and (*c*) 1-mm section thickness and pitch of 2 for evaluation of the segmental and subsegmental bronchi. For the purpose of clarity, the trachea and main-stem and lobar bronchi will be further referred to as central bronchi, whereas the segmental and subsegmental bronchi will be referred to as peripheral bronchi. For each patient, the duration of the spiral sequence resulted from a compromise between adequate coverage of the z axis and the patient's ability to maintain apnea, leading to scanning of a volume varying from 40 to 120 mm^3. Patients routinely received hyperventilation before scanning to assist them in holding their breath during the entire scanning time. All the examinations were performed during inspiration. When hilar vascular structures were to be evaluated during the same acquisition (n = 22), 120–140 mL of a 15%–30% iodinated contrast agent was administered at a rate of 4–5 mL/sec by using a power injector.

Image reconstruction.—Transverse CT scans were reconstructed at 2-mm intervals for tracheal indications and at 1-mm intervals for central and peripheral bronchial examinations, by means of a 180° linear interpolation algorithm. For diagnostic purposes, two series of CT scans were systematically generated: (*a*) mediastinal images, reconstructed with a soft reconstruction kernel and obtained with mediastinal window settings (width, 350 HU; level, 50 HU) and (*b*) lung images, reconstructed with a high reconstruction kernel and obtained with lung window settings (width, 1,600 HU; level, −600 HU).

For the purpose of generating volume-rendered images, a third series of transverse CT scans was systematically reconstructed with a soft reconstruction kernel from each data set, at 1-mm intervals for data sets acquired with 2 mm or thicker sections or at 0.5-mm intervals for data sets acquired with 1-mm section thickness. To include the entire data set in the final reconstruction, care was taken to select a field of view with a size equal to or larger than the z-axis coverage; otherwise, part of the volume surveyed was excluded from the volume-rendered image. The next step consisted of manually drawing the contours of the airway(s) of interest on each CT scan to erase all the regions outside the defined area. This was performed by a technologist who then transferred the images from the main console to a Magic View workstation (Siemens Medical Systems) on which volume-rendered images were generated by means of the Siemens software.

To generate bronchographic images, parameter selection was based on the results of a preliminary determination of the optimal image display parameters (11). According to this study, the following parameters were successively considered. (*a*) The selection of the trapezoid position, which consisted of the selection of a window width and a window level: The window width was positioned to select the voxels located at the interface between the aeric column and the airway wall. Each selection was depicted on a minimum intensity projection image of the edited data set to verify that a continuous rim of peripheral voxels had been selected. The window level was systematically chosen at the midpoint of the window width range. (*b*) In contrast to the trapezoid position, which was individually determined, the remaining volume-rendering parameters were systematically selected: a triangular trapezoid shape, 70% parenchymal opacification, and use of the unshaded volume-rendering algorithm.

According to the orientation of the airway of interest, the following images were created. (*a*) In case of vertical or oblique airways, four views were obtained about the z axis at 45° increments (ie, lateral view, right [or left] oblique view, frontal view, left [or right] oblique view) and completed, when necessary, by adding views at smaller increments about the z axis. (*b*) In case of horizontal airways, images about the x axis were generated from an inferosuperior projection. The overall duration of the procedure

TABLE 1
Overall Quality of Bronchographic Images

Group	Image Quality Grade 3 (excellent)*	2 (good)†	1 (poor)‡
1 (n = 47)	32	13	2
2 (n = 15)	11	4	0
3 (n = 12)	11	1	0
Total (n = 74)	54 (73%)	18 (24%)	2 (3%)

* Sharp interfaces with no motion artifacts.
† Small stair-step artifacts.
‡ Visually disruptive stair-step artifacts.

TABLE 2
Accuracy of Transverse CT Scans and Bronchographic Images in Detection of Airway Stenosis (group 1)

Image	No. of True-Positive Findings	No. of False-Positive Findings	No. of True-Negative Findings	No. of False-Negative Findings	Accuracy (%)
Transverse CT scans (n = 47)	30	0	13	4	91.5*
Bronchographic volume-rendered images (n = 47)	32	0	13	2	95.7†

* 95% confidence interval, 79.2%, 97.9%.
† 95% confidence interval, 85.4%, 99.5%.

varied between 15 and 45 minutes, mainly depending on the duration of the editing step. The latter procedure lasted several minutes for the trachea, a maximum of 10 minutes for the main-stem and lobar bronchi, and between 15 and 25 minutes for the segmental and subsegmental bronchi. Whereas automatic editing was possible for central bronchi, manual drawing of the contour of the peripheral airway(s) of interest was required on every CT scan, which explains the variation in the duration of the editing step. All the images were then obtained with variable window settings directly selected from the workstation (window width, varying between 4,000 and 2,000 HU; window level, varying between 1,000 and 200 HU).

Study Design

Transverse CT scans and volume-rendered images were interpreted separately and in random order by means of independent reading by two experienced radiologists (M.R.J., J.R.) to assess image quality and presence of airway abnormality. The readers knew the group to which the study belonged, although they were blinded to clinical and endoscopic data. Whenever an airway lesion was detected, images were assessed for lesion morphology and extent as further detailed. Any discordant interpretation between the two readers led to a consensus reading. Scoring of image quality was based on a three-point scale: 1, poor quality (severe respiratory-motion artifacts on transverse CT scans or visually disruptive stair-step artifacts on volume-rendered images); 2, good quality (minimal motion artifacts or small stair-step artifacts); and 3, excellent quality (sharp interfaces with no motion artifacts).

In group 1, the images were analyzed for the presence of airway stenosis. A shelf was defined as a small, thin (1–2-mm-thick) eccentric protrusion into the lumen at the site of an anastomosis that did not result in narrowing of the underlying airway. The site and length of airway narrowing were recorded, as was the shape of the stenotic segment. (*a*) Symmetric airway narrowing was defined as any concentric luminal deformity, and (*b*) asymmetric airway narrowing was defined on the basis of one or more eccentric luminal deformities. The severity of airway narrowing was determined after comparison with the diameter of the adjacent normal airway and was expressed as a percentage airway stenosis. When the reduction in airway diameter was less than 30%, it was graded as mild stenosis; between 30% and 50%, moderate; greater than 50%, severe. In a comparison of the respective value of transverse CT scans and volume-rendered images in the evaluation of airway stenosis, a difference greater than 20 mm in the evaluation of stenosis length and a difference greater than 20% in the severity of airway stenosis were considered to be discordant results. The presence of additional abnormalities surrounding the stenotic area was systematically recorded on images obtained with both modalities.

In group 2, the airway anatomy was assessed to determine the bronchial branching pattern in patients suspected of having congenital airway anomalies. In patients with known or suspected of having fistulous tract of infectious or tumoral origin, the goal of the spiral CT evaluation was to assess the presence and the morphologic characteristics of the corresponding airway anomalies. In group 3, two categories of diagnostic information were evaluated: (*a*) the presence of cylindric bronchiectasis in patients with a normal chest radiograph and (*b*) the extent of bronchiectasis in the presurgical evaluation of varicose bronchiectasis. Bronchiectasis was diagnosed on transverse CT scans and volume-rendered reconstructions on the basis of the presence of an internal diameter greater than that of the adjacent pulmonary artery and the lack of progressive tapering of the bronchial lumina (12).

The value of volume-rendered images in understanding lesion morphology and in aiding the ability to judge lesion extent were evaluated on the scale defined by Zeiberg et al (13): 1, poor or misleading (the volume-rendered images provided misleading information when compared with findings on the transverse CT scans); 2, minimal value (the findings on the volume-rendered images were concordant but added no complementary value to findings on the transverse CT scans); 3, moderate value (the volume-rendered images improved confidence in the interpretation of findings on the transverse CT scans); 4, good (the volume-rendered images provided some supplemental information to findings on the transverse CT scans); and 5, highly valuable (the volume-rendered images provided information that could correct potential interpretive errors on the basis of viewing only transverse CT scans).

Fiberoptic Endoscopy

Fiberoptic endoscopic examinations were always performed within 10 days of

CT, with a fiberoptic bronchoscope (Olympus Models, New Hyde Park, NY). For the purpose of this study, the official report of the bronchoscopic examination was used as the interpretation. Bronchoscopic findings were used as proof when the accuracy of imaging in detection of airway stenosis was calculated.

RESULTS

Image Quality

All the patients were able to maintain apnea during the entire spiral sequence; in the absence of respiratory motion artifacts, all transverse CT scans were considered as interpretable. The overall quality of bronchographic images is summarized in Table 1. Fifty-four reconstructions (73%) showed sharp interfaces with no motion artifacts (grade 3 image quality), 18 (24%) showed small stair-step artifacts (grade 2), and two (3%) were not compatible with a confident analysis of airway caliber owing to the presence of marked stair-step artifacts (grade 1). In the latter two cases, marked artifacts were observed at the level of the lower third of the trachea and the left main bronchus and were attributed to aortic motion.

Evaluation of Volume-rendered Images

Group 1 (n = 47).—Interpretation of transverse CT scans revealed 30 stenoses, whereas 17 airways were considered as normal. Airway lesions were present in the trachea ($n = 18$) and main-stem ($n = 4$), lobar ($n = 5$), and segmental ($n = 3$) bronchi. For the purpose of comparison with bronchoscopic findings, the shelves ($n = 8$) were considered as normal airways. Transverse CT scans produced 30 true-positive findings, four false-negative findings, no false-positive findings, and 13 true-negative findings of stenotic lesions (accuracy, 91.5%; Table 2). The false-negative findings were observed at the level of three main-stem bronchi and one segmental bronchus that showed mild stenosis.

On bronchographic images, two reconstructions were considered as noninterpretable due to the presence of marked motion artifacts; 32 stenoses were identified at the level of the trachea ($n = 18$) and main-stem ($n = 6$), lobar ($n = 5$), and segmental ($n = 3$) bronchi, and 13 airways were graded as normal. The bronchographic images produced 32 true-positive findings, two false-negative findings (ie, the two noninterpretable reconstructions), no false-positive finding, and 13 true-negative findings of stenotic lesions (accuracy, 95.7%; Table 2).

The value of volume-rendered images was interpreted as grade 1 in two cases, grade 2 in 27 cases, grade 3 in none, grade 4 in 16 cases, and grade 5 in two cases.

The two grade 1 cases consisted of images of bronchial anastomoses after left lung transplantation with marked artifacts due to aortic motion. These artifacts precluded confident interpretation of the anastomotic sites, whereas these areas were interpreted as normal on transverse CT scans, which were otherwise considered to be of good quality.

In the 16 grade 4 cases, the supplemental information provided with volume-rendered images included (*a*) a confident recognition of three tracheal stenoses (Fig 1) and one main-stem bronchial stenosis (in every case, a reduction of less than 30% in the airway diameter was identified by the two readers on the broncho-

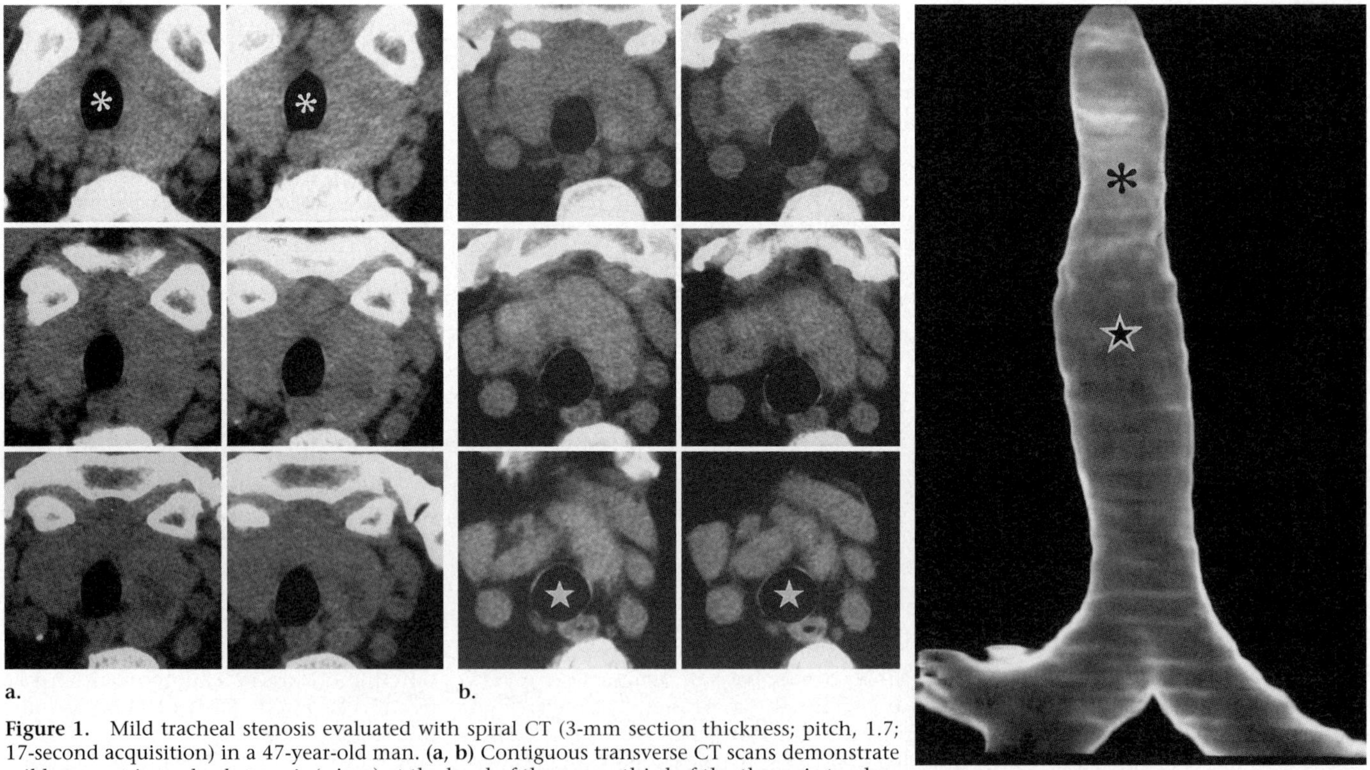

a. b. c.

Figure 1. Mild tracheal stenosis evaluated with spiral CT (3-mm section thickness; pitch, 1.7; 17-second acquisition) in a 47-year-old man. **(a, b)** Contiguous transverse CT scans demonstrate mild symmetric tracheal stenosis (* in **a**) at the level of the upper third of the thoracic trachea secondary to the presence of a heterogeneous thyroid goiter. **(c)** The presence of a mild reduction in the tracheal diameter (*) is easier to detect on the anteroposterior view of the bronchographic volume-rendered image than in **a** and **b** (trapezoid position, −800 to −300 HU). In **b** and **c**, ★ indicates normal tracheal caliber.

graphic images, whereas interobserver disagreement was found on transverse CT scans; in each of these three cases, the volume-rendered findings were concordant with fiberoptic bronchoscopic interpretations) and (*b*) a more precise evaluation of the shape (n = 7), length (n = 7), and/or degree (n = 2) of airway stenosis at the level of the trachea (n = 11) and the main-stem (n = 2) and lobar (n = 1) bronchi.

In the two grade 5 cases, volume-rendered images enabled recognition of anastomotic stenoses that were missed by the two readers on transverse CT scans (Fig 2). In both cases, a reduction of less than 30% in the airway diameter was observed on volume-rendered images, in concordance with fiberoptic bronchoscopic findings. In three patients, tracheal diverticuli were identified on transverse CT scans, and none were recognized on volume-rendered images, which showed only minimal mural irregularities. No anastomotic dehiscence was found with either imaging modality.

Group 2 (n = 15).—Among the 10 patients suspected of having congenital airway anomalies, volume-rendered images provided diagnostic information similar to that provided on transverse CT scans in three cases (ie, grade 2 value for volume-rendered images) and improved confidence in the interpretation with transverse CT scans in six patients (ie, grade 3 value for volume-rendered images). The information obtained on both transverse CT scans and volume-rendered images can be summarized as follows: (*a*) identification of a right tracheal bronchus, supplying the right upper lobe, of normal caliber (two of three cases), and (*b*) identification of the ectopic origin of the anterior segmental bronchus of the right upper lobe, originating from the right bronchus intermedius, of normal caliber (one of three cases).

In six patients, volume-rendered images improved confidence in the interpretation of the transverse CT scans, enabling the readers to identify the following abnormalities: (*a*) In three patients, volume-rendered images confirmed the presence of a right (one case) and left (two cases) tracheal bronchus. In addition, these images allowed confident analysis of the bronchial branching patterns from the ectopic bronchus (ie, a right tracheal bronchus supplying the entire right upper

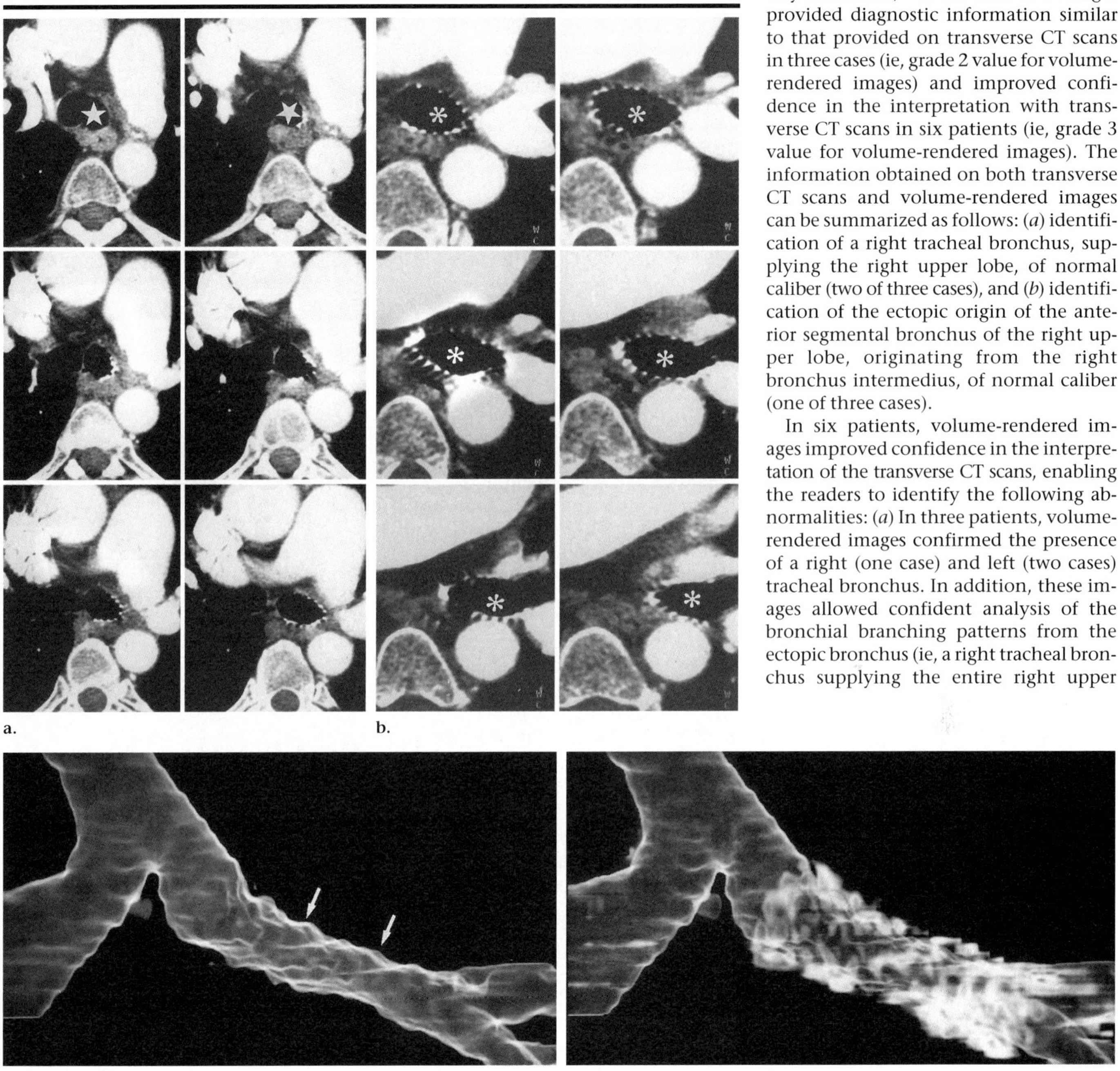

a. b. c. d.

Figure 2. Spiral CT follow-up (2-mm section thickness; pitch, 2; 22-second acquisition) of an ischemic stenosis in the left main bronchus treated with an endoprosthesis after left-side single-lung transplantation in a 51-year-old woman. **(a, b)** Contiguous transverse CT scans demonstrate a left main bronchus of normal diameter at the level of its initial portion (★ in **a**) and the level of the bronchial stent (* in **b**). **(c)** Anteroposterior view of the bronchographic volume-rendered image demonstrates a mild reduction in the airway diameter at the level of the anastomotic site (arrows) (trapezoid position, −600 to −350 HU). **(d)** Selection of a second trapezoid (trapezoid position, 100 to 400 HU) enables concurrent depiction of the airways and the metallic bronchial stent on the volume-rendered image.

lobe [one case] and a left upper lobe bronchus supplying the apicoposterior segment of the left upper lobe [two cases]). In one patient, the origin of one left tracheal bronchus showed severe stenosis. (*b*) In three patients suspected of having bronchial atresia, volume-rendered images confirmed the incompleteness of the bronchial tree suspected on transverse CT scans (absence of the upper division of the left upper lobe bronchus [$n = 1$], absence of the left apicoposterior segmental bronchus [$n = 1$], absence of the right paracardiac segmental bronchus [$n = 1$]), thus leading the readers to support the diagnosis of congenital airway anomaly (Fig 3).

In one patient with a previous history of left diaphragmatic hernia and a small left lung, volume-rendered images enabled a confident demonstration of the completeness of the left bronchial tree. On the basis of this morphologic information, which was unavailable on transverse CT scans, it was possible to exclude left lobar agenesis and to suggest left lung hypoplasia (ie, grade 5 value for volume-rendered images). Bronchial anatomy was confirmed with endoscopic findings in every case.

In four of the five patients in group 2 evaluated for fistulous tracts, transverse CT scans and volume-rendered images provided similar diagnostic information (ie, grade 2 value for volume-rendered images). In the remaining patient, volume-rendered images enabled the identification of a subcarinal fistula between the right and left main-stem bronchi that was missed on transverse CT scans (ie, grade 5 value for volume-rendered images; Fig 4). Interobserver agreement was found in the interpretation of all the volume-rendered images from group 2. Analysis of transverse CT scans led to interobserver discordance in the assessment of abnormal bronchial branching patterns ($n = 2$) and stenosis of the origin of a tracheal bronchus ($n = 1$).

Group 3 (n = 12).—In six patients with recurrent respiratory infections and suspicion for focal cylindric bronchiectasis on thin-section CT scans, volume-rendered images demonstrated the lack of progressive tapering at the level of segmental bronchi of the right upper ($n = 1$), right middle ($n = 1$), and right and left lower ($n = 4$) lobes. The supplemental information provided with volume-rendered images allowed the diagnosis of focal cylindric bronchiectasis and the coding of these images with a grade 4 value (Fig 5). In these six patients, fiberopticbronchoscopic studies failed to help identify segmental cylindric bronchiectasis.

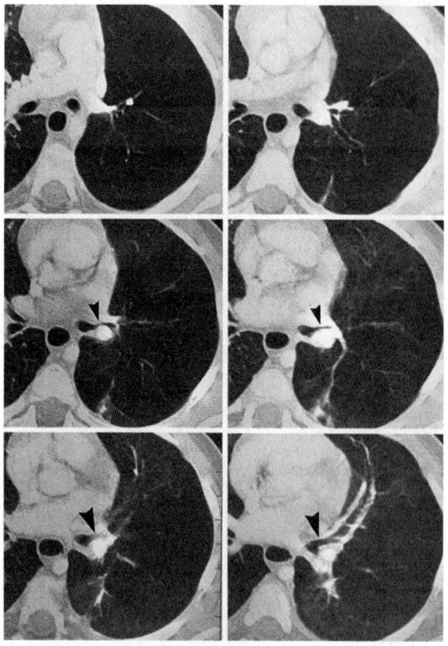

a.

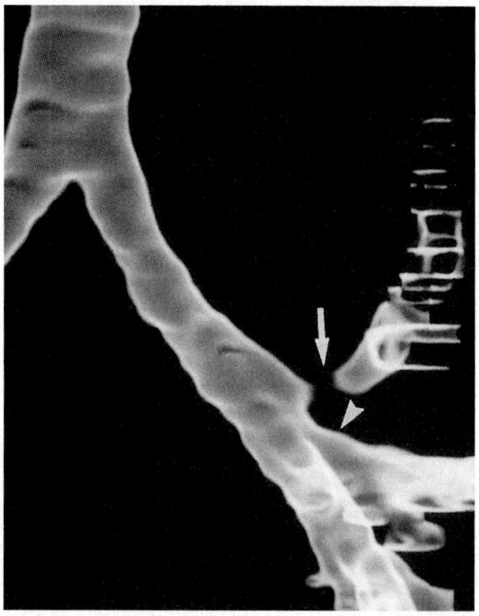

b.

Figure 3. Spiral CT evaluation (2-mm section thickness; pitch, 2; 13-second acquisition) was performed with general anesthesia in a 2-year-old child presenting with the symptoms of left upper lobe emphysema at chest radiography (not shown). **(a)** Contiguous transverse CT scans confirm left upper lobe emphysematous changes and suspected stenosed bronchus (small arrowhead) supplying the upper portion of the left upper lobe and arising separately from the lingular bronchus (large arrowhead). **(b)** Anteroposterior view of the bronchographic volume-rendered image confirms the presence of a severely stenosed bronchus (arrow) supplying the upper portion of the left upper lobe. This bronchus arises from the distal part of the left main bronchus, separately from the lingular bronchus (arrowhead), and corresponds to a stenosed left tracheal bronchus. The pseudo-occluded appearance is due to partial volume effect at the level of the stenotic area (trapezoid position, −450 to −150 HU).

In the presurgical evaluation of focal varicose bronchiectasis ($n = 6$), the extent of bronchiectasis was analyzed on transverse CT scans and volume-rendered images. Concordant findings between both imaging modalities were observed in five patients (ie, grade 2 value for volume-rendered images) with lobar ($n = 1$) and segmental ($n = 4$) bronchiectasis. In one patient with left upper lobe bronchiectasis diagnosed on transverse CT scans, volume-rendered images demonstrated the concurrent presence of bronchiectasis in the apical segment of the left lower lobe that had not been confidently recognized on transverse CT scans. This additional information led to coding of the volume-rendered images with a grade 4 value. In group 3, interobserver agreement was found in the interpretation of all the volume-rendered images and in that for all but two transverse CT scans.

Value of Volume-rendered Images

The value of the volume-rendered images in the entire study group is summarized in Table 3. When compared with transverse CT scans, (*a*) the volume-rendered image quality was not compatible with the interpretation of the airway caliber in two cases (3%) (ie, misleading information when compared with the transverse CT scans, or grade 1). (*b*) Findings on the volume-rendered images were concordant but added no complementary value to those on the transverse CT scans (grade 2) in 39 cases (53%). (*c*) The volume-rendered images improved confidence in the interpretation of findings on transverse CT scans (grade 3) in six cases (8%). (*d*) The volume-rendered images provided some supplemental information to that on the transverse CT scans (grade 4) in 23 cases (31%). (*e*) The volume-rendered images provided information that could correct potential interpretive errors from viewing only transverse CT scans (grade 5) in four cases (5%). Concordant interpretation between the two readers was a constant finding with volume-rendered images ($\kappa = 1$), whereas interobserver disagreement was found in the interpretation of transverse CT scans in seven cases ($\kappa = 0.71$).

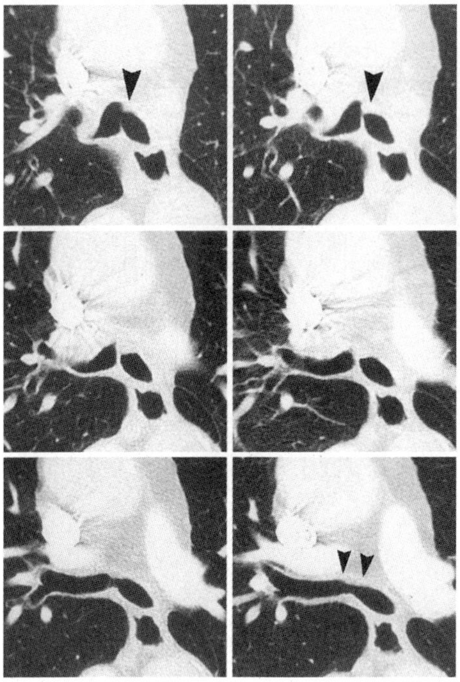

a.

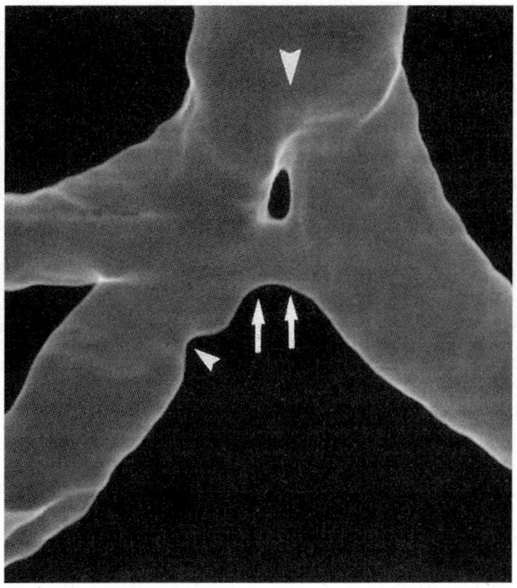

b.

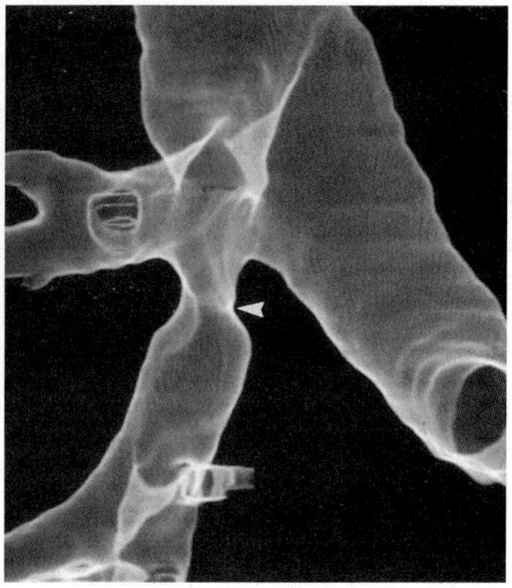

c.

Figure 4. Spiral CT evaluation (2-mm section thickness; pitch, 1.5; 18-second acquisition) of a tuberculous fistulous tract in a 75-year-old man. **(a)** Contiguous transverse CT scans of the carinal region were interpreted as normal. The fistulous tract between the right and left main bronchi (small arrowheads), observed 10 mm below the carina (large arrowheads), was missed by both readers and was erroneously interpreted as a normal carina. **(b)** Anteroposterior view of the bronchographic volume-rendered image, which enables correction of the interpretive error with **a**, demonstrates a large fistulous tract (arrows) between the right and left main bronchi, 10 mm below the carina (large arrowhead) (trapezoid position, −600 to −150 HU). Note the presence of a mild mural irregularity (small arrowhead) at the level of the initial portion of the right bronchus intermedius, 5 mm below the level of the fistulous tract. **(c)** Left posterior oblique view of the bronchographic volume-rendered image provides a synthetic analysis of the asymmetric stenosis (arrowhead) of the proximal right bronchus intermedius.

DISCUSSION

Findings in the present study confirm the ability of the volume-rendering algorithm to generate bronchographic images from data sets obtained in clinical practice inasmuch as the latter were obtained during strict apnea. With regard to the overall reconstruction quality, it is noticeable that the image quality of 97% of the 74 bronchographic images was graded as good or excellent owing to their visual similarity with conventional bronchograms. Nevertheless, 3% of the volume-rendered reconstructions showed disruptive stair-step artifacts at the level of the lower third of the trachea and left main bronchus. In the absence of respiratory motion artifacts on the corresponding transverse CT scans and the exclusive location of these artifacts on airways in close contact with the aortic arch, vascular motion was considered as the most likely explanation. These volume-rendered images were not compatible with a confident analysis of the airway caliber, which led the readers to grade them as noninterpretable.

With regard to the volume rendering parameter selection, these clinical results confirm the validity of those previously determined on the basis of spiral CT examinations of normal airway (11). Whereas every volume-rendered reconstruction required the selection of a triangular trapezoid shape, 70% parenchymal opacification, and use of the unshaded algorithm, findings in the present study confirm the benefit of depicting the voxel selection on a minimum intensity projection image of the edited data set before generating the volume-rendered reconstruction. This step allowed the radiologist to verify that a continuous rim of peripheral voxels had been selected for the final image and, thus, allowed individual adjustment of the optimal trapezoid position selection.

TABLE 3
Value of Bronchographic Images in the Population Studied

Finding	Grade 1 (poor or misleading information)	Grade 2 (minimal value)	Grade 3 (moderate value)	Grade 4 (supplemental information)	Grade 5 (highly valuable information)
Airway stenosis (group 1, $n = 47$)	2	27	0	16	2
Complex airway anatomy (group 2, $n = 15$)	0	7*	6†	0	2‡
Bronchiectasis (group 3, $n = 12$)	0	5	0	7	0
Total ($n = 74$)	2 (3%)	39 (53%)	6 (8%)	23 (31%)	4 (5%)

* Congenital, three; acquired, four.
† Congenital, six; acquired, none.
‡ Congenital, one; acquired, one.

Owing to the ability of the volume-rendering algorithm to create images similar to conventional bronchograms without the administration of contrast medium, we attempted to evaluate the clinical usefulness of this technique as a complement to transverse CT in patients suspected of having congenital or acquired airway lesions. Among group 1 patients, the accuracy of demonstration of the presence of airway stenosis was 95.7% with volume-rendered images versus

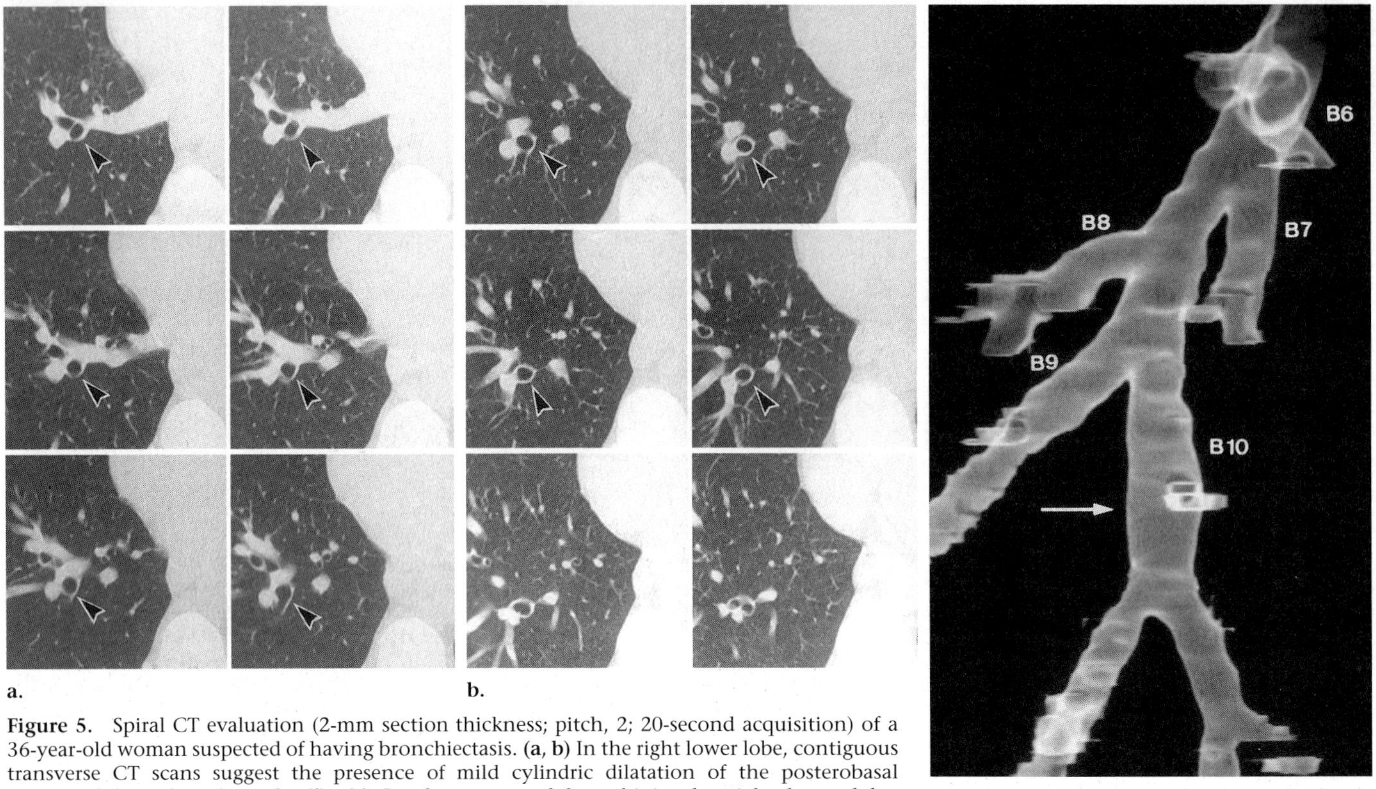

a. b. c.

Figure 5. Spiral CT evaluation (2-mm section thickness; pitch, 2; 20-second acquisition) of a 36-year-old woman suspected of having bronchiectasis. **(a, b)** In the right lower lobe, contiguous transverse CT scans suggest the presence of mild cylindric dilatation of the posterobasal segmental bronchus (arrowhead). **(c)** In the segmental bronchi in the right lower lobe, anteroposterior volume-rendered bronchographic image (trapezoid position, −750 to −600 HU) demonstrates the lack of progressive tapering of the posterobasal segmental bronchus (*B10*, arrow) and enables the assessment of focal cylindric bronchiectasis. *B6* = apical, *B7* = paracardiac (mediobasal), *B8* = anterobasal, *B9* = laterobasal segmental bronchi.

91.5% with transverse CT scans. Except for the two noninterpretable reconstructions, a confident analysis of the airway diameter was possible on bronchographic images, providing 32 true-positive and 13 true-negative results. It is noticeable that mild abnormalities in airway diameter were identified on every volume-rendered image, in agreement with fiberoptic bronchoscopic findings, whereas two mild bronchial anastomotic stenoses were missed on transverse CT scans. In both cases, a diameter reduction of less than 30% in the right and left main bronchus was not detected on transverse scans owing to the oblique orientation of the airway relative to the scanning plane. Conversely, the synthetic view provided with volume-rendered images enabled confident recognition of mild airway changes in every case.

In the 16 patients from group 1, the volume-rendered images provided supplemental information to that on the transverse CT scans, enabling a more precise evaluation of the shape, length, and/or degree of central airway stenosis. These results are in agreement with previous reports on the complementarity between transverse CT scans and 3D reformations in the morphologic evaluation of airway stenosis (2,14–16). In four cases in group 1, the volume-rendered images enabled a confident recognition of mild tracheal and main-stem bronchial stenoses by both readers, whereas interobserver disagreement was found with corresponding transverse CT scans. As previously emphasized in the literature, transverse imaging has limitations inherent in its representation of reality as a stack of transverse sections, which explains why the craniocaudal extent of tracheal disease is frequently underestimated and why mild airway changes may be missed (5,16–20).

Among the 15 patients in group 2 evaluated for complex airway anatomy, the volume-rendered images provided supplemental or highly valuable information in eight patients (53%). In six patients, an abnormal bronchial branching pattern was clearly depicted on the corresponding bronchographic images, which may allow the noninvasive assessment of congenital bronchial anomalies. In two patients, the 3D depiction of the bronchial tree with bronchographic images allowed the readers to correct interpretive errors as a result of viewing only transverse CT sections. In one patient with a history of left diaphragmatic hernia and a small left lung, the confident recognition of a complete left bronchial tree enabled the assessment of left lung hypoplasia rather than left lobar agenesis or aplasia, which is known to be potentially complicated by recurrent bronchial infections due to the presence of a bronchial cul-de-sac. In a second patient suspected of having a fistulous tract of infectious origin, the bronchographic images enabled the identification of a subcarinal fistula between the right and left main-stem bronchi, which was missed by both readers on transverse CT scans. Whereas retrospective analysis of the transverse CT scans demonstrated the fistulous tract, the latter was initially mistaken for the carina on the successive CT sections. In group 2, interobserver agreement was found in the analysis of all volume-rendered images, whereas discordant interpretations between the two readers were found in three cases of congenital bronchial anomaly on transverse CT scans.

As previously emphasized by Lacrosse et al (5), the mental reconstruction process required to integrate spatially partial data collected from multiple sections may become arduous when complex tracheobronchial deformities are encountered. In such cases, transverse CT scans may be insufficient, and our results suggest a potential application for volume-rendered reconstructions of the bronchial tree.

Despite the limited number of pediatric cases in the present study, we point out the superiority of spiral CT over conventional tracheobronchography in the evaluation of congenital anomalies of the airways. As previously emphasized by Manson et al (21), tracheobronchography is quite invasive and can carry an important risk in pediatric cases. This risk is greatest in conditions that compromise the tracheal lumen, such as congenital tracheal stenosis. Moreover, airway lesions may not be isolated anomalies, and it is important to emphasize the possibility offered by spiral CT to simultaneously provide bronchographic images as well as angiographic reconstructions, thus enabling the evaluation of complex malformations in a single examination and avoiding unnecessary invasive procedures.

With regard to the evaluation of bronchiectasis, findings in the present study confirm that varicose bronchiectasis is easily recognized on transverse CT scans and that 3D reconstructions are of limited clinical value. Nevertheless, to allow the clinician to obtain a bronchographic view of airway abnormalities, volume rendering could be used. Among the group 3 patients, a potential application for bronchographic images was observed in the diagnosis and assessment of the severity and extent of cylindric bronchiectasis. As previously emphasized in the literature, there are limitations to the thin-section technique in the identification of mild bronchial enlargement at the level of bronchi located perpendicular or oblique to the axial plane of thin-section CT scans (12,22,23). Conversely, the lack of progressive tapering, which characterizes cylindric bronchiectasis, was easily detected on a bronchographic image and enabled a confident diagnosis of cylindric bronchiectasis in six patients from group 3.

To reduce the number of false-negative CT results in the identification of cylindric bronchiectasis, volumetric CT acquisition has been recently evaluated (22). Although this technique allowed a more accurate assessment of the extent of bronchiectasis, it was found to result in an increase in the patient's total radiation exposure and was recommended for patients in whom thin-section CT scans were difficult to interpret. In agreement with the conclusions of Lucidarme et al (22), our results suggest that any spiral CT data set acquired for such an indication could be used to generate not only transverse CT scans but also complementary volume-rendered images of the bronchial tree whenever necessary.

Whereas volume rendering has the potential to create diagnostically useful images of the peripheral bronchial tree, a few technical details should be emphasized. Owing to the necessity to acquire data sets with thin sections to generate high-quality reconstructions of peripheral airways, the z-axis coverage will be limited to a few centimeters. A careful selection of the volume to be surveyed is mandatory to include the airway of interest within it. Among the successive steps in the creation of a volume-rendered reconstruction of the bronchial tree, it is important to emphasize the potential drawbacks inherent in the editing step. Whereas a simple editing process is usually necessary for central airways, the creation of volume-rendered reconstructions of the peripheral airways requires precise manual drawing of the contours of the airway(s) of interest on each CT scan. This time-consuming process is aimed at erasing all the regions outside the defined area to obtain reconstructions of the peripheral airways without the superimposition of structures of similar attenuation value that are also present within the volume surveyed. Whenever this editing process is inaccurately performed, one may obtain a volume-rendered reconstruction of an artificially incomplete bronchial tree which could, in turn, influence the interpretation of the volume-rendered image. However, the simultaneous interpretation of the 3D reconstructions and the transverse CT scans usually precludes any interpretive error. From a practical standpoint, a precise knowledge of the normal airway anatomy, as well as the understanding of morphologic characteristics of the lesion to be reconstructed, are mandatory to ensure accurate editing.

One limitation of the volume-rendering technique was the inability to detect tracheal diverticuli on the bronchographic images, which were depicted as only mild mural irregularities. Depending on the size of the diverticuli, this limitation could be explained on the basis of the threshold values selected and, also, the presence of narrow diverticular necks. Moreover, the present implementation did not allow the user to actively display the 3D data set, thus precluding adjustment of the image display parameters as quickly as is available with real-time interactive rendering (24).

The volume-rendered images improved the recognition of mild cylindric bronchiectasis and stenosis and helped identification of congenital or acquired complex airway anatomy. Whereas the 3D reconstruction contained no more information than the corresponding series of transverse scans, our results confirm that spatial relationships are more easily appreciated by the viewer on a 3D display than on a series of sections, and the bronchographic images provided the reader with diagnostically and/or morphologically useful information in 36% of the examinations. On the basis of our findings, the main indications for volume-rendered images of the bronchial tree are the assessment and/or evaluation of airway stenosis and mild bronchiectasis, as well as the interpretation of complex airway lesions. Whereas several studies have already demonstrated a complementarity between transverse CT scans and 3D reconstructions, further evaluation remains mandatory to determine the respective advantages of the most currently available reconstruction techniques in the evaluation of airway lesions, namely shaded surface display, minimum intensity projection, and volume rendering.

Acknowledgments: We are grateful to the following CT technologists: Dominique Dumont, Jean-Pierre Guillot, Olivier Lescieux, Abdel Naili, Bertrand Stock, Martine Wywijas. They helped us generate the volume-rendered bronchographic images.

References

1. Fram EK, Godwin JD, Putman CE. Three-dimensional display of the heart, aorta, lungs and airway using CT. AJR 1982; 139:1171–1176.
2. Ney DR, Fishman EK, Magid D, Drebin RA. Volumetric rendering of computed tomographic data: principles and techniques. IEEE Comput Graphics Appl 1990; 10:24–32.
3. Kitaoka H, Yumoto T. Three-dimensional CT of the bronchial tree: a trial using an inflated fixed lung specimen. Invest Radiol 1990; 25:813–817.
4. Newmark GM, Conces DJ, Kopecky KK. Spiral CT evaluation of the trachea and bronchi. J Comput Assist Tomogr 1994; 18:552–554.
5. Lacrosse M, Trigaux JP, Van Beers BE, Weymants P. 3D spiral CT of the tracheal bronchial tree. J Comput Assist Tomogr 1995; 19:341–347.
6. Tello R, Kruskal J, Dupuy D, Costello PH. In vivo three-dimensional evaluation of the tracheobronchial tree. J Thorac Imaging 1995; 10:291–293.
7. LoCicero J, Costello PH, Campos CT, et al. Spiral CT with multiplanar and three-dimensional reconstructions accurately predicts tracheobronchial pathology. Ann Thorac Surg 1996; 62:811–817.
8. Kauczor HU, Wolcke B, Fischer B, Mildenberger P, Lorenz J, Thelen M. Three-

dimensional helical CT of the tracheobronchial tree: evaluation of imaging protocols and assessment of suspected stenoses with bronchoscopic correlation. AJR 1996; 167:419–424.
9. Remy-Jardin M, Remy J, Deschildre F, Artaud D, Ramon PH, Edme JL. Obstructive lesions of the central airways: evaluation by using spiral CT with multiplanar and three-dimensional reformations. Eur Radiol 1996; 6:807–816.
10. Johnson PT, Heath DG, Kuszyk BS, Fishman EK. CT angiography: thoracic vascular imaging with interactive volume rendering technique. J Comput Assist Tomogr 1997; 21:110–114.
11. Remy-Jardin M, Remy J, Artaud D, Fribourg M, Naili A. Tracheobronchial tree: assessment with volume rendering—technical aspects. Radiology 1998; 208:393–398.
12. Kang EY, Miller RR, Muller NL. Bronchiectasis: comparison of preoperative thin-section CT and pathologic findings in resected specimens. Radiology 1995; 195: 649–654.
13. Zeiberg AS, Silverman PM, Sessions RB, Troost TH, Davros WJ, Zeman RK. Helical (spiral) CT of the upper airway with three-dimensional imaging: technique and clinical assessment. AJR 1996; 166:293–299.
14. Ney DR, Kuhlman JE, Hruban RH, Ren H, Hutchins GM, Fishman EK. Three-dimensional CT-volumetric reconstruction and display of the bronchial tree. Invest Radiol 1990; 25:736–742.
15. Whyte RI, Quint LE, Kazerooni EA, Cascade PN, Iannettoni MD, Orringer MB. Helical computed tomography for the evaluation of tracheal stenosis. Ann Thorac Surg 1995; 60:27–31.
16. Quint LE, Whyte RI, Kazerooni EA, et al. Stenosis of the central airways: evaluation by using helical CT with multiplanar reconstructions. Radiology 1995; 194:871–877.
17. Shepard JO, McLoud TC. Imaging the airways: computed tomography and magnetic resonance imaging. Clin Chest Med 1991; 12:151–168.
18. Dennie CJ, Coblentz CL. The trachea: normal anatomic features, imaging and cases of displacement. J Can Assoc Radiol 1993; 44:81–89.
19. Morency G, Chalaoui J, Samson L, Sylvestre J. Malignant neoplasms of the trachea. J Can Assoc Radiol 1989; 40:198–200.
20. Spinarzi DL, Shepard JO, McLoud TC, Grillo HC, Dedrick G. CT of adenoid cystic carcinoma of the trachea. AJR 1986; 146:1129–1132.
21. Manson D, Babyn P, Filler R, Holowka S. Three-dimensional imaging of the pediatric trachea in congenital tracheal stenosis. Pediatr Radiol 1994; 24:175–179.
22. Lucidarme O, Grenier PH, Coche E, Lenoir S, Aubert B, Beigelman C. Bronchiectasis: comparative assessment with thin-section CT and helical CT. Radiology 1996; 200:673–679.
23. Lynch DA, Newell JD, Tschomper BA, Cink TM, Newman LS, Bethel R. Uncomplicated asthma in adults: comparison of CT appearance of the lungs in asthmatic and healthy subjects. Radiology 1993; 188:829–833.
24. Johnson PT, Heath DG, Cabral B, Fishman EK. Three-dimensional CT: real-time interactive volume rendering. AJR 1996; 167: 581–583.

Geoffrey D. Rubin, MD
Ann N. Leung, MD
Valerie J. Robertson, MD
Paul Stark, MD

Index terms:
Computed tomography (CT), artifact
Computed tomography (CT), technology
Mediastinum, CT, 67.12115
Lung, CT, 60.12115

Radiology 1998; 208:771–776

[1] From the Department of Radiology, S-072B, Stanford University School of Medicine, Stanford, CA 94305-5105 (G.D.R., A.N.L., V.J.R., P.S.), and the Veterans Administration Palo Alto Health Care System, Calif (P.S.). Received November 24, 1997; revision requested January 5, 1998; revision received March 16; accepted April 28. **Address reprint requests to** G.D.R.

Author contributions:
Guarantor of integrity of entire study, G.D.R.; study concepts, G.D.R.; study design, G.D.R., A.N.L.; literature research, G.D.R.; clinical studies, G.D.R, A.N.L., V.J.R., P.S.; data acquisition, V.J.R.; data analysis, G.D.R.; statistical analysis, G.D.R.; manuscript preparation and editing, G.D.R.; manuscript review, G.D.R., A.N.L., P.S.

Thoracic Spiral CT: Influence of Subsecond Gantry Rotation on Image Quality [1]

PURPOSE: To determine if the lower milliampere second setting and shorter acquisition time of subsecond spiral computed tomography (CT) affects the image quality of thoracic CT scans.

MATERIALS AND METHODS: In 92 consecutive outpatients referred for thoracic CT, spiral CT (120 kV, 292 mA) was performed with 1-second (n = 45) or 0.75-second (n = 47) scanning time. An equal percentage of patients (70%) in each group received intravenous contrast medium. At six mediastinal and six lung zones, degradation due to motion and noise, respectively, were graded independently on a four-point scale by three blinded radiologists. Statistically significant differences were determined with a two-tailed t test.

RESULTS: Mediastinal image quality was significantly better on 0.75-second scans than on 1-second scans ($P < .001$). Regions with the greatest improvement in image quality were around the aortic root, cardiac ventricles, and aortic arch. Lung image quality was also better on 0.75-second scans than on 1-second scans ($P = .04$). On 0.75- and 1-second scans, respectively, motion-related artifacts were found to degrade image quality 6.2 and 8.7 times more than noise-related artifacts in the mediastinum and 2.6 and 3.9 times more in the lungs.

CONCLUSION: Subsecond spiral CT is associated with improved clarity and diminished motion artifacts on mediastinal and pulmonary images when compared with 1-second spiral CT.

When spiral computed tomography (CT) was introduced by Kalender and colleagues (1,2) in 1990, the minimum gantry rotation period was 1 second. This value remained fixed until the introduction of the Somatom Plus 4 spiral CT scanner (Siemens Medical Systems, Erlangen, Germany) in 1995; this scanner offered a minimum gantry rotation period of 750 msec. Subsecond scanning offers several potential advantages over 1-second scanning. These include greater temporal resolution and faster scanning, which can be used to achieve (a) greater coverage per unit time without a reduction in spatial resolution or (b) improved longitudinal spatial resolution for a fixed coverage per unit time. Specifically, in the case of a gantry rotation period of 0.75 second, the longitudinal coverage is 33% greater for a fixed section thickness and pitch. A 15-cm-long scan with 3-mm collimation and pitch of 1.7 could be completed in 22.5 seconds with a 0.75-second gantry rotation period rather than in 30 seconds with a 1-second gantry rotation period, preserving longitudinal spatial resolution and shortening acquisition time. Use of a shorter acquisition time might be preferable for patients unable to sustain a 30-second breath hold or those in need of a reduced dose of iodinated contrast medium. Alternatively, if breath-hold duration and iodine dose are less critical, subsecond scanning can be used to improve longitudinal spatial resolution. A 30-second, 15-cm scan could be obtained with a table speed of 3.75 mm per gantry rotation with a 0.75-second gantry rotation period versus 5 mm per rotation with a 1-second period. With these table speeds, scanning with a pitch less than or equal to 2 would allow selection of a 2-mm section thickness and a pitch of 1.9 for the 0.75-second gantry rotation period and a 3-mm section thickness and a pitch of 1.7 for the 1-second period. As a result, the effective section thickness, defined as the full width at half maximum of the section profile, would be approximately 2.5 mm with a 0.75-second gantry rotation period versus 3.6 mm with a 1-second period, with 180° linear interpolation (3). This represents a 44% increase in longitudinal spatial resolution.

Two parameters that influence image quality and might be affected by variations in gantry rotation period are motion and noise. The greater temporal resolution of subsecond scanning may improve image quality by diminishing motion artifacts; however, images obtained with a subsecond gantry rotation period will be noisier unless the tube current is increased to maintain the same photon statistics. The purpose of this investigation was to determine the effect that a subsecond gantry rotation period has on spiral CT image quality. Further, because the temporal resolution of reconstructed CT scans acquired with a subsecond gantry rotation period approximates the cardiac cycle duration, we further sought to determine the influence of heart rate on image quality.

MATERIALS AND METHODS

Patients

Between September 1995 and December 1995, 92 consecutive outpatients (43 male and 49 female patients; age range, 5–84 years; mean age, 50.30 years) referred to undergo thoracic CT were enrolled in our study. Institutional review board approval and written informed consent were not necessary for this study. Patients undergoing concomitant abdominal, pelvic, or neck CT had been excluded from the study. Indications for the CT examinations included staging or follow-up of neoplasia, infectious survey in immunocompromised hosts, characterization of chest radiographic abnormalities, and the diagnosis or assessment of diffuse lung disease. None of the patients received mechanical ventilation. The patients were randomly assigned to two groups: either 0.75-second gantry rotation period (n = 47; mean age, 49.9 years ± 18.8 [standard deviation]) or 1-second period (n = 45; mean age, 50.9 years ± 16.5). Metal clips, radiopaque intrathoracic catheters, or both were present in 47% of patients in each study group. A summary of the indications for CT and the distribution of lesions detected is provided in Table 1. Abnormalities were present on 79% of studies obtained with a 0.75-second gantry rotation period and 76% with a 1-second period.

Image Acquisition

All scans were obtained during suspended ventilation with a Somatom Plus 4 CT scanner with 120 kV, 292 mA, 8-mm section thickness, and a pitch of 1.0–1.5, selected to image from the thoracic inlet through the lung bases during a single 25–35-second breath hold. Images were reconstructed with a bone reconstruction kernel, 30–36-cm field of view, and 180° linear interpolation algorithm at 8-mm intervals. Twenty images were photographed onto each sheet of film by using mediastinal (level, 40 HU; width, 400 HU) and lung (level, −700 HU; width, 1,500 HU) window settings.

Fourteen patients in each group were examined without intravenous contrast medium. When contrast medium was administered, 90 mL of Isovue 300 (Bracco Diagnostics, Princeton, NJ) was injected at a rate of 2.5 mL/sec. Scanning commenced 25 seconds after the initiation of injection of the contrast medium into an antecubital vein.

A pulse oximeter was used to measure each patient's heart rate immediately before, during, and immediately after completion of scanning.

Image Analysis

Three independent and blinded thoracic radiologists (G.D.R., A.N.L., P.S.) with at least 10 years of radiology experience reviewed each scan in random order to assign a numerical image quality score to each of 12 regions—six mediastinal and six pulmonary. Image quality was assessed on a four-point scale for the presence of motion artifact, noise, or both: 1, poor image quality; 2, fair; 3, good; 4, very good. Additionally, the reviewers identified whether they thought that motion, noise, or both were responsible for important image degradation in the mediastinum and lungs. Prior to formal scoring of the CT scans obtained in the patients enrolled in this study, the three reviewers observed seven CT scans obtained in patients not in the study population and assigned a score in consensus to ensure consistency in use of the grading scheme.

Data Analysis

Scores from each reviewer were averaged across each study group for each of the 12 anatomic regions. Cumulative pulmonary and mediastinal scores were calculated for each reviewer by separately averaging the six pulmonary and six mediastinal results from each reviewer. For each reviewer, the statistical significance of differences between group scores was calculated with a two-tailed t test.

TABLE 1
Indications for and Findings at Spiral CT

Data	Gantry Rotation Period (sec) 0.75 (n = 47)	1.0 (n = 45)
Indication for CT		
Evaluation of chest radiographic abnormality	14	17
Lymphoma	16	8
Lung cancer	2	6
Primary mediastinal neoplasm	7	2
Extrathoracic neoplasm	7	8
Diffuse lung disease	1	4
CT finding		
Pulmonary lesions	13	17
Mediastinal mass	12	7
Chest wall or pleural mass	3	2
Combination of locations	9	8
Total		
Positive	37	34
Negative	10	11

Note.—Numbers are the number of patients.

To assess the influence of heart rate on image quality, we defined a "cardiac-scan index" as the ratio of the time required to acquire views for a transverse spiral CT section to the duration of the cardiac cycle (in heart beats per section), as follows: gantry rotation period (in seconds per gantry rotation) divided by cardiac cycle, where the cardiac cycle was calculated as 1/mean heart rate (in beats per second). The mean heart rate was determined as an equal weighting of heart rate values obtained immediately before, during, and immediately after the acquisition. An index of 1.0 corresponds to a cardiac cycle that occurs in the same amount of time required to collect data for a single transverse section. To calculate the cardiac-scan index, we assumed that the temporal resolution of a reconstructed transverse section is the gantry rotation period, which corresponds to the amount of data (360°) required to create a transverse section of the gantry center with a 180° linear interpolation algorithm. This is only an approximation of the true temporal resolution, which is a complex function that is spatially variant from the gantry center to the periphery, because of the weighting of projection data obtained at different times. Nevertheless, this approximation does not substantially influence our results, as the relative relationship between cardiac-

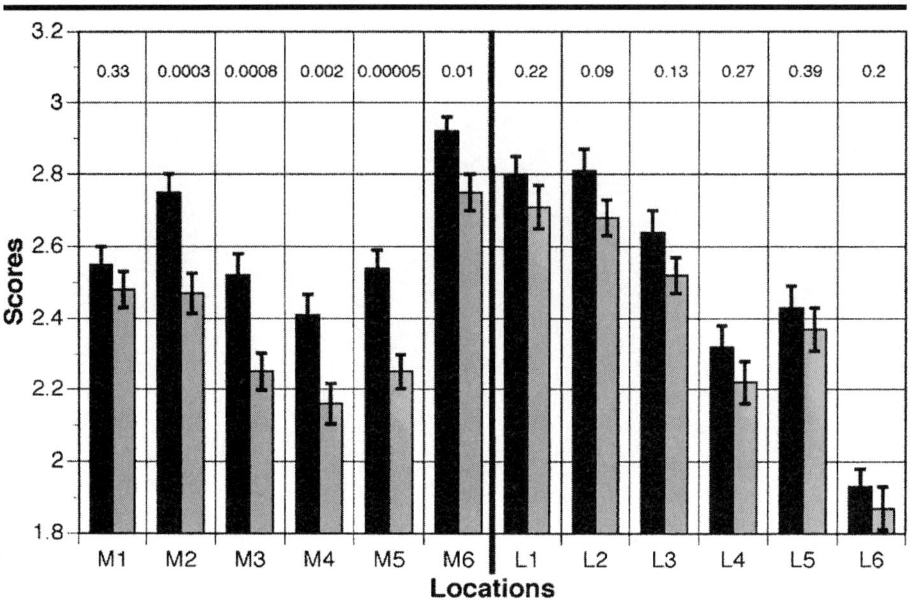

Figure 1. Image quality scores for each of six mediastinal and six pulmonary locations averaged across all reviewers and all patients who underwent spiral CT with 0.75- (black bars) and 1-second (gray bars) gantry rotation periods. Numbers above the value bars are *P* values from two-tailed *t* tests comparing mean scores from 0.75- and 1-second gantry rotation periods for each location. Error bars indicate the standard error of the mean. *M1* = thoracic inlet; *M2* = aortic arch; *M3* = right pulmonary artery; *M4* = aortic root; *M5* = center of cardiac ventricles; *M6* = diaphragm; *L1* = right, *L2* = left lung above the carina; *L3* = right, *L4* = left lung between the carina and the inferior pulmonary veins; *L5* = right, *L6* = left lung below the inferior pulmonary veins.

scan index and image quality score will not change, but the absolute relationship might vary 10%–20%.

Scatterplots of cardiac-scan index versus mean mediastinal and pulmonary image quality scores were created, and linear regression analysis was applied.

RESULTS

Mediastinal and pulmonary regional scores for each gantry rotation period, averaged across the three reviewers, are presented in Figure 1. In general, image degradation to the greatest extent occurred closer to the base of the heart in the mediastinum and closer to the left ventricle in the lungs. Within the mediastinum, image quality was worst at the aortic root, and it improved progressively at the right pulmonary artery and middle ventricular level, the thoracic inlet, and the aortic arch, with the best overall image quality at the diaphragm. A comparative example of image quality at the right pulmonary artery level obtained in two different patients is presented in Figure 2. Within the lungs, image quality was worst in the left lower lung (below the inferior pulmonary veins), and it improved progressively at the left middle lung (between the carina and the inferior pulmonary veins), the right lower lung (below the inferior pulmonary veins), and the right middle lung (between the carina and the inferior pulmonary veins), with the best overall image quality in the right and left upper lungs (above the carina). Mean image quality scores were better for the 0.75-second gantry rotation period at all mediastinal and pulmonary locations, but differences achieved statistical significance ($P < .01$) only from the aortic arch to the middle ventricular levels.

Results with contrast material–enhanced scans were pooled for all three reviewers and all mediastinal locations and then compared to results with nonenhanced scans. Contrast enhancement resulted in significantly better image quality with a 1-second gantry rotation period ($P < .001$). Although the image quality scores were better for contrast-enhanced scans with a 0.75-second gantry rotation period, this difference did not achieve statistical significance ($P = .07$). The 0.75-second gantry rotation period was superior to the 1-second gantry rotation period for both nonenhanced and contrast-enhanced scans (both, $P < .001$). Notably, the magnitude of this improvement for the 1-second period was more than twice that for the 0.75-second period.

As shown in Table 2, when scores for all mediastinal and pulmonary locations were pooled for the three reviewers for the 0.75- and 1-second gantry rotation periods, respectively, the mean mediastinal image quality scores were 2.62 and 2.40, and the mean pulmonary image quality scores were 2.48 and 2.40. The overall image quality of mediastinal images was superior with the 0.75-second period as compared to that with the 1-second period ($P < .001$). The overall image quality of lung scans was better with the 0.75-second period as compared to that with the 1-second period, but the difference barely achieved statistical significance ($P = .04$). Analysis of the mean image quality scores for individual reviewers, however, showed that statistical significance of differences for the mediastinal locations was achieved for only reviewers 1 and 2. There was even less uniformity for the pulmonary locations: Although reviewers 1 and 3 found image quality with the 0.75-second gantry rotation period to be superior, differences achieved statistical significance for only reviewer 1.

The relative frequency with which noise, motion, or both were considered to influence image quality for mediastinal and pulmonary scans is presented in Table 3. In the mediastinum with the 0.75- and 1-second gantry rotation periods, respectively, motion influenced image quality 6.2 and 8.7 times more frequently than noise, and in the lungs, 2.6 and 3.9 times more frequently. For both mediastinal and pulmonary locations, differences in the relative influence of noise or motion with 0.75- and 1-second periods were not significant ($P > .2$), but the greater frequency with which motion was identified as an important limitation of image quality was significant with both periods ($P < .001$).

There was poor correlation between the cardiac-scan index and mean mediastinal or pulmonary image quality (r^2 = 0.12 and 0.06, respectively; Fig 3).

DISCUSSION

Our results suggest that image quality at spiral CT with a subsecond gantry rotation period, particularly for mediastinal assessment, is better than that at spiral CT with a 1-second gantry rotation period. Image quality scores from mediastinal locations were superior with the 0.75-second period for all three reviewers, but differences achieved statistical significance for only two (Table 2). The advantage with subsecond rotation for lung images is less certain. Differences in the image quality of lung scans were significantly better with 0.75-second rotation for only one reviewer. The scores of reviewer 3 suggest superiority of 0.75-second rotation for lung images, but the difference did not achieve statistical significance. Further, scores for reviewer 2 with 0.75-second rotation were worse than those with 1-second rotation. Although this difference was less significant than that for the other two reviewers (P = .34), who preferred 0.75-second rotation, an element of uncertainty is introduced as to the absolute superiority of lung imaging with 0.75-second compared with 1-second rotation.

Our results further suggest that image quality at spiral CT with a subsecond gantry rotation period is significantly better than that at spiral CT with 1-second rotation because of a reduction in motion-induced artifacts rather than a reduction in noise, but they also suggest that motion-induced effects are the main limitation on image quality at thoracic CT (Table 3). In a comparison of image quality at conventional CT with either full (360° or 1-second) reconstructions versus segmented or half-scan (225° or 0.6 second of data) reconstructions, obtained in patients receiving mechanical ventilation, overall image quality was superior with segmented reconstruction (4). This was attributed to diminished motion artifacts with segmented reconstruction, despite the observation that noise was substantially increased with this reconstruction technique. In our study, noise did not negatively affect image quality to the extent that it did in the study by Posniak and colleagues (4). This may be attributable to differences in tube current, detector efficiency, or effective exposure duration (0.6 vs 0.75 second). Another interesting difference between findings in their study and ours is that diminished motion effects were greatest on lung images in theirs and on mediastinal images in ours. This may be explained by the greater motion effects present in their population of patients undergoing active mechanical ventilation in contrast to our population of patients holding their breath, in whom the greatest source of motion in the thorax originated from the heart.

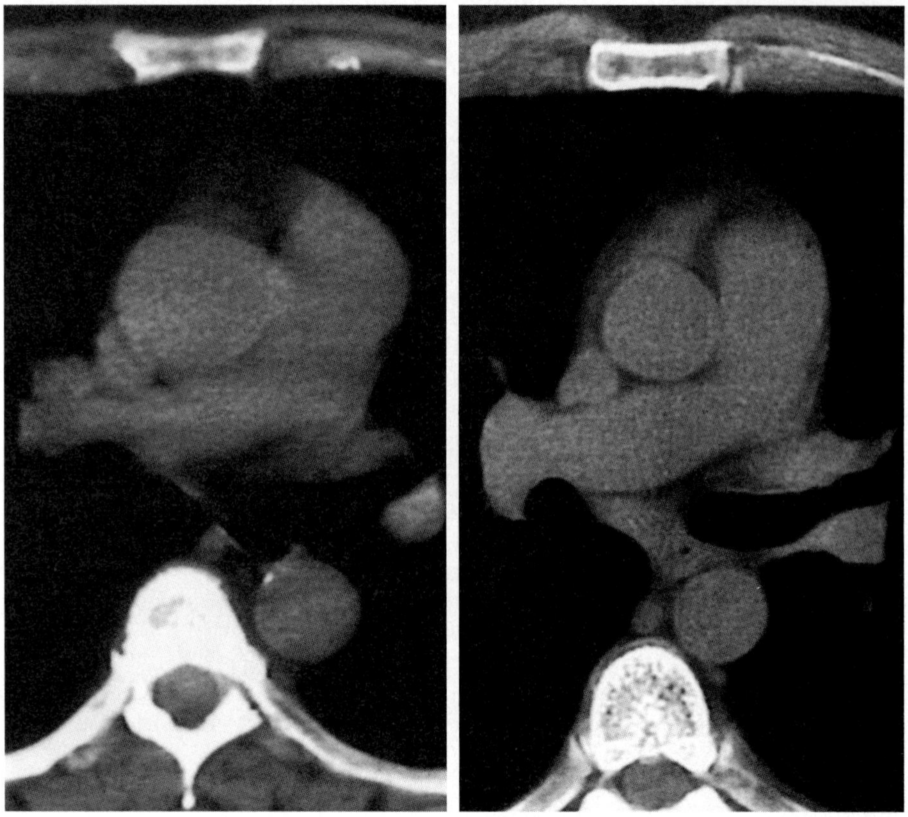

a. b.

Figure 2. (**a**) Spiral CT scan of the right pulmonary artery obtained with a 1-second gantry rotation period. The image quality scores of the three reviewers were 1, 2, and 1. (**b**) In a different patient, spiral CT scan of the right pulmonary artery was obtained with a 0.75-second gantry rotation period. The image quality scores of the three reviewers were 4, 4, and 3.

TABLE 2
Mean Image Quality Scores for Reviewers 1–3

Location and Gantry Rotation Period (sec)	Reviewer 1	Reviewer 2	Reviewer 3	All
Mediastinum				
0.75	2.75	2.48	2.62	2.62
1.0	2.33	2.34	2.53	2.40
P value	<.001	<.001	.13	<.001
Lungs				
0.75	2.61	2.11	2.71	2.48
1.0	2.42	2.17	2.63	2.40
P value	.004	.34	.07	.04

Note.—Data were averaged over all patients and locations for each gantry rotation period and both mediastinal and lung regions. *P* values were calculated with a two-tailed *t* test.

We therefore sought to investigate if a relationship existed between motion artifacts and the duration of the cardiac cycle. We hypothesized that when image acquisition is less than the duration of the cardiac cycle, motion-induced artifacts might diminish, particularly if cardiac systole does not occur during the entire time of image acquisition. This notion was previously suggested by findings in a study of motion-related CT artifacts (5). In the study by Ritchie and co-workers (5), the minimum scanning time required to totally eliminate cardiac-related motion artifacts with a third-generation conventional CT scanner was calculated as 19.1 msec. Whereas this value is 39 times shorter than that with a 0.75-second scanner and reconstruction with a 180° linear interpolation algorithm, it was calculated on the basis of maximum cardiac and juxtacardiac pulmonary vessel velocities (systole) and addressed only the complete elimination of motion-related artifacts and not potential artifact diminution as a function of scanning time.

Cardiac systole typically occupies 40%

TABLE 3
Relative Frequency of Influence of Noise or Motion on Image Quality

Location and Gantry Rotation Period (second)	Noise	Motion	Motion vs Noise	*P* Value
Mediastinum				
0.75	14%	83%	6.2	<.001
1.0	10%	87%	8.7	<.001
P value	.5	.5		
Lungs				
0.75	25%	66%	2.6	<.001
1.0	19%	74%	3.9	<.001
P value	.3	.2		

Note.—*P* values were calculated with a two-tailed *t* test.

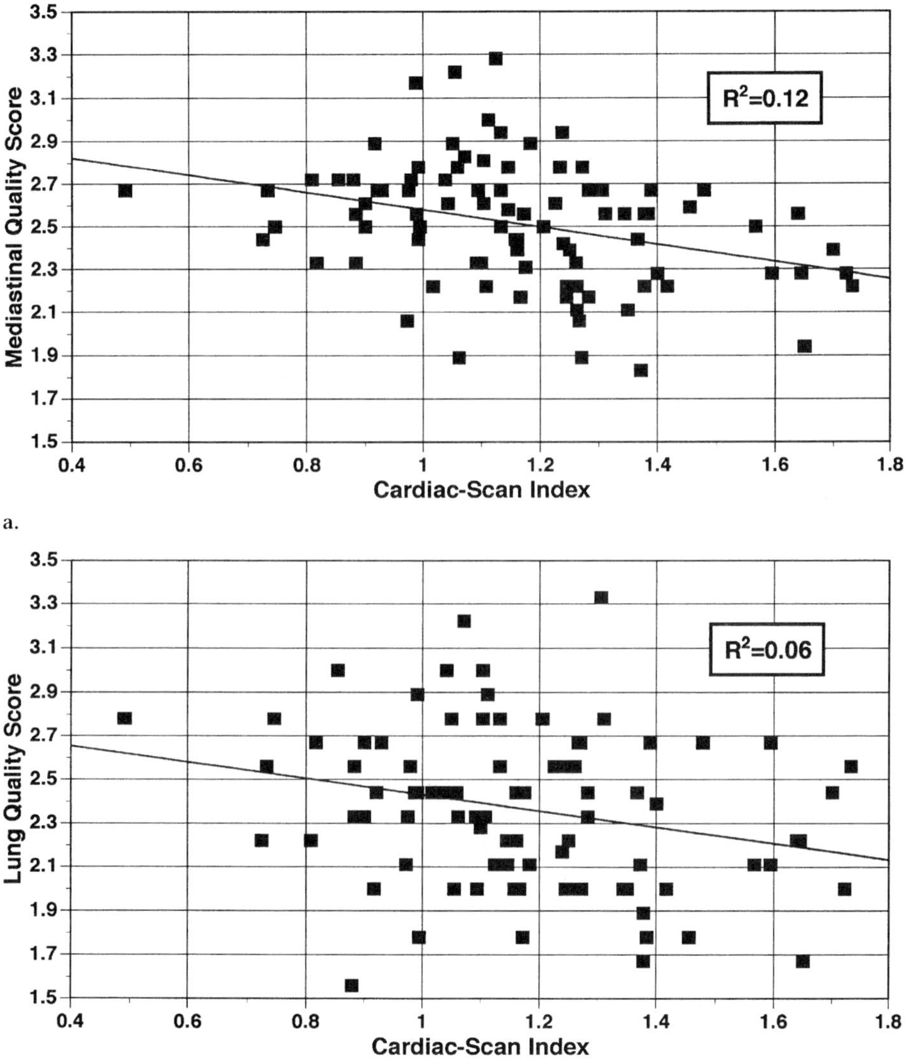

Figure 3. Scatterplots of cardiac-scan index versus image quality scores for **(a)** mediastinal and **(b)** lung scans.

of the cardiac cycle (6), and 0.75 second corresponds to a heart rate of 80 beats per minute. Therefore, with a gantry rotation period of 0.75 second and 180° linear interpolation, the heart rate would need to be less than 60% of 80 beats per minute, or 48 beats per minute, to complete a 360° gantry rotation entirely within diastole; with a gantry rotation period of 1 second and 180° linear interpolation, the heart rate would need to be 36 beats per minute or less.

Overall, we found no correlation between image quality and heart rate; however, only one patient had a cardiac-scan index less that 0.6. His mediastinal and pulmonary image quality scores were 2.67 and 2.22, respectively. These values are not significantly greater than the mean values for all patients who underwent scanning with a 0.75-second gantry rotation period (2.62 and 2.40, respectively). The image quality might have been better had the reconstructions been retrospectively selected to use projections acquired during diastole alone (7). This would have required prospective registration of electrocardiographic tracings and scan data.

Nevertheless, if retrospective reconstruction techniques are to be developed that compensate for cardiac motion by reconstructing cross sections acquired entirely within diastole (retrospective cardiac gating), then the temporal resolution of CT scans must fall. This could be accomplished with spiral CT scanners with the capacity for a shorter gantry rotation period (substantially below 0.75 second) or with electron-beam CT. Alternatively, the cardiac-scan index could be reduced by means of half-scan interpolation (4), although spiral artifacts would become more prominent, potentially limiting the clinical usefulness of this approach. If half-scan interpolation (8) had been available on our scanner, the temporal resolution of reconstructed sections acquired with 0.75-second gantry rotation would have been 0.47 second, and a cardiac-scan index of 0.6 or less would have been achieved in 36% of our cases. To achieve a cardiac-scan index of less than 0.6 with use of 180° linear interpolation in 50% of our patients, the gantry rotation period would need to be less than 0.44 second; to include 90% of our patients (median heart rate, 82.5 beats per minute; 90th percentile heart rate, 101 beats per minute), it would need to be less than 0.36 second. With use of half-scan interpolation, the gantry rotation period would need to be less than 0.70 and 0.58 second for 50% and 90% of our patients, respectively.

Several limitations of this study are noteworthy. First, this comparison of gantry rotation periods could be achieved only by comparing two distinct patient groups. Although the patients were randomized according to the temporal order in which the studies were performed—and there was no significant difference in patient age, examination indication, final diagnosis, or the presence of indwelling catheters and clips between the two groups—we did not control for other variables, including body habitus. Second, these results were obtained with only one CT scanner by using our routine acquisition and reconstruction protocol. The generalizability of our results to other scanners and imaging protocols is speculative. Finally, our analysis of image quality does not assess the influence of subsecond gantry rotation period on diagnostic accuracy.

In summary, with 292 mA, we found no degradation in image quality with a 0.75-second gantry rotation period, despite a lower patient dose. Overall image quality improvement with a subsecond gantry rotation period was greater in the mediastinum than in the lungs, but differences achieved statistical significance in both anatomic regions. Subsecond (0.75-second) spiral CT in the mediastinum and lungs offers greater patient coverage, higher spatial resolution, and diminished scanning duration when compared with 1-second spiral CT. On the basis of results in this study, an additional advantage of subsecond scanning is improved thoracic image quality as a result of diminished motion artifacts, particularly in regions closest to the heart. However, current acquisition speeds are not fast enough to eliminate all motion-induced artifacts nor will they permit reconstruction of cross sections acquired entirely within diastole for the majority of patients.

Acknowledgment: The authors thank Sandy Napel, PhD, for his expert critique of this manuscript.

References

1. Kalender WA, Seissler W, Klotz E, Vock P. Spiral volumetric CT with single-breath-hold technique, continuous transport, and continuous scanner rotation. Radiology 1990; 176:181–190.
2. Kalender WA, Vock P, Polacin A, Soucek M. Spiral CT: a new volume scanning technique. I. Principles and methodology. Röntgenpraxis 1990; 43:3–10.
3. Polacin A, Kalender WA, Marchal G. Evaluation of section sensitivity profiles and image noise in spiral CT. Radiology 1992; 185:29–35.
4. Posniak HV, Olson MC, Demos TC, Pierce KL, Kalbhen CL. CT of the chest and abdomen in patients on mechanical pulmonary ventilators: quality of images made at 0.6 vs 1.0 sec. AJR 1994; 163:1073–1077.
5. Ritchie CJ, Godwin JD, Crawford CR, Stanford W, Anno H, Kim Y. Minimum scan speeds for suppression of motion artifacts in CT. Radiology 1992; 185:37–42.
6. Wiggers C. Studies on the consecutive phases of the cardiac cycle. I. The duration of the consecutive phases of the cardiac cycle and the criteria for their precise determination. Am J Physiol 1921; 56:415–438.
7. Napel SA, Rubin GD, Drangova M, Jeffrey RB. Retrospective minimization of vascular motion artifacts for spiral CT angiography (abstr). Radiology 1994; 193(P):139.
8. Crawford CR, King KF. Computed tomography scanning with simultaneous patient translation. Med Phys 1990; 17:967–982.

Invasive Pulmonary Aspergillosis: Prediction at Thin-Section CT in Patients with Neutropenia—A Prospective Study[1]

Hyung Jin Won, MD
Kyung Soo Lee, MD
Jung-Eun Cheon, MD
Jung Hwa Hwang, MD
Tae Sung Kim, MD
Hong Ghi Lee, MD
Joungho Han, MD

Index terms:
Aspergillosis, 60.2056
Lung, CT, 60.1211
Lung, hemorrhage, 60.4123
Lung, infection, 60.2056
Mucormycosis, 60.2059

Radiology 1998; 208:777–782

[1] From the Departments of Radiology (H.J.W., K.S.L., J.E.C., J.H.H., T.S.K.), Medicine (H.G.L.), and Diagnostic Pathology (J.H.), Samsung Medical Center, College of Medicine, Sung Kyun Kwan University, 50 Ilwon-Dong, Kangnam-Ku, Seoul 135-230, South Korea. Received November 25, 1997; revision requested February 18, 1998; revision received March 5; accepted April 17. **Address reprint requests to** K.S.L.

Author contributions:
Guarantor of integrity of entire study, K.S.L.; study concepts and design, K.S.L.; definition of intellectual content, H.J.W., K.S.L.; literature research, H.J.W., J.E.C.; clinical studies, H.J.W., J.E.C., J.H.H., T.S.K.; data acquisition, H.J.W., J.H.H., T.S.K., H.G.L., J.H.; data analysis, T.S.K., J.H.H.; statistical analysis, H.J.W., K.S.L.; manuscript preparation, H.J.W.; manuscript editing, K.S.L.; manuscript review, H.J.W., K.S.L.

PURPOSE: To evaluate prospectively the usefulness of thin-section computed tomography (CT) in the prediction of biopsy-proved invasive pulmonary aspergillosis in patients with neutropenia.

MATERIALS AND METHODS: In 11 consecutively seen neutropenic patients, 12 open-lung biopsies were performed prospectively for suspected angioinvasive (n = 10) or airway-invasive (n = 2) pulmonary aspergillosis. Thin-section CT findings in the patients with angioinvasive pulmonary aspergillosis were reviewed, and the findings were compared with those of other diseases.

RESULTS: Five of 12 biopsy specimens were positive for angioinvasive pulmonary aspergillosis; none was positive for airway-invasive pulmonary aspergillosis. In five (50%) of 10 cases, suspicion of angioinvasive pulmonary aspergillosis proved to be correct. The most common CT findings were segmental areas of consolidation plus ground-glass attenuation (four of five cases [80%]) and at least one nodule surrounded by a halo (two of five cases [40%]). Segmental areas of consolidation plus ground-glass attenuation were seen as isolated findings in three and mixed findings with nodules that have a surrounding halo in one case. In two patients, at least one nodule with a halo was an isolated finding in one patient and a mixed finding in one patient. Mucormycosis, organizing pneumonia, and pulmonary hemorrhage produced similar findings.

CONCLUSION: At thin-section CT, segmental areas of consolidation plus ground-glass attenuation or at least one nodule with the halo sign were seen in patients with invasive pulmonary aspergillosis. The findings were nonspecific, however, and can be seen in neutropenic patients with mucormycosis, organizing pneumonia, or pulmonary hemorrhage.

Invasive pulmonary aspergillosis is a frequent serious complication in immunocompromised patients. Conditions that predispose patients to it include acute leukemia with neutropenia, use of corticosteroids and other immunosuppressive agents, organ transplantation, and lymphoreticular or hematologic malignancy (1). The increasing number of patients with myelosuppression parallels the increasing frequency (14%–23%) of invasive pulmonary aspergillosis and the high rate of mortality due to the disease (2). Early diagnosis of invasive pulmonary aspergillosis is important, since early institution of amphotericin B therapy has been reported to improve survival rates (2–4).

Nodules surrounded by areas of ground-glass attenuation (the halo sign) during the neutropenic period and air crescents that surround soft-tissue lesions (the crescent sign) during convalescence from neutropenia have been regarded as specific for invasive pulmonary aspergillosis (5–10). Recently, segmental areas of consolidation with or without nodules with the halo sign have also been reported to indicate invasive pulmonary aspergillosis (11–13). In addition, invasive aspergillosis of the airways can appear in patients with neutropenia as areas of peribronchial consolidation or as centrilobular nodules (14).

To our knowledge, except for one study of invasive aspergillosis of the airways (14), studies of angioinvasive pulmonary aspergillosis have been retrospective and have been based on the analysis of computed tomographic (CT) findings of the cases that were proved partly by means of histopathologic analysis (5,6,8–10,12,13). The aim of this study was to evaluate prospectively the usefulness of thin-section CT in the prediction of biopsy-proved invasive pulmonary aspergillosis in neutropenic patients and to compare the findings of the disease with those of other diseases.

MATERIALS AND METHODS

From October 1995 to September 1997, 12 open-lung biopsies in 11 consecutively seen neutropenic patients with chest abnormalities at CT were performed because of the suspicion of either angio- or airway-invasive pulmonary aspergillosis. One patient underwent two biopsies at different locations, thus the total of 12 biopsies in 11 patients. Lung biopsy was performed by means of video-assisted thoracoscopic surgery in nine cases and open thoracotomy (including one wedge resection) in three. At CT before the biopsy, angioinvasive pulmonary aspergillosis was suspected in 10 cases and airway-invasive aspergillosis was suspected in two. When CT scans showed segmental areas of consolidation plus ground-glass attenuation or at least one nodule with the halo sign, the findings were regarded as compatible with angioinvasive pulmonary aspergillosis (5–13). Findings of peribronchial consolidation or centrilobular nodules were presumed to represent airway-invasive aspergillosis (14).

The patients were six men and five women aged 17–59 years (mean, 44 years). All patients had, in addition to fever, symptoms and signs of pulmonary infection, including cough, sputum, or hemoptysis. Underlying diseases in the patients were acute myelogenous leukemia in eight and non-Hodgkin lymphoma in three. One of the patients with acute myelogenous leukemia had undergone bone marrow transplantation. All patients had neutropenia at the time of open-lung biopsy (Table).

Thin-section CT scans were obtained with a HiSpeed Advantage scanner (GE Medical Systems, Milwaukee, Wis) in all patients. Scanning parameters were 140 kVp, 220 mA, and 1-second scanning time. The scans were obtained with 1-mm collimation at 10-mm intervals through the thorax during full inspiration. The images were reconstructed by using a bone algorithm. Scans were viewed at standard mediastinal windows (level, 20 HU; width, 400 HU) and lung windows (level, −700 HU; width, 1,500 HU). Ten patients (including one patient who underwent two open-lung biopsies) underwent CT within 5 days of histopathologic diagnosis, and one patient underwent CT within 10 days. The findings seen at CT were used prospectively by the surgeon as a guide to the optimal site of biopsy.

The CT scans were analyzed by two radiologists (H.J.W., K.S.L.), and decisions about the findings were reached by means of consensus. The pattern, distribution, and extent of pulmonary abnormalities were analyzed. The pattern was classified as consolidation, ground-glass attenuation, nodules, or reticular lesions. Consolidation was further subcategorized as segmental, peribronchial, or patchy. Segmental consolidation was regarded as present when the lesion assumed a pleural-based wedge shape. It was regarded as peribronchial when the lesion existed along the bronchovascular bundles. Distribution was regarded as patchy when the lesion could not be classified as either segmental or peribronchial.

In all patients, special stainings (with methenamine silver stain and periodic acid–Schiff reaction) were performed in addition to routine hematoxylin-eosin staining. The special stains were used mainly to search for specific microorganisms. Because biopsy sites were determined preoperatively, direct one-to-one correlation between a CT pattern of abnormalities at biopsy sites and the histopathologic findings was possible.

RESULTS

Initial CT findings (n = 12) in the 11 patients were at least one segmental area of consolidation plus ground-glass attenuation (n = 4); segmental areas of consolidation, ground-glass attenuation, and nodules with the halo sign (n = 2); one nodule with the halo sign (n = 2); poorly defined centrilobular nodules (n = 2); multiple nodules with the halo sign (n = 1); and segmental areas of consolidation, ground-glass attenuation, and poorly defined centrilobular nodules (n = 1) (Table). The results of open-lung biopsy included angioinvasive pulmonary aspergillosis (n = 5), organizing pneumonia (n = 2), mucormycosis (n = 2), pulmonary hemorrhage (n = 2), and bronchiolitis obliterans organizing pneumonia (cryptogenic organizing pneumonia, n = 1) (Table).

CT and Histopathologic Findings of Invasive Pulmonary Aspergillosis

In five (50%) of 10 cases, suspicion of angioinvasive pulmonary aspergillosis proved to be correct. The most common CT findings of angioinvasive pulmonary aspergillosis were segmental areas of consolidation plus ground-glass attenuation (four of five cases [80%]) (Fig 1) and at least one nodule surrounded by a halo (two of five cases [40%]) (Fig 2). Segmental areas of consolidation plus ground-glass attenuation were seen as an isolated finding in three cases and were mixed with nodules surrounded by a halo in one case. At least one nodule with a halo was seen in one patient as an isolated finding and in one patient as a mixed finding.

The predominant abnormalities at histopathologic examination, regardless of thin-section CT findings of a segmental area of consolidation plus ground-glass attenuation or a nodule surrounded by a halo, consisted of hemorrhagic infarction with angioinvasion (Fig 1). Colonization with *Aspergillus* organisms was identified in the walls of small- to medium-sized pulmonary arteries. Thrombus formation with vascular occlusion in the arteries was also seen. Less common histopathologic findings were fibrinoid necrosis, organizing pneumonia, and diffuse alveolar damage. At correlation of CT and histopathologic findings, consolidated or nodular lesions represented coagulation fungal necrosis, whereas surrounding areas of ground-glass attenuation represented intraalveolar hemorrhage (Table).

Other Diseases that Simulated Invasive Pulmonary Aspergillosis

At CT, mucormycosis simulated the findings of angioinvasive pulmonary aspergillosis in two patients: one with a nodule with the halo sign and the other with a segmental area of consolidation plus ground-glass attenuation (Fig 3). At histopathologic examination, the disease consisted of hemorrhagic infarction with necrotizing inflammation. Mucormycotic organisms were seen in alveolar spaces as well as in vascular walls (Fig 3). Organizing pneumonia simulated the findings of invasive aspergillosis in two patients: one with segmental areas of consolidation, ground-glass attenuation, and poorly defined centrilobular nodules with the halo sign and the other with multiple, poorly defined nodules with the halo sign. Intrapulmonary hemorrhage simulated the findings of invasive pulmonary aspergillosis in one patient with findings of mul-

Thin-Section CT and Histopathologic Findings in 11 Neutropenic Patients

Patient No./Age (y)/Sex	Underlying Disease	Neutrophil Count* (no./mL)	Thin-Section CT Findings	CT Findings at Biopsy Site	Histopathologic Findings	Histopathologic Diagnosis
1/51/M	AML	100	Multiple segmental areas of consolidation plus GGA, nodules with halo	Consolidation plus GGA	Hemorrhagic infarction, vascular invasion by *Aspergillus* species	Invasive aspergillosis
2/56/F	AML	320	Multiple segmental areas of consolidation plus GGA	Consolidation plus GGA	Intraalveolar hemorrhage and fibrinous exudate, vascular invasion by *Aspergillus* species	Invasive aspergillosis
3/55/M	NHL	300	Multiple segmental areas of consolidation plus GGA	Consolidation plus GGA	Diffuse alveolar damage and hemorrhagic infarction, vascular invasion by *Aspergillus* species	Invasive aspergillosis
4/37/F	AML and BMT	50	Segmental area of consolidation plus GGA	Consolidation plus GGA	Coagulation necrosis with fungal species, hemorrhagic infarction	Invasive aspergillosis
5/17/F	AML	300	Single nodule with halo → nodule with air crescent, pneumomediastinum, and interstitial emphysema	Nodule with air crescent	Organizing pneumonia with chronic active inflammation and fibrinoid necrosis, aspergillus fungal ball	Invasive aspergillosis → aspergilloma
		200	Single nodule with halo	Nodule with halo	Fungal organism floating on background area of coagulation necrosis	Mucormycosis
6/32/M	NHL	300	Segmental area of consolidation plus GGA	Consolidation plus GGA	Hemorrhagic infarction with necrotizing inflammation, mucormycosis in alveolar spaces and walls of blood vessels	Mucormycosis
7/58/M	AML	200	Multiple segmental areas of consolidation plus GGA, poorly defined centrilobular nodules with halo	Centrilobular nodules with halo	Organizing pneumonia with microfoci of intraalveolar hemorrhage	Organizing pneumonia
8/54/F	AML	150	Multiple nodules with halo	Nodule with halo	Organizing pneumonia with focal abscess formation	Organizing pneumonia
9/33/F	AML	240	Poorly defined multiple centrilobular nodules	Centrilobular nodule	Hemosiderin-laden macrophage with chronic interstitial inflammation	Pulmonary hemorrhage
10/31/M	NHL	345	Multiple segmental areas of consolidation plus GGA, poorly defined centrilobular nodules	Segmental consolidation plus GGA	Intraalveolar hemorrhage, edema, and fibrinoid exudate, chronic interstitial inflammation	Pulmonary hemorrhage
11/24/M	AML	435	Poorly defined centrilobular nodules	Centrilobular nodule	Obliterative bronchiolitis with granulation polyp	Bronchiolitis obliterans organizing pneumonia (cryptogenic organizing pneumonia)

Note.—AML = acute myelogenous leukemia, BMT = bone marrow transplantation, GGA = ground-glass attenuation, NHL = non-Hodgkin lymphoma.
* Absolute number of polymorphonuclear leukocytes.

tiple segmental areas of consolidation plus ground-glass attenuation and poorly defined centrilobular nodules.

In the two patients with findings of poorly defined centrilobular nodules only in whom airway-invasive aspergillosis was initially presumed, the diseases turned out to be pulmonary hemorrhage in one and bronchiolitis obliterans organizing pneumonia (cryptogenic organizing pneumonia) in one (Table).

DISCUSSION

The spectrum of pulmonary involvement with *Aspergillus* infection is various and depends largely on the patient's underlying pulmonary and immune status. Invasive pulmonary aspergillosis occurs in immunosuppressed patients. Clinically, patients with invasive pulmonary aspergillosis present with fever, dyspnea, nonproductive cough, and, frequently, pleuritic chest pain. On occasion, massive hemoptysis may occur. The reported mortality rate of the disease varies from 30% to 90%. Amphotericin B is the most effective antifungal treatment and is most successful if initiated early (15).

The radiologic characteristics of invasive pulmonary aspergillosis have been extensively described. The findings include nodules, masslike infiltrates, and subsegmental and segmental consolidation (1,5–7,16). Findings of recent studies suggest that CT may allow early recognition of invasive pulmonary aspergillosis by depicting a characteristic halo of ground-glass attenuation (CT halo sign) around the nodule (5–10).

Although findings of the CT halo sign have been regarded as indicative of invasive pulmonary aspergillosis (5–10), the sensitivity and specificity of the sign in neutropenic patients has not been tested. The most common CT finding of invasive pulmonary aspergillosis in our study was the presence of segmental consolidation

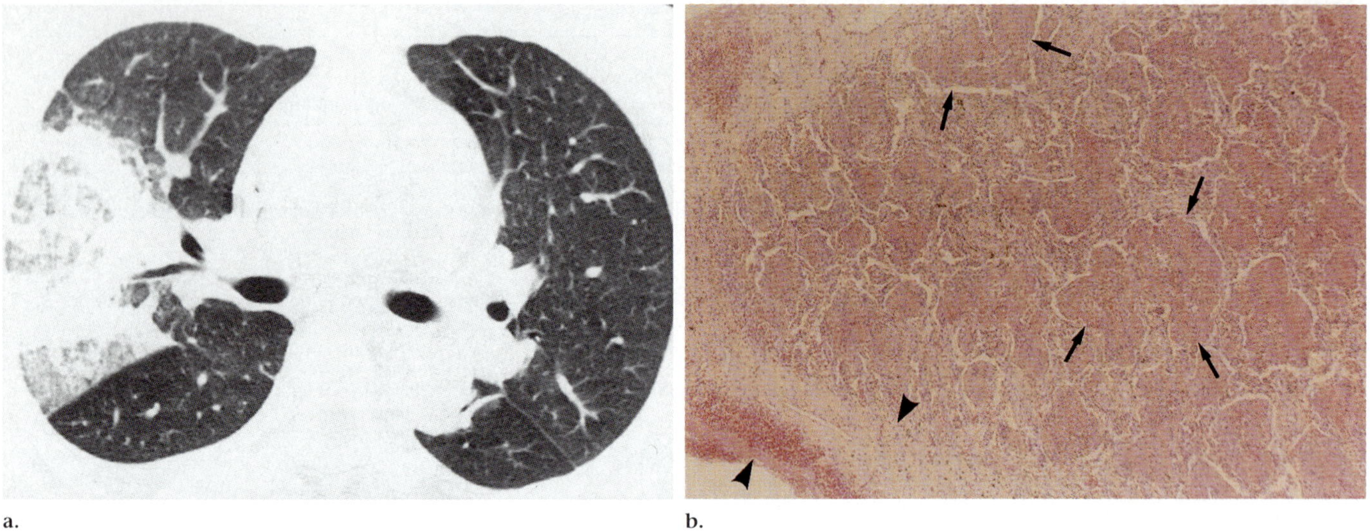

Figure 1. Patient 2. Invasive pulmonary aspergillosis in a 56-year-old woman with acute myelogenous leukemia. **(a)** Thin-section CT scan (1-mm collimation) obtained at the subcarinal level shows a segmental area of consolidation plus areas of ground-glass attenuation in the posterior segment of the right upper lobe. **(b)** Photomicrograph of a biopsy specimen obtained in the right upper lobe reveals widespread intraalveolar (arrows) fibrin mixed with acute inflammatory cells, macrophages, and red blood cells. These findings suggest previous hemorrhagic infarction. Pleural thickening (arrowheads) is also seen in **b**. Vascular invasion by *Aspergillus* species was seen (not shown). (Hematoxylin-eosin stain; original magnification, ×100.)

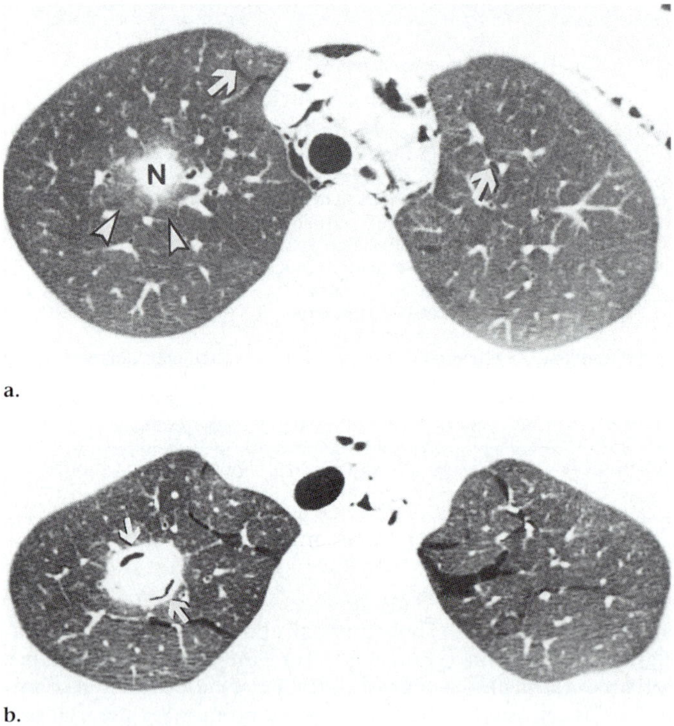

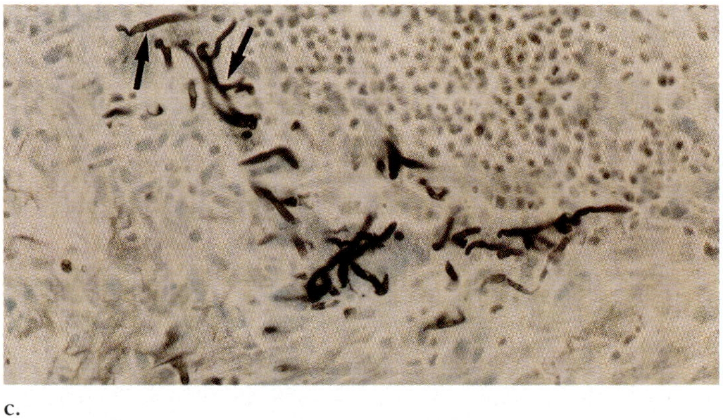

Figure 2. Patient 5. Invasive pulmonary aspergillosis in a 17-year-old girl with acute myelogenous leukemia. **(a)** Thin-section CT scan (1-mm collimation) obtained at the level of the thoracic inlet shows a small nodule (*N*) with a surrounding halo (arrowheads) in the right upper lobe. Interstitial emphysema in both upper lobes (arrows), pneumomediastinum, and subcutaneous emphysema in the left chest wall are also seen. **(b)** Follow-up CT scan obtained at a slightly higher level than that in **a** after amphotericin B therapy demonstrates an enlarged nodule with an air-crescent sign (arrows). Interstitial emphysema and pneumomediastinum are still visible. **(c)** Photomicrograph of a pathologic specimen obtained at surgical resection demonstrates microfoci of fungal septate hyphae (arrows) branching at an acute angle. This pattern is morphologically consistent with *Aspergillus* species. (Methenamine silver stain; original magnification, ×400.)

plus surrounding ground-glass attenuation (four of five cases [80%]). At least one nodule surrounded by a halo was seen in two patients (40%). Therefore, we think segmental areas of consolidation plus ground-glass attenuation, either alone or mixed with nodules surrounded by a halo, are findings of invasive pulmonary aspergillosis.

As confirmed in our study, it is not strange that mucormycosis can occur with the CT halo sign. Because Mucorales organisms have the same propensity as *Aspergillus* to invade blood vessels and thus to result in vascular thrombosis, mucormycosis can lead to lung infarction and resultant segmental areas of consolidation plus ground-glass attenuation or a nodule surrounded by a halo at thin-section CT. In our study, organizing pneumonia and pulmonary hemorrhage simulated the findings of invasive pulmonary aspergillosis: segmental areas of consolidation plus ground-glass attenuation or at least one nodule with the halo sign.

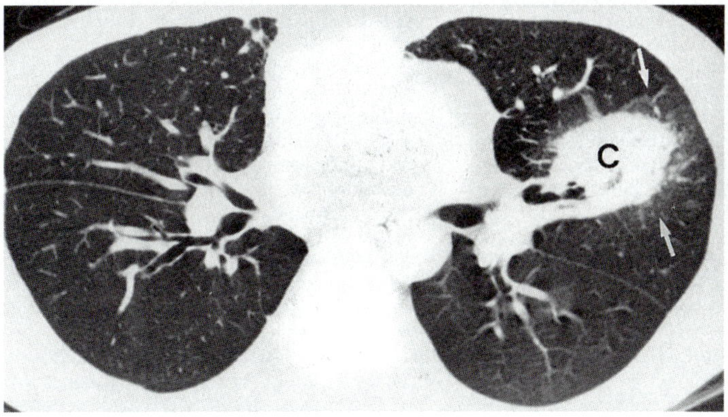

a.

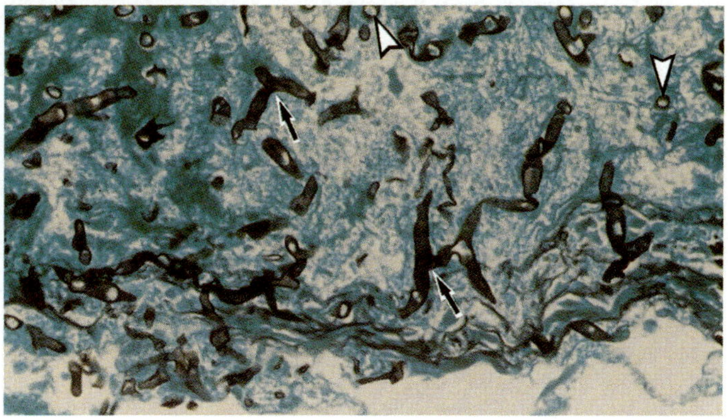

c.

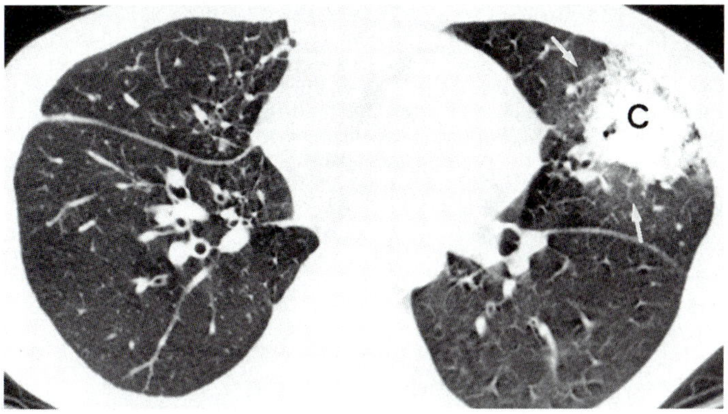

b.

Figure 3. Patient 6. Mucormycosis in a 32-year-old man with non-Hodgkin lymphoma. **(a)** Thin-section CT scan (1.0-mm collimation) obtained at the subcarinal level shows an area of consolidation (*C*), with surrounding areas of ground-glass attenuation (arrows) in the left upper lobe. **(b)** CT scan obtained 30 mm lower than **a** demonstrates a segmental area of consolidation (*C*) and areas of ground-glass attenuation (arrows). **(c)** Photomicrograph of a biopsy specimen demonstrates a mixture of hyphae (arrows) and yeast (arrowheads), which is morphologically consistent with mucormycosis. (Methenamine silver stain; original magnification, ×400.)

The most common manifestation of invasive pulmonary aspergillosis is hemorrhagic infarction. Two histopathologic patterns are known to be associated with hemorrhagic infarction. One is a fairly well defined nodule with a surrounding hemorrhagic rim, and the other is a wedge-shaped, hemorrhagic, pleural-based consolidation similar to a thromboembolic infarct (17,18). Although the former pattern has been documented as more common (17,18), the latter pattern can be as common as the former, as seen in our study. A majority of findings of consolidation were associated with a surrounding halo of ground-glass attenuation at CT.

At correlation of CT and histopathologic findings in the present study, both patterns appeared with coagulation necrosis in the center and adjacent intraalveolar hemorrhage due to hemorrhagic infarction. There was extensive vascular permeation and apparent occlusion of small- to medium-sized arteries by fungal hyphae, with or without thrombus formation. Given that the underlying pathologic condition was hemorrhagic infarction due to vascular invasion, segmental consolidation and ground-glass attenuation were not strange findings of invasive pulmonary aspergillosis.

Although positive findings of sputum cultures in neutropenic patients were suggested to be highly predictive of invasive aspergillosis in one study (19), it is generally believed that findings of sputum cultures are rarely positive in the early period of the disease (3,20). Serologic tests are unreliable (21). Lavage fluid yields a high percentage of true-positive results but a small percentage of false-positive results (22). Therefore, definitive diagnosis of invasive pulmonary aspergillosis requires tissue examination. Most articles in which invasive pulmonary aspergillosis is described, however, are based on cases of the disease diagnosed, in part, at histopathologic examination. Our study was performed prospectively and on the basis of histopathologically diagnosed cases of invasive pulmonary aspergillosis.

In spite of the radiographic distinction of the air crescent sign, its late appearance in the course of infection (during recovery) substantially limits its usefulness for diagnostic purposes (18). At follow-up CT in two patients in our series, the air crescent sign was seen in one patient. In the other patient, the area of consolidation increased in extent in spite of amphotericin B therapy. At histopathologic correlation in the specimen that showed the air crescent sign (patient 5), a central rounded area represented necrotic lung tissue with fungal colonization, a finding consistent with a previous report (6).

Our study has several limitations. Although prospective, the number of patients is small, and we did not perform open-lung biopsy in all neutropenic patients with abnormalities at chest radiography or CT. Furthermore, to attain CT-histopathologic correlation, our study included only patients in whom both CT and open-lung biopsy were performed. Therefore, there could be a selection bias. Selection bias can be substantiated by the inclusion in our series of only two cases of bacterial infection (organizing pneumonia).

In conclusion, segmental areas of consolidation plus ground-glass attenuation or at least one nodule with the halo sign are seen in biopsy-proved cases of invasive pulmonary aspergillosis. The findings at CT represent hemorrhagic necrosis with angioinvasion. Thin-section CT findings of invasive pulmonary aspergillosis are nonspecific, however, and similar findings can be seen in patients with neutropenia and mucormycosis, organizing pneumonia, or pulmonary hemorrhage. Therefore, for definitive diagnosis of invasive pulmonary aspergillosis, tissue biopsy—including open-lung biopsy or core biopsy performed with the percutaneous technique—is mandatory.

References

1. Gefter WB. The spectrum of pulmonary aspergillosis. J Thorac Imaging 1992; 7:56–74.

2. Burch PA, Karp JE, Merz WG, Kuhlman JE, Fishman EK. Favorable outcome of invasive aspergillosis in patients with acute leukemia. J Clin Oncol 1987; 5:1985–1993.
3. Fisher BD, Armstrong D, Yu B, Gold JWM. Invasive aspergillosis: progress in early diagnosis and treatment. Am J Med 1981; 71:571–577.
4. Aisner J, Schimpff SC, Wiernik PH. Treatment of invasive aspergillosis: relation of early diagnosis and treatment to response. Ann Intern Med 1977; 86:539–543.
5. Kuhlman JE, Fishman EK, Siegelman SS. Invasive pulmonary aspergillosis in acute leukemia: characteristic findings on CT, the CT halo sign, and the role of CT in early diagnosis. Radiology 1985; 157:611–614.
6. Curtis AMB, Smith GJW, Ravin CE. Air crescent sign of invasive aspergillosis. Radiology 1979; 133:17–21.
7. Fraser RS, Pare JAP, Fraser RG, Pare PD. Infectious disease of the lungs. In: Fraser RS, ed. Synopsis of diseases of the chest. 2nd ed. Philadelphia, Pa: Saunders, 1994.
8. Kuhlman JE, Fishman EK, Burch PA, Karp JE, Zerhouni EA, Siegelman SS. Invasive pulmonary aspergillosis in acute leukemia: the contribution of CT to early diagnosis and aggressive management. Chest 1987; 92:95–99.
9. Kuhlman JE, Fishman EK, Burch PA, Karp JE, Zerhouni EA, Siegelman SS. CT of invasive pulmonary aspergillosis. AJR 1988; 150:1015–1020.
10. Blum U, Windfuhr M, Buitrago-Tellez C, Sigmund G, Herbst EW, Langer M. Invasive pulmonary aspergillosis: MRI, CT, and plain radiographic findings and their contribution for early diagnosis. Chest 1994; 106:1156–1161.
11. Brown MJ, Miller RR, Müller NL. Acute lung disease in the immunocompromised host: CT and pathologic findings. Radiology 1994; 190:247–254.
12. Feuerstein IM, Ng J, Chow C, Courcoutsakis NA, Decarlo E, Holland S. The appearance of aspergillus fumigatus infection in patients with chronic granulomatous disease (abstr). AJR 1997; 168(P):72.
13. Bray A, Pirronti T, Sallustio G, Marano P. Clinicoradiological patterns of invasive pulmonary aspergillosis (abstr). Radiology 1997; 205(P):673.
14. Logan PM, Primack SL, Miller RR, Müller NL. Invasive aspergillosis of the airways: radiographic, CT, and pathologic findings. Radiology 1994; 193:383–388.
15. Aquino SL, Kee ST, Warnock ML, Gamsu G. Pulmonary aspergillosis: imaging findings with pathologic correlation. AJR 1994; 163:811–815.
16. Orr DP, Myerowitz RL, Dubois PJ. Pathoradiologic correlation of invasive pulmonary aspergillosis in the compromised host. Cancer 1978; 41:2028–2039.
17. Hruban RH, Meziance MA, Zerhouni EA, Wheeler PS, Dumler JS, Hutchins GM. Radiologic-pathologic correlation of the CT halo sign in invasive pulmonary aspergillosis. J Comput Assist Tomogr 1987; 11:534–536.
18. Gefter WB, Albelda SM, Talbot GH, Gerson SL, Cassileth PA, Miller WT. Invasive pulmonary aspergillosis and acute leukemia: limitations in the diagnostic utility of the air crescent sign. Radiology 1985; 157:605–610.
19. Yu VL, Muder RR, Porsattar A. Significance of isolation of aspergillus from the respiratory tract in diagnosis of invasive pulmonary aspergillosis: results from a three-year prospective study. Am J Med 1986; 81:249–254.
20. Young RC, Bennett JE, Vogel CL, Carbone PP, De Vita VT. Aspergillosis: the spectrum of the disease in 98 patients. Medicine 1970; 49:147–173.
21. Weiner MH, Talbot GH, Gerson SL, Filice G, Cassileth PA. Antigen detection in the diagnosis of invasive aspergillosis. Ann Intern Med 1983; 99:772–782.
22. Andrews CP, Weiner MH. Aspergillus antigen detection in broncho-alveolar lavage fluid from patients with invasive aspergillosis and aspergillomas. Am J Med 1983; 73:372–380.

Debra M. Lau, MD
Marilyn J. Siegel, MD
Charles F. Hildebolt, PhD, DDS
Alan H. Cohen, MD

Index terms:
Bronchi, CT, 60.12118
Bronchiectasis, 60.26
Bronchiolitis obliterans, 60.2191
Lung, transplantation, 60.458

Radiology 1998; 208:783–788

[1] From the Mallinckrodt Institute of Radiology (D.M.L., M.J.S., C.F.H.) and the Department of Pediatrics (A.H.C.), Washington University School of Medicine, 510 S Kingshighway Blvd, St Louis, MO 63110. Received December 22, 1997; revision requested January 26, 1998; final revision received April 15; accepted May 8. **Address reprint requests to** M.J.S.

Bronchiolitis Obliterans Syndrome: Thin-Section CT Diagnosis of Obstructive Changes in Infants and Young Children after Lung Transplantation[1]

PURPOSE: To characterize the thin-section computed tomographic (CT) appearance of bronchiolitis fibrosa obliterans syndrome in infants and young children after lung transplantation.

MATERIALS AMD METHODS: Thin-section CT studies in six patients with bronchiolitis obliterans syndrome (age range, 2 months to 5½ years) and in 15 control patients without obstructive airway disease (age range, 2 months to 7 years) who underwent bilateral lung transplantation were retrospectively reviewed. The thin-section CT scans were obtained during quiet sleep at a median of 24 months (range, 6–36 months) after transplantation. The CT studies were evaluated for mosaic perfusion, bronchial dilatation, bronchial wall thickening, and mucous plugging. Final diagnoses in all patients were based on pulmonary function test results.

RESULTS: Thin-section CT findings in the six patients with clinically proved bronchiolitis obliterans syndrome were mosaic perfusion in five (83%), bronchial dilatation in three (50%), and bronchial wall thickening in one (17%). Of the 15 control patients with normal pulmonary function test results, six (40%) had mosaic perfusion; none had bronchial dilatation or bronchial wall thickening. Mucous plugging was not seen in either group. Only the association of bronchial dilatation with bronchiolitis obliterans syndrome was significant ($P = .02$).

CONCLUSION: Infants and young children with bronchiolitis obliterans syndrome after lung transplantation are more likely to have CT abnormalities than those with normal pulmonary function test results.

Author contributions:
Guarantors of integrity of entire study, D.M.L., M.J.S.; study concepts, M.J.S.; study design, M.J.S., D.M.L.; definition of intellectual content, D.M.L., M.J.S.; literature research, M.J.S., D.M.L., A.H.C.; clinical studies, A.H.C., M.J.S., D.M.L.; data analysis, M.J.S., D.M.L., C.F.H.; statistical analysis, C.F.H.; manuscript preparation, D.M.L., M.J.S.; manuscript editing, D.M.L., M.J.S., C.F.H.; manuscript review, D.M.L., M.J.S., C.F.H., A.H.C.

"Bronchiolitis fibrosa obliterans syndrome" refers to lung graft deterioration due to progressive airway disease for which no other cause has been identified, while the term "bronchiolitis obliterans" refers to a histologically proved diagnosis (1,2). Diagnosis of bronchiolitis obliterans syndrome does not require histologic proof but is based on functional evidence of irreversible airflow obstruction generated from pulmonary function tests.

Transbronchial biopsy and chest radiography are part of the routine monitoring of lung transplant recipients. However, transbronchial biopsy and chest radiography have been shown to be both insensitive and nonspecific for the diagnosis of bronchiolitis obliterans (3,4). Computed tomography (CT) during inspiration and expiration has been used increasingly in the evaluation of small airway disease in older children and adults who are able to suspend respiration for the examination (5,6). To our knowledge, the value of thin-section CT findings in young children who are unable to suspend respiration has not yet been reported.

The purpose of this study was to identify whether there are CT findings that suggest the development of bronchiolitis obliterans in children and infants who cannot hold their breath. We compared thin-section CT findings with the results of pulmonary function testing to determine the best CT indexes of airflow obstruction, the hallmark of bronchiolitis obliterans.

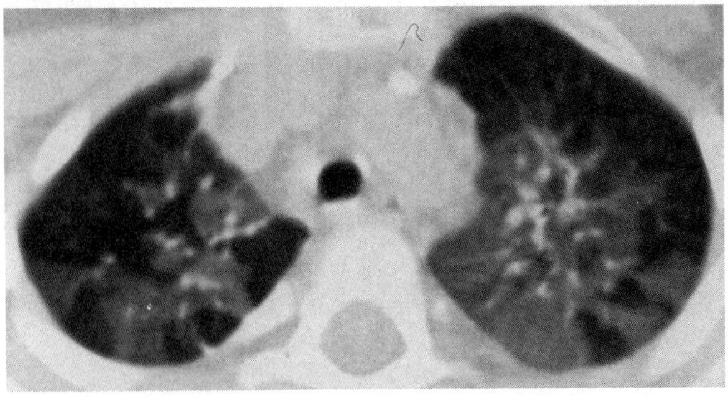

Figure 1. Mosaic perfusion in bronchiolitis obliterans. Thin-section CT scan in a 3-year-old girl with posttransplantation bronchiolitis obliterans demonstrates focal, patchy areas of decreased attenuation and vascularity scattered between areas of increased attenuation and perfusion.

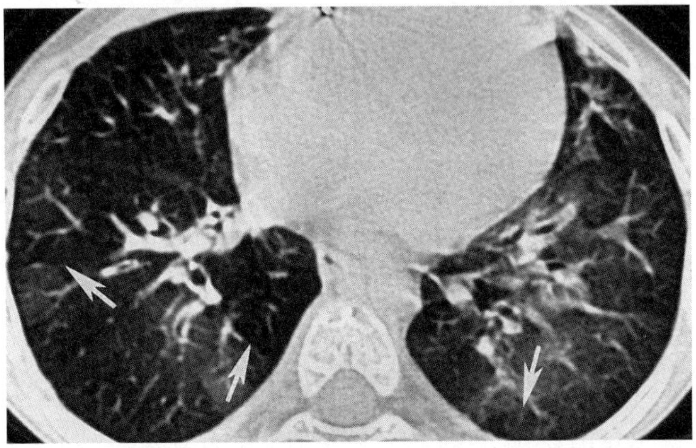

Figure 2. Subtle mosaic perfusion (arrows) in bronchiolitis obliterans. Thin-section CT scan obtained in a 3-year-old girl during quiet respiration demonstrates less obvious areas of mixed attenuation in both lower lobes.

MATERIALS AND METHODS

The medical records and imaging studies of infants and young children who underwent bilateral lung transplantation between January 1991 and January 1997 were reviewed. Patients were included in the study if they underwent thin-section CT without breath holding at least 6 months after transplantation. We chose 6 months as the earliest time for review of the CT findings to minimize the possibility of early postoperative complications, such as acute graft rejection or infection.

The protocol at our institution requires the routine monitoring of all lung transplant recipients by means of chest radiography and CT at 3, 6, and 12–15 months after transplantation, and then yearly. The timing of the CT studies is designed to correspond to the timing of the pulmonary function monitoring. Additional studies are performed when patients are symptomatic and clinical suspicion of acute infection or rejection exists. Patients who received a unilateral lung transplant or a heart-lung transplant were excluded.

There were 21 bilateral-lung transplant recipients who met the entry criteria. The study population comprised 12 male patients and nine female patients aged 2 months to 6–8½ years (median, 19 months) at the time of transplantation. The indications for transplantation were pulmonary hypertension with or without congenital heart disease ($n = 6$), pulmonary venous obstruction ($n = 4$), inadequate pulmonary arterial supply ($n = 2$), pulmonary alveolar proteinosis ($n = 2$), idiopathic pulmonary fibrosis ($n = 2$), cystic fibrosis ($n = 2$), bronchopulmonary dysplasia ($n = 2$), and interstitial pneumonitis ($n = 1$).

Clinical Testing

Final diagnoses were based on the results of pulmonary function testing, which all patients underwent. Six (29%; age range, 2 months to 5½ years) of the 21 patients were able to perform voluntary respiratory maneuvers in a reproducible manner with the use of a spirometer. Fifteen patients (71%; age range, 2 months to 7 years) were too young to cooperate in spontaneous pulmonary function testing and underwent infant respiratory testing by means of the open-circuit nitrogen washout test technique (7,8). All pulmonary function tests were administered within 48 hours of CT scanning.

The diagnosis of airway obstruction in older children who were able to undergo spirometry was based on measurement of the forced expiratory volume in the 1st second (1,2). After exclusion of other conditions that could reduce the forced expiratory volume in the 1st second, such as airway infection or acute graft rejection, a fractional decline of 20% from previous baseline studies obtained at least 1 month before was considered diagnostic of bronchiolitis obliterans syndrome. Infants were considered to have airway obstruction if they had a functional residual capacity greater than or equal to 125% of the predicted value (8,9) along with a diminished maximum volume of functional residual capacity (10,11).

Flexible fiberoptic bronchoscopy, transbronchial biopsy, and bronchoalveolar lavage were performed a minimum of four times within the first 3 months after transplantation. Thereafter, they were performed every 3 months until the 1st year after transplantation, when they were then performed a minimum of every 6–12 months. Additional bronchoscopy was performed if clinical findings were suggestive of acute rejection or substantial lower respiratory infection.

All patients received standard posttransplantion immunosuppression with cyclosporine, azathioprine, and prednisone (12).

Thin-Section CT

CT scans were obtained with a Somatom Plus S-Scanner or Somatom Plus 4 Scanner (Siemens, Erlangen, Germany).

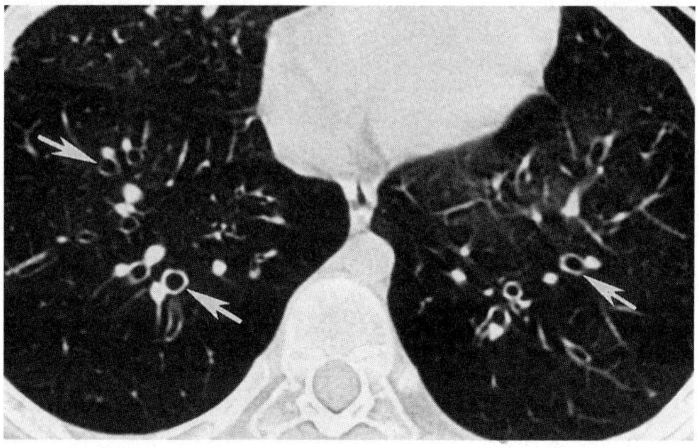

Figure 3. Bronchial dilatation in bronchiolitis obliterans. Thin-section CT scan in a 5½-year-old boy demonstrates that bronchial diameters (arrows) are greater than those of the adjacent vessels. Mild bronchial wall thickening is also present.

Contiguous routine 4- or 8-mm-thick scans were obtained with 4- or 8-mm/sec table feed, 120 kVp, 180 mAs, and 1-second scanning time from the lung apex to the diaphragm. Thin-section scans were obtained with 2-mm collimation at 10-mm intervals throughout the lungs during quiet respiration without breath holding. The thin-section CT scans were obtained during quiet sleep at a median of 24 months (range, 6–36 months) after transplantation. Although some patients were able to cooperate for spirometric examination, none was able to suspend respiration for CT examination. The scans were reconstructed by using a high-spatial-frequency algorithm. The images were photographed at window levels of −600 to −700 HU and window widths of 1,000 to 1,500 HU. The thin-section CT studies were obtained within 48 hours of the pulmonary function tests and within 72 hours of flexible fiberoptic bronchoscopy and transbronchial biopsy.

The thin-section CT scans were retrospectively reviewed by two radiologists (D.M.L., M.J.S.) blinded to the patient's respiratory status and posttransplantation diagnosis. The CT scans were evaluated for the presence and distribution of features suggestive of small airway disease: (*a*) mosaic perfusion; (*b*) bronchial abnormalities at a subsegmental level, which were bronchial dilatation and bronchial wall thickening; and (*c*) mucous plugging.

The definition of mosaic perfusion was based on criteria established by Austin et al (13). In their definition, mosaic perfusion was described as alternating areas of varied lung attenuation that are presumed to be due to regional differences in perfusion (13). Bronchial dilatation was considered present when the bronchial diameter was greater than the diameter of the accompanying pulmonary artery or when bronchi were clearly identified in the periphery of the lung within 1 cm of the pleura. The diagnosis of bronchial wall thickening was established subjectively when the walls of the bronchi were thicker than the walls of other bronchi in the same cross section. The extent of mosaic perfusion, bronchial dilatation, and bronchial wall thickening was graded on a three-point scale as follows: 1, disease in one lobe; 2, disease in two or three lobes; and 3, disease in four or five lobes.

Statistical Analysis

Because of small sample sizes, differences in proportions were tested with the Fisher exact test, for which exact probabilities were calculated (14). Sensitivities, specificities, odds ratios, and 95% CIs were also calculated. A P value of less than .05 indicated a statistically significant difference. Statistical analyses were performed with JMP (SAS Institute, Cary, NC) and STATXACT-TURBO (Cytel, Cambridge, Mass).

RESULTS

Clinical Findings

Six of the 21 patients evaluated had clinical evidence of bronchiolitis obliterans as compared with findings of baseline studies. Five of the six patients with bronchiolitis obliterans had greater than 125% functional residual capacity (range, 126%–227%) and decreased maximal velocity at functional residual capacity, as measured with serial infant pulmonary function tests. The remaining patient, who was able to undergo spirometry, had findings of severe obstruction by 6 months after transplantation. None of the six patients had evidence of bronchiolitis obliterans at transbronchial biopsy, and the diagnosis was based solely on the results of pulmonary function testing. The median postoperative time until the onset of bronchiolitis obliterans syndrome was 24 months (range, 6–36 months).

Of the 15 control patients, five were able to undergo spirometry and 10 were examined by means of serial infant pulmonary function tests. None of these patients had evidence of airflow obstruction. Transbronchial biopsy performed at the time of the pulmonary function tests also demonstrated no evidence of bronchiolitis obliterans. Final clinical findings in these patients were bronchitis or normal airways.

CT Findings

Pulmonary abnormalities were detected at thin-section CT in five of the six patients with bronchiolitis obliterans syndrome. Mosaic perfusion was the most frequent finding and was present in five (83%) of six patients (Figs 1, 2). It involved one lobe in one patient, two to three lobes in one patient, and all the lobes in three patients.

The second most frequent finding was bronchial dilatation, occurring in three (50%) of six patients (Fig 3). All three patients with bronchial dilatation also had mosaic perfusion. Bronchial dilatation affected two to three lobes in all three patients. Although the bronchi were dilated in three patients, the bronchial walls were thickened in only one patient (Fig 4). No patients had identifiable mucus plugging. Two patients with bronchiolitis obliterans had one abnormal CT finding, two had two findings, and one had three findings.

Mosaic perfusion was the only finding noted in the control group, occurring in six (40%) of the 15 patients (Fig 5). Bronchial dilatation, wall thickening, or mucus plugging was not seen in any of the control patients.

The CT findings of mosaic perfusion, wall thickening, and bronchial dilatation were more frequent in the infants and children with obstructive changes than in the control patients. The sensitivity of bronchial dilatation for the diagnosis of bronchiolitis obliterans was 50% (three of six); the specificity was 100% (15 of

15). The sensitivity of mosaic perfusion for the diagnosis of bronchiolitis obliterans was 83% (five of six), but the specificity was only 60% (nine of 15) (Table). The sensitivity and specificity of bronchial wall thickening were 17% (one of six) and 100% (15 of 15), respectively. The association of the clinical diagnosis of bronchiolitis obliterans with the CT finding of bronchial dilatation was significant (P = .02). The associations for mosaic perfusion and wall thickening were not significant (P = .15 and P = .29, respectively).

DISCUSSION

Bronchiolitis obliterans is a late complication of lung transplantation and heart-lung transplantation and is characterized by obstructive airway disease. Histopathologically, a severe fibrosing inflammatory process affects the terminal and respiratory bronchioles, which results in the airway scarring and obstruction that characterizes the disease (15). Bronchiolitis obliterans is believed to be the consequence of repeated episodes of rejection and has been treated by augmenting immunosuppression. The prevalence of bronchiolitis obliterans in long-term transplant recipients is approximately 50% (15,16). The diagnosis of bronchiolitis obliterans, referred to clinically as "bronchiolitis obliterans syndrome," is difficult because it manifests as nonspecific signs and symptoms. Despite the difficulty of clinical diagnosis, the early detection and initiation of therapy are critical in improving outcome. This has prompted frequent evaluation by means of pulmonary function tests, transbronchial biopsy, and radiologic or CT examination.

The clinical diagnosis of bronchiolitis obliterans is established when pulmonary function test results indicate obstructive small airway disease in the absence of other causes 3 or more months after transplantation (1,2). A diminishment in the forced expiratory volume in the 1st second by more than 20% is considered a reliable predictor of bronchiolitis obliterans. However, such alterations in pulmonary function test results do not provide the specificity required to discriminate between infection and rejection. Discrimination between these two conditions is often accomplished with a combination of negative biopsy results for infection, clinical course, and lesion response to adjustments in steroidal or immunosuppressive therapy. The absence of other disease processes is considered supportive evidence of bronchiolitis obliterans. Transbronchial biopsy results alone are not reliable for the diagnosis of bronchiolitis obliterans because of the patchy distribution of the disease (17,18).

Plain radiographic studies are generally normal or nonspecific and have not proved helpful in differentiating between bronchiolitis obliterans and other parenchymal complications associated with lung transplantation in children and infants. Radiographic findings that have been reported include air-space or interstitial disease and pleural effusion (3,4).

CT is considered superior to chest radiography in discriminating between normal and abnormal lung parenchyma and in delineating bronchial size. Although chest CT is considered of value in adults with lung transplants, the data on its value in diagnosing bronchiolitis obliterans in children and infants are sparse. Lynch et al (19) reported on six children with postinfectious bronchiolitis obliterans. The most frequent findings were focal areas of decreased lung opacity and bronchial dilatation, occurring in 83% (five of six) and 66% (four of six) of their subjects, respectively. Medina et al (20) reported the thin-section CT findings in six children with bronchiolitis obliterans after lung transplantation. In that series, ground-glass opacities were found in four (67%) and bronchial dilatation in one (17%) of the six patients. That study (20) focused on the acute pulmonary complications after transplantation, and the mean time between transplantation and CT was 6 months. There were no CT findings that separated bronchiolitis obliterans from acute rejection or allograft infection.

The demonstration of bronchial dilatation, bronchial wall thickening, mosaic perfusion, and air trapping at CT are believed to be highly suggestive of bronchiolitis obliterans in adult lung transplant recipients. Bronchial dilatation has been reported in both heart-lung transplant recipients and lung transplant recipients. Morrish et al (4) examined four patients with bronchiolitis obliterans after lung transplantation. They found peripheral bronchial dilatation on thin-section CT scans in all recipients. Later, Lentz et al (5) examined seven heart-lung transplant patients with bronchiolitis obliterans; six (86%) had bronchial dilatation at the time airway obstruction was diagnosed. These authors (5) also noted that the lower lobe bronchi were involved more often than the upper lobe bronchi and that the percentage of dilated bronchi increased with the severity of pulmonary dysfunction. More recently,

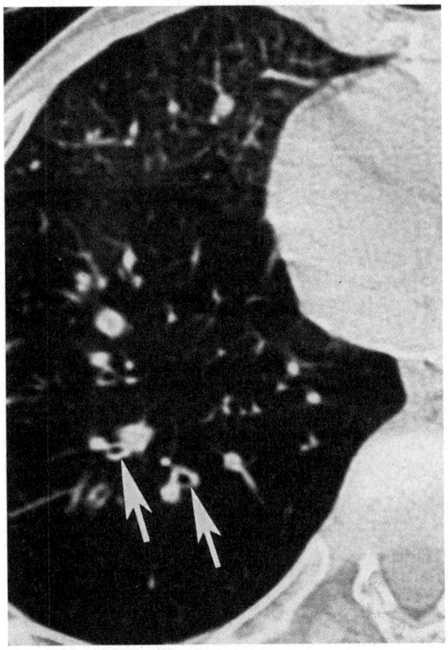

Figure 4. Bronchial wall thickening. Thin-section CT scan in a 5½-year-old patient demonstrates wall thickening of several bronchi (arrows) in the right lower lobe.

Worthy et al (6) reported on 15 patients with histopathologically proved bronchiolitis obliterans after lung transplantation. Bronchial dilatation had a sensitivity of 80% (12 of 15) and a specificity of 78% (14 of 18) for the diagnosis of bronchiolitis obliterans. However, none of these studies included young children and infants.

In our series, study patients had significantly more bronchial dilatation than did control patients (P = .02). The sensitivity in our study (50% [three of six]) was generally lower than what has been reported; however, the specificity in our study (100% [15 of 15]) was higher.

The difference between the sensitivity and specificity in our study and those previously reported may be the result of sample size differences or the non–breath-hold CT technique. None of the control patients had bronchial dilatation; thus, the calculation of an odds ratio involved division by zero, producing an infinite odds ratio.

In light of the results of other researchers (6), the specificity in our study is likely inflated. If in our study bronchial dilatation had been found in one of the control patients (that is, if specificity had been 93% instead of 100%), our results still would have been significant with an odds ratio of 14 (95% CI: 1.1, 185.6). This suggests that bronchiolitis obliterans is at

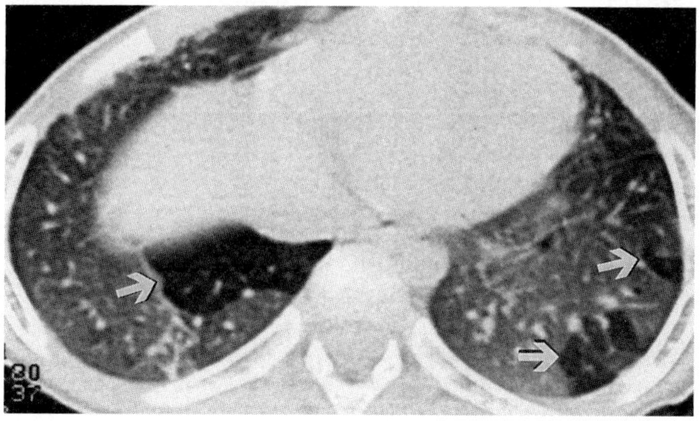

Figure 5. Mosaic perfusion (arrows) in a 3½-year-old girl with chronic bronchitis after lung transplantation. Thin-section CT demonstrates areas of scattered, mixed attenuation accompanied by a decrease in vessel caliber. The presence of mosaic perfusion is not specific for bronchiolitis obliterans.

Sensitivities, Specificities, and 95% CIs

CT Finding	Sensitivity (%)	Specificity (%)
Mosaic perfusion	83 (43, 100)	60 (35, 80)
Bronchial dilatation*	50 (10, 90)	100 (75, 100)
Wall thickening	17 (0, 57)	100 (75, 100)

Note.—Numbers in parentheses are 95% CIs.
* Statistically significant association ($P = .02$, Fisher exact test).

least 14 times more likely if bronchial dilatation is identified. Thus, the presence of bronchial dilatation is highly suggestive of bronchiolitis obliterans.

Mosaic perfusion has been described in transplant recipients with bronchiolitis obliterans, as well as in patients with bronchiolitis obliterans due to other causes (6,21,22). The low-attenuation areas seen with mosaic perfusion are presumed to reflect air trapping and hypoxic vasoconstriction due to obstructed small airways, while the higher attenuation regions are thought to represent relatively normal areas of lung with or without compensatory hyperemia (23). Mosaic perfusion is distinct from mosaic attenuation, which refers to attenuation changes but not to secondary vascular changes.

Sweatman et al (22) performed conventional CT at 10-mm collimation in 15 adult patients with bronchiolitis obliterans due to causes other than lung transplantation and reported mosaic perfusion in 13 patients (87%). Similar thin-section CT findings were reported by Padley et al (21) in 15 (83%) of 18 patients. Medina et al (20) reported the presence of mosaic perfusion in four (67%) of six patients. However, as mentioned above, Medina et al's study described the more acute posttransplantation complications in the immediate 6 months after transplantation. On the other hand, Worthy et al (6) reported on 15 patients with histopathologically proved bronchiolitis obliterans after lung transplantation and found mosaic perfusion in only six (40%). Mosaic perfusion was identified in only four (22%) of 18 control subjects, leading to a specificity of 78% (14 of 18).

In our study, mosaic perfusion was observed more often in infants and children with bronchiolitis obliterans (83%) than in control patients (40%). This difference was not statistically significant ($P = .15$), and the resultant odds ratio was 7.5. If these interrelationships held and the sample size were doubled, these results (including the odds ratio) would be significant. Although the association of mosaic perfusion with bronchiolitis obliterans may not be as strong as that of bronchial dilatation, mosaic perfusion should still be regarded as suspicious for bronchiolitis obliterans.

Bronchial wall thickening has been reported as a finding of bronchiolitis obliterans at thin-section CT; however, it is not a frequent observation. Worthy et al (6) observed bronchial wall thickening in 27% ($n = 4$) of 15 patients with bronchiolitis obliterans and in none of the control subjects, leading to a specificity of 100% (18 of 18). In our study, bronchial wall thickening was noted in only one patient with bronchiolitis obliterans and in none of the control patients.

Expiratory scans help accentuate subtle areas of mosaic perfusion, but they do not appear to increase sensitivity. Worthy et al (6) observed air trapping in 80% of patients with bronchiolitis obliterans and in only 6% of the control population, resulting in a specificity of 94% (15 of 16). In that study, all patients with air trapping also had mosaic perfusion. Unfortunately, the detection of air trapping requires expiratory CT, which is not possible in infants and young children who cannot hold their breath.

Similar to reported results in adults, mosaic perfusion, bronchial dilatation, and bronchial wall thickening are seen more often in infants and young children with bronchiolitis obliterans than in control patients. In our study, bronchial dilatation was significantly associated with bronchiolitis obliterans syndrome, and mosaic perfusion was suggestive of this syndrome. Although the sample size was small, our findings support the continued use of thin-section CT as an adjunctive study to confirm the diagnosis of bronchiolitis obliterans syndrome. Further prospective studies with larger numbers of patients are warranted to evaluate the cardinal findings of obstruction in infants and young children.

References

1. Cooper JD, Billingham M, Egan T, et al. A working formulation for the standardization of nomenclature and for clinical staging of chronic dysfunction in lung allografts. J Heart Lung Transplant 1993; 12:713–716.
2. Yousem SA, Berry GJ, Brunt EM, et al. A working formulation for the standardization of nomenclature in the diagnosis of heart and lung rejection: lung rejection study group. J Heart Lung Transplant 1990; 9:593–601.
3. Medina LS, Siegel MJ, Bejarano PA, Glazer HS, Anderson DJ, Mallory GB. Pediatric lung transplantation: radiographic-histopathologic correlation. Radiology 1993; 187:807–810.
4. Morrish WF, Herman SJ, Weisbrod GL, Chamberlain DW. Bronchiolitis obliterans after lung transplantation: findings at chest radiography and high-resolution CT. Radiology 1991; 179:487–490.
5. Lentz D, Bergin CJ, Berry GH, Stoehr C, Theodore J. Diagnosis of bronchiolitis obliterans in heart-lung transplantation patients: importance of bronchial dilatation on CT. AJR 1992; 159:463–467.
6. Worthy SA, Park CS, Kim JS, Müller NL. Bronchiolitis obliterans after lung transplantation: high-resolution CT findings in 15 patients. AJR 1997; 169:673–677.
7. Gerhardt T, Hehre D, Bancalari E, Watson H. A simple method for measuring functional residual capacity by N2 washout in small animals and newborn infants. Pediatr Res 1985; 19:1165–1169.
8. Hanson JS, Shinozaki T. Hybrid computer studies of ventilatory distribution and lung volume. I. Normal newborn infants. Pediatrics 1970; 46:900–914.
9. Gerhardt T, Reifenberg L, Hehre D, et al.

Functional residual capacity in normal neonates and children up to 5 years of age determined by a N_2 washout method. Pediatr Res 1986; 20:668–671.
10. Godfrey S, Bar-Yishay E, Arad I, Landau LI, Taussig LM. Flow-volume curves in infants with lung disease. Pediatrics 1983; 72:517–522.
11. Taussig LM, Landau LI, Godfrey S, Arad I. Determinants of forced expiratory flows in newborn infants. J Appl Physiol 1982; 53:1220–1227.
12. Spray T. Pediatric lung transplantation. Semin Thorac Cardiovasc Surg 1992; 4:113–121.
13. Austin JHM, Müller NL, Friedman PJ, et al. Glossary of terms for CT of the lungs: recommendations of the Nomenclature Committee of the Fleischner Society. Radiology 1996; 200:327–331.
14. Siegel S, Castellan NJ. Nonparametric statistics for the behavioral sciences. 2nd ed. New York, NY: McGraw-Hill, 1988; 103–111.
15. Keller CA, Cagle PT, Brown RW, Noon G, Frost AE. Bronchiolitis obliterans in recipients of single, double, and heart-lung transplantation. Chest 1995; 107:973–980.
16. Keenan RJ, Bruzzone P, Paradis IL, et al. Similarity of pulmonary rejection patterns among heart-lung and double-lung transplant recipients. Transplantation 1991; 51:176–180.
17. Kramer MR, Stoehr C, Whang JL, et al. The diagnosis of obliterative bronchiolitis after heart-lung and lung transplantation: low yield of transbronchial lung biopsy. J Heart Lung Transplant 1993; 12:675–681.
18. Chamberlain D, Maurer J, Chaparro C, Idolor L. Evaluation of transbronchial lung biopsy specimens in the diagnosis of bronchiolitis obliterans after lung transplantation. J Heart Lung Transplant 1994; 13:963–971.
19. Lynch DA, Brasch RC, Hardy KA, Webb WR. Pediatric pulmonary disease: assessment with high-resolution ultrafast CT. Radiology 1990: 176:243–248.
20. Medina LS, Siegel MJ, Glazer HS, et al. Diagnosis of pulmonary complications associated with lung transplantation in children: value of CT versus histopathologic studies. AJR 1994; 162:969–974.
21. Padley SPG, Adler BD, Hansell DM, Müller NL. Bronchiolitis obliterans: high resolution CT findings and correlation with pulmonary function tests. Clin Radiol 1993; 47:236–240.
22. Sweatman MC, Millar AB, Strickland B, Turner-Warwick M. Computed tomography in adult obliterative bronchiolitis. Clin Radiol 1990; 41:116–119.
23. Eber CD, Stark P, Bertozzi P. Bronchiolitis obliterans on high-resolution CT: a pattern of mosaic oligemia. J Comput Assist Tomogr 1993; 17:853–856.

Vascular Lesions in Children: Percutaneous MR Imaging–guided Interstitial Nd:YAG Laser Therapy—Preliminary Experience[1]

Frank K. Wacker, MD
Dietmar Cholewa, MD
Andre Roggan, PhD
Andreas Schilling, MD
Jürgen Waldschmidt, MD
Karl-Jürgen Wolf, MD

Index terms:
Angioma, 9*.31[2], **.362[3]
Blood vessels, abnormalities, 9*.14
Interventional procedures, in infants and children, 9*.1269
Lasers, interstitial therapy, 9*.1269
Magnetic resonance (MR), guidance, 9*.1269, **.121411, **.121416
Magnetic resonance (MR), temperature monitoring, 9*.1269
Skin, diseases, 40.362, 9*.362, **.362

Radiology 1998; 208:789–794

Abbreviation:
ILT = interstitial laser therapy

[1] From the Departments of Radiology (F.K.W., A.S., K.J.W.) and Pediatric Surgery (D.C., J.W.) and the Laser Medicine Technology Center (A.R.), Benjamin Franklin Hospital, Free University Berlin, Hindenburgdamm 30, D-12200 Berlin, Germany. From the 1996 RSNA scientific assembly. Received November 19, 1997; revision requested February 6, 1998; revision received March 23; accepted April 23. **Address reprint requests to** F.K.W. (e-mail: *wacker@ukbf.fu-berlin.de*)

[2] 9* Vascular system, location unspecified

[3] ** Multiple body systems

PURPOSE: To investigate the use of magnetic resonance (MR) imaging to guide interstitial laser therapy of deep hemangiomas and vascular malformations in children.

MATERIALS AND METHODS: Sixteen children aged 3 months to 16 years with symptomatic vascular lesions underwent percutaneous laser treatment. MR imaging guidance of the laser applicator and online thermomonitoring with MR imaging were performed with a 0.2-T open MR system. Follow-up studies were performed 2 days and 6 weeks after thermotherapy.

RESULTS: Interactive positioning of the laser applicator was possible in all patients. Online thermomonitoring was possible in 122 of 137 therapy spots (89%). There was a good correlation between volumes of coagulated tissue on intraprocedural T1-weighted images and volumes of coagulated tissue on follow-up T2-weighted images. At 6-week follow-up, MR imaging demonstrated a reduction in lesion size in 10 patients (mean reduction, 72%) and an increase in lesion size in two patients (mean increase, 134%). Clinical symptoms improved in 14 of 16 patients (88%).

CONCLUSION: MR imaging–guided laser therapy appears to be a safe and potentially effective minimally invasive treatment for selected children with vascular lesions.

Hemangiomas and vascular malformations are among the most difficult therapeutic dilemmas in medicine. The patients present with a myriad of clinical symptoms. Therapeutic intervention should be considered in all patients with such complications as ulceration, infection, hemorrhage, consumption coagulopathy (Kasabach-Merritt syndrome), rapid growth, compression of vital structures, and high-output cardiac failure. Even after therapy, recurrence is a common problem in these patients. They typically seek help from a number of physicians. Therapy varies with the type and size of the lesion and should involve a multidisciplinary approach that includes drug treatment, embolization techniques, surgical resection, and laser therapy (1–9).

Laser-induced thermotherapy has proved to be effective in the management of hemangiomas and vascular malformations (1,3,6,9). The advantage of this technique is the precise delivery of energy to tissue with minimal damage to adjacent structures. For relatively superficial lesions, palpation or ultrasonography (US) is sufficient to guide the laser applicator (6,8,10). However, there are situations in which the lesion cannot be safely and effectively managed with these guidance techniques. Moreover, a display of the spatial temperature distribution within and around the lesion is often necessary when vital structures are involved. Magnetic resonance (MR) imaging provides both optimal soft-tissue contrast with exact demonstration of the lesion and surrounding structures and the possibility of monitoring temperature changes (11–15).

The purpose of our study was to investigate the use of guidance with an open, low-field-strength MR imager in interstitial laser therapy (ILT) of vascular malformations.

Author contributions:
Guarantors of integrity of entire study, J.W., K.J.W.; study concepts, F.K.W., D.C.; study design, F.K.W., D.C., A.R., A.S.; definition of intellectual content, J.W., K.J.W.; literature research, F.K.W., D.C.; clinical studies, F.K.W., D.C.; experimental studies, A.R.; data acquisition, F.K.W., D.C., A.S.; data analysis, F.K.W., A.S., A.R.; statistical analysis, A.S., A.R.; manuscript preparation, F.K.W., D.C.; manuscript editing, F.K.W., A.S.; manuscript review, K.J.W., J.W.

MATERIALS AND METHODS

From March 1996 to July 1997, 329 children were referred to our hospital for treatment of vascular lesions. At an interdisciplinary clinical conference, treatment guidelines were recommended on the basis of the sizes and locations of the lesions and the clinical symptoms. Laser therapy is a common part of our treatment regimen because many such patients are referred by other hospitals, where they could not be treated with conventional methods. MR imaging guidance was selected for ILT when other guidance methods were not appropriate because of poor sonographic visualization of the lesion or limited access to it.

Sixteen patients aged 3 months to 16 years with symptomatic vascular lesions were treated with MR imaging–guided ILT. All parents gave written informed consent for participation in the study, and the Declaration of Helsinki principles were followed. The lesions were classified as hemangiomas in four patients and vascular malformations in 12 on the basis of the patient history, results of clinical examination, and histologic findings (16). Patient data, lesion locations and types, symptoms, and prior therapies are given in Table 1.

ILT was performed jointly by radiologists and pediatric surgeons (F.K.W., D.C.). For all patients, general anesthesia was induced on the imaging table in the MR imaging suite. Such anesthesia was absolutely necessary because laser-induced thermotherapy is painful and the patients were relatively young. Before laser treatment, all patients received antibiotics (50 mg/kg cefotiam hydrochloride [Spizef; Takeda Pharma, Aachen, Germany] and 5 mg/kg gentamicin sulfate [Refobacin; Merck, Darmstadt, Germany]).

TABLE 1
Patient and Lesion Characteristics

Patient No./ Age/Sex	Lesion Location	Lesion Type*	Symptoms and Other Problems	Therapies prior to MR Imaging–guided ILT
1/8 y/F	Thigh	Venous	Pain, palsy	US-guided ILT
2/14 y/M	Thigh	Venous	Pain	US-guided ILT, direct embolization
3/2 y/F	Retroperitoneum	Mixed (venous and lymphatic)	Severe scoliosis, pain	Steroids, resection
4/16 y/F	Buttocks	Venous	Palsy	US-guided ILT
5/9 y/M	Thigh	Arteriovenous	Pain, weakness	ILT
6/6 y/M	Thigh	Venous	Pain	ILT
7/12 y/F	Retroperitoneum	Mixed (mainly lymphatic)	Bleeding	Rectoscopic mucosal laser therapy, endoscopic US–guided ILT, systemic steroid therapy
8/3 y/F	Posterior to sternum	Hemangioendothelioma (Kaposi sarcoma–like)	Kasabach-Merritt syndrome, pleural effusion	Thoracoscopic laser therapy, embolization, systemic steroid therapy, interferon
9/4 mo/F	Neck	Hemangioma	Stridor	Tracheoscopic laser therapy
10/1 y/F	Neck	Hemangioma	Bleeding	Embolization
11/5 y/M	Thigh	Venous	Pain	US-guided ILT
12/14 y/F	Anterior to sacrum	Mixed (venous and lymphatic)	Bleeding	Rectoscopic ILT
13/8 mo/F	Retroperitoneum	Lymphatic	Urinary stasis	Steroids
14/2 y/M	Buttocks	Venous	Palsy	Direct embolization
15/6 y/M	Neck and face	Hemangioma	Stridor	ILT
16/4 y/F	Thigh	Hemangioma	Pain, weakness	US-guided ILT

* Based on histologic findings or best clinical diagnosis.

MR Imaging

MR imaging before, during, and after ILT was performed with a 0.2-T imager (Magnetom Open; Siemens, Erlangen, Germany) and a large standard surface coil. The open design of the imager allowed complete monitoring throughout the procedure. Before therapy, conventional T1-weighted spin-echo images (repetition time msec/echo time msec = 450/5, 256^2 matrix, 7–10-mm section thickness, two signals acquired) and T2-weighted fast spin-echo images (5,000/117, 256^2 matrix, 7–10-mm section thickness, one signal acquired) in the axial and sagittal or coronal planes were obtained in all patients. After initial imaging, the optimal entry point and angle to the lesion were determined with an external marker at the entry site and a biplanar short gradient-echo (fast low-angle shot) sequence (66/9, 80° flip angle, 256^2 matrix, 10-mm section thickness, one signal acquired) performed adjacent to the axis of the needle. After marking of the skin, the entry site was sterilely prepared and the walls of the coil were sterilely draped. Follow-up MR imaging with the same T1- and T2-weighted sequences was performed immediately (n = 15), 48 hours (n = 7), and 6 weeks (n = 12) after ILT. No other therapy was performed during the 6-week follow-up.

Laser-induced Thermotherapy

A 14-gauge titanium alloy needle (Somatex, Berlin, Germany) was advanced under MR imaging guidance until the tip was in the lesion. For interactive imaging, the gradient-echo sequence was used, with a 10-second measuring time and three sections obtained parallel to the course of the needle. The middle section was acquired to cover the guidance plane; the two parallel sections were acquired to detect any needle deviation. The success of targeting was confirmed by acquiring an additional section along the needle orthogonal to the guidance plane. After positioning of the needle, a sterile light fiber 600 μm in diameter was introduced and the needle was withdrawn.

A neodymium:yttrium-aluminum-garnet laser unit (Medilas 5100; Dornier Medizintechnik, Germering, Germany) (1.064-nm wavelength, 4–8 W of power) installed outside the MR imaging suite was connected to the fiber. Multifocal ILT (four to 19 therapy spots per patient) was performed in all patients. The mean application time per therapy spot was 293 seconds. Application of energy was terminated when the size of the area with low signal intensity was constant on four subsequent control images. There was usually a single entrance point; after application at each therapy spot, the fiber was partially withdrawn at 2-cm intervals until the border of the lesion was reached. The fiber was then repeatedly advanced together with the needle in a radial-like fashion in several steps and at various angles.

To monitor ILT, T1-weighted gradient-echo (132/9, 80° flip angle, 256^2 matrix, 10-mm section thickness, one signal acquired, 19-second measuring time) and

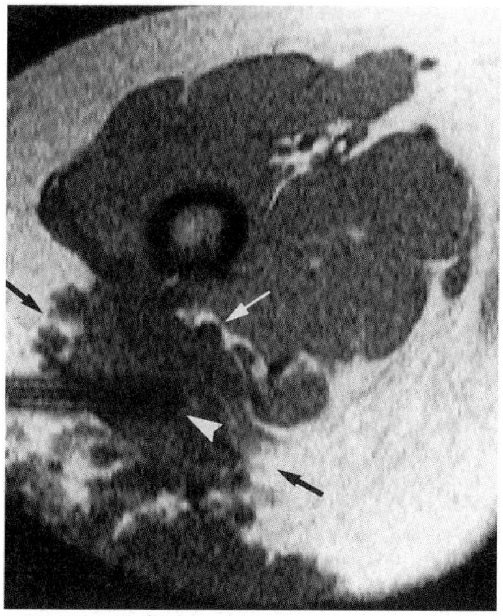

Figure 1. Gluteal angioma. Axial gradient-echo MR image (66/9) obtained through the thigh during ILT shows the susceptibility artifact produced by the needle, which has been advanced into the lesion (black arrows). The relationship of the needle tip (arrowhead) to the sciatic nerve (white arrow) is clearly demonstrated.

fast spin-echo (540/24, echo train length of five, 256^2 matrix, 10-mm section thickness, one signal acquired, 18-second measuring time) images were repeatedly acquired during energy application and 60 and 180 seconds afterward. These sequences were selected on the basis of the temporal resolution of each sequence. The sequence parameters were optimized in a pilot study in explanted pig livers, in which reversible and irreversible signal intensity changes during energy application were correlated with macroscopic changes in liver tissue.

Image Analysis

With commercially available image evaluation software, the total volumes of the lesions were determined before and 6 weeks after therapy by interactively defining the respective irregular regions of interest on a section-by-section basis on T2-weighted images. The T1-weighted images acquired during therapy were analyzed for zones of signal intensity changes. The maximum area of reduced signal intensity was measured in the central section during energy application and compared with the remaining area of decreased signal intensity on posttherapy T1-weighted control images and with the area on posttherapy T2-weighted images. The analysis was performed by two independent, unblinded observers (F.K.W., A.S.). Linear regression analysis was used to compare the areas of reversible signal intensity loss on T1-weighted images with the areas of decreased signal intensity on posttherapy T2-weighted images.

RESULTS

Needle Positioning

Visualization of the susceptibility-induced signal void caused by the needle was sufficient for needle positioning in all patients (Figs 1, 2). Coaxial placement of the laser fiber was possible without any problems. Needle repositioning could be performed on the basis of the thermal effects shown on previous MR images. Because we had no electronic tracking system and the image update time was relatively long, a mean of 49 seconds (range, 15–180 seconds) was needed to find the needle after repositioning.

Monitoring of ILT

In 96 of the 137 therapy spots, the zone of low signal intensity gradually increased on intraprocedural T1-weighted images (maximum diameter, 25 mm) (Fig 2). Seventy-four of these 96 therapy spots showed a slow, homogeneous decrease in signal intensity over time. In 22 of these 96 therapy spots, there was a central area of marked signal intensity loss at the fiber tip that remained stable during and after energy application and could be well identified on follow-up T1-weighted images (Fig 2). In 26 of 137 therapy spots, marked, irreversible signal intensity loss over time was seen at the fiber tip with no peripheral reaction. No signal intensity change was seen in 15 of 137 therapy spots.

ILT was stopped when signal intensity changes were seen adjacent to the carotid artery ($n = 3$), aorta ($n = 1$), vena cava ($n = 2$), or sciatic nerve ($n = 3$). Areas of decreased signal intensity that slowly enlarged during energy application diminished after the laser was shut off; on 3-minute follow-up T1-weighted images, the diameters of these areas were 32%–76% of the maximum diameters on intraprocedural images. There was excellent correlation between the maximum areas on intraprocedural T1-weighted images and posttherapy T2-weighted images (Fig 3).

Clinical and Follow-up Results

The average lesion volume before ILT was 563 cm^3 (range, 88–1,478 cm^3) (Table 2). Analysis of interobserver reproducibility of the measurements yielded an average difference of 8.4% for lesion volume. MR images obtained immediately after ILT showed an increase in lesion size compared with the size on pretherapy images. The increase was most marked on the T2-weighted fast spin-echo images, which showed a mean volume increase of 16.2% ± 9.4 (Fig 4).

At 6-week follow-up, lesion size was reduced in 10 of 12 patients in whom such follow-up was performed (mean reduction, 72.1% ± 13.5). In two of these 10 patients, the symptoms completely resolved after therapy. Subsequent US- or palpation-guided ILT of superficial parts of the lesion was performed in five of the 10 patients and surgery with or without laser therapy was performed in three of the 10 patients after the 6-week follow-up. In two of 12 patients, lesion size was increased at 6-week follow-up (mean increase, 133.5% ± 1.5).

One of the latter two patients had a rapidly proliferating hemangioendothelioma with associated lymphaticlike vessels; her clinical problems—recurrent pleural effusions and Kasabach-Merritt syndrome—improved after the first laser therapy. She underwent steroid therapy in the acute phase of her illness, followed by repeated thoracoscopic laser therapy. The other patient had a massive mixed (lymphatic and venous) malformation and underwent ablative surgery. Both of these patients are still under observation because cure or lesion control has not been achieved.

Complications occurred in two patients. One had a small, superficial area of skin sloughing, which healed with conservative treatment. One patient who underwent ILT of the neck developed pneumonia due to aspiration after tube removal.

DISCUSSION

Hemangiomas and vascular malformations have a variety of anatomic and histologic forms (16). Therapy of these lesions is based on lesion type and symptoms, which may vary with the type and size of the lesion. Management of these lesions can be difficult. There are several therapeutic options; no one method is suitable for treating all lesion types (2,4–7). Steroids have been shown to inhibit angiogenesis, but many hemangiomas are not treatable with steroids (2). Surgical resection can be curative, especially for smaller lesions. Large lesions or lesions that involve vital structures are often not suitable for complete resection (5).

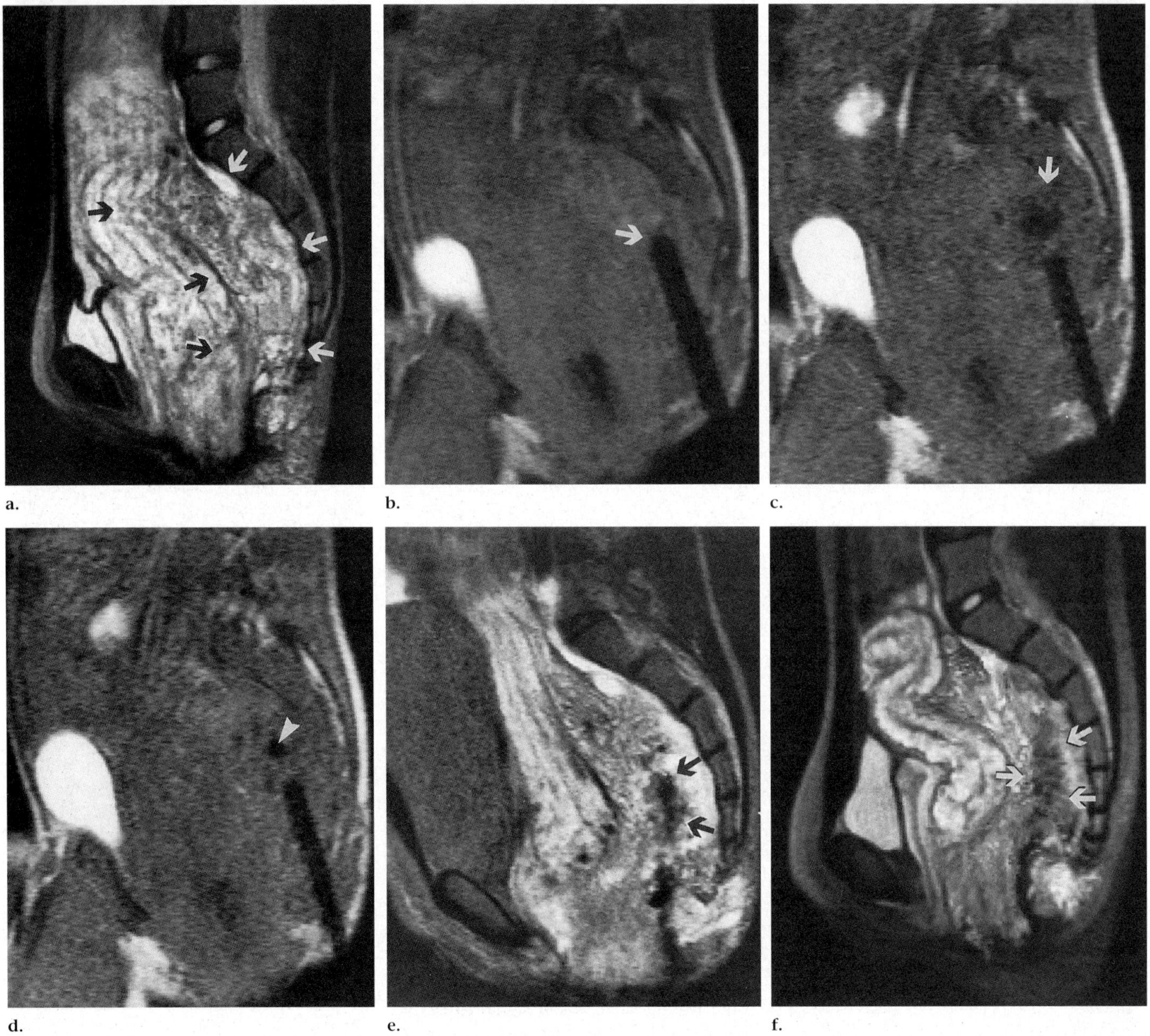

Figure 2. Mixed venous and lymphatic pelvic vascular lesion with presacral mass effect and involvement of the rectum. **(a)** Pretherapy sagittal T2-weighted MR image (5,000/117) shows the lesion (arrows). **(b)** T1-weighted gradient-echo MR image (66/9) shows exact positioning of the needle (arrow). **(c)** T1-weighted gradient-echo MR image (132/9) obtained during ILT shows the maximum area of temperature-induced signal intensity change (arrow). **(d)** T1-weighted gradient-echo MR image (132/9) obtained 3 minutes after ILT shows the central area of irreversible signal intensity loss (arrowhead) adjacent to the fiber tip. **(e)** Control T2-weighted MR image (5,000/117) obtained after ILT shows large zones of low signal intensity (arrows) that represent coagulation necrosis. **(f)** Control T2-weighted MR image (5,000/117) obtained 6 weeks after ILT still shows low-signal-intensity zones (arrows) in the lesion. The presacral mass effect is reduced.

Transcatheter arterial embolization has been used for sole, palliative, and combined (with surgery) therapy of vascular malformations (7,17). The outcome depends on the blood supply to and the blood flow in the lesion (5). Malformations with limited arterial access due to prior surgery or embolization, high-flow lesions with a large venous component, capillary or cavernous hemangiomas, and lymphangiomas may be difficult to embolize. Alternative approaches, such as transvenous embolization and direct injection techniques, have been suggested for inaccessible transarterial malformations (5,17). However, it may be difficult to determine the extent, vascular supply, and nidus of a lesion, especially with a direct injection technique. Both conventional and alternative embolization techniques require fluoroscopic guidance. Complications include catheter adhesion to the vessel wall, alcohol intoxication, ischemia, and permanent skin, nerve, or muscle damage (4,5,18).

Percutaneous ILT of hemangiomas and vascular malformations has several advantages over alternative methods (2,9). It can shrink and cause fibrosis in vascular malformations, rendering subsequent sur-

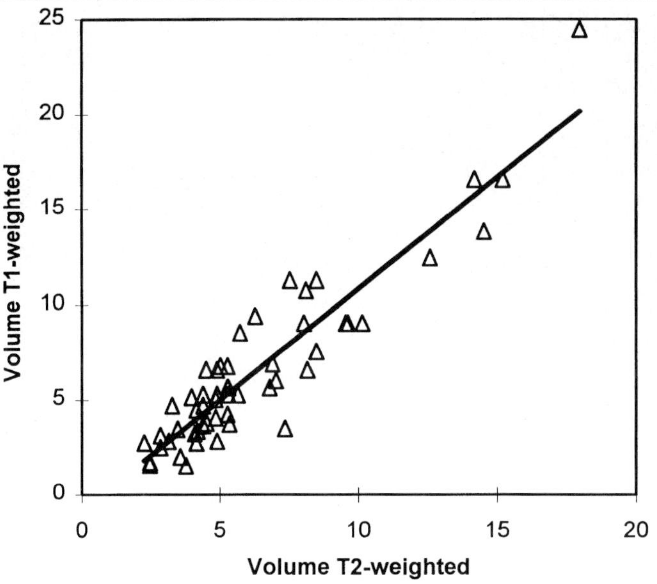

Figure 3. Graph of the diameters (in millimeters) of coagulated tissue volumes on intraprocedural T1-weighted images versus posttherapy T2-weighted images. Slope = 1.17, r = .9266.

TABLE 2
Treatment Summary and Results of Follow-Up

Patient No.	Lesion Volume (cm³) Before ILT	6-week Follow-up	No. of Therapy Spots	Volume Treated (cm³)*	Clinical Outcome
1	712	. . .	6	38 (5.3)	Partial improvement
2	339	121	8	33 (9.7)	Substantial improvement
3	1,478	1,951	6	118 (8.0)	No improvement, continued proliferation
4	670	526	6	86 (12.8)	Substantial improvement
5	88	71	6	37 (42.0)	Substantial improvement
6	201	166	4	28 (13.9)	Partial improvement
7	862	694	16	57 (6.6)	Partial improvement
8	106	143	7	28 (26.4)	Partial improvement, continued proliferation
9	283	200	4	36 (12.7)	Partial improvement
10	818	. . .	7	92 (11.2)	Substantial improvement
11	210	. . .	4	35 (16.7)	Partial improvement
12	1,257	987	19	97 (7.7)	No improvement
13	987	. . .	13	128 (13.0)	Substantial improvement
14	200	149	11	68 (34.0)	Substantial improvement
15	652	400	11	133 (20.4)	Partial improvement
16	143	111	9	77 (53.8)	Partial improvement

* Numbers in parentheses are percentages of untreated lesion volume.

gical excision easier or even unnecessary (6,8). The neodymium:yttrium-aluminum-garnet laser is well suited for interstitial application because it has a greater penetration depth than the argon or carbon dioxide laser. The applied laser energy is mainly converted to heat in the tissue. Thermocoagulation induces a series of microthromboses or infarcts at multiple levels in the lesion (19). The resulting thermal damage is similar to that of surgical resection, but there is only slight damage to the skin surface and the bleeding risk is minimized by coagulation (9,10,19). Unlike with open surgery, sensitive neighboring structures can be protected by using a reliable guidance procedure.

US guidance has proved effective in treating superficial lesions (8,10). However, the soft-tissue resolution of US is relatively poor and does not allow detailed assessment of soft-tissue contrast and tissue changes during laser therapy (15,20,21). With excellent soft-tissue contrast and no exposure to ionizing radiation, MR imaging is the imaging modality of choice for diagnosing deep vascular lesions in children (7,22). It has also proved effective in monitoring thermal changes (13–15,23). Until recently, imager access was poor, which hindered MR imaging–guided positioning and monitoring during therapeutic procedures. Newer, more open magnet designs have facilitated access and thus improved intraprocedural MR imaging. We have shown that MR imaging can be used to localize lesions, guide the laser applicator under near–real-time imaging, and monitor thermal changes with temperature-sensitive methods.

Cost is a major drawback of use of MR imaging to noninvasively monitor temperature during ILT due to the treatment time of 1–3 hours. Despite the cost, MR imaging guidance can be justified relative to less costly methods because of the safety and efficaciousness of the former. Other guidance methods should be considered only if they can provide an optimal overview of the lesion, needle, and adjacent structures. In larger lesions, conventional guidance methods can be combined with MR imaging guidance, with the latter used only in problematic or inaccessible parts of the lesion.

The limitations of MR imaging as a tissue thermometer are well known (11,24,25). Nevertheless, some of the major effects of thermal interaction can be detected with a T1-weighted sequence. Irreversible signal intensity loss can be interpreted as a combination of tissue water loss and altered tissue water mobility due to surrounding central charring and thermonecrosis; the surrounding reversible signal intensity loss is mostly the effect of a rise in temperature (11,12). The assumption that online monitoring with T1-weighted imaging allows estimation of the extent of coagulation necrosis is supported by the good correlation between maximum thermal lesion areas on intraprocedural T1-weighted images and those on postprocedural T2-weighted images. MR imaging currently seems to be the most reliable imaging method for thermomonitoring (12,14,15,21,25). This method may be further improved with temperature-sensitive MR imaging methods (23,24,26), which are not yet available for 0.2-T imagers.

Another drawback of the ILT technique currently in use is that the volume effect is relatively small with conventional applicators. In larger lesions, MR imaging–guided repositioning may be somewhat time-consuming even with an open system that allows interactive MR imaging–guided positioning. The target volume can be enlarged with multispot application (27), but this technique increases the risk of scarring and the invasiveness of the method, especially in hypervascular lesions. Cooled laser applicators that allow substantially higher laser energy may reduce this problem. Perfusion is another problem in ILT of well-vascularized lesions (24). Controlling temperature is difficult because of the strong dependence of temperature on the blood perfusion rate,

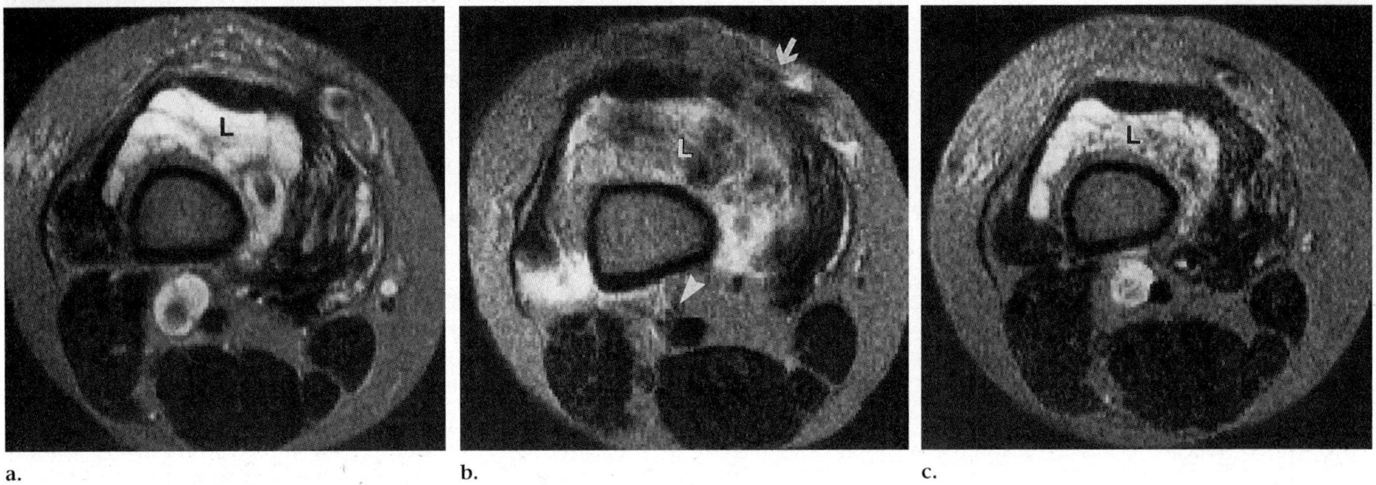

Figure 4. Axial T2-weighted fast spin-echo MR images (5,000/117) of a vascular lesion in the distal thigh. **(a)** Image obtained immediately before ILT shows the lesion (*L*). **(b)** Immediately after ILT, there is swelling of the lesion (*L*) with reduced blood flow in the popliteal vein (arrowhead) and a superficial draining vein (arrow). **(c)** Six weeks after ILT, substantial shrinkage of the lesion (*L*) is seen; blood flow is still reduced compared with that on the pretherapy image (**a**).

which varies considerably within a well-vascularized lesion. Therefore, angiography and embolization have to be considered for all lesions with evidence of high-flow regions on pretherapy images.

Our preliminary results indicate that an open MR imager can be used to guide ILT of hemangiomas and vascular malformations in children. Tissue changes during laser therapy can be monitored with MR imaging. In combination with other therapies, such as steroids and embolization, MR imaging–guided ILT may replace ILT guided by more invasive methods.

References

1. Rosenfeld H, Sherman R. Treatment of cutaneous and deep vascular lesions with the Nd:YAG laser. Lasers Surg Med 1986; 6:20–23.
2. Enjolras O, Riche MC, Merland JJ, Escande JP. Management of alarming hemangiomas in infancy: a review of 25 cases. Pediatrics 1990; 85:491–498.
3. Landthaler M, Hohenleutner U. Laser treatment of congenital vascular malformations. Int Angiol 1990; 9:208–213.
4. Ashinoff R, Berenstein A, Geronemus RG. Arteriovenous malformation treated with embolization and laser therapy. Arch Dermatol 1991; 127:642–644.
5. Gomes AS. Embolization therapy of congenital arteriovenous malformations: use of alternate approaches. Radiology 1994; 190:191–198.
6. Apfelberg DB. Intralesional laser photocoagulation: steroids as an adjunct to surgery for massive hemangiomas and vascular malformations. Ann Plast Surg 1995; 35:144–148.
7. Yakes WF, Rossi P, Odink H. How I do it: arteriovenous malformation management. Cardiovasc Intervent Radiol 1996; 19:65–71.
8. Waldschmidt J, Cholewa D, Hoffmann K, Schier F. Die behandlung von lymphangiomen im kindesalter mit dem Nd:YAG-laser. In: Waidelich W, Staehler G, Waidelich R, eds. Laser in der medizin. Berlin, Germany: Springer-Verlag, 1996; 355–359.
9. Achauer BM, Chang CJ, Vander Kam VM. Management of hemangioma of infancy: review of 245 patients. Plast Reconstr Surg 1997; 99:1301–1308.
10. Werner JA, Lippert BM, Hoffmann P, Rudert H. Nd:YAG laser therapy of voluminous hemangiomas and vascular malformations. Adv Otorhinolaryngol 1995; 49:75–80.
11. Jolesz FA, Bleier AR, Jakab P, Ruenzel PW, Huttl K, Jako GJ. MR imaging of laser-tissue interactions. Radiology 1988; 168:249–253.
12. Kahn T, Bettag M, Ulrich F, et al. MRI-guided laser-induced interstitial thermotherapy of cerebral neoplasms. J Comput Assist Tomogr 1994; 18:519–532.
13. Matsumoto R, Mulkern RV, Hushek SG, Jolesz FA. Tissue temperature monitoring for thermal interventional therapy: comparison of T1-weighted MR sequences. JMRI 1994; 4:65–70.
14. Vogl TJ, Mack MG, Müller P, et al. Recurrent nasopharyngeal tumors: preliminary clinical results with interventional MR imaging–controlled laser-induced thermotherapy. Radiology 1995; 196:725–733.
15. Vogl TJ, Weinhold N, Müller PK, et al. Erste klinische erfahrungen zur MR gesteuerten laserinduzierten thermotherapy (LITT) von lebermetastasen im präoperativen einsatz. ROFO 1996; 164:413–421.
16. Mulliken JB, Glowacki J. Hemangiomas and vascular malformations in infants and children: a classification based on endothelial characteristics. Plast Reconstr Surg 1982; 69:412–422.
17. Dubois J, Garel L, Abela A, Laberge L, Yazbeck S. Lymphangiomas in children: percutaneous sclerotherapy with an alcoholic solution of zein. Radiology 1997; 204:651–654.
18. Behnia R. Systemic effects of absolute alcohol embolization in a patient with a congenital arteriovenous malformation of the lower extremity. Anesth Analg 1995; 80:415–417.
19. Mueller G. In vitro studies using a diode laser (850 nm) for laser induced thermotherapy (LITT). Endosc Surg 1993; 1:1–5.
20. Amin Z, Donald JJ, Masters A, et al. Hepatic metastases: interstitial laser photocoagulation with real-time US monitoring and dynamic CT evaluation of treatment. Radiology 1993; 187:339–347.
21. Mumtaz H, Hall-Craggs MA, Witherspoon A, et al. Laser therapy for breast cancer: MR imaging and histopathologic correlation. Radiology 1996; 200:651–658.
22. Stoever B, Laubenberger J, Niemeyer C, Stahl F, Brandis M, Langer M. Haemangiomatosis in children: value of MRI during therapy. Pediatr Radiol 1995; 25:123–126.
23. Kahn T, Harth T, Schwabe B, Schwarzmaier HJ, Mödder U. MR-tomographische temperaturquantifizierung bei 1.5 T in vitro: vergleich von schnellen parameterbildern und einer phasensensitiven sequenz. ROFO 1997; 167:187–193.
24. Le Bihan D, Delannoy J, Levin RL. Temperature mapping with MR imaging of molecular diffusion: application to hyperthermia. Radiology 1989; 171:853–857.
25. Gewiese B, Beuthan J, Fobbe F, et al. Magnetic resonance imaging–controlled laser-induced interstitial thermotherapy. Invest Radiol 1994; 29:345–351.
26. Young I, Hand J, Kühne S. Modeling and observation of temperature changes in vivo using MRI. Magn Reson Med 1994; 32:358–369.
27. Matsumoto R, Selig AM, Colucci VM, Jolesz FA. Interstitial Nd:YAG laser ablation in normal rabbit liver: trial to maximize the size of laser-induced lesions. Lasers Surg Med 1992; 12:650–658.

Barbara S. Hertzberg, MD
Mark A. Kliewer, MD
James D. Bowie, MD
Patricia J. McNally, BS, RDMS

Index terms:
Fetus, abnormalities, 856.876
Fetus, gastrointestinal tract, 856.876
Fetus, US, 856.1298, 856.12983
Gallbladder, US, 762.1298, 762.12983

Radiology 1998; 208:795–798

[1] From the Department of Radiology, Duke University Medical Center, Box 3808, Rm 24259 Red Zone South, Durham, NC 27710. Received January 30, 1998; revision requested March 19; revision received April 8; accepted May 8. **Address reprint requests to** B.S.H.

Author contributions:
Guarantor of integrity of entire study, B.S.H.; study concepts, B.S.H., M.A.K.; study design, B.S.H.; definition of intellectual content, B.S.H., M.A.K., J.D.B.; literature research, B.S.H., M.A.K.; clinical studies, B.S.H., M.A.K., J.D.B., P.J.M.; data acquisition, B.S.H., M.A.K., J.D.B., P.J.M.; data analysis, B.S.H.; manuscript preparation and editing, B.S.H., M.A.K., J.D.B.; manuscript review, B.S.H., M.A.K., J.D.B., P.J.M.

Enlarged Fetal Gallbladder: Prognostic Importance for Aneuploidy or Biliary Abnormality at Antenatal US[1]

PURPOSE: To test the strength of the association of cholecystomegaly with aneuploidy and biliary abnormality and to assess the prognostic importance of the detection of an enlarged fetal gallbladder at antenatal ultrasonography (US).

MATERIALS AND METHODS: Gallbladder size was prospectively evaluated during 842 consecutive second- and third-trimester US examinations in 775 fetuses. The area of the gallbladder was calculated on the image that depicted the maximal gallbladder size, and the actual gallbladder area was compared with the gallbladder area expected on the basis of the gestational age. Fetuses with an enlarged gallbladder were followed up.

RESULTS: Forty-three fetuses had an enlarged gallbladder (area more than 2 SDs above the mean for gestational age). Outcome was normal in 38 of the 39 fetuses who could be followed up. With the exception of a single baby with an isolated ventricular septal defect, which closed spontaneously, none of the babies with an enlarged fetal gallbladder had structural anatomic defects or evidence of aneuploidy or a biliary tract abnormality.

CONCLUSION: Identification of an enlarged gallbladder at antenatal US does not appear to be associated with a substantially increased risk of chromosomal aneuploidy or biliary tract malformation.

It has been well documented that the fetal gallbladder can be depicted by means of antenatal ultrasonography (US) in the majority of fetuses during the second and third trimesters of pregnancy (1–4). The gallbladder typically changes in size in a predictable fashion with advancing gestational age, although on occasion an unusually large gallbladder, a finding termed "cholecystomegaly," is found. The enlarged fetal gallbladder has been proposed as a marker for aneuploidy and for biliary abnormality (3,5–7). If this association is true, then a systematic assessment of gallbladder size might arguably be an important and useful addition to fetal anatomic US surveys, at least in select cases. The goal of this study was to prospectively test in a large number of fetuses the strength of the association of cholecystomegaly with aneuploidy and biliary abnormality and to ascertain the prognostic importance of the discovery of an unusually large fetal gallbladder.

MATERIALS AND METHODS

The fetal gallbladder was evaluated prospectively during 842 consecutive second- and third-trimester US examinations performed at our institution. A total of 775 fetuses were scanned, as in some fetuses more than one US examination was performed during the course of the study. Indications for US varied but most commonly were either estimation of gestational age, evaluation of fetal anatomy, or assessment of fetal growth.

The upper abdomen of each fetus was carefully scrutinized in an effort to image the gallbladder. Color Doppler US was used as needed to confirm the identification of the gallbladder and to distinguish it from intraabdominal blood vessels, such as the portal or

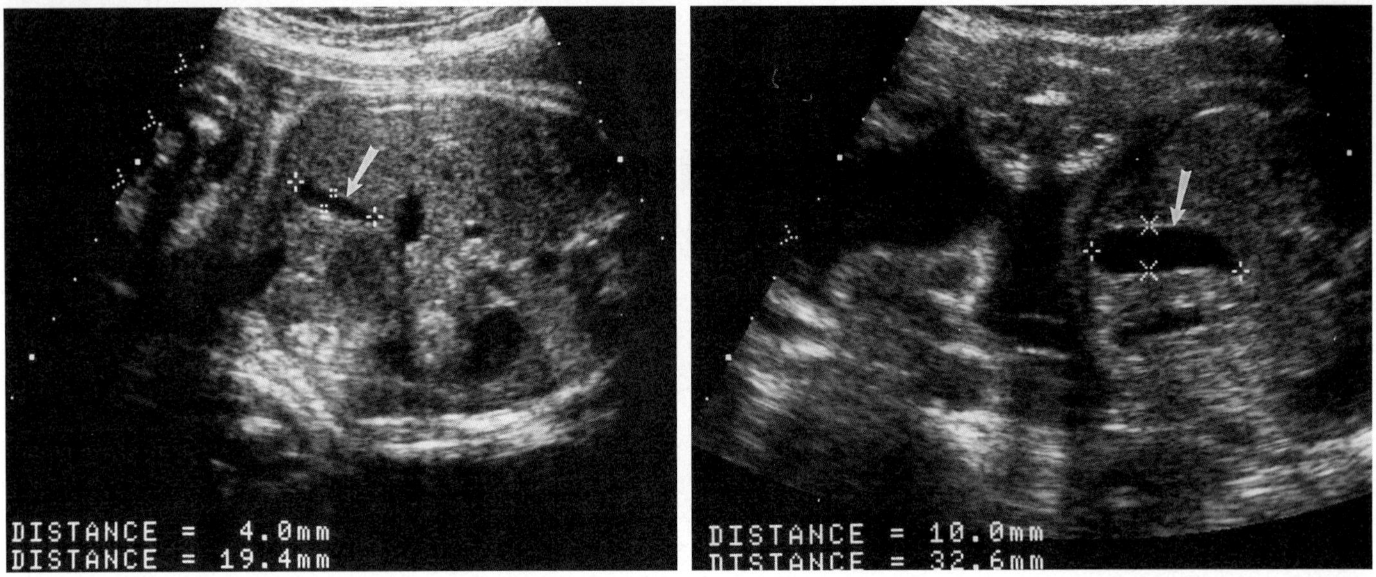

a. b.

Axial US scans of a fetal abdomen depict **(a)** a normal gallbladder (arrow) and **(b)** an enlarged gallbladder (arrow) at 31 weeks gestational age. The length and width of the gallbladder have been measured with electronic calipers.

hepatic veins. If the gallbladder was not identified at the time of the initial search, the fetal abdomen was intermittently rescanned during the course of the US examination in a continued attempt to depict it.

When the gallbladder was seen, it was evaluated prospectively for internal echoes consistent with gallstones. The scanning plane was adjusted to depict the maximal length and width of the gallbladder demonstrable on a single image. Electronic measurement calipers were positioned on the anterior and posterior surfaces of the gallbladder wall to measure its maximal length. Another set of electronic calipers was positioned on the medial and lateral surfaces of the gallbladder wall perpendicular to the long axis of the gallbladder at the level of maximal gallbladder width (Figure). The area of the gallbladder in this plane was then calculated by using the formula for the area of an ellipse: $\pi \times$ length $\times$ width $\div$ 2.

Fetuses were stratified into seven subgroups on the basis of estimated gestational age at the time of US scanning. The mean gallbladder area and SD for each gestational age subgroup were calculated from a data set of 477 fetal gallbladder measurements collected in an earlier large series whose findings were previously published by our laboratory (1) (Table 1). None of the fetuses from the study used to establish gallbladder size standards were included in the current study.

The gallbladder area for each fetus in the current study was compared with the expected gallbladder area for that gestational age subgroup. Fetal gallbladders were considered to be enlarged if their area measured more than 2 SDs above the mean area for the corresponding gestational age subgroup (Table 1).

Follow-up was performed, when possible, in all fetuses with an enlarged gallbladder. Follow-up involved review of pediatric and delivery records, amniocentesis reports, and, when needed, telephone conversations with parents or physicians. For the purposes of this study, outcome was considered normal if the infant was healthy except for the usual childhood illnesses or if the only complications were attributable to prematurity or trauma.

All scans were obtained by using a transabdominal US approach, with a model XP (Acuson, Mountain View, Calif) or HDI (Advanced Technology Laboratories, Bothell, Wash) unit. Linear and curvilinear transducers were used with frequencies ranging from 2.5 to 5.0 MHz. Transducer configuration and scanning frequency were selected to optimize depiction of the fetal gallbladder. All studies were performed by sonologists and sonographers experienced in fetal US.

TABLE 1
Mean Area of Gallbladder and Mean Area Plus 2 SDs according to Estimated Gestational Age

Estimated Gestational Age	Mean Area (mm^2)	Mean Area (mm^2) +2 SD*
12–15 wk 6 d	8.0	17.5
16–19 wk 6 d	17.6	43.9
20–23 wk 6 d	36.3	69.6
24–27 wk 6 d	66.1	134.0
28–31 wk 6 d	78.6	174.4
32–35 wk 6 d	90.5	169.9
36 wk to term	88.3	171.0

Note.—Mean area calculated from 477 fetal gallbladder measurements obtained in a series with previously published findings (1).
* This is the threshold for an enlarged gallbladder.

RESULTS

The gallbladder was seen on 81.9% (n = 690) of 842 US scans, which is similar to the 82.5% rate (477 of 578 US scans) of visualization in the prior study (1) from our laboratory. Table 2 shows the number of fetuses with enlarged gallbladders (area greater than 2 SDs above the mean) as a function of gestational age. An enlarged gallbladder was seen on 43 US scans (5.1%) obtained in 43 fetuses. Enlarged gallbladders were most frequently detected at 20–24 weeks gestational age.

Amniocentesis had been performed in five of the 43 fetuses with an enlarged gallbladder. The karyotype was normal in all five of these fetuses. Antenatal US did

TABLE 2
Fetuses with Enlarged Gallbladders according to Estimated Gestational Age

Estimated Gestational Age	No. of Fetuses with Enlarged Gallbladders*
12–15 wk 6 d (*n* = 26)	2 (8)
16–19 wk 6 d (*n* = 227)	5 (2.2)
20–23 wk 6 d (*n* = 146)	15 (10.3)
24–27 wk 6 d (*n* = 129)	6 (4.7)
28–31 wk 6 d (*n* = 166)	5 (3.0)
32–35 wk 6 d (*n* = 106)	6 (5.7)
36 wk to term (*n* = 42)	4 (10)
All ages (*N* = 842)	43 (5.1)

* Number in parentheses is the percentage.

not depict structural fetal abnormalities in any of the 43 fetuses with an enlarged gallbladder. Polyhydramnios was seen in two pregnancies in which the fetus had an enlarged gallbladder, and subchorionic hematoma was seen in one.

Postnatal follow-up was performed in 39 of the 43 fetuses with an enlarged gallbladder. In the remaining four fetuses, delivery was performed at a different institution, and we were unable to locate the mother for postnatal follow-up. Mean gestational age at the time of delivery was 38.1 weeks (range, 28–41 weeks). The mean duration of follow-up was 8.2 months (range, 1 day to 18 months). Outcome was normal in 38 of the 39 fetuses with follow-up, including the two pregnancies with polyhydramnios and the one with a subchorionic hematoma. One neonate had a membranous ventricular septal defect identified postnatally, but this baby was asymptomatic and had no other abnormalities and no physical features of aneuploidy. The ventricular septal defect closed spontaneously by 11 months of age, and the baby was growing normally, attaining normal developmental milestones at the time of the most recent follow-up examination at 15 months of age.

Echogenic foci consistent with gallstones were seen on three of the 842 US scans. All three fetuses with gallstones were at 28–32 weeks gestational age when the stones were identified. None of the fetuses with gallstones had an enlarged gallbladder. The mean gallbladder area for the three fetuses with gallstones was 69.3 mm^2, compared with a mean gallbladder area of 78.6 mm^2 for fetuses at 28–32 weeks gestational age.

Gallstones were not identified in any of the 43 fetuses with an enlarged gallbladder.

DISCUSSION

Although recent reports have suggested that fetal cholecystomegaly is a potential marker of fetal aneuploidy or a biliary system abnormality (3,5), findings in our larger prospective series do not support this contention. Follow-up findings in 39 fetuses with an enlarged gallbladder (area of more than 2 SDs greater than the area expected for the gestational age) did not reveal evidence of aneuploidy or biliary tract abnormality. In contrast, a previous report (5) had described eight fetuses with cholecystomegaly (also identified by using the 2-SD criterion), and three (38%) of these eight subsequently were shown to have trisomy 13, 18, or 21.

The strikingly different results between the current and previous study (5) might be explained by the retrospective nature of the previous study. In that study (5), additional anomalies were concurrently identified with US in the aneuploid fetuses. Perhaps the presence of these abnormalities led to closer examination of the fetuses in these cases, which would constitute what has been termed "work-up bias" (8). Evaluation of the gallbladder is not a routine feature of the standard obstetric US examination, so an enlarged gallbladder could conceivably have been present but not recognized or reported in many normal fetuses scanned during the same period. In contrast, the gallbladders of all fetuses presenting for second- and third-trimester US were evaluated in our study, regardless of other US findings; thus, our study is less prone to bias and more likely to provide a representative sample of all fetuses with an enlarged gallbladder.

There is little pre- or postnatal evidence that supports a link between an enlarged gallbladder and trisomy 21 or trisomy 18. Fetuses and infants with trisomy 21 can certainly exhibit a multitude of malformations in various body systems, but we could find no report of an association of trisomy 21 with gallbladder anomalies (9–11). As defined, fetal cholecystomegaly is a relatively frequent finding, seen in approximately 5% of fetuses in the current study. Trisomy 21 is also relatively frequent, so we suspect that the finding of fetal cholecystomegaly in a single fetus with trisomy 21 in the prior study (5) may be coincidental. Trisomy 18 also does not appear to be associated with cholecystomegaly: Indeed, the gallbladder abnormality reported in infants with trisomy 18 is hypoplasia, not enlargement (11). Only trisomy 13 has been reported to be associated with an abnormally large gallbladder in children (11).

A potential weakness of the current study is that only a minority of the fetuses with an enlarged gallbladder actually underwent karyotyping. All fetuses who did undergo amniocentesis had a normal karyotype. Furthermore, it seems extremely unlikely that any of the remaining fetuses had a chromosomal abnormality, as none of the babies (with the exception of the single infant with an asymptomatic membranous ventricular septal defect, which resolved spontaneously) had congenital abnormalities or physical features of aneuploidy after birth.

These study findings likewise call into question the contention that a large fetal gallbladder indicates a bile duct abnormality (3). None of the fetuses with a large gallbladder in this study had evidence of obstructive jaundice or any other anomaly of the biliary system after birth. Similarly, although recent reports have suggested an association between cholecystomegaly and fetal gallstones or sludge (6,7), we found that the three fetuses with gallstones in the current study had normal-sized gallbladders. Multiple other reports (12–19) of fetal gallstones did not mention the finding of cholecystomegaly, although none of these reports specifically addressed the issue of gallbladder size. We suspect that there is a wide range of gallbladder sizes in fetuses with gallstones, including contracted, normal-sized, and enlarged gallbladders.

In summary, fetal cholecystomegaly does not appear to be associated with a substantially increased risk for chromosomal aneuploidy or a particular anatomic malformation. The majority of fetuses with an unusually large gallbladder will have a normal outcome, and the isolated finding of an enlarged fetal gallbladder should not be considered an indication for fetal karyotyping. As with gallstones or nonvisualization of the fetal gallbladder, US identification of fetal cholecystomegaly appears to have limited prognostic importance.

Acknowledgments: The authors thank Mitzi K. Daniels for assistance with data entry and Susan M. Murray for assistance with manuscript preparation.

References

1. Hertzberg BS, Kliewer MA, Maynor C, et al. Nonvisualization of the fetal gallbladder: frequency and prognostic importance. Radiology 1996; 199:679–682.
2. Chan L, Rao BK, Jiang Y, Endicott B, Wapner RJ, Reece EA. Fetal gallbladder growth and development during gestation. J Ultrasound Med 1995; 14:421–425.
3. Goldstein I, Tamir A, Weisman A, Jakobi P, Copel JA. Growth of the fetal gallbladder in normal pregnancies. Ultrasound Obstet Gynecol 1994; 4:289–293.

4. Bronshtein M, Weiner Z, Abramovici H, Filmar S, Erlik Y, Blumenfeld Z. Prenatal diagnosis of gallbladder anomalies: report of 17 cases. Prenat Diagn 1993; 13:851–861.
5. Sepulveda W, Nicolaidis P, Hollingsworth J, Fisk NM. Fetal cholecystomegaly: a prenatal marker of aneuploidy. Prenat Diagn 1995; 15:193–197.
6. Petrikovsky B, Klein V, Holsten N. Sludge in fetal gallbladder: natural history and neonatal outcome. Br J Radiol 1996; 69: 1017–1018.
7. Petrikovsky B, Klein VR. Cholecystomegaly and fetal gallstones (letter). Prenat Diagn 1995; 15:875–880.
8. Begg CB. Biases in the assessment of diagnostic tests. Stat Med 1987; 6:411–423.
9. Nyberg DA, Resta RG, Luthy DA, Hickok DE, Mahony BS, Hirsch JH. Prenatal sonographic findings of Down syndrome: review of 94 cases. Obstet Gynecol 1990; 76:370–377.
10. Taybi H, Lachman RS, eds. Radiology of syndromes, metabolic disorders, and skeletal dysplasias. St Louis, Mo: Mosby–Year Book, 1990.
11. Jones KL, ed. Chromosomal abnormality syndromes. In: Smith's recognizable patterns of human malformation. Philadelphia, Pa: Saunders, 1988; 10–25.
12. Nishi T. Ultrasonographic diagnosis of fetal cholelithiasis. J Obstet Gynaecol Res 1997; 23:251–254.
13. Brown DL, Teele RL, Doubilet PM, DiSalvo DN, Benson CB, Van Alstyne GA. Echogenic material in the fetal gallbladder: sonographic and clinical observations. Radiology 1992; 182:73–76.
14. Devonald KJ, Ellwood DA, Colditz PB. The variable appearances of fetal gallstones. J Ultrasound Med 1992; 11:579–585.
15. Klingensmith WC III, Cioffi-Ragan DT. Fetal gallstones. Radiology 1988; 167:143–144.
16. Kiserud T, Gjelland K, Bogno H, Waardal M, Reigstad H, Rosendahl K. Echogenic material in the fetal gallbladder and fetal disease. Ultrasound Obstet Gynecol 1997; 10:103–106.
17. Stringer MD, Lim P, Cave M, Martinez D, Lilford RJ. Fetal gallstones. J Pediatr Surg 1996; 31:1589–1591.
18. Suchet IB, Labatte MF, Dyck CS, Salgado LA. Fetal cholelithiasis: a case report and review of the literature. JCU 1993; 21:198–202.
19. Abbitt PL, McIlhenny J. Prenatal detection of gallstones. JCU 1990; 18:202–204.

Gao-Jun Teng, MD[2]
Michael A. Bettmann, MD
P. Jack Hoopes, DVM, PhD
Robert J. Wagner, MA
Byeong-Ho Park, MD[3]
Li Yang, MD, PhD[4]
Brian R. Baxter, MD

Transjugular Intrahepatic Portosystemic Shunt: Effect of Bile Leak on Smooth Muscle Cell Proliferation[1]

Index terms:
Liver, interventional procedure, 761.1269, 958.123
Shunts, portosystemic, 958.453
Stents and prostheses, 958.1268

Radiology 1998; 208:799–805

Abbreviations:
PTFE = polytetrafluoroethylene
SMC = smooth muscle cell
TIPS = transjugular intrahepatic portosystemic shunt

[1] From the Department of Radiology, Dartmouth-Hitchcock Medical Center, One Medical Center Dr, Lebanon, NH 03756. Received October 31, 1997; revision requested January 5, 1998; final revision received April 27; accepted May 11. **Address reprint requests to** M.B.

[2] Current address: Nanjing Railway Medical College, Nanjing, China.

[3] Current address: Dong-A Medical Center, Pusan, Korea.

[4] Current address: General Military Hospital of PLA, Beijing, China.

PURPOSE: To evaluate the effect of bile on smooth muscle cell (SMC) proliferation in vitro and in vivo in a porcine transjugular intrahepatic portosystemic shunt (TIPS) model.

MATERIALS AND METHODS: In vitro, SMCs explanted from porcine thoracic aorta were cultured with standard techniques. After initial pilot studies, they were subcultured in one of three groups: 1% porcine serum plus 1% bile, 10% porcine serum plus 1% bile, and 10% porcine serum. Cells were harvested at 3, 10, or 14 days, and DNA, protein, and disintegrations per minute (an indicator of proliferation) were measured. In vivo, TIPS creation was successful in 45 swine. All pigs were euthanized at 10–16 days. The proliferative response within the stent was histologically quantified and correlated for evidence of bile leak.

RESULTS: In pilot studies, 2.5%–10.0% bile solutions caused 100% SMC mortality by 3 days. In the presence of 1% bile (with or without porcine serum), both DNA and protein production decreased significantly compared with that in porcine serum alone ($P < .05$). In vivo, 13 of 45 specimens (29%) showed bile leak at gross or microscopic examination. SMC proliferation was less overall in animals with versus those without bile leak (difference not significant).

CONCLUSION: These data suggest that the proliferative response in a TIPS is not primarily due to bile leak. Bile leak may promote thrombosis, but it appears to inhibit myointimal proliferation.

Transjugular intrahepatic portosystemic shunts (TIPS) are widely used for portal decompression in the setting of portal hypertension complicated by variceal hemorrhage or intractable ascites (1,2). Long-term primary patency of TIPS is disappointing, however, with rates of 31%–42%, 51%–60%, and 12% at 1, 2, and 3 years, respectively (3,4). Current interventional techniques performed to treat TIPS occlusion or stenosis are thrombolysis, balloon dilation, and placement of an additional stent. The efficacy of limited TIPS then is due to the high frequency and poor understanding of TIPS stenosis.

TIPS restenosis in humans is caused primarily by proliferation of myofibroblastic tissue (pseudointimal proliferation) (5–8). This pseudointimal proliferation results from smooth muscle cell (SMC) proliferation and collagen deposition by these SMCs, thereby producing a "neoarterialisation" of the TIPS (9). Similar histologic characteristics have been previously described in a TIPS porcine model, although the proliferation is much faster and more extensive than that seen in humans (8,10–12).

The mechanism for proliferation within a TIPS may differ from that after arterial stent placement. A TIPS stent bridges the liver parenchyma between a portal vein branch and a hepatic vein, whereas a vascular stent remains intraluminal. Nonetheless, after TIPS creation, to our knowledge, substantial hepatocyte ingrowth into the stent has been identified in only one early study in pigs (10). Several investigators, however, have demonstrated bile duct transection and bile extravasation into a TIPS in both humans and swine (6–8,11,13). This biliary involvement is thought to play a role in pseudointimal

Author contributions:
Guarantors of integrity of entire study, M.A.B., G.J.T.; study concepts, G.J.T., M.A.B., B.H.P.; study design, G.J.T., M.A.B.; definition of intellectual content, G.J.T., M.A.B., P.J.H.; literature research, G.J.T.; experimental studies, G.J.T., R.J.W., L.Y., B.H.P.; data acquisition, G.J.T., P.J.H., R.J.W.; data analysis, G.J.T.; statistical analysis, G.J.T.; manuscript preparation, G.J.T., B.R.B.; manuscript editing, M.A.B.; manuscript review, M.A.B.

proliferation in a TIPS. Stout et al (13) reported a case with a 6.5-month-old TIPS specimen in which biliary epithelial proliferation had formed large cystlike spaces within the pseudointima. Saxon et al (8) described substantial biliary fistulas in seven of nine porcine TIPS and in seven of eight human TIPS with documented severe parenchymal tract stenosis or occlusion. Conversely, these authors observed no substantial biliary injury in patent, nonstenotic parenchymal tracts (13 in humans, and two in pigs).

Currently, the effect of bile leak and bile on pseudointimal proliferation in a TIPS remains unclear. We therefore evaluated the effect of bile on the SMC proliferative response by performing studies in vitro and in an in vivo TIPS porcine model.

MATERIALS AND METHODS

Culture of SMCs

Isolation of porcine SMCs.—Porcine SMCs were harvested from the thoracic aorta of a 25-kg pig by using a previously established explantation method (14). Cells were cultured to the third passage from primary cultures in medium-199 supplemented with 0.2 mmol/mL L-glutamine, 100 U of penicillin, 100 g/mL streptomycin, and 10% fetal bovine serum. (Sigma Chemical, St Louis, Mo) incubated at 37°C in humidified 5% CO_2 and 95% air.

Preparation of bile.—Bile was aspirated from a 27-kg pig under aseptic conditions, filtered by using a 0.45-μm syringe filter (Uniflo; Schleicher and Schuell, Keene, NH), and frozen at −70°C until used.

To determine the appropriate concentration of bile as a culture medium, 10%, 5%, 2.5,% and 1% bile solutions were each used as the culture medium in a pilot study.

Medium preparation.—Three test media were used. On the basis of results in the pilot studies, bile at a concentration of 1% was used in medium-199 plus 10% porcine serum; the three higher concentrations were found to be lethal to SMCs. The three experimental media groups were the following: group 1, medium-199 plus 1% porcine serum plus 1% bile; group 2, medium-199 plus 10% porcine serum plus 1% bile; group 3, medium-199 plus 10% porcine serum.

SMC Culture in Experimental Media

Three days before the experiment, the 10% phosphate-buffered saline solution in the growth medium was replaced with medium containing 10% porcine serum (Sigma Chemical). SMC cultures were established in each group by plating cells at a density of 1 × 10^5 in each well of a six-well plate (Falcon multiwell tissue culture plate; Becton Dickinson, Lincoln Park, NJ). Twenty-four hours after the SMCs were plated, the growth medium was replaced with appropriate experimental growth medium. The medium was changed every 48 hours until harvesting. The SMCs were harvested on days 3, 10, and 14 (six wells per day per group), and results for each of the three groups were compared.

SMC Harvest

The SMCs were harvested by adding 4.5 mL of 0.3-N KOH to each well. SMC protein and DNA were precipitated with 1.5 mL of 0.9-N HCL and 25% trichloroacetic acid solution at 4C° for 24 hours. The precipitate was pelleted and the supernatant discarded. The pellet was resuspended in 1.0 mL of 0.1-N KOH. Aliquots (0.1 mL) of sample were used for DNA assessment, protein assays, and tritiated-thymidine counting.

SMC, DNA, and Protein Assays

Differences in SMC density in each group were measured by using a standard DNA quantification fluorometric technique (15). Aliquots (0.1 mL) of sample were added to 3 mL of fluorometric buffer (100 mmol of NaCl; 10 mmol of ethylenediaminetetraacetic acid, or EDTA; 10 mmol of tromethamine, or tris, 7.0; and 100 hg/mL of fluorescent dye [bisBenzimide, Hoechst No. 33258; Sigma Chemical]) and read in a fluorospectrophotometer (Perkin-Elmer, Norwalk, Conn) with wave-length settings of 365 nm for excitation and 450 nm for emission. Quantification was achieved by comparing sample results with a standard curve generated from calf thymus DNA (Sigma Chemical).

Total protein in the cultured SMCs was measured by using a bicinchoninic acid spectrophotometric assay (BCA Protein Assay Reagent; Pierce, Rockford, Ill) (16). Samples were compared with a standard curve generated from purified bovine serum albumin (Pierce).

Uptake of Tritiated Thymidine

Cellular proliferation was determined by measuring the incorporation of tritiated thymidine. Proliferation rates were quantified by measuring the hydrogen-3-thymidine uptake after a pulse (2 μCi [0.074 MBq] per milliliter per well) 2 hours before harvest. A 0.1-mL aliquot of sample was added to 4 mL of scintillation fluid (Ecolite; IGN, Coasta Mesa, Calif) and disintegrations per minute were counted in a B-scintillation counter (TM Analytic, Elk Grove Village, Ill). Disintegrations per minute were standardized to DNA.

Porcine TIPS Model

TIPS stents were placed in 45 normal (ie, no portal hypertension) domestic swine, each weighing 20–30 kg. In conjunction with other studies to evaluate the effects of different stents, three stent designs were used: in 10 pigs, a tantalum balloon-expandable stent (8 mm [diameter] × 6 cm [length], Cordis, Miami, Fla); in 13 pigs, a stainless steel balloon-expandable stent (8 × 6 mm, Cordis); and in 22 pigs, a Wallstent (8 mm × 6 cm, Schneider, Minneapolis, Minn). The technique and instrumentation used to create the TIPS was similar to that used in humans. Instruments included a coaxial puncture needle (AngioDynamics, Queensbury, NY) and a 9-F sheath and metal cannula (Cook, Bloomington, Ind). The TIPS stent was dilated with a balloon to a final diameter of 8 (n = 19) or 10 (n = 26) mm, as a function of pig size and adequacy of flow.

With anesthesia, before euthanasia, direct portography was performed via a catheter placed in the portal vein by means of direct visualization. Pigs were then euthanized by means of intravenous injection of 15 mL of 30% KCl at 10 (n = 1), 11 (n = 1), 12 (n = 1), 14 (n = 38), and 16 (n = 4) days after TIPS creation. Euthanasia performed before 14 days was due to complicating factors, such as infection. Although data from all pigs were included, analysis of the results focused on findings obtained at 14 days ± 2.

All protocols related to pigs in this study were approved by the Dartmouth Medical School Animal Care and Use Committee.

Necropsy was performed immediately after euthanasia. The TIPS and involved tissue were evaluated by means of gross examination at necropsy, particularly for bile staining in the stent, and preserved for histologic assessment. In all cases, sections were obtained longitudinally or transversely after gross inspection from the areas of apparent bile leak or focal stenosis. After fixation in buffered 4% formaldehyde solution for at least 24 hours, cross sections were routinely cut in each specimen from the central, hepatic, and portal vein regions of the stent. The metal of the Wallstents was removed before embedding. The metal of the Cordis stents was removed after they were embedded by using a hand saw, and the

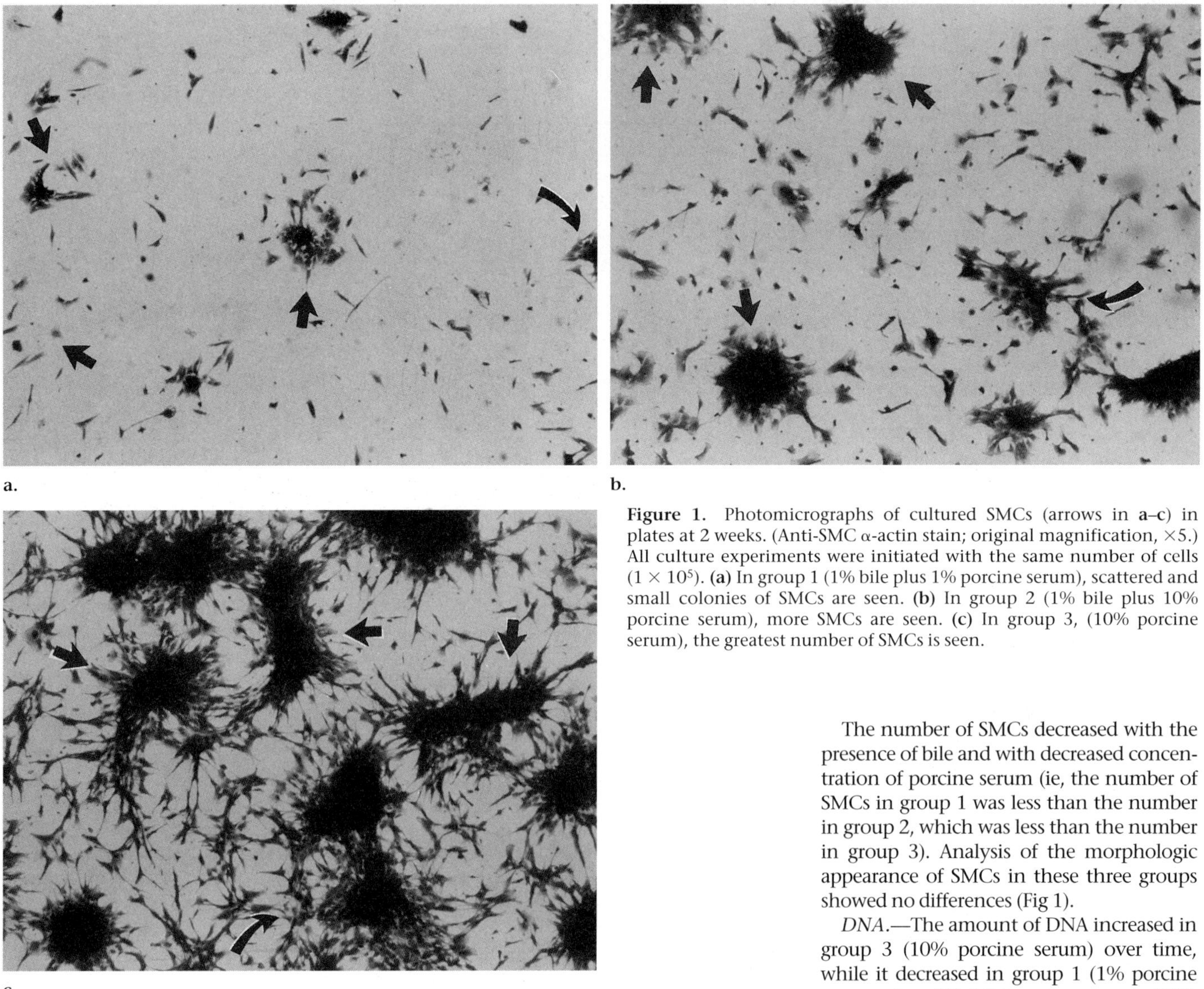

a. b. c.

Figure 1. Photomicrographs of cultured SMCs (arrows in **a–c**) in plates at 2 weeks. (Anti-SMC α-actin stain; original magnification, ×5.) All culture experiments were initiated with the same number of cells (1×10^5). **(a)** In group 1 (1% bile plus 1% porcine serum), scattered and small colonies of SMCs are seen. **(b)** In group 2 (1% bile plus 10% porcine serum), more SMCs are seen. **(c)** In group 3, (10% porcine serum), the greatest number of SMCs is seen.

specimens were subsequently reembedded in JB-4. The tissues were then cut 5-μm thick and stained with modified Giemsa and basic fuchsin. Frozen sections were obtained in three specimens, and immunocytochemistry staining was performed with anti-SMC α-actin to identify SMC in the proliferative reaction.

TIPS stent patency was determined at venography (performed by means of premortal direct catheterization of the portal vein) and autopsy. Histologic quantification included measurement of the thickness of the area from the stent to the lumen (excluding thrombus) and determination of the ratio of the proliferation area to the total lumen area (total area of myointimal proliferation as a percentage of the circular area delineated by the stent mesh). Measurements were performed with standard planimetric techniques. In each pig, samples were taken from the same three areas within the stent: the hepatic venous end, the portal venous end, and the middle.

Values are expressed as the mean plus or minus the standard error of the mean. Analysis of variance, *F* test, and Student *t* test were used for the quantitative data, and χ^2 test was used for the qualitative data. Significance was established by means of a two-tailed test, with *P* less than .05 indicating a statistically significant difference.

RESULTS

In Vitro SMC Studies

In the pilot study, all SMCs cultured in media containing 10% or 5% bile died within 1 day, and all those in 2.5% bile died by day 3.

The number of SMCs decreased with the presence of bile and with decreased concentration of porcine serum (ie, the number of SMCs in group 1 was less than the number in group 2, which was less than the number in group 3). Analysis of the morphologic appearance of SMCs in these three groups showed no differences (Fig 1).

DNA.—The amount of DNA increased in group 3 (10% porcine serum) over time, while it decreased in group 1 (1% porcine serum plus 1% bile) and group 2 (10% porcine serum plus 1% bile). The difference was significant ($P < .05$) among the three groups at all three harvest points (Table 1).

Protein.—In group 1, the amount of protein sharply decreased at 10 days and decreased to zero at 14 days. In group 2, it increased from 3 to 10 days and then decreased remarkably by day 14. In group 3, it increased markedly from days 3 to 10, then decreased moderately at day 14. Compared with findings in the control group (group 3), the amount of protein was significantly less in groups 1 and 2 (each with 1% bile) at all three harvest points ($P < .0001$, Table 1).

Disintegrations per minute.—There were no differences in uptake of H-3-thymidine among all the samples.

In Vivo Studies

Immediately after placement, a patent stent was demonstrated angiographically in all pigs. Pressure gradients were invariably 1–5 mm Hg.

Overall, TIPS malfunction, defined as no flow demonstrated at direct portography, occurred in 33 of 45 pigs (73%). This correlated histologically with either complete obstruction or severe stenosis. A patent stent was seen in 12 pigs (27%). Bile staining in thrombus was identified at autopsy in 13 pigs (29%); in all of these, malfunction had been seen at portography. Five of these pigs had fistulas between the biliary tract and the stent that were seen at venography immediately before sacrifice (Fig 2). No bile leak was evident in the 12 patent stents or in 20 of the 33 malfunctioning stents. Massive thrombus was the primary cause of occlusion in the five TIPS with bile leak. In contrast, pseudointimal proliferative response was the primary contributor to TIPS malfunction in the absence of bile leak. In a subsample, the proliferative reaction was seen to be composed primarily of myofibroblastic cells that morphologically resemble SMCs (confirmed with anti-SMC α-actin staining). Overall, histologic findings in the proliferative reaction were similar in pigs with and those without bile leak, but there was less cellularity and more thrombus in the pigs with bile leak. Additionally, there were few or no endothelial cells covering the luminal surface in pigs with a bile leak. The presence or absence of bile leak did not correlate significantly with the diameter of the original stent (Table 2), although there was a trend toward increased leak in 10-mm-diameter stents (38% vs 16%).

Ingrowth of new bile ducts into the proliferative tissue was histologically verified in eight of the 13 TIPS with bile leak. Histologically, the new bile ducts appeared to have tall columnar epithelium that resembled the bile epithelium seen in adjacent liver. No bile duct cysts were observed in the new bile ducts. These ducts caused 15%–25% of the total occlusion of the TIPS in three of eight pigs with verified ingrowth of new bile ducts (Fig 2e). Such ingrowth was present sporadically and did not contribute significantly to obstruction of the stent in the remaining five pigs.

A single layer of endothelial-like cells was evident in 17 of 32 pigs (53%) without bile leak, whereas no endothelial cells were evident in the 13 pigs with a leak. Ten of the 12 pigs with patent stents had a continuous monolayer of endothelial-like cells covering the luminal surface of the stent. Scattered or discontinuous endothelial-like cells were present in 12 of 22 pigs with occluded stents without bile leak.

Quantification of the proliferative reaction within the TIPS is shown in Table 3. The thickness of proliferation and the ratio of proliferation area to total lumen area in representative stent areas (portal, middle, and hepatic venous regions) in pigs with bile leak were lower than those in pigs without a leak. The differences, however, were not statistically significant.

The number of pigs euthanized at time points other than at 14 days (n = 7) was small, but there were no apparent differences in the components of the occlusive process.

Regarding differences between stents, a bile leak occurred in three of 10 (30%) Cordis tantalum stents, in three of 13 (23%) Cordis stainless steel stents, and in seven of 22 (32%) Wallstents (differences were not statistically significant). Among the 12 patent stents, a Wallstent was in six pigs (six of 22 stents, 27% patent), a Cordis tantalum stent in two pigs (two of 10 stents, 20% patent), and a Cordis stainless steel stent in four pigs (four of 13 stents, 31% patent) (differences were not statistically significant).

TABLE 1
Quantification of DNA and Total Protein in Cultured SMCs

Exposure (d)	Quantity (μg/mL) per Group: 1	2	3	P Value (F test)
DNA				
3	1.40 ± 0.37	1.83 ± 0.31	2.08 ± 0.38	<.05
10	0.22 ± 0.03	1.72 ± 0.12	3.15 ± 0.17	<.01†
14	0.08 ± 0.00	0.44 ± 0.20	3.38 ± 0.44	<.02†
Total protein				
3	124.28 ± 10.14	150.64 ± 4.02	180.18 ± 17.67	<.0001‡
10	31.15 ± 8.99	204.12 ± 10.00	279.24 ± 4.09	<.0001‡
14	0.00 ± 0.00	40.81 ± 15.83	198.12 ± 16.31	<.0001‡

Note.—Group 1, 1% bile plus 1% porcine serum; group 2, 1% bile plus 10% porcine serum; group 3, 10% porcine serum. Data are the mean ± standard error of the mean.

* Group 1 versus group 3, $P < .05$; group 1 versus group 2, difference not significant; group 2 versus group 3, difference not significant.

† $P < .05$ among all groups compared with each other.

‡ $P < .01$ among all groups compared with each other.

TABLE 2
Bile Leak Correlated with Balloon Diameter at TIPS Creation

No. of Pigs	Diameter (mm) of Balloon	No. With Bile Leak*
19	8	3 (16)
26	10	10 (38)

Note.—The difference was not significant (χ^2 test).

* Numbers in parentheses are percentages.

DISCUSSION

The high prevalence of TIPS malfunction, with associated recurrent variceal bleeding or ascites, is the major problem with the overall usefulness of the procedure (4,17). Treatment options for malfunction include balloon dilation and placement of additional stents, but these repeat interventions may be inconvenient, costly, and of limited safety and efficacy. Clearly, to prevent TIPS malfunction, the restenosis process must be fully understood. Unfortunately, it has been easier to document the prevalence, time course, and histologic findings of shunt malfunction than the etiology. Currently, there is little understanding of TIPS stenosis or occlusion at the cellular or molecular biologic level.

Findings in histopathologic studies (5–12) in humans and swine demonstrate myofibroblastic or SMC proliferation as the main histologic feature of TIPS stenosis. Thrombus formation and inflammatory reaction have also been described. These findings suggest that TIPS malfunction is multifactorial. There is some evidence, seconded by opinion, that bile duct injury and bile leak may play a role in TIPS malfunction (6,8,11–13).

Bile duct lacerations and bile staining of surrounding pseudointima in patients after TIPS creation were first mentioned, to our knowledge, by LaBerge and her colleagues (6). They suggested that bile duct transection is a cause of TIPS occlusion and that bile may play a role in pseudointimal proliferation. In addition, Nishimine et al (11) demonstrated that the prevalence of early TIPS malfunction in pigs was decreased by using a stent-graft covered with polytetrafluoroethyl-

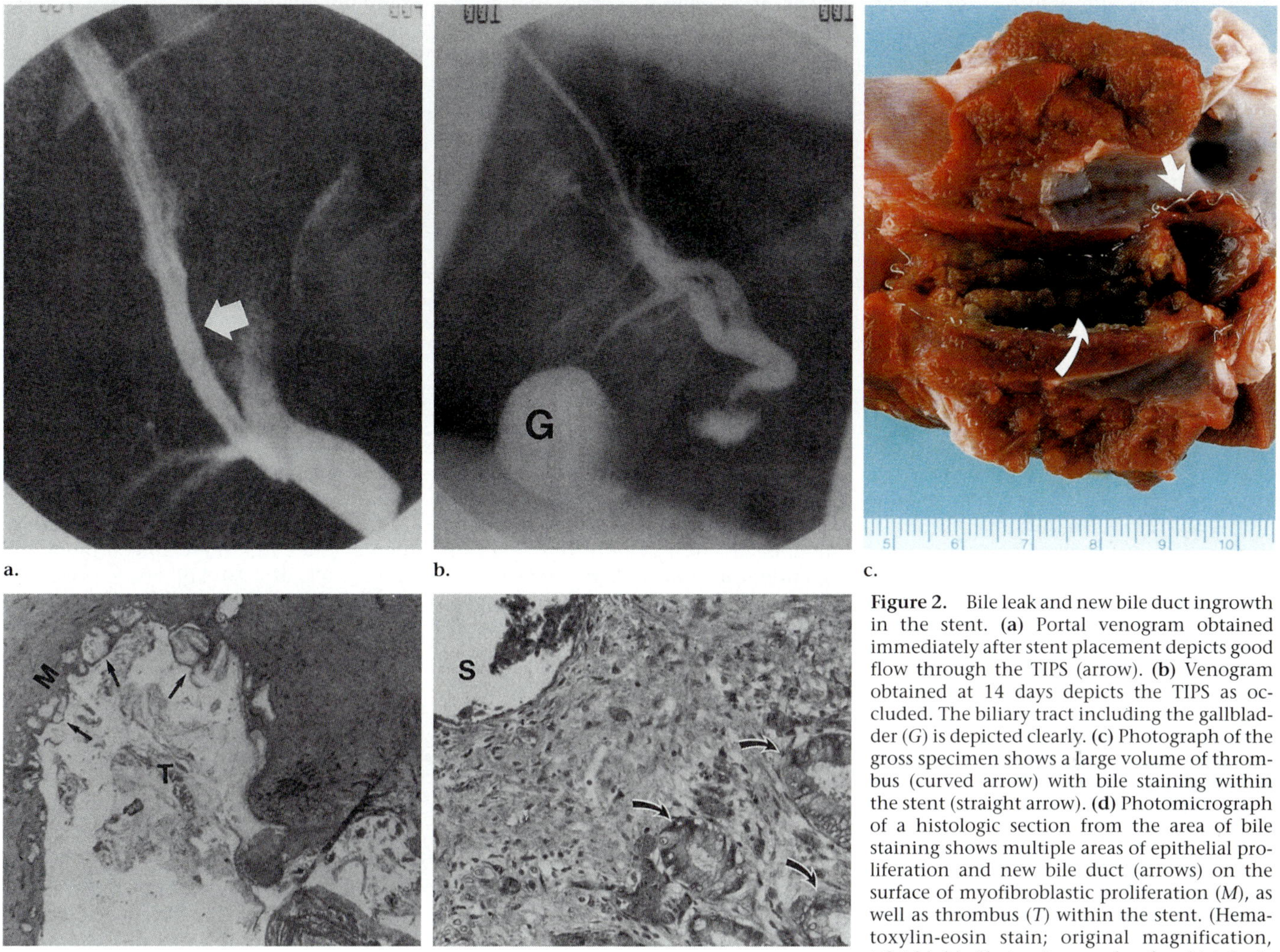

a. b. c. d. e.

Figure 2. Bile leak and new bile duct ingrowth in the stent. **(a)** Portal venogram obtained immediately after stent placement depicts good flow through the TIPS (arrow). **(b)** Venogram obtained at 14 days depicts the TIPS as occluded. The biliary tract including the gallbladder (*G*) is depicted clearly. **(c)** Photograph of the gross specimen shows a large volume of thrombus (curved arrow) with bile staining within the stent (straight arrow). **(d)** Photomicrograph of a histologic section from the area of bile staining shows multiple areas of epithelial proliferation and new bile duct (arrows) on the surface of myofibroblastic proliferation (*M*), as well as thrombus (*T*) within the stent. (Hematoxylin-eosin stain; original magnification, ×3.12.) **(e)** Photomicrograph of a histologic section from the area of epithelial proliferation of new bile duct (arrows) shows histologic characteristics of the biliary tract under a stent hole (*S*). (Hematoxylin-eosin stain; original magnification, ×250.)

TABLE 3
Quantification of Histologically Proved Proliferative Reaction within the TIPS: Bile Leak versus No Bile Leak

Venous Region	Thickness* (mm)		*P* Value (*t* test)	Percentage of Proliferation Area to Total Area		*P* Value (*t* test)
	Bile Leak	No Bile Leak		Bile Leak	No Bile Leak	
Hepatic	1.60 ± 0.15	1.65 ± 1.18	.93	47.86 ± 27.61	51.43 ± 28.33	.70
Middle	1.18 ± 0.50	1.71 ± 0.86	.08	40.47 ± 13.75	55.81 ± 23.51	.06
Portal	1.92 ± 0.91	2.27 ± 1.19	.42	59.65 ± 22.57	67.60 ± 28.92	.40
Average	1.47 ± 0.93	1.87 ± 1.10	.18	49.23 ± 23.18	54.45 ± 27.68	.10

Note.—Data are the mean ± standard error of the mean.
* Distance from stent to lumen, including proliferation but excluding thrombus.

ene (PTFE), leading to the theory that intimal hyperplasia was partially related to bile leak into the stent. Findings in a recently reported case demonstrated biliary epithelial proliferation with formation of large cystlike spaces within the pseudointima at the site of TIPS stenosis (13). Stout et al (13) speculated that biliary secretions may stimulate pseudointimal hyperplasia or that cysts themselves may contribute to stenosis (13). In contrast, our data do not support the theory that bile acts as a mitogen for SMC migration and proliferation and the resultant pseudointimal proliferation after TIPS creation. Findings in our in vitro study, despite some limitations, show that bile concentrations between 2.5% and 10% kill SMCs and that 1% bile concentration inhibits SMC proliferation.

There are limitations to this in vitro study. SMCs from healthy porcine aorta rather than from cirrhotic human liver were used, and a limited range of bile concentrations was examined. Further, the effects of bile in vivo may be modulated by local factors. Nevertheless, the observed direct effects of bile on SMC growth do not support prior hypotheses. To our knowledge, however, this is the first attempt to identify the in vitro effects of bile on SMC.

These in vitro results disagree with previous speculation concerning the role of bile leak in TIPS stenosis (6,11), but they are consistent with the in vivo results of our study. The interaction between bile leak and TIPS patency in this study, however, may shed some light on the disparity between clinical conclusions and our in vitro and in vivo findings. The frequency of TIPS malfunction in our porcine model is higher in the group with a bile leak than in the group without a leak, owing to increased thrombus formation in the former. Thrombus was the primary cause of TIPS malfunction in the group with bile leak, whereas myofibroblastic tissue was the major cause of malfunction in the group without bile leak. In a recent study, in humans and swine, Saxon et al (8) concluded that bile duct transection and bile leak are causally associated with TIPS parenchymal tract abnormalities. Those authors suggested that proliferative cholangiocytes that line the newly placed stent may migrate into the lumen and form a direct communication between the bile duct and TIPS lumen. It has been shown that mucin secretion from metaplastic biliary epithelial cells is strongly thrombogenic (18) and may cause early thrombosis of the TIPS; the cholangiocyte proliferative response itself may contribute to delayed stenosis of the TIPS (8). Our data strongly support the hypothesis that bile has a prothrombotic effect in the TIPS. The contribution of cholangiocytes to TIPS malfunction, however, appears to be less important than that suggested in previous investigations (8,13). In our in vivo study, new bile duct proliferation contributing to approximately 15%–25% of the total proliferative response was found in only three of the eight pigs with new bile duct ingrowth. Thus, it is likely that biliary epithelial proliferation will become an important cause of TIPS malfunction only if there is, over time, substantial regression of the myofibroblastic tissue. Although the duration of follow-up in this study was shorter than that in previous studies (8,13), this seems unlikely to happen. A time point of 10–16 days after TIPS creation was chosen for euthanasia in our study, as in our prior in vivo study (12), and necropsy findings showed that marked myofibroblastic proliferation, with occlusion of the TIPS in most animals, occurred by about 14 days.

Endothelialization of the lumen of the TIPS is presumably critical for a durable shunt (8). It is well known that endothelial cells play a key role in regulation of coagulation, anticoagulation, and fibrinolysis, as well as in the myofibroblastic arterial response to injury (19). Removal of the endothelium during angioplasty results in platelet adhesion and aggregation and thrombus formation (20). Currently, to our knowledge, little is known about the effect of bile on endothelium. In our study, as in previous studies (6,8), endothelialization of the TIPS was absent in the presence of a bile leak. Previous research in dogs has demonstrated that endothelial cells from liver sinusoids swell when examined with scanning electron microscopy 24 hours after intravenous injection of bile (21). We therefore believe that a bile leak may predispose to TIPS malfunction by encouraging thrombus formation while decreasing myofibroblastic occlusion by inhibiting SMC proliferation.

Nishimine et al (11) suggested that stent design may alter the rate of bile duct transection during placement, as they observed no bile leak with Z stents (Cook, Bloomington, Ind) but did note it with Wallstents. In our study, there was no significant difference in the frequency of bile leak among the three stent designs evaluated (we did not use Z stents). Conversely, and probably not surprisingly, our data suggest that bile leak may correlate with use of larger stents, which lead to increased biliary injury. Currently, the TIPS diameter optimal for long-term patency is not known (22,23), and it generally is dependent on pressure gradient rather than other considerations. Nevertheless, it is probably worth attempting to use the smallest stent diameter possible to achieve the target pressure gradient of 5–12 mm Hg.

Determination of disintegrations per minute in this study was performed to help detect the proliferation of SMCs. Unexpectedly, the results showed no difference in uptake of H-3-thymidine. Probable explanations include the short incorporation time (15 minutes) used in this study and the possibility that the difference in the uptake among the three groups is not large enough to be detected with our technique.

Transection of bile ducts and consequent bile leak are probably inevitable during TIPS creation. It is, therefore, important to consider means to block the effect of bile on the TIPS. A mechanical method, a PTFE-covered stent-graft, appeared to be useful in swine, presumably by separating the bile from the lumen of the TIPS to a certain extent (11). Ferral et al (24) found improved TIPS patency in humans by using a covered stent-graft, but theirs was a single-armed study with relatively few patients. Further prospective, controlled investigations with long-term follow-up are necessary to clarify efficacy. In addition to technical limitations inherent in the construction and deployment of covered stents, it is uncertain that PTFE-covered stent-grafts can totally exclude bile leak from the TIPS lumen. It is, therefore, critical to investigate other approaches, such as locally released pharmaceuticals or radiation therapy, to solve the problem of TIPS malfunction. However, our quantified in vitro and in vivo results suggest that at least a two-pronged approach is necessary; use of pharmaceuticals that target myofibroblastic proliferation may be insufficient to prevent failure. Development of techniques to address bile-induced TIPS thrombosis or to improve endothelialization may help prevent TIPS malfunction.

In conclusion, findings in our study demonstrate that high concentrations of bile (2.5%–10.0%) kill aortic SMCs in culture, whereas SMCs are inhibited by 1% bile. Additionally, decreased SMC proliferation in TIPS appears to be associated with the presence of bile. The presence of bile leak correlated significantly with TIPS malfunction in swine but as a result of thrombus formation rather than of myofibroblastic proliferation. The effect of bile on thrombus formation may be secondary to mucin secretion from epithelial duct cells, or, perhaps more important, it may inhibit the endothelialization process after TIPS creation. New bile duct ingrowth into the proliferative reaction contributed a relatively small component to the occlusion and in only a small percentage of swine. Questions remain regarding the effects of low (<1%) concentrations of bile and the role of bile composition on SMCs or endothelium.

Practical application: Findings in this study suggest that bile leak may play a role in TIPS occlusion due to thrombus formation. Bile, however, does not stimulate but rather appears to inhibit occlusion by myofibroblastic proliferation. As early occlusion of TIPS in humans is rare, bile leak in TIPS is probably not a detrimental occurrence and may, in theory, actually aid patency. This, however, remains to be proved in the clinical setting.

References

1. Richter GM, Noldge G, Palmaz JC, et al. Transjugular intrahepatic portacaval stent shunt: preliminary clinical results. Radiology 1990; 174:1027–1030.
2. Ochs A, Rossle M, Haag K, et al. The transjugular intrahepatic portosystemic stent-shunt procedure for refractory ascites. N Engl J Med 1995; 332:1192–1197.
3. Haskal ZJ, Cope C, Shlansky-Goldberg R, et al. Three-year outcome in patients un-

dergoing TIPS placement (abstr). JVIR 1996; 7(suppl):152.
4. LaBerge JM, Somberg KA, Lake JR, et al. Two-year outcome following transjugular intrahepatic portosystemic shunt for variceal bleeding: results in 90 patients. Gastroenterology 1995; 108:1143–1151.
5. LaBerge JM, Ferrell LD, Ring EJ, et al. Histopathologic study of transjugular intrahepatic portosystemic shunts. JVIR 1991; 2:549–556.
6. LaBerge JM, Ferrell LD, Ring EJ, Gordon RL. Histopathologic study of stenotic and occluded transjugular intrahepatic portosystemic shunts. JVIR 1993; 4:779–786.
7. Lehr S, Haskal ZJ, Furth EE, Gannon F. Histopathologic analysis of the biologic response to transjugular intrahepatic portosystemic shunts and proposal of a pathogenic model (abstr). JVIR 1997; 8(suppl):180.
8. Saxon RR, Mende-Hartvig J, Corless CL, et al. Bile duct injury as a major cause of stenosis and occlusion in transjugular intrahepatic portosystemic shunts: comparative histopathologic analysis in humans and swine (abstr). JVIR 1996; 7(suppl): 487.
9. Sanyal AJ, Contos MJ, Graham MF. Pathogenesis of TIPS stenosis: neoarterialisation and collagen deposition by smooth muscle cells (abstr). Hepatology 1995; 22(suppl):255.
10. Rosch J, Uchida BT, Putnam JS, et al. Experimental intrahepatic portacaval anastomosis: use of expandable Gianturco stents. Radiology 1987; 162:481–485.
11. Nishimine K, Saxon RR, Kichiawa K, et al. Improved transjugular intrahepatic portosystemic shunt patency with PTFE-covered stent-grafts: experimental results in swine. Radiology 1995; 196:341–347.
12. Teng GJ, Bettmann MA, Hoopes PJ, et al. Transjugular intrahepatic portosystemic shunt in a porcine model: histological characteristics. Presented at the 46th Annual Meeting of the Association of University Radiologists, New Orleans, La, March 25–29, 1998.
13. Stout LC, Lyon RE, Murray GB, Barth MH. Pseudointimal biliary epithelial proliferation and Azhn's infarct associated with a 6½-month-old transjugular intrahepatic portosystemic shunt. Am J Gastroenterol 1995; 90:126–130.
14. Fillinger MF, O'Connor SE, Wagner RJ, et al. The effect of endothelial cell-culture on SMC proliferation. J Vasc Surg 1993; 17:1058–1067.
15. Brunk OF, Jones KC, James TW. Assay for nanogram quantities of DNA in cellular homogenates. Anal Biochem 1979; 92: 497–500.
16. Smith PV, Krohn RI, Hermanson CT, et al. Measurement of protein using bicinchoninic acid. Anal Biochem 1985; 150:76–85.
17. Rossle M, Haag K, Ochs A, et al. The transjugular intrahepatic portosystemic stent-shunt procedure for variceal bleeding. N Engl J Med 1995; 330:165–171.
18. Edwards RL, Sliver J, Richles FR. For the Registry of the Subcommittee on Haemostasis and Malignancy of the Scientific and Standardization Committee, International Society on Thrombosis and Haemostassis. Human tumor procoagulants. Thromb Haemost 1993; 69:205–213.
19. Shireman PK, Pearce WH. Endothelium cell function: biologic and physiologic functions in health and diseases. AJR 1996; 166:7–13.
20. Schwartz RS, Holmes DR Jr, Topol EJ. The restenosis paradigm revised: an alternative proposal for cellular mechanisms (editorial). J Am Coll Cardiol 1992; 20:1284–1293.
21. Kang QS. Intravenous injection of autologous bile in dogs. Dissertation. College of Medicine, Cheom-Buk National University, Takgu, Korea, 1995.
22. Valji K, Bookstein JJ, Roberts AC, et al. Overdilation of Wallstent to optimize portal decompression during transjugular intrahepatic portosystemic shunt placement. Radiology 1994; 191:173–176.
23. Kuhn-Fulton J, Trerotola SO, Harris VJ, et al. Transjugular intrahepatic portosystemic shunt procedure: efficacy of 10-mm versus 12-mm Wallstents. Radiology 1996; 199:658–664.
24. Ferral H, Alcantare A, Kimura Y, Castaneda WR. Transjugular intrahepatic portosystemic shunts: a comparative study using covered and noncovered stents (abstr). JVIR 1997; 8(suppl):181.

Tracy Q. Callister, MD
Bruce Cooil, PhD
Sai P. Raya, PhD
Nicholas J. Lippolis, MD
Donald J. Russo, MD
Paolo Raggi, MD

Coronary Artery Disease: Improved Reproducibility of Calcium Scoring with an Electron-Beam CT Volumetric Method[1]

Index terms:
Arteriosclerosis, 54.76
Calcium
Computed tomography (CT), electron beam, 54.12119
Coronary vessels, calcification, 54.76
Coronary vessels, CT, 54.12111. 54.12119

Radiology 1998; 208:807–814

Abbreviations:
CVS = calcium volumetric score
TCS = traditional calcium score

[1] From the EBT Research Foundation, 64 Valleybrook Dr, Hendersonville, TN 37075 (T.Q.C., S.P.R., N.J.L., D.J.R., P.R.), and the Department of Statistics, Vanderbilt University, Nashville, Tenn (B.C.). Received December 23, 1997; revision requested February 17, 1998; revision received March 6; accepted April 23. **Address reprint requests to** P.R.

S.P.R. is the president of SciImage, Los Altos, Calif, which developed the software used in this study.

See also the editorial by Flamm (pp 571–572) in this issue.

PURPOSE: To assess the variability and reproducibility of a volumetric calcium score calculated with electron-beam computed tomographic (CT) scans of coronary arteries.

MATERIALS AND METHODS: Two sets of electron-beam CT scans were obtained in patients with coronary calcification (group A) or known risk factors for coronary arterial disease (group B). The second set of scans was obtained after a brief interval (group A, n = 52) or after 1 year with no risk modification (group B, n = 27). Traditional (plaque area and attenuation) and volumetric calcium scores were calculated for each patient and lesion.

RESULTS: The median percentage change for individual lesions in group A was 13% for the volumetric and 19% for the traditional score. The overall reduction in error with the volumetric score was 40% ($P < .001$). The median percentage change for group A patient totals was 9% for the volumetric and 15% for the traditional score ($P < .001$). In group B patients, the median volumetric score increased by 44% after 1 year.

CONCLUSION: The volumetric score showed better reproducibility than the traditional score, and its variability was considerably less than the score increase in untreated patients after 1 year. The reproducibility of the volumetric method makes it useful for assessing the progression of coronary arterial disease on serial electron-beam CT studies.

Electron-beam computed tomography (CT) is an extremely sensitive tool for the identification of coronary arterial calcification, which is known to be a marker of coronary arterial disease (1–7). The study of the progression and regression of established coronary atherosclerosis may be one of the most interesting clinical applications of this technology, but thus far this application has been hampered by the limited reproducibility of the calcium score currently in use (7).

To calculate the traditional calcium score (TCS) described by Agatston et al (2), the computer software multiplies the area of a calcified plaque by an assigned coefficient selected on the basis of the highest attenuation measured in the area. Minimal variations in estimated plaque attenuation or area on serial studies obtained in the same patient can result in substantially different score calculations.

In this study, we analyzed the applicability of a volumetric calcium scoring method to electron-beam CT. The score is calculated on the basis of isotropic interpolation, which has been in use in the field of medical imaging for several years (8–11). The value obtained with this method represents a volume and not an abstract number derived from the multiplication of the attenuation and area of a calcified plaque and may have an important application in the study of the progression of atherosclerotic coronary arterial disease.

To analyze the reproducibility of this method, 52 patients underwent two scanning procedures within a few minutes of each other. Twenty-seven additional patients under-

Author contributions:
Guarantors of integrity of entire study, P.R., T.Q.C., B.C.; study concepts, S.P.R., T.Q.C.; study design, P.R., T.Q.C.; definition of intellectual content, P.R.; literature research, N.J.L.; clinical studies, P.R.; experimental device, S.P.R., P.R.; data acquisition, D.J.R., N.J.L.; data analysis, N.J.L., P.R.; statistical analysis, B.C.; manuscript preparation, P.R.; manuscript editing, T.Q.C.; manuscript review, S.P.R., D.J.R.

went two scanning procedures at a 1-year interval without having received any therapy for coronary arterial disease or having made changes to their diet or smoking habits. Our goal was twofold: to assess whether this volumetric method results in improved interscan reproducibility compared with that of the TCS and to verify that the measurement error of the volumetric method is substantially smaller than the increase in plaque size measured after a 1-year follow-up. If our hypothesis should prove to be correct, this volumetric scoring method could be used reliably in follow-up studies of the progression of coronary arterial disease.

TABLE 1
Average TCS and CVS Levels per Lesion by Artery in Group A

Variable and Coronary Artery	No. of Lesions	Minimum	Maximum	25th Percentile	Median	75th Percentile	Mean*
TCS†							
Left anterior descending	112	0.7	546	8	27	63	65 (10)
Right	35	0.5	844	5	20	61	99 (34)
Left circumflex	28	0.7	84	3	11	29	19 (4)
CVS‡							
Left anterior descending	112	0.6	401	7	20	53	49 (8)
Right	35	0.9	628	5	18	60	78 (25)
Left circumflex	28	0.8	65	3	11	26	16 (3)

* Number in parentheses is the standard error of the mean.
† Variable is the mean TCS calculated from the first and second scans.
‡ Variable is the mean CVS calculated from the first and second scans.

MATERIALS AND METHODS

Patients

All patients had measurable coronary arterial calcifications on the initial electron-beam CT scan. Two separate groups of patients were studied: Patients in group A ($n = 52$) underwent two studies within a few minutes of each other after brief ambulation between the studies. The group A patients were consecutive patients referred by primary care physicians for screening purposes. Patients in group B (n = 27), who had known risk factors for coronary arterial disease, underwent two scanning procedures separated by 1 year; during that interval, the patients undertook no risk modification.

To ensure the continuity and homogeneity of the interpretations of findings, a single expert investigator (T.Q.C.) reviewed all scans. The study was conducted according to standard ethical criteria for clinical research and was approved by our internal review board. Written informed consent was obtained from each patient after the nature of the study had been fully explained.

CT Procedures

All patients underwent electron-beam CT with an Imatron C-100 scanner (Imatron, South San Francisco, Calif). Imaging was performed with a 100-msec acquisition time and a 3-mm section thickness. A total of 40 sections were obtained during two breath-holding periods. Scanning was electrocardiographically triggered at 80% of the R-R interval. All areas of calcification within the borders of a coronary artery and that had a minimal attenuation of 130 HU were analyzed. Images were obtained with a 30-cm² field of view (pixel size, 0.586 mm). To avoid scoring miscalculations, scans with artifacts produced by motion, breathing, cardiac arrhythmias, or erroneous electrocardiographic gating were excluded from the study. The TCS and the calcium volumetric score (CVS) were calculated for each individual calcified plaque and for each patient. Analyses of calcified plaques were performed with the aid of software (NetraMD; ScImage, Los Altos, Calif) installed on a workstation.

Calculation of the TCS

The TCS was calculated according to the method described by Agatston et al (2). This score was derived by placing an area of interest over each calcified coronary artery focus that had a minimal attenuation of 130 HU. The computer software measured the plaque area and the maximal attenuation within each region of interest. A score was then calculated by multiplying the measured area by an attenuation coefficient based on the peak CT number (coefficient 1 for peak attenuation = 131–200 HU; coefficient 2 for peak attenuation = 201–300 HU; coefficient 3 for peak attenuation = 301–400 HU; coefficient 4 for peak attenuation ≥ 401 HU). The sum of the individual scores measured within the borders of each coronary artery was used to compute the final TCS.

Calculation of the CVS

The method of isotropic interpolation is described in depth in several specialized publications (8–11). Here, we give a simplified description of the method as it is applied to the extraction of a CVS from electron-beam CT scans. The voxel size on electron-beam CT scans obtained with a 3-mm section thickness and a typical field of view of 30 cm² (pixel size = 0.586 mm) corresponds to $0.586 \times 0.586 \times 3 = 1.03$ mm³.

With the technique of isotropic interpolation, the input data set is sampled at several intermediate cross sections between the original sections (10). For the purpose of calculating the CVS, the size of the intermediate cross sections is chosen to correspond to the size of the pixel in use. In the example given above the voxel size is now $0.586 \times 0.586 \times 0.586 = 0.201$ mm³.

The smaller size of the interpolated voxel allows a more precise volume reconstruction of the structure under analysis compared with that possible with the original voxels. By using a linear intensity distribution calculated on the basis of the plaque attenuation measured at the level of the reference section and the distance of the voxel from the reference section, each interpolated voxel is assigned a numeric value. All voxels with a value greater than 130 are used in the final three-dimensional reconstruction of the calcified plaque. The reconstruction is performed automatically by the software according to a fast, three-dimensional region-growing algorithm, and the plaque is viewed as a series of interconnected voxels with a value greater than 130. The final score is presented as a whole number to facilitate comparison with the TCS, although it actually is a volume estimated as a fraction of a cubic centimeter. For the purpose of presenting it as a whole number, the measured CVS is multiplied by 1,000.

Statistical Analysis

As the basic measure of the relative accuracy of the CVS and the TCS, we used the absolute difference between scan measurements relative to their mean: $|x_1 - x_2| / [(x_1 + x_2)/2] \times 100$, where x_1 is the measurement from the first scan and x_2 is the measurement from the second scan; we

TABLE 2
Variability in the Replication of CVS and TCS: Lesion-by-Lesion Analysis in Group A

Variable	No. of Lesions	Minimum	Maximum	25th Percentile	Median	75th Percentile	Mean*
Percentage change in CVS	175	0	200	4	13	28	22 (2)
Percentage change in TCS	175	0	200	9	19	46	35 (3)
Percentage change in TCS minus percentage change in CVS	175	−55	133	−2	7	21	13 (2)

Note.—Equations for calculating percentage change in CVS and TCS are given in the text.
* Number in parentheses is the standard error of the mean.

refer to this as the percentage change (12,13). For both the CVS and the TCS, the distributions of the percentage change values across lesions and across patients were very positively skewed. Consequently, the range and quartiles (50th [median], 25th, and 75th percentiles) of each distribution provide useful descriptive statistics of the relative accuracy of each measure. To study the relative accuracy of the two methods, we analyzed the differences between the percentage change in the TCS and that in the CVS by lesion and by patient total for group A patients. Finally, we compared the replication error in the measurement of the CVS in group A patients with the change in the CVS in group B patients during the 1-year follow-up. We used analyses of variance to analyze the average difference in the accuracy between the TCS and the CVS per lesion and per patient. The Wilcoxon rank-sum statistic was used to make inferences about median differences in accuracy. To accommodate the positive skew in the distribution of percentage change values, the Mood test was used to analyze the overall median relative accuracy of the CVS. Finally, nonparametric tolerance limits were constructed to interpret the relevance of various levels of the relative change in a patient's CVS.

RESULTS

Table 1 provides a descriptive summary of the distribution of TCS and CVS levels across lesions by type of artery in group A patients, where the level per lesion is the average of the measurements from each of the two scans. Of the 175 lesions, 112 (64%) were in the left anterior descending coronary artery, 35 (20%) were in the right coronary artery, and 28 (16%) were in the left circumflex coronary artery. The distributions of the TCS and CVS levels across lesions were positively skewed so that the mean levels were uniformly higher than the median levels in each artery, and the largest values of both the TCS and the CVS were in the left anterior descending and right coronary arteries.

Group A Lesions: CVS and TCS Reproducibility

Table 2 illustrates the greater overall precision of the CVS relative to that of the TCS by showing the comparison of the distributions of the percentage change in the two types of measurement between scans obtained in group A patients. This table shows that the mean percentage change in the CVS (22%) was substantially lower than that of the TCS (35%) and indicates that there was a 37% overall reduction in error. This comparison of means is misleading given that the distribution of values was positively skewed. However, the findings were confirmed by use of the median percentage change in the CVS across lesions, which was 32% lower than that of the TCS. The median percentage change in both measures was relatively constant across types of artery (for the left anterior descending, right coronary, and left circumflex arteries, respectively, the percentage change in CVS was 14%, 11%, and 14% and that in TCS was 21%, 18%, and 18%). These median values were not significantly different across artery type (P = .65 for CVS and P = .76 for TCS; Mood test for equality).

These summary statistics underemphasize the greater precision of the CVS compared with that of the TCS. To document the statistical significance of the greater precision of CVS measurements, we analyzed the distribution of differences in percentage change values between the TCS and the CVS by lesions. The percentage change in the TCS between scans was larger than that in the CVS for 123 (70%) of the 175 lesions. The median difference by lesion in percentage change values between the TCS and the CVS (ie, [median percentage change in TCS − median percentage change in CVS] × 100) was 7% (95% confidence interval: 4%, 11%) and did not change significantly in an artery-by-artery analysis (P = .66). Thus, the CVS measurements were significantly more precise than those of the TCS (P < .001, Wilcoxon rank-sum test), and this result was consistent across arteries.

Figure 1 shows the regression line for relative change in the CVS versus the corresponding relative change in the TCS for the 175 lesions. (Note that in this case we used the relative change in each measurement, $(x_2 - x_1)/[(x_1 + x_2)/2]$, rather than the absolute percentage change). This analysis indicates that the average variability of the CVS was only 53% as large as that of the TCS.

Figure 2 is a plot of the percentage change in CVS values versus $\ln[1 + [(CVS_1 + CVS_2)/2]]$. This plot shows that the relative accuracy of the CVS improves as the mean CVS per lesion increases. For 120 lesions with an average CVS of greater than 7.5, the median percentage change in the CVS was 8%, whereas the median percentage change for the entire sample was 13% (median improvement, 38%).

Finally, we used analyses of variance to test for patient and artery effects. In one analysis, the effect of "artery" was nested within the "patients" factor. This is appropriate if one assumes that artery effects are potentially different for each patient. For the other analysis, we used type of artery as a covariate with two degrees of freedom. This latter design assumes that the artery effect would be relatively constant across patients. Both analyses indicated that there were no significant differences among arteries or patients with respect to the relative precision of the CVS and TCS (for all effects, P > .6).

Group A Patients: Reproducibility of Total CVS and TCS

Among the 52 patients in group A, the median value of the average CVS and TCS across patients was 58 and 64, respectively. Thirty-nine (75%) of these patients had a mean CVS of less than 210 and a mean TCS of less than 336. The mean percentage change was 18% for CVS and 29% for TCS (22% and 35%, respectively, across lesions), which represents a 38% overall reduction in error. The median percentage change was 9% for the total CVS (25th percentile, 4%; 75th percentile, 20%) and 15% for the total TCS (25th percentile, 9%; 75th percentile, 37%). This measurement error was smaller than that in the analysis of individual lesions, where the median percentage change was 13%

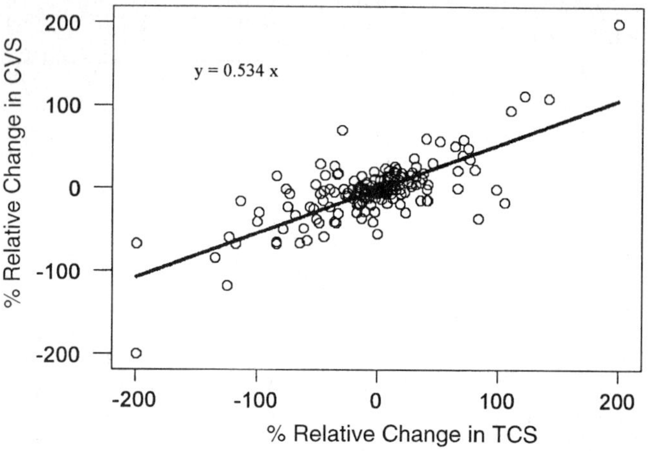

Figure 1. Graph shows the results of the regression of relative changes in the CVS versus relative changes in the TCS per lesion. On average, the variability of the CVS was only 53% as large as that of the TCS.

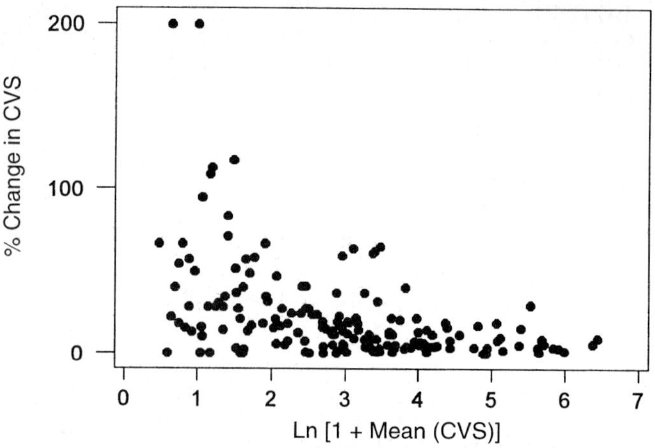

Figure 2. Plot shows the percentage change in the CVS versus ln[1 + [(CVS_1 + CVS_2)/2)] (*Ln[1 + Mean (CVS)]*) per lesion. A value of 2.1 on the x axis corresponds to a CVS of 7.5.

and 19% for CVS and TCS, respectively. The greater accuracy of the total patient scores was expected, because in relative terms sums are usually more stable than individual measurements.

The relative error in CVS measurements was smaller than that in TCS measurements in 38 (73%) of the 52 patient totals. The mean difference in percentage change between the TCS and the CVS patient totals was 12% ± 3 (standard error of the mean), and the median difference was 8% (95% confidence interval: 4%, 14%). This difference between the TCS and the CVS for patient totals was significant ($P < .001$, Wilcoxon rank-sum test).

As was the case with the analysis of individual plaques, there was a tendency for the precision of the repeated measurements of the total CVS to improve above a threshold level, which in this case was established at 30 (Fig 3, Table 3). Accordingly, we conducted a separate analysis of the reproducibility of the CVS in 35 patients with an average CVS greater than 30. We found that the median percentage change in the CVS was 6% (25th percentile, 2%; 75th percentile, 12%), whereas the corresponding median in the entire sample was 9%, as was reported earlier in this article.

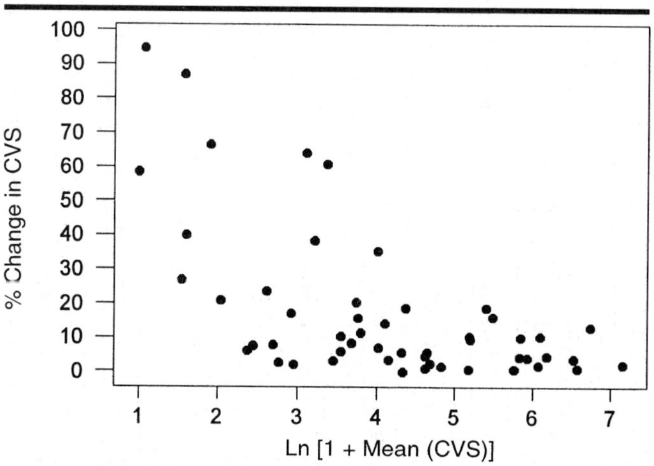

Figure 3. Plot shows the percentage change in CVS versus ln[1 + [(CVS_1 + CVS_2)/2]] (*Ln[1 + Mean (CVS)]*) per patient. A value of 3.4 on the x axis corresponds to a CVS of 30.

Subtraction of the Attenuation Cofactor from the TCS

One of the main reasons for the poor reproducibility of the TCS may be the inclusion in its calculation of an arbitrary attenuation cofactor. To verify this hypothesis, we used the results in 17 group A patients to compare the interscan variability of the CVS, the TCS, and a modified TCS in which the attenuation cofactor was eliminated. These patients were selected because they showed a substantial change in peak plaque attenuation between the first and second CT examinations, with a marked increase in the calculated total TCSs obtained 5 minutes apart. The median percentage change in the CVS, the TCS, and the modified TCS was 13%, 40%, and 25%, respectively. This indicates that a 15% absolute improvement in the percentage change in the TCS (with an improvement in the relative discrepancy between the TCS and the CVS from 68% to 48%) can be obtained simply by eliminating the attenuation cofactor. Of note, the median percentage change for both the CVS and the TCS was higher in this group of patients than in the entire cohort, which probably indicates a selection of particularly difficult cases and the statistical effect of the small number of patients in the subgroup. However, the expected frequency of the occurrence of peak attenuation changes in practice cannot be predicted.

Group B Patients: Relative Change in the CVS

For group B patients, the relative change in CVS was calculated with respect to the initial baseline CVS measurement by using [(CVS_2 − CVS_1)/CVS_1] × 100. All patients in this group had an initial CVS of greater than 30. The variability of the CVS observed in the replication study with patients in group A was small relative to the average change in CVS mea-

TABLE 3
Comparison of CVS between Group A and Group B Patients with CVS Greater than 30

Group	No. of Patients	Minimum	Maximum	25th Percentile	Median	75th Percentile	Mean*
A							
Mean CVS >30†	35	0	36	2	6.0	12	8.0 (1.0)
First CVS >30‡	35	−30	23	−4	−0.7	9	0.8 (2.0)
B‡	27	6	116	21	44.0	82	52.0 (7.0)

* Number in parentheses is the standard error of the mean.
† The measure was $|CVS_1 - CVS_2| / [(CVS_1 + CVS_2)/2] \times 100$, where CVS_1 and CVS_2 are the CVSs from the first and second scans, respectively.
‡ The measure was $[(CVS_2 - CVS_1)/CVS_1] \times 100$, where CVS_1 and CVS_2 are the CVSs from the first and second scans, respectively.

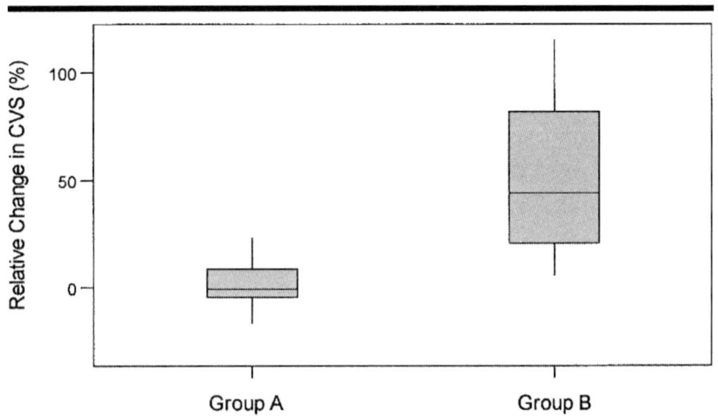

Figure 4. Graph shows the relative percentage change in the CVS in group A patients with an initial CVS greater than 30 and that in the group B patients.

sured in group B patients at the end of the 1-year follow-up. In fact, all patients in group B showed a sizable progression, with an average change of 52% ± 7 and a median change of 44% (95% confidence interval: 28%, 69%). Thus, the median change in the CVS in group B was seven times as large as that in the subsample of 17 group A patients with a mean CVS level greater than 30 (Table 3, Fig 4).

In Table 3, two sets of measurements for the replication of the CVS are given: (*a*) the percentage change calculated according to the method of Bland and Altman (13), which is used throughout this article, and (*b*) the change in the CVS relative to its initial measurement (as described in the preceding paragraph). The latter provides a closer comparison with the method used for the calculation of the change in the CVS in group B patients.

We did not assess the progression of the TCS relative to the average replication error of this method. During the course of our study, it became clear that the CVS was a much more precise measurement than the TCS, and we decided not to use the latter for the purpose of completing the follow-up analysis in group B patients. There are two recent reports (14,15) of the progression of the TCS as measured from follow-up electron-beam CT scans. A study (14) with 3.5-year follow-up results in 81 patients demonstrated an average 24% yearly increase in the TCS. Another study (15) with 29 consecutive patients showed an average increase in the TCS of 59% ± 59 in patients with severe coronary arterial stenosis at angiography and an average increase in the TCS of 11% ± 24 in patients with mild to moderate disease at 1 year. Given the wide interscan variability demonstrated by the TCS in our study (mean variability, 35% ± 3) we considered the precision of this measurement insufficient for estimation of the progression of coronary arterial disease.

Analysis of Tolerance Limits for Error in Measurement of Total CVS Change

The variation in CVS measurements obtained in group A patients represents the reproducibility error, whereas the variation in CVS measurements obtained in group B patients represents actual disease progression, with some replication error. To determine the level of change in the CVS that is indicative of true progression of atherosclerotic disease (rather than simple replication error), we analyzed the tolerance limits of the replication error in the CVS in group A patients with a baseline CVS greater than 30. We concluded that a change of more than 15% is infrequent in patients in whom there has been no atherosclerotic progression. In fact, the replication error exceeded 15% in only four (11%) of 35 patients. Of note, 23 (85%) of the group B patients showed an increase in their CVS above this level at 1 year. Furthermore, a replication error greater than 23% will occur in only 3% of cases, on average. Finally, there is a 2.5% probability that more than 10% of the patients with stabilized coronary arterial disease will show an increase in the CVS greater than 23%.

DISCUSSION

In this study, we assessed the value of a volumetric score—the CVS—to improve the reproducibility of serial electron-beam CT measurements. We carefully excluded from the analysis all cases with misregistration artifacts, because we were interested in the actual reproducibility of this method and its comparison with the traditional scoring method under ideal circumstances. The volumetric method demonstrated superior reproducibility compared with that of the TCS, at both the level of the individual lesion and the level of the total patient score. Reproducibility of the CVS improved even further in patients with a CVS greater than 30. Of note, the variability of the CVS was substantially smaller than the measured increase in the CVS found in untreated patients at the end of 1 year. There are several considerations that help explain our findings.

The main limitations of the TCS reside in the fact that the third spatial dimension of a calcified plaque is not taken into consideration and in the introduction of an arbitrary attenuation scaling factor. Hence, a minimal variation in the area or attenuation of a plaque may cause substantial variability in scoring between repeated CT studies.

The aging of an atherosclerotic plaque entails progressive accumulation of calcium and fibrous tissue (7,16,17). This process may translate into an increase in plaque attenuation over time, with a sub-

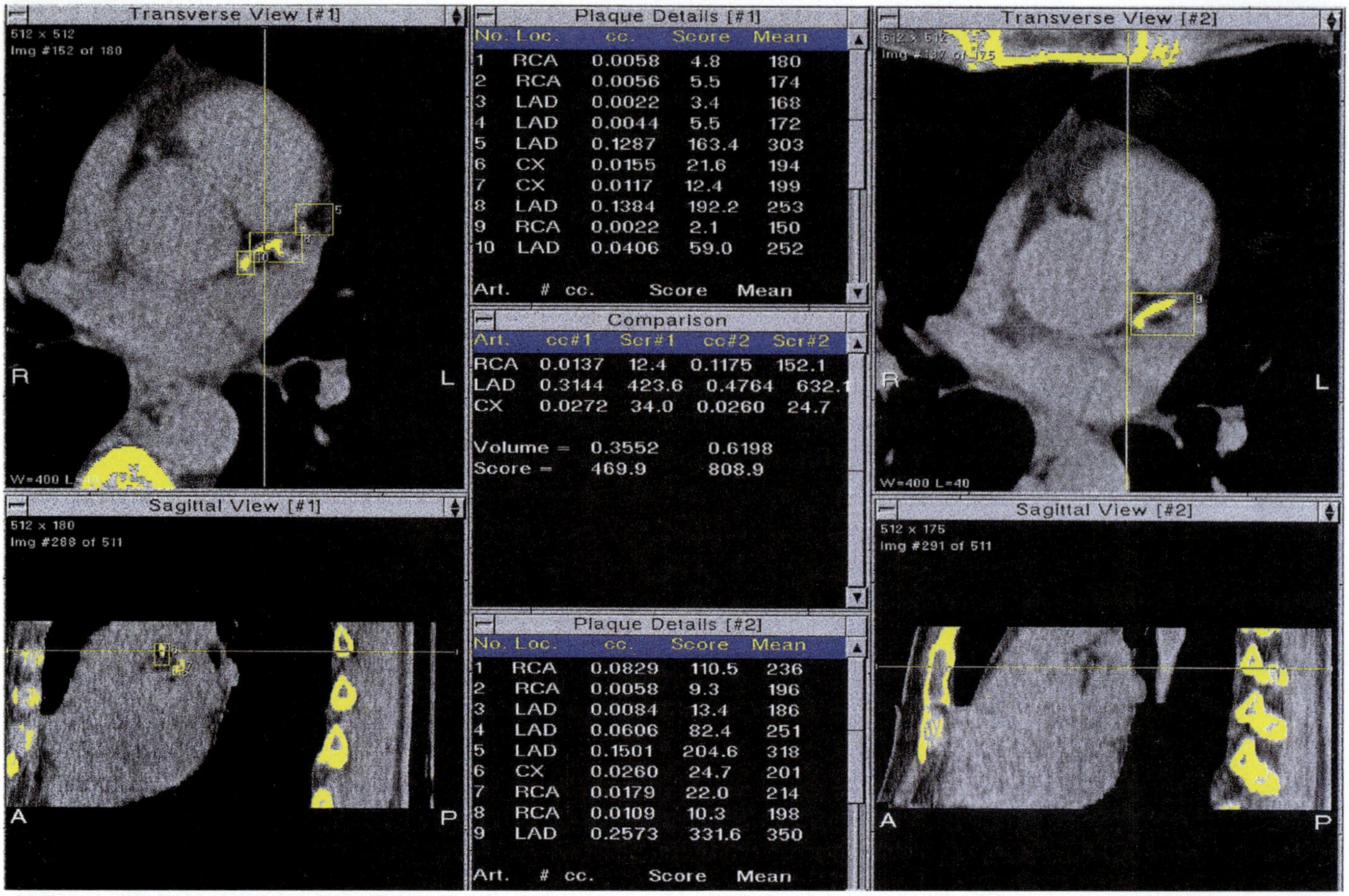

Figure 5. Calcified plaque analysis in the same patient performed with electron-beam CT scans obtained 1 year apart (April 1996 and April 1997). The software automatically highlights in yellow all areas with an attenuation greater than 130 HU. The analysis is conducted with the transverse views (upper right and upper left); the sagittal views (lower right and lower left) allow the interpreting physician to examine the acquired three-dimensional data sets for the presence of motion artifacts. In this case, there were no motion artifacts. A detailed enumeration of each individual plaque detected in the coronary arteries is shown (upper middle and lower middle), with the CVS expressed in cubic centimeters (*cc*). The TCS is reported in the "Score" column, and the mean attenuation of each plaque is reported in the "Mean" column. For comparison with the TCS, the CVS is multiplied by 1,000. A summary of the two studies obtained at a 1-year interval (center) is shown for both the individual artery and the total score. There was progression of disease, with good agreement between the CVS and the TCS. *cc#1* = CVS from April 1996, *cc#2* = CVS from April 1997, *CX* = left circumflex coronary artery, *LAD* = left anterior descending coronary artery, *RCA* = right coronary artery, *Scr#1* = TCS from April 1996, *Scr#2* = TCS from April 1997.

sequent increase in the TCS (18). Because of the use of scalar attenuation coefficients with a sudden shift of the weighting for small changes in attenuation (ie, a coefficient of 2 for an attenuation of 299 HU and a coefficient of 3 for an attenuation of 302 HU), an increase in the TCS may not necessarily indicate an increase in plaque size but rather a simple increase in plaque attenuation. The results of our limited analysis of the reproducibility of the TCS after elimination of the attenuation cofactor support this opinion, although the CVS still showed superior results.

The volumetric score we propose is not directly affected by either the area or the peak attenuation of a plaque, although the minimal attenuation of 130 HU necessary for an interpolated voxel to be included in the reconstructed plaque is determined on the basis of the attenuation in the reference section.

The results of previous analyses (19–22) of the reproducibility of the TCS have confirmed the large interscan variability of this measure. To evaluate the interscan reproducibility of this method, some investigators (19) limited their analysis of calcified coronary arterial plaques to the proximal 12 sections of a 20-section study. With this approach, the core question behind the need for a reproducible test is not addressed: Can the calcium score be used for follow-up studies? If this is the goal, one cannot afford to miss new, small, or peripheral lesions that may be important in future measurements. Other investigators (20) have used log-transform calculations to mathematically (but not practically) reduce the apparent, wide interscan variability of the TCS. Wang et al (12) concluded that the TCS is not accurate enough to use for serial studies in the same patient. In an attempt to improve the reproducibility of the TCS, Wang et al suggested the acquisition of thicker (6-mm) sections. Yet, although such a method could eliminate some of the motion artifacts, it would probably further impair the reproducibility and reliability for serial follow-up studies. In fact, it is conceivable that resorting to thicker sections may result in the neglect of small, new, and softer plaques that may grow to more sizable dimensions in the future.

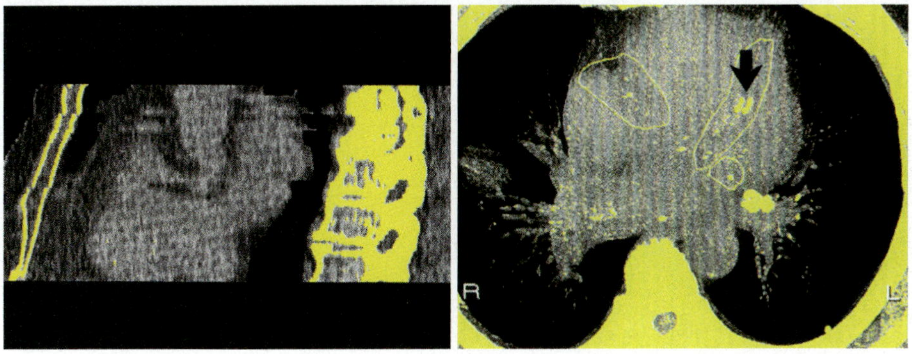

a. b.

Figure 6. (**a**) Sagittal and (**b**) axial electron-beam CT scans in one patient show irregular cardiac borders, indicating the presence of marked motion artifacts. Because of shifting during the examination, a lesion in the middle part of the left anterior descending artery is reproduced twice (arrow in **b**) on the axial view. This "twinning" phenomenon can cause substantial measurement error. As in Figure 5, the yellow highlighting is added automatically by the software to all areas with an attenuation greater than 130 HU.

Because both high sensitivity for the detection of calcified plaques and high calcium score reproducibility are necessary to follow the evolution of coronary atherosclerotic disease, a 6-mm section thickness may not be advisable. This opinion was indirectly supported by the recent observations of Broderick et al (23). They demonstrated improved reproducibility of coronary arterial calcium scoring with the use of helical CT scans by using a volumetric method and lowering to 90 HU the threshold limit for the detection of a calcified plaque.

Several other factors that affect reproducibility should be taken into account. Of importance is the effect of partial volume averaging. The shape of a voxel obtained with electron-beam CT with a 30-cm^2 field of view is that of a parallelepiped with very uneven dimensions of $0.56 \times 0.56 \times 3$ mm. This limits the reliable reproduction of the same plaque when it is imaged in different spatial planes. Further, a newly forming plaque often has an attenuation near to or lower than the minimal necessary attenuation of 130 HU, and bordering voxels may contain only the margins of a forming plaque. This is of great consequence in the calculation of the TCS, because the voxels that contain only part of a calcified plaque may be included in or discarded from the calculation of a final score simply on the basis of the detected average attenuation over the entire voxel. Finally (and always related to the effect of partial volume averaging), a very small plaque may cover one or two voxels at the first examination and three or four voxels at the second, just by virtue of a difference in the patient's position between examinations. A change of a few voxels with regard to such small values may result in a magnified error when mathematic calculations are applied to relative percentage changes. In fact, we demonstrated a greater interscan variability below a minimal threshold score both at the level of the individual lesion and at the level of the total patient score.

Other factors known to affect score reproducibility, such as motion and arrhythmia artifacts, were carefully avoided in our study. However, motion artifacts remain important drawbacks of the current technology (7). Our software allows on-screen visualization of the entire three-dimensional data set and simultaneous analysis of a calcified plaque. This allows the interpreting physician to quickly assess the quality of the acquired data for the presence of motion artifacts before beginning the analysis (Figs 5, 6). More reliable electrocardiographic-triggering mechanisms and faster acquisition times will probably yield further improvements.

The CVS is based on a pathophysiologically sound concept, and in our experience it showed excellent reproducibility. The application of the CVS will render electron-beam CT a highly reliable method for the study of the progression of established coronary atherosclerosis. Our analysis allowed us to determine which level of change in the CVS can be considered to be reliable evidence of the true progression of disease rather than mere replication error, thus providing important information for the practicing physician. Caution should be used when interpreting the small changes in calcified plaques observed on longitudinal studies as representative of clinically relevant disease progression. However, a measured change in the CVS in the range of 15% or greater at the end of follow-up has a high likelihood of representing true progression of disease.

References

1. Blankenhorn DH. Coronary arterial calcification: a review. Am J Med Sci 1961; 42:1–49.
2. Agatston AS, Janowitz WR, Hildner FJ, Zusmer NR, Viamonte M Jr, Detrano R. Quantification of coronary artery calcium using ultrafast computed tomography. J Am Coll Cardiol 1990; 15:827–832.
3. Agatston AS, Janowitz WR. Coronary calcification: detection by ultrafast computed tomography. In: Stanford W, Rumberger JA, eds. Ultrafast computed tomography in cardiac imaging: principle and practice. Mt Kisco, NY: Futura, 1992; 77–95.
4. Stanford W, Thompson BH, Weiss RM. Coronary artery calcification: clinical significance and current methods of detection. AJR 1993; 161:1139–1146.
5. Fallavollita J, Brody A, Bunnell I, Kumar K, Canty J. Fast computed tomography detection of coronary calcification in the diagnosis of coronary artery disease. Circulation 1994; 89:285–290.
6. Mautner GC, Mautner SL, Froehlich J, et al. Coronary artery calcification: assessment with electron-beam CT and histomorphometric correlation. Radiology 1994; 192:619–623.
7. Wexler L, Brundage B, Crouse J, et al. Coronary artery calcification: pathophysiology, epidemiology, imaging methods, and clinical implications—a statement for health professionals from the American Heart Association. Circulation 1996; 94: 1175–1192.
8. Levine D. Multidimensional reconstruction by set-valued approximations. IMA J Numer Anal 1986; 6:173–184.
9. Raya SP, Udupa JK. Shape-based interpolation of multidimensional objects. IEEE Trans Med Imaging 1990; 9:32–42.
10. Raya SP, Udupa JK, Barrett WA. A PC-based imaging system: algorithms, software, and hardware considerations. Comput Med Imaging Graphics 1990; 14:353–370.
11. Raya SP. Low-level segmentation of 3D magnetic resonance brain images: a rule-based system. IEEE Trans Med Imaging 1990; 9:327–337.
12. Wang S, Detrano RC, Secci A, et al. Detection of coronary calcification with electron-beam computed tomography: evaluation of interexamination reproducibility and comparison of three image-acquisition protocols. Am Heart J 1996; 132:550–558.
13. Bland J, Altman D. Statistical methods for assessing agreement between two methods of clinical measurements. Lancet 1986; 1:307–310.
14. Maher JE, Bielak LF, Raz JA, Sheedy PF, Schwartz RS, Peyser PA. Progression of coronary artery calcification (abstr). In: Advances in electron beam computed tomography: 1997—an international scientific symposium. Iowa City, Iowa: University of Iowa Press, 1997; 6.
15. Möhlenkamp S, Pump H, Schimpf S, et al. The progression of calcified plaques dif-

fers in patients with obstructive coronary artery disease: a one year follow-up study by EBCT (abstr). In: Advances in electron beam computed tomography: 1997—an international scientific symposium. Iowa City, Iowa: University of Iowa Press, 1997; 7.
16. Stary HC. The sequence of cell and matrix changes in atherosclerotic lesions of coronary arteries in the first forty years of life. Eur Heart J 1990; 11(suppl E):3–19.
17. Doherty TM, Detrano RC. Coronary arterial calcification as an active problem: a new perspective of an old problem. Calcif Tissue Int 1994; 54:224–230.
18. Janowitz WR, Agatston AS, Viamonte M Jr. Comparison of serial evaluation of calcified coronary artery plaque by ultrafast computed tomography in persons with and without obstructive coronary artery disease. Am J Cardiol 1991; 68:1–6.
19. Hernigou A, Challande P, Boudeville JC, Sene V, Grataloup C, Plainfosse MC. Reproducibility of coronary calcification detection with electron-beam computed tomography. Eur Radiol 1996; 6:210–216.
20. Kajinami K, Seki H, Takekoshi N, Mabuchi H. Quantification of coronary artery calcification using ultrafast computed tomography: reproducibility of measurements. Coron Artery Dis 1993; 4:1103–1108.
21. DeVries S, Wolfkiel C, Shah V, Chomka E, Rich S. Reproducibility of coronary artery calcium scoring with ultrafast CT. Am J Cardiol 1995; 75:973–975.
22. Bielak LF, Kaufmann RB, Moll PP, McCollough CH, Schwartz RS, Sheedy PF II. Small lesions in the heart identified at electron-beam CT: calcification or noise? Radiology 1994; 192:631–636.
23. Broderick LS, Shemesh J, Wilensky RL, et al. Measurement of coronary artery calcium with dual-slice helical CT compared with coronary angiography: evaluation of CT scoring methods, interobserver variations, and reproducibility. AJR 1996; 167: 439–444.

Gregory F. F. Evans, MD
Ronald G. Haller, MD
Philip S. Wyrick, MD
Robert W. Parkey, MD
James L. Fleckenstein, MD

Submaximal Delayed-Onset Muscle Soreness: Correlations between MR Imaging Findings and Clinical Measures[1]

Index terms:
Athletic injuries, 41.491
Extremities, edema, 41.491
Extremities, injuries, 41.491
Muscles, injuries, 41.491

Radiology 1998; 208:815–820

Abbreviations:
CK = creatine kinase
DOMS = delayed-onset muscle soreness
MVC = maximal voluntary contraction
STIR = short inversion time inversion recovery

[1] From the Departments of Radiology (G.F.F.E., R.W.P., J.L.F.) and Neurology (R.G.H., P.S.W.), University of Texas Southwestern Medical Center, 5323 Harry Hines Blvd, Dallas, TX 75235-8896, and the Institute for Exercise and Environmental Health, Presbyterian Medical Center, Dallas (G.F.F.E., R.G.H., P.S.W., R.W.P., J.L.F.). Received October 10, 1997; revision requested December 19; final revision received April 16, 1998; accepted May 8. Supported in part by Specialized Center of Research and Training grant NRA-92-OSSA-12 from the National Aeronautics and Space Administration and a grant from Procter & Gamble. **Address reprint requests to** J.L.F.

Author contributions:
Guarantors of integrity of entire study, J.L.F., G.F.F.E.; study concepts, J.L.F.; study design, J.L.F., R.G.H., R.W.P.; definition of intellectual content, J.L.F., G.F.F.E., R.G.H.; literature research, J.L.F., G.F.F.E.; experimental studies, J.L.F., P.S.W., G.F.F.E.; data acquisition, J.L.F., G.F.F.E., R.G.H., P.S.W.; data analysis, G.F.F.E., P.S.W.; statistical analysis, J.L.F.; manuscript preparation, J.L.F., G.F.F.E., P.S.W.; manuscript editing and review, J.L.F., R.G.H., P.S.W.

PURPOSE: To assess correlations between muscle edema on magnetic resonance (MR) images and clinical indexes of muscle injury in delayed-onset muscle soreness (DOMS) produced by submaximal exercise protocols.

MATERIALS AND METHODS: Sixteen subjects performed 36 elbow flexions ("biceps curls") at one of two submaximal workloads that emphasized eccentric contractions. Changes in MR imaging findings, plasma levels of creatine kinase, and pain scores were correlated.

RESULTS: Both exercise protocols produced DOMS in all subjects. The best correlation was between change in creatine kinase level and volume of muscle edema on MR images, regardless of the workload. Correlations tended to be better with the easier exercise protocol.

CONCLUSION: Whereas many previous studies of DOMS focused on intense exercise protocols to ensure positive results, the present investigation showed that submaximal workloads are adequate to produce DOMS and that correlations between conventionally measured indexes of injury may be enhanced at lighter exercise intensities.

Muscle pain is a frequent result of physical exertion. Such pain occurring hours to days after exercise is termed delayed-onset muscle soreness (DOMS) (1,2). DOMS is particularly associated with eccentric (lengthening) muscle contractions (3–18) and is linked to ultrastructural damage (3–5); increased plasma levels of muscle proteins, especially creatine kinase (CK) (3,6–16,19–24); and edemalike changes in muscle on magnetic resonance (MR) images (3,6,7,25–27). Although soreness would seem to be an undesirable aspect of exercise, eccentric muscle contractions are an effective means of building muscle mass (28). In addition, one episode of DOMS appears to confer a "protective" effect on muscle, in that subsequent bouts of DOMS are less severe than preceding ones (8,9,19–21). This observation helps explain why DOMS tends to be especially severe in those who might benefit most from exercise: the deconditioned. DOMS is associated with sustained decrements in strength (8) and may be of sufficient severity to discourage subsequent exercise, thereby eliminating the health benefit of any newfound exercise program. DOMS can be a cause of serious morbidity, including renal failure from myoglobinuria in extreme, "boot camp" situations (22). Given the concurrent risks and benefits of exercise with eccentric muscle contractions and the incomplete understanding of the pathophysiology, DOMS has been the subject of innumerable published studies over the years, as reviewed elsewhere (1,2).

In the scientific study of DOMS, highly intense exercise protocols have frequently been used to ensure measurable DOMS-related changes (4–6,8–15,17,19,20,23,25). Focus on submaximal exercise is much less common, usually being restricted to protracted bouts of low-intensity contractions (18,22,23) or downhill running (3,16,21). Although high-intensity exercise protocols have yielded useful information, it would be ideal if the counterproductive aspects of attendant excessive soreness could be eliminated. Furthermore, it would be desirable to identify the minimum amount of soreness that remains associated with objective measures of tissue injury, such as an elevated CK level. Given that MR imaging is highly sensitive to muscle edema associated with DOMS (3,6,7,25–27), we proposed to use this tool to objectify muscle damage resulting from exercise that was less intense than in previous studies. If useful in this application, inclusion of edema on MR images as a criterion important to the evaluation of DOMS would potentially alleviate the need for unduly injurious exercise protocols. Hence, we established guidelines for submaximal, eccentric-weighted muscle contractions that reliably cause DOMS. We then analyzed the effects of decreasing the workload on correlations between the various indicators of tissue injury, including proton T1 and T2, volume of muscle edema, CK level, and pain.

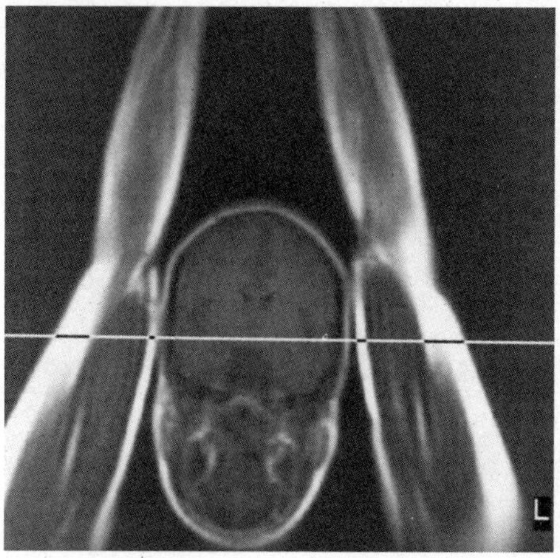

a.

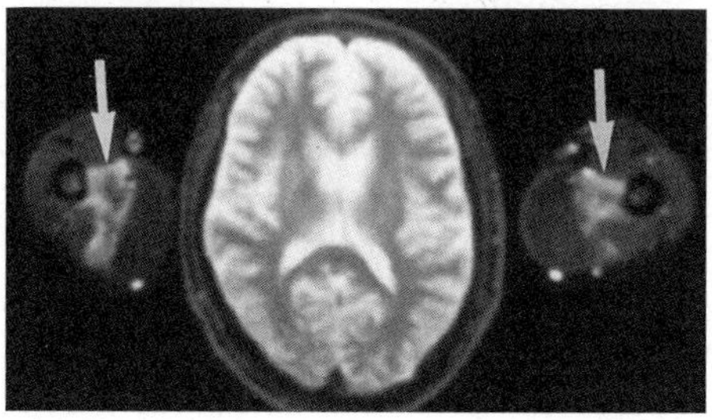

b.

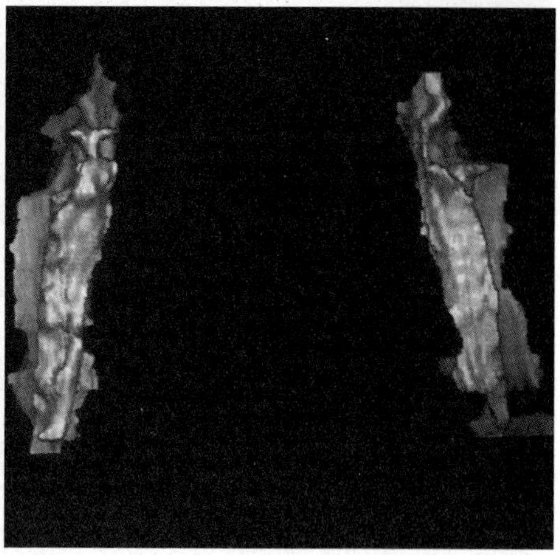

c.

Figure 1. Method of obtaining MR imaging data on edematous muscles in subjects with DOMS. **(a)** Coronal localizing T1-weighted MR image (repetition time msec/echo time msec = 300/15) shows a subject with the shoulders abducted and the arms alongside the head. The line denotes the site of the axial section used for obtaining T1 and T2 measurements. **(b)** Axial short inversion time inversion-recovery (STIR) MR image (2,000/52, 165-msec inversion time) obtained in the same volunteer 48 hours after exercise at 80% MVC force shows obvious hyperintensity in both brachialis muscles (arrows). **(c)** Rendered three-dimensional image from contiguous axial STIR images shows edematous muscle.

MATERIALS AND METHODS

The institutional review board at our institution approved the study, and all subjects provided written informed consent. The subjects were eight men and eight women; all were healthy and took no medications. Each denied performing regular exercise, defined as once a week or more often, or any substantial physical activity (including weight training) in the previous 6 months. Subjects were matched for sex and then randomly assigned to one of two groups. One group performed muscle contractions at 80% of their maximal voluntary contraction (MVC) force; the other group performed contractions at 60% MVC force. There was no statistically significant difference between the groups in terms of age (80% MVC force, 29.0 years ± 5.9; 60% MVC force, 28.6 years ± 8.4), weight (80% MVC force, 172.0 lb ± 24.9 [77.4 kg ± 11.2]; 60% MVC force, 179.5 lb ± 46.0 [80.8 kg ± 20.7]), or height (80% MVC force, 171.8 cm ± 14.6; 60% MVC force, 175.5 cm ± 9.4).

Exercise consisted of elbow flexion (ie, "biceps curls") and was monitored in all subjects by one investigator (P.S.W.). It was performed with a commercially available device (Lifecircuit; Life-Fitness, Irvine, Calif) that exercises both arms at the same time and permits precise setting of the resistance at a fixed percentage of the individual's MVC force. During the concentric (shortening) portion of the curl, the resistance was set at 60% or 80% of the subject's MVC force in an effort to provide one light workload and one moderately more difficult. To accentuate the efficiency of producing DOMS at submaximal workloads, resistance during the eccentric portion of the curl was set at 140% of the resistance during the concentric portion; this setting was the maximal multiple of the concentric force permitted by the device. Each subject performed 36 muscle contractions in three sets of 12 repetitions, with 2 minutes of rest between each set.

Subjects were first instructed in appropriate use of the exercise device during a coaching set of curls. The unit was adjusted for the subject's body, then the subject performed three concentric MVCs, with 2-minute recovery periods between trials. The maximum force value of these three contractions was considered to be the subject's MVC force for the purpose of adjustments in concentric versus eccentric force.

Pain assessment was performed in a manner similar to that described by Tiidus and Ianuzzo (23). The volunteers subjectively assessed the pain experienced during elbow extension, during elbow straightening, and on palpating the sore muscle using an analog scale that ranged from 0 (no pain) to 10 (extremely strong pain) (23). Assessments were made immediately before and after the exercise and at each mealtime and at bedtime for the following 7 days. MR imaging was performed and blood was drawn for determination of CK level before and 48 hours after the exercise. No subject took medication for the pain.

MR imaging was performed with a 1.5-T unit (ACS 3.1; Philips Medical Systems, Shelton, Conn). For analysis of T1 and T2, a single 10-mm-thick axial section was obtained at the midarm before exercise and an axial section directed to the point of maximum soreness was obtained after exercise (Fig 1). The single-section approach was used to eliminate the possibility of saturation transfer from adjacent sections, as may occur in multisection acquisitions. The concatenated sequence included repetition times of 4,000 and 2,000 msec; echo times of 22, 44, 66, 88, 110, 132, 156, and 178 msec; and an inversion time of 400 msec. The matrix was 128 × 128, the field of view was 45 cm, and two signals were acquired. For volumetric studies, a contiguous (interleaved) multisection STIR sequence was used (2,000/52, 165-msec inversion time, 256 × 256 matrix, 45-cm field of view, four signals acquired, 10-mm section thickness, echo train length of four).

The MR imaging data were analyzed by one investigator (G.F.F.E.). Regions of in-

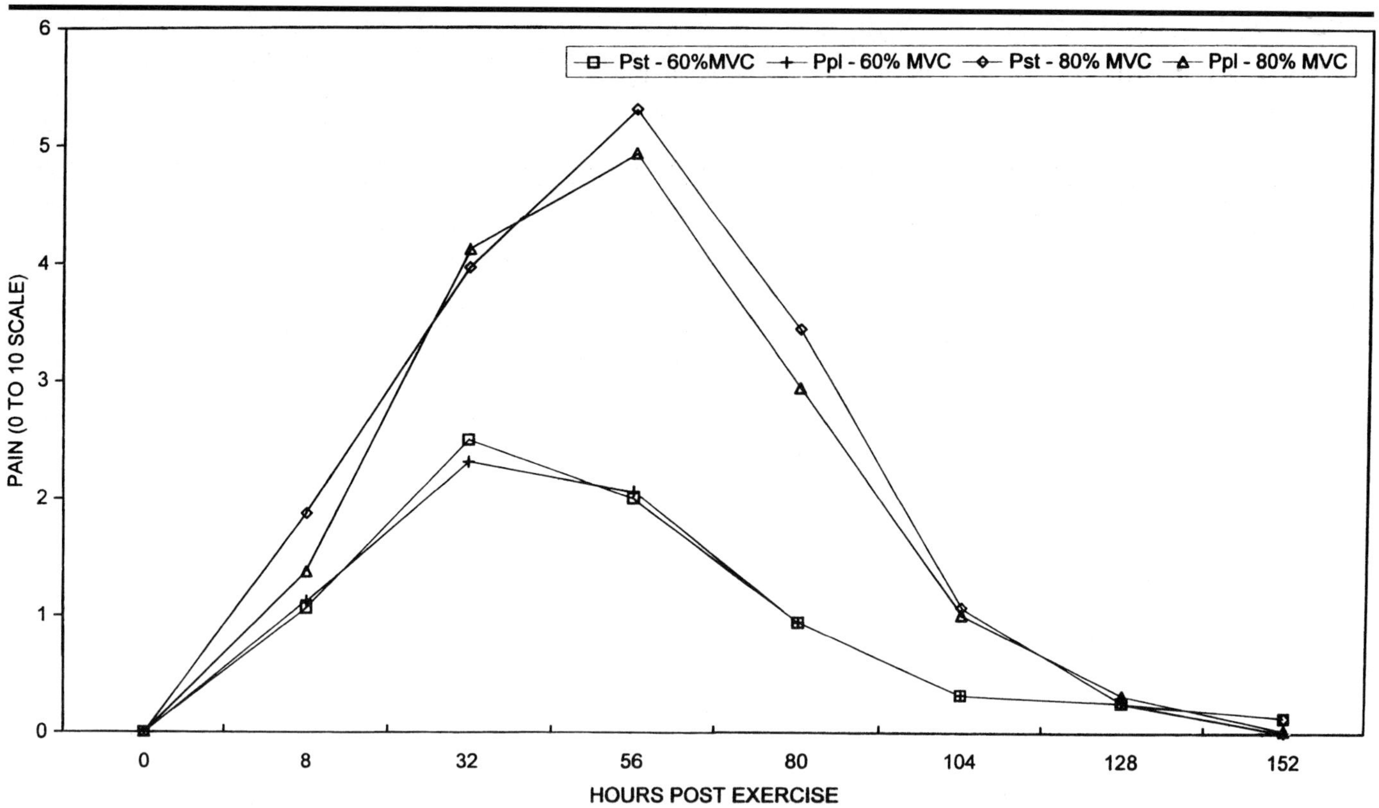

Figure 2. Mean pain scores for the 60% MVC force and 80% MVC force groups over 7 days after exercise. The pain scores tend to peak around 48 hours, the time when follow-up MR imaging was performed and CK levels were obtained for correlation with the pain scores. Error bars are omitted. *Ppl* = pain during palpation, *Pst* = pain during straightening.

terest were selected in brachialis muscle for estimation of relaxation times. The reliability of relaxation time estimation in similarly sized muscles with the same device was previously determined in a study of various soft-tissue measurements (coefficient of variation of the method = 2.8% for muscle T1 and 5.0% for muscle T2) (29).

The axial STIR images obtained 48 hours after exercise were used to render three-dimensional images and calculate the volume of muscle edema (Fig 1). Three-dimensional volume rendering was performed on an independent workstation (I.S.G. Technologies, Mississauga, Canada) by using the 3DGV option of the Computer Assisted Medical Reconstruction and Analysis S200 software package, version 4.1. The rendering procedure consisted of a fixed threshold and "seed"-planting technique similar to those we previously used to produce three-dimensional muscle volume data sets (30). Images were viewed at a level of 305 and width of 700, and three-dimensional reconstruction of edematous muscle was accomplished by automated selection of pixels with signal intensity over a threshold of 152; areas of high signal intensity not related to muscle (ie, veins) were manually eliminated. The threshold of 152 was selected after extensive trial and error revealed that this value allowed reliable detection of edematous muscle with a minimum of operator interaction. Three-dimensional rendered images reconstructed from the successive two-dimensional axial images yielded volume values, which were multiplied by the section thickness to provide each subject's volume of edematous muscle. Although we did not perform reliability tests in this study, we previously determined the reliability of individual cross-sectional area measurements of the biceps muscle (coefficient of variation of the method = 1.8%) (28). In that study, we also compared the volume of a cadaveric biceps muscle determined with MR imaging and that calculated by means of water volume displacement; the techniques varied by 3.7%.

Statistical analysis was begun by computing global variables for pain during straightening, pain during palpation, change in CK level, volume of muscle edema, change in T1, and change in T2. Pain during straightening and pain during palpation were summarized as the sums of the subjects' values over the 7-day postexercise period. Change in CK level was calculated as the multiple of the baseline CK value at 48 hours. Volume of muscle edema was determined by summing the values from the left and right sides in each subject. Changes in T1 and T2 were defined by the percentage change from day 0 to day 2. The strengths of the relationships between these indexes were calculated as Spearman correlations. The Student *t* test was used to judge the significance of the correlations being different from zero. Correlations between the DOMS indexes were calculated for both MVC force groups and for the combined data. All measures were also assessed for a sex-dependent effect.

RESULTS

All subjects reported experiencing DOMS, although the degree of DOMS was highly variable. Individual pain scores ranged from 0 to 9. Mean pain scores over 7 days for both groups are shown in Figure 2. The maximum individual pain score ranged from 1 to 9. Similarly high variability was observed in the other measurements (Table 1). Statistically significant correlations between various parameter pairs are shown in Table 2. When all data were combined without regard to exercise intensity, change in CK level correlated with change in T1, change in T2, pain during straightening, pain during palpation, and volume of muscle edema. No pain measure correlated with any MR imaging measure except for volume of muscle edema, which correlated with pain during straightening.

Compared with the 60% MVC force protocol, the 80% MVC force protocol effected significantly greater change in T2, volume of muscle edema, and pain during straightening. Change in T1, change in CK level, and pain during palpation did not differ significantly between the two protocols. At the more intense exercise level (80% MVC force), change in CK level correlated only with change in T2 and volume of muscle edema. Pain measures did not correlate significantly with any other measure at this level. At the lower exercise intensity (60% MVC force), volume of muscle edema correlated with change in CK level, pain during straightening, and pain during palpation. Pain during straightening also correlated with change in CK level.

No sex-dependent variation was found for any quantity or correlation.

TABLE 1
DOMS Parameters at Two Submaximal Levels of Exercise Intensity

Parameter	60% MVC Force	80% MVC Force	*P* Value*
Change in T1 (%)	3.0 ± 9.0	20.0 ± 21.0	NS
Change in T2 (%)	16.0 ± 17.0	59.0 ± 50.0	<.05
Volume of muscle edema (cm³)	92.1 ± 116.7	390.4 ± 370.4	<.05
Change in CK level	4.4 ± 9.5	38.8 ± 46.6	NS
Pain during straightening†	8.0 ± 8.6	18.4 ± 6.8	<.002
Pain during palpation†	6.8 ± 7.1	13.3 ± 9.5	NS

Note.—Numbers are the mean ± standard deviation.
* NS = not significant.
† Sum of pain scores over 7 days.

TABLE 2
Correlations between Clinical Measures of DOMS

Parameter by Patient Group	Pain during Straightening	Pain during Palpation	Change in CK Level
All patients (*n* = 16)			
Change in T1	NS	NS	.52 (*P* = .0374)
Change in T2	NS	NS	.76 (*P* = .0007)
Change in CK level	.79 (*P* = .0003)	.51 (*P* = .0427)	NA
Volume of muscle edema	.60 (*P* = .0133)	NS	.75 (*P* = .0009)
60% MVC force (*n* = 8)			
Change in T1	NS	NS	NS
Change in T2	NS	NS	NS
Change in CK level	.78 (*P* = .0215)	NS	NA
Volume of muscle edema	.77 (*P* = .0245)	.77 (*P* = .0245)	.76 (*P* = .02274)
80% MVC force (*n* = 8)			
Change in T1	NS	NS	NS
Change in T2	NS	NS	.76 (*P* = .0280)
Change in CK level	NS	NS	NA
Volume of muscle edema	NS	NS	.74 (*P* = .0366)

Note.—Only those correlation coefficients that were statistically significant are provided. NA = not applicable, NS = not significant.

DISCUSSION

Our data indicate that muscle edema and DOMS can result from exercise protocols that involve only 36 submaximal contractions. It therefore appears unnecessary to expose deconditioned muscle to more intense exercise or a greater duration of physical stress to elicit DOMS-related objective measures. In addition, decreasing the intensity of the submaximal workload was associated with a greater number of statistically significant correlations between the various parameters.

There was a good correlation (r = .79) between change in CK level and pain during DOMS. This result contrasts with the lack of such correlations in the vast majority of DOMS studies, which generally employ highly vigorous exercise to ensure that muscle soreness develops (4–6,8–15,17,19,20,23,25). Our finding is not unique, however, with a similar result occurring in another study that also employed submaximal workloads to generate DOMS (23). A close relationship between pain and change in CK level was documented in that study at 35% and 70% of maximum effort, but no correlation was found at maximal exercise intensity. However, this observation was not discussed, presumably because the degree of muscle soreness produced by the lower exercise levels was minimal compared with the marked soreness produced by the higher exercise levels. Our results indicate that although DOMS induced by submaximal exercise may be mild compared with that induced by severe exercise, the associated edemalike changes on MR images are readily apparent and easily quantitated. The ability of MR imaging to demonstrate muscle edema in DOMS produced by submaximal effort confirms a potential role for MR imaging in future studies of ways to avoid substantial tissue injury.

Our study showed a statistically significant correlation between the volume of edematous muscle and change in CK level (r = .75). This result is logical because the more muscle that is damaged, the more edema and elevation in CK level one might expect. However, previous studies showed no correlation between change in CK level and the mass of muscle involved in the exercise (9–11,19). These observations and the fact that elevations of CK level are highly variable after a standard exercise protocol led to the conclusion that CK level is an inadequate indicator of muscle damage (9,11). Plasma inhibitors of CK activity were even sought to explain such findings, although none was found (9). However, in previous studies, only indirect measures of muscle mass were correlated with postexercise elevations of CK level.

In those earlier studies, one exercising limb was compared with two (10) or more (19) limbs. Absence of an increase in CK level commensurate with the number of stressed limbs was used to infer that change in CK level does not correlate with the mass of muscle involved in the exercise. However, those studies varied the amount of muscle exercised, which is not necessarily the amount of muscle injured by the exercise. Nevertheless, the amount of muscle injured was assumed to vary directly with the amount of muscle used. That this may not be a valid assumption is supported by the high intrasubject variations in elevated CK level in these studies, with right-left differences as high as threefold. Unequal elevations of CK level arising from performance of identical work by right and left limbs could simply have reflected more voluminous injury in one limb. Had MR imaging been used in those studies, documentation of the volume of muscle rendered edematous by eccentric work would have eliminated the reliance on possibly erroneous assumptions regarding the symmetry or universality of muscle injury patterns. On the basis of our results, change in CK level is supported as an objective indicator of the mass of muscle adversely affected by the exercise.

The volume of edematous muscle not only correlated with change in CK level, it also correlated with pain. This finding supports the possibility that pain is a cumulative phenomenon, becoming more severe as more fibers are disrupted. The fact that the correlations between pain and change in CK level and between pain and volume of muscle edema did not occur with the more intense exercise protocol suggests that a threshold exists beyond which a greater volume of damaged muscle and related CK release no longer elicits the same pain triggers as at lower levels of fiber disruption. The fact that volume of muscle edema and change in CK level continued to correlate at the more intense exercise level suggests that they may remain linked despite the disappearance of a correlation with pain.

Although changes in muscle proton relaxation times, especially T2, correlated with change in CK level, they did not correlate with pain. Because volume of muscle edema did correlate with pain, at least at the more modest exercise intensity, volume of muscle edema appears to be the more important MR imaging parameter to monitor in future studies on prevention of DOMS, such as drug studies. When this finding is coupled with the fact that change in T2 correlated with change in CK level at the more intense exercise level, one might conclude that change in T2 is a redundant measure in DOMS studies. However, reports that the muscle proton T2 elevations associated with DOMS persist for much longer than pain or change in CK level (6,7,25) indicate a compelling phenomenon that merits further attention.

Limitations of our study include the small number of subjects and limited range of exercise intensities. More individuals of both sexes exercising at a larger variety of intensities would allow better definition of the effect of workload on relationships between DOMS-related parameters. Another potential shortcoming was that all subjects underwent MR imaging and measurement of CK level only at 48 hours after exercise. The time at which CK level, pain, and MR imaging changes peak depends in part on the severity of DOMS. With increasing severity of DOMS, the rise in CK level is later, higher, and more protracted (8,12,23). Furthermore, the time courses of change in CK level, pain, and MR imaging changes vary somewhat. For example, in severe DOMS, change in CK level has been shown to lag slightly behind changes in pain and MR imaging changes (6). However, because we wished to evaluate submaximal DOMS and therefore less severe and earlier patterns of injury, we chose to repeat MR imaging and measurement of CK level only at 48 hours. Finally, only one imaging section was used to characterize the T1 and T2 of painful muscles. Because pain was the primary symptom investigated, the point of maximal pain was chosen as the site of proton relaxation measurements. Slightly different results could be anticipated if different section locations were used.

Despite these potential limitations, we conclude that extreme exercise intensity is not required to yield discrete volumes of DOMS-related muscle edema. Submaximal workloads are adequate to produce DOMS, and correlations between conventionally measured indexes of injury may be enhanced at more modest workloads. The fact that volume of muscle edema correlated with elevation of CK level substantiates the value of this muscle enzyme as a quantitative indicator of muscle damage in DOMS. The statistically significant correlations between volume of edematous muscle and pain at reduced workloads suggest that the changes produced by such exercise protocols may reflect early but important pathophysiologic events that have been unappreciated. This finding suggests a need for investigation of even milder exercise protocols.

Acknowledgments: We thank Dorothy Smith, Alison Russell, Virginia Reed Vaughn, and Mark Daugherty for their technical expertise. We also acknowledge Bally Life Fitness for a discount on the exercise device employed.

References

1. Armstrong RB. Mechanisms of exercise-induced delayed onset muscle soreness: a brief review. Med Sci Sports Exerc 1984; 16:529–538.
2. Cleak MJ, Eston RG. Delayed onset muscle soreness: mechanisms and management. J Sports Sci 1992; 10:325–341.
3. Nurenberg P, Giddings CJ, Stray-Gundersen J, Fleckenstein JL, Gonyea WJ, Peshock RM. MR imaging–guided muscle biopsy for correlation of increased signal intensity with ultrastructural change and delayed-onset muscle soreness after exercise. Radiology 1992; 184:865–869.
4. Newham DJ, McPhail G, Mills KR, Edwards RHT. Ultrastructural changes after concentric and eccentric contractions of human muscle. J Neurol Sci 1983; 61:109–122.
5. Friden J, Sjostrom M, Ekblom B. Myofibrillar damage following intense eccentric exercise in man. Int J Sports Med 1983; 4:170–176.
6. Fleckenstein JL, Weatherall PT, Parkey RW, Payne JA, Peshock RM. Sports-related muscle injuries: evaluation with MR imaging. Radiology 1989; 172:793–798.
7. Nosaka K, Clarkson PM. Changes in indicators of inflammation after eccentric exercise of the elbow flexors. Med Sci Sports Exerc 1996; 28:953–961.
8. Newham DJ, Jones DA, Clarkson PM. Repeated high-force eccentric exercise: effects on muscle pain and damage. J Appl Physiol 1987; 63:1381–1386.
9. Clarkson PM, Ebbeling C. Investigation of serum creatine kinase variability after muscle-damaging exercise. Clin Sci 1988; 75:257–261.
10. Nosaka K, Clarkson PM. Relationship between post-exercise plasma CK elevation and muscle mass involved in the exercise. Int J Sports Med 1992; 13:471–475.
11. Clarkson PM, Byrnes WJ, McCormick KM, Tercet LP, White JS. Muscle soreness and serum creatine kinase activity following isometric, eccentric, and concentric exercise. Int J Sports Med 1986; 7:152–155.
12. Newham DJ, Jones DA, Edwards RHT. Large delayed plasma creatine kinase changes after stepping exercise. Muscle Nerve 1983; 6:380–385.
13. Rodenburg JB, Bar PR, De Boer RW. Relations between muscle soreness and biochemical and functional outcomes of eccentric exercise. J Appl Physiol 1993; 74: 2976–2983.
14. Friden J, Sfakianos PN, Hargens AR. Blood indices of muscle injury associated with eccentric muscle contractions. J Orthop Res 1989; 7:142–145.
15. Jones DA, Newham DJ, Clarkson PM. Skeletal muscle stiffness and pain following eccentric exercise of the elbow flexors. Pain 1987; 30:233–242.
16. Newham DJ, Jones DA, Edwards RHT. Plasma creatine kinase changes after eccentric and concentric contractions. Muscle Nerve 1986; 9:59–63.
17. Bobbert MF, Hollander AP, Huijing PA. Factors in delayed onset muscular soreness of man. Med Sci Sports Exerc 1986; 18:75–81.
18. Friden J, Sfakianos PN, Hargens AR. Muscle soreness and intramuscular fluid pressure: comparison between eccentric and concentric load. J Appl Physiol 1986; 61: 2175–2179.
19. Graves JE, Clarkson PM, Litchfield P, Kirwan JP, Norton JP. Serum creatine kinase activity following repeated bouts of isometric exercise with different muscle groups. Eur J Appl Physiol 1987; 56:657–661.

20. Clarkson PM, Litchfield P, Graves J, Kirwan J, Byrnes WJ. Serum creatine kinase activity following forearm flexion isometric exercise. Eur J Appl Physiol 1985; 53:368–371.
21. Byrnes WJ, Clarkson PM, White JS, Hsieh SS, Frykman PN, Maughan RJ. Delayed onset muscle soreness following repeated bouts of downhill running. J Appl Physiol 1985; 59:710–715.
22. Ross JH, Attwood EC, Atkin GE, Villar RN. A study on the effects of severe repetitive exercise on serum myoglobin, creatine kinase, transaminases, and lactate dehydrogenase. Q J Med 1983; 206:268–273.
23. Tiidus PM, Ianuzzo CD. Effects of intensity and duration of muscular exercise on delayed soreness and serum enzyme activities. Med Sci Sports Exerc 1983; 15:461–465.
24. Van Der Meulen JH, Kuipers H, Drukker J. Relationship between exercise-induced muscle damage and enzyme release in rats. J Appl Physiol 1991; 71:999–1004.
25. Shellock FG, Fukunaga T, Mink JH, Edgerton VR. Exertional muscle injury: evaluation of concentric versus eccentric actions with serial MR imaging. Radiology 1991; 179:659–664.
26. Fleckenstein JL, Shellock FG. Exertional muscle injuries: magnetic resonance imaging evaluation. Top Magn Reson Imaging 1991; 3:50–70.
27. Fleckenstein JL, Weatherall PT, Bertocci LA, et al. Locomotor system assessment by muscle magnetic resonance imaging. Magn Reson Q 1991; 7:79–103.
28. Roman WJ, Fleckenstein J, Stray-Gundersen J, Always SE, Peshock R, Gonyea WJ. Adaptations in the elbow flexors of elderly males after heavy-resistance training. J Appl Physiol 1993; 74:750–754.
29. Meler JD, Solomon MA, Steele JR, Yancy CW, Parkey RW, Fleckenstein JL. The MRI appearance of volume overload in the lower extremities. J Comput Assist Tomogr 1997; 21:969–973.
30. McColl RW, Fleckenstein JL, Bowers J, Theriault G, Peshock RM. Three-dimensional reconstruction of skeletal muscle from MRI. Comput Med Imaging Graph 1992; 16:363–371.

Henk-Jan van der Woude, MD
Koenraad L. Verstraete, MD
Pancras C. W. Hogendoorn, MD
Anthonie H. M. Taminiau, MD
Jo Hermans, PhD
Johan L. Bloem, MD

Musculoskeletal Tumors: Does Fast Dynamic Contrast-enhanced Subtraction MR Imaging Contribute to the Characterization?[1]

Index terms:
Bone neoplasms, MR, 40.121412, 40.30
Magnetic resonance (MR), contrast enhancement, 48.12143
Magnetic resonance (MR), rapid imaging, 48.12146
Magnetic resonance (MR), vascular studies, 48.12142
Muscles, neoplams, 40.30
Neoplasms, blood supply, 48.31, 48.32, 48.36, 48.37

Radiology 1998; 208:821–828

Abbreviations:
NPV = negative predictive value
PPV = positive predictive value

[1] From the Departments of Radiology (H.J.v.d.W., K.L.V., J.L.B.), Pathology (P.C.W.H.), Orthopedic Surgery (A.H.M.T.), and Medical Statistics (J.H.), Leiden University Medical Center, Albinusdreef 2, PO Box 9600, NL-2300 RC Leiden, The Netherlands, and the Department of Diagnostic Radiology, University Hospital Ghent, Belgium (K.L.V.). Received October 31, 1997; revision requested, January 7, 1998; revision received March 13; accepted April 17. **Address reprint requests to** H.V.

PURPOSE: To prospectively analyze the value of fast, dynamic, subtraction magnetic resonance (MR) imaging in the characterization of musculoskeletal tumors.

MATERIALS AND METHODS: In 175 consecutive patients with a musculoskeletal mass, dynamic contrast-enhanced subtraction MR imaging was performed after administration of 0.1 mmol per kilogram of body weight gadopentetate dimeglumine or gadoteridol. A turbo gradient-echo technique was used, with a temporal resolution of 1–3 seconds. The interval between arterial and early tumor enhancement, the pattern (peripheral or diffuse) of enhancement, and the progression of tumor enhancement, as visualized on time–signal intensity curves, were assessed. MR enhancement features were related to the histopathologic diagnoses.

RESULTS: Differentiation of benign from malignant soft-tissue masses was possible with a sensitivity of 91% and specificity of 72% based on start of enhancement, a sensitivity of 73% and specificity of 97% based on peripheral or diffuse enhancement, and a sensitivity of 86% and specificity of 81% based on progression of enhancement. Benign bone tumors could not be accurately differentiated from malignant bone tumors on the basis of the three defined parameters (sensitivity, 63%–76%; specificity, 50%–76%).

CONCLUSION: Dynamic, contrast-enhanced, subtraction MR images may be useful to differentiate malignant from benign soft-tissue masses.

Author contributions:
Guarantors of integrity of entire study, H.J.v.d.W., J.L.B., P.C.W.H.; study concepts, H.J.v.d.W., K.L.V., J.L.B., P.C.W.H.; study design, H.J.v.d.W., K.L.V., J.L.B., J.H.; definition of intellectual content, H.J.v.d.W., K.L.V., P.C.W.H., J.L.B.; literature research, H.J.v.d.W.; clinical studies, H.J.v.d.W., K.L.V., A.H.M.T., P.C.W.H., J.L.B.; data acquisition, H.J.v.d.W., K.L.V.; data analysis, H.J.v.d.W., K.L.V., P.C.W.H., J.L.B.; statistical analysis, J.H.; manuscript preparation, H.J.v.d.W., J.L.B.; manuscript editing, J.L.B.; manuscript review, H.J.v.d.W., K.L.V., P.C.W.H., J.L.B., A.H.M.T., J.H.

The use of unenhanced or contrast material–enhanced magnetic resonance (MR) imaging to characterize musculoskeletal tumors has yielded controversial results (1–11). Various studies designed to differentiate between benign and malignant masses were based on the evaluation of morphologic parameters, such as size, demarcation of margins, involvement of adjacent vital structures, signal homogeneity, and measurements of relaxation times (2,7,10,12–14). In a recent study, the use of a gadolinium contrast agent was found not to contribute to the differential diagnosis or patient care in 89% of patients (11). In dynamic gradient-echo MR studies, slope values, reflecting the increase of signal intensity after the administration of a contrast agent as a function of time, have also been used in assessing the malignant potential of musculoskeletal tumors (1,4–6). These studies resulted in statistically significant differences in slope values between benign and malignant tumors; however, sensitivity and specificity were adversely affected by slope values of poorly vascularized malignant tumors and highly vascularized benign tumors (such as giant cell tumor and eosinophilic granuloma) (4–6). Sampling errors in large, heterogeneously enhancing tumors are another problem of single-section gradient-echo images. Dynamic, contrast-enhanced, rapid-acquisition, spin-echo MR imaging has been used to defeat this limitation; however, qualitative analysis of enhancement patterns in a rather

TABLE 1
Diagnoses in 175 Patients with Musculoskeletal Masses

Benign Soft-Tissue Masses	No. of Patients (n = 32)	Malignant Soft-Tissue Masses	No. of Paients (n = 22)	Benign Bone Tumors	No. of Patients (n = 50)	Low-Grade Malignant Bone Tumors	No. of Patients (n = 26)	High-Grade Malignant Bone Tumors	No. of Patients (n = 45)
Lipoma	6	Small cell liposarcoma	1	Osteochondroma	9	Chondrosarcoma	12	Osteosarcoma	23
Schwannoma	7	Liposarcoma	1	Giant cell tumor	9	Chordoma	3	Undifferentiated carcinoma	1
Abscess	1	Leiomyosarcoma	3	Osteoma	1	Primary bone lymphoma	2	Malignant fibrous histiocytoma	6
Ganglion	3	Undifferentiated sarcoma	3	Solitary bone cyst	3	Adamantinoma of long bone	6	High-grade chondrosarcoma	2
Aggressive fibromatosis	5	Soft-tissue osteosarcoma	3	Aneurysmal bone cyst	5	Juxtacortical osteosarcoma	2	Ewing sarcoma	9
Arteriovenous malformation	1	Synovial sarcoma	6	Fibrous dysplasia	5	Low-grade malignant fibrous histiocytoma	1	Metastases	4
Benign fibrous histiocytoma	1	Rhabdomyosarcoma	2	Eosinophilic granuloma	3				
Synovial chondromatosis	1	Malignant fibrous histiocytoma	2	Enchondroma	6				
Hemangioma	2			Epidermoid cyst	1				
Myositis ossificans	1	Neurofibrosarcoma	1	Desmoplastic fibroma	1				
Neurofibromatosis	1			Abscess	1				
Pseudolymphoma	1			Osteoid osteoma	2				
Hematoma	1			Osteoblastoma	1				
Lipoblastoma	1			Osteomyelitis	2				
				Chondroblastoma	1				

small population did not demonstrate statistically significant differences in enhancement patterns between benign and malignant tumors (3). The advantage of multisection imaging with this method is at the cost of temporal resolution. There is no consensus about the temporal resolution required to differentiate benign from malignant tumors by using dynamic contrast-enhanced MR imaging (15).

In the present prospective study, a fast, dynamic, contrast-enhanced gradient-echo MR subtraction technique was used to differentiate malignant from benign musculoskeletal tumors and/or to restrict the differential diagnosis. The study focused on the start of initial tumor enhancement relative to arterial enhancement and on the qualitative evaluation of the pattern and progression of initial enhancement.

The hypothesis was that rapidly progressive enhancement (type I curve) with early start of tumor enhancement (≤6 seconds after arterial enhancement) and peripheral enhancement represent (high-grade) malignancy of either bone or soft tissue. Conversely, late (>6 seconds after arterial enhancement) or no enhancement (types II and III curves) and diffuse enhancement may represent benign tumors.

MATERIALS AND METHODS

Patients

Between January 1994 and December 1996, 175 consecutive patients with a musculoskeletal tumor or tumorlike mass were examined with MR imaging. The ages of the patients ranged from 9 to 76 years (mean, 34.6 years). The diagnoses are summarized in Table 1. Because our institute functions as a referral center for diagnosis and treatment of musculoskeletal tumors, possible referral bias may have occurred. Tumors were categorized as malignant (high or low grade for bone tumors) or benign. Diagnoses were histologically confirmed with material obtained from trocar biopsy or resection of the tumor.

MR Imaging

After giving informed consent, all patients were examined with a standard imaging protocol and a 0.5-T MR system (model T5-II; Philips Medical Systems, Shelton, Conn). The study was approved by the local medical ethics committee. A surface coil was used, except in a few patients with large tumors for whom a body coil was applied. Unenhanced T1-weighted spin-echo MR images with a short repetition time and a short echo time (repetition time msec/echo time msec = 600/20) and T2-weighted turbo spin-echo images with long repetition times and long echo times (3,000–7,000/120–150; echo train length of eight) in two orthogonal planes were used to localize the tumor and to determine intra- and extramedullary extension. T2-weighted images were always combined with fat-selective presaturation. On the basis of these findings, two longitudinal or transverse sections that displayed the largest and most representative tumor dimensions were selected for a dynamic contrast-enhanced study. In small intraosseous tumors, only one section was selected.

Dynamic imaging was performed with a T1-weighted, fast, magnetization-prepared, gradient-echo sequence. The following imaging parameters were used: 15/6.8, 30° flip angle, 741-msec preparatory pulse delay time, 10-mm section thickness, one signal acquired per data line, 128 × 256 matrix size, 200–450-mm field of view. This sequence was identified as our optimal sequence with regard to temporal and spatial resolution as obtained from in vitro gradient-echo studies on a phantom with a series of increasing concentrations of gadoteridol (ProHance; Bracco Diagnostics, Milan, Italy). In this setting, the temporal resolution was 1.5

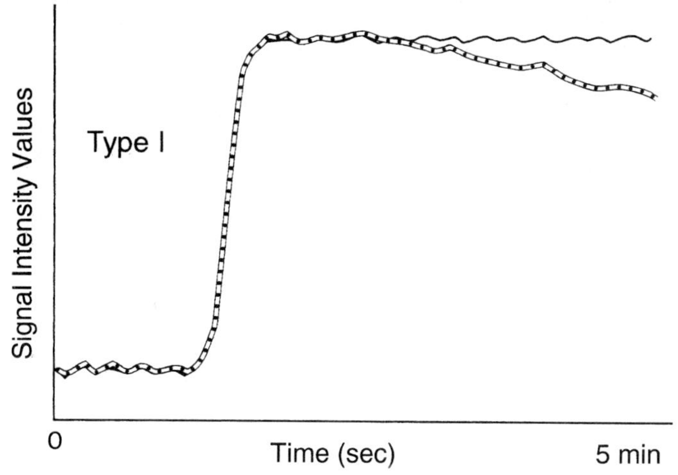

a.

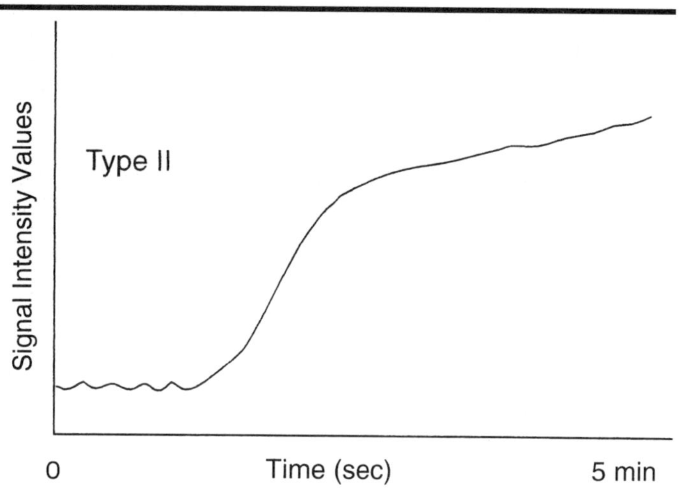

b.

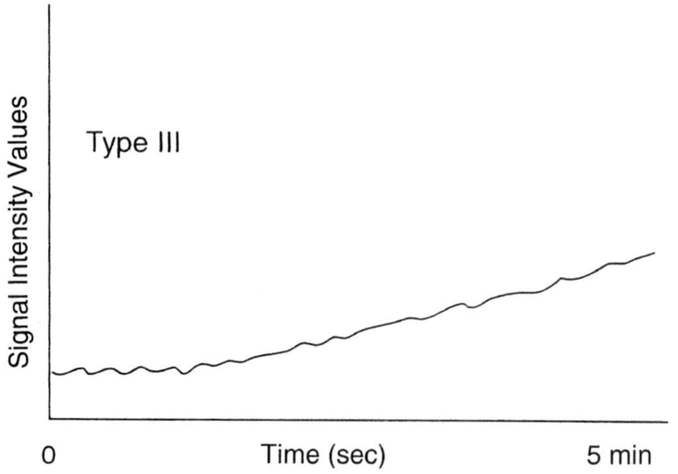

c.

Figure 1. Three types of time–signal intensity curves (adapted, with permission, from Verstraete KL. Academic thesis. University of Ghent, Belgium, 1994.) **(a)** Type I curve: early onset of enhancement followed by rapidly progressive linear increase of signal intensity (represented by a steep slope, parallel to the arterial curve) to an early maximum followed by a distinct transition to a stable level of signal intensity (biphasic curve), or decrease of signal intensity (washout of contrast agent). **(b)** Type II curve: steady increase or flattening of the curve after the steepest part of the time–signal intensity curve. **(c)** Type III curve: linear enhancement with a very low slope, representing slow or absent enhancement, similar to a curve representing normal muscle.

seconds for single-section studies and 3 seconds for dynamic studies comprising two parallel sections. Forty-seven to 64 (in single-section studies) acquisitions were obtained after the administration by manual injection (at a rate of approximately 5 mL/sec) of an intravenous bolus of 0.1 mmol per kilogram of body weight gadopentetate dimeglumine (Magnevist; Schering, Berlin, Germany) in 155 patients or gadoteridol in 20 patients. The manual injection was started after the fourth dynamic acquisition (5–6 seconds after initiation of the dynamic sequence), immediately followed by a saline flush of 20 mL at the same injection rate. The duration of the dynamic studies was 5 minutes at maximum.

In each patient, all contrast-enhanced dynamic images were subtracted from the first unenhanced gradient-echo image by using the subtraction function available as standard software on the MR unit. Regions of interest of each tumor were selected by two observers (H.J.v.d.W., K.L.V.) in concert and manually delineated with a cursor on the display screen in one selected image. The same region of interest was automatically plotted on all images of the same sequence. Subsequently, the dynamic enhancement of the entire tumor and selected parts of the tumor were automatically plotted as a function of time. In addition, time–signal intensity curves were obtained from an artery depicted within the plane of dynamic imaging and from normal muscle.

The following parameters were determined in each patient on the series of subtraction images and time–signal intensity curves by two observers (H.J.v.d.W., K.L.V.) in concert:

Start of enhancement.—Arrival of the bolus of contrast medium in an artery in the plane of dynamic imaging and the interval between arterial enhancement and onset of tumor enhancement were visually assessed on the series of subtraction images. Early tumor enhancement was defined as 6 seconds or less after arterial enhancement (16–18).

Pattern of initial enhancement.—The pattern of enhancement, assessed on the subtraction images of the dynamic imaging sequence (maximum acquisition time, 5 minutes), was categorized as peripheral, diffuse and/or homogeneous, or absent.

Progression of enhancement.—The progression of enhancement in each patient was classified according to the shape of the time–signal intensity curves described in Figure 1 (18,19).

Sensitivity, specificity, positive predictive value (PPV), and negative predictive value (NPV) were calculated to evaluate whether the above-mentioned individual dynamic features allowed us to differentiate between malignant and benign tumors.

RESULTS

Start of Enhancement

Benign versus malignant soft-tissue masses.—Twenty of 22 soft-tissue sarcomas enhanced early (Table 2) (Figs 2, 3). Enhancement started late (>6 seconds) in an intermediate grade malignant myxoid liposarcoma with round-cell features and one undifferentiated soft-tissue sarcoma.

Eight of 32 benign soft-tissue masses enhanced early, whereas the other 24 showed late start of enhancement, if any (Table 2) (Fig 4). Benign masses that demonstrated early enhancement occurred in three patients with aggressive fibromatosis, three patients with schwannoma, one patient with synovial chondromatosis, and one patient with a pseudolymphoma (*Nocardia* infection). According to these data, sensitivity to distinguish malignant from benign soft-tissue masses was 91%, specificity was 72%, PPV was 71%, and NPV was 92% (Table 3).

Benign versus malignant bone tumors.—Forty-three of 45 high-grade bone tumors enhanced early (Table 2). Enhancement of two malignant fibrous histiocytomas started 6–9 seconds after arterial enhancement. Four (two adamantinomas of long bone, two grade I–II chondrosarcomas) of 26 low-grade malignant bone tumors enhanced early, whereas enhancement in the other 22 started after 6 seconds. Early enhancement was also observed in 22 of 50 benign bone masses (Table 2). The latter group consisted of all nine giant cell tumors (Fig 5), all five aneurysmal bone cysts, two eosinophilic granulomas, two osteoid osteomas, one osteoblastoma, one fibrous dysplasia, one abscess, and one chondroblastoma. Twenty-eight of 50 benign tumors showed late or no enhancement (Table 2). Start of enhancement was not an accurate parameter to discriminate between malignant and benign bone tumors (Table 3). A sensitivity of 95% and specificity of 56% were found when this parameter was used to differentiate high-grade malignant from benign bone tumors (PPV, 66%; NPV, 93%). Very low sensitivity (15%) and specificity (56%) were found when benign tumors were compared with low-grade malignant bone tumors (PPV, 15%; NPV, 56%).

Peripheral, Diffuse, or No Enhancement

Benign versus malignant soft-tissue masses.—All 22 malignant and 20 of 32 benign soft-tissue masses enhanced (Table 2). Sixteen of 22 soft-tissue sarcomas enhanced peripherally during the early dynamic sequence (Table 2) (Fig 2). Five of six synovial sarcomas and one malignant fibrous histiocytoma enhanced homogeneously (Fig 3). Peripheral enhancement was noticed in only one benign soft-tissue mass (abscess). Thus, initial peripheral enhancement was a specific sign (specificity, 97%; PPV, 94%) for differentiating malignant from benign soft-tissue tumors (Table 3).

TABLE 2
Results of Characterization of Musculoskeletal Masses according to Different Enhancement Parameters

Parameter	Test*	Soft-Tissue Masses: Benign (*n* = 32)	Soft-Tissue Masses: Malignant (*n* = 22)	Bone Tumors: Benign (*n* = 50)	Bone Tumors: Low-Grade Malignant (*n* = 26)	Bone Tumors: High-Grade Malignant (*n* = 45)
Start of enhancement	≤6 sec (M)	8 (25)	20 (91)	22 (44)	4 (15)	43 (96)
	>6 sec (B)	24 (75)	2 (9)	28 (56)	22 (85)	2 (4)
Pattern of enhancement						
	Peripheral (M)	1 (3)	16 (73)	12 (24)	10 (38)	35 (78)
	Diffuse (B)	19 (59)	6 (27)	19 (38)	16 (62)	10 (22)
	No enhancement (B)	12 (38)	0 (0)	19 (38)	0 (0)	0 (0)
Progression of enhancement	Type I (M)	6 (19)	19 (86)	25 (50)	6 (23)	44 (98)
	Type II/III (B)	26 (81)	3 (14)	25 (50)	20 (77)	1 (2)

Data are the number of patients. Numbers in parentheses are percentages.
* B = parameter indicating benignancy, M = parameter indicating malignancy.

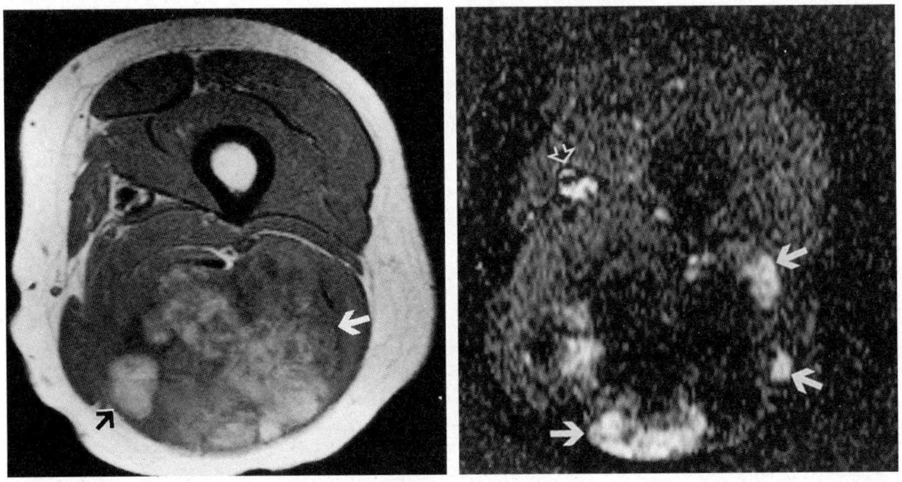

a. b.

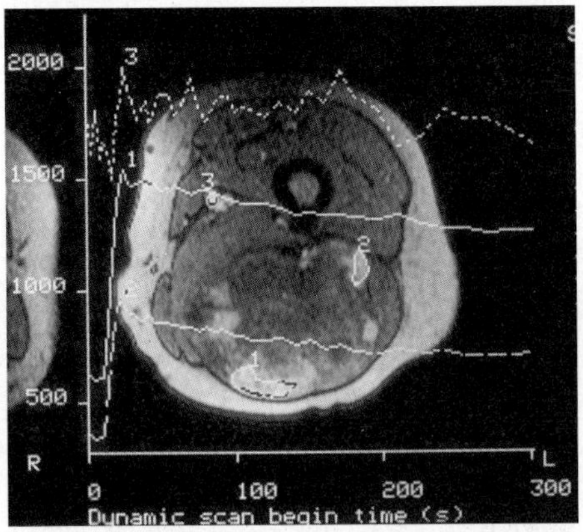

c.

Figure 2. Case of a 23-year-old woman with a large soft-tissue mass of the posterior upper leg. Early and peripheral enhancement are consistent with malignancy. Histologic diagnosis was soft-tissue osteosarcoma. **(a)** Transverse T1-weighted spin-echo MR image (600/20) shows the mass (white arrow) is inhomogeneous with areas of slightly increased signal intensity and fluid-fluid levels (black arrow), consistent with hemorrhage. **(b)** Early (20 seconds after bolus injection, 3 seconds after arterial [open arrow] enhancement) dynamic, contrast-enhanced subtraction image demonstrates enhancing areas in the periphery (arrows). **(c)** Time–signal intensity curves, superimposed on a dynamic, contrast-enhanced, gradient-echo MR image (15/6.8, 30° flip angle) before subtraction, show rapidly progressive enhancement of the peripheral tumor areas (*1* and *2*) with early washout (type I curve), indicating malignancy. *3* = blood vessel.

Benign versus malignant bone tumors.—All 71 malignant and 31 of 50 benign bone tumors enhanced (Table 2). Initial peripheral enhancement was found in 35 of 45 high-grade malignant bone tumors. In 10 of 26 low-grade malignant bone tumors, enhancement was also peripheral but started usually at the end of the dynamic sequence. In 12 of 31 enhancing benign tumors, enhancement was periph-

TABLE 3
Characterization of Musculoskeletal Masses according to Three Different Enhancement Parameters

Parameter	Test Characteristic	Soft-Tissue Masses (malignant vs benign)	Bone Tumors (malignant vs benign)
Start of enhancement	Sensitivity (%)	91 (71, 99)	66 (54, 77)
	Specificity (%)	72 (57, 89)	56 (41, 70)
	PPV (%)	71 (51, 87)	68 (56, 79)
	NPV (%)	92 (75, 99)	54 (39, 68)
Pattern of enhancement	Sensitivity (%)	73 (50, 89)	63 (51, 75)
	Specificity (%)	97 (84, 100)	76 (62, 87)
	PPV (%)	94 (71, 100)	79 (66, 89)
	NPV (%)	84 (68, 94)	59 (46, 71)
Progression of enhancement	Sensitivity (%)	86 (65, 97)	70 (58, 81)
	Specificity (%)	81 (64, 93)	50 (35, 65)
	PPV (%)	76 (55, 91)	68 (56, 78)
	NPV (%)	90 (73, 98)	53 (38, 68)

Note.—Numbers in parentheses are the 95% confidence interval.

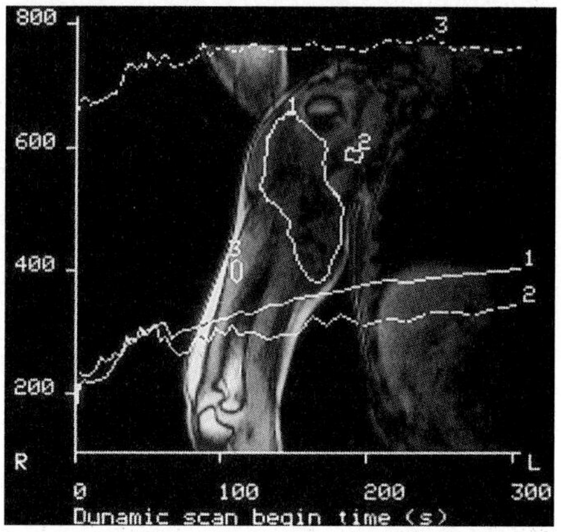

Figure 4. Case of a 12-year-old child with a large soft-tissue mass of the upper arm. Late, gradual, and homogeneous enhancement are consistent with a benign mass. Histologic diagnosis was neurofibromatosis. Time–signal intensity curve, superimposed on a dynamic contrast-enhanced gradient-echo image (15/6.8, 30° flip angle) in a sagittal plane, of the mass (*1*) displays gradual enhancement (type III). Enhancement was homogeneous. *2* and *3* = muscle.

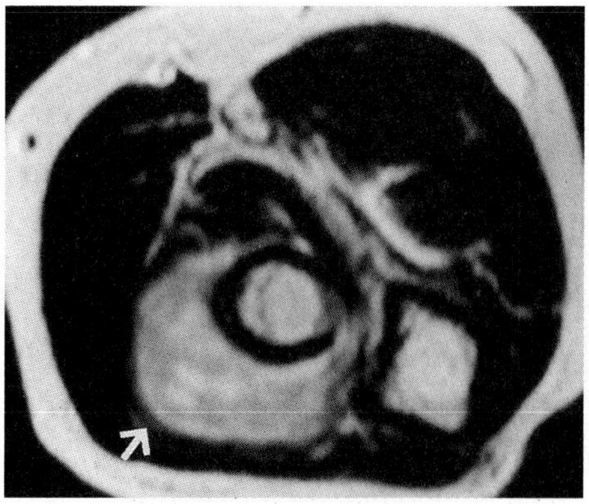

a.

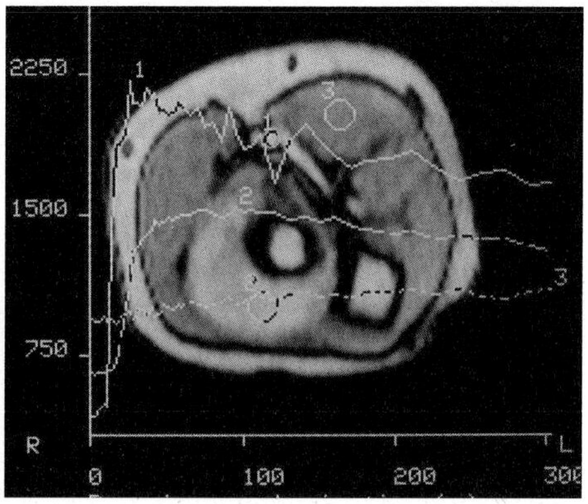

c.

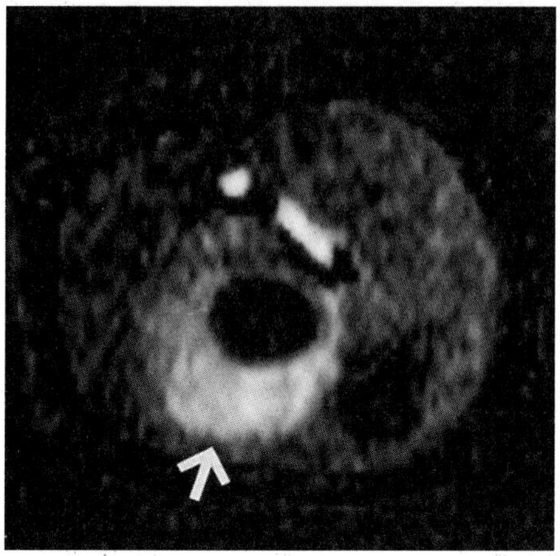

b.

Figure 3. Case of a 16-year-old girl with a soft-tissue mass in the lower arm. Early and rapid progression of enhancement are consistent with malignancy, despite initial homogeneous enhancement. Histologic diagnosis was synovial sarcoma. **(a)** Axial T2-weighted turbo spin-echo image (5,065/150) shows a homogeneous relatively well-defined soft-tissue mass (arrow) of high signal intensity, abutting the cortical bone (signal void). **(b)** Dynamic contrast-enhanced subtraction image reveals early, homogeneous enhancement of the soft-tissue mass (arrow). Image was acquired at 6 seconds after arterial enhancement. **(c)** Time–signal intensity curves, superimposed on a fast gradient-echo MR image (15/6.8, 30° flip angle), of artery (*1*), soft-tissue tumor component (*2*), and normal muscle (*3*), display rapidly progressive enhancement of tumor, followed by an early plateau phase and washout (type I curve).

eral. These data resulted in relatively low sensitivity (63%) and specificity (76%) for discrimination between malignant and benign bone tumors (Table 3).

Progression of Enhancement

Benign versus malignant soft-tissue tumors.—A type I curve was seen in 19 of 22 soft-tissue sarcomas (Table 2). The exceptions were one synovial sarcoma, one undifferentiated sarcoma, and one small cell liposarcoma. Six (three aggressive fibromatoses, one benign fibrous histiocytoma, one synovial chondromatosis, and one pseudolymphoma) of 32 benign soft-tissue masses also showed a type I curve. A type II curve was shown in two schwannomas and in two aggressive fibromatoses, whereas a type III curve was found in the remaining 22 benign soft-tissue tumors (Fig 4). Sensitivity, specificity, and PPV did not reach 90%; only NPV was 90% (Table 3).

Benign versus malignant bone tumors.—Forty-four of 45 high-grade bone sarcomas revealed a type I curve with an early plateau phase in 27 tumors and washout in 17 tumors (Table 2). One malignant fibrous histiocytoma showed a type II curve. Only six (five adamantinomas of long bone, one chondrosarcoma) of 26 low-grade malignant bone tumors showed a type I curve. A type I curve was also observed in 25 of 50 benign bone tumors (including giant cell tumor [Fig 5], aneurysmal bone cyst, eosinophilic granuloma, osteoid osteoma, osteoblastoma, chondroblastoma). Early washout as part of the type I curve was seen in eight of nine giant cell tumors, in two of five fibrous dysplasias, in one of five aneurysmal bone cysts, in the one chondroblastoma, and in the one osteoblastoma.

Twenty-five benign tumors revealed gradual or absent dynamic enhancement (type III curve). A sensitivity of 98% and specificity of 50% were found when this parameter was used to differentiate high-grade malignant from benign bone tumors (Table 3). Low sensitivity and specificity were found when benign tumors were compared with low-grade malignant bone tumors (Table 3). Sensitivity and specificity were 70% and 50% when all malignant bone tumors were compared with benign bone tumors (Table 3).

Combination of Parameters

On the basis of the good results of single parameters in patients with soft-tissue masses, we also assessed sensitivity, specificity, and predictive values of three sets, each consisting of two combined parameters (Table 4). Specificity and PPV did not increase (Tables 3, 4); only sensitivity and NPV increased secondary to a decrease of false-negative test results (Tables 3, 4).

TABLE 4
Characterization of Soft-Tissue Masses according to Combined Parameters

Test Characteristic	Start of Enhancement and Pattern of Enhancement	Start of Enhancement and Progression of Enhancement	Pattern of Enhancement and Progression of Enhancement
Sensitivity (%)	96	91	91
Specificity (%)	72	72	78
PPV (%)	70	69	74
NPV (%)	96	92	93

Note.—Criteria indicating presence of malignant lesions: ≤6 seconds, peripheral enhancement, type I curve; criteria indicating presence of benign lesions: >6 seconds, diffuse enhancement, type II/III curve.

DISCUSSION

The three defined enhancement parameters cannot be used to accurately differentiate benign from malignant bone masses and therefore do not add to the diagnostic power of conventional radiographs. Conversely, soft-tissue masses could be characterized fairly accurately on the basis of early enhancement (sensitivity, 91%; specificity, 72%), pattern of enhancement (sensitivity, 73%; specificity, 97%), and progression of enhancement (sensitivity, 86%; specificity, 81%). For all practical purposes, initial enhancement at the periphery of a soft-tissue mass indicated malignancy (specificity, 97%; PPV, 94%), whereas absence of enhancement or late and diffuse enhancement indicated presence of a benign soft-tissue mass (sensitivity, 96%; NPV, 96%). Sensitivity and NPV of all three combinations of parameters were over 90% (Table 4). Absence of enhancement during the 5-minute acquisition indicated presence of a benign soft-tissue mass (NPV, 100%). Unfortunately, only 38% of benign tumors exhibited this feature (Table 2). The relevance of early peripheral enhancement in soft-tissue sarcomas in our study is in accord with the results of the recent study by Ma et al (20), who used a rim-to-center enhancement ratio to differentiate between benign and malignant musculoskeletal masses.

Synovial sarcoma cannot be identified by using these practical guidelines. Five of six synovial sarcomas displayed diffuse (Fig 3) instead of peripheral enhancement. However, the other two parameters indicated malignancy; enhancement of all six synovial sarcomas started within 6 seconds after arterial enhancement, and five of these tumors had a type I curve. There were three other soft-tissue sarcomas with incidental benign enhancement characteristics. One of two malignant fibrous histiocytomas enhanced diffusely, but in addition to a type I enhancement curve, start of enhancement was within 6 seconds after arterial enhancement. One liposarcoma with small cell features exhibited two benign parameters (late start of enhancement, type III curve) and one malignant parameter (peripheral enhancement). Peripheral enhancement was also the only malignant sign in an undifferentiated soft-tissue sarcoma. This tumor displayed a type II curve, and enhancement started more than 6 seconds after arterial enhancement. We did not find specific reasons why these eight sarcomas displayed one or more benign parameters.

There were nine benign soft-tissue masses exhibiting at least one enhancement characteristic that might falsely indicate the presence of malignancy. Three of seven benign schwannomas showed early enhancement; however, in all masses, diffuse enhancement and type II curves were found. Three of five aggressive fibromatoses depicted early enhancement with a type I curve. None of these masses enhanced peripherally. Moreover, the appearance of aggressive fibromatosis on T2-weighted images is rather typical (21). One benign fibrous histiocytoma showed a type I curve; however, enhancement was diffuse and started after 6 seconds. Synovial chondromatosis also has a typical morphologic appearance on MR images and radiographs. The one synovial chondromatosis displayed early enhancement with a type I curve; enhancement was, however, only focal. One soft-tissue abscess showed peripheral enhancement; however, enhancement started late with a type II curve. Also, clinical features usually assist in making a diagnosis of soft-tissue abscess. In one patient, a soft-tissue mass of the popliteal fossa displayed very early marked, but diffuse, enhancement (type I curve). Malignancy was suspected. In addition, the mass completely encased the neurovascular bundle. However, histologic diagnosis and bacterial culture revealed *Nocardia* infection (pseudolymphoma).

In clinical practice, it would also be useful to be able to distinguish low-grade malignant bone tumors from benign bone tumors. Unfortunately, in our study, early dynamic enhancement features did not allow differentiation between benign tumors and low-grade malignant bone tumors (sensitivity, 15%; specificity, 56%). Absence of enhancement during the 5-minute acquisition time was the only parameter indicating presence of a benign bone tumor (sensitivity, 100%; NPV, 100%). This observation, however, has limited value since only 38% of benign bone tumors showed absence of enhancement. Also, some potentially malignant tumors such as sclerotic osteosarcoma may share this feature with benign tumors.

Even when high-grade malignant bone tumors were included, poor discrimination between benign and malignant bone tumors was found (Table 2). The combination of early start of tumor enhancement and rapid progression of enhancement to an early plateau with or without washout of contrast medium (type I curve) was found in almost all patients with high-grade bone sarcomas and metastases, but also in patients with certain benign bone tumors, including all patients with giant cell tumor (Fig 5) or aneurysmal bone cyst, and in patients with osteoblastoma, osteoid osteoma, eosinophilic granuloma, or, incidentally, fibrous dysplasia. Furthermore, late start of enhancement and/or gradual or slow progression of enhancement occurred in various benign bone tumors but also in low-grade malignant bone tumors. Owing to these overlapping results, a sensitivity in the range

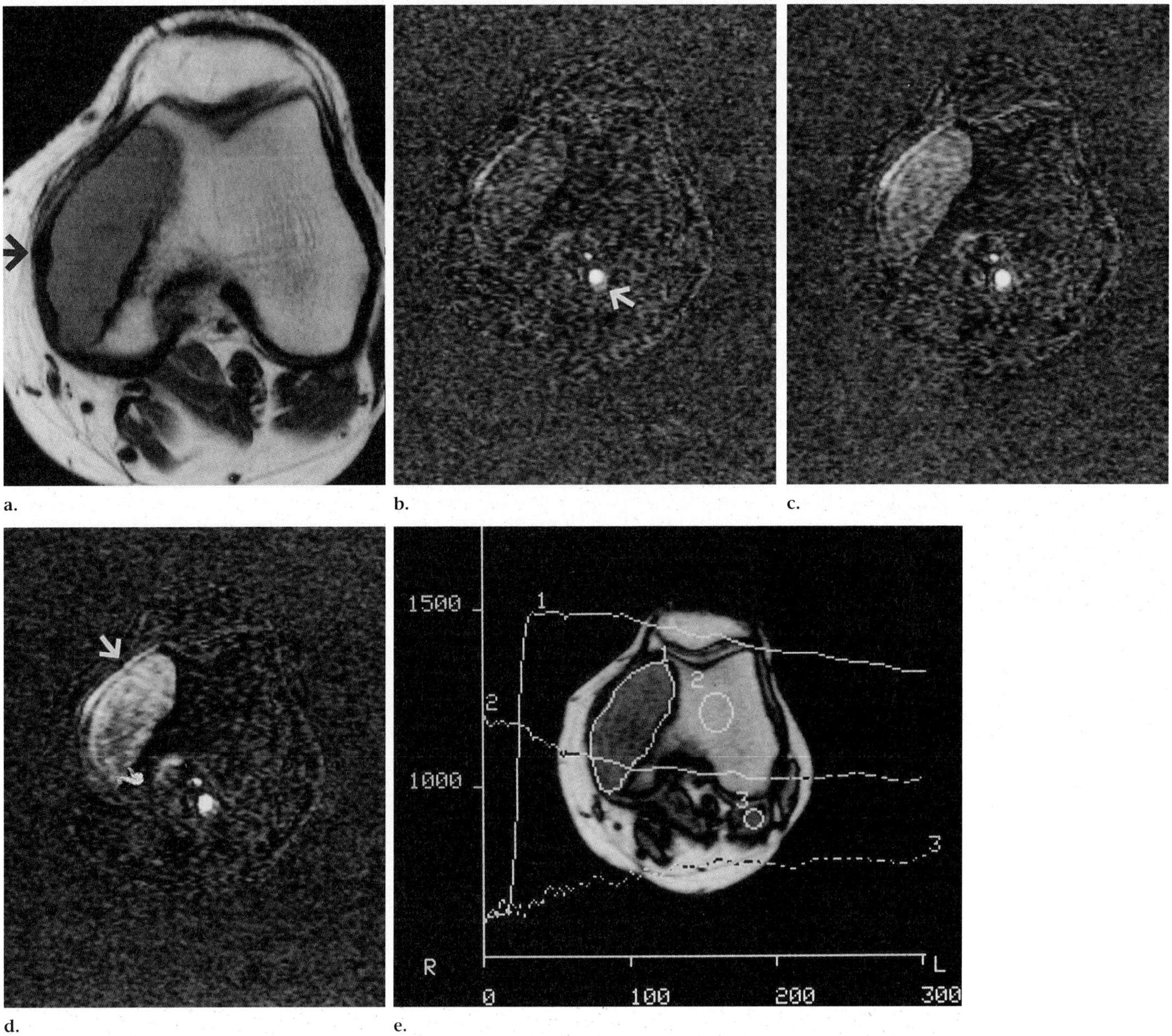

Figure 5. Case of a 27-year-old woman with intraosseous tumor of the medial femoral condyle. Early and rapidly progressive enhancement suggests malignancy. Histologic diagnosis was giant cell tumor. **(a)** Axial T1-weighted spin-echo image (600/20) reveals a sclerotically demarcated, somewhat lobulated tumor (arrow) with intermediate signal intensity. There is no soft-tissue extension. **(b–d)** Dynamic contrast-enhanced subtraction images obtained **(b)** at arrival of the bolus of contrast material in an artery (arrow) in the plane of dynamic imaging, **(c)** 3 seconds after arterial enhancement, and **(d)** 6 seconds after arterial enhancement. The sequence of dynamic images shows early, relatively homogeneous, and marked enhancement of the mass (arrow in **d**). **(e)** Corresponding time–signal intensity curves, superimposed on a dynamic contrast-enhanced gradient-echo image (15/6.8, 30° flip angle), display early and rapidly progressive enhancement of the entire tumor (*1*, type I curve), relative to bone marrow (*2*) and normal muscle (*3*). An early plateau phase is appreciated, followed by early washout. This is in accord with a highly cellular and vascularized tumor.

of 64%–70% and a specificity in the range of 50%–61% were found. This is in accord with results in several other dynamic MR studies that focused on the discrimination between benign and malignant musculoskeletal tumors on the basis of measurements of slope values of time–signal intensity curves (1,4–6). This again stresses the central role of radiographs in making the differential diagnosis of bone tumors.

Results of the present study implicate that the early enhancement characteristics determined with fast dynamic MR imaging reflect the biologic activity, such as cellularity, cell turnover time, and (neo)vascularity, rather than the malignant potential or histologic composition of bone tumors. Our findings subscribe the correlation between rate of contrast enhancement and tumor microvessel density that has been found in recent studies on the enhancement of breast lesions (22). This is also illustrated by the different enhancement patterns that can be encountered within certain groups of histologic diagnoses, such as fibrous dysplasia, eosinophilic granuloma, and osteomyelitis. A chronic inert status is reflected by a gradual or even absent dynamic enhancement pattern, as opposed to rapidly progressive enhancement in cases of biologic activity.

When a dynamic sequence with a high temporal resolution is used, arrival of the contrast material at the tumor can always be visualized, and the interval between arterial and tumor enhancement can be determined. We consider a temporal resolution in the 1–3-second range necessary, both to distinguish between true tumor extension and perineoplastic edema and to restrict the differential diagnosis of musculoskeletal, in particular soft-tissue, tumors (15,16). Arterial enhancement and not the start of bolus injection is the preferred reference, since this reduces the influence of the mode of contrast agent delivery and/or patient-related factors, such as the cardiovascular function and location of the tumor in the body (eg, neck, lower leg). Although we think that the manual injections had no implications on the results, use of a programmed power injector would further decrease the potential variability in injection rate, which may be introduced by administering the bolus of contrast material manually. The limitation of single or double section selection for dynamic imaging in voluminous, heterogeneous tumors can be overcome, as there are now fast sequences (including echo-planar imaging) available that allow imaging of large volumes with a temporal resolution of 3 seconds or less (22). Dynamic imaging of the entire tumor volume would also expand the potential use to targeting biopsies in soft-tissue masses and to identifying small residual or recurrent tumor foci present after different modes of therapy (18,19). Assistance in needle guiding is particularly helpful in large, heterogeneous tumors composed of necrotic and/or hemorrhagic parts.

Accurate MR diagnosis may also have an influence on patient care when MR findings contradict biopsy results. When our results can be confirmed, it may even become possible to identify subcategories in which small tumors can be excised primarily (without biopsy), on the basis of MR findings. Prospective studies that include larger numbers of patients are warranted to allow analyses of subcategories of soft-tissue tumors on the basis of MR findings.

In conclusion, fast, dynamic, contrast-enhanced subtraction MR imaging is a readily available technique that may be useful in the differentiation between benign and malignant soft-tissue masses.

References

1. Erlemann R, Reiser MF, Peters PE, et al. Musculoskeletal neoplasms: static and dynamic Gd-DTPA-enhanced MR imaging. Radiology 1989; 171:767–773.
2. Berquist TH, Ehman RL, King BF, Hodgman CG, Ilstrup DM. Value of MR imaging in differentiating benign from malignant soft-tissue masses: study of 95 lesions. AJR 1990; 155:1251–1255.
3. Mirowitz SA, Totty WG, Lee JKL. Characterization of musculoskeletal masses using dynamic Gd-DTPA enhanced spin-echo MRI. J Comput Assist Tomogr 1992; 16:120–125.
4. Verstraete KL, Dierick A, De Deene Y, et al. First-pass images of musculoskeletal lesions: a new and useful diagnostic application of dynamic contrast-enhanced MRI. Magn Reson Imaging 1994; 12:687–702.
5. Verstraete KL, De Deene Y, Roels H, Dierick A, Uyttendaele D, Kunnen M. Benign and malignant musculoskeletal lesions: dynamic contrast-enhanced MR imaging—parametric "first-pass" images depict tissue vascularization and perfusion. Radiology 1994; 192:835–843.
6. Verstraete KL, Vanzieleghem B, De Deene Y, et al. Static, dynamic and first-pass MR imaging of musculoskeletal lesions by use of gadodiamide injection. Acta Radiol 1995; 36:27–36.
7. Totty WG, Murphy WA, Lee JKT. Soft-tissue tumors: MR imaging. Radiology 1986; 160:135–141.
8. Kransdorf MJ, Jelinek JS, Moser RP. Soft tissue masses: diagnosis using MR imaging. AJR 1989; 153:541–547.
9. Hermann G, Abdelwahab IF, Miller T, Klein MJ, Lewis MM. Tumour and tumour-like conditions of the soft tissue: magnetic resonance imaging features differentiating benign from malignant masses. Br J Radiol 1992; 65:14–20.
10. Crim JR, Seeger LL, Yao L, Chandnani V, Eckardt JJ. Diagnosis of soft-tissue masses with MR imaging: can benign masses be differentiated from malignant ones? Radiology 1992; 185:581–586.
11. May DA, Good RB, Smith DK, Parsons TW. MR imaging of musculoskeletal tumors and tumor mimickers with intravenous gadolinium: experience with 242 patients. Skeletal Radiol 1997; 26:1–15.
12. Kransdorf MJ. Magnetic resonance imaging of musculoskeletal tumors. In: Syllabus for the categorial course on imaging of cancers. Reston, Va: American College of Radiology, 1992.
13. Sundaram M, McGuire MH, Schajowicz F. Soft-tissue masses: histologic basis for decreased signal (short T2) on T2-weighted images. AJR 1987; 148:1247–1250.
14. Pettersson H, Slone RM, Spanier S, Gillespy T III, Fitzsimmons JR, Scott KN. Musculoskeletal tumors: T1 and T2 relaxation times. Radiology 1988; 167:783–785.
15. Fletcher BD, Reddick WE, Taylor JS. Dynamic MR imaging of musculoskeletal neoplasms. Radiology 1996; 200:869–872.
16. van der Woude HJ, Bloem JL, Verstraete KL, Taminiau AHM, Nooy MA, Hogendoorn PCW. Osteosarcoma and Ewing's sarcoma after neoadjuvant chemotherapy: value of dynamic MR imaging in detecting viable tumor before surgery. AJR 1995; 165:593–598.
17. Verstraete KL, van der Woude HJ, Hogendoorn PCW, de Deene Y, Kunnen M, Bloem JL. Dynamic contrast-enhanced MRI in the musculoskeletal system. JMRI 1996; 6:311–321.
18. van der Woude HJ, Verstraete KL, Hogendoorn PCW, Taminiau AHM, Bloem JL. Fast dynamic contrast-enhanced subtraction MR imaging in characterization and follow-up of patients with musculoskeletal tumors (abstr). Radiology 1995; 197(P):463.
19. Verstraete KL, Achten E, Dierick A, et al. Dynamic contrast-enhanced MRI of musculo-skeletal neoplasms: different types and slopes of time-intensity curves (abstr). In: Book of abstracts: Society of Magnetic Resonance in Medicine 1992. Berkeley, Calif: Society of Magnetic Resonance in Medicine, 1992; 2609.
20. Ma LD, Frassica FJ, McCarthy EF, Bluemke DA, Zerhouni EA. Benign and malignant musculoskeletal masses: MR imaging differentiation with rim-to-center differential enhancement ratios. Radiology 1997; 202:739–744.
21. De Schepper AM, Vandevenne JE. Tumors of fibrous tissue. In: De Schepper AM, ed. Imaging of soft tissue tumors. Berlin, Germany: Springer-Verlag, 1997; 147–172.
22. Passe TJ, Bluemke DA, Siegelman SS. Tumor angiogenesis: tutorial on implications for imaging. Radiology 1997; 203:593–600.

Letters to the Editor

The Meaning of Words

From:
John R. Wilcox, Jr, MD
Department of Radiology, Naval Medical Center
620 John Paul Jones Circle, Portsmouth, VA 23708

Editor:
The opinions expressed in the Perspectives article "Customers and Providers" in the January 1998 issue of *Radiology* (1) develop a position that seems unnecessarily argumentative. The topics discussed involve two important and fundamentally different philosophic issues. The first is "the meaning of words," and the second is "the sacred versus the secular."

It takes a broad-based vocabulary to be able to communicate subtlety, and subtle distinctions are essential when dealing with an enterprise as complex as modern health care. The word "patient," as it refers to someone "waiting to receive treatment" (2), precisely communicates the image of someone waiting to be examined and treated by a physician. The use of the word is ancient, and its meaning is well understood. This word emphasizes the importance of the physician and the appropriateness of waiting to receive treatment. However, if I were trying to emphasize the dependence of the physician on those seeking the treatment, the word "patient" would miss the mark. There is a dependency that exists between the physician and the person seeking treatment. The word "customer" implies this dependency and, as such, is a good and useful word. To create a diatribe over the use of "customer" when it attempts only to describe another dimension in the provision of medical care does not seem reasonable.

Another issue raised by Dr Friedenberg is more contentious: that involves the sacred versus the secular. In the statement, "The term is another by-product of the administrative takeover of medicine by businessmen" (1), Dr Friedenberg seems to imply that businessmen are less honorable, less caring, and less responsible than physicians and, furthermore, that medicine is not a business. Although modern European-style medicine has close ties to the monastic tradition of the Middle Ages and its development of the hospital, in the United States medicine is an enterprise licensed by the various states as a business, just as is the case with any other activity requiring licensing. The "priesthood" does not require licensing and is not a business. The difference is that medicine is mercantile and the priesthood is religious. Medicine in the United States is not, and never has been, to any substantial degree, part of the sacred vocations. But more important is the fact that virtue and honor exist both within the sacred and the secular. The implication that the businessman by nature is less virtuous than the physician and cares less about the people and the services he or she provides is not true. I call to mind one particularly honorable carpenter from Palestine. Both offer services, both charge fees, some are honorable and some are not, but both are involved in mercantile activities.

Proper use of words makes for effective communication. The words: "patient," "customer," "physician," and "provider" are all good and proper words used to describe different attributes of a complex enterprise.

References
1. Friedenberg RM. Customers and providers. Radiology 1998; 206: 16.
2. Fowler FG, Fowler HW. Pocket Oxford Dictionary of Current English. Oxford, England: Clarendon, 1984.

Dr Friedenberg responds:

Dr Wilcox of course realizes that opinions expressed in Perspectives are personal and the reader has the right to disagree. The words "patient" and "physician" have time-honored meanings and imply a relationship that transcends the business of medicine. There is no denying that a patient is a customer or that a physician is a provider. However, the word "physician" has been used since the time of Socrates and has always implied a very special relationship between individuals. Why not call a priest a provider? I believe it would degrade the priesthood, as it does the medical profession. I guess I just would like to consider the practice of medicine a profession first, a business second. The use of "provider" and "customer" reverses that order.

Richard M. Friedenberg, MD
Department of Radiological Sciences, RT 140, University of California Irvine Medical Center
101 The City Drive, Orange, CA 92868-3298

Aunt Minnie

From:
Rita L. Teele, MD,* and N. Thorne Griscom, MD†
Department of Radiology, Christchurch School of Medicine, University of Otago, Private Bag 4710, Christchurch, New Zealand*
Department of Radiology, Boston Children's Hospital, 300 Longwood Avenue, Boston, MA 02115†

Editor:
It is unusual to send a letter about a book review, but when one's family is concerned, the genealogic record should be accurate!

In his review of *Aunt Minnie's Atlas and Imaging-specific Diagnosis* (1) in the July 1997 issue of *Radiology*, Leonard Berlin wrote "we do know that it was Felson who created the not-so-sophisticated but oft-used method of radiographic interpretation commonly referred to as the 'Aunt Minnie approach'."

We have it on the best authority, Ben Felson himself, that Aunt Minnie likely came from Boston (or perhaps from Philadelphia) and not from Cincinnati. He stated in the preface to his 1960 book *Chest Roentgenology* (2) that "the latter method has been aptly termed—I think first by Neuhauser—the 'Aunt Minnie approach'."

We do not know Aunt Minnie's ancestry—neither of us thought to ask Ed Neuhauser, Chief of Radiology at Boston Children's Hospital, while he was alive—but we are delighted that she has been cloned and is recognized around the world from New England to New Zealand.

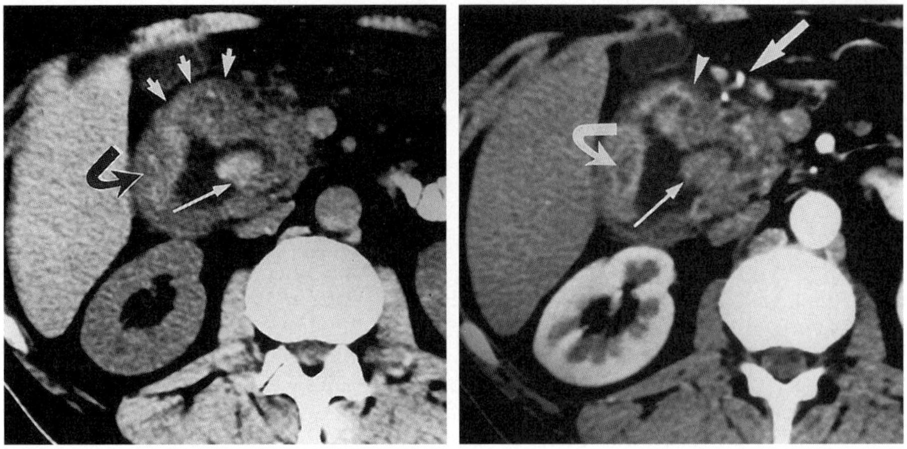

a. b.

Cystic dystrophy of the duodenal wall. **(a)** Unenhanced CT scan demonstrates a markedly thickened duodenal wall (short straight arrows), predominantly on the pancreatic side of the duodenum. Within the thickened duodenal wall, the cystic formation contains a hyperattenuating area (long straight arrow). Note the duodenal lumen (curved arrow). **(b)** Early-phase, contrast material–enhanced CT scan demonstrates no enhancement of the hyperattenuating area (thin straight arrow). Smaller cysts (arrowhead) are also demonstrated within the thickened duodenal wall. Note the duodenal lumen (curved arrow) and the displaced gastroduodenal artery (thick straight arrow).

References

1. Berlin L. Aunt Minnie's atlas and imaging-specific diagnosis (book review). Radiology 1997; 204:278.
2. Felson B. Fundamentals of chest roentgenology. Philadelphia, Pa: Saunders, 1960.

Dr Berlin responds:

I am pleased that Drs Teele and Griscom have clarified the facts surrounding the origin of the "not-so-sophisticated but oft-used method of radiographic interpretation commonly referred to as the 'Aunt Minnie approach'." It has finally been resolved that the term was created by Dr Neuhauser but popularized by Dr Felson. What remains to be determined, but, alas, may never be, is the question of whether either, both, or neither Dr Neuhauser nor Dr Felson actually had an aunt named Minnie. Perhaps one day we may yet find the answer to this great radiologic mystery. Are there any radiologic history sleuths out there who can help?

I suspect that Drs Felson and Neuhauser, who probably every day compete at tennis in the heavenly recreation center or try to "one-up" each other in "film interpretation" sessions that take place at the periodic heavenly conventions attended by past radiologic luminaries, are thoroughly enjoying this renewed notoriety about Aunt Minnie brought on by the book written by Drs Ford and Pope, the book review, and the subsequent letters published in *Radiology*. I can see them now, looking down on us, smiling from ear to ear.

Leonard Berlin, MD
Department of Radiology, Rush North Shore Medical Center
9600 Gross Point Road, Skokie, IL 60076

CT Features of Cystic Dystrophy of the Duodenal Wall

From:
Lionel Arrivé, MD, and Jean-Pierre Saint-Maurice, MD
Department of Radiology, Hôpital Saint-Antoine
184 Rue du Faubourg Saint-Antoine, 75771 Paris 12, France

Editor:
We read with interest the recent article by Procacci and colleagues (1) in the December 1997 issue of *Radiology* that describes the radiologic characteristics of 10 cases of cystic dystrophy of the duodenal wall. We recently observed a case of cystic dystrophy of the duodenal wall with computed tomographic (CT) and histopathologic features different from those reported by Procacci and colleagues.

A 36-year-old man presented with epigastric pain and vomiting. CT demonstrated a marked thickening of the pancreatic side of the second portion of the duodenum. Within the thickened wall, an elongated cystic lesion contained several hyperattenuating areas at unenhanced CT that were not enhanced after contrast material injection (Figure). A pancreaticoduodenectomy specimen showed an uneven thickening of the duodenal wall that was predominant on the pancreatic side of the duodenum. A true abscess was located within the thickened wall and contained thick yellow material and large protein plugs. At microscopy, the epithelium was completely eroded, with an important amount of surrounding inflammatory granulation tissue. Nodules of aberrant pancreatic tissue were also demonstrated within the duodenal wall.

We assume that hyperattenuating areas within the cystic lesion may be related to proteinaceous material contained within the abscess. Such hyperattenuating areas should be differentiated from blood-related hyperattenuating areas observed in duodenal hematoma. A case of abscess formation within cystic dystrophy of the duodenal wall has already been reported on (2); however, in this case, no specific CT feature was observed.

References

1. Procacci L, Graziani R, Zamboni G, et al. Cystic dystrophy of the duodenal wall: radiologic findings. Radiology 1997; 205: 741–747.
2. Vullierme MP, Vilgrain V, Fléjou JF, Zins M, Bernades P, Nahum H. Dystrophie kystique gastroduodénale sur pancréas aberrant: aspect échographique et tomodensitométrique. Rev Im Med 1993; 51:307–313.

Dr Procacci and colleagues respond:

We thank Drs Lionel Arrivé and Jean-Pierre Saint-Maurice for their interest in our article (1) in the December 1997 issue of *Radiology.* Their case adds to our understanding of the spectrum of clinical presentations related to cystic dystrophy of the duodenal wall, in that they have described abscess formation as a complication hitherto not recognized by us. We are encouraged by their corroboration of our observations of intramural cyst and displacement of the gastroduodenal artery as direct and indirect signs of cystic dystrophy of the duodenal wall.

Drs Arrivé and Saint-Maurice describe hyperattenuating regions within the cystic masses. We have not observed this finding and concur with their speculation on the cause of this abnormality. We are not sure that the presence of hyperattenuating regions in these lesions is pathognomonic for abscess formation. Once again, radiologic findings must be correlated with the clinical condition of the patient.

Reference

1. Procacci C, Graziani R, Zamboni G, et al. Cystic dystrophy of the duodenal wall: radiologic findings. Radiology 1997; 205:741–747.

Carlo Procacci, Rossella Graziani, Giuseppe Zamboni, Giorgio Cavallini, Paolo Pederzoli, Alessandro Guarise, Giuseppe Bogina, Carlo Biasiutti, Giovanni Carbognin, Ivo Andrea Bergamo-Andreis, and Gianfranco Pistolesi
Department of Radiology, University of Verona, Italy

Comparing Test Bolus Injections with Full Bolus Injections during MR Angiography

From:
George X. Zaleski, MD, and Brian Funaki, MD
Department of Radiology, University of Chicago Hospitals, 5841 S Maryland, Chicago, IL 60637

Editor:
We read with interest the recent article on test bolus examination at dynamic gadolinium-enhanced magnetic resonance (MR) angiography by Kim and colleagues (1) in the January 1998 issue of *Radiology* and found it to be a thought-provoking and useful article. However, we have a few ideas on their injection protocols as they relate to both the test and full bolus injections of gadopentetate dimeglumine during MR angiography. Because Drs Kim and colleagues injected different total volumes during the test and full bolus injections, we are concerned that the center (or peak) of the time-concentration curve for enhancement could be different after each injection. The test bolus consisted of 1–2 mL of gadopentetate dimeglumine, followed by a flush of 5 mL of physiologic saline solution. During this test bolus injection, the center of the time-concentration curve remains within the brachial vein or perhaps the axillary vein. The 1–2-mL test volume and 5-mL flush generally do not displace the blood volume of the brachial vein or the axillary veins. However, during the full bolus injection, the contrast agent may reach the right atrium and circulation earlier than expected from the test injection results. This is due to the differences in the total volumes injected during each phase of the study.

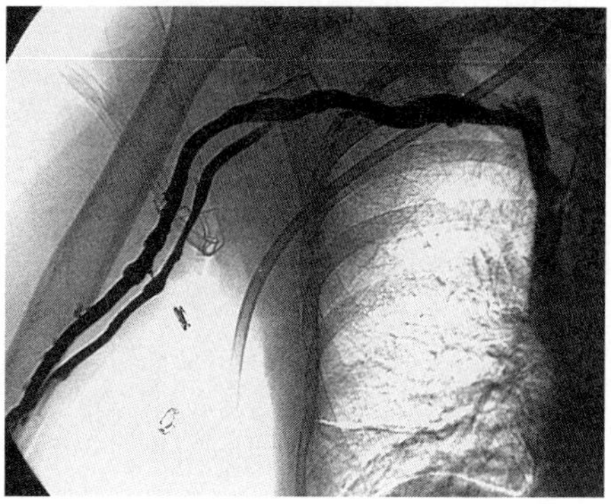

Figure 1. Venogram obtained during injection of 14 mL of iodinated contrast agent into the brachial vein.

Specifically, the center of the time-concentration curve during the full bolus injection will be located approximately "10 mL" further than the test bolus because of differences in the total volumes injected. If, for example, the patient has a small venous capacity, the center of the full bolus injection can be located past the right atrium. On the other hand, if the patient has a larger venous capacity, the center of the full bolus injection could still be within the brachial vein (Fig 1). However, in both patients, small test injections will have the center of the time-concentration curves within the peripheral veins. It is unlikely that the center of the time-concentration curve of the small test injection will match the center of the time-concentration curve of the larger full bolus injection.

To minimize this error, did the authors consider using a test bolus of 28 mL (total volume of gadopentetate dimeglumine needed for a 70-kg patient)? Other methods, such as flushing one-half of the full-bolus volume (14 mL) after injection of contrast agent, may also place the peak of the time-concentration curve for the small-volume test bolus injection closer to where the peak would be for the large-volume full bolus injection.

Reference

1. Kim JK, Farb RI, Wright GA. Test bolus examination in the carotid artery at dynamic gadolinium-enhanced MR angiography. Radiology 1998; 206:283–289.

Dr Kim and colleagues respond:

We appreciate the attention paid by Drs Zaleski and Funaki to our recent article (1) and are grateful for the opportunity to clarify this portion of our article. Drs Zaleski and Funaki point out that a 5-mL physiologic saline solution flush for the test bolus, as described, would not have been sufficient either to push the test bolus into the right atrium or to be a fair analogue to the larger full bolus. We agree with this and did indeed consider this factor during the development of our technique. Our article described a flow-insensitive MR test bolus detection technique performed before a full bolus injection of gadopentetate dimeglumine to image the carotid arteries. The described 5 mL of physiologic saline solution represented the known volume of saline solution residing

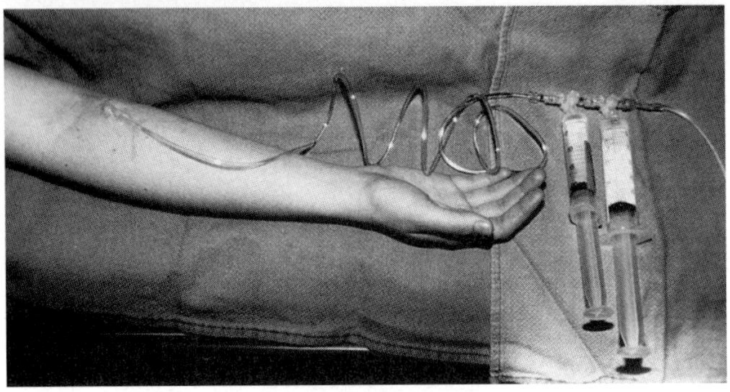

Figure 2. Photograph of intravenous tubing setup.

within the injection tubing between the saline solution syringe and the small test bolus of contrast agent in the line just before the intravenous site (Fig 2). Our article left the mistaken impression that this was the entirety of the saline solution bolus used to follow the test bolus. In actuality, approximately 20 mL of saline solution was present in the saline solution syringe before the test bolus injection, all of which was pushed into the patient. A total of approximately 25 mL of saline solution was therefore pushed into each patient for the test bolus. This approach closely approximated the transit time of the leading edge of the full bolus from the injection site to the carotid arteries. As a result, we attained consistent images of first-pass enhancement of the carotid arteries, as described in our article. Test bolus examinations in more than 20 subsequent patients have also given similar results.

In recent months, we have extended our approach to contrast agent–enhanced three-dimensional MR angiography of the carotid arteries to include (*a*) flow-regulated injection of contrast agent and saline solution at 2 mL per second (Spectris MR Injector; MedRad, Pittsburgh, Pa) and (*b*) our own interactive, automated trigger sequence for three-dimensional MR angiography. Automated flow regulation ensures a smaller variability in the injection rate than can be provided with manual injection. Automated triggering permits a more accurate detection of the arrival of contrast agent at a target site. The trigger sequence that we have developed uses flow-insensitive bolus detection, as described for the test bolus technique. The use of a test bolus examination, while more complex than an automatically triggered examination, still provides sufficiently accurate information for capture of the first pass of gadolinium-based contrast agent at the carotid arteries.

Reference

1. Kim JK, Farb RI, Wright GA. Test bolus examination in the carotid artery at dynamic gadolinium-enhanced MR angiography. Radiology 1998; 206:283–289.

Jae K. Kim, MD, PhD,*,† Richard I. Farb, MD,† Graham A. Wright, PhD *,‡

Departments of Imaging Research,* Medical Imaging,† and Medical Biophysics‡, Sunnybrook Health Science Centre
2075 Bayview Avenue, Toronto, Ontario, M4N 3M5 Canada

Normal Endometrial Signals at Color and Spectral Doppler US

From:
Michael Applebaum, MD
Diagnostic Ultrasound, Water Tower Place
845 North Michigan Avenue, Suite 935E, Chicago, IL 60611

Editor:
In their article "Uterine Arteriovenous Malformations: Gray-Scale and Doppler US Features with MR Imaging Correlation" in the January 1998 issue of *Radiology,* Huang et al (1) stated that "Normal endometrial color signals are rarely encountered with current equipment."

I must take exception to that comment.

Normally, endometrial color signals are frequently encountered with currently available equipment, depending, among other things, on the day of the menstrual cycle and the patient's age. In fact, the absence of a signal is abnormal (again, depending on the day of the menstrual cycle, the patient's age, etc) (2–10).

One would expect that endometrial color signals would be rarely encountered if (*a*) one is not trying to demonstrate them, (*b*) one is not using the technique necessary to demonstrate them, (*c*) one's equipment is not capable of demonstrating them, (*d*) one's equipment in one's hands is not capable of demonstrating them, (*e*) one examines the patient during the wrong time of the menstrual cycle (not around midcycle), and (*f*) one does not consider that they are demonstrable.

To claim that "normal endometrial color signals are rarely encountered" and shortchange the capabilities of "current equipment" in a study where no apparent consideration was paid to time of cycle and whose focus was not endometrial interrogation seems overly broad. (By implication, does this mean that abnormal signals are frequently encountered?)

References

1. Huang MW, Muradali D, Thurston WA, Burns PA, Wilson SR. Uterine arteriovenous malformations: gray-scale and Doppler US features with MR imaging correlation. Radiology 1997; 206:115–123.
2. Fleischer AC, Applebaum M, Parsons AK. Transvaginal sonography of the normal endometrium. In: Fleischer AC, Kurjak A, Granberg S, eds. Ultrasound and the endometrium. New York, NY: Parthenon, 1997; 1–16.
3. Applebaum M. The menstrual cycle, menopause, ovulation induction and in vitro fertilization. In: Copel JA, Reed KL, eds. Doppler ultrasound in obstetrics and gynecology. New York, NY: Raven, 1995; 71–86.
4. Zaidi J, Campbell S, Pittrof R, Tan SL. Endometrial thickness, morphology, vascular penetration and velocimetry in predicting implantation in an in vitro fertilization program. Ultrasound Obstet Gynecol 1995; 6:191–198.
5. Applebaum M. The uterine biophysical profile. Ultrasound Obstet Gynecol 1995; 5:67–68.
6. Applebaum M. The uterine biophysical profile (UBP). In: Allahbadia G, ed. Endosonography in obstetrics and gynecology. Mulund (West), India: Rotunda Medical Technologies, 1997; 343–352.
7. Applebaum M. The "steel" or "Teflon" endometrium: ultrasound visualization of endometrial vascularity in IVF patients and outcome. In: The Third World Congress of Ultrasound in Obstetrics and Gynecology. London, England: Parthenon, 1993; 10.

8. Applebaum M. Ultrasound visualization of endometrial vascularity in normal premenopausal women. In: The Third World Congress of Ultrasound in Obstetrics and Gynecology. London, England: Parthenon, 1993; 11.
9. Applebaum M. Ultrasound visualization of endometrial vascularity in normal pre-menopausal women. Presented at the 2nd Conference on the Endometrium, Bologna, Italy, September 20–22, 1993.
10. Applebaum M. The "steel" or "Teflon" endometrium: ultrasound visualization of endometrial vascularity in IVF patients and outcome. Presented at the 2nd Conference on the Endometrium, Bologna, Italy, September 20–22, 1993.

Drs Wilson and Burns respond:

We thank Dr Applebaum for his timely letter to the editor pointing out the ability of current ultrasonographic (US) equipment to display blood flow information in the normal endometrium on both color and spectral Doppler images. At approximately the time that our article "Uterine Arteriovenous Malformations: Gray-Scale and Doppler US Features with MR Imaging Correlation" appeared in press, we were fortunate enough to install several state-of-the-art US machines in our own department. As is frequently the case, each generation of equipment does offer improved sensitivity and capability of demonstrating blood flow. We also are frequently demonstrating normal endometrial Doppler signals.

We are grateful to Dr Applebaum for bringing this point to light.

Reference

1. Huang MW, Muradali D, Thurston WA, Burns PA, Wilson SR. Uterine arteriovenous malformations: gray-scale and Doppler US features with MR imaging correlation. Radiology 1997; 206:115–123.

Stephanie R. Wilson, MD,* and Peter M. Burns, MD†
Department of Diagnostic Imaging, The Toronto Hospital
200 Elizabeth Street, Toronto, Ontario, M5G 2C4 Canada*

Department of Imaging Research, Sunnybrook Health Sciences Centre
2075 Bayview Avenue, Toronto, Ontario, M4N 4M5 Canada†

Residual Metal Shavings and Fragments Associated with Large-Core Biopsy Needles: A Follow-up

From:
Charles A. Finder, MD, Richard W. Kisielewski, MS, and Anita M. Kedas, PhD
U.S. Food and Drug Administration, Center for Devices and Radiological Health, HFZ-240
1350 Piccard Drive, Rockville, MD 20850
The opinions or assertions presented herein are the private views of the authors and are not to be construed as conveying either an official endorsement or criticism by the U.S. Department of Health and Human Services, the Public Health Service, or the Food and Drug Administration.

Editor:
As a follow-up to our letter (1) in the August 1996 issue of *Radiology*, we report here on our analysis of large-core biopsy needles with respect to postfire fragmentation and the production of metal shavings.

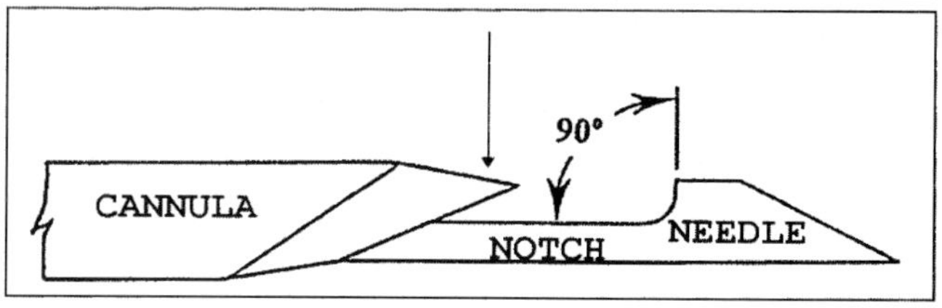

Diagram demonstrates the large-core biopsy needle with a 90° notch angle. The residual metal shavings and fragments are formed when the lead cutting edge of the outer cannula (arrow) strikes the top of the 90° notch angle.

Large-core biopsy with stereotactic guidance has been used extensively to evaluate palpable breast lesions detected with screening mammography (2–4). Adverse event reports submitted to the U.S. Food and Drug Administration, Rockville, Md, have contained claims that metal shavings and fragments have been detected in organ tissue, core samples, or both after large-core biopsy with side-notch needles. Reports of residual metal shavings and fragments were commonly associated with multiple firings of an automatic core biopsy device with 14-gauge biopsy needles. With the exception of two references to kidney tissue, all reports received referred to breast tissue. Whether this was due to the limited support given to the needle by the surrounding breast tissue or to the ability of today's screen-film mammography to demonstrate small metal fragments is unclear.

In response to these reported adverse events, we tested 43 different side-notch core biopsy needles. The needles were tested by firing them either into gelatin-filled test cells (simulating breast tissue) or into air-filled test tubes. We found that 10 models produced metal shavings or fragments when fired multiple times in either gelatin or air. The factor most commonly associated with this problem was a 90° front notch angle (Figure). None of the needles with a notch angle greater than 90° produced shavings or fragments, while 10 of the 14 needles with 90° notch angles did. Of the 90° notch angle needles tested, one produced fragments after just two firings; two others, after four firings. In our experiment, all the metal shavings or fragments could be identified as arising from the lead cutting edge of the outer cannula and are believed to be caused by the striking of this portion of the cannula against the top of the 90° notch angle (Figure). The largest metal fragment identified measured 1.5×0.45 mm.

Several manufacturers have or are in the process of modifying their needles to increase this angle to greater than 90°. Some manufacturers continue to produce the 90° notch angle biopsy needles. We urge those physicians who use needles with 90° notch angles to avoid dry firings or multiple firings in tissue and to closely monitor all their core biopsy procedures to identify needle damage or fragmentation.

If a practitioner becomes aware of a medical device–related problem, he or she is encouraged to report the problem to the Food and Drug Administration via MedWatch, a voluntary reporting program. The American Medical Association, Chicago, Ill, is an active supporter of this program.

Voluntary reports or requests for report forms should he

directed as follows: Medical Product Reporting Program, MedWatch, HF-2, Food and Drug Administration, 5600 Fishers Ln, Rockville, MD 20857; phone, 1-800-FDA-1088.

References

1. Kedas AM, Byrd LJ, Kisielewski RW. Residual metal shavings and fragments associated with large-core breast biopsy (letter). Radiology 1996; 200:585.
2. Parker SH, Lovin JD, Jobe WE, et al. Stereotactic breast biopsy with a biopsy gun. Radiology 1990; 176:741–747.
3. Parker SH, Lovin JD, Jobe WE, Burke BJ, Hopper KD, Yakes WF. Nonpalpable breast lesions: stereotactic automated large-core biopsies. Radiology 1991; 180:403–407.
4. Dronkers DJ. Stereotaxic core biopsy of breast lesions. Radiology 1992; 183:631–634.

Errata

"Lumbar Spine: Quantitative and Qualitative Assessment of Positional (Upright Flexion and Extension) MR Imaging and Myelography." Radiology 1998; 207:391–398.

On page 391, the last sentence of the Abstract should read as follows: "In a selected patient population, only small changes in the sagittal diameter of the dural sac and foraminal size can be expected between various body positions, and the information gained **in addition to that from** standard MR imaging is limited."

"Brachytherapy for Prophylaxis of Restenosis after Long-Segment Femoropopliteal Angioplasty: Pilot Study." Radiology 1998; 208:173–179.

The caption for Figure 2 should read as follows:

Figure 2. Graphs show **(a)** ABI **(b)** PVR versus time before and after angioplasty. Mean (bold dashed line) and individual values for the 10 patients are graphed. **Values below the dotted line at an ABI of 1.0 in a are abnormal, and values above the dotted line at a PVR of 2.4 in b are indicative of at least 50% stenosis.**

Abstracts of Current Literature

Gastrointestinal System

Cost Analysis of Alternative Approaches to Colorectal Screening in Familial Adenomatous Polyposis. David M. Cromwell, Richard D. Moore, Jill D. Brensinger, et al. *Gastroenterology* 1998; 114:893–901. (D.M.C., Department of Medicine, Johns Hopkins School of Medicine, 1830 E Monument St, #8061, Baltimore, MD 21287)

Background and Aims: The commercial availability of gene testing for familial adenomatous polyposis (FAP) represents an important advance in screening for inherited colon cancer. The authors investigated the financial impact of this diagnostic tool on colorectal screening for FAP. *Methods:* Decision analysis was used to compare per-person costs with third-party payers of three colorectal screening strategies used to diagnose FAP in at-risk persons. The strategies included conventional serial flexible sigmoidoscopy and two APC gene testing approaches. *Results:* For one at-risk relative who begins screening at age 12 years, average screening costs are $2,625 for genotyping the proband first, $2,674 for genotyping the at-risk relative first, and $3,208 for conventional sigmoidoscopy. The cost advantage of genotyping increases as the pedigree size increases. For a pedigree of five at-risk relatives, sigmoidoscopy would have to cost less than $85.60 (professional plus facility fee) for conventional screening to compete with genotyping. The cost advantage of genotyping is diminished for at-risk relatives who begin FAP screening at older ages. *Conclusions:* The choice of least expensive FAP screening strategy depends on the cost of flexible sigmoidoscopy, patient age when screening starts, and pedigree size. Genotyping can substantially reduce the cost of FAP screening and, when possible, should start with the proband.
Authors' Abstract

The Inaccuracy of Duplex Ultrasonography in Predicting Patency of Transjugular Intrahepatic Portosystemic Shunts. Charles A. Owens, Christopher Bartolone, David L. Warner, et al. *Gastroenterology* 1998; 114:975–980. (Thomas J. Layden, Section of Digestive and Liver Diseases, University of Illinois at Chicago Medical Center, 840 S Wood St, Rm 718E, Chicago, IL 60612-7323)

Background and Aims: To the authors' knowledge, a prospective, double-blinded study with preset sonographic criteria has not been performed to assess the accuracy of duplex ultrasonography (US) in determining the patency of transjugular intrahepatic portosystemic shunts (TIPS). The purpose of this study was to determine the sensitivity and specificity of duplex US in predicting shunt malfunction by using accepted preset sonographic criteria. *Methods:* Sixty US and venographic follow-up comparisons were made in 38 patients with cirrhosis who had undergone TIPS placement for variceal bleeding ($n = 28$) or intractable ascites ($n = 10$). US results were analyzed by one of two board-certified ultrasonographers without knowledge of venographic findings. *Results:* In the 31 occluded ($n = 8$) or stenotic ($n = 23$) shunts, US accurately demonstrated a shunt malfunction (occlusion or stenosis) in only 11 studies and incorrectly indicated patency in 20. In comparison with venography, US had a sensitivity of 35% and a specificity of 83% in predicting TIPS stenosis or occlusion. *Conclusions:* These results suggest that duplex sonography is not a sensitive test in predicting the presence of a hemodynamically significant stenosis and that shunt status should be assessed with venography and direct portal pressure measurements until a more reliable and proved noninvasive US criterion is devised.
Authors' Abstract

"Salvage" Transjugular Intrahepatic Portosystemic Shunts: Gastric Fundal Compared with Esophageal Variceal Bleeding. Tai Nin Chau, David Patch, Yu Wai Chan, et al. *Gastroenterology* 1998; 114:981–987. (Andrew Kenneth Burroughs, Department of Liver Transplantation and Hepatobiliary Medicine, Royal Free Hospital, Pond St, Hampstead, London NW3 2QG, England)

Background and Aims: The optimal emergency treatment for gastric fundal variceal bleeding is still unclear. In this study, the efficacy of the transjugular intrahepatic portosystemic stent/shunt (TIPS) in patients with uncontrolled gastric fundal variceal bleeding was compared with the efficacy in esophageal variceal bleeding. *Methods:* One hundred twelve consecutive patients with uncontrolled variceal bleeding required emergency TIPS, 84 with esophageal varices unresponsive to endoscopic and vasoconstrictor therapy and 28 with gastric fundal varices unresponsive to vasoconstrictor therapy. Clinical and biochemical data were retrieved, and the two groups were compared. *Results:* Variceal bleeding was controlled in all patients after TIPS except for one in each group. There were no significant differences between the two groups in terms of markers of disease severity, severity of bleeding, or portal hemodynamics. During a median follow-up of 7 months, 20 in the esophageal varices group (24%) and eight in the gastric fundal varices group (29%) developed clinical rebleeding. Most early rebleeding (within 7 days after TIPS) was related to esophageal ulceration secondary to previous sclerotherapy. Rates of mortality were similar in both groups. *Conclusions:* These results suggest that emergency TIPS is equally effective in the immediate short-term control of gastric fundal variceal bleeding compared and variceal bleeding.
Authors' Abstract

Clinical Events after Transjugular Intrahepatic Portosystemic Shunt: Correlation with Hemodynamic Findings. Marta Casado, Jaume Bosch, Juan Carlos García-Pagán, et al. *Gastroenterology* 1998; 114:1296–1303. (J.B., Hepatic Hemodynamic Laboratory, Liver Unit, Hospital Clinic, Villarroel 170, 08036 Barcelona, Spain)

Background and Aims: Transjugular intrahepatic portosystemic shunt (TIPS) procedures are increasingly being used, but the relationship between the hemodynamic effects of TIPS and the clinical events at follow-up remains undefined. Hence, the authors investigated the hemodynamic correlations of portal hypertension–related events after a TIPS procedure. *Methods:* Prospective follow-up was performed in 122 patients with cirrhosis who underwent a TIPS procedure because of variceal hemorrhage. *Results:* The portacaval pressure gradient (PPG) significantly decreased after the TIPS procedure (from 19.7 mm Hg ± 4.6 [standard deviation] to 8.6 mm Hg ± 2.7; $P > .001$), but increased thereafter and at rebleeding ($n = 25$) was more than 12 mm Hg in all patients (18.4 mm Hg ± 4.6). Twenty-six patients developed ascites; the PPG (measured in 19) was always more than 12 mm Hg. Increasing the PPG to more than 12 mm Hg occurred very frequently (83% at 1 year). Within 1 year, 77% of patients underwent balloon angioplasty or repeated stent placement. However, 80% had again a PPG of more than 12 mm Hg 1 year after reintervention. Hepatic encephalopathy developed in 31% of patients at 1 year; 21 of 23 patients had a PPG of less than 12 mm Hg. *Conclusions:* Total protection from the risk of recurrent complications of portal hypertension after a TIPS procedure requires that the PPG be decreased and maintained at less than 12 mm Hg. However, reintervention will be required in most patients within 1 year and again the 2nd year. On the other hand, such portal decompression is associated with an increased risk of hepatic encephalopathy.
Authors' Abstract

Clinical Course of Colorectal Crohn's Disease: A 35-Year Follow-up Study of 507 Patients. Annika Lapidus, Olle Bernell, Göran Hellers, et al. *Gastroenterology* 1998; 114:1151–1160. (A.L., Department of Gastroenterology, Karolinska Institute, Huddinge University Hospital, S-141 86 Huddinge, Sweden)

Background and Aims: Crohn's disease confined to the colon and rectum is an increasing clinical entity. The aim of this study was to assess the features and clinical course of colorectal Crohn's disease. *Methods:* This was a retrospective cohort study of 507 patients in whom colonic or rectal Crohn's disease had been diagnosed between 1955 and 1989. *Results:* Colonic distribution was segmental in 40%, total in 31%, and left-sided in 26%. Perianal/rectal fistulas occurred in 37%. In patients who attained clinical remission, the 5-year cumulative relapse rate after diagnosis was 67% (95% confidence interval [CI], 62%, 72%). At the initial presentation of Crohn's disease, the frequency of major surgery decreased from 24% to 14% ($P < .005$) over time. Still, the overall long-term probability of major surgery after 10 years was unaltered (49% vs 47%). The presence of fistulas increased the probability of

surgical resection (relative risk [RR], 1.7 [95% CI, 1.3, 2.2]), whereas left-sided disease was associated with a decrease (RR, 0.6 [95% CI, 0.4, 0.8]). Twenty-four percent of the patients developed inflammation in the small bowel. The cumulative risk for a permanent ileostomy was 25% (95% CI, 21%, 29%) 10 years after diagnosis. *Conclusions:* Colorectal Crohn's disease is an increasing entity carrying substantial morbidity. Half of the patients will undergo surgical resection within the first 10 years, and half of those will ultimately undergo ileostomy. Changed management at diagnosis has not affected the long-term probability of resection.
Authors' Abstract

Successful Treatment of Retractile Mesenteritis with Oral Progesterone. Roberto Mazure, Pablo Fernández Marty, Sonia Niveloni, et al. *Gastroenterology* 1998; 114:1313–1317. (Julio C. Bai, Uriburu 346, [1846] Adrogué, Buenos Aires, Argentina)

Retractile mesenteritis is a rare inflammatory mesenteric disorder that involves the intestine secondarily. The natural history of this process is diverse, but most patients require some empiric therapeutic measures. Up to now, pharmacologic therapy has included corticosteroids, colchicine, and immunosuppressive drugs. Although these drugs are successful in most patients, some have been refractory to these therapies and, in others, the beneficial effects were counterbalanced by adverse reactions. Many patients require surgery, but most have poor results. This report describes a 42-year-old man with histologically proved retractile mesenteritis refractory to surgical intervention who had a good response to oral progesterone (10 mg/d for 6 months) with complete disappearance of tumor mass and clinical symptoms. No adverse effects were detected. Current knowledge about the mechanism by which progesterone affects fibrogenesis is scanty. It seems likely that progesterone downregulates proliferation and metabolism of fibroblasts and fibrogenesis.
Authors' Abstract

Breast

Sentinel Lymph Node Biopsy in Breast Cancer: Initial Experience at Memorial Sloan-Kettering Cancer Center. Brian J. O'Hea, Arnold D. K. Hill, Ayda M. El-Shirbiny, et al. *J Am Coll Surg* 1998; 186:423–427. (Hiram S. Cody III, Breast Service, Department of Surgery, Memorial Sloan-Kettering Cancer Center, 1275 York Ave, New York, NY 10021)

Background: Sentinel node biopsy has emerged as a potential alternative to routine axillary dissection in clinically node-negative breast cancer. *Study Design:* From September 1995 to June 1996 at Memorial Sloan-Kettering Cancer Center, 60 patients with clinically node-negative cancer underwent sentinel node biopsy, which was immediately followed by standard axillary dissection. Both blue dye and a radioisotope were used to identify the sentinel node. Sentinel node biopsy results were compared with standard axillary dissection results for their ability to accurately reflect the final pathologic status of the axillary nodes. *Results:* The sentinel node was successfully identified with lymphoscintigraphy in 75% (42 of 56), with blue dye in 75% (44 of 59), with the isotope in 88% (52 of 59), and with the combination of blue dye and the isotope in 93% (55 of 59) of all 59 evaluable patients. Of the 55 patients in this study whose sentinel nodes were identified, 20 (36%) were histologically positive. The sentinel node was falsely negative in three patients, yielding an accuracy of 95%. Sentinel node biopsy was more accurate for T1 (98%) than for T2-T3 tumors (82%). *Conclusions:* Lymphatic mapping is technically feasible, reliably identifies a sentinel node in most cases, and appears more accurate for T1 tumors than for larger lesions. Blue dye and the radioisotope are complementary techniques, and the overall success of the procedure is maximized when the two are used together.
Authors' Abstract

A Comparative Analysis of Lobular and Ductal Carcinoma of the Breast: Presentation, Treatment, and Outcomes. David J. Winchester, Helena R. Chang, Theresa A. Graves, et al. *J Am Coll Surg* 1998; 186:416–422. (David P. Winchester, Evanston Hospital, 2650 Ridge Ave, Burch 105, Evanston, IL 60201)

Background: Compared with invasive ductal carcinoma, invasive lobular carcinoma of the breast is considered by many to be a more indistinct and multicentric form of cancer that is detected later and is treated less optimally by breast-preservation techniques. This study analyzed the presentation, treatment trends, and survival rates in women who had invasive lobular and ductal breast carcinoma. The objective was to determine the utility of breast-preservation therapy for invasive lobular carcinoma by analyzing historic data on tumor features and survival. *Study Design:* Data on 291,273 women diagnosed with invasive carcinoma between 1985 and 1993 were obtained from the National Cancer Data Base. Analysis included the patient's age at diagnosis; tumor histology, anatomic site, diameter, grade, and stage; treatment; and disease status 5 years after diagnosis. *Results:* The mean patient age at diagnosis was 61.0 years for invasive ductal carcinoma, 63.0 years for invasive lobular carcinoma, and 60.6 years for tumors with combined histology. The anatomic location, tumor diameter, and tumor grade were similar for each histotype. Breast-preservation therapy was less frequent for invasive lobular carcinoma. The 5-year overall survival and local disease-free survival rates for women treated with breast preservation were similar for invasive ductal carcinoma (84% overall survival; 97% disease-free survival) and invasive lobular carcinoma (87% overall survival; 98% disease-free survival). *Conclusions:* Invasive lobular carcinoma manifests with a similar age distribution, anatomic subsite, diameter, and grade as invasive ductal carcinoma. Breast preservation is selected less commonly for women who have invasive lobular carcinoma, but this choice of therapy does not compromise the disease-free or overall survival status of this group of patients.
Authors' Abstract

Genitourinary System

Inconclusive Clinical and Ultrasound Evaluation of the Scrotum: Impact of Magnetic Resonance Imaging on Patient Management and Cost. Alexander D. Serra, Hedvig Hricak, Fergus V. Coakley, et al. *Urology* 1998; 51:1018–1021. (F.V.C., Department of Radiology, University of California—San Francisco, Box 0628, L-308, 505 Parnassus Ave, San Francisco, CA 94143-0628)

Objectives: To determine the diagnostic utility and net cost of magnetic resonance (MR) imaging in the management of clinically and sonographically inconclusive scrotal lesions. *Methods:* A multicenter retrospective review identified 34 patients with lesions diagnosed by means of scrotal MR imaging following inconclusive clinical and ultrasound (US) evaluation. The final diagnoses were based on surgery (n = 18) or clinical and US follow-up (n = 16). Final diagnoses of 29 testicular lesions were as follows: orchitis (n = 11), infarct (n = 6), neoplasm (n = 6), rupture (n = 3), torsion (n = 2), and radiation fibrosis (n = 1). The final diagnoses of five extratesticular lesions were as follows: epididymitis (n = 2), epididymal abscess (n = 2), and neoplasm (n = 1). Management plans prior to and after MR imaging findings were formulated by a general urologist and a urologic oncologist. The costs of the pre- and post-MR imaging management plans were estimated by using the Medicare reimbursement schedule. *Results:* The leading US diagnosis was correct for 10 of 34 patients (29%), and the leading MR imaging diagnosis was correct for 31 of 34 patients (91%). MR imaging improved the management plan of the general urologist and urologic oncologist in 19 patients (56%) and 17 patients (50%), respectively. MR imaging worsened the management plan of both clinicians in one patient. Management was unchanged in all other patients. The overall net cost savings were $543–$730 per patient for the urologic oncologist and the general urologist, respectively, and $3,833 per patient originally scheduled for surgery. *Conclusions:* Use of MR imaging after inconclusive clinical and US evaluation of scrotal lesions may improve management, decrease the number of surgical procedures, and result in net cost savings.
Authors' Abstract

Outpatient Ultrasound-guided Palladium 103 Brachytherapy for Localized Adenocarcinoma of the Prostate: A Preliminary Report of 434 Patients. Jerrold Sharkey, Stanley D. Chovnick, Raymond J. Behar, et al. *Urology* 1998; 51:796–803. (J.S., Urology Health Center, 5652 Meadow Ln, New Port Richey, FL 34652)

Objectives: To assess the effectiveness of palladium-103 brachytherapy in stage T1 and T2 adenocarcinoma of the prostate. *Methods:* Charts of 474 patients treated between 1991

and 1996 with transperineal real-time ultrasound-guided Pd-103 implants were reviewed to assess posttreatment prostate-specific antigen (PSA) levels and follow-up biopsy results. Of 474 patients, 434 had sufficient data for this report. The implant technique used allows precise placement of seeds and accurate dose delivery of the entire prostate. Preoperative neoadjuvant leuprolide and flutamide were given selectively to reduce prostates larger than 50 cm^3 and for lesions with a Gleason grade of more than 7. *Results:* Of 434 patients, successful cancer control was demonstrated in 81% of patients by a decrease in PSA levels to less than 1.5 ng/mL at 1 year. Biopsy results were negative in 88% of patients 1 year after the procedure and in 89% at 2 years. Analysis of the data suggests that patients with pretreatment PSA levels less than 10 ng/mL had the best outcomes. There were no disease-related deaths; the predominant morbidity was short-term bladder and bowel irritation without permanent sequelae. Incontinence occurred in less than 5% of patients who had undergone prior transurethral resection of the prostate. Impotence occurred in less than 15% of patients. *Conclusions:* The technique used in this study proved effective in reducing PSA levels to less than 1.5 ng/mL and in producing negative biopsies 1 and 2 years postoperatively. Results are comparable to those of external-beam radiation therapy, demonstrating a significant reduction in morbidity.
Authors' Abstract

A High-Efficiency Microwave Thermoablation System for the Treatment of Benign Prostatic Hyperplasia: Results of a Randomized, Sham-controlled, Prospective, Double-Blind, Multicenter Clinical Trial. Thayne R. Larson, Michael L. Blute, Reginald C. Bruskewitz, et al. *Urology* 1998; 51:731–742. (T.R.L., Department of Urology, Mayo Clinic, 13400 E Shea Blvd, Scottsdale, AZ 85259)

Objectives: To determine the effectiveness, safety, and impact on patient quality of life of a novel transurethral microwave thermoablation system for the treatment of benign prostatic hyperplasia (BPH). *Methods:* A total of 169 patients with BPH were randomized to undergo a 1-hour microwave (n = 125) or sham (n = 44) procedure performed with the Urologix Targis thermoablation system on an outpatient basis, without general or regional anesthesia. Symptoms, flow rates, and quality of life scores were determined before the study procedure and periodically thereafter up to 6 months. *Results:* The mean American Urological Association (AUA) score in the microwave group diminished 50% ($P < .001$) by the 6-month evaluation (10.5; 95% confidence interval [CI], 9.2, 11.8) compared with baseline values (20.8; 95% CI, 19.8, 21.9). The sham group also exhibited lower postprocedural AUA scores; however, the magnitude of the postprocedural decline in AUA score in the microwave group was significantly greater ($P < .01$) than that in the sham group. Half the microwave group had an AUA score of less than 9 by 6 months, and the decrease in symptoms was similar among patients with initially moderate versus initially severe symptoms. The mean peak urinary flow rate (Qmax) in the microwave group increased by 51% ($P < .001$) within 6 months to 11.8 mL/sec (95% CI, 10.7, 13.0 mL/sec) versus a pretreatment value of 7.8 mL/s (95% CI, 7.4, 8.2 mL/sec). The magnitude of the postprocedural increase in Qmax was significantly greater in the microwave than the sham group ($P < .05$). In nearly half the microwave group (47%), Qmax increased by 50% or more within 6 months compared with 24% of the sham group. Microwave treatment resulted in a significantly greater ($P < .05$) positive impact on patient quality of life than did the sham procedure. By 6 months, the quality of life score in microwave-treated patients (2.2; 95% CI, 1.9, 2.4) averaged 48% lower ($P < .001$) than that at baseline (4.2; 95% CI, 4.0, 4.4). Significantly greater durability of treatment effects was also evident with microwave than with sham treatment, as judged by the higher proportion of microwave-treated patients (98.4%) requiring no further treatment during the 6-month study period versus 83.3% of sham control patients ($P < .001$). Microwave treatment was well tolerated, and complications were generally minor, readily manageable, and transitory. *Conclusions:* The microwave thermoablation system proved to be an effective and safe treatment modality for BPH, with a positive impact on patient quality of life.
Authors' Abstract

Anatomy of Radical Prostatectomy as Defined by Magnetic Resonance Imaging. Robert P. Myers, Donald R. Cahill, Richard M. Devine, et al. *J Urol* 1998; 159:2148–2158. (R.P.M., Department of Urology, Mayo Clinic, 200 First Street SW, Rochester, Minnesota 55905)

Purpose: The authors examined and defined anatomic structures relevant to radical prostatectomy by using magnetic resonance (MR) imaging. *Materials and Methods:* Before radical prostatectomy, 15 men underwent high-resolution MR imaging studies of their pelvic floors (fast spin-echo, T2 weighting of 3–4-mm contiguous or overlapping sections) in axial, coronal, and sagittal planes. *Results:* Pubovesical ligaments, rather than the commonly reported puboprostatic ligaments, were observed attaching the bladder-prostate unit to the pubis. The authors suggest that the part of the urethra that extends from the apex of the prostate to the bulb of the penis, which is surrounded by the striated sphincter, should be termed the sphincteric urethra rather than the membranous urethra. Further, the authors found no evidence that supports the traditional concept of a urogenital diaphragm. The lower part of the striated urethral sphincter was flanked on its sides by the anterior recesses of the ischioanal fossae. The portion of the levator ani, which the authors have termed the puboanalis sling, flanked the apex of the prostate. The most anteromedial portion of this sling inserts into the perineal body and should be termed the puboperinealis. The terminal part of the gastrointestinal tract (the part continued beyond the levator ani) should be termed the anal canal, not the rectum, as used frequently in the urologic literature. Therefore, the initial plane of dissection in radical perineal prostatectomy passes along the anterior portion of the anal canal, not the rectum. *Conclusion:* The authors used MR imaging to study male pelvic floor and perineal anatomy without the artifact of dissection. This study allowed them to devise a more precise nomenclature with respect to radical prostatectomy and, in so doing, to provide a better understanding of both the retropubic and the perineal operations.
Authors' Abstract

Cardiovascular System

Clinical Consequences of Periprosthetic Leak after Endovascular Repair of Abdominal Aortic Aneurysm. Jon S. Matsumura, Wesley S. Moore, for the Endovascular Technologies Investigators. *J Vasc Surg* 1998; 27:606–613. (W.S.M., Department of Surgery, UCLA School of Medicine, Box 956904, Los Angeles, CA 90095-6904)

Purpose: The study was conducted to evaluate risk factors, natural history, and clinical consequences of a periprosthetic leak after endovascular repair of an abdominal aortic aneurysm. *Methods:* The authors reviewed the initial and follow-up data, including angiograms, contrast-enhanced computed tomographic (CT) scans, abdominal duplex scans, and plain abdominal radiographs for all patients undergoing tube graft repair with the endovascular graft system (early prototype) between February 10, 1993, and January 24, 1995. *Results:* Sixty-eight patients underwent placement or attempted placement of a tube graft implant at 13 centers in the United States. Nine patients required conversion to open repair, leaving 59 patients with functioning grafts for evaluation. The mean follow-up time was 27 months ± 8 (range, 2–48 months). Twenty-eight (47%) of 59 patients had initial periprosthetic leaks (six proximal, 14 distal, three proximal and distal, five indeterminate) on their first postoperative CT scans. Fourteen (50%) of the initial 28 leaks sealed spontaneously. Two other patients had their leaks sealed by endovascular means, leaving 12 patients with persistent leaks for follow-up evaluation. Four patients developed late leaks between 18 and 24 months of follow-up: one who had a spontaneously sealed initial leak, one with a second leak, and two who developed late leaks. Of the 16 patients with sealed leaks, 10 had aneurysm size reduction during follow-up. Three aneurysm sacs enlarged before spontaneous sealing but have not been followed up for enough time to document the size change since the seal. One patient died of respiratory failure 5 months after graft implantation. One patient whose leak was sealed by intervention has not yet undergone CT for evaluation. In one patient with a sealed leak whose aneurysm had initially shrunk, the area reopened and progressed to a nonfatal rupture that was surgically corrected. There were two late deaths from unrelated causes. Twelve patients in the

sealed group are alive and well. Of the 12 patients with persistent leaks, five underwent open surgical repair without complication, and one underwent successful endovascular repair with a second graft. Six patients continue to live with their initial grafts and have an average aneurysm sac enlargement of 0.1 cm per year. *Conclusions:* Although initial periprosthetic leaks were common with the use of this early prototype, 50% spontaneously sealed. The subsequent clinical course of patients with persistently sealed leaks was no different from that of patients who had no leaks. However, continued CT surveillance is warranted because, in one patient with an initially sealed leak, the area reopened and progressed to nonfatal rupture. Another two patients without initial leaks developed late leaks. In a small group of selected patients with continued leaks, their aneurysms appeared to enlarge at a rate considerably slower than would have been expected in patients with untreated aneurysm, suggesting that even in those with a persistent leak after endovascular repair there may have been some beneficial hemodynamic modification.
Authors' Abstract

Natural History of the Residual Infrarenal Aorta after Infrarenal Abdominal Aortic Aneurysm Repair. David A. Lipski, Calvin B. Ernst. *J Vasc Surg* 1998; 27:805–812. (C.B.E., Allegheny University of Health Sciences, Broad and Vine, Mail Stop 468, Philadelphia, PA 19102-1192)

Purpose: The authors determined the natural history of the residual native infrarenal aortic segment after conventional abdominal aortic aneurysm (AAA) repair. *Methods:* For the retrospective arteriographic case series, 800 hundred translumbar aortograms (TLAs) were obtained in 272 patients before and after conventional AAA repair. The main outcome measures were changes in the aortographic diameter and the length of the infrarenal aortic segment, corrected and uncorrected for magnification by normalization to the first lumbar vertebral body height. *Results:* The mean follow-up time from the preoperative TLA to the most recent postoperative TLA was 42 months (range, 1–257 months). Vertebral body height did not change (P = .35). The length of the native infrarenal aorta cephalad to the proximal anastomosis increased a mean of 3 mm, from 23 to 26 mm (P = .001). However, in 115 patients (43%), this aortic segment elongated more than 5 mm, and in 63 patients (24%), it elongated more than 10 mm. The native residual infrarenal aorta above the proximal anastomosis dilated a mean of 1 mm, from 23 to 24 mm (P = .001), but in 21 patients (8%), it dilated more than 5 mm. There was a weak positive correlation between the increase in residual native aortic diameter and duration of follow-up. There was a negative correlation between this increase and the initial size. The diameters of the proximal anastomosis and proximal graft did not change. Marked variability in the changes in aortic dimensions was observed. *Conclusions:* A mean period of 42 months after conventional AAA repair, the native infrarenal aortic segment elongates and dilates. Although such enlargement is statistically significant, the average increase appears to be small. However, residual aortic cuff diameter increased more than 5 mm and neck length more than 10 mm in a significant number of patients, with potentially serious implications for endovascular treatment of AAA.
Authors' Abstract

Musculoskeletal System

Estimates of the Prevalence of Arthritis and Selected Musculoskeletal Disorders in the United States. Reva C. Lawrence, Charles G. Helmick, Frank C. Arnett, et al. *Arthritis Rheum* 1998; 41:778–799. (R.C.L., National Institutes of Health, National Institute of Arthritis and Musculoskeletal and Skin Diseases, Bldg 45, Rm 5AS-13, Bethesda, MD 20892)

Objective: To provide a single source for the best available estimates of the national prevalence of arthritis in general and of selected musculoskeletal disorders (osteoarthritis, rheumatoid arthritis, juvenile rheumatoid arthritis, the spondylarthropathies, systemic lupus erythematosus, scleroderma, polymyalgia rheumatica/giant cell arteritis, gout, fibromyalgia, and low back pain). *Methods:* The National Arthritis Data Workgroup reviewed data from available surveys, such as the National Health and Nutrition Examination Survey series. For overall national estimates, the authors used surveys based on representative samples. Because data based on national population samples are unavailable for most specific musculoskeletal conditions, the authors derived data from various smaller survey samples from defined populations. Prevalence estimates from these surveys were linked to 1990 U.S. Bureau of the Census population data to calculate national estimates. The authors also estimated the expected frequency of arthritis in the year 2020. *Results:* Current national estimates are provided, with important caveats regarding their interpretation, for self-reported arthritis and selected conditions. An estimated 15% of Americans (40 million) had some form of arthritis in 1995. By the year 2020, an estimated 18.2% (59.4 million) will be affected. *Conclusion:* Given the limitations of the data on which they are based, this report provides the best available prevalence estimates for arthritis and other rheumatic conditions overall, and for selected musculoskeletal disorders, in the U.S. population.
Authors' Abstract

Pediatrics

Renal Angiomyolipoma in Children: Diagnostic Difficulty in 3 Patients. Zaven Tchaprassian, Guendalina Mognato, Guglielmo Paradias, et al. *J Urol* 1998; 159:1654–1656. (From the Department of Pediatric Surgery, University of Padua, Italy)

Purpose: Because angiomyolipoma is less common in children than in adults, its diagnosis in children can be difficult. The authors present three cases of pediatric angiomyolipoma in which diagnostic problems resulted due to the presenting characteristics. *Materials and Methods:* The authors describe three children with unilateral renal angiomyolipoma. Computed tomography (CT) and ultrasound (US) revealed three large renal masses, 20, 7, and 8 cm in diameter. A correct diagnosis was not made preoperatively in any case by means of CT, US, or fine-needle biopsy. Wilms tumor was suspected in the first patient who received preoperative chemotherapy. Imaging was inconclusive in the other two cases. *Results:* All patients underwent surgical exploration and subsequent nephrectomy due to the large size of the tumor. At follow-up 33, 23, and 13 months postoperatively, all children were well, without signs of recurrence. *Conclusions:* It has been reported that the demonstration of fat at renal US and CT indicates angiomyolipoma in 95% of the cases. Most radiologists rely solely on CT demonstration of lipid density in the renal mass to diagnose angiomyolipoma, but the identification at imaging of lipid tissue may be difficult in small tumors. In the authors' cases, the fat content of the tumors was less than 10% despite the large size. This low fat content results in misdiagnosis, since fatty tissue is also present in other renal tumors, such as lipoma, liposarcoma, teratoma, and Wilms tumors. The authors recommend conservative surgery in pediatric patients with angiomyolipoma, when tumor size permits, to avoid chemotherapy.
Authors' Abstract

Minimal Head Trauma in Children Revisited: Is Routine Hospitalization Required? Sean P. Roddy, Stephen M. Cohn, Beth A. Moller, et al. *Pediatrics* 1998; 101:575–577. (S.M.C., Division of Trauma and Surgical Critical Care, Department of Surgery, University of Miami School of Medicine, PO Box 016960 [D-40], Miami, FL 33101)

Treatment of minor head injuries has been debated. The definition of a minor head injury includes patients with a Glasgow Coma Scale (GCS) score of at least 13 and a history of loss of consciousness or amnesia for the event. It is estimated that more than 100,000 children per year sustain head injuries warranting hospital admission in the United States, and 90% have a GCS score of at least 13. Adjuncts, including non–contrast material–enhanced head computed tomography (CT), have been introduced to improve detection of subtle intracranial pathology in patients after minor closed head trauma. CT scans in cases of minor head injuries has revealed acute lesions in up to 20% of the adult population, and it has been estimated that 2.6% of patients with a GCS score of 15 will require neurosurgical intervention. Early diagnosis of intracranial hemorrhage has been shown to result in an improved outcome. The objective of this study was to review pediatric trauma admissions during a 3-year period in children with a normal head CT scan, normal neurologic examination findings, and an admission GCS score of 15, to determine whether admission for isolated head trauma was obligatory. The records of children admitted to a level I trauma center were reviewed. The children had an initial GCS score of 15, normal neurologic findings, and a normal head CT scan. Children with associated injuries requiring admission were excluded. Sixty-two patients were studied (mean age, 7 years; 65% boys). The mechanisms of injury were vehicular crash in most children, and the main length of stay was 1.2 days. There was a prolonged hospitalization in nine patients. No child developed important central nervous system sequelae. The total charges for the hospitalizations were $177,874. The conclusions indicated that children undergoing emergency department work-up of occult head injuries with normal findings at neurologic examination and a normal head CT scan do not seem to be at risk for important central nervous system sequelae. These patients could be discharged home with parental supervision, avoiding hospitalization. This study confirms that mandatory admission in such cases is not warranted.

Beverly P. Wood, MD
Childrens Hospital, Los Angeles, Calif

Adverse Asthma Outcomes among Children Hospitalized with Asthma in California. Daphne Calmes, Barbara D. Leake, David M. Carlisle. *Pediatrics* 1998; 101:845–850. (D.C., Department of Pediatrics, King-Drew Medical Center, 12021 S Wilmington Ave, Los Angeles, CA 90059)

Asthma is the most common chronic respiratory disease of children and adolescents, affecting 2–5 million children in the United States. Despite substantial advances in medical management, the burden of childhood asthma on the American health care system is increasing, and by 1990 asthma-related costs were estimated to be nearly $6.2 billion, with the greatest proportion of this expense being allocated for hospital care. Hospitalization rates for children have increased to 26 hospitalizations per 10,000 children per year, with children aged 0–4 years affected most notably. In this study, administrative data were used to determine whether adverse asthma outcomes for pediatric asthma hospitalizations were related to specific clinical and nonclinical patient characteristics. Pediatric asthma-related hospital discharges from 1986 to 1993 in California were examined. There were a total of 113,974 eligible patients with asthma-related discharge. Adverse outcomes such as incubation, cardiopulmonary arrest, and death were measured, and it was found that adverse asthma outcomes occurred in 0.48% of subjects. The frequency of adverse asthma outcomes increased during the 1990s compared with 1986. Adverse outcomes were more likely to occur in children aged 5–11 years and 12–17 years compared with those aged 0–4 years. Asian Pacific American children were more likely than were white children to experience an adverse outcome. Children with a secondary diagnosis of pneumonia also were more likely to experience an adverse asthma outcome.

Beverly P. Wood, MD
Childrens Hospital, Los Angeles, Calif

Cystic Fibrosis: When Should High-Resolution Computed Tomography of the Chest Be Obtained? Francesca Santamaria, Giacomo Grillo, Guido Guidi, et al. *Pediatrics* 1998; 101: 908–913. (F.S., Department of Pediatrics, Federico II University, Via Pansini 5, 80131 Naples, Italy)

Pulmonary disease is the main cause of morbidity in cystic fibrosis, with progressive lung destruction from chronic obstruction and infection of the respiratory tract leading to severe pulmonary disease and eventual death. The assessment of the severity of pulmonary involvement in cystic fibrosis includes clinical, functional, and radiologic evaluation. Among imaging techniques, conventional chest radiography has been used to assess the extent of lung injury, and radiologic scoring systems are used for clinical studies. However, conventional radiology is sensitive only to advanced lung abnormalities and is insensitive to early changes. This study compares conventional chest radiography and high-resolution computed tomography (CT) of the lung in a group of patients with cystic fibrosis. Clinical score and pulmonary function tests were performed, and the results were related to both radiographic and CT findings. Thirty patients with cystic fibrosis (aged 6.75–24 years) were assessed, and it was found that conventional chest radiographic scores correlated highly with high-resolution CT and clinical scores, whereas total CT scores were not related to clinical scores. Of all the specific CT findings, only bronchiectasis appeared to be related significantly to the clinical score. Most pulmonary function tests were related to radiographic and total CT scores but not to CT scoring of specific changes. Forced vital capacity and radiographic scores appeared to be the best predictors of the CT score. In patients with mild lung disease, high-resolution CT demonstrated bronchiectasis and air trapping in 57% and 71% of cases, respectively. In patients with more abnormal chest radiographs, bronchiectasis and air trapping were demonstrated at CT in all cases. The conclusion is that high-resolution CT of the chest is most useful in the identification of early lung abnormalities in patients with cystic fibrosis with mild respiratory symptoms, whereas for established disease conventional chest radiography is still the first-line imaging technique. The advantage of detecting early changes with cystic fibrosis imaging awaits additional confirmation. In addition to concerns about the high cost of the procedure, the high radiation dose compared with conventional chest radiography and the need for cooperation to minimize motion artifact suggest that the cost-benefit ratio should be considered in each individual case before a decision to perform high-resolution CT of the chest.

Beverly P. Wood, MD
Childrens Hospital, Los Angeles, Calif

Health and Developmental Outcomes at 18 Months in Very Preterm Infants with Bronchopulmonary Dysplasia. Marie-Claude Grégoire, Francine Lefebvre, Jacqueline Glorieux. *Pediatrics* 1998; 101:856–860. (F.L., Department of Pediatrics, Hôpital Ste-Justine, 3175 Chemin Côte-Ste-Catherine, Montreal, Quebec, Canada H3T 1C5)

Since its description in 1967, the accepted definition of bronchopulmonary dysplasia (BPD) was oxygen dependency for more than 28 days after mechanical ventilation and persistent increased opacities on chest radiographs. The original cohort had no infants less than 31 weeks gestation and only one weighing less than 1,500 g. Currently there are large numbers of extremely preterm infants surviving who need oxygen for more than 28 days, and it is uncertain whether the original BPD criteria apply to these infants. Oxygen dependency at 28 days is not a good predictor of persistent pulmonary problems at 1 year of age in infants weighing less than 1,500 g and born at less than 30 weeks gestation. It has been suggested that the use of oxygen dependency at 36 weeks gestational age to define which infants are at high risk for long-term pulmonary problems is more useful. The purpose of this study was to clarify the effect on outcome in an extremely premature population when BPD is defined as oxygen dependency for more than 28 days or at 36 weeks gestational age. The hypothesis was that in very preterm children oxygen dependency at 28 days but not persisting beyond 36 weeks gestational age would not increase future health or developmental problems. A total of 217 infants born at 24–28 weeks gestation were classified into three groups: neonatal comparison group, oxygen for less than 28 days of life; BPD group 1, oxygen for more than 28 days but not at 36 weeks gestational age; and BPD group 2, oxygen at more than 36 weeks gestational age. Outcome measures were growth, persistent respiratory problems, surgery, hospitalization, and neurodevelopmental impairment. There were no differences among the three groups in weight, height, head circumference, or total number of days of rehospitalization for any causes or in the rate of rehospitalization to the intensive care unit, persistent pulmonary problems, cerebral palsy, or sensory impairment. Children in BPD group 2 needed more hernia repair and had more days of readmission for respiratory problems. They had a lower mean developmental quotient. Intraparenchymal cerebral lesions, high familial adversity, and prolonged ventilation were the most important factors influencing the developmental outcome. The results demonstrated that for extremely premature babies, BPD as traditionally defined does not adversely affect outcome. Oxygen dependency at 36 weeks gestational age is associated with developmental delay at 18 months by means of the effect of prolonged ventilation.

Beverly P. Wood, MD
Childrens Hospital, Los Angeles, Calif

Management of Acute Gastroenteritis in Children in Israel. Raanan Shamir, Ilan Zahavi, Tova Abramowich, et al. *Pediatrics* 1998; 101: 892–894. (Gabriel Dinari, Division of Gastroenterology and Nutrition, Schneider Children's Medical Center, 14 Kaplan St, Petah Tikva 49202, Israel)

Diarrheal diseases continue to be a leading cause of death worldwide, with up to 5 million deaths annually. Morbidity and mortality in industrialized countries are much lower but are still substantial. Each year 220,000 children under 5 years of age are hospitalized in the United States with acute gastroenteritis, and 300–500 children die of diarrhea and dehydration. Deaths from gastroenteritis account for about 10% of preventable causes of postnatal deaths. This present study was designed to examine the knowledge and practice among pediatricians of the revised American Academy of Pediatrics (AAP) guidelines of 1996, the effect of medical school on the physicians' practice, and the effect of the type of practice on the management of gastroenteritis. A multiple-choice questionnaire was distributed at two pediatrics meetings, and 87 pediatricians completed the questionnaire. They were aware of 73% of the current AAP guidelines and followed 60% of them. Most pediatricians used oral rehydration solutions for the treatment of dehydration and gastroenteritis, but 60% believed that full-strength feedings are inappropriate in the presence of gastroenteritis, and 67% do not recommend full-strength formulas. Thirty-seven percent of the pediatricians stopped feeding temporarily in the presence of gastroenteritis in contradiction to the 1996 AAP guidelines. Indications suggest that pediatricians in Israel, regardless of country of origin, medical school, or place of practice, are aware of the correct use of oral rehydration solution but do not follow nutritional practices as recommended by the AAP.
Beverly P. Wood, MD
Childrens Hospital, Los Angeles, Calif

Long-term Outcome after Neonatal Meconium Obstruction. Julie R. Fuchs, Jacob C. Langer. *Pediatrics* 1998; 101(4); *http://www.pediatrics.org/cgi/content/full/101/4/e7*. (From the Department of Surgery, Washington University School of Medicine, St Louis, Mo)

Meconium obstruction in the newborn is a spectrum of disease that includes meconium ileus and meconium plug syndrome. Meconium ileus is the presenting symptom in 10%–15% of these patients. This study was designed to determine whether neonates with cystic fibrosis who present with meconium obstruction have a different long-term outcome than those who do not. To control for the effect of cystic fibrosis on outcome, the authors sought to determine long-term outcome in patients with neonatal meconium obstruction who did not have cystic fibrosis. Charts of all newborns with meconium ileus between 1966 and 1992 were reviewed (group 1); two control groups were also studied: cystic fibrosis patients without meconium ileus (group 2), and infants with meconium plug syndrome (group 3). The mean follow-up was 12.6 years ± 6, 12.6 years ± 6, and 9.3 years ± 4 in groups 1, 2, and 3, respectively. Patients without cystic fibrosis demonstrated better growth and functional status and a lower incidence of pulmonary and gastrointestinal problems. Although the presence of meconium ileus among cystic fibrosis patients was associated with an earlier diagnosis, there were no significant differences between groups 1 and 2 with respect to hepatobiliary, nutritional, functional, or respiratory status. Meconium ileus was associated with a higher risk of meconium ileus equivalent (20% vs 6%), although the difference was not statistically significant. Long-term surgical complications were seen in 27% of the children with meconium ileus, and no long-term surgical complications occurred in group 2 or 3. At the time of the study, 12 of the group 1 patients had died; nine had uncomplicated and three had complicated meconium ileus. The study indicates that long-term outcome is similar in cystic fibrosis patients who present with meconium ileus and those who do not aside from a slightly higher frequency of meconium ileus equivalent and a significantly higher rate of surgical complications.
Beverly P. Wood, MD
Childrens Hospital, Los Angeles, Calif

A Randomized Comparison of Surfactant Dosing via a Dual-lumen Endotracheal Tube in Respiratory Distress Syndrome. Adolf Valls-i-Soler, Begoña Fernández-Ruanova, Jon López-Heredia y Goya, et al. *Pediatrics* 1998; 101(4); *http://www.pediatrics.org/cgi/content/full/101/4/e4*. (From the Department of Pediatrics, Hospital de Cruces, Osakidetza, Basque University School of Medicine, Bilbao, Spain)

A trial of a dual-lumen endotracheal tube for delivery of surfactant was undertaken, assuming that avoiding interruption of mechanical ventilation would help avoid a decrease in oxygen saturation or a decrease in transcutaneous partial oxygen pressure and consequent bradycardia during the bolus injection. One hundred ninety-eight infants with respiratory distress syndrome who received mechanical ventilation were randomly assigned to receive 200 mg/kg of Curosurf by means of either bolus instillation or a simplified dosing technique in which the full dose is administered in 1 minute via a dual-lumen endotracheal tube. Two additional doses were delivered at 12 and 24 hours by means of the same method. Fewer episodes of hypoxia and a smaller decrease in heart rate and oxygen saturation were observed in the dual-lumen group. There were no differences between groups in the frequency of air leaks, intraventricular hemorrhage, patent ductus arteriosus, bronchopulmonary dysplasia, or survival. The study indicates that a simplified 1-minute Curosurf dosing procedure in which a dual-lumen endotracheal tube is used without fractional doses reduces the number of dosing-related adverse transient episodes of hypoxia.
Beverly P. Wood, MD
Childrens Hospital, Los Angeles, Calif

Publishers' Row

A "printed parallel" of Publishers' Row at the RSNA annual meeting, listing *current* imaging texts available either in book or videocassette form. Complete addresses and phone numbers of publishers are included as a service to readers who wish to obtain texts or further information.

NOTE:
The first group of publishers are offering a 10% discount to* Radiology *readers. To obtain your discount, please mention that the book or tape was listed in* Radiology*'s Publishers' Row when ordering. (Check publisher's listing for any specific discount codes.)

BLACKWELL SCIENCE, INC.
350 Main Street
Malden, MA 02148-5018 USA
(800) 215-8250
(781) 388-8250
Telefax (781) 388-8255

(10% Discount)

Advances in MRI
L. Heuser and M. Oudkerk
1996 • Hardcover • 176 pages • $95.00

Atlas of Breast Imaging
Marla Jones
1997 • Hardcover • 272 pages • $95.00

Atlas of Diagnostic Radiology in Gastroenterology
Ramsay Valiance
Dec 1998 • Hardcover • 480 pages • $245.00

Atlas of Infertility: Diagnostic and Therapeutic Imaging
Amy Thurmond
1997 • Hardcover • 128 pages • $75.00

Atlas of Mammography: New Early Signs in Breast Cancer
P. Gamagami
1996 • Hardcover • 350 pages • $185.00

Atlas of Ultrasound Color Flow Imaging
Barry Goldberg
1997 • Hardcover • 338 pages • $140.00

Atlas of Ultrasound and Ductal Echography of Breast
M. Teboul
1995 • Hardcover • 416 pages • $295.00

Cerebral and Spinal Computed Tomography
Sebastian Lange, MD
1997 • CD-ROM • $295.00

Cerebral and Spinal Computed Tomography 3rd ed
Thomas Grumme
Oct 1998 • Hardcover • $195.00

Chesney's Care of the Patient in Diagnostic Radiography
P. Culmer
1995 • Paper • 416 pages • $34.95

Chesney's Equipment for Student Radiographers. 4th ed
P.H. Carter
1994 • Paper • 336 pages • $38.95

Chesney's Radiographic Imaging. 2nd ed
J.L. Ball
1995 • Paper • 448 pages • $46.95

Complications in Diagnostic and Interventional Radiology
G. Ansell
1996 • Hardcover • 556 pages • $265.00

A Comprehensive Approach to Stereotactic Breast Biopsy
Laurie Fajardo
1996 • Hardcover • 375 pages • $95.00

Diagnostic Imaging. 4th ed
Peter Armstrong
1998 • Hardcover • 456 pages • $85.00

Dictionary of Ultrasound
S. Schering
1997 • Paper • 168 pages • $38.95

Dictionary of Ultrasound CD-ROM
S. Schering
1997 • Windows • $125.00

Essential Physics for Radiographers. 3rd ed
John Ball
1997 • Paper • 352 pages • $39.95

Gynecologic, Obstetric, and Breast Radiology: A Text/Atlas of Imaging in Women
A. Thurmond
1996 • Hardcover • 928 pages • $235.00

Handbook of MRI Techniques
Catherine Westbrook
1994 • Paper • 256 pages • $29.95

Imaging in Muscuoloskeletal and Sports Medicine
Brian Halpern
1997 • Hardcover • 250 pages • $125.00

Imaging in Spinal Trauma in Children
L.R. Kuhns
1997 • Hardcover • 272 pages • $95.00

The Invisible Light: 100 Years of Medical Radiology
A.M.K. Thomas, editor
1995 • Paper • 120 pages • $19.95

Lecture Notes on Radiology
P.R. Patel
1997 • Paper • 256 pages • $29.95

MRI Atlas of the Chest and Neck
John Markisz
1997 • Hardcover • 256 pages • $125.00

MRI in Practice. 2nd ed
Catherine Westbrook
1997 • Paper • 320 pages • $44.95

MRI in Prostate Cancer
Gerrit Jager
Jun 1998 • Paper • 144 pages • $44.95

Nuclear Medicine Physics
Rachel Powsner
Aug 1998 • Paper • 256 pages • $39.95

Orthopaedic Radiology. 2nd ed
Peter Renton
Oct 1998 • Hardcover • 528 pages • $135.00

Radiology in Medical Diagnostics
Gerd Rosenbusch
1995 • Hardcover • 650 pages • $110.00

The Rational Use of MRI
P.A. Rinck
1996 • Hardcover • 300 pages • $135.00

Review Questions for Computed Tomography
Euclid Seeram
1997 • Paper • 250 pages • $21.95

Review Questions for MRI
William Kaut
1995 • Paper • 144 pages • $24.95

Techniques in Diagnostic Imaging. 3rd ed
Graham Whitehouse
1996 • Hardcover • 526 pages • $175.00

Transcranial Doppler Sonography
Ulrich Bogdahn
Aug 1998 • Hardcover • 440 pages • $195.00

Ultra Fast Magnetic Resonance Imaging
M. Oudkerk
1998 • Hardcover • 400 pages • $135.00

Whole Body Computed Tomography CD-ROM
Otto Henning Wegener
1995 • Windows • $199.95

BUTTERWORTH-HEINEMANN

225 Wildwood Avenue
Woburn, MA 01801
(800) 366-2665
Telefax (800) 446-6520

(10% Discount - Quote: Code MS12)

Human Cross-Sectional Anatomy Pocket Atlas: Body Sections and CT Images
Harold Ellis, Bari M. Logan, and Adrian Dixon
1994 • Paper • 184 pages • $31.50

Magnetic Resonance Imaging in Obstetrics and Gynecology
Martin C. Powell, Brian S. Worthington, and Malcolm Symonds
1994 • Hardcover • 192 pages • $112.50

CRC PRESS, INC.

2000 Corporate Boulevard NW
Boca Raton, FL 33431
(800) 272-7737
(407) 994-0563 (Florida only)

(10% Discount)

Cancer Therapy with Radiolabeled Antibodies
David M. Goldenberg
1994 • Hard/Sewn • 336 pages • $242.00
• Cat. No. 5112

Handbook of Biological Effects of Electromagnetic Fields. 2nd ed
1995 • Hard/Sewn • 672 pages • $125.00
• Cat. No. 641

Handbook of Radiobiology. 2nd ed
Kedar N. Prasad
1995 • $110.00 • Cat. No. 2501

Handbook of Targeted Delivery of Imaging Agents
Vladimir P. Torchilin and Mannfred A. Hollinger
1995 • Hard/Sewn • 752 pages • $125.00
• Cat. No. 8308

The Image Processing Handbook. 2nd ed
John C. Russ
1994 • Hard/Sewn • 668 pages • $89.95
• Cat. No. 2516

Imaging Atlas of the Normal Gallbladder and Its Variants
Jon W. Meilstrup, MD
1994 • Hard/Sewn • 128 pages • $133.00
• Cat. No. 4788

Non-Invasive Thermometry of the Human Body
1995 • Hard/Sewn • 288 pages • $157.00
• Cat No. 4738

Quantitative Dynamic Telethermometry in Medical Diagnosis and Management
Michael Anbar
1994 • Hard/Sewn • 240 pages • $91.00
• Cat. No. 4409

Radiation and the Gastrointestinal Tract
Andre Dubois, Gregory King, and David R. Livengood
1994 • Adhesive • 297 pages • $169.95
• Cat. No. 7667

The Science of Phototherapy
Leonard I. Grossweiner
1994 • Adhesive • 256 pages (approx)
• $139.00 • Cat. No. 4980

Sites of Drug Action in the Brain
Anat Biegon and Nora D. Volkow
1995 • Hard/Sewn • $157.95
• Cat. No. 7653

DAVIES PUBLISHING, INC.

32 South Raymond Avenue
Pasadena, CA 91105
(818) 792-3046
Telefax (818) 792-5308

(10% Discount)

Instructional Videotape Series
Keith Mauney, RN
- **Cardiac Anatomy and Physiology for the Echocardiographer**
  1995 • 2.5 hours • $175.00
- **Cardiovascular Physiology: The Entire Story**
  1995 • 7 hours • $295.00
- **Introduction to Electrophysiology: ECG Rhythm Analysis Workshop**
  1995 • 4 hours • $175.00
- **Statistics for the Nonstatistician**
  1995 • 90 minutes • $79.00
- **Vascular Physiology: The Complete Picture**
  1995 • 4 hours • $275.00

Introduction to Vascular Scanning: A Guide for the Complete Beginner. 2nd ed
Donald Ridgway, RVT
1998 • Paper • 290 pages • $59.95

Preparation Agenda for Study Success Audiocassettes with Workbook
Lori Green, RT, RDMS, RVT, editor
— Abdomen, OB/GYN, General Physics, Vascular Technology, Vascular Physics, Cardiac Physics, Cardiac Technology
1994 • $95.00 • ($89.50 each 2 or more)

Registry Review Flashcards with Audiocassettes
Lori Green, RT, RDMS, RVT, and Lori Sens, RT, RDMS, RVT
— Adult Echo, Ultrasound Physics, Abdomen, OB/GYN, Vascular Technology, Cardiac Physics, and Vascular Physics
1995 • $57.50

Techniques of Abdominal Vascular Imaging
Marsha M. Neumyer, BS, RVT, Brian Thiele, MD, and D. Eugene Strandness, Jr, MD
1996 • 50 minutes • $125.00

Ultrasound Videotape Series
Lori Green, RT, RDMS, RVT, and Lori Sens, RT, RDMS, RVT
- **Emergency Medicine Ultrasound**
  1997 • 3 hours • $299.00
- **Introduction to Adult Echocardiography**
  1994 • 90 minutes • $225.00
- **Introduction to Cardiac Doppler/Color Flow Ultrasound**
  1994 • 55 minutes • $140.00
- **Introduction to Carotid Duplex/Color Flow Imaging**
  1994 • 1 hour • $125.00
- **Introduction to Gynecological Sonography**
  1995 • 45 minutes • $125.00
- **Introduction to Obstetrical Sonography**
  1994 • 45 minutes • $125.00
- **Introduction to Ultrasound Physics**
  1996 • 45 minutes • $125.00
- **Introduction to Venous Duplex/Color Flow Imaging**
  1994 • 1 hour • $125.00

Venous Imaging Techniques, 2nd ed
Steven A. Talbot, RVT, and Mark A. Oliver, MD, RVT
1998 • 70 minute videotape • $99.00

Vascular Laboratory Operations Manual: A Guide to Survival. 2nd ed
Claudia B. Rumwell, RN, RVT, editor
1998 • Looseleaf • 405 pages • $295.00

Vascular Laboratory Policies and Procedures Manual
Claudia B. Rumwell, RN, RVT, Michalene McPharlin, RN, RVT, D. Eugene Strandness, Jr, MD, and Edward G. Grant, MD, editors
1995 • Looseleaf with IBM Computer Disks
• 450 printed pages • $795.00

Vascular Physics Review
Barton A. Bean, RVT, editor
1997 • Paper • 180 pages • $55.00

Vascular Technology: An Illustrated Review for the Registry Exam
Claudia Rumwell, RN, RVT, and Michalene McPharlin, RN, RVT
1996 • Paper • 267 pages • $57.50

Vascular Technology Review, 4th ed
Barton A. Bean, RVT
1998 • Paper • 210 pages • $55.00

FUTURA PUBLISHING COMPANY, INC.

135 Bedford Road
P.O. Box 418
Armonk, NY 10504-0418
(800) 877-8761
(914) 273-1014
Telefax (914) 273-1015

(10% Discount)

Advances in Neuro-Oncology II
Paul L. Kornblith, MD, and Michael D. Walker, MD, editors
1997 • Hardcover • 584 pages • $125.00

Application of Magnetic Resonance to the Study of Lung
Antonio G. Cutillo, MD
1996 • Hardcover • 624 pages • $98.00

Atlas of Three-Dimensional Echocardiography
Navin C. Nanda, MD
1998 • Hardcover • In preparation
• Price not set

Breast Cancer: Controversies in Management
Leslie Wise, MD, and Houston Johnson, Jr, MD
1994 • Hardcover • 608 pages • $105.00

Congenital Heart Disease: Textbook of Angiocardiography (2 volume set)
Robert M. Freedom, MD, FRCP(C), J. B. Mawson, MB, CHB, Shi Joon Yoo, MD, and Leland N. Benson, MD, FRCP(C)
1997 • Hardcover • 1,552 pages • $275.00

Congenital Heart Disease Visualized. Echocardiography with Pathology Correlation on CD-ROM
Girish S. Shirali, MD, Frank Lombano, Daniel A. Dyar, MA, RDCS, Ranae L. Larsen, MD, Debra L. Kearney, MD, and J. Timothy Bricker, MD
1997 • CD-ROM • IBM PC/MAC • $225.00

Current and Future Applications of Magnetic Resonance in Cardiovascular Disease
Charles B. Higgins, MD, Joanne S. Ingwall, PhD, and Gerald M. Pohost, MD, editors
1998 • Hardcover • 576 pages • $130.00

Functional Neuroimaging
Roger E. Kelley
1994 • Hardcover • 488 pages • $98.00

Guidebook to Endovascular Coronary Diagnostic Techniques
Herbert J. Geschwind, MD, and Morton J. Kern, MD, editors
1997 • Hardcover • 576 pages • $125.00

Handbook of Echo-Doppler Interpretation
Edmund Kenneth Kerut, MD, Elizabeth F. McIlwain, MHS, RDCS, and Gary D. Plotnick, MD, FACC, editors
1996 • Paper • 288 pages • $39.00

High Dose Rate Brachytherapy
Subir Nag, MD
1994 • Hardcover • 480 pages • $69.00

Interactive Echocardiography: A Clinical Atlas of CD-ROM
Th. Binder, MD, G. Rehak, G. Porenta, MD, M. Zangeneh, MD, H. Baumgartner, MD, and G. Maurer, MD
1997 • CD-ROM • IBM PC/MAC • $175.00

New Developments in Cardiac Nuclear Imaging
Ami E. Iskandrian, MD, FACC, FACP, and Mario S. Verani, MD
1998 • Hardcover • 300 pages • $85.00

Noninvasive Imaging of Congenital Heart Disease
Alvin J. Chin, MD
1994 • Hardcover • 400 pages • $128.00

Principles and Practice of Brachytherapy
Subir Nag, MD, editor
1997 • Hardcover • 752 pages • $160.00

Quantitative Cerebral Blood Flow Measurements Using Stable Xenon/CT: Clinical Applications
Masamichi Tomonaga, MD, Akira Tanaka, MD, and Howard Yonas, MD, editors
1995 • Hardcover • 368 pages • $75.00

Three-Dimensional Echocardiography
Natesa G. Pandian, MD, Jos R.T.C. Roelandt, MD, and Navin C. Nanda, MD
1998 • Hardcover • In preparation
• Price not set

Three-Dimensional Echocardiography in Congenital Heart Disease
Gerald R. Marx, MD and Michael Vogel, MD
1998 • Hardcover • In preparation
• Price not set

Vascular Brachytherapy, 2nd Ed
Ron Waksman, MD
1998 • Hardcover • Price not set

Venous Thromboembolism: An Evidence-Based Atlas
Russell D. Hull, MBBS, Gary E. Raskob, MSc, and Graham F. Pineo, MD, editors
1996 • Hardcover • 464 pages • $149.00

WARREN H. GREEN, INC.

8356 Olive Boulevard
St. Louis, MO 63132
(314) 991-1335

(10% Discount)

Acupuncture in Obstetrics and Gynecology
Drs. Tureanu, V&L
1997 • Paper • 344 pages • In preparation

Atlas of the Corpus Collosum
R. N. Sener, MD
1996 • Hardcover • In preparation

Medical Administration: Management Techniques
A. Everette James, Jr, MD
1994 • Paper • 158 pages • $24.95

MR Angiography Applications in Pediatric Intracranial Vascular Lesions
R. Sener
1996 • Hardcover • 112 pages • $32.50

Musculoskeletal Manifestations of AIDS
Jamshid Tehranzadeh, MD, and Lynne S. Steinbach, MD
1994 • Paper • 181 pages • $37.50

Origins, Icons and Illusions
Harold R. Booher, PhD
1997 • In preparation

S. KARGER PUBLISHERS, INC.

26 West Avon Road
P.O. Box 529
Farmington, CT 06085
(860) 675-7834
Telefax (860) 675-7302

(10% Discount - shown below)

Intraoperative Radiation Therapy in the Treatment of Cancer (Frontiers of Radiation Therapy and Oncology, Vol 31)
J.M. Vaeth, editor
1997 • Hardcover • 280 pages • $224.25

Musculoskeletal Imaging Diagnostic and Therapeutic Procedures
J.C. Hodge, editor
1997 • Soft Cover • 250 pages • $88.25

Radiotherapy of Ocular Disease (Frontiers of Radiation Therapy and Oncology, Vol 30)
T. Wiegel, N. Bornfeld, M. H. Foerster, and W. Hinkelbein, editors
1997 • Hardcover • 302 pages • $172.50

KLUWER ACADEMIC PUBLISHERS

101 Philip Drive • Assinippi Park
Norwell, MA 02061
(781) 871-6600
Telefax (781) 871-6528
E-mail: kluwer@wkap.com
http://www.wkap.nl

(10% Discount)

Adenosine, Cardioprotection and Clinical Application
Robert M. Mentzer, Jr, Masafumi Kitakaze, James M. Downey, and Masatsugu Hori
1997 • Hardcover • 256 pages • $50.00

Advances in Echo Imaging Using Contrast Enhancement. 2nd ed
Navin C. Nanda, Reinhard Schlief, and Barry B. Goldberg
1997 • Hardcover • 408 pages • $155.00

Advances in Imaging Techniques in Ischemic Heart Disease
Ernst E. van der Wall, Thomas H. Marwick, and Johan H. C. Reiber
1995 • Hardcover • 168 pages • $69.00

Advances in Radiation Therapy
Bharat B.Mittal, James A. Purdy and K.K. Ang
1998 • Hardcover • 320 pages • $298.00

Advances in X-Ray Contrast Collected Papers
P. Dawson and W. Clauss
1998 • Paperback • 120 pages • $50.00

Biological Models in Radiopharmaceutical Development
Richard M. Lambrecht
1996 • Hardcover • 288 pages • $136.00

Californium-252: Isotope for 21st Century Radiotherapy
Proceedings of the NATO Advanced Research Workshop, Detroit, USA, April 24–27, 1996
Jacek G. Wierzbicki
1997 • Hardcover • 324 pages • $170.00

Cardiac Positron Emission Tomography
Markus Schwaiger
1996 • Hardcover • 416 pages • $275.00

Cardiac Positron Emission Tomography: Viability, Perfusion, Receptors, and Cardiomyopathy
Ernst E. van der Wall, Paul K. Blanksma, Menco G. Niemeyer, and Anne M.J. Paans
1995 • Hardcover • 276 pages • $120.00

Cardiovascular Imaging
Johan H.C. Reiber and Ernst E. Van der Wall
1996 • Hardcover • 600 pages • $218.00

The Clinical Applications of SPET
P.H. Cox and M. Pillay
1995 • Hardcover • 288 pages • $110.50

Clinical PET
R. Bares and G. Lucignani
1996 • Hardcover • 152 pages • $63.50

Contrast Agents in Liver Imaging
Th. Balzer, H. P. Neindorf, and B. Hamm
1995 • Hardcover • 112 pages • $80.50

Coronary Pressure
Nico H.J. Pijis and Bernard De Bruyne
1995 • Hardcover • 112 pages • $142.00

Coronary Stenosis Morphology: Analysis and Implication
Lloyd Klein
1997 • Hardcover • 392 pages • $187.00

Current Directions in Radiopharmaceutical Research and Development
Stephen J. Mather
1996 • Hardcover • 260 pages • $141.00

Diagnosis and Treatment of Genitourinary Malignancies
Kenneth J. Pienta
1996 • Hardcover • 280 pages • $236.50

Echocardiography and Cardiovascular Function
Tools for the Next Decade
Julio E. Pérez and Roberto M. Lang
1997 • Hardcover • 288 pages • $95.00

Imaging and Intervention in Cardiology
Christoph A. Nienaber and Udo Sechtem
1996 • Hardcover • 548 pages • $295.00

The Imaging of Infection and Inflammation
Peter H. Cox and John R. Buscombe
1998 • Hardcover • 240 pages • $146.00

Myocardial Viability: Detection and Clinical Relevance
Abdulmassih S. Iskandrian and Ernst E. van der Wall
1994 • Hardcover • 212 pages • $135.00

Peritoneal Carcinomatosis: Principles of Management
Paul H. Sugarbaker
1996 • Hardcover • 464 pages • $291.50

PET for Drug Development and Evaluation
D. Comar
1995 • Hardcover • 384 pages • $131.00

Progress in Quantitive Coronary Arteriography
Johan H.C. Reiber and Patrick W. Serruys
1994 • Hardcover • 432 pages • $228.50

SPECT Imaging of the Brain
R. Duncan
1997 • Hardcover • 260 pages • $169.00

Stress Echocardiography
Thomas H. Marwick
1994 • Hardcover • 192 pages • $112.00

Systemic Manifestations of IBD
The Pending Challenge for Subtle Diagnosis and Treatment
B. Lembcke, W. Kruis, and R.B. Sartor
1998 • Hardcover • 416 pages • $175.00

Three-dimensional Image Reconstruction in Radiology
Pierre Grangeat and Jean-Louis Amans
1996 • Hardcover • 328 pages • $147.50

What's New in Cardiovascular Imaging?
Johan H.C. Reiber and Ernst E. van der Wall
1998 • Hardcover • 438 pages • $159.00

Ultrasound Angioplasty
Robert J. Siegel
1997 • Hardcover • 304 pages • $225.50

NUCLEAR ASSOCIATES

100 Voice Road
P.O. Box 349
Carle Place, NY 11514-0349
(516) 741-6360
Telefax (516) 741-5414
Toll free (in USA) 1-888-466-8257
E-mail address: sales@nucl.com
Worldwide Web: http://www.victoreen.com

(10% Discount)

The Basics of Film Processing in Medical Imaging
Arthur G. Haus and Susan M. Jaskulski
1997 • Softcover • 340 pages • $69.00

Mammography Quality Assurance Manual for MQSA
1996 • Three-ring binder • 150 pages • $295.00

Nuclear Medicine Procedure Manual
1997/98 • Three-ring binder • 150 pages • $355.00 (print and digital version)

Radiation in the Medical Environment
1997 • Videotape & manual • 21 minutes • $125.00

Radiologic Quality Control Manual
1994 • Binder/paper • 250+ pages • $75.00

Radiation Protection Standards
1994 • Videotape • 40 minutes • VHS format • $295.00

Radiation Protection Standards Revisited
1997 • Videotape • 39 minutes • VHS format • $295.00

Radiation Safety and Common Sense
1995 • Videotape • 26 minutes • VHS format • $195.00

Ultrasound Quality Control—Basic Texts
1997 • Paper • 27 pages

NOTE: FOLLOWING PUBLISHERS ARE NOT INCLUDED IN THE 10% DISCOUNT

ALMQVIST & WIKSELL INTERNATIONAL

P.O. Box 4627
Karlbergsvägen 77-81 (visiting address)
S-11691 Stockholm, Sweden
Phone: 46 8 728 25 00
Telefax: 46 8 33 87 07

Lung Cancer: The Art of Detection by Conventional Radiography. 1st ed
Alfred Szamosi
1995 • Hardcover • 116 pages • SEK 280.00 (approx. $40.00)

AMERICAN COLLEGE OF RADIOLOGY

1891 Preston White Drive
Reston, VA 20191
(800) ACR-7762 (Publications Sales)
(703) 648-8900

Chest Disease. 5th Series
Barry A. Siegel, MD, Anthony V. Proto, MD, editors, and Robert H. Choplin, MD, section editor
1996 • Hardcover • 600 pages • $150.00 (members) • $220.00 (nonmembers) • $125.00 (residents)

Diagnostic Ultrasonography. 2nd Series
Barry A. Siegel, MD, David H. Stephens, MD, editors, and Thomas L. Lawson, MD, section editor
1994 • Hardcover • 940 pages • $150.00 (members) • $220.00 (nonmembers) • $125.00 (residents)

Emergency Radiology. 2nd Series
Barry A. Siegel, MD, Anthony V. Proto, MD, Marilyn J. Siegel, MD, David H. Stephens, MD, editors, and Kent R. Donovan, MD, section editor
1997 • Hardcover • 850 pages • $150 (members) • $220 (nonmembers) • $125 (residents)

Gastrointestinal Disease. 5th Series
Barry A. Siegel, MD, David H. Stephens, MD, editors, and Dennis M. Balfe, MD, section editor
1995 • Hardcover • 650 pages • $150.00 (members) • $220.00 (nonmembers) • $125.00 (residents)

Musculoskeletal Disease
Barry A. Siegel, MD, David H. Stephens, MD, editors, and William A. Murphy, Jr, MD, section editor
1994 • Hardcover • 900 pages • $150.00 (members) • $220.00 (nonmembers) • $125.00 (residents)

Neuroradiology. 2nd Series
Barry A. Siegel, MD, Anthony V. Proto, MD, editors, and Eric J. Russell, MD, section editor
1998 • Hardcover • 650 pages • $150.00 (members) • $220.00 (nonmembers) • $125.00 (residents)

APPLETON & LANGE

P.O. Box 120041
Stamford, CT 06912-0041
(800) 423-1359
(203) 406-4500

Applications Manual for Radiographic Anatomy and Positioning
Diane H. Gronefeld, MEd, RT(R), and Mary L. Madigan, RT(R) (M)
1998 • Paper • 302 pages • $29.95

Competency Manual for Radiographic Anatomy and Positioning
Andrea Gauthier Cornuelle, MS, RT(R)
1998 • Paper • 399 pages • $29.95

Current Review of MRI
Javier Beltran, MD
1996 • Casebound • 400 pages • $110.00

Fundamentals of Obstetrics and Gynecologic Ultrasound
E. Albert Reece, MD, et al
1994• Casebound • 272 pages • $95.00

Pocket Manual for Radiographic Anatomy and Positioning
Mary L. Madigan, RT(R) (M), et al
1998 • Paper • 297 pages • $21.95

Radiographic Anatomy and Positioning: An Integrated Approach
Andrea Gauthier Cornuelle, MS, RT(R) and Diane H. Gronefeld, MEd, RT(R)
1998 • Casebound • 565 pages • $95.00

Sonography in Obstetrics and Gynecology. 5th ed
Arthur C. Fleischer, MD, et al
1996 • Casebound • 1,052 pages • $165.00

Technical Magnetic Resonance Imaging
John A. Markisz, MD, PhD, and Michael G. Aquilia, RT
1996 • Paper • 260 pages • $37.50

Ultrasonography of the Prenatal and Neonatal Brain
Ilan E. Timor-Tritsch, MD, et al
1996 • Casebound • 418 pages • $145.00

CHANNING L. BETE CO., INC.

200 State Road
South Deerfield, MA 01373
(800) 628-7733
(413) 665-7611
Telefax (800) 499-6464

Scriptographic™ Booklets for Educating Radiology Patients

Classic Style – For Adults:
- About Colorectal Cancer (12823) Revised 5/98
- About Contrast Radiology (12088)
- About Mammography (14175 Revised 4/97, Eng., 37119 Revised 4/97, Spanish)
- CT Scans (12898 Eng., 37333 Spanish)
- Diagnostic X-ray (38612) Revised 4/98
- Magnetic Resonance Imaging (14803 Revised 7/97, Eng., 37168 Revised 7/97, Spanish)
- Nuclear Medicine (39180) Revised10/97
- Open MRI (39149)
- Radiation Therapy (38281)
- Ultrasound (38802 Eng., 39032 Spanish) 1995/96• Paper• 16 pages
- Angiography (39735)
- Magnetic Resonance Angiography (39727) 1997 • Paper • 16 pages

Low Reading Level Titles:
- Mammography (41210 Revised 3/98, Eng., 41277 Revised 3/98, Spanish)
- Prostate Cancer (41293 Eng., 41749 Spanish) 1996 • Paper • 8 pages

New Full Color Titles:
- Looking At Ultrasound—What You Can Expect (71977)Revised 4/98
- Mammograms—A Picture of Breast Health (71969)Revised 2/98
- MRI—Keeping an Eye on Your Health (45419)
- CT Scans—A Closer Look (45427) 1997 • Paper • 8 pages

New Realistic Graphics:
- Breast Cancer (44347)
- CT Scans (42226) Revised 4/98
- MRI (42234)
- Mammography (70185)
- Nuclear Medicine (71514)
- Ultrasound (45468)
- Your Mammography Results (44362) 1995/96 • Paper • 8–16 pages
- Bone Densitometry Testing (31427)
- Breast Self Exam Folder (31393)
- Mammography Folder (31401) Revised 4/98 1997 • 8 1/2" x 14" tri-fold Paper

Children's Booklets:
- CT Scan Coloring Book (56622)
- MRI Coloring Book (56630) Revised 4/95 1994 • Paper • 8 pages

(Quantity discount pricing)
Sample copy available upon request.

CHURCHILL LIVINGSTONE INTERNATIONAL

A Division of Harcourt Brace
Order Department
6277 Sea Harbor Drive
Orlando, FL 32887
(800) 545-2522
(800) 433-0001 (Florida)

Bones and Joints: A Guide for Students. 3rd ed
Christine Gunn
1997 • Paper • 168 pages • $24.00

Diagnostic Radiology. 3rd ed
Ronald G. Grainger and David V. Allison, editors
1997 • Hardcover • 2,944 pages • $495.00 (3-vol set)

Essentials of Neuroimaging. 2nd ed
J. Robert Kirkwood
1996 • Hardcover • 736 pages • $142.00

Fetal Heart Scanning A Teaching Video
Lindsey D. Allan
1995 • Videotape • 1 hour • VHS/PAL • $115.00 (includes 8-page booklet)

Imaging Children
Helen Carty, Donald Shaw, Francis Brunelle, and Brian Kendall, editors
1995 • Hardcover • 2,038 pages • $380.00 • (2-vol set)

Imaging of Abdominal and Pelvic Anatomy
Francis S. Weill and Mike Manco-Johnson, editors
1998 • Hardcover • 368 pages • $135.00

Imaging, Radiography (Colour Guide)
D. N. Redhead
1995 • Paper • 110 pages • $16.95

Interpreting CT Head Scans. A Basic Guide to Image Analysis
Lynda Albertyn and Randall Brown
1996 • Paper • 162 pages • $39.00

Interventional Breast Procedures
D. David Dershaw
1996 • Hardcover • 179 pages • $78.00

Interventional Radiology Procedure Manual
Michael A. Braun, Robert L. Vogelzang, and Albert A. Nemcek, Jr
1997 • Hardcover • 256 pages (approx) • $75.00

Mayo Clinical Manual of Nuclear Medicine
Michael K. O'Connor
1996 • Paper • 592 pages • $89.00

MCQ Companion to Grainger & Allison's Diagnostic Radiology. Vol 1
John Cockburn and Adam Mitchell; Philip Gishen, editor; Ronald G. Grainger and David V. Allison, series editors
1998 • Paper • 320 pages (approx) • $35.00 • In preparation

MCQ Tutor in Radiology. Part 1 FRCR
Andrea L. Brown, Lesley A. Apthorp, Uday S. Bhonsle, and Gerald de Lacey
1996 • Paper • 227 pages • $25.00

MRI of Head and Neck Anatomy
William T. C. Yuh, E. Turgut Tali, Adel K. Afifi, Kayihan Sahinoglu, Feng Gao, and Ronald A. Bergman
1994 • Hardcover • 384 pages • $205.00

Musculoskeletal Ultrasound (Clinics in Diagnostic Ultrasound)
Bruno D. Fornage, editor
1995 • Hardcover • 246 pages • $95.00

Nuclear Medicine in Clinical Diagnosis and Treatment
I. P. Murray and P. J. Ell, editors
1999 • Hardcover • 1,776 pages • $395.00 • (2-vol set)

Picture Tests in Imaging (Colour Guide)
Jeremy Hughes and Michael Hughes
1997 • Paper • 158 pages (approx) • $15.95

Principles of Radiological Physics. 3rd ed
Donald T. Graham
1996 • Paper • 667 pages • $56.00

Radiographic Imaging. A Practical Approach. 2nd ed
Derrick P. Roberts, Nigel L. Smith, and C. Gunn
1995 • Hardcover • 232 pages • $61.00

Radiology and Imaging for Medical Students. 6th ed
David Sutton
1994 • Paper • 270 pages • $41.00

Radiology Image Bank
— Disk 1: Head, Neck, and Central Nervous System
— Disk 2: Thorax and Contained Viscera
— Disk 3: Abdomen and Viscera
— Disk 4: Pelvis and Obstetrical
— Disk 5: Orthopaedic
1996 • Win CD-ROM • $210 each
• 5-Disk Set $1,000.00

Radiotherapy. Principles to Practice A Manual for Quality in Treatment Delivery
Sue E. Griffiths and Chris A. Short
1994 • Hardcover • 298 pages • $83.00

Sectional Anatomy by MRI. 2nd ed
Georges Y. El-Khoury, Ronald A. Bergman, and William J. Montgomery
1995 • Hardcover • 776 pages • $295.00

Skeletal Anatomy. 3rd ed
Glenda J. Bryan
1996 • Paper • 250 pages • $44.00

Textbook of Fetal Abnormalities
P. Twining, J. McHugo, and D. Pilling, editors
1998 • Hardcover • 668 pages (approx)
• $240.00 (tentative) • In preparation

Textbook of Radiology and Imaging. 6th ed
David Sutton, editor
1998 • Hardcover • 1,600 pages (approx)
• (2-vol set) • $349.00 • In preparation

Thoracic Imaging (Rad Notes)
Jeffrey Klein, Alexander Baxter, and Eric Oestele
1996 • Win or Mac CD-ROM • $99.00

Thoracic Imaging Professional Version (Rad Notes)
Jeffrey Klein, Alexander Baxter, and Eric Oestele
1996 • Mac CD-ROM • $155.00

Ultrasound Diagnosis of Breast Disease
Eriko Tohno, David O. Cosgrove, and John P. Sloane
1994 • Hardcover • 207 pages • $126.00

Ultrasound in fetal Syndromes
Beryl R. Benacerraf, MD
1998 • Hardcover • 464 pages • $125.00

Ultrasound of Superficial Structures High Frequencies, Doppler and Interventional Procedures
Luigi Solbiati and Giorgio Rizzatto, editors
1995 • Hardcover • 416 pages • $205.00

Ultrasound in Gastroenterology (Clinics in Diagnostic Ultrasound)
Paul A. Dubbins and A. E. A. Joseph
1994 • Hardcover • 215 pages • $109.00

Ultrasound in Gynecology
Steven R. Goldstein and Ilan Timor-Tritsch
1995 • Hardcover • 344 pages • $110.00

Ultrasound of the Breast
Jack Jellins, A. Patricia Romilly-Harper, and Kenneth J. W. Taylor, editors
1998 • Hardcover • 300 pages (approx)
• $85.00 (tentative) • In preparation

Venous Access Management
Timothy C. McCowan and Timothy C. Goertzen
1998 • Hardcover • 304 pages (approx)
• $125.00 (tentavive) • In preparation

Walter's & Miller's Textbook of Radiotherapy, Radiation Physics, Therapy and Oncology 5th ed
C. K. Bomford, Ian H. Kunkler, and Susan B. Sherriff
1994 • Paper • 608 pages • $88.00

DEAN BOOKS COMPANY

P.O. Box 346
Jericho, New York 11753
(516) 338-4594
Telefax (516) 694-5434
www/mribook.com

The Pioneers of NMR and Magnetic Resonance in Medicine. The Story of MRI
James Mattson and Merrill Simon, editors
1996 • Hardcover • 838 pages • Library Edition $75.00 • Leatherbound $150.00

INTERNATIONAL COMMISSION ON RADIATION UNITS AND MEASUREMENTS (ICRU)

7910 Woodmont Avenue
Suite 800
Bethesda, MD 20814
(301) 657-2652
Toll Free (North America) 1-800-229-2652
Telefax (301) 907-8768
Worldwide Web: http://www.icru.org

Conversion Coefficients for Use in Radiological Protection Against External Radiation
ICRU Report 57
1997 • Paper • 238 pages (approx) • In press

Dose and Volume Specification for Reporting Interstitial Therapy
ICRU Report 58
1997 • Paper • 34 pages • $35.00

Dosimetry of External Beta Rays for Radiation Protection
ICRU Report 56
1996 • Paper • 135 pages • $60.00

Gamma Ray Spectrometry in the Environment
ICRU Report 53
1995 • Paper • 84 pages • $50.00

Medical Imaging—The Assessment of Image Quality
ICRU Report 54
1996 • Paper • 114 pages • $60.00

Particle Counting in Radioactivity Measurements
ICRU Report 52
1994 • Paper • 80 pages • $50.00

Secondary Election Spectra from Charged Particle Interactions
ICRU Report 55
1996 • Paper • 113 pages • $65.00

KRAMES/STAYWELL

1100 Grundy Lane
San Bruno, CA 94066-3030
(800) 333-3032

Diagnostic and treatment educational materials for the radiology patient

$20 for package of 50 brochures:
— Abdominal Sonogram (#91037)
— Abdominal Sonogram\Spanish Version (#91067)
— Abdominal Ultrassound (#93012)
— Barium Enema (#9464)
— Bone Density Studies (#93011)
— Bone Scan (#93015)
— Breast Health Brochure (#91143)
— Breast Health Brochure\Spanish Version (#91433)
— Cardiac Nuclear Imaging (#91931)
— Carotid Angiography (#9774)
— Computed Tomography (#9462)
— Doppler Ultrasound (#93014)
— HSG-Hysterosalpingogram (#9395)
— Intravenous Pyelogram (#9467)
— Lower GI Endoscopy brochure (#91090)
— Magnetic Resonance Imaging (#9463)
— Mammography (#9466)
— Mammography\Spanish Version (#9349)
— Mammography\USPSTF Guidelines (#9399)
— Nuclear Medicine Scan (#93016)
— Pelvic Sonogram brochure (#91036)
— Pelvic Sonogram brochure\Spanish Version (#91066)
— Pelvic Ultrasound (#93013)
— Peripheral Angiography (#9773)
— Peripheral Angioplasty (#9775)
— Upper GI Endoscopy brochure (#91089)
— Upper GI Endoscopy brochure\Spanish Version (#91610)
— Upper GI Series (#9465)
— X-Ray (#93010)

1 page • Pad of 50 tear sheets • $12.50/pad:
— Caring for Your Skin and Nails (#5470)
— Controlling Nausea and Vomiting (#5463)
— Coping with Hair Loss (#5466)
— Managing Fatigue (#5468)
— Managing Lymphedema (#5462)
— Preventing Bleeding (#5467)
— Preventing Infections (#5469)
— Relieving Mouth Sores and Dry Mouth (#5464)
— Treating Diarrhea and Constipation (#5465)

Other brochures and booklets:

— Bladder Cancer booklet (#1783), 16 pages/$1.35
— Breast Health booklet (#1349), 16 pages/$1.35
— Breast Lumps booklet (#1019), 16 pages, $1.35
— Breast Lumps booklet (#1060), 16 pages, $1.35
— Breast Surgery booklet (#1291), 16 pages, $1.25
— Breast Surgery booklet/Spanish version (#1823), 16 pages, $1.25 each
— Chemotherapy booklet (#1994), 16 pages, $1.50
— Computed Tomography booklet (#5009), 8 pages, $0.70
— Magnetic Resonance Imaging booklet (#5008), 8 pages, $0.70
— Mammography booklet (#5010), 8 pages, $0.70
— Prostate Cancer booklet (#1375), 16 pages $1.35
— Prostate Health: Screening for Cancer booklet (#1335), 8 pages, $1.10
— Radiation Therapy booklet (#1338), 8 pages $1.35 each
— Ultrasound booklet ($5013), 8 pages, $0.70
— Upper GI Endoscopy booklet (#5006), 8 pages, $0.70

(Quantity discount pricing. Sample copies available upon professional request. All publications in full color. Other titles available.)

LIPPINCOTT WILLIAMS & WILKINS

P.O. Box 1600
Hagerstown, MD 21741-1600
(800)777-2295
(301)714-2300
Telefax (301)824-7390

Abdominal and Pelvic Ultrasound on CD-ROM with CT and MR Correlation
R. Brooke Jeffrey, Jr, MD
1996 • CD-ROM • 330 cases • $350.00

Abrams' Angiography, Volumes I, II, and III. 4th ed
Stanley Baum, MD
1996 • 3,000 pages • 3-volume set • $495.00

An Atlas of Imaging of the Paranasal Sinuses
Lalitha Shankar, Kathryn Evans, Michael Hawke, and Heinz Stammberger
1994 • Hardcover • 208 pages • $150.00

Atlas of Intravascular Ultrasound
John McB. Hodgson and Helen M. Sheehan, editors
1994 • Hardcover • 352 pages • $138.00

Breast Imaging
Daniel B. Kopans, MD
1997 • 750 pages • $95.00

Breast Imaging Companion
Gilda Cardenosa, MD
1997 • Hardcover • 456 pages • $63.00

Breast Specimen Radiography
Eva Rubin, MD and Jean F. Simpson, MD
Nov 1997 • Hardcover • 304 pages • $100.00

Cancer: Principles and Practice of Oncology. 5th ed
Vincent T. Devita, Jr, MD, Samuel Hellman, MD, and Steven A. Rosenberg, MD, PhD
1997 • Hardcover • 3,456 pages • single volume, $225.00 • double volume, $255.00 • single and CD-ROM, $325.00 • double and CD-ROM, $355.00 • CD-ROM, $250.00

Cardiac SPECT Imaging
E. Gordon DePuey, Daniel S. Berman, and Ernest V. Garcia, editors
1995 • 304 pages • $151.00

Cerebral SPECT Imaging. 2nd ed
Ronald L. Van Heertum and Ronald S. Tikofsky, editors
1995 • Hardcover • 240 pages • $157.00

Clinical Applications of Doppler Ultrasound. 2nd ed
Kenneth J. W. Taylor, Peter N. Burns, and Peter N. T. Wells
1995 • Hardcover • 416 pages • $139.00

Clinical Computed Tomography for the Technologist. 2nd ed
Lee C. Chiu, James D. Lipcamon, and Victoria S. Yiu-Chiu
1995 • 224 pages • $69.00

Clinical Gynecologic Imaging
Arthur C. Fleischer, MD, Marcia C. Javitt, MD, R. Brooke Jeffrey, Jr, MD, and Howard W. Jones III, MD
1997 • Hardcover • 448 pages • $156.00

Clinical Imaging: An Atlas of Differential Diagnosis. 3rd ed
Ronald L. Eisenberg, MD
1997 • Hardcover • 1,264 pages • $185.00

Clinical SPECT Imaging
Elissa Lipcon Kramer and Joseph J. Sanger, editors
1995 • Hardcover • 272 pages • $140.00

Color Flow and Power Doppler Ultrasound Teaching File
R. Brooke Jeffrey and Philip W. Ralls
October 1997 • Hardcover • 280 pages • $135.00

Color Flow and Power Doppler Ultrasound Teaching File on CD-ROM
R. Brooke Jeffrey and Philip W. Ralls
1997 • 125 cases • $295.00

Computed Body Tomography with MRI Correlation. 3rd ed
Joseph K. T. Lee, Stuart S. Sagel, Robert J. Stanley, and Jay P. Herken
1997 • 2,000 pages • $260.00
(2-vol set)

CT and Sonography of the Acute Abdomen. 2nd ed
R. Brooke Jeffrey and Philip W. Ralls
1996 • Hardcover • 384 pages • $157.00

Diagnostic Obstetrical Ultrasound
John P. McGahan and Manuel Porto
1994 • Hardcover • 544 pages • $105.00

Diagnostic Ultrasound: A Logical Approach
John P. McGahan, MD, and Barry B. Goldberg, MD
1997 • Hardcover • 1,312 pages • $195.00

Diagnostic Ultrasound on CD-ROM
John P. McGahan, MD, and Barry B. Goldberg, MD
December 1997 • $195.00

Diagnostic Ultrasound Applied to Obstetrics and Gynecology. 3rd ed
Rudy E. Sabbagha
1994 • Hardcover • 752 pages • $131.00

Differential Diagnosis of Tumor-like Lesions of Bones and Joints
Adam Greenspan, MD, and Wolfgang Remagen, MD
1997 • Hardcover • 480 pages • $225.00

Diffusion and Perfusion Magnetic Resonance Imaging: Applications to Functional MRI
Denis Le Bihan, editor
1995 • Paper • 408 pages • $172.00

Diseases of the Breast
Jay R.Harris, Marc Lippman, Monica Morrow, and Samuel Hellman
1996 • Hardcover • 1,072 pages • $178.00

Doppler Ultrasound in Obstetrics and Gynecology
Joshua A. Copel and Kathryn L. Reed, editors
1995 • Hardcover • 368 pages • $142.00

Duke Radiology Case Review
James M. Provenzale, MD, and Rendon C. Nelson, MD
1997 • Hardcover • 640 pages • $75.00

The Echo Manual
Jae K. Oh, MD, James B. Seward, MD, and A. Jamil Tajik, MD
1994 • Paper • 272 pages • $94.95

Endoluminal Vascular Protheses
Timothy A.M. Chuter, Carlos E. Donayre, and Rodney A. White
1995 • Hardcover • 352 pages •$85.00

Essays from the Heart
J. Willis Hurst
1995 • Hardcover • 192 pages • $69.00

Essentials of Cardiac Imaging, 2nd ed
James T. T. Chen, MD
1997 • Hardcover • 400 pages • $138.50

Functional Imaging: Principles and Methods
Gustav K. Von Schulthess, MD, PhD, and Jurgen Hennig, PhD
1997 • Hardcover • 480 pages • $158.00

Gastrointestinal Radiology. 3rd ed
Ronald L. Eisenberg
1995 • Hardcover • 1,216 pages • $183.00

Handbook of Interventional Radiologic Procedures. 2nd ed
Krishna Kandarpa, MD, and John E. Aruny, MD
1995 • Paper • 508 pages • $41.00

Helical (Spiral) Computed Tomography
Paul M. Silverman, MD
April 1998 • Paper • 180 pages • $48.00

High Resolution CT of the Chest: A Comprehensive Atlas
Eric J. Stern and Stephen J. Swenson
1996 • 304 pages • $124.00

High-Resolution CT of the Lung. 2nd ed
W. Richard Webb, Nestor L. Muller, and David P. Naidich, editors
1996 • 336 pages • $146.00

Imaging Atlas of Orthopedic Appliances and Prostheses
Thomas H. Berquist
1995 • Hardcover • 2,866 pages • $215.00

Imaging of Bone Tumors
George B. Greenfield and John Arrington
1995 • Hardcover • 512 pages (approx) • $135.00

Imaging in Infertility and Reproductive Endocrinology
Richard Jaffe, Roger A. Person, and Jacques S. Abramowicz
1995 • Hardcover • 448 pages • $137.00

Imaging of Head Trauma
Alisa D. Gean
1994 • Hardcover • 592 pages • $135.00

Imaging of the Pediatric Head, Neck and Spine
Mauricio Castillo, MD, and Suresh Murkherji, MD
1996 • Hardcover • 768 pages • $165.00

Imaging of the Scrotum
Hedvig Hricak, MD, Bernd Hamm, and Boyhun Kim
1995 • Hardcover • 288 pages • $153.00

Imaging of Vertebral Trauma. 2nd ed
Richard H. Daffner
1996 • Hardcover • 304 pages • $131.00

Interpretation of ERCP
Andrew J. Taylor, MD, and Anthony G. Bohorfoush III, MD
1997 • Hardcover • 352 pages • $102.00

Magnetic Resonance Bioeffects, Safety, and Patient Management. 2nd ed
Frank G. Shellock, PhD, and Emanuel Kanal, MD
1997 • 332 pages • $47.00

Magnetic Resonance in Epilepsy
Rubin I. Kuzniecky and Graeme D. Jackson
1995 • Hardcover • 368 pages • $120.00

Magnetic Resonance Imaging in Orthopaedics and Sports Medicine. 2nd ed
David W. Stoller
1997 • 1,408 pages • $261.00

Magnetic Resonance Imaging in Orthopaedics and Sports Medicine on CD-ROM
David W. Stoller
1997 • $411.00 (Text and CD-ROM)

Magnetic Resonance Imaging of the Body. 3rd ed
Charles B. Higgins, Hedvig Hricak, and Clyde A. Helms
1997 • 1,616 pages • $261.00

Magnetic Resonance Imaging of the Brain and Spine. 2nd ed
Scott W. Atlas
1996 • Hardcover • 1,696 pages • $270.00

Magnetic Resonance Imaging of the Elbow
Russell C. Fritz
September 1997 • Hardcover • 150 pages • $95.00

Mammography on CD-ROM Diagnosis and Intervention
Ralph L.Smathers, MD, editor
1997 • CD-ROM • 200+ cases • $320.00

Manual of Obstetric and Gynecologic Ultrasound
Richard Jaffe, MD, and Jacques S. Abramowicz, MD
1997 • Paper • 324 pages • $49.95

Manual of Radiology: Acute Problems and Essential Procedures
John Eng, MD, editor
1997 • Paper • 368 pages • $38.00

Mastering MRI
An Educational and Reference Series on CD-ROM
William G.Bradley, Jr, MD and John V. Crues III, MD, editors
1996 • 2 CD-ROM disks • $250.00

MRI and CT of the Spine: Case Study Approach. 2nd ed
Robert Kricun and Morrie E. Kricun
1994 • Hardcover • 416 pages • $146.00

MR Angiography. A Teaching File
Michael Brant-Zawadski, MD, Orest B. Boyko, MD, PhD, Maureen C. Jensen, MD, and Gary D. Gillian, RT
1994 • Hardcover • 256 pages • $79.00

MRI Contrast Enhancement in the Central Nervous System: A Case Study Approach
Robert C. Brasch, editor, Burton P. Drayer, Victor M. Haughton, J. Randy Jinkins, Kevin Nelson, and Gordon Sze, associate editors
1994 • Hardcover • 352 pages • $115.00

MRI of the Cardiovascular System (MRI Teaching File)
Andre J. Duerinckx, Charles B. Higgins, and Roderic I. Pettigrew, editors
1994 • Hardcover • 304 pages • $76.00

MRI of the Central Nervous System
William G.Bradley, Jr, MD, PhD, FACR
1996 • CD-ROM • PC version • $250.00

MRI of the Knee. 2nd ed
Peter L. Munk and Clyde A. Helms, editors
1996 • Hardcover • 384 pages • $142.00

MRI of the Musculoskeletal System. 2nd ed
A Teaching File
Andrew L. Deutsch and Jerrold H. Mink, editors
1997 • Hardcover • 768 pages • $156.00

MRI of the Musculoskeletal System. 3rd ed
Thomas A. Berquist
1996 • Hardcover • 1,008 pages • $170.00

MRI of the Musculoskeletal System on CD-ROM
John V. Crues III, MD
1996 • CD-ROM • PC version • $250.00

MRI of the Spine
Thomas E. St Amour, MD, PhD, Steven C. Hodges, MD, Robert W. Laakman, MD, and David E. Tamas, MD
1994 • Hardcover • 864 pages • $211.00

MRI Survival Guide
Jim D. Cardoza and Robert J. Herfkens
1994 • Hardcover • 240 pages • $63.00

Multidisciplinary Atlas of Breast Surgery
David W. Kinne, MD
1997 • Hardcover • 256 pages • $157.00

Neoplasms of the Digestive Tract: Imaging, Staging and Management
Morton A. Meyers, MD
1997 • Hardcover • 624 pages • $172.00

Neurodiagnostic Imaging: Pattern Analysis and Differential Diagnosis
J. Randy Jinkins and Claudia da Costa Leite
October 1997 • Hardcover • 1,200 pages • $220.00

Neuroradiology Companion: Methods, Guidelines, and Imaging Fundamentals
Mauricio Castillo
1995 • Paper • 384 pages • $54.00

Nuclear Medicine Annual, 1998
Leonard M. Freeman, MD
1998 • 320 pages • $112.00

On-Call Radiology
Mark Mittleman and Marc R. Hamet
1997 • Paper • 225 pages • $39.00

Paul and Juhl's Essentials of Radiologic Imaging. 7th ed
John H. Juhl, Andrew B. Crummy, and Janet E. Kuhlman, MD
1998 • Hardcover • 1,408 pages • $149.00

Pediatric Images
Casebook of Differential Diagnosis
Eugene Blank
1997 • Hardcover • 1,264 pages • $192.00

Pediatric Neuroimaging. 2nd ed
A. James Barkovich
1995 • Hardcover • 688 pages • $175.00

Pediatric Neuroradiology
William S. Ball, Jr
1997 • Hardcover • 816 pages • $182.00

Pediatric Radiation Oncology. 2nd ed
Edward C. Halperin, Louis S. Constine, Nancy J. Tarbell, and Larry E. Kun
1994 • Hardcover • 640 pages • $124.00

Pediatric Sonography. 2nd ed
Marilyn J. Siegel, editor
1995 • Hardcover • 612 pages • $164.00

Pocket Atlas of MRI Body Anatomy
Thomas H. Berquist, MD
1995 • Paper • 112 pages • $16.95

Pocket Atlas of MRI Musculoskeletal Anatomy
Thomas H. Berquist, MD
1995 • Paper • 112 pages • $16.95

Pocket Atlas of Obstetric Ultrasound
Gary A. Thieme, John C. Hobbins, and Michael Manco-Johnson
1996 • Paper • 96 pages • $16.95

Pocket Guide to MR Procedures and Metallic Objects. Update 1994
Frank G. Shellock
1995 • Paper • 88 pages • $16.95

Posttherapeutic Neurodiagnostic Imaging
J. Randy Jinkins, MD, FACR
1997 • Hardcover • 320 pages • $131.00

A Practical Guide to Echocardiography and Cardiac Doppler Ultrasound. 2nd ed
Ibrahim A. Jawad
1996 • Paper • 432 pages • $43.00

Practical Guide to Ultrasound in Obstetrics and Gynecology. 2nd ed.
Eric E. Sauerbrei, Khanh T. Nguyen, and Robert L. Nolan
1997 • Paper • 736 pages • $52.95

Practical MRI: A Teaching File
Jeffrey J. Brown and Franz J. Wippold III
1995 • Hardcover • 544 pages • $135.00

Practical Pediatric Imaging: Diagnostic Radiology of Infants and Children. 3rd ed
Donald R. Kirks and N. Thorne Griscom
1997 • Hardcover • 1,600 pages • $225.00

Practical Sonography in Obstetrics and Gynecology. 2nd ed
John W. Seeds, Nancy C. Chescheir, and Ronald V. Wade
1996 • Hardcover • 320 pages • $72.00

Primer of Noninvasive Vascular Technology
Terrance D. Case, MEd, RVT
1994 • Paper • 336 pages • $50.00

Principles and Practice of Radiation Oncology. 2nd ed
Carlos A. Perez and Luther W. Brady
1997 • 2,240 pages • $215.00

Producing Quality Radiographs. 2nd ed
Angeline M. Cullinan and John E. Cullinan
1994 • Hardcover • 352 pages • $51.00

Radiobiology for the Radiologist. 4th ed
Eric J. Hall
1994 • Hardcover • 496 pages • $87.00

Radiographic Positioning. 2nd ed
Ronald Eisenberg, Cynthia Dennis, and Chris R. May
1995 • Hardcover • 432 pages • $74.00

Radiographic Positioning Pocket Manual
Cynthia Dennis, Chris R. May, and Ronald L. Eisenberg
1995 • Spiralbound • 288 pages • $28.95

Radiology: Diagnosis-Imaging-Intervention
Clinical text in five volumes
Editor-in-Chief: Juan M. Taveras, MD
1996 • Looseleaf with annual updates • 6,505 pages • $620.00

Radiology On-Call Survival Guide
Brian Funaki and Martin J. Lipton
1996 • Paper • 256 pages • $35.00

Radiology on CD-ROM
Editor-in-Chief: Juan M. Taveras, MD
1996 • Annual Updates • 6,505 pages • $650.00

Radiology 101
William E. Erkonen, MD
July 1998 • Paper • 480 pages • $34.95

Radiology Pocket Reference
Eisenberg and Margulis
1995 • Paper • 480 pages • $42.00

Shoulder Magnetic Resonance Imaging
Lynn S. Steinback, Phillip F.J. Tirman, Charles G. Peterfy, and John F. Feller
1998 • Hardcover • 288 pages • $149.00

Skull and Spine Imaging: An Atlas of Differential Diagnosis
Ronald L. Eisenberg, MD
1994 • Hardcover • 320 pages • $110.50

Sonography of the Abdomen
R. Brooke Jeffrey, Jr, and Philip W. Ralls
1995 • Hardcover • 432 pages • $167.00

Spiral CT of the Body: A Teaching File
R. Brooke Jeffrey, Jr, and Elliot K. Fishman, editors
1997 • Hardcover • 336 pages • $152.00

Spiral CT of the Chest and Abdomen
R. Brooke Jeffrey, Jr, and Elliot K. Fishman
CD-ROM • 150 cases • PC version • $295.00

Spiral CT: Principles, Techniques and Clinical Applications. 2nd ed
Elliot K. Fishman, MD
June 1998 • Hardcover • 448 pages • $125.00

A Text Atlas of Urogenital Ultrasound
Dennis Cochlin, Paul Dubbins, Barry Goldberg, and Archie Alexander
1995 • Hardcover • 448 pages • $150.00

Textbook of Nuclear Medicine
Michael A. Wilson, MD, editor
1997 • Hardcover • 688 pages • $95.00

Three-Dimensional CT Angiography
Hideo Adachi and Jun Nagai, editors
1995 • Hardcover • 248 pages • $162.00

Thyroid Disease: Endocrinology, Surgery, Nuclear Medicine, and Radiotherapy. 2nd ed
Steven A. Falk, MD, FACS, editor
1997 • Hardcover • 704 pages • $146.00

Transvaginal Sonography: A Clinical Analysis. 2nd ed
Arthur C. Fleischer and Donald M. Keppel
1995 • Hardcover • 448 pages • $99.00

Trauma Radiology Companion: Methods, Guidelines, and Imaging Fundamentals
Eric J. Stern, et al
1997 • Paper • 400 pages • $65.00

Tumor Board Case Management
David P. Winchester, MD, FACS, editor
1997 • Hardcover • 788 pages • $105.00

Ultrasound Exam Review: Sonographer's Self-Assessment Guide. 2nd ed
Marveen Craig
1994 • Paper • 304 pages • $38.00

Ultrasound of the Prostate: Imaging in the Diagnosis and Therapy of Prostatic Disease. 2nd ed
Matthew D. Rifkin, MD, editor
1997 • Hardcover • 480 pages • $142.00

University of California San Francisco Radiology CD-ROM series includes:
Abdominal Imaging: Genitourinary Radiology
Abdominal Imaging: Gastrointestinal Radiology
Interventional Radiology
Upper Abdominal Ultrasonographic Anatomy
1997 • CD-ROM • $295.00

MCGRAW-HILL
11 West 19th St—2nd Floor
New York, NY 10011
(800) 262-4729

Cardiac Nuclear Medicine. 3rd ed
Myron C. Gerson, MD
1997 • Hardcover • 688 pages • $120.00

Differential Diagnosis in Neuroradiology
J. Randy Jinkins, MD
1998 • Hardcover • 400 pages • $98.00

Harrison's Principles of Internal Medicine. 14th ed
Anthony Fauci, MD, Eugene Braunwald, MD, and Kurt J. Isselbacher, MD, et al
1998 • Hardcover • 2,688 pages • $99.00 (1-vol ed) • $129.00 (2-vol set)

Head and Neck Imaging
Lalitha Shankar, MD, FRCP
1998 • Hardcover • 550 pages • $98.00 (tentative)

Helical/Spinal CT: A Practical Approach
Robert K. Zeman, MD, James A. Brink, MD, Philip Costello, MD, et al
1995 • Hardcover • 256 pages • $95.00

Magnetic Resonance Angiography: A Practical Approach
E. Kent Yucel, MD
1995 • Hardcover • 217 pages • $79.00

Mammographic Interpretation: A Practical Approach. 2nd ed
Marc J. Homer, MD
1997 • Hardcover • 320 pages • $98.00

Mammography for Radiologic Technologist. 2nd ed
Gini Wentz, RT, and Ward C. Parsons, MD
1997 • Paper • 158 pages • $39.00

MRI for Technologists
Peggy Woodward, BS, RT(R), and Roger D. Freimark, RT
1995 • Paper • 480 pages • $48.00

Neuroimaging: A Companion to Adams and Victor's Principles of Neurology
Jack O. Greenberg, MD
1995 • Hardcover • 614 pages • $125.00

Oncological Imaging: A Clinical Perspective
Claudia G. Berman, MD, Norman J. Brodsky, MD, and Robert A. Clark, MD
1997 • Hardcover • 700 pages • $110.00

Principles of Shoulder Imaging
David J. Sartoris, MD
1995 • Hardcover • 464 pages • $110.00

Radiation Therapy Planning. 2nd ed
Gunilla C. Bentel, MD
1996 • Hardcover • 643 pages • $68.00

Radiology
Margery Manuli, MD
1998 • Paper • 456 pages • $40.00

Review of Thoracic Imaging and Chest Disease
Richard M. Slone, MD, and Fernando Gutierrez, MD
1998 • Paper • 500 pages • $59.00

Shoulder Arthroscopy
Stephen J. Snyder, MD
1994 • Hardcover • 288 pages • $149.00

Transesophageal Echocardiography
Gerald Maurer, MD
1994 • Hardcover • 304 pages • $149.00

Ultrasound: A Pattern Approach
Patricia L. Abbitt
1995 • Hardcover • 496 pages • $125.00

MEDICAL PHYSICS PUBLISHING

4513 Vernon Blvd.
Madison, WI 53705-4964
(800) 442-5778
(608) 262-4021
Telefax (608) 265-2121
email: mpp@medicalphysics.org

Applications of New Technology: External Dosimetry
Jack Higginbotham, editor
1996 • Hardcover • 464 pages • $69.95

Applied Physics for Radiation Oncology
Robert Stanton and Donna Stinson
1996 • Paper $53.95 • Hardcover $68.95 • 375 pages

The Basics of Film Processing in Medical Imaging
Arthur Haus and Susan Jaskulski
1997 • Paper, $69.95 • Hardcover, $85.95 • 340 pages

Brachytherapy Physics: 1994 AAPM Summer School Proceedings
Jeff Williamson, Bruce Thomadsen, and Ravinder Nath, editors
1995 • Paper • 715 pages • $79.95

Exposure of the Pregnant Patient to Diagnostic Radiations
A Guide to Medical Management. 2nd ed
Louis Wagner, Richard Lester, and Luis Saldana
1997 • Hardcover • 280 pages • $69.95

The Fundamentals of Diagnostic Radiology—CD-ROM
Cupido Daniels, editor
1997 • CD-ROM • Individual: $99.00 • Institution $195.00

Good Practices in Health Physics
Gregory R. Komp and Michael A. Thompson, editors
1998 • Paper • 288 pages • $35.95

Internal Radiation Dosimetry
Otto Raabe, editor
1994 • Paper • 667 pages • $48.95

Introduction to Clinical Radiation Oncology. 3rd ed
Lawrence R. Coia and David J. Moylan
1998 • Paper • 580 pages • $48.95

Mammography Quality Control: The Why and How Book
Calvin P. Myers
1997 • Paper • 50 pages • $19.95

Management and Administraation of Radiation Safety Programs
Charles E. Roessler, editor
1998 • Hardcover • 603 pages • $69.95

Medical Physicists and Malpractice
Robert Shalek and David Gooden
1996 • Paper $21.00 • Hardcover $27.00 • 140 pages

My Life with Radiation—Hiroshima + 50
Ralph E. Lapp
Cogito Books 1995 • Paper • $17.95

The Nuclear Imaging Tutor—CD-ROM
Developed by the Medical College of Georgia
Casimir Eubig
1998 • CD-ROM • Individual: $85.95 • Institution $289.95

Physical Principles of Medical Imaging. 2nd ed
Perry Sprawls
1995 • Hardcover • 656 pages • $69.95

The Physics of Radiotherapy X-Rays from Linear Accelerators
Peter Metcalfe, Tomas Kron, and Peter Hoban
1997 • Paper $98.95 • Hardcover $119.95 • 500 pages

A Practical Manual of Brachytherapy
Bernard Pierquin and Ginette Marinello, editors
1997 • Hardcover • 300 pages • $109.95

Practical Radiography
H. Snowden Ward
1995 • Paper • 112 pages • $16.95

A Primer on Theory and Operation of Linear Accelerators in Radiation Therapy. 2nd ed
C. J. Karzmark and R. J. Morton
1998 • Paper • 64 pages • $26.95

The Q Book: The Physics of Radiotherapy X-Rays: Problems and Solutions
Peter Metcalfe, Tomas Kron, and Peter Hoban
1998 • Paperback • 100 pages • $33.95

Radiation Protection at Nuclear Reactors
Constantine J. Maletskos
1995 • Hardcover • 624 pages • $69.95

RadReview: Diagnostic Radiological Physics Examination and Study Guide
Perry Sprawls, compiler
1995 • Paper • 80 pages • $23.95

RAPHEX 94
Radiological Physics Examination
Radiological and Medical Physics Society of New York (RAMPS)
1994 • Practice Exam and Answer booklets • $25.00

Shielding Techniques for Radiation Oncology Facilities
Patton H. McGinley
1998 • Hardcover • 150 pages • $62.95

Therapy Physics Review Part 1: Basic Physics Examination and Study Guide
Bhudatt Paliwal
1996 • Paper • 65 pages • $24.95

MOSBY, INC.

11830 Westline Industrial Drive
St. Louis, MO 63146
(800) 633-6699
(314) 872-8370

Atlas and Text of Clinical Imaging
Jamie Weir, MB, BS, and Allison Murray, MB, ChB
1998 • paper • 256 pages • $33.95

Atlas of Normal Roentgen Variants That May Simulate Disease. 6th ed
Theodore E. Keats, MD
1996 • Hardcover • 1,042 pages • $235.00

Atlas of Ultrasound Color Flow Imaging
Barry A. Goldberg, MD, Daniel A. Merton, BS, RDMS, and Colin R. Deane, PhD
1997 • Hardcover • 304 pages • $140.00

Breast Diseases: A Year Book Quarterly
S. Eva Singletary, MD
1998 • Paper • 200 pages • $27.00 single copy, $47.00 student yearly rate (USA), $79.00 individual yearly rate (USA), $118.00 institutional rate (USA)

Cardiac Radiology: The Requisites
Stephen W. Miller, MD
1996 • Hardcover • 466 pages • $84.95

Chest Radiology: Plain Film and Differential Diagnoses. 4th ed
James C. Reed, MD
1996 • Hardcover • 496 pages • $95.00

Computed Tomography and MRI of the Whole Body. 3rd ed
John R. Haaga, MD, Charles Lanzieri, MD, Elias Zerhouni, MD, and David Sartoris, MD
1994 • Hardcover • 2,000 pages • $305.00

A Concise Textbook of Clinical Imaging. 2nd ed
David Sutton, MD, and Jermey W. R. Young, MD
1995 • Hardcover • 944 pages • $145.00

Diagnosis and Detection of Breast Disease
Deborah E. Powell, MD, and Carol B. Stelling, MD
1994 • Hardcover • 465 pages • $99.00

Diagnostic Imaging of Child Abuse. 2nd ed
Paul K. Kleinman, MD
1998 • 528 pages • $95.00

Diagnostic Imaging Expert: A CD-ROM Reference and Review
Ralph Weissleder, MD, PhD, Jack Wittenberg, MD, Mark Rieumont, MD, and Genevieve Bennett, MD
1997 • $230.00

Diagnostic Ultrasound. 2nd ed
Carol M. Rumack, MD, J. William Charboneau, MD, and Stephanie R. Wilson, MD
1997 • Hardcover • 1,940 pages • $250.00 • (2 vol-set)

Functional Brain Imaging
William W. Orrison, Jr, MD
1994 • Hardcover • 400 pages • $95.00

Functional Computed Tomography
Kenneth A. Miles, MBBS, MSc, FRCR, MD, Peter Dawson, MRCR, FRCR, and Martin Blomley, MBB, MRCP
1997 • Hardcover • 192 pages • $155.00

Gamuts in Nuclear Medicine
Frederic L. Datz, MD
1994 • Hardcover • 505 pages • $45.95

Genitourinary Radiology—The Requisites
Ronald J. Zagoria, MD, and Glenn A. Tung, MD
1997 • Hardcover • 432 pages • $79.95

Handbook of Head and Neck Imaging. 2nd ed
H. Ric Harnsberger, MD
1995 • Paper • 576 pages • $49.95

Handbook of Interventional Radiology and Angiography. 2nd ed
Myron Wojtowycz, MD
1995 • Hardcover • 448 pages • $45.00

Handbook of Neuroradiology: Brain and Skull. 2nd ed
Anne G. Osborn, MD, and Karen Tong, MD
1996 • Paper • 736 pages • $45.95

Handbook of Pediatric Radiology
Vesna Martich Kriss, MD
1997 • 457 pages • $39.95

Handbook of Skeletal Radiology. 2nd ed
B. J. Manaster
1996 • Paper • 420 pages • $42.95

Handbook of Syndromes and Metabolic Disorders: Radiologic and Clinical Manifestations
Hooshang Taybi, MD
1997 • 504 pages • $39.95

Head and Neck Imaging. 3rd ed
Peter M. Som, MD, and Hugh D. Curtin, MD
1995 • Hardcover • 1,698 pages • $315.00 • (2 vol-set)

Head and Neck Imaging: Case Review
David M. Yousem, MD
1998 • 256 pages • $39.95

Imaging Atlas of Human Anatomy. 2nd ed
Jamie Weir, MB, BS, and Peter Abrahams, MB, MS
1997 • Paper • 216 pages • $37.95

Imaging Atlas of Human Anatomy CD-ROM Version 2.0
Jamie Weir, MB, BS, and Peter Abrahams, MB, MS
1997 • $69.95

Imaging Diseases of the Chest. 2nd ed
Peter Armstrong, MD, Alan Wilson, MD, Paul Dee, MD, and David Hansell, MD
1994 • Hardcover • 971 pages • $215.00

Intravascular Ultrasound
Raimund Erbel, Jos R.T.C. Roelandt, Junbo Ge and Günther Görge
1997 • Hardcover • 296 pages • $120.00

Interventional MRI
Robert Lufkin, MD
1998 • 384 pages • $129.00

Invasive Ultrasound
William R. Lees, FRCR, FRACR (Hon) and Edward A. Lyons, FRCP(C), FACR
1996 • Hardcover • 294 pages • $134.00

Magnetic Resonance Angiography of the Head & Neck: A Teaching File
Jeffrey Ross, MD
1994 • Hardcover • 424 pages • $99.00

Magnetic Resonance Imaging. 3rd ed
David D. Stark, MD, and William G. Bradley, Jr., MD, PhD
1998 • 2,800 pages • $399.00 • (3-vol set)

Margulis and Burhenne's Alimentary Tract Radiology. 5th ed
Patrick C. Freeny, MD, and Giles Stevenson, MD
1994 • Hardcover • 2,016 pages • $380.00 (2-vol set)

MRI of the CNS: A Teaching File
Douglas H. Yock, MD
1994 • Hardcover • 752 pages • $139.00

MR Imaging of the Female Pelvis
Clare M. C. Tempany, MD
1994 • Hardcover • 500 pages • $125.00

MRI Manual. 2nd ed
Robert B. Lufkin, MD
1997 • Paper • 480 pages • $64.95

Musculoskeletal Imaging: The Requisites
David J. Sartoris, MD
1995 • Hardcover • 432 pages • $84.95

Neuroradiology: The Requisites
Robert I. Grossman, MD, and David M. Yousem, MD
1994 • Hardcover • 560 pages • $89.00

Nuclear Cardiology: State of the Art and Future Directions. 2nd ed
Barry L. Zaret, MD, and George A. Beller, MD
1998 • Hardcover • 448 pages • $99.00

Nuclear Medicine: Principles and Practice
Robert E. Henkin, MD, et al
1995 • Hardcover • 1,856 pages • $300.00

Nuclear Medicine: The Requisites
James E. Thrall, MD, and Harvey A. Ziessman, MD
1994 • Hardcover • 384 pages • $84.95

Pediatric Radiology—The Requisites. 2nd ed
Johan G. Blickman, MD
1997 • Hardcover • 340 pages • $79.00

Pitfalls, Variants and Artifacts in Body MRI
Scott A. Mirowitz, MD
1996 • Hardcover • 544 pages • $140.00

Primer of Diagnostic Imaging. 2nd ed
Ralph Weissleder, MD, PhD, Mark Rieumont, MD, and Jack Wittenberg, MD
1996 • Paper • 992 pages • $89.95

Questions and Answers in Nuclear Medicine
Robert H. Wagner, MD, Stephen M. Karesh, PhD, and James R. Halama, PhD
1998 • 300 pages • $39.00

Radiation Therapy Physics. 2nd ed
William R. Hendee, MD, and Geoffrey S. Ibbott, MD
1996 • Hardcover • 576 pages • $74.95

Radiology: An Illustrated History (Commemorative Edition)
Ronald L. Eisenberg, MD
1994 • Leather-bound, foil-stamped • 606 pages • $158.00

Radiology of Syndromes, Metabolic Disorders, and Skeletal Dysplasias. 4th ed
Hooshang Taybi, MD, and Ralph Lachman, MD
1995 • Hardcover • 1,157 pages • $210.00

Skeletal Nuclear Medicine
B. David Collier, Jr, MD, Ignac Fogelman, MD, and Leonard Rosenthall, MD
1996 • Hardcover • 512 pages • $179.00

Structural Fetal Abnormalities
Roger C. Sanders, MD
1995 • Hardcover • 296 pages • $62.95

Textbook of Metallic Stents
Andreas Adam, MB, BS(Hons), FRCP, FRCR, Professor Robert F. Dondelinger, and Peter Mueller, PhD
1997 • Hardcover • 248 pages • $130.00

Thoracic Radiology—The Requisites
Theresa C. McCloud, MD
1997 • Hardcover • 544 pages • $79.00

Ultrasound: The Requisites
Alfred B. Kurtz, MD, and William B. Middleton, MD
1995 • Hardcover • 548 pages • $89.95

1998 Year Book of Diagnostic Radiology
Ann Osborne, MD, editor
1998 • Hardcover • 600 pages • $79.00

1997 Year Book of Neuroradiology
Anne G. Osborn, MD, editor
1997 • Hardcover • 300 pages • $94.95

1998 Year Book of Nuclear Medicine
Alexander Gottschalk, MD, editor
1998 • Hardcover • 420 pages • $86.00

1997 Year Book of Ultrasound
Christopher R. B. Merritt, MD, editor
1997 • Hardcover • 350 pages • $95.00

MT. HOPE PUBLISHING CO., INC.

c/o The Elizabeth Wende Breast Clinic
1351 Mt. Hope Avenue, Suite 110
Rochester, NY 14620
(800) 681-6011
(716) 442-2190
Telefax (716) 442-1837

Breast Cancer: A Practical Guide to Diagnosis. Vol 1—Procedures
Wende Logan-Young, MD, and Nancy Hoffman, MS
1994 • Hardcover • 432 pages • $110.00 (plus shipping)

NATIONAL COUNCIL ON RADIATION PROTECTION AND MEASUREMENTS (NCRP)

7910 Woodmont Avenue, Ste 800
Bethesda, MD 20814
(301) 657-2652
Toll Free (North America) 800-229-2652
Telefax (301) 907-8768
Worldwide Web: http://www.ncrp.com

Acceptability of Risk from Radiation—Application to Human Space Flight Symposium Proceedings 3 on May 29, 1996
Paper • 197 pages • $30.00

Considerations Regarding the Unintended Radiation Exposure of the Embryo, Fetus or Nursing Child
NCRP Commentary No. 9
1994 • Paper • 19 pages • $20.00

Deposition, Retention and Dosimetry of Inhaled Radioactive Substances
NCRP Report No. 125
1997 • Paper • 252 pages • $40.00

Dose Control at Nuclear Power Plants
NCRP Report No. 120
1994 • Paper • 138 pages • $30.00

Dose Limits for Individuals Who Receive Exposure from Radionuclide Therapy Patients
NCRP Commentary No. 11
1995 • Paper • 19 pages • $20.00

Environmental Dose Reconstruction and Risk Implications Proceedings of the Thirty-First Annual Meeting on April 12–13, 1995 (1996) (Including Taylor Lecture No. 19)
NCRP Proceedings No. 19
1996 • Paper • 373 pages • $50.00

A Guide For Uncertainty Analysis In Dose and Risk Assessments Related to Environmental Contamination
NCRP Commentary No. 14
1996 • Paper • 54 pages • $20.00

Implications of New Data on Radiation Cancer Risk, Proceedings of the Thirty-Second Annual Meeting on April 3-4, 1996 (Including Taylor Lecture No. 20)
NCRP Proceedings No. 18
1997 • Paper • 315 pages • $45.00

An Introduction to Efficacy in Diagnostic Radiology
NCRP Commentary No. 13
1995 • Paper • 29 pages • $20.00

Mice, Myths, and Men
R. J. Michael Fry
1994 • Paper • 61 pages • $25.00

Operational Radiation Safety Program
NCRP Report No. 127 • 1998 • In press

A Practical Guide to the Determination of Human Exposure to Radiofrequency Fields
NCRP Report No. 119
1994 • Paper • 233 pages • $40.00

Principles and Applications of Collective Dose in Radiation Protection
NCRP Report No. 121
1995 • Paper • 106 pages • $25.00

Screening Models for Releases of Radionuclides to Atmosphere, Surface Water, and Ground, Vols I & II
NCRP Report No. 123
1996 • Paper • Vol I, 316 pages; Vol II, 205 pages • $75.00

Sources and Magnitude of Occupational and Public Exposures from Nuclear Medicine Procedures
NCRP Report No. 124
1996 • Paper • 77 pages • $25.00

Uncertainties in Fatal Cancer Risk Estimates Used in Radiation Protection
NCRP Report No. 126
1997 • Paper • 112 pages • $25.00

Use of Personal Monitors to Estimate Effective Dose Equivalent and Effective Dose to Workers for External Exposure to Low-LET Radiation
NCRP Report No. 122
1995 • Paper • 64 pages • $25.00

PERGAMON AN IMPRINT OF ELSEVIER SCIENCE

655 Avenue of the Americas
New York, NY 10010-5107
Tel: (212) 633-3730
Toll Free (North America) 1-888-4ES-INFO (437-4636)
FAX: (212) 633-3680
Worldwide Web: http://www.elsevier.com

Age-dependent Doses to Members of the Public from Intake of Radionuclides: Part 2
ICRP Publication #67
1994 • Paper • 120 pages • $115.50

Age-dependent Doses to Members of the Public from Intake of Radionuclides: Part 3. Ingestion Dose Coefficients.
ICRP Publication #69
1995 • Paper • 74 pages • $69.00

Age-dependent Doses to Members of the Public from Intake of Radionuclides: Part 4. Inhalation Dose Coefficients
ICRP Publication #71
1996 • Paper • 410 pages • $124.50

Age-dependent Doses to the Members of the Public from Intake of Radionuclides: Part 5. Compilation of Ingestion and Inhalation Coefficients
ICRP Publication #72
1997 • Paper • 94 pages • $69.00

Conversion Coefficients for use in Radiological Protection against External Radiation
ICRP Publication #74
1996 • Paper • 220 pages • $138.00

Dose Coefficients for Intakes of Radionuclides by Workers
ICRP Publication #68
1995 • Paper • 110 pages • $61.00

General Principles for the Radiation Protection of Workers
ICRP Publication #75
1997 • Paper • 61 pages • $73.00

Human Respiratory Tract Model for Radiological Protection
ICRP Publication #66
1995 • Paper • 300 pages • $184.00

Protection from Potential Exposures: Application to Selected Radiation Sources
ICRP Publication #76
1997 • Paper • 61 pages • $73.00

Protection Against Radon-222 at Home and at Work
ICRP Publication #65
1994 • Paper • 48 pages • $58.00

Radiation Protection: Basic Anatomical and Physiological Data
ICRP Publication #70
1996 • Paper • 96 pages (approx) • $62.50

Radiological Protection and Safety in Medicine
ICRP Publication #73
1996 • Paper • 50 pages • $69.00

Radiology of Carpal Instability: A Practical Approach
W. R. Obermann
1994 • Hardcover • 200 pages • $228.00

PLENUM PUBLISHING CORPORATION

233 Spring Street
New York, NY 10013-1578
(212) 620-8000
Telefax (212) 647-1898
Worldwide Web: http://www.plenum.com

Biological Effects of Magnetic and Electromagnetic Fields
Shoogo Ueno, editor
1997 • Hardcover • 253 pages • $79.50

Cancer Neutron Capture Therapy
Yutaka Mishima, editor
1996 • Hardcover • Proceedings • $175.00

Chemists' Views of Imaging Centers
Ali M. Emran, editor
1995 • Hardcover • 552 pages • $139.50

Magnetic Resonance Scanning and Epilepsy
S. D. Shorvon, D. R. Fish, G. M. Bydder, H. Stefan, and F. Andermann, editors
(Volume 264 in NATO ASI Series A, Life Sciences)
1994 • Hardcover • 334 pages • $105.00

Neuroimaging I: Basic Science
Erin D. Bigler, editor
Set price with Neuroimaging II: $125.00
1996 • Hardcover • 334 pages • $75.00

Neuroimaging II: Clinical Applications
Erin D. Bigler, editor
Set price with Neuroimaging I: $125.00
1996 • Hardcover • 382 pages • $75.00

Radiofrequency Radiation Standards: Biological Effects, Dosimetry, Epidemiology, and Public Health Policy
B. Jon Klauenberg, Martino Grandolfo, and David N. Erwin
(Volume 274 in NATO ASI Series A, Life Sciences)
1995 • Hardcover • 470 pages • $135.00

Radiolabeled Blood Elements: Recent Advances in Techniques and Applications
J. Martin-Comin, M. L. Thakur, C. Piera, M. Roca, and F. Lomeña, editors
(Volume 262 in NATO ASI Series A, Life Sciences)
1994 • Hardcover • 382 pages • $125.00

SAN FRANCISCO PRESS, INC.

Box 426800
San Francisco, CA 94142-6800
(510) 524-1000

Electron Microscopy Safety Handbook
V. C. Barber and J. A. Mascorro, editors
1994 • Hardcover • 64 pages • $15.00

Microscopy and Microanalysis 1995
G. W. Bailey, M. H. Ellisman, R. A. Henniger, N. J. Zaluzec, editors
1995 • Hardcover • 1,096 pages • $50.00

Microscopy and Microanalysis 1996
G. W. Bailey, J. M. Corbett, R. Dimlich, J. R. Michael, N. J. Zaluzec, editors
1996 • Hardcover • 1,060 pages • $90.00

W. B. SAUNDERS/HBJ

Order Department
6277 Sea Harbor Drive
Orlando, FL 32887
(800) 545-2522
(800) 433-0001 (Florida)

(Publisher's prices)

Arthritis in Black and White. 2nd ed
Anne C. Brower, MD, and Donald J. Flemming, MC, CDR, MC, USNR
1996 • Hardcover • 448 pages • $83.00

Atlas of Clinical Diagnosis
M. Afzal Mir, DCH, FRCP
1995 • Paper • 276 pages • $45.00

Atlas of CT Pathology
Deborah L. Durham, BS, RT(R)
1996 • Hardcover • 208 pages • $42.00

Atlas of MR Pathology
Deborah L. Durham, BS, RT(R)
1996 • Hardcover • 208 pages • $42.00

Atlas of Neuroradiology
Steven J. Willing, MD
1995 • Hardcover • 400 pages • $145.00

Atlas of Nuclear Medicine
Marc Coel, MD, and Jimmy Leung, MD
1996 • Hardcover • 756 pages • $235.00

Basic Atlas of Sectional Anatomy with Correlated Imaging. 3rd ed
Walter J. Bo, PhD, et al
1998 • Hardcover • 560 pages (approx) • $120.00

Bone and Joint Imaging. 2nd ed
Donald Resnick, MD
1996 • Hardcover • 1,360 pages • $195.00

Clinical Magnetic Resonance Imaging. 2nd ed
Robert E. Edelman, MD, John R. Hesselink, MD, and Michael Zlatkin, MD
1996 • Hardcover • 2,352 pages • $325.00 • (2-vol set)

Computed Tomography: A Study Guide and Review
Euclid Seeram, RT(R), BSc, MSc
1997 • Paper • 220 pages • $37.00

Current Oral and Maxillofacial Imaging
Thomas F. Razmus, BS, DDS, MS, and Gail F. Williamson, RDH, MS
1996 • Hardcover • 320 pages • $37.00

Diagnosis of Bone and Joint Disorders. 3rd ed
Donald Resnick, MD
1994 • Hardcover • 4,496 pages • $699.00
• (6-vol set)
• CD-ROM • $1,500.00 Multi-User
• $725.00 Single-User

Diagnosis of Diseases of the Breast
Lawrence W. Bassett, MD, Valerie Jackson, MD, Richard Gold, MD, and Yao Si Fu, MD
1996 • Hardcover • 624 pages • $152.00

Diagnostic Imaging Review
Gordon Gamsu, MD, and Maitray Patel, MD
1998 • Hardcover • 720 pages (approx) • $89.00

Diagnostic Sonography: Principles and Clinical Applications. 2nd ed
Arthur Fleischer, MD, and Donna Kepple, RDMS
1995 • Hardcover • 800 pages • $184.00

Diagnostic Ultrasound. 5th ed
Frederick Kremkau, PhD
1998 • Hardcover • 640 pages (approx) • $49.95

Encyclopedia of Radiographic Positioning
Steven B. Dowd, EdD, RTCR, and Bettye Wilson, MEd, RTCR, RDMS
1995 • Hardcover • 1,249 pages • $145.00 • (2-vol set)

Essentials of Nuclear Medicine Imaging. 4th ed
Fred A. Mettler, Jr, MD, and Milton J. Guiberteau, MD
1998 • Hardcover • 512 pages (approx) • $69.00 (approx)

Essentials of Radiology
Fred A. Mettler, MD, MPH
1995 • Paper • 464 pages • $39.95

Essentials of Ultrasound
Michael R. Williamson, MD
1995 • Hardcover • 274 pages • $49.95

Fetal Echocardiography
Julia Drose, RT(R), RDMS, RDCS
1998 • Hardcover • 350 pages (approx) • $65.00

Fetal Sonography
Terry J. Dubose, BBS, AS, RDMS, RRT
1995 • Hardcover • 536 pages • $75.00

Fundamentals of Body CT, 2nd ed.
W. Richard Webb, MD, William E. Brant, MD, and Clyde A. Helms, MD
1997 • Paper • 352 pages (approx) • $49.00

Fundamentals of Chest Radiology
Andrew Meholic, MD, and Loren Ketai, MD
1996 • Paper • 256 pages • $39.95

Fundamentals of Emergency Radiology
Philip W. Wiest, MD, and Paul B. Roth, MD
1996 • Paper • 192 pages • $39.95

Fundamentals of Neuroimaging
Blaine L. Hart, MD, Edward C. Benzel, MD, and Corey C. Ford, MD
1996 • Paper • 216 pages • $39.00

Fundamentals of Skeletal Radiology. 2nd ed
Clyde A. Helms, MD
1994 • Paper • 256 pages • $41.00

Imaging of Soft Tissue Tumors
Mark Kransdorf, MD, and Mark D. Murphey, MD
1996 • 448 pages • $152.00

Imaging of the Hand and Wrist
Louis A. Gilula, MD, and Yuming Yin, MD
1995 • Hardcover • 640 pages • $135.00

Imaging Pharmaceuticals and Their Administration
Marianne Tortorici, EdD, RT(R)
1996 • Paper • 176 pages • $26.00

Internal Derangements of Joints: Emphasis on MR Imaging
Donald Resnick, MD, and Heung Sik Kang, MD
1997 • Hardcover • 992 pages (approx) • $235.00

Interventional Neuroradiology
J.J. Connors and Joan C. Wojak
1998 • Hardcover • 800 pages (approx) • $125.00

Introduction to Health Care Delivery and Radiology Administration
Stephen S. Hiss, RT, MS
1997 • Paper • 285 pages • $26.00

Introduction to Ultrasound
William J. Zwiebel, MD, and Roya Sohaey, MD
1997 • Hardcover • 400 pages (approx) • $89.00 (approx) • In preparation

Law and Ethics in Diagnostic Imaging and Therapeutic Radiology: With Risk Management and Safety Applications
Ann M. Obergfell, JD, RT(R)
1995 • Hardcover • 256 pages • $27.00

Manual of Neonatal Emergency X-ray Interpretation
P.W.D. Meerstadt and C. Guyll
1995 • Paper • 304 pages • $33.95

Marcus Cardiac Imaging: A Companion to Braunwald's Heart Disease. 2nd ed
David J. Skorton, MD, Heinrich Schelbert, MD, Gerald Wolf, PhD, MD, and Bruce Brundage, MD
1996 • Hardcover • 1,336 pages • $215.00

Medical Effects of Ionizing Radiation. 2nd ed
Fred A. Mettler, Jr, MD, and Robert D. Moseley, Jr, MD
1995 • Hardcover • 464 pages • $140.00

MRI of the Brain: Normal Anatomy and Normal Variants
Vimal H. Patel, MD, and Lawrence Friedman, MD
1996 • Hardcover • 496 pages • $89.00

Neuroimaging (2 volume set)
William W. Orrison, Jr., MD
1998 • Hardcover • 1,984 pages (approx) • $415.00 (approx)

Neuroradiology. 3rd ed
Ruth G. Ramsey, MD
1994 • Hardcover • 1,044 pages • $175.00

Orthopaedic Radiography
Bruce W. Long, MS, RT(R), and John A. Rafert, MS, RT(R)
1994 • Hardcover • 560 pages • $75.00

Pediatric Imaging
Cecilie Godderidge, BS, FCR, RT
1995 • Hardcover • 288 pages • $49.95

Pediatric Nuclear Imaging
John H. Miller, MD, FACR, and Michael J. Gelfand, MD
1994 • Hardcover • 393 pages • $115.00

Practical Pediatric Radiology. 2nd ed
Saskia von Waldenburg Hilton, MD, and David K. Edwards, MD
1994 • Hardcover • 592 pages • $150.00

Principles and Clinical Applications of MRI Technology
Luann Culbreth, RT(R), Med
1998 • Hardcover • 480 pages (approx) • $65.00 (approx)

Principles of Nuclear Medicine. 2nd ed
Henry N. Wagner, MD, Zsolt Szabo, MD, and Julia W. Buchanan, BS
1995 • Hardcover • 1302 pages • $249.00

Radiographic Critique
Kathy McQuillen-Martensen, RT(R)
1996 • Hardcover • 448 pages • $52.50

Radiographic Pathology
Terri Ann Linn-Watson, MEd, RT, RDMS
1996 • Hardcover • 320 pages • $45.00

Radiology: MGH Clinical Review
Daniel Rosenthal, MD, Felix S. Chew, MD, William E. Palmer, MD, Daniel P. Barboriak, MD, and Andrew E. Rosenberg, MD
1994 • Paper • 464 pages • $58.00

Radiology of the Kidney and Urinary Tract. 3rd ed
Alan J. Davidson, MD and David S. Hartman, MD
1999 • Hardcover • 830 pages • $150.00 (approx)

Registry Review for Computed Tomography
Daniel N. DeMaio, RT(R)
1996 • Paper • 232 pages • $26.00

Review of Neuroradiology
Val M. Runge, MD
1995 • Paper • 224 pages • $45.00

Review of Radiology. 2nd ed
Carl E. Ravin, MD, Cirrelda Cooper, MD, and Richard Leder, MD
1994 • Paper • 480 pages • $57.95

Synopsis of Diseases of the Chest. 2nd ed
Robert G. Fraser, MD, J.A.P. Paré, MD, Richard S. Fraser, MD, and P.D. Paré, MD
1994 • Hardcover • 752 pages • $105.00

Teaching Atlas of Hand Radiology: A Self-Assessment Text
S. Gilani and B. Wignall
1995 • Paper • 216 pages • $29.00

Textbook of Diagnostic Imaging. 2nd ed
Charles E. Putman, MD, and Carl E. Ravin, MD
1994 • Hardcover • 2,368 pages • $310.00 • (2-vol set)

Textbook of Gastrointestinal Radiology
Richard M. Gore, MD, Marc S. Levine, MD, and Igor Laufer, MD
1994 • Hardcover • 2,896 pages • $340.00 • (2-vol set)

Textbook of Interventional Cardiology. 2nd ed
Eric J. Topol, MD
1994 • Hardcover • 1,503 pages • $220.00

Textbook of Radiation Oncology
Steven A. Leibel, MD, and Theodore L. Phillips, MD
1998 • Hardcover • 1,376 pages • $225.00

Ultrasonography: An Introduction to Normal Structure and Function
Reva A. Curry, PhD, RDMS, RT(R), and Betty Bates Tempkin, RDMS, RT(R)
1995 • Hardcover • 496 pages • $71.00

Ultrasonography in Obstetrics and Gynecology. 3rd ed
Peter W. Callen, MD
1994 • Hardcover • 736 pages • $89.95

Ultrasound in Emergency Medicine
Michael Heller and Dietrich Jehle
1995 • Hardcover • 256 pages • $58.00

Ultrasound Pathology: A Comparative Approach
Felicia Jones, RDMS, RVT
1998 • Hardcover • 600 pages (approx) • $60.00 (approx)

Ultrasound Scanning: Principles and Protocols. 2nd ed
Betty Bates Tempkin, RT(R), RDMS
1998 • Hardcover • 510 pages (approx) • $55.00 (approx)

SOCIETY OF NUCLEAR MEDICINE

Book Order Department
Matthews Medical Book Company
11559 Rock Island Court
Maryland Heights, MO 63043
Tel: (800)633-2665 or (314)432-1401
Fax: (800)421-8816 or (314)432-7044

Diagnostic Patterns in Nuclear Medicine
Edward B. Silberstein, MD
1998 • Paper • 250 pages • $45.00 (Introductory Price)

Internet Guide for Allied Health Professionals
Jerry V. Glowniak, MD
1997 • Paper • 94 pages • $20 (members) • $28 (nonmembers)

MIRD Cellular S Values
SNM MIRD Committee
1997 • Hardcover • 183 pages • $45 (members) • $63 (nonmembers)

The Nuclear Medicine Handbook for Achieving Compliance with NRC Regulations
Jeffrey S. Mason, Katherine M. Elliott, and Alisha Mitro
1997 • Paper • 120 pages • $25 (members) • $35 (nonmembers)

Nuclear Medicine: Self-Study Program III: Cardiology, Topic Booklet 1 Physical and Technical Aspects of Nuclear Cardiology
Elias H. Botvinick, MD
1997 • Paper • 95 pages • $25

Nuclear Medicine: Self-Study Program III: Cardiology, Topic Booklet 2 Pharmacological Stress Scintigraphy and Associated Topics
Elias H. Botvinick, MD
1998 • Paper • 195 pages • $35.00 (Introductory price)

Nuclear Medicine: Self-Study Program II: Instrumentation.
Barry A. Siegel, MD, Peter T. Kirchner, MD, and L. Stephen Graham, PhD, editors
1996 • Paper • 90 pages • $45 (members) • $63 (nonmembers) • $40 (residents/technologists)

Nuclear Medicine: Self-Study Program IV: Oncology, Topic Booklet 1 Overview of Nuclear Medicine Oncology
E. Edmund Kim, MD, and Thomas P. Haynie, MD, editor
1997 • Paper • 50 pages • $15.00

Nuclear Medicine: Self-Study Program IV: Oncology, Topic Booklet 2 Conventional Tumor Imaging
Patrice K. Rehm, MD and Thomas P. Haynie, MD, editor
1997 • Paper • 50 pages • $20.00

Preparation for Examinations in Nuclear Medicine Technology
Ann M. Steves, CNMT
1997 • Paper • 106 pages • $18 (members) • $25.00 (nonmembers)

Radionuclides in Nephrourology
Andrew Taylor, MD, Joseph V. Nally, MD, and Henrik S. Thomsen, MD
1997 • Paper • 222 pages • $50 (members) • $57 (nonmembers)

Review of Nuclear Medicine Technology. 2nd ed
Ann M. Steves, MS, CNMT
1996 • Paper • 141 pages • $30 (members) • $42 (nonmembers)

SPECT: A Primer. 3rd ed
Robert J. English, CNMT
1995 • Paper • 223 pages • $30 (members) • $42 (nonmembers)

Nuclear Medicine Patient Pamphlets:
—The Benefits of Nuclear Medicine
—Cardiac Nuclear Imaging: Stress-Rest Test
—Nuclear Medicine Breast Imaging
—Nuclear Medicine Prostate Cancer Imaging
—Nuclear Medicine Imaging for Ovarian and Colorectal Cancer
—Nuclear Medicine Liver and Hepatobiliary Imaging
—Nuclear Medicine Bone Imaging
—Nuclear Medicine Renal Imaging in Children
—Nuclear Medicine Brain Imaging
—Guidelines for Patients Receiving Radioiodine Treatment
—Precauciones para pacientes que reciben tratamineto con radioyodo
(Spanish version of the above- mentioned pamplet)
.40¢ copy/ minimum order 50

SPRINGER-VERLAG NEW YORK, INC.

175 Fifth Avenue
New York, NY 10010
(800) SPRINGER (US and Canada)
(212) 460-1500

Modern Imaging of the Alimentary Tube
Alexander R. Margulis
1997 • Hardcover • 300 pages • $159.00

Atlas of Bone Scintigraphy in the Pathological Paediatric Skeleton
I. Gordon, S. Fischer, and K. Hahn
1996 • Hardcover • 343 pages • $150.00

Biliary Tract Radiology
P. Rossi and M. Bezzi
1997 • Hardcover • 427 pages • $236.00

Blood Perfusion and Microenvironment of Human Tumors: Implications for Clinical Radiooncology
M. Molls and P. Vaupel
1997 • Hardcover • 238 pages • $116.00

Carcinoma of the Bladder: Innovations in Management
Zbigniew Petrovich, Luc Baert, and Luther W. Brady
1997 • 350 pages • $161.00 (tentative)

Carcinoma of the Prostate: Innovations in Management
Zbigniew Petrovich, Luv Baert, and Luther W. Brady
1998 • Hardcover • 326 pages • $160.00

Childhood Tuberculosis: Modern Imaging and Clinical Concepts
Bryan J. Cremin and Douglas H. Jamieson
1996 • Hardcover • 122 pages • $108.00

Combined Scintigraphic and Radiographic Diagnosis of Bone and Joint Diseases
Y. W. Bahk
1995 • Hardcover • 241 pages • $206.00

Contrast-Enhanced MRI of the Breast
Sylvia Heywang-Köbrunner and Ranier Beck
1996 • Hardcover • 229 pages • $115.00

The Cranial Nerves. 2nd ed
André Leblanc
1995 • Hardcover • 300 pages • $289.00

Diagnosis and Therapy of Spinal Tumors
Paul R. Algra, J. Valk, and J.J. Heimans
1998 • Hardcover • 300 pages • $169.00

Doppler Ultrasound in Obstetrics and Gynecology
Dev Maulik
1997 • Hardcover • 624 pages • $159.00

Dynamic Radiology of the Abdomen. 4th ed
Morton A. Meyers
1994 • Hardcover • 593 pages • $169.00

Essentials of Ultrasonography: A Practical Guide
D. Pickuth
1995 • Hardcover • 323 pages • $81.95

Gamut Index of Skeletal Dysplasias
Peter Beighton and Kaz Kozlowski
1995 • Paper • 300 pages • $53.95

Gamuts in Radiology on CD-ROM
Maurice M. Reeder and William G. Bradley, Jr
1997 • CD-ROM for Windows and Macintosh • $185.00

Handbook of Transcranial Doppler
John P. McCartney, Kathleen M. Thomas-Lukes, and Camilo R. Gomez
1997 • Paper • 92 pages • $39.95

The Human Brain and Spinal Cord. 2nd ed
Lennart Heimer
1995 • Paper • 506 pages • $59.95

The Human Brain Stem and Cerebellum
Henri M. Duvernoy
1995 • Hardcover • 430 pages • $235.00

Imaging of Soft Tissue Tumors
A. M. Deschepper, P. M. Parizel, F. Ramon, L. Debeuckleer, and J. E. Vandevenne
1997 • Hardcover • 390 pages • $198.00

Interventional Magnetic Resonance Imaging
J.F. Debatin and Gerhard Ada
1998 • Hardcover • 319 pages • $165.00

Late Sequelae in Oncology
J. Dunst and R. Sauer
1995 • Hardcover • 311 pages • $145.00

Lower Genitourinary Radiology
Syed Zafar Hasan Jafri, Marco A. Amendola, and Ananias C. Diokno
1998 • Hardcover • 578 pages • $195.00

Magnetic Resonance Angiography
Ingolf P. Arlart, Georg M. Bongartz, and Guy Marchal
1996 • Hardcover • 350 pages • $239.00

Pelvic MRI
Andreas Heuck and Maximilian Reiser
1998 • 368 pages • $198.00

Magnetic Resonance Imaging: Theory and Practice
M. T. Vlaardingerbroek and J. A. D. Boer
1996 • Hardcover • 384 pages • $98.50

Magnetic Resonance of Myelin, Myelination and Myelin Disorders. 2nd ed
M.S. van der Knaap and J. Valk
1995 • Hardcover • 558 pages • $298.00

Mediastinal Tumors
D. E. Wood, C. R. Thomas, Jr.
1995 • Hardcover • 131 pages • $98.00

MR Cholangiopancreatography: Techniques, Results, and Clinical Indications
P. Pavone and R. Passariello, A. Laghi, and C. Catalano
1997 • Hardcover • 150 pages • $115.00

MRI: A Conceptual Overview
S. S. Rajan
1998 • Paper • 167 pages • $34.95

MRI for Radiographers
Philip English, and C. Moore
1995 • Paper • 187 pages • $107.00

MRI Physics for Radiologists A Visual Approach. 3rd ed
Alfred L. Horowitz
1995 • Paper • 187 pages • $38.00

MRI Study Guide for Technologists
Kenneth S. Meacham
1995 • Paper • 184 pages • $32.95

Muscle Imaging in Health and Disease
James Fleckenstein, John V. Crues III, and Carl D. Reimers
1996 • Hardcover • 461 pages • $155.00

Neuroimaging: Clinical and Physical Principles
R. A. Zimmerman, W. A. Gibby, and R. F. Carmody
1998 • Hardcover • 1488 pages (approx) • $195.00 (tentative)

Pediatric Nuclear Medicine. 2nd ed
S. T. Treves
1995 • Hardcover • 598 pages • $139.00

Pediatric Radiology. 2nd ed
Jack O. Haller and Thomas L. Slovis
1995 • Hardcover • 217 pages • $82.00

Pediatric Skeletal Scintigraphy
L. P. Connolly and S. T. Treves
1998 • Hardcover • 286 pages • $135.00

Phlebography and Sonography of the Veins
W. Hach and Viola Hach-Wunderle
1997 • Hardcover • 300 pages • $225.00

Radiation Therapy in Pediatric Oncology
J. Robert Cassady
1994 • Hardcover • 398 pages • $115.00

Radiation Therapy of Benign Diseases A Clinical Guide. 2nd ed
Stanley E. Order and Sarah S. Donaldson
1998 • 250 pages • $129.00

Radiation Oncology of Gynecological Cancers
H.W. Vahrson
1998 • 485 pages • $265.00

Radiological Diagnosis of Breast Diseases
M. Friedrich and Edward Sickles
1997 • Hardcover • 387 pages • $236.00

Radiological Imaging of Sports Injuries
Carlo Masciocchi
1998 • 295 pages • $139.00

Radiology of Female Pelvic Organs
Erich K. Lang
1998 • Hardcover • 250 pages • $180.00 (tentative)

Radiology of Trauma
M. Heller and A. Fink
1997 • Hardcover • 406 pages • $236.00

Spiral CT of the Chest
M. Rémy-Jardin and J. Rémy
1997 • Hardcover • 341 pages • $198.00

Thermoradiotherapy and Thermochemotherapy: Volumes I & II
Seegenschmidt, Fessenden, and Vernon
1995 • Hardcover • Vol I: 495 pages • Vol II: 420 pages • Vol I: $210.00 • Vol II: $189.00

Ultrasound Diagnosis of Digestive Diseases. 4th ed
Francis S. Weil, M. Lafortune, G. Schmutz, P.J. Valette, and Y. Menu
1996 • Hardcover • 743 pages • $198.00

Diagnostic of Vascular Disease
P. Lanzer and M. Lipton
1997 • Hardcover • 362 pages • $159.00

Vascular Disease in Neonates, Infants, and Children: Interventional Neuroradiology Management
P. Lasjuanias
1997 • Hardcover • 707 pages • $239.00

THIEME
333 Seventh Avenue
New York, NY 10001
(800) 782-3488
212-760-0888
Fax: 212-947-1112
e-mail: custserv@thieme.com
www.thieme.com

Acute Abdomen
G. P. Krestin and P. L. Choyke
1996 • Paper • 304 pages • $59.00

Atlas of Brain Function
William W. Orrison, Jr.
1995 • Paper • 184 pages • $49.00

Atlas of Musculoskeletal Imaging
Thomas L. Pope, Jr., and Steven Loehr
1999 • Hardcover • 448 (tentative) pages • $69.00 (tentative)

The Augmented Breast: Radiologic and Clinical Perspectives
David P. Gorozyca and R. James Brenner
1997 • Hardcover • 240 pages • $95.00

Bone and Joint Disorders: Conventional Radiologic Differential Diagnosis
F. A. Burgener and M. Kormano
1997 • Hardcover • 336 pages • $79.00

Breast Ultrasound
C. Sohn, J. Blohmer, and U. M. Hamper
1999 • Hardcover • 184 (tentative) pages • $59.00 (tentative)

CD•ROM Atlas of Neurofunctional Systems
H. J. Kretschmann and W. Weinrich
1999 • CD•ROM • $98.00 (tentative)

Clinical Radiology and Endoscopy of the Colon
J. Reeders and G. Rosenbusch
1994 • Hardcover • 598 pages • $199.00

Color Duplex Sonography
K. J. Wolf and F. Fobbe
1995 • Hardcover • 320 pages • $159.00

Diagnosis of Genitourinary Disease
M. I. Resnick and R. Older
1997 • Hardcover • 688 pages • $149.00

Diagnostic Breast Imaging
Sylvia H. Heywang•Koebrunner, Ingrid Schreer, and D. David Dershaw
1997 • Hardcover • 428 pages • $99.00

Differential Diagnosis in Computed Tomography
F. A. Burgener and M. Kormano
1996 • Hardcover • 528 pages • $165.00

Differential Diagnosis in Chest X•Rays
F. Burgener and M. Kormano
1997 • Hardcover • 192 pages • $69.00

Differential Diagnosis in Conventional Gastrointestinal Radiology
F. Burgener and M. Kormano
1997 • Hardcover • 240 pages • $79.00

Differential Diagnosis in Head and Neck Imaging
T. Vogl
1999 • Hardcover • 400 pages • $139.00 (tentative)

The Electronic Clinical Brain Atlas
Wieslaw L. Nowinski, R. Nick Bryan, and Raghu Raghavan
1998 • CD•ROM • Manual 50 (tentative) pages • $349.00

Differential Diagnosis in Pediatric Radiology
Klaus•Dietrich Ebel, Eberhard Willich, Ernst Richter, and Johan G. Blickmann
199g • Hardcover • 824 pages • $179.00 (tentative)

Essential Radiology: Clinical Presentation Pathophysiology Imaging
Richard B. Gunderman
1998 • Paper • 592 pages • $45.00

Essentials of Pediatric Radiology
Edward M. Burton and Alan S. Brody
1999 • Hardcover • 480 (tentative) pages • $89.00 (tentative)

The Female Infertility Ultrasound Scan
T. Bourne and F. Degenhardt
1997•CD•ROM•$89.00

Hepatobiliary and Pancreatic Radiology
G. Scott Gazelle, Sanjay Saini, and Peter R. Mueller
1998•Hardcover•912 pages•$169.00

Imaging of the Globe and Orbit
Norbert Hosten and Norbert Bornfeld
1998•Hardcover•208 pages•$79.00

Imaging of the Head and Neck
G. E. Valvassori, B. L. Carter, and F. Mafee
1995•Hardcover•548 pages•$209.00

Imaging of the Temporal Bone, 3rd edition
Joel D. Swartz and H. Ric Harnsberger
1998•Hardcover•512 pages•$129.00

Intramedullary Spinal Cord Tumors
G. Fischer and J. Brotchi
1996•Hardcover•128 pages•$119.00

Manual of GI Fluoroscopy
B. R. Javors
1996•Paper•224 pages•$31.00

Manual of Nuclear Medicine Imaging
Christopher C. Kuni and René P. du Cret
1997•Paper•336 pages•$35.00

Minimally Invasive Therapy of the Brain
Antonio DeSalles and Robert Lufkin
1997•Hardcover•292 pages•$189.00

Minimally Invasive Therapy of the Liver and Biliary System
J. G. McNulty
1994•Hardcover•219 pages•$115.00

Nuclear Medicine (CD•ROM)
Rodney Hicks
1997 • CD•ROM • $298.00

Nuclear Medicine
J. C. Harbert, W. C. Eckelman, and R. D. Neumann
1996•Hardcover•1272 pages•$199.00

Nuclear Medicine Board Review
Richard Goldfarb, Lionel Zuckier, Steven Parmett, and Jeffrey Cooper
1998•Paper•160 pages•$19.95

Ophthalmic Ultrasound
Cathy W. DiBernardo, Andrew P. Schachat, and Sharon Fekrat
1998•Hardcover•160 pages•$69.00

Pediatric Radiology Casebase
Joanna J. Seibert and Charles A. James
1998 • Paper • 560 pages • $59.00

Pediatric Radiology: Casebase on CD•ROM
Joanna J. Seibert and Charles A. James
1999•CD•ROM•$149.00

Peripheral Musculoskeletal Ultrasound Atlas
R. F. Dondelinger, S. Marcelis, B. Daenen, and M. A. Ferrara
1996•Hardcover•213 pages•$115.00

Pocket Atlas of Cross•Sectional Anatomy, Vol. 1: Head, Neck, Spine and Joints (new edition)
Torsten B. Moeller and Emil Reif
1999•Paper•255 pages•$28.50 (tentative)

Pocket Atlas of Cross•Sectional Anatomy, Vol. 2: Thorax, Abdomen, and Pelvis
Torsten B. Moeller and Emil Reif
1994•Paper•254 pages•$28.50

Pocket Atlas of Radiographic Positioning
Torsten B. Moeller and Emil Reif
1997•Paper•296 pages•$19.90

Principles of Genitourinary Radiology
Z. L. Barbaric
1994•Hardcover•520 pages•$99.00

Radiology of Chest Diseases
Sebastian Lange and Geraldine Walsh
1998•Hardcover•392 pages•$79.00

Teaching Atlas of Breast Ultrasound
Dagmar Leucht and Helmut Madjar
1996•Hardcover•264 pages•$99.00

Teaching Atlas of Interventional Radiology
Saadoon Kadir
1999•Hardcover•524 (tentative) pages•$89.00 (tentative)

Teaching Atlas of Spine Imaging
Ruth G. Ramsey
1999•Hardcover•800 (tentative) pages• $125.00 (tentative)

Teaching Atlas of Urologic Radiology
Sebastian Lange
1995•Hardcover•312 pages•$99.00

Ultrasound Teaching Manual
Matthias Hofer
1999 • Paper • 64 (tentative) pages • $19.95 (tentative)

Vascular Diagnosis with Ultrasound
Michael Hennerici and Doris Neuerburg•Heusler
1998•Hardcover•520 pages•$149.00

Vascular Intervention: A Clinical Approach
Bruce A. Perler and Gary J. Becker
1998•Hardcover•768 pages•$129.00

Vasculature of the Brain and Cranial Base
Walter Grand and L. N. Hopkins
1999•Hardcover•248 (tentative) pages• $149.00 (tentative)

Venous Interventional Radiology: With Clinical Perspectives
Scott J. Savader and Scott O. Trerotola
1996•Hardcover•511 pages•$125.00

CHARLES C THOMAS, PUBLISHER

2600 S. First Street
Springfield, IL 62794-9265
(217) 789-8980
(800) 258-8980
Telefax (217) 789-9130

Fuchs's Radiographic Exposure, Processing and Quality Control. 6th ed
Quinn B. Carroll
1998•Hardcover•588 pages•$49.95

The Fundamentals of X-ray and Radium Physics. 8th ed
Joseph Selman
1994• Hardcover• 656 pages• $49.95

Manual of Gastrointestinal Fluoroscopy: Performance of Procedures
David J. Ott, David W. Gelfand, and Michael Y.M. Chen
1996 • Hardcover • 194 pages • $52.95

X-Ray Repair
Joseph P. Panichello
1998•Hardcover•310 pages•$59.95

WICK PUBLISHING, INC.

4720 East Oxford Avenue
Englewood, CO 80110
(303) 782-5208

Nuclear Medicine Procedure Manual–1997–98
Wm. C. Klingensmith III, MD, Dennis Eshima, PhD, and John Goddard, PhD, editors
1997–98 • Binder/Software disk • 500 pages • $225.00/$195.00

JOHN WILEY & SONS, INC.

605 Third Avenue
New York, NY 10158-0012
In the U.S., call toll-free 1-800-879-4539; Fax 732-302-2300.
In Canada call toll-free 1-800-567-4797; Fax 416-236-8743.
In Mexico, Central, and South America call 732-469-4400; Fax 732-302-2300.
Outside North, South, Central America call +44-1243-843294; Fax +44-1243-770460.

Prices subject to change. Prices may be higher outside the U.S.

Atlas of Human Cross-Sectional Anatomy: With CT and MR Images. 3rd ed
Donald R. Cahill, Matthew J. Orlando, and Gary M. Miller
1995 • Hardcover • 328 pages • $199.95

Basic Ultrasound
Hylton B. Meire and Pat Farrant
1995•Paper•234 pages•$59.90

Biomedical Imaging: Visualization, and Analysis
Richard A. Robb
June 1999 • Hardcover • 288 pages (approx) • $89.00 (tentative)

Clinical Applications of MR Spectroscopy
Suresh K. Mukherji, editor
1998 • Hardcover • 336 pages • $95.00

Clinical MR Spectroscopy: First Principles
Nouha Salibi and Mark A. Brown
1997 • Paperback • 236 pages • $39.95

Clinical Radiation Oncology: Indications, Techniques and Results. 2nd ed.
C. C. Wang, editor
March 1999 • Hardcover • 480 pages (approx) • $129.00 (tentative)

Cybersurgery: Advanced Technologies for Surgical Practice
Richard M. Satava and Jonathan M. Sackier, editors
1997 • Hardcover • 218 pages • $69.95

Guidelines and Gamuts in Musculoskeletal Ultrasound
Rethy Chhem and Etienne Cardinal
November 1998 • Hardcover • 300 pages (approx) • $100.00 (tentative)

Hepatobiliary and Pancreatic Surgery: Imaging Strategies and Surgical Decision-Making
Stephen R. T. Evans and Susan M. Ascher, Editors
October 1997 • Hardcover • 589 pages • $129.95

Imaging Handbook for House Officers
Paul M. Silverman and Douglas J. Quint, editors
1996 • Paperback • 455 pages • $38.00

Magnetic Resonance Imaging: Mathematical Foundations and Applications
Walter Schempp
September 1998 • Hardcover • 324 pages (approx) • $125.00 (tentative)

MRI: Basic Principles and Applications
Mark A. Brown and Richard C. Semelka
1995 • Paper • 158 pages • $34.95

MRI of the Abdomen and Pelvis: A Text-Atlas
Richard C. Semelka Susan M. Ascher, and Caroline Reinhold
1997 • Hardcover • 744 pages • $195.00

PACS: Basic Principles and Applications
H. K. Huang
November 1998 • Paperback • 416 pages (approx) • $49.95 (tentative)

PACS: Picture Archiving and Communication Systems in Biomedical Imaging
H. K. Huang
1996 • Hardcover • 489 pages • $160.00

Physics and Instrumentation of Diagnostic Medical Ultrasound, 2nd ed.
Peter Fish, editor
Septemer 1999 • Paper • 200 pages (approx.) • $44.95 (tentative)

Radiation Therapy for Head and Neck Neoplasms, 3rd ed
C. C. Wang
1996 • Hardcover • 400 pages • $109.95

Three-Dimensional Biomedical Imaging: Principles and Practice
Richard A. Robb
1995 • Hardcover • 320 pages • $165.00
November 1997 • Paperback • 320 pages • $69.95

Ultrasound in Surgical Practice: Basic Principles and Clinical Applications
Jay K. Harness, editor
March 1999 • Paperback • 225 pages (approx) • $34.95 (tentative)

Ultrasound of the Prostate, 2nd ed
Bruno D. Fornage and Soren Torp-Pedersen, editors
June 1999 • Hardcover • 350 pages
• $115.00 pre-publication (tentative)
• $145.00 after publication (tentative)

WILLIAMS & WILKINS

351 W. Camden St.
Baltimore, MD 21201-2436
(410) 528-4000
(800) 638-0672
Telefax (800) 447-8438

Atlas of Radiologic Anatomy. 5th ed
Lothar Wicke, MD and Anna N. Taylor, PhD
1997 • Hardcover • 304 pages • $42.95

Atlas of Vascular Anatomy: An Angiographic Approach
Renan Uflacker, MD
1996 • Hardcover • 500 pages • $199.00

Aunt Minnie's Atlas of Imaging-Specific Diagnosis
Kenneth L. Ford, MD, and Thomas L. Pope, Jr, MD
1997 • Hardcover • 320 pages • $85.00

Basic Principles of Radiographic Exposure
Dianne DeVos, RRT
1995 • Paper • 165 pages • $29.00

Breast Imaging: A Teaching File
Gilda Cardenosa, MD
1999 • Hardcover • 425 pages • $89.00

Cardiac Catheterization, Angiography and Intervention. 5th ed
Donald S. Baim, MD, and William Grossman, MD
1996 • Hardcover • 698 pages • $90.00

Comprehensive Review for the Radiology Registry
Mark F. Pierce, RT, (R)(CT)
1998 • Paper • 250 pages • $29.95

CD Roentgen: Interactive Radiology Teaching File
Michael P. McDermott, MD, and Thorsten L. Krebs, MD
1997 • CD-ROM • $175.00

Clinical Cases in Neuroradiology
James M. Provenzale, MD, and Juan M. Taveras, MD
1994 • Hardcover • 319 pages • $89.00

CT and MRI of the Abdomen and Pelvis: A Teaching File
Pablo R. Ros, MD, and Sylvester Lee, ME
1997 • Hardcover • 384 pages • $89.00

Dahnert's Electronic Radiology Review
John Eng, MD, and Eric Tamm, MD
1997 • Mac Disk, Windows Disk, and CD-ROM • $89.00

Diagnostic Nuclear Medicine. 3rd ed
Martin P. Sandler, MD, Alex Gottschalk, MD, Edward Coleman, MD, and Paul Holfe, MD
1996 • Hardcover • 1,600 pages • $279.00

Differential Diagnosis in Pediatric Radiology. 2nd ed
Leonard E. Swischuk, MD
1995 • Casebound • 480 pages • $99.00

Emergency Imaging of the Acutely Ill or Injured Child. 3rd ed
Leonard E. Swischuk, MD
1994 • Casebound • 768 pages • $129.00

The Essential Physics of Medical Imaging
Jerrold T. Bushberg, PhD, J. Anthony Seibert, PhD, Edwin M. Liedholdt, Jr, PhD, and John M. Boone, PhD
1994 • Casebound • 752 pages • $79.00

Essentials of Skeletal Radiology. 2nd ed
Terry R. Yochum, BS, DC, and Lindsay J. Rowe, BappSc (Chiro)
1996 • Hardcover • 1,800 pages • $225.00 • (2-vol set)

Fundamentals of Diagnostic Radiology. 2nd ed
William E. Brant, MD, and Clyde A. Helms, MD
1998 • Hardcover • 1,600 pages • $149.00

The Handbook of Health Physics and Radiological Health. 3rd ed
Bernard Shleien, PharmD, Lester A. Slaback, Jr, and Brian Birky
1997 • Hardcover • 700 pages • $115.00

High Resolution Atlas of Cranial Neuroanatomy
Charles L. Truwit, MD
1994 • Casebound • 624 pages • $169.00

Hysterosalpingography. 2nd ed
David J. Ott, MD, Jamil A. Fayez, MD, and Ronald J. Zagoria, MD
1998 • Hardcover • 160 pages • $89.00

Imaging in Ob/Gyn: A Teaching File
Patricia L. Abbitt, MD
1997 • Hardcover • 394 pages • $89.00

Imaging of the Newborn, Infant, and Young Child
Leonard E. Swischuk, MD
1997 • Hardcover • 1,304 pages • $175.00

Imaging of the Spine: A Teaching File
Mauricio Castillo, MD, and John H. Harris, Jr., MD, DSc
1998 • Hardcover • 400 pages • $89.00

Interventional Radiology Advisor CD-ROM
Steven V. Lossef, MD
1998•CD-ROM•$99.00

Interventional Radiology. 3rd ed
Wilfrido R. Castaneda-Zuniga, MD, MSc, and S. Murthy Tadavarthy, MD
1996• Hardcover• 1,956 pages (2 vol set) • $275.00

Introduction to Computed Tomography
Lois R. Romans, RT(R)
1996 • Paper • 228 pages • $27.00

Introductory Physics of Nuclear Medicine. 5th ed
Ramesh Chandra, PhD
1997• Paper• 256 pages• $39.00

Levitt and Tapley's Technological Basis of Radiation Therapy. 3rd ed
Seymour H. Levitt, MD, Roger A. Potish, MD, and Faiz M. Khan, MD
1998 • Hardcover • 420 pages • $89.00

MRI: The Basics
Ray H. Hashemi, MD, and William G. Brodley, MD
1996 • Paper • 336 pages • $45.00

MRI and CT of the Head and Spine. 2nd ed
C. Barrie Grossman, MD
1996 • Hardcover • 704 pages • $139.00

MRI and CT of the Spine
Krishna C.V.G. Rao, MD, John P. Williams, MD, Benjamin C.P. Lee, MD, and John L. Sherman
1994 • Casebound • 560 pages • $145.00

Neuroradiology. 3rd ed
Juan Taveras, MD
1996 • Hardcover • 1,216 pages • $189.00

Nuclear Medicine: A Teaching File
Reza Habibian, MD
1998 • Hardcover • 576 pages • $95.00

The Physics of Radiation Therapy. 2nd ed
Faiz M. Khan, PhD
1994 • Casebound • 576 pages • $95.00

Practical Neuroangiography
P. Pearce Morris, MD
1997• Hardcover• 400 pages• $109.00

Primer of Sectional Anatomy with MRI and CT Correlation. 2nd ed
Charles P. Barrett, PhD, Steven J. Poliakoff, MD, Lawrence E. Holder, MD, and Lawrence Anderson, MD
1994• Paper• 160 pages• $27.00

Principles and Practice of Echocardi-ography. 2nd ed
Arthur E. Weyman, MD
1994• Hardcover• 1,335 pages• $195.00

A Radiologic Approach to Diseases of the Chest. 2nd ed
Irwin M. Freundlich, MD, and David G. Bragg, MD
1996• Hardcover• 896 pages• $139.00

Radiologic Interventions: Embolotherapy
Douglas M. Coldwell, PhD, MD
1997•Hardcover•256 pages•$59.00

Radiologic Interventions: Non-Cardiac Thoracic Interventions
Alan Matsumoto, MD
1997 • Hardcover • 384 pages $89.00

Radiologic Interventions: Uroradiology
Marc P. Banner, MD, FACR
1997•Hardcover•232 pages•$69.00

The Radiology of Acute Cervical Spine Trauma. 3rd ed
John H. Harris, Jr, MD, and Stuart E. Mirvis, MD
1996 • Hardcover • 560 pages • $95.00

Radiology Review Manual. 3rd ed
Wolfgang Dahnert, MD
1996• Paper• 879 pages• $89.00

Radiotherapy for Head and Neck Cancers: Indications and Techniques
K. Kian Ang, MD, PhD, Johannes H.A.M. Kaanders, MD, and Lester J. Peters, MD
1994 • Hardcover • 141 pages • $85.00

Review of Radiological Physics
Walter Huda, PhD, and Richard M. Sloan, MD
1995 • Paper • 278 pages • $31.00

Review Questions and Explanations in Computed Tomography
Lois R. Romans, RT(R)
1996 • Paper • 300 pages • $24.95

Skeletal Radiology: The Bare Bones. 2nd ed
Felix S. Chew, MD
1996 • Hardcover • 336 pages • $89.00

Skeletal Radiology Interactive: The Bare Bones CD-ROM
Felix S. Chew, MD
1997• Hybrid CD-ROM (both Mac and PC compatible) • $149.00 (approx)

Stedman's Radiology and Oncology Words. 2nd ed
1995 • Paper • 689 pages • $34.95

Textbook of Uroradiology. 2nd ed
N. Reed Dunnick, MD, Carl M. Sandler, MD, Jeffrey H. Newhouse, MD, and E. Stephen Amis, Jr, MD
1996• Hardcover• 650 pages• $125.00

Treatment Planning in Radiation Oncology
Faiz M. Khan, PhD, and Roger A. Potish, MD
1997 • Hardcover • 608 pages • $80.00

Understanding Helical Scanning
Cheryl Blanck
1998•Paper•120 pages•$24.95

Workbook for Quality Mammography. 2nd ed
Carolyn Kimme-Smith, PhD, Lawrence W. Bassett, MD, and Richard H. Gold, MD
1996• Paper• 238 pages• $42.95

Classified Services

POLICY

As a service to its readers, *Radiology* accepts classified advertising, and every effort is made to ensure that the ads are relevant to the practice of radiology. Acceptable categories include positions available, positions sought, fellowships, announcements of postgraduate courses or symposia, practices for sale, medical facilities for rent or sale, used radiologic equipment and apparatus for sale, medical employment bureau advertising, academic posts to be filled, available posts for interns and residents, and malpractice insurance. We retain the right to refuse any advertisement considered not relevant, and respondents are advised to investigate each offer since we cannot assume responsibility for the offers or claims of advertisers.

RATES (per month, per insertion)

Line ads in *Radiology* (no agency commission)

50 words or less $90.00

51–100 words $135.00

Each word over 100—$1.00 per word.

Box Number—$30.00 additional per each insertion (this service is optional).

TERMS

Payment must accompany order.* Make checks payable to **Radiological Society of North America.** We accept American Express, VISA, Mastercard, and Diners Club for classified ads. Call for details. Send payment to:

RSNA, Radiology Classified Ad Department
Accounts Payable, 2021 Spring Road, Suite 600
Oak Brook, IL 60523-1860 USA.

*Purchase Order Numbers are accepted with prior approval.

Please mark each issue:

❒ Jan ❒ Feb ❒ Mar ❒ Apr ❒ May ❒ June
❒ July ❒ Aug ❒ Sept ❒ Oct ❒ Nov ❒ Dec

Send invoice and tearsheet to:

____

____

____

____

Advertisers who cancel ads will not receive refunds.

DEADLINE

Copy must be received by the **20th of the second month preceding issue.** Please submit copy typed and double-spaced. Initials or abbreviations equal one word. Telephone numbers with area code equal one word.

CLASSIFIED DISPLAY ADVERTISING

Black and white frequency rates are based on the total number of insertions used within a 12-month period from date of first insertion.

Ad Space	Size	1X	6X	12X
1 page	7" x 9-1/2"	$2250	2170	2090
2/3 pg vert	4-1/2" x 9-1/2"	$1900	1830	1760
1/2 pg horzt	7" x 4-1/2"	$1350	1300	1250
1/2 pg vert	3-3/8" x 9-1/2"	$1350	1300	1250
1/2 pg island	4-1/4" x 7-1/2"	$1350	1300	1250
1/3 pg vert	2-1/4" x 9-1/2"	$1085	1045	1005
1/3 pg square	4-1/2" x 4-1/2"	$1085	1045	1005
1/4 page	3-3/8" x 4-1/2"	$ 850	820	790
1/6 page	2-1/4" x 4-1/2"	$ 605	585	565
1/9 page	2-1/4" x 3"	$ 420	400	380

Preferred materials are composite negatives, right-reading, emulsion side down. (Conversion materials such as positive film, repro proofs, and camera-ready artworks are acceptable at additional charge.)

Customer supplied negative: cost as noted
Customer supplied mechanical: add 10%
Customer supplied copy to be set and ad prepared: add 20%

Call Production Department for additional information. Address for correspondence, insertion orders, copy, proofs, box number, and payment:

***Radiology* Advertising Production Office**
2021 Spring Road, Suite 600
Oak Brook, IL 60523-1860

To respond to a box number ad, send your CV and/or any other information to the above address; on the front of the envelope, please indicate the appropriate box number.

For further information:
Carissa Mucccianti, *Advertising Coordinator*
630.571.7817
630.571.7837 (fax)

Positions Available

ENDOWED PROFESSORSHIP OF RADIOLOGY AND BIOMEDICAL ENGINEERING - COLUMBIA UNIVERSITY—The Departments of Radiology and Biomedical Engineering at Columbia University in the city of New York are searching for a Professor to serve as Scientific and Academic Director of our Magnetic Resonance Research and Teaching Programs. The appointment of this endowed professorship will be in the Departments of Radiology and Biomedical Engineering. Academic responsibilities include teaching and advising undergraduate and graduate students in the biomedical imaging track in the newly announced Department of Biomedical Engineering. The Director also will be expected to participate in and organize a multidisciplinary research effort in close collaboration with colleagues in both the medical and engineering faculties. The position is supported by office and laboratory space in the Hatch Magnetic Resonance Center at the health sciences campus and by additional space in the School of Engineering on the Morningside campus. These two sites are three miles apart and are linked by ATM. The goals are to develop an outstanding medical research program, an outstanding teaching program in biomedical engineering and to gain extramural support to lead these efforts and associated faculty. A variety of equipment is available at the Hatch Center including a 4.2 Telsa 105cm bore MR system for human and basic research studies as well as access to three state-of-the-art clinical 1.5T MRI systems for correlative studies. The staff currently consists of four PhDs, support personnel, and an administrative director. Candidates must have a PhD and/or MD or equivalent. Salary will be commensurate with experience and qualifications. Please send resume to Philip O. Alderson, MD, Professor and Chairman, Department of Radiology, College of Physicians and Surgeons of Columbia University, 177 Fort Washington Ave, MHB 2-131, New York, NY 10032. Columbia University is an affirmative action/equal opportunity employer. Women and minorities are encouraged to apply. Application deadline is November 30, 1998.

THE DEPARTMENT OF RADIOLOGY OF THE UNIVERSITY OF MISSOURI-KANSAS CITY—Is seeking a staff radiologist with subspecialty training or interest in musculoskeletal radiology, GI/GU, mammography or ultrasound. Contact Dr Martin L. Goldman; 816-556-3926. EOE.

BEAUTIFUL NORTH GEORGIA—Major Lake community of 10,000 one-hour North of Atlanta near major university and North Georgia Mountains. Staff positions available to cover 150-bed facilities. Imaging services include MRI, CT, ultrasound, nuclear medicine, and mammography. Direct contract with the hospital system offering competitive salary, production incentive, and benefit package including retirement plan. Call David King (King Search, Inc) at 800-990-0780, 770-886-0780 or fax 770-886-9522. Send CV to King Search & Consulting, Inc, 1380 Zephyr Ct, Cumming, GA 30041.

VASCULAR AND INTERVENTIONAL RADIOLOGIST—The University of Michigan is expanding its well-established interventional division, and has two faculty positions available. Applicants must be ABR certified, fellowship trained, and CAQ eligible. The division performs a wide range of percutaneous vascular, biliary, and GI/GU procedures. All faculty participate in an active teaching program and in research. Interested individuals should contact M. Victoria Marx, MD, Division Director, Vascular and Interventional Radiology, UH B1D502, University of Michigan Medical Center, 1500 E Medical Center Dr, Ann Arbor, MI, 48109-0030. Phone 734-936-4478, fax 734-936-7948, e-mail *mvmarx@umich.edu*. A non-discriminatory, affirmative action employer.

NIGHT-TIME RADIOLOGIST/MID-ATLANTIC REGION—Hospital based radiology group desires energetic individual to provide night coverage for main hospital and teleradiology services for two other affiliated hospitals. Candidate must possess general diagnostic, MRI, nuclear medicine, musculoskeletal, CT, ultrasound and basic angiography skills. Will provide a total of 26 weeks of coverage annually. Attractive compensation package. Please send CV to Box R-086.

TRAUMA AND EMERGENCY RADIOLOGIST/ GENERAL RADIOLOGIST—The University of Texas Southwestern Medical Center in affiliation with Parkland Hospital in Dallas, TX, is seeking a Board certified radiologist to join a large academic practice including a level 1 trauma center. The position will include clinical and teaching responsibilities in a large residency program. Fellowship training in trauma/emergency radiology, musculoskeletal, abdominal imaging or neuroradiology desirable. Salary and academic rank commensurate with experience. Please send cover letter and CV to Julie Champine, MD, Department of Radiology, UT Southwestern Medical Center, 5323 Harry Hines Blvd, Dallas, TX 75235-8896; 214-648-6423, fax 214-648-2678. The University of Texas Southwestern Medical Center is an equal opportunity employer.

GULF COAST FLORIDA OPPORTUNITIES (2)—Picture yourself practicing quality interventional radiology in a beautiful SW Florida gulf coast resort community. A progressive, hospital-based four man practice with outpatient office seeks a Board certified, fellowship trained interventionalist with body MR skills to join them on their partnership track. A second position is available for a part-time, Board certified general diagnostic radiologist with basic interventional skills. This flexible, employee position will include some evening and weekend call. Both positions offer an opportunity to work with top notch radiologists in a state-of-the-art environment and receive a generous remuneration and benefits package. You will enjoy sun, sand, blue skies and the Gulf of Mexico year around. For more information, contact Peggy Cavalancia at Gable Healthcare Group, 800-430-4424, fax your CV 954-942-0302 or e-mail us at *ghcg@aol.com*.

OKLAHOMA CITY—Join a large multi-specialty group and replace a radiologist. Existing department with established referral pattern (four other radiologists). Do full radiology including interventional cases. A $180,000 base salary + benefits + production incentive. Employee under salary the initial 2-years and then partnership. Live next to The University of Oklahoma and even get involved with their residency program (optional). Call David 800-677-7987 ext 8-065 or fax your CV 800-440-2676; e-mail *dbgmsg@aol.com*.

SOUTHERN LOUISIANA—Community of 104,000 population needs a particular type of radiologist (a women's health specialist). Work alongside another bright radiologist (1:2). No MRI or interventional work involved. Primarily breast biopsy and mammography. Believe it or not, this is big business in this community! Salary of $180,000 + health, life, dental, malpractice insurance + no buy-in or restrictive covenant involved! Easy access to New Orleans, LSU, and has a major airport! Call David at 800-677-7987 ext 8-064 or fax 800-440-2676; e-mail *dbgmsg@aol.com*.

PENSACOLA, FL - INTERVENTIONAL—Radiologist needed to join department of 11 radiologists in premier 150+ physician multi-specialty group. Enjoy a four-day work week, call 1:6 with teleradiology, competitive salary, full benefits, and future partnership. Dynamic city on gulf coast offers great schools and year-round recreational and cultural amenities. Call Kathy Jordan, 800-765-3055, ID#5958RA, fax 314-726-3009, e-mail *kjordan@cejka.com*.

THE DEPARTMENT OF RADIOLOGY—At the University of Pittsburgh School of Medicine is recruiting for the position of a general radiologist. This is a non-tenure stream position with an expected hiring date in the fall of 1998. The position requires a Board certified radiologist who has substantial experience in general radiology, with a subspecialty interest being desirable. The physician should be licensed (or eligible for licensure) to practice medicine in the Commonwealth of Pennsylvania. Additionally, the individual should have an academic orientation with a strong background in clinical service. The University of Pittsburgh Health System comprises tertiary hospitals and community hospitals, and provides premier programs in patient care, biomedical and health services research, and teaching that will contribute to the prevention, diagnosis, and treatment of human disease and disability. Interested candidates should submit a curriculum vitae to Manuel L. Brown, MD, Vice Chairman, Department of Radiology, University of Pittsburgh Medical Center, 200 Lothrop St, Pittsburgh, PA 15213. The University of Pittsburgh is an affirmative action, equal opportunity employer.

THE DEPARTMENT OF RADIOLOGY—At the University of Pittsburgh School of Medicine is recruiting for the position of abdominal imager. The Division of Abdominal Imaging is nationally renowned for its research and clinical services, and has state-of-the-art equipment in all modalities that includes CT, MRI, fluoroscopy, and ultrasound. The department also has a PET facility with three PET tomographs, including a combined PET-CT tomograph dedicated to research such as oncologic diagnosis. This is a non-tenure stream position with an expected hiring date in the fall of 1998. The position requires a Board certified radiologist who has completed an abdominal imaging fellowship or who has substantial experience in abdominal imaging. The physician should be licensed (or eligible for licensure) to practice medicine in the Commonwealth of Pennsylvania. Additionally, the individual should have an academic orientation with a strong background in clinical service. The University of Pittsburgh Health System comprises tertiary hospitals and community hospitals, and provides premier programs in patient care, biomedical and health services research, and teaching that will contribute to the prevention, diagnosis, and treatment of human disease and disability. Interested candidates should submit a curriculum vitae to Manuel L. Brown, MD, Vice Chairman, Department of Radiology, University of Pittsburgh Medical Center, 200 Lothrop St, Pittsburgh, PA 15213. The University of Pittsburgh is an affirmative action, equal opportunity employer.

INTERVENTIONAL RADIOLOGIST—Well-established group in southern Oregon seeks fellowship trained, Board certified interventionalist to join busy practice of 13 members in a regional referral center. Expertise needed in both vascular and non-vascular studies, but proficiency expected in other modalities of radiology. Generous compensation package with 2-years to partnership. Outstanding lifestyle with numerous cultural and recreational activities available in a beautiful area. Send a current CV to Seth M. Hofstetter, MD, 842 E Main St, Medford, OR 97504.

MRI-ANGIOGRAPHY OPPORTUNITY—Department of Veterans Affairs, Central Texas Veterans Health Care System (CTVHCS), in Temple, TX in affiliation with Texas A&M Health Science Center has an immediate position for BE/BC radiologist with experience or recent training in MRI and angiography to work at Temple, TX. The position will include some general radiology and teaching of residents/medical students. Applicants should be qualified for academic appointment. Citizenship or permanent resident status required. Excellent benefits package. Competitive salary. Central Texas enjoys moderate climate, recreational and cultural activities. No state income tax and is ideally located between Dallas and Austin. Fax CV to Mary Doerfler, Physician Recruiter, CTVHCS, 1901 S First St, Temple, TX 76504; fax 254-899-4007, voice 254-899-4049. Applicants are subject to drug testing. Equal opportunity employer.

THE DEPARTMENT OF RADIOLOGY—At the University of Pittsburgh School of Medicine is recruiting for the position of Chief of the Division of Neuroradiology. This is a non-tenure stream position with an expected hiring date in the fall of 1998. The position requires a Board certified radiologist who has completed a neuroradiology fellowship and has substantial experience in neuroradiology. The individual should have significant academic and research accomplishments. Prior leadership experience in a formal administrative role is preferred. The University of Pittsburgh Radiology Department has a state-of-the-art functional neuroimaging facility including a PET center with three PET tomographs with a focus of research in neuropsychiatric disease and a MR research faculty with a dedicated 1.5T and a 3.0T magnets. The division is comprised of 10 neuroradiologists and offers a 2-year fellowship program. The physician should be licensed (or eligible for licensure) to practice medicine in the Commonwealth of Pennsylvania. The University of Pittsburgh Health System comprises tertiary hospitals and community hospitals, and provides premier programs in patient care, biomedical and health services research, and teaching that will contribute to the prevention, diagnosis, and treatment of human disease and disability. Interested candidates should submit a curriculum vitae to Manuel L. Brown, MD, Vice Chairman, Department of Radiology, University of Pittsburgh Medical Center, 200 Lothrop St, Pittsburgh, PA 15213. The

University of Pittsburgh is an affirmative action, equal opportunity employer.

RADIOLOGIST/ABDOMINAL/THORACIC IMAGING—The Department of Radiology at the Louisiana State University Medical Center has a full-time position available in the abdominal/thoracic imaging section at the rank of Assistant Professor (tenure-track or clinical-track), Associate Professor (tenured or clinical-track), or Professor (tenured or clinical-track) beginning immediately. At the Assistant Professor level, minimum requirements are Board certification in radiology, a minimum of 1-year post residency specialty training or experience in abdominal/thoracic imaging and a demonstrated involvement in quality research accepted or published in peer reviewed journals. Appointment at the rank of Associate Professor requires Board certification in radiology, minimum of 4-years post residency training or experience in abdominal/thoracic imaging, a professional distinction in research and writing, and a demonstrated effectiveness in teaching and advising. Appointment at the rank of Professor requires Board certification in radiology, a minimum of 6-years post residency specialty training or experience in abdominal/thoracic imaging, a national reputation in research and writing, and evidence of leadership in candidate's professional field in addition to other qualifications listed for Assistant and Associate Professor status. Responsibilities will include all facets of abdominal/thoracic imaging as well as graduate and undergraduate medical instruction. For tenure-track and tenured positions, research performance will be strongly encouraged and evaluated. Salary is negotiable and competitive, and is dependent upon scholarly productivity and post MD experience. Applicants must be licensed or able to obtain a license to practice medicine in the state of Louisiana prior to appointment date. Send letters to Dr Wilfrido R. Castaneda, Professor, Department of Radiology, LSU Medical Center, 1542 Tulane Ave, Room 307, New Orleans, LA 70112. The Louisiana State University Medical Center is an equal opportunity educator and employer.

MUSCULOSKELETAL RADIOLOGIST—The University of Utah Department of Radiology seeks a Board certified radiologist with experience and expertise in musculoskeletal radiology at the Assistant, Associate or Professor rank. Outpatient and inpatient facilities are state-of-the-art. Minimum requirements for this position are Board certification in radiology and 1-year of post-residency sub-specialty training. Applicants must demonstrate a record of continuous involvement in research, publication, and teaching. Salary is competitive. Applicant must be able to obtain a license to practice medicine in the state of Utah prior to the starting date. Please forward CV, and a letter describing background. Interest and the names and addresses of references to Dr William Orrison, Chair, Department of Radiology, 1A71 School of Medicine, University of Utah, Salt Lake City, UT 84132. The University of Utah is an equal opportunity/affirmative action employer and encourages applications from women and minorities.

RAPIDLY EXPANDING 12-MEMBER OUTPATIENT PRACTICE—Operating three of the nations largest state-of-the-art imaging centers seeks two additional Board certified, fellowship trained radiologists. Our facilities include six MRI, four CT, and two angio suites. These positions currently involve no call, no weekends, and no angio coverage. Please send your CV to Dr David Haas, 2950 S Maryland Parkway, Las Vegas, NV 89109.

RADIOLOGIST - CROSS CANCER INSTITUTE EDMONTON, ALBERTA—The Cross Cancer Institute, a division of the Alberta Cancer Board, is seeking a radiologist to join our four person team within the Department of Oncologic Imaging. The Cross Cancer Institute is a comprehensive tertiary care cancer center providing oncologic consultative expertise and medical management for a referral base of 1.5 million. Our radiology positions are site specific and joint appointed through the University of Alberta. The successful candidate could participate in MRI, CT, US, x-rays and biopsy/interventional duties. The position would be professionally satisfying with minimum on call, no travel, daily interesting cases, and friendly interactions with the entire medical staff. Protected time for research could be provided. A dual certification in nuclear medicine would be an asset but is not a requirement. Address inquiries to Steven Halls, MD, Cross Cancer Institute, Department of Oncologic Imaging, 11560 University Ave, Edmonton, Alberta, Canada T6G 1Z2, Phone 403-432-8554, fax 403-432-8552; *steven.halls@cancerboard.ab.ca*.

NUCLEAR MEDICINE SPECIALIST - CROSS CANCER INSTITUTE EDMONTON, ALBERTA—The Cross Cancer Institute, a division of the Alberta Cancer Board, is seeking a specialist in nuclear medicine within our Department of Oncologic Imaging. The Cross Cancer Institute is a comprehensive tertiary care cancer center pro-

Medical Center, PO Box 23089, Savannah, GA 31403; 912-350-7394, or e-mail *mmcrad@g-net.net.*

ABDOMINAL RADIOLOGIST—The College of Physicians and Surgeons of Columbia University has an unexpected opening for an experienced radiologist to join our multi-modality (MRI, CT, ultrasound, fluoroscopy, and radiography) abdominal division. The primary duties for this position will be to establish a center of excellence in gastrointestinal and hepatobiliary radiology, including promotion and development of the newest imaging techniques. Appropriate experience and /or fellowship training required. Salary and academic rank will commensurate with experience and qualifications. Board certification and NYS medical license required; narcotics license desirable. Please send resume to Philip O. Alderson, MD, Chairman, Department of Radiology, Columbia-Presbyterian Medical Center, 177 Fort Washington Ave, New York, NY 10032. Columbia University is an affirmative action/ equal opportunity employer. Women and minorities are encouraged to apply.

RADIOLOGY RESIDENCY—Unexpected openings for two 1st-year diagnostic radiology residents (PGY 2) starting on July 1, 1999 in a fully accredited residency program. Sisters of Charity Medical Center-St. Vincent's Campus (a New York Medical College affiliate), located in a suburban setting, is a 400-bed tertiary hospital and level 1 trauma center. Applications for July 2000 are also being accepted via the ERAS system. Please call 718-876-3153 or send CV (fax 718-876-1869) to Sisters of Charity Medical Center, St. Vincent's Campus, Department of Radiology, attn Megan McGill, 355 Bard Ave, Staten Island, NY 10310. EOE.

INTERVENTIONAL RADIOLOGIST—Outstanding opportunity available for a Board certified/ Board eligible interventional radiologist to join a busy well-established five person single specialty group. Practice is located in a beautiful, upper midwest suburban area with excellent, nationally ranked schools and universities. Tremendous recreational and cultural activities available. Attractive salary and compensation package with many additional benefits. Opportunity for partnership. Please contact Cindy Cummings of Christopher and Long for additional information at 888-821-1667 or fax your CV to 800-800-2661.

THE DEPARTMENT OF RADIOLOGY AT THE UNIVERSITY OF FLORIDA - ULTRASOUND FACULTY POSITION—The department is actively recruiting for a tenure track faculty member for our Body/Abdominal Imaging Division in the College of Medicine. Appointment will be at the Instructor, Assistant Professor, Associate Professor, or Professor level, as credentials permit. Minimum requirements include a fellowship trained MD with Board certification (or Board eligibility) by the American Board of Radiology. Applicants must be eligible for licensure in the state of Florida. Salary is negotiable. The department is looking for a radiologist with special interest in ultrasonography. This person would be involved with development of a high-end ultrasound service with expectations to perform ultrasound contrast research. Participation in the other facets of the body imaging service is required. Active industry links and research are to be encouraged. The successful candidate will demonstrate skills in clinical care, teaching, as well as clinical research interest. The following systems are available in the department; color-flow doppler, three Toshiba vascular labs (one biplane and two single plane), one angio suite with Phillips C-arm and Camtronics video plus digital, a 1.5T GE MRI with phased contrast and spectroscopy, a Siemens 1.5T vision MRI, a siemens open MRI, a GE 3T MRI research unit, two GE Highlight Advantage CT scanners, ISG 3-D workstations, and ICU electronic image display stations, with an advanced PACS system for display and retrievals throughout the department. Application deadline for this position is October 30, 1998 with a start date soon thereafter. Applicants should send a CV to Patricia L. Abbitt, MD, Professor, Department of Radiology, University of Florida, College of Medicine, Box 100374, Gainesville, FL 32610-0374. An affirmative action equal employment employer.

VA PITTSBURGH HEALTHCARE SYSTEM, PITTSBURGH, PA—Imaging group of seven physicians is seeking a general radiologist. Advanced MRI musculoskeletal training desirable but not required. Locum tenens candidates will be considered. Our institution is the tertiary referral medical center amount five VA center's in western Pennsylvania and West Virginia as well as for liver transplantation. It is close to and affiliated with the University of Pittsburgh School of Medicine. State-of-the-art equipment in all modalities. Please send CV to Herbert A. Klein, MD, PhD (132N-U), VA Pittsburgh Healthcare System, University Drive, Pittsburgh, PA 15240 or fax to 412-688-6907.

INTERVENTIONAL RADIOLOGIST (ABR, CAQ, SCVIR)—Desires small-midsize practice position. Fellowship trained. Experienced in a wide range of invasive procedures. Able to do general including MRI, US, CT, NM. Will work to build a practice or assume an existing practice. Voice 248-549-2785; fax 248-544-9946; e-mail *tbechtel@cris.com*.

FLORIDA, WEST COAST RADIOLOGY PRACTICE—Seeking general radiologist. Competence in full range of diagnostic radiology modalities required. Board certified/eligible. Private office and two hospital locations. Excellent benefits and compensation. Respond to Radiology Associates, Executive Director, PO Box 1175, New Port Richey, FL 34656-1175.

THORACIC RADIOLOGIST—The Department of Radiology at Indiana University School of Medicine is pleased to announce the availability of a tenure or clinical track faculty position in thoracic radiology. Candidates must be Board certified in diagnostic radiology and have fellowship training or substantial equivalent experience in thoracic radiology. Responsibilities will include clinical care, teaching and research. Salary and academic rank will be commensurate with experience and qualifications. Interested applicants should send their curriculum vitae to Dewey J. Conces, Jr, MD, Department of Radiology, Indiana University Hospital, Room 0279, 550 N University Blvd, Indianapolis, IN 46202-5253 or e-mail*dconces@iupui.edu*. Indiana Unversity is an equal opportunity/affirmative action employer.

RADIOLOGIST—Multi-modality imaging center (including MRI) in western suburb has opening for a full-time radiologist. Responsibilities also include overseeing marketing development & practice expansion. Fax CV to 713-526-8875.

PEDIATRIC INTERVENTIONAL RADIOLOGIST—The Department of Radiology, Indiana University School of Medicine has an immediate opening for a full-time pediatric radiologist to develop an interventional radiology service at a 200-bed children's hospital. Riley Hospital for Children is the only pediatric children's hospital in Indiana. This is a tenure track faculty position at the rank of Assistant Professor to Professor. Responsibilities will include clinical care, teaching and research. Minimum requirements include MD with Board certification in radiology and eligiblity for licensure in Indiana. The ideal candidate will be CAQ-eligible/certified in both interventional and pediatric radiology. This is an opportunity for an interested candidate to join a vibrant interventional radiology service performing over 6,000 procedures annually. Intersted candidates should send their curriculum vitae to John A. Smith, MD, Department of Radiology, Riley Hospital for Chidren, 702 Barnhill Dr, Indianapolis, IN 46202-5200; phone 317-274-2951; fax 317-274-2920. Indidana University is an equal opportunity/affirmative action employer.

NEURORADIOLOGIST—Large radiology practice is seeking a Board certified, fellowship trained neuroradiologist for a full-time position in a rapidly expanding practice. A strong background in neuroangiography, myleography, CT and MRI is required. Applicants should possess skills and be comfortable with general radiology, including fluoroscopy, ultrasound, and mammography. This is a dynamic group practice in a very desirable location with an excellent opportunity for a long term career. Position available starting December 1998. Please reply with CV to Radiology Associates of Burlington County, 227 Madison Ave, Mt. Holly, NJ 08060 or fax to 609-261-4180.

DIRECTOR OF MEDICAL IMAGING—Denver Health Medical Center is recruiting a Director of the Department of Medical Imaging. Applicants should have Board certification in radiology, 5-years of management experience, and a demonstrated track record in academic radiology. Because DHMC is a regional level 1 trauma center, specialty interests in trauma are desirable but not mandatory. Denver Health is a vertically integrated health system affiliated with the University of Colorado School of Medicine with shared housestaff and faculty. Applications are encour-

---

RADIOLOGY

Marshfield Clinic has an immediate opening for an individual with special interest or fellowship training in **angio/interventional radiology.**

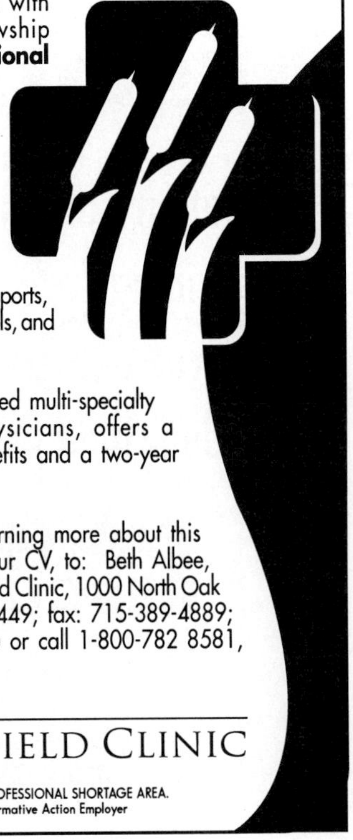

This is a full service practice located at Marshfield Clinic-Lakeland Center in Minocqua, Wisconsin. Minocqua is a beautiful northern Wisconsin community that boasts of year 'round sports, water activities, excellent schools, and a healthy environment.

Marshfield Clinic, a renowned multi-specialty clinic with over 500 physicians, offers a competitive salary and benefits and a two-year partnership track.

If you are interested in learning more about this opportunity, please send your CV, to: Beth Albee, Physician Recruiter, Marshfield Clinic, 1000 North Oak Avenue, Marshfield, WI 54449; fax: 715-389-4889; e-mail: albeee@mfldclin.edu or call 1-800-782 8581, extension 94451.

MARSHFIELD CLINIC

SORRY. NOT A HEALTH PROFESSIONAL SHORTAGE AREA.
An Equal Opportunity/Affirmative Action Employer

RADIOLOGIST

Gundersen Lutheran is seeking a board certified/board eligible Radiologist who has completed a fellowship in Magnetic Resonance Imaging to add to our rapidly expanding department. A new Siemens 1.5 T Vision unit and open system have just recently been installed.

Gundersen Lutheran is a large multi-specialty group practice with over 320 physicians located in La Crosse, WI. It's main campus is attached to a 402 bed acute care hospital. The Gundersen Lutheran system includes 36 regional community clinics based throughout western Wisconsin, eastern Minnesota and northeastern Iowa. Gundersen Lutheran is a modern state-of-the-art facility that has a service area for a population base of over 530,000. Gundersen Lutheran is also the designated western campus of the University of Wisconsin Medical School.

La Crosse, Wisconsin, nestled between towering bluffs, is located where the Mississippi, La Crosse, and Black Rivers merge. The area was untouched by the glaciers, leaving many hills and valleys. The metropolitan area of La Crosse, with its 100,000 people, offers exceptional year round opportunities for recreational activities. The area also offers outstanding public and private schools, low crime rates, and cultural activities.

We offer competitive salaries and excellent fringe benefits. Interested candidates should send a letter of application and curriculum vitae to Frank Perez-Guerra, Director, Recruitment, Retention, and Resource Planning, Gundersen Lutheran, 1836 South Avenue, La Crosse, WI 54601; or call 800-362-9567, Ext. 6325.

Gundersen Lutheran

Equal Opportunity Employer

Portland metropolitan area and Salem providing quality care to over 430,000 plan members in Oregon and Washington. Ours is a collegial and stimulating practice in one of the most success-

ful managed care programs in the country. In addition to a lifestyle inherent to the beautiful Pacific Northwest, we offer a predictable work schedule, and a competitive salary and benefit package which includes professional liability coverage, a comprehensive pension program, sabbatical leave and more. For additional information please forward CV to R.A. Clark, Director, Physician Resources, Northwest Permanente, PC, 500 NE Multnomah, Suite 100, Portland, OR 97232-2099. EOE.

NEURORADIOLOGIST—Mallinckrodt Institute of Radiology (MIR) seeks Board certified neuroradiologist with neuroradiology fellowship and interest in spine for 100-bed community hospital in West St. Louis County. Expertise in myelography, pain mgt, MR brain and spine required. This 100-bed hospital specializing in orthopedic and spine surgery is staffed by four MIR diagnostic radiologists. Position available July 1999; position carries clinical appointment at Washington University School of Medicine. Academic time at MIR possible. Send inquiries and CV to Robert Levitt, MD, FACR, Chief of Radiology, Barnes Jewish West County Hospital, 12634 Olive Blvd, St. Louis, MO 63141 or fax 314-996-8515.

GENERAL RADIOLOGIST NEEDED—To join strong, progressive 20-member group in the greater Cincinnati area. Special interest in nuclear medicine, body imaging, and/or mammography would be helpful. Board certification required. Fellowship preferred but not required. Nonvascular interventional skills required. This is a partnership track position. Please send CV to Mr Joe Roesel, MD, PO Box 17630, 170 Barnwood Dr, Edgewood, KY 41017; e-mail *DLubbers@msn.com*.

MAGNETIC RESONANCE IMAGING (MRI) SPECTROSCOPIST—The Department of Radiology is seeking to recruit a PhD spectroscopist at the rank of Assistant Professor. The applicant should have some expertise in clinical MR spectroscopic studies. The successful candidate will be expected to participate in providing a clinical service in MR spectroscopy as well as developing new human spectroscopic studies at both 1.5 and 4 T. Candidates will be expected to develop an independently funded program of research. Start-up support will be provided. Applications should include a curriculum vitae, a statement of research interests and the names and addresses of three references. Applications should be sent to Mitchell D. Schnall, MD, PhD, MRI Section, Department of Radiology, University of Pennsylvania, 3400 Spruce St, Philadelphia, PA 19104. The University of Pennsylvania is an equal opportunity/affirmative action employer. Qualified female and minority candidates are encouraged to apply.

STAFFORD SPRINGS, CT—General radiology position, part-time (five days/week, four-six hours/day, flexible schedule) located at Johnson Memorial Hospital, a pleasant 100-bed community hospital with all imaging modalities including US, CT, and MRI. No call, holidays, or weekends. Please send CV with references to Steven Urbanski, MD, Department of Radiology, Johnson Memorial Hospital, Box 860, Stafford Springs, CT 06076.

PORTLAND, OR—Immediate opening for a partnership track position in a state-of-the-art community hospital-based practice. Seeking BC radiologist with fellowship training and/or special interest in ultrasound and cross-sectional imaging with ability to participate in all diagnostic modalities. Excellent interpersonal skills required. Competitive financial and benefits package. A liberal vacation plan allows quality family and personal time. Send CV to Mark D. Kettler, MD, Department of Medical Imaging, Adventist Medical Center, 10123 SE Market , Portland, OR 97216.

INTERVENTIONAL RADIOLOGIST—Recently fellowship trained interventionalist needed to join two others in active interventional practice. An 11-person group practicing at 400-bed Rapid City Regional Hospital with state-of-the-art equipment. Partnership track with generous compensation and time off. Family oriented and friendly, Rapid City is a town of 65,000 located at the edge of the beautiful Black Hills in western South Dakota. There are excellent schools with a local university and many outdoor opportunities. Start no later than summer 1999. Reply to William Zavitz, MD, 716 Quincy St, Rapid City, SD 57701; 605-341-8200; fax 605-342-3930.

DIRECTOR, THORACIC RADIOLOGY—The Georgetown University Medical Center Department of Radiology seeks a section head for its thoracic radiology practice. The practice will be centered at Georgetown University Hospital in the District of Columbia where there are excellent collaborative programs in thoracic and cardiovascular surgery, critical care medicine, pulmonology, and oncology at the Lombardi Cancer Center. The clinical practice includes radiography, MRI (Siemens Vision) and CT (General Electric spiral CT). Extensive research facilities are available at the Georgetown Imaging Science and Information Systems (ISIS) Center. In addition to the hospital practice, there are suburban offices in Washington, Virginia and Maryland. The appointment will be at the Assistant, Associate or full Professor level in the clinician educator track at Georgetown University. Please direct inquiries to Michael J. Pentecost, MD, Professor and Chairman, Department of Radiology, Georgetown University Medical Center, 3800 Reservoir Rd NW, Washington, DC 20007.

THE UNIVERSITY OF MIAMI/JACKSON MEMORIAL MEDICAL CENTER—Seeks fellowship trained musculoskeletal radiologist. Experience in MR related to sports medicine and oncological orthopedics is required. Invasive procedural experience in biopsies, aspirations and interventional spine diagnosis is preferred. Board certification and Florida license required. CV to Dr Robert Quencer, Department of Radiology, UMSM, 1150 NW 14th St, #511, Miami, FL 33136-2116.

THE DEPARTMENT OF RADIOLOGY AT THE UNIVERSITY OF ALABAMA AT BIRMINGHAM—Is actively recruiting an interventional radiologist. The section of Vascular and Interventional Radiology provides services for 1,100-beds at the University and Verteran's Administration Hospitals and performs over 5,500 procedures per year. Currently there are three full-time faculty members. Facilities include a Siemens Multistar TOP and two Philips angio suites currently under construction. Applicants must be Board certified in diagnostic radiology, have a CAQ in vascular and interventional radiology (or eligible for a CAQ), and eligible for licensure in the state of Alabama. Duties include medical student and resident teaching, radiology service and clinical research. Academic rank and tenure status will depend upon qualifications and experience. Interested candidates should submit their CV to Robert J. Stanley, MD, Department of Radiology, University of Alabama at Birmingham, AL 35233.

Classified Services

The University of Alabama at Birmingham is an affirmative action/equal opportunity employer.

FACULTY POSITION, GENERAL RADIOLOGY, CREIGHTON UNIVERSITY, OMAHA, NE—The Department of Radiology at Creighton University, Omaha, NE is seeking a general radiologist to add to its faculty. Applicants should be BC/BE with skills in general radiology with experience in mammography or neuroradiology a plus. No interventional radiology required. The department has state-of-the-art CT, MRI, and fluoroscopy and offer the ability to pursue individual interests in clinical practice, teaching or research. The Omaha area has a population of 500,000 and offers big-city amenities with small town friendliness and hospitality. Faculty appointment commensurate with experience. Please respond with CV to Dr Charles Lerner, Creighton University, Department of Radiology, 301 N 30th St, Omaha, NE 68131-2197; telephone 402-449-4540; fax 402-449-4271.

EMERGENCY RADIOLOGY—The Department of Radiology at the Hospital of the University of Pennsylvania is seeking applicants for a faculty position as an emergency radiologist in the clinician-educator non-tenure track at the rank of Assistant or Associate Professor. Must be Board certified and have training and/or competence in CT/ultrasound. This section, in conjunction with the Department of Emergency Medicine, has been completely modernized with the latest technology, including CT and ultrasound. The radiology component additionally includes soft-copy workstations and computed radiography equipment, all integrated into a PACS environment. The position will involve resident supervision and teaching. Schedules will involve evening and overnight coverage. Competitive compensation is available for qualified applicants. Please send resume to Ruben Mezrich, MD, PhD, Chief, Section of Emergency Radiology, Department of Radiology, University of Pennsylvania Medical Center, 3400 Spruce St, Philadelphia, PA 19104. The University of Pennsylvania is an affirmative action, equal opportunity employer.

NEURORADIOLOGIST—The College of Physicians and Surgeons of Columbia University is searching for a junior level radiologist in our neuroradiology division. Salary and academic rank will be commensurate with experience and qualifications. Responsibilities include patient care, active participation in resident and fellowship education and participation in clinical and/or basic research. Requirements include Board certification in diagnostic radiology and at least 2-years of neuroradiology experience, expertise in neuro-interventional procedures, hands-on experience in CT and MRI scanning and angiographic procedures. NYS medical license required; narcotics license desirable. Please direct inquiries to Philip O. Alderson, MD, Chairman, Columbia University, Department of Radiology, 177 Fort Washington Ave, New York, NY 10032. Columbia University is an affirmative action/equal opportunity employer. Women and minorities are encouraged to apply.

THE DEPARTMENT OF RADIOLOGY, VIRGINIA COMMONWEALTH UNIVERSITY, MEDICAL COLLEGE OF VIRGINIA CAMPUS, RICHMOND, VA—Seeks candidates for several faculty positions in diagnostic radiology. These include positions in musculoskeletal/emergency radiology, angiography/interventional radiology, abdominal imaging, and chest radiology. ABR certification or eligibility required. Fellowship training and interest in teaching and research are preferred. MCV Hospital is a 1,058-bed facility and a level 1 trauma center. Individuals should have experience working in a culturally diverse environment. Academic rank and salary commensurate with experience. For position description, or to submit CV, write or phone BJ Manaster, MD, PhD, Department of Radiology, PO Box 980470, Richmond, VA 23298-0470; 804-828-6600; 804-828-6129 fax. VCU/MCV is an equal opportunity/affirmative action employer. Women, minorities, and persons with disabilities are encouraged to apply.

RADIOLOGIST—Opportunity for well-trained ambitious womens imager to join 12 person private practice in western Connecticut. Must have excellent clinical, leadership, and managerial skills to lead service in community teaching hospital and outpatient offices. Send CV to Donald Hulnick, MD, Department of Radiology, 24 Hospital Ave, Danbury, CT 06810; fax 203-431-4045.

FACULTY OPPORTUNITY - BODY IMAGING—The Department of Radiology at The Mount Sinai Medical Center, New York, NY, is seeking a full-time faculty member to serve in the Body Imaging Section. The applicant must be a Board certified radiologist with experience in body imaging including CT, US, MRI, and biopsy procedures. Special consideration will be given to candidates with expertise in cardiac MRI or musculoskeletal imaging. Faculty title and salary are commensurate with experience. Interested candidates should send their CV to Dr Robert S. Shapiro, Director of Body Imaging, The Mount Sinai Medical Center, One Gustave L. Levy Place, New York, NY 10029-6574; phone 212-241-7427; fax 212-427-8137. We are an equal opportunity employer fostering diversity in the workplace.

DIAGNOSTIC RADIOLOGY RESIDENCY—Unexpected opening for a 1st-year radiology resident (PGY-2) at The Mercy Hospital of Pittsburgh. Mercy Hospital is a major urban medical-surgical and level 1 trauma referral facility for adult and pediatric patients. Applicants must have completed a clinical base year of training in an ACGME or AOA approved program and be able to begin training on July 1, 1999. William R. Poller, MD, Chairperson and Radiology Residency Program Director. For more information, contact Sandy Balon, Residency Program Assistant, 412-232-7910 or e-mail *diagnostic.radiology.residency@mercy.pmhs.org*.

GENERAL RADIOLOGIST—Bassett Healthcare is seeking two BC/BE general radiologists. One of the candidates should be certified by the ABNM or ABR with special competency in nuclear medicine and would serve as Section Chief of Nuclear Medicine. Responsibilities for both will include general diagnostic radiology, mammography, MRI, CT, US, and ideally basic angiography/interventional, along with student/resident teaching. Bassett Healthcare is a regional referral center and a teaching affiliate of Columbia University. It is located in a beautiful family-oriented mountain/lake region with an abundance of year-around recreational and cultural activities. We offer a competitive salary with incentives, paid malpractice excellent benefits, and education/travel allowance. Please send CV and correspondence to Denise B. Harter, Medical Staff Recruiter, Bassett Healthcare, One Atwell Rd, Cooperstown, NY 13326; fax 607-547-3844, or for more information please call 607-547-6982.

BOARD-CERTIFIED RADIOLOGIST—Rapidly growing multi-state Mobil practice looking for radiologist with basic angio/interventional skills. State license required in at least one of the following states: Pennsylvania, New Jersey, Mary-

secondary to both retiring members as well as an expanding service area. We are group of 17 radiologists in northeast Pennsylvania covering two hospitals in Scranton, one hospital in Wilkes Barre, one hospital in Nanticoke, as well as an MRI center which houses two 1.5 Tesla magnets as well as an open 0.3 Tesla magnet. We are currently targeting fellowship trained or an equivalent experienced radiologist. Competitive salary and benefits are being offered for this excellent opportunity. Reply to Radiological Consultants, Inc, c/o John J. Culliney, MD, 751 Keystone Industrial Park, Dunmore, PA 18512. Phone 717-346-8272 or fax CV to 717-346-4872.

ESTABLISHED PRACTICE IN SOUTHERN CALIFORNIA—Is seeking a Board certified, fellowship trained breast imaging radiologist and general diagnostic radiologist. Our practice is located in a beautiful coastal community with both hospital and free-standing imaging center business. Please mail your CV to Digital & Radiologic Imaging Associates, Inc, 26161 Marguerite Parkway, Suite D, Mission Viejo, CA 92691; attn: Kerry Jones.

RADIOLOGIST-BREAST IMAGING—The Department of Diagnostic Radiology and Nuclear Medicine at Rush Medical College and Rush-Presbyterian-St. Luke's Medical Center is seeking a Board certified radiologist with fellowship training or equivalent subspecialty experience in breast imaging. The department has dedicated outpatient facilities for breast imaging including a stereotactic unit for needle biopsy. Rank and salary are commensurate with experience. Interested parties should contact Peter Jokich, MD, Director of the Section of Breast Imaging, Department of Diagnostic Radiology and Nuclear Medicine, Rush-Presbyterian-St. Luke's Medical Center, 1653 W Congress Parkway, Chicago, IL 60612. Rush is an equal opportunity/affirmative employer.

WOMEN'S CENTER RADIOLOGIST—Suburban Atlanta, GA. Progressive 13-member subspecialized group seeking mammographer. State-of-the-art women's facility is on main hospital campus with large interventional mammography, obstetrical and neonatal services. Please send replies to Robert Eisenberg, MD, Promina Gwinnett Health System, 1000 Medical Center Blvd, Lawrenceville, GA 30045-7694; 770-995-4440.

OPEN RANK—The University of Arizona Department of Radiology is seeking a Board certified/eligible academic radiologist for Section Chief of Body Imaging, Assistant Professor, Associate Professor or Professor, TT/NTE. Required, fellowship training in MRI, demonstrated knowledge of MRI and CT technology and application and eligibility for medical licensure in the state of Arizona. This position will open July 1, 1998. Review applications will commence September 1, 1998 and continue until the position is filled. The applicant must be able to obtain an Arizona license prior to the starting date. Letters of inquiry and CV should be sent to Theron W Ovitt, MD, Chair, Department of Radiology, AHSC, PO Box 245067, Tucson, AZ 85724-5067. For more information see web site *http://w3.arizona.edu/~ahschr/jobs.htm.* The University of Arizona is an EEO/AA employer. M/W/D/V.

THE UNIVERSITY OF MISSISSIPPI MEDICAL CENTER—Department of Radiology is seeking a general radiologist with interest in mammography. Some fellowship training preferred. The department currently has four mammographic units, stereotactic biopsy and breast ultrasound. Compensation will be based on qualifications and productivity. Interested parties should contact Dr Brent Harrison at 601-984-2515. EOE, M/F/D/V.

RADIOLOGIST—TTUHSC at El Paso, Department of Radiology seeks a Board eligible or certified radiologist with fellowship training in body imaging. This is an interesting and challenging position in a county hospital that is the trauma center for a community of 650,000 and the primary inpatient and outpatient care giver for a large indigent and underserved population of 250,000. Our equipment is current with a new MRI, second CT scanner, and combined cardiovascular machine soon to be installed. Our mammography program is a center of excellence. Our ultrasound and mammography sections are ACR accredited. This is an ideal position for a recent trainee who desires to affiliate with a medical school and become a part of an active clinical service. Salary is commensurate with training and experience. Benefits including retirement are generous. El Paso is a delightful city of 650,000 with a year-round warm dry climate and the ease of

ing applications for a interventional radiologist. Candidates must be eligible for or certified by the American Board of Radiology and also be eligible for or have passed the CAQ examination. Candidate must possess strong clinical skills and communication abilities. The hospital is affiliated with Allegheny University of the Health Sciences. The department offers a private practice opportunity. The hospital has strong history of excellence in gastroenterology, oncology, orthopedics and cardiology. The department is outfitted with state-of-the-art equipment. In addition, there is a free standing imaging center. Philadelphia offers numerous cultural, historical and recreational activities. Please send letter of interest and current curriculum vitae to Arthur P. Staddon, MD, Radiology Search Committee, AUH-Graduate, 1840 S St, 2nd Fl, Philadelphia, PA 19146.

RADIOLOGY DEPARTMENT CHAIRMAN—Allegheny University - Graduate Hospital is seeking applications for the Chair of the Department of Radiology. Candidates must be certified by the American Board of Radiology and should possess strong clinical skills with excellent organizational and management abilities. The hospital is affiliated with Allegheny University of the Health Sciences. The department offers a private practice opportunity. The hospital has a strong history of excellence in gastroenterology, oncology, orthopedics and cardiology. The department is outfitted with state-of-the-art equipment. In addition, there is a free-standing outpatient imaging center. Philadelphia offers numerous cultural, historical and recreational activities. Please send letter of interest and current curriculum vitae to Arthur P. Staddon, MD, Radiology Search Committee, AUH-Graduate, 1840 S St, 2nd Fl, Philadelphia, PA 19146.

OREGON - GENERAL RADIOLOGIST—Wanted for job sharing position. Work 26 weeks per year. Flexible schedule. Low stress practice with up-to-date equipment in pleasant SW Oregon town. No mammography/angiography; very limited interventional; average two call-backs per month. Fax CV and references to L. Taylor 541-440-1368.

NORTH FLORIDA GULF COAST—An eight man group seeks Board certified candidate with fellowship training in MRI with interest in musculoskeletal imaging. Practice includes four MRI units. Partnership track and excellent benefits. Respond to Box R-084.

FLORIDA GULF COAST GROUP—Seeks Board certified fellowship trained neuroradiologist. Practice includes both hospital and outpatient centers. Partnership track and excellent benefits. Respond to Box R-085.

NIGHT RADIOLOGISTS—Bay Imaging Consultants Medical Group, Inc, a large San Francisco Bay area private practice radiology group with multiple outpatient and hospital sites, is seeking night radiologists for the night rotation. The night rotation is comprised of 12-hour rotations from 7:00pm to 7:00am. Must be Board certified. Competitive salary. Start date as soon as possible. Please submit your CV, a cover letter and the names of three references to Human Resources, 175 Lennon Ln, Suite 100, Walnut Creek, CA 94598. EOE.

BOARD CERTIFIED RADIOLOGISTS—Rapidly growing group in northeastern Pennsylvania seeks two aggressive Board certified radiologists with fellowship trainining in nuclear medicine and body imaging/MRI. State-of-the-art equipment including: GE LCA digital angio suite, GE Spiral CT with SUN workstation, two digital fluoroscopy suites, ATL HDI 5000 and Ultramark 9, Siemans Dual Head E Cam, fixed GE MRI, stereotactic breast. Outstanding opportunity to practice general radiology and to build the practice in your area of expertise. Excellent financial package with early partnership. Address inquiries to David Fontaine, MD, Chairman, 717-621-4420. Fax CV to 717-621-4582.

CONNECTICUT - TWO RADIOLOGISTS NEEDED— Fellowship-trained neuroradiologist with CAQ eligibility and fellowship-trained body imaging specialist sought by growing, progressive, subspecialty-oriented group of 15 radiologists. Yale-affiliated, community hospital-based

FACULTY POSITION BREAST IMAGING AND MAMMOGRAPHY

The Department of Radiology at MetroHealth Medical Center, a Case Western Reserve University affiliated teaching hospital, invites applications from interested, qualified radiologists for a faculty position in Breast Imaging. The ideal candidate will be Board certified and have fellowship experience in Breast Imaging and Mammography. Additional experience in Cross-Sectional Imaging will be an advantage. A faculty appointment will be made commensurate with the candidate's experience and qualifications.

MHMC is a 746-bed trauma center providing tertiary care and general hospital services to the Cleveland metropolitan area. The medical center is committed to providing excellence in care with a highly qualified, interdisciplinary, hospital-based medical staff. The Department of Radiology is an active, expanding department, providing general and specialized services using state-of-the-art equipment. The Breast Imaging Center has four modern mammography units and is equipped for stereotactic localization and needle biopsy, as well as Ultrasound and MR Imaging.

The position provides an excellent opportunity for professional development, collaborative and/or individual research, as well as medical student and resident education.

Interested candidates should forward curriculum vitae and other pertinent information to:

Errol M. Bellon, MD
Chairman, Department of Radiology
MetroHealth Medical Center
2500 MetroHealth Drive
Cleveland, OH 44109-1998
Telephone: 216-778-4020

MetroHealth Medical Center and Case Western Reserve University are Equal Opportunity Employers.

DARTMOUTH-HITCHCOCK MEDICAL CENTER

Division Head Department of Radiology

The Department of Radiology at Dartmouth-Hitchcock Medical Center is recruiting a division head for its body cross-sectional imaging division. The successful candidate should be capable of leading a small division in body MRI and CT into the next century and will be involved in the day-to-day workload in these modalities. Candidates should be knowledgeable in functional and vascular imaging and will perform image-guided invasive procedures including biopsies and drainages. Experience in cardiac MR desirable. There are additional duties in routine imaging as well as non-interventional call. A vigorous interest in teaching at all levels is essential. Research skills and interest congruent with body imaging are also essential.

The successful candidate must collaborate well in a multispecialty academic faculty setting. This 400 bed and ambulatory center contains a modern full service department with state-of-the-art MRI and CT as well as MR research facilities. Candidates should be board certified in diagnostic radiology, fellowship trained and have at least 2 years post-fellowship experience. Please send CVs to: **Peter K. Spiegel, M.D., Professor and Chairman, Department of Radiology, Dartmouth-Hitchcock Medical Center, 1 Medical Center Drive, Lebanon, NH, 03756. http://www.hitchcock.org**

The Dartmouth-Hitchcock Medical Center is an equal opportunity/ affirmative action employer and encourages applications from women and members of minority groups.

Dartmouth-Hitchcock Medical Center

private practice with residents and separate outpatient facilities. Positions available now, but will wait for the right people. Responsibilities divided between subspecialty areas and general office and hospital radiology. Excellent opportunities with expectation for partnership. Send CV to Alan Kaye, MD, 777 Commerce Dr, Fairfield, CT 06432, or fax to 203-384-4363.

INTERVENTIONALIST NEEDED—Looking for young superstar interventionalist to earn his/her way into full partnership in the premier radiology group in the mid-Hudson Valley. Maintain skills in all aspects of imaging with state-of-the-art equipment and expert colleagues while helping to lead the interventional department of a 300-bed tertiary care hospital. Many outpatient offices also including multiple MRI/CT sites. Send CV or call V. Gaines, MD, Department Imaging, Vassar Brothers Hospital, Reade Place, Poughkeepsie, NY 12601; 914-431-5644.

IMMEDIATE OPENING FOR TWO RADIOLOGISTS WITH CROSS-SECTIONAL IMAGING BACKGROUND, FELLOWSHIP PREFERRED BUT NOT A REQUIREMENT—Large progressive group near metropolitan Chicago in northwest Indiana. Covering four hospitals, several clinics and a free-standing imaging center, four MRIs, several CTs, state-of-the-art ultrasound and in-home PET scanner. Please send CV to Radiologic Associates of Northwest Indiana, Inc, 825 E. Lincolnway, Valparaiso, IN 46383 or call Dr James Forde at 219-464-4891.

NEURORADIOLOGIST—Georgetown University has a unique opportunity to join an academic radiology group in Washington, DC. The neuroradiology section includes four faculty and four fellows. Excellent collaborative research opportunities exist with the Georgetown Imaging Science and Information Systems group, the Georgetown Institute for Cognitive and Computational Sciences, and the neighboring National Institutes of Health in Bethesda, MD. The candidate should exhibit special interest and knowledge in neuro MRI. Experience with non-anatomic or functional MRI and background in research are desirable. Working skills in traditional invasive techniques (diagnostic angiography, myelography, etc), Board certification, and a certificate of added qualification in neuroradiology (or eligibility) are required. The Department of Radiology operates two 1.5T Siemens magnets (Vision), three advanced GE CT scanners (two helical) and a new Siemens Neurostar angio/interventional suite. The position is expected to be filled on or before July 1, 1999. Interested parties should contact Michael J. Pentecost, MD, Professor and Chairman, Department of Radiology, Georgetown University Medical Center, 3800 Reservoir Rd, NW, Washington, DC, e-mail *pentecom@gunet.georgetown.edu*, fax 202-687-1804.

DIAGNOSTIC RADIOLOGIST, ISLAND OF GUAM—Immediate opening available in a recently opened private imaging office. GE spiral CT, Accuson sonography and general radiography support a full cancer treatment center as well as outpatient referrals. Opportunity for cross coverage with an affiliated Maui, HI based diagnostic radiology group. Partnership track, apartment and auto provided. Please send CV and direct inquiries ro Mr Nick Gladdis, Administrative Director, 221 Mahalani St, Wailuku, HI 96793; phone 808-242-2054, fax 808-242-1940, e-mail *mrc@maui.net*.

MAUI, HI—Hospital based radiology group seeks Board certified radiologist for evening and night coverage position. This 200-bed facility includes diagnostic radiology, interventional/angiography, nuclear medicine, computerized tomography, ultrasound and magnetic resonance. Basic angiography/interventional skills are a plus. As part of the interview process candidates will be required to spend a minimum of one week in locum tenens position in the hospital environment. Please send CV and direct inquiries to Mr Nick Gladdis, Administrative Director, 221 Mahalani St, Wailuku, HI 96793; phone 808-242-2054, fax 808-242-1940, e-mail *mrc@maui.net*.

SE MICHIGAN—Progressive group seeks Board certified body imager with special expertise in vascular ultrasound to head up ultrasound department at new suburban hospital. Practice includes busy MR center as well as general radiology. A 440-bed hospital located between Detroit and Flint, with state-of-the-art equipment. Completely filmless digital department. Partnership track is available. Generous compensation and vacation package. Send or fax CV to Eugene Brown, MD, 10775 S Saginaw St, Suite D, Grand Blanc, MI 48439; fax 810-695-6615.

PUGET SOUND BASED RADIA MEDICAL IMAGING—A 32-member radiologist practice serving five hospitals, one large multi-specialty clinic and various outpatient radiology sites, is seeking a Board certified general radiologist with cross-

RADIOLOGIST

Gundersen Lutheran is seeking a board certified/board eligible Radiologist who has completed a fellowship in Mammography or who has extensive experience in Mammography, including Mammography intervention.

Gundersen Lutheran is a large multi-specialty group practice with over 320 physicians located in La Crosse, WI. It's main campus is attached to a 402 bed acute care hospital. The Gundersen Lutheran system includes 36 regional community clinics based throughout western Wisconsin, eastern Minnesota and northeastern Iowa. Gundersen Lutheran is a modern state-of-the-art facility that has a service area for a population base of over 530,000. Gundersen Lutheran is also the designated western campus of the University of Wisconsin Medical School.

La Crosse, Wisconsin, nestled between towering bluffs, is located where the Mississippi, La Crosse, and Black Rivers merge. The area was untouched by the glaciers, leaving many hills and valleys. The metropolitan area of La Crosse, with its 100,000 people, offers exceptional year round opportunities for recreational activities. The area also offers outstanding public and private schools, low crime rates, and cultural activities.

We offer competitive salaries and excellent fringe benefits. Interested candidates should send a letter of application and curriculum vitae to Frank Perez-Guerra, Director, Recruitment, Retention, and Resource Planning, Gundersen Lutheran, 1836 South Avenue, La Crosse, WI 54601; or call 800-362-9567, Ext. 6325.

Equal Opportunity Employer

Gundersen Lutheran

Check out RSNA Link

for additional classified advertising opportunities

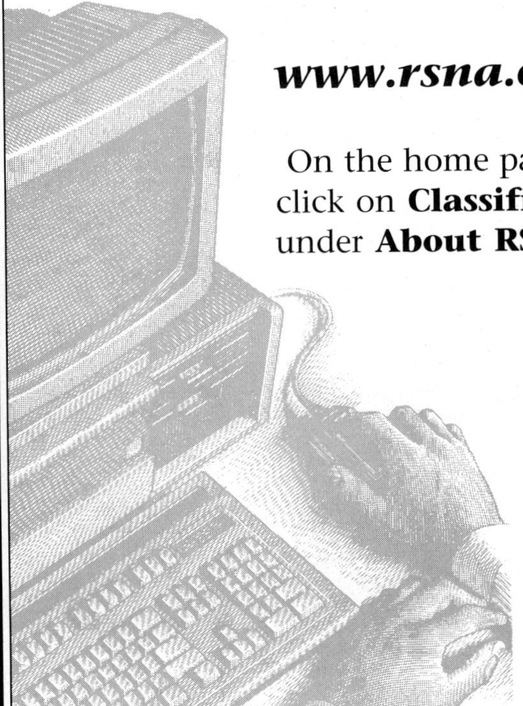

www.rsna.org

On the home page, click on **Classifieds** under **About RSNA** sectional imaging experience. Candidates with fellowship training are preferred. Implementation of 24-hour emergency services coverage via a teleradiology network and elevated exam volumes have increased the need for radiologists. If you are interested in working with a progressive practice, developing and promoting your area of subspecialization, sharing evenings and night work rotation, and living in an environment that allows access to a multitude of metropolitan and outdoor activities, please forward your curriculum vitae to Sanjiv Parikh, MD, Radia Medical Imaging, 3822 Colby Ave, Everett, WA 98201. Fax 425-339-8322.

FLORIDA - GENERAL RADIOLOGIST—Central Florida West Coast group seeks BE/BC radiologist. Interventional fellowship and/or body imaging fellowship desirable. Competitive compensation/benefits. CVs may be faxed to 813-898-4505.

SOUTH FLORIDA, IMMEDIATE OPENINGS—Desirable private practice with two hospitals in need of fellowship trained MRI radiologist, fellowship trained interventional radiologist, and a fellowship trained pediatric radiologist. The successful candidates must be willing to do general radiology as well. Excellent positions for excellent individuals. Please send CVs to fax 561-488-8347.

PUGET SOUND BASED RADIA MEDICAL IMAGING—A 32-member radiologist practice serving five hospitals, one large multispecialty clinic and various outpatient radiology sites, is seeking a Board certified general radiologist subspecializing in nuclear medicine with Board certification. Practice at a progressive 200-bed community hospital with state-of-the-art equipment. Practice involves developing and promoting nuclear medicine, working in other areas, sharing evening and night work rotation. Live in an environment that allows access to a multitude of metropolitan and outdoor activities, good schools and cultural diversity. Please forward your CV to Sanjiv Parikh, MD, c/o Cheryl West, Radia Medical Imaging, 3822 Colby Ave, Everett, WA 98201.

LEXINGTON, KY—BC/BE diagnostic radiologist for salaried position in a six person radiology group. No weekend, on-call or holiday responsibilities. Expertise in general radiology, mammography, CT, nuclear medicine, and ultrasound required. Interest in women's imaging is a plus. MRI and angiography are a plus, but not required. Competitive salary and benefits. Please send CV to Scott Stevens, MD, Radiology, 1740 S Nicholasville Rd, Lexington, KY 40503.

ABR CERTIFIED RADIOLOGIST—Needed for nighthawk coverage in Raleigh, NC metropolitan area. Responsibilities include general, nuclear medicine, CT, ultrasound, and basic MR. Excellent salary, generous benefits and time off. Please send CV to William H. Johnson, Administrator at Wake Radiology, PO Box 19366, Raleigh, NC 27619.

A 14-MEMBER RADIOLOGY GROUP—Seeking two Board certified radiologists: one with fellowship training in musculoskeletal or MRI with strong general radiology skills; and one general radiologist. Please reply to B.L. Storm, MD, PO Box 12219, Tallahassee, FL 32317-2219. Office telephone 850-942-4497; fax 850-942-1610.

NEW ORLEANS, LA—Outstanding opportunity for Board certified radiologist with recent fellowship in interventional radiology. Practice includes state-of-the-art interventional suite, 1.5T MRI, CT/US, mammography, nuclear medicine and general diagnostic. Candidate will spend 50% of time in interventional and rest in imaging and diagnostic radiology. Progressive group in acute care hospital and one outpatient clinic with teleradiology call coverage. Generous salary and benefits with opportunity for full partnership. Generous salary and benefits with opportunity for full partnership. Please reply with CV to PO Box 1827, Harvey, LA 70058.

VASCULAR/INTERVENTIONAL RADIOLOGIST—The Department of Radiology at Saint Louis University Health Sciences Center is seeking an ABR eligible or certified, fellowship trained vascular/interventional radiologist for a full-time, faculty position open in July, 1998. The rapidly expanding practice has a case load including diagnostic angiography (including pulmonary angiography), angioplasty, central venous access, thrombolysis, embolization, IVC Filter placement, biliary and uroradiology, TIPS, percutaneous biopsy and percutaneous gastrostomy. A broad range of teaching and research opportunities is available. Appointment is anticipated at the Assistant Professor level. For information, contact Thomas Bocchini, MD, Chief, Section of Interventional Radiology, Department of Radiology, Saint Louis University Health Sciences Center, 3635 Vista at Grand Boulevard, St. Louis, MO 63110-0250. Phone 314-268-5784; fax 314-268-5116. Saint Louis University Health Sciences Center is an equal opportunity employer M/F/D/V.

THE RADIOLOGY GROUP—Affiliated with the Stratford General Hospital and environs is seeking a radiologist to join their group. The successful individual must have experience with numerous modalities including ultrasound, mammography, CT and interventional procedures. The interested candidate should send his/her CV to Dr. Yale A. Erenberg, Radiologist in Chief, c/o Department of Medical Imaging, Stratford General Hospital, 46 General Hospital Dr, Stratford, Ontario N5A 2Y6. Phone 519-272-8210 ext 2278, fax 519-272-8221.

ASHEVILLE, NC— A third board certified radiologist is needed for night, weekend day, and holiday call coverage of 21 person group practice in major referral center. Salaried position with excellent time off and benefits package in beautiful mountain vacation area. Send CV to Ms. Sue Spivey, P.O. Box 2959, Asheville, NC 28802

DIAGNOSTIC RADIOLOGIST—Broadly trained general radiologist needed to join two others in hospital practice in Fremont, OH, 35 miles from Toledo. Practice performs approximately 33,000 studies per year, including MRI, CT, US, nuclear, and interventional/angio. Fellowship training is not required but is welcome. Additional coverage in an outpatient center in Toledo is also required. Generous vacation allowance and compensation package. Please send CV to Dr. Daniel Dessner, Toledo Radiological Associates, Inc, 4841 Monroe Street, Suite 103, Toledo, OH 43623, or fax to 419-479-6078.

HARTFORD, CT—Large, private radiology group in Hartford, CT is seeking well-trained individual for full-time, partnership tract position. The practice includes Hartford Hospital (a large community hospital with Level 1 Trauma Center with an independent radiology residency program) and three suburban offices. Please send CV to Steven K. Sussman, MD, Jefferson X-Ray Group, 85 Seymour St, Suite 200, Hartford, CT 06106.

Position Sought

EXPERIENCED ABR-CERTIFIED—Fellowship-trained (neuroradiology), ASNR senior member seeks full-time position. Neuroradiology, general radiology, or interventional or some combination. Administrative experience. Available 1/1/99. Prefer midwest, but other locations considered. Reply to Box R-083.

Fellowships

FELLOWSHIP ABDOMINAL IMAGING AND INTERVENTIONS—The Department of Radiology, Massachusetts General Hospital and Harvard Medical School, offers a 2-year fellowship in abdominal imaging and interventional radiology beginning July 1, 2000. Training covers all aspects of abdominal imaging (fluoroscopy, ultrasound, CT and MR) and nonvascular interventions in the GI/GU tract. This is an accredited interventional fellowship which includes elective time to allow a fellow to take the vascular/interventional CAQ exam. Ample time is made available for both clinical and laboratory research in the above areas the 2nd-year. Candidates should be ABR eligible or ABR certified. Address inquiries to Peter R. Mueller, MD, Department of Radiology, EL 234, Massachusetts General Hospital, 55 Fruit St, Boston, MA 02114. An equal opportunity employer.

BREAST IMAGING—A 1-year fellowship available July 1st of every year or two six month position one starting July 1st and the other starting January 2nd. Exposure to all aspects of clinical/academic breast imaging. Appointment to the faculty will be at the level of an instructor. Participation in research/teaching. Send cover letter and CV to Pamela Otto, MD, Assistant Professor, Director of Education, Mammography. The University of Texas Health Science Center at San Antonio, 7703 Floyd Curl Dr, San Antonio, TX 78284-7800. The University of Texas Health Science Center at San Antonio is an affirmative action/equal opportunity employer.

NEURORADIOLOGY FELLOWSHIPS AVAILABLE JULY 1999 AND JULY 2000—The Department of Radiology at the Medical College of Wisconsin offers a 1- or 2-year fellowship in neuroradiology. The fellowship provides extensive experience in interpretation of MR spectroscopy and functional MRI, in addition to the conventional imaging studies performed in most neuroradiology sections. Imaging facilities include three state-of-the-art CT scanners with helical capabilities, three Signa MR scanners and access to an experimental 3.0T imager, three up-to-date angiographic suites with state-of-the-art digital capabilities. Staffing includes six neuroradiologists with excellent academic credentials. Two of the staff perform interventional neuroradiologic procedures. All have specialized areas of expertise in neuroradiology. Fellows have the opportunity to pursue research interests in anatomy, pathology, and functional imaging. On call responsibilities are shared between staff and fellows. Contact David Daniels, MD by phone 414-259-3122 or e-mail *ddaniels@mcw.edu*. The Medical College of Wisconsin is an equal opportunity/affirmative action employer.

CROSS-SECTIONAL IMAGING FELLOWSHIP, ST. LUKE'S MEDICAL CENTER, MILWAUKEE, WI—The Department of Radiology at St. Luke's Medical Center (a 711-bed advanced tertiary care teaching hospital), Milwaukee, WI, is soliciting applications for a 1-year fellowship in cross-sectional imaging, beginning July 1, 1999. The program will consist of rotations in ultrasound, computed tomography, and magnetic resonance imaging. Both body imaging and neurospinal imaging will be provided, as well as neurovascular and peripheral vascular MRA. Elective and research time are included. Equipment includes six Acuson colorflow doppler scanners, one GE 9800 CT, two GE CTi helical scanners and one GE high speed helical scanner with two Advantage Windows work stations, and two GE Signa 1.5T and 1.0T MR. Fellows will receive extensive hands-on experience in all ultrasound and CT guided interventional procedures. Applicants should be ABR eligible or certified. Requests for applications and additional information should be sent to Peter Bessette, MD, Department of Radiology, St. Luke's Medical Center, PO Box 2901, Milwaukee, WI 53201-2901.

FELLOWSHIP IN ULTRASOUND AND BODY CT/MR—There are 1-year fellowships in ultrasound and body CT/MRI beginning July 1999 and July 2000 that are being offered by The New York Hospital-Cornell Medical Center. The department provides state-of-the-art equipment, including Acuson and ATL ultrasound with color doppler and power doppler, GE 9800 spiral CT with Windows work station, and GE Signa 1.5 Telsa MR with fast spin echo and angiographic capabilities. A very wide variety of ultrasound examinations include abdominal, obstetrics and gynecology, duplex and color doppler, small parts, peripheral vascular, carotid, transvaginal, and transrectal. CT and MR examinations include neck, chest, cardiovascular, abdomen, pelvis, and extremities. The fellow receives extensive hands-on experience in ultrasound and CT guided biopsy procedures. In addition, the fellow participates in resident and medical student teaching and interdepartmental conferences. There are also opportunities for clinical research. Applicants should be ABR eligible or certified. Send CV to William A. Rubenstein, MD, Department of Radiology, New York Hospital-Cornell Medical Center, 525 E 68th St, New York, NY 10021; phone 212-747-2561, fax 212-746-8590.

FELLOWSHIP IN NEURORADIOLOGY—A 1- or 2-year neuroradiology fellowship position is available for the 1998, 1999, 2000 academic year. The program features state-of-the-art facilities including echoplanar MRI, ultra high gradient (40 mT/M), high speed MR unit, helical CT, Cine CT, PET/SPECT, and digital biplane angiography. The neuroradiology program has a strong, practical orientation and provides excellent research opportunities in a busy tertiary care center in a cooperative multidisciplinary environment. Candidates must have completed an accredited residency program and be Board certified or eligible in diagnostic radiology. Women and members of minority groups are encouraged to apply. For information and application contact William T.C. Yuh, MD, Director, MRI, and Neuroradiology Sections, Department of Radiology/MRI Center, University of Iowa Hospitals and Clinics, Iowa City, IA, 52242; phone 319-356-3767; fax 319-353-6275. The University of Iowa is an affirmative action/equal opportunity employer.

HENRY FORD HOSPITAL HAS AN UNEXPECTED OPENING FOR CROSS-SECTIONAL FELLOWSHIP STARTING JULY 1, 1999—The fellowship consists of MRI - body and neuro, including MRA, spiral CT, including abscess drainage and biopsy, and abdominal, vascular, obstetrical and pelvic ultrasound. Equipment includes three MRI scanners, five CT machines, and numerous ultrasound units. Please direct inquiries to Michael A. Sandler, MD, Department of Diagnostic Radiology, Henry Ford Hospital, Detroit, MI; 313-876-1355; fax 313-876-1106.

NEURORADIOLOGY FELLOWSHIP OPPORTUNITY—The Neuroradiology Division of the Johns Hopkins University Department of Radiology has an unexpected fellowship position for July 1, 1998. This is a 2-year fellowship, ideal for candidates interested in developing a research track record as well as acquiring and refining sophisticated clinical neuroradiologic skills. Clinical equipment includes seven 1.5T MRI systems, two biplane angiography suites, and seven CT scanners. A whole body PET scanner and cyclotron are also available within the department. Research opportunities exist in interventional neuroradiology, acute stroke imaging, image guided surgery, neuroreceptor and

12th Annual Fellowship Award in Cardiac Imaging and Invasive Cardiology

Bracco Diagnostics and The Society for Cardiac Angiography & Interventions invite the submission of applications for the 12th Annual Award of the Bracco/SCA&I Fellowship Program for Research in Cardiac Imaging and Invasive Cardiology for 1999-2000.

The purpose of the awards is to encourage meaningful scientific investigation of cardiovascular imaging and invasive techniques and to foster new insights into patient care. The program grants two fellowships to physicians-in-training with demonstrated medical excellence whose research promises diagnostic advancement and contributions to cardiovascular imaging and invasive techniques. The awards are limited to a maximum of $25,000 each.

A description of the fellowship, eligibility requirements, and application materials can be obtained by contacting:

Bracco/SCA&I Fellowship Program Awards Committee
Frank Hildner, M.D., Chairman
c/o SCAI, Attn: M.A. Dilday
4101 Lake Boone Trail, Suite 201
Raleigh, North Carolina 27607
Telephone: 919-787-5181 / Fax: 919-787-4916

Applications must be received at the Awards Committee office no later than Wednesday, January 20, 1999. Those selected for the 1999-2000 Awards will be notified in early March and will be honored at the 22nd Annual Meeting of the Society for Cardiac Angiography and Interventions, May 11-15, 1999, in Monterey, California.

cerebral blood flow imaging, metabolic and morphologic assessment of brain tumors, and functional neuroimaging (fMRI and PET). Interested individuals should call David M. Yousem, MD, newly appointed Director of Neuroradiology; 215-662-3066; fax 215-662-3283; beeper 215-980-4661 or e-mail *yousem@oasis.rad.upenn .edu.* Please fax your curriculum vitae and two letters of recommendation to his attention at above number.

NEURORADIOLOGY FELLOWSHIP - UNIVERSITY OF MICHIGAN—Opening for an additional 1999-2000 fellow. Call Dr Gebarski 734-936-4484.

FELLOWSHIPS AT YALE UNIVERSITY—The Department of Diagnostic Radiology at Yale University School of Medicine offer the following fellowships: abdominal imaging - four positions: balanced position CT/US/MR, CT focus, US focus, MR focus. Each focused position includes rotations through all three imaging services; contact Morton Burrell, MD. Thoracic imaging - one position: includes plain film interpretation, lung biopsies, CT and MRI; contact Ann McB. Curtis, MD. Breast imaging - one position: includes breast biopsies, (stereotactic and ultrasound guided), breast ultrasound, breast MRI, and nuclear breast imaging; contact Irena Tocino, MD. Neuroradiology - three 2-year positions offered each year. Contact Gordon Sze, MD. Vascular and interventional - three positions each year; contact Jeffrey Pollak, MD. Pediatric radiology (ACGME accredited) - one position each year; contact Marc S. Keller, MD. Interested applicants should send their CV and three letters of recommendation to the appropriate program director at PO Box 208042 (333 Cedar St), New Haven, CT 06520.

NUCLEAR MEDICINE RESIDENCY/FELLOWSHIP—The Harvard Medical School, Joint Program in Nuclear Medicine invites applications for the 1-year fellowship and 2-year residency positions beginning July 1st, 1999 and 2000. Please direct your inquiries to Kathy Fantegrossi, Program Coordinator, Joint Program in Nuclear Medicine, Children's Hospital, 300 Longwood Ave, Boston, MA 02115 or by e-mail at *fantegrossik@a1.tch.harvard.edu.*

ABDOMINAL IMAGING FELLOWSHIP—The Department of Radiology at the University of Texas Health Science Center at San Antonio is seeking candidates for a 1-year abdominal imaging fellowship beginning July, 2000. The program provides training in abdominal CT, MRI, sonography, nonvascular intervention and GI/GU fluoroscopy. One month of elective time is allowed. Rotations are at the University Hospital (600-beds) and the Audie Murphy VA Hospital (450-beds). The hospitals are regional referral centers for trauma, oncology, surgery, general medicine and organ transplantations. The image equipment is state-of-the-art with four helical CT units, one GE Signa MR unit with fast scanning and angio capabilities (another to be installed in 1999), seven color Doppler ultrasound units and four fluoroscopy rooms (2 digital). For further information, please contact Gerald D. Dodd, III, MD, Professor, Department of Radiology, UT Health Science Center at San Antonio, 7703 Floyd Curl Dr, San Antonio, 7703 Floyd Curl Dr, San Antonio, TX 78284-7800; 210-567-6470. The University of Texas Health Science Center at San Antonio is an equal opportunity/affirmative action employer.

FELLOWSHIPS IN RADIOLOGY, MEMORIAL SLOAN-KETTERING CANCER CENTER—The Department of Radiology at Memorial Sloan-Kettering Cancer Center offers fellowships beginning 7/1/00. Body Imaging - 1-year. Extensive clinical experience in body CT (25,000 cases/year), body MRI (1,800 cases/year) and ultrasound (5,000 cases/year). Equipment includes two GE HighSpeed (helical) Advantage CTs; two GE HiLite Advantage CTs; GE 1.5T Signa MRI; Picker 1.0T MRI; and three Acuson XP units with color doppler. Research is integral part of program. Director David Panicek, MD. Breast Imaging - 6 months (plus 6 months of body imaging). There are 60,000 mammograms, 500 preoperative needle localizations, 150 stereotaxic biopsies, and 1,400 breast sonograms and sonographically-guided breast biopsies performed yearly. Equipment includes nine dedicated mammography machines and a stereotactaxic biopsy table. Director David Dershaw, MD. Other fellowships include nuclear medicine (2-years; contact Steven Larson, MD at MSKCC), and combined New York Hospital/MSKCC fellowships in neuroradiology (2-years; contact Michael Deck, MD at NYH) and vascular/interventional radiology (1-year; contact Thomas Sos, MD, at NYH). Excellent opportunities for research exist at this Cornell University Medical College affiliate, with competitive salary and benefits. Request application from David Panicek, MD, Department of Radiology, Memorial Sloan-Kettering Cancer

NATIONAL INSTITUTES OF HEALTH

Fellowships in Imaging Sciences Program at the National Institutes of Health

The Radiological and Imaging Sciences Program at the National Institutes of Health (NIH) is accepting applications for two-year fellowship positions beginning July 1999 and July 2000. This fellowship training program provides opportunities in clinical and basic imaging research available in the Departments of Diagnostic Radiology, Nuclear Medicine, Positron Emission Tomography, and the Laboratory of Diagnostic Radiology Re-search. The training program emphasizes research in all aspects of clinical and imaging sciences and image processing. Fellows can choose to work in areas of research including: Neuroimaging, Interventional, Oncological, Vascular, and Metabolic Imaging using various imaging techniques as well as basic areas of research in Magnetic Resonance Imaging and Spectroscopy, MR Microscopy, unique PET Radioligands as probes for receptors, specific uptake and metabolic pathways, Contrast Agent develop-ment and evalu-ation for Molecular Imaging, Tissue Perfusion and Metabolism, and innovative image processing and visual-ization algorithms. Qualified applicants will be able to have clini-cal exposure to a unique research patient population found at the NIH. Fellows in the Imaging Sciences Program have access to state-of-the-art imaging and computer facilities dedicated to research found in the Clinic Center, In Vivo NMR Research Center, and basic science laboratories including both "hot" and "cold" wet chemistry labs and tissue culture facilities.

Applicants should hold an M.D. or Ph.D. degree and should have completed clinical training in Diagnostic Radiology, Nuclear Medicine or related fields. Applicants from individuals currently in U.S. residency programs may also be considered for research fellowship positions. U.S. citizenship or permanent residents will receive preference for these full-time appointments.

Candidates should submit a Curriculum Vitae, at least 3 letters of reference, and a statement of research interest to:

Joseph A. Frank, M.D.
Chief
Laboratory of Diagnostic Radiology Research
National Institutes of Health
900 Rockville Pike, Building 10, Room B1N256
Bethesda, Maryland 20892-1074
Fax: 301-402-3216
E-mail: jafrank@helix.nih.gov

Equal Opportunity Employer

RSNA®

RSNA Executive Offices • 2021 Spring Road, Suite 600
Oak Brook, IL 60523 • (630) 571-2670

Bulletin Board September 1998

✓ More "Hot Topics" for 1998 Meeting

✓ PAC System Course to be Offered at RSNA'98

✓ Review Your Membership Directory Listing

■ The ongoing "Hot Topics" presentation was developed in 1991 by William A. Murphy, Jr, MD, then chairman of the RSNA Program Committee, to gather the most recent scientific information for the RSNA Scientific Assembly and Annual Meeting.

"Hot Topics" will again be a part of the 1998 meeting. If you have performed research that was too recent to be submitted by the April 15 deadline, please call (630) 571-7877 to request an application for your "hot topic." The deadline for submissions is November 1, 1998.

■ A new course titled "Advanced Course in Configuring a PAC (picture archiving and communications) System for Interested Radiologists and Managers" will be offered at RSNA '98. This course was not listed in the Refresher Course Enrollment, Scientific Program, Advance Registration, and Housing Registration booklet.

The course will be conducted in conjunction with, but separate from, the PAC system workstation workshop Refresher Course. The objective of the course is to introduce the attendee to issues surrounding effective configuration of a PAC system. Specific topics to be covered include network issues, DICOM protocol, application entities, acquisition from imaging devices, demographics, RIS/HIS interfaces, database integrity, folder/workflow manager concepts, setting autorouting and prefetching rules, "hanging" or image sequencing protocols, archive management, backup, and quality assurance. Strongly suggested prerequisites for attending the "Advanced Course in Configuring a PAC System for Interested Radiologists and Managers" are as follows: Attendees should possess a basic familiarity with a PAC system and workstation concepts or should have attended the workstation workshop in prior years or at RSNA '98.

Taught by David E. Arvin, PhD, Janice C. Honeyman, PhD, Katherine P. Andriole, PhD, and Ronald L. Arenson, MD, the "Advanced Course" is scheduled to take place Monday, Nov 30, 10:30 AM–12:00 NOON (course 030); Tuesday, Dec 1, 1:00 PM–2:30 PM (course 031); and Wednesday, Dec 2, 10:30 AM–12:00 NOON (course 032). Seating will be limited to 75 people. Attendees may earn 1½ hours of category 1 credit.

If you would like to register for the "Advanced Course," enter the course number, 030, 031, or 032, on the *info*RAD course enrollment form, which is located in your Refresher Course Enrollment, Scientific Program, Advance Registration, and Housing Registration booklet. You may also register online at *www.rsna.org/RSNA2/rsna98/advanceregistration/welcometochicago.html*. Click on "*info*RAD Plan of Presentation" and look for the PACS Advanced Course icon.

Information about the "Advanced Course in Configuring a PAC System for Interested Radiologists and Managers" can be found in future issues of *RSNA News*.

■ RSNA members should review their listings in the 1998 RSNA Membership Directory and submit changes and corrections to the Manager of Membership Records, RSNA, 2021 Spring Road, Suite 600, Oak Brook, IL 60523. Changes received by the end of the year will be included in the 1999 directory.

■ The following is a list of applicants for RSNA membership, published as provided by the bylaws of the Society. Society members are asked to review these names. Should a member have a question concerning the eligibility of an applicant, within 30 days of the publication of this list, the member should request that the applicant's membership be withheld pending investigation and reconsideration by the Membership and Credentials Board. Please mark your signed letter of protest "Confidential" and address it to Secretary-Treasurer, RSNA, 2021 Spring Road, Suite 600, Oak Brook, IL 60523. Please note that listed here are only the locations in which the prospective members reside and the counselors for those areas.

ALABAMA
Counselor: Leon W. Bell III, MD
D. S. Kelly, MD, Gadsden

CALIFORNIA
Counselors: Deborah S. Ablin, MD
Gary R. Hansen, MD
Eric W. Olcott, MD
Zbigniew Petrovich, MD
Dolores H. Pretorius, MD
Morton Wexler, MD
William C. Buss, MD, Redlands
Grant R. Lindee, MD, Santa Rosa
Sonja M. Moelleken, MD, San Francisco
Todd D. Spencer, MD, Madera
Shendee Teng, MD, Los Angeles

COLORADO
Counselor: Michael A. Foster, MD
Rondle M. Moubry, MD, MS, Alamosa

DISTRICT OF COLUMBIA
Counselor: Edward N. Smith, Jr, MD
Bradley J. Snyder, MD, Washington

FLORIDA
Counselor: John A. Arrington, MD
Maria C. Fonseca De Chacon, MD, Miami
Douglas M. Roy, MD, Winter Haven
Richard L. Stern, MD, Fort Pierce
Michael S. Thorpe, MD, Coral Gables

GEORGIA
Counselor: Robert F. Long, MD
Oliver A. Sorsdahl, MD, Atlanta

KENTUCKY
Counselor: Dwight B. Short, MD
Dean F. Leslie, MD, Louisville

LOUISIANA
Counselor: David R. Hunter, MD
Maria R. Beltran, MD, Lafayette

MARYLAND
Counselor: Douglas R. Brunner, MD
Bijan Keramati, MD, Ellicott City

MICHIGAN
Counselors: Judith M. Bender, MD
Walter W. Laidlaw, MD
Carmen Endress, MD, Bloomfield Hills
Paula K. Maas, MD, Holland
Rennard B. Tucker, MD, Detroit

MISSOURI
Counselors: David P. Diemer, MD
George D. Dixon, MD
Martin L. Goldman, MD, Kansas City
Bruce L. Hedgepeth, MD, Springfield

NEBRASKA
Counselor: Kevin R. Gillespie, MD
Mary S. Davey, MD, Omaha

NEW YORK
Counselors: Mario A. Grosso, MD
David M. Panicek, MD
Arthur J. Segal, MD
Nobufusa Furukawa, MD, Rochester
Ceceleta Y. Maitland, MD, Brooklyn
Leonard B. Resnikoff, MD, Staten Island
Paul B. Rolen, MD, MS, New York
Edward M. Smith, ScD, Rochester

NORTH CAROLINA
Counselor: James A. Fagan, MD
Michelle L. Rivera, MD, Durham
John W. Wu, MD, Winston-Salem

OHIO
Counselors: Michael A. Geisinger, MD
Jonathan S. Moulton, MD
Kameswararao Chalasani, MD, New Philadelphia
Lawrence S. Richman, MD, Akron
Michael J. Seider, PhD, MD, Akron

PENNSYLVANIA
Counselors: Nilima Dash, MD
Kathryn A. Evers, MD
John E. Madewell, MD
Frank L. D'Amelio, MD, Waynesboro
Kenneth A. Edgar, MD, Bridgeville
Lara A. Hardesty, MD, Pittsburgh
Craig C. Trent, MD, Grove City

PUERTO RICO
Counselor: Rene Dietrich, MD
Julio A. Calcano Perez, MD, Caguas

RHODE ISLAND
Counselor: Barbara Schepps, MD
James C. Bass, MD, East Greenwich

TENNESSEE
Counselor: Joseph J. Busch, MD
Joseph B. Cornett, MD, Nashville
Clark M. Pollitt, MD, Springfield
Leland Y. Tsao, MD, Nashville

TEXAS
Counselors: Karl A. Glastad, MD
Franz J. Hallermann, MD
Timothy W. Lillick, MD
Cody B. DuVall, MD, Lufkin
Patrick K. Elvin, MD, Corpus Christi
Sunjay Verma, MD, Midland

AIR FORCE
Counselor: Thomas G. Johnson, MD
Sonia G. Britton, MD, Panama

MEXICO
Counselors: Jose H. Arredondo, MD
Manuel A. Cabal, MD
Jose M. Cardoso, MD
Miguel A. Carrillo, MD
Ramon R. Ponte, MD
Francisco J. Reynaga-Garcia, MD
Cecilia M. Ortiz, MD, Mexico City

CANADA

QUEBEC
Counselors: Pierre M. Bourgouin, MD
Gilles Hudon, MD
Raquel Del Carpio-O'Donovan, MD, Montreal

CORRESPONDING
Osbert N. Adjei, MBChB, PhD, Saudi Arabia
Jordi Aldoma Puigdomenech, MD, Spain
Georgina M. Allen, BM, United Kingdom
Abdullah M. Attar IV, MD, Saudi Arabia
Vincente Belloch, MD, Spain
Leslie C. Berman, MBBCh, Mmed, South Africa
Paolo Campioni, MD, Italy
Rosa B. Castro, MD, Brazil
Roger J. Chinn, MBBS, United Kingdom
Salvador D'Andrea Neto, MD, Brazil
Roger P. Davies, MBBS, United Kingdom
Helmut Dinkloh, MD, Germany
Heinz Domes, MD, Austria
Mikael N. Enblom, MD, Sweden
Olivier J. Ernst, MD, France
Liana M. Falcon, MD, Peru
Gideon Flusser, MD, Israel
Hiroyuki Horikoshi, Sr, MD, Japan
Wen-Tao Huang, PhD, Taiwan ROC
Ian M. Kelly, MBBCh, United Kingdom
Shigeru Kiryu, MD, Japan
Richard I. Kitney, PhD, Dsc, United Kingdom
Martin H. Kolb, MD, Germany
Andreas L. Kotziamanis, MD, Cyprus
Juan Mazzucco, Sr, MD, Argentina
Armenio Mekhitarian, MD, Brazil
Sandra M. Morales Sanchez, MD, Spain
Sojiro Morita, MD, PhD, Japan
Katsuhito L. Murata, MD, PhD, Japan
Ziv Neeman, MD, Israel
Martti S. Pamilo, MD, PhD, Finland
Klaus Rudisser, MD, Germany
Edgardo Santa Cruz, MD, Argentina
Jiyeol Shin, MD, South Korea
Suren S. Surenthiran, MBBS, United Kingdom
Zhenyan Yang, MD, People's Rep of China
Masashi Yukihiro, MD, PhD, Japan
Cheng Zhou, MD, People's Rep of China
Chun-Wu Zhou, MD, People's Rep of China
Martin Zwaan, MD, Germany

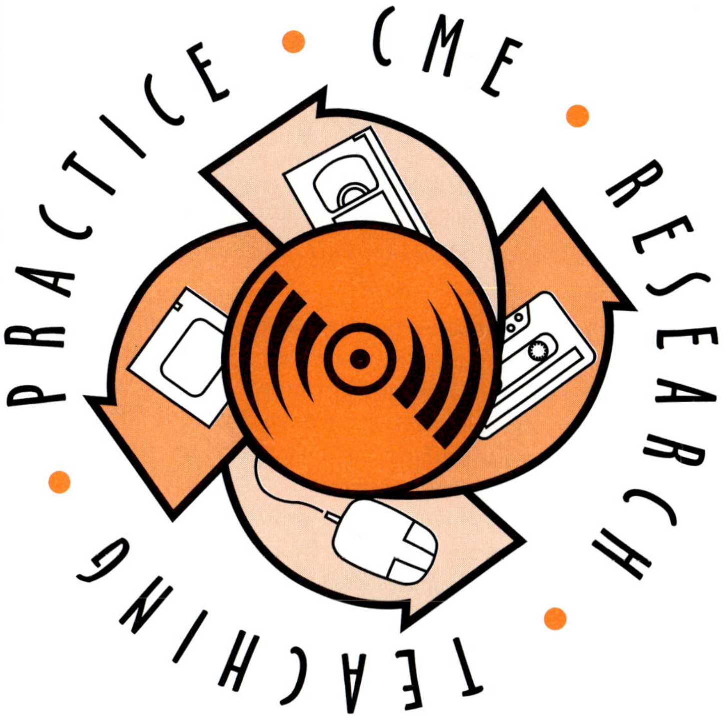

Ultrasound

Learning Center Resources

September 1998

RSNA® | Radiological Society of North America
Founded in 1915

Featured Topics

- Ultrasound Evaluation of the Kidney
- Color Doppler US: Pediatric Extracranial Applications
- Ultrasound Artifacts
- Ultrasound Equipment Selection

New Service

The entire 1997–1998 Learning Center Resources Catalog is now available on the RSNA Link, the Web site of the Radiological Society of North America, on the Internet.

You can reach us through the World Wide Web (WWW) by entering the uniform resource locator: http://www.rsna.org

We invite you to browse through the catalog, search for specific courses of interest, then simply order via our fax or 800 phone number.

ch and store for your future use.

The following 23 Ultrasound titles are now available in the Learning Center Resources Library. All videotapes are available for purchase or rental (U.S., Canada, and Mexico). All video programs may be purchased in NTSC, PAL, and SECAM television standards. Slides and audiotapes are available for purchase only.

For more information, call or fax the RSNA Learning Center Resources at the numbers listed on the order form. To order by mail, use the form on the back.

New!

Ultrasound Evaluation of the Kidney *RSP 621*

Neil T. Wolfman, MD
Mitchell E. Tublin, MD

This program reviews the most important applications of US of the genitourinary tract and compares US with other modalities. Special attention is given to hydronephrosis, renovascular disease, and renal failure in the native kidney. This course also covers US in acute treatment of the transplant, with emphasis on primary vascular and other complications.

120 slides/audiotape *M$140, N$160*
VHS *M$140, N$160*

New!

Genitourinary US: The Scrotum and Prostate *RSP 622*

Franklin N. Tessler, MD, CM
Matthew D. Rifkin, MD

This program addresses new and controversial aspects of scrotal US, including (1) detection and clinical significance of testicular microlithiasis, (2) the testicular mass, (3) color and spectral Doppler studies of the acute scrotum, and (4) high-frequency scrotal US. The use of US of the prostate in evaluation of prostatic cancer, benign prostatic hyperplasia, and other abnormalities is also addressed.

101 slides/audiotape *M$140, N$160*
VHS *M$140, N$160*

New!

Color Doppler US: Pediatric Extracranial Applications *RSP 626*

Marta Hernanz-Schulman, MD

This course will familiarize radiologists with clinically useful extracranial applications of Doppler techniques in pediatric patients. Vascular applications are presented with, particular emphasis on applications of power Doppler US. *Learning objectives:* (1) To learn applications of extracranial Doppler sonography in children. (2) To learn the advantages of power Doppler sonography.

[illegible] slides/audiotape *M$140, N$160*
VHS *M$140, N$160*

New!

US Artifacts *RSP 660*

Donovan M. Bakalyar, PhD
Lance V. Hefner, MS
Frederick W. Kremkau, PhD
Beatrice L. Madrazo, MD

This course teaches the student how to recognize the presence of artifacts, understand their underlying causes, and alter the scanning procedure in order to avoid them. It is composed of lectures on the basic physics of US, gray-scale and vascular artifacts, and a clinical review of common artifacts. *Learning objectives:* (1) To detail the origin and appearance of US artifacts. (2) To offer techniques to aid in the recognition of artifacts. (3) To provide methods to minimize the effect of artifacts.

VHS *M$205, N$225*
Not available in slide/audiotape

New!

Physics Tutorial on Equipment Selection: Ultrasound *RSP 665*

James A. Zagzebski, PhD
J. Brian Fowlkes, PhD
Brian S. Garra, MD
Lori Brennan, BS, RDMS

Equipment Performance: Low- to High-End Scanners

James A. Zagzebski, PhD

An overview of US equipment is presented with explanation of design factors, including transducer sensitivity and bandwidth, array element and channel number density, and beam-former technology. New generations of US test devices are described, along with examples from different imaging systems. (J.A.Z. provides some consulting to RMI.)

Technical Specification and Acceptance Testing of Equipment: What Is Image Quality?

J. Brian Fowlkes, PhD

Technical specifications of US equipment can provide valuable information for purchase of imaging systems and provide a basis for some of the acceptance testing. Examples are given of various levels of specifications and acceptance testing and their uses and assessment of their image quality.

RSP 665 continued on next page...

M/N = Member/Nonmember prices
To order call 800-272-2920 or FAX 708-409-9703

Selection of Ultrasound Imaging Equipment: A Physician's Perspective
Brian S. Garra, MD

Today, declining reimbursement may make buying the "latest and greatest" instrument every few years financially impossible. Physicians must balance cost and capabilities against the intended use of the machine and expected level of reimbursement. This section considers the specter of mandatory US accreditation and the development of performance criteria and discusses how the above factors affect decision-making at a practical level.

Selection of Ultrasound Imaging Equipment: A Sonographer's Perspective
Lori Brennan, BS, RDMS

Managed-care contracts, provider consolidation, and cost containment have complicated purchase of US equipment. The successful proposal requires careful analysis and preparation. Equipment productivity, flexibility, and operational issues are presented from a sonographer's perspective.
VHS *M$205, N$225*
Not available in slide/audiotape

US and US-guided Interventional Procedures Involving the Breast *RSP 478*
Paula Gordon, MD
VHS *M$205, N$225*
Not available in slide/audiotape

Musculoskeletal US *RSP 533*
Marnix van Holsbeeck, MD
130 slides/audiotape *M$205, N$225*
VHS *M$205, N$225*

Obstetric US: Fetal CNS *RSP 540*
Alfred B. Kurtz, MD
42 slides/audiotape *M$140, N$160*
VHS *M$140, N$160*

Obstetric US: Growth Parameters and Growth Retardation *RSP 541*
Barbara S. Hertzberg, MD
53 slides/audiotape *M$140, N$160*
VHS *M$140, N$160*

Obstetric US: Fetal Echocardiography *RSP 544*
Douglas L. Brown, MD
61 slides/audiotape *M$140, N$160*
VHS *M$140, N$160*

Ultrasound Evaluation of the Hepatobiliary Tract *RSP 8001*
Philip W. Ralls, MD
Michelle L. Robbin, MD
Faye C. Laing, MD
135 slides/audiotape *M$205, N$225*
VHS *M$205, N$225*

Diagnostic Ultrasound in the Evaluation of Leg Pain *RSP 8002*
Edward I. Bluth, MD
William J. Zwiebel, MD
79 slides/audiotape *M$140, N$160*
VHS *M$140, N$160*

Duplex and Color Doppler US of Masses in the Groin and Scrotum *RSP 8003*
A. Thomas Stavros, MD
Barbara A. Carroll, MD
98 slides/audiotape *M$140, N$160*
VHS *M$140, N$160*

Ultrasound Evaluation of Shoulder and Arm Pain *RSP 8004*
Janis G. Letourneau, MD
Marnix T. van Holsbeeck, MD
83 slides/audiotape *M$140, N$160*
VHS *M$140, N$160*

Ultrasound Assessment of Renal Failure, Hematuria, and Hypertension *RSP 8005*
Robert L. Bree, MD
John J. Cronan, MD
Laurence Needleman, MD
119 slides/audiotape *M$205, N$225*
VHS *M$205, N$225*

Diagnostic Ultrasound of the Acute Abdomen and Pelvis *RSP 8006*
John S. Pellerito, MD
Sharlene A. Teefey, MD
W. Dennis Foley, MD
139 slides/audiotape *M$140, N$160*
VHS *M$140, N$160*

Ultrasound Assessment of Gestational Age and Fetal Growth *RSP 8007*
Alfred B. Kurtz, MD
Francis P. Hadlock, MD
53 slides/audiotape *M$140, N$160*
VHS *M$140, N$160*

Sonographic Evaluation of First-Trimester and Third-Trimester Bleeding *RSP 8008*
Arthur C. Fleischer, MD
Barbara S. Hertzberg, MD
VHS *M$140, N$160*
Not available in slide/audiotape

The Role of Diagnostic Ultrasound in Screening for Fetal Abnormalities *RSP 8009*
Mark A. Kliewer, MD
Dolores H. Pretorius, MD
Ruth B. Goldstein, MD
123 slides/audiotape *M$140, N$160*
VHS *M$140, N$160*

Ultrasound Evaluation of the Carotid Arteries and the Palpable Neck Mass *RSP 8010*
Carl C. Reading, MD
Joseph F. Polak, MD, MPH
103 slides/audiotape *M$140, N$160*
VHS *M$140, N$160*

Pediatric Ultrasound: Clinical Questions, Practical Answers *RSP 8011*
Richard D. Bellah, MD
Carol M. Rumack, MD
Henrietta Rosenberg, MD
102 slides/audiotape *M$140, N$160*
VHS *M$140, N$160*

Gynecologic Ultrasound *RSP 8012*
Peter H. Arger, MD
Andrew M. Fried, MD
Edward A. Lyons, MD
Beverly G. Coleman, MD
160 slides/audiotape *M$205, N$225*
VHS *M$205, N$225*

Diagnostic Ultrasound of the Abdomen and Pelvis *RSP 8013*
Harris L. Cohen, MD
R. Brooke Jeffrey, Jr, MD
101 slides/audiotape *M$140, N$160*
VHS *M$140, N$160*

Place Stamp Here

TO: RSNA LEARNING CENTER RESOURCES
PO BOX 5316
OAK BROOK, IL 60522-5316
USA

FOLD HERE

PRACTICE • CME • RESEARCH • TEACHING

Order Form

You may mail or fax this form. To fax your order, dial 708-409-9703. Please print.

☐ *RSNA Member* ☐ *Nonmember*

NAME

RSNA MEMBER # (REQUIRED FOR MEMBER PRICING)

ADDRESS

CITY

STATE/COUNTRY

ZIP

PHONE

FAX

Order Information (for purchase and rentals)

Course Number	*Showing Date (Rental Only)*	*Format (Purchase Only)*	*Price*

FOLD HERE

Check one:

☐ *Rental*

☐ *Purchase*

Subtotal ______

Shipping & Handling ______

Total ______

Shipping Information

United States

1 program = $7

2 – 3 programs = $10

4 – 6 programs = $20

7 programs and up = $30

Rental

No charge for shipping to renter. Renter is responsible for return shipping charges.

Outside United States

1 program = $10

Each additional program = $5

All orders from outside the U.S. must be prepaid, either by MasterCard, VISA, AMEX or Diner's Club or a check in U.S. dollars, drawn on a U.S. bank.

Payment Information

☐ Payment by check

☐ Payment by credit card: ☐ VISA ☐ MasterCard ☐ AMEX ☐ Diner's Club

CARD NUMBER

SIGNATURE

EXP. DATE

For faster service, phone 800-272-2920 or fax 708-409-9703.

TEAR HERE

RAD 9.98

Foto Comm Corporation is the distributor of RSNA Learning Center Resources.